	HydrOXYzine	Meperidine	Metoc[illegible]	[illegible]	[illegible]	[illegible]	[illegible]	[illegible]	[illegible]	[illegible]	[illegible]	P[illegible]	Ranitidine	Scopolamine Hbr	Secobarbital	Thiethylperazine
	C	C	C	C	[illegible]	[illegible]	[illegible]	[illegible]	C	C	C	C	C	C	I	
	C	C	C	C	C		C	I	C	C		C		C	I	C
	C	C	C	C	C		C	I	C	C	C	C	C	C	I	
								I							I	
	I	I	I		I	I	I	I	I	I	I	I		I	I	I
	I	C	C	I	C		C	I	C	I	I	I	C	C	I	
	C	C	C	C	C		C	I	C	C	C	C	C	C	I	
	C	C	C		C	C	C	I	C	C	C	C		C	I	
	C	C	C		C		C	I	C	C	C	C	C	C	I	
	C	C			C		I	I		C	C	C	C	C	I	
		I			I		I					I				
		C	C		C	C	C	I		C	C	C	I	C	I	
	C		C		I		C	I	C	C	C	C	C	C	I	
	C	C			C		C		C	C	C	C	C	C	I	
	C		C		C	C		I	I	I	C	C	I	C		C
	C	I	C				C	I	C	C	C	C	C	C	I	
	C							I		C		*	C	C	I	C
	C	C	C		C			I	C	C	C	C	C	C	I	
	I	I			I	I	I		I	I	I	I		C	I	
		C	C		C		C	I		C		C	C	C	I	I
	C	C	C		C	C	C	I	C		C	C	C	C	I	
	C	C	C		C		C	I		C		C		C	I	
	C	C	C		C	C	C	I	C	C	C		C	C	I	
		C	C	I	C	C	C		C	C		C		C		C
	C	C	C		C	C	C	C	C	C	C	C	C		I	
	I	I	I		I	I	I	I	I	I	I	I		I		I
						C			I				C		I	

Parenteral compatibility occurs when two or more drugs are successfully mixed without liquefaction, deliquescence, or precipitation.

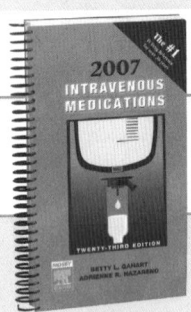

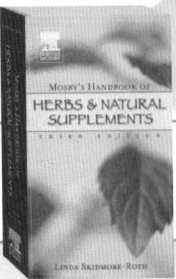

http://evolve.elsevier.com/nursingdrugupdates/Skidmore/NDG

Mosby's Drug Guide for Nurses, Seventh Edition, Companion CD-ROM

Use *Mosby's Drug Guide for Nurses, Seventh Edition, Companion CD-ROM* to find drug information fast! This four-in-one CD-ROM provides you with complete information and NCLEX® questions for 65 key drugs, a calculation tutorial, a drug card creator, and calculators.

This Companion CD-ROM includes:

- **NCLEX® Questions for 65 Key Drugs**
  Includes complete information for the 65 key drugs in the book, matched with 260 NCLEX®-style questions.
- **Calculation Tutorial**
  Provides calculations and conversions paired with practice problems and answers.
- **Drug Card Creator**
  Features a blank drug card template that is fully customizable and printable.
- **Calculators**
  Contains 30 handy clinical calculators, including several IV and PO dosage calculators, and an IV dose rate calculator.

Contact Us

For further information, visit us at http://us.elsevierhealth.com or call us at (800) 545-2522.

Mini CD-ROM

This mini CD-ROM will work in your CD-ROM drive. Place it on the inner ring of the tray, as shown, and follow the on-screen installation instructions.

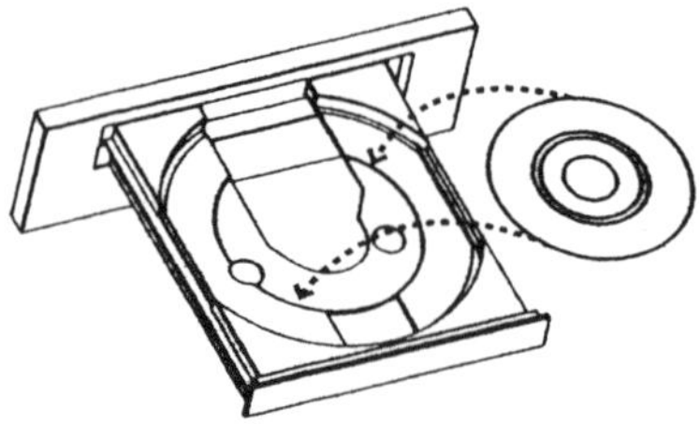

This mini-CD does not work in:
Floppy Drives
Slot Drives
Zip Drives
Stereos
Insert this mini-CD into your CD-ROM drive as shown at left.

Important

No credit or refund will be issued on this book if the CD envelope has been opened, torn, or otherwise tampered with.

Companion CD-ROM for *Mosby's Drug Guide for Nurses,* Seventh Edition

MINIMUM SYSTEM REQUIREMENTS AND SOFTWARE REQUIREMENTS FOR THIS COMPANION CD-ROM:
To use this electronic resource, your computer should meet the following minimum requirements:

This CD will run on both PC and Mac.

Windows® 98se, 2000, or XP
Pentium® II 400 MHz or faster processor
At least 64 MB RAM recommended
10 MB free hard disk space
48× or faster CD-ROM drive
800 × 600 monitor with True Color

Macintosh®
OS X or greater
Power Macintosh
At least 64 MB RAM recommended
1 GHz+ PowerPC G4
10 MB free hard disk space
48× or faster CD-ROM drive
800 × 600 monitor with millions of colors

HOW TO RUN THE PROGRAM

Windows®
1. Start Microsoft Windows and insert the CD-ROM. The program should run automatically.
2. To manually run the program, double click on your CD-ROM drive. Double click on "Skidmore.exe" to start with the CD-ROM still in the drive.

Macintosh®
1. Insert the CD-ROM into the drive.
2. Double click on the CD-ROM icon on your desktop and double click on the file called "Skidmore.osx" (Flash file) to start the program.

TECHNICAL SUPPORT
Technical support for this product is available between 7:30 AM and 7 PM CST, Monday through Friday. Before calling, be sure that your computer meets the minimum system requirements to run this software. Inside the United States and Canada, call 1-800-692-9010. Outside North America, call 314-872-8370. You may also fax your questions to 314-523-4932, or contact Technical Support through e-mail: technical.support@elsevier.com.

9996025764

Mosby's Drug Guide for Nurses

Mosby's Drug Guide for Nurses

SEVENTH EDITION

Linda Skidmore-Roth, RN, MSN, NP
Consultant
Littleton, Colorado

Formerly, Nursing Faculty
New Mexico State University
Las Cruces, New Mexico
El Paso Community College
El Paso, Texas

MOSBY
ELSEVIER

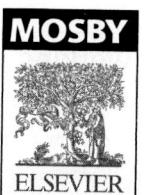

MOSBY
ELSEVIER

11830 Westline Industrial Drive
St. Louis, Missouri 63146

MOSBY'S DRUG GUIDE FOR NURSES, SEVENTH EDITION

ISBN-13: 978-0-323-05332-7
ISBN-10: 0-323-05332-7

NOTICE

Knowledge and best practice in this field are constantly changing. As new research and experience broaden our knowledge, changes in practice, treatment and drug therapy may become necessary or appropriate. Readers are advised to check the most current information provided (i) on procedures featured or (ii) by the manufacturer of each product to be administered, to verify the recommended dose or formula, the method and duration of administration, and contraindications. It is the responsibility of the practitioner, relying on their own experience and knowledge of the patient, to make diagnoses, to determine dosages and the best treatment for each individual patient, and to take all appropriate safety precautions. To the fullest extent of the law, neither the Publisher nor the Editor assumes any liability for any injury and/or damage to persons or property arising out of or related to any use of the material contained in this book.

The Publisher

ISBN-13: 978-0-323-05332-7
ISBN-10: 0-323-05332-7

Executive Publisher: Darlene Como
Managing Editor: Tamara Myers
Developmental Editor: Laura M. Selkirk
Publishing Services Manager: Melissa Lastarria
Project Manager: Joy Moore
Design Direction: Mark Oberkrom

Printed in the United States of America

Last digit is the print number: 9 8 7 6 5 4 3 2 1

Consultants

Victoria Agyekum, RN, MSN
Department Head
Savannah Technical College
Savannah, Georgia

Timothy L. Brenner, PharmD
Assistant Professor
University of Arizona College of Pharmacy
Tucson, Arizona

Jennifer Chan, PharmD
Clinical Assistance Professor of Pharmacy and Pharmacology
University of Texas Health Science Center
San Antonio, Texas

Bruce D. Clayton, BS, PharmD, RPh
Professor of Pharmacy Practice
College of Pharmacy and Health Sciences
Butler University
Indianapolis, Indiana

Daryl D. DePestel, PharmD
Clinical Assistant Professor/Infectious Diseases
University of Michigan Health System
Ann Arbor, Michigan

Amanda Gross, RPh
Pharmacist
University Hospital
Denver, Colorado

Dana H. Hamamura, PharmD
Clinical Pharmacist
University of Colorado Hospital
Denver, Colorado

Cynthia M. Harvey, RN, CLNC
Merit Quest Legal Nurse Consulting, LLC
St. Louis, Missouri

Peter Huynh, PharmD
Diabetes Fellow
Washington State University
Spokane, Washington

Amy E. Miller, PharmD
Assistant Professor of Clinical Pharmacy
Philadelphia College of Pharmacy
University of the Sciences in Philadelphia
Philadelphia, Pennsylvania

Teresa L. Moore, PharmD
Camilla, Georgia

Lisa Nagle, CMA
Program Director – Medical Assisting
Augusta Technical College
Augusta, Georgia

Randolph E. Regal, BS, PharmD, RPh
Clinical Assistant Professor
College of Pharmacy
University of Michigan Hospital
Ann Arbor, Michigan

Roberta J. Secrest, PhD, PharmD, RPh
Eli Lilly and Company
Indianapolis, Indiana

Stephen M. Setter, PharmD, CDE, CGP, DVM
Assistant Professor of Pharmacotherapy
Washington State University
Elder Services/Visiting Nurses Association
Spokane, Washington

John J. Smith, EdD
Director – Health Sciences
Corinthian Colleges, Inc.
Santa Ana, California

Travis Sonnett, PharmD
Clinical Research Associate/Geriatric Resident
Washington State University
Spokane, Washington

Patricia R. Teasley, MSN, RN, APRN, BC
Professor, Nursing Department
Central Texas College
Killeen, Texas

Cheryle I. Whitney, RN, MSN
President
ciwhitney & associates, LLC
The Woodlands, Texas

Preface

Mosby's Drug Guide for Nurses, seventh edition, is the most in-depth handbook available for nursing students! Since its first publication in 1996, more than 100 U.S. and Canadian pharmacists and consultants have reviewed the book's content closely. Today, *Mosby's Drug Guide for Nurses* is more up-to-date than ever—with features that make it easy to find critical information fast!

NEW FACTS

This edition features more than 2000 new drug facts, including:

- new drugs and new dosage information
- newly researched adverse effects
- the latest precautions, interactions, and contraindications
- IV therapy updates
- revised nursing considerations
- updated patient/family education guidelines
- updates on key new drug research

NEW FEATURES

- A color insert featuring drug mechanisms and sites of action illustrations, as well as a photo atlas of drug administration
- Appendix A, "Selected new drugs," provides detailed monographs for 13 drugs and a brief monograph for 1 rarely used drug recently approved by the FDA. (See Table of Contents for a complete list.) Included are monographs for:
  - abatacept (Orencia) for treatment of rheumatoid arthritis
  - exenatide (Byetta) for treatment of type 2 diabetes mellitus
  - pramlintide (Symlin) for treatment of type 1 and type 2 diabetes mellitus
- In addition to the Appendix A monographs, approximately 20 common clinical drugs, including fluticasone and docetaxel, have been added to the book.
- A handy, removable card that includes a Safe Medication Administration Guide, the Nomogram for Calculation of Body Surface Area, and BMI and Body Surface Area equations.
- Appendix B, "Recent FDA drug approvals," lists generic/trade names and uses for six of the most recently approved drugs.
- An updated Companion CD-ROM that now features drug information for the 65 key drugs in the book, along with over 250 NCLEX®-style questions for those 65 key drugs; a comprehensive calculation tutorial; a drug card creator; and dosage calculators.

ORGANIZATION

This handbook is organized into five main sections:

- Four-color insert of drug mechanisms and drug administration
- Individual drug monographs (in alphabetical order by generic name)
- Drug Categories
- Appendixes
- Disorders Index

The guiding principle behind this book is to provide fast, easy access to drug information and nursing considerations. Every detail—from the cover, binding, and paper to the typeface, two-color design, and appendixes—has been carefully chosen with the user in mind.

Here's what you'll find in each section of the handbook:

Color Insert

Mechanisms and Sites of Action

These 16 detailed, four-color illustrations are added to help enhance the understanding of the mechanisms or sites of action for the following drugs and drug classes:

- ACE inhibitors
- adrenocortical steroids
- anticholinergic bronchodilators
- antidepressants
- antidiabetic agents
- antifungal agents
- antiinfective agents
- antiretroviral agents
- benzodiazepines
- diuretics
- drugs used to treat GERD
- laxatives
- narcotic agonist-antagonist analgesics
- narcotic analgesics
- phenytoin
- sympatholytics

Photo Atlas of Drug Administration

This practical resource for students and practitioners lists standard precautions and provides 30 full-color illustrations depicting the physical landmarks and administration techniques used for **IV**, IM, SUBCUT, and ID drug delivery.

Individual Drug Monographs

This book includes monographs for more than 4000 generic and trade medications—those most commonly administered by students. Common trade names are given for all drugs regularly used in the United States and Canada, with drugs available only in Canada identified by a maple leaf icon (✤).

Each monograph provides the following information, whenever possible, for safe, effective administration of each drug:

High-alert status: Identifies drugs with the most potential to cause harm to patients if administered incorrectly.

"Tall Man" lettering: Uses the capitalization of distinguishing letters to avoid medication errors and is required by the FDA for drug manufacturers.

Key drug status: Identifies drugs of special prominence within their functional class, often encountered by students during clinicals; denoted with a special icon (🔑).

Pronunciation: Helps the nurse master complex generic names.

Rx, OTC: Identifies prescription or over-the-counter drugs.

Functional and chemical classifications: Helps the nurse recognize similarities and differences among drugs in the same functional but different chemical classes.

Pregnancy category: FDA pregnancy categories A, B, C, D, or X are noted at the beginning of the monographs, as well as under Precautions or Contraindications depending on FDA category. Appendix J provides a detailed explanation of each category.

Controlled substance schedule: Includes schedules for the United States and Canada.

Do not confuse: Presents drug names that might easily be confused, within each appropriate monograph.

Action: Describes pharmacologic properties concisely.

Therapeutic outcome: Details all possible results of medication use.

Uses: Lists the conditions the drug is used to treat.

Investigational uses: Describes drug uses that may be encountered in practice but are not yet FDA approved.

Dosages and routes: Lists all available and approved dosages and routes for adult, pediatric, and elderly patients.

Available forms: Includes tablets, capsules, extended-release, injectables (**IV**, IM, SUBCUT), solutions, creams, ointments, lotions, gels, shampoos, elixirs, suspensions, suppositories, sprays, aerosols, and lozenges.

Adverse effects: Groups these reactions by alphabetical body system, with common side effects *italicized* and life-threatening reactions in **bold** type for emphasis.

Contraindications: Lists conditions under which the drug absolutely should not be given, including FDA pregnancy safety categories D or X.

Precautions: Lists conditions that require special consideration when the drug is prescribed, including FDA pregnancy safety categories A, B, and C.

Pharmacokinetics/pharmacodynamics: Features a quick-reference chart of concise facts of pharmacokinetics (absorption, distribution, metabolism, excretion, half-life) and pharmacodynamics (onset, peak, duration).

Interactions: Lists confirmed drug, food, herb, and lab test interactions.

Nursing considerations: Identifies key nursing considerations for each step of the nursing process: Assessment, Nursing Diagnoses, Implementation, Patient/Family Education, and Evaluation, including positive therapeutic outcomes. Instructions for giving drugs by various routes (e.g., **IV**, PO, IM, SUBCUT, topically, rectally) appear under Implementation, with route subheadings in bold.

Compatibilities: Lists syringe, Y-site, and additive compatibilities and incompatibilities. If no compatibilities are listed for a drug, the necessary compatibility testing has not been done and that compatibility information is unknown. To ensure safety, assume that the drug may not be mixed with other drugs unless specifically stated.

Nursing Alert icon ◆: Highlights situations in which the patient potentially could be at risk.

Treatment of overdose: Lists drugs and treatments for overdoses where appropriate.

Drug Categories

The Drug Categories section, following the individual drug monographs, provides general information about the various functional classes to promote learning about the similarities and differences among drugs in the same functional class. It summarizes action, uses, adverse effects, contraindications, precautions, pharmacokinetics, interactions, and nursing considerations for each functional class.

Appendixes

Selected new drugs: Includes comprehensive information on 14 key drugs approved by the FDA during the past 12 months.

Recent FDA drug approvals: Summarizes basic information, such as generic name, trade name and uses, for drugs so recently approved by the FDA that complete information was not yet available when this book went to press.

High-alert drugs: Lists the 103 drugs in *Mosby's Drug Guide for Nurses* that cause significant harm to patients if administered incorrectly.

Ophthalmic, otic, nasal, and topical products: Provides essential information for more than 150 ophthalmic, otic, nasal, and topical products commonly used today, grouped by chemical drug class.

Combination products: Provides details on the forms and uses of more than 700 combination products.

Rarely used drugs: Provides concise monographs for 88 infrequently used drugs, including dosage and routes, uses, and contraindications.

Less frequently used antihistamines: Includes names, uses, doses, forms, interactions, and contraindications.

Vaccines and toxoids: Features an easy-to-use table with generic and trade names, uses, dosages and routes, and contraindications for 29 key vaccines and toxoids.

Herbal products: Features basic usage information on more than 47 common herbs and natural supplements.

FDA pregnancy categories: Explains the five FDA pregnancy categories.

Controlled substance chart: Covers the drug schedules for the United States, with examples.

Commonly used abbreviations: Lists abbreviations alphabetically with their meanings.

High-alert Canadian medications: Lists the drugs that the Institute for Safe Medication Practices Canada considers high alert because of their potential to cause significant harm to patients.

Canadian controlled substance chart: Covers the drug schedules for Canada, with examples.

Canadian recommended immunization schedules for infants and children: Convenient, up-to-date reference table for Canadian patients.

Disorders Index

This book includes both a general index and a disorders index, both of which are updated and expanded in this edition. Dovetailing with the content nursing students encounter in medical-surgical courses, the disorders index lists major disorders and major drugs used in their management. The page number for each drug listed follows.

The following sources were consulted in the preparation of this edition:

Blumenthal M: *The complete German Commission E monographs: therapeutic guide to herbal medicines,* Austin, 2002, American Botanical Council.

Drug information: Bethesda, American Hospital Formulary Service.

Facts and comparisons: St Louis, updated monthly.

Gahart BL: *Intravenous medications,* ed 22, St Louis, 2006, Mosby.

Hardman JG, et al: *Goodman and Gilman's the pharmacological basis of therapeutics,* ed 10, New York, 2002, McGraw-Hill.

McKenry LM, Salerno E: *Mosby's pharmacology in nursing,* ed 21, St Louis, 2003, Mosby.

Mediphor Editorial Group: *Drug interaction facts,* Philadelphia, updated quarterly, Lippincott Williams & Wilkins.

Review of natural products: Philadelphia, updated monthly, *Facts and Comparisons.*

Acknowledgments

I am indebted to the nursing and pharmacology consultants who reviewed the manuscript and pages and thank them for their criticism and encouragement. I would also like to thank Darlene Como, Tamara Myers, and Laura Selkirk, my editors, whose active encouragement and enthusiasm have made this book better than it might otherwise have been. I am likewise grateful to Joy Moore and Graphic World Inc. for the coordination of the production process and assistance with the development of the new edition.

Linda Skidmore-Roth

Contents

Color Insert — Mechanisms and Sites of Action, 1
Photo Atlas of Drug Administration, 18

Individual Drug Monographs, 33

Drug Categories, 991

Appendixes

A. Selected New Drugs, 1027
abatacept
entecavir
exenatide
galsulfase
insulin, inhaled
mecasermin
nelarabine
pramlintide
pregabalin
ramelteon
rotavirus vaccine
sorafenib
tigecycline
tipranavir
B. Recent FDA Drug Approvals, 1041
C. High-Alert Drugs, 1042
D. Ophthalmic, Nasal, Topical, and Otic Products, 1044
E. Combination Products, 1056
F. Rarely Used Drugs, 1086
G. Less Frequently Used Antihistamines, 1102
H. Vaccines and Toxoids, 1105
I. Herbal Products, 1111
J. FDA Pregnancy Categories, 1116
K. Controlled Substance Chart, 1117
L. Commonly Used Abbreviations, 1118
M. High-Alert Canadian Medications, 1121
N. Canadian Controlled Substance Chart, 1123
O. Canadian Recommended Immunization Schedules for Infants and Children, 1125

Disorders Index, 1127

General Index, 1131

Mechanisms and Sites of Action

Plate 1: Sites of Action—ACE Inhibitors
Plate 2: Mechanisms of Action—Adrenocortical Steroids
Plate 3: Sites and Mechanisms of Action—Anticholinergic Bronchodilators
Plate 4: Mechanisms of Action—Antidepressants
Plate 5: Mechanisms of Action—Antidiabetic Agents
Plate 6: Sites and Mechanisms of Action—Antifungal Agents
Plate 7: Sites and Mechanisms of Action—Antiinfective Agents
Plate 8: Mechanisms and Sites of Action—Antiretroviral Agents
Plate 9: Mechanisms of Action—Benzodiazepines
Plate 10: Sites of Action—Diuretics
Plate 11: Sites of Action—Drugs Used to Treat GERD
Plate 12: Mechanisms of Action—Laxatives
Plate 13: Mechanisms of Action—Narcotic Agonist-Antagonist Analgesics
Plate 14: Mechanisms of Action—Narcotic Analgesics
Plate 15: Mechanisms of Action—Phenytoin
Plate 16: Sites of Action—Sympatholytics

Photo Atlas of Drug Administration*

Plate 17: Needles
Plate 18: Needle with Plastic Guard
Plate 19: Preparing an Injection from a Vial
Plate 20: Administering an Injection
Plate 21: Subcutaneous Injection
Plate 22: Intradermal Injection
Plate 23: Subcutaneous Injection Sites
Plate 24: Deltoid Intramuscular Injection
Plate 25: Vastus Lateralis Intramuscular Injection
Plate 26: Ventrogluteal Intramuscular Injection
Plate 27: Z-track Method of Injection
Plate 28: Comparison of Needle Angles
Plate 29: Administering Medication by IV Bolus
Plate 30: Administering Medication by Piggyback
Plate 31: Adding Medications to IV Fluid Containers
Plate 32: Standard Precautions

*All color plates of drug administration are from Potter PA and Perry AG: *Fundamentals of Nursing*, ed 6, St. Louis, 2004, Mosby, except where noted.

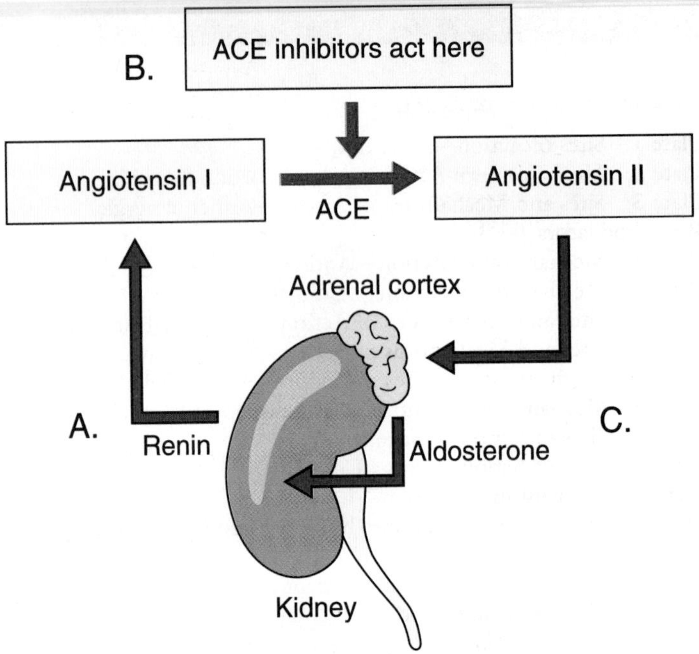

Plate 1 The renin-angiotensin-aldosterone system plays a major role in regulating BP. Any condition that decreases renal blood flow, reduces BP, or stimulates $beta_1$-adrenergic receptors prompts the kidneys to release renin **(A).** Renin acts on angiotensinogen, which is converted to angiotensin I, a weak vasoconstrictor. Angiotensin-converting enzyme (ACE) converts angiotensin I to angiotensin II, which causes systemic and renal blood vessels to constrict **(B).** Systemic vasoconstriction increases peripheral vascular resistance, raising the BP. Renal vasoconstriction decreases glomerular filtration, resulting in sodium and water retention and increasing blood volume and BP. In addition, angiotensin II also acts on the adrenal cortex causing it to release aldosterone **(C).** This makes the kidneys retain additional sodium and water, which further increases the BP. ACE inhibitors, such as captopril, enalapril, and lisinopril, block the action of ACE. As a result, angiotensin II can't form, which prevents systemic and renal vasoconstriction and the release of aldosterone. (From Prosser S, Worster B, Dewar K: *Applied Pharmacology for Nurses and Other Health Care Professionals,* St. Louis, 2000, Mosby.)

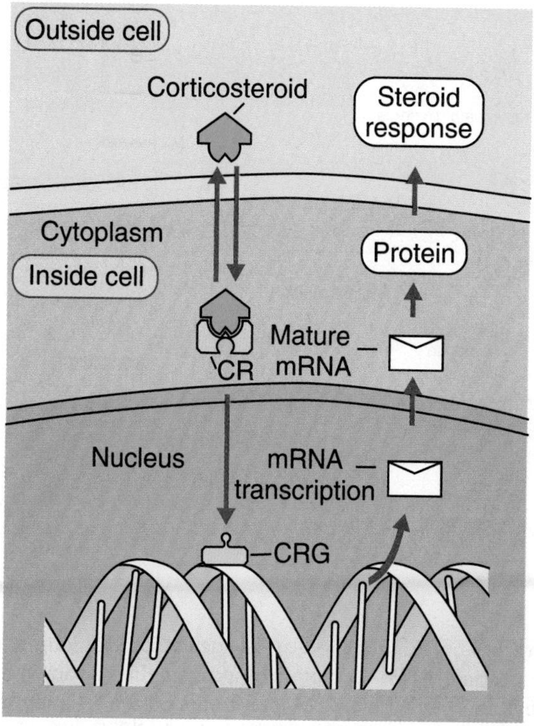

Plate 2 Adrenocortical steroids (also called corticosteroids) are available in many forms, such as predniSONE, and produce a wide range of effects, such as immunosupression and anti-inflammation. Here's how these drugs work at the cellular level.

Corticosteroids are hormones that are naturally produced by the body (endogenous hormones). Synthetic corticosteroids work much the same as the endogenous hormones. When a corticosteroid enters a cell, it binds to corticosteroid receptors (CRs) in the cell's cytoplasm, forming a complex. The complex moves to the nucleus where it causes the transcription of corticosteroid responsive genes (CRGs) to messenger ribonucleic acid (mRNA), eventually translating to a protein that produces a steroid response in target tissues. (From Taylor: *Mosby's Crash Course Pharmacology*, St. Louis, 1998, Mosby.)

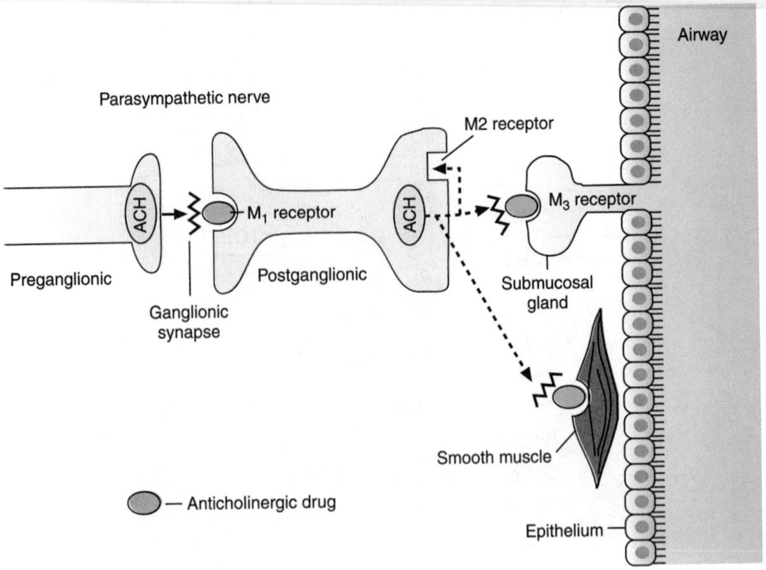

Plate 3 Anticholinergic bronchodilators, such as ipratropium, work by blocking muscarinic-1 (M_1) receptors on postganglionic parasympathetic nerve endings and muscarinic-3 (M_3) receptors on the cell membranes of bronchial smooth muscles and submucosal glands. Normally, stimulation of the M_1 and M_3 receptors by acetylcholine (ACH) causes bronchoconstriction and mucus secretion from submucosal glands. Anticholinergic bronchodilators block these specific muscarinic receptors from the effects of acetylcholine, causing bronchial smooth muscle relaxation, bronchodilation, and decreased mucus production. (From Rau J: *Respiratory Care Pharmacology*, ed 6, St. Louis, 2002, Mosby.)

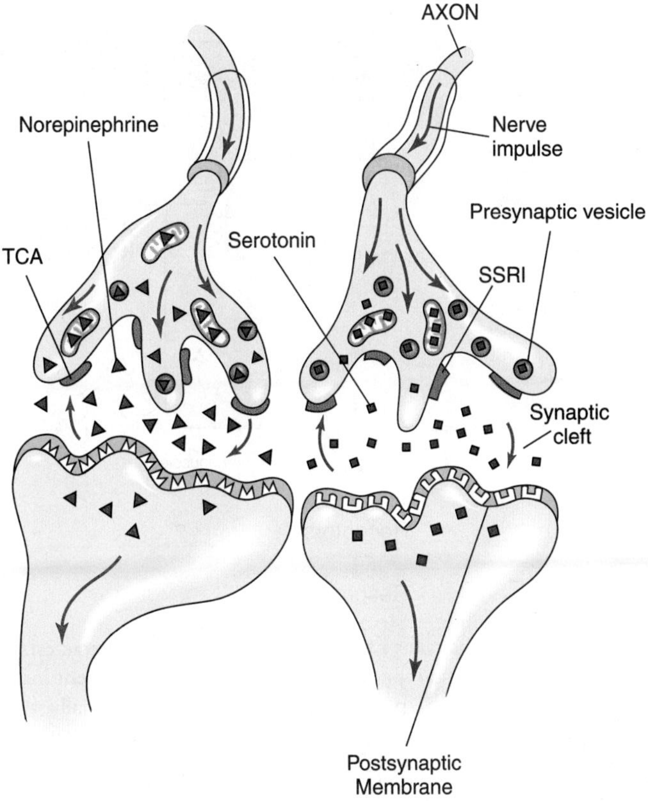

Plate 4 Depression is thought to occur when levels of neurotransmitters, such as norepinephrine and serotonin, are reduced at postsynaptic receptor sites. These neurotransmitters affect a wide array of functions, including mood, obsessions, appetite, and anxiety. Antidepressants work by increasing the availability of these neurotransmitters at postsynaptic membranes and by enhancing and prolonging their effects. As a result, these agents improve mood, reduce anxiety, and minimize obsessions.

Antidepressants typically are classified as tricyclic antidepressants (TCAs), monoamine oxidase inhibitors (not shown), selective serotonin reuptake inhibitors (SSRIs), and atypical antidepressants (not shown). TCAs, such as amitriptyline and desipramine, primarily block norepinephrine reuptake at presynaptic membranes, thereby increasing the norepinephrine concentration at synapses and making more available at postsynaptic receptors **(A).**

SSRIs, such as fluoxetine and paroxetine, selectively inhibit serotonin uptake at presynaptic membranes. This action leads to increased serotonin availability at postsynaptic receptors **(B).** (From Gutierrez K: *Pharmacotherapeutics: Clinical Decision Making in Nursing,* Philadelphia, 1999, Saunders.)

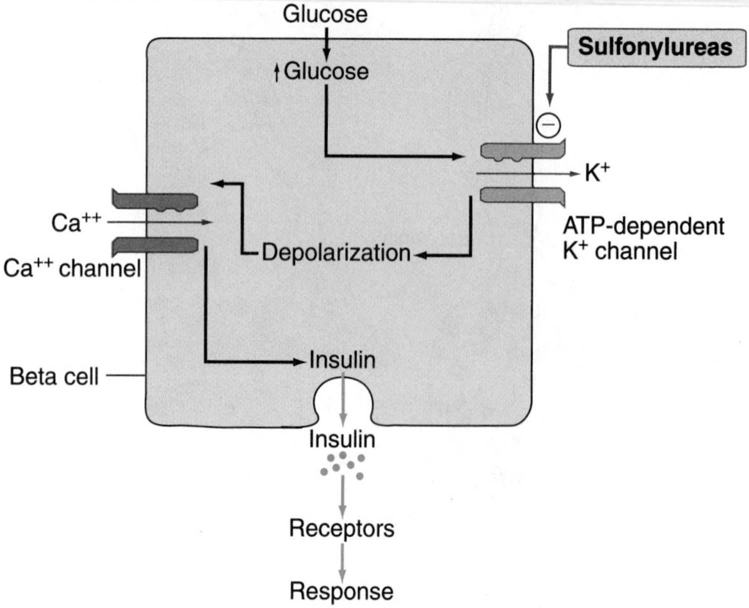

Plate 5 Diabetes mellitus takes two forms: type 1 diabetes characterized by a complete lack of insulin and type 2 diabetes marked by insufficient insulin secretion, insulin resistance in peripheral tissues, or both. Normally, the beta cells in the pancreatic islets of Langerhans are responsible for secreting insulin. When glucose levels rise in the beta cell, it triggers adenosine triphosphate (ATP)-dependent potassium (K^+) channels in the membranes of beta cells to close. Then the beta cells depolarize and calcium (Ca^{++}) enters the cell through Ca^{++} channel, and insulin is released from the cell. When circulating insulin engages with insulin receptors on cell membranes, it facilitates the movement of glucose into the cell, among other actions.

Type 1 diabetes is treated with the use of exogenous insulin, which mimics natural insulin in the body. Insulin takes many forms with varying degrees of onset, peak and duration, including rapid, regular, intermediate, and long-acting.

Type 2 diabetes is usually treated with oral agents. Sulfonylureas, such as glyburide for example, block ATP-dependent K^+ channels in the cell membranes of beta cells, ultimately resulting in the release of insulin. (From Taylor: *Mosby's Crash Course Pharmacology,* St. Louis, 1998, Mosby.)

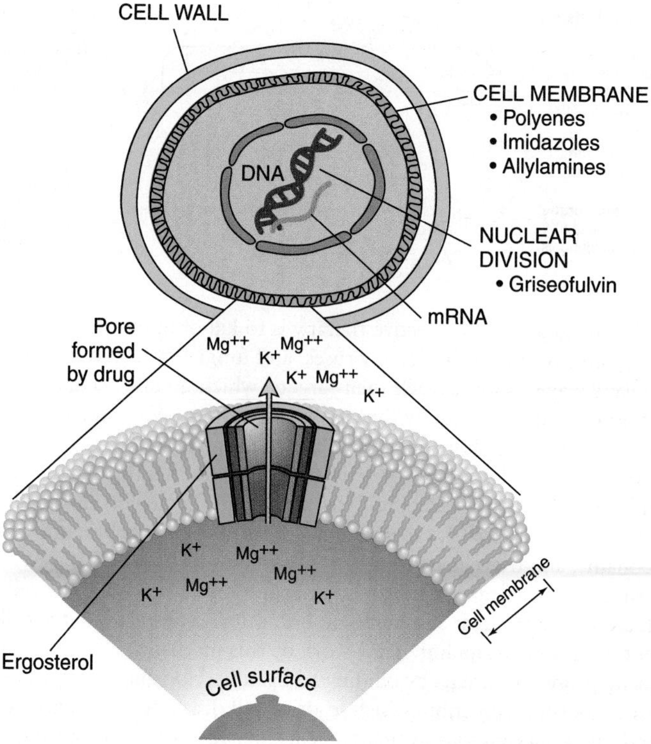

Plate 6 Antifungal agents primarily affect fungi at one of two sites: the cell membrane or the cell nucleus. Most of these agents, such as polyene, imidazole, and allylamine antifungals, act on the fungal cell membrane. Polyene antifungals, such amphotericin B, bind to ergosterol and increase cell membrane permeability. Imidazole antifungals, such as fluconazole and ketoconazole, interfere with ergosterol synthesis by inhibiting the cytochrome P_{450} enzyme system, altering the cell membrane, and inhibiting fungal growth. Allylamine antifungals, such as terbinafine, inhibit the enzyme squaline epoxidase, which disrupts ergosterol production—and cell membrane integrity. When cell membrane permeability increases, cellular components, including potassium (K^+) and magnesium (Mg^{++}), leak out. Loss of these cellular components leads to cell death.

Another antifungal agent, griseofulvin directly affects the fungal nucleus, interfering with mitosis. By binding to structures in the mitotic spindle, it prevents cells from dividing, which eventually leads to their death. (From Gutierrez K: *Pharmacotherapeutics: Clinical Decision Making in Nursing*, Philadelphia, 1999, Saunders.)

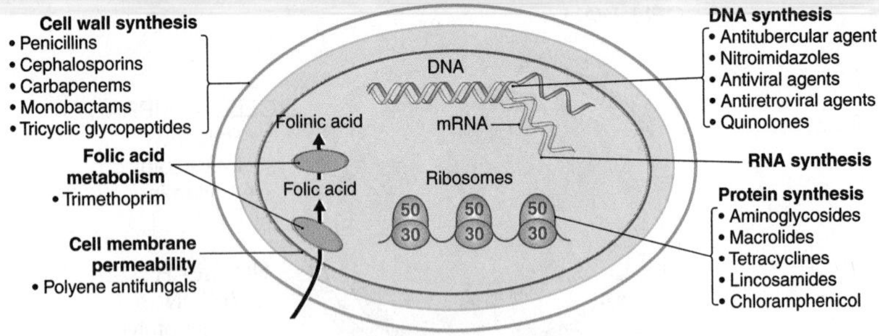

Plate 7 The goal of anti-infective therapy is to kill or inhibit the growth of microorganisms, such as bacteria, viruses, and fungi. To achieve this goal, anti-infective agents must reach their targets, which usually occurs through absorption and distribution by the circulatory system. When the target is reached, a drug can kill or suppress microorganisms by:

- inhibiting cell wall synthesis or activating enzymes that disrupt the cell wall, which leads to cellular weakening, lysis, and death. Penicillins (ampicillin), cephalosporins (cefazolin), carbapenems (imipenem), monobactams (aztreonam), and tricyclic glycopeptides (vancomycin) act in this way.
- altering cell membrane permeability through direct action on the cell wall, which allows intracellular substances to leak out and destabilizes the cell. Polyene antifungals (amphotericin) work by this mechanism.
- altering protein synthesis by binding to bacterial ribosomes (50/30) or affecting ribosomal function, which leads to cell death or slowed growth respectively. Aminoglycosides (gentamicin), macrolides (erythromycin), tetracyclines (doxycycline), lincosamides (clindamycin), and the miscellaneous anti-infective chloramphenicol use the action.
- inhibiting DNA or RNA, including messenger RNA (mRNA), by synthesis by binding to nucleic acids or interacting with enzymes required for their synthesis. Antitubercular agents (rifampin), nitroimidazoles (metronidazole), antiviral agents (acyclovir), antiretroviral agents (stavudine), and quinolones (ciprofloxacin) act like this.
- inhibiting the metabolism of folic acid and folinic acid or other cellular components that are essential for bacterial cell growth. The miscellaneous anti-infective trimethoprim employs this mechanism of action. (From Page C, et al: *Integrated Pharmacology,* ed 2, St. Louis, 2002, Mosby.)

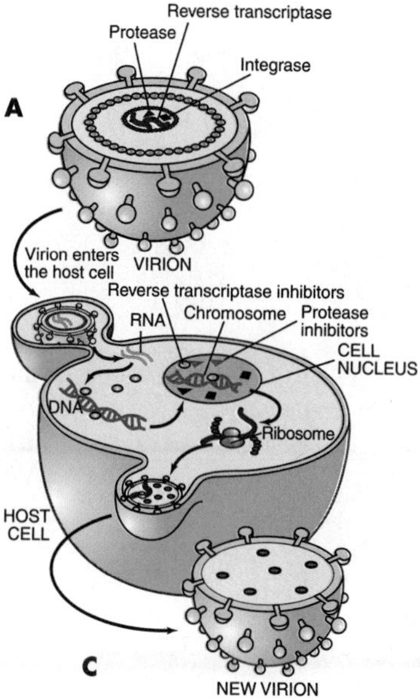

Plate 8 When viruses reproduce, the infectious viral particle or virion **(A)** enters the host cell. The virion attaches to the cell's surface and then inserts itself into the host cell **(B).** Once inside, the virion uncoats, and the enzyme reverse transcriptase makes two copies of the viral RNA: one copy is identical; the other is a mirror image. These two copies form double-stranded viral DNA that enters the host cell's nucleus, where it inserts itself into the host cell's DNA with the help of the enzyme integrase. Then viral DNA reprograms the host cell to produce additional viral RNA, which begins the process of forming new viruses. Specifically, messenger RNA (mRNA) instructs ribosomal RNA (rRNA) to produce a new chain of proteins and enzymes that are used to form new viruses. Protease cuts the chains, creating individual proteins. These combine with new RNA to create new virions, which bud and are released from the host cell **(C).**

Antiretroviral agents target specific enzymes during viral reproduction. Nucleoside reverse transcriptase inhibitors, such as stavudine, interfere with the action of reverse transcriptase by mimicking naturally occurring nucleosides. Nucleotide reverse transcriptase inhibitors, such as tenofovir, block reverse transcriptase by competing with the natural substrate deoxyadenosine triphosphate and by causing DNA chain termination. Nonnucleoside reverse transcriptase inhibitors, such as delavirdine, work by directly binding to reverse transcriptase. As a result, no viral DNA is available to insert itself into the host cell's DNA. Protease inhibitors, such as indinavir, bind to and interefere with the action of protease, thus, the new chain of proteins formed by rRNA can't be cut into individual proteins to make new viruses. (From Gutierrez K: *Pharmacotherapeutics: Clinical Decision Making in Nursing,* Philadelphia, 1999, Saunders.)

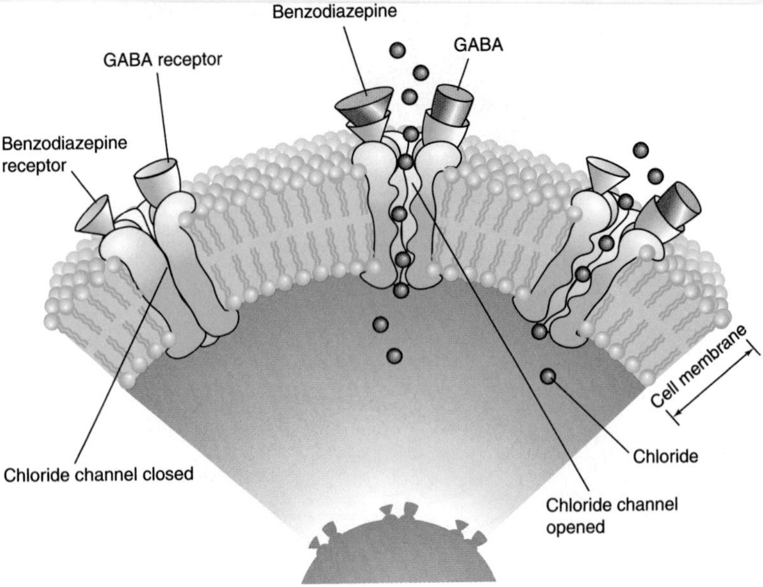

Plate 9 Benzodiazepines reduce anxiety by stimulating the action of the inhibitory neurotransmitter, gamma-aminobutyric acid (GABA), in the limbic system. The limbic system plays an important role in the regulation of human behavior. Dysfunction of GABA neurotransmission in the limbic system may be linked to the development of certain anxiety disorders.

The limbic system contains a highly dense area of benzodiazepine receptors that may be linked to the antianxiety effects of benzodiazepines. These benzodiazepine receptors are located on the surface of neuronal cell membranes and are adjacent to GABA receptors. The binding of a benzodiazepine to its receptor enhances the affinity of a GABA receptor for GABA. In the absence of a benzodiazepine, the binding of GABA to its receptor causes the chloride channel in the cell membrane to open, which increases the influx of chloride into the cell. This influx of chloride results in hyperpolarization of the neuronal cell membrane and reduces the neuron's ability to fire, which is why GABA is considered an inhibitory neurotransmitter.

A benzodiazepine acts only in the presence of GABA. When it binds to a benzodiazepine receptor, it prolongs the time that the chloride channel remains open. This results in greater depression of neuronal function and a reduction in anxiety. (From Gutierrez K: *Pharmacotherapeutics: Clinical Decision Making in Nursing*, Philadelphia, 1999, Saunders.)

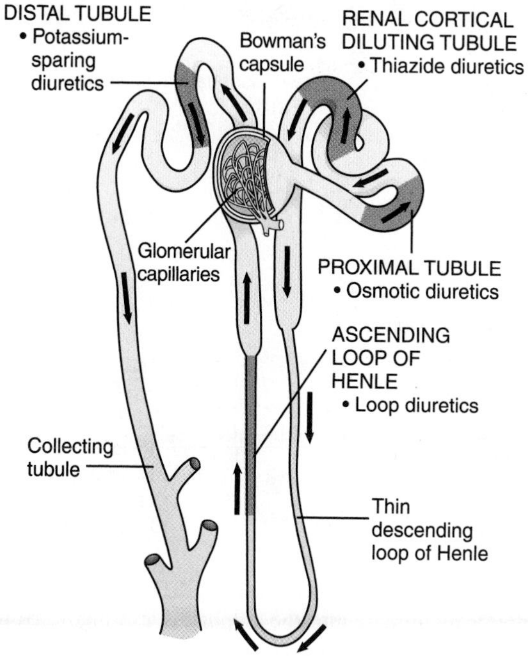

Plate 10 Diuretics act primarily to increase water and sodium excretion by the kidneys, thereby increasing urine output. In the process, chloride, potassium, and other electrolytes may also be excreted. Most diuretics act by blocking sodium, water, and chloride reabsorption by peritubular capillaries in the nephrons. As a result, water and electrolytes remain in the convoluted tubules to be excreted as urine. The increased water and electrolyte excretion reduces blood volume—and ultimately blood pressure.

Diuretics belong to four major subclasses:

1. Thiazide diuretics, such as hydrochlorothiazide, act in the early portion of the distal convoluted tubule, called the cortical diluting segment. These drugs block sodium, chloride, and water reabsorption and promote their excretion along with potassium.
2. Loop diuretics, such as furosemide, act primarily in the thick ascending limb of the loop of Henle, blocking sodium, water, and chloride reabsorption. Then these substances are excreted along with potassium.
3. Potassium-sparing diuretics, such as spironolactone, act in the late portion of the distal convoluted tubule and collecting tubule. Here, they inhibit the action of aldosterone, leading to sodium excretion and potassium retention. Although triamterene and amiloride, two other potassium-sparing diuretics, act at the same site, they don't affect aldosterone. Instead, these drugs directly block the exchange of sodium and potassium, leading to decreased sodium reabsorption and decreased potassium excretion.
4. Osmotic diuretics, such as mannitol, work in the proximal convoluted tubule. As their name implies, these diuretics increase the osmotic pressure of the glomerular filtrate, inhibiting the passive reabsorption of water, sodium, and chloride. (From Gutierrez K: *Pharmacotherapeutics: Clinical Decision Making in Nursing,* Philadelphia, 1999, Saunders.)

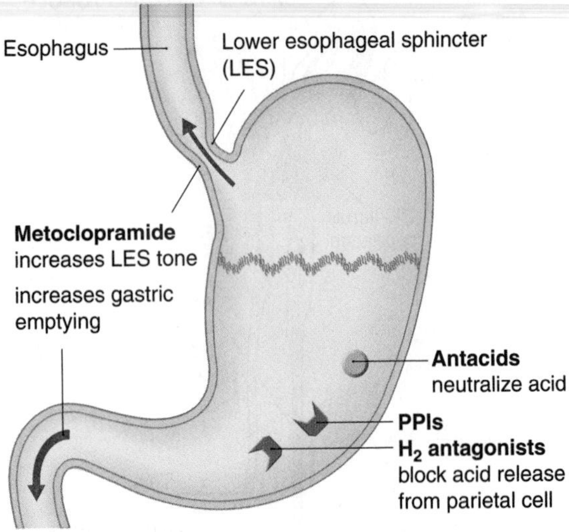

Plate 11 Gastroesophageal reflux disease (GERD) occurs when acidic stomach contents regurgitate into the esophagus, causing heartburn. The disorder may result from a weakness or incompetence of the lower esophageal sphincter (LES). Because the malfunctioning LES makes the reflux leave the esophagus and re-enter the stomach slowly, the esophageal mucosa is exposed to the acid for a long time. Because the enzymatic action of parietal cells in the stomach makes the reflux highly acidic, GERD causes irritation and possible erosion of the esophageal mucosa.

Treatment of GERD can employ drugs from several classes: histamine (H_2) antagonists, proton pump inhibitors (PPIs), the miscellaneous GI agent metoclopramide, and antacids. H_2 antagonists, such as cimetidine, act in parietal cells of the stomach. Normally, H_2-receptor stimulation results in gastric acid secretion. By blocking these receptors, H_2 antagonists decrease the amount and acidity of gastric secretion, including secretion that occurs with fasting, food consumption at night, and stomach distension.

PPIs, such as esomeprazole, also suppress gastric acid secretion. However, they do it by inhibiting the hydrogen-potassium-adenosine triphsophatase enzyme system, which is located on the surface of parietal cells and controls their gastric acid secretion. PPIs block acid secretion that results from fasting or abdominal distension caused by food ingestion.

Metoclopramide increases the tone and motility of the upper GI tract. It works by stimulating the release of acetylcholine from GI nerve endings, which improves LES tone and leads to decreased reflux. The drug also stimulates gastric emptying, which reduces gastric contents.

Antacids, such as aluminum hydroxide, act primarily in the stomach by chemically combining with the hydrogen ions (H^+) in gastric acid and raising the pH of gastric contents. They don't prevent reflux. However, they make the reflux less acidic, so it causes less damage to the esophageal mucosa. (From Page C, et al: *Integrated Pharmacology*, ed 2, St. Louis, 2002, Mosby.)

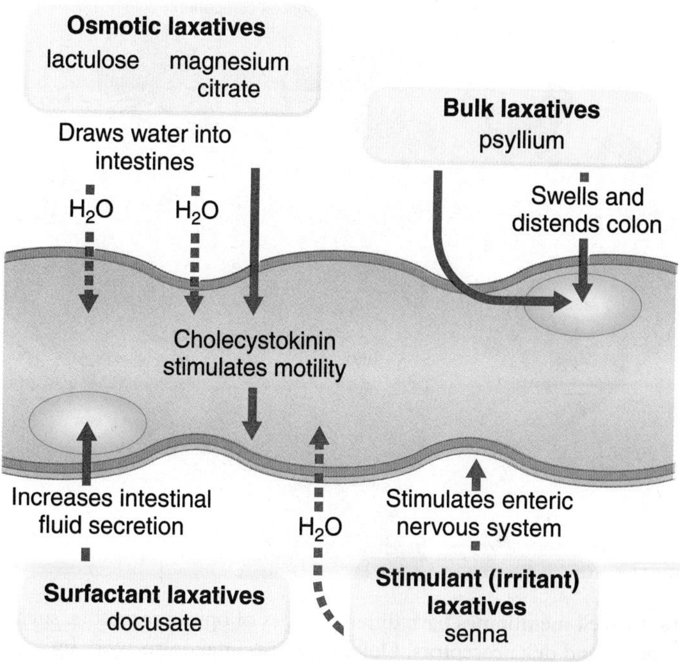

Plate 12 Laxatives ease or stimulate defecation. Typically, they're classified by their mechanism of action as bulk-forming, osmotic, stimulant, or surfactant laxatives.

Bulk-forming laxatives, such as psyllium, act in the small and large bowel. Because ingredients in these laxatives are undigestible, they remain within the stool and increase the fecal mass by drawing in water. These agents also enhance bacterial growth in the colon, further adding to the fecal mass.

Osmotic laxatives, such as lactulose, draw water into the intestinal lumen, causing the fecal mass to soften and swell. This osmotic action may be enhanced by the metabolism of colonic bacteria to lactate and other organic acids. These acids decrease colonic pH and increase colonic motility.

Stimulant (or irritant) laxatives, such as senna, act on the intestinal wall to increase water and electrolytes in the intestinal lumen. In addition, they directly irritate the colon, increasing motility.

Surfactant laxatives (or fecal softeners), such as docusate, reduce the surface tension of the stool, allowing water to enter it. These laxatives may also help to increase water and electrolyte excretion into the intestinal lumen, softening and increasing the fecal mass. (From Page C, et al: *Integrated Pharmacology*, ed 2, St. Louis, 2002, Mosby.)

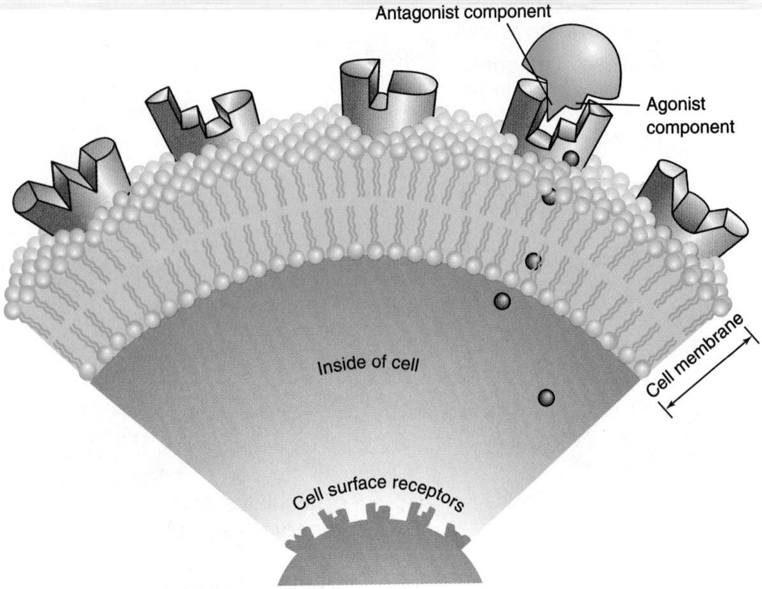

Plate 13 Cell membranes have different types of opioid receptors, such as mu, kappa, and delta receptors. Opioid agonist-antagonists work by stimulating one type of receptor, while simultaneously blocking another type. As agonists, they work primarily by activating kappa receptors to produce analgesia and such other effects as CNS and respiratory depression, decreased GI motility, and euphoria. As antagonists, they compete with opioids at mu receptors, helping to reverse or block some of the other effects of agonists. (From Gutierrez K: *Pharmacotherapeutics: Clinical Decision Making in Nursing,* Philadelphia, 1999, Saunders.)

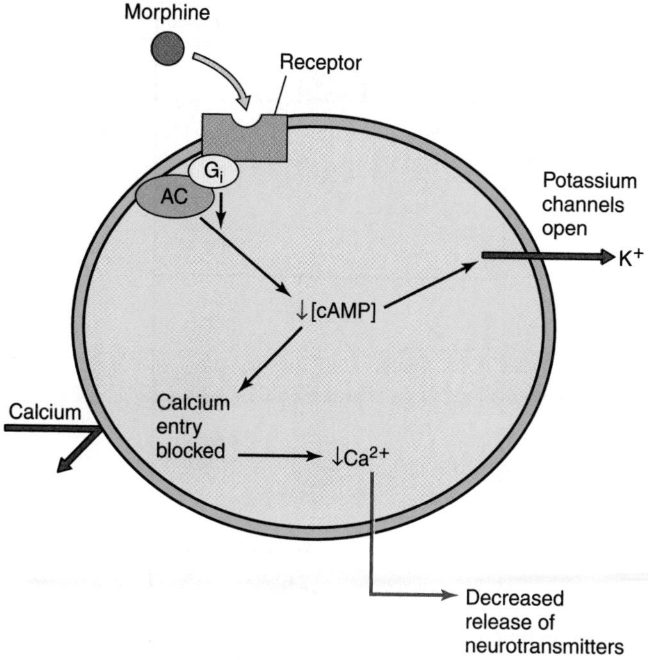

Plate 14 Narcotic analgesics bind to three types of opioid receptors: mu, kappa, and delta receptors. They produce analgesia primarily by activating mu receptors. However, they also engage with and activate kappa and delta receptors, producing other effects, such as sedation and vasomotor stimulation.

When morphine or another narcotic analgesic binds to opioid receptors, activation occurs. The receptors send signals to the enzyme adenyl cyclase (AC) to slow activity by way of G proteins (G_i). Decreased adenyl cyclase activity causes less cyclic adenosine monophosphate (cAMP) to be produced. A secondary messenger substance, cAMP is important for regulating cell membrane channels. A reduced cAMP level allows fewer potassium ions to leave the cell and blocks calcium ions from entering the cell. This ion imbalance—especially the reduced intracellular calcium level—ultimately decreases the release of neurotransmitters from the cell, thereby blocking or reducing pain impulse transmission. (From Brody TM, Larner J, Minneman KP: *Human Pharmacology: Molecular to Clinical,* ed 3, St. Louis, 1998, Mosby.)

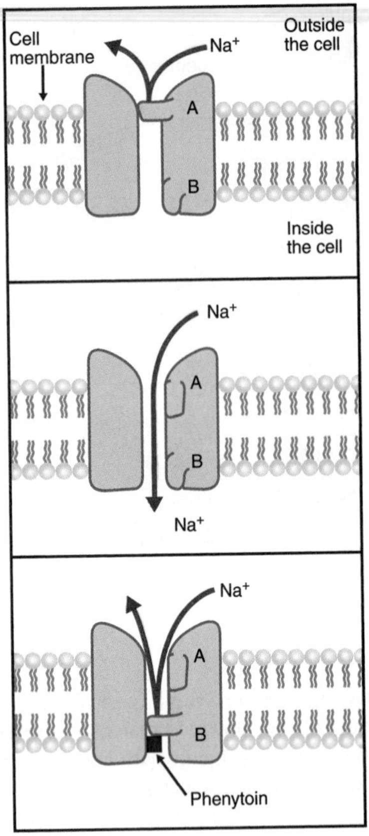

Plate 15 Phenytoin, which is used to treat tonic-clonic seizures, acts in the motor cortex and brain stem where the tonic phase of tonic-clonic seizures originates. By altering sodium transport across neuronal cell membranes, phenytoin stabilizes the cell membrane, reduces repetitive firing of the neurons, and halts or limits the spread of seizures. The first illustration shows a neuronal cell membrane in its resting state. The activation gate **(A)** of the sodium channel in the cell membrane is closed and blocks sodium (Na^+) from entering the cell. In the second illustration, a nerve impulse has caused depolarization and opening of the activation gate, allowing Na^+ to move into the cell. In the third illustration, depolarization continues and an inactivation gate **(B)** moves into the channel. This prevents Na^+ from moving into the cell. Phenytoin prolongs the inactivated state of the sodium channel by preventing reopening of the inactivation gate. By further preventing Na^+ from entering the cell, phenytoin slows impulse transmission, and thus slows the rate at which neurons fire. (From Brody TM, Larner J, Minneman KP: *Human Pharmacology: Molecular to Clinical,* ed 3, St. Louis, 1998, Mosby.)

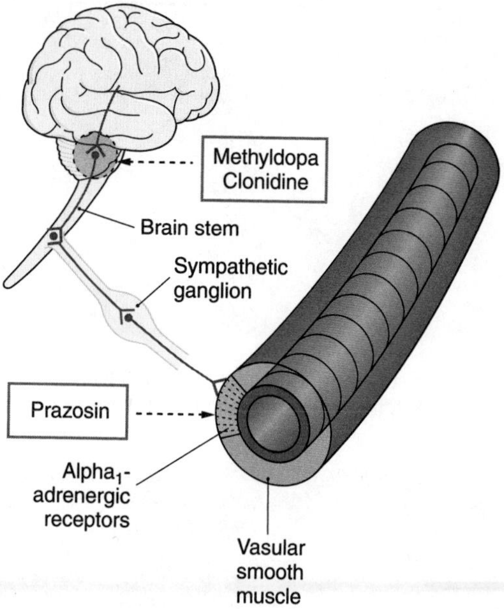

Plate 16 Sympatholytics inhibit sympathetic nervous system (SNS) activity, which plays a major role in regulating BP. Normally when the SNS is stimulated, nerve impulses travel from the cardiovascular center of the CNS to the sympathetic ganglia. From there, the impulses travel along postganglionic fibers to specific effector organs, such as the heart and blood vessels. SNS stimulation also triggers the release of norepinephrine, which acts primarily at alpha-adrenergic receptors.

Sympatholytics fall into two subclassees: central-acting alpha$_2$ agonists and peripheral-acting alpha$_1$-adrenergic antagonists. Central-acting alpha$_2$ agonists, such as methyldopa and clonidine, stimulate alpha$_2$-adrenergic receptors in the cardiovascular center of the CNS and reduce activity in the vasomotor center of the brain, interfering with sympathetic stimulation of the heart and blood vessels. This causes blood vessel dilation and decreased cardiac output, which leads to reduced BP.

Peripheral-acting alpha$_1$-adrenergic antagonists, such as prazosin, inhibit the stimulation of alpha$_1$-adrenergic receptors by norepinephrine in vascular smooth muscle, interfering with SNS-induced vasoconstriction. As a result, the blood vessels dilate, reducing peripheral vascular resistance and venous return to the heart. These effects, in turn, lead to decreased BP. (From Prosser S, Worster B, Dewar K: *Applied Pharmacology for Nurses and Other Health Care Professionals,* St. Louis, 2000, Mosby.)

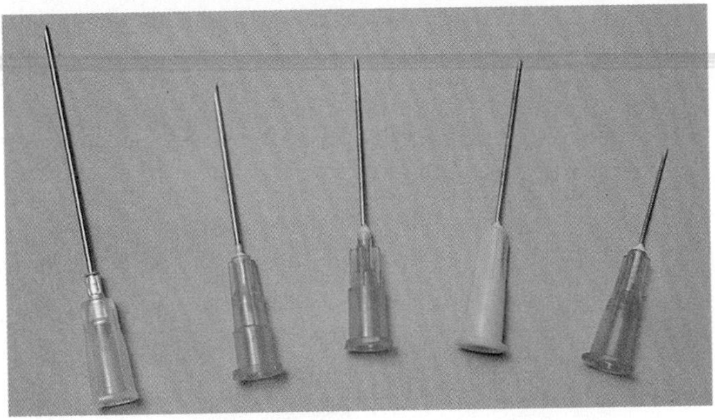

Plate 17 Needles. Left to right: 19 gauge, 1½-inch length; 20 gauge, 1-inch length; 21 gauge, 1-inch length; 23 gauge, 1-inch length; and 25 gauge, ⅝-inch length.

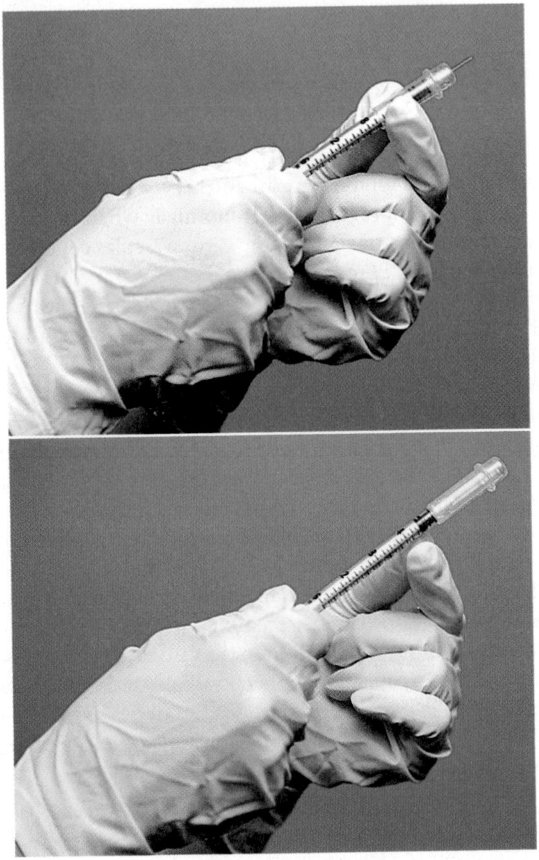

A

B

Plate 18 Needle with plastic guard to prevent needle sticks. **A,** Position of guard before injection. **B,** After injection, the guard locks in place, covering the needle.

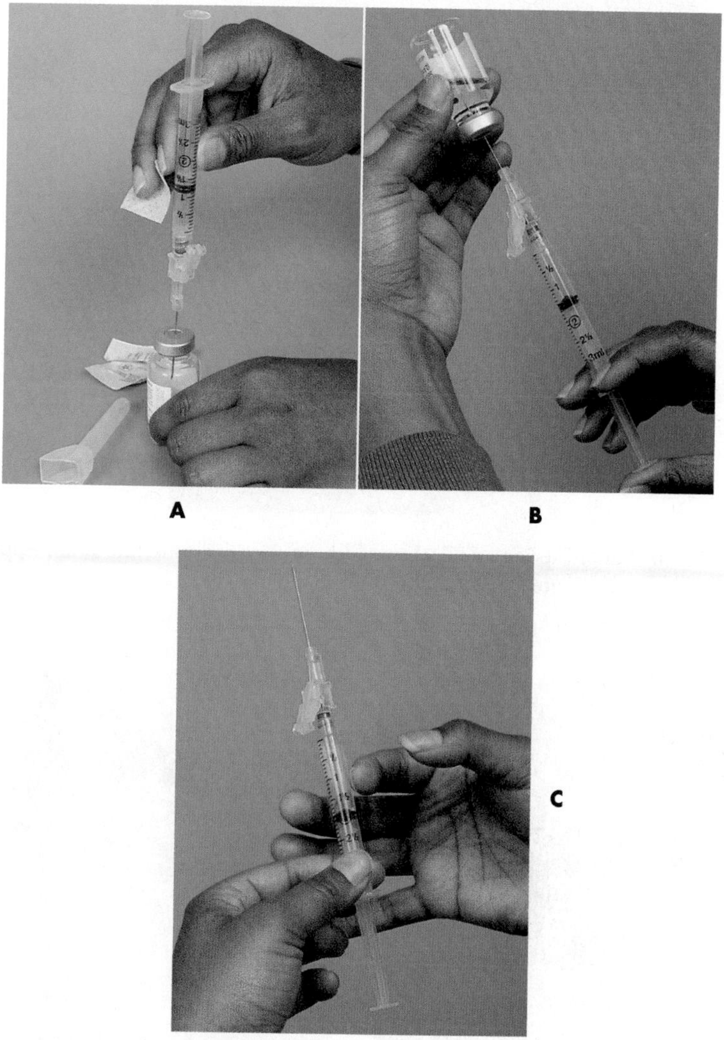

Plate 19 Preparing an injection from a vial. Remove needle cap from syringe. Pull back on the plunger to draw amount of air into syringe equivalent to volume of medication to be aspirated from vial. **A,** Insert tip of needle, with bevel pointing up, through center of rubber seal. Apply pressure on tip of needle during insertion. **B,** Allow air pressure to fill syringe gradually with medication. Pull back slightly on plunger if necessary. **C,** Remove remaining air from syringe by holding it and needle upright. Tap barrel to dislodge air bubbles. Draw back slightly on plunger and then push plunger upward to eject air. Do not eject fluid.

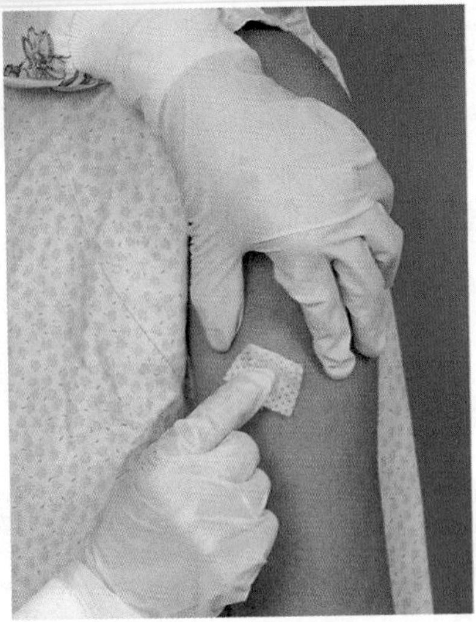

Plate 20 Administering an injection. Cleanse site with antiseptic swab. Apply swab at center of site and rotate outward in circular direction for about 5 cm (2 in).

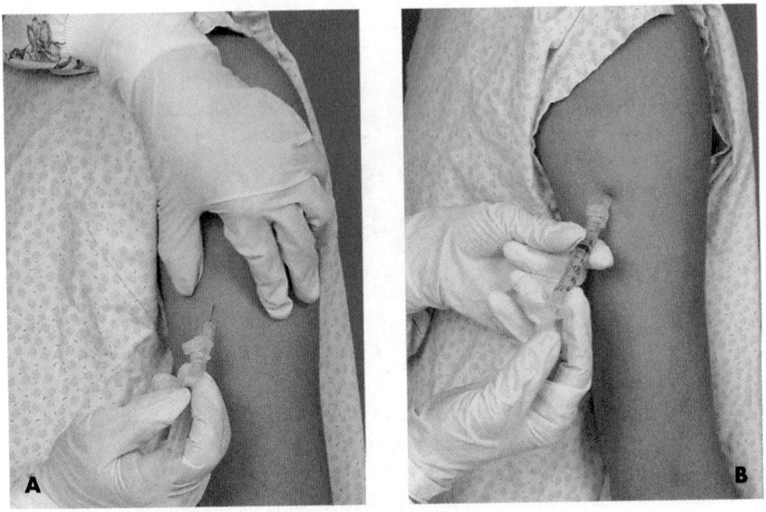

Plate 21 **A,** For a subcutaneous injection, hold the syringe between the thumb and forefinger of the dominant hand as a dart, with the palm down. **B,** After injecting the needle at a 45- to 90-degree angle, grasp lower end of syringe barrel with nondominant hand to end of plunger. Avoid moving syringe while slowly pulling back on plunger to aspirate drug. If blood appears in syringe, remove needle, discard medication and syringe, and repeat procedure. *Exception:* do not aspirate when giving heparin.

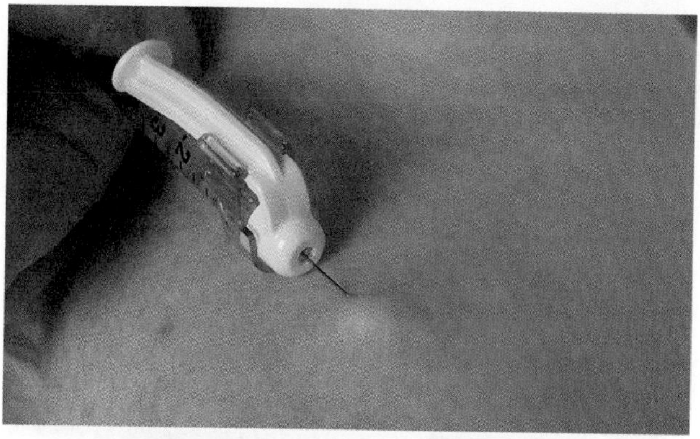

Plate 22 For an intradermal injection, note formation of small bleb approximately 6 mm (¼ in) in diameter at injection site.

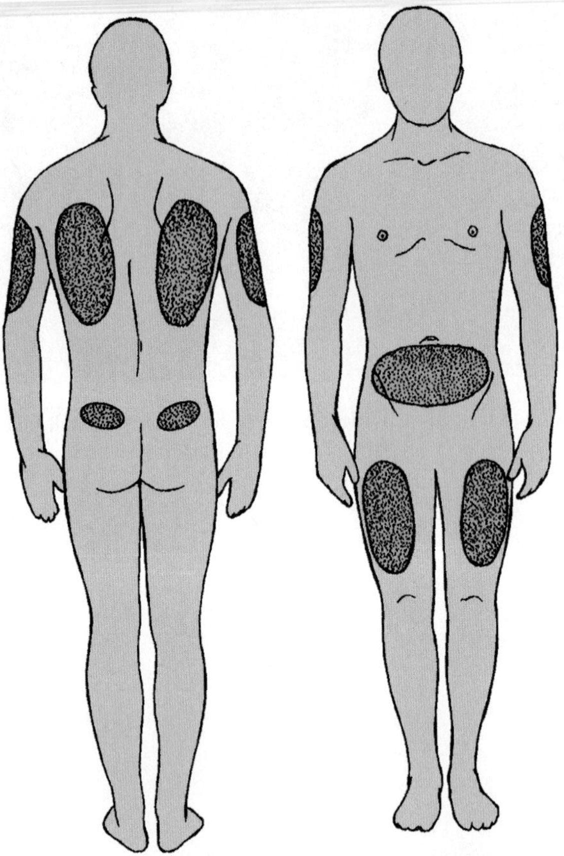

A

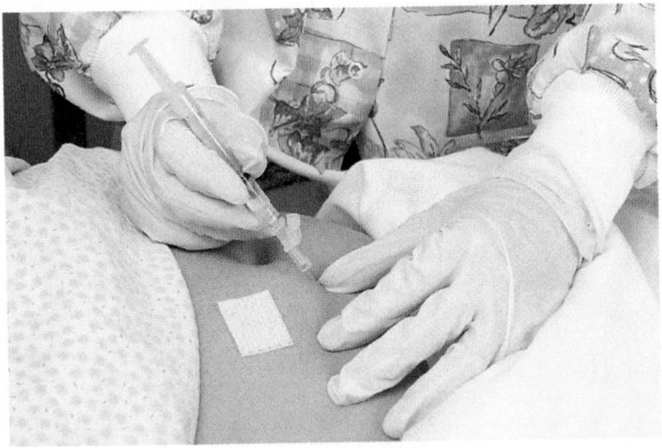

B

Plate 23 **A,** Sites recommended for subcutaneous injections. **B,** Giving subcutaneous injection in the abdomen.

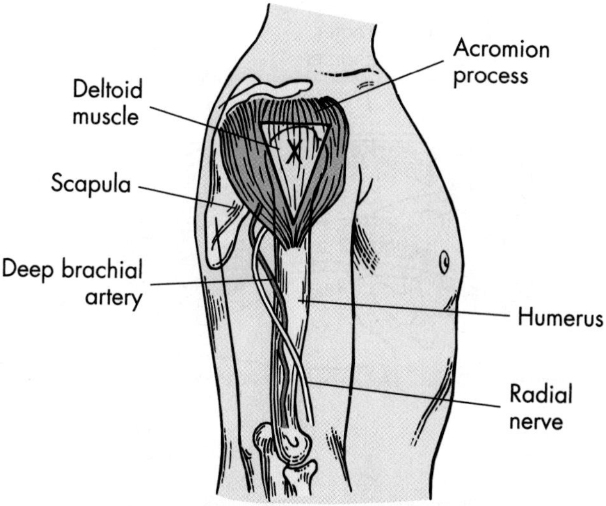

A

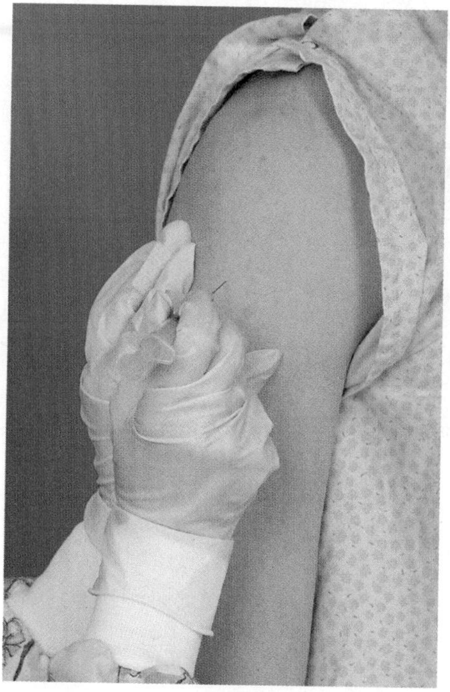

B

Plate 24 **A,** Landmarks for IM injection into the deltoid muscle. **B,** Giving IM injection in deltoid muscle.

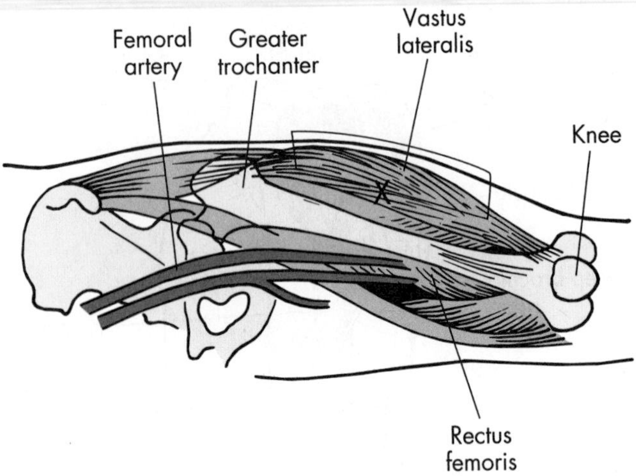

A

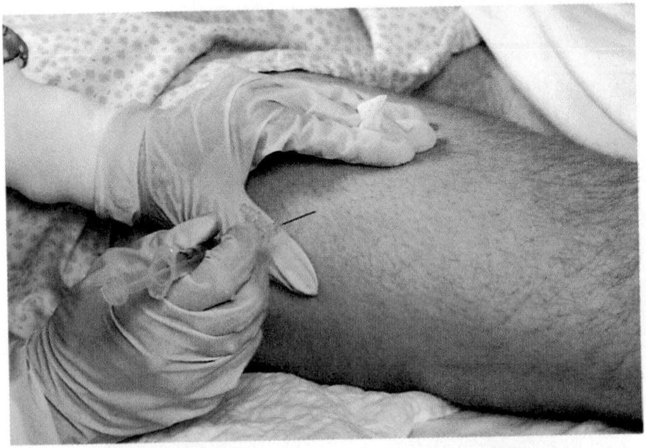

B

Plate 25 **A,** Landmarks for IM injection in vastus lateralis. **B,** Giving IM injection in vastus lateralis site.

A

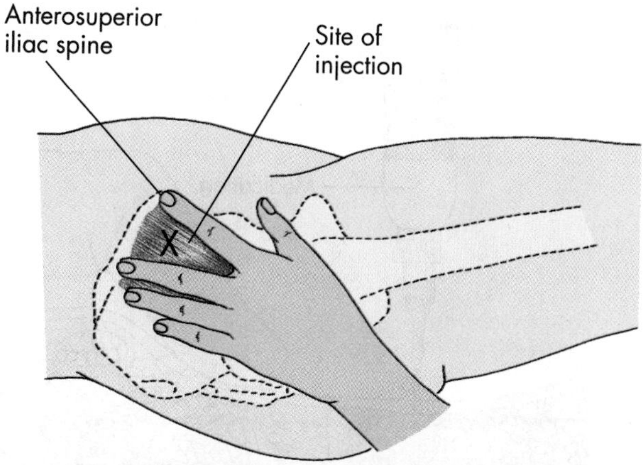

B

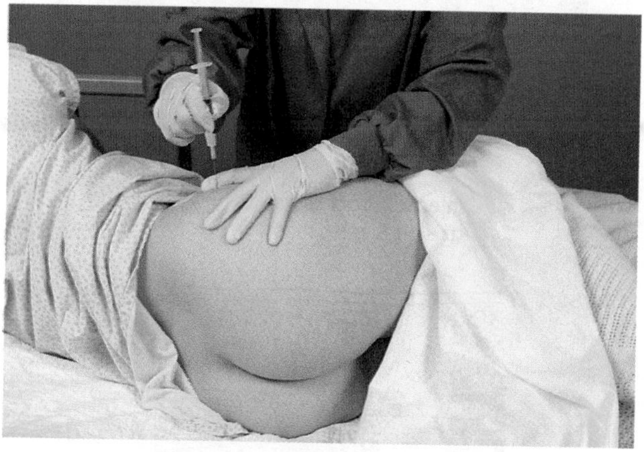

Plate 26 **A,** Anatomical view of ventrogluteal site. **B,** Giving IM injection into ventrogluteal muscle to avoid major nerves and blood vessels.

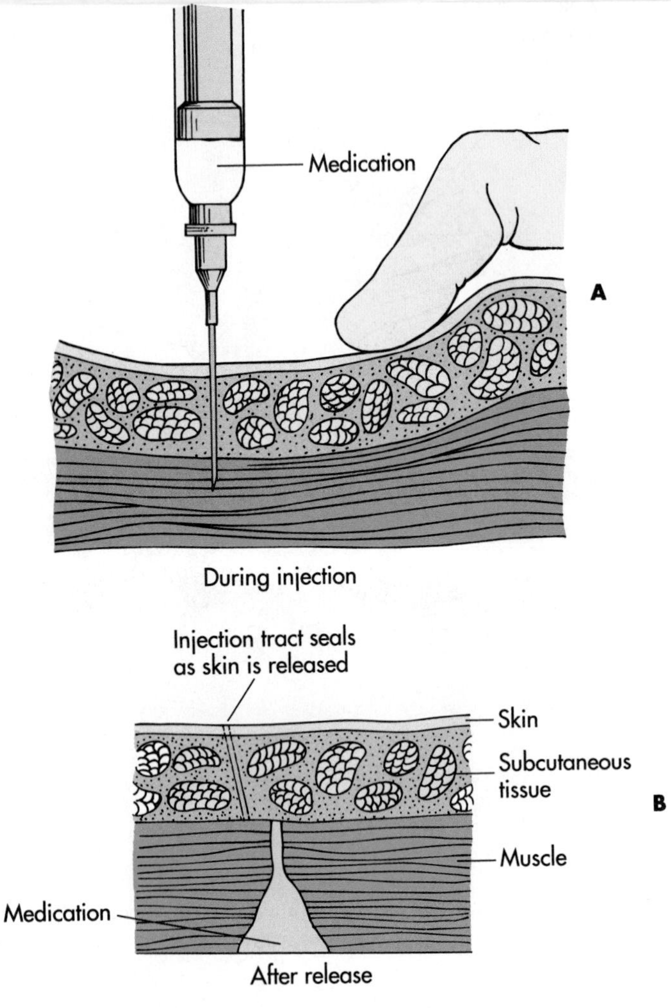

Plate 27 Z-track method of injection. **A,** Pulling on overlying skin during IM injection moves tissues to prevent later tracking. **B,** The Z-track left after injection prevents the deposit of medication through sensitive tissue.

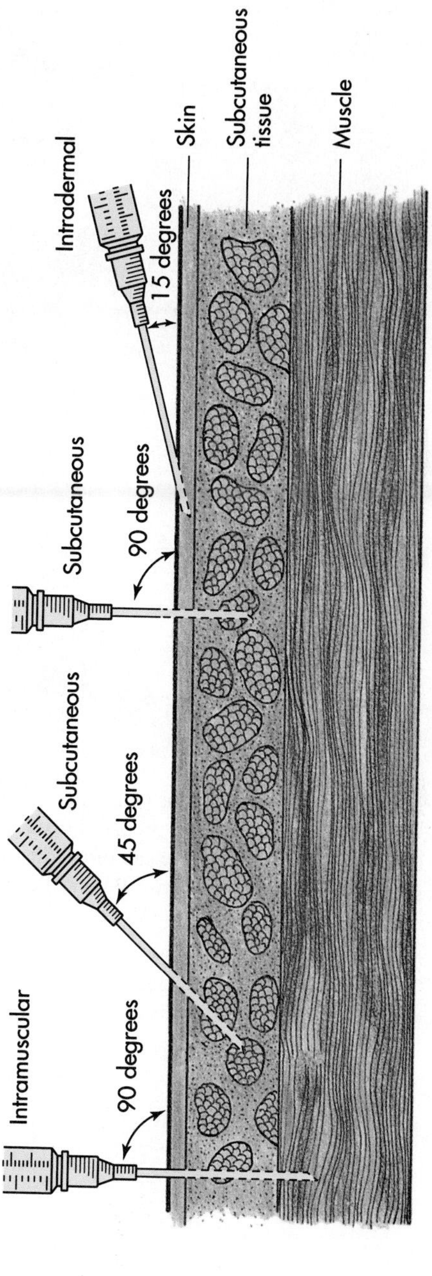

Plate 28 Comparison of angles of insertion for IM (90 degrees), SUBCUT (45 degrees and 90 degrees), and ID (15 degrees) injections.

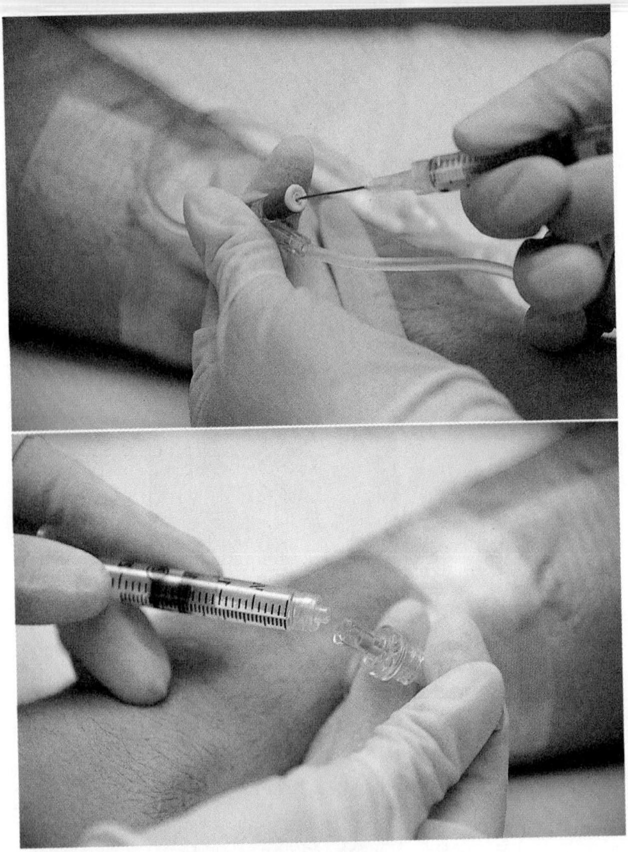

A

B

Plate 29 Administering medication by IV bolus (push). **A,** Needle system: insert small-gauge needle of syringe containing prepared drug through center of injection port. **B,** Needleless system: Remove cap of needleless injection port. Connect tip of syringe directly. (From Potter PA and Perry AG: *Fundamentals of Nursing,* ed 5, St. Louis, 2001, Mosby.) *Continued*

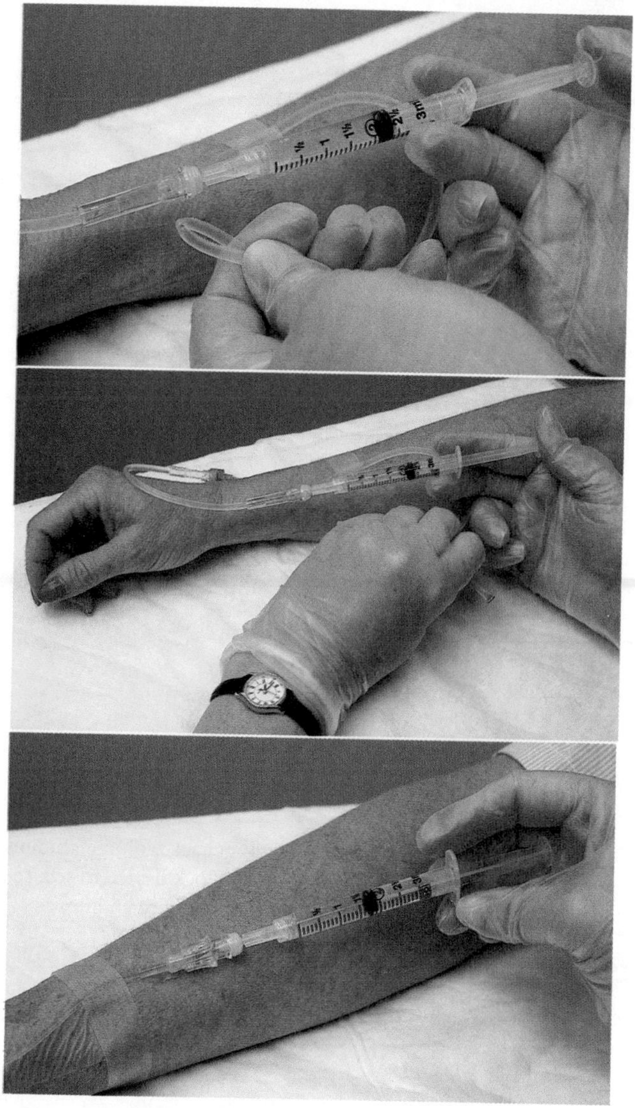

C

D

E

Plate 29 **C,** Occlude IV line by pinching tubing just above injection port. Pull back gently on syringe's plunger to aspirate blood return. **D,** After noting blood return, continue to occlude tubing and inject medication slowly over several minutes (read directions on drug package). Use watch to time administration. **E,** IV lock: Insert needle of syringe containing prepared drug through center of diaphragm.

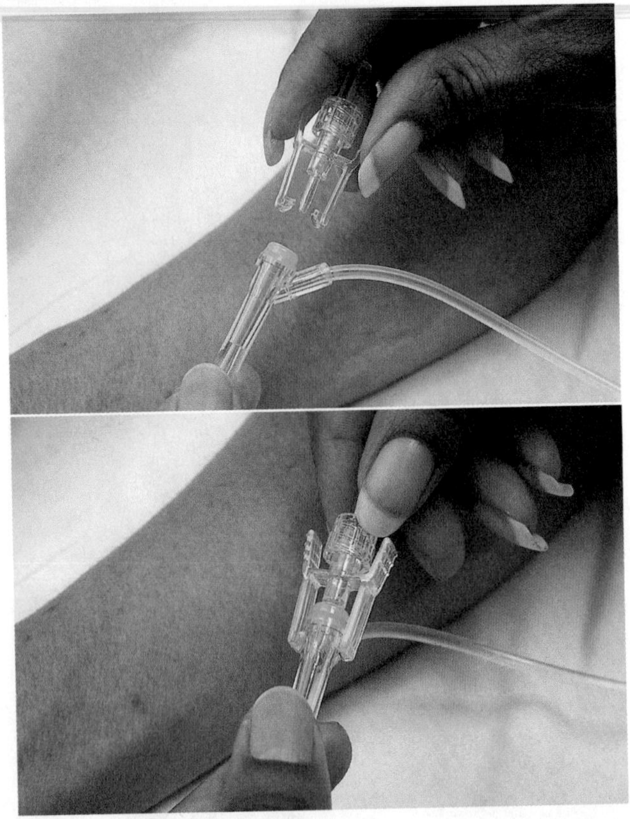

Plate 30 Administering IV medication by piggyback, volume administration sets of miniinfusors (syringe pump). Use needle-lock device to secure needle of secondary piggyback line through injection port of main line.

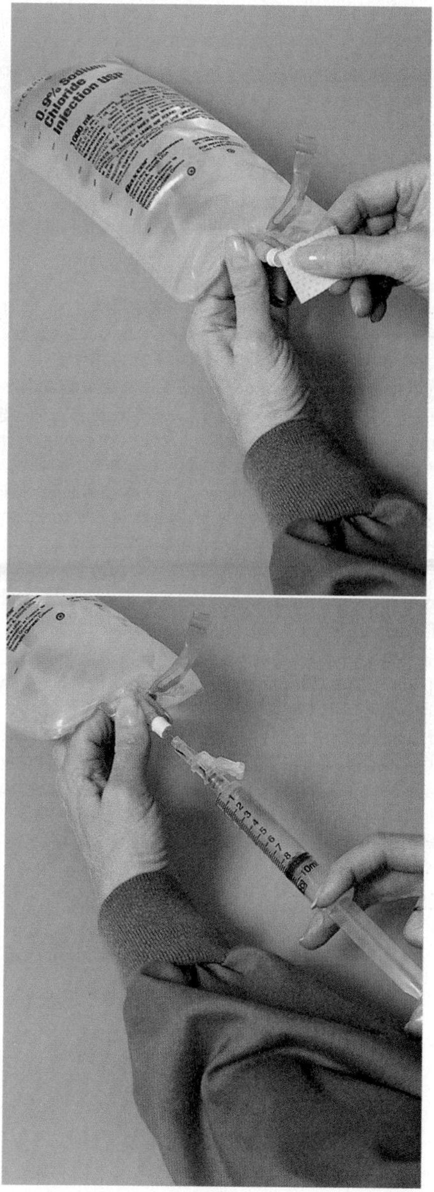

A

B

Plate 31 Adding medications to IV fluid containers. **A,** Wipe off port or injection site with alcohol or antiseptic swab. **B,** Remove needle cap from syringe and insert needle of syringe through center of injection port or site, and inject medication.

Plate 32
STANDARD PRECAUTIONS

The following precautions are used in the care of all patients regardless of their diagnosis or disease. They are also applied when handling or cleaning equipment or supplies that are potentially contaminated.

1. Wear gloves any time that you may contact blood, any moist body fluid (except sweat), secretions, excretions, nonintact skin, or mucous membranes.
2. Remove your gloves, wash your hands, and reapply clean gloves if your gloves become soiled with infective material.
3. Even if you are wearing gloves, remove them, wash your hands, and apply clean gloves *immediately before* contact with mucous membranes or nonintact skin.
4. Wear a protective cover gown of waterproof material if your clothing is likely to have substantial contact with infective material or if splashing of body fluids is likely.
5. Wear a face shield or goggles to protect your eyes if splashing of secretions is likely.
6. Any time a face shield or goggles is worn, wear a surgical mask to protect the mucous membranes of your nose and mouth. A surgical mask may be worn during certain sterile procedures without protective eyewear. However, protective eyewear is *never* worn without a surgical mask.
7. Handle needles, razors, broken glass, and other sharp objects with care. Needles should never be recapped. All sharps should be disposed of in a puncture-resistant sharps container.
8. Wash your hands before and after each patient contact.
9. Wash your hands before you apply and after you remove gloves. Do not assume that handwashing is unnecessary because gloves were worn. Do not wash your hands with gloves on them.
10. Gloves are used for the care of one patient only, then discarded.
11. Follow your facility policy for disposal of gloves and other contaminated items. These items are generally not disposed of in open trash containers. Facilities have designated disposal sites for these biohazardous waste materials.
12. Use resuscitation barrier devices as an alternative to mouth-to-mouth resuscitation.
13. Linen should be handled in a manner that prevents contamination of the outside of the container. Linen from isolation rooms was previously double bagged. Double bagging is no longer recommended, since all linen is handled as potentially infectious. Double bag linen only if the outside of the bag becomes contaminated during the bagging process.

abacavir (Rx)
(aba-ka'veer)
Ziagen
Func. class.: Antiretroviral
Chem. class.: Nucleoside reverse transcriptase inhibitor (NRTI)

Pregnancy category C

Action: A synthetic, nucleoside analog with inhibitory action against HIV. Inhibits replication of HIV by incorporating into cellular DNA by viral reverse transcriptase, thereby terminating the cellular DNA chain

Therapeutic Outcome: Decreased symptoms of HIV

Uses: In combination with other antiretroviral agents for HIV-1 infection

Dosage and routes
Adult: PO 300 mg bid or 600 mg daily with other antiretrovirals
Adolescents and children ≥3 mo: PO 8 mg/kg bid, max 300 mg bid with other antiretrovirals

Hepatic dose
Adult: PO (oral/sol) (Child-Pugh 5-6) 200 mg bid

Available forms: Tabs 300 mg; oral sol 20 mg/ml

Adverse effects
CNS: *Fever, headache, malaise, insomnia,* paresthesia
GI: *Nausea, vomiting, diarrhea, anorexia, cramps, abdominal pain, increased AST, ALT,* ***hepatotoxicity***
HEMA: **Granulocytopenia, anemia,** lymphopenia
INTEG: Rash, urticaria
META: **Lactic acidosis**
MISC: Increased CPK, **fatal hypersensitivity reactions**
RESP: Dyspnea

Contraindications: Hypersensitivity, lactic acidosis

Precautions: Pregnancy **C**, granulocyte count <1000/mm^3 or Hgb <9.5 g/dl, lactation, children, severe renal disease, impaired hepatic function

Pharmacokinetics

Absorption	Well absorbed (PO)
Distribution	50% plasma protein binding
Metabolism	To inactive metabolite
Excretion	Kidneys, feces
Half-life	1½-2 hr

Pharmacodynamics
Unknown

Interactions
Individual drugs
Alcohol: increased abacavir levels; do not use with alcohol
Ribavirin: possible lactic acidosis
Methadone: decreased levels of methadone

NURSING CONSIDERATIONS
Assessment
- Assess for lactic acidosis (elevated lactate levels, increased liver function tests) and severe hepatomegaly with steatosis; discontinue treatment and do not restart
- Assess for fatal hypersensitivity reactions: fever, rash, nausea, vomiting, fatigue, cough, dyspnea, diarrhea, abdominal discomfort; treatment should be discontinued and not restarted
- Assess for pancreatitis: abdominal pain, nausea, vomiting, elevated liver enzymes; drug should be discontinued because condition can be fatal
- Monitor CBC, differential, platelet count qmo; withhold drug if WBC is <4000/mm^3 or platelet count is <75,000/mm^3; notify prescriber of results; monitor viral load and CD4 counts during treatment
- Monitor renal function studies; BUN, serum uric acid, urine CCr before, during therapy; these may be elevated throughout treatment
- Monitor temp q4h, may indicate beginning of infection
- Monitor liver function tests before, during therapy (bilirubin, AST, ALT, amylase, alkaline phosphatase, creatine phosphokinase, creatinine prn or qmo)

Nursing diagnoses
- Infection, risk for (uses)
- Injury, risk for (adverse reactions)
- Knowledge, deficient (teaching)

Implementation
PO route
- Give on empty stomach, q12h around the clock
- Give in combination with other antiretrovirals with or without food

• Store in cool environment; protect from light, do not freeze

Patient/family education

• Advise patient to report signs of infection: increased temp, sore throat, flulike symptoms; to avoid crowds and those with known infections
• Instruct patient to report signs of anemia: fatigue, headache, faintness, shortness of breath, irritability
• Advise patient to report bleeding; avoid use of razors or commercial mouthwash
• Inform patient that drug is not a cure but will control symptoms
• Inform patient that major toxicities may necessitate discontinuing drug
• Instruct patient to use contraception during treatment
• Caution patient to avoid OTC products or other medications without approval of prescriber
• Caution patient not to have any sexual contact without use of a condom, needles should not be shared, blood from infected individual should not come in contact with another's mucous membranes
• Give Medication Guide and Warning Card; discuss points on guide
• Advise patient to stop drug if skin rash, fever, cough, shortness of breath, GI symptoms occur, notify prescriber immediately; advise all health care providers that allergic reactions have occurred with this drug

Evaluation

Positive therapeutic outcome

• Decreased infection; symptoms of HIV

abarelix (Rx)

(a-ba-rel'iks)

Plenaxis

Func. class.: Gonadotropin releasing hormone antagonist

Chem. class.: Synthetic decapeptide

Pregnancy category X

Action: Inhibitor of pituitary gonadotropin secretion; inhibits LH, FSH, thereby reducing testosterone

Therapeutic Outcome: Reduction in tumor size

Uses: Palliative treatment of prostate cancer

Dosage and routes

Adult: IM 100 mg in buttock on day 1,15,29 (week 4) and every 4 wk, thereafter

Available forms: Powder for inj 113 mg

Adverse effects

CNS: *Headache, dizziness, fatigue, sleep disturbance*

ENDO: Breast enlargement, nipple tenderness

GI: *Nausea, constipation, diarrhea*

GU: *Dysuria, frequency, retention, UTI*

INTEG: Pain on inj; local site reactions

MISC: *Pain including back pain, hot flashes*

SYST: **Anaphylaxis, systemic allergic reaction,** decreased bone density (long-term treatment)

Contraindications: Pregnancy **X**, hypersensitivity, latex allergy, lactation, children

Pharmacokinetics

Absorption	Unknown
Distribution	Protein binding 96-99%
Metabolism	Unknown
Excretion	Urine
Half-life	Depends on dosage

Pharmacodynamics

Unknown

Interactions: None known

NURSING CONSIDERATIONS

Assessment

• Assess patient for anaphylaxis: swelling of face, throat, eyes, tongue, chest tightness, difficulty breathing; hypotension, fainting, shock; if these occur, usually occur within ½ hr of administration
• Monitor blood studies: ALT, AST, GGT, alk phosphatase

Nursing diagnoses

• Injury, risk for (adverse reactions)
• Infection, risk for (adverse reactions)
• Knowledge, deficient (teaching)

Implementation

• Reconstitute 1 vial with provided diluent (50 mg/ml)
• Prior to reconstitution gently shake vial; hold at 45-degree angle and tap lightly to break caking; withdraw 2.2 ml of 0.9% NaCl inj using 18G, 1½ inch needle and 3 ml syringe enclosed, discard remaining, unused diluent
• Keeping vial upright, insert needle all the way in the vial and inject diluent quickly; withdraw needle, removing 2.2 ml of air; shake for several seconds; allow vial to stand for 2 min; tap to remove foam, swirl.
• Store between 59-80° F; use within 1 hr of reconstitution

Patient/family education

- Instruct patient to notify prescriber if family members have QTc interval prolongation
- Instruct patient to notify prescriber immediately of chest, throat tightness, flushing, lightheadedness, shortness of breath
- ❗ Inform patient that chances of serious or life-threatening allergic reaction may increase with each injection

Evaluation

Positive therapeutic outcome

- Reduction in growth of tumor

abatacept

Orencia

See Appendix A, Selected New Drugs

acarbose (Rx)

(a-kar'bose)

Prandese 🍁, Precose

Func. class.: Oral antidiabetic

Chem. class.: α-Glucosidase inhibitor

Pregnancy category B

Do Not Confuse:

Precose/PreCare

Action: Delays the digestion of ingested carbohydrates, results in a smaller rise in blood glucose after meals; does not increase insulin production

Therapeutic Outcome: Decreased blood glucose levels in diabetes mellitus

Uses: Type 2 diabetes mellitus, alone or in combination with a sulfonylurea

Dosage and routes

Initial dose

Adult: PO 25 mg tid with first bite of meal

Maintenance dose

Adult: PO may be increased to 50-100 mg tid; dosage adjustment at 4-8 wk intervals

Adult <60 kg: PO not to exceed 100 mg tid

Available forms: Tabs 25, 50, 100 mg

Adverse effects

GI: *Abdominal pain, diarrhea, flatulence, increased serum transaminase level*

Contraindications: Hypersensitivity, diabetic ketoacidosis, cirrhosis, inflammatory bowel disease, colonic ulceration, partial intestinal obstruction, chronic intestinal disease, serum creatinine >2 mg/dl

Precautions: Pregnancy **B,** renal disease, lactation, children, hepatic disease

Pharmacokinetics

Absorption	Unknown
Distribution	Unknown
Metabolism	GI tract
Excretion	Kidneys as intact drug
Half-life	Elimination 2 hr

Pharmacodynamics

Peak 1 hr

Interactions

Individual drugs

Digoxin: decreased acarbose effect

Insulin, phenytoin: increased hypoglycemia

Isoniazid, nicotinic acid, thyroid: increased hyperglycemia

Drug classifications

Calcium channel blockers, corticosteroids, diuretics, estrogens, oral contraceptives, phenothiazines, progestins, sympathomimetics: increased hyperglycemia

Digestive enzymes, intestinal absorbents, thiazide diuretics, loop diuretics, corticosteroids: decreased effect of acarbose

Sulfonylureas, insulin: increased hypoglycemia

Drug/herb

Alfalfa, aloe, basil, bay, bilberry, bitter melon, black cohosh, buchu, burdock, chromium, coenzyme Q10, coriander, eyebright (po), fenugreek, garlic, ginseng, glucomannan, glucosamine, goat's rue, gymnema, horehound, horse chestnut, jambul, myrrh, myrtle, raspberry, Siberian ginseng: increased hypoglycemia

Bee pollen, blue cohosh, broom, chromium, elecampane, eucalyptus, gotu kola, senega: decreased antihypoglycemia

Drug/lab test

Increased: AST, bilirubin

Decreased: calcium, vit B_6

NURSING CONSIDERATIONS

Assessment

- Assess for hypoglycemia (weakness, hunger, dizziness, tremors, anxiety, tachycardia, sweating), hyperglycemia; even though this drug does not cause hypoglycemia, if on a sulfonylurea or insulin, hypoglycemia may be additive; if hypoglycemia occurs, treat with glucose or if severe, **IV** dextrose or IM glucagon
- Monitor 1 hr postprandial for establishing effectiveness, then glycosylated Hgb q3 mo
- Monitor AST, ALT q3 mo × 1 yr, and periodically thereafter, if elevated dose may need to be

reduced or discontinued; obtain glycosylated Hgb periodically

Nursing diagnoses

- Nutrition: more than body requirements, imbalanced (uses)
- Nutrition: less than body requirements, imbalanced (adverse reactions)
- Knowledge, deficient (teaching)
- Noncompliance (teaching)

Implementation

- Give tid with first bite of each meal
- Provide storage in tight container in cool environment

Patient/family education

- Teach patient the symptoms of hypoglycemia, hyperglycemia and what to do about each
- Instruct that medication must be taken as prescribed; explain consequences of discontinuing the medication abruptly; that insulin may need to be used during stress such as trauma, surgery, fever
- Tell patient to avoid OTC medications, herbal products unless approved by prescriber
- Teach patient that diabetes is a life-long illness; drug will not cure condition
- Instruct patient to carry/wear emergency ID as diabetic
- Teach patient that diet and exercise regimen must be followed

Evaluation

Positive therapeutic outcome

- Improved signs, symptoms of diabetes mellitus (decreased polyuria, polydipsia, polyphagia; clear sensorium, absence of dizziness, stable gait)

acebutolol (Rx)

(a-se-byoo′ toe-lole)

Monitan ♣, Sectral

Func. class.: Antihypertensive

Chem. class.: Selective β_1-blocker; group II antidysrhythmic (II)

Pregnancy category B

Action: Competitively blocks stimulation of β-adrenergic receptors within vascular smooth muscle (decreases rate of SA node discharge, increases recovery time), slows conduction of AV node resulting in decreased heart rate (negative chronotropic effect), which decreases O_2 consumption in myocardium because of β_1-receptor antagonism, also decreases renin-aldosterone-angiotensin system at high doses, inhibits β_2-receptors in bronchial system (high doses)

Therapeutic Outcome: Decreased B/P, heart rate, AV conduction, control of dysrhythmias

Uses: Mild to moderate hypertension, sinus tachycardia, persistent atrial extrasystoles, tachydysrhythmias, management of PVCs

Investigational uses: Prophylaxis of MI, treatment of angina pectoris, tremor, mitral valve prolapse, thyrotoxicosis, idiopathic hypertrophic subaortic stenosis

Dosage and routes

Hypertension

Adult: PO 400 mg daily or in 2 divided doses; may be increased to desired response; maintenance 200-1200 mg daily in 2 divided doses

Ventricular dysrhythmia

Adult: PO 200 mg bid, may increase gradually; usual range 600-1200 mg daily; should be tapered over 2 wk before discontinuing

Elderly: PO not to exceed 800 mg daily

Renal dose

Adult: PO CCr 25-50 ml/min, reduce dose by 50%; if <25 ml/min reduce dose by 75%

Available forms: Caps 200, 400 mg; tabs 100, 200, 400 mg ♣

Adverse effects

CNS: *Insomnia, fatigue, dizziness, mental changes,* memory loss, hallucinations, depression, lethargy, drowsiness, strange dreams, catatonia

CV: **Profound hypotension, bradycardia, CHF,** cold extremities, postural hypotension, **2nd- or 3rd-degree heart block**

EENT: Sore throat; dry, burning eyes

ENDO: Increased hypoglycemic response to insulin

GI: *Nausea, diarrhea,* vomiting, **mesenteric arterial thrombosis, ischemic colitis,** flatulence

GU: *Impotence,* decreased libido, dysuria, nocturia

HEMA: **Agranulocytosis, thrombocytopenia, purpura**

INTEG: Rash, flushing, pruritus, sweating, alopecia, dry skin

MISC: Facial swelling, weight gain, decreased exercise tolerance

MS: Joint pain, cramping

RESP: **Bronchospasm,** dyspnea, wheezing, cough

Contraindications: Hypersensitivity to β-blockers, cardiogenic shock, heart block

(2nd or 3rd degree), sinus bradycardia, CHF, cardiac failure

Precautions: Pregnancy **B**, major surgery, lactation, diabetes mellitus, renal disease, thyroid disease, COPD, asthma, well-compensated heart failure, hepatic disease, peripheral vascular disease, children

Pharmacokinetics

Absorption	Well absorbed
Distribution	Crosses placenta, minimal CNS; protein binding 26%
Metabolism	Liver to diacetolol
Excretion	Urine
Half-life	8-13 hr diacetolol, 3-4 hr acebutolol

Pharmacodynamics

	PO (ANTIHYPERTENSIVE)	PO (ANTIDYSRHYTHMIAS)
Onset	1-1½ hr	1 hr
Peak	2-4 hr	4-6 hr
Duration	12-24 hr	10-12 hr

Interactions

Individual drugs

Alcohol (large amounts), cimetidine, diltiazem, hydrALAZINE, prazosin: increased hypotension
Calcium, cholestyramine, colestipol: decreased antihypertensive effect
Cimetidine, diltiazem, hydrALAZINE, prazosin: bradycardia
Ergots: increased peripheral ischemia
Insulin: increased hypoglycemia
Thyroid: decreased effectiveness
Verapamil: increased myocardial depression

Drug classifications

Antidiabetics, oral: increased hypoglycemic effect
Antihypertensives: increased hypertension
Calcium channel blockers, diuretics, nitrates: increased hypotension
Calcium channel blockers, cardiac glycosides, diuretics: bradycardia
NSAIDs: decreased antihypertensive effect
Theophyllines, β_2-agonists: decreased bronchodilatation

Drug/herb

Aconite: increased toxicity, death
Aloe, buckthorn bark/berry, cascara sagrada bark, rhubarb root, senna leaf/fruits: increased acebutolol effect
Astragalus, cola tree: increased or decreased antihypertensive effect
Barberry, betony, black catechu, black cohosh, bloodroot, broom, burdock, cat's claw, dandelion, figwort, fumitory, goldenseal, Irish moss, Jamaican dogwood, kelp, khella, kudzu, licorice, mistletoe, parsley: increased antihypertensive effect
Coltsfoot, guarana, khat, licorice: decreased antihypertensive effect
Horehound: increased serotonin effect

Drug/lab test

False positive: antinuclear antibodies titer
Increased: serum lipoprotein levels, BUN, potassium, triglyceride, uric acid, LDH, AST, ALT, blood glucose, alkaline phosphatase

NURSING CONSIDERATIONS

Assessment

- Monitor B/P during beginning treatment, periodically thereafter; pulse q4h; note rate, rhythm, quality; apical/radial pulse before administration; notify prescriber of any significant changes (pulse <50 bpm)
- Check for baselines in renal, liver function tests before therapy begins
- Assess for edema in feet, legs daily, monitor I&O, daily weight; check for jugular vein distention, crackles bilaterally, dyspnea (CHF)
- Monitor skin turgor, dryness of mucous membranes for hydration status, especially elderly

Nursing diagnoses

- Cardiac output, decreased (side effects)
- Injury, risk for (side effects)
- Knowledge, deficient (teaching)
- Noncompliance (teaching)

Implementation

PO route

- Given ac, at bedtime; tablet may be crushed or swallowed whole; give with food to prevent GI upset; reduced dosage in renal dysfunction; check pulse before giving, hold dose and notify prescriber if pulse is <60 bpm
- Store protected from light, moisture; place in cool environment

Patient/family education

- ❗ Teach patient not to discontinue drug abruptly, severe cardiac reactions may occur, taper over 2 wk; may cause precipitate angina if stopped abruptly
- Advise patient that drug may mask signs of hypoglycemia or alter blood glucose levels
- Teach patient not to use OTC products containing α-adrenergic stimulants (such as nasal decongestants, cold preparations); to avoid alcohol, smoking; to limit sodium intake as prescribed
- Teach patient how to take pulse and B/P at home, advise when to notify prescriber

• Instruct patient to comply with weight control, dietary adjustments, modified exercise program
• Tell patient to carry/wear emergency ID to identify drug(s) that patient is taking, allergies; tell patient that drug controls symptoms but does not cure
• Caution patient to avoid hazardous activities if dizziness or drowsiness is present; that drug may cause sensitivity to cold
• Teach patient to report symptoms of CHF: difficult breathing, especially on exertion or when lying down, night cough, swelling of extremities or bradycardia, dizziness, confusion, depression, fever
• Teach patient to take drug as prescribed, not to double or skip doses; take any missed doses as soon as remembered if several hours until next dose
• Advise patient to continue with required lifestyle changes (exercise, diet, weight loss, stress reduction)

Evaluation

Positive therapeutic outcome

• Decreased B/P in hypertension (after 1-2 wk)
• Absence of dysrhythmias

Treatment of overdose: Lavage, **IV** atropine for bradycardia, **IV** theophylline for bronchospasm, digitalis, O_2, diuretic for cardiac failure, hemodialysis, **IV** glucose for hypoglycemia, **IV** diazepam (or phenytoin) for seizures

acetaminophen ⊶ (OTC)

(a-seat-a-mee'noe-fen)

Abenol ✤, Acephen, Aceta, Actimol, Aminofen, Apacet, APAP, Apo-Acetaminophen ✤, Arthritis Foundation Pain Reliever Aspirin-Free, Aspirin-Free Anacin, Aspirin-Free Pain Relief, Atasol ✤, Banesin, Children's Feverall, Dapa, Dapacin, Datril, Exdol ✤, FemEtts, Genapap, Genebs, Halenol, Liquiprin, Mapap, Maranox, Meda, Neopap, Oraphen-PD, Panadol, Redutemp, Robigesic ✤, Rounax ✤, Silapap, Tapanol, Tempra, Tylenol

Func. class.: Nonopioid analgesic

Chem. class.: Nonsalicylate, paraaminophenol derivative

Pregnancy category B

Action: May block pain impulses peripherally that occur in response to inhibition of prostaglandin synthesis; does not possess antiinflammatory properties; antipyretic action results from inhibition of prostaglandins in the CNS (hypothalamic heat-regulating center)

Therapeutic Outcome: Decreased pain, fever

Uses: Mild to moderate pain or fever

Dosage and routes

Adult and child >12 yr: PO/REC 325-650 mg q4h prn, max 4 g/day
Child: PO 10-15 mg/kg q4h
Child 6-12 yr: REC 325 mg q4-6h, max 2-6 g/day
Child 3-6 yr: REC 125 mg q4-6h, max 720 mg/day
Child 1-3 yr: REC 80 mg q4h
Child 3-11 mo: REC 80 mg q6h

Available forms: Rec supp 80, 120, 125, 325, 600, 650 mg; chewable tabs 80, 160 mg; caps 500 mg; elix 120, 160, 325 mg/5 ml; liq 160 mg/5 ml, 500 mg/15 ml; sol 100 mg/1 ml, 120 mg/2.5 ml; tabs 160, 325, 500, 650 mg; granules 80 mg/pkg or cup

Adverse effects

CNS: Stimulation, drowsiness
GI: Nausea, vomiting, abdominal pain; **hepatotoxicity, hepatic seizure (overdose)**
GU: **Renal failure** (high, prolonged doses)
HEMA: **Leukopenia, neutropenia, hemolytic anemia (long-term use), thrombocytopenia, pancytopenia**
INTEG: Rash, urticaria
SYST: **Hypersensitivity**
TOXICITY: **Cyanosis, anemia, neutropenia, jaundice, pancytopenia, CNS stimulation, delirium followed by vascular collapse, convulsions, coma, death**

Contraindications: Hypersensitivity; intolerance to tartrazine (yellow dye #5), alcohol, table sugar, saccharin, depending on product

Precautions: Pregnancy **B**, anemia, hepatic disease, renal disease, chronic alcoholism, elderly, lactation

Pharmacokinetics	
Absorption	Well absorbed (PO), variable (REC)
Distribution	Widely distributed; crosses placenta in low concentrations
Metabolism	Liver 85%-95%; metabolites are toxic at high levels
Excretion	Kidneys—metabolites, breast milk
Half-life	3-4 hr

A

Pharmacodynamics

	PO	REC
Onset	½-1 hr	½-1 hr
Peak	1-3 hr	1-3 hr
Duration	3-4 hr	3-4 hr

Interactions

Individual drugs

Alcohol, carbamazepine, diflunisal, isoniazid, rifabutin, rifampin, sulfinpyrazone: increased hepatotoxicity; decreased effect
Colestipol, cholestyramine: decreased absorption of acetaminophen
Warfarin: hypoprothrombinemia; long-term use, high doses of acetaminophen
Zidovudine: increased bone marrow suppression

Drug classifications

Barbiturates, hydantoins: decreased effect; increased hepatotoxicity
NSAIDs, salicylates: increased renal adverse reactions

Drug/lab test

Interference: Chemstrip G, Dextrostix, Visidex II, 5-HIAA

NURSING CONSIDERATIONS

Assessment

- Monitor liver function studies: AST, ALT, bilirubin, creatinine before therapy if long-term therapy is anticipated; may cause hepatic toxicity at doses >4 g/day with chronic use
- Monitor renal function studies: BUN, urine creatinine, occult blood; albumin indicates nephritis
- Monitor blood studies: CBC, pro-time if patient is on long-term therapy
- Check I&O ratio; decreasing output may indicate renal failure (long-term therapy)
- Assess for fever and pain: type of pain, location, intensity, duration, temperature, diaphoresis
- Assess for chronic poisoning: rapid, weak pulse; dyspnea; cold, clammy extremities; report immediately to prescriber
- Assess hepatotoxicity: dark urine, clay-colored stools, yellowing of skin and sclera; itching, abdominal pain, fever, diarrhea if patient is on long-term therapy
- Assess allergic reactions: rash, urticaria; if these occur, drug may have to be discontinued

Nursing diagnoses

- Pain, acute (uses)
- Pain, chronic (uses)
- Mobility, physical, impaired (uses)
- Injury, risk for (side effects)
- Knowledge, deficient (teaching)

Implementation

PO route

- Administer to patient crushed or whole; chewable tabs may be chewed
- Give with food or milk to decrease gastric symptoms; give 30 min before or 2 hr after meals; absorption may be slowed

Patient/family education

- Teach patient not to exceed recommended dosage; acute poisoning with liver damage may result; acute toxicity includes symptoms of nausea, vomiting, and abdominal pain; prescriber should be notified immediately
- Tell patient to read label on other OTC drugs; many contain acetaminophen and may cause toxicity if taken concurrently
- Teach patient to recognize signs of chronic overdose: bleeding, bruising, malaise, fever, sore throat
- Inform patient that urine may become dark brown as a result of phenacetin (metabolite of acetaminophen)
- Tell patient to notify prescriber for pain or fever lasting more than 3 days

Evaluation

Positive therapeutic outcome

- Decreased pain
- Decreased fever

Treatment of overdose: Drug level q4h, gastric lavage, activated charcoal; administer oral acetylcysteine to prevent hepatic damage (*see acetylcysteine monograph,* p. 42)

acetaZOLAMIDE (Rx)

(a-set-a-zole′-a-mide)

Apo-Acetazolamide ✦, acetaZOLAMIDE, Damazide, Diamox, Diamox Sequels

Func. class.: Diuretic carbonic anhydrase inhibitor; antiglaucoma agent, antiepileptic

Chem. class.: Sulfonamide derivative

Pregnancy category C

Do Not Confuse:

acetaZOLAMIDE/acetoHEXAMIDE, Diamox/Dobutrex, Diamox/Trimox

Action: Decreases the aqueous humor in the eye, which lowers intraocular pressure by the inhibition of carbonic anhydrase; also inhibits carbonic anhydrase activity in proximal renal tubules to decrease reabsorption of water, sodium, potassium, bicarbonate; decreases carbonic anhydrase in CNS, increasing seizure threshold; prevents uric acid or cysteine buildup in the renal system by the decrease in pH causing alkaline urine

Therapeutic Outcome: Decreased intraocular pressure; control of seizures; prevention and treatment of acute mountain sickness; prevention of uric acid/cysteine renal stones; decreased edema in lung tissue and peripherally; decreased B/P

Uses: Open-angle glaucoma, narrow-angle glaucoma (preoperatively if surgery delayed), epilepsy (petit mal, grand mal, mixed), edema in CHF, drug-induced edema, acute mountain sickness

Investigational uses: Prevention of uric acid/cysteine renal stones, decrease CSF production in infants with hydrocephalus

Dosage and routes

Closed angle glaucoma

Adult: PO/IM/**IV** 250 mg q4h or 250 mg bid, to be used for short-term therapy

Open angle glaucoma

Adult: PO/IM/**IV** 250 mg-1 g/day in divided doses for amounts over 250 mg or 500 mg SR bid

Edema in CHF

Adult: IM/**IV** 250-375 mg/day in AM

Child: IM/**IV** 5 mg/kg/day in AM

Seizures

Adult: PO/IM/**IV** 8-30 mg/kg/day in 1-4 divided doses, usual range 375-1000 mg/day

Child: PO/IM/**IV** 8-30 mg/kg/day in divided doses tid or qid, or 300-900 mg/m^2/day, not to exceed 1 g/day

Mountain sickness

Adult: PO 250 mg q8-12h

Renal stones

Adult: PO 250 mg at bedtime

Infants with hydrocephalus

Infant: **IV** 5 mg/kg/day q6h, may be increased up to 100 mg/kg/day if tolerated

Available forms: Tabs 125, 250 mg; ext rel caps 500 mg; inj 500 mg

Adverse effects

CNS: Drowsiness, paresthesia, anxiety, depression, headache, dizziness, confusion, stimulation, fatigue, **seizures,** sedation, nervousness

EENT: Myopia, tinnitus

ENDO: Hyperglycemia

GI: Nausea, vomiting, anorexia, constipation, diarrhea, melena, weight loss, **hepatic insufficiency,** taste alterations

GU: Frequency, hypokalemia, polyuria, **uremia,** glucosuria, hematuria, dysuria, crystalluria, renal calculi

HEMA: **Aplastic anemia, hemolytic anemia, leukopenia, agranulocytosis, thrombocytopenia, purpura, pancytopenia**

INTEG: Rash, pruritus, urticaria, fever, **Stevens-Johnson syndrome,** photosensitivity

META: *Hypokalemia, hyperchloremic acidosis*

Contraindications: Hypersensitivity to sulfonamides, severe renal disease, severe hepatic disease, electrolyte imbalances (hyponatremia, hypokalemia), hyperchloremic acidosis, Addison's disease, long-term use in narrow-angle glaucoma

Precautions: Pregnancy **C,** hypercalciuria, lactation, respiratory acidosis, COPD

Pharmacokinetics

Absorption	GI tract—65% if fasting, 75% with food; **IV**—complete
Distribution	Crosses placenta; widely distributed
Metabolism	None
Excretion	Kidneys, unchanged (80% within 24 hr); breast milk
Half-life	2½-5½ hr

Pharmacodynamics

	PO	PO–EXT REL	IV
Onset	1½ hr	2 hr	2 min
Peak	2-4 hr	3-6 hr	15 min
Duration	8-12 hr	18-24 hr	4-5 hr

Interactions

Individual drugs

CycloSPORINE: increased toxicity

Diflunisal: increased side effects

Lithium: increased excretion of lithium

Methenamine: decreased acetaZOLAMIDE effect

Primidone: decreased primidone level

Drug classifications

Amphetamines: increased action

Anticholinergics: increased anticholinergic action

Salicylates: increased toxicity

Procainamide: increased action of procainamide

Quinidine: increased action of quinidine

Drug/lab test

Decreased: thyroid iodine uptake

False positive: urinary protein, 17-hydroxysteroids

NURSING CONSIDERATIONS

Assessment

- Assess patient for tinnitus, hearing loss, ear pain; periodic testing of hearing is needed

when high doses of this drug are given by **IV** route
• Monitor manifestations of hypokalemia: *RENAL:* acidic urine, reduced urine osmolality, nocturia, polyuria, polydipsia; *CARDIAC:* hypotension, broad T wave, U wave, ectopy, tachycardia, weak pulse; *NEURO:* muscle weakness, altered LOC, drowsiness, apathy, lethargy, confusion, depression; *GI:* anorexia, nausea, cramps, constipation, distention, paralytic ileus; *RESP:* hypoventilation, respiratory muscle weakness
• Monitor for CNS, GI, cardiovascular, integumentary, neurologic manifestations of hypocalcemia: *CNS:* personality changes, anxiety, disturbances, depression, psychosis, nausea, vomiting; *GI:* constipation, abdominal pain from muscle spasm; *CV:* decreased contractility, decreased cardiac output, hypotension, lengthened ST segment, prolonged QT interval; *INTEG:* scaling eczema, alopecia, hyperpigmentation; *NEURO:* tetany, muscle twitching, cramping, grimacing, seizure, altered deep tendon reflexes, spasm
• Monitor for manifestations of hypomagnesemia: *CNS:* agitation; *NEURO:* muscle twitching, paresthesias, hyperactive reflexes, positive Babinski's reflex, dysphagia, nystagmus, seizures, tetany; *GI:* nausea, vomiting, diarrhea, anorexia, abdominal distention; *CARDIAC:* ectopy, tachycardia, broad, flat, or inverted T waves, depressed ST segment, prolonged QT, decreased cardiac output, hypotension
• Monitor for manifestations of hyponatremia: *CV:* increased B/P, cold, clammy skin, hypovolemia or hypervolemia, vomiting, diarrhea, abdominal cramps; *NEURO:* lethargy, increased intracranial pressure, confusion, headache, seizures, coma, fatigue, tremors, hyperreflexia
• Monitor for manifestations of hyperchloremia: *NEURO:* weakness, lethargy, coma; *RESP:* deep, rapid breathing
• Assess fluid volume status: I&O ratio and record, count or weigh diapers as appropriate, distended neck veins, crackles in lung, color, quality and sp gr of urine, skin turgor, adequacy of pulses, moist mucous membranes, bilateral lung sounds, peripheral pitting edema; dehydration symptoms of decreasing output, thirst, hypotension, dry mouth, and mucous membranes should be reported
• Monitor electrolytes: potassium, sodium, calcium, magnesium; also include BUN, blood pH, ABGs, uric acid, CBC, blood glucose
• Assess B/P before and during therapy with patient lying, standing, and sitting as appropriate; orthostatic hypotension can occur rapidly
• Monitor blood, urine glucose in diabetic patients; glucose levels may be increased
• Assess for eye pain, change in vision when using drug for intraocular pressure
• Assess neurologic status when using drug for seizures
• Assess for decreased symptoms of acute mountain sickness: headache, nausea, vomiting, dizziness, fatigue, drowsiness, shortness of breath, insomnia
• Assess for cross-sensitivity between other sulfonamides and this drug

Nursing diagnoses

- Sensory perception, disturbed (uses)
- Fluid volume, deficient (side effects)
- Fluid volume, excess (uses)
- Knowledge, deficient (teaching)

Implementation

• Give in AM to avoid interference with sleep
• Administer fluids 2-3 L/day to prevent renal calculi, unless contraindicated
• Potassium replacement if potassium level is <3.0 ml/dl

PO route

• Do not crush or chew ext rel caps; caps may be opened and sprinkled on food
• Give with food, if nausea occurs, crush tabs and mix with sweet substance to counteract bitter taste

IV route

• Do not use solution that is yellow or has a precipitate or crystals
• Dilute 500 mg of drug/5 ml or more sterile water for inj: use within 24 hr

IV, direct route

• Give over 1 min or more

Intermittent IV infusion route

• May be added to NS, D_5W, $D_{10}W$, 0.45% NaCl; give over 4-8 hr

Additive compatibilities: Cimetidine, ranitidine

Additive incompatibilities: Multivitamins

Patient/family education

• Teach patient to take the medication early in the day to prevent nocturia
• Instruct patient to take with food or milk if GI symptoms of nausea and anorexia occur
• Teach patient to maintain a record of weight on a weekly basis and notify prescriber of weight loss of >5 lb
• Caution patient that this drug causes a loss of potassium, so food rich in potassium should

be added to the diet; refer to a dietician for assistance in planning

- Advise patient to wear protective clothing and sunscreen in the sun to prevent photosensitivity
- Teach patient not to use alcohol or any OTC medications without prescriber's approval; serious drug reactions may occur
- Emphasize the need to contact prescriber immediately if muscle cramps, weakness, nausea, dizziness, or numbness occurs
- Teach patient to take own B/P and pulse and record
- Teach patient to continue taking medication even if feeling better; this drug controls symptoms but does not cure the condition
- Teach patient to see ophthalmologist periodically; glaucoma is a slow process
- Advise patient to increase fluids to 2-3 L/day if not contraindicated
- Instruct patient to report nausea, vertigo, rapid weight gain, change in stools

Evaluation

Positive therapeutic outcome

- Decreased intraocular pressure
- Decreased edema
- Decreased seizures
- Prevention of mountain sickness
- Prevention of uric acid/cysteine stones

Treatment of overdose: Lavage if taken orally, monitor electrolytes, administer dextrose in saline, monitor hydration, CV, renal status

acetylcysteine 🔑 (Rx)

(a-se-teel-sis'tay-een)

Acetadote, Mucomyst, Mucosil, Parvolex ♣

Func. class.: Mucolytic; antidote—acetaminophen

Chem. class.: Amino acid L-cysteine

Pregnancy category B

Action: Decreases viscosity of secretions in respiratory tract by breaking disulfide links of mucoproteins; increases hepatic glutathione, which is necessary to inactivate toxic metabolites in acetaminophen overdose

Therapeutic Outcome: Decreased hepatotoxicity from acetaminophen overdose (PO); decreased viscosity of mucus in respiratory disorders (inh)

Uses: Acetaminophen toxicity; bronchitis; pneumonia; cystic fibrosis; emphysema; atelectasis; tuberculosis; complications of thoracic surgery and cardiovascular surgery; diagnosis in bronchial lab tests

Investigational uses: Prevention of contrast media nephrotoxicity

Dosage and routes

Mucolytic

Adult and child: INSTILL 1-2 ml (10%-20% sol) q1-4h prn, or 3-5 ml (20% sol) or 6-10 ml (10% sol) tid or qid; nebulization (face, mask, mouthpiece, tracheostomy) 1-10 ml of a 20% sol or 2-20 ml of a 10% sol q2-6h; nebulization (tent, croupette) may require large dose, up to 300 ml/treatment

Acetaminophen toxicity

Adult and child: PO 140 mg/kg, then 70 mg/kg q4h × 17 doses to total 1330 mg/kg; **IV** loading dose 150 mg/kg over 15 min (dilution 150 mg/kg in 200 ml of D_5); maintenance dose 1:50 mg/kg over 4 hr (dilution 50 mg/kg in 500 ml D_5); maintenance dose 2:100 mg/kg over 16 hr (dilution 100 mg/kg in 1000 ml D_5)

Available forms: Oral sol 10%, 20%; inj 20% (200 mg/ml)

Adverse effects

CNS: *Dizziness, drowsiness,* headache, fever, chills

CV: Hypotension

EENT: *Rhinorrhea,* tooth damage

GI: *Nausea,* stomatitis, constipation, vomiting, anorexia, **hepatotoxicity**

INTEG: Urticaria, rash, fever, clamminess

RESP: **Bronchospasm,** burning, **hemoptysis,** chest tightness

Contraindications: Hypersensitivity, increased intracranial pressure, status asthmaticus

Precautions: Pregnancy **B,** hypothyroidism, Addison's disease, CNS depression, brain tumor, asthma, hepatic disease, renal disease, COPD, psychosis, alcoholism, seizure disorders, lactation

Pharmacokinetics

Absorption	Extensive (PO), locally (inh)
Distribution	Unknown
Metabolism	Liver
Excretion	Kidneys
Half-life	5.6 hr (adult), 11 hr (newborn)

Pharmacodynamics

	PO	INH
Onset	Unknown	1 min
Peak	Unknown	Unknown
Duration	Up to 4 hr	5-10 min

Interactions
Individual drugs
Iron, copper, rubber: do not use with acetylcysteine
Amphotericin B, chlortetracycline, chymotrypsin, erythromycin lactobionate, hydrogen peroxide, iodized oil, oxytetracycline, sodium ampicillin, tetracycline, trypsin: do not mix with antibiotics

NURSING CONSIDERATIONS
Assessment
Mucolytic use
- Assess cough: type, frequency, character, including sputum
- Assess characteristics, rate, rhythm of respirations, increased dyspnea, sputum; discontinue if bronchospasm occurs; ABGs for increased CO_2 retention in asthma patients
- Monitor VS, cardiac status including checking for dysrhythmias, increased rate, palpitations

Antidotal use
- Assess liver function tests, acetaminophen levels, pro-time, glucose, electrolytes; inform prescriber if dose is vomited or vomiting is persistent; provide adequate hydration; decrease dosage in hepatic encephalopathy
- Assess for nausea, vomiting, rash; notify prescriber if these occur

Nursing diagnoses
- Injury, risk for (uses) (antidote)
- Gas exchange, impaired (uses) (mucolytic)
- Airway clearance, ineffective (uses) (mucolytic)
- Poisoning, risk for (uses) (antidote)
- Knowledge, deficient (teaching)

Implementation
- Give decreased dosage to elderly patients; their metabolism may be slowed; give gum, hard candy, frequent rinsing of mouth for dryness of oral cavity
- Use only if suction machine is available

PO route: *Antidotal use*
- Lavage, then give within 24 hr; give with cola or soft drink to disguise taste; can be given with H_2O through tubes; use within 1 hr

Inhalation route: *Mucolytic use*
- Use ac ½-1 hr for better absorption, to decrease nausea; only after patient clears airway by deep breathing, coughing
- Give by syringe 2-3 doses of 1-2 ml of 20% or 2-4 ml of 10% sol; 20% sol diluted with NS or water for injection; may give 10% sol undiluted
- Store in refrigerator: use within 96 hr of opening
- Provide assistance with inhaled dose: bronchodilator if bronchospasm occurs; wash face and rinse mouth after use to remove sticky feeling
- Use mechanical suction if cough insufficient to remove excess bronchial secretions

Patient/family education
Mucolytic use
- Tell patient to avoid driving or other hazardous activities until patient is stabilized on this medication; avoid alcohol, other CNS depressants; will enhance sedating properties of this drug
- Teach patient that unpleasant odor will decrease after repeated use; that discoloration of solution after bottle is opened does not impair its effectiveness; avoid smoking, smoke-filled rooms, perfume, dust, environmental pollutants, cleaners

Evaluation
Positive therapeutic outcome
- Absence of purulent secretions when coughing (mucolytic use)
- Clear lung sounds bilaterally (mucolytic use)
- Absence of hepatic damage (acetaminophen toxicity)
- Decreasing blood toxicology (acetaminophen toxicity)

activated charcoal (OTC)
Actidose-Aqua, Charco-Aid 2000, CharcoCaps, Liqu-Char
Func. class.: Antiflatulent/antidote

Pregnancy category C

Action: Binds poisons, toxins, irritants; increases adsorption in GI tract; inactivates toxins and binds until excreted

Therapeutic Outcome: Prevention of toxicity and death resulting from absorption of drugs

Uses: Poisoning

Dosage and routes
Poisoning
Children should not get more than 1 dose of products with sorbitol
Adult and child: PO 30-100 g or 1 g/kg, minimum dosage 30 g/250 ml of water; may give 20-40 g q6h for 1-2 days in severe poisoning

Available forms: Powder 15, 25 🍁, 30, 40, 120, 125, 240 g/container; oral susp 12.5 g/60 ml, 15 g/72 ml, 15 g/120 ml, 25 g/120 ml, 30 g/120 ml, 50 g/240 ml; 🍁 15 g/120

ml, 25 g/125 ml, 50 g/225 ml, 50 g/250 ml; tabs/caps should not be used in poisonings

Adverse effects

GI: *Nausea, black stools,* vomiting, constipation, diarrhea

Contraindications: Hypersensitivity to this drug, unconsciousness, semiconsciousness, poisoning of cyanide, mineral acids, alkalis, gag reflex, depression, ethanol intoxication

Precautions: Pregnancy **C**

Pharmacokinetics	
Absorption	None
Distribution	None
Metabolism	None
Excretion	Feces (unchanged)
Half-life	Unknown

Pharmacodynamics	
Onset	1 min
Peak	Unknown
Duration	4-12 hr

Interactions

Individual drugs

Acetylcysteine: inactivation

NURSING CONSIDERATIONS

Assessment

- Assess neurologic status including LOC, pupil reactivity, cough reflex, gag reflex, and swallowing ability before administration; do not give if neurologic status is impaired; aspiration may occur unless a protected airway is present
- Assess toxin, poison ingested, time of ingestion, and amount
- Monitor respiration, pulse, B/P to determine charcoal effectiveness if taken for barbiturate/opioid poisoning

Nursing diagnoses

- Injury, risk for (uses)
- Poisoning, risk for (uses)
- Knowledge, deficient (teaching)

Implementation

- Give after inducing vomiting unless vomiting contraindicated (i.e., cyanide or alkalies); mix with 8 oz of water or fruit juice to form thick syrup; do not use dairy products to mix charcoal; repeat dose if vomiting occurs soon after dose
- Space at least 2 hr before or after other drugs, or absorption will be decreased; use a laxative to promote elimination; constipation occurs often
- If patient unable to swallow, dilute to a less thick sol; keep container tightly closed to prevent absorption of gases
- Give through a nasogastric tube if patient unable to swallow

Patient/family education

- Tell patient stools will be black
- Teach patient about overdose/poison prevention and about keeping poison control chart available

Evaluation

Positive therapeutic outcome

- Alert, PERL (poisoning)
- Absence of distention
- Absence of odor in wounds

acyclovir ⊶ (Rx)

(ay-sye′kloe-veer)

Avirax ✤, Zovirax

Func. class.: Antiviral

Chem. class.: Acylic purine nucleoside analog

Pregnancy category B

Action: Interferes with DNA synthesis by conversion to acyclovir triphosphate, causing decreased viral replication, time of lesional healing

Therapeutic Outcome: Decreased amount and time of healing of lesions

Uses: Mucocutaneous herpes simplex virus, herpes genitalis (HSV-1, HSV-2), herpes zoster; simple mucocutaneous herpes simplex in immunocompromised clients with initial herpes genitalis; herpes simplex encephalitis, cytomegalovirus, HSV after transplant

Dosage and routes

Renal dose

Adult and child: PO/**IV** CCr >50 ml/min 100% dose q8h; CCr 25-50 ml/min 100% dose q12h; CCr 10-25 ml/min 100% dose q24h; CCr 0-10 ml/min 50% of dose q24h

Herpes simplex

Adult and child >12 yr: **IV** inf 5 mg/kg over 1 hr q8h × 5 days

Child <12 yr: **IV** inf 250 mg/m^2 or 30 mg/kg/day divided q8h over 1 hr × 5 days

Genital herpes

Adult: PO 200 mg q4h 5 times a day while awake × 5 days to 6 mo depending on whether initial, recurrent, or chronic; **IV** 5 mg/kg q8hr × 5 days

Adult and child: TOP apply to all lesions q3h while awake, 6 times a day × 1 wk

Herpes simplex encephalitis
Adult: **IV** 10 mg/kg over 1 hr q8h × 10 days
Child 3 mo-12 yr: **IV** 20 mg/kg q8h × 10 days
Child birth-3 mo: **IV** 10 mg/kg q8h × 10 days

Herpes zoster
Adult: PO 800 mg q4h while awake × 7-10 days; **IV** 5 mg/kg q8h

Varicella-zoster
Adult: PO 1000 mg q6h × 5 days or 600-800 mg q4h (5×/day while awake); **IV** 500 mg/m^2 q8h or 10 mg/kg q8h × 7 days
Child: PO 10-20 mg/kg (max 800 mg) qid × 5 days; **IV** 500 mg/m^2 q8h or 10 mg/kg q8h × 7 days

Mucosal/cutaneous herpes simplex infections in immunosuppressed patients
Adult and child >12 yr: **IV** 5 mg/kg q8h × 7 days
Child <12 yr: **IV** 10 mg/kg q8h × 7 days

Chickenpox
Adult and child >40 kg: PO 800 mg qid × 5 days
Child 2 yr or older <40 kg: PO 20 mg/kg qid × 5 days

Available forms: Caps 200 mg; tabs 400, 800 mg; inj **IV** 500 mg; top ointment 5% (50 mg/g); oral susp

Adverse effects
CNS: Tremors, confusion, lethargy, hallucinations, **seizures,** *dizziness, headache,* encephalopathic changes
EENT: Gingival hyperplasia
GI: Nausea, vomiting, diarrhea, increased ALT, AST, abdominal pain, glossitis, colitis
GU: **Oliguria, proteinuria, hematuria,** vaginitis, moniliasis, **glomerulonephritis, acute renal failure,** changes in menses, polydipsia
HEMA: **Thrombotic thrombocytopenia purpura, hemolytic uremic syndrome** (immunocompromised patient)
INTEG: Rash, urticaria, pruritus, pain or phlebitis at **IV** site, unusual sweating, alopecia
MS: Joint pain, leg pain, muscle cramps

Contraindications: Hypersensitivity

Precautions: Pregnancy **B,** lactation, hepatic disease, renal disease, electrolyte imbalance, dehydration

Pharmacokinetics

Absorption	Minimal (PO)
Distribution	Widely distributed, crosses placenta, CSF concentration 50% plasma
Metabolism	Liver, minimal
Excretion	Kidneys, 95% unchanged
Half-life	2.0-3.5 hr, increased in renal disease

Pharmacodynamics

	PO	IV	TOP
Onset	Unknown	Rapid	Unknown
Peak	1½-2½	Infusion's end	Unknown

Interactions
Individual drugs
Interferon: increased synergistic effect
Probenecid: increased neurotoxicity, nephrotoxicity
Zidovudine: increased CNS side effects

NURSING CONSIDERATIONS

Assessment

- Monitor for signs of infection, type of lesions, area of body covered, purulent drainage
- Check I&O ratio; report hematuria, oliguria, fatigue, weakness; may indicate nephrotoxicity; check for protein in urine during treatment
- Monitor any patient with compromised renal system, since drug is excreted slowly in poor renal system function; toxicity may occur rapidly
- Monitor liver studies: AST, ALT
- Monitor blood studies: WBC, RBC, Hct, Hgb, bleeding time; blood dyscrasias may occur; drug should be discontinued
- Monitor renal studies: urinalysis, protein, BUN, creatinine, CCr; increased BUN, creatinine indicates renal failure and nephrotoxicity
- Obtain C&S before drug therapy; drug may be taken as soon as culture is taken; repeat C&S after treatment; determine the presence of other sexually transmitted diseases
- Monitor bowel pattern before, during treatment; if severe abdominal pain with bleeding occurs, drug should be discontinued
- Assess allergies before treatment, reaction of each medication; place allergies on chart in bright red letters; allergic reaction: burning, stinging, swelling, redness, rash, vulvitis, pruritus

Nursing diagnoses

- Infection, risk for (uses)
- Knowledge, deficient (teaching)

Implementation

PO route

- Do not break, crush, or chew caps
- Give with food to lessen GI symptoms; may give without regard to meals with 8 oz of water
- Store at room temperature in dry place
- May be taken orally before infection occurs or when itching or pain occurs, usually before eruptions
- Must be taken in equal intervals around the clock
- Shake suspension before use

Topical route

- Use finger cot or rubber glove to prevent further infection
- Enough medication to cover lesions completely
- After cleansing with soap and water before each application, dry well

IV route

- Provide increased fluids to 3 L/day to decrease crystalluria
- Give by int inf after reconstituting with 10 ml sterile water for injection/500 mg of drug (50 mg/ml); shake; dilute in 0.9% NaCl, LR, D_5W, D_5/0.25% NaCl, D_5/0.45% NaCl, D_5/0.9% NaCl (7 mg/ml); give over at least 1 hr (constant rate) by infusion pump to prevent nephrotoxicity; do not reconstitute with sol containing benzyl alcohol or parabens; check infusion site for redness, pain, induration; rotate sites
- Lower dosage in acute or chronic renal failure
- Store at room temperature for up to 12 hr after reconstitution; if refrigerated, sol may show a precipitate that clears at room temperature, yellow discoloration does not affect potency

Y-site compatibilities: Allopurinol, amikacin, ampicillin, amphotericin B cholesteryl sulfate complex, cefamandole, cefazolin, cefonicid, cefoperazone, ceforanide, cefotaxime, cefoxitin, ceftazidime, ceftizoxime, ceftriaxone, cefuroxime, cephapirin, chloramphenicol, cimetidine, clindamycin, co-trimoxazole, dexamethasone sodium phosphate, dimenhyDRINATE, diphenhydrAMINE, doxycycline, DOXOrubicin, erythromycin, famotidine, filgrastim, fluconazole, gallium, gentamicin, granisetron, heparin, hydrocortisone sodium succinate, hydromorphone, imipenem/cilastatin, lorazepam, magnesium sulfate, melphalan, methylPREDNISolone sodium succinate, metoclopramide, metronidazole, multivitamin infusion, nafcillin, oxacillin, paclitaxel, penicillin G potassium, pentobarbital, perphenazine, piperacillin, potassium chloride, propofol, ranitidine, remifentanil, sodium bicarbonate, tacrolimus, teniposide, tetracycline, theophylline, thiotepa, ticarcillin, tobramycin, trimethoprim-sulfamethoxazole, vancomycin, zidovudine

Y-site incompatibilities: DOBUTamine, DOPamine, ondansetron, verapamil

Additive compatibilities: Fluconazole

Additive incompatibilities: Blood products, protein-containing solutions, DOBUTamine, DOPamine

Patient/family education

PO route

- Teach patient that drug may be taken orally before infection occurs or when itching or pain occurs, usually before eruptions; that partners need to be told that patient has herpes; they can become infected, so condoms must be worn to prevent reinfections; that drug does not cure infection, just controls symptoms and does not prevent infection to others
- Tell patient to report sore throat, fever, fatigue; may indicate superinfection; that drug must be taken in equal intervals around the clock to maintain blood levels for duration of therapy
- Tell patient to notify prescriber of side effects: bruising, bleeding, fatigue, malaise; may indicate blood dyscrasias
- Tell patient to seek dental care during treatment to prevent gingival hyperplasia
- Teach female patients with genital herpes to have regular Pap smears to prevent undetected cervical cancer

Topical route

- Tell patient not to use in eyes; for use when there is no evidence of infection; apply with glove to prevent further infection
- Instruct patient to avoid use of OTC creams, ointments, lotions unless directed by prescriber; may cause reinfection, delayed healing
- Teach patient to use asepsis (hand washing) before, after each application and avoid contact with eyes; to adhere strictly to prescribed regimen to maximize successful treatment outcome

Evaluation

Positive therapeutic outcome

- Absence of itching, painful lesions
- Crusting and healed lesions

Treatment of overdose: Discontinue drug, hemodialysis, resuscitate if needed

adalimumab (Rx)

(add-a-lim'yu-mab)

Humira

Func. class.: Antirheumatic agent (disease modifying), immunomodulator

Pregnancy category B

Do Not Confuse:
Humira/Humalin

Action: A form of human IgG1 monoclonal antibody specific for human tumor necrosis factor (TNF). Elevated levels of TNF are found in patients with rheumatoid arthritis

Therapeutic Outcome: Decreased pain, inflammation in joints, better ROM

Uses: Reduction in signs and symptoms and inhibiting progression of structural damage in patients with moderate to severe active rheumatoid arthritis in patients ≥18 years of age who have not responded to other disease-modifying agents

Dosage and routes

Adult: **SUBCUT** 40 mg every other wk

Available forms: Inj 40 mg/0.8 ml

Adverse effects

CNS: Headache
EENT: Sinusitis
GI: Abdominal pain, nausea
INTEG: Rash, *inj site reaction*
MISC: Flulike symptoms, UTI, hypertension, back pain, lupuslike syndrome
RESP: *URI*

Contraindications: Hypersensitivity, active infections

Precautions: Pregnancy **B**, lactation, children, elderly, CNS demyelinating disease, lymphoma, latent TB

Pharmacokinetics

Absorption	Unknown
Distribution	Unknown
Metabolism	Unknown
Excretion	Unknown
Half-life	Terminal 2 wk

Pharmacodynamics

Unknown

Interactions

Drug classification

Vaccines: do not give concurrently; immunization should be brought up to date before treatment

NURSING CONSIDERATIONS

Assessment

- Assess for pain, stiffness, ROM, swelling of joints during treatment
- Check for inj site pain, swelling; usually occur after 2 inj (4-5 days)
- Check for infections, stop treatment if present, some serious infections, including sepsis, may occur; patients with active infections should not be started on this drug

Nursing diagnoses

- Pain, chronic (uses)
- Mobility, physical, impaired (uses)
- Activity intolerance (uses)
- Knowledge, deficient (teaching)

Implementation

- Do not admix with other sol or medications, do not use filter, protect from light

Patient/family education

- Teach patient about self-administration if appropriate: inj should be made in thigh, abdomen, upper arm; rotate sites at least 1 inch from old site; do not inject in areas that are bruised, red, hard
- Advise patient that if medication is not taken when due, inject next dose as soon as remembered and inject next dose as scheduled

Evaluation

Positive therapeutic outcome

- Decreased inflammation, pain in joints

adefovir dipivoxil (Rx)

(add-ee-foh'veer)

Hepsera

Func. class.: Antiviral

Pregnancy category C

Action: Inhibits hepatitis B virus DNA polymerase by competing with natural substrates and by causing DNA termination after its incorporation into viral DNA; causes viral DNA death

Therapeutic Outcome: Improving liver function tests, lessening symptoms of chronic hepatitis B

Uses: Chronic hepatitis B

Dosage and routes

Adult: **PO** 10 mg daily, optimal duration unknown

Renal dose

Adult: **PO** CCr ≥50 ml/min 10 mg q24h; CCr 20-49 ml/min 10 mg q48h; CCr 10-19 ml/min

10 mg q72h; hemodialysis 10 mg q7 days following dialysis

Available forms: Tabs 10 mg

Adverse effects

CNS: ***Headache***

GI: ***Dyspepsia,*** abdominal pain

Contraindications: Hypersensitivity

Precautions: Pregnancy **C,** lactation, children, severe renal disease, impaired hepatic disease, elderly

Pharmacokinetics	
Absorption	Rapidly from GI tract
Distribution	Unknown
Metabolism	Unknown
Excretion	Kidneys 45%
Half-life	7.48 hr

Pharmacodynamics	
Onset	Unknown
Peak	1¾
Duration	Unknown

Interactions

Individual drugs

Acetaminophen, aspirin, indomethacin: increased granulocytopenia

Acetaminophen, acyclovir, adriamycin, amphotericin B, cimetidine, dapsone, DOXOrubicin, fluconazole, flucytosine, ganciclovir, indomethacin, interferon, morphine, pentamidine, phenytoin, probenecid, trimethoprim, vinBLAStine, vinCRIStine: increased serum concentrations, toxicity

Drug classifications

Benzodiazepines, nucleoside analogs (experimental), sulfonamides: increased serum concentrations, toxicity

NURSING CONSIDERATIONS

Assessment

- Assess for nephrotoxicity: increasing CCr, BUN
- Assess for HIV before beginning treatment because HIV resistance may occur in chronic hepatitis B patients
- Assess for lactic acidosis, severe hepatomegaly with stenosis
- Assess elderly patients more carefully; may develop renal, cardiac symptoms more rapidly
- Assess for exacerbations of hepatitis after discontinuing treatment, monitor liver function tests

Nursing diagnoses

- Infection, risk for (uses)
- Knowledge, deficient (teaching)

Implementation

- Give by mouth without regard to food
- Store in cool environment; protect from light

Patient/family education

- Advise patient that optimal duration of treatment is unknown
- Advise patient to avoid use with other medications unless approved by prescriber
- Advise patient to notify prescriber of decreased urinary output

Evaluation

Positive therapeutic outcome

- Decreased symptoms of chronic hepatitis B, improving liver function tests

! HIGH ALERT

adenosine (Rx)

(ah-den'oh-seen)

Adenocard, Adenoscan

Func. class.: Antidysrhythmic—miscellaneous

Chem. class.: Endogenous nucleoside

Pregnancy category C

Do Not Confuse:

Adenocard/adenosine

Action: Slows conduction through AV node, can interrupt reentry pathways through AV node, and can restore normal sinus rhythm in patients with supraventricular tachycardia (SVT)

Therapeutic Outcome: Normal sinus rhythm in patients diagnosed with SVT

Uses: SVT, as a diagnostic aid to assess myocardial perfusion defects in CAD

Dosage and routes

Antidysrhythmic

Adult: **IV** bol 6 mg; if conversion to normal sinus rhythm does not occur within 1-2 min, give 12 mg by rapid **IV** bol; may repeat 12 mg dose again in 1-2 min

Infants and children: 0.05 mg/kg; if not effective, increase dose by 0.05 mg/kg q2 min to a max of 0.25 mg/kg or 12 mg

Diagnostic use

Adult: **IV** 140 mcg/kg/min × 6 min

Available forms: Inj 3 mg/ml (vial); 6 mg/2 ml (vial)

Adverse effects

CNS: Lightheadedness, dizziness, arm tingling, numbness, apprehension, blurred vision, headache

CV: Chest pain/pressure, **atrial tachydysrhythmias,** sweating, palpitations, hypotension, *facial flushing*
GI: *Nausea,* metallic taste, throat tightness, groin pressure
RESP: *Dyspnea, chest pressure,* hyperventilation

Contraindications: Hypersensitivity, 2nd- or 3rd-degree heart block, AV block, sick sinus syndrome, atrial flutter, atrial fibrillation

Precautions: Pregnancy **C**, lactation, children, asthma, elderly

Pharmacokinetics

Absorption	Complete bioavailability
Distribution	Erythrocytes, cardiovascular endothelium
Metabolism	Liver, converted to inosine and adenosine monophosphate
Excretion	Kidneys
Half-life	10 sec

Pharmacodynamics

Onset	Rapid
Peak	Unknown
Duration	1-2 min

Interactions

Individual drugs

Caffeine, theophylline: decreased effects of adenosine
Carbamazepine: increased heart block
Digoxin: increased ventricular fibrillation
Dipyridamole: increased effects of adenosine

Smoking

Increased: tachycardia

Drug/herb

Aconite: increased toxicity, death
Aloe, broom, chronic buckthorn use, cascara sagrada (chronic use), figwort, fumitory, goldenseal, kudzu, licorice, rhubarb, senna: increased effect
Coltsfoot, guarana: decreased effect
Horehound: increased serotonin effect

NURSING CONSIDERATIONS

Assessment

- Monitor I&O ratio, electrolytes (potassium, sodium, chloride)
- Assess cardiopulmonary status: pulse, respiration, ECG intervals (PR, QRS, QT); check for transient dysrhythmias (PVCs, PACs, sinus tachycardia, AV block)
- Assess respiratory status: rate, rhythm, lung fields for crackles, watch for respiratory depression; bilateral crackles may occur in CHF patient; if increased respiration, increased pulse occurs, drug should be discontinued
- Assess CNS effects: dizziness, confusion, paresthesias; drug should be discontinued

Nursing diagnoses

- Cardiac output, decreased (uses)
- Gas exchange, impaired (adverse reactions)
- Knowledge, deficient (teaching)

Implementation

IV, direct (bolus) route

- Give **IV** bol undiluted; give 6 mg or less by rapid inj; if using an **IV** line, use port near insertion site, flush with 0.9% NaCl (50 ml); warm to room temperature before giving

Continuous infusion route

- Give 30-ml vial undiluted via peripheral vein

Solution compatibilities: D_5LR, D_5W, LR, 0.9% NaCl

- Store at room temperature; sol should be clear; discard unused drug

Patient/family education

- Tell patient to report facial flushing, dizziness, sweating, palpitations, chest pain
- Instruct patient to rise from sitting or standing slowly to prevent orthostatic hypotension

Evaluation

Positive therapeutic outcome

- Normal sinus rhythm
- Diagnosis of perfusion defect

alatrofloxacin (Rx)

(ah-lat-troh-floks'ah-sin)
Trovan IV

trovafloxacin (Rx)

(troh-vah-floks'ah-sin)
Trovan (oral)
Func. class.: Antiinfective
Chem. class.: Fluoroquinolone

Pregnancy category C

Do Not Confuse:
Trovan/Tenormin

Action: Interferes with conversion of intermediate DNA fragments into high molecular weight DNA in bacteria; DNA gyrase inhibitor

Therapeutic Outcome: Bacterial action against the following: nosocomial pneumonia: *Escherichia coli, Pseudomonas aeruginosa, Haemophilus influenzae, Staphylococcus aureus;* community-acquired pneumonia: *Staphylococcus pneumoniae, Haemophilus influenzae, Staphylococcus aureus, Klebsiella pneumoniae, Mycoplasma pneumoniae,*

Mycoplasma catarrhalis, Legionella pneumophilia, Chlamydia pneumoniae

Uses: Nosocomial pneumonia, community-acquired pneumonia, chronic bronchitis, acute sinusitis, complicated intraabdominal infections, gyn/pelvic infection, skin/skin structure infections, UTIs, chronic bacterial prostatitis, urethral gonorrhea in males, PID, cervicitis caused by susceptible organisms

Dosage and routes

Alatrofloxacin

Serious infections

Adult: **IV** 300 mg q24h

Other infections

Adult: **IV** 200 mg q24h

Perioperative prophylaxis

Adult: 200 mg ½-4 hr before surgery

Trovafloxacin

Gonorrhea

Adult: PO 100 mg as a single dose

Other infections

Adult: PO 100-200 mg q24h

Perioperative prophylaxis

Adult: PO 200 mg ½-4 hr before surgery

Available forms: Conc sol for inj 5 mg/ml (200 mg/40 ml, 300 mg/60 ml) (alatrofloxacin); tabs 100, 200 mg (trovafloxacin)

Adverse effects

CNS: Headache, *dizziness,* insomnia, anxiety, psychosis, **seizures**

GI: Nausea, flatulence, vomiting, diarrhea, abdominal pain, **pseudomembranous colitis, hepatotoxicity, fatal hepatitis**

GU: Vaginitis, crystalluria, increased BUN, creatinine

HEMA: Anemia, **thrombocytopenia, leukopenia,** decreased Hgb; Hct, increased platelets

INTEG: Rash, pruritus, photosensitivity

MS: Arthralgia, myalgia

SYST: **Anaphylaxis, Stevens-Johnson syndrome**

Contraindications: Hypersensitivity to quinolones, seizure disorders, cerebral atherosclerosis, photosensitivity

Precautions: Pregnancy **C**, lactation, children

Pharmacokinetics	
Absorption	Unknown
Distribution	Unknown
Metabolism	Liver
Excretion	Kidneys, unchanged
Half-life	Unknown

Pharmacodynamics	
Onset	Unknown
Peak	Unknown
Duration	Unknown

Interactions

Individual drugs

Citric acid/sodium citrate, iron, sucralfate: decreased absorption

CycloSPORINE: increased nephrotoxicity

Morphine **IV**: decreased absorption of trovafloxacin

Theophylline: increased theophylline level, toxicity

Warfarin: increased warfarin level

Drug classifications

Antacids with aluminum/magnesium: decreased absorption

Drug/herb

Do not use acidophilus concurrently with antiinfectives

Cola tree: increased antiinfective effect

NURSING CONSIDERATIONS

Assessment

- Assess for previous sensitivity reaction to fluoroquinolones
- Monitor for signs and symptoms of infection: characteristics of sputum, WBC >10,000/mm^3, fever; obtain baseline information before and during treatment
- Obtain C&S before beginning drug therapy to identify if correct treatment has been initiated
- Assess for allergic reactions: rash, urticaria, pruritus, chills, fever, joint pain; may occur a few days after therapy begins; epINEPHrine and resuscitation equipment should be available for anaphylactic reaction
- Assess bowel pattern daily; if severe diarrhea occurs, drug should be discontinued
- Assess for overgrowth of infection, perineal itching, fever, malaise, redness, pain, swelling, drainage, rash, diarrhea, change in cough, sputum
- Identify urine output; if decreasing, notify prescriber (may indicate nephrotoxicity); also check for increased BUN, creatinine
- Assess for CNS disorders; other fluoroquinolones cause seizures, stimulation
- Monitor blood studies: AST, ALT, CBC, Hct, bilirubin, LDH, alkaline phosphatase, Coombs' test monthly if patient is on long-term therapy
- Monitor electrolytes: potassium, sodium, chloride monthly if patient is on long-term therapy

- Assess for hepatotoxicity, use only for serious or life-threatening infection

Nursing diagnoses
- Infection, risk for (uses)
- Diarrhea (side effects)
- Injury, risk for (side effects)
- Knowledge, deficient (teaching)
- Noncompliance (teaching)

Implementation
PO route
- May be taken with or without food
- Separate sucralfate, antacids by ≥4 hr
- Increased fluid intake 2 L/day to prevent crystalluria

Intermittent IV infusion route
- Check for irritation, extravasation, phlebitis daily
- Dilute with compatible solution to a concentration of 1-2 mg/ml, run over 1 hr

Y-site compatibilities: Amikacin, cycloSPORINE, DOPamine, droperidol, fentanyl, gentamicin, ketorolac, lorazepam, midazolam, nitroglycerin, ondansetron, tobramycin, vancomycin

Incompatibilities: Do not use with magnesium in the same **IV** line

Solution compatibilities: D_5, ½% NaCl, D_5/0.2% NaCl, LR

Patient/family education
- Teach patient to report sore throat, bruising, bleeding, joint pain; may indicate blood dyscrasias (rare)
- Advise patient to avoid hazardous activities until response is known
- Advise patient to contact prescriber if vaginal itching, loose foul-smelling stools, furry tongue occur, may indicate superinfection; report itching, rash, pruritus, urticaria
- Advise patient to rinse mouth frequently, use sugarless candy or gum for dry mouth
- Instruct patient to take all medication prescribed for the length of time ordered; drug must be taken around the clock to maintain blood levels; not to give medication to others; to avoid other medication unless approved by prescriber; not to use theophyllines, toxicity may occur
- Advise patient to notify prescriber of diarrhea with blood or pus, may indicate pseudomembranous colitis
- Advise patient to use sunscreen to prevent photosensitivity
- Teach patient to increase fluid intake to 2 L/day to prevent crystalluria

Evaluation
Positive therapeutic outcome
- Absence of signs/symptoms of infection (WBC <10,000/mm^3, temp WNL)
- Reported improvement in symptoms of infection

albumin, normal serum 5%/25% (Rx)
(al-byoo'min)

Albuminar 5%, Albutein 5%, Buminate 5%, Plasbumin 5%, Albuminar 25%, Albutein 25%, Buminate 25%, Plasbumin 25%

Func. class.: Blood derivative—volume expander

Chem. class.: Placental human plasma

Pregnancy category C

Action: Exerts colloidal oncotic pressure, which expands volume of circulating blood by pulling fluid from extravascular to intravascular spaces, and maintains cardiac output

Therapeutic Outcome: Restoration of plasma volume by extravascular to intravascular fluid shift

Uses: Restores plasma volume in burns, hyperbilirubinemia, shock, hypoproteinemia, prevention of cerebral edema, cardiopulmonary bypass procedures, ARDS, hemorrhage; also replacement in nephrotic syndrome, hepatic failure

Dosage and routes
Burns

Adult: **IV** dose to maintain plasma albumin at 30-50 g/L, use 5% sol initially, then 25% sol after 24 hr

Shock

Adult: **IV** 500 ml of 5% sol q30 min, as needed

Child: 0.5-1 g/kg/dose

Hypoproteinemia

Adult: **IV** 1000-2000 ml of 5% sol daily, not to exceed 5-10 ml/min or 25-100 g of 25% sol daily, not to exceed 3 ml/min, titrated to patient response

Hyperbilirubinemia/erythroblastosis fetalis

Infant: **IV** 1 g of 25% sol/kg before transfusion

Available forms: Inj 50, 250 mg/ml (5%, 25%)

Adverse effects

CNS: Fever, chills, flushing, headache
CV: **Fluid overload,** hypotension, erratic pulse, tachycardia
GI: Nausea, vomiting, increased salivation
INTEG: Rash, urticaria
RESP: Altered respirations, **pulmonary edema**

Contraindications: Hypersensitivity, CHF, severe anemia, renal insufficiency

Precautions: Pregnancy **C,** decreased salt intake, decreased cardiac reserve, lack of albumin deficiency, hepatic disease, renal disease

Pharmacokinetics	
Absorption	Complete bioavailability
Distribution	Intravascular spaces
Metabolism	Liver
Excretion	Unknown
Half-life	Unknown

Pharmacodynamics	
Onset	15-30 min
Peak	Unknown
Duration	Unknown

Interactions: None known
Drug/lab test
Increased: alkaline phosphatase

NURSING CONSIDERATIONS

Assessment

- Monitor blood studies: Hct, Hgb; if serum protein declines, dyspnea, hypoxemia can result; check for decreasing B/P, erratic pulse, respiration
- ◆ Monitor CVP: pulmonary wedge pressure will increase if overload occurs; I&O ratio: urinary output may decrease; CVP reading: distended neck veins indicate circulatory overload; shortness of breath, anxiety, insomnia, expiratory crackles, frothy blood-tinged sputum, cough, cyanosis indicate pulmonary overload
- Assess for allergy: fever, rash, itching, chills, flushing, urticaria, nausea, vomiting, hypotension; requires discontinuation of infusion, use of new lot if therapy reinstituted; premedicate with diphenhydrAMINE

Nursing diagnoses

- Fluid volume, deficit (uses)
- Injury, risk for (uses)
- Fluid volume, excess (adverse reactions)
- Knowledge, deficient (teaching)

Implementation

IV route

- Check type of albumin; some are stored at room temperature, some need to be refrigerated; use only amber-colored sol without precipitate; solution should be clear
- Give **IV** slowly to prevent fluid overload; 5% may be given undiluted; 25% may be given diluted (D_5W, 0.9% NaCl) or undiluted; give over 4 hr, use infusion pump
- Provide adequate hydration before, during administration; whole blood may need to be given to prevent anemia; monitor hydration during treatment

Y-site compatibilities: Diltiazem
Solution compatibilities: LR, NaCl, Ringer's, D_5W, $D_{10}W$, $D_{2½}W$, dextrose/saline, dextran$_6$ D_5, dextran$_6$ NaCl 0.9%, dextrose/Ringer's, dextrose/LR

Patient/family education

- Explain use, reason for albumin; provide information on what to report to prescriber (hypersensitivity, fluid overload)

Evaluation

Positive therapeutic outcome

- Increased B/P, decreased edema (shock, burns)
- Increased serum albumin levels
- Increased plasma protein (hypoproteinemia)

albuterol (Rx)

(al-byoo'ter-ole)
AccuNeb, Airet, albuterol, Gen-Salbutamol ✦, Novo-Salmol ✦, Proventil, Salbutamol, Ventodisk, Ventolin
Func. class.: Bronchodilator
Chem. class.: Adrenergic β_2-agonist, sympathomimetic, bronchodilator

Pregnancy category C

Do Not Confuse:
Ventolin/Vantin, Proventil/ Prinivil, albuterol/ atenolol, Volmax/Flomax, Sambutamol/ salmeterol

Action: Causes bronchodilatation by action on β_2 (pulmonary) receptors by increasing levels of cyclic adenosine monophosphate (cAMP), which relaxes smooth muscle; produces bronchodilatation; CNS, cardiac stimulation, increased diuresis, and increased gastric acid secretion; longer acting than isoproterenol

Therapeutic Outcome: Increased ability to breathe because of bronchodilatation

Uses: Prevention of exercise-induced asthma, acute bronchospasm, bronchitis, emphysema, bronchiectasis, reversible airway obstruction

Investigational uses: Hyperkalemia in dialysis patients

Dosage and routes

To prevent exercise-induced bronchospasm

Adult: INH (metered dose inhaler) 2 puffs 15 min before exercising

Other respiratory conditions

Adult and child ≥12 yr: INH (metered dose inhaler) 2 puffs q4h; **PO** 2-4 mg tid-qid, not to exceed 8 mg; NEB/IPPB 2.5 mg tid-qid

Elderly: PO 2 mg tid-qid, may increase gradually to 8 mg tid-qid

Child 2-12 yr: INH (metered dose inhaler) 0.1 mg/kg tid (max 2.5 mg tid-qid); NEB/IPPB 0.1-0.15 mg/kg/dose tid-qid or 1.25 mg tid-qid for child 10-15 kg or 2.5 mg tid-qid >15 kg

Adult and child >4 yr: INH cap (Rotahaler inhalation) 200 mcg cap inhaled q4-6h; may use 15 min before exercise

Available forms: Aerosol 90, 100 mcg/actuation; tabs 2, 4 mg; oral sol 2 mg/5 ml, ✤ ext rel 4, 8 mg; inh sol 0.83, 0.5, 1, 2, 5 mg/ml; powder for inh (Ventodisk) 200, 400 mcg; inh caps 200 mcg; 100 mcg/spray, 80 inh/canister, 200 inh/canister

Adverse effects

CNS: *Tremors, anxiety,* insomnia, headache, dizziness, stimulation, *restlessness,* hallucinations, flushing, irritability

CV: *Palpitations, tachycardia, hypertension,* angina, hypotension, dysrhythmias

EENT: Dry nose, irritation of nose and throat

GI: *Heartburn, nausea, vomiting*

MISC: Flushing, sweating, anorexia, bad taste/smell changes

MS: Muscle cramps

RESP: Cough, wheezing, dyspnea, **bronchospasm,** dry throat

Contraindications: Hypersensitivity to sympathomimetics, tachydysrhythmias, severe cardiac disease, heart block

Precautions: Pregnancy **C,** lactation, cardiac disorders, hyperthyroidism, diabetes mellitus, hypertension, prostatic hypertrophy, narrow-angle glaucoma, seizures, exercise-induced bronchospasm (aero-sol) in children <12 yr, hypoglycemia

Pharmacokinetics

Absorption	Well absorbed (PO)
Distribution	Unknown
Metabolism	Liver extensively, tissues
Excretion	Unknown, breast milk
Half-life	3-4 hr

Pharmacodynamics

	PO	PO–EXT REL	INH
Onset	½ hr	½ hr	5-15 min
Peak	2½ hr	2-3 hr	1-1½ hr
Duration	4-6 hr	12 hr	4-6 hr

Interactions

Drug classifications

Adrenergics: increased action of albuterol; do not use together

β-Adrenergic blockers: block therapeutic effect

Antidepressants (tricyclic): increased chance of hypertension, do not use together

Bronchodilators (aerosol): increased action of bronchodilator

Diuretics (potassium-losing): increased ECG changes/hypokalemia

MAOIs: increased chance of hypertensive crisis, do not use together

Oxytocics: severe hypotension, do not use together

Theophylline: toxicity

Drug/herb

Black tea, green tea, cola nut, guarana: increased stimulation

Drug/food

Caffeine products, chocolate: increased stimulation

NURSING CONSIDERATIONS

Assessment

- Assess respiratory function: vital capacity, forced expiratory volume, ABGs, lung sounds; heart rate, rhythm; B/P, sputum (baseline and during therapy)
- Determine that patient has not received theophylline therapy before giving dose, to prevent additive effect; client's ability to self-medicate
- Monitor for evidence of allergic reactions; paradoxic bronchospasm; withhold dose; notify prescriber if bronchospasm occurs

Nursing diagnoses

- Airway clearance, ineffective (uses)
- Gas exchange, impaired (uses)
- Knowledge, deficient (teaching)

Implementation

PO route

- Do not break, crush, or chew ext rel tabs
- Give PO with meals to decrease gastric irritation; oral sol for children (no alcohol, sugar)
- In elderly patients, a spacing device is advised

Aerosol route

- Give after shaking metered dose inhaler; have patient exhale and place mouthpiece in mouth, inhale slowly while depressing inhaler, hold breath, remove inhaler, exhale slowly; allow at least 1 min between inhalations
- Store in light-resistant container; do not expose to temperatures > 86° F (30° C)

Nebulizer/IPPB route

- Dilute 5 mg/ml sol/2.5 ml 0.9% NaCl for inhalation; other solutions do not require dilution for nebulizer O_2 flow or compressed air 6-10 L/min

Patient/family education

- Tell patient not to use OTC medications before consulting prescriber; excess stimulation may occur; instruct patient to use this medication before other medications and allow at least 5 min between each to prevent overstimulation; to limit caffeine products such as chocolate, coffee, tea, and cola
- Teach patient to use inhaler; review package insert with patient; to avoid getting aerosol in eyes or blurring may result; to wash inhaler in warm water and dry daily; to rinse mouth after using; to avoid smoking, smoke-filled rooms, persons with respiratory infections
- (Alert) Teach patient that if paradoxic bronchospasm occurs to stop drug immediately and notify prescriber
- Instruct patient on administration of dose, not to use more than prescribed; serious side effects may occur; if taking PO regularly and dose is missed, take when remembered; space other doses on new time schedule; do not double doses
- In elderly patients, a spacing device is advised

Evaluation

Positive therapeutic outcome

- Absence of dyspnea and wheezing after 1 hr
- Improved airway exchange
- Improved ABGs

Treatment of overdose: Administer a β_1-adrenergic blocker

! HIGH ALERT

aldesleukin (Rx)

(al-dess-loo'kin)

interleukin-2, IL-2, Proleukin

Func. class.: Miscellaneous antineoplastics

Chem. class.: Interleukin-2, human recombinant, cytotine

Pregnancy category C

Do Not Confuse: aldesleukin/oprelvekin, Proleukin/Oprelvekin, Proleukin/Prokine

Action: Enhancement of lymphocyte mitogenesis and stimulation of IL-2–dependent cell lines; enhancement of lymphocyte cytotoxicity; induction of killer cell activity; induction of interferon-γ production; results in activation of cellular immunity and cytokines and inhibition of tumor growth

Therapeutic Outcome: Prevention of rapid growth of malignant cells

Uses: Metastatic renal cell carcinoma in adults, phase II for HIV in combination with zidovudine, melanoma

Investigational uses: Kaposi's sarcoma given with zidovudine, metastatic melanoma given with cyclophosphamide, non-Hodgkin's lymphoma given with lymphokine-activated killer cells, AIDS (phase I) given with zidovudine

Dosage and routes

Adult: **IV** inf 600,000 international units/kg (0.037 mg/kg) over 15 min q8h × 14 doses; off 9 days; repeat schedule for another 14 doses, for a maximum of 28 doses/course

Available forms: Powder for inj 2.2 million international units/vial

Adverse effects

CNS: Mental status changes, dizziness, sensory dysfunction, syncope, motor dysfunction, fever, chills, headache, impaired memory, depression, sleep disturbances, hallucinations, rigors, neuropathy

CV: Hypotension, sinus tachycardia, dysrhythmias, bradycardia, PVCs, PACs, myocardial ischemia, **myocardial infarction, cardiac arrest,** capillary leak syndrome, **CVA**

EENT: Reversible visual changes

GI: Nausea, vomiting, *diarrhea,* stomatitis, anorexia, GI bleeding, dyspepsia, constipation, **intestinal perforation/ileus,** jaundice, ascites

GU: **Oliguria/anuria, proteinuria, hematuria,** dysuria, **renal failure**

HEMA: *Anemia,* **thrombocytopenia, leukopenia, coagulation disorders, leukocytosis, eosinophilia**
INTEG: Pruritus, *erythema, rash,* dry skin, **exfoliative dermatitis,** purpura, petechiae, urticaria
MS: Arthralgia, myalgia
RESP: Pulmonary congestion, dyspnea, **pulmonary edema, respiratory failure,** tachypnea, pleural effusion, wheezing, **apnea**
SYST: Infection

Contraindications: Hypersensitivity, abnormal thallium stress test or pulmonary function tests, organ allografts

Precautions: Pregnancy **C,** CNS metastases, bacterial infections, renal/hepatic, cardiac/pulmonary disease, lactation, children, anemia, thrombocytopenia

Pharmacokinetics

Absorption	Complete bioavailability
Distribution	Rapid extracellular, intravascular
Metabolism	Kidneys (convoluted tubules)
Excretion	Kidneys
Half-life	85 min

Pharmacodynamics

Onset	4 wk
Duration	≤12 mo

Interactions

Individual drugs

Indomethacin, methotrexate, asparaginase, DOXOrubicin: increased toxicity
Radiation: increased bone marrow suppression

Drug classifications

Aminoglycosides, antineoplastics: increased toxicity
Antihypertensives: increased hypotension
Antineoplastics: increased bone marrow suppression
Glucocorticosteroids: decreased tumor effectiveness
Psychotropics: unpredictable reactions

Drug/lab test

Increased: bilirubin, BUN, serum creatinine, transaminase, alkaline phosphatase, hypomagnesemia, acidosis hypocalcemia, hypophosphatemia, hypokalemia, hyperuricemia, hypoalbuminemia, hypoproteinemia, hyponatremia, hyperkalemia, alkalosis (toxic effect of drug)

NURSING CONSIDERATIONS

Assessment

- Monitor CBC, differential, platelet count weekly; withhold drug if WBC is <2000/mm^3 or platelet count is <75,000/mm^3; notify prescriber of these results; transfusion of RBCs, platelets may be required
- ❗ Identify capillary leak syndrome (CLS), including a drop in mean arterial pressure (2-12 hr after initiating therapy); hypotension and hypoperfusion will occur; if B/P <90 mm Hg, monitor ECG, CVP in cardiac patients
- Monitor renal function studies: BUN, serum uric acid, urine CCr, electrolytes before, during therapy; I&O ratio; report fall in urine output to <30 ml/hr
- Monitor temperature q4h; fever may indicate beginning infection
- Check liver function tests before, during therapy: bilirubin, AST, ALT, alkaline phosphatase, LDH as needed or monthly
- Monitor ECG; watch for ST-T wave changes, low QRS and T, possible dysrhythmias (sinus tachycardia, PVCs)
- Monitor baselines in pulmonary function; document FEV >2 L or ≥75% before therapy; check daily VS, pulse oximetry, dyspnea, crackles, ABGs, watch for respiratory failure, intubate if necessary
- Obtain stress thallium study before therapy; document normal ejection fraction, unimpaired wall motion
- Assess for bleeding: hematuria, guaiac, bruising or petechiae, mucosa, or orifices q8h
- Assess for GI symptoms: frequency of stools, cramping
- Assess for acidosis, signs of dehydration: rapid respirations, poor skin turgor, decreased urine output, dry skin, restlessness, weakness
- Assess for cardiac status: B/P, pulse, character, rhythm, rate, ABGs, ECG
- Assess for infection: sore throat; antibiotics may be prescribed prophylactically

Nursing diagnoses

- Injury, risk for (adverse reactions)
- Body image, disturbed (adverse reactions)
- Infection, risk for (adverse reactions)
- Knowledge, deficient (teaching)

Implementation

Intermittent IV infusion route

- Give by intermittent **IV** inf after diluting 22 million international units (1.3 mg)/1.2 ml sterile (1.1 mg/ml) H_2O for inj at side of vial and swirl, do not shake; dilute dose with 50 ml D_5W and give over 15 min; use plastic bag; do not use an in-line filter; give through Y-tube or 3-way stopcock

- Give DOPamine 1-5 kg/min before onset of hypotension; decreased dose preserves kidney output
- Give hydrocortisone, dexamethasone, or sodium bicarbonate (1 mEq/1 ml) for extravasation, apply ice compresses
- Store in refrigerator any diluted drug; do not freeze; administer within 48 hr; bring to room temperature before infusing; discard unused portion

Y-site compatibilities: Amikacin, **IV** fat emulsion, gentamicin, morphine, piperacillin, potassium chloride, ticarcillin, tobramycin, TPN #145, amphotericin B, calcium gluconate, diphenhydrAMINE, DOPamine, fluconazole, foscarnet, heparin, magnesium sulfate, metoclopramide, ondansetron, ranitidine, trimethoprim/sulfamethoxazole

Patient/family education

- Teach patient to avoid use of products containing aspirin or ibuprofen, razors, commercial mouthwash because bleeding may occur; to report symptoms of bleeding, hematuria, tarry stools
- Tell patient to report signs of anemia: fatigue, headache, irritability, faintness, shortness of breath
- Tell patient to report any changes in breathing or coughing even several months after treatment
- Advise patient that contraception will be necessary during treatment; teratogenesis may occur
- Teach patient to report signs/symptoms of infection: fever, chills, sore throat; patient should avoid crowds or persons with known infections
- Advise patient to avoid alcohol, NSAIDs, salicylates; GI bleeding may occur
- Advise patient that visual problems may occur but are reversible

Evaluation

Positive therapeutic outcome

- Decreased spread of malignancy

alemtuzumab (Rx)

(al-em-tuz'uh-mab)

Campath

Func. class.: Antineoplastic—miscellaneous

Chem. class.: Monoclonal antibody

Pregnancy category C

Action: Composed of recombinant DNA-derived humanized monoclonal antibody (campath-1H), binds to CD52 antigen that is present on surface of B and T lymphocytes, causes lysis of leukemic cells

Therapeutic Outcome: Decreased in number of white blood cells

Uses: B-cell chronic lymphocytic leukemia that has been treated with alkylating agents

Dosage and routes

Adult: **IV** 3 mg over 2 hr daily; when tolerated, increase to 10 mg; when 10 mg tolerated, increase to 30 mg daily; maintenance is 30 mg/day 3×/wk on alternate days for 12 wk, titration usually takes 3-7 days, max single dose 30 mg; max weekly dose 90 mg

Available forms: Sol for inj 30 mg/3 ml

Adverse effects

CNS: *Dizziness,* insomnia, depression, headache, tremor, somnolence, fatigue

CV: *Hypotension, tachycardia, hypertension, edema, chest pain, supraventricular tachycardia*

GI: *Anorexia, diarrhea,* constipation, *nausea, stomatitis, vomiting, abdominal pain, dyspepsia*

HEMA: **Anemia, neutropenia, thrombocytopenia, pancytopenia,** purpura, epistaxis

INTEG: *Rash,* local reaction, pruritus

MISC: Rigors, fever

RESP: Cough, pneumonia, rhinitis, **bronchospasm,** dyspnea, pharyngitis

Contraindications: Hypersensitivity, active systemic infection, immunodeficiency

Precautions: Pregnancy **C,** lactation, children

Pharmacokinetics	
Absorption	Unknown
Distribution	Unknown; steady state 6 wk
Metabolism	Unknown
Excretion	Unknown
Half-life	12 days

Pharmacodynamics	
Onset	Unknown
Peak	Unknown
Duration	Unknown

Interactions

Drug classifications

Live virus vaccines: do not administer

Drug/lab test

Diagnostic tests using antibodies

NURSING CONSIDERATIONS

Assessment

- Assess CBC, platelets qwk or more often if myelosuppression occurs; assess $CD4^+$

after therapy until recovery of >200 cells/mcL
- Assess for symptoms of infection; chills, fever, headache, may be masked by drug fever; do not administer drug if infection is present
- Assess CNS reaction: LOC, mental status, dizziness, confusion
- Assess cardiac status: lung sounds; ECG before and during treatment, especially in those with cardiac disease
- Assess for bone marrow depression: bruising, bleeding, blood in stools, urine, sputum, emesis

Nursing diagnoses
- Infection, risk for (adverse reactions)
- Injury, risk for (adverse reactions)
- Nutrition: less than body requirements, imbalanced (side effects)
- Body image, disturbed (adverse reactions)
- Knowledge, deficient (teaching)

Implementation
IV route
- Do not give **IV** push or bolus
- Withdraw amount needed; do not shake ampule; use 5 µm filter prior to dilution, check for particulate matter and discoloration; inject into 100 ml sterile 0.9% NaCl or D_5W, invert to mix, do not add other drugs or infuse in same **IV** tubing
- Store reconstituted sol for ≤8 hr at room temp, do not freeze; protect from light

Patient/family education
- Instruct patient to take acetaminophen for fever
- Advise patient to avoid hazardous tasks, since confusion, dizziness may occur
- Instruct patient to report signs of infection: sore throat, fever, diarrhea, vomiting

Evaluation
Positive therapeutic outcome
- Decreased in production of malignant lymphocytes

alendronate (Rx)
(al-en'droe-nate)
Fosamax
Func. class.: Bone-resorption inhibitor
Chem. class.: Bisphosphonate
Pregnancy category C

Do Not Confuse:
Fosamax/Flomax

Action: Absorbs calcium phosphate crystal in bone and may directly block dissolution of hydroxyapatite crystals of bone; inhibits normal and abnormal bone resorption

Therapeutic Outcome: Decreased symptoms of osteoporosis, Paget's disease

Uses: Treatment and prevention of osteoporosis in postmenopausal women, Paget's disease, treatment of corticosteroid-induced osteoporosis in postmenopausal women not receiving estrogen, or in men who are continuing corticosteroid treatment with low bone mass

Dosage and routes
Osteoporosis in postmenopausal women
Adult and elderly: PO 10 mg daily or 70 mg qwk

Paget's disease
Adult and elderly: PO 40 mg daily × 6 mo, consider retreatment for relapse

Prevention of osteoporosis
Adult: PO 5 mg daily or 35 mg qwk

Corticosteroid-induced osteoporosis in postmenopausal women (not receiving estrogen)
Adult: PO 10 mg daily

Corticosteroid-induced osteoporosis in men or premenopausal women (not receiving estrogen)
Adult: PO 5 mg daily

Available forms: Tabs 5, 10, 35, 40, 70 mg; oral sol 70 mg

Adverse effects
CNS: Headache
GI: Abdominal pain, anorexia, constipation, nausea, vomiting, esophageal ulceration, acid reflux, dyspepsia
META: Anemia, hypokalemia, hypomagnesemia, hypophosphatemia, hypocalcemia
MS: Bone pain

Contraindications: Hypersensitivity to bisphosphonates, delayed esophageal emptying, inability to sit or stand for 30 min, hypocalcemia

Precautions: Pregnancy **C**, children, lactation, CCr <35 ml/min, esophageal disease, ulcers, gastritis

Pharmacokinetics

Absorption	Unknown
Distribution	Mainly to bones
Metabolism	Unknown
Excretion	Via kidneys
Half-life	Unknown

Pharmacodynamics

Unknown

Interactions

Individual drugs

Ranitidine (**IV**): increased alendronate effect

Drug classifications

Antacids, calcium supplements: decreased absorption

NSAIDs, salicylates: increased GI reactions

Drug/food

Caffeine, food, orange juice: decreased drug absorption

NURSING CONSIDERATIONS

Assessment

- Hormonal status if a woman, prior to treatment
- For osteoporosis: bone density testing
- For Paget's disease: increased skull size, bone pain, headache
- Monitor renal studies and Ca, P, Mg, K
- Assess for hypercalcemia: paresthesia, twitching, laryngospasm, Chvostek's, Trousseau's signs
- Monitor alkaline phosphatase; level of 2× upper limit of normal is indicated for Paget's disease

Nursing diagnoses

- Injury, risk for (uses)
- Knowledge, deficient (teaching)

Implementation

- Give PO for 6 mo to be effective in Paget's disease; take with 8 oz of water 30 min before 1st food, beverage, or medication of the day
- Patient to remain upright for 30 min after dose to prevent esophageal irritation
- Store in cool environment out of direct sunlight

Patient/family education

- Teach patient to remain upright for 30 min after dose to prevent esophageal irritation; if dose is missed, skip dose, do not double doses or take later in day
- Teach patient to take in AM, only before food, other meds, to take with 6-8 oz of water (not mineral water)
- To take calcium, vit D if instructed by provider
- To use weight-bearing exercise to increase bone density
- Teach patient to let provider know if pregnancy is planned or suspected or if nursing

Evaluation

Positive therapeutic outcome

- Increased bone mass, absence of fractures

alfuzosin (Rx)

(al-fyoo'zoe-sin)

Uroxatral

Func. class.: Antiadrenergic

Chem. class.: Quinazolone

Pregnancy category B

Action: Binds preferentially to α_{1A}-adrenoceptor subtype located mainly in the prostate

Therapeutic Outcome: Resolution of symptoms of benign prostatic hyperplasia

Uses: Symptoms of benign prostatic hyperplasia; has not been studied for and is not indicated for the treatment of high blood pressure

Dosage and routes

Adult: PO ext rel 10 mg daily, taken after same meal each day

Available forms: Ext rel tabs 10 mg

Adverse effects

CNS: ***Dizziness, headache,*** fatigue

CV: Postural hypotension (dizziness, lightheadedness, fainting) within a few hours of administration, chest pain, tachycardia

GI: Nausea, abdominal pain, dyspepsia, constipation

GU: Impotence, priaprism

INTEG: Rash

MISC: Body pain in general

RESP: Upper respiratory tract infection, pharyngitis, bronchitis, sinusitis

Contraindications: Hypersensitivity, moderate to severe hepatic impairment, not indicated for use in women or children

Precautions: Pregnancy **B**, lactation, coronary artery disease, coronary insufficiency, mild hepatic disease, mild/moderate/severe renal disease, history of QT prolongation or coadministration with medications known to prolong QT interval

Pharmacokinetics

Absorption	Unknown
Distribution	Moderately protein bound (82%-90%)
Metabolism	Liver (by CYP3A4 enzyme)
Excretion	Urine
Half-life	10 hr

Pharmacodynamics

Onset	Unknown
Peak	Unknown
Duration	Unknown

Interactions

Individual drugs

Alcohol: possible increased effects of alfuzosin, doxazosin, itraconazole, ketoconazole, prazosin, ritonavir, terazosin: do not take concurrently

Drug classifications

CYP3A4 inhibitors: do not take concurrently

NURSING CONSIDERATIONS

Assessment

- Assess for prostatic hyperplasia: change in urinary patterns, baseline and throughout treatment
- Monitor CBC with differential and liver function tests; B/P and heart rate
- Monitor BUN, uric acid, urodynamic studies (urinary flow rates, residual volume)
- Monitor I&O ratios, weight daily, edema; report weight gain or edema

Nursing diagnoses

- Urinary elimination, impaired (uses)
- Knowledge, deficient (teaching)

Implementation

- Swallow tabs whole; do not break, crush, or chew tabs
- Store in tight container in cool environment

Patient/family education

- Advise not to drive or operate machinery for 4 hr after first dose or after dosage increase

Evaluation

Positive therapeutic outcome

- Decreased symptoms of benign prostatic hyperplasia

alitretinoin (Rx)

(al-ee-tret'i-noyn)

Panretin

Func. class.: Retinoid, 2nd generation

Pregnancy category D

Action: Controls cellular differentiation and proliferation of neoplastic and healthy cells by binding to retinoid receptors

Therapeutic Outcome: Decreased size and number of lesions

Uses: Kaposi's sarcoma cutaneous lesions

Dosage and routes

Adult: TOP apply enough gel to cover lesions with a generous coating, allow to dry for 3-5 min before covering with clothing, do not apply near mucosal areas, apply as long as benefit occurs, do not rub gel into lesion

Available forms: Top gel 0.1%

Adverse effects

INTEG: Rash, stinging, pain, warmth, redness, erythema, blistering, crusting, peeling, dermatitis, pain

Contraindications: Pregnancy **D**, hypersensitivity to retinoids

Precautions: Lactation, eczema, sunburn, elderly, cutaneous T-cell lymphoma

Pharmacokinetics

Absorption	Small amounts
Distribution	Unknown
Metabolism	Unknown
Excretion	Kidneys
Half-life	Unknown

Pharmacodynamics

Unknown

Interactions

Individual drugs

DEET: do not use around DEET (an insect repellant)

NURSING CONSIDERATIONS

Assessment

- Assess part of body involved, including time involved, what helps or aggravates condition, cysts, dryness, itching
- Assess for dermal toxicity that may start as erythema, then edema; drug may need to be discontinued and restarted

Nursing diagnoses

- Skin integrity, impaired (uses)
- Body image, disturbed (uses)
- Knowledge, deficient (teaching)

Implementation

- Apply bid initially to lesions, can be increased to tid-qid according to tolerance, discontinue for a few days if severe reactions occur
- Store at room temp
- Wash hands after application

Patient/family education

- Instruct patient to avoid application on normal skin, and to avoid getting cream in eyes, nose, other mucous membranes
- Advise patient to avoid sunlight, sunlamps or

to use protective clothing or sunscreen to prevent burns
- Advise patient that treatment may cause warmth, stinging; dryness; peeling will occur
- Caution patient that drug does not cure condition; only relieves symptoms; that therapeutic results may be seen in 2-3 wk but may not be optimal until after 6 wk

Evaluation
Positive therapeutic outcome
- Decreased in size and number of lesions

allopurinol (Rx)
(al-oh-pure'i-nole)
alloprim, allopurinol, Apo-Allopurinol ✤, Lopurin, Purinol ✤, Zyloprim
Func. class.: Antigout drug
Chem. class.: Xanthine enzyme inhibitor
Pregnancy category C

Do Not Confuse:
allopurinol/apresoline, Lopurin/Lupron

Action: Inhibits the enzyme xanthine oxidase, reducing uric acid synthesis

Therapeutic Outcome: Decreasing serum uric acid levels, decreasing joint pain

Uses: Chronic gout, hyperuricemia associated with malignancies, recurrent calcium oxalate calculi, Chagas disease, cutaneous/visceral leishmaniasis, uric acid calculi

Investigational uses: Stomatitis (mouthwash)

Dosage and routes
Increased uric acid levels in malignancies
Adult: **IV** inf 200-400 mg/m^2/day, max 600 mg/day
Child: **IV** inf 200 mg/m^2/day, initially

Gout/hyperuricemia
Adult: PO 200-600 mg daily depending on severity, not to exceed 800 mg/day
Child 6-10 yr: 300 mg daily
Child <6 yr: 150 mg daily

Impaired renal function
Adult: PO CCr 20-30 ml/min: 200 mg daily
Adult: PO CCr <20 ml/min: 100 mg daily
Adult: **IV** CCr 10-20 ml/min: 200 mg/day; CCr 3-10 ml/min 100 mg/day; CCr <3 ml/min 100 mg/day at intervals

Recurrent calculi
Adult: PO 200-300 mg daily

Uric acid nephropathy prevention
Adult and child >10 yr: PO 600-800 mg daily × 2-3 days

Stomatitis
Adult: Mouthwash dose varies, do not swallow mouthwash

Available forms: Tabs, scored, 100, 300 mg; inj 500 mg/vial

Adverse effects
CNS: *Headache,* drowsiness, neuritis, paresthesia
EENT: Retinopathy, cataracts, epistaxis
GI: *Nausea, vomiting, anorexia, malaise,* metallic taste, cramps, peptic ulcer, diarrhea, stomatitis
HEMA: **Agranulocytosis, thrombocytopenia, aplastic anemia, pancytopenia, leukopenia, bone marrow suppression, eosinophilia**
INTEG: Fever, chills, dermatitis, pruritus, purpura, erythema, ecchymosis, alopecia
MISC: Myopathy, arthralgia, hepatomegaly, **cholestatic jaundice, renal failure, exfoliative dermatitis**

Contraindications: Hypersensitivity

Precautions: Pregnancy **C,** lactation, renal disease, hepatic disease, children

Pharmacokinetics	
Absorption	80%
Distribution	Widely distributed
Metabolism	Liver to oxypurinol
Excretion	Kidneys
Half-life	2-3 hr, terminal 18-30 hr

Pharmacodynamics	PO	IV
Onset	Unknown	Unknown
Peak	2-4 hr	Unknown
Duration	Unknown	Unknown

Interactions
Individual drugs
Ammonium chloride potassium/sodium phosphate, vit C: increased kidney stone formation
Ampicillin, amoxicillin, bacampicillin: increased risk of rash
Azathioprine: increased action of azathioprine
Chlorpropamide: increased action of chlorproPAMIDE
Cyclophosphamide: increased action of cyclophosphamide
Hydantoin: increased action of hydantoin

Mercaptopurine: increased action of mercaptopurine
Probenecid: decreased effects of probenecid
Theophylline: increased action of theophylline

Drug classifications

ACE inhibitors: increased action of ACE inhibitors
Aluminum salts: decreased effects of allopurinol
Anticoagulants (oral): increased action of oral anticoagulants
Antineoplastics: increased bone marrow suppression
Diuretics (thiazide): increased allopurinol toxicity

NURSING CONSIDERATIONS

Assessment

- Assess for pain including location, characteristics, onset/duration, frequency, quality, intensity or severity of pain, precipitating factors
- Monitor uric acid levels q2 wk; normal uric acid levels are 6 mg/dl or less; check I&O ratio; increase fluids to 2 L/day to prevent stone formation, toxicity
- Monitor CBC, AST, BUN, creatinine before starting treatment, monthly; check blood glucose in diabetic patients receiving oral antidiabetic agents
- Monitor nutritional status: discourage organ meat, sardines, salmon, legumes, gravies (high-purine foods), alcohol

Nursing diagnoses

- Nutrition: more than body requirements, imbalanced (uses)
- Knowledge, deficient (teaching)

Implementation

PO route

- Give with meals to prevent GI symptoms; crush and mix with food or fluids for patients with swallowing difficulties
- Increased fluid intake to 2 L/day
- Give a few days before antineoplastic therapy if using for hyperuricemia associated with malignancy

IV infusion route

- Reconstitute 30-ml vial with 25 ml of sterile water for inj; dilute to desired conc with 0.9% NaCl for inj or D_5 for inj, begin inf within 10 hr

Solution incompatibilities: Amikacin, amphotericin B, carmustine, cefotaxime, chlorproMAZINE, cilastatin, cimetidine, clindamycin, cytarabine, dacarbazine, DAUNOrubicin, diphenhydrAMINE, DOXOrubicin, doxycycline, droperidol, floxuridine, gentamicin, haloperidol, hydrOXYzine, idarubicin, imipenem, mechlorethamine, meperidine, metoclopramide, methylPREDNISolone, minocycline, nalbuphine, netilmicin, ondansetron, prochlorperazine, promethazine, sodium bicarbonate, streptozocin, tobramycin, vinorelbine

Patient/family education

- Tell patient to increase fluid intake to 2 L/day; to avoid taking large doses of vit C; kidney stone formation may occur; to maintain a diet enhancing urine alkalinity (e.g., milk, other dairy products); if taking for calcium oxalate stones, reduce dairy products, refined sugar, sodium, meat
- Tell patient to report skin rash, stomatitis, malaise, fever, aching; drug should be discontinued
- Advise patient to avoid hazardous activities if drowsiness or dizziness occurs; response may take several days to determine
- Tell patient to avoid alcohol, caffeine; these substances increase uric acid levels and decrease allopurinol levels
- Teach patient to report side effects and adverse reactions to prescriber, including rash, itching, nausea, vomiting

Evaluation

Positive therapeutic outcome

- Decreased pain in joints
- Decreased stone formation in kidney
- Decreased uric acid level to 6 mg/dl

almotriptan (Rx)

(al-moh-trip'tan)
Axert
Func. class.: Antimigraine agent
Chem. class.: 5-HT_1 receptor agonist

Pregnancy category C

Action: Binds selectively to the vascular 5-HT_1 receptor subtype, exerts antimigraine effect; causes vasoconstriction in cranial arteries

Therapeutic Outcome: Absence of migraines

Uses: Acute treatment of migraine with or without aura

Dosage and routes

Adult: PO may use 6.25 mg dose initially, but 12.5 mg is more effective; may repeat dose after 2 hr; do not give more than 2 doses/24 hr or 4 treatment cycles within any 30-day period

Hepatic/renal dose

Adult: PO 6.25 mg initially, max 12.5 mg

Available forms: Tabs 6.25, 12.5 mg

Adverse effects

CV: Flushing, palpitations, tachycardia, **coronary artery vasospasm, MI, ventricular fibrillation, ventricular tachycardia**
EENT: Throat, mouth, nasal discomfort; vision changes
GI: Nausea, xerostomia
INTEG: Sweating
MS: Weakness, neck stiffness, myalgia
NEURO: Tingling, hot sensation, burning, feeling of pressure, tightness, numbness, dizziness, sedation, headache, anxiety, fatigue, cold sensation
RESP: Chest tightness, pressure

Contraindications: Cluster headache, hemiplegia, vascular migraine, ischemic heart disease, peripheral vascular syndrome; concurrent use of ergotamine-containing preparations, uncontrolled hypertension, basilar or hemiplegic migraine; concurrent MAOI therapy or within 2 wk

Precautions: Pregnancy **C**, postmenopausal women, men >40 yr, risk factors for coronary artery disease, hypercholesterolemia, obesity, diabetes, impaired hepatic or renal function, lactation, children <18 yr, elderly

Pharmacokinetics

Absorption	Well absorbed (~70%)
Distribution	35% protein bound
Metabolism	Liver (metabolite); metabolized by MAO-A, CYP2D6, CYP3A4
Excretion	Urine, feces
Half-life	3-4 hr

Pharmacodynamics

Onset	Unknown
Peak	1-3 hr
Duration	3-4 hr

Interactions

Individual drugs

Ergot: increased vasospastic effects
Ketoconazole: increased plasma concentration of almotriptan

Drug classifications

5-HT_1 agonists, ergot derivatives: increased vasospastic effects
MAOIs: increased almotriptan effect
CYP2D6 inhibitors: increased almotriptan effect

Drug/herb

Butterbur: increased almotriptan effect

NURSING CONSIDERATIONS

Assessment

- Assess B/P, signs/symptoms of coronary vasospasms
- Assess for tingling, hot sensation, burning, feeling of pressure, numbness, flushing
- Assess for stress level, activity, recreation, coping mechanisms
- Assess neurologic status: LOC, blurring vision, nausea, vomiting, tingling in extremities preceding headache
- Assess for ingestion of tyramine-containing foods (pickled products, beer, wine, aged cheese), food additives, preservatives, colorings, artificial sweeteners, chocolate, caffeine, which may precipitate these types of headaches

Nursing diagnoses

- Pain, acute (uses)
- Knowledge, deficient (teaching)

Implementation

- Swallow tabs whole; do not break, crush, or chew tabs
- Provide quiet, calm environment with decreased stimulation from noise, bright light, excessive talking

Patient/family education

- Instruct patient to use contraception while taking drug, notify prescriber if pregnancy is planned or suspected, avoid breastfeeding
- Advise patient to have dark, quiet environment available
- Inform patient that drug does not prevent or reduce number of migraine attacks
- Advise patient to report chest pain, drowsiness, dizziness, tingling, flushing, pressure

Evaluation

Positive therapeutic outcome

- Decreased in severity of migraine

Treatment of overdose: Gastric lavage followed by activated charcoal; clinical and ECG monitoring for ≥20 hr after overdose

alprazolam (Rx)

(al-pray'zoe-lam)

Apo-Alpraz ✤, Novo-Alprazol ✤, Nu-Alpraz ✤, Xanax, Xanax XR

Func. class.: Antianxiety/sedative/hypnotic
Chem. class.: Benzodiazepine

Pregnancy category D

Controlled substance schedule IV

Do Not Confuse:
alprazolam/lorazepam, Xanax/Lanoxin, Xanax/Tylox, Xanax/Zantac

Action: Depresses subcortical levels of CNS, including limbic system, reticular formation; potentiates GABA (γ-aminobutyric acid)

Therapeutic Outcome: Decreased anxiety

Uses: Anxiety, panic disorders, anxiety with depressive symptoms

Investigational uses: Depression, social phobia, premenstrual syndrome, dysphoric disorders

Dosage and routes

Anxiety disorder

Adult: PO 0.25-0.5 mg tid, not to exceed 4 mg/day in divided doses

Elderly: PO 0.125-0.25 mg bid; increase by 0.125 mg as needed

Panic disorder

Adult: PO 0.5 mg tid, may increase, max 10 mg/day; ext rel tabs (Xanax XR) give daily in AM 0.5-1 mg initially, maintenance 1-10 mg daily

Premenstrual dysphoric disorders

Adult: PO 0.25 mg bid-qid, starting on day 16-18 of menses, taper over 2-3 days when menses occurs

Social phobia

Adult: PO 2-8 mg/day

Hepatic dose

Reduce dose by 50%

Available forms: Tabs 0.25, 0.5, 1, 2 mg; oral sol 0.1, 1 mg/ml; ext rel tabs (Xanax XR) 0.5, 1, 2, 3 mg

Adverse effects

CNS: *Dizziness, drowsiness,* confusion, headache, anxiety, tremors, stimulation, fatigue, depression, insomnia, hallucinations

CV: *Orthostatic hypotension,* **ECG changes, tachycardia,** hypotension

EENT: *Blurred vision,* tinnitus, mydriasis

GI: Constipation, dry mouth, nausea, vomiting, anorexia, diarrhea

INTEG: Rash, dermatitis, itching

Contraindications: Pregnancy **D**, hypersensitivity to benzodiazepines, narrow-angle glaucoma, psychosis, lactation, addiction

Precautions: Elderly, debilitated, hepatic disease

Pharmacokinetics	
Absorption	Slow, complete
Distribution	Widely distributed; crosses placenta; crosses blood-brain barrier
Metabolism	Liver, to active metabolites
Excretion	Kidneys, breast milk
Half-life	12-15 hr

Pharmacodynamics	
Onset	1 hr
Peak	1-2 hr
Duration	4-6 hr, therapeutic response 2-3 days

Interactions

Individual drugs

Alcohol: increased CNS depression

Cimetidine, disulfiram, erythromycin, fluoxetine, isoniazid, ketoconazole, levodopa, metoprolol, propoxyphene, propranolol, valproic acid: increased action of alprazolam

Levodopa: decreased action of levodopa

Rifampin: decreased action of alprazolam

Drug classifications

A substrate of CYP3A4

Anticonvulsants, antihistamines: increased CNS depression

Barbiturates: decreased action of alprazolam

Contraceptives (oral): increased action of alprazolam

Sedative/hypnotics: increased CNS depression

Xanthines: decreased sedation

Drug/herb

Cat's claw, chamomile, cowslip, echinacea, goldenseal, hops, kava, licorice, Queen Anne's lace, skullcap, St. John's wort, valerian, wild cherry: increased CNS depression

Drug/food

Grapefruit juice: increased drug level

Drug/lab test

Increased: ALT, AST, alkaline phosphatase

NURSING CONSIDERATIONS

Assessment

- Assess mental status: mood, sensorium, anxiety, affect, sleeping pattern, drowsiness, dizziness, especially elderly; physical dependency, withdrawal symptoms: anxiety, panic attacks, agitation, seizures, headache, nausea, vomiting, muscle pain, weakness; suicidal tendencies; indications of increasing tolerance and abuse; withdrawal seizures may occur after rapid decrease in dose or abrupt discontinuation; short duration of action makes it the drug of choice in the elderly

• Monitor B/P (with patient lying, standing), pulse; if systolic B/P drops 20 mm Hg, hold drug, notify prescriber
• Monitor blood studies: CBC during long-term therapy; blood dycrasias have occurred rarely; decreased hematocrit, neutropenia may occur
• Monitor hepatic studies: AST, ALT, bilirubin, creatinine LDH, alkaline phosphatase, if on long-term treatment
• Monitor I&O; indicate renal dysfunction if on long-term treatment

Nursing diagnoses

• Anxiety (uses)
• Injury, risk for (adverse reactions)
• Knowledge, deficient (teaching)

Implementation

• Give with food or milk for GI symptoms; tab may be crushed, if patient is unable to swallow medication whole, and mixed with foods or fluids; may divide total daily dose into more times/day, if anxiety occurs between doses
• Give sugarless gum, hard candy, frequent sips of water for dry mouth

Patient/family education

• Tell patient that drug may be taken with food or fluids, and tabs may be crushed or swallowed whole
• Tell patient not to use for everyday stress or longer than 4 mo unless directed by prescriber; not to take more than prescribed amount; may be habit forming; not to double doses or skip doses; memory impairment is a sign of long-term use
• Tell patient to avoid OTC preparations unless approved by prescriber; alcohol and CNS depressants will increase CNS depression
• Tell patient to avoid driving, activities that require alertness, since drowsiness may occur; to avoid alcohol ingestion or other psychotropic medications; to rise slowly or fainting may occur, especially elderly; that drowsiness may worsen at beginning of treatment
• Tell patient not to discontinue medication abruptly after long-term use; withdrawal symptoms include vomiting, cramping, tremors, seizures

Evaluation

Positive therapeutic outcome

• Decreased anxiety, restlessness, sleeplessness (short-term treatment only)

Treatment of overdose: Lavage, VS, supportive care, flumazenil

! HIGH ALERT

alteplase (Rx)

(al-ti-plaze′)

Activase, Activase rt-PA ✤, Lysatec rt-PA ✤, Cathflo, tissue plasminogen activator, t-PA

Func. class.: Thrombolytic enzyme

Chem. class.: Tissue plasminogen activator (TPA)

Pregnancy category C

Do Not Confuse:

alteplace/Altace

Action: Produces fibrin conversion of plasminogen to plasmin; able to bind to fibrin, convert plasminogen in thrombus to plasmin, which leads to local fibrinolysis, limited systemic proteolysis

Therapeutic Outcome: Lysis of thrombi in MI, pulmonary emboli (life threatening)

Uses: Lysis of obstructing thrombi associated with acute MI; conditions requiring thrombolysis (e.g., PE, DVT, unclotting arteriovenous shunts, acute ischemic CVA)

Investigational uses: Unstable angina, occluded central venous catheters

Dosage and routes

Pulmonary embolism

Adult: **IV** 100 mg over 2 hr, then heparin

Acute ischemic stroke

Adult: **IV** 0.9 mg/kg, max 90 mg; give as inf over 1 hr, give 10% of dose **IV** BOL over 1st min

Myocardial Infarction (standard infusion)

Adult >65 kg: **IV** a total of 100 mg; 6-10 mg given **IV** bol over 1-2 min, 60 mg given over 1st hr, 20 mg given over 2nd hr, 20 mg given over 3rd hr; or 1.25 mg/kg given over 3 hr for <65 kg patient

Adult <65 kg: **IV** 0.75 mg over 1st hr, 0.075-0.125 mg/kg given **IV** bol over first 1-2 min, 0.25 mg/kg over 2nd hr, 0.25 mg/kg over 3rd hr to a total dose of 1.25 mg/kg, max 100 mg total

Myocardial Infarction (accelerated infusion)

Adult: **IV** bol 15 mg; then 0.75 mg/kg over ½ hr; then 0.5 mg/kg over 1 hr, usually given with heparin

Occluded central venous catheters

Adult: 2 mg/2 ml infused in each port of dual lumen catheter; dwell time varies widely

Available forms: Powder for inj 50 mg (29 million international units/vial), 100 mg (58 million international units/vial)

Adverse effects

CV: **Sinus bradycardia, ventricular tachycardia, accelerated idioventricular rhythm, bradycardia**
INTEG: Urticaria, rash
SYST: **GI, GU, intracranial, retroperitoneal bleeding, surface bleeding, anaphylaxis**

Contraindications: Hypersensitivity, active internal bleeding, recent CVA, severe uncontrolled hypertension, intracranial/intraspinal surgery/trauma, aneurysm, brain tumor

Precautions: Pregnancy **C**, lactation, children, elderly, neurologic deficits, mitral stenosis, recent GI, GU bleeding

Pharmacokinetics

Absorption	Complete
Distribution	Unknown
Metabolism	>80% liver
Excretion	Kidneys
Half-life	35 min

Pharmacodynamics

Onset	Immediate
Peak	30-45 min
Duration	4 hr

Interactions

Individual drugs

Abciximab, aspirin, clopidrogrel, dipyridamole, eptifibatide, heparin, plicamycin, ticlopidine, tirofiban, valproic acid: increased bleeding

Drug classifications

Anticoagulants (oral), cephalosporins (some), NSAIDs, salicylates: increased bleeding

Drug/herb

Agrimony, alfalfa, angelica, anise, basil, bay, bilberry, black haw, bogbean, bromelain, buchu, chondroitin, cinchona bark, dong quai, fenugreek, feverfew, garlic, ginger, ginkgo, ginseng, horse chestnut, Irish moss, kelp, kelpware, khella, lovage, lungwort, meadowsweet, motherwort, mugwort, nettle, papaya, parsley (large amounts), pau d'arco, pineapple, poplar, prickly ash, safflower, saw palmetto, tonka bean, turmeric, wintergreen, yarrow: increased risk of bleeding
Chamomile, coenzyme Q10, flax, glucomannan, goldenseal, guar gum: decreased anticoagulant effect

Drug/lab test

Increased: PT, APTT, TT

NURSING CONSIDERATIONS

Assessment

- Monitor VS q15 min, B/P, pulse, respirations (including peripheral), neurologic signs, temp at least q4h; temp >104° F (40° C) indicates internal bleeding; monitor rhythm closely; ventricular dysrhythmias may occur with hyperfusion; monitor heart, breath sounds, neurologic status, and peripheral pulses
- Assess for bleeding during 1st hr of treatment and 24 hr after procedure: hematuria, hematemesis, bleeding from mucous membranes, epistaxis, ecchymosis, puncture sites; guaiac all body fluids and stools; obtain blood studies (Hct, platelets, PTT, PT, TT, APTT) before starting therapy; PT or APTT must be less than 2 times control before starting therapy; TT or PT q3-4h during treatment; obtain CPK-MB to identify drug effectiveness
- Assess hypersensitivity: fever, rash, facial swelling, dyspnea, itching, chills; mild reaction may be treated with antihistamines; report to prescriber
- Monitor ECG; on monitor, watch for segment changes, changes in rhythm: sinus bradycardia, ventricular tachycardia, accelerated idioventricular rhythm may occur due to reperfusion, cardiac enzymes, radionuclide myocardial scanning/coronary angiography

Nursing diagnoses

- Pain, chronic (uses)
- Tissue perfusion, ineffective (uses)
- Injury, risk for (adverse reactions)

Implementation

Intermittent IV infusion route

- Give after reconstituting with provided diluent; add appropriate amount of sterile water for injection (no preservatives); 20-mg vial/20 ml or 50-mg vial/50 ml (1 mg/ml); mix by slow inversion or dilute with 0.9% NaCl, D_5W to a concentration of 0.5 mg/ml further dilution; 1.5 to <0.5 mg/ml may result in precipitation of drug; use 18G needle; flush line with NaCl after administration; use reconstituted **IV** sol within 8 hr or discard, within 6 hr of coronary occlusion for best results
- Do not use 150 mg or more total dose; intracranial bleeding may occur
- Give heparin therapy after thrombolytic therapy is discontinued and when TT, ACT, and APTT less than 2 times control (about 3-4 hr)
- Avoid invasive procedures, inj, rec temp; apply pressure for 30 sec to minor bleeding sites; 30 min to sites of atrial puncture, fol-

lowed by pressure dressing; inform prescriber if this does not attain hemostasis; apply pressure dressing
- Store powder at room temperature or refrigerate; protect from excessive light

Y-site compatibilities: Lidocaine, metoprolol, propranolol
Y-site incompatibilities: DOBUTamine, DOPamine, heparin, nitroglycerin
Additive compatibilities: Lidocaine, morphine, nitroglycerin

Patient/family education
- Teach patient reason for alteplase, signs and symptoms of bleeding, allergic reactions, when to notify prescriber

Evaluation
Positive therapeutic outcome
- Lysis of pulmonary thrombi
- Adequate hemodynamic state
- Absence of congestive heart failure

aluminum hydroxide (OTC)
AlternaGEL, Alu-Cap, Alugel ✦, Aluminet, Aluminett, aluminum hydroxide, Alu-Tab, Amphojel, Basalgel, Basaljel, Dialume
Func. class.: Antacid, hypophosphatemic, antiulcer
Chem. class.: Aluminum product, phosphate binder

Pregnancy category C

Action: Neutralizes gastric acidity, binds phosphates in GI tract; these phosphates are excreted

Uses: Peptic, gastric, duodenal ulcers; hyperphosphatemia in chronic renal failure; reflux esophagitis, hyperacidity, heartburn, stress ulcer prevention in critically ill, GERD

Investigational uses: GI bleeding

Therapeutic Outcome: Decreased acidity, healing of ulcers; decreased phosphate levels in chronic renal failure

Dosage and routes
Adult: SUSP 5-10 ml 1 hr pc, at bedtime; PO 600 mg 1 hr pc, at bedtime; chewed, max 6 times per day

GI bleeding
Infant: PO 2-5 ml/dose q1-2h
Child: PO 5-15 ml/dose q1-2h

Hyperphosphatemia in renal failure
Adult: SUSP 500 mg-2 g bid-qid

Available forms
Caps 475, 500 mg; tabs 300, 500, 600 mg; susp 320 mg/5 ml, 450 mg/5 ml, 600 mg/5 ml; 675 mg/5 ml

Adverse effects
GI: *Constipation,* anorexia, **obstruction,** fecal impaction
META: *Hypophosphatemia,* hypercalciuria

Contraindications: Hypersensitivity to this drug or aluminum products

Precautions: Pregnancy **C,** elderly, fluid restriction, decreased GI motility, GI obstruction, dehydration, renal disease, sodium-restricted diets

Pharmacokinetics	
Absorption	Not usually absorbed
Distribution	Widely distributed if absorbed; crosses placenta
Metabolism	Unknown
Excretion	Feces, kidneys (small amounts), breast milk
Half-life	Unknown

Pharmacodynamics	
Onset	20-40 min
Peak	½ hr
Duration	1-3 hr

Interactions
Individual drugs
Allopurinol: decreased allopurinol effect
Amprenavir: decreased amprenavir effect
Ciprofloxacin: decreased ciprofloxacin effect
Delavirdine: decreased delavirdine effect
Diflunisal: decreased diflunisal effect
Digitalis: decreased digitalis effect
Gabapentin: decreased gabapentin effect
Gatifloxacin: decreased gatifloxacin effect
Isoniazid: decreased isoniazid effect
Ketoconazole: decreased ketoconazole effect
Penicillamine: decreased penicillamine effect
Phenytoin: decreased phenytoin effect
Quinidine: decreased quinidine effect
Ticlopidine: decreased ticlopidine effect
Warfarin: decreased warfarin effect

Drug classifications
Cephalosporins: decreased cephalosporin effect
Corticosteroids: decreased corticosteroid effect
Digitalis: decreased digitalis effect
H_2 antagonists: decreased H_2 antagonist effect
Iron salts: decreased iron salt effect
Phenothiazines: decreased phenothiazine effect

Tetracyclines: decreased tetracycline effect
Thyroid hormones: decreased thyroid effect

Drug/herb

Buckthorn, cascara sagrada, castor, Chinese rhubarb: decreased action of these herbs

NURSING CONSIDERATIONS

Assessment

- Assess pain symptoms: location, duration, intensity, alleviating precipitating factors
- Monitor phosphate levels, since drug is bound in GI system; urinary pH, calcium, electrolytes; hypophosphatemia: anorexia, weakness, fatigue, bone pain, hyperreflexia
- Monitor constipation; increase bulk in diet if needed

Nursing diagnoses

- Pain, chronic (uses)
- Constipation (adverse reactions)
- Knowledge, deficient (teaching)

Implementation

- 2 tsp (10 ml) will neutralize 20 mEq of acid; 2 tabs will neutralize 16 mEq of acid

PO route

- Give laxatives or stool softeners if constipation occurs, especially elderly
- Give after shaking liquid; follow with water to facilitate passage
- Tab may be chewed if patient is unable to swallow; drink 8 oz of water after chewing; or by nasogastric tube if patient unable to swallow
- Give with 8 oz of water for hyperphosphatemia unless contraindicated
- Give 1 hr before or after other medications to prevent poor absorption
- Give 15 ml 30 min pc and at bedtime (esophagitis)

NG tube route

- May be given as prescribed q1-2h and given by gastric tube after diluting with water (peptic ulcer)

Patient/family education

- Instruct patient to increase fluids to 2000 ml/day unless contraindicated
- Instruct patient to avoid phosphate-containing foods (most dairy products, eggs, fruits, carbonated beverages) during drug therapy; to add cheese, corn, pasta, plums, prunes, lentils after drug (hypophosphatemia)
- Instruct patient not to use for prolonged periods if serum phosphate is low or if on a low-sodium diet; CHF patients should check for sodium content and use sodium-reduced products
- Instruct patient that stools may appear white or speckled; constipation may result; to report black tarry stools, which indicate gastric bleeding
- Instruct patient to check with prescriber after 2 wk of self-prescribed antacid use; may be used for 4-6 wk after symptoms subside or as prescribed
- Instruct patient to separate other medications by 2 hr

Evaluation

Positive therapeutic outcome

- Absence of pain, decreased acidity
- Increased pH of gastric secretions
- Decreased phosphate levels

amantadine (Rx)

(a-man'ta-deen)

amantadine HCl, Symadine, Symmetrel

Func. class.: Antiviral, antiparkinsonian agent

Chem. class.: Tricyclic amine

Pregnancy category C

Do Not Confuse:
amantadine/ranitidine, amantadine/rimantidine, Symmetrel/Synthroid

Action: Prevents uncoating of nucleic acid in viral cell, preventing penetration of virus to host; causes release of dopamine from neurons

Therapeutic Outcome:
Resolution of infection, lessening of parkinsonism symptoms

Uses: Prophylaxis or treatment of influenza type A, extrapyramidal reactions, parkinsonism

Investigational uses: Neuroleptic malignant syndrome, cocaine dependency, enuresis

Dosage and routes

Influenza type A

Adult and child >12 yr: PO 200 mg/day in single dose or divided bid; max 400 mg/day

Elderly: PO No more than 100 mg/day

Child 9-12 yr: PO 100 mg bid

Child 1-9 yr: PO 5 mg/kg/day divided bid-tid, not to exceed 150 mg/day

Extrapyramidal reaction/ parkinsonism

Adult: PO 100 mg bid, up to 400 mg/day in EPS; give for 1 wk, then 100 mg as needed up to 400 mg in parkinsonism

MS-associated fatigue (off-label)

Adult: PO 200 mg daily or 100 mg bid

Neuroleptic malignant syndrome (off-label)
Adult: PO 100 mg bid × 3 wk

Renal dose
Adult: PO CCr 40-50 ml/min 100 mg/day; CCr 30 ml/min 200 mg 2×/wk; CCr 20 ml/min 100 mg 3×/wk; CCr 10 ml/min 100 mg alternating with 200 mg q7days

Available forms: Caps 100 mg; syr 50 mg/5 ml

Adverse effects
CNS: *Headache, dizziness,* drowsiness, fatigue, *anxiety,* psychosis, *depression, hallucinations,* tremors, ***seizures,*** confusion, *insomnia*
CV: *Orthostatic hypotension,* ***CHF***
EENT: Blurred vision
GI: *Nausea, vomiting,* constipation, dry mouth
GU: *Frequency, retention*
HEMA: Leukopenia
INTEG: Photosensitivity, dermatitis

Contraindications: Hypersensitivity, lactation, child <1 yr, eczematic rash

Precautions: Pregnancy **C**, epilepsy, CHF, orthostatic hypotension, psychiatric disorders, hepatic disease, renal disease, peripheral edema, elderly

Pharmacokinetics	
Absorption	Unknown
Distribution	Crosses placenta
Metabolism	Not metabolized
Excretion	Urine unchanged (90%), breast milk
Half-life	24 hr

Pharmacodynamics	
Onset	48 hr
Peak	Unknown
Duration	Unknown

Interactions
Individual drugs
Atropine: increased anticholinergic response
Triamterene, hydrochlorothiazide: decreased excretion of amantadine
Drug classifications
CNS stimulants: increased CNS stimulation
Anticholinergics (other): increased anticholinergic response
Drug/herb
Belladonna, henbane: increased anticholinergic response
Pheasant's eye, quinine, scopolia root: increased action/side effects
Kava: decreased action

NURSING CONSIDERATIONS
Assessment
- Monitor I&O ratio; report frequency, hesitancy
- Assess CHF, confusion, mottling of skin
- Assess bowel pattern before, during treatment
- Assess skin eruptions, photosensitivity after administration of drug
- Assess respiratory status: rate, character, wheezing, tightness in chest
- Assess allergies before initiation of treatment, reaction of each medication
- Assess signs of infection

Nursing diagnoses
- Infection, risk for (uses)
- Knowledge, deficient (teaching)

Implementation
- Give before exposure to influenza; continue for 10 days after contact
- Give at least 4 hr before bedtime to prevent insomnia
- Give after meals for better absorption, to decrease GI symptoms
- Give in divided doses to prevent CNS disturbances: headache, dizziness, fatigue, drowsiness
- Store in tight, dry container
- Caps may be opened and mixed with food

Patient/family education
- Advise patient to change body position slowly to prevent orthostatic hypotension
- Teach about aspects of drug therapy: need to report dyspnea, weight gain, dizziness, poor concentration, dysuria, behavioral changes
- Advise patient to avoid hazardous activities if dizziness, blurred vision occurs
- Advise patient to take drug exactly as prescribed; parkinsonian crisis may occur if drug is discontinued abruptly; do not double dose; if a dose is missed, do not take within 4 hr of next dose
- Teach to avoid alcohol

Evaluation
Positive therapeutic outcome
- Absence of fever, malaise, cough, dyspnea in infection; tremors, shuffling gait in Parkinson's disease

Treatment of overdose: Withdraw drug, maintain airway, administer epiNEPHrine, aminophylline, O_2, IV corticosteroids, physostigmine

amifostine (Rx)

(a-mi-foss'teen)

Ethyol

Func. class.: Cytoprotective agent for cisplatin

Pregnancy category C

Action: Binds and detoxifies damaging metabolites of cisplatin by converting this drug by alkaline phosphatase in tissue to an active free thiol compound

Therapeutic Outcome: Decreased toxic reaction from cisplatin

Uses: Used to reduce renal toxicity when cisplatin is given in ovarian cancer, reduces xerostomia (dry mouth) in radiation therapy for head, neck cancer

Dosage and routes

Reduction of renal damage with cisplatin

Adult: **IV** 910 mg/m^2 daily, within ½ hr before chemotherapy; give over 15 min; may reduce dose to 740 mg/m^2 if higher dose is poorly tolerated

Xerostomia

Adult: **IV** 200 mg/m^2 daily over 3 min as inf 15-30 min before radiation therapy

Available forms: Powder for inj lyophilized 500 mg/vial

Adverse effects

CNS: Dizziness, somnolence
CV: Hypotension
EENT: Sneezing
GI: Nausea, vomiting, hiccups
INTEG: Flushing, feeling of warmth
MISC: Hypocalcemia, rash, chills

Contraindications: Hypersensitivity to mannitol, aminothiol; hypotension, dehydration, lactation

Precautions: Pregnancy **C**, elderly, CV disease, children

Pharmacokinetics

Absorption	Complete
Distribution	Unknown
Metabolism	To free thiol compound
Excretion	Unknown
Half-life	5-8 min

Pharmacodynamics

Unknown

Interactions

Drug classfications

Antihypertensives: increased hypotension

NURSING CONSIDERATIONS

Assessment

- Assess for xerostomia: mouth lesion, dry mouth during therapy
- Assess fluid status before administration; administer antiemetic before administration to prevent severe nausea and vomiting; also, dexamethasone 20 mg **IV** and a serotonin antagonist such as ondansetron, dolasetron, or granisetron
- Monitor calcium levels before and during treatment, may cause hypocalcemia; calcium supplements may be given for hypocalcemia
- Monitor blood pressure before and q5 min during infusion; antihypertensive should be discontinued 24 hr prior to infusion if severe hypotension occurs, give **IV** 0.9% NaCl to expand fluid volume, place in modified Trendelenburg position

Nursing diagnoses

- Injury, risk for (uses)
- Knowledge, deficient (teaching)

Implementation

Intermittent IV infusion route

- Give by **IV** intermittent inf after reconstituting with 9.5 ml of sterile 0.9% NaCl, further dilute with 0.9% NaCl to a concentration of 5-40 mg/ml, give at a rate over 15 min within ½ hr of chemotherapy
- Patient to be in supine position during infusion

Y-site compatibilities: Amikacin, aminophylline, ampicillin, ampicillin/sulbactam, aztreonam, bleomycin, bumetanide, buprenorphine, butorphanol, calcium gluconate, carboplatin, carmustine, cefazolin, cefonicid, cefotaxime, cefotetan, cefoxitin, ceftazidime, ceftizoxime, ceftriaxone, cefuroxime, cimetidine, ciprofloxacin, clindamycin, cyclophosphamide, cytarabine, dacarbazine, dactinomycin, DAUNOrubicin, dexamethasone, diphenhydrAMINE, dobutamine, DOPamine, DOXOrubicin, doxycycline, droperidol, enalaprilat, etoposide, famotidine, floxuridine, fluconazole, fludarabine, fluorouracil, furosemide, gallium, gentamicin, granisetron, haloperidol, heparin, hydrocortisone, hydromorphone, idarubicin, ifosfamide, imipenem-cilastatin, leucovorin, lorazepam, magnesium sulfate, mannitol, mechlorethamine, meperidine, mesna, methotrexate, methylPREDNISolone, metoclopramide, metronidazole, mezlocillin, mitomycin, mitoxantrone, morphine, nalbuphine, netilmicin, ondansetron, piperacillin, plicamycin, potassium chloride, promethazine, ranitidine, sodium bicarbonate, streptozocin, teniposide, thiotepa, ticarcillin, ticarcillin/clavulanate, tobramycin, trimethoprim/sulfamethoxazole, trimetrexate, vancomycin, vinBLAStine, vinCRIStine, zidovudine

Additive incompatibilities: Do not mix with other drugs or solutions

Patient/family education

- Teach reason for medication and expected results
- Teach that side effects may cause severe nausea, vomiting, decreased B/P, chills, dizziness, somnolence, hiccups, sneezing

Evaluation

Positive therapeutic outcome

- Absence of renal damage

amikacin (Rx)

(am-i-kay'sin)

amikacin sulfate, Amikin

Func. class.: Antibiotic

Chem. class.: Aminoglycoside

Pregnancy category D

Do Not Confuse:

Amikin/Amicar

Action: Interferes with protein synthesis in bacterial cell by binding to ribosomal subunit, which causes misreading of genetic code; inaccurate peptide sequence forms in protein chain, causing bacterial death

Therapeutic Outcome: Bactericidal effects for the following organisms: *Pseudomonas aeruginosa, Escherichia coli, Enterobacter, Acinetobacter, Providencia, Citrobacter, Staphylococcus, Serratia, Proteus*

Uses: Severe systemic infections of CNS, respiratory, GI, urinary tract, bone, skin, soft tissues

Investigational uses: *Mycobacterium avium* complex (intrathecal or intraventricular) in combination; aerosolization

Dosage and routes

Severe systemic infections

Adult and child: **IV** inf 15 mg/kg/day in 2-3 divided doses q8-12h in 100-200 ml D_5W over 30-60 min, not to exceed 1.5 g; decreased dosages are needed in poor renal function as determined by blood levels, renal function studies; IM 15 mg/kg/day in divided doses q8-12h; daily or extended internal dosing as an alternative dosing regimen

Infants: **IV**/IM 10 mg/kg initially, then 7.5 mg/kg q12h

Neonates: IM/**IV** inf 10 mg/kg initially, then 7.5 mg/kg q12h

Premature neonates: **IV** 10 mg/kg initially, then 7.5 mg/kg q8-12h

Severe urinary tract infections

Adults: IM 250 mg bid

Renal dose

Adult: **IV**/IM 7.5 mg/kg initially, then increased as determined by blood levels, renal function studies

Available forms: Inj IM, **IV** 50, 250 mg/ml

Adverse effects

CNS: Confusion, depression, numbness, tremors, **seizures,** muscle twitching, **neurotoxicity,** dizziness, vertigo, tinnitus

CV: Hypotension or hypertension, palpitations

EENT: Ototoxicity, deafness, visual disturbances

GI: *Nausea, vomiting, anorexia,* increased ALT, AST, bilirubin, hepatomegaly, **hepatic necrosis,** splenomegaly

GU: **Oliguria, hematuria, renal damage, azotemia, renal failure, nephrotoxicity**

HEMA: **Agranulocytosis, thrombocytopenia, leukopenia, eosinophilia, anemia**

INTEG: *Rash,* burning, urticaria, dermatitis, alopecia

Contraindications: Pregnancy **D,** mild to moderate infections, hypersensitivity to aminoglycosides, sulfites

Precautions: Neonates, mild renal disease, myasthenia gravis, lactation, hearing deficits, parkinsonism, elderly

Pharmacokinetics

Absorption	Well absorbed (IM), completely absorbed (**IV**)
Distribution	Widely distributed in extracellular fluids, poor in CSF; crosses placenta
Metabolism	Minimal; liver
Excretion	Mostly unchanged (79%) in kidneys, removed by hemodialysis
Half-life	2-3 hr, prolonged up to 7 hr in infants; increased in renal disease

Pharmacodynamics

	IM	IV
Onset	Rapid	Rapid
Peak	15-30 min	1-2 hr

Interactions

Individual drugs

Dimenhydrinate, ethacrynic acid: increased masking of ototoxicity
Indomethacin: increased serum trough and peak

Drug classifications

Aminoglycosides, diuretics (loop): increased ototoxicity
Aminoglycosides: increased neurotoxicity, nephrotoxicity
Anesthetics, nondepolarizing neuromuscular blockers: increased neuromuscular blockade, respiratory depression
Cephalosporins: inactivation of amikacin, nephrotoxicity
Penicillins: inactivation of amikacin

Drug/herb

Lysine (large amounts): increased toxicity
Acidophilus: do not use with antiinfectives

Drug/lab test

Increased: BUN, ALT, AST, bilirubin, LDH, alkaline phosphatase, creatinine
Decreased: calcium, sodium, potassium, magnesium

NURSING CONSIDERATIONS

Assessment

- Assess patient for previous sensitivity reaction
- Assess patient for signs and symptoms of infection, including characteristics of wounds, sputum, urine, stool, WBC >10,000/mm^3, earache, temp; obtain baseline information before and during treatment
- Obtain C&S tests before beginning drug therapy to identify if correct treatment has been initiated
- Assess for allergic reactions: rash, urticaria, pruritus
- Identify urine output; if decreasing, notify prescriber (may indicate nephrotoxicity); also notify prescriber of increased BUN and creatinine, urine CCr <80 ml/min; lower dosage should be given in renal impairment; urinalysis daily for protein, cells, casts, nephrotoxicity may be reversible if drug stopped at first sign
- Monitor blood studies: AST, ALT, CBC, Hct, bilirubin, LDH, alkaline phosphatase; Coombs' test monthly if patient is on long-term therapy
- Monitor electrolytes: potassium, sodium, chloride, magnesium monthly if patient is on long-term therapy
- Assess bowel pattern daily; if severe diarrhea occurs, drug should be discontinued
- Monitor for bleeding: ecchymosis, bleeding gums, hematuria, stool guaiac daily if on long-term therapy
- Assess for overgrowth of infection: perineal itching, fever, malaise, redness, pain, swelling, drainage, rash, diarrhea, change in cough, sputum
- Obtain weight before treatment; calculation of dosage is usually based on ideal body weight, but may be calculated on actual body weight
- Monitor VS during infusion, watch for hypotension, change in pulse
- Assess **IV** site for thrombophlebitis including pain, redness, swelling q30 min; change site if needed; apply warm compresses to discontinued site
- Obtain serum peak, drawn 30-60 min after **IV** infusion or 60 min after IM injection; trough level drawn just before next dose; 20-30 mcg/ml, trough 4-8 mcg/ml, blood level should be 2-4 times bacteriostatic level
- Urine pH if drug is used for UTI; urine should be kept alkaline
- ❗ Deafness by audiometric testing, ringing, roaring in ears, vertigo; assess hearing before, during, after treatment
- Dehydration: high sp gr, decrease in skin turgor, dry mucous membranes, dark urine
- Vestibular dysfunction: nausea, vomiting, dizziness, headache; drug should be discontinued if severe

Nursing diagnoses

- Infection, risk for (uses)
- Diarrhea (side effects)
- Knowledge, deficient (teaching)
- Injury, risk for (side effects)

Implementation

IM route

- Give deeply in large muscle mass, rotate inj sites

Intermittent IV infusion route

- Dilute 500 mg of drug in 100-200 ml of **IV** D_5W, D_5NaCl, or 0.9% NaCl and give over ½-1 hr; flush after administration with D_5W or 0.9% NaCl

Syringe compatibilities: Clindamycin, doxapram

Y-site compatibilities: Acyclovir, amifostine, amiodarone, amsacrine, aztreonam, cisatracurium, cyclophosphamide, dexamethasone, diltiazem, enalaprilat, esmolol, filgrastim, fluconazole, fludarabine, foscarnet, furosemide, granisetron, idarubicin, IL-2, labetalol, lorazepam, magnesium sulfate, melphalan, midazolam, morphine, ondansetron, paclitaxel, perphenazine, remifentanil, sargramostim, teniposide, thiotepa, TPN #54, #61, #91, #203, #204, #212, vinorelbine, warfarin, zidovudine

Patient/family education

- Teach patient to report sore throat, bruising, bleeding, joint pain; may indicate blood dyscrasias (rare)
- Advise patient to contact prescriber if vaginal itching, loose foul-smelling stools, furry tongue occur; may indicate superinfection
- Advise patient to report hypersensitivity: rash, itching, trouble breathing, facial edema and notify prescriber

Evaluation

Positive therapeutic outcome

- Absence of signs/symptoms of infection: WBC <10,000/mm^3, temp WNL; absence of red draining wounds; absence of earache
- Reported improvement in symptoms of infection

Treatment of overdose: Withdraw drug; administer epINEPHrine, O_2, hemodialysis, exchange transfusion in the newborn; monitor serum levels of drug; may give ticarcillin or carbenicillin

amiloride (Rx)

(a-mill'oh-ride)

Amiloride HCl, Midamor

Func. class.: Potassium-sparing diuretic

Chem. class.: Pyrazine

Pregnancy category B

Action: Acts primarily on proximal distal tubule by inhibiting reabsorption of sodium and water and increasing potassium retention and conserving hydrogen ions

Therapeutic Outcome: Diuretic and antihypertensive effect while retaining potassium

Uses: Diuretic-induced hypokalemia; used with other agents to treat edema, hypertension

Dosage and routes

Adult: PO 5 mg daily; may be increased to 10-20 mg daily if needed

Available forms: Tabs 5 mg

Adverse effects

CNS: *Headache,* dizziness, fatigue, weakness, paresthesias, tremor, depression, anxiety

CV: Orthostatic hypotension, dysrhythmias, angina

EENT: Loss of hearing, tinnitus, blurred vision, nasal congestion, increased intraocular pressure

ELECT: **Hyperkalemia**

GI: *Nausea, diarrhea,* dry mouth, *vomiting, anorexia,* cramps, constipation, abdominal pain, jaundice, bleeding

GU: *Polyuria,* dysuria, frequency, impotence

HEMA: **Aplastic anemia, neutropenia**

INTEG: *Rash, pruritus,* alopecia, urticaria

MS: Cramps, joint pain

RESP: Cough, dyspnea, shortness of breath

Contraindications: Anuria, hypersensitivity, hyperkalemia, impaired renal function

Precautions: Pregnancy **B,** dehydration, diabetes, acidosis, lactation, elderly

Pharmacokinetics	
Absorption	Variable (10%-15%)
Distribution	Widely distributed
Metabolism	Unchanged in urine (50%), in feces (40%)
Excretion	Renal; breast milk
Half-life	6-9 hr

Pharmacodynamics	
Onset	2 hr
Peak	6-10 hr
Duration	24 hr

Interactions

Individual drugs

Lithium: increased lithium toxicity

Drug classifications

ACE inhibitors, diuretics (potassium-sparing), potassium products, salt substitutes: increased hyperkalemia

Antihypertensives: increased action

NSAIDs: decreased effectiveness of amiloride

Drug/herb

Arginine: fatal hypokalemia

Bearberry, gossypol: increased hypokalemia

Cucumber, dandelion, horsetail, licorice, nettle, pumpkin, Queen Anne's lace: increased amiloride effect

Khella: increased hypotension

St. John's wort: increased severe photosensitivity

Drug/food

Potassium foods: increased hyperkalemia

Drug/lab test

Interference: GTT

NURSING CONSIDERATIONS

Assessment

- Monitor manifestations of hyperkalemia: *MS:* fatigue, muscle weakness; *CARDIAC:*

dysrhythmias, hypotension; *NEURO:* paresthesias, confusion; *RESP:* dyspnea

- Monitor for manifestations of hyponatremia: *CV:* increased B/P, cold, clammy skin, hypovolemia or hypervolemia; *GI:* anorexia, nausea, vomiting, diarrhea, abdominal cramps; *NEURO:* lethargy, increased ICP, confusion, headache, seizures, coma, fatigue, tremors, hyperreflexia
- Monitor for manifestations of hyperchloremia: *NEURO:* weakness, lethargy, coma; *RESP:* deep rapid breathing
- Assess fluid volume status: I&O ratios and record, weight, distended red veins, crackles in lung, color, quality, and sp gr of urine, skin turgor, adequacy of pulses, moist mucous membranes, bilateral lung sounds, peripheral pitting edema; dehydration symptoms of decreasing output, thirst, hypotension, dry mouth and mucous membranes should be reported
- Monitor electrolytes: potassium, sodium, calcium, magnesium; also include BUN, ABGs, uric acid, CBC, blood glucose
- Assess B/P before and during therapy with patient lying, standing, and sitting as appropriate; orthostatic hypotension can occur rapidly

Nursing diagnoses

- Fluid volume, deficient (side effects)
- Fluid volume, excess (uses)
- Knowledge, deficient (teaching)

Implementation

- Give in AM to avoid interference with sleep
- With food; if nausea occurs, absorption may be increased

Patient/family education

- Teach patient to take medication early in the day to prevent nocturia
- Instruct patient to take with food or milk if GI symptoms of nausea and anorexia occur
- Teach patient to maintain a weekly record of weight and notify prescriber of weight loss >5 lb
- Caution patient that this drug causes an increase in potassium levels, so foods high in potassium should be avoided; refer to dietician for assistance, planning
- Caution patient not to exercise in hot weather or stand for prolonged periods since orthostatic hypotension will be enhanced
- Teach patient not to use alcohol or any OTC medications without prescriber's approval; serious drug reactions may occur
- Emphasize the need to contact prescriber immediately if muscle cramps, weakness, nausea, dizziness, or numbness occurs
- Teach patient to take own B/P and pulse and record
- Advise patient that dizziness and confusion may occur; avoid driving or other hazardous activities if alertness is decreased
- Teach patient to continue taking medication even if feeling better; this drug controls symptoms but does not cure the condition
- Advise patient with hypertension to continue other medical treatment (exercise, weight loss, relaxation techniques, cessation of smoking)

Evaluation

Positive therapeutic outcome

- Prevention of hypokalemia (diuretic use)
- Decreased edema
- Decreased B/P
- Increased diuresis

Treatment of overdose: Lavage if taken orally; monitor electrolytes; administer **IV** fluids; monitor hydration, CV, renal status

amino acid (Rx)

(a-mee'noe)

Injection: FreAmine, HepatAmine

Solution: Aminess, Aminosyn, BranchAmin, FreAmine III, NephrAmine, Novamine, ProcalAmine, RenAmin, Travasol, Trophamine

Func. class.: Caloric agent

Chem. class.: Nitrogen product

Pregnancy category C

Action: Needed for anabolism to maintain structure; decreases catabolism, promotes healing

Therapeutic Outcome: Positive nitrogen balance, decreased catabolism

Uses: Hepatic encephalopathy, cirrhosis, hepatitis, nutritional support in cancer trauma, intestinal obstruction, short bowel syndrome, severe malabsorption

Dosage and routes

Amino acid injection

Adult: **IV** 80-120 g/day; 500 ml of amino acids/500 ml D_{50} given over 24 hr

Amino acid solution

Adult: **IV** 1-1.5 g/kg/day titrated to patient's needs

Child: **IV** 2-3 g/kg/day titrated to patient's needs

Available forms: Inj **IV** 2.75%, 3.5%, 4.25%, 5%, 5.5%, 6%, 8.5%, 10%, 11.4%, 15% amino acids

Adverse effects

CNS: *Dizziness, headache,* confusion, **loss of consciousness**
CV: Hypertension, **CHF, pulmonary edema**
ENDO: *Hyperglycemia, rebound hypoglycemia, electrolyte imbalances, hyperosmolar syndrome, hyperosmolar hyperglycemic nonketotic syndrome,* alkalosis, acidosis, hypophosphatemia, hyperammonemia, dehydration, hypocalcemia
GI: Nausea, vomiting, liver fat deposits, abdominal pain
GU: Glycosuria, osmotic diuresis
INTEG: Chills, flushing, warm feeling, rash, urticaria, extravasation necrosis, phlebitis at inj site

Contraindications: Hypersensitivity, severe electrolyte imbalances, anuria, severe liver damage, maple syrup urine disease, PKU

Precautions: Pregnancy **C**, renal disease, children, diabetes mellitus, CHF

Pharmacokinetics

Absorption	Complete bioavailability
Distribution	Widely distributed
Metabolism	Anabolism
Excretion	Kidney to urea nitrogen
Half-life	Unknown

Pharmacodynamics

Unknown

Interactions
Drug classifications

Tetracycline: decreased protein-sparing effects

NURSING CONSIDERATIONS
Assessment

- Monitor electrolytes (potassium, sodium, calcium, chloride, magnesium), blood glucose, ammonia, phosphate, ketones; renal, liver function studies: BUN, creatinine, ALT, AST, bilirubin; urine glucose q6h using Chemstrips, which are not affected by infusion substances; if BUN increases over 15%, therapy may need to be discontinued
- Check inj site for extravasation: redness along vein, edema at site, necrosis, pain; for a hard, tender area
- Monitor respiratory function q4h: auscultate lung fields bilaterally for crackles; monitor respirations for quality, rate, rhythm that indicates fluid overload
- Monitor temperature q4h for increased fever, indicating infection; if infection is suspected, infusion is discontinued and tubing, bottle, catheter tip cultured; blood catheter may be obtained
- ❗ Monitor for impending hepatic coma: asterixis, confusion, fetor, lethargy
- Hyperammonemia: nausea, vomiting, malaise, tremors, anorexia, convulsions; increased ammonia, ketone levels may occur

Nursing diagnoses

- Nutrition: less than body requirements, imbalanced (uses)
- Injury, risk for (uses, adverse reactions)
- Infection, risk for (adverse reactions)
- Knowledge, deficient (teaching)

Implementation
Continuous IV route

- Give up to 40% protein and dextrose (up to 12.5%) via peripheral vein; stronger solutions require central **IV** administration; TPN only mixed with dextrose to promote protein synthesis
- Use immediately after mixing in pharmacy under strict aseptic technique using laminar flowhood; use infusion pump, in-line filter (0.22 μm) unless mixed with fat emulsion and dextrose (3 in 1)
- ❗ Use careful monitoring technique; do not speed up infusion; pulmonary edema, glucose overload will result
- Storage depends on type of solution; consult manufacturer
- Change dressing and **IV** tubing to prevent infection q24-48h or q5-7 days if transparent dressing is used

Y-site compatibilities: Amikacin, aminophylline, amoxicillin, ampicillin, ascorbic acid inj, atracurium, azlocillin, aztreonam, bumetanide, buprenorphine, calcium gluconate, carboplatin, cefamandole, cefazolin, cefonicid, cefoperazone, cefotaxime, cefotetan, cefoxtin, ceftazidime, ceftizoxime, ceftriaxone, cefuroxime, cephalothin, cephapirin, chloramphenicol, chlorproMAZINE, cimetidine, clindamycin, clonazepam, dexamethasone, diazepam, digoxin, diphenhydrAMINE, DOBUTamine, DOPamine, doxycycline, droperidol, enalaprilat, epINEPHrine, erythromycin lactobionate, famotidine, fentanyl, flucloxacillin, fluconazole, folic acid, foscarnet, gentamicin, granisetron, haloperidol, heparin, hydrocortisone, hydromorphone, hydrOXYzine, idarubicin, ifosfamide, IL-2, imipenem/cilastatin, insulin (regular), isoproterenol, kanamycin, leucovorin, levorphanol, lidocaine, lorazepam, magnesium sulfate, mannitol, meperidine, mesna, methicillin, metronidazole, mezlocillin, miconazole, morphine, moxalactam, multivitamins, nafcillin, netilmicin, nitroglycerin, norepINEPHrine, octreotide, ofloxacin, ondansetron, oxacillin, paclitaxel, penicillin G, penicillin G potassium, pentobarbital, phenobarbital, piperacillin, potassium chloride, prochlorperazine, ranitidine, salbutamol, sargramostim, tacrolimus, thiotepa, ticarcillin, ticarcillin/clavulanate, tobramycin, trimethoprim/sulfamethoxazole, urokinase, vancomycin, vecuronium, zidovudine

Y-site incompatibilities: Cephradine

Additive compatibilities: Amikacin, aminophylline, aztreonam, calcium gluconate, cefamandole, cefazolin, cefepime, cefotaxime, cefoxitin, cefsulodin, ceftazidime, ceftriaxone, cefuroxime, cimetidine, clindamycin, cyanocobalamin, cyclophosphamide, cycloSPORINE, cytarabine, DOPamine, epoetin, erythromycin, famotidine, folic acid, fosphenytoin, furosemide, heparin, insulin (regular), isoproterenol, lidocaine, meperidine, metaraminol, methicillin, methotrexate, methyldopate, methylPREDNISolone, metoclopramide, morphine, nafcillin, netilmicin, nizatidine, norepINEPHrine, ondansetron, oxacillin, penicillin G potassium, penicillin G sodium, phytonadione, polymyxin B, sodium bicarbonate, tacrolimus, tobramycin, vancomycin

Patient/family education

- Teach reason for use of amino acids as part of nutrition (TPN)
- Instruct patient to report at once to prescriber if chills, sweating are experienced

Evaluation

Positive therapeutic outcome

- Weight gain
- Decreased jaundice in liver disorders
- Increased LOC

aminocaproic acid (Rx)

(a-mee-noe-ka-proe′ik)

Amicar, epsilon-aminocaproic acid

Func. class.: Hemostatic, fibrinolysis inhibitor

Chem. class.: Synthetic monoaminocarboxylic acid

Pregnancy category C

Action: Inhibits fibrinolysis by inhibiting plasminogen

Therapeutic Outcome: Decreased fibrinolysis, decreased bleeding, increased clot formation

Uses: Severe hemorrhage from hyperfibrinolysis, adjunctive therapy in hemophilia

Investigational uses: Prevention of recurrent subarachnoid hemorrhage; prevention of bleeding following oral surgery (hemophiliacs); severe hemorrhage following thrombolytic agents

Dosage and routes

Acute bleeding from elevated fibrinolytic activity

Adult: PO 5 g 1st hr, then 1-1.25 g qhr × 8 hr or hemorrhage controlled; or 6 g given over 24 hr in prostate surgery, max 30 g/day; **IV** 4-5 g over 1st hr, then 1 g/hr × 8 hr or hemorrhage controlled, or 6 g given over 24 hr in prostate surgery, max 30 g/day

Child: PO/**IV** 100 mg/kg or 3 g/m^2 over 1st hr, then CONT INF 33.3 mg/kg/hr or 1 g/m^2/hr, max 18 g/m^2/24 hr

Subarachnoid hemorrhage

Adult: **IV** 36 g/day × 10 days, then PO 3 g q2hr (36 g/day), continue for 21 days after bleeding stops, then 2 g q2hr (24 g/day) × 3 days, then 1 g q2hr (12 g/day) × 3 day

Available forms: **IV** inj 250 mg/ml; tabs 500 mg; syr 1.25 mg/ml

Adverse effects

CNS: *Headache, dizziness,* malaise, fatigue, hallucinations, delirium, psychosis, **convulsions**, weakness

CV: **Dysrhythmias**, orthostatic hypotension, bradycardia (**IV**)

EENT: *Tinnitus, nasal congestion*

GI: Nausea, vomiting, abdominal cramps, diarrhea

GU: Dysuria, frequency, oliguria, **renal failure**, ejaculatory failure, menstrual irregularities

HEMA: Thrombosis

INTEG: *Rash*

Contraindications: Hypersensitivity, new burns

Precautions: Pregnancy **C**, neonates/infants, mild or moderate renal disease, hepatic disease, thrombosis, cardiac disease, DIC, upper urinary tract bleeding

Pharmacokinetics	
Absorption	Well absorbed (PO)
Distribution	Widely distributed
Metabolism	Unknown
Excretion	Kidneys, unchanged
Half-life	Unknown

Pharmacodynamics	
	PO/IV
Onset	Unknown
Peak	2 hr
Duration	Unknown

Interactions
Drug classifications
Estrogens: increased hypercoagulation
Conjugated clotting factors: increased thrombosis risk
Drug/lab test
Increased: potassium, CPK, AST, aldolase, serum potassium

NURSING CONSIDERATIONS
Assessment
- Monitor I&O ratios if urinary output decreases; notify prescriber and stop drug
- Monitor blood studies: coagulation factors, platelets, protamine coagulation factors, platelets, protamine coagulation test for extravascular clotting, thrombophlebitis; creatinine phosphokinase; check for thromboembolic symptoms (leg pain, redness, positive Homans' sign), edema, dyspnea, chest pain
- Monitor B/P, pulse, respiratory status; watch for increasing B/P and pulse
- Assess for allergy: fever, rash, itching, jaundice
- Monitor myopathy: if weakness, fever, myoglobinemia, or oliguria, discontinue drug; watch for increased CPK, AST, aldolase
- Assess for bleeding q15 min: mucous membranes, epistaxis, ecchymosis, petechiae, hematuria, hematemesis
- Monitor neurologic status (LOC, pupils, motor status) in subarachnoid hemorrhage

Nursing diagnoses
- Tissue perfusion, ineffective (uses)
- Injury, risk for (uses, adverse reactions)
- Knowledge, deficient (teaching)

Implementation
IV route
- Give **IV** after dilution with 4-5 g/250 ml NS, D_5W, LR; give over 1 hr; may give by cont inf after loading dose(s); use inf pump; do not give by direct **IV**; stabilize catheter to prevent thrombophlebitis

Continuous IV route
- May be diluted in 50-100 ml of diluent and run at 1 g/hr by inf pump
- Store in tight container in cool environment; do not freeze; do not mix with other drugs

Additive incompatibilities: Do not mix with other drugs in sol or syringe

Patient/family education
- Instruct patient to report any signs of bleeding (gums, under skin, urine, stools, emesis) or myopathy
- Instruct patient to change position slowly to decrease orthostatic hypotension
- Teach patient proper administration for 8-10 days following dental procedure in hemophilia
- Instruct patient to inform physicians and dentists that drug is being taken

Evaluation
Positive therapeutic outcome
- Decreased bleeding
- Absence of rebleeding (subarachnoid hemorrhage)

aminophylline (theophylline ethylenediamine) (Rx)
(am-in-off'i-lin)
Phyllocontin, Truphylline
Func. class.: Bronchodilator, spasmolytic
Chem. class.: Xanthine, ethylenediamine
Pregnancy category C

Action: Exact mechanism unknown; relaxes smooth muscle of respiratory system by blocking phosphodiesterase, which increases cyclic AMP; increased cyclic AMP alters intracellular calcium ion movements; produces bronchodilatation, increased pulmonary blood flow, relaxation of respiratory tract

Therapeutic Outcome: Increased ability to breathe

Uses: Bronchial asthma, bronchospasm associated with chronic bronchitis, emphysema, bradycardia

Investigational uses: Apnea in infancy for respiratory/myocardial stimulation, Cheyne-Stokes respirations as a respiratory stimulant

Dosage and routes
Adult: PO 6 mg/kg, then 3 mg/kg q6h × 2 doses, then 3 mg/kg q8h maintenance, max 900 mg/day or 13 mg/kg; PO in CHF 6 mg/kg, then 2 mg/kg q8h × 2 doses, then 1-2 mg/kg q12h maintenance; **IV** 4.7 mg/kg, then 0.55 mg/kg/hr × 12 hr, then 0.36 mg/kg/hr maintenance, **IV** in CHF 4.7 mg/kg, then 0.39 mg/kg/hr × 12 hr, then 0.08-0.16 mg/kg/hr maintenance

Elderly and in cor pulmonale: PO 6 mg/kg, then 2 mg/kg q6h × 2 doses, then 2

mg/kg q8h maintenance; **IV** 4.7 mg/kg, then 0.47 mg/kg/hr × 12 hr, then 0.24 mg/kg/hr maintenance
Child 9-16 yr: PO 6 mg/kg, then 3 mg/kg q4h × 3 doses, then 3 mg/kg q6h maintenance, max 18 mg/kg/day 12-16 yr, or 20 mg/kg/day 9-12 yr; **IV** 4.7 mg/kg, then 0.79 mg/kg/hr × 12 hr, then 0.63 mg/kg/hr maintenance
Child 6 mo-9 yr: PO 4 mg/kg q4h × 3 doses, then 4 mg/kg q6h maintenance, max 24 mg/kg/day; **IV** 4.7 mg/kg, then 0.95 mg/kg/hr × 12 hr, then 0.79 mg/kg/hr maintenance
Infants 6-52 wk: Dose (0.2 × age in wk) ÷ 5 × kg = 24 hr dose in mg

Premature <24 day postnatal: 1 mg/kg q12h initially

>24 days postnatal: 1.5 mg/kg q12hr

Neonates up to 40 wk premature postconception age: PO/**IV** 1 mg/kg q12hr

Neonates at birth or 40 wk postconception age: PO/**IV** >8 wk postnatal 1-3 mg/kg q6h; 4-8 wk postnatal 1-2 mg/kg q8h; up to 4 wk postnatal 1-2 mg/kg q12h

Hepatic disease
Adult: PO 6 mg/kg, then 2 mg/kg q8h × 2 doses, then 1-2 mg/kg q12h maintenance; **IV** 4.7 mg/kg, then 0.39 mg/kg/hr × 12 hr, then 0.08-0.16 mg/kg/hr maintenance

Available forms: Inj 250 mg/10 ml, 500 mg/20 ml, 100 mg/100 ml in 0.45% NaCl; 200 mg/100 ml in 0.45% NaCl; rec supp 250 mg, 500 mg; oral liq 105 mg/5 ml; tabs 100, 200 mg; cont rel tabs 225, 350 mg

Adverse effects

CNS: Anxiety, restlessness, insomnia, *dizziness,* **seizures,** headache, lightheadedness, muscle twitching
CV: *Palpitations, sinus tachycardia,* hypotension, flushing, dysrhythmias
GI: *Nausea, vomiting,* diarrhea, dyspepsia, anal irritation (suppositories), epigastric pain
GU: Urinary frequency, SIADH
INTEG: Flushing, urticaria
RESP: Tachypnea, increased respiratory rate

Contraindications: Hypersensitivity to xanthines, tachydysrhythmias, active peptic ulcer disease

Precautions: Pregnancy **C**, elderly, CHF, cor pulmonale, hepatic disease, diabetes mellitus, hyperthyroidism, hypertension, seizure disorder, irritation of the rectum or lower colon, children, lactation, alcoholism

Pharmacokinetics

Absorption	Well absorbed (PO), slow (PO–ext rel), erratic (rec)
Distribution	Widely distributed; crosses placenta
Metabolism	Liver to caffeine
Excretion	Kidneys
Half-life	3-12 hr, increased in renal disease, CHF, elderly patients, smokers

Pharmacodynamics

	PO	PO–EXT REL	IV
Onset	15-60 min	Unknown	Immediate
Peak	1-2 hr	4-7 hr	Infusion's end
Duration	6-8 hr	8-12 hr	6-8 hr

Interactions

Individual drugs
Allopurinol (high doses), cimetidine, clarithromycin, erythromycin, mexiletine, fluvoxamine, disulfiram, interferon: decreased metabolism, increased toxicity of aminophylline
Carbamazepine, isoniazid: increased or decreased aminophylline levels
Halothane: increased risk of dysrhythmias
Ketoconazole, phenytoin, rifampin: decreased aminophylline effect
Lithium: decreased effect of lithium
Drug classifications
Antibiotics (macrolide), calcium channel blockers, diuretics (loop), corticosteroids, fluoroquinolones, influenza vaccines, benzodiazepines, oral contraceptives: increased aminophylline levels
Barbiturates, β-adrenergic blockers: decreased effect of aminophylline
Corticosteroids, influenza vaccines: increased aminophylline toxicity
Diuretics (loop): may increase or decrease aminophylline levels
Dose-dependent reversal of neuromuscular blockade
Fluoroquinolones: decreased metabolism, increased toxicity
Sympathomimetics: increased CNS, increased CV, adverse reactions
Tetracyclines: increased adverse reactions
Smoking
Increased metabolism, decreased effect
Drug/herb
Ginseng, horsetail, Siberian ginseng, cola tree, guarana, tea (black, green), yerba maté: increased effects
St. John's wort: decreased effects

Drug/food
Xanthines: increased effect
Low-carbohydrate, high-protein diet, charcoal-broiled beef: increased elimination
High-carbohydrate, low protein diet: decreased elimination
Drug/lab test
Increased: plasma free fatty acids

NURSING CONSIDERATIONS
Assessment
- Monitor theophylline blood levels (therapeutic level is 10-20 mcg/ml); toxicity may occur with small increase above 20 mcg/ml, especially elderly; determine whether theophylline was given recently (24 hr); check for toxicity: nausea, vomiting, anxiety, restlessness, insomnia, tachycardia, dysrhythmias, seizures; notify prescriber immediately
- Monitor I&O; diuresis will occur; dehydration may result in elderly or children in whom diuresis is great
- Monitor respiratory rate, rhythm, depth; auscultate lung fields bilaterally; notify prescriber of abnormalities; check ECG for tachycardia, PVCs, PACs in patients with cardiac problems
- Monitor allergic reactions: rash, urticaria; if these occur, drug should be discontinued, prescriber notified

Nursing diagnoses
- Airway clearance, ineffective (uses)
- Activity intolerance (uses)
- Injury, risk for (uses, adverse reactions)
- Knowledge, deficient (teaching)

Implementation
- Give around the clock to maintain blood (theophylline) levels
- If switching from **IV** to PO, give controlled-release dose at time of **IV** infusion discontinuation; if giving tab (immediate release), discontinue **IV** and wait >4 hr
- If GI upset occurs, take with 8 oz of water or food
- Increase fluids to 2 L/day

PO route
- Do not break, crush, or chew enteric-coated or cont rel tabs
- Avoid giving with food

Rectal route
- Rec dose if patient is unable to take PO; retain rec dose for ½ hour

IV route
- May be diluted for **IV** inf in 100-200 ml in D_5W, $D_{10}W$, $D_{20}W$, 0.9% NaCl, 0.45% NaCl, LR
- Give loading dose over ½ hr, max rate of inf 25 mg/min, use infusion pump; after loading dose, give by cont inf
- Avoid IM inj; pain and tissue damage may occur
- Only clear sol; flush **IV** line before dose; store diluted sol for 24 hr if refrigerated

Syringe compatibilities: Heparin, metoclopramide, pentobarbital, thiopental

Y-site compatibilities: Allopurinol, amifostine, amphotericin B sulfate complex, inamrinone, aztreonam, ceftazidime, cimetidine, cladribine, DOXOrubicin liposome, enalaprilat, esmolol, famotidine, filgrastim, fluconazole, fludarabine, foscarnet, gallium, granisetron, heparin sodium with hydrocortisone sodium succinate, labetalol, melphalan, meropenem, netilmicin, paclitaxel, pancuronium, piperacillin/tazobactam, potassium chloride, propofol, ranitidine, remifentanil, sargramostim, tacrolimus, teniposide, thiotepa, tolazoline, vecuronium

Y-site incompatibilities: DOBUTamine, hydrALAZINE, ondansetron

Additive compatibilities: Amobarbital, bretylium, calcium gluconate, chloramphenicol, cibenzoline, cimetidine, dexamethasone, diphenhydrAMINE, DOPamine, erythromycin lactobionate, esmolol, floxacillin, flumazenil, furosemide, heparin, hydrocortisone, lidocaine, mephentermine, meropenem, methyldopate, metronidazole/sodium bicarbonate, nitroglycerin, pentobarbital, phenobarbital, potassium chloride, ranitidine, secobarbital, sodium bicarbonate, terbutaline

Additive incompatibilities: Ascorbic acid, bleomycin, cephalothin, cefotaxime, chlorproMAZINE, cimetidine, clindamycin, codeine, dimenhyDRINATE, DOBUTamine, DOXOrubicin, doxycycline, epINEPHrine, erythromycin gluceptate, hydrALAZINE, hydrOXYzine, insulin, isoproterenol, meperidine, methicillin, morphine, nafcillin, nitroprusside, norepinephrine, oxytetracycline, papaverine, penicillin G, pentazocine, phenobarbital, phenytoin, prochlorperazine, promazine, promethazine, sulfiSOXAZOLE, tetracycline, vancomycin

Patient/family education
- Teach patient to take doses as prescribed, not to skip dose; to check OTC medications, current prescription medications for epHEDrine, which will increase CNS stimulation; advise patient not to drink alcohol or caffeine products (tea, coffee, chocolate, colas), which will increase action
- Teach patient to avoid hazardous activities; dizziness may occur

- Teach patient if GI upset occurs, to take drug with 8 oz of water or food; absorption may be decreased
- Teach patient to remain in bed 15-20 min after rec supp is inserted to prevent removal
- Instruct patient to avoid smoking because it increases metabolism; decreases blood levels and terminal half-life; dosage may need to be increased
- Teach patient to obtain blood levels of drug every few months to prevent toxicity; not to change brands, since effect may not be the same
- Teach patient to increase fluids to 2 L/day to decrease viscosity of secretions
- Advise patient to report toxicity: nausea, vomiting, anxiety, insomnia, rapid pulse, seizures, flushing, headache, diarrhea

Evaluation

Positive therapeutic outcome

- Decreased dyspnea
- Respiratory stimulation in infants
- Clear lung fields bilaterally

! HIGH ALERT

amiodarone (Rx)

(a-mee-oh′da-rone)

Cordarone, Pacerone

Func. class.: Antidysrhythmic (Class III)

Chem. class.: Iodinated benzofuran derivative

Pregnancy category D

Do Not Confuse:
amiodarone/inamrinone, Cordarone/Inocor

Action: Prolongs action potential duration and effective refractory period, slows sinus rate with increasing PR and QT intervals, noncompetitive α- and β-adrenergic inhibition; increases PR and QT intervals, decreases sinus rate, decreases peripheral vascular resistance

Therapeutic Outcome: Decreased amount and severity of ventricular dysrhythmias

Uses: Severe ventricular tachycardia, supraventricular tachycardia, ventricular fibrillation or atrial fibrillation not controlled by 1st-line agents

Dosage and routes

Ventricular dysrhythmias

Adult: PO loading dose 800-1600 mg/day for 1-3 wk; then 600-800 mg/day × 1 mo; maintenance 400 mg/day; **IV** loading dose (first rapid) 150 mg over the first 10 min then slow 360 mg over the next 6 hr; maintenance 540 mg given over the remaining 18 hr, decrease rate of the slow infusion to 0.5 mg/min

Child: PO loading dose 10-15 mg/kg/day in 1-2 divided doses for 4-14 days then 5 mg/kg/day (not recommended in children)

Child/infant: **IV**/Intraosseous 5 mg/kg as a bolus (PALS guidelines)

Perfusion tachycardia: **IV** 5 mg/kg loading dose given over 20-60 min

Supraventricular tachycardia

Adult: PO 600-800 mg/day × 7 days or until desired response, then 400 mg/day × 21 days, then 200-400 mg/day maintenance

Child: PO 10 mg/kg/day (800 mg/1.72 m^2/day) × 10 days or until desired response, then 5 mg/kg/day (400 mg/1.72 m^2/day) × 21-28 days, then 2.5 mg/kg/day (200 mg/1.72 m^2/day) (not recommended in children)

Available forms: Tabs 200, 400 mg; inj 50 mg/ml

Adverse effects

CNS: *Headache, dizziness,* involuntary movement, tremors, peripheral neuropathy, malaise, fatigue, ataxia, paresthesias, insomnia

CV: *Hypotension,* **bradycardia, sinus arrest, CHF, dysrhythmias, SA node dysfunction**

EENT: Blurred vision, halos, photophobia, **corneal microdeposits,** dry eyes

ENDO: Hyperthyroidism or hypothyroidism

GI: Nausea, vomiting, diarrhea, abdominal pain, anorexia, constipation, **hepatotoxicity**

INTEG: Rash, photosensitivity, blue-gray skin discoloration, alopecia, spontaneous ecchymosis, **toxic epidermal necrolysis**

MISC: Flushing, abnormal taste or smell, edema, abnormal salivation, coagulation abnormalities

MS: Weakness, pain in extremities

RESP: **Pulmonary fibrosis,** pulmonary inflammation, **adult respiratory distress syndrome, gasping syndrome in neonates**

Contraindications: Pregnancy **D,** sinus node dysfunction; 2nd- or 3rd-degree AV block; neonates, infants, bradycardia, lactation

Precautions: Goiter, Hashimoto's thyroiditis, electrolyte imbalances, CHF, severe hepatic, respiratory disease, children

Pharmacokinetics

Absorption	Slow, variable (PO) up to 65%
Distribution	Body tissues; crosses placenta
Metabolism	Liver
Excretion	Bile, kidney (minimal)
Half-life	15-100 days

Pharmacodynamics

	PO
Onset	1-3 wk
Peak	Unknown
Duration	Up to months

Interactions

Individual drugs

CycloSPORINE, dextromethorphan, digoxin, disopyramide, flecainide, mexiletine, procainamide, quinidine, warfarin: increased blood levels, increased toxicity
Phenytoin: increased blood levels
Theophylline: increased levels
Warfarin: increased bleeding

Drug classifications

β-Adrenergic blockers, calcium channel blockers: increased bradycardia

Drug/herb

Aconite: increased toxicity, death
Aloe, broom, buckthorn (chronic use), cascara sagrada (chronic use), Chinese rhubarb, figwort, fumitory, goldenseal, kudzu, licorice, senna: increased effect
Coltsfoot: decreased effect
Horehound: increased serotonin effect

Drug/lab test

Increased: T_4

NURSING CONSIDERATIONS

Assessment

- Monitor I&O ratio; monitor electrolytes: potassium, sodium, chloride
- Monitor chest x-ray, thyroid function tests
- Monitor liver function studies: AST, ALT, bilirubin, alkaline phosphatase
- Monitor ECG continuously to determine drug effectiveness; measure PR, QRS, QT intervals; check for PVCs, other dysrhythmias; monitor B/P continuously for hypotension, hypertension; check for rebound hypertension after 1-2 hr
- Monitor for dehydration or hypovolemia
- Assess for CNS symptoms: confusion, psychosis, numbness, depression, involuntary movements; if these occur, drug should be discontinued
- Assess for hypothyroidism: lethargy, dizziness, constipation, enlarged thyroid gland, edema of extremities, cool, pale skin
- Monitor hyperthyroidism: restlessness, tachycardia, eyelid puffiness, weight loss, frequent urination, menstrual irregularities, dyspnea, warm, moist skin
- (Alert) Assess for pulmonary toxicity including ARDS, pulmonary fibrosis: dyspnea, fatigue, cough, fever, chest pain; drug should be discontinued if these occur
- Monitor cardiac rate, respiration: rate, rhythm, character, chest pain, ventricular tachycardia, supraventricular tachycardia or fibrillation
- Assess sight and vision before treatment and throughout therapy; microdeposits on the cornea may cause blurred vision, halos, and photophobia

Nursing diagnoses

- Cardiac output, decreased (uses)
- Gas exchange, impaired (adverse reactions)
- Knowledge, deficient (teaching)

Implementation

Start with patient hospitalized and monitored

PO route

- Give reduced dosage slowly with ECG monitoring only
- Loading dose with food to decrease nausea

Intermittent IV infusion route

- 1000 mg/24 hr during loading/maintenance
- Initial loading: add 3 ml (150 mg) 100 ml D_5W (1.5 mg/ml) give over 10 min
- Loading inf: add 18 ml (900 mg) 500 ml D_5W (1.8 mg/ml) give over next 6 hr
- Maintenance inf: Give remainder of loading inf 540 mg over 18 hr (0.5 mg/min)

Continuous infusion route

- After 24 hr, give 1-6 mg/ml at 0.5 mg/ml, max 30 mg/min

Y-site compatibilities: Amikacin, bretylium, clindamycin, DOBUTamine, DOPamine, doxycycline, erythromycin, esmolol, gentamicin, insulin (regular), isoproterenol, labetalol, lidocaine, metaraminol, metronidazole, midazolam, morphine, nitroglycerin, norepinephrine, penicillin G potassium, phentolamine, phenylephrine, potassium chloride, procainamide, tobramycin, vancomycin

Additive compatibilities: DOBUTamine, lidocaine, potassium chloride, procainamide, verapamil

Solution compatibilities: D_5W, 0.9% NaCl

Patient/family education

- Instruct patient to report side effects immediately to prescriber

- Instruct patient that skin discoloration is usually reversible, but skin may turn bluish on neck, face, arms when used for long periods
- Advise patient that dark glasses may be needed for photophobia
- Instruct patient to use sunscreen and protective clothing to prevent burning associated with photosensitivity
- Instruct patient to take medication as prescribed, not to double doses
- Instruct patient to complete follow-up appointment with health care provider including pulmonary function studies, chest x-ray, ophthalmic examinations

Evaluation

Positive therapeutic outcome

- Decreased ventricular tachycardia
- Decreased supraventricular tachycardia or fibrillation

Treatment of overdose: Administer O_2, artificial ventilation, ECG, DOPamine for circulatory depression, diazepam or thiopental for seizures, isoproterenol

amitriptyline (Rx)

(a-mee-trip'ti-leen)

amitriptyline HCl, Apo-Amitriptyline ♣, Endep, Levate ♣, Novotriptyn ♣

Func. class.: Antidepressant—tricyclic

Chem. class.: Tertiary amine

Pregnancy category C

Do Not Confuse:
amitriptyline/nortriptyline, Elavil/Mellaril, Elavil/Oruvail

Action: Blocks reuptake of norepinephrine, serotonin into nerve endings that increase action of norepinephrine, serotonin in nerve cells

Uses: Major depression

Investigational uses: Chronic pain management, prevention of cluster/migraine headaches, fibromyalgia

Therapeutic Outcome: Decreased symptoms of depression after 2-3 wk

Dosage and routes

Depression

Adult: PO 75 mg/day in divided doses; may increase to 150 mg daily, not to exceed 300 mg/day; IM 20-30 mg qid, or 80-120 mg at bedtime

Elderly/Adolescent: PO 30 mg/day in divided doses; may be increased to 100 mg/day

Cluster/migraine headaches

Adult: PO 50-150 mg/day

Chronic pain

Adult: PO 75-150 mg/day

Fibromyalgia

Adult: PO 10-50 mg nightly

Available forms: Tabs 10, 25, 50, 75, 100, 150 mg; inj IM 10 mg/ml; syr 10 mg/5 ml

Adverse effects

CNS: *Dizziness, drowsiness,* confusion, headache, anxiety, tremors, stimulation, weakness, insomnia, nightmares, EPS (elderly), increased psychiatric symptoms, **seizures**

CV: *Orthostatic hypotension,* **ECG changes, tachycardia, hypertension,** palpitations, dysrhythmias

EENT: *Blurred vision,* tinnitus, mydriasis, ophthalmoplegia

GI: *Constipation, dry mouth,* weight gain, nausea, vomiting, **paralytic ileus,** increased appetite, cramps, epigastric distress, jaundice, **hepatitis,** stomatitis

GU: *Urinary retention*

HEMA: **Agranulocytosis, thrombocytopenia, eosinophilia, leukopenia**

INTEG: Rash, urticaria, sweating, pruritus, photosensitivity

Contraindications: Hypersensitivity to tricyclic antidepressants, recovery phase of myocardial infarction, narrow-angle glaucoma

Precautions: Pregnancy **C,** suicidal patients, seizure disorders, prostatic hypertrophy, schizophrenia, psychosis, severe depression, increased intraocular pressure, urinary retention, cardiac disease, hepatic/renal disease, hyperthyroidism, electroshock therapy, elective surgery, child <12 yr, elderly

Pharmacokinetics

Absorption	Well absorbed
Distribution	Widely distributed; crosses placenta
Metabolism	Liver, extensively
Excretion	Kidneys, breast milk
Half-life	10-46 hr

Pharmacodynamics

	PO/IM
Onset	45 min
Peak	2-12 hr
Duration	Unknown

Interactions
Individual drugs
Alcohol: increased CNS depression
Carbamazepine: increased amitriptyline levels, increased toxicity
Cimetidine, fluoxetine: increased levels, increased toxicity
Clonidine: decreased effects
Guanethidine: decreased effects
Drug classifications
Antidepressants, antidysrhythmics IC, phenothiazines: increased amitriptyline levels, toxicity
Antihypertensives: blocked response to antihypertensives
Antithyroid agents: increased risk of agranulocytosis
Barbiturates, benzodiazepines, CNS depressants, opioids, sedative/hypnotics, sympathomimetics (direct acting): increased CNS effects
MAOIs: hypertensive crisis, seizures, hyperpyretic crisis
Oral contraceptives: increased effects, toxicity
Sympathomimetics (indirect acting): decreased effects
Smoking
Increased metabolism, decreased effects
Drug/herb
Belladonna, henbane, jimsonweed, scopolia: increased anticholinergic effect
Chamomile, hops, kava, lavender, skullcap, valerian: increased CNS depression
SAM-e, St. John's wort: serotonin syndrome
Scopolia: increased amitriptyline action
Yohimbe: increased hypertension
Drug/lab test
Increased: blood glucose, alkaline phosphatase

NURSING CONSIDERATIONS
Assessment
- Monitor B/P (with patient lying, standing), pulse q4h; if systolic B/P drops 20 mm Hg, hold drug, notify prescriber; take VS q4h in patients with cardiovascular disease
- Monitor blood studies: CBC, leukocytes, differential, cardiac enzymes if patient is receiving long-term therapy
- Monitor hepatic studies: AST, ALT, bilirubin
- Check weight weekly; appetite may increase with drug
- Assess ECG for flattening of T wave, bundle branch block, AV block, prolongation of QTc interval, dysrhythmias in cardiac patients
- Assess for EPS primarily in elderly: rigidity, dystonia, akathisia
- Assess mental status: mood, sensorium, affect, suicidal tendencies; increase in psychiatric symptoms: depression, panic
- Monitor urinary retention, constipation; constipation is more likely to occur in children or elderly
- Assess for withdrawal symptoms: headache, nausea, vomiting, muscle pain, weakness; do not usually occur unless drug was discontinued abruptly
- Identify alcohol consumption; if alcohol is consumed, hold dose until morning

Nursing diagnoses
- Coping, ineffective (uses)
- Injury, risk for (side effects)
- Knowledge, deficient (teaching)
- Noncompliance (teaching)

Implementation
PO route
- Give with food or milk for GI symptoms
- Crush if patient is unable to swallow medication whole
- Give dosage at bedtime if oversedation occurs during day; may take entire dose at bedtime; elderly may not tolerate once/day dosing
- Store at room temp; do not freeze

Patient/family education
- Teach patient that therapeutic effects may take 2-3 wk
- Instruct patient to use caution in driving or other activities requiring alertness because of drowsiness, dizziness, blurred vision; to avoid rising quickly from sitting to standing, especially elderly
- Advise patient to avoid alcohol ingestion, other CNS depressants; overheating
- Teach patient not to discontinue medication quickly after long-term use; may cause nausea, headache, malaise
- Advise patient to wear sunscreen or large hat, since photosensitivity occurs; hyperthermia can occur
- Teach patient to increase fluids, bulk in diet if constipation, urinary retention occur, especially elderly
- Teach patient to use gum, hard sugarless candy, or frequent sips of water for dry mouth
- Instruct patient to use contraception during treatment

Evaluation
Positive therapeutic outcome
- Decreased depression
- Absence of suicidal thoughts

Treatment of overdose: ECG monitoring, lavage, administer anticonvulsant, sodium bicarbonate

amlodipine (Rx)

(am-loe'di-peen)

Norvasc

Func. class.: Antianginal, calcium channel blocker, antihypertensive

Chem. class.: Dihydropyridine

Pregnancy category C

Do Not Confuse: amlodipine/amiloride, Norvasc/Navane

Action: Inhibits calcium ion influx across cell membrane during cardiac depolarization; produces relaxation of coronary vascular smooth muscle, peripheral vascular smooth muscle; dilates coronary vascular arteries; increases myocardial oxygen delivery in patients with vasospastic angina

Therapeutic Outcome: Decreased angina pectoris, dysrhythmias, B/P

Uses: Chronic stable angina pectoris, hypertension, vasospastic angina (Prinzmetal's angina); may coadminister with other antihypertensives, antianginals

Dosage and routes

Angina

Adult: PO 5-10 mg daily

Hypertension

Adult: PO 5 mg daily initially, max 10 mg/day

Hepatic dose/Elderly

Adult: PO 25 mg/day, may increase to 10 mg/day (antihypertensive); 5 mg/day, may increase to 10 mg/day (antianginal)

Available forms: Tabs 2.5, 5, 10 mg

Adverse effects

CNS: Headache, fatigue, dizziness, asthenia, anxiety, depression, insomnia, paresthesia, somnolence

CV: Dysrhythmia, peripheral edema, bradycardia, hypotension, palpitations, syncope, chest pain

GI: Nausea, vomiting, diarrhea, gastric upset, constipation, flatulence, anorexia, gingival hyperplasia, dyspepsia, dysphagia

GU: Nocturia, polyuria, sexual difficulties

INTEG: Rash, pruritus, urticaria, hair loss

MISC: Flushing, sexual difficulties, muscle cramps, cough, weight gain, tinnitus, epistaxis

Contraindications: Sick sinus syndrome, 2nd- or 3rd-degree heart block, hypersensitivity, severe aortic stenosis, obstructive coronary artery disease

Precautions: Pregnancy **C**, CHF, hypotension, hepatic injury, lactation, children, elderly

Pharmacokinetics

Absorption	Well absorbed up to 90%
Distribution	Crosses placenta, protein binding 95%
Metabolism	Liver, extensively
Excretion	Kidneys to metabolites (90%)
Half-life	30-50 hr; increased in elderly, hepatic disease

Pharmacodynamics

Onset	Unknown
Peak	6-10 hr
Duration	24 hr

Interactions

Individual drugs

Alcohol: increased hypotension

Diltiazem: increased amlodipine

Lithium: increased neurotoxicity

Drug classifications

Antihypertensives, nitrates: increased hypotension

NSAIDs: decreased antihypertensive effect

Drug/herb

Barberry, betel palm, burdock, goldenseal, khat, khella, lily of the valley, plantain: increased effect

Yohimbe: decreased effect

Drug/food

Grapefruit juice: increased hypotension

NURSING CONSIDERATIONS

Assessment

- Assess fluid volume status: I&O ratio and record, weight, distended red veins, crackles in lung, color, quality and sp gr of urine, skin turgor, adequacy of pulses, moist mucous membranes, bilateral lung sounds, peripheral pitting edema; dehydration symptoms of decreasing output, thirst, hypotension, dry mouth and mucous membranes should be reported
- Monitor B/P and pulse; if B/P drops, call prescriber
- Monitor ALT, AST, bilirubin daily; if these are elevated, hepatotoxicity is suspected
- Monitor if platelet count is $<150,000/mm^3$; drug is usually discontinued and another drug started
- Monitor cardiac status: B/P, pulse, respiration, ECG

Nursing diagnoses
- Cardiac output, decreased (uses)
- Knowledge, deficient (teaching)

Implementation
- Give once a day, without regard to meals

Patient/family education
- Advise patient to avoid hazardous activities until stabilized on drug, dizziness is no longer a problem
- Instruct patient to avoid alcohol and OTC drugs unless directed by prescriber
- Advise patient to comply in all areas of medical regimen: diet, exercise, stress reduction, smoking cessation, drug therapy; to notify prescriber of irregular heartbeat, shortness of breath, swelling of feet and hands, severe dizziness, constipation, nausea, hypotension
- Teach patient to use as directed even if feeling better; may be taken with other cardiovascular drugs (nitrates, β-blockers)

Evaluation
Positive therapeutic outcome
- Decreased anginal pain
- Decreased B/P
- Increased exercise tolerance

Treatment of overdose: Defibrillation, β-agonists, **IV** calcium inotropic agents, diuretics, atropine for AV block, vasopressor for hypotension

amoxapine (Rx)
(a-mox'a-peen)

amoxapine, Asendin

Func. class.: Antidepressant

Chem. class.: Dibenzoxazepine derivative, secondary amine

Pregnancy category C

Do Not Confuse:
amoxapine/amoxicillin, amoxapine/Amoxil

Action: Blocks reuptake of norepinephrine, serotonin into nerve endings, thereby increasing action of norepinephrine, serotonin in nerve cells

Therapeutic Outcome: Decreased symptoms of depression after 2-3 wk

Uses: Depression

Dosage and routes
Adult: PO 50 mg tid; may increase to 100 mg tid on 3rd day of therapy; not to exceed 300 mg/day unless lower doses have been given for at least 2 wk; may be given daily dose at bedtime; not to exceed 600 mg/day in hospitalized patients

Elderly: PO 25 mg at bedtime, may increase by 25 mg/wk, up to 150 mg/day in divided doses

Available forms: Tabs 25, 50, 100, 150 mg

Adverse effects
CNS: *Dizziness, drowsiness,* confusion, headache, anxiety, tremors, stimulation, weakness, insomnia, nightmares, EPS (elderly), increased psychiatric symptoms, paresthesia, impairment of sexual functioning, **neuroleptic malignant syndrome**

CV: *Orthostatic hypotension, ECG changes, tachycardia,* hypertension, palpitations

EENT: *Blurred vision,* tinnitus, mydriasis, ophthalmoplegia

GI: *Dry mouth, constipation,* nausea, vomiting, **paralytic ileus,** increased appetite, cramps, epigastric distress, jaundice, **hepatitis,** stomatitis, weight gain

GU: Urinary retention, **acute renal failure**

HEMA: **Agranulocytosis, thrombocytopenia, eosinophilia, leukopenia**

INTEG: Rash, urticaria, sweating, pruritus, photosensitivity

META: Increased prolactin levels

Contraindications: Hypersensitivity to tricyclic antidepressants, recovery phase of myocardial infarction, seizure disorders, prostatic hypertrophy, narrow-angle glaucoma

Precautions: Pregnancy **C,** suicidal patients, severe depression, increased intraocular pressure, urinary retention, cardiac disease, hepatic disease, hyperthyroidism, electroshock therapy, elective surgery, elderly

Pharmacokinetics	
Absorption	Well absorbed
Distribution	Widely distributed; crosses placenta
Metabolism	Liver, extensively
Excretion	Kidneys, breast milk
Half-life	8 hr

Pharmacodynamics	
Onset	1-2 wk
Peak	2-6 wk
Duration	6-12 wk

Interactions
Individual drugs
Alcohol: increased CNS depression

Cimetidine, fluoxetine, fluvoxamine, parox-

A

etine, sertraline: increased amoxapine levels, increased toxicity of amoxapine
Clonidine, epINEPHrine, norepinephrine: increased hypertensive effect
Guanethidine: decreased effects of amoxapine

Drug classifications

Barbiturates, benzodiazepines, CNS depressants: increased CNS depression
Contraceptives (oral): increased effects, toxicity of amoxapine
MAOIs: hypertensive crisis, seizures, hyperpyretic crisis

Drug/herb

Chamomile, hops, kava, lavender, skullcap, St. John's wort, valerian: increased CNS depression
Belladonna, corkwood, henbane, jimsonweed: increased anticholinergic effect
Scopolia: increased amoxapine action

Drug/lab test

Increased: blood glucose, LFTs
Decreased: blood glucose, UBC

NURSING CONSIDERATIONS

Assessment

- Monitor B/P (with patient lying, standing), pulse q4h; if systolic B/P drops 20 mm Hg hold drug, notify prescriber; take vital signs q4h in patients with cardiovascular disease
- Monitor blood studies: CBC, leukocytes, differential, cardiac enzymes if patient is receiving long-term therapy
- Monitor blood level: therapeutic 20-100 ng/ml
- Monitor hepatic studies: AST, ALT, bilirubin
- Check weight weekly; appetite may increase with drug
- Assess ECG for flattening of T wave, bundle branch block, AV block, dysrhythmias in cardiac patients
- Assess for EPS primarily in elderly: rigidity, dystonia, akathisia
- Assess mental status: mood, sensorium, affect, suicidal tendencies; increase in psychiatric symptoms: depression, panic; confusion (elderly)
- Monitor urinary retention, constipation; constipation is more likely to occur in children and elderly
- Assess for withdrawal symptoms: headache, nausea, vomiting, muscle pain, weakness; do not usually occur unless drug was discontinued abruptly
- Identify alcohol consumption; if alcohol is consumed, hold dose until morning

Nursing diagnoses

- Coping, ineffective (uses)
- Injury, risk for (side effects)
- Knowledge, deficient (teaching)
- Noncompliance (teaching)

Implementation

- Give with food or milk for GI symptoms
- Crush if patient is unable to swallow medication whole
- Store at room temp; do not freeze

Patient/family education

- Teach patient that therapeutic effects may take 2-3 wk
- Instruct patient to use caution in driving or other activities requiring alertness because of drowsiness, dizziness, blurred vision; to avoid rising quickly from sitting to standing, especially elderly
- Teach patient to avoid alcohol ingestion, other CNS depressants, may potentiate effects
- Teach patient not to discontinue medication quickly after long-term use: may cause nausea, headache, malaise
- Teach patient to wear sunscreen or large hat, since photosensitivity occurs
- Teach patient to increase fluids, bulk in diet if constipation, urinary retention occur, especially elderly
- Advise patient to take gum, hard sugarless candy, or frequent sips of water for dry mouth

Evaluation

Positive therapeutic outcome

- Decreased depression
- Absence of suicidal thoughts

Treatment of overdose: ECG monitoring, induce emesis, lavage, activated charcoal, administer anticonvulsant

amoxicillin (Rx)

(a-mox-i-sill'in)

amoxicillin, Amoxil, Apo-Amoxi ♣, Novamoxin ♣, Nu-Amoxi ♣, Trimox, Wymox

Func. class.: Antiinfective, antiulcer
Chem. class.: Aminopenicillin

Pregnancy category B

Do Not Confuse:
amoxicillin/amoxapine, Amoxil/amoxapine, Amoxil/amoxicillin, Trimox/Diamox, Trimox/Tylox, Wymox/Tylox

Action: Interferes with cell wall replication of susceptible organisms by binding to the bacterial cell wall; the cell wall, rendered osmotically unstable, swells and bursts from osmotic pressure

Therapeutic Outcome: Bactericidal effects for the following organisms: effective for gram-positive cocci *(Streptococcus pyogenes, Streptococcus faecalis, Streptococcus pneumoniae)*, gram-negative cocci *(Neisseria gonorrhoeae, Neisseria meningitidis, Escherichia coli)*, gram-negative bacilli *(Haemophilus influenzae, Proteus mirabilis, Salmonella)*, in combination for *Helicobacter pylori*

Uses: Infections of respiratory tract, skin, skin structures, genitourinary tract, otitis media, meningitis, septicemia, sinusitis, and bacterial endocarditis prophylaxis

Investigational uses: Lyme disease

Dosage and routes

Renal disease

Adult: PO CCr 10-50 ml/min dose q12h; CCr <10 ml/min dose q24h

Systemic infections

Adult: PO 750 mg-1.5 g daily in divided doses q8h

Child: PO 20-50 mg/kg/day in divided doses q8h

Gonorrhea/urinary tract infections

Adult: PO 3 g given with 1 g probenecid as a single dose; followed by tetracycline or erythromycin

Chlamydia trachomatis

Adult: PO 500 mg/day × 1 wk

Bacterial endocarditis prophylaxis

Child: PO 50 mg/kg/hr before and 25 mg/kg 6 hr after procedure

Helicobacter pylori

Adult: PO 1000 mg bid given with lansoprazole 30 mg bid, clarithromycin 500 mg bid × 2 wk; or 1000 mg bid given with omeprazole 20 mg bid, clarithromycin 500 mg bid × 2 wk; or 1000 mg tid given with lansoprazole 30 mg tid × 2 wk

Available forms: Caps 250, 500 mg; chewable tabs 125, 200, 250, 400 mg; tabs 500, 875 mg; susp pedidrops 50 mg/ml; susp 125, 200, 250, 400 mg/5 ml

Adverse effects

CNS: Headache, fever, **seizures**

GI: *Nausea, vomiting, diarrhea,* increased AST, ALT, abdominal pain, glossitis, colitis, **pseudomembranous colitis**

HEMA: Anemia, increased bleeding time, **bone marrow depression, granulocytopenia**

INTEG: *Urticaria, rash*

SYST: **Anaphylaxis, respiratory distress, serum sickness**

Contraindications: Hypersensitivity to penicillins

Precautions: Pregnancy **B,** hypersensitivity to cephalosporins, neonates, renal disease

Pharmacokinetics	
Absorption	Well absorbed (90%)
Distribution	Readily in body tissues, fluids, CSF; crosses placenta
Metabolism	Liver (30%)
Excretion	Breast milk, kidney, unchanged (70%)
Half-life	1-1.3 hr

Pharmacodynamics	
Onset	½ hr
Peak	2 hr

Interactions

Individual drugs

Probenecid: increased amoxicillin levels, decreased renal excretion

Warfarin: increased anticoagulant effects

Drug classifications

Anticoagulants (oral): increased anticoagulant effects

Contraceptives (oral): decreased contraceptive effectiveness

Drug/herb

Acidophilus: do not use with antiinfectives

Khat: decreased absorption, separate by 2 hr

Drug/lab test

False positive: urine glucose, urine protein, direct Coombs' test

NURSING CONSIDERATIONS

Assessment

- Assess patient for previous sensitivity reaction to penicillins or other cephalosporins; cross-sensitivity between penicillins and cephalosporins is common
- Assess patient for signs and symptoms of infection, including characteristics of wounds, sputum, urine, stool, WBC >10,000/mm^3, earache, fever; obtain baseline information and monitor symptoms during treatment
- Obtain C&S before beginning drug therapy to identify if correct treatment has been initiated
- Assess for allergic reactions during treatment: rash, urticaria, pruritus, chills, fever, joint pain; angioedema may occur a few days after therapy begins; epINEPHrine and resuscitation equipment should be available for anaphylactic reactions

- Identify urine output; if decreasing, notify prescriber (may indicate nephrotoxicity); also, increased BUN, creatinine, urinalysis, protein, blood
- Monitor blood studies: AST, ALT, CBC, Hct, bilirubin, LDH, alkaline phosphatase, Coombs' test monthly if patient is on long-term therapy
- Monitor electrolytes: potassium, sodium, chloride monthly if patient is on long-term therapy
- Assess bowel pattern daily; diarrhea, cramping, blood in stools; if severe diarrhea occurs, notify prescriber; drug should be discontinued; pseudomembranous colitis may occur
- Monitor for bleeding: ecchymosis, bleeding gums, hematuria, stool guaiac daily if on long-term therapy
- Assess for overgrowth of infection: perineal itching, fever, malaise, redness, pain, swelling, drainage, rash, diarrhea, change in cough, sputum

Nursing diagnoses

- Infection, risk for (uses)
- Diarrhea (side effects)
- Injury, risk for (side effects)
- Knowledge, deficient (teaching)
- Noncompliance (teaching)

Implementation

PO route

- Give in even doses around the clock; if GI upset occurs, give with food; drug must be given for 10-14 days to ensure organism death and prevent superinfection; store in tight container
- The caps may be opened and contents taken with fluids
- Shake susp well before each dose, may be used alone or mixed in drinks, use immediately; susp may be stored in refrigerator for 14 days

Patient/family education

- ◆ Teach patient to report sore throat, bruising, bleeding, joint pain; may indicate blood dyscrasias (rare)
- Advise patient to contact prescriber if vaginal itching, loose foul-smelling stools, diarrhea, sore throat, fever, fatigue, furry tongue occur; may indicate superinfection or agranulocytopenia
- Instruct patient to take all medication prescribed for the length of time ordered; not to double dose; chew form is available
- Advise patient to notify prescriber of diarrhea with blood or pus, which may indicate pseudomembranous colitis

Evaluation

Positive therapeutic outcome

- Absence of signs/symptoms of infection (WBC <10,000/mm^3, temp WNL, absence of red draining wounds or earache)
- Prevention of endocarditis
- Resolution of ulcer symptoms

Treatment of anaphylaxis: Withdraw drug, maintain airway, administer epINEPHrine, aminophylline, O_2, **IV** corticosteroids

amoxicillin/clavulanate (Rx)

(a-mox-i-sill'in)

Augmentin, Augmentin ES-600, Augmentin XR, Clavulin ♣

Func. class.: Broad-spectrum antiinfective (extended spectrum)

Chem. class.: Aminopenicillin-β-lactamase inhibitor

Pregnancy category B

Action: Interferes with cell wall replication of susceptible organisms; the cell wall, rendered osmotically unstable, swells and bursts from osmotic pressure; combination increases spectrum of activity, β-lactamase resistance

Therapeutic Outcome: Bactericidal effects for the following organisms: *Escherichia coli, Proteus mirabilis, Haemophilus influenzae, Streptococcus faecalis, Streptococcus pneumoniae;* and β-lactamase–producing organisms: *Neisseria gonorrhoeae, Neisseria meningitidis, Shigella, Salmonella, Enterococcus, Streptococcus*

Uses: Infections of respiratory tract, skin, skin structures, genitourinary tract; otitis media, meningitis, septicemia, sinusitis, and endocarditis prophylaxis

Dosage and routes

Adult: PO 250-500 mg q8h or 500-875 mg q12h depending on severity of infection

Child ≤40 kg: PO 20-40 mg/kg/day in divided doses q8h or 25-45 mg/kg/day in divided doses q12h

Renal dose

Adult: PO CCr 10-30 ml/min dose q12h; CCr <10 ml/min dose q24h

Available forms: Tabs 250, 500, 875 mg/125 mg clavulanate; chewable tabs 125, 200, 250, 400 mg; powder for oral susp 125, 200, 250, 400 mg/5 ml; (XR) ext rel tabs 1000 mg amoxicillin/62.5 mg clavulanate; (ES) powder for oral susp 600 mg amoxicillin; 42.9 mg clavulanate 5 ml

Adverse effects

CNS: Headache, fever, **seizures**
GI: *Nausea, diarrhea, vomiting,* increased AST, ALT, abdominal pain, glossitis, colitis, black tongue, **pseudomembranous colitis**
GU: **Oliguria, proteinuria, hematuria,** *vaginitis, moniliasis,* **glomerulonephritis**
HEMA: Anemia, **bone marrow depression, granulocytopenia, leukopenia, eosinophilia, thrombocytopenic purpura**
INTEG: Rash, urticaria
META: Hyperkalemia, hypokalemia, alkalosis, hypernatremia
SYST: **Anaphylaxis, respiratory distress, serum sickness, superinfection**

Contraindications: Hypersensitivity to penicillins; neonates

Precautions: Pregnancy **B,** lactation, hypersensitivity to cephalosporins; neonates; renal disease

Pharmacokinetics

Absorption	Well absorbed (90%)
Distribution	Readily in body tissues, fluids, CSF; crosses placenta
Metabolism	Liver (30%)
Excretion	Breast milk; kidney, unchanged (70%), removed by hemodialysis
Half-life	1-1.3 hr

Pharmacodynamics

Onset	½ hr
Peak	2 hr

Interactions

Individual drugs

Probenecid: increased amoxicillin levels
Warfarin: increased anticoagulant effect

Drug classifications

Anticoagulants (oral): increased anticoagulant effects
Contraceptives (oral): decreased contraceptive effectiveness

Drug/herb

Acidophilus: do not use with antiinfectives
Khat: decreased absorption, separate by 2 hr

Drug/lab test

False positive: urine glucose, urine protein, direct Coombs' test

NURSING CONSIDERATIONS

Assessment

- Assess patient for previous sensitivity reaction to penicillins or other cephalosporins; cross-sensitivity between penicillins and cephalosporins is common
- Assess patient for signs and symptoms of infection, including characteristics of wounds, sputum, urine, stool, WBC >10,000/mm^3, earache, fever; obtain baseline information and during treatment
- Complete C&S before beginning drug therapy to identify if correct treatment has been initiated
- Assess for anaphylaxis: rash, urticaria, pruritus, chills, dyspnea, laryngeal edema, fever, joint pain; angioedema may occur a few days after therapy begins; epINEPHrine and resuscitation equipment should be available for anaphylactic reaction
- Identify urine output; if decreasing, notify prescriber (may indicate nephrotoxicity)
- Monitor renal studies: urinalysis, protein, blood, BUN, creatinine
- Monitor blood studies: AST, ALT, CBC, Hct, bilirubin, LDH, alkaline phosphatase, Coombs' test monthly if patient is on long-term therapy
- Monitor electrolytes: potassium, sodium, chloride monthly if patient is on long-term therapy
- Assess bowel pattern daily; diarrhea, cramping, blood in stools, report to prescriber; if severe diarrhea occurs, drug should be discontinued; may indicate pseudomembranous colitis
- Monitor for bleeding: ecchymosis, bleeding gums, hematuria, stool guaiac daily if on long-term therapy
- Assess for overgrowth of infection: perineal itching, fever, malaise, redness, pain, swelling, drainage, rash, diarrhea, change in cough, sputum

Nursing diagnoses

- Infection, risk for (uses)
- Injury, risk for (side effects)
- Diarrhea (side effects)
- Knowledge, deficient (teaching)
- Noncompliance (teaching)

Implementation

PO route

- Give in even doses around the clock; if GI upset occurs, give with food; drug must be taken for 10-14 days to ensure organism death and prevent superinfection; store in tight container; cap can be opened and mixed with food or liq; chewable tabs should be chewed
- Administer only as directed; 2 250-mg tabs not equivalent to 1 500-mg tab due to strength of clavulanate
- Shake susp well before each dose; may be used alone or mixed in drinks, use imme-

diately; susp may be stored in refrigerator for 10 days

Patient/family education

- Teach patient to report sore throat, bruising, bleeding, joint pain; may indicate blood dyscrasias (rare)
- Advise patient to contact prescriber if vaginal itching, loose foul-smelling stools occur; may indicate superinfection
- Instruct patient to take all medication prescribed for the length of time prescribed
- Advise patient to notify prescriber of diarrhea with blood or pus, which may indicate pseudomembranous colitis
- Advise patient to use alternative contraceptive measures if using oral contraceptives

Evaluation

Positive therapeutic outcome

- Absence of signs/symptoms of infection (WBC <10,000/mm^3, temp WNL)
- Reported improvement in symptoms of infection

Treatment of anaphylaxis: Withdraw drug, maintain airway, administer epINEPHrine, aminophylline, O_2, **IV** corticosteroids

amphotericin B deoxycholate (Rx)

(am-foh-tehr'ih-sin de-ox-ee-kohl'ate)

Fungizone

amphotericin B cholesteryl (Rx)

Amphotec

amphotericin B lipid based (Rx)

Abelcet

amphotericin B liposome (Rx)

AmBisome

Func. class.: Antifungal

Chem. class.: Amphoteric polyene

Pregnancy category B

Action: increased cell membrane permeability in susceptible organisms by binding sterols in fungal cell membrane; decreases potassium, sodium, and nutrients in cell

Therapeutic Outcome: Fungistatic against histoplasmosis, blastomycosis, coccidioidomycosis, cryptococcosis, aspergillosis, phycomycosis, candidiasis, sporotrichosis

Uses: Treatment of severe, possibly fatal fungal infections (**IV**); treatment of topical fungal infections (top)

Investigational uses: Candiduria (bladder irrigation)

Dosage and routes

Deoxycholate

Adult: **IV** Give test dose of 1 mg (not required); then 0.25 mg/kg, increase daily slowly to 0.5 mg/kg, may give 1 mg/kg/day or 1.5 mg/kg/day, alternate day dosing may be used

Child: **IV** 0.25 mg/kg infused initially, increase by 0.25 mg/kg every other day to max of 1 mg/kg/day

Adult and child: TOP apply 2-4 × daily

Adult and child: 1 ml qid

(Amphotec)

Adult and child: **IV** 3-4 mg/kg/day, max 7.5 mg/kg/day

(Abelcet)

Adult and child: **IV** 5 mg/kg/day as a 1 mg/ml inf given 2.5 mg/kg/hr

(AmBisome)

Fungal infections

Adult and child: **IV** 3-5 mg/kg q24h

Visceral leishmaniasis: 3 mg/kg q24h days 1-5

Available forms: Amphotericin deoxycholate: inj 50-mg vial, oral susp 100 mg/ml; cream, ointment, lotion 3%; amphotericin B cholesteryl powder: for inj 50 mg/20 ml, 100 mg/50 ml; amphotericin B lipid based: susp for inj 100 mg/20-ml vial; amphotericin B lipid complex: susp for inj 100 mg/20 ml vial; amphotericin B liposome: powder for inj 50 mg vial

Adverse effects

CNS: *Headache, fever, chills,* peripheral nerve pain, paresthesias, peripheral neuropathy, **seizures,** dizziness

EENT: Tinnitus, deafness, diplopia, blurred vision

GI: *Nausea, vomiting, anorexia,* diarrhea, cramps, **hemorrhagic gastroenteritis, acute liver failure**

GU: *Hypokalemia,* axotemia, hyposthenuria, **renal tubular acidosis,** nephrocalcinosis, **permanent renal impairment, anuria, oliguria**

HEMA: Normochromic and normocytic anemia, **thrombocytopenia, agranulocytosis, leukopenia, eosinophilia,** hypokalemia, hyponatremia, hypomagnesemia

INTEG: *Burning, irritation,* pain, necrosis at inj site with extravasation, flushing, dermatitis, skin rash (top route)
MS: *Arthralgia, myalgia,* generalized pain, weakness, weight loss

Contraindications: Hypersensitivity, severe bone marrow depression

Precautions: Pregnancy **B,** renal disease, lactation

Pharmacokinetics

Absorption	Complete bioavailability (**IV**), rapidly absorbed (top)
Distribution	Body tissues
Metabolism	Liver
Excretion	Kidneys, detectable for several weeks
Half-life	Initial 24-48 hr, terminal 15 days

Pharmacodynamics

	IV	TOP
Onset	Immediate	Unknown
Peak	1-2 hr	Unknown

Interactions
Individual drugs
Cisplatin, cycloSPORINE, polymyxin B, vancomycin: increased nephrotoxicity
Digitalis: increased hypokalemia
Drug classifications
Diuretics, nephrotoxic antibiotics: increased nephrotoxicity
Glucocorticoids, thiazides, skeletal muscle relaxants: increased hypokalemia
Drug/herb
Acidophilus: do not use with antiinfectives
Gossypol: increased risk of nephrotoxicity

NURSING CONSIDERATIONS
Assessment
- Monitor VS q15-30 min during first inf; note changes in pulse, B/P
- Monitor blood studies: Hgb, Hct, potassium, sodium, calcium, magnesium q2 wk; BUN, creatinine weekly; decreased Hgb, Hct, and magnesium are common with increased potassium
- Monitor weight weekly; if weight increases over 2 lb/wk, edema is present; renal damage should be considered
- Monitor for renal toxicity: increasing BUN, serum creatinine; if BUN is >40 mg/dl or if serum creatinine >3 mg/dl, drug may be discontinued or dosage reduced; I&O ratio: watch for decreasing urinary output, change in sp gr; discontinue drug to prevent permanent damage to renal tubules; provide hydration of 2-3 L/day
- Monitor for hepatotoxicity: increasing AST, ALT, alkaline phosphatase, bilirubin
- Monitor for allergic reaction: dermatitis, rash; drug should be discontinued, antihistamines (mild reaction) or epINEPHrine (severe reaction) administered; check inj site for thrombophlebitis
- Monitor for hypokalemia: anorexia, drowsiness, weakness, decreased reflexes, dizziness, increased urinary output, increased thirst, paresthesias; if these occur, drug should be decreased or discontinued and potassium administered

Topical route
- Monitor for allergic reaction: burning, stinging, swelling, redness

Nursing diagnoses
- Infection, risk for (uses)
- Injury, risk for (adverse reaction)
- Knowledge, deficient (teaching)

Implementation
Topical route
- Provide enough medication to cover lesions completely; do not cover with occlusive dressing; apply liberally and rub thoroughly into affected area; administer after cleansing with soap, water before each application, dry well (as ordered), wear gloves during application
- Store at room temp in dry place

Deoxycholate
Intermittent IV infusion route
- Give after diluting 50 mg in 10 ml sterile water (no preservatives) (5 mg-1 ml); shake well, further dilute with 500 ml of D_5W to concentration of 0.1 mg/ml; do not use other diluents or sol; use large needle (20G); change needle for each step; wear gloves
- Use test dosage of 1 mg/20 ml D_5W; give over 10-30 min; if no reaction, drug is administered as ordered
- Administer **IV** using in-line filter (mean pore diameter >1 μm) using distal veins; check for extravasation, necrosis q8h; use an infusion pump; administer over 6 hr; rapid inf may result in circulation collapse; may also be given through central line
- Give acetaminophen and diphenhydrAMINE 30 min before inf to reduce fever, chills, headache
- Give drug only after C&S confirm organism, drug needed to treat condition; make sure drug is used in life-threatening infections
- Store protected from moisture and light;

diluted sol is stable for 24 hr at room temp, 1 wk refrigerated
Syringe compatibilities: Heparin
Y-site compatibilities: Aldesleukin, diltiazem, DOXOrubicin liposome, famotidine, remifentanil, tacrolimus, teniposide, thiotepa, zidovudine
Y-site incompatibilities: Enalaprilat, fludarabine, foscarnet, ondansetron
Additive compatibilities: Fluconazole, heparin, hydrocortisone, methylPREDNISolone, sodium bicarbonate
Solution compatibilities: D_5W

Cholesteryl Liposomal complex

IV route

- Reconstitute with 12 ml sterile water/50 ml vial (4 mg/ml), shake, use 5 micron filter, dilute in D_5W (1-2 mg/ml), give over 2 hr

Lipid complex

IV route

- Shake vial until dissolved, withdraw dose using 18G needle, replace needle from syringe with drug using 5 micron filter needle (use needle for 4 vials or less), empty contents in **IV** of D_5W (1 mg/ml), give at 2.5 mg/kg/hr, use infusion pump

Patient/family education

Topical route

- Teach patient that skin and clothing may become discolored; to use asepsis (hand washing) before, after each application to prevent further infection
- Instruct patient to apply with glove to prevent further infection; not to cover with occlusive dressing; to continue even if condition improves
- Teach patient to avoid use of OTC creams, ointments, lotions, unless directed by prescriber
- Instruct patient to report increased itching, burning, rash, redness; ointment may irritate most hairy areas; to report if condition worsens

IV route

- Advise patient that long-term therapy may be needed to clear infection (2 wk-3 mo depending on type of infection)
- Teach patient side effects and when to notify prescriber

Evaluation

Positive therapeutic outcome

- Decreased in size, number of lesions (top)
- Decreased fever, malaise, rash
- Negative C&S for infecting organism

ampicillin (Rx)

(am-pi-sill'in)

Ampicin ✤, Marcillin, Nu-Ampi ✤, NovoAmpicillin ✤, Omnipen, Penbriten ✤, Polycillin, Principen, Totacillin

Func. class.: Broad-spectrum antiinfective
Chem. class.: Aminopenicillin

Pregnancy category B

Do Not Confuse:
Omnipen/imipenem

Action: Interferes with cell wall replication of susceptible organisms; the cell wall, rendered osmotically unstable, swells, and bursts from osmotic pressure

Therapeutic Outcome: Bactericidal effects for the following organisms: effective for gram-positive cocci *(Streptococcus pyogenes, Streptococcus faecalis, Streptococcus pneumoniae)*, gram-negative cocci *(Neisseria gonorrhoeae, Neisseria meningitidis)*, gram-negative bacilli *(Haemophilus influenzae, Proteus mirabilis, Salmonella, Shigella, Listeria monocytogenes)*, gram-positive bacilli

Uses: Infections of respiratory tract, skin, skin structures, genitourinary tract; otitis media, meningitis, septicemia, sinusitis, and endocarditis prophylaxis

Investigational uses: C-section patients that are high risk for developing infection

Dosage and routes

Renal dose

CCr 10-30 ml/min dose q8-12h; <10 ml/min dose q12h

Systemic infections

Adult and child ≥40 kg (88 lb): PO 1-2 g daily in divided doses q6h; **IV**/IM 2-8 g daily in divided doses q4-6h
Child <40 kg: PO 25-100 mg/kg/day in divided doses q6h; **IV**/IM 25-50 mg/kg/day in divided doses q8h

Bacterial meningitis

Adult: **IV** 8-14 g/day in divided doses q3-4h × 3 days
Child: **IV** 100-200 mg/kg/day in divided doses q3-4h

Gonorrhea

Adult and child ≥ 45 kg (99 lb): PO 3.5 g given with 1 g probenecid as a single dose or IM/**IV** 500 mg q6h (≥40 kg); IM/**IV** 50 mg/kg/day in divided doses q6-8h (<40 kg)

Available forms: Powder for inj 125, 250, 500 mg, 1, 2, 10 g; **IV** inf 500 mg, 1, 2 g; caps 250, 500 mg; powder for oral susp, 125, 250, 500 mg/5 ml

Adverse effects

CNS: Lethargy, hallucinations, anxiety, depression, twitching, **coma, seizures**

GI: *Nausea, vomiting, diarrhea,* **pseudomembranous colitis**

GU: Oliguria, proteinuria, hematuria, *vaginitis, moniliasis,* **glomerulonephritis**

HEMA: Anemia, increased bleeding time, **bone marrow depression, granulocytopenia**

INTEG: *Rash,* urticaria

SYST: **Anaphylaxis, serum sickness**

Contraindications: Hypersensitivity to penicillins

Precautions: Pregnancy **B**, lactation, hypersensitivity to cephalosporins; neonates; renal disease

Pharmacokinetics

Absorption	Moderate, duodenum (35%-50%)
Distribution	Readily in body tissues, fluids, CSF; crosses placenta
Metabolism	Liver (30%)
Excretion	Breast milk; kidney unchanged (70%), removed by dialysis
Half-life	50-110 min

Pharmacodynamics

	PO	IM	IV
Onset	Rapid	Rapid	Rapid
Peak	2 hr	1 hr	Infusion's end

Interactions

Individual drugs

Allopurinol: increased ampicillin-induced skin rash

Probenecid: increased ampicillin levels, decreased renal excretion

Drug classifications

Contraceptives (oral): decreased contraceptive effectiveness

Drug/herb

Acidophilus: do not use with antiinfectives

Khat: decreased absorption, separate by 2 hr

Drug/lab test

Increased: AST, ALT

Decreased: conjugated estrone in pregnancy, conjugated estriol

False positive: urine glucose, urine protein, direct Coombs' test

NURSING CONSIDERATIONS

Assessment

- Assess patient for previous sensitivity reaction to penicillins or other cephalosporins; cross-sensitivity between penicillins and cephalosporins is common
- Assess patient for signs and symptoms of infection, including characteristics of wounds, sputum, urine, stool, WBC >10,000/mm^3, earache, fever; obtain baseline information and during treatment
- Obtain C&S before beginning drug therapy to identify if correct treatment has been initiated
- Assess for allergic reactions: rash, urticaria, pruritus, chills, fever, joint pain; angioedema may occur a few days after therapy begins; epINEPHrine and resuscitation equipment should be on unit for anaphylactic reaction; also, check for ampicillin rash: pruritic, red, raised
- ⚠ Identify urine output; if decreasing, notify prescriber (may indicate nephrotoxicity)
- Monitor renal studies: urinalysis, protein, blood, BUN, creatinine
- Monitor blood studies: AST, ALT, CBC, Hct, bilirubin, LDH, alkaline phosphatase, Coombs' test monthly if patient is on long-term therapy
- Monitor electrolytes: potassium, sodium, chloride monthly if patient is on long-term therapy
- Assess bowel pattern daily; if severe diarrhea occurs, drug should be discontinued; may indicate pseudomembranous colitis
- Monitor for bleeding: ecchymosis, bleeding gums, hematuria, stool guaiac daily if on long-term therapy
- Assess for overgrowth of infection: perineal itching, fever, malaise, redness, pain, swelling, drainage, rash, diarrhea, change in cough, sputum

Nursing diagnoses

- Infection, risk for (uses)
- Injury, risk for (side effects)
- Diarrhea (side effects)
- Knowledge, deficient (teaching)
- Noncompliance (teaching)

Implementation

PO route

- Give in even doses around the clock; drug must be taken for 10-14 days to ensure organism death and prevent superinfection; store caps in tight container
- Tabs may be crushed or caps opened and mixed with water
- Shake susp well before each dose; store in refrigerator for 2 wk or 1 wk at room temp

IM route

- Reconstitute with 125 mg/0.9-1.2 ml; 250 mg/0.9-1.9 ml; 500 mg/1.2-1.8 ml; 1 g/2.4-7.4 ml; 2 g/6.8 ml
- Give deep in large muscle mass

IV route

- Reconstitute with 125 mg/0.9-1.2 ml; 250 mg/0.9-1.9 ml; 500 mg/1.2-1.8 ml; 1 g/2.4-7.4 ml; 2 g/6.8 ml
- Give by direct **IV** over 3-5 min in lower dosages (125-500 mg) or over 15 min in higher dosages (1-2 g)
- Give by intermittent inf after diluting with 0.9% NaCl, LR, D_5W, $D_5/0.45\%$ NaCl; use 50 ml of sol and dilute to concentration of <30 mg/ml

Syringe compatibilities: Chloramphenicol

Syringe incompatibilities: Erythromycin, gentamicin, kanamycin, lincomycin, metoclopramide, oxytetracycline, streptomycin, tetracycline

Y-site compatibilities: Acyclovir, amifostine, allopurinol, aztreonam, cyclophosphamide, DOXOrubicin liposome, enalaprilat, esmolol, famotidine, filgrastim, fludarabine, foscarnet, granisetron, heparin, regular insulin, labetalol, magnesium sulfate, melphalan, meperidine, morphine, multivitamins, oflaxacin, perphenazine, phytonadione, potassium chloride, propofol, remifentanil, thiotepa, tolazoline, vit B with C

Y-site incompatibilities: Calcium gluconate, epINEPHrine, fluconazole, hetastarch, hydromorphone, hydrALAZINE, ondansetron, sargramostim, verapamil, vinorelbine

Additive incompatibilities: Amikacin, aztreonam, chlorproMAZINE, DOPamine, gentamicin, hydrALAZINE, hydrocortisone, prochlorperazine

Additive compatibilities: Cefotiam, clindamycin, erythromycin, floxacillin, furosemide, tacrolimus, teniposide, theophylline, verapamil

Patient/family education

- Teach patient to report sore throat, bruising, bleeding, joint pain; may indicate blood dyscrasias (rare)
- Advise patient to contact prescriber if vaginal itching, loose foul-smelling stools, furry tongue occur; may indicate superinfection
- Instruct patient to take all medication prescribed for the length of time ordered
- Advise patient to notify prescriber of diarrhea with blood or pus, which may indicate pseudomembranous colitis
- Tab may be crushed; cap may be opened and mixed with water

Evaluation

Positive therapeutic outcome

- Absence of signs/symptoms of infection (WBC <10,000, temp WNL)
- Reported improvement in symptoms of infection

Treatment of anaphylaxis: Withdraw drug, maintain airway, administer epINEPHrine, aminophylline, O_2, **IV** corticosteroids

ampicillin/sulbactam (Rx)

(am-pi-sill'in/sul-bak'tam)

Unasyn

Func. class.: Broad-spectrum antiinfective

Chem. class.: Aminopenicillin

Pregnancy category B (ampicillin)

Action: Interferes with cell wall replication of susceptible organisms; the cell wall, rendered osmotically unstable, swells and bursts from osmotic pressure; this combination extends the spectrum of activity and inhibits β-lactamase that may inactivate ampicillin

Therapeutic Outcome: Bactericidal against *Pneumococcus, Enterococcus, Streptococcus, Escherichia coli, Proteus mirabilis, Neisseria meningitidis, Neisseria gonorrhoeae, Shigella, Salmonella,* and *Haemophilus influenzae* organisms; use only with β-lactamase–producing strain of infection

Uses: Skin and structure infections, intraabdominal infections, gynecologic infections, soft tissue infections, otitis media, sinusitis, meningitis, septicemia

Dosage and routes

Adult and child >40 kg: **IV**/IM 1 g ampicillin and 0.5 g sulbactam or 2 g ampicillin, and 1 g sulbactam q6h, not to exceed 4 g/day sulbactam

Child <40 kg: **IV** 100-200 mg/kg/day (ampicillin component) divided q6h, max 8 g/day

Renal dose

Adult ≥40 kg: IM/**IV** CCr 15-29 ml/min dose q12h; CCr 5-14 ml/min dose q24h

Available forms: Powder for inj 1.5 g (1 g ampicillin, 0.5 g sulbactam), 3 g (2 g ampicillin, 1 g sulbactam), 10 g (10 g ampicillin, 5 g sulbactam)

Adverse effects

CNS: Lethargy, hallucinations, anxiety, depression, twitching, **coma, seizures**

GI: *Nausea, vomiting, diarrhea,* increased AST, ALT, abdominal pain, glossitis, colitis, **pseudomembranous colitis**

GU: Oliguria, proteinuria, hematuria, *vaginitis, moniliasis,* **glomerulonephritis**, dysuria

HEMA: Anemia, increased bleeding time, **bone marrow depression, granulocytopenia**

SYST: **Anaphylaxis, serum sickness**

Contraindications: Hypersensitivity to penicillins, ampicillin, or sulbactam

Precautions: Pregnancy **B,** lactation, hypersensitivity to cephalosporins, neonates, renal disease

Pharmacokinetics

Absorption	Well absorbed (IM)
Distribution	Readily in body tissues, fluids, CSF; crosses placenta
Metabolism	Liver (10%-50%)
Excretion	Breast milk; kidney unchanged (75%)
Half-life	50-110 min (ampicillin)

Pharmacodynamics

	IM	IV
Onset	Rapid	Immediate
Peak	1 hr	Infusion's end

Interactions

Individual drugs

Allopurinol: ampicillin-induced skin rash

Probenecid: increased ampicillin levels, decreased renal excretion

Drug classifications

Contraceptives (oral): decreased contraceptive effectiveness

Drug/herb

Acidophilus: do not use with antiinfectives

Khat: decreased absorption, separate by 2 hr

Drug/lab test

False positive: urine glucose, urine protein

NURSING CONSIDERATIONS

Assessment

- Assess patient for previous sensitivity reaction to penicillins or cephalosporins; cross-sensitivity between penicillins and cephalosporins is common
- Assess patient for signs and symptoms of infection; including characteristics of wounds, sputum, urine, stool, WBC >10,000/mm^3, earache, fever; obtain baseline information and during treatment
- Complete C&S before beginning drug therapy to identify if correct treatment has been initiated
- Assess for allergic reactions: rash, urticaria, pruritus, chills, fever, joint pain; angioedema may occur a few days after therapy begins; epINEPHrine and resuscitation equipment should be on unit for anaphylactic reaction
- (Alert) Identify urine output; if decreasing, notify prescriber (may indicate nephrotoxicity)
- Assess renal studies: urinalysis, protein, BUN, creatinine
- Monitor blood studies: AST, ALT, CBC, Hct, bilirubin, LDH, alkaline phosphatase, Coombs' test monthly if patient is on long-term therapy
- Monitor electrolytes: potassium, sodium, chloride monthly if patient is on long-term therapy
- Assess bowel pattern daily; if severe diarrhea occurs, drug should be discontinued; may indicate pseudomembranous colitis
- Monitor for bleeding: ecchymosis, bleeding gums, hematuria, stool guaiac daily if on long-term therapy
- Assess for superinfection: perineal itching, fever, malaise, redness, pain, swelling, drainage, rash, diarrhea, change in cough, sputum

Nursing diagnoses

- Infection, risk for (uses)
- Diarrhea (adverse reactions)
- Injury, risk for (adverse reactions)
- Knowledge, deficient (teaching)
- Noncompliance (teaching)

Implementation

IM route

- Reconstitute by adding 3.2 ml/1.5 g or 6.4 ml/3 g; use sterile water, 0.5% or 2% lidocaine; give within 1 hr of preparation; give deep in large muscle mass
- Give after C&S completed; on empty stomach

IV route

- Give **IV** after diluting 1.5 g/3.2 ml sterile H_2O for inj; or 3 g/6.4 ml (250 mg ampicillin/125 mg sulbactam); allow to stand until foaming stops; give directly over 15-30 min; dilute further in 50 ml or more of D_5W, D_5/10.45% NaCl, 10% invert sugar in water, LR, 6% sodium lactate, isotonic NaCl; administer within 1 hr after reconstitution; give as an intermittent inf over 15-30 min

Y-site compatibilities: Amifostine, aztreonam, cefepime, enalaprilat, famotidine, filgrastim, fluconazole, fludarabine, granisetron, heparin, regular insulin, meperidine, morphine, paclitaxel, remifentanil, tacrolimus, teniposide, theophylline, thiotepa
Y-site incompatibilities: Idarubicin, ondansetron, sargramostim
Additive compatibilities: Aztreonam
Additive incompatibilities: Aminoglycosides

Patient/family education
- Teach patient to report sore throat, bruising, bleeding, joint pain, persistent diarrhea; may indicate blood dyscrasias (rare) or superinfection
- Advise patient to contact prescriber if vaginal itching, loose foul-smelling stools, furry tongue occur; may indicate superinfection
- Instruct patient to use another form of contraception other than oral contraceptives
- To report immediately pseudomembranous colitis: fever, diarrhea with pus, blood, or mucus; may occur up to 4 wk after treatment
- To wear or carry emergency ID if allergic to penicillin products

Evaluation
Positive therapeutic outcome
- Absence of signs/symptoms of infection (WBC <10,000/mm^3, temp WNL, absence of red draining wounds, earache)
- Reported improvement in symptoms of infection

Treatment of overdose: Withdraw drug, maintain airway, administer epINEPHrine, aminophylline, O_2, **IV** corticosteroids for anaphylaxis

amprenavir (Rx)
(am-pren′-a-ver)
Agenerase
Func. class.: Antiretroviral
Chem. class.: Protease inhibitor
Pregnancy category C

Action: Inhibits HIV-1 protease

Therapeutic Outcome: Prevents maturation of the infectious virus

Uses: HIV-1 in combination with other antiretroviral agents

Dosage and routes
Caps and solution are not interchangeable
Adult: PO (cap) 1200 mg bid; sol 1400 mg bid
Child >50 kg: PO (cap) 1200 mg bid
Child <50 kg: PO (cap) 20 mg/kg bid or 15 mg/kg tid, max 2400 mg/day; PO (oral sol) 22.5 mg/kg bid or 17 mg/kg tid daily, max 2800 mg/day

Amprenavir/Ritonavir regimen
Adult: PO 600 mg amprenavir, 100 mg ritonavir bid or 1200 mg amprenavir, 200 mg ritonavir bid

Hepatic dose
Child: PO (Child-Pugh score 5-8) 450 mg bid (caps), 513 mg bid (sol) in combination; (Child-Pugh score 9-12) 300 mg bid (caps) 342 mg bid (sol) in combination

Available forms: Cap 50 mg; oral sol 15 mg/ml

Adverse effects
CNS: *Paresthesia*
ENDO: New-onset diabetes, hyperglycemia, exacerbation of preexisting diabetes mellitus, hypertriglyceridemia
GI: *Diarrhea, abdominal pain, nausea,* **hepatotoxicity**
HEMA: **Acute hemolytic anemia**
INTEG: *Rash,* **Stevens-Johnson syndrome**

Contraindications: Hypersensitivity; oral sol: renal failure

Precautions: Pregnancy **C,** liver/renal disease, lactation, children, hemophilia, sulfonamide sensitivity, elderly

Pharmacokinetics	
Absorption	Rapidly
Distribution	90% Protein Binding
Metabolism	Unknown
Excretion	Unknown
Half-life	7-10½ hr

Pharmacodynamics
Unknown

Interactions
Individual drugs
Alprazolam, atorvastatin, carbamazepine, clonazepam, clozapine, dapsone, diazepam, diltiazem, fentanyl, flurazepam, niCARdipine, NIFEdipine, pimozide, triazolam, verapamil: toxicity may occur
Amiodarone, lidocaine, quinidine: serious life-threatening reactions
Bepridil, loratadine, lovastatin, midazolam: do not use together; toxicity may occur
Cimetidine, indinavir, ritonavir: increased amprenavir levels

Clarithromycin, erythromycin, itraconazole, ketoconazole: increased amprenavir levels; toxicity may occur
Carbamazepine, didanosine, efavirenz, nevirapine, phenobarbital, rifamycin: decreased amprenavir levels
Methadone: decreased methadone effect
Warfarin: increased serious life-threatening interactions

Drug classifications
Antacids: decreased amprenavir levels
Antidepressants (tricyclics): increased serious life-threatening reactions
Contraceptives (oral): decreased effects of oral contraceptives
Ergots: do not use together; toxicity may occur

Drug/herb
St. John's wort: decreased amprenavir level

Drug/food
Increased: bioavailability after high-fat meal

Drug/lab test
Increased: glucose, cholesterol, triglycerides

NURSING CONSIDERATIONS

Assessment
- Assess for renal/hepatic failure, pregnancy, or those receiving disulfiram, metronidazole; oral sol contains propylene glycol in greater quantities
- Assess signs of infection, anemia
- Monitor liver studies: ALT, AST; viral load, CD4 count throughout treatment
- Monitor C&S before drug therapy; drug may be taken as soon as culture is taken; repeat C&S after treatment; determine the presence of other sexually transmitted diseases
- Assess bowel pattern before, during treatment; if severe abdominal pain with bleeding occurs, drug should be discontinued; monitor hydration
- Assess skin eruptions, rash, urticaria, itching
- Assess allergies before treatment, reaction of each medication; place allergies on chart

Nursing diagnoses
- Infection, risk for (uses)
- Knowledge, deficient (teaching)

Implementation
- Caps and oral sol are not interchangeable on a mg/mg basis

Patient/family education
- Advise patient to take as prescribed with or without food, avoid high-fat foods; if dose is missed, take as soon as remembered up to 1 hr before next dose; do not double dose, do not share with others
- Advise patient that drug must be taken in equal intervals around the clock to maintain blood levels for duration of therapy
- Advise patient to use nonhormonal method of contraception during treatment, use condoms
- Advise patient to notify prescriber of diarrhea, nausea, vomiting, rash
- Teach patient that drug does not cure AIDS or prevent transmission to others, only controls symptoms

Evaluation
Positive therapeutic outcome
- Increasing CD4 counts
- Decreased viral load
- Resolution of HIV

anagrelide (Rx)
(a-na'gre-lide)
Agrylin
Func. class.: Antiplatelet
Chem. class.: Imidazoquinazolinone
Pregnancy category C

Action: Reduces platelet count (mechanism not clear) and prevents early platelet shape changes in response to aggregating agents thus inhibiting platelet aggregation

Therapeutic Outcome: Inhibition of platelet aggregation

Uses: Essential thrombocythemia

Dosage and routes
Adult: PO 0.5 mg qid or 1 mg bid, may be adjusted after 1 wk, max 10 mg/day or 2.5 mg single dose; maintenance: titrate to lowest dose to maintain platelets <600,000

Available forms: Caps 0.5, 1.0 mg

Adverse effects
CNS: *Headache, dizziness,* **seizures,** paresthesia, **CVA**, fever
CV: *Postural hypotension,* tachycardia, palpitations, **CHF, MI,** cardiomyopathy, cardiomegaly, **complete heart block, atrial fibrillation, arrhythmia,** chest pain
GI: Diarrhea, abdominal pain, nausea, flatulence, vomiting, anorexia, constipation, pancreatitis
GU: Dysuria
HEMA: Anemia, **thrombocytopenia,** ecchymosis, lymphadenoma
INTEG: *Rash*, photosensitivity
MISC: Edema, pain, fever
MS: Asthenia, back pain
RESP: Dyspnea

Contraindications: Hypersensitivity, hypotension

Precautions: Pregnancy **C**, lactation, child <16 yr, cardiac, renal, hepatic disease

Pharmacokinetics	
Absorption	Unknown
Distribution	Unknown
Metabolism	Liver, extensively
Excretion	Feces/urine
Half-life	1.3 hr

Pharmacodynamics	
Onset	Unknown
Peak	1 hr
Duration	>24 hr

Interactions

Individual drugs

Abciximab, aspirin, eptifibatide, tirofiban, ticlopidine: increased bleeding risk
Sucralfate: decreased absorption, decreased plasma concentrations

Drug classifications

Anticoagulants, NSAIDs, thrombolytics: increased bleeding risk

Drug/herb

Bogbean, dong quai, feverfew, ginger, ginkgo: increased effect
Bilberry, saw palmetto: decreased effect
Green tea: increased bleeding risk

Drug/food

Decreased: absorption

NURSING CONSIDERATIONS

Assessment

- Monitor B/P, pulse baseline and during treatment until stable; take B/P with patient lying, standing; orthostatic hypotension is common
- Assess cardiac status: chest pain, what aggravates or ameliorates condition
- Monitor platelet counts q2 days × 1 wk, and qwk thereafter, response should begin after 1-2 wk; Hgb, WBC

Nursing diagnoses

- Cardiac output, decreased (uses)
- Knowledge, deficient (teaching)

Implementation

- May give with food, monitor closely for dosage adjustment, there is better absorption on empty stomach
- Store at room temp

Patient/family education

- Teach patient that this medication is not a cure.
- Advise patient that drug may have to be taken continuously in evenly spaced doses only as directed; if a dose is missed, take one when remembered up to 4 hr; do not double doses
- Inform patient that it is necessary to quit smoking to prevent excessive vasoconstriction
- Advise patient to rise slowly from sitting or lying down to prevent orthostatic hypotension
- Caution patient not to use alcohol or OTC medication unless approved by prescriber
- Caution patient to avoid hazardous activities until stabilized on medication; dizziness may occur
- Teach patient to report cardiac reactions, increased bruising/bleeding
- Advise patient to use contraception (female, child-bearing age)

Evaluation

Positive therapeutic outcome

- Absence of thrombocythemia

anakinra (Rx)

(an-ah-kin'rah)

Kineret

Func. class.: Antirheumatic agent (disease modifying), immunomodulator

Chem. class.: Recombinant form of human interleukin-1 receptor antagonist (IL-1Ra)

Pregnancy category B

Action: A form of human interleukin-1 receptor antagonist (IL-1Ra) produced by DNA technology; blocks activity of IL-1, resulting in decreased cartilage degradation and decreased bone resorption

Therapeutic Outcome: Decreased pain, inflammation

Uses: Reduction in signs and symptoms of moderate to severe active rheumatoid arthritis in patients 18 years of age or older who have not responded to other disease-modifying agents

Dosage and routes

Adult: SUBCUT 100 mg daily

Available forms: Sol for inj, 100 mg/ml

Adverse effects

CNS: Headache
EENT: Sinusitis
GI: Abdominal pain, nausea, diarrhea
HEMA: **Neutropenia**
INTEG: Rash, *inj site reaction*
MISC: Flulike symptoms
MS: *Worsening of RA, arthralgia*
RESP: *URI*

Contraindications: Hypersensitivity to *Escherichia coli*–derived proteins or this product, sepsis

Precautions: Pregnancy **B,** lactation, children, renal impairment, elderly

Pharmacokinetics

Absorption	Well absorbed (SC)
Distribution	Unknown
Metabolism	Unknown
Excretion	Unknown
Half-life	4-6 hr

Pharmacodynamics

Onset	Unknown
Peak	3-7 hr
Duration	Unknown

Interactions
Drug classifications
Etanercept, TNF blocking agents: increased risk of severe infection
Vaccines: do not coadminister; immunizations should be brought up to date before treatment
Drug/herb
Arginine: increased gastric irritation
Bilberry, saw palmetto: decreased effect
Bogbean, dong quai, feverfew, ginger, ginkgo: increased effect

NURSING CONSIDERATIONS
Assessment
- Assess pain, stiffness, ROM, swelling of joints during treatment
- Assess for inj site pain, swelling; usually occur after 2 inj (4-5 days)
- Assess for infections, stop treatment if present

Nursing diagnoses
- Pain, chronic (uses)
- Mobility, physical, impaired (uses)
- Injury, risk for (side effects)
- Knowledge, deficient (teaching)

Implementation
- Do not use if cloudy or discolored or if particulate is present, protect from light
- Do not admix with other sol or medications, do not use filter

Patient/family education
- Teach patient about self-administration if appropriate: inj should be made in thigh, abdomen, upper arm; rotate sites at least 1 in from old site
- Advise patient to notify prescriber if pregnancy is planned or suspected, avoid breastfeeding

Evaluation
Positive therapeutic outcome
- Decreased inflammation, pain in joints

anastrozole (Rx)
(an-ass-stroh'zole)
Arimidex
Func. class.: Antineoplastic
Chem. class.: Aromatase inhibitor

Pregnancy category D

Action: Lowers serum estradiol concentrations; many breast cancers have strong estrogen receptors

Therapeutic Outcome: Prevention of rapidly growing malignant cells

Uses: Advanced breast carcinoma that has not responded to other therapy in estrogen-receptor-positive patients (usually postmenopausal)

Dosage and routes
Adult: PO 1 mg daily

Available forms: Tabs 1 mg

Adverse effects
CNS: Hot flashes, headache, light-headedness, depression, dizziness, confusion, insomnia, anxiety
CV: Chest pain, hypertension, thrombophlebitis, edema
GI: Nausea, vomiting, altered taste leading to anorexia, diarrhea, constipation, abdominal pain, dry mouth
GU: Vaginal bleeding, pruritus vulvae, vaginal dryness, pelvic pain
***HEMA:* UTI, leukopenia**
INTEG: *Rash*
MS: Bone pain, myalgia, asthenia
RESP: Cough, sinusitis, dyspnea

Contraindications: Pregnancy **D,** hypersensitivity

Precautions: Lactation, children, elderly, liver disease, renal disease

Pharmacokinetics

Absorption	Adequately absorbed
Distribution	Unknown
Metabolism	Liver
Excretion	Feces, urine
Half-life	50 hr

Pharmacodynamics

Onset	Unknown
Peak	4-7 hr
Duration	Unknown

Interactions

Drug/lab test

Increased: GGT, AST, ALT, alkaline phosphatase, cholesterol, LDL

NURSING CONSIDERATIONS

Assessment

- Monitor CBC, differential, platelet count weekly; withhold drug if WBC is <4000/mm^3 or platelet count is <75,000/mm^3; notify prescriber of results; monitor calcium levels (hypercalcemia is common)
- Assess for tumor flare: increase in bone, tumor pain during beginning treatment; give analgesics as ordered to decrease pain
- Assess for bleeding: hematuria, guaiac, bruising or petechiae, mucosa or orifices, q8h; no rec temp

Nursing diagnoses

- Injury, risk for (adverse reactions)
- Knowledge, deficient (teaching)

Implementation

- Do not break, crush, or chew enteric products
- Give with food or fluids for GI upset; repeat dose may be needed if vomiting occurs
- Store in light-resistant container at room temp

Patient/family education

- Instruct patient to report any complaints, side effects to health care prescriber; if dose is missed, do not double next dose
- Advise patient that vaginal bleeding, pruritus, hot flashes, can occur, and are reversible after discontinuing treatment
- Inform patient about who should be told about tamoxifen therapy
- Advise patient to report vaginal bleeding immediately; that tumor flare—increase in size of tumor, increased bone pain—may occur and will subside rapidly; may take analgesics for pain
- Caution patient to use sunscreen and protective clothing to prevent burns because photosensitivity is common
- Teach patient that hair loss may occur during treatment; a wig or hairpiece may make patient feel better; new hair may be different in color, texture after completion of therapy
- Inform patient that rash or lesions are temporary and may become large during beginning therapy

Evaluation

Positive therapeutic outcome

- Decreased spread of malignant cells in breast cancer

! HIGH ALERT

anistreplase (Rx)

(an-is-tre-plaze′)

anisoylated plasminogen, APSAC, Eminase

Func. class.: Thrombolytic enzyme

Chem. class.: Plasminogen activator

Pregnancy category C

Action: Promotes thrombolysis by promoting conversion of plasminogen to plasmin; complex is a combination of plasminogen and streptokinase

Therapeutic Outcome: Thrombolysis in coronary arteries

Uses: Management of acute MI; for lysis of coronary artery thrombi

Dosage and routes

Adult: **IV** inj 30 units over 4-5 min as soon as possible after onset of symptoms

Available forms: Powder, lyophilized 30 units/vial

Adverse effects

CNS: Headache, fever, sweating, agitation, dizziness, paresthesia, tremor, vertigo, **intracranial hemorrhage**

CV: Hypotension, **dysrhythmias,** conduction disorders

GI: Nausea, vomiting

HEMA: Decreased Hct, **GI, GU, intracranial, retroperitoneal,** surface bleeding; **thrombocytopenia**

INTEG: Rash, urticaria, phlebitis at site, itching, flushing

MS: Low back pain, arthralgia

RESP: Altered respirations, dyspnea, **bronchospasm, lung edema**

SYST: **Anaphylaxis (rare)**

Contraindications: Hypersensitivity, active internal bleeding, intraspinal or intracranial surgery, neoplasms of CNS, severe, uncontrolled hypertension, cerebral embolism, thrombosis, hemorrhage, hypersensitivity to this drug or streptokinase, recent trauma/history of CVA

Precautions: Pregnancy **C,** arterial emboli from left side of heart, ulcerative colitis/enteritis, renal disease, hepatic disease, hypocoagulation, COPD, subacute bacterial endocarditis, rheumatic valvular disease, intraarterial diagnostic procedure or surgery (10 days), recent major surgery, lactation, elderly

Pharmacokinetics

Absorption	Complete bioavailability
Distribution	Unknown
Metabolism	Binds to plasmin
Excretion	Kidneys
Half-life	105 min

Pharmacodynamics

Onset	Unknown
Peak	45 min
Duration	Unknown

Interactions

Individual drugs

Abciximab, aspirin, clopidogrel, dipyridamole, eptifibatide, heparin, plicamycin, ticlopidine, tirofiban, valproic acid: increased bleeding risk

Aminocaproic acid, aprotinen, tranexamic acid: decreased action of anistreplase

Drug classifications

Anticoagulants, antiplatelets, cephalosporins (some), NSAIDs: increased bleeding risk

Drug/herb

Agrimony, alfalfa, angelica, anise, basil, bay, bilberry, black haw, bogbean, bromelain, buchu, chondroitin, cinchona bark, dong quai, fenugreek, feverfew, garlic, ginger, ginkgo, ginseng, horse chestnut, Irish moss, kelp, kelpware, khella, lovage, lungwort, meadowsweet, motherwort, mugwort, nettle, papaya, parsley (large amounts), pau d'arco, pineapple, poplar, prickly ash, safflower, saw palmetto, tonka bean, turmeric, wintergreen, yarrow: increased risk of bleeding

Chamomile, coenzyme Q10, flax, glucomannan, goldenseal, guar gum: decreased anticoagulant effect

Drug/lab test

Increased: PT, APTT, TT

Decreased: fibrinogen, plasminogen

NURSING CONSIDERATIONS

Assessment

- Monitor VS, B/P, pulse, respirations, neurologic signs, temp at least q4h, temp >104° F (40° C) or indicators of internal bleeding
- Assess for hypersensitivity: fever, rash, itching, chills; mild reaction may be treated with antihistamines; hypersensitivity reactions/dyspnea, wheezing, facial swelling should be treated with epINEPHrine
- ❗ Monitor bleeding during 1st hr of treatment (hematuria, hematemesis, bleeding from mucous membranes, epistaxis, ecchymosis), continue to monitor for 24 hr after treatment; blood studies (Hct, platelets, PTT, PT, TT, APTT) before starting therapy; PT or APTT must be less than 2 × control before starting therapy; TT or PT q3-4h during treatment
- Monitor ECG, treat bradycardia, ventricular changes; assess neurologic status, neurologic change may indicate intracranial bleeding; cardiac enzymes, radionuclide, myocardial scanning/coronary angiography

Nursing diagnoses

- Tissue perfusion, ineffective (uses)
- Injury, risk for (uses, adverse reactions)
- Knowledge, deficient (teaching)

Implementation

- Give heparin therapy after thrombolytic therapy is discontinued, TT or APTT less than 2 × control (about 3-4 hr)
- Avoid invasive procedures: inj, rec temp; about 10% of patients have high streptococcal antibody titers, requiring increased loading doses
- Treat fever with acetaminophen
- Provide pressure for 30 sec to minor bleeding sites, 30 min to sites of arterial puncture followed by dressing; inform prescriber if hemostasis not attained; apply pressure dressing

IV, direct route

- Give after reconstituting single-dose vial/5 ml sterile water for inj (not bacteriostatic water), and roll (not shake) to enhance reconstitution, try to minimize foaming; give over 2-5 min by direct **IV**, give within ½ hr of reconstitution or discard, do not add other meds to vial or syringe; give within 6 hr of thrombi identification for best results; cryoprecipitate or fresh frozen plasma if bleeding occurs; store powder in refrigerator; use within 30 min after reconstitution

Incompatibilities: Do not mix with other drugs in sol or syringe

Patient/family education

- Teach patient action of drug and expected outcome; alert patient to possible hypersensitivity reactions and symptoms to report
- Advise patient bed rest is needed during entire course of treatment; handle patient as little as possible during therapy

Evaluation

Positive therapeutic outcome

- Absence of thrombolysis in MI
- Improved ventricular function

! HIGH ALERT

antihemophilic factor VIII (AHF) (Rx)

(an-tee-hee-moe-fill'ik)

Alphanate, antihemophilic factor, Bioclate, Helixate FS, Hemofil M, Humate-P, Hyate:C, Koate-DVI, Kogenate, Kogenate FS, Monoclate-P, Recombinate, ReFacto

Func. class.: Hemostatic, blood factor

Chem. class.: Factor VIII

Pregnancy category C

Action: Necessary for clotting. Activates factor X in conjunction with activated factor IX; transforms prothrombin to thrombin

Therapeutic Outcome: Control of hemorrhage or excessive bleeding in factor VIII deficiency

Uses: Hemophilia A, patients with acquired circulating factor VIII inhibitors, factor VIII deficiency

Dosage and routes

Depends on severity of deficiency and level of antihemophilic factor

Massive hemorrhage

Adult and child: **IV** 40-50 units/kg, then 20-25 units/kg q8-12h

Bleeding (overt)

Adult and child: **IV** 15-25 units/kg, then 8-15 units/kg q8-12h × 4 days

Hemorrhage near vital organs

Adult and child: **IV** 15 units/kg, then 8 units/kg q8h × 2 days, then 4 units/kg q8h × 2 days

Minor hemorrhage

Adult and child: **IV** 8-10 units/kg q24h × 2-3 days or 8 units/kg q12h × 2 days, then q24h × 2 days

Joint bleeding

Adult and child: **IV** 5-10 units/kg q8-12h × 1-2 days

Available forms: Inj 250, 500, 1000, 1500 units/vial (number of units noted on label)

Adverse effects

CNS: Headache, *lethargy, chills, fever, flushing*

CV: *Hypotension,* tachycardia

GI: Nausea, vomiting, abdominal cramps, jaundice, constipation, diarrhea, anorexia, **viral hepatitis**

HEMA: **Thrombosis, hemolysis, risk of hepatitis B, HIV**

INTEG: Rash, flushing, *urticaria,* stinging at inj site

MISC: **Anaphylaxis,** blurred vision

RESP: **Bronchospasm**, rhinitis, dyspnea, nosebleeds

Contraindications: Hypersensitivity to mouse, hamster, bovine, porcine protein, lactation, HIV, viral infection

Precautions: Pregnancy **C,** neonates/infants, hepatic disease, blood types A, B, AB, factor VIII inhibitor

Pharmacokinetics	
Absorption	Complete availability
Distribution	Plasma
Metabolism	Not metabolized
Excretion	No excretion
Half-life	Biphasic 4 hr, 15 hr

Pharmacodynamics	
Onset	Immediate
Peak	Unknown
Duration	12 hr

Interactions

Drug classifications

Anticoagulants, NSAIDs, salicylates: increased bleeding

NURSING CONSIDERATIONS

Assessment

- Monitor blood studies (coagulation factors assay by % normal): 5% prevents spontaneous hemorrhage, 30%-50% for surgery, 80%-100% for severe hemorrhage; blood group of patient, donors (if applicable; most factor VIII not from specific blood group donors)
- Monitor I&O, urine color; notify prescriber if urine becomes orange, red; change in urine color signifying hemolytic reaction; patients other than blood type O are more at risk
- Monitor pulse: discontinue infusion if significant increase
- Obtain test for factor VIII inhibitors before starting treatment, may require concomitant antiinhibitor coagulant complex therapy; Hct, Coombs' test with blood types A, B, AB
- Assess for allergy: fever, rash, itching, jaundice, wheezing, tachycardia, nausea, vomiting; give diphenhydrAMINE (Benadryl);

continue therapy if reaction is mild, discontinue if severe; notify prescriber

- ⚠ Monitor bleeding at ankles, knees, elbows, other joints; check for rebleeding after 15-30 min

Nursing diagnoses

- Tissue perfusion, ineffective (uses)
- Injury, risk for (uses, adverse reactions)
- Knowledge, deficient (teaching)

Implementation

IV route

- Administer **IV** slowly; use plastic syringe to reconstitute and administer; do not use glass, drug adheres to glass; use another needle as a vent when reconstituting; rotate gently to mix
- Administer after dilution with warm NS, D_5W, LR; give within 3 hr

IV infusion route

- Administer by **IV** inf: give at ≤2 ml/min if concentration exceeds 34 units/ml; or over 3 min if concentration is less than 34 units/ml; filter before using
- Store in refrigerator; do not freeze; after reconstitution, do not refrigerate; give within 3 hr

Additive compatibilities: Do not mix with other drugs in sol or syringe

Patient/family education

- Advise patient to report any signs of bleeding: gums, under skin, urine, stools, emesis; review methods to prevent bleeding; to be checked q2-3mo for HIV screen
- Instruct patient to avoid salicylates/NSAIDs; increases bleeding tendencies, decreases clotting
- Instruct patient to prepare, administer factor VIII concentrates at first sign of danger
- Instruct patient to advise health professionals of treatment for hemophilia
- Advise patient that immunization for hepatitis B may be given first
- Instruct patient to report hives, urticaria, chest tightness, hypotension; may be monoclonal antibody–derived factor VII; signs of viral hepatitis, AIDS
- Advise patient to carry/wear emergency ID describing disease process, drugs used

Evaluation

Positive therapeutic outcome

- Absence of bleeding
- Prevention of rebleeding

apomorphine (Rx)

(a-poe-mor′feen)

Apokyn

Func. class.: Antiparkinson agent

Chem. class.: Dopamine-receptor agonist, non-ergot

Pregnancy category C

Action: Selective agonist for D_2 subfamily receptors (presynaptic/postsynaptic sites); binding at D_3 receptor may contribute to antiparkinson effects

Therapeutic Outcome: Decrease in on/off periods in Parkinsonism

Uses: Parkinsonism: for acute, intermittent treatment of hypomobility (off) episodes in advanced parkinsonism

Dosage and routes

Adult: SUBCUT 0.2 ml (2 mg) titrate upward, max 0.6 ml (6 mg), administer a test dose of 0.2 ml (2 mg) and closely monitor B/P; to be used concomitantly with antiemetic

Renal dose

Reduce test dose and starting dose to 0.1 ml (1 mg)

Available forms: Inj 10 mg/ml

Adverse effects

CNS: *Agitation,* psychosis, hallucination, depression, dizziness, headache, confusion, **sleep attacks,** yawning, dykinesias, drowsiness, somnolence

CV: *Orthostatic hypotension,* edema, syncope, tachycardia

EENT: Blurred vision, rhinorrhea, sweating

GI: *Nausea,* vomiting, *anorexia,* constipation, dysphagia, dry mouth

GU: Impotence, urinary frequency

HEMA: **Hemolytic anemia, leukopenia, agranulocytosis**

Contraindications: Hypersensitivity

Precautions: Pregnancy **C,** renal, hepatic, cardiac disease, MI with dysrhythmias, affective disorders, psychosis, preexisting dyskinesias, elderly

Pharmacokinetics

Absorption	Unknown
Distribution	Unknown
Metabolism	Minimal
Excretion	Unknown
Half-life	Unknown

Pharmacodynamics

Unknown

Interactions

Individual drugs

Ondansetron, granisetron, dolasetron (5HT3 antagonists): do not give concurrently, profound hypotension may occur

Levodopa, cimetidine, ranitidine, diltiazem, triamterene, verapamil, quinidine: increased apomorphine levels

Levodopa: increased effect of levodopa

Drug classifications

DOPamine antagonists, phenothiazines, metoclopramide, butyrophenones: decreased apomorphine levels

Drug/herb

Chaste tree fruit, kava: decreased effect of apomorphine

NURSING CONSIDERATIONS

Assessment

- Assess B/P supine/standing predose, and 20, 40, 60 min post dose
- Monitor renal, hepatic, cardiac studies baseline
- Assess for involuntary movements in parkinsonism: akinesia, tremors, staggering gait, muscle rigidity, drooling
- Assess mental status: affect, mood, behavioral changes, depression; complete suicide assessment
- Assess for risk of QT prolongation, this drug may increase QT prolongation and possibility of prodysrrthmias

Nursing diagnoses

- Mobility, impaired (uses)
- Injury, risk for (uses)
- Knowledge, deficient (teaching)
- Noncompliance (teaching)

Implementation

- Adjust dosage to patient response
- Do not give **IV**
- Use a test dose of 0.2 ml (2 mg), those that tolerate this dose, but achieve no response, give 0.4 ml (4 mg) at the next "off"
- Give antiemetic usually trimethobenzemide 300 mg tid PO 3 day prior to beginning apomorphine and continue for 2 months
- Provide assistance with ambulation during beginning therapy
- Store at 77° F, excursion permitted to 59°-86° F

Patient/family education

- Instruct patient to notify prescriber if pregnancy is planned or suspected

Evaluation

Positive therapeutic outcome

- Decrease in end of dose wearing off and unpredictable on/off episodes

aprepitant (Rx)

(ap-re'pi-tant)

Emend

Func. class.: Antiemetic—miscellaneous

Pregnancy category B

Action: Selective antagonist of human substance P/neurokinin 1 (NK_1) receptors

Therapeutic Outcome: Decreased nausea, vomiting during chemotherapy

Uses: Prevention of nausea, vomiting associated with cancer chemotherapy including high-dose cisplatin; used in combination with other antiemetics

Dosage and routes

Adult: PO day 1 (1 hr prior to chemotherapy) aprepitant 125 mg with 12 mg dexamethasone PO, with 32 mg ondansetron **IV**; day 2 aprepitant 80 mg with 8 mg dexamethasone PO; day 3 aprepitant 80 mg with 8 mg dexamethasone PO; day 4 only dexamethasone 8 mg PO

Available forms: Caps 80, 125 mg

Adverse effects

CNS: *Headache, dizziness,* insomnia, anxiety, depression, confusion, peripheral neuropathy

CV: Bradycardia, DVT, hypertension

GI: *Diarrhea, constipation,* abdominal pain, anorexia, gastritis, increased AST, ALT, *nausea,* vomiting, heartburn

GU: Increased BUN, serum creatine, proteinuria, dysuria

HEMA: Anemia, **thrombocytopenia, neutropenia**

MISC: Asthenia, fatigue, dehydration, fever, hiccups, tinnitus

Contraindications: Hypersensitivity

Precautions: Pregnancy **B,** lactation, children, hepatic disease, elderly

Pharmacokinetics

Absorption	Unknown
Distribution	95% protein bound
Metabolism	Liver (CYP3A4 enzymes to an active metabolite)
Excretion	Not in kidneys
Half-life	10-12 hr

Pharmacodynamics

Onset	Unknown
Peak	Unknown
Duration	Unknown

Interactions
Individual drugs
Paroxetine: decreased action of both drugs
Drug classifications
CYP2C9 substrates (phenytoin, TOLBUTamide, warfarin) oral contraceptives: decreased action
CYP3A4 inhibitors (clarithromycin, diltiazem, itraconazole, ketoconazole, nefazodone, nelfinavir, ritonavir, troleandomycin): increased aprepitant action
CYP3A4 inducers (carbamazepine, phenytoin, rifampin): decreased aprepitant action
CYP3A4 substrates (alprazolam, cisapride, dexamethasone, docetaxel, etoposide, ifosfamide, irinotecan, methylPREDNISolone, midazolam, paclitaxel, pimozide, triazolam, vinBLAStine, vinCRIStine, vinorelbine): increased action

NURSING CONSIDERATIONS
Assessment
- Assess for absence of nausea, vomiting during chemotherapy
- Advise those on warfarin to have clotting monitored closely during 2-wk period following administration of aprepitant

Nursing diagnoses
- Knowledge, deficient (teaching)

Implementation
- Give PO on 3-day schedule
- Take 1st dose 1 hr prior to chemotherapy
- Store at room temperature

Patient/family education
- Teach to report diarrhea, constipation
- Advise to take only as prescribed
- Advise to report all medication to prescriber prior to taking this medication
- Instruct to use nonhormonal form of contraception while taking this agent

Evaluation
Positive therapeutic outcome
- Absence of nausea, vomiting during cancer chemotherapy

! HIGH ALERT

argatroban (Rx)
(are-ga-troe'ban)
Argatroban
Func. class.: Anticoagulant
Chem. class.: Thrombin inhibitor
Pregnancy category B

Do Not Confuse:
argatroban/Aggrastat

Action: Direct inhibitor of thrombin that is derived from L-arginine; it reversibly binds to the thrombin active site

Therapeutic Outcome: Absence or decrease of thrombosis

Uses: Thrombosis, prophylaxis or treatment; anticoagulation prevention/treatment of thrombosis in heparin-induced thrombocytopenia; percutaneous coronary intervention (PCI)

Dosage and routes
Heparin-induced thrombocytopenia or heparin-induced thrombocytopenia and thrombosis syndrome
Adult: **IV** 2 mcg/kg/min (1 mg/ml) give at 6 ml/hr for 50 kg of weight, at 8 ml/hr for 70 kg of weight, at 11 ml/hr for 90 kg of weight, at 13 ml/hr for 110 kg of weight, at 16 ml/hr for 130 kg of weight

Percutaneous coronary intervention (PCI) in HIT
Adult: **IV** inf 25 mcg/kg/min and a bolus of 350 mcg/kg given over 3-5 min, check ACT 5-10 min after bolus is completed, proceed if ACT >300 sec

Hepatic dose
Adult: **Cont Inf** 0.5 mcg/kg/min, adjust rate based on APTT

Available forms: Inj 100 mg/ml (must dilute 100-fold)

Adverse effects
CNS: Fever
CV: **Atrial fibrillation, ventricular tachycardia, coronary thrombosis, MI myocardial ischemia, coronary occlusion, bradycardia**, chest pain, hypotension
GI: Nausea, vomiting, abdominal pain, diarrhea, **GI bleeding**
GU: *Hematuria,* abnormal kidney function, UTI
HEMA: **Hemorrhage, thrombocytopenia**
RESP: Pneumonia, dyspnea, coughing
SYST: **Sepsis**

Contraindications: Hypersensitivity, overt major bleeding

Precautions: Pregnancy **B**, intracranial bleeding, renal function impairment, lactation, children, hepatic disease

Pharmacokinetics

Absorption	Unknown
Distribution	To extracellular fluid, 54% plasma protein binding
Metabolism	Liver
Excretion	Feces
Half-life	39-51 min

Pharmacodynamics

Unknown

Interactions

Drug classifications

Antiplatelets, anticoagulants, thrombolytics: increased risk of bleeding

Drug/herb

Agrimony, alfalfa, angelica, anise, basil, bay, bilberry, black haw, bogbean, bromelain, buchu, chondroitin, cinchona bark, dong quai, fenugreek, feverfew, garlic, ginger, ginkgo, ginseng, horse chestnut, Irish moss, kelp, kelpware, khella, lovage, lungwort, meadowsweet, motherwort, mugwort, nettle, papaya, parsley, pau d'arco, pineapple, poplar, prickly ash, safflower, saw palmetto, tonka bean, turmeric, wintergreen, yarrow: increased risk of bleeding

Chamomile, coenzyme Q10, flax, glucomannan, goldenseal, guar gum: decreased anticoagulant effect

NURSING CONSIDERATIONS

Assessment

- Obtain baseline APTT before treatment; do not start treatment if APTT ratio ≥2.5, then APTT 4 hr after initiation of treatment and at least daily thereafter; if APTT above target, stop inf for 2 hr, then restart at 50%, take APTT in 4 hr; if below target, increase inf rate by 20%, take APTT in 4 hr, do not exceed inf rate of 0.21 mg/kg/hr without checking for coagulation abnormalities
- Monitor APTT, which should be 1.5-3 × control
- Assess for bleeding gums, petechiae, ecchymosis, black tarry stools, hematuria/epistaxis, B/P, vaginal bleeding and possible hemorrhage
- Fever, skin rash, urticaria

Nursing diagnoses

- Cardiac output, decreased (uses)
- Diarrhea (adverse reactions)
- Knowledge, deficient (teaching)

Implementation

- Avoid all IM inj that may cause bleeding

IV infusion route

- Dilute in 0.9% NaCl, D_5, LR to a final conc 1 mg/ml; dilute each 2.5-ml vial 100-fold by mixing with 250 ml of diluents, mix by repeated inversion of the diluent bag for 1 min; may be slightly hazy
- Dosage adjustment may be made after review of APTT, not to exceed 10 mcg/kg/min

Patient/family education

- Advise patient to use soft-bristle toothbrush to avoid bleeding gums, avoid contact sports, use electric razor, avoid IM inj
- Instruct patient to report any signs of bleeding: gums, under skin, urine, stools

Evaluation

Positive therapeutic outcome

- Absence or decrease of thrombosis

aripiprazole (Rx)

(a-rip-ip-pra'zol)

Abilify

Func. class.: Antipsychotic/neuroleptic

Pregnancy category C

Action: Exact mechanism unknown; may be mediated through both dopamine type 2 (D_2) and serotonin type 2 ($5\text{-}HT_2$) antagonism

Therapeutic Outcome: Decreased excitement, hallucinations, delusions, paranoia, reorganization of patterns of thought, speech

Uses: Schizophrenia

Dosage and routes

Adult: **PO** 10-15 mg/day; if needed, dosage may be increased to 30 mg daily after 2 wk; maintenance 15 mg/day, periodically reassess

Available forms: Tabs 5, 10, 15, 20, 30 mg

Adverse effects

CNS: *Drowsiness, insomnia, agitation, anxiety, headache,* **seizures, neuroleptic malignant syndrome**, *lightheadedness, akathisia, asthenia, tremor*

CV: Orthostatic hypotension, **tachycardia**

EENT: Blurred vision, rhinitis

GI: Constipation, *nausea,* vomiting, jaundice, weight gain

Contraindications: Hypersensitivity, lactation, seizure disorders

Precautions: Pregnancy **C**, children, renal disease, hepatic disease, elderly

Pharmacokinetics

Absorption	Unknown
Distribution	Protein binding, 90%
Metabolism	Liver, extensively to major active metabolism
Excretion	Unknown
Half-life	Unknown

Pharmacodynamics

Unknown

Interactions

Individual drugs

Alcohol: increased sedation
Carbamazepine: decreased effects of aripiprazole; increased dose
Erythromycin, fluoxetine, ketoconazole, quinidine, paroxetine: increased effects of aripiprazole, reduce dose
Famotidine, valproate: decreased aripiprazole level
Lithium: increased extrapyramidal symptoms (EPS)

Drug classifications

Antipsychotics: increased extrapyramidal symptoms
CNS depressants: increased sedation
CYP3A4/CYP2D6 inhibitors: increased effects of aripiprazole, reduce dose
CYPA34 inducers: decreased effects of aripiprazole; increase dose

Drug/herb

Betel palm, kava: increased EPS
Cola tree, hops, nettle, nutmeg: increased neuroleptic effect

NURSING CONSIDERATIONS

Assessment

- Assess mental status before initial administration
- Check for swallowing of PO medication; check for hoarding or giving of medication to other patients
- Monitor I&O ratio; palpate bladder if urinary output is low
- Monitor bilirubin, CBC, liver function tests qmo
- Assess affect, orientation, LOC, reflexes, gait, coordination, sleep pattern disturbances
- Monitor B/P standing and lying; also pulse, respirations; take q4h during initial treatment; establish baseline before starting treatment; report drops of 30 mm Hg; watch for ECG changes
- Assess for dizziness, faintness, palpitations, tachycardia on rising
- Assess for extrapyramidal symptoms, including akathisia (inability to sit still, no pattern to movements), tardive dyskinesia (bizarre movements of the jaw, mouth, tongue, extremities), pseudoparkinsonism (rigidity, tremors, pill rolling, shuffling gait)
- (Alert) Assess for neuroleptic malignant syndrome: hyperthermia, increased CPK, altered mental status, muscle rigidity
- Assess skin turgor daily
- Assess for constipation, urinary retention daily; if these occur, increase bulk and water in diet

Nursing diagnoses

- Thought processes, disturbed (uses)
- Sensory perception, disturbed (uses)
- Noncompliance (teaching)
- Knowledge, deficient (teaching)

Implementation

- Administer reduced dose in elderly
- Decreased stimulus by dimming lights, avoiding loud noises
- Supervise ambulation until patient is stabilized on medication; do not involve in strenuous exercise program because fainting is possible; patient should not stand still for a long time
- Store in tight, light-resistant container

Patient/family education

- Advise patient that orthostatic hypotension may occur and to rise from sitting or lying position gradually
- Advise patient to avoid hot tubs, hot showers, tub baths; hypotension may occur
- Instruct patient to avoid abrupt withdrawal of this drug; extrapyramidal symptoms may result; drug should be withdrawn slowly
- Teach patient to avoid OTC preparations (cough, hayfever, cold) unless approved by prescriber, because serious drug interactions may occur; avoid use with alcohol, CNS depressants; increased drowsiness may occur
- Advise patient to avoid hazardous activities if drowsy or dizzy
- Explain importance of compliance with drug regimen
- Advise patient, family to report impaired vision, tremors, muscle twitching, urinary retention
- Instruct patient to take extra precautions to stay cool in hot weather, that heat stroke may occur

Evaluation

Positive therapeutic outcome

- Decreased in emotional excitement, hallucinations, delusions, paranoia; reorganization of patterns of thought, speech

Treatment of overdose: Lavage if orally ingested; provide airway; *do not induce vomiting*

! HIGH ALERT

arsenic trioxide (Rx)

Trisenox

Func. class.: Antineoplastic-miscellaneous

Pregnancy category D

Action: Not understood, causes morphologic changes and DNA fragmentation

Therapeutic Outcome: Decreased in malignant cells

Uses: Acute promyelocytic leukemia

Dosage and routes

Induction

Adult: **IV** 0.15 mg/kg/day until bone marrow remission, max 60 doses

Consolidation treatment

Wait 3-6 wk after completion of induction

Adult: **IV** 0.15 mg/kg/day × 25 doses over a period of up to 5 wk

Available forms: Inj 1 mg/ml

Adverse effects

CNS: *Anxiety, confusion, insomnia,* headache, paresthesia, depression, dizziness, tremor, **seizures,** agitation, **coma,** weakness

CV: *Hypotension, hypertension,* prolonged QT interval, other ECG changes, chest pain, *tachycardia,* torsades de pointes

GI: *Abdominal pain, constipation, diarrhea, dyspepsia,* fecal incontinence, **GI hemorrhage,** dry mouth, *nausea, vomiting, anorexia*

GU: Vaginal hemorrhage, **renal failure,** incontinence

HEMA: Leukocytosis, anemia, **thrombocytopenia, neutropenia,** DIC

META: Increased ALT/AST, hyperkalemia, hypokalemia, hypomagnesemia, hyperglycemia

MISC: Weight gain or decrease, fatigue, severe edema, rigors, herpes simplex/zoster

RESP: **Pleural effusion,** dyspnea, cough, epistaxis, hypoxia, sinusitis, wheezing, crackles, tachypnea

Contraindications: Pregnancy **D,** hypersensitivity

Precautions: Elderly, lactation, children

Pharmacokinetics

Absorption	Unknown
Distribution	Stored in liver, kidney, heart, lung, hair, nails
Metabolism	Liver
Excretion	Kidneys
Half-life	Unknown

Pharmacodynamics

Unknown

Interactions: None known

NURSING CONSIDERATIONS

Assessment

- Monitor for APL differentiation syndrome: fever, dyspnea, pulmonary infiltrates, pleural or pericardial effusions, weight gain; this condition can be fatal; give high-dose steroids
- Assess for ECG changes: QT interval prolongation, complete AV block; obtain baseline ECG prior to drug therapy
- Monitor electrolytes: potassium, calcium, magnesium, creatine

Nursing diagnoses

- Infection, risk for (adverse reactions)
- Nutrition: less than body requirements, imbalanced (adverse reactions)
- Knowledge, deficient (teaching)

Implementation

IV route

- Dilute with 100-250 ml D_5 or 0.9% NaCl immediately after withdrawing from ampule, give over 1-2 hr; may give over 4 hr if reactions occur

Patient/family education

- Teach patient to report planned or suspected pregnancy
- Inform patient that fertility impairment has not been studied

Evaluation

Positive therapeutic outcome

- Decreased in malignant cells

Treatment of overdose: Dimercaprol 3 mg/kg IM q4h, then 250 mg penicillamine PO, max 4×/day (≤1 g/day)

ascorbic acid (vitamin C) (OTC, Rx)

(as-kor'bic)

Apo-C ♣, ascorbic acid, Ascorbicap, C-Span, Cebid, Cecon, Cecore 500, Cemill, Cenolate, Cetane, Cevalin, Cevi-Bid, Ce-Vi-Sol, Flavorcee, Mega-C/A Plus, Ortho/CS, Sunkist

Func. class.: Vitamin C, water-soluble vitamin

Pregnancy category C

Action: Needed for wound healing, collagen synthesis, antioxidant, carbohydrate metabolism, protein, lipid synthesis, prevention of infection

Therapeutic Outcome: Replacement and supplementation of vit C

Uses: Vit C deficiency, scurvy, delayed wound and bone healing, chronic disease, urine acidification, before gastrectomy; increased need: lactation, pregnancy, hyperthyroidism, emotional stress, trauma, burns, acidification of urine, dietary supplement

Investigational uses: Common cold prevention

Dosage and routes

RDA

Neonates and up to 6 mo: 30 mg/day
Infants 6 mo-1 yr: 35 mg/day
Child 1-3 yr: 40 mg/day
Child 4-10 yr: 45 mg/day
Child 11-14 yr: 50 mg/day
Adult and child ≥14 yr: 50-200 mg/day
Pregnancy: 70 mg/day
Lactation: 90 mg/day

Scurvy

Adult: PO/SUBCUT/IM/**IV** 100 mg-500 mg daily × 2 wk, then 50 mg or more daily
Child: PO/SUBCUT/IM/**IV** 100-300 mg daily × 2 wk, then 35 mg or more daily

Wound healing/chronic disease/fracture

May be given with zinc
Adult: SUBCUT/IM/**IV**/PO 200-500 mg daily for 1-2 mo
Child: SUBCUT/IM/**IV**/PO 100-200 mg added doses for 1-2 mo

Urine acidification

Adult: 4-12 g daily in divided doses
Child: 500 mg q6-8h

Available forms: Tabs 25, 50, 100, 250, 500, 1000, 1500 mg; effervescent tabs 1000 mg; chewable tabs 100, 250, 500 mg; timed release tabs 500, 750, 1000, 1500 mg; timed release caps 500 mg; crystals 4 g/tsp; powder 4 g/tsp; liq 35 mg/0.6 ml; sol 100 mg/ml; syr 20 mg/ml, 500 mg/5 ml; inj SUBCUT, IM, **IV** 100, 250, 500 mg/ml

Adverse effects

CNS: Headache, insomnia, dizziness, fatigue, flushing
GI: Nausea, vomiting, diarrhea, anorexia, heartburn, cramps
GU: Polyuria, urine acidification, oxalate or urate renal stones, dysuria
HEMA: **Hemolytic anemia in patients with G6PD**
INTEG: Inflammation at inj site

Contraindications: Tartrazine, sulfite sensitivity; G6PD deficiency

Precautions: Pregnancy **C,** gout, diabetes, renal calculi (large doses)

Pharmacokinetics	
Absorption	Readily absorbed (PO)
Distribution	Widely distributed; crosses placenta
Metabolism	Oxidation
Excretion	Kidneys, inactive; breast milk
Half-life	Unknown

Pharmacodynamics
Unknown

Interactions: None known

Drug/lab test

False positive: negatives in glucose tests (Clinitest, Tes-Tape)
False negative: occult blood (large dose), urine bilirubin, leukocyte determination

NURSING CONSIDERATIONS

Assessment

- Assess nutritional status for inclusion of foods high in vit C: citrus fruits, cantaloupe, tomatoes
- Assess for vit C deficiency before, during, and after treatment; scurvy (gingivitis, bleeding gums, loose teeth); poor bone development
- Monitor I&O ratio, polyuria; in patients receiving large doses renal stones may occur
- Monitor ascorbic acid levels throughout treatment if continued deficiency is suspected
- Assess inj sites for inflammation, pain, redness

Nursing diagnoses

- Nutrition: less than body requirements, imbalanced (uses)
- Knowledge, deficient (teaching)

Implementation

PO route

- Swallow timed rel tabs or caps whole; do not break, crush, or chew
- Mix oral sol with foods or fluids

IM route

- Not to be diluted; give deep in large muscle mass

IV, direct route

- Give undiluted by *direct* **IV** 100 mg over at least 1 min, rapid inf may cause fainting

Intermittent IV infusion route

- Give by intermittent inf after diluting with D_5W, $D_{10}W$, 0.9% NaCl, 0.45% NaCl, LR, Ringer's sol, dextrose/saline, dextrose/Ringer's combinations; temperature will increase pressure in ampules; wrap with gauze before breaking

Syringe compatibilities: Metoclopramide, aminophylline, theophylline

Syringe incompatibilities: Cefazolin, doxapram

Additive compatibilities: Amikacin, calcium chloride, calcium gluceptate, calcium gluconate, cephalothin, chloramphenicol, chlorproMAZINE, colistimethate, cyanocobalamin, diphenhydrAMINE, heparin, kanamycin, methicillin, methyldopate, penicillin G potassium, polymyxin B, prednisoLONE, procaine, prochlorperazine, promethazine, verapamil

Additive incompatibilities: Bleomycin, cephapirin, nafcillin, sodium bicarbonate, warfarin

Y-site compatibilities: Warfarin

Patient/family education

- Teach patient necessary foods to be included in diet that are rich in vit C: citrus fruits, cantaloupe, tomatoes, chili peppers (red)
- Teach patient that smoking decreases vit C levels; not to exceed prescribed dose; increases will be excreted in urine, except time release
- Teach patient not to exceed RDA recommended dose, urinary stones may occur
- Teach patient using ascorbic acid for acidification of urine to test urine pH periodically

Evaluation

Positive therapeutic outcome

- Absence of anorexia, irritability, pallor, joint pain, hyperkeratosis, petechiae, poor wound healing
- Reversal of scurvy: bleeding gums, gingivitis, loose teeth

! HIGH ALERT

asparaginase (Rx)

(a-spar'a-gin-ase)

Elspar, Kidrolase ♣

Func. class.: Antineoplastic

Chem. class.: Escherichia coli enzyme

Pregnancy category C

Action: Indirectly inhibits protein synthesis in tumor cells; without amino acids, DNA, RNA synthesis is halted; asparagine, protein synthesis is halted; G_1 phase of cell cycle specific; a nonvesicant

Therapeutic Outcome: Prevention of rapidly growing malignant cells in leukemia

Uses: Acute lymphocytic leukemia in combination with other antineoplastics unresponsive to other agents

Dosage and routes

In combination

Adult/child: **IV** 1000 international units/kg/day × 10 days given over 30 min; IM 6000 international units/m^2/day

Sole induction

Adult/child: **IV** 200 international units/kg/day × 28 days

Desensitization

Adult/child: **IV**/ID test dose of 2 international units ID, then 1 international unit, then double dose q10 min, until total dose is administered or reaction occurs

Available forms: Inj 10,000 international units with mannitol

Adverse effects

CNS: Neuritis, dizziness, headache, **coma,** depression, fatigue, confusion, hallucinations, lethargy, drowsiness, agitation, parkinsonism-like syndrome, **seizures**, chills, fever

CV: Chest pain

ENDO: Hyperglycemia

GI: *Nausea, vomiting, anorexia, cramps, stomatitis,* diarrhea, weight loss, **hepatotoxicity, pancreatitis**

GU: Urinary retention, **renal failure,** glycosuria, polyuria, azotemia, proteinuria, uric acid neuropathy

HEMA: **Thrombocytopenia, leukopenia, myelosuppression, anemia, decreased clotting factors** (V, VII, VIII, IX), decreased fibrinogen

INTEG: *Rash,* urticaria, perspiration
RESP: **Fibrosis, pulmonary infiltrate**
SYST: **Anaphylaxis**

Contraindications: Hypersensitivity, infants, lactation, pancreatitis

Precautions: Pregnancy **C**, renal disease, hepatic disease

Pharmacokinetics

Absorption	Complete bioavailability (**IV**)
Distribution	Intravascular spaces
Metabolism	Unknown
Excretion	Reticuloendothelial system
Half-life	8-30 hr (**IV**), 39-49 hr (IM)

Pharmacodynamics

	IV	IM
Onset	Immediate	Immediate
Peak	14-24 hr	Unknown
Duration	3-5 wk	3-5 wk

Interactions

Individual drugs

Methotrexate: blocked action of methotrexate
VinCRIStine, predniSONE: increased toxicity

Drug classifications

Live virus vaccines: decreased response of vaccines

Drug/lab test

Increased: uric acid
Decreased: thyroid function tests

NURSING CONSIDERATIONS

Assessment

- Assess for signs and symptoms of pancreatitis (nausea, vomiting, severe abdominal pain), anaphylaxis (bronchospasm, dyspnea), cyanosis; monitor amylase, glucose; more toxic in adults than children
- Assess symptoms indicating severe allergic reaction: rash, pruritus, urticaria, purpuric skin lesions, itching, flushing; joint pain, bronchospasm, hypotension; epINEPHrine and emergency equipment should be nearby
- Monitor for frequency of stools, characteristics: cramping, acidosis; signs of dehydration: rapid respirations, poor skin turgor, decreased urine output, dry skin, restlessness, weakness
- Monitor CBC, differential, platelet count weekly; withhold drug if WBC is $<4000/mm^3$ or platelet count is $<100{,}000/mm^3$, notify prescriber of results; also monitor PT, PTT, and TT, which may be increased
- Monitor pulmonary function tests, chest x-ray studies before, during therapy; chest x-ray film should be obtained q2 wk during treatment
- Monitor renal function studies: BUN, serum uric acid, ammonia urine CCr, electrolytes before, during therapy
- Check I&O ratio; report fall in urine output of 30/ml/hr
- Monitor temp q4h; elevated temp may indicate beginning infection
- Obtain liver function tests before, during therapy (bilirubin, AST, ALT, LDH) as needed or monthly
- Monitor RBC, Hct, Hgb, since these may be decreased; serum, urine glucose levels
- Assess for bleeding: hematuria, guaiac, bruising or petechiae, mucosa, or orifices q8h
- (Alert) Assess for dyspnea, crackles, nonproductive cough, chest pain, tachypnea, fatigue, increased pulse, pallor, lethargy, or swelling around eyes or lips; anaphylaxis may occur
- Assess for yellowing of skin and sclera, dark urine, clay-colored stools, itchy skin, abdominal pain, fever, diarrhea

Nursing diagnoses

- Injury, risk for (uses, adverse reactions)
- Body image, disturbed (adverse reactions)

Implementation

- Give after intradermal skin testing and desensitization, give 0.1 ml (2 international units) intradermally after reconstituting with 5 ml sterile H_2O or 0.9% NaCl for inj; then add 0.1 ml of reconstituted drug to 9.9 ml diluent (20 international units/ml); observe for 1 hr, check for wheal
- Use allopurinol or sodium bicarbonate to reduce uric acid levels, alkalinization of urine

IM route

- Reconstitute with 2 ml 0.9% NaCl/10,000 international units/vial, refrigerate, use within 8 hr, discard sooner if sol becomes cloudy

IV route

- Give by **IV** inf using 21-, 23-, 25-gauge needle; administer by slow **IV** inf via Y-tube or 3-way stopcock of flowing D_5W or 0.9% NaCl inf over 30 min after diluting 10,000 international units/5 ml of sterile H_2O or 0.9% NaCl (no preservatives) (2000 international units/ml); use of filter may be necessary if fibers are present

Y-site compatibilities: Methotrexate, sodium bicarbonate

Patient/family education

- Teach patient to report any complaints or side effects to nurse or physician

- Teach patient to report any changes in breathing or coughing
- Advise patient not to receive vaccinations while taking this drug
- Advise patient to use contraception, since drug is teratogenic

Evaluation

Positive therapeutic response

- Decreased replication of leukemia cells

Treatment of anaphylaxis: Administer epINEPHrine, diphenhydrAMINE, **IV** corticosteroids, O_2

aspirin (OTC)

(as'pir-in)

acetylsalicylic acid, Acuprin, Apo-ASA ✤, Apo-Asen ✤, Arthrinol ✤, Arthrisin ✤, Artria S.R., A.S.A., Aspergum, Aspirin ✤, Aspir-Low, Aspirtab, Astrin ✤, Bayer Aspirin, Coryphen ✤, Easprin, Ecotrin, 8-Hour Bayer Timed Release, Empirin, Entrophen ✤, Halfprin, Norwich Extra-Strength, Novasen ✤, PMS-ASA ✤, Sloprin, St. Joseph Children's Supasa ✤, Therapy Bayer, ZORprin

Func. class.: Nonopioid analgesic

Chem. class.: Salicylate

Pregnancy category D (3rd trimester)

Action: Blocks pain impulses in CNS, reduces inflammation by inhibition of prostaglandin synthesis; antipyretic action results from vasodilatation of peripheral vessels; decreases platelet aggregation

Therapeutic Outcome: Decreased pain, inflammation, fever; absence of MI, transient ischemic attacks, thrombosis

Uses: Mild to moderate pain or fever including rheumatoid arthritis, osteoarthritis, thromboembolic disorders, transient ischemic attacks in men, rheumatic fever, post-MI, prophylaxis of MI

Investigational uses: Prevention of cataracts (long-term use), prevention of pregnancy loss in women with clotting disorders

Dosage and routes

Arthritis

Adult: PO 2.6-5.2 g/day in divided doses q4-6h

Child: PO 90-130 mg/kg/day in divided doses q4-6h

Kawasaki disease

Child: PO 80-120 mg/kg/day in 4 divided doses, maintenance 3-8 mg/kg/day as a single dose × 8 wk

MI, stroke prophylaxis

Adult: PO 81-650 mg/day

Pain/fever

Adult: PO/REC 325-650 mg q4h prn, not to exceed 4 g/day

Child: PO/REC 40-100 mg/kg/day in divided doses q4-6h prn

Acute rheumatic fever

Adult: PO 5-6 g/day initially

Child: PO 100 mg/kg/day × 2 wk, then 75 mg/kg/day × 4-6 wk

Thromboembolic disorders

Adult: PO 325-650 mg/day or bid

Transient ischemic attacks

Adult: PO 650 mg bid or 350 mg qid

Available forms: Tabs 81, 162.5, 325, 500, 650, 975 mg; chewable tabs 80, 81 mg; supp 60, 120, 125, 130, 150, 160, 195, 200, 300, 320, 325, 600, 640, 650 mg, 1.2 g; cream; gum 227 mg; dispersible tabs 325, 500 mg; delayed release, enteric coated tabs 80, 165, 300, 325, 500, 600, 650, 975 mg; ext rel 325, 650, 800 mg; del rel caps 325, 500 mg

Adverse effects

CNS: Stimulation, drowsiness, dizziness, confusion, **seizures,** headache, flushing, hallucinations, **coma**

CV: Rapid pulse, pulmonary edema

EENT: Tinnitus, hearing loss

ENDO: Hypoglycemia, hyponatremia, hypokalemia

GI: *Nausea, vomiting,* **GI bleeding,** diarrhea, heartburn, anorexia, **hepatitis**

HEMA: **Thrombocytopenia, agranulocytosis, leukopenia, neutropenia, hemolytic anemia,** increased pro-time, PTT, bleeding time

INTEG: *Rash,* urticaria, bruising

RESP: Wheezing, hyperpnea

SYST: **Reye's syndrome (children), anaphylaxis, laryngeal edema**

Contraindications: Pregnancy **D** (3rd trimester), hypersensitivity to salicylates, tartrazine (FDC yellow dye #5), GI bleeding, bleeding disorders, children <12 yr, children with flulike symptoms, lactation, vit K deficiency, peptic ulcer, NSAIDs

Precautions: Anemia, hepatic disease, renal disease, Hodgkin's disease, pre/postoperatively, gastritis, asthmatic patients with nasal polyps or aspirin sensitivity

Pharmacokinetics

Absorption	Well absorbed, small intestine (PO); erratic (enteric); slow (rec)
Distribution	Rapidly, widely distributed; crosses placenta
Metabolism	Liver, extensively
Excretion	Inactive metabolites, kidney; breast milk
Half-life	15-20 min (low doses); 30 hr (high doses)

Pharmacodynamics

	PO	REC
Onset	15-30 min	Slow
Peak	1-2 hr	4-5 hr
Duration	4-6 hr	6-7 hr

Interactions

Individual drugs

Alcohol, cefamandole, clopidogrel, eptifibatide, heparin, plicamycin, ticlopidine, tirofiban: increased risk of bleeding
Ammonium chloride, nizatidine: increased salicylate level
Insulin, methotrexate, phenytoin, valproic acid, warfarin: increased effects of each specific drug
Nitroglycerin: increased hypotension
PABA: increased toxic effects
Probenecid: decreased effects of probenecid
Spironolactone, sulfinpyrazone: decreased effects

Drug classifications

ACE inhibitors: decreased antihypertensive effect
Antacids, corticosteroids, steroids, urinary alkalizers: decreased effects of aspirin
Anticoagulants, thrombolytics: increased risk of bleeding
Carbonic anhydrase inhibitors: increased toxic effects
Diuretics (loop), sulfonylamides, NSAIDs, β-blockers: decreased effect of each specific drug
NSAIDs, antiinflammatories, steroids: increased gastric ulcers
Penicillins, thrombolytic agents: increased effects of each specific drug
Salicylates: decreased blood glucose levels
Urinary acidifiers: increased salicylate levels

Drug/herb

Anise, basil, bilberry, bogbean, chamomile, chondroitin, clove, fenugreek, feverfew, garlic, ginger, ginkgo, ginseng (*Panax*), horse chestnut, Irish moss, licorice, pansy, kelpware: increased risk of bleeding
Arginine, gossypol: gastric irritation
Chamomile, coenzyme Q10, flax, glucomannan, goldenseal, guar gum: decreased anticoagulant effect

Drug/food

Foods acidifying urine may increase aspirin levels

Drug/lab test

Increased: coagulation studies, liver function studies, serum uric acid, amylase, CO_2, urinary protein
Decreased: serum potassium, PBI, cholesterol
Interference: urine catecholamines, pregnancy test, urine glucose tests (Clinistix, Tes-Tape)

NURSING CONSIDERATIONS

Assessment

- Assess for pain: character, location, intensity, ROM before and 1 hr after administration
- Monitor liver function studies: AST, ALT, bilirubin, creatinine if patient is on long-term therapy
- Monitor renal function studies: BUN, urine creatinine if patient is on long-term therapy
- Monitor blood studies: CBC, Hct, Hgb, pro-time if patient is on long-term therapy
- Check I&O ratio; decreasing output may indicate renal failure (long-term therapy)
- ◆ Assess hepatotoxicity: dark urine, clay-colored stools, yellowing of the skin and sclera, itching, abdominal pain, fever, diarrhea if patient is on long-term therapy
- Assess for allergic reactions: rash, urticaria; if these occur, drug may have to be discontinued; patients with asthma, nasal polyps, allergies; severe allergic reactions may occur
- Assess for ototoxicity: tinnitus, ringing, roaring in ears; audiometric testing needed before, after long-term therapy
- Monitor salicylate level: therapeutic level 150-300 mcg/ml for chronic inflammation
- Assess for visual changes: blurring, halos; corneal, retinal damage
- Check edema in feet, ankles, legs
- Identify prior drug history; there are many drug interactions

Nursing diagnoses

- Pain, acute (uses)
- Pain, chronic (uses)
- Mobility, physical, impaired (uses)
- Injury, risk for (side effects)
- Knowledge, deficient (teaching)

Implementation

PO route

- Do not break, crush, or chew enteric product

- Administer to patient crushed or whole; chewable tab should be chewed
- Give with food or milk to decrease gastric symptoms; separate by 2 hr of enteric product; absorption may be slowed
- Give antacids 1-2 hr after enteric products
- Give with 8 oz of water and have patient sit upright for 30 min after dose; discard tabs if vinegar-like smell is present; avoid if allergic to tartrazine
- Give ½ hr before planned exercise

Patient/family education

- Teach patient to report any symptoms of hepatotoxicity, renal toxicity, visual changes, ototoxicity, allergic reactions, bleeding (long-term therapy)
- Instruct patient to take with 8 oz of water and sit upright for 30 min after dose to facilitate drug passing into the stomach; to discard tabs if vinegar-like smell is present; to avoid if allergic to tartrazine
- Instruct patient not to exceed recommended dosage; acute poisoning may result
- Advise patient to read label on other OTC drugs; many contain aspirin
- Inform patient that the therapeutic response takes 2 wk (arthritis)
- Teach patient to report tinnitus, confusion, diarrhea, sweating, hyperventilation
- Advise patient to avoid alcohol ingestion; GI bleeding may occur
- Advise patient with allergies, nasal polyps, asthma, that allergic reactions may develop
- Instruct patient to read labels on other OTC drugs: may contain salicylates
- Teach patient not to give to children or teens with flulike symptoms or chicken pox; Reye's syndrome may develop

Evaluation

Positive therapeutic outcome

- Decreased pain
- Decreased inflammation
- Decreased fever
- Absence of MI
- Absence of transient ischemic attacks, thrombosis

Treatment of overdose: Lavage, activated charcoal, monitor electrolytes, VS

atazanavir (Rx)

(at-a-za-na'veer)

Reyataz

Func. class.: Antiretroviral

Chem. class.: Protease inhibitor

Pregnancy category B

Action: Inhibits human immunodeficiency virus (HIV-1) protease, which prevents maturation of the infectious virus

Therapeutic Outcome: Decreasing symptoms of HIV

Uses: HIV-1 infection in combination with other antiretroviral agents

Dosage and routes

Antiretroviral-naive patients

Adult: PO 400 mg daily

Antiretroviral-experienced patients

Adult: PO 300 mg daily and ritonavir 100 mg daily

Hepatic dose

Adult: PO (Child-Pugh B) 300 mg daily; (Child-Pugh C) do not use

Available forms: Caps 100, 150, 200 mg

Adverse effects

CNS: Headache, depression, dizziness, insomnia, peripheral neuropathy

GI: *Diarrhea, abdominal pain, nausea,* vomiting, **hepatotoxicity**

INTEG: *Rash,* **Stevens-Johnson syndrome**, *photosensitivity*

MISC: Fatigue, fever, arthralgia, back pain, cough, lipodystrophy, pain, gynecomastia

Contraindications: Hypersensitivity

Precautions: Pregnancy **B,** liver disease, lactation, children, elderly

Pharmacokinetics	
Absorption	Rapid, increased with food
Distribution	86% protein bound
Metabolism	Liver extensively
Excretion	27% excreted unchanged in urine/feces (minimal)
Half-life	7 hr

Pharmacodynamics	
Onset	Unknown
Peak	2 hr
Duration	Unknown

Interactions

Individual drugs

CycloSPORINE, irinotecan, midazolam, pimozide, sildenafil, sirolimus, tacrolimus, triazolam, warfarin: increased levels resulting in increased toxicity
Didanosine, efavirenz, rifampin: decreased atazanavir levels
Indinavir: increased hyperbilirubinemia

Drug classifications

Antacids, H_2-receptor antagonists, proton pump inhibitors: decreased atazanavir levels
Antidepressants (tricyclics), antidysrhythmics, ergots, calcium channel blockers, HMG-CoA reductase inhibitors: increased levels resulting in increased toxicity
Contraceptives (oral): increased effects

Drug/herb

St. John's wort: decreased atazanavir levels

Drug/lab test

Increased: AST, ALT, total bilirubin, amylase, lipase

NURSING CONSIDERATIONS

Assessment

- ❗ Assess for hepatic failure
- Assess for signs of infection, anemia
- Monitor liver function studies: ALT, AST, bilirubin
- Monitor bowel pattern before, during treatment; if severe abdominal pain with bleeding occurs, drug should be discontinued; monitor hydration
- Monitor viral load, CD4 count throughout treatment
- Assess skin eruptions, rash, urticaria, itching
- Identify allergies before treatment, reaction of each medication; place allergies on chart

Nursing diagnoses

- Injury, risk for (uses, adverse reactions)
- Knowledge, deficient (teaching)

Implementation

- Administer with food

Patient/family education

- Advise to take as prescribed with other antiretrovirals as prescribed; if dose is missed, take as soon as remembered up to 1 hr before next dose; do not double dose; do not share with others
- Teach that drug must be taken daily to maintain blood levels for duration of therapy
- Teach that photosensitivity may occur; use protective clothing or stay out of the sun
- Instruct to notify prescriber if diarrhea, nausea, vomiting, rash occur; dizziness, light-headedness, ECG may be altered
- Inform that drug interacts with many drugs and St. John's wort; advise prescriber of all drugs, herbal products used
- Advise that redistribution of body fat may occur; the effect is not known
- Teach that drug does not cure HIV-1 infection or prevent transmission to others, only controls symptoms
- Advise that if taking sildenafil with atazanavir, there may be an increased risk of sildenafil-associated adverse events, including hypotension and prolonged penile erection; notify physician promptly of these symptoms

Evaluation

Positive therapeutic outcome

- Increasing CD4 counts; decreased viral load, resolution of symptoms of HIV-1 infection

atenolol (Rx)

(a-ten'oh-lole)

Apo-Atenolol ✤, atenolol, Novo-Atenol ✤, Tenormin

Func. class.: Antihypertensive

Chem. class.: β-Blocker; β_1-, β_2-blocker (high doses)

Pregnancy category D

Do Not Confuse:

atenolol/albuterol/Altenol, Tenormin/thiamine/Imuran/Trovan

Action: Competitively blocks stimulation of β-adrenergic receptor within vascular smooth muscle; produces negative chronotropic activity, positive inotropic activity (decreases rate of SA node discharge, increases recovery time), slows conduction of AV node, decreases heart rate, decreases O_2 consumption in myocardium; also decreases renin-aldosterone-angiotensin system at high doses, inhibits β_2-receptors in bronchial system at higher doses

Therapeutic Outcome: Decreased B/P, heart rate, prevention of angina pectoris, MI

Uses: Mild to moderate hypertension; prophylaxis of angina pectoris; suspected or known MI (**IV** use)

Investigational uses: Dysrhythmia, mitral valve prolapse, pheochromocytoma, hypertrophic cardiomyopathy, vascular headaches, thyrotoxicosis, tremors, alcohol withdrawal

Dosage and routes

Adult: **IV** 5 mg; repeat in 10 min if initial

dose is well tolerated, then start PO dose 10 min after last **IV** dose

Adult: PO 50 mg daily, increasing q1-2 wk to 100 mg daily; may increase to 200 mg daily for angina or up to 100 mg for hypertension

Elderly: PO 25 mg/day initially

Renal dose

Adult: PO CCr 15-35 ml/min, max 50 mg/day; CCr <15 ml/min max 25 mg/day; hemodialysis 25-50 mg after dialysis

MI-Renal dose

Adult: **IV** 5 mg, then 5 mg over 10 min, then after 10 min give PO dose

Available forms: Tabs 25, 50, 100 mg; 500 inj mcg/ml

Adverse effects

CNS: *Insomnia, fatigue, dizziness, mental changes,* memory loss, hallucinations, depression, lethargy, drowsiness, strange dreams, catatonia

CV: **Profound hypotension, bradycardia, CHF,** *cold extremities, postural hypotension, 2nd- or 3rd-degree heart block*

EENT: Sore throat, dry burning eyes, blurred vision, stuffy nose

ENDO: Increased hypoglycemic response to insulin

GI: *Nausea, diarrhea,* vomiting, **mesenteric arterial thrombosis, ischemic colitis**

GU: Impotence, decreased libido

HEMA: **Agranulocytosis, thrombocytopenia, purpura**

INTEG: Rash, fever, alopecia

RESP: **Bronchospasm,** dyspnea, wheezing, pulmonary edema

Contraindications: Pregnancy **D,** hypersensitivity to β-blockers, cardiogenic shock, 2nd- or 3rd-degree heart block, sinus bradycardia, CHF, cardiac failure, Raynaud's disease, pulmonary edema

Precautions: Major surgery, lactation, diabetes mellitus, renal disease, thyroid disease, CHF, COPD, asthma, well-compensated heart failure, dialysis, myasthenia gravis

Pharmacokinetics

Absorption	50%-60% (PO)
Distribution	Crosses placenta; protein binding (5%-15%)
Metabolism	Not metabolized
Excretion	Breast milk, kidneys (50%), feces (50%—unabsorbed drug)
Half-life	6-9 hr

Pharmacodynamics

	PO	IV
Onset	1 hr	Rapid
Peak	2-4 hr	5 min
Duration	24 hr	Unknown

Interactions

Individual drugs

Digoxin, diltiazem, hydralazine, methyldopa, prazosin, reserpine, verapamil: increased hypotension, bradycardia

Drug classifications

Anticholinergics, cardiac glycosides, antihypertensives: increased hypotension, bradycardia

Sympathomimetics (cough, cold preparations): mutual inhibition

Drug/herb

Aconite: increased toxicity, death

Betel palm, butterbur, cola tree, figwort, fumitory, guarana, hawthorn, jaborandi tree, lily of the valley, motherwort, plantain: increased atenolol effect

Coenzyme Q10, yohimbe: decreased atenolol effect

Drug/lab test

Increased: uric acid, potassium, triglyceride, blood glucose, BUN, ANA titer

NURSING CONSIDERATIONS

Assessment

- Monitor B/P during beginning treatment, periodically thereafter; pulse q4h; note rate, rhythm, quality: apical/radial pulse before administration; notify prescriber of any significant changes (pulse <50 bpm)
- Check for baselines in renal, liver function tests before therapy begins
- Assess for edema in feet, legs daily; monitor I&O, daily weight; check for jugular vein distention, crackles bilaterally, dyspnea (CHF)

Nursing diagnoses

- Cardiac output, decreased (uses)
- Injury, risk for (side effects)
- Knowledge, deficient (teaching)
- Noncompliance (teaching)

Implementation

PO route

- Given ac, at bedtime; tablet may be crushed or swallowed whole; give with food to prevent GI upset; reduced dosage in renal dysfunction; take at same time each day
- Store protected from light, moisture; place in cool environment

IV route

- Give **IV** direct over 5 min or diluted in 10-50 ml D_5W, 0.9% NaCl, and give at prescribed rate

Y-site compatibilities: Meperidine, meropenem, morphine

Patient/family education

- ❗ Teach patient not to discontinue drug abruptly; taper over 2 wk; may cause precipitate angina if stopped abruptly, take at same time each day
- Teach patient not to use OTC products containing α-adrenergic stimulants (such as nasal decongestants, OTC cold preparations); to limit alcohol, smoking; to limit sodium intake as prescribed
- Teach patient how to take pulse and B/P at home; advise when to notify prescriber
- Instruct patient to comply with weight control, dietary adjustments, modified exercise program
- Advise patient to carry/wear emergency ID for drugs, allergies, conditions being treated; tell patient drug controls symptoms but does not cure
- Caution patient to avoid hazardous activities if dizziness, drowsiness is present
- Teach patient to report symptoms of CHF: difficult breathing, especially on exertion or when lying down, night cough, swelling of extremities or bradycardia, dizziness, confusion, depression, fever
- Teach patient to take drug as prescribed, not to double doses, skip doses; take any missed doses as remembered if at least 6 hr until next dose
- Advise patient that drug may mask symptoms of hypoglycemia in diabetic patients
- Advise patient to use contraception while taking this drug

Evaluation

Positive therapeutic outcome

- Decreased B/P in hypertension (after 1-2 wk)
- Absence of dysrhythmias
- Absence of MI
- Decreased angina

Treatment of overdose: Lavage, **IV** atropine for bradycardia, **IV** theophylline for bronchospasm, digitalis, O_2, diuretic for cardiac failure, hemodialysis, **IV** glucose for hyperglycemia, **IV** diazepam (or phenytoin) for seizures

atomoxetine (Rx)

(at-o-mox'eh-teen)

Strattera

Func. class.: Psychotherapeutic—miscellaneous

Pregnancy category C

Action: A selective norepinephrine reuptake inhibitor. May inhibit the presynaptic norepinephrine transporter. Exact mechanism of action is unknown

Therapeutic Outcome: Decreased hyperactivity, impulsivity, increased attention, organization, ability to complete tasks

Uses: Attention deficit hyperactivity disorder

Dosage and routes

Child ≤70 kg: **PO** 0.5 mg/kg, increase after 3 days to a target daily dose of 1.2 mg/kg in AM or evenly divided doses AM, late afternoon; max 1.4 mg/kg/day or 100 mg daily, whichever is less

Adult/child >70 kg: **PO** 40 mg daily, increase after 3 days to a target daily dose of 80 mg in AM or evenly divided doses AM, late afternoon; max 100 mg daily

Hepatic dose

(Child-Pugh B) reduce dose by 50%
(Child-Pugh C) reduce dose by 75%

Available forms: Caps 10, 18, 25, 40, 60 mg

Adverse effects

CNS: *Insomnia,* dizziness, headache, irritability, crying, mood swings, fatigue
CV: *Palpitations,* hot flushes
ENDO: Growth retardation
GI: Dyspepsia, nausea, anorexia, dry mouth, weight loss, vomiting, diarrhea, constipation
GU: Urinary hesitancy, retention, dysmenorrhea, erectile disturbance, ejaculation failure, impotence, prostatitis, abnormal orgasm
INTEG: **Exfoliative dermatitis,** sweating
MISC: Cough, rhinorrhea, dermatitis, ear infection

Contraindications: Hypersensitivity, narrow-angle glaucoma

Precautions: Pregnancy **C,** hypertension, lactation, children >6 yr; hepatic, cardiac, or cerebrovascular disease

Pharmacokinetics	
Absorption	Unknown
Distribution	Protein binding, 98%
Metabolism	Liver
Excretion	Kidneys
Half-life	Unknown

A

Pharmacodynamics

Unknown

Interactions

Individual drug

Albuterol: increased cardiovascular effects

Drug classifications

CYP2D6 inhibitors: increased effects of atomoxetine
MAOIs, vasopressors: hypertensive crisis
Pressor agents: increased cardiovascular effects

NURSING CONSIDERATIONS

Assessment

- Monitor VS, B/P; check patients with cardiac disease more often for increased B/P
- Monitor height, growth rate q3mo in children; growth rate may be decreased
- Assess mental status: mood, sensorium, affect, stimulation, insomnia, aggressiveness
- Assess appetite, sleep, speech patterns
- Assess for attention span, decreased hyperactivity in ADHD persons

Nursing diagnoses

- Thought processes, disturbed (uses)
- Coping, ineffective (uses)
- Family coping, impaired (uses)
- Knowledge, deficient (teaching)

Implementation

- Provide gum, hard candy, frequent sips of water for dry mouth

Patient/family education

- Advise patient to avoid OTC preparations unless approved by prescriber
- Advise patient to avoid alcohol ingestion
- Advise patient to avoid hazardous activities until stabilized on medication
- Advise patient to get needed rest; patients will feel more tired at end of day

Evaluation

Positive therapeutic outcome

- Decreased hyperactivity (ADHD)

atorvastatin (Rx)

(a-tore′va-stat-in)

Lipitor

Func. class.: Antilipidemic
Chem. class.: HMG-CoA reductase inhibitor

Pregnancy category X

Action: Inhibits HMG-CoA reductase enzyme, which reduces cholesterol synthesis

Therapeutic Outcome: Decreased cholesterol levels and LDLs, increased HDLs

Uses: As an adjunct in primary hypercholesterolemia (types Ia, Ib), dysbetalipoproteinemia, elevated triglyceride levels

Dosage and routes

Adult: PO 10-20 mg daily, usual range 10-80, dosage adjustments may be made in 2-4 wk intervals, max 80 mg/day; patients requiring >45% reduction in LDL may be started at 40 mg daily

Available forms: Tabs 10, 20, 40, 80 mg

Adverse effects

CNS: Headache, asthenia
EENT: Lens opacities
GI: *Abdominal cramps, constipation, diarrhea, heartburn,* nausea, dyspepsia, *flatus,* **liver dysfunction,** pancreatitis, increased serum transaminase
GU: Impotence
INTEG: Rash, pruritus, alopecia
MISC: Hypersensitivity
MS: Myalgia, **rhabdomyolysis,** arthralgia
RESP: Pharyngitis, sinusitis

Contraindications: Pregnancy **X,** hypersensitivity, lactation, active liver disease

Precautions: Past liver disease, alcoholism, severe acute infections, trauma, severe metabolic disorders, electrolyte imbalance

Pharmacokinetics

Absorption	Unknown
Distribution	Unknown
Metabolism	Liver
Excretion	Bile, feces, kidneys
Half-life	14 hr

Pharmacodynamics

Unknown

Interactions

Individual drugs

Clofibrate, cycloSPORINE, erythromycin, gemfibrozil, niacin: increased risk of rhabdomyolysis
Colestipol: decreased action of atorvastatin
Digoxin: increased action of digoxin
Warfarin: increased action of warfarin

Drug classifications

Antifungals (azole): possible rhabdomyolysis
Contraceptives (oral): increased action

Drug/herb

Glucomannan: increased effect
Gotu kola: decreased effect

Drug/food
Possible toxicity when used with grapefruit juice
Food increases blood levels
Drug/lab test
Increased: bilirubin, alkaline phosphatase
Interference: thyroid function tests

NURSING CONSIDERATIONS
Assessment
- Assess nutrition: fat, protein, carbohydrates; nutritional analysis should be completed by dietician before treatment
- Assess for muscle pain, tenderness, obtain CPK if these occur, drug may need to be discontinued
- Monitor bowel pattern daily; diarrhea may be a problem
- Monitor triglycerides, cholesterol at baseline and throughout treatment; LDL and VLDL should be watched closely; if increased, drug should be discontinued
- Monitor liver function studies q1-2 mo during the first 1½ yr of treatment; AST, ALT, liver function tests may be increased
- Monitor renal studies in patients with compromised renal system: BUN, I&O ratio, creatinine
- Assess eyes via ophthalmic exam 1 mo after treatment begins, annually

Nursing diagnoses
- Diarrhea (adverse reactions)
- Knowledge, deficient (teaching)
- Noncompliance (teaching)

Implementation
- Administer total daily dose at any time of day
- Store in cool environment in airtight, light-resistant container

Patient/family education
- Inform patient that compliance is needed for positive results to occur, not to double doses
- Teach patient that risk factors should be decreased: high-fat diet, smoking, alcohol consumption, absence of exercise
- Advise patient to notify prescriber if the GI symptoms of diarrhea, abdominal or epigastric pain, nausea, vomiting; chills, fever, sore throat; muscle pain, weakness occur
- Advise patient that treatment will take several years
- Advise patient that blood work and eye exam will be necessary during treatment
- Advise not to take if pregnant
- Advise patient to stay out of the sun, use protective clothing, or use sunscreen to prevent photosensitivity (rare)

Evaluation
Positive therapeutic outcome
- Decreased cholesterol levels, serum triglyceride
- Improved ratio of HDLs

atovaquone (Rx)
(a-toe'va-kwon)
Mepron
Func. class.: Antiprotozoal
Chem. class.: Aromatic diamide derivative; analog of ubiquinone
Pregnancy category C

Do Not Confuse:
Mepron (U.S.)/Mepron (meprobamate in Australia)

Action: Interferes with DNA/RNA synthesis in protozoa, specifically ATP and nucleic acid synthesis

Therapeutic Outcome: Antiprotozoal for *Pneumocystis jiroveci* only

Uses: *P. jiroveci* infections in patients intolerant of trimethoprim/sulfamethoxazole (co-trimoxazole)

Dosage and routes
Acute, mild, moderate Pneumocystis jiroveci *pneumonia (PCP)*
Adult and adolescents 13-16 yr: PO 750 mg bid with food tid for 21 days
Pneumocystis jiroveci *pneumonia prophylaxis*
Adult and adolescents: PO 1500 mg daily with meal

Available forms: Susp 750 mg/5 ml

Adverse effects
CNS: *Dizziness, headache, anxiety,* insomnia
CV: Hypotension
GI: *Nausea, vomiting, diarrhea,* anorexia, increased AST and ALT, acute pancreatitis, constipation, abdominal pain
HEMA: Anemia, **leukopenia, neutropenia**
INTEG: Pruritus, urticaria, *rash,* oral monilia
META: Hyperkalemia, hypoglycemia, hyponatremia

Contraindications: Hypersensitivity or history of developing life-threatening allergic reactions to any component of the formulation, benzyl alcohol sensitivity

Precautions: Pregnancy **C,** blood dyscrasias, hepatic disease, diabetes mellitus, lactation, children, elderly, GI disease, respiratory insufficiency

Pharmacokinetics

Absorption	Poor; increased when taken with fatty foods
Distribution	Unknown
Metabolism	Hepatic recycling
Excretion	Feces, unchanged (94%)
Half-life	2-3 days

Pharmacodynamics

Onset	Unknown
Peak	1-8 hr

Interactions

Individual drugs

Rifampin, rifabutin: decreased effectiveness of atovaquone

Drug classifications

Use cautiously with highly protein-bound drugs with narrow therapeutic indices

NURSING CONSIDERATIONS

Assessment

- Assess for *Pneumocystis jiroveci:* monitor WBC, bilateral lung sounds, sputum for C&S; these should be checked before, periodically during, and after treatment; after collection of 1st sputum, therapy may begin
- Monitor for symptoms of hyponatremia: *CV:* increased B/P, cold, clammy skin, hypovolemia or hypervolemia; *GI:* anorexia, nausea, vomiting, diarrhea, abdominal cramps; *NEURO:* lethargy, increased ICP, confusion, headache, seizures, coma, fatigue, tremors, hyperreflexia
- Monitor for symptoms of hypoglycemia/hyperglycemia in diabetic patients
- Monitor blood studies: blood glucose, CBC, platelets; I&O ratio; ECG for cardiac dysrhythmias, check B/P; liver function studies: AST, ALT
- Monitor for signs of infection; anemia; monitor bowel pattern before, during treatment
- Monitor respiratory status: rate, character, wheezing, dyspnea
- Assess for dizziness, confusion, hallucination
- Assess for allergies before treatment, reaction of each medication; place allergies on chart; notify all people giving drugs

Nursing diagnoses

- Infection, risk for (uses)
- Diarrhea (adverse reactions)
- Knowledge, deficient (teaching)

Implementation

- Give with food (preferably fatty); increased absorption of the drug and higher plasma concentrations will occur; give tid × 3 wk

Patient/family education

- Instruct patient to take with food, preferably fatty foods, to increase plasma concentrations
- Advise patient to take drug exactly as prescribed

Evaluation

Positive therapeutic outcome

- Decreased temperature
- Ability to breathe
- Three negative sputum cultures

! HIGH ALERT

atropine (Rx)

(a'troe-peen)

atropine sulfate, Atro-Pen, Sal-Tropine

Func. class.: Antidysrhythmic, anticholinergic parasympatholytic, mydriatic

Chem. class.: Belladonna alkaloid

Pregnancy category C

Do Not Confuse:
atropine/Akarpine

Action: Blocks acetylcholine at parasympathetic neuroeffector sites; increases cardiac output, heart rate by blocking vagal stimulation in heart; dries secretions, decreases sweating, salivation in low doses; mydriasis, increased heart rate and cycloplegia occur at moderate doses; motility of GI, GU systems at high dose

Therapeutic Outcome: Drying of secretions, increased heart rate, cycloplegia, mydriasis

Uses: Bradycardia, bradydysrhythmia, reversal of anticholinesterase agents, insecticide poisoning, blocking cardiac vagal reflexes, decreasing secretions before surgery, antispasmodic with GU and biliary surgery, bronchodilator; ophthalmically for cycloplegia, mydriasis

Dosage and routes

Bradycardia/ bradydysrhythmias

Adult: **IV** bol 0.5-1 mg given q3-5 min, not to exceed 2 mg

Child: **IV** bol 0.01-0.03 mg/kg up to 0.4 mg or 0.3 mg/m^2; may repeat q4-6h, min dose 0.1 mg to avoid paradoxical reaction

Organophosphate poisoning

Adult and child: IM/**IV** 2 mg qh until muscarinic symptoms disappear; may need 6 mg qh

Atro-pen
Adult and child 90 lb, usually >10 yr: 2 mg
Child 40-90 lb, usually 4-10 yr: 1 mg
Child 15-40 lb, 6 mo-4 yr: 0.05 mg

Presurgery
Adult and child >20 kg: SUBCUT/IM/**IV** 0.4-0.6 mg before anesthesia
Child 12-16 kg: SUBCUT/IM 0.3 mg 1 hr preop
Child 7-9 kg: SUBCUT/IM 0.2 mg 1 hr preop
Child 3 kg: SUBCUT/IM 0.1 mg 1 hr preop

Cycloplegic refraction
Adult: OPHTH 1-2 gtt of 1% sol 1 hr before exam
Child: OPHTH 1-2 gtt of 0.5% sol bid-tid for up to 3 days before and 1 hr after exam

GI disorders
Adult: PO 0.3-1.2 mg q4-6h

Available forms: Inj 0.05, 0.1, 0.3, 0.4, 0.5, 0.8, 1 mg/ml; tabs 0.4 mg; inj prefilled autoinjectors (Atro-Pen) 0.5, 1, 2 mg

Adverse effects

CNS: Headache, dizziness, involuntary movement, confusion, psychosis, anxiety, coma, flushing, drowsiness, insomnia, weakness, delirium (elderly)
CV: Hypotension, paradoxic bradycardia, angina, PVCs, hypertension, tachycardia, ectopic ventricular beats
EENT: Blurred vision, photophobia, glaucoma, eye pain, pupil dilatation, nasal congestion
GI: Dry mouth, nausea, vomiting, abdominal pain, anorexia, constipation, paralytic ileus, abdominal distention, altered taste
GU: Retention, hesitancy, impotence, dysuria
INTEG: Rash, urticaria, contact dermatitis, dry skin, flushing
MISC: Suppression of lactation, decreased sweating

Contraindications: Hypersensitivity to belladonna alkaloids, angle closure glaucoma, GI obstructions, myasthenia gravis, thyrotoxicosis, ulcerative colitis, prostatic hypertrophy, tachycardia/tachydysrhythmias, asthma, acute hemorrhage, hepatic disease, myocardial ischemia

Precautions: Pregnancy **C**, renal disease, lactation, CHF, tachydysrhythmias, hyperthyroidism, COPD, hepatic disease, child <6 yr, hypertension, elderly, intraabdominal infections, Down syndrome, spastic paralysis, gastric ulcer

Pharmacokinetics

Absorption	Well absorbed (PO, SUBCUT, IM)
Distribution	Crosses blood-brain barrier, placenta
Metabolism	Liver
Excretion	Kidneys, unchanged (70%-90%); breast milk
Half-life	13-40 hr

Pharmacodynamics

	PO	IM/ SUBCUT	IV	OPHTH
Onset	½ hr	15 min	2-4 min	½ hr
Peak	½-1 hr	30 min	2-4 min	30-60 min
Duration	4-6 hr	4-6 hr	4-6 hr	1-2 wk

Interactions

Individual drugs
Amantadine: increased anticholinergic effect
Ketoconazole, levodopa: decreased absorption
Potassium chloride (oral): increased GI lesions

Drug classifications
Antacids: decreased absorption of atropine
Antidepressants (tricyclic), antiparkinson agents: increased anticholinergic effect

Drug/herb
Aconite: increased toxicity, death
Aloe, buckthorn (chronic use), cascara sagrada (chronic use), figwort, fumitory, goldenseal, jimsonweed, kudzu, licorice, rubarb, scopolia, senna: increased effect
Black root: forms insoluble complex
Coltsfoot: decreased effect
Horehound: increased serotonin effect

NURSING CONSIDERATIONS

Assessment

- Monitor I&O ratio; check for urinary retention and daily output in elderly or postoperative patients
- Monitor ECG for ectopic ventricular beats, PVC, tachycardia in cardiac patients
- Monitor for bowel sounds; check for constipation; abdominal distention and constipation may occur
- Monitor respiratory status: rate, rhythm, cyanosis, wheezing, dyspnea, engorged neck veins
- Monitor for increased intraocular pressure: eye pain, nausea, vomiting, blurred vision, increased tearing; discontinue use if pain occurs (optic)
- Monitor cardiac rate: rhythm, character, B/P continuously
- Monitor allergic reaction: rash, urticaria

Nursing diagnoses
- Cardiac output, decreased (uses)
- Sensory perception, disturbed (adverse reactions)
- Constipation (adverse reactions)
- Knowledge, deficient (teaching)

Implementation
PO route
- PO 30 min ac
- Give increased bulk, water in diet if constipation occurs (anticholinergic effect)

IM route
- Expect atropine flush 15-20 min after inj; it may occur in children and is not harmful

Ophthalmic route
- Place pressure on lacrimal sac for 1 min; do not touch dropper to eye

IV route
- Give **IV** undiluted or diluted with 10 ml sterile H_2O; give at a rate of 0.6 mg/min; give through Y-tube or 3-way stopcock; do not add to **IV** sol; may cause paradoxic bradycardia lasting 2 min

Syringe compatibilities: Benzquinamide, butorphanol, chlorproMAZINE, cimetidine, dimenhyDRINATE, diphenhydrAMINE, droperidol, fentanyl, glycopyrrolate, heparin, hydromorphone, hydrOXYzine, meperidine, metoclopramide, midazolam, milrinone, morphine, nalbuphine, pentazocine, perphenazine, prochlorperazine, promazine, promethazine, propiomazine, ranitidine, scopolamine, sufentanil, vit B with C

Y-site compatibilities: Amrinone, etomidate, famotidine, heparin, hydrocortisone sodium succinate, meropenem, nafcillin, potassium chloride, sufentanil, vit B/C

Additive compatibilities: Dobutamine, furosemide, meropenem, netilmicin, sodium bicarbonate, verapamil

Patient/family education
- Advise patient not to perform strenuous activity in high temperatures; heat stroke may result
- Instruct patient to take as prescribed; not to skip doses
- Instruct patient to report change in vision; blurring or loss of sight; trouble breathing; sweating; flushing, chest pain, allergic reactions, constipation, urinary retention
- Caution patient not to operate machinery if drowsiness occurs
- Advise patient not to take OTC products without approval of physician

Ophthalmic route
- Teach patient method of instillation
- Instruct patient that blurred vision will decrease with repeated use of drug; to omit next instillation if side effects are present
- Instruct patient not to perform hazardous tasks until able to see
- Advise patient to wait 5 min to use other drops; not to blink more than usual; use sunglasses to protect eyes

Evaluation
Positive therapeutic outcome
- Decreased dysrhythmias
- Increased heart rate
- Decreased secretions, GI, GU spasms
- Bronchodilatation
- Decreased in inflammation (iritis) or cycloplegic refraction (ophthalmic)

Treatment of overdose: O_2, artificial ventilation, ECG; administer DOPamine for circulatory depression; administer diazepam or thiopental for convulsion; assess need for antidysrhythmics

attapulgite (OTC)
(at-a-pull'gite)

Diar Aid, Diasorb, Fowler's Diarrhea Tablets ✤, Hydrated Magnesium Silicate, Kaopectate, Kaopectate Advanced Formula, Kaopectate Maximum Strength, Parepectolin, Rheaban, St. Joseph Antidiarrheal

Func. class.: Antidiarrheal

Chem. class.: Hydrous magnesium aluminum silicate

Pregnancy category C

Action: Decreases gastric motility, water content of stool; adsorbent, demulcent

Therapeutic Outcome: Decreased diarrhea

Uses: Diarrhea (cause undetermined), mild to moderate

Dosage and routes
Adult: PO 60-120 ml (45-90 ml conc) after each loose bowel movement

Child >12 yr: PO 60 ml after each loose bowel movement

Child 6-12 yr: PO 30-60 ml (30 ml conc) after each loose bowel movement

Child 3-6 yr: PO 15-30 ml (15 ml conc) after each loose bowel movement

Available forms: Susp kaolin 0.87 g/5 ml, pectin 43 mg/5 ml; kaolin 0.98 g/5 ml, pectin 21.7 mg/5 ml

Adverse effects
GI: Constipation (chronic use)

Precautions: Pregnancy **C**

Pharmacokinetics

Absorption	Not absorbed
Distribution	Unknown
Metabolism	Unknown
Excretion	Unknown
Half-life	Unknown

Pharmacodynamics

Unknown

Interactions
All drugs: decreased action of all other drugs

Drug/herb

Nutmeg: increased effect

NURSING CONSIDERATIONS
Assessment
- Assess bowel pattern before, during, and after treatment; check for rebound constipation
- Monitor for dehydration in children

Nursing diagnoses
- Diarrhea (uses)
- Constipation (adverse reactions)
- Knowledge, deficient (teaching)

Implementation
- For 48 hr only after each diarrhea stool
- Shake well before administration

Patient/family education
- Advise patient not to exceed recommended dosage; notify prescriber if symptoms continue
- Instruct patient to shake well before administration

Evaluation
Positive therapeutic outcome
- Decreased diarrhea

! HIGH ALERT

azacitidine (Rx)
(a-za-sie-ti'deen)

Vidaza

Func. class.: Antineoplastic hormone

Chem. class.: DNA demethylation agent

Pregnancy category D

Action: Cytotoxic by producing damage to double-strand DNA during DNA synthesis

Therapeutic Outcome: Improved blood counts in refractor anemia

Uses: Myelodysplastic syndrome (MDS)

Dosage and routes
Adult: SUBCUT 75 mg/m^2 daily × 7 days, q4 wk, premedicate with antiemetic, dose may be increased to 100 mg/m^2 if no response is seen after 2 treatment cycles, minimum treatment 4 cycles

Available forms: Powdered for inj, lyophilized 100 mg

Adverse effects
CNS: Anxiety, depression, dizziness, fatigue, headache

CV: Cardiac murmur, hypotension, tachycardia

GI: **Diarrhea**, nausea, vomiting, anorexia, constipation, abdominal pain, distention, tenderness, hemorrhoids, mouth hemorrhage, tongue ulceration, stomatitis, dyspepsia, **hepatotoxicity, hepatic coma**

GU: **Real failure, renal tubular acidosis**, dysuria, UTI

HEMA: **Leukopenia, anemia, thrombocytopenia, neutropenia**, ecchymosis

INTEG: Irritation at site, rash, sweating, pyrexia

META: Hypokalemia

Contraindications: Pregnancy **D**, hypersensitivity to this drug or mannitol, advanced malignant hepatic tumors

Precautions: Lactation, children, elderly, renal and hepatic disease; a man should not father a child while taking this drug

Pharmacokinetics

Absorption	Rapid
Distribution	Unknown
Metabolism	Liver
Excretion	Urine
Half-life	35-49 min

Pharmacodynamics

Onset	Unknown
Peak	½ hr
Duration	Unknown

Interactions: None known

NURSING CONSIDERATIONS
Assessment
- Assess for CNS symptoms: fever, headache, chills, dizziness
- Monitor hematologic response with patients with baseline WBC = to 3 × 10^9/L, absolute

neutrophil count (ANC) = 1.5×10^9/L, and platelets = 75×10^9/L, adjust dose; ANC < 0.5 $\times 10^9$/L, platelets < 25×10^9/L, give 50% dose next course; ANC 0.5 – 1.5×10^9/L, platelets 25 – 50×10^9/L, give 67% next course

- Assess buccal cavity q8h for dryness, sores, or ulceration, white patches, oral pain, bleeding, dysphagia
- Assess for signs of bone marrow depression: bruising, bleeding, blood in stools, urine, sputum, emesis

Nursing diagnoses

- Injury, risk for (adverse reactions)
- Body image, disturbed (adverse reactions)
- Infection, risk for (adverse reactions)
- Knowledge, deficient (teaching)

Implementation

- Administer antiemetics and dexamethasone 10 mg at least ½ hr before antineoplastics

IV route

- Reconstitute with 4 ml sterile water for inj (25 mg/ml), inject dilutent slowly into vial, invert vial 2-3 times and gently rotate, sol will be cloudy, use immediately, divide doses greater than 4 ml into 2 syringes, resuspend the contents 2-3 times and gently roll syringe between the palms for 30 sec immediately prior to administration
- Rotate injection site
- Increase patient's fluid intake to 2-3 L/day to prevent dehydration, unless contraindicated
- Assist patient with rinsing of mouth tid-qid with water, club soda; brushing of teeth bid-tid with soft brush or cotton-tipped applicator for stomatitis; use unwaxed dental floss
- Provide a nutritious diet with iron, vitamin supplement, low fiber, few dairy products

Patient/family education

- Instruct patient to avoid foods with citric acid or hot or rough texture if stomatitis is present; to drink adequate fluids
- Instruct patient to report stomatitis; any bleeding, white spots, ulcerations in mouth; tell patient to examine mouth daily, report symptoms
- Advise patient to use contraception during therapy
- Advise patient not to father a child while receiving this drug

Evaluation

Positive therapeutic outcome

- Improvement in blood counts in refractory anemia, or refractory anemia with excess blasts

azathioprine (Rx)

(ay-za-thye'oh-preen)

Imuran

Func. class.: Immunosuppressant

Chem. class.: Purine antagonist

Pregnancy category D

Do Not Confuse:

Imuran/Imferon/Elmiron/IMDUR/Enduron/Tenormin

Action: Produces immunosuppression by inhibiting purine synthesis, DNA, RNA in cells

Therapeutic Outcome: Absence of graft rejection, slowing of rheumatoid arthritis

Uses: Renal transplants to prevent graft rejection, often used with corticosteroids, cytotoxics; refractory rheumatoid arthritis, refractory ITP, glomerulonephritis, nephrotic syndrome, bone marrow transplant

Investigational uses: Myasthenia gravis, chronic ulcerative colitis, Crohn's disease, Behçet's syndrome

Dosage and routes

Renal dose

CCr 10-50 ml/min 75% of dose; CCr <10 ml/min 50% of dose

Prevention of rejection

Adult and child: PO, **IV** 3-5 mg/kg/day, then maintenance (PO) of at least 1-2 mg/kg/day

Refractory rheumatoid arthritis

Adult: PO 1/mg/kg/day; may increase dosage after 2 mo by 0.5 mg/kg/day; not to exceed 2.5 mg/kg/day

Available forms: Tabs 50 mg; inj **IV** 100 mg

Adverse effects

GI: Nausea, vomiting, stomatitis, esophagitis, **pancreatitis, hepatotoxicity, jaundice**

HEMA: **Leukopenia, thrombocytopenia, anemia, pancytopenia**

INTEG: Rash, alopeia

MISC: Raynaud's symptoms, **serum sickness**

MS: Arthralgia, muscle wasting

Contraindications: Pregnancy **D,** hypersensitivity, lactation

Precautions: Severe renal disease, severe hepatic disease, elderly

Pharmacokinetics

Absorption	Readily (PO)
Distribution	Crosses placenta
Metabolism	Liver to mercaptopurine
Excretion	Kidney, minimal
Half-life	3 hr

Pharmacodynamics

	PO	IV
Onset	Unknown	Unknown
Peak	4 hr	Unknown
Duration	Unknown	Unknown

Interactions

Individual drugs

Do not admix with other drugs
Cotrimoxazole: increased leukopenia
Allopurinol: increased action of azathioprine
CycloSPORINE: increased myelosuppression
Warfarin: decreased action of warfarin

Drug classifications

ACE inhibitors: increased leukopenia
Antineoplastics: increased myelosuppression
Vaccines: decreased immune response

Drug/herb

Astragalus, echinacea, melatonin, safflower: increased immunosuppression
Ginseng, maitake, mistletoe, schisandra, St. John's wort, turmeric: decreased effect

Drug/lab test

Increased: liver function tests
Decreased: uric acid
Interference: CBC, diff count

NURSING CONSIDERATIONS

Assessment

- Assess symptoms of rheumatoid arthritis: pain in joints, stiffness, poor range of motion, inflammation before and during treatment
- Monitor blood studies: Hgb, WBC, platelets during treatment monthly; if leukocytes are <3000/mm^3 or platelets <100,000/mm^3, drug should be discontinued or reduced; decreased Hgb level may indicate bone marrow suppression
- Monitor liver function studies: alkaline phosphatase, AST, ALT, amylase, bilirubin; and for hepatotoxicity: dark urine, jaundice, itching, light-colored stools; drug should be discontinued
- Monitor I&O, weight daily, report decreasing urine output, toxicity may occur
- Assess for infection: increased temp, WBC; sputum, urine

Nursing diagnoses

- Mobility, impaired (uses)
- Infection, risk for (uses)
- Knowledge, deficient (teaching)

Implementation

PO route

- Give all medications PO if possible, avoiding IM inj, since bleeding may occur
- Give with meals to reduce GI upset; nausea is common
- For several days before transplant surgery, patients should be placed in protective isolation

IV route

- Prepare in biologic cabinet using gown, gloves, mask; give after diluting 100 mg/10 ml of sterile water for inj; rotate to dissolve; may further dilute with 50 ml or more saline or glucose in saline given over >30 min (intermittent inf)

Solution compatibilities: D_5W, NaCl 0.9%, NaCl 0.45%

Patient/family education

- Teach patient to take as prescribed, do not miss doses, if dose is missed on daily regimen, skip dose, if on multiple dosing/day, take as soon as remembered
- Teach patient that therapeutic response may take 3-4 mo in rheumatoid arthritis, to continue with prescribed exercise, rest, other medications; that drug is needed for life in renal transplant
- Instruct patient to report fever, rash, severe diarrhea, chills, sore throat, fatigue, since serious infections may occur; or clay-colored stools and cramping (hepatotoxicity)
- Advise patient to use contraceptive measures during treatment for 12 wk after ending therapy; drug is teratogenic
- Advise patient to avoid vaccinations
- Tell patient to avoid crowds and persons with known infections to reduce risk of infection
- Instruct patient not to use OTC medications without approval of prescriber
- Advise patient to use soft-bristled toothbrush to prevent bleeding

Evaluation

Positive therapeutic outcome

- Absence of graft rejection
- Immunosuppression in autoimmune disorders
- Increased joint mobility without pain in rheumatoid arthritis

azelastine (Rx)

(ay'ze-lass-teen)

Optivar

Func. class.: Leukotriene synthesis inhibitor

Chem. class.: Phthalazinone derivative

Pregnancy category C

Do Not Confuse:
Zithromax/Zinacef/azithromycin/erythromycin

Action: Inhibits the synthesis and release of leukotrienes; antagonizes action of acetylcholine, histamine, serotonin

Therapeutic Outcome: Decreased nasal stuffiness, itching, swollen eyes

Uses: Seasonal allergic rhinitis

Dosage and routes

Adult and child ≥12 yr: Nasal 2 sprays/nostril bid

Available forms: Spray 137 mcg/actuation

Adverse effects

CNS: Sedation (more common with increased dosages), drowsiness

MISC: Weight increase, myalgia

Contraindications: Hypersensitivity

Precautions: Pregnancy **C**

Pharmacokinetics	
Absorption	Unknown
Distribution	Unknown
Metabolism	Liver, extensively
Excretion	Feces
Half-life	25-42 hr

Pharmacodynamics	
Onset	Unknown
Peak	4-5 hr
Duration	Unknown

Interactions

Individual drugs

Alcohol: increased CNS depression

Drug classifications

CNS depressants, opioids, sedative/hypnotics: increased CNS depression

NURSING CONSIDERATIONS

Assessment

- Assess respiratory status: rate, rhythm, increase in bronchial secretions, wheezing, chest tightness; provide fluids to 2 L/day to decrease secretion thickness

Nursing diagnoses

- Airway clearance, ineffective (uses)
- Knowledge, deficient (teaching)
- Noncompliance (teaching, overuse)

Implementation

- Remove cap/safety clip from spray pump
- Prime pump if using for first time, push 4 times quickly, away from face, blow your nose, then place tip of pump into one nostril, while holding other nostril closed, tilt head forward, and spray into nostril
- Put cover/safety clip back on

Patient/family education

- Teach patient all aspects of drug uses; to notify prescriber if confusion, sedation occur; to avoid driving and other hazardous activity if drowsiness occurs; to avoid alcohol and other CNS depressants that may potentiate effect
- Caution patient not to exceed recommended dosage; dysrhythmias may occur

Evaluation

Positive therapeutic outcome

- Absence of runny or congested nose

azithromycin (Rx)

(ay-zi-thro-my'sin)

Zithromax

Func. class.: Antiinfective

Chem. class.: Macrolide (azalide)

Pregnancy category B

Do Not Confuse:
azithromycin/erythromycin
zithromax/zinacef

Action: Binds to 50S ribosomal subunits of susceptible bacteria and suppresses protein synthesis; much greater spectrum of activity than erythromycin

Therapeutic Outcome: Bacteriostatic against the following susceptible organisms: *Moraxella catarrhalis, Streptococcus pneumoniae, Streptococcus pyogenes, Staphylococcus aureus, Haemophilus influenzae, Clostridium, Legionella pneumophila, Chlamydia trachomatis, Mycoplasma;* no effect on methicillin-resistant *S. aureus;* in children: acute otitis media *(H. influenzae, M. catarrhalis, S. pneumoniae)* PO, acute pharyngitis/tonsillitis (group A streptococcal) PO; acute skin/soft tissue infections (PO); community-acquired pneumonia *(C. pneumoniae, H. influenzae, M. pneumoniae, S. pneumoniae)* PO; pharyngitis/tonsillitis *(S. pyogenes)*

Uses: Mild to moderate infections of the upper respiratory tract, lower respiratory tract; uncomplicated skin and skin structure infections, nongonococcal urethritis, or cervicitis; prophylaxis of disseminated *Mycobacterium avium* complex (MAC)

Investigational uses: Bacterial endocarditis prevention, chlamydial infections, gonococcocal infections, prophylaxis after sexual assault

Dosage and routes

Most infections

Adult: PO 500 mg on day 1, then 250 mg daily on days 2-5 for a total dose of 1.5 g

Child 2-15 yr: PO 10 mg/kg on day 1, then 5 mg/kg × 4 days

Pharyngitis/tonsillitis

Adult: PO 12 mg/kg daily × 5 days

Pelvic inflammatory disease

Adult: PO/**IV** 500 mg **IV** q24h × 2 doses, then 500 mg PO q24h × 7-10 days

Cervicitis, chlamydia, chancroid, nongonococcal urethritis

Adult: PO 1 g single dose

Gonorrhea

Adult: PO 2 g single dose

Endocarditis, prophylaxis

Adult: PO 500 mg 1 hr prior to procedure

Child: PO 15 mg/kg 1 hr prior to procedure

Community-acquired pneumonia

Adult: PO/**IV** 500 mg **IV** q24h × 2 doses, then 500 mg PO q24h × 7-10 days

Disseminated MAC infections

Adult: PO 600 mg/day in combination with ethambutol

Lower respiratory tract infections, acute skin/soft tissue infections, acute pharyngitis/tonsillitis

Child: PO 3-day regimen, 10 mg/kg daily × 3 days

Acute otitis media

Child: PO 30 mg/kg as a single dose or 10 mg/kg daily × 3 days or 10 mg/kg as a single dose on day 1, max 500 mg/day, then 5 mg/kg on days 2-5, max 250 mg/day

Prevention of acute otitis media

Child: PO 10 mg/kg qwk × 6 mo

Available forms: Tabs 250, 600 mg; powder for inj 500 mg; powder for oral susp 1 g/packet; susp 100, 200 mg/5 ml

Adverse effects

CNS: Dizziness, headache, vertigo, somnolence

CV: Palpitations, chest pain

GI: *Nausea, vomiting, diarrhea,* **hepatotoxicity,** abdominal pain, stomatitis, heartburn, dyspepsia, flatulence, melena, **cholestatic jaundice, pseudomembranous colitis**

GU: Vaginitis, moniliasis, nephritis

INTEG: Rash, urticaria, pruritus, photosensitivity

SYST: **Angioedema**

Contraindications: Hypersensitivity to azithromycin, erythromycin, or any macrolide

Precautions: Pregnancy **B,** lactation, hepatic/renal/cardiac disease, elderly, child <6 mo for otitis media, child <2 yr for pharyngitis, tonsillitis

Pharmacokinetics

Absorption	Rapid, (PO) up to 50%
Distribution	Widely distributed
Metabolism	Unknown, minimal metabolism
Excretion	Unchanged (bile); kidneys, minimal
Half-life	11-70 hr

Pharmacodynamics

	PO	IV
Onset	Unknown	Unknown
Peak	2-4 hr	End of infusion
Duration	24 hr	24 hr

Interactions

Individual drugs

Bromocriptine, carbamazepine, cycloSPORINE, digoxin, disopyramide, methylPREDNISolone, phenytoin, theophylline, triazolam: increased effects of specific drugs

Pimozide: fatal reaction

Triazolam: decreased clearance of triazolam

Drug classifications

Aluminum, magnesium antacids: decreased levels of azithromycin

Anticoagulants (orals): increased effect of oral anticoagulants

Oral contraceptives: increased effects

Drug/herb

Acidophilus: do not use with antiinfectives

Drug/lab test

Increased: bilirubin, alkaline phosphatase, CPK, BUN, creatinine, AST, ALT

NURSING CONSIDERATIONS

Assessment

- Assess for signs and symptoms of infection: drainage, fever, increased WBC >10,000/mm^3, urine culture positive, sore throat, sputum culture positive

- Monitor respiratory status: rate, character, wheezing, tightness in chest; discontinue drug if these occur
- Monitor allergies before treatment, reaction of each medication; place allergies on chart, notify all people giving drugs; skin eruptions, itching
- Monitor I&O ratio, renal studies; report hematuria, oliguria in renal disease; check urinalysis, protein, blood
- Monitor liver studies: AST, ALT, bilirubin, LDH, alkaline phosphatase; CBC with differential
- Monitor C&S before drug therapy; drug may be taken as soon as culture is taken; C&S may be repeated after treatment
- Monitor bowel pattern before, during treatment
- Assess for superinfection: sore throat, mouth, tongue; fever, fatigue, diarrhea, anogenital pruritus

Nursing diagnoses
- Infection, risk for (uses)
- Diarrhea (adverse reactions)
- Knowledge, deficient (teaching)

Implementation
PO route
- Provide adequate intake of fluids (2 L) during diarrhea episodes
- Give with a full glass of water; give susp 1 hr before or 2 hr pc; tabs may be taken without regard to food; do not give with fruit juices
- Store at room temperature
- Reconstitute 1 g packet for susp with 60 ml water, mix, rinse glass with more water and have patient drink to consume all medication; packets not for pediatric use
- Do not take aluminum/magnesium-containing antacids or food simultaneously with this drug

IV route
- Reconstitute 500 mg drug/4.8 ml sterile water for inj (100 mg/ml), shake, dilute with ≥250 ml 0.9% NaCl, 0.45% NaCl, or LR to 1-2 mg/ml; diluted solution is stable for 24 hr or 7 days if refrigerated
- Give 500 mg or more/1 hr, never give IM or as a bol

Patient/family education
- Instruct patient to report sore throat, black furry tongue, fever, loose foul-smelling stool, vaginal itching, discharge, fatigue; may indicate superinfection
- Caution patient not to take aluminum/magnesium-containing antacids or food simultaneously with this drug; blood levels of azithromycin will be decreased
- Instruct patient to notify prescriber of diarrhea stools, dark urine, pale stools, yellow discoloration of eyes or skin, severe abdominal pain; cholestatic jaundice is a severe adverse reaction
- Teach patient complete dosage regimen; to notify prescriber if symptoms continue
- Teach patient that if pregnancy is suspected to notify prescriber
- Inform patient that sunburns may occur; wear protective clothing and sunscreen

Evaluation
Positive therapeutic outcome
- C&S negative for infection
- WBC within 5000-10,000/mm^3

baclofen (Rx)
(bak'loe-fen)

Lioresal

Func. class.: Skeletal muscle relaxant, central acting

Chem. class.: GABA, chlorophenyl derivative

Pregnancy category C

Action: Inhibits synaptic responses in CNS by stimulating GABAb receptor subtype, which decreases neurotransmitter function; decreasing frequency, severity of muscle spasms

Therapeutic Outcome: Decreased spasticity of muscles

Uses: Spinal cord injury, spasticity in multiple sclerosis

Investigational uses: Trigeminal neuralgia

Dosage and routes
Adult: PO 5 mg tid × 3 days, then 10 mg tid × 3 days, then 15 mg tid × 3 days, then 20 mg tid × 3 days, then titrated to response; not to exceed 80 mg/day

Adult: Intrathecal Use implantable intrathecal inf pump; 100-800 mcg/day infusion, screening trial of 3 separate bol

Child: Intrathecal Use implantable intrathecal infusion pump 25-1200 mcg/day infusion

Available forms: Tabs 10, 20 mg; intrathecal inj 10 mg/20 ml (500 mcg/ml), 10 mg/5 ml (2000 mcg/ml)

Adverse effects
CNS: *Dizziness, weakness, fatigue, drowsiness,* headache, disorientation, insomnia, paresthesias, tremors

CV: Hypotension, chest pain, palpitations, edema

EENT: Nasal congestion, blurred vision, mydriasis, tinnitus
GI: ***Nausea,*** constipation, vomiting, increased AST, alkaline phosphatase, abdominal pain, dry mouth, anorexia
GU: Urinary frequency
INTEG: Rash, pruritus

Contraindications: Hypersensitivity

Precautions: Pregnancy **C**, renal disease, hepatic disease, stroke, seizure disorder, diabetes mellitus, children, elderly

Pharmacokinetics

Absorption	Well (PO)
Distribution	Widely, crosses placenta
Metabolism	Liver, partially
Excretion	Kidney, unchanged 70%-80%
Half-life	2½-4 hr

Pharmacodynamics

	PO/IT
Onset	0.5-1 hr
Peak	4 hr
Duration	4-8 hr

Interactions
Individual drugs
Alcohol: CNS depression
Drug classifications
Antidepressants, antihistamines, opioids, sedative/hypnotics, tricyclics: increased CNS depression
MAOIs: increased hypotension, CNS depression
Drug/herb
Chamomile, hops, kava, valerian: increased CNS depression
Drug/lab test
Increase: AST, ALT, alkaline phosphatase, blood glucose

NURSING CONSIDERATIONS
Assessment
- Monitor B/P, weight, blood glucose, and hepatic function periodically
- Check for increased seizure activity in patients with epilepsy; this drug decreases seizure threshold, monitor ECG
- Check I&O ratio; check for urinary retention, frequency, hesitancy
- Allergic reactions: rash, fever, respiratory distress; severe weakness, numbness in extremities
- Assess CNS depression: dizziness, drowsiness, psychiatric symptoms
- Check dosage, as individual titration is required

Nursing diagnoses
- Mobility, physical, impaired (uses)
- Injury, risk for (adverse reactions)
- Knowledge, deficient (teaching)

Implementation
PO route
- Give with meals for GI symptoms; gum, frequent sips of water for dry mouth
- Store in airtight container at room temperature

IT route
- Titration is based on response
- Test dose: Dilute to a concentration of 50 mcg/ml, give over 1 min or more
- Observe for decrease in muscle spasticity
- If response is not adequate, give 2 additional test doses (75 mcg/1.5 ml and 100 mcg/2 ml)

Patient/family education
- Give test doses 24 hr apart
- Advise patient not to discontinue medication quickly; hallucinations, spasticity, tachycardia will occur; drug should be tapered off over 1-2 wk

IT route
- Advise patient not to take with alcohol, other CNS depressants
- Caution patient to avoid altering activities while taking this drug; to avoid hazardous activities if drowsiness or dizziness occur
- Advise patient to avoid using OTC medication (cough preparations, antihistamines) unless directed by prescriber

Evaluation
Positive therapeutic outcome
- Decreased pain, spasticity

Treatment of overdose: Induce emesis if conscious patient, lavage, dialysis

balsalazide (Rx)
(ball-sal′a-zide)
Colazal
Func. class.: GI antiinflammatory
Chem. class.: Salicylate derivative
Pregnancy category B

Action: Delivered intact to the colon, bioconverted to 5-ASA

Therapeutic Outcome: Decreased inflammation in colon

Uses: Active, mild to moderate ulcerative colitis

B

Dosage and routes

Adult: PO 2.25 g (3 tabs) tid × 8 wk, may take up to 12 wk

Available forms: Tabs 750 mg

Adverse effects

CNS: Headache, insomnia, fatigue, fever, dizziness

EENT: Dry mouth, dry eyes, rhinitis, sinusitis, watery eyes, blurred vision

GI: Nausea, vomiting, abdominal pain, diarrhea, rectal bleeding, flatulence, dyspepsia, dry mouth, constipation

MS: Arthralgia, back pain, myalgia

SYST: **Anaphylaxis**

Contraindications: Hypersensitivity to salicylates

Precautions: Pregnancy **B**, child <14 yr, lactation, pyloric stenosis

Pharmacokinetics

Absorption	Low, variable
Distribution	Plasma protein binding 99%
Metabolism	Unknown
Excretion	Kidneys, as metabolites
Half-life	Unknown

Pharmacodynamics

Unknown

Interactions: None known

Drug/lab test

Increased: AST, ALT, GGT, LDH, bilirubin, alkaline phosphatase

False positive: urinary glucose test

NURSING CONSIDERATIONS

Assessment

- Monitor kidney function studies: BUN, creatinine, urinalysis (long-term therapy)
- Assess for allergic reaction: rash, dermatitis, urticaria, pruritus, dyspnea,bronchospasm

Nursing diagnoses

- Injury, risk for (uses)
- Knowledge, deficient (teaching)

Implementation

- Give with food in evenly divided doses
- Use with resuscitative equipment available; severe allergic reactions may occur
- Give total daily dose evenly spaced to minimize GI intolerance
- Store in tight, light-resistant container at room temp

Patient/family education

- Advise patient to notify prescriber if symptoms do not improve, if rash, hives, or respiratory problems occur

Evaluation

Positive therapeutic outcome

- Absence of fever, mucus in stools, resolution of symptoms of ulcerative colitis

! HIGH ALERT

basiliximab (Rx)

(bas-ih-liks'ih-mab)

Simulect

Func. class.: Immunosuppressant

Chem. class.: Murine/human monoclonal antibody (interleukin-2) receptor antagonist

Pregnancy category B

Action: Binds to and blocks the IL-2 receptor, which is selectively expressed on the surface of activated T-lymphocytes; impairs the immune system to antigenic challenges

Therapeutic Outcome: Prevention of graft rejection

Uses: Acute allograft rejection in renal transplant patients when used with cycloSPORINE and corticosteroids

Dosage and routes

Adult: **IV** 20 mg × 2 doses; 1st dose within 2 hr before transplant surgery; 2nd dose given 4 days after transplantation

Child 2-15 yr: **IV** 12 mg/m^2 × 2 doses; 1st dose within 2 hr before transplant surgery; 2nd dose given 4 days after transplantation

Available forms: Powder for inj 20 mg

Adverse effects

CNS: *Pyrexia, chills, tremors, headache, insomnia, weakness*

CV: *Chest pain,* angina, **cardiac failure,** hypotension, hypertension, edema

GI: *Vomiting, nausea, diarrhea,* constipation, abdominal pain, GI bleeding, gingival hyperplasia, stomatitis

INTEG: *Acne*

META: Acidosis, hypercholesterolemia, hyperuricemia, hyperkalemia, hypocalcemia, hypokalemia, hypophosphatemia

MISC: Infection, moniliasis, **anaphylaxis**

MS: Arthralgia, myalgia

RESP: *Dyspnea, wheezing, cough,* **pulmonary edema**

Contraindications: Hypersensitivity, exposure to viral infections, lactation

Precautions: Pregnancy **B,** infections, elderly, children

Pharmacokinetics

Absorption	Unknown
Distribution	Unknown
Metabolism	Unknown
Excretion	Unknown
Half-life	7 days (adult) 9½ days (child)

Pharmacodynamics

Onset	Unknown
Peak	½ hr (adults)
Duration	Unknown

Interactions

Drug classifications

Immunosuppressants: increased immunosuppression

Drug/herb

Astragalus, echinacea, melatonin, safflower: increased immunosuppression

Ginseng, maitake, mistletoe, schisandra, St. John's wort, turmeric: decreased effect

Drug/lab test

Increased: BUN, cholesterol, uric acid, creatinine, potassium, calcium, blood glucose, Hgb, Hct

Decreased: Hgb, Hct, platelets, magnesium, phosphate

NURSING CONSIDERATIONS

Assessment

- Assess for infection, increased temp, WBC, sputum, urine
- Monitor blood studies: Hgb, WBC, platelets during treatment qmo; if leukocytes are <3000/mm^3, drug should be discontinued
- Monitor liver function studies: alkaline phosphatase, AST, ALT, bilirubin
- Assess hepatotoxicity: dark urine, jaundice, itching, light-colored stools; drug should be discontinued
- ◆ Assess for anaphylaxis, hypersensitivity: dyspnea, wheezing, rash, pruritus, hypotension, tachycardia; if severe hypersensitivity reactions occur, drug should not be used again

Nursing diagnoses

- Infection, risk for (adverse reactions)
- Knowledge, deficient (teaching)

Implementation

- Administer all medications PO if possible; avoid IM inj, since infection may occur

IV route

- After adding 5 ml sterile water for inj, shake gently to dissolve, reconstitute to a vol of 50 ml with 0.9% NaCl or D_5, gently invert bag, do not shake, do not admix

Patient/family education

- Instruct patient to report fever, chills, sore throat, fatigue, since serious infection may occur; avoid crowds, persons with known upper respiratory infections; use contraception during treatment

Evaluation

Positive therapeutic outcome

- Absence of graft rejection

beclomethasone (Rx)

(be-kloe-meth′a-sone)

Beclodisk ✤, Becloforte Inhaler ✤, Beclovent, Beclovent Rotocaps ✤, QVAR, Vanceril, Vanceril Double Strength

Func. class.: Synthetic glucocorticoid (long acting)

Chem. class.: Beclomethasone diester

Pregnancy category C

Do Not Confuse:
Vanceril/Vancenase

Action: Antiinflammatory; vasoconstrictive properties; also immunosuppressive

Therapeutic Outcome: Decreased inflammation and normal immunity

Uses: Seasonal, perennial allergic rhinitis, nasal polyps, chronic steroid-dependent asthma

Dosage and routes

Adult and child >12 yr: INH 2-4 puffs bid-qid (42 mcg/actuations), max 20 inh/day; inh 2 puffs bid, max 10 inh/day (84 mcg/actuation)

Child 6-12 yrs: INH 1-2 puffs tid-qid (42 mcg/actuation); 2 puffs bid, max 5 inh/day (84 mcg/actuation)

Available forms: Aero for inh 40, 80, 250✤ mcg /activation; inh cap 100✤, 200 mcg

Adverse effects

CNS: *Headache,*

EENT: *Candidal infection, hoarseness,* sore throat

GI: Dry mouth, dyspepsia

MISC: **Angioedema adrenal insufficiency,** facial edema, Churg-Strauss syndrome

RESP: **Bronchospasm,** wheezing, cough

Contraindications: Hypersensitivity, status asthmaticus (primary treatment), nonasthmatic bronchial disease, bacterial, fungal, viral infections of mouth, throat, lungs

Precautions: Pregnancy **C**, children <12, nasal disease/surgery, lactation

Pharmacokinetics

Absorption	Locally only
Distribution	Not distributed
Metabolism	Lungs, liver (by CYP3A)
Excretion	Feces, urine
Half-life	2.8 hr

Pharmacodynamics

	INH	NASAL
Onset	10 min	10 min
Peak	Unknown	Unknown
Duration	Unknown	Unknown

NURSING CONSIDERATIONS

Assessment

- Assess adrenal suppression: 17-KS, plasma cortisol for decreased levels, adrenal function periodically for HPA axis suppression during prolonged therapy; monitor growth and development
- Assess blood studies, neutrophils, decreased platelets; WBC with diff baseline and q3 mo, if neutrophils <1000/mm^3, discontinue treatment
- Check nasal passages during long-term treatment for changes in mucus; check for burning, stinging; assess for glucocorticoid withdrawal: dizziness, hypotension, fatigue, muscle/joint pain; notify prescriber immediately
- Assess respiratory status: rest, rhythm, characteristics; auscultate lung bilaterally before and throughout treatment
- Assess for fungal infections in mucous membranes

Nursing diagnoses

- Airway clearance, ineffective (uses)
- Oral mucous membrane, impaired (adverse reactions)
- Knowledge, deficient (teaching)
- Noncompliance (teaching)

Implementation

- Give PO, using a spacer device for proper dose
- Use after cleaning aerosol top daily with warm water; dry thoroughly
- Store in cool environment; do not puncture or incinerate container

Inhalation route

- Shake inhaler, invert, tilt head backward, insert nozzle into nostril, away from septum; hold other nostril closed and depress activator, inhale through nose, exhale through mouth

Patient/family education

- Teach patient to gargle/rinse mouth after each use to prevent oral fungal infections
- Teach patient that in times of stress, systemic corticosteroids may be needed to prevent adrenal insufficiency; do not discontinue oral drug abruptly, taper slowly
- Teach patient to continue using product even if mild nasal bleeding occurs; is usually transient
- Teach patient method of instillation after providing written instructions from manufacturer
- Teach patient to clear nasal passages before administration; use decongestant if needed

Evaluate

Positive therapeutic outcome

- Decrease in runny nose, improved symptoms of bronchial asthma

benazepril (Rx)

(ben-a′za-pril)

Lotensin

Func. class.: Antihypertensive

Chem. class.: ACE inhibitor

Pregnancy category
C (1st trimester),
D (2nd/3rd trimesters)

Do Not Confuse:
Lotensin/Lioresal, Lotensin/Loniten

Action: Selectively suppresses renin-angiotensin-aldosterone system; inhibits ACE, preventing conversion of angiotensin I to angiotensin II

Therapeutic Outcome: Decreased B/P in hypertension

Uses: Hypertension, alone or in combination with thiazide diuretics

Dosage and routes

Adult: PO 10 mg daily initially, then 20-40 mg/day divided bid or daily (without a diuretic); 5 mg PO daily (with a diuretic)

Renal dose

Adult: PO 5 mg daily with CCr <30 ml/min; increase as needed to maximum of 40 mg/day

Elderly: PO 5-10 mg/day initially

Available forms: Tabs 5, 10, 20, 40 mg

Adverse effects

CNS: Anxiety, hypertonia, insomnia, paresthesia, headache, dizziness, fatigue
CV: Hypotension, postural hypotension, syncope, palpitations, angina
GI: Nausea, constipation, vomiting, gastritis, melena
GU: Increased BUN, creatinine, decreased libido, impotence, urinary tract infection
INTEG: Rash, flushing, sweating
META: Hyperkalemia, hyponatremia
MISC: **Angioedema**
MS: Arthralgia, arthritis, myalgia
RESP: Cough, asthma, bronchitis, dyspnea, sinusitis

Contraindications: Pregnancy **D** (2nd/3rd trimesters), hypersensitivity to ACE inhibitors, lactation, children

Precautions: Pregnancy **C** (1st trimester), impaired renal/liver function, dialysis patients, hypovolemia, blood dyscrasias, CHF, COPD, asthma, elderly, bilateral renal artery stenosis

Pharmacokinetics	
Absorption	<40%
Distribution	Unknown; crosses placenta
Metabolism	Liver metabolites; protein binding 97%
Excretion	Kidney, breast milk (minimal)
Half-life	10-11 hr (metabolite); increased in renal disease

Pharmacodynamics	
Onset	Unknown
Peak	½-1 hr
Duration	Unknown

Interactions

Individual drugs

Alcohol: increased hypotension (large amounts)
Digoxin, lithium: increased serum levels

Drug classifications

Antihypertensives, diuretics, nitrates, phenothiazines: increased hypotension
Diuretics (potassium-sparing), potassium supplements: increased hyperkalemia

Drug/herb

Aconite: increased toxicity, death
Astragalus, cola tree: increased or decreased antihypertensive effect
Barberry, betony, black catechu, black cohosh, bloodroot, broom, burdock, cat's claw, dandelion, goldenseal, Irish moss, Jamaican dogwood, kelp, khella, mistletoe, parsley: increased antihypertensive effect
Coltsfoot, guarana, khat, licorice, pineapple, yohimbe: decreased antihypertensive effect

Drug/lab test

Increased: AST, ALT, alkaline phosphatase, bilirubin, uric acid, blood glucose
False positive: ANA titer
Positive: ANA titer

NURSING CONSIDERATIONS

Assessment

- Monitor blood studies: neutrophils, decreased platelets
- Monitor B/P at peak/trough level of drug, check for orthostatic hypotension, syncope; if changes occur, dosage change may be required
- Monitor renal studies: protein, BUN, creatinine; watch for increased levels that may indicate nephrotic syndrome and renal failure; monitor urine for protein; monitor renal symptoms: polyuria, oliguria, frequency, dysuria
- Establish baselines in renal, liver function tests before therapy begins
- Check potassium levels throughout treatment, although hyperkalemia rarely occurs
- Assess for allergic reactions: rash, fever, pruritus, urticaria; drug should be discontinued if antihistamines fail to help

Nursing diagnoses

- Cardiac output, decreased (uses)
- Injury, risk for (side effects)
- Knowledge, deficient (teaching)
- Noncompliance (teaching)

Implementation

- Store in air-tight container at 86° F (30° C) or less
- Severe hypotension may occur after 1st dose of this medication; decreased hypotension may be prevented by reducing or discontinuing diuretic therapy 3 days before beginning benazepril therapy

Patient/family education

- Instruct patient not to discontinue drug abruptly; advise patient to tell all persons associated with care
- Teach patient not to use OTC products (cough, cold, allergy) unless directed by prescriber; serious side effects can occur; xanthines such as coffee, tea, chocolate, cola can prevent action of drug
- Emphasize the importance of complying with dosage schedule, even if feeling better; to continue with medical regimen to decrease B/P: exercise, cessation of smoking, decreasing stress, diet modifications

• Emphasize the need to rise slowly to sitting or standing position to minimize orthostatic hypotension; not to exercise in hot weather because increased hypotension can occur
• Teach patient to notify prescriber of mouth sores, sore throat, fever, swelling of hands or feet, irregular heartbeat, chest pain, coughing, shortness of breath
• Caution patient to report excessive perspiration, dehydration, vomiting, diarrhea; may lead to fall in B/P
• Caution patient that drug may cause dizziness, fainting, light-headedness; may occur during 1st few days of therapy; to avoid activities that may be hazardous
• Teach patient how to take B/P; teach normal readings for age-group; ensure patient takes own B/P
• Advise patient to notify prescriber of pregnancy, drug will need to be discontinued

Evaluation
Positive therapeutic outcome
• Decreased B/P in hypertension

Treatment of overdose: 0.9% NaCl **IV** inf, hemodialysis

benzonatate (Rx)
(ben-zoe'na-tate)
Tessalon
Func. class.: Antitussive
Chem. class.: Tetracaine derivative
Pregnancy category C

Action: Inhibits cough reflex by anesthetizing stretch receptors in respiratory system, direct action on cough center in medulla

Therapeutic Outcome: Decreased cough

Uses: Nonproductive cough

Dosage and routes
Adult and child ≥10 yr: PO 100 mg tid, max 600 mg/day

Available forms: Caps 100 mg

Adverse effects
CNS: *Dizziness, drowsiness,* headache
CV: Increased B/P, chest tightness, numbness
EENT: Nasal congestion, burning eyes
GI: *Nausea,* constipation, upset stomach
INTEG: Urticaria, rash, pruritus

Contraindications: Hypersensitivity

Precautions: Pregnancy **C**, lactation

Pharmacokinetics	
Absorption	Unknown
Distribution	Unknown
Metabolism	Unknown
Excretion	Unknown
Half-life	Unknown

Pharmacodynamics	
Onset	15-20 min
Peak	Unknown
Duration	3-8 hr

NURSING CONSIDERATIONS
Assessment
• Cough: type, frequency, character, including sputum

Nursing diagnoses
• Airway clearance, ineffective (uses)
• Knowledge, deficient (teaching)

Implementation
• Do not break, crush, or chew caps; will anesthetize mouth
• Increase fluids to liquefy sputum
• Chest percussion to bring up secretion if needed
• Store in tight, light-resistant containers

Patient/family education
• Teach patient to avoid driving, other hazardous activities until patient is stabilized on this medication
• Teach patient to avoid smoking, smoke-filled rooms, perfumes, dust, environmental pollutants, cleaners
• Advise patient that cough lasting over 1 wk should be checked by prescriber

Evaluation
Positive therapeutic outcome
• Absence of cough

benztropine (Rx)
(benz'troe-peen)
Apo-Benztropin ✱, benztropine mesylate, Cogentin
Func. class.: Cholinergic blocker, antiparkinson agent
Chem. class.: Tertiary amine
Pregnancy category C

Action: Blockade of central acetylcholine receptors in the CNS, neurotransmitters are balanced

Therapeutic Outcome: Decreased involuntary movements

Uses: Parkinsonian symptoms, extrapyramidal symptoms (EPS) associated with neuroleptic drugs, acute dystonia

Dosage and routes

Drug-induced extrapyramidal symptoms

Adult: IM/**IV** 1-4 mg daily/bid; give PO dose as soon as possible; PO 1-2 mg bid/tid; increase by 0.5 mg q5-6 days

Child: IM/**IV** 0.02-0.05 mg/kg/dose 1-2 × 1 day

Elderly: PO 0.5 mg daily/bid, increase by 0.5 mg q5-6 days

Parkinsonian symptoms

Adult: PO 1-2 mg daily, in divided doses; increased 0.5 mg q5-6 days titrated to patient response; max 6 mg daily

Acute dystonic reactions

Adult: IM/**IV** 1-2 mg, may increase to 1-2 mg bid (PO)

Available forms: Tabs 0.5, 1, 2 mg; inj IM, **IV** 1 mg/ml

Adverse effects

CNS: Confusion, anxiety, restlessness, irritability, delusions, hallucinations, headache, sedation, depression, incoherence, dizziness, memory loss; delirium (elderly)

CV: Palpitations, tachycardia, hypotension, bradycardia

EENT: Blurred vision, photophobia, dilated pupils, difficulty swallowing, dry eyes, mydriasis, increased intraocular tension, angle closure glaucoma

GI: *Dryness of mouth, constipation,* nausea, vomiting, abdominal distress, **paralytic ileus,** epigastric distress

GU: Hesitancy, retention, dysuria

INTEG: Rash, urticaria, dermatoses

MISC: Increased temperature, flushing, decreased sweating, **hyperthermia, heat stroke,** numbness of fingers

MS: Muscular weakness, cramping

Contraindications: Hypersensitivity, narrow angle glaucoma, myasthenia gravis, GI/GU obstruction,child <3 yr, peptic ulcer, megacolon, prostate hypertrophy

Precautions: Pregnancy **C**, elderly, lactation, tachycardia, liver, kidney disease, drug abuse history, dysrhythmias, hypotension, hypertension, psychiatric patients, children

Pharmacokinetics

Absorption	Well (PO, IM), completely (**IV**) absorbed
Distribution	Unknown
Metabolism	Unknown
Excretion	Unknown
Half-life	Unknown

Pharmacodynamics

	IM/IV	PO
Onset	15 min	1 hr
Peak	Unknown	Unknown
Duration	6-10 hr	6-10 hr

Interactions

Individual drugs

Disopyramide, quinidine: increased anticholinergic effects

Drug classifications

Antidepressants (tricyclic), antihistamines, phenothiazines: increased anticholinergic effects

Antidiarrheals: decreased absorption

Drug/herb

Butterbur, jimsonweed: increased benztropine effect

Black catechu: increased constipation

Kava, jaborandi, pill-bearing spurge: decreased benztropine effect

NURSING CONSIDERATIONS

Assessment

- Monitor I&O ratio; retention commonly causes decreased urinary output, distention, frequency, incontinence
- Assess for parkinsonism, EPS: shuffling gait, muscle rigidity, involuntary movements, loss of balance, pill rolling, muscle spasms, drooling before and during treatment
- Monitor for urinary hesitancy, retention; palpate bladder if retention occurs
- Monitor for constipation, cramping, pain in abdomen, abdominal distention; increase fluids, bulk, exercise if this occurs
- Assess for tolerance over long-term therapy; dosage may have to be increased or changed
- Assess for mental status: affect, mood, CNS depression, worsening of mental symptoms during early therapy
- Assess for benztropine "buzz" or "high," patients may imitate EPS

Nursing diagnoses

- Mobility, impaired (uses)
- Knowledge, deficient (teaching)
- Noncompliance (teaching)

Implementation

PO route

- Give with or after meals to prevent GI upset; may give with fluids other than water; hard candy, frequent drinks, gum to relieve dry mouth
- Give at bedtime to avoid daytime drowsiness in patient with parkinsonism
- May be crushed and mixed with food
- Store at room temperature

IM route

- Give in large muscle mass for dystonic symptoms

IV route

- Give parenteral dose with patient recumbent to prevent postural hypotension; give undiluted 1 mg/1 min

Syringe compatibilities: ChlorproMAZINE, fluphenazine, metoclopramide, perphenazine, thiothixene

Y-site compatibilities: Fluconazole, tacrolimus

Patient/family education

- Teach patient to use caution in hot weather; drug may increase susceptibility to stroke since perspiration is decreased; patient should remain indoors
- Advise patient not to discontinue this drug abruptly; to taper off over 1 wk to prevent withdrawal symptoms (insomnia, involuntary movements, anxiety, tachycardias)
- Caution patient to avoid driving or other hazardous activities; drowsiness, dizziness may occur
- Teach patient to avoid OTC medication: cough, cold preparations with alcohol, antihistamines unless directed by prescriber; increased CNS depression may occur
- Advise patient to rise from sitting or recumbent position slowly to minimize orthostatic hypotension
- Teach patient to use gum, hard candy, frequent sips of water to decrease dry mouth; if dry mouth continues, saliva substitutes may be prescribed
- Instruct patient that doses should not be doubled, but missed dose may be taken up to 2 hr before next dose
- Advise patient to use good oral hygiene, use frequent sips of water, sugarless gum for dry mouth

Evaluation

Positive therapeutic outcome

- Absence of involuntary movements (pill rolling, tremors, muscle spasms)

betamethasone (Rx)

(bay-tah-meth′ah-sone)

Betnelan ♣, Betnesol ♣, Celestone, Cel-U-Jec, Selestoject ♣

Func. class.: Corticosteroid, synthetic; glucocorticoid, long acting

Pregnancy category C

Action: Decreases inflammation by suppression of migration of polymorphonuclear leukocytes, fibroblasts, reversal of increased capillary permeability and lysosomal stabilization

Therapeutic Outcome: Decreased inflammation and normal immunity

Uses: Immunosuppression, severe inflammation, prevention of neonatal respiratory distress syndrome (by administration to mother), chronic asthma, rhinitis (inh); psoriasis, eczema, contact dermatitis, pruritus (top)

Dosage and routes

Adult: PO 0.6-7.2 mg daily; IM/**IV** 0.6-7.2 mg daily in joint or soft tissue (sodium phosphate)

Child: PO 17.5 mcg/kg/day in 3 divided doses; IM 17.5 mcg/kg/day in 3 divided doses every 3rd day or 5.8-8.75 mcg/kg/day as a single dose (adrenal insufficiency)

Child: PO 62.5-250 mcg/kg/day in 3 divided doses; IM 20.8-125 mcg/kg/day of the base q12-24h (other uses)

Adult and child: TOP apply to affected area qid

Adult: INH 2-4 puffs tid-qid; not to exceed 20 inh/day

Child 6-12 yr: INH 1-2 puffs tid-qid; not to exceed 10 inh/day

Adult and child >12 yr: INSTILL 1-2 sprays in each nostril bid-qid

Available forms: Tabs 500, 600 mcg; effervescent tabs 500 mcg ♣; syr 600 mcg/5 ml; ext rel tab 1 mg; sol for inj (phosphate) 3 mg/ml; susp for inj (phosphate/acetate) 6 mg/ml

Adverse effects

CNS: *Depression, flushing, sweating,* headache, bruising, mood changes

CV: *Hypertension,* **circulatory collapse, thrombophlebitis, embolism,** tachycardia, **necrotizing angiitis, CHF**

EENT: Fungal infections, increased intraocular pressure, blurred vision

GI: *Diarrhea, nausea, abdominal distention,* **GI hemorrhage,** increased appetite, **pancreatitis**

HEMA: **Thrombocytopenia**
INTEG: ***Acne, poor wound healing, bruising,*** petechiae
MS: Fractures, osteoporosis, weakness

Contraindications: Psychosis, hypersensitivity, idiopathic thrombocytopenia, acute glomerulonephritis, amebiasis, fungal infections, nonasthmatic bronchial disease, child <2 yr, AIDS, TB

Precautions: Pregnancy **C**, diabetes mellitus, glaucoma, osteoporosis, seizure disorders, ulcerative colitis, CHF, myasthenia gravis, renal disease, esophagitis, peptic ulcer

Pharmacokinetics

Absorption	Well absorbed (PO); systemic (top)
Distribution	Crosses placenta
Metabolism	Liver, extensively
Excretion	Kidney, breast milk
Half-life	3-5 hr, adrenal suppression 3-4 days

Pharmacodynamics

	PO	IM	IV	TOP
Onset	1-2 hr	Unknown	Rapid	Unknown
Peak	2 hr	4-8 hr	4-8 hr	Unknown
Duration	3 days	1-1½ days	1-1½ days	Unknown

Interactions
Individual drugs
Alcohol, indomethacin: increased GI bleeding
Amphotericin B, mezlocillin, ticarcillin: increased hypokalemia
Insulin: increased need for insulin
Isoniazid: decreased effect
Phenytoin, rifampin: decreased action; increased metabolism

Drug classifications
Anticoagulants: decreased effect
Barbiturates: decreased action; increased metabolism
Hypoglycemic agents: increased need for hypoglycemic agents
NSAIDs, salicylates: increased GI bleeding
Toxoids/vaccines: decreased immune response

Drug/herb
Aloe, buckthorn, cascara sagrada, Chinese rhubarb, senna: increased hypokalemia
Goldenseal, hawthorn, hops, lemon balm, licorice, lily of the valley, mistletoe, perilla, pheasant's eye, squill: increased corticosteroid effect

Drug/food
Grapefruit juice should be avoided

Drug/lab test
Increased: cholesterol, sodium, blood glucose, uric acid, calcium, urine glucose
Decreased: calcium, potassium, T_4, T_3, thyroid ^{131}I uptake test, urine 17-OHCS, 17-KS, PBI
False negative: skin allergy tests

NURSING CONSIDERATIONS
Assessment
Systemic route
- Monitor potassium, blood glucose, urine glucose while on long-term therapy; hypokalemia and hyperglycemia; check weight daily; notify prescriber of weekly gain >5 lb
- Monitor B/P q4h, pulse; notify prescriber if chest pain occurs
- Monitor I&O ratio; be alert for decreasing urinary output and increasing edema
- Check plasma cortisol levels during long-term therapy (normal level: 138-635 nmol/L [SI units] when drawn at 8 AM); adrenal function periodically for HPA axis suppression
- Assess for symptoms of infection: increased temperature, WBC even after withdrawal of medication; drug masks infection symptoms
- Assess for symptoms of potassium depletion: paresthesias, fatigue, nausea, vomiting, depression, polyuria, dysrhythmias, weakness
- Monitor for edema, hypertension, cardiac symptoms
- Assess for mental status: affect, mood, behavioral changes, aggression

Topical route
- Check temperature; if fever develops, drug should be discontinued
- Assess for systemic absorption: increased temperature, inflammation, irritation

Nursing diagnoses
- Infection, risk for (adverse reactions)
- Knowledge, deficient (teaching)
- Noncompliance (teaching)

Implementation
PO route
- Give with food or milk to decrease GI symptoms

IM route
- Give IM inj deep in large mass, rotate sites, avoid deltoid, use 21-G needle; in one dose in AM to prevent adrenal suppression; avoid SUBCUT administration; may damage tissue

Inhalation route
- Give inh with water to decrease possibility of fungal infections; titrated dose; use lowest effective dose
- Use after cleaning aerosol top daily with warm water; dry thoroughly
- Store in cool environment; do not puncture or incinerate container

Topical route
- Apply only to affected areas; do not get in

eyes; apply medication, then cover with occlusive dressing (only if prescribed), seal to normal skin, change q12h; systemic absorption may occur

- Apply only to dermatoses; do not use on weeping, denuded, or infected area
- Cleanse before applying drug; use treatment for a few days after area has cleared
- Store at room temperature

IV route

- Give **IV** (only sodium phosphate product); give over >1 min; may be given by **IV** inf in compatible sol after shaking susp (parenteral)
- Give titrated dose; use lowest effective dose

Y-site compatibilities: Heparin, hydrocortisone, potassium chloride, vit B/C

Patient/family education

Systemic route

- Advise patient that long-term therapy may be needed to clear infection (1-2 mo depending on type of infection); that emergency ID as steroid user should be carried or worn; dosage adjustment may be needed
- Instruct patient to notify prescriber if therapeutic response decreases; caution patient not to discontinue abruptly; adrenal crisis can result
- Instruct patient to avoid OTC products: salicylates, alcohol in cough products, cold preparations unless directed by prescriber
- Teach patient all aspects of drug usage, including cushingoid symptoms
- Teach patient symptoms of adrenal insufficiency: nausea, anorexia, fatigue, dizziness, dyspnea, weakness, joint pain

Topical route

- Caution patient to avoid sunlight on affected area; burns may occur

Evaluation

Positive therapeutic outcome

- Ease of respirations, decreased inflammation (systemic)
- Absence of severe itching, patches on skin, flaking (top)

bethanechol (Rx)

(be-than′e-kol)

bethanechol chloride, Duvoid, Urebeth, Urecholine

Func. class.: Urinary tract stimulant, cholinergic

Chem. class.: Synthetic choline ester

Pregnancy category C

Action: Stimulates muscarinic acetylcholine receptors directly; mimics effects of parasympathetic nervous system stimulation; stimulates gastric motility, micturition; increases lower esophageal sphincter pressure

Therapeutic Outcome: Absence of continued urinary retention

Uses: Urinary retention (postoperative, postpartum), neurogenic atony of bladder with retention

Dosage and routes

Adult: PO 25-50 mg bid-qid; SUBCUT 5-10 mg tid-qid prn

Child: PO 0.6 mg/kg/day divided in 3-4 doses/day; SUBCUT 0.06 mg/kg tid or 0.15 mg/kg qid

Test dose

Adult: SUBCUT 2.5 mg repeated 15-30 min intervals × 4 doses to determine effective dose

Gastric atony, ileus (off label)

Adult: PO 10-20 mg tid-qid before meals in incomplete retention; SUBCUT 10-20 mg tid-qid if retention is complete

Available forms: Tabs 5, 10, 25, 50 mg; inj SUBCUT 5 mg/ml

Adverse effects

CNS: Dizziness

CV: Hypotension, bradycardia, orthostatic hypotension, reflex tachycardia, **cardiac arrest, circulatory collapse**

EENT: Miosis, increased salivation, lacrimation, blurred vision

GI: *Nausea, bloody diarrhea, belching, vomiting, cramps, fecal incontinence*

GU: Urgency

INTEG: Rash, urticaria, flushing, increased sweating

RESP: **Acute asthma, dyspnea, bronchoconstriction**

Contraindications: Hypersensitivity, severe bradycardia, asthma, severe hypotension, hyperthyroidism, peptic ulcer, parkinsonism, seizure disorders, CAD, COPD, coronary occlusion, mechanical obstruction, peritonitis, recent urinary or GI surgery, GI/GU obstruction

Precautions: Pregnancy **C**, hypertension, lactation, child <8 yr

Pharmacokinetics

Absorption	Poorly absorbed (PO); well absorbed (SUBCUT)
Distribution	Does not cross blood-brain barrier
Metabolism	Unknown
Excretion	Kidneys
Half-life	Unknown

Pharmacodynamics

	PO	SUBCUT
Onset	30-90 min	5-15 min
Peak	1 hr	15-30 min
Duration	1-6 hr	2 hr

Interactions

Individual drugs

Donepezil: increased action of bethanechol
Procainamide, quinidine: decreased action of bethanechol

Drug classifications

Anticholinergics: decreased action
Cholinergic agonists, anticholinesterase agents: increased action, increased toxicity
Ganglionic blockers: increased severe hypotension

Drug/herb

Jaborandi: increased cholinergic effect
Jimsonweed, scopolia: decreased effects

Drug/lab test

Increased: AST, lipase/amylase, bilirubin, BSP

NURSING CONSIDERATIONS

Assessment

- Monitor B/P, pulse, respirations; observe after parenteral dose for 1 hr
- Check I&O ratio; check for urinary retention or incontinence; if bladder emptying does not occur, notify prescriber; catheterization may be needed
- Assess for bradycardia, hypotension, bronchospasm, headache, dizziness, seizures, sweating, cramping, respiratory depression; drug should be discontinued if toxicity occurs; atropine administration

Nursing diagnoses

- Urinary elimination, impaired (uses)
- Injury, risk for (adverse reactions)
- Knowledge, deficient (teaching)

Implementation

PO route

- Give increased doses if tolerance occurs as prescribed
- To avoid nausea and vomiting, take on an empty stomach; 1 hr ac or 2 hr pc
- Store at room temperature

SUBCUT route

- Alert: Give parenteral dose by SUBCUT route; use of IM, **IV** may result in cardiac arrest or cholinergic crisis (diarrhea with blood, cramping, hypotension, circulatory collapse)
- Alert: Administer only with atropine sulfate available for cholinergic crisis; give only after all other cholinergics have been discontinued
- Do not use sol with a precipitate, or if discolored

Patient/family education

- Instruct patient to take drug exactly as prescribed; 1 hr ac or 2 hr pc; do not double doses; if dose is missed take within 1 hr of scheduled dose
- Caution patient to make position changes slowly; orthostatic hypotension may occur
- Instruct patient to report cramping, diarrhea with blood, flushing to prescriber

Evaluation

Positive therapeutic outcome

- Absence of urinary retention
- Absence of abdominal distention

Treatment of overdose: Administer atropine 0.6-1.2 mg **IV** or IM (adult)

! HIGH ALERT

bevacizumab (Rx)

(beh-va-kiz'you-mab)

Avastin

Func. class.: Antineoplastic—miscellaneous
Chem. class.: Monoclonal antibody

Pregnancy category C

Action: DNA-derived monoclonal antibody selectively binds to and inhibits activity of human vascular endothelial growth factor to reduce microvascular growth and inhibition of metastatic disease progression

Therapeutic Outcome: Decreased tumor size

Uses: Metastatic carcinoma of the colon or rectum in combination with 5-FU **IV**

Investigational uses: Adjunctive in breast, renal cancer

Dosage and routes

Adult: **IV** inf 5 mg/kg q14 days given over 90 min; if well tolerated, the next infusion may be given over 60 min; if 60 min infusions are well tolerated, subsequent infusions may be given over 30 mins.

Available forms: Inj 25 mg/ml

Adverse effects

CNS: Asthenia, dizziness
CV: **Deep vein thrombosis**, hypertension, hypotension, **hypertensive crisis**
GI: Nausea, vomiting, anorexia, diarrhea, constipation, abdominal pain, colitis, stomatitis, **GI hemorrhage**
GU: Proteinuria, urinary frequency/urgency, **nephrotic syndrome**
HEMA: **Leukopenia, neutropenia, thrombocytopenia**
META: Bilirubinemia, hypokalemia
MISC: **Exfoliative dermatitis, hemorrhage**
RESP: Dyspnea, upper respiratory infection

Contraindications: Hypersensitivity

Precautions: Pregnancy **C**, lactation, children, elderly, CHF, blood dyscrasias, cardiovascular disease, hypertension

Pharmacokinetics	
Absorption	Unknown
Distribution	Unknown
Metabolism	Unknown
Excretion	Unknown
Half-life	20 days

Pharmacodynamics	
Onset	Unknown
Peak	Unknown
Duration	Steady state 100 days

Interactions: None known

NURSING CONSIDERATIONS

Assessment

- Monitor B/P q 3-4 wk
- Assess for symptoms of infection; may be masked by drug
- Monitor CNS reaction: dizziness, confusion
- Assess for GI perforation, serious bleeding, nephrotic syndrome, hypertensive crisis, drug should be discontinued permanently; proteinuria, or surgery, drug should be discontinued temporarily

Nursing diagnoses

- Injury, risk for (adverse reactions)
- Body image, disturbed (adverse reactions)
- Infection, risk for (adverse reactions)
- Knowledge, deficient (teaching)

Implementation

IV route

- Do not give by **IV** bolus, or **IV** push
- Give as **IV** infusion over 90 min for first dose and 60 min thereafter, if well tolerated

Patient/family education

- Instruct patient to avoid hazardous tasks, since confusion, dizziness may occur
- Instruct patient to report signs of infection: sore throat, fever, diarrhea, vomiting
- Advise patient not to become pregnant while taking this drug, or for several months after discontinuing treatment
- Advise patient to notify prescriber if pregnant or planning a pregnancy

Evaluation

Positive therapeutic outcome

- Decrease in size of tumors

bexarotene (Rx)

(bex-air′-oo-teen)

Targretin

Func. class.: Retinoid, 2nd generation

Pregnancy category X

Action: Selectively binds and activates retinoid X receptors (RXRs) that are partially responsible for cellular proliferation and differentiation; inhibits some tumor cells

Therapeutic Outcome: Decreased size and number of lesions

Uses: Cutaneous T-cell lymphoma

Investigational uses: Breast cancer

Dosage and routes

Adult: PO 300 mg/day/mm^2, may increase to 400 mg/day with proper monitoring

Available forms: Caps 75 mg

Adverse effects

CNS: Headache, fatigue, lethargy
GI: Nausea, abdominal pain, diarrhea, **acute pancreatitis**
HEMA: **Leukopenia, neutropenia, anemia**
INTEG: Rash, asthenia, dry skin
SYST: Infection, hypothyroidism

Contraindications: Pregnancy **X,** hypersensitivity to retinoids

Precautions: Lactation, sunburn, hepatic, renal disease, children

Pharmacokinetics

Absorption	Unknown
Distribution	Unknown
Metabolism	Unknown
Excretion	Kidneys
Half-life	Unknown

Pharmacodynamics

Unknown

Interactions

Individual drugs

Phenytoin: decreased bexarotene levels
Tamoxifen: decreased action of tamoxifen
Vitamin A: limit intake to ≤15,000 international units/day

Drug classifications

Antidiabetics: increased action of antidiabetics
Azole antiinfectives: increased bexarotene levels
Barbiturates, rifampin: decreased bexarotene levels
Oral contraceptives: decreased action of oral contraceptives

Drug/food

Grapefruit juice: increased bexarotene levels

NURSING CONSIDERATIONS

Assessment

- Assess part of body involved, including time involved, what helps or aggravates condition, cysts, dryness, itching
- Assess cholesterol, HDL, triglycerides; these may be elevated
- Monitor CBC for leukopenia, neutropenia, anemia

Nursing diagnoses

- Skin integrity, impaired (uses)
- Body image, disturbed (uses)
- Knowledge, deficient (teaching)

Implementation

- Administer with food

Patient/family education

- Advise patient to avoid sunlight, sunlamps or to use protective clothing or sunscreen to prevent burns
- Instruct patient to avoid pregnancy while taking this drug and ≥1 mo after discontinuing therapy
- Teach patient to limit vit A to ≤15,000 international units/day to prevent toxicity
- Advise diabetic patients on insulin to watch for hypoglycemia

Evaluation

Positive therapeutic outcome

- Decrease in size and number of lesions

bicalutamide (Rx)

(bi-kal-yut'ah-mide)

Casodex

Func. class.: Antineoplastic hormone
Chem. class.: Nonsteroidal antiandrogen

Pregnancy category X

Action: Competitively inhibits the action to androgens by binding to cytosol androgen receptors in target tissue

Therapeutic Outcome: Prevention of growth of malignant cells

Uses: Prostate cancer in combination with luteinizing hormone-releasing hormone (LHRH) analog

Dosage and routes

Adult: PO 50 mg daily with LHRH

Available forms: Tabs 50 mg

Adverse effects

CV: Hot flashes, hypertension, chest pain, **CHF,** edema
CNS: Dizziness, paresthesia, insomnia, anxiety, neuropathy, headache
GI: *Diarrhea, constipation, nausea,* vomiting, increased liver enzyme test, anorexia, dry mouth, melena, abdominal pain
GU: Nocturia, **hematuria,** UTI, impotence, gynecomastia, urinary incontinence, frequency, dysuria, retention, urgency, breast tenderness, decreased libido
INTEG: Rash, sweating, dry skin, pruritus, alopecia
MISC: Infection, anemia, dyspnea, bone pain, headache, asthenia, *back pain,* flulike symptoms

Contraindications: Pregnancy **X,** hypersensitivity

Precautions: Renal, hepatic disease, elderly, lactation

Pharmacokinetics

Absorption	Well absorbed
Distribution	Unknown
Metabolism	Liver
Excretion	Urine, feces
Half-life	5.2 days

Pharmacodynamics

Onset	Unknown
Peak	31½ hr
Duration	Unknown

Interactions
Drug classifications
Anticoagulants: increased anticoagulation
Drug/lab test
Increased: AST, ALT, bilirubin, BUN, creatinine
Decreased: Hgb, WBC

NURSING CONSIDERATIONS
Assessment
- Assess for diarrhea, constipation, nausea, vomiting
- Assess for hot flashes, gynecomastia; assure patient that these are common side effects
- Monitor prostate specific antigen (PSA) liver function studies

Nursing diagnoses
- Injury, risk for (uses, adverse reactions)
- Knowledge, deficient (teaching)

Implementation
- Give at same time each day (for both drugs) either AM or PM with or without food
- Give only with LHRH treatment

Patient/family education
- Teach patient to recognize and report signs of anemia, hepatotoxicity, renal toxicity
- Advise patient that hair may be lost, but is reversible after therapy is discontinued
- Advise patient not to use other products unless approved by prescriber
- Advise patient to use contraception

Evaluation
Positive therapeutic outcome
- Decreased tumor size, spread of malignancy

biperiden (Rx)
(bye-per′i-den)
Akineton
Func. class.: Antiparkinsonian agent, anticholinergic
Pregnancy category C

Action: Centrally acting competitive anticholinergic; blocks cholinergic responses in the CNS

Therapeutic Outcome: Decreased involuntary movements

Uses: Parkinsonian symptoms, extrapyramidal symptoms (EPS) secondary to neuroleptic drug therapy

Dosage and routes
Extrapyramidal symptoms
Adult: PO 2 mg daily-tid; IM/**IV** 2 mg q30 min, if needed, not to exceed 8 mg/24 hr

Child: IM 40 mcg/kg or 1.2 mg/m^2, may repeat q½h

Parkinsonian symptoms
Adult: PO 2 mg tid-qid; max 16 mg/24 hr or 4 treatment cycles within any 30-day period

Available forms: Tabs 2 mg; inj IM/**IV** 5 mg/ml (lactate)

Adverse effects
CNS: Confusion, anxiety, restlessness, irritability, delusions, hallucinations, headache, sedation, depression, incoherence, dizziness, euphoria, tremors, memory loss
CV: Palpitations, tachycardia, postural hypotension, bradycardia
EENT: *Blurred vision,* photophobia, dilated pupils, difficulty swallowing, mydriasis, increased intraocular tension, angle closure glaucoma
GI: *Dryness of mouth, constipation,* nausea, vomiting, abdominal distress, **paralytic ileus**
GU: Hesitancy, retention, dysuria
INTEG: Rash, urticaria, dermatoses
MISC: Increased temperature, flushing, decreased sweating, **hyperthermia, heat stroke,** numbness of fingers
MS: Weakness, cramping

Contraindications: Hypersensitivity, narrow-angle glaucoma, myasthenia gravis, GI/GU obstruction, megacolon, stenosing peptic ulcers, prostatic hypertrophy

Precautions: Pregnancy **C,** elderly, lactation, tachycardia, dysrhythmias, liver, kidney disease, drug abuse, hypotension, Cognitive impairment, Alzheimer's disease, hypertension, cognitive impairments, Alzheimer's disease, psychiatric patients, children <8 yr

Pharmacokinetics

Absorption	Well absorbed (PO, IM)
Distribution	Unknown
Metabolism	Unknown
Excretion	Unknown
Half-life	18-24 hr

Pharmacodynamics

	IM/IV	PO
Onset	15 min	1 hr
Peak	Unknown	Unknown
Duration	6-10 hr	6-10 hr

Interactions
Individual drugs
Alcohol: increased sedation
Amantadine, quinidine: increased anticholinergic effects

Haloperidol: increased schizophrenic symptoms

Drug classifications

Antacids, antidiarrheals: decreased biperiden absorption
Antidepressants (tricyclic), antihistamines, phenothiazines: increased anticholinergic effects

Drug/herb

Black catechu: increased constipation
Butterbur, jimsonweed: increased biperiden effect
Kava, jaborandi, pill-bearing spurge: decreased biperiden effect

NURSING CONSIDERATIONS

Assessment

- Monitor I&O ratio; retention commonly causes decreased urinary output, distention, frequency, incontinence
- Assess for parkinsonism, EPS: shuffling gait, muscle rigidity, involuntary movements, pill rolling, muscle spasms, drooling before and during treatment
- Assess patient response if anticholinergics are given
- Monitor for urinary hesitancy, retention; palpate bladder if retention occurs
- Monitor for constipation, cramping, pain in abdomen, abdominal distention; increase fluids, bulk, exercise if this occurs
- Assess for tolerance over long-term therapy; dosage may have to be increased or changed
- Assess for mental status: affect, mood, CNS depression, worsening of mental symptoms during early therapy

Nursing diagnoses

- Mobility, impaired (uses)
- Knowledge, deficient (teaching)

Implementation

PO route

- Give with food or pc to prevent GI upset; may give with fluids other than water; hard candy, frequent drinks, gum to relieve dry mouth
- Give at bedtime to avoid daytime drowsiness in patients with parkinsonism
- Store at room temp

IV route

- Give parenteral dose with patient recumbent to prevent postural hypotension; give undiluted 2 mg or less over 1 min or more

Patient/family education

- Teach patient to use caution in hot weather; drug may increase susceptibility to heat stroke since perspiration is decreased; patient should remain indoors
- Teach patient not to discontinue this drug abruptly; to taper off over 1 wk to prevent withdrawal symptoms (insomnia, involuntary movements, anxiety, tachycardias)
- Teach patient to avoid driving or other hazardous activities; drowsiness, dizziness may occur
- Teach patient to avoid OTC medication: cough, cold preparations with alcohol, antihistamines unless directed by prescriber; increased CNS depression may occur
- Caution patient to rise from sitting or recumbent position slowly to minimize orthostatic hypotension
- Teach patient to use gum, hard candy, frequent sips of water to decrease dry mouth; if dry mouth continues, saliva substitutes may be prescribed
- Instruct patient that doses should not be doubled, but missed dose may be taken up to 2 hr before next dose

Evaluation

Positive therapeutic outcome

- Absence of involuntary movements (pill rolling, tremors, muscle spasms)

bisacodyl (OTC)

(bis-a-koe'dill)

Bisc-Evac, Bisaco-Lax, Bisacolax ✦, Bisco-Lax, Carter's Little Pills, Dacodyl, Deficol, Dulcagen, Dulcolax, Feen-a-Mint, Fleet Laxative, Laxit ✦, Modane, Reliable Gentle Laxative, Therelax

Func. class.: Laxative, stimulant
Chem. class.: Diphenylmethane

Pregnancy category C

Action: Acts directly on intestine by increasing motor activity; thought to irritate colonic intramural plexus; increases water in the colon

Therapeutic Outcome: Decreased constipation

Uses: Short-term treatment of constipation, bowel or rectal preparation for surgery, examination

Dosage and routes

Adult ≥12 yr: PO 5-15 mg in PM or AM; may use up to 30 mg for bowel or rec preparation; REC 10 mg (single dose)
Child 2-11 yr: PO 5-10 mg as a single dose; REC 10 mg as a single dose, do not use oral rate
Child <2 yr: REC 5 mg as a single dose; do not use oral rate

B

Available forms: Enteric coated tabs 5 mg; supp 5, 10 mg; rec sol 10 mg/37 ml; enema 0.33 mg/ml, 10 mg/5 ml; powder for rec sol 1.5 mg bisacodyl/2.5 g tannic acid

Adverse effects

CNS: Muscle weakness
GI: *Nausea, vomiting, anorexia, cramps,* diarrhea, rectal burning (supp)
META: Protein-losing enteropathy, alkalosis, hypokalemia, **tetany,** electrolyte and fluid imbalances

Contraindications: Hypersensitivity, rectal fissures, abdominal pain, nausea, vomiting, appendicitis, acute surgical abdomen, ulcerated hemorrhoids, acute hepatitis, fecal impaction, intestinal/biliary tract obstruction

Precautions: Pregnancy **C**, lactation

Pharmacokinetics

Absorption	Poor
Distribution	Unknown
Metabolism	Liver, minimally
Excretion	Kidneys
Half-life	Unknown

Pharmacodynamics

	PO	RECT
Onset	6-10 hr	15-60 min
Peak	Unknown	Unknown
Duration	Unknown	Unknown

Interactions

Drug classifications

Antacids, gastric acid pump inhibitors, H_2-blockers: increased gastric irritation

Drug/herb

Flax, lily of the valley, pheasant's eye, senna, squill: increased laxative action

Drug/food

Milk: increased gastric irritation

NURSING CONSIDERATIONS

Assessment

- Monitor blood, urine electrolytes if used often by patient; check I&O ratio to identify fluid loss
- Assess cramping, rectal bleeding, nausea, vomiting; if these symptoms occur, drug should be discontinued; identify cause of constipation; identify whether fluids, bulk, or exercise missing from lifestyle

Nursing diagnoses

- Constipation (uses)
- Diarrhea (side effects)
- Knowledge, deficient (teaching)
- Noncompliance (teaching)

Implementation

PO route

- Swallow tabs whole; do not break, crush, or chew
- Give alone with water only for better absorption; do not take within 1 hr of antacids, milk
- Administer in AM or PM (oral dose)

Rectal route

- Lubricate before insertion, patient should retain for ½ hr

Patient/family education

- Discuss with the patient that adequate fluid and bulk consumption is necessary
- Advise patient that normal bowel movements do not always occur daily
- Teach patient not to use in presence of abdominal pain, nausea, vomiting; tell patient to notify prescriber if constipation unrelieved or if symptoms of electrolyte imbalance occur: muscle cramps, pain, weakness, dizziness, excessive thirst

Evaluation

Positive therapeutic outcome

- Decreased constipation within 3 days

bismuth subsalicylate (OTC)

(bis′meth sub-sa-li′si-late)

Bismatrol, Bismatrol Extra Strength, Bismed, Pepto-Bismol, Pepto-Bismol Maximum Strength, Pink Bismuth, PMS-Bismuth Subsalicylate

Func. class.: Antidiarrheal
Chem. class.: Salicylate

Pregnancy category C

Action: Inhibits prostaglandin synthesis responsible for GI hypermotility; stimulates absorption of fluid and electrolytes; antimicrobial, antisecretory effects

Therapeutic Outcome: Absence of loose, watery stools

Uses: Diarrhea (cause undetermined); prevention of diarrhea when traveling; may be included to treat *Helicobacter pylori*

Dosage and routes

Antidiarrheal

Adult: PO 524 mg q½h or 1048 mg q1h, max 4.2 g/24 hr
Child 9-12 yr: PO 15 ml; 262 mg q½-1h, max 2.1 g/24 hr

Child 6-9 yr: PO 174.6 mg q½-1h, max 1.4 g/24 hr
Child 3-6 yr: PO 88 mg q½-1h, max 704 mg/24 hr

Available forms: Tabs 262 mg; chewable tabs 262, 300 mg; susp 262, 524 mg/15 ml

Adverse effects

CNS: Confusion, twitching
EENT: Hearing loss, tinnitus, metallic taste, blue gums, black tongue (chew tabs)
GI: Increased fecal impaction (high doses), dark stools, constipation
HEMA: Increased bleeding time

Contraindications: Child <3 yr; impaction, children, teens with flulike symptoms, hypersensitivity (aspirin), history of GI bleeding, renal disease

Precautions: Pregnancy **C,** anticoagulant therapy, elderly, lactation, gout, diabetes mellitus, immobility

Pharmacokinetics	
Absorption	Salicylate >90%
Distribution	None
Metabolism	None
Excretion	Feces (unchanged)
Half-life	Unknown

Pharmacodynamics	
Onset	1 hr
Peak	2 hr
Duration	4 hr

Interactions

Individual drugs

Aminosalicylic acid: increased side effects, increased toxicity
Tetracycline: decreased absorption

Drug classifications

Anticoagulants (oral): increased effect of anticoagulants
Antidiabetics (oral): increased effect of antidiabetics
Salicylates: increased risk of salicylate toxicity

Drug/herb

Nutmeg: increased antidiarrheal effect
Sarsaparilla: increased bismuth absorption

Drug/lab test

Interference: radiographic studies of GI system

NURSING CONSIDERATIONS

Assessment

- Monitor skin turgor; dehydration may occur in severe diarrhea; monitor electrolytes (potassium, sodium, chloride) if diarrhea is severe or continues long term
- Assess bowel pattern (frequency, consistency, shape, volume, color) before drug therapy, after treatment; check weight, bowel sounds; identify factors contributing to diarrhea (bacteria, diet, medications, tube feedings)

Nursing diagnoses

- Diarrhea (uses)
- Constipation (adverse reactions)
- Knowledge, deficient (teaching)

Implementation

- Shake susp before use; chewable tabs should not be swallowed whole

Patient/family education

- Teach patient to stop use if symptoms do not improve within 2 days or become worse, or if diarrhea is accompanied by high fever
- Teach patient to increase fluids for rehydration
- Tell patient to chew or dissolve chewable tabs in mouth; do not swallow whole; shake susp before using
- Tell patient to avoid other salicylates unless directed by prescriber; not to give to children because of possibility of Reye's syndrome
- Tell patient that stools may turn gray; tongue may darken; impaction may occur in debilitated patients

Evaluation

Positive therapeutic outcome

- Decreased diarrhea

bisoprolol (Rx)

(bis-oh'pro-lole)
Zebeta
Func. class.: Antihypertensive
Chem. class.: β_1-Blocker (selective)
Pregnancy category C

Do Not Confuse:

Zebeta/Diabeta/Zetia

Action: Preferentially and competitively blocks stimulation of β_1-adrenergic receptor within cardiac muscle (decreases rate of SA node discharge, increases recovery time), slows conduction of AV node, decreases heart rate, which decreases O_2 consumption in myocardium; decreases renin-aldosterone-angiotensin system; inhibits β_2-receptors in bronchial and vascular smooth muscle at high doses

Therapeutic Outcome: Decreased B/P, heart rate

Uses: Mild to moderate hypertension

Investigational uses: Stable angina pectoris, stable CHF

Dosage and routes

Renal/hepatic dose

Adult: PO 2.5 mg, titrate upward

Hypertension

Adult: PO 5 mg daily; may increase if necessary to 20 mg once daily; may need to reduce dose in presence of renal or hepatic impairment

Available forms: Tabs 5, 10 mg

Adverse effects

CNS: Vertigo, headache, insomnia, fatigue, dizziness, mental changes, memory loss, hallucinations, depression, lethargy, drowsiness, strange dreams, catatonia, peripheral neuropathy
CV: **Ventricular dysrhythmias, profound hypotension, bradycardia, CHF,** cold extremities, postural hypotension, 2nd- or 3rd-degree heart block
EENT: Sore throat, dry burning eyes
ENDO: Increased hypoglycemic response to insulin
GI: Nausea, diarrhea, vomiting, **mesenteric arterial thrombosis,** ischemic colitis, flatulence, gastritis, gastric pain
GU: Impotence, decreased libido
HEMA: **Agranulocytosis, thrombocytopenia,** purpura, **eosinophilia**
INTEG: Rash, flushing, alopecia, pruritus, sweating
MISC: Facial swelling, weight gain, decreased exercise tolerance
MS: Joint pain, arthralgia
RESP: **Bronchospasm,** dyspnea, wheezing, cough, nasal stuffiness

Contraindications: Hypersensitivity to β-blockers, cardiogenic shock, heart block (2nd or 3rd degree), sinus bradycardia, CHF, cardiac failure

Precautions: Pregnancy **C,** major surgery, lactation, children, diabetes mellitus, renal or hepatic disease, thyroid disease, COPD, asthma, well-compensated heart failure, aortic or mitral valve disease, peripheral vascular disease, myasthenia gravis

Pharmacokinetics	
Absorption	Well absorbed
Distribution	Unknown; protein binding (30%)
Metabolism	Liver, inactive metabolites
Excretion	Urine, unchanged (50%)
Half-life	9-12 hr

Pharmacodynamics	
Onset	Unknown
Peak	2-4 hr
Duration	24 hr

Interactions

Individual drugs

Guanethidine, reserpine: increased hypotension

Drug classifications

Calcium channel blockers: increased myocardial depression
Ergots: increased peripheral ischemia
NSAIDs: decreased antihypertensive effects

Drug/herb

Aconite: increased toxicity, death
Betel palm, butterbur, cola tree, figwort, fumitory, guarana, hawthorn, lily of the valley, motherwort, plantain: increased β-blocking effect
Coenzyme Q10, yohimbe: decreased β-blocking effect

Drug/lab test

Increased: AST, ALT, blood glucose, BUN, uric acid, potassium, lipoprotein, ANA titer
Interference: glucose/insulin tolerance tests

NURSING CONSIDERATIONS

Assessment

- Monitor B/P during beginning treatment, periodically thereafter; pulse q4h: note rate, rhythm, quality; apical/radial pulse before administration; notify prescriber of any significant changes (pulse <50 bpm)
- Check for baselines in renal, liver function tests before therapy begins
- Assess for edema in feet, legs daily, monitor I&O, daily weight; check for jugular vein distention, crackles, bilaterally, dyspnea (CHF)
- Monitor skin turgor, dryness of mucous membranes for hydration status, especially elderly

Nursing diagnoses

- Cardiac output, decreased (uses)
- Injury, risk for (side effects)
- Knowledge, deficient (teaching)
- Noncompliance (teaching)

Implementation

- Give daily; give with food to prevent GI upset; may be crushed
- Store protected from light, moisture; place in cool environment

Patient/family education

- Teach patient not to discontinue drug abruptly; may cause precipitate angina if stopped abruptly, evaluate noncompliance
- Teach patient not to use OTC products containing α-adrenergic stimulants (such as nasal decongestants, cold preparations); to avoid alcohol, smoking and to limit sodium intake as prescribed
- Teach patient how to take pulse and B/P at home; advise when to notify prescriber
- Instruct patient to comply with weight control, dietary adjustments, modified exercise program
- Tell patient to carry/wear emergency ID to identify drug being taken, allergies; tell patient drug controls symptoms but does not cure
- Caution patient to avoid hazardous activities if dizziness, drowsiness present
- Teach patient to take drug as prescribed, not to double doses, skip doses; take any missed doses as soon as remembered if at least 8 hr until next dose
- Advise patient to report bradycardia, dizziness, confusion, depression, fever, cold extremities
- Teach patient if diabetic, may mask signs of hypoglycemia, or alter blood glucose levels

Evaluation

Positive therapeutic outcome

- Decreased B/P in hypertension (after 1-2 wk)

Treatment of overdose: Lavage, **IV** atropine for bradycardia, **IV** theophylline for bronchospasm, digitalis, O_2, diuretic for cardiac failure, hemodialysis, **IV** glucose for hypoglycemia, **IV** diazepam (or phenytoin) for seizures

! HIGH ALERT

bivalirudin (Rx)

(bye-val-i-rue′din)

Angiomax

Func. class.: Anticoagulant

Chem. class.: Thrombin inhibitor

Pregnancy category B

Action: Direct inhibitor of thrombin that is highly specific

Therapeutic Outcome: Anticoagulation in percutaneous transluminal coronary angioplasty (PTCA)

Uses: Unstable angina in patients undergoing PTCA

Dosage and routes

Adult: **IV** bol 0.75 mg/kg, then **IV** inf 1.75 mg/kg/hr for 4 hr; another **IV** inf may be used at 0.2 mg/kg/hr for ≤20 hr; this drug is intended to be used with aspirin (325 mg daily) adjusted to body weight

Renal dose

Adult: **IV** GFR 30-59 ml/min give 1.75 mg/kg/h; GFR 10-29 ml/min give 1 mg/kg/h; dialysis-dependent patients give 0.25 mg/kg/h

Available forms: Inj, lyophilized 250 mg vial

Adverse effects

CNS: *Headache, insomnia, anxiety, nervousness*

CV: *Hypo/hypertension, bradycardia*

GI: *Nausea, vomiting, abdominal pain, dyspepsia*

HEMA: **Hemorrhage**

MISC: Pain at inj site, pelvic pain, urinary retention, fever

MS: *Back pain*

Contraindications: Hypersensitivity, active bleeding

Precautions: Pregnancy **B,** renal function impairment, lactation, children, hepatic disease, elderly

Pharmacokinetics	
Absorption	Unknown
Distribution	No protein binding
Metabolism	Unknown
Excretion	Kidneys
Half-life	25 min

Pharmacodynamics	
Duration	1 hr

Interactions

Drug classifications

Anticoagulants, thrombolytics: increased risk of bleeding

Drug/herb

Agrimony, alfalfa, angelica, anise, bilberry, black haw, bogbean, buchu, chondroitin, dong quai, fenugreek, feverfew, garlic, ginger, ginkgo, ginseng, horse chestnut, Irish moss,

kelp, kelpware, khella, lovage, lungwort, meadowsweet, motherwort, mugwort, nettle, papaya, parsley (large amounts), pau d'arco, pineapple, poplar, prickly ash, safflower, saw palmetto, tonka bean, turmeric, wintergreen, yarrow: increased risk of bleeding
Chamomile, coenzyme Q10, flax, glucomannan, goldenseal, guar gum: decreased anticoagulant effect

NURSING CONSIDERATIONS
Assessment
- Assess for fall in B/P or Hct that may indicate hemorrhage
- Assess for fever, skin rash, urticaria
- Assess bleeding: check arterial and venous sites, IM inj sites, catheters; all punctures should be minimized

Nursing diagnoses
- Cardiac output, decreased (uses)
- Knowledge, deficient (teaching)

Implementation
- Prior to PTCA, give with aspirin, 325 mg

IV direct 1 mg/kg as a bolus; then intermittent infusion

Intermittent IV infusion route
- To each 250-mg vial add 5 ml of sterile water for inj, swirl until dissolved, further dilute reconstituted vial with 50 ml of D_5W or 0.9% NaCl (5 mg/ml); the dose is adjusted to body weight, run at 2.5 mg/kg/hr, do not admix before or during administration
- Give reduced dose in renal impairment

Patient/family education
- Explain reason for drug and expected results

Evaluation
Positive therapeutic outcome
- Anticoagulation in PTCA

! HIGH ALERT

bleomycin (Rx)
(blee-oh-mye'sin)
Blenoxane
Func. class.: Antineoplastic, antibiotic
Chem. class.: Glycopeptide

Pregnancy category D

Action: Inhibits synthesis of DNA, RNA, protein; derived from *Streptomyces verticillus;* replication is decreased by binding to DNA, which causes strand splitting; phase specific in the G_2 and M phases; a nonvesicant

Therapeutic Outcome: Prevention of rapidly growing malignant cells

Uses: Cancer of head, neck, penis, cervix, vulva of squamous cell origin, Hodgkin's disease, lymphosarcoma, reticulum cell sarcoma, testicular carcinoma, malignant pleural effusion

Dosage and routes
Adult and child: SUBCUT/**IV**/IM 0.25-0.5 units/kg q1-2 wk or 10-20 units/m^2; then 1 unit/day or 5 units/wk; may also be given by cont inf; do not exceed total dose, 400 units in lifetime

Malignant pleural effusion
Adult: 60 units diluted in 100 ml of 0.9% NaCl intrapleural inj given through a thoracotomy tube following drainage of excess pleural fluid and complete lung expansion, remove after 4 hr

Available forms: Powder for inj 15, 30 units/vial

Adverse effects
CNS: Pain at tumor site, headache, confusion
CV: Hypotension, peripheral vasoconstriction
GI: *Nausea, vomiting, anorexia, stomatitis, weight loss,* ulceration of mouth, lips
HEMA: Hypotension, peripheral vasoconstriction
IDIOSYNCRATIC REACTION: Hypotension, confusion, fever, chills, wheezing
INTEG: *Rash, hyperkeratosis, nail changes, alopecia,* pruritus, acne, striae, peeling, hyperpigmentation
RESP: **Fibrosis,** pneumonitis, wheezing, **pulmonary toxicity**
SYST: **Anaphylaxis,** radiation recall, Raynaud's phenomenon

Contraindications: Pregnancy **D,** hypersensitivity, prior idiosyncratic reaction

Precautions: Renal, hepatic, respiratory disease, patients >70 yr old

Pharmacokinetics

Absorption	Well absorbed (IM, SUBCUT, intrapleural, intraperitoneal)
Distribution	Widely distributed
Metabolism	Liver, 30%
Excretion	Kidneys, unchanged (50%)
Half-life	2 hr; increased in renal disease

Pharmacodynamics
Unknown

Interactions

Individual drugs

Fosphenytoin, phenytoin: decreased phenytoin levels

Radiation: increased toxicity, bone marrow suppression

Drug classifications

Anesthetics (general), antineoplastics: increased toxicity

NURSING CONSIDERATIONS

Assessment

- Assess buccal cavity q8h for dryness, sores or ulceration, white patches, oral pain, bleeding, dysphagia; obtain prescription for viscous lidocaine (Xylocaine)
- ❗ Assess symptoms indicating anaphylaxis: rash, pruritus, urticaria, purpuric skin lesions, itching, flushing, wheezing, hypotension; have emergency equipment available
- Monitor CBC, differential, platelet count weekly; withhold drug if WBC $<4000/mm^3$ or platelet count $<100,000/mm^3$; notify prescriber of results if WBC $<20,000/mm^3$, platelets $<150,000/mm^3$
- Monitor temp q4h (may indicate beginning of infection)
- Monitor liver function tests before and during therapy (bilirubin, AST, ALT, LDH) as needed or monthly
- Assess for bleeding: hematuria, stool guaiac, bruising or petechiae, mucosa or orifices q8h; inflammation of mucosa, breaks in skin
- Identify dyspnea, crackles, unproductive cough, chest pain, tachypnea
- Identify effects of alopecia on body image; discuss feelings about body changes; if edema in feet, joint pain, stomach pain, shaking present, prescriber should be notified; identify inflammation of mucosa, breaks in skin

Nursing diagnoses

- Injury, risk for (adverse reactions)
- Body image, disturbed (adverse reactions)
- Infection, risk for (adverse reactions)
- Knowledge, deficient (teaching)

Implementation

- Avoid contact with skin, very irritating; wash completely to remove
- Give fluids **IV** or PO before chemotherapy to hydrate patient
- Give antacid before oral agent; give antiemetic 30-60 min before giving drug to prevent vomiting and prn and antibiotics for prophylaxis of infection
- Provide liq diet: carbonated beverages, gelatin may be added if patient is not nauseated or vomiting
- Rinsing of mouth tid-qid with water, club soda; brushing of teeth bid-qid with soft brush or cotton-tipped applicators for stomatitis; use unwaxed dental floss

IM/SUBCUT route

- IM test dose in lymphoma
- Reconstitute with 1-5 ml sterile water for inj; D_5W, 0.9% NaCl, rotate inj sites

IV route

- Drug should be prepared by experienced personnel using proper precautions
- Two test doses 2-5 units before initial dose in lymphoma; monitor for anaphylaxis
- Give by direct **IV** after reconstituting 15 units or less/5 ml or more of D_5W or 0.9% NaCl; give 15 units or less/10 min through Y-tube or 3-way stopcock initial dose; monitor for anaphylaxis

Intermittent IV infusion route

- Administer after diluting 50-100 ml 0.9% NaCl, D_5W and giving at prescribed rate

Intrapleural route

- Give 60 units/50-100 ml of 0.9% NaCl, administered by physician through thoracotomy tube

Syringe compatibilities: Cisplatin, cyclophosphamide, DOXOrubicin, droperidol, fluorouracil, furosemide, heparin, leucovorin, methotrexate, metoclopramide, mitomycin, vinBLAStine, vinCRIStine

Y-site compatibilities: Allopurinol, amisostine, aztreonam, cisplatin, cyclophosphamide, DOXOrubicin, DOXOrubicin liposome, droperidol, filgrastim, fludarabine, fluorouracil, granisetron, heparin, leucovorin, melphalan, methotrexate, metoclopramide, mitomycin, ondansetron, paclitaxel, piperacillin/tazobactam, sargramostim, teniposide, thiotepa, vinBLAStine, vinCRIStine, vinorelbine

Additive compatibilities: Amikacin, cephapirin, dexamethasone, diphenhydrAMINE, fluorouracil, gentamicin, heparin, hydrocortisone, phenytoin, streptomycin, tobramycin, vinBLAStine, vinCRIStine

Additive incompatibilities: Aminophylline, ascorbic acid inj, carbenicillin, cefazolin, cephalothin, diazepam, hydrocortisone, methotrexate, mitomycin, nafcillin, penicillin G sodium, terbutaline

Solution compatibilities: 0.9% NaCl

Patient/family education

- Teach patient to avoid use of products containing aspirin or ibuprofen, razors, commercial mouthwash; bleeding may occur; to report symptoms of bleeding (hematuria, tarry stools)

• Instruct patient to report signs of anemia (fatigue, headache, irritability, faintness, shortness of breath)
• Instruct patient to report any changes in breathing or coughing even several months after treatment; to avoid crowds and persons with respiratory tract or other infections
• Inform patient that hair may be lost during treatment; a wig or hairpiece may make patient feel better; new hair may be different in color, texture
• Caution patient not to have any vaccinations without the advice of the prescriber; serious reactions can occur
• Advise patient contraception is needed during treatment and for several months after completion of therapy

Evaluation

Positive therapeutic outcome
• Prevention of rapid division of malignant cells

bortezomib (Rx)

(bor-tez′oh-mib)
Velcade
Func. class.: Antineoplastic—miscellaneous
Chem. class.: Proteasome inhibitor

Pregnancy category D

Action: Reversible inhibitor of chymotrypsin-like activity in mammalian cells; causes a delay in tumor growth

Therapeutic Outcome: Decreased growth and spread of malignant cells.

Uses: Multiple myeloma when at least two other treatments have failed.

Dosage and routes

***Adult:* IV** BOL 1.3 mg/m^2/dose 2×/wk for 2 wk (days 1, 4, 8, 11) followed by 10-day rest period (days 12 to 21); max 8 cycles

Neuropathic pain
Grade 1 with pain or grade 2: Reduce to 1 mg/m^2; Grade 2 with pain or grade 3: Hold drug until toxicity resolves, then start at 0.7 mg/m^2 qwk; Grade 4 hematologic toxicities, withhold use

Available forms: Lyophilized powder for inj 3.5 mg

Adverse effects

CNS: Anxiety, insomnia, dizziness, headache, peripheral neuropathy, rigors, paresthesia
CV: Hypotension, edema
GI: Abdominal pain, constipation, diarrhea, dyspepsia, nausea, vomiting, anorexia
HEMA: Anemia, **neutropenia, thrombocytopenia,**
MISC: Dehydration, weight loss, herpes zoster, rash, pruritus, blurred vision
MS: Fatigue, malaise, weakness, arthralgia, bone pain, muscle cramps, myalgia, back pain
RESP: Cough, pneumonia, dyspnea, URI

Contraindications: Pregnancy **D**, hypersensitivity to this drug, boron, or mannitol

Precautions: Peripheral neuropathy, elderly, hepatic, renal disease, hypotension, lactation, children

Pharmacokinetics

Absorption	Unknown
Distribution	Protein binding 83%
Metabolism	P450 enzymes (3A4, 2D6, 2C19, 2C9, 1A2)
Excretion	Unknown
Half-life	9-15 hr

Pharmacodynamics

Onset	Unknown
Peak	Unknown
Duration	Unknown

Interactions

Individual drugs
Amiodarone, isoniazid, nitrofurantoin: increased peripheral neuropathy
Bortezomib: increased exposure to CYP450 2C19 substrates

Drug classifications
Antihypertensives: increased hypotension
Antivirals, statins: increased peripheral neuropathy
Drugs that induce or inhibit CYP450 3A4: increased toxicity or decreased efficacy
Oral hypoglycemics: increased hypo/hyperglycemia

NURSING CONSIDERATIONS

Assessment

• Assess hematologic status: platelets, CBC throughout treatment
• Monitor for extravasation at inj site

Nursing diagnoses

• Injury, physical (uses, adverse reactions)
• Knowledge, deficient (teaching)

Implementation

• Reconstitute each vial with 3.5 ml 0.9% NaCl
• Use protective clothing during handling, preparation; avoid contact with skin

Patient/family education

- Teach to use contraception while on this drug, avoid breastfeeding
- Advise to monitor blood glucose levels if diabetic
- Instruct to contact prescriber if new or worsening peripheral neuropathy, severe vomiting, diarrhea
- Advise to avoid driving, operating machinery until effect is known
- Advise to avoid using other medications unless approved by prescriber

Evaluation

Positive therapeutic outcome

- Improvement of multiple myeloma symptoms

bosentan (Rx)

(boh-sen-tan)

Tracleer

Func. class.: Vasodilator

Chem. class.: Endothelin receptor antagonist

Pregnancy category X

Action: Peripheral vasodilation occurs via antagonism of the effect of endothelin on endothelium and vascular smooth muscle

Therapeutic Outcome: Decreased pulmonary arterial hypertension

Uses: Pulmonary arterial hypertension with class III, IV symptoms

Investigational uses: Septic shock to improve microcirculatory blood flow

Dosage and routes

Adult >40 kg and >12 yr: PO 62.5 mg bid × 4 wk, then 125 mg bid

Adult <40 kg and >12 yr: PO 62.5 mg bid

Available forms: Tabs 62.5, 125 mg

Adverse effects

CNS: Headache, flushing, fatigue

CV: *Hypotension,* palpitations, edema of lower limbs

GI: Abnormal liver function, dyspepsia, **hepatotoxicity**

INTEG: Pruritus

MISC: Anemia

Contraindications: Pregnancy **X**, hypersensitivity, CVA, CAD

Precautions: Mitral stenosis, elderly, lactation, impaired hepatic function, children

Pharmacokinetics

Absorption	50% absorbed
Distribution	Protein binding >98%
Metabolism	Liver (metabolites); metabolized CYP2C9, CYP3A4, and possibly CYP2C19; steady state 3-5 days
Excretion	Biliary
Half-life	5 hr

Pharmacodynamics

Onset	Unknown
Peak	Unknown
Duration	Unknown

Interactions

Individual drugs

CycloSPORINE A, glyBURIDE: do not coadminister

CycloSPORINE A, ketoconazole: increased bosentan level

CycloSPORINE: decreased cycloSPORINE level

GlyBURIDE: glyBURIDE level decreased significantly, bosentan also decreased, increased liver function tests

Simvastatin: decreased effects

Warfarin: decreased anticoagulation

Drug classifications

Contraceptives (hormonal), statins: decreased effects

Drug/lab test

Increased: ALT, AST

Decreased: Hgb, Hct

NURSING CONSIDERATIONS

Assessment

- Assess B/P, pulse during treatment until stable
- Assess hepatic tests: AST, ALT, bilirubin; liver enzymes may increase; if ALT/AST >3 and ≤5 × ULN, confirm lab value, decrease dose or interrupt treatment and monitor AST/ALT q2wk; if >8 × ULN, stop treatment
- Assess blood studies: Hct, Hgb may be decreased
- Assess hepatic involvement: vomiting, jaundice; drug should be discontinued

Nursing diagnoses

- Tissue perfusion, ineffective (uses)
- Knowledge, deficient (teaching)

Implementation

- Store at room temp

Patient/family education

- Instruct patient to report jaundice, dark urine, joint pain, fatigue, malaise, bruising, easy bleeding; may indicate blood dyscrasias

• Caution patient to avoid pregnancy; to use nonhormonal form of contraception

Evaluation

Positive therapeutic outcome

• Decrease in pulmonary hypertension

! HIGH ALERT

bretylium (Rx)

(bre-til'ee-um)

Bretylate, bretylium tosylate, Bretylol

Func. class.: Antidysrhythmic (Class III)

Chem. class.: Quaternary ammonium compound

Pregnancy category C

Action: After a transient release of norepinephrine, inhibits further release by postganglionic nerve endings; prolongs action potential, duration, and effective refractory period

Therapeutic Outcome: Absence of dysrhythmias

Uses: Life-threatening ventricular tachycardia, cardioversion, ventricular fibrillation; for short-term use only

Dosage and routes

Renal dose

Adult: **IV** CCr 10-50 ml/min 25%-50% dose; CCr <10 ml/min avoid use

Severe ventricular fibrillation

Adult: **IV** bol 5 mg/kg; increase to 10 mg/kg repeated q15 min, up to 30 mg/kg; **IV** inf 1-2 mg/min or give 5-10 mg/kg over 10 min q6h (maintenance)

Ventricular tachycardia

Adult: **IV** inf 500 mg diluted in 50 ml D_5W or NS; infuse over 10-30 min; may repeat in 1 hr; maintain with 1-2 mg/min or 5-10 mg/kg over 10-30 min q6h; IM 5-10 mg/kg undiluted; repeat in 1-2 hr if needed; maintain with same dose q6-8h

Child: 2-5mg/kg/dose

Available forms: Inj 50 mg/ml; 1, 2, 4 mg/ml prefilled syringes

Adverse effects

CNS: *Syncope, dizziness,* confusion, psychosis, anxiety

CV: *Hypotension, postural hypotension, bradycardia,* angina, PVCs, substernal pressure, transient hypertension, precipitation of angina

GI: *Nausea, vomiting*

RESP: **Respiratory depression**

Contraindications: Hypersensitivity, digitalis toxicity, aortic stenosis, pulmonary hypertension, children

Precautions: Pregnancy **C**, renal disease, lactation, children

Pharmacokinetics

Absorption	Complete bioavailability (**IV**)
Distribution	Unknown
Metabolism	Not metabolized
Excretion	Kidneys, unchanged
Half-life	4-17 hr

Pharmacodynamics

	IV	IM
Onset	5 min	½-2 hr
Peak	Infusion's end	Unknown
Duration	6-24 hr	6-24 hr

Interactions

Individual drugs

Caffeine: decreased effects of bretylium

Carbamazepine: increased heart block

Dopamine, norepinephrine: increased pressor effects

Drug classifications

Cardiac glycosides: increased toxicity

Sympathomimetics: increased sympathomimetic effect

Drug/herb

Aconite: increased toxicity, death

Aloe, broom, buckthorn (chronic use), cascara sagrada (chronic use), Chinese rhubarb, figwort, fumitory, goldenseal, kudzu, licorice: increased effect

Coltsfoot: decreased effect

Horehound: increased serotonin effect

NURSING CONSIDERATIONS

Assessment

• Monitor ECG continuously to determine drug effectiveness; measure PR, QRS, QT intervals; check for PVCs, other dysrhythmias; monitor B/P continuously for hypotension, hypertension; check for rebound hypertension after 1-2 hr

Nursing diagnoses

• Cardiac output, decreased (uses)
• Gas exchange, impaired (adverse reactions)
• Knowledge, deficient (teaching)

Implementation

IM route

• Give in large muscle mass, rotate sites to prevent necrosis

IV, direct route

- Give **IV** bol undiluted; give 6 mg or less over 1 min; if using an **IV** line, use port near insertion site, flush with NS (50 ml)

Intermittent IV infusion route

- Give by intermittent inf after diluting 500 mg/50 ml or more with 0.9% NaCl, D_5W, D_5/0.45% NaCl, D_5/0.9% NaCl, LR, ⅙ mol/L sodium lactate; run over >8 min

Continuous infusion route

- Give by cont inf diluted in sol; give 1-2 mg/min; use inf site
- Store at room temp; sol should be clear

Additive compatibilities: Aminophylline, atracurium, calcium chloride, calcium gluconate, digoxin, DOPamine, esmolol, regular insulin, lidocaine, potassium chloride, quinadine verapamil

Y-site compatibilities: Amiodarone, inamrinone, cisatracurium, diltiazem, DOBUTamine, famotidine, isoproterenol, ranitidine, remifentanil

Additive incompatibilities: Phenytoin

Evaluation

Positive therapeutic outcome

- Decreased B/P, dysrhythmias, heart rate; normal sinus rhythm

bromocriptine (Rx)

(broe-moe-krip'teen)

Alti-Bromocriptine ✦, Apo-Bromocriptine ✦, Parlodel

Func. class.: Antiparkinsonian agent; DOPamine receptor agonist

Chem. class.: Ergot alkaloid derivative

Pregnancy category B

Do Not Confuse:
Parlodel/pindolol/Provera

Action: Inhibits prolactin release by activating postsynaptic dopamine receptors; activation of striatal dopamine receptors may be reason for improvement in Parkinson's disease

Therapeutic Outcome: Decreased involuntary movements in Parkinson's disease; decreased lactation; decreased hormone levels in acromegaly; absence of amenorrhea in hyperprolactinemia

Uses: Adjunct with levodopa in Parkinson's disease, amenorrhea/galactorrhea caused by hyperprolactinemia, acromegaly

Investigational uses: Pituitary adenomas, neuroleptic malignant syndrome

Dosage and routes

Hyperprolactinemia

Adult: PO 1.25-2.5 mg with meals; may increase by 2.5 mg q3-7 days; usual dosage 5-7.5 mg

Acromegaly

Adult: PO 1.25-2.5 mg/day × 3 days at bedtime may increase by 1.25-2.5 mg q3-7 days; usual range 20-30 mg/day; max 100 mg/day

Parkinson's disease

Adult: PO 1.25 mg bid with meals; may increase q2-4 wk by 2.5 mg/day; not to exceed 100 mg/day

Pituitary adenoma

Adult: PO 1.25 mg bid-tid, may increase over several weeks

Neuroleptic malignant syndrome (off-label)

Adult: PO 5 mg daily, max 20 mg/day

Cocaine withdrawal

Adult: PO 0.625 mg qid × 42 days

Alcoholism (off-label)

Adult: PO 7.5 mg/day

Mastalgia

Adult: PO 2.5-7.5 bid, starting 10-14 days prior to menses, discontinue when menses begins

Available forms: Caps 5 mg; tabs 2.5 mg

Adverse effects

CNS: *Headache,* depression, restlessness, anxiety, nervousness, confusion, **seizures,** hallucinations, *dizziness,* fatigue, drowsiness, abnormal involuntary movements, psychosis

CV: *Orthostatic hypotension,* decreased B/P, palpitations, extrasystole, **shock,** dysrhythmias, bradycardia, **MI**

EENT: Blurred vision, diplopia, burning eyes, nasal congestion

GI: *Nausea, vomiting, anorexia,* cramps, constipation, diarrhea, dry mouth, GI hemorrhage

GU: Frequency, retention, incontinence, diuresis

INTEG: *Rash on face, arms,* alopecia, coolness, pallor of fingers, toes

Contraindications: Hypersensitivity to ergot, severe ischemic disease, severe peripheral vascular disease

Precautions: Pregnancy **B,** lactation, hepatic disease, renal disease, children, pituitary tumors

B

Pharmacokinetics	
Absorption	Poorly absorbed
Distribution	Unknown
Metabolism	Liver, completely
Excretion	85%-98% feces
Half-life	4 hr (initial); 50 hr (terminal)

Pharmacodynamics	
Onset	½-1½ hr
Peak	1-3 hr
Duration	8-12 hr

Interactions

Individual drugs

Alcohol: increased disulfiram-like reaction
Haloperidol, loxapine, methyldopa, metoclopramide, reserpine: decreased levels of bromocriptine
Levodopa: increased neurologic effects

Drug classifications

Analgesics (opioid), antihistamines, sedative/hypnotics: increased CNS depression
Antihypertensives: increased hypotension
Contraceptives (oral), estrogens, MAOIs, phenothiazines, progestins: decreased levels of bromocriptine

Drug/herb

Chaste tree fruit, kava: decreased bromocriptine effect
Horehound: increased serotonin effect

Drug/lab test

Increased: growth hormone, AST, ALT, BUN, CK, uric acid, alkaline phosphatase

NURSING CONSIDERATIONS

Assessment

- Assess symptoms of Parkinson's disease (EPS): shuffling gait, muscle rigidity, involuntary movements, pill rolling, muscle spasms, drooling before and during treatment
- Assess for resolution of symptoms of neuroleptic malignant syndrome: decreased temp, seizures, sweating, pulse
- Monitor for change in size of soft tissue volume in acromegaly
- Monitor B/P; establish baseline, compare with other readings; this drug decreases B/P; patient should remain recumbent for 2-4 hr after first dose; supervise ambulation

Nursing diagnoses

- Mobility, impaired (uses)
- Knowledge, deficient (teaching)

Implementation

- Give with meals or milk to prevent GI symptoms; crush tab if patient has swallowing difficulty
- Give at bedtime so dizziness, orthostatic hypotension do not occur
- Store at room temp in air-tight container

Patient/family education

- Advise patient to change position slowly to prevent orthostatic hypotension
- Tabs may be crushed and mixed with food
- Caution patient to use contraceptives during treatment with this drug; pregnancy may occur; to use methods other than oral contraceptives
- Teach patient that therapeutic effect for Parkinson's disease may take 2 mo: galactorrhea, amenorrhea
- Caution patient to avoid hazardous activity if dizziness, drowsiness occurs during treatment start-up
- Advise patient to avoid alcohol and OTC medication unless approved by prescriber
- Teach patients with acromegaly to notify prescriber immediately if severe headache, nausea, vomiting, blurred vision occur; indicates change in enlargement of tumor
- Advise patient to report symptoms of MI immediately

Evaluation

Positive therapeutic outcome

- Parkinson's disease: decreased dyskinesia, decreased slow movements, decreased drooling
- Decreased breast engorgement with accompanied pain, tenderness
- Acromegly: decreased growth hormone levels

brompheniramine (OTC, Rx)

(brome-fen-eer'a-meen)

Bidhist, Bromfenac, brompheniramine, Brove X, Brove X CT, Chlorphed, Dehist, Dimetane, Dimetane Extentabs, Dimetapp Allergy Liqui-Gels, Lo Hist 12 Hour, Lodrane 24, Lodrane XR, Nasahist-B, VaZol

Func. class.: Antihistamine
Chem. class.: Alkylamine, H_1-receptor antagonist

Pregnancy category C

Action: Acts on blood vessels, GI, respiratory system by competing with histamine for H_1-receptor site; decreases allergic response by blocking histamine

Therapeutic Outcome: Absence of allergy symptoms and rhinitis

Uses: Allergy symptoms, rhinitis, allergic dermatoses, nasal allergies, hypersensitivity reactions including blood transfusion reactions, anaphylaxis

Dosage and routes

Adult and child >12 yr: PO 4-8 mg bid-qid, not to exceed 36 mg/day; time rel 6-12 mg bid-tid, not to exceed 36 mg/day

Child 6-12 yr: PO 2 mg bid-qid, not to exceed 12 mg/day

Child 2-6 yr: 1 mg tid-qid (not to exceed 6 mg/day)

Child <2 yr: PO 0.5 mg/kg/day in divided doses (qid)

Available forms: Tabs 4 mg; elix 2 mg/5 ml; caps 4 mg; chew tab 12 mg; ext rel tab 6 mg; ext rel cap 12 mg; liquid 8 mg, 12 mg/5 ml

Adverse effects

CNS: *Dizziness, drowsiness,* poor coordination, fatigue, anxiety, euphoria, confusion, paresthesia, neuritis
CV: Hypotension, palpitations, tachycardia
EENT: Blurred vision, dilated pupils, tinnitus, nasal stuffiness, dry nose, throat, mouth
GI: Nausea, vomiting, anorexia, constipation, diarrhea
GU: Retention, dysuria, frequency, impotence
HEMA: **Thrombocytopenia, agranulocytosis, hemolytic anemia** (rare)
INTEG: Photosensitivity
RESP: Increased thick secretions, wheezing, chest tightness

Contraindications: Hypersensitivity to H_1-receptor antagonists, acute asthma attack, lower respiratory tract disease, child <2 yr

Precautions: Pregnancy **C**, increased intraocular pressure, renal disease, cardiac disease, hypertension, bronchial asthma, seizure disorder, stenosed peptic ulcers, hyperthyroidism, prostatic hypertrophy, bladder neck obstruction, angle closure glaucoma

Pharmacokinetics

Absorption	Well absorbed (PO, IM)
Distribution	Widely distributed; crosses blood-brain barrier
Metabolism	Liver, extensively
Excretion	Kidneys, metabolite; breast milk (minimal)
Half-life	12-34 hr

Pharmacodynamics

	PO	SUBCUT/IM	IV
Onset	15-30 min	30 min	Immediate
Peak	2-5 hr	Unknown	Unknown
Duration	6-12 hr	8-12 hr	8-12 hr

Interactions

Individual drugs

Alcohol: increased CNS depression
Aminophylline, insulin, pentobarbital: drugs are incompatible

Drug classifications

Barbiturates, opiates, sedative/hypnotics, tricyclics: increased CNS depression
MAOIs: increased anticholinergic effect

Drug/herb

Corkwood, henbane leaf: increased anticholinergic effect
Hops, Jamaican dogwood, khat, senega: increased antihistamine effect
Kava: increased CNS depression

Drug/lab test

Interference: skin allergy tests (discontinue antihistamines before testing)

NURSING CONSIDERATIONS

Assessment

- Assess respiratory status: rate, rhythm, increase in bronchial secretions, wheezing, chest tightness; provide fluids to 2 L/day to decrease secretion thickness
- Monitor I&O ratio: be alert for urinary retention, frequency, dysuria, especially elderly; drug should be discontinued if these occur
- Monitor CBC during long-term therapy; blood dyscrasias may occur but are rare

Nursing diagnoses

- Airway clearance, ineffective (uses)
- Injury, risk for (side effects)
- Knowledge, deficient (teaching)
- Noncompliance (teaching, overuse)

Implementation

- May give with food to prevent GI upset; absorption is not altered by food
- Store in tight, light-resistant container

Patient/family education

- Teach patient all aspects of drug use; to notify prescriber if confusion, sedation, hypotension occur; to avoid driving or other hazardous activity if drowsiness occurs; to avoid alcohol or other CNS depressants that may potentiate effect
- Instruct patient not to exceed recommended dosage; dysrhythmias may occur

- Teach patient hard candy, gum, frequent rinsing of mouth may be used for dryness

Evaluation

Positive therapeutic outcome

- Absence of runny or congested nose, rashes

Treatment of overdose: Administer lavage, vasopressors, barbiturates (short acting)

budesonide (Rx)

(byoo-des′oh-nide)

Entocort EC, Pulmicort, Rhinocort Aqua

Func. class.: Glucocorticoid

Pregnancy category C

Action: Prevents inflammation by depression of migration of polymorphonuclear leukocytes, fibroblasts, reversal of increased capillary permeability and lysosomal stabilization; does not suppress hypothalamus and pituitary function

Uses: Rhinitis; prophylaxis for asthma; Crohn's disease

Dosage and routes

Rhinitis (Rhinocort, Rhinocort Aqua)

Adult and child >6 yr: SPRAY/INH 2 sprays in each nostril AM, PM or 4 sprays in each nostril AM; max 256 mcg/day

Asthma

Adult and child ≥6 yr: INH 400-600 mcg/day

Crohn's disease

Adult: PO 9 mg daily AM × 8 wk

Available forms: Dry powder for INH (Pulmicort turbuhaler) 200 mcg/metered dose; inh susp 0.25 mg/2 ml, 0.5 mg/2 ml; cap 3 mg; (Rhinocort Aqua) 32 mcg/spray; caps (Entocort EC) 3 mg

Adverse effects

CNS: *Headache,* insomnia, hypertonia, syncope

EENT: *Sinusitis, pharyngitis,* rhinitis

ENDO: Adrenal insufficiency, growth suppression in children

GI: Dry mouth, dyspepsia, nausea, vomiting, abdominal pain,

MISC: Ecchymosis, fever, *hypersensitivity,* flulike symptoms

MS: Back pain, myalgias, fractures

RESP: Nasal irritation, cough, nasal bleeding, *respiratory infections,* ***bronchospasm***

Contraindications: Hypersensitivity, status asthmaticus

Precautions: Pregnancy **C,** inhaled form (B); lactation, children, TB, fungal, bacterial, systemic viral infections, ocular herpes simplex, nasal septal ulcers; hepatic disease (caps)

Pharmacokinetics	
Absorption	39%
Distribution	In airways, protein binding 85-90%
Metabolism	Liver
Excretion	In urine (60%), small amounts in feces
Half-life	2-3.6 hr

Pharmacodynamics	
Onset	Respules 2-8 days, Rhinocort Aqua 10 hr, Turbuhaler 24 hr
Peak	Respules 4-6 wk, Rhinocort Aqua 2 wk, Turbuhaler 1-2 wk

Interactions

Avoid using with drugs metabolized by CYP3A4 inhibition

Cimetidine, ketoconazole: decreased budesonide metabolism

Drug/herb

Aloe, buckthorn, Chinese rhubarb, senna: increased hypokalemia

Drug/food

Avoid taking with grapefruit juice (capsule PO)

NURSING CONSIDERATIONS

Assessment

- Assess respiratory status: rate, rhythm, increase in bronchial secretions, wheezing, chest tightness; provide fluids to 2 L/day to decrease thickness of secretions; check for oral candidiasis
- For bronchospasm, stop treatment and give bronchodilator
- With viral infections, corticosteroid use can mask infections
- For increased intraocular pressure, discontinue use if increase occurs

Nursing diagnoses

- Ineffective airway clearance (uses)
- Risk for injury (uses)
- Knowledge deficient (teaching)

Implementation

PO route (Crohn's disease)

- Swallow caps whole; do not break, crush, or chew

• May repeat 8-wk course if needed; may taper to 6 mg/day for 2 wk before cessation

INH route (asthma)

• Use scissors to open pouch
• Use Turbuhaler upright to load, prime when using first time, turn grip to the right, then left to click in place; to provide dose turn to right, then to the left, click in place. Place mouthpiece between lips, inhale forcefully, do not exhale through Turbuhaler, rinse after use
• Store at 59°-86° F (15°-30° C); keep away from heat, open flame

Patient/family education

• Teach patient to notify prescriber of pharyngitis, nasal bleeding
• Instruct patient not to exceed recommended dose; adrenal suppression may occur
• Teach patient to carry/wear emergency ID identifying steroid use
• Instruct patient to read and follow package directions
• Instruct patient to prevent exposure to infections, especially viral
• Advise to use good oral hygiene if using by nebulizer or inhaler

Evaluation

Positive therapeutic outcome

• Absence of asthma, rhinitis

bumetanide (Rx)

(byoo-met'a-nide)

Bumex

Func. class: Loop diuretic, antihypertensive
Chem. class.: Sulfonamide derivative

Pregnancy category C

Do Not Confuse:

Bumex/Buprenex/Permax

Action: Acts on the ascending loop of Henle in the kidney to inhibit the reabsorption of the electrolytes sodium and chloride, causing excretion of sodium, calcium, magnesium, chloride, water, and some potassium; also decreases reabsorption of sodium and chloride and increases the excretion of potassium in the distal tubule of the kidney; responsible for antihypertensive effect and peripheral vasodilatation

Therapeutic Outcome: Decreased edema in lung tissue and peripherally; decreased B/P

Uses: Edema in congestive heart failure, nephrotic syndrome, ascites caused by hepatic disease, hepatic cirrhosis

Investigational uses: May be used alone or as adjunct with antihypertensives such as spironolactone, triamterene

Dosage and routes

Adult: PO 0.5-2 mg daily may give 2nd or 3rd dose at 4-5 hr intervals; not to exceed 10 mg/day; may be given on alternate days or intermittently; **IV**/IM 0.5-1 mg/day; may give 2nd or 3rd dose at 2-3 hr intervals; not to exceed 10 mg/day

Child: PO/IM/**IV** 0.02-0.1 mg/kg q12h, max 10 mg/day

Available forms: Tabs 0.5, 1, 2 mg; inj 0.25 mg/ml

Adverse effects

CNS: Headache, fatigue, weakness, vertigo
CV: *Hypotension,* chest pain, ECG changes, **circulatory collapse,** dehydration
EENT: Ear pain, tinnitus, blurred vision, loss of hearing
ELECT: *Hypokalemia, hypochloremic alkalosis, hypomagnesia, hyperuricemia, hypocalcemia, hyponatremia*
ENDO: *Hyperglycemia*
GI: *Nausea,* diarrhea, dry mouth, vomiting, anorexia, cramps, **acute pancreatitis,** upset stomach, abdominal pain, **jaundice**
GU: *Polyuria,* **renal failure,** *glycosuria*
HEMA: **Thrombocytopenia**
INTEG: *Rash, pruritus, purpura,* **Stevens-Johnson syndrome**, sweating, photosensitivity
MS: Muscular cramps, stiffness, arthritis, tenderness

Contraindications: Hypersensitivity to sulfonamides, anuria, severe electrolyte deficiency, hepatic coma

Precautions: Pregnancy **C,** diabetes mellitus, dehydration, severe renal disease, lactation, ascites, hepatic cirrhosis

Pharmacokinetics

	PO/IM
Absorption	Rapidly, completely absorbed
	PO/IM/IV
Distribution	Crosses placenta, protein binding >91%
Metabolism	Liver (30%-40%)
Excretion	Breast milk, urine (50% unchanged), feces (20%)
Half-life	1-1½ hr; 6-15 hr neonates

Pharmacodynamics

	PO	IM	IV
Onset	½-1 hr	40 min	5 min
Peak	1-2 hr	1-2 hr	½ hr
Duration	3-6 hr	4-6 hr	3-6 hr

Interactions
Individual drugs
Alcohol: increased orthostatic hypotension
Digitalis: increased toxicity
Ethacrynic acid: combination may cause increased chance of dysrhythmias (do not use together)
Indomethacin: decreased diuretic and antihypertensive effects of bumetanide
Lithium: decreased renal clearance causing increased toxicity
Metolazone: increased diuresis, electrolyte loss
Probenecid: decreased diuretic effect
Drug classifications
Aminoglycosides: increased ototoxicity
Glucocorticoids, potassium-wasting drugs: increased hypokalemia
NSAIDs: decreased diuretic effect
Drug/herb
Aloe, cucumber, dandelion, horsetail, pumpkin, Queen Anne's lace: increased diuretic effect
Khella: increased hypotensian
St. John's wort: severe photosensitivity
Drug/lab test
Increased: urinary phosphate

NURSING CONSIDERATIONS
Assessment
- Assess patient for tinnitus, hearing loss, ear pain; periodic testing of hearing is needed when high doses of this drug are given by **IV** route
- Monitor for manifestations of hypokalemia: *RENAL:* acidic urine, reduced urine osmolality, nocturia, polyuria, polydipsia; *CV:* hypotension, broad T wave, U wave, ectopy, tachycardia, weak pulse; *NEURO:* muscle weakness, altered LOC, drowsiness, apathy, lethargy, confusion, depression; *GI:* anorexia, nausea, cramps, constipation, distention, paralytic ileus; *RESP:* hypoventilation, respiratory muscle weakness
- Monitor for manifestations of hypocalcemia: *CNS:* personality changes, anxiety, disturbances, depression, psychosis; *GI:* nausea, vomiting, constipation, abdominal pain from muscle spasm; *CV:* decreased contractility, decreased cardiac output, hypotension, lengthened ST segment, prolonged QT interval; *INTEG:* scaling eczema, alopecia, hyperpigmentation; *NEURO:* tetany, muscle twitching, cramping, grimacing, seizure, altered deep tendon reflexes, spasm
- Monitor for manifestations of hypomagnesemia: *CNS:* agitation; *NEURO:* muscle twitching, paresthesias, hyperactive reflexes, positive Babinski's reflex, dysphagia, nystagmus, seizures, tetany; *GI:* nausea, vomiting, diarrhea, anorexia, abdominal distention; *CV:* ectopy, tachycardia, broad, flat, or inverted T waves, depressed ST segment, prolonged QT, decreased cardiac output, hypotension
- Monitor for manifestations of hyponatremia: *CV:* increased B/P, cold, clammy skin, hypovolemia or hypervolemia; *GI:* anorexia, nausea, vomiting, diarrhea, abdominal cramps; *NEURO:* lethargy, increased ICP, confusion, headache, seizures, coma, fatigue, tremors, hyperreflexia
- Monitor for manifestations of hyperchloremia: *NEURO:* weakness, lethargy, coma; *RESP:* deep rapid breathing
- Assess fluid volume status: I&O ratio and record, distended red veins, crackles in lung, color, quality and sp gr of urine, skin turgor, adequacy of pulses, moist mucous membranes, bilateral lung sounds, peripheral pitting edema; dehydration symptoms of decreasing output, thirst, hypotension, dry mouth and mucous membranes should be reported; if urinary output decreases or azotemia occurs, drug should be discontinued
- Monitor electrolytes: potassium, sodium, calcium, magnesium; also include BUN, blood pH, ABGs, uric acid, CBC, blood glucose
- Assess B/P before and during therapy with patient lying, standing, and sitting as appropriate; orthostatic hypotension can occur rapidly
- Monitor for digoxin toxicity (anorexia, nausea, vomiting, confusion, paresthesia, muscle cramps) in patients taking digoxin; lithium toxicity in those taking lithium

Nursing diagnoses
- Urinary elimination, impaired (side effects)
- Fluid volume, deficient (side effects)
- Fluid volume, excess (uses)
- Knowledge, deficient (teaching)

Implementation
- Give in AM to avoid interference with sleep
- Potassium replacement if potassium level is <3.0 mg/dl whole, or use oral solutions; drug may be crushed if patient is unable to swallow

PO route

- With food, if nausea occurs; absorption may be reduced; the safest dosage schedule is on alternate days

IV route

- Do not use solution that is yellow or has a precipitate or crystals

IV, direct route

- Give undiluted through Y-tube or 3-way stopcock; give 20 mg or less/min

Intermittent IV infusion route

- May be added to 0.9% NaCl, D_5W, $D_{10}W$, $D_{20}W$, invert sugar 10% in electrolyte #1, LR, sodium lactate ⅙ mol/L; use within 24 hr to ensure compatibility; give through Y-tube or 3-way stopcock; give at 4 mg/min or less; use infusion pump

Syringe compatibility: Doxapram

Y-site compatibilities: Allopurinol, amifostine, aztreonam, cefepime, cisatracurium, cladribine, diltiazem, filgrastim, granisetron, lorazepam, morphine, piperacillin/tazobactam, propofol, remifantanil, teniposide, thiotepa, vinorelbine

Additive compatibilities: Floxacillin, furosemide

Patient/family education

- Teach patient to take the medication early in the day to prevent nocturia
- Instruct the patient to take with food or milk if GI symptoms of nausea and anorexia occur
- Teach patient to maintain weekly record of weight and notify prescriber of weight loss of >5 lb
- Caution the patient that this drug causes a loss of potassium, so food rich in potassium should be added to the diet; refer to a dietician for assistance in planning
- Caution the patient not to exercise in hot weather or stand for prolonged periods since orthostatic hypotension will be enhanced
- Teach patient not to use alcohol or any OTC medications without prescriber's approval; serious drug reactions may occur
- Emphasize the need to contact prescriber immediately if muscle cramps, weakness, nausea, dizziness, or numbness occurs
- Teach patient to take own B/P and pulse and record
- Caution the patient that orthostatic hypotension may occur; patient should rise slowly from sitting or reclining positions and lie down if dizziness occurs
- Teach patient to continue taking medication even if feeling better; this drug controls symptoms but does not cure the condition
- Advise the patient with hypertension to continue other medical treatment (exercise, weight loss, relaxation techniques, cessation of smoking)

Evaluation

Positive therapeutic outcome

- Decreased edema
- Decreased B/P
- Increased diuresis

buprenorphine (Rx)

(byoo-pre-nor'feen)

Buprenex

Func. class.: Opioid analgesic, partial agonist

Chem. class.: Thebaine derivative

Pregnancy category C

Controlled substance schedule V

Do Not Confuse:

Buprenex/Bumex

Action: Inhibits ascending pain pathways in limbic system, thalamus, midbrain, hypothalamus by binding to opiate receptor sites; this alters pain perception and response; generalized CNS depression

Therapeutic Outcome: Relief of pain

Uses: Moderate to severe pain

Dosage and routes

Adult: IM/**IV** 0.3 mg q6h prn; may repeat dose after ½ hr; reduce dosage in elderly, may repeat after ½ hr; epidural 60-180 mcg over 48 hr

Child 2-12 yr: IM/**IV** 2-6 mcg/kg q4-6h

Elderly: PO 0.15 mg q6h prn

Available forms: Inj 0.3 mg/ml (1-ml vials)

Adverse effects

CNS: *Drowsiness, dizziness, confusion, headache, sedation, euphoria,* **increased intracranial pressure,** amnesia

CV: Palpitations, bradycardia, change in B/P, tachycardia

EENT: Tinnitus, blurred vision, *miosis,* diplopia

GI: *Nausea,* vomiting, anorexia, constipation, cramps, dry mouth

GU: Increased urinary output, dysuria, urinary retention

INTEG: *Rash,* urticaria, bruising, flushing, diaphoresis, pruritus

RESP: **Respiratory depression,** dyspnea, hypo-/hyperventilation

Contraindications: Hypersensitivity

Precautions: Pregnancy **C**, addictive personality, lactation, increased intracranial pressure, MI (acute), severe heart disease, respiratory depression, hepatic disease, renal disease, hypothyroidism, Addison's disease, addiction (opioid)

Pharmacokinetics

Absorption	Well absorbed (IM)
Distribution	Crosses placenta
Metabolism	Liver, extensively
Excretion	Kidneys, feces, breast milk
Half-life	2½-3½ hr

Pharmacodynamics

	IM	IV
Onset	10-15 min	Immediate
Peak	1 hr	5 min
Duration	4 hr	2-5 hr

Interactions

Individual drugs

Alcohol: increased respiratory depression, hypotension, sedation

Drug classifications

Antihistamines, CNS depressants, sedative/hypotension: increased respiratory depression, hypotension

MAOIs: do not use within 2 wk

Opioids: increased CNS depression

Drug/herb

Corkwood: increased anticholinergic effect

Jamaican dogwood, kava, lavender, mistletoe, nettle, pokeweed, poppy, senega, valerian: increased CNS depression

NURSING CONSIDERATIONS

Assessment

- Assess pain characteristics: location, intensity, type, severity before medication administration and after treatment
- Monitor VS after parenteral route; note muscle rigidity, drug history, liver, kidney function tests, respiratory dysfunction: respiratory depression, character, rate, rhythm; notify prescriber if respirations are <10/min
- Monitor CNS changes: dizziness, drowsiness, hallucinations, euphoria, LOC, pupil reaction; withdrawal in opioid-dependent persons; if dependence occurs within 2 wk of discontinuing drug, withdrawal symptoms will occur
- Monitor allergic reactions: rash, urticaria

Nursing diagnoses

- Pain, acute (uses)
- Pain, chronic
- Sensory perception, disturbed (adverse reactions)
- Breathing pattern, ineffective (adverse reactions)
- Knowledge, deficient (teaching)

Implementation

- Give by inj (IM, **IV**), only with resuscitative equipment available; give slowly to prevent rigidity

IM route

- Give deep in large muscle mass; rotate sites of inj

IV route

- Give **IV** direct undiluted over 3-5 min (0.3 mg/2 min); give slowly

Syringe compatibility: Midazolam

Y-site compatibilities: Allopurinol, amifostine, aztreonam, cefepime, cisatracurium, cladribine, filgrastim, granisetron, melphalan, piperacillin/tazobactam, propofol, remifentanil, teniposide, thiotepa, vinorelbine

Additive compatibilities: Atropine, bupivacaine, diphenhydrAMINE, droperidol, glycopyrrolate, haloperidol, hydrOXYzine, promethazine, scopolamine

Additive incompatibilities: Diazepam, floxacillin, furosemide, lorazepam

Patient/family education

- Instruct patient to report any symptoms of CNS changes, allergic reactions
- Caution patients to avoid CNS depressants: alcohol, sedative/hypnotics for at least 24 hr after taking this drug
- Discuss with patient that dizziness, drowsiness, and confusion are common; to avoid getting up without assistance, to avoid hazardous activities
- Discuss in detail all aspects of the drug
- Instruct patient to change position slowly to prevent orthostatic hypotension
- Teach patient to turn, cough, deep breathe after surgery to prevent atelectasis

Evaluation

Positive therapeutic outcome

- Relief of pain

buPROPion (Rx)
(byoo-proe'pee-on)
buPROPion, Wellbutrin, Wellbutrin SR, Zyban
Func. class.: Antidepressant—miscellaneous, smoking deterrent
Chem. class.: Aminoketone

Pregnancy category B

Do Not Confuse:
buPROPion/busPIRone, Zyban/Diovan/Zagam

Action: Inhibits reuptake of dopamine, serotonin, norepinephrine

Therapeutic Outcome: Decreased symptoms of depression after 2-3 wk

Uses: Depression (Wellbutrin), smoking cessation (Zyban)

Dosage and routes
Depression
Adult: PO 100 mg bid initially, then increase after 3 days to 100 mg tid if needed; may increase after 1 mo to 150 mg tid; SR 150 mg bid, initially 150 mg AM, increase to 300 mg/day if initial dose is tolerated
Elderly: PO 50-100 mg/day, may increase by 50-100 mg q3-4 days

Smoking cessation
Adult: PO 150 mg bid, begin with 150 mg daily × 3 days then 300 mg/day continue for 7-12 wk, not to exceed 300 mg/day

Available forms: Tabs 75, 100 mg; sus rel tabs (Zyban) 100, 150, 200 mg; ext rel tab (XL) 150, 300 mg

Adverse effects
CNS: *Headache, agitation, confusion,* **seizures,** delusions, *insomnia, sedation, tremors,* dizziness, akinesia, bradykinesia
CV: **Dysrhythmias,** *hypertension,* palpitations, *tachycardia,* hypotension, **complete AV block**
EENT: *Blurred vision, auditory disturbance*
GI: *Nausea, vomiting, dry mouth,* anorexia, diarrhea, increased appetite, *constipation*
GU: Impotence, frequency, retention, *menstrual irregularities*
INTEG: *Rash,* pruritus, *sweating*
MISC: *Weight loss or gain*

Contraindications: Hypersensitivity, eating disorders, seizure disorder

Precautions: Pregnancy **B,** renal and hepatic disease, recent MI, cranial trauma, lactation, children <18 yr, seizure disorders, elderly

Pharmacokinetics

Absorption	Well absorbed; bioavailability poor
Distribution	Unknown
Metabolism	Liver extensively
Excretion	Kidneys
Half-life	14 hr, steady state 1½-5 wk

Pharmacodynamics

Onset	Up to 4 wk
Peak	Unknown
Duration	Unknown

Interactions
Individual drugs
Alcohol, levodopa, theophylline: increased risk of seizures
Carbamazepine, cimetidine, phenobarbitol, phenytoin: decreased buPROPion effect
Cimetidine: increased levels
Ritonavir: increased buPROPion toxicity

Drug classifications
Antidepressants, benzodiazepines, MAOIs, steroids (systemic): increased risk of seizures
Barbiturates, CYP450 drugs: decreased buPROPion effects
CNS depressants: increased effects
MAOIs: acute toxicity
Phenothiazines: increased toxicity, risk of seizures

Drug/herb
Belladonna, corkwood, jimsonweed: increased anticholinergic effect
Hops, kava, lavender: increased CNS depression

NURSING CONSIDERATIONS
Assessment
- Monitor B/P (with patient lying, standing), pulse q4h; if systolic B/P drops 20 mm Hg hold drug, notify prescriber; take vital signs q4h in patients with cardiovascular disease
- Assess smoking cessation progress after 7-12 wk, if progress has not been made, drug should be discontinued
- Assess for increased risk of seizures; if patient has used CNS depressant or CNS stimulants, dosage of buPROPion should not be exceeded
- Monitor blood studies: CBC, leukocytes, differential, cardiac enzymes if patient is receiving long-term therapy
- Monitor hepatic studies: AST, ALT, bilirubin if on long-term treatment
- Check weight weekly; appetite may increase with drug

- Assess ECG for flattening of T wave, bundle branch block, AV block, dysrhythmias in cardiac patients
- Assess for EPS primarily in elderly: rigidity, dystonia, akathisia
- Assess mental status: mood, sensorium, affect, suicidal tendencies; increase in psychiatric symptoms: depression, panic
- Monitor urinary retention, constipation; constipation is more likely to occur in children or elderly
- Identify alcohol consumption; if alcohol was consumed, hold dose

Nursing diagnoses
- Coping, ineffective (uses)
- Injury, risk for (side effects)
- Knowledge, deficient (teaching)
- Noncompliance (teaching)

Implementation
- Give with food or milk for GI symptoms
- Give sugarless gum, hard candy, or frequent sips of water for dry mouth
- Store at room temp; do not freeze

Patient/family education
- Teach patient that therapeutic effects may take 2-3 wk; not to increase dose without prescriber's approval; that treatment for smoking cessation lasts 7-12 wk
- Teach patient to use caution in driving or other activities requiring alertness because of drowsiness, dizziness, blurred vision; to avoid rising quickly from sitting to standing, especially elderly
- Teach patient to avoid alcohol ingestion; alcohol may increase risk of seizures, obtain approval for other drugs
- Teach patient to increase fluids, bulk in diet if constipation, urinary retention occur, especially elderly; notify prescriber immediately if retention occurs
- Teach patient to take gum, hard sugarless candy, or frequent sips of water for dry mouth
- Advise patient not to use with nicotine patches unless directed by prescriber, may increase B/P
- Teach patient that risk of seizures increases when dose is exceeded, or if patient has seizure disorder
- Teach patient to notify prescriber if pregnancy is suspected or planned

Evaluation
Positive therapeutic outcome
- Decrease in depression
- Absence of suicidal thoughts
- Smoking cessation

Treatment of overdose: ECG monitoring, induce emesis, lavage, activated charcoal, administer anticonvulsant

busPIRone (Rx)
(byoo-spye'rone)
BuSpar
Func. class.: Antianxiety, sedative
Chem. class.: Azaspirodecanedione
Pregnancy category B

Do Not Confuse:
busPIRone/buPROPion

Action: Acts by inhibiting the action of serotonin (5-HT) by binding to serotonin and dopamine receptors; also increases norepinephrine metabolism; has shown little potential for abuse

Therapeutic Outcome: Decreased anxiety

Uses: Management and short-term relief of generalized anxiety disorders

Dosage and routes
Adult: PO 5 mg tid; may increase by 5 mg/day q2-3 days; not to exceed 60 mg/day

Available forms: Tabs 5, 7.5, 10, 15, 30 mg

Adverse effects
CNS: *Dizziness, headache, depression, stimulation, insomnia, nervousness, lightheadedness, numbness, paresthesia, incoordination, tremors,* excitement, involuntary movements, confusion, akathisia, nightmares
CV: *Tachycardia, palpitations,* hypotension, hypertension, **CVA, CHF, MI**
EENT: *Sore throat, tinnitus, blurred vision, nasal congestion,* red, itching eyes, change in taste, smell
GI: *Nausea, dry mouth, diarrhea, constipation,* flatulence, increased appetite, rectal bleeding
GU: Frequency, hesitancy, menstrual irregularity, change in libido
INTEG: *Rash,* edema, pruritus, alopecia, dry skin
MISC: *Sweating,* fatigue, weight gain, fever
MS: *Pain, weakness,* muscle cramps, spasms
RESP: Hyperventilation, chest congestion, shortness of breath

Contraindications: Hypersensitivity, child <18 yr

Precautions: Pregnancy **B**, lactation, elderly, impaired hepatic/renal function

Pharmacokinetics

Absorption	Rapidly absorbed
Distribution	Unknown
Metabolism	Liver, extensively
Excretion	Feces
Half-life	2-3 hr

Pharmacodynamics

Unknown

Interactions

Individual drugs

Alcohol: increased CNS depression
Carbamazepine, dexamethasone, phenobarbitol, phenytoin, rifampin: decreased busPIRone effect
Erythromycin, itraconazole, ketoconazole, nefazodone, ritonavir: increased busPIRone levels

Drug classifications

CYP450 drugs: increased busPIRone levels
Drugs induced by CYP3A4: decreased busPIRone action
MAOIs: increased B/P, do not use together
Psychotropics: increased CNS depression

Drug/herb

Cowslip, kava, Queen Anne's lace, valerian: increased CNS depression

Drug/food

Grapefruit juice: increased busPIRone effect

NURSING CONSIDERATIONS

Assessment

- Assess anxiety reaction: inability to sleep, apprehension, dread, foreboding, or uneasiness related to unidentified source of danger
- Assess for previous drug dependence or tolerance; if patient is drug dependent or tolerant, amount of medication should be restricted
- Monitor B/P (lying, standing), pulse; if systolic B/P drops 20 mm Hg, hold drug, notify prescriber; check I&O; may indicate renal dysfunction
- Monitor mental status: mood, sensorium, affect, sleeping patterns, drowsiness, dizziness, suicidal tendencies
- Assess for CNS reaction, some reactions may be unpredictable

Nursing diagnoses

- Anxiety (uses)
- Knowledge, deficient (teaching)
- Noncompliance (teaching)

Implementation

- Give with food or milk for GI symptoms; sugarless gum, hard candy, frequent sips of water for dry mouth
- May be crushed

Patient/family education

- Teach patient that drug may be taken with food; if dose is missed take as soon as remembered; do not double doses
- Caution patient to avoid OTC preparations unless approved by the prescriber; to avoid alcohol ingestion and other psychotropic medications unless prescribed; that 1-2 wk of therapy may be required before therapeutic effects occur
- Caution patient to avoid driving and activities requiring alertness since drowsiness may occur; until medication response is known, tell patient that drowsiness may worsen at beginning of treatment
- Instruct patient not to discontinue medication abruptly after long-term use; if dose is missed, do not double
- Advise patient to rise slowly or fainting may occur, especially in elderly

Evaluation

Positive therapeutic outcome

- Increased well-being
- Decreased anxiety, restlessness, sleeplessness, dread

Treatment of overdose: Gastric lavage, VS, supportive care

! HIGH ALERT

busulfan (Rx)

(byoo-sul'fan)

Busulfex, Myleran

Func. class.: Antineoplastic alkylating agent
Chem. class.: Nitrosourea

Pregnancy category D

Do Not Confuse:
Myleran/Leukeran

Action: Changes essential cellular ions to covalent bonding with resultant alkylation; this interferes with normal biologic function of DNA; activity is not phase specific; action is due to myelosuppression

Therapeutic Outcome: Prevention of rapid growth of malignant cells in chronic myelocytic leukemia

Uses: Chronic myelocytic leukemia

B

Dosage and routes
Chronic myelocytic (granulocytic) leukemia
Adult: PO 4-8 mg/day initially until WBC levels fall to 15,000/mm^3; then drug is stopped until WBC levels rise over 50,000/mm^3; then 1-3 mg/day

Child: PO 0.06-0.12 mg/kg or 1.8-4.6 mg/m^2/day; dosage is titrated to maintain WBC levels at 20,000/mm^3, but never <10,000 mm^3

Allogenic hemopoietic stem cell transplantation in chronic myelogenous leukemia
Adult: **IV** 0.8 mg/kg q6h × 4 days (total 16 doses); give cyclophosphamide **IV** 60 mg/kg over 1 hr daily for 2 days, starting after 16th dose of busulfan

Available forms: Tabs 2 mg; sol for inj 6 mg/ml

Adverse effects
PO route

CV: *Hypotension,* **thrombosis,** *chest pain,* **tachycardia, atrial fibrillation, heart block,** pericardial effusion, **cardiac tamponade** (high dose with cyclophosphamide)

GI: Anorexia, constipation, dry mouth, nausea, vomiting, *diarrhea*

GU: Impotence, sterility, amenorrhea, gynecomastia, **renal toxicity,** hyperuremia, adrenal insufficiency–like syndrome

RESP: **Alveolar hemorrhage,** atelectasis, cough, hemoptysis, hypoxia, pleural effusion, pneumonia, sinusitis, **pulmonary fibrosis**

IV route

CNS: **Cerebral hemorrhage, coma, seizures,** *anxiety, depression, dizziness, headache,* encephalopathy, weakness, mental changes

CV: *Hypotension,* **thrombosis,** *chest pain,* **tachycardia, atrial fibrillation, heart block**

EENT: *Pharyngitis, epistaxis, cataracts*

GI: *Diarrhea, nausea, vomiting, weight loss*

HEMA: **Thrombocytopenia, leukopenia, pancytopenia, severe bone marrow depression**

INTEG: Dermatitis, hyperpigmentation, alopecia

MISC: **Chromosomal aberrations**

RESP: Irreversible pulmonary fibrosis: pneumonitis

Contraindications: Pregnancy **D** (3rd trimester), radiation, chemotherapy, lactation, blastic phase of chronic myelocytic leukemia, hypersensitivity

Precautions: Child-bearing age men and women, leukopenia, thrombocytopenia, anemia, hepatotoxicity, renal toxicity

Pharmacokinetics

Absorption	Rapidly absorbed
Distribution	Unknown; crosses placenta
Metabolism	Liver, extensively
Excretion	Kidneys, breast milk
Half-life	2.5 hr

Pharmacodynamics
Unknown

Interactions
Individual drugs
Acetaminophen, itraconazole: decreased busulfan clearance

Cyclophosphamide: cardiac tamponade

Phenytoin: decreased busulfan level

Radiation: increased toxicity, bone marrow suppression

Thioguanine: hepatotoxicity

Drug classifications
Anticoagulants, salicylates: increased risk of bleeding

Antineoplastics: increased toxicity, bone marrow suppression

Live virus vaccines: decreased antibody reaction

Drug/lab test
False positive: breast, bladder, cervix, lung cytology tests

NURSING CONSIDERATIONS
Assessment
- Monitor CBC, differential, platelet count weekly; withhold drug if WBC <4000/mm^3 or platelets <75,000/mm^3; notify prescriber of results if WBC <15,000/mm^3, platelets <150,000/mm^3; institute thrombocytopenia precautions
- Monitor pulmonary function tests, chest x-ray films before, during therapy; chest film should be obtained q2 wk during treatment; check for dyspnea, crackles, nonproductive cough, chest pain, tachypnea; pulmonary fibrosis may occur up to 10 yr after treatment with busulfan
- Assess for increased uric acid levels, swelling, joint pain primarily in extremities; patient should be well hydrated to prevent urate deposits
- Monitor renal function studies: BUN, serum uric acid, urine CCr before, during therapy; I&O ratio; report fall in urine output of 30 ml/hr; check for decreased hyperuricemia

- Monitor for cold, fever, sore throat (may indicate beginning infection); identify edema in feet, joint or stomach pain, shaking; prescriber should be notified
- Assess for bleeding: hematuria, guaiac, bruising or petechiae, mucosa or orifices q8h; no rectal temps

Nursing diagnoses

- Injury, risk for (adverse reactions)
- Body image, disturbed (adverse reactions)
- Infection, risk for (adverse reactions)
- Knowledge, deficient (teaching)

Implementation

- Give 1 hr before or 2 hr pc to lessen nausea and vomiting; give at same time daily
- Increased fluid intake to 2-3 L/day to prevent urate deposits, calculus formation
- Administer antibiotics for prophylaxis of infection; may be prescribed since infection potential is high
- Store in tight container

IV route

- Prepare in biologic cabinet using gloves, gown, mask; dilute with 10 times volume of drug using D_5W or 0.9% NaCl (0.5 mg/ml); when withdrawing drug, use needle with 5-micron filter provided, remove amount needed, remove filter, and inject drug into diluent; always add drug to diluent, not vice versa; stable for 8 hr at room temp using D_5W or 0.9% NaCl; give by central venous catheter over 2 hr q6h × 4 days, use infusion pump, do not admix
- Give antiemetic before **IV** route
- Give phenytoin before **IV** to prevent seizures in those with seizure disorders

Patient/family education

- Teach patient to avoid use of products containing aspirin or ibuprofen, razors, commercial mouthwash since bleeding may occur; to report symptoms of bleeding (hematuria, tarry stools)
- Instruct patient to report signs of anemia (fatigue, headache, irritability, faintness, shortness of breath)
- Instruct patient to report any changes in breathing or coughing even several months after treatment; to avoid crowds and persons with respiratory tract or other infections
- Teach patient that hair loss may occur; discuss the use of wigs or hair pieces
- Caution patient not to have any vaccinations without the advice of the prescriber; serious reactions can occur
- Advise patient that contraception is needed during treatment and for several months after the completion of therapy

Evaluation

Positive therapeutic outcome

- Decreased leukocytes to normal limits
- Absence of sweating at night
- Increased appetite, increased weight

butorphanol (Rx)

(byoo-tor′fa-nole)

Stadol, Stadol NS

Func. class.: Opiate analgesic

Chem class: Opioid antagonist, partial agonist

Pregnancy category C

Controlled substance schedule IV

Do Not Confuse:

Stadol/Haldol/Sotalol

Action: Inhibits ascending pain pathways in limbic system, thalamus, midbrain, hypothalamus by binding to opiate receptor sites; this alters pain perception and response

Therapeutic Outcome: Relief of pain

Uses: Moderate to severe pain, analgesia during labor, sedation preoperatively

Investigational uses: Migraine headache, pain

Dosage and routes

Adult: IM 1-4 mg q3-4h prn; **IV** 0.5-2 mg q3-4h prn; nasal spray in 1 nostril q3-4h; may give another dose 1-1½ hr later; may repeat q3-4h

Elderly: **IV** ½ adult dose at 2× the interval

Intranasal: May repeat q1-2h

Renal dose

Adult: **IV**/IM CCr 10-50 ml/min 75% dose; CCr <10 ml/min 50% dose

Severe pain

Adult: Intranasal 1 spray in each nostril q3-4h

Available forms: Inj 1, 2 mg/ml; intranasal 10 mg/ml

Adverse effects

CNS: *Drowsiness, dizziness, confusion, headache, sedation, euphoria, weakness, hallucinations*

CV: Palpitations, bradycardia, hypotension

EENT: Tinnitus, blurred vision, miosis, diplopia, nasal congestion

GI: *Nausea, vomiting, anorexia, constipation, cramps*

GU: Increased urinary output, dysuria, urinary retention

INTEG: Rash, urticaria, bruising, flushing, diaphoresis, pruritus
RESP: **Respiratory depression,** pulmonary hypertension

Contraindications: Hypersensitivity to this drug or preservative, addiction (opioid), CHF, MI

Precautions: Pregnancy **C,** addictive personality, lactation, increased intracranial pressure, respiratory depression, hepatic disease, renal disease, child <18 yr

Pharmacokinetics

Absorption	Well absorbed (IM, nasal); complete (**IV**)
Distribution	Crosses placenta
Metabolism	Liver, extensively
Excretion	Feces (10%-15%); kidneys, unchanged (small amounts)
Half-life	3-4 hr

Pharmacodynamics

	IM	IV	NASAL
Onset	10-30 min	1 min	15 min
Peak	½ hr	5 min	1-2 hr
Duration	3-4 hr	2-4 hr	4-5 hr

Interactions
Individual drugs
Alcohol: increased respiratory depression, hypotension, sedation
Drug classifications:
Antipsychotics, CNS depressants, opioids, sedative/hypnotics, skeletal muscle relaxants: increased respiratory depression, hypotension
MAOIs: do not use 2 wk before butorphanol, fatal reaction
Drug/herb
Chamomile, kava, Jamaican dogwood, lavender, mistletoe, nettle, pokeweed, poppy, senega, skullcap, valerian: increased CNS depression
Corkwood: increased anticholinergic effect

NURSING CONSIDERATIONS
Assessment
- Monitor VS after parenteral route; note muscle rigidity, drug history, liver, kidney function tests, respiratory dysfunction: respiratory depression, character, rate, rhythm; notify prescriber if respirations are <10/min
- Monitor CNS changes: dizziness, drowsiness, hallucinations, euphoria, LOC, pupil reaction
- Monitor allergic reactions: rash, urticaria

Nursing diagnoses
- Pain, acute (uses)
- Pain, chronic (uses)
- Sensory perception, disturbed (adverse reactions)
- Injury, risk for (adverse reactions)
- Knowledge, deficient (teaching)

Implementation
- Store in light-resistant container at room temp

IM route
- Give deeply in large muscle mass; rotate inj sites

Intranasal route
- Give 1 spray in nostril
- Remove clip and cover, prime before using until spray appears; pump must be reprimed q48h; close nostril with finger and spray once quickly; have patient sniff

IV route
- Give **IV** undiluted at a rate of ≤2 mg/>3-5 min; titrate to patient response

Syringe compatibilities: Atropine, chlorproMAZINE, cimetidine, diphenhydrAMINE, droperidol, fentanyl, hydrOXYzine, meperidine, methotrimeprazine, metoclopramide, midazolam, morphine, pentazocine, perphenazine, prochlorperazine, promethazine, scopolamine, thiethylperazine

Syringe incompatibilities: DimenhyDRINATE, pentobarbital

Y-site compatibilities: Allopurinol, amifostine, azetreonam, cefepime, cisatracurium, cladribine, DOXOrubicin liposome, enalaprilat, esmolol, filgrastim, fludarabine, granisetron, labetalol, melphalan, paclitaxel, piperacillin/tazobactam, propofol, remifentanil, sargramostim, teniposide, thiotepa, vinorelbine

Patient/family education
- Instruct patient to report any symptoms of CNS changes, allergic reactions; to avoid CNS depressants: alcohol, sedative/hypnotics for at least 24 hr after taking this drug
- Discuss with patient that dizziness, drowsiness, and confusion are common; to avoid getting up without assistance
- Discuss in detail all aspects of the drug

Nasal route
- Teach patient to blow nose to clear both nostrils before using
- Patient should replace clip and cover after use; caution patient not to shake medication

Evaluation
Positive therapeutic outcome
- Pain relief

Treatment of overdose: Narcan 0.2-0.8 **IV**, O_2, **IV** fluids, vasopressors

cabergoline (Rx)

(ka-ber'goe-leen)

Dostinex

Func. class: Antihyperprolactinemic

Chem. class: Dopamine antagonist

Pregnancy category C

Action: Inhibits prolactin by dopamine antagonisim

Therapeutic Outcome: Decreased levels of prolactin

Uses: Hyperprolactinemia, idiopathic or pituitary

Dosage and routes

Adult: PO 0.25 two times each week, may increase q4 wk to max 1 mg two times each week

Available forms: Tabs 0.5 mg

Adverse effects

CNS: ***Dizziness, headache,*** fatigue, anxiety, weakness, paresthesia

CV: Postural hypotension

GI: ***Constipation, nausea,*** vomiting, anorexia, abdominal pain

GU: Dysmenorrhea, breast tenderness/pain

OTHER: Hot flashes

Contraindications: Pregnancy **C**, hypersensitivity to this product or ergots, lactation, severe, uncontrolled hypertension

Precautions: Liver disease, children

Pharmacokinetics	
Absorption	Well
Distribution	Widely
Metabolism	Liver, extensively
Excretion	Kidneys
Half-life	64-68.5 hr

Pharmacodynamics	
Onset	Unknown
Peak	Up to 4 weeks
Duration	Unknown

Interactions

Drug classifications

Antihypertensive: increased hypotension

Butyrophenones, phenothiazines: decreased effect of cabergoline

Drug/lab test

Decreased: serum prolactin levels

NURSING CONSIDERATIONS

Assessment

- Monitor B/P before treatment and often thereafter. Check for postural hypotension, assist with ambulation if needed
- Monitor serum prolactin levels qmo until normal (<20 mcg/L in women, <15 mcg/L in men)

Nursing diagnoses

- Injury, risk for (adverse reactions)
- Knowledge, deficient (teaching)

Implementation

- Give PO with or without food

Patient/family education

- Advise patient to use as directed, not to skip doses
- Teach patient not to operate machinery or drive if dizziness occurs
- Inform patient to use nonhormonal type of contraception while taking this product; not to breastfeed
- Teach patient to change positions slowly to prevent postural hypotension
- Advise patient to report severe nausea, vomiting, severe headache with blurred vision, if using for pituitary tumor

Evaluation

Positive therapeutic outcome

- Decreased prolactin levels

calcitonin (human) (Rx)

(kal-sih-toh'nin)

Cibacalcin

calcitonin (salmon) (Rx)

Calcimir, Miacalcin, Miacalin Nasal Spray, Osteocalcin, Salmonine

Func. class.: Parathyroid agents (calcium regulator)

Chem. class.: Polypeptide hormone

Pregnancy category C

Action: Decreases bone resorption, blood calcium levels by direct action on bone, GI system, and kidney; increases deposits of calcium in bones; renal excretion of calcium occurs; opposes parathyroid hormone

Therapeutic Outcome: Lowered calcium level, decreasing symptoms of Paget's disease

Uses: Paget's disease, postmenopausal osteoporosis, hypercalcemia

Dosage and routes

Human

Paget's disease

Adult: SUBCUT 0.5 mg/day initially; may require 0.5 mg bid × 6 mo, then decrease until symptoms reappear

Salmon

Postmenopausal osteoporosis

Adult: SUBCUT/IM 100 international units/day; nasal 200 international units (1 spray) alternating nostrils daily, activate pump before 1st dose

Paget's disease

Adult: SUBCUT/IM 100 international units daily, maintenance 50-100 international units daily or every other day

Hypercalcemia

Adult: SUBCUT/IM 4 international units/kg q12h, increase to 8 international units/kg q6h if response is unsatisfactory

Available forms: Human: Inj (SUBCUT) 500 mg/vial; Salmon: Inj 100 international units, 200 international units/ml, nasal spray 200 international units/actuation

Adverse effects

CNS: Headache, **tetany,** chills, weakness, dizziness, fever
CV: Chest pressure
EENT: Nasal congestion, eye pain
GI: Nausea, diarrhea, vomiting, anorexia, abdominal pain, salty taste, epigastric pain
GU: Diuresis, nocturia, urine sediment, frequency
INTEG: Rash, flushing, pruritus of earlobes, edema of feet, inj site reaction
MS: Swelling, tingling of hands
RESP: Dyspnea
SYST: **Anaphylaxis**

Contraindications: Hypersensitivity

Precautions: Pregnancy **C,** renal disease, children, lactation, osteogenic sarcoma, pernicious anemia

Pharmacokinetics

Absorption	Completely absorbed
Distribution	Unknown
Metabolism	Rapid; kidneys, tissue, blood
Excretion	Kidneys, inactive metabolite
Half-life	1 hr

Pharmacodynamics

	SUBCUT
Onset	15 min
Peak	4 hr
Duration	8-24 hr

Interactions: None known

NURSING CONSIDERATIONS

Assessment

- Assess for GI symptoms, polyuria, flushing, head swelling, tingling, headache; may indicate hypercalcemia; nervousness, irritability, twitching, seizures, spasm, paresthesia indicate hypocalcemia during beginning of treatment
- Identify nutritional status; check diet for sources of vit D (milk, some seafood), calcium (dairy products, dark green vegetables), phosphates
- Monitor BUN, creatinine, uric acid, chloride, electrolytes, urine pH, urinary calcium, magnesium, phosphate, urinalysis (calcium should be kept at 9-10 mg/dl; vit D 50-135 international units/dl), alkaline phosphatase baseline and q3-6 mo; check urine sediment for casts throughout treatment; monitor urine hydroyproline in Paget's disease
- Assess for increased drug level, since toxic reactions occur rapidly; have parenteral calcium or gluconate on hand if calcium level drops too low; check for tetany (irritability, paresthesia, nervousness, muscle twitching, seizure, tetanic spasm)

Nursing diagnoses

- Injury, risk for (adverse reactions)
- Pain, chronic (uses)
- Knowledge, deficient (teaching)

Implementation

- Store at <77° F (25° C); protect from light

SUBCUT route (human)

- Give by SUBCUT route only; rotate inj sites; use within 6 hr of reconstitution; give at bedtime to minimize nausea, vomiting

IM route (salmon)

- After test dose of 10 international units/ml, 0.1 ml intradermally; watch 15 min; give only with epINEPHrine and emergency meds available
- IM inj in deep muscle mass slowly; rotate sites

Nasal route

- Use alternating nostrils for nasal spray

Patient/family education

- Teach method of inj if patient will be responsible for self-medication
- Instruct patient to notify prescriber for

hypercalcemic relapse: renal calculi, nausea, vomiting, thirst, lethargy, deep bone or flank pain

- Teach patient that warmth and flushing occur and last 1 hr
- Provide a low-calcium diet as prescribed (Paget's disease, hypercalcemia)
- Advise patients with osteoporosis to increase calcium and vit D in diet and to continue with moderate exercise to prevent continued bone loss
- Advise patients to report difficulty swallowing or change in side effects to prescriber immediately

Evaluation

Positive therapeutic outcome

- Calcium levels 9-10 mg/dl
- Decreasing symptoms of Paget's disease, including pain
- Decreased bone loss in osteoporosis

calcitriol (Rx)

(kal-si-tree'ole)

Calcijex, Rocaltrol, (1,25-dihydroxycholecalciferol) Vitamin D_3

Func. class.: Parathyroid agent (calcium regulator)

Chem. class.: Vitamin D hormone

Pregnancy category C

Do Not Confuse:

calcitriol/Calciferol

Action: Increases intestinal absorption of calcium, provides calcium for bones, increases renal tubular resorption of phosphate

Therapeutic Outcome: Calcium at normal level

Uses: Hypocalcemia in chronic renal disease, hyperparathyroidism, pseudohypoparathyroidism

Dosage and routes

Hypocalcemia

Adult: **IV** 0.5 mcg tid, initially; may increase by 0.25-0.5 mcg/dose q2-4 wk; 0.5-3 mcg tid maintenance

Predialysis

Adult: PO 0.25 mcg/day, max 0.5 mcg/day
Child: PO 0.25 mcg/day, max 0.5 mcg/day
Child <3 yr: PO 10-15 mcg/kg/day

Hypocalcemia during chronic dialysis

Adult: PO 0.5-3 mcg/day
Child: PO 0.25-2 mcg/day

Renal osteodystrophy

Adult: PO 0.25 mcg every other day-3 mcg/day
Child: PO 0.014-0.041 mcg/kg/day

Hypoparathyroidism

Adult: PO 0.25-2.7 mcg/day
Child: PO 0.04-0.08 mcg/kg/day

Available forms: Caps 0.25, 0.5 mcg; inj 1 mcg, 2 mcg/ml

Adverse effects

CNS: Drowsiness, headache, vertigo, fever, lethargy
CV: Palpitations
EENT: Blurred vision, photophobia
GI: Nausea, diarrhea, vomiting, jaundice, anorexia, dry mouth, constipation, cramps, metallic taste
GU: Polyuria, hypercalciuria, hyperphosphatemia, hematuria, thirst
MS: Myalgia, arthralgia, decreased bone development, weakness

Contraindications: Hypersensitivity, hyperphosphatemia, hypercalcemia, vit D toxicity

Precautions: Pregnancy **C**, renal calculi, lactation, CV disease

Pharmacokinetics	
Absorption	Well absorbed
Distribution	To liver, crosses placenta
Metabolism	Liver
Excretion	Bile
Half-life	3-6 hr, undergoes hepatic recycling, excreted in bile

Pharmacodynamics	
Onset	2-6 hr
Peak	10-12 hr
Duration	Up to 5 days

Interactions

Individual Drugs

Cholestyramine, mineral oil: decreased absorption of calcitriol
Phenytoin: increased vit D metabolism
Verapamil: increased dysrhythmias

Drug classifications

Antacids: increased hypermagnesemia
Diuretics (thiazide), calcium supplements: increased hypercalcemia
Cardiac glycosides: increased dysrhythmias
Vitamin D products: increased toxicity
Vitamins (fat-soluble): decreased calcitriol absorption

Drug/food
Large amounts of high-calcium foods may cause hypercalcemia
Drug/lab test
False: increased cholesterol
Interference: alkaline phosphatase, electrolytes

NURSING CONSIDERATIONS
Assessment
- Assess GI symptoms, polyuria, flushing, head swelling, tingling, headache; may indicate hypercalcemia
- Identify nutritional status; check diet for sources of vit D (milk, some seafood), calcium (dairy products, dark green vegetables), phosphates
- Monitor BUN, creatinine, uric acid, chloride, electrolytes, urine pH, urinary calcium, magnesium, phosphate, urinalysis (calcium should be kept at 9-10 mg/dl; vit D 50-135 international units/dl), alkaline phosphatase baseline and q3-6 mo
- ❗ Assess for increased drug level, since toxic reactions occur rapidly; have calcium chloride on hand if calcium level drops too low; check for tetany

Nursing diagnoses
- Injury, risk for (adverse reactions)
- Pain, chronic (uses)
- Knowledge, deficient (teaching)

Implementation
PO route
- Do not break, crush, or chew caps
- Give with meals for GI symptoms

IV route
- Give by direct **IV** over 1 min

Patient/family education
- Teach patient the symptoms of hypercalcemia (renal stones, nausea, vomiting, anorexia, lethargy, thirst, bone or flank pain) and about foods rich in calcium
- Advise patient to avoid products with sodium: cured meats, dairy products, cold cuts, olives, beets, pickles, soups, meat tenderizers in chronic renal failure
- Advise patient to avoid products with potassium: oranges, bananas, dried fruit, peas, dark green leafy vegetables, milk, melons, beans in chronic renal failure
- Advise patient to avoid OTC products containing calcium, potassium, or sodium in chronic renal failure
- Instruct patient to avoid all preparations containing vit D
- Instruct patient to monitor weight weekly

Evaluation
Positive therapeutic outcome
- Calcium levels 9-10 mg/dl

C

calcium carbonate (Rx) (PO-OTC, IV-Rx)
Alka-Mints, Amitone, Apo-Cal ♣, BioCal, Calcarb, Calci-Chew, Calcilac, Calcite ♣, Calglycine ♣, Cal-Plus, Calsan ♣, Caltrate 600, Caltrate Jr., Chooz, Dicarbosil, Equilet, Gencalc, Liquid-Cal, Liquid-Cal-600, Maalox Antacid Caplets, Mallamint, Mylanta Lozenges ♣, Nephro-Calci, Nu-Cal ♣, Os-Cal 500, Oysco 500, Oystercal 500, Oyst-Cal 500, Rolaids Calcium Rich, Titralac, Tums, Tums E-X Extra Strength

Func. class.: Antacid, calcium supplement
Chem. class.: Calcium product

calcium acetate
(kal'see-um ass'e-tate)
Calphron, PhosLo

Pregnancy category C

Action: Neutralizes gastric acidity

Therapeutic Outcome: Neutralized gastric acidity; calcium at normal levels

Uses: Antacid, calcium supplement; not suitable for chronic therapy, hyperphosphatemia, hypertension in pregnancy, osteoporosis, prevention/treatment of hypocalcemia, hyperparathyroidism

Dosage and routes
Antacid
Adult: PO 0.5-1.5 g or 2 pieces of gum 1 hr pc and at bedtime

Hyperphosphatemia
Adult: PO 1 g or more in divided doses

Hypertension in pregnancy
Adult: PO 500 mg tid during 3rd trimester

Prevention of hypocalcemia, depletion, osteoporosis
Adult: PO 1-2 g daily

Available forms: Calcium carbonate; chewable tabs 350, 420, 450, 500, 750, 1000, 1250 mg; tabs 500, 600, 650, 1000, 1250 mg; gum 300, 450, 500 mg; susp 1250 mg/5 ml; lozenges 600 mg; caps 1250 mg; powder 6.5 g/packet; calcium acetate: tabs 250 mg (65 mg Ca), 667 mg (169 mg Ca), 668 mg (169 mg Ca), 1 g (250 mg Ca); caps 333.5, 500, 667 mg (125 mg Ca); gelcaps 667 mg

Adverse effects

GI: *Constipation,* anorexia, nausea, vomiting, flatulence, diarrhea, rebound hyperacidity, eructation

Contraindications: Hypersensitivity, hypercalcemia, hyperparathyroidism, bone tumors

Precautions: Pregnancy **C**, elderly, fluid restriction, decreased GI motility, GI obstruction, dehydration, renal disease, lactation

Pharmacokinetics	
Absorption	⅓ absorbed by small intestine
Distribution	Unknown
Metabolism	Unknown
Excretion	Feces, urine, crosses placenta
Half-life	Unknown

Pharmacodynamics	
Onset	20 min
Peak	Unknown
Duration	20-180 min

Interactions

Individual drugs

Quinidine: increased quinidine levels

Drug classifications

Amphetamines: increased levels of amphetamines

Calcium channel blockers, iron products, salicylates, tetracyclines: decreased levels of each specific drug

Ketoconazole: decreased ketoconazole levels

Quinolone antiinfectives: decreased levels of antiinfectives

Drug/herb

Lily of the valley, pheasant's eye, shark cartilage, squill: increased side effect, action

Drug/lab test

False increase: increased chloride

False decrease: decreased magnesium, oxylate, lipase

False positive: benzodiazepines

NURSING CONSIDERATIONS

Assessment

- Monitor Ca^+ (serum, urine), Ca^+ should be 8.5-10.5 mg/dl, urine Ca^+ should be 150 mg/day, monitor weekly
- ◆ Assess for milk-alkali syndrome: nausea, vomiting, disorientation, headache
- Assess for constipation; increase bulk in the diet if needed
- Assess for hypercalcemia: headache, nausea, vomiting, confusion

Nursing diagnoses

- Nutrition, imbalanced, less than body requirements (uses)
- Knowledge, deficient (teaching)

Implementation

PO route

- Administer as antacid 1 hr pc and at bedtime
- Administer as supplement 1½ hr pc and at bedtime
- Administer only with regular tablets or capsules; do not give with enteric-coated tablets
- Administer laxatives or stool softeners if constipation occurs

Patient/family education

- Advise patient to increase fluids to 2 L unless contraindicated, to add bulk to diet for constipation; notify prescriber of constipation
- Advise patient not to switch antacids unless directed by prescriber, not to use as antacid for >2 wk without approval by prescriber
- Teach patient that therapeutic dose recommendations are figured as elemental calcium

Evaluation

Positive therapeutic outcome

- Absence of pain, decreased acidity

calcium chloride
calcium gluceptate
calcium gluconate
calcium lactate

(PO-OTC, **IV**-Rx)

Func. class.: Electrolyte replacement—calcium product

Pregnancy category C

Action: Cation needed for maintenance of nervous, muscular, skeletal systems, enzyme reactions, normal cardiac contractility, coagulation of blood; affects secretory activity of endocrine, exocrine glands

Therapeutic Outcome: Calcium at normal level, absence of increased magnesium, potassium

Uses: Prevention and treatment of hypocalcemia, hypermagnesemia, hypoparathyroidism, neonatal tetany, cardiac toxicity caused by hyperkalemia, lead colic, hyperphosphatemia, vit D deficiency, osteoporosis prophylaxis, calcium antagonist toxicity (calcium channel blocker toxicity)

Dosage and routes

Calcium chloride

Adult: **IV** 500 mg-1 g q1-3 days as indicated by serum calcium levels; give at <1 ml/min; IAV 200-800 mg injected in ventricle of heart
Child: **IV** 25 mg/kg over several min

Calcium gluceptate

Adult: **IV** 5-20 ml; IM 2-5 ml
Newborn: 0.5 ml/100 ml of blood transfused

Calcium gluconate

Adult: PO 0.5-2 g bid-qid; **IV** 0.5-2 g at 0.5 ml/min (10% sol); max **IV** dose 3 g
Child: PO/**IV** 500 mg/kg/day in divided doses

Calcium lactate

Adult: PO 325 mg-1.3 g tid with meals
Child: PO 500 mg/kg/day in divided doses

Available forms: Many; check product listings

Adverse effects

CV: Shortened QT interval, heart block, hypotension, bradycardia, dysrhythmias; **cardiac arrest (IV)**
GI: Vomiting, nausea, constipation
HYPERCALCEMIA: Drowsiness, lethargy, muscle weakness, headache, constipation, **coma,** anorexia, nausea, vomiting, polyuria, thirst
INTEG: Pain, burning at **IV** site, severe venous thrombosis, necrosis, extravasation

Contraindications: Hypercalcemia, digitalis toxicity, ventricular fibrillation, renal calculi

Precautions: Pregnancy **C,** lactation, children, renal disease, respiratory disease, cor pulmonale, digitalized patient, respiratory failure

Pharmacokinetics

Absorption	Complete bioavailability (**IV**)
Distribution	Readily extracellular; crosses placenta
Metabolism	Liver
Excretion	Feces (80%), kidney (20%), breast milk
Half-life	Unknown

Pharmacodynamics

	PO	IV
Onset	Unknown	Immediate
Peak	Unknown	Rapid
Duration	Unknown	½-1½ hr

Interactions

Individual drugs

Atenolol: decreased effects of atenolol
Digitalis glycosides: increased dysrhythmias
Phenytoin: decreased absorption of phenytoin when calcium is taken PO
Tetracycline: decreased absorption of tetracycline (PO)
Verapamil: decreased effects of verapamil; increased toxicity

Drug classifications

Antacids: milk-alkali syndrome (renal disease)
Diuretics (thiazide): increased hypercalcemia
Fluoroquinolones: decreased absorption of fluoroquinolones when calcium is taken PO
Iron salts: decreased absorption of iron when calcium is taken PO

Drug/herb

Lily of the valley, pheasant's eye, shark cartilage, squill: increased side effects, action

Drug/lab test

False: decreased magnesium, decreased 17-OHCS, increased 11-OHCS

NURSING CONSIDERATIONS

Assessment

- Monitor ECG for decreased QT interval and T-wave inversion: in hypercalcemia, drug should be reduced or discontinued
- Monitor calcium levels during treatment (9-10 mg/dl is normal level)
- Assess cardiac status: rate, rhythm, CVP (PWP, PAWP if being monitored directly)

Nursing diagnoses

- Injury, risk for (uses, adverse reactions)
- Knowledge, deficient (teaching)

Implementation

PO route

- Give PO with or following meals to enhance absorption
- Store at room temp

IV route

- Administer **IV** undiluted or diluted with equal amounts of 0.9% NaCl for inj to a 5% sol; give 0.5-1 ml/min
- Give through small-bore needle into large vein; if extravasation occurs, necrosis will result (**IV**); IM inj may cause severe burning, necrosis, and tissue sloughing; warm sol to body temp before administering (only gluconate/gluceptate)
- Provide seizure precautions: padded side rails, decreased stimuli (noise, light); place airway suction equipment, padded mouth gag if calcium levels are low
- Patient should remain recumbent 30 min after IV dose

C

Calcium chloride
Syringe compatibilities: Milrinone
Y-site compatibilities: Amrinone, dobutamine, epINEPHrine, esmolol, morphine, paclitaxel
Additive compatibilities: Amikacin, amphotericin B, ampicillin, ascorbic acid, bretylium, ceftriaxone, cephapirin, chloramphenicol, DOPamine, hydrocortisone, isoproterenol, lidocaine, methicillin, norepinephrine, penicillin G potassium, penicillin G sodium, pentobarbital, phenobarbital, verapamil, vit B/C
Calcium gluceptate
Additive compatibilities: Ascorbic acid inj, isoproterenol, lidocaine, norepinephrine, phytonadione, sodium bicarbonate
Calcium gluconate
Syringe compatibilities: Aldesleukin, allopurinol, amifostine, aztreonam, cefazolin, cefepime, ciprofloxacin, cladribine, DOBUTamine, enalaprilat, epINEPHrine, famotidine, filgrastim, granisetron, heparin/hydrocortisone, labetalol, melphalan, midazolam, netilmicin, piperacillin/tazobactam, potassium chloride, prochlorperazine, propofol, sargramostim, tacrolimus, teniposide, thiotepa, tolazoline, vinorelbine, vit B/C
Additive compatibilities: Amikacin, aminophylline, ascorbic acid inj, bretylium, cephapirin, chloramphenicol, corticotropin, dimenhyDRINATE, erythromycin, furosemide, heparin, hydrocortisone, lidocaine, magnesium sulfate, methicillin, norepinephrine, penicillin G potassium, penicillin G sodium, phenobarbital, potassium chloride, tobramycin, vancomycin, verapamil, vit B/C

Patient/family education

- Caution patient to add food high in vit D content; to add calcium-rich foods to diet: dairy products, shellfish, dark green leafy vegetables; decrease oxalate-rich and zinc-rich foods: nuts, legumes, chocolate, spinach, soy
- Advise patient to prevent injuries, avoid immobilization

Evaluation

Positive therapeutic outcome

- Decreased twitching, paresthesias, muscle spasms
- Absence of tremors, convulsions, dysrhythmias, dyspnea, laryngospasm, negative Chvostek's sign, negative Trousseau's sign

calcium polycarbophil (OTC)

(pol-i-kar'boe-fil)
Equalactin, Fiberall, FiberCon, Fiber-Lax, Mitrolan
Func. class.: Laxative, bulk-forming
Pregnancy category C

Action: Attracts water, expands in intestine to increase peristalsis; also absorbs excess water in stool; decreases diarrhea

Therapeutic Outcome: Absence of constipation or diarrhea in irritable bowel syndrome

Uses: Constipation, irritable bowel syndrome (diarrhea), acute, nonspecific diarrhea

Dosage and routes

Adult: PO 1 g daily-qid prn, not to exceed 6 g/24 hr
Child 6-12 yr: PO 500 mg bid prn, not to exceed 3 g/24 hr
Child 3-6 yr: PO 500 mg bid prn, not to exceed 1.5 g/24 hr

Available forms: Chewable tabs 500, 1000 mg; tabs 500 mg

Adverse effects

GI: **Obstruction,** abdominal distention, flatus, laxative dependence

Contraindications: Hypersensitivity, GI obstruction

Precautions: Pregnancy **C,** lactation

Pharmacokinetics	
Absorption	None
Distribution	None
Metabolism	Unknown
Excretion	Feces
Half-life	Not known

Pharmacodynamics	
Onset	12-24 hr
Peak	1-3 days
Duration	Unknown

Interactions

Drug/herb
Flax, lily of the valley, pheasant's eye, senna, squill: increased side effects, action

NURSING CONSIDERATIONS

Assessment

- Monitor blood, urine electrolytes if used often by patient; check I&O ratio to identify fluid loss

• Assess cramping, rectal bleeding, nausea, vomiting; if these symptoms occur, drug should be discontinued; identify cause of constipation; identify whether fluids, bulk, or exercise is missing from lifestyle

Nursing diagnoses
• Constipation (uses)
• Diarrhea (side effects)
• Knowledge, deficient (teaching)
• Noncompliance (teaching)

Implementation
• Give alone for better absorption; give after mixing with water immediately before use; administer with 6-8 oz of water or juice followed by another 8 oz of fluid
• Administer in AM or PM

Patient/family education
• Discuss with the patient that adequate fluid consumption is necessary; not to use laxatives long-term, laxative dependence will result
• Teach patient that normal bowel movements do not always occur daily
• Teach patient not to use in presence of abdominal pain, nausea, vomiting; tell patient to notify prescriber if constipation is unrelieved or if symptoms of electrolyte imbalance occur: muscle cramps, pain, weakness, dizziness, excessive thirst

Evaluation
Positive therapeutic outcome
• Decreased constipation within 3 days
• Decreased diarrhea in colitis within 1 wk

candesartan (Rx)
(can-deh-sar'tan)
Atacand
Func. class.: Antihypertensive
Chem. class.: Angiotensin II receptor (Type AT_1)

Pregnancy category
C (1st trimester),
D (2nd/3rd trimesters)

Action: Blocks the vasoconstrictor and aldosterone-secreting effects of angiotensin II; selectively blocks the binding of angiotensin II to the AT_1 receptor found in tissues

Therapeutic Outcome: Decreased B/P

Uses: Hypertension, alone or in combination

Dosage and routes
Adult: PO (single agent) 16 mg daily initially in patients who are not volume depleted, range 8-32 mg/day; with diuretic or volume depletion 2-32 mg/day as a single dose or divided bid

Renal dose
Adult: PO Give lowest possible dose

Available forms: Tabs 4, 8, 16, 32 mg

Adverse effects
CNS: *Dizziness,* fatigue, headache
CV: Chest pain, peripheral edema
EENT: Sinusitis, rhinitis, pharyngitis
GI: *Diarrhea,* nausea, abdominal pain, vomiting
GU: **Renal failure**
MS: Arthralgia, pain
RESP: *Cough, upper respiratory infection*
SYST: **Angioedema**

Contraindications: Pregnancy **D** (2nd/3rd trimesters), hypersensitivity

Precautions: Pregnancy **C** (1st trimester), hypersensitivity to ACE inhibitors, lactation, children, elderly

Pharmacokinetics	
Absorption	Well absorbed
Distribution	Bound to plasma proteins
Metabolism	Extensive
Excretion	Feces, urine, breast milk
Half-life	9 hr

Pharmacodynamics	
Onset	Unknown
Peak	2 hr
Duration	24 hr

Interactions
Drug/herb
Aconite: increased toxicity, death
Astragalus, cola tree: increased or decreased antihypertensive effect
Barberry, betony, black catechu, black cohosh, bloodroot, broom, burdock, cat's claw, dandelion, goldenseal, Irish moss, Jamaican dogwood, kelp, khella, mistletoe, parsley, Queen Anne's lace, rue: increased antihypertensive effect
Coltsfoot, guarana, khat, licorice: decreased antihypertensive effect

NURSING CONSIDERATIONS
Assessment
• Assess B/P, pulse q4h; note rate, rhythm, quality
• Monitor electrolytes: potassium, sodium, chloride; total CO_2
• Obtain baselines in renal, liver function tests before therapy begins

- Assess blood studies: BUN, creatinine, liver function tests before treatment
- Monitor for edema in feet, legs daily
- Assess for skin turgor, dryness of mucous membranes for hydration status; for angioedema: facial swelling, dyspnea
- Assess for pregnancy, this drug can cause fetal death when given in pregnancy
- Assess for adverse reactions, especially in renal disease

Nursing diagnoses
- Fluid volume, deficient (side effects)
- Noncompliance (teaching)
- Knowledge, deficient (teaching)

Implementation
- Administer without regard to meals

Patient/family education
- Teach patient not to take the drug if breast-feeding or pregnant, or have had an allergic reaction to this drug
- If a dose is missed, instruct patient to take as soon as possible, unless it is within an hour before next dose
- Advise patient to comply with dosage schedule, even if feeling better
- Teach patient to notify prescriber of fever, swelling of hands or feet, irregular heartbeat, chest pain
- Advise patient excessive perspiration, dehydration, diarrhea may lead to fall in blood pressure—consult prescriber if these occur
- Inform patient that drug may cause dizziness, fainting; lightheadedness may occur
- Caution patient to rise slowly to sitting or standing position to minimize orthostatic hypotension
- Advise patient to avoid all OTC medications unless approved by prescriber; to inform all health care providers of medication use
- Teach proper technique for obtaining B/P and acceptable parameters

Evaluation
Positive therapeutic outcome
- Decreased B/P

capecitabine (Rx)
(cap-eh-sit'ah-bean)
Xeloda
Func. class.: Antineoplastic, antimetabolite
Chem. class.: Fluoropyrimidine carbamate

Pregnancy category D

Do Not Confuse:
Xeloda/Xenical

Action: Competes with physiologic substrate of DNA synthesis, thus interfering with cell replication in the S phase of cell cycle (before mitosis); drug is converted to 5-fluorouracil (5-FU)

Therapeutic Outcome: Decreasing symptoms of breast cancer

Uses: Monotherapy for paclitaxel-anthracycline-resistant metastatic breast, colorectal cancer; treatment of patients with colorectal cancer who have undergone complete resection of their primary tumor

Dosage and routes:
Adult: PO 2500 mg/m^2/day in 2 divided doses q12h at end of meal × 2 wk, then 1 wk rest period; given in 3 wk cycles; may be combined with Docetaxel, when capecitalane dose is lowered; follow the NCIC (National Cancer Institute of Canada) common toxicity criteria

Available forms: Tabs 150, 500 mg

Adverse effects
CNS: Dizziness, headache, *paresthesia, fatigue,* insomnia
GI: *Nausea, vomiting, anorexia, diarrhea, stomatitis, abdominal pain, constipation, dyspepsia,* **intestinal obstruction**
HEMA: **Neutropenia, lymphopenia, thrombocytopenia,** anemia
INTEG: *Hand and foot syndrome,* dermatitis, nail disorder
MISC: Hyperbilirubinemia, eye irritation, edema, myalgia, limb pain, *pyrexia,* dehydration

Contraindications: Pregnancy **D**, hypersensitivity to 5-FU, infants, severe renal impairment (CCr <30 ml/min)

Precautions: Renal disease, hepatic disease, lactation, children, elderly

Pharmacokinetics	
Absorption	Readily, food decreased
Distribution	Unknown
Metabolism	Liver, extensively
Excretion	Kidneys
Half-life	45 min

Pharmacodynamics	
Onset	Unknown
Peak	1½ hr
Duration	Unknown

Interactions

Individual drugs

Leucovorin: increased toxicity
Phenytoin: increased phenytoin level
Warfarin: increased risk of bleeding

Drug classifications

Antacids (aluminum, magnesium): increased capecitabine

NURSING CONSIDERATIONS

Assessment

- Assess buccal cavity q8h for dryness, sores or ulceration, white patches, pain, bleeding, dysphagia; obtain prescription for viscous lidocaine (Xylocaine)
- Assess symptoms indicating severe allergic reation: rash, pruritus, urticaria, purpuric skin lesions, itching, flushing; drug should be discontinued
- Monitor CBC, differential, platelet count weekly; withhold drug if WBC $<4000/mm^3$ or platelet count is $<100,000/mm^3$; notify prescriber of results if WBC $<20,000/mm^3$, platelet count $<150,000/mm^3$
- Monitor temp q4h (may indicate beginning of infection)
- Assess for hand/foot syndrome: paresthesia, tingling, painful/painless swelling, blistering, erythema with severe pain of hands/feet
- Assess for toxicity: severe diarrhea, nausea, vomiting, stomatitis
- Assess GI symptoms: frequency of stools, cramping; if severe diarrhea occurs, fluids/electrolytes may need to be given
- Monitor liver function tests before and during therapy (bilirubin, AST, ALT, LDH) as needed or monthly; note jaundice of skin or sclera, dark urine, clay-colored stools, itchy skin, abdominal pain, fever, diarrhea
- Assess for bleeding: hematuria, stool guaiac, bruising or petechiae, mucosa or orifices q8h; inflammation of mucosa, breaks in skin

Nursing diagnoses

- Injury, risk for (adverse reactions)
- Body image, disturbed (adverse reactions)
- Infection, risk for (adverse reactions)
- Knowledge, deficient (teaching)

Implementation

- Give antiemetic 30-60 min before giving drug to prevent vomiting and prn; give antibiotics for prophylaxis of infection
- Provide liq diet: carbonated beverages; gelatin may be added if patient is not nauseated or vomiting
- Help patient to rinse mouth tid-qid with water or club soda, brush teeth bid-qid with soft brush or cotton-tipped applicators for stomatitis, use unwaxed dental floss

Patient/family education

- Contraceptive measures are recommended during therapy; drug is teratogenic to fetus
- Advise patient to avoid use of products containing aspirin or ibuprofen, razors, commercial mouthwash, since bleeding may occur; to report symptoms of bleeding (hematuria, tarry stools)
- Instruct patient to report signs of anemia (fatigue, headache, irritability, faintness, shortness of breath)
- Advise patient not to become pregnant while taking this drug; to avoid using while lactating
- Advise patient not to double dose, if dose is missed
- Advise patient to report immediately severe diarrhea, vomiting, stomatitis, fever ≥100° F, hand/foot syndrome, anorexia

Evaluation

Positive therapeutic outcome

- Prevention of rapid division of malignant cells

captopril (Rx)

(kap'toe-pril)

Capoten, Novo-Captopril ♣

Func. class.: Antihypertensive

Chem. class.: Angiotensin-converting enzyme (ACE) inhibitor

Pregnancy category
C (1st trimester),
D (2nd/3rd trimesters)

Do Not Confuse:
Captopril/Capitrol/Carvedilol

Action: Selectively suppresses renin-angiotensin-aldosterone system; inhibits ACE; prevents conversion of angiotensin I to angiotensin II

Therapeutic Outcome: Decreased B/P in hypertension; decreased preload, afterload in CHF

Uses: Hypertension, CHF, left ventricular dysfunction (LVD) after MI, diabetic nephropathy

Dosage and routes

Malignant hypertension

Adult: PO 25 mg increasing q2h until desired response; not to exceed 450 mg/day

Hypertension

Adult: Initial dose: PO 25 mg bid-tid; may

increase to 50 mg bid-tid at 1-2 wk intervals; usual range 25-150 mg bid-tid; max 450 mg
Child: PO 0.3-0.5 mg/kg/dose, titrate up to 6 mg/kg/day in 2-4 divided doses
Neonate: PO 10 mcg (0.01 mg)/kg bid-tid, may increase as needed

CHF
Adult: PO 12.5 mg bid-tid; may increase to 50 mg bid-tid; after 14 days may increase to 150 mg tid if needed

LVD After MI
Adult: PO 50 mg tid, may begin treatment 3 days after MI; give 6.25 mg as a single dose, then 12.5 mg tid, increase to 25 mg tid for several days, then 50 mg tid

Diabetic nephropathy
Adult: PO 25 mg tid

Renal dose
Adult: PO 6.25-12.5 mg bid-tid
Child: PO 150 mcg (0.15)/kg tid

Available forms: Tabs 12.5, 25, 50, 100 mg

Adverse effects
CNS: Fever, chills
CV: *Hypotension,* postural hypotension, *tachycardia,* angina
GI: Loss of taste, liver function tests
GU: Impotence, dysuria, nocturia, **proteinuria, nephrotic syndrome, acute reversible renal failure,** polyuria, oliguria, frequency
HEMA: **Neutropenia, agranulocytosis, pancytopenia, thrombocytopenia,** anemia
INTEG: Rash
MISC: **Angioedema,** hyperkalemia
RESP: **Bronchospasm,** *dyspnea, cough*

Contraindications: Pregnancy **D** (2nd/3rd trimesters), hypersensitivity, lactation, heart block, children, potassium-sparing diuretics, bilateral renal artery stenosis

Precautions: Pregnancy **C** (1st trimester), dialysis patients, hypovolemia, leukemia, scleroderma, LE, blood dyscrasias, CHF, diabetes mellitus, renal disease, thyroid disease, COPD, asthma

Pharmacokinetics

Absorption	Well absorbed
Distribution	Widely distributed; crosses placenta, excreted in breast milk, small amounts
Metabolism	Liver (50%)
Excretion	Kidneys, unchanged (50%)
Half-life	2 hr increase in renal disease

Pharmacodynamics

Onset	¼-1 hr
Peak	1 hr
Duration	6-12 hr

Interactions
Individual drugs
Alcohol (acute ingestion): increased hypotension (large amounts)
Digoxin, lithium: increased serum levels, toxicity
Insulin: increased hypoglycemia
Drug classifications
Antacids, NSAIDs: decreased captopril effect
Antidiabetics (oral): increased hypoglycemia
Antihypertensives, diuretics, nitrates, phenothiazines: increased hypotension
Diuretics (potassium-sparing), potassium supplements: increased toxicity, do not use
Sympathomimetics: do not use
Drug/herb
Aconite: increased toxicity, death
Astragalus, cola tree: increased or decreased antihypertensive effect
Barberry, betony, black catechu, black cohosh, bloodroot, broom, burdock, cat's claw, dandelion, goldenseal, Irish moss, Jamaican dogwood, kelp, khella, mistletoe, parsley: increased antihypertensive effect
Coltsfoot, guarana, khat, licorice: decreased antihypertensive effect
Drug/lab test
Increased: AST, ALT, alkaline phosphatase, bilirubin, uric acid, glucose
False positive: urine acetone, ANA titer

NURSING CONSIDERATIONS
Assessment
- May be crushed and mixed with food
- Monitor blood studies: decreased platelets; WBC with diff baseline and periodically q3 mo, if neutrophils <1000/mm^3, discontinue treatment
- Monitor B/P, check for orthostatic hypotension, syncope; if changes occur, dosage change may be required
- Monitor renal studies: protein, BUN, creatinine; watch for increased levels that may indicate nephrotic syndrome and renal failure; monitor renal symptoms: polyuria, oliguria, frequency, dysuria
- Establish baselines in renal, liver function tests before therapy begins and check periodically; monitor for increased liver function studies; watch for increased uric acid, glucose
- Check potassium levels throughout treatment, although hyperkalemia rarely occurs

- Check for edema in feet, legs daily; monitor weight daily in CHF
- Assess for allergic reactions: rash, fever, pruritus, urticaria; drug should be discontinued if antihistamines fail to help

Nursing diagnoses
- Cardiac output, decreased (uses)
- Injury, risk for (side effects)
- Knowledge, deficient (teaching)
- Noncompliance (teaching)

Implementation
- Store in air-tight container at 86° F (30° C) or less
- Severe hypotension may occur after 1st dose of this medication; decreasing hypotension may be prevented by reducing or discontinuing diuretic therapy 3 days before beginning captopril therapy
- Administer 1 hr ac or 2 hr pc
- May crush tab and dissolve in water, give within ½ hr, make sure tab is completely dissolved

Patient/family education
- Caution patient not to discontinue drug abruptly; advise patient to tell all persons associated with care
- Teach patient not to use OTC products (cough, cold, allergy) unless directed by prescriber; serious side effects can occur; xanthines such as coffee, tea, chocolate, cola can prevent action of drug
- Teach patient importance of complying with dosage schedule, even if feeling better; to continue with medical regimen to decrease B/P: exercise, cessation of smoking, decreasing stress, diet modifications
- Emphasize the need to rise slowly to sitting or standing position to minimize orthostatic hypotension; not to exercise in hot weather or increased hypotension can occur
- Teach patient to notify prescriber of mouth sores, sore throat, fever, swelling of hands or feet, irregular heartbeat, chest pain, coughing, shortness of breath
- Caution patient to report excessive perspiration, dehydration, vomiting, diarrhea; may lead to fall in B/P
- Caution patient that drug may cause dizziness, fainting, lightheadedness; may occur during 1st few days of therapy; to avoid activities that may be hazardous
- Teach patient how to take B/P, and teach normal readings for age-group; ensure patient takes regularly
- Advise patient to tell prescriber if pregnancy is suspected or planned

Evaluation
Positive therapeutic outcome
- Decreased B/P in hypertension

Treatment of overdose: 0.9% NaCl **IV** infusion, hemodialysis

C

carbamazepine (Rx)
(kar-ba-maz′e-peen)

Apo-Carbamazepine ✦, Atretol, Carbatrol, Epitol, Equetro, Novo-Carbamaz ✦, Tegretol, Tegretol CR ✦, Tegretol-XR

Func. class.: Anticonvulsant

Chem. class.: Iminostilbene derivative

Pregnancy category D

Do Not Confuse:
Tegretol/Toradol

Action: Exact mechanism unknown; appears to decrease polysynaptic responses and block posttetanic potentiation

Therapeutic Outcome: Absence of seizures; decreased trigeminal neuralgia pain

Uses: Tonic-clonic, complex-partial, mixed seizures; trigeminal neuralgia, bipolar disorder

Investigational uses: Diabetes insipidus, neurogenic pain, schizophrenia, psychotic behavior with dementia, rectal administration, diabetic neuropathy, restless legs syndrome

Dosage and routes
Seizures

Adult and child >12 yr: PO 200 mg bid; may be increased by 200 mg/day in divided doses q6-8h; maintenance 800-1200 mg/day; maximum 1600 mg/day (adult); max child 12-15 yr 1000 mg/day; max child >15 yr 1200 mg/day; adjustment is needed to minimum dose to control seizures; ext rel give bid; rec administration of oral susp 200 mg/10 ml or 6 mg/kg as a single dose

Child 6-12 yr: PO tabs 100 mg bid or susp 50 mg qid; may increase by <100 mg qwk, max 1000 mg/day; ext rel tabs daily-bid

Child <6 yr: PO 10-20 mg/kg/day in 2-3 divided doses, may increase qwk

Trigeminal neuralgia

Adult: PO 100 mg/bid; may increase 100 mg q12h until pain subsides; not to exceed 1200 mg/day; maintenance is 200-400 mg bid

Bipolar disorder

Adult: PO (Equetro only) 200 mg bid, may

adjust dose by 200 mg daily to desired response; max 1600 mg/day

Available forms: Chewable tabs 100, 200 mg; tabs 200 mg; oral susp 100 mg/5 ml; ext rel tabs 100, 200, 400 mg; ext rel caps (Carbatrol) 200, 300 mg

Adverse effects

CNS: *Drowsiness,* dizziness, confusion, fatigue, **paralysis,** headache, hallucinations, **worsening of seizures,** unsteadiness, speech disturbances
CV: **Hypertension, CHF,** hypotension, aggravation of CAD, dysrhythmias, **AV block**
EENT: Tinnitus, dry mouth, blurred vision, diplopia, nystagmus, conjunctivitis
ENDO: Syndrome of inappropriate antidiuretic hormone (SIADH) (elderly)
GI: *Nausea, constipation, diarrhea,* anorexia, vomiting, abdominal pain, stomatitis, glossitis, increased liver enzymes, **hepatitis**
GU: Frequency, retention, albuminuria, glycosuria, impotence, increased BUN, **renal failure**
HEMA: **Thrombocytopenia, agranulocytosis, leukocytosis, aplastic anemia, eosinophilia,** increased protime
INTEG: *Rash,* **Stevens-Johnson syndrome,** urticaria, photosensitivity
RESP: Pulmonary hypersensitivity (fever, dyspnea, pneumonitis)

Contraindications: Pregnancy **D,** hypersensitivity to carbamazepine or tricyclic antidepressants, bone marrow depression, concomitant use of MAOIs

Precautions: Glaucoma, hepatic disease, renal disease, cardiac disease, psychosis, lactation, child <6 yr

Pharmacokinetics	
Absorption	Slow; completely absorbed
Distribution	Widely distributed; protein binding 76%
Metabolism	Extensively, liver
Excretion	Urine, feces, breast milk
Half-life	14-16 hr or more

Pharmacodynamics	
Onset	2-4 day
Peak	4-8 hr
Duration	Unknown

Interactions

Individual drugs

Benzodiazepines: decreased effect of benzodiazepine, verapamil
Cisplatin, danazol, DOXOrubicin, felbamate, phenobarbitol, phenytoin, primidone, rifampin, theophylline: decreased carbamazepine levels
Clarithromycin, verapamil: increased toxicity
Contraceptives (oral): decreased effect of oral contraceptives
Doxycycline: decreased effect of doxycycline
Felbamate, fluoxetine, fluroxamine: increased carbamazepine effect
Lithium: increased CNS toxicity
Phenobarbital: increased effect
Phenytoin: increased and decreased plasma levels; decreased carbamazepine plasma levels
Thyroid hormones: decreased effect of thyroid hormones
Valproic acid: decreased plasma levels; increased half-life of carbamazepine
Warfarin: decreased effect of warfarin

Drug classifications

Barbiturates: decreased serum levels of carbamazepine
◆ MAOIs: fatal reaction; do not use together

Drug/herb

Ginkgo, quinine: increased anticonvulsant action
Ginseng, santonica: decreased anticonvulsant action

Drug/food

Grapefruit juice: increased peak concentration of carbamazepine

NURSING CONSIDERATIONS

Assessment

- Assess for seizures: character, location, duration, intensity, frequency, presence of aura
- Assess for trigeminal neuralgia: facial pain including location, duration, intensity, character, activity that stimulates pain
- Monitor liver function tests (AST, ALT) and urine function tests, BUN, urine protein periodically during treatments
- Assess blood studies: RBC, Hct, Hgb, reticulocyte counts qwk for 4 wk then q3-6mo if on long-term therapy; if myelosuppression occurs, drug should be discontinued
- Check blood levels during treatment or when changing dose; therapeutic level 4-12 mcg/ml
- Assess for blood dyscrasias: fever, sore throat, bruising, rash, jaundice, epistaxis (long-term treatment only)
- Assess seizure activity including type, aura, location, duration, and character; provide seizure precaution

Nursing diagnoses

- Injury, risk for (side effects)
- Knowledge, deficient (teaching)

Implementation
- Do not break, crush, or chew ext rel tabs and caps
- Ext rel caps may be opened and beads mixed with food
- Chewable tabs should be chewed, not swallowed whole
- Give with food for GI symptoms
- Shake oral susp before use
- Mix an equal amount of water, D_5W, 0.9% NaCl when giving by NG tube, flush tube with 100 ml of above sol

Patient/family education
- Teach patient to carry/wear emergency ID stating patient's name, drugs taken, condition, prescriber's name, phone number
- Caution patient to avoid driving, other activities that require alertness until stabilized on medication
- Teach patient not to discontinue medication quickly after long-term use
- Teach patient to use a nonhormonal type of contraception to prevent harm to the fetus
- Advise patient to use sunscreen to prevent burns
- Teach patient to take exactly as prescribed; do not double or omit doses
- Teach patient to report immediately chills, rash, light-colored stools, dark urine, yellowing of skin/eyes, abdominal pain, sore throat, mouth, ulcers, bruising, blurred vision, dizziness

Evaluation
Positive therapeutic outcome
- Decreased seizure activity

Treatment of overdose: Lavage, VS

carbidopa-levodopa (Rx)
(kar-bi-doe'pa lee-voe-doe'pa)

Atamet, carbidopa/levodopa, Sinemet, Sinemet CR

Func. class.: Antiparkinsonism agent

Chem. class.: Catecholamine

Pregnancy category C

Action: Decarboxylation of levodopa to periphery is inhibited by carbidopa; more levodopa is made available for transport to brain and conversion to dopamine in the brain

Therapeutic Outcome: Absence of involuntary movements

Uses: Parkinsonism, restless legs syndrome, chronic manganese intoxication, cerebral arteriosclerosis

Investigational uses: Restless legs syndrome

Dosage and routes
Beginning therapy for those not taking levodopa

Adult: PO 25 mg carbidopa/100 mg levodopa tid-qid, may increase daily or every other day to desired response; ext rel tabs carbidopa 5 mg/levodopa 200 mg bid

For those not taking levodopa ER

Adult: PO 50 mg carbidopa/200 mg levodopa bid

For those taking levodopa ER

Adult: Begin treatment with 10% more levodopa/day given PO q4-8h, may increase or decrease dose q3 days

For those taking levodopa <1.5 g/day

Adult: PO 25 mg carbidopa/100 mg levodopa tid-qid, may increase daily to desired response

For those taking levodopa >1.5 g/day

Adult: PO 25 mg carbidopa/250 mg levodopa tid-qid, may increase daily to desired response

Restless legs syndrome (RLS) (off-label)

Adult: PO carbidopa 25 mg/levodopa 100 mg

Available forms: Tabs 10/100, 25/100, 25 mg carbidopa/250 mg levodopa; ext rel tab 25 mg/100 mg, 50 mg/200 mg carbidopa/levodopa (Sinemet CR)

Adverse effects
CNS: *Involuntary choreiform movements, hand tremors, fatigue, headache, anxiety, twitching, numbness, weakness, confusion, agitation, insomnia, nightmares,* psychosis, hallucination, hypomania, severe depression, dizziness

CV: *Orthostatic hypotension,* tachycardia, hypertension, palpitation

EENT: Blurred vision, diplopia, dilated pupils

GI: *Nausea, vomiting, anorexia, abdominal distress, dry mouth, flatulence, dysphagia, bitter taste, diarrhea, constipation*

HEMA: **Hemolytic anemia, leukopenia, agranulocytosis**

INTEG: Rash, sweating, alopecia

MISC: Urinary retention, incontinence, weight change, dark urine

Contraindications: Hypersensitivity, narrow-angle glaucoma, malignant melanoma, history of malignant melanoma, or undiagnosed skin lesions resembling melanoma

Precautions: Pregnancy **C,** renal disease, cardiac disease, hepatic disease, respiratory disease, MI with dysrhythmias, wide angle glaucoma, convulsions, peptic ulcer, lactation

Pharmacokinetics

Absorption	Well absorbed (PO); ER dose slow
Distribution	Widely distributed
Metabolism	Liver, extensively
Excretion	Kidneys, metabolites
Half-life	Levodopa (1 hr); carbidopa (1-2 hr)

Pharmacodynamics

	PO	PO-ER
Onset	Unknown	Unknown
Peak	1 hr	2½ hr
Duration	6-24 hr	Unknown

Interactions

Individual drugs

Metoclopramide: increased effects of levodopa

Papaverine, pyridoxine: decreased effects of levodopa

Drug classifications

Antacids: increased effects of levodopa

Anticholinergics, benzodiazepines, hydantoins: decreased effects of levodopa

MAOIs: hypertensive crisis

Drug/herb

Kava, octacosanol: increased Parkinson's symptoms

Indian snakeroot: decreased action; increased extrapyramidal symptoms

Drug/food

Protein: decreased absorption of levodopa

Pyridoxine: decreased levodopa effect

Drug/lab test

Increased: AST, ALT, bilirubin, LDH, alkaline phosphatase, BUN

Decreased: VMA, BUN, creatinine

False increase: uric acid, urine protein

False positive: urine ketones (dipstick)

False negative: urine glucose

NURSING CONSIDERATIONS

Assessment

- Assess B/P, respiration, orthostatic B/P
- Monitor I&O ratio; retention commonly causes decreased urinary output, distention, frequency, incontinence; palpate bladder if retention occurs
- Assess for muscle twitching, blepharospasm that may indicate toxicity
- Monitor renal, liver, hematopoietic studies, also for diabetes, acromegaly during long-term therapy
- Assess for parkinsonism: shuffling gait, muscle rigidity, involuntary movements, pill rolling, muscle spasms, drooling before and during treatment
- Monitor for constipation, cramping, pain in abdomen, abdominal distention; increase fluids, bulk, exercise if this occurs
- Assess for tolerance over long-term therapy; dose may have to be increased or changed
- Assess for mental status: affect, mood, CNS depression, worsening of mental symptoms during early therapy

Nursing diagnoses

- Mobility, physical, impaired (uses)
- Knowledge, deficient (teaching)

Implementation

PO route

- Swallow ext rel tabs whole; do not break, crush, or chew
- Give drug until NPO before surgery; check with prescriber for continuing drug
- Adjust dosage depending on patient response
- Give with meals or pc to prevent GI symptoms; limit protein taken with drug
- Give only after MAOIs have been discontinued for 2 wk; if previously on levodopa, discontinue for at least 8 hr before change to levodopa-carbidopa

Patient/family education

- Teach patient to change positions slowly to prevent orthostatic hypotension
- Teach patient to report side effects: twitching, eye spasms, grimacing, protrusion of tongue, personality changes that indicate overdose
- Instruct patient to use drug exactly as prescribed; if drug is discontinued abruptly, parkinsonian crisis may occur; do not double doses; take missed dose as soon as remembered up to 2 hr before next dose
- Teach patient that urine, sweat may darken and is harmless
- Advise patient to use physical activities to maintain mobility and lessen spasms
- Instruct patient that OTC medications should not be used unless approved by prescriber
- Advise patient that drowsiness, dizziness are common; to avoid hazardous activities until response is known
- Explain that sips of water, hard candy, or gum may lessen dry mouth
- Teach patient to take with meals to prevent GI symptoms; to limit protein intake, which impairs drug's absorption

Evaluation
Positive therapeutic outcome
- Decrease in akathisia
- Improved mood
- Decreased involuntary movements

! HIGH ALERT

carboplatin (Rx)
(kar'boe'pla-tin)

Paraplatin, Paraplatin-AQ ♣

Func. class.: Antineoplastic alkylating agent

Chem. class.: Platinum coordination compound

Pregnancy category D

Do Not Confuse:
carboplatin/cisplatin
Paraplatin/platinol

Action: Produces interstrand DNA cross-links and to a lesser extent DNA-protein cross-links; activity is not cell cycle phase specific

Therapeutic Outcome: Prevention of rapidly growing malignant cells

Uses: Initial treatment of ovarian cancer in combination with other agents; palliative treatment of recurrent ovarian carcinoma after treatment with other antineoplastic agents, including cisplatin

Dosage and routes
(single agent)

Adult: **IV** inf initially 300 mg/m^2 given with cyclophosphamide, q4-6 wk; refractory tumors 360 mg/m^2 single dose, may repeat q4 wk, as needed; do not repeat until neutrophils >2000 mm^3 and platelets ≥100,000/mm^3

Renal dose

Adult: **IV** CCr 41-59 ml/min 250 mg/m^2, CCr 16-40 ml/min 200 mg/m^2; do not use in Ccr <15 ml/min

Available forms: Inj 50, 150, 450, 600 mg/vial

Adverse effects
CNS: **Seizures, central neurotoxicity,** peripheral neuropathy, dizziness, confusion

CV: Cardiac abnormalities

EENT: Tinnitus, hearing loss, ***vestibular toxicity,*** visual changes

GI: Severe nausea, vomiting, diarrhea, weight loss, mucositis, anorexia, constipation, taste change

GU: **Renal tubular damage,** renal insufficiency, impotence, sterility, amenorrhea, gynecomastia

HEMA: **Thrombocytopenia, leukopenia, pancytopenia, neutropenia, anemia,** bleeding

INTEG: Alopecia, dermatitis, rash, erythema, pruritus, urticaria

META: Hypomagnesemia, hypocalcemia, hypokalemia, hyponatremia, hyperuremia

SYST: **Anaphylaxis**

Contraindications: Pregnancy **D**, hypersensitivity to this drug, platinum products, mannitol; severe bone marrow depression, significant bleeding, aluminum products used to prepare or adminster carboplatin

Precautions: Radiation therapy within 1 mo, chemotherapy within 1 mo, lactation, liver disease

Pharmacokinetics	
Absorption	Complete
Distribution	Unknown
Metabolism	Liver
Excretion	Kidneys
Half-life	Initial 1-2 hr; postdistribution 2½-6 hr; increased in renal disease

Pharmacodynamics	
Onset	½ hr
Peak	Unknown
Duration	4-6 hr

Interactions
Individual drugs

Amphotericin B: increased nephrotoxicity or ototoxicity
Aspirin: increased risk of bleeding
Radiation: increased toxicity, bone marrow suppression

Drug classifications

Aminoglycosides: increased nephrotoxicity
Aminoglycosides: ototoxicity
Antineoplastics, bone marrow–suppressing drugs: increased bone marrow suppression
Myelosuppressives: increased myelosuppression
NSAIDs: increased risk of bleeding

Drug/lab test

Increased: AST, BUN, alkaline phosphatase, bilirubin, creatinine

NURSING CONSIDERATIONS
Assessment
- Monitor CBC, differential, platelet count weekly; withhold drug if neutrophil count is

<2000/mm^3 or platelet count is <100,000/mm^3; notify prescriber of results if WBC <20,000/mm^3, platelets <150,000/mm^3
- Assess for anaphylaxis: pruritus, wheezing, tachycardia; notify physician after discontinuing drugs; resuscitation equipment should be available
- Monitor renal function studies: BUN, creatinine, serum uric acid, urine CCr before and during therapy; I&O ratio; report fall in urine output to <30 ml/hr
- Monitor temp q4h (may indicate beginning of infection)
- Monitor liver function tests before and during therapy (bilirubin, AST, ALT, LDH) as needed or monthly; note jaundice of skin or sclera, dark urine, clay-colored stools, itchy skin, abdominal pain, fever, diarrhea
- Assess for bleeding: hematuria, stool guaiac, bruising or petechiae, mucosa or orifices q8h; inflammation of mucosa, breaks in skin
- Identify dyspnea, crackles, unproductive cough, chest pain, tachypnea
- Identify effects of alopecia on body image; discuss feelings about body changes

Nursing diagnoses
- Injury, risk for (adverse reactions)
- Body image, disturbed (adverse reactions)
- Infection, risk for (adverse reactions)
- Knowledge, deficient (teaching)

Implementation
- Antiemetic 30-60 min before giving drug to prevent vomiting, and prn

IV route
- Give **IV** after diluting 10 mg/ml of sterile water for inj, D_5W, 0.9% NaCl (10 mg/ml); then further dilute with the same sol 1-4 mg/ml; give over 15 min or more (intermittent inf)
- Give **IV** inf over 5-6 hr; do not use needles or **IV** administration sets containing aluminum; may cause precipitate or loss of potency; diuretic (furosemide 40 mg **IV**) after inf
- Store protected from light at room temp; reconstituted sol is stable for 8 hr at room temp

Y-site compatibilities: Allopurinol, amifostine, aztreonam, cefepime, cladribine, DOXOrubicin liposome, filgrastim, fludarabine, granisetron, melphalan, ondansetron, paclitaxel, piperacillin/tazobactam, propofol, sargramostim, teniposide, thiotepa, vinorelbine

Additive compatibilities: Cisplatin, etoposide, floxuridine, ifosfamide, ifosfamide/etoposide, paclitaxel

Additive incompatibilities: Fluorouracil, mesna

Solution compatibilities: D_5/0.2% NaCl, D_5/0.45% NaCl, D_5/0.9% NaCl, 0.9% NaCl, D_5W, sterile water for inj

Solution incompatibilities: Sodium bicarbonate

Patient/family education
- Advise patient to report ringing/roaring in the ears, numbness, tingling in face, extremities, weight gain
- Teach patient to avoid use of products containing aspirin or ibuprofen, NSAIDs, alcohol, razors, commercial mouthwash, since bleeding may occur; to report symptoms of bleeding (hematuria, tarry stools)
- Instruct patient to report signs of anemia (fatigue, headache, irritability, faintness, shortness of breath); sore throat, bleeding, bruising, chills, back pain, blood in stools, dyspnea
- Instruct patient to report any changes in breathing or coughing even several months after treatment; to avoid crowds and persons with respiratory tract or other infections
- Advise patient that hair may be lost during treatment; a wig or hairpiece may make patient feel better; new hair may be different in color, texture
- Caution patient not to have any vaccinations without the advice of the prescriber; serious reactions can occur
- Teach patient that contraception is needed during treatment and for several months after the completion of therapy; not to breastfeed during treatment; to notify prescriber if pregnancy is planned or suspected

Evaluation
Positive therapeutic outcome
- Prevention of rapid division of malignant cells

carboprost (Rx)
(kar'boe-prost)
Hemabate, Prostin/15M ✤
Func. class.: Oxytocic, abortifacient
Chem. class.: Prostaglandin
Pregnancy category C

Action: Stimulates uterine contractions, causing complete abortion in approximately 16 hr

Therapeutic Outcome: Loss of fetus; decreased postpartum bleeding

Uses: Abortion between 13-20 wk gestation; postpartum hemorrhage caused by uterine atony not controlled by other methods

Dosage and routes

To induce abortion

Adult: IM 250 mcg, then 250 mcg q1½-3½h, may increase to 500 mcg if no response, not to exceed 12 mg total dose

Postpartum hemorrhage

Adult: IM 250 mcg, repeat at 15-90 min intervals, max total dosage 2 mg

Available forms: Inj 250 mcg/ml

Adverse effects

CNS: *Fever, chills,* headache

GI: *Nausea, vomiting, diarrhea*

Contraindications: Hypersensitivity, severe hepatic disease, severe renal disease, PID, respiratory disease, cardiac disease

Precautions: Pregnancy **C**, asthma, anemia, jaundice, diabetes mellitus, seizure disorders, past uterine surgery

Pharmacokinetics	
Absorption	Well absorbed (nasal)
Distribution	Widely distributed (extracellular fluid)
Metabolism	Liver—rapidly
Excretion	Kidneys
Half-life	3-9 min

Pharmacodynamics	
Onset	Unknown
Peak	16 hr
Duration	Unknown

Interactions

Drug classifications

Oxytocics: increased effects

NURSING CONSIDERATIONS

Assessment

- Monitor B/P, pulse; watch for change that may indicate hemorrhage
- Monitor respiratory rate, rhythm, depth; notify physician of abnormalities
- For length, duration of contraction; notify physician of contractions lasting over 1 min or absence of contractions
- Assess for incomplete abortion, pregnancy must be terminated by another method; drug is teratogenic

Nursing diagnoses

- Knowledge, deficient (teaching)

Implementation

- Give IM inj in deep muscle mass; rotate inj sites if additional doses are given
- Have crash cart available on unit

Patient/family education

- Advise patient to report increased blood loss, abdominal cramps, increased temperature or foul-smelling lochia

Evaluation

Positive therapeutic outcome

- Loss of fetus
- Control of bleeding

carisoprodol (Rx)

(kar-i-soe-proe′dole)

carisoprodol, Soma, Vanadom

Func. class.: Skeletal muscle relaxant, central acting

Chem. class.: Meprobamate congener

Pregnancy category C

Do Not Confuse:

Soma/Soma compound

Action: Depresses CNS by blocking interneuronal activity in descending reticular formation of spinal cord, producing sedation

Therapeutic Outcome: Relaxation of skeletal muscles

Uses: Relieving pain, stiffness in musculoskeletal disorders

Dosage and routes

Adult and child >12 yr: PO 350 mg tid and at bedtime

Child 6-12 yr: PO 6.25 mg/kg qid

Available forms: Tabs 350 mg

Adverse effects

CNS: *Dizziness, weakness, drowsiness,* headache, tremor, depression, insomnia, ataxia, irritability

CV: Postural hypotension, tachycardia

EENT: Diplopia, temporary loss of vision

GI: Nausea, vomiting, hiccups, epigastric discomfort

HEMA: Eosinophilia

INTEG: Rash, pruritus, fever, facial flushing, **erythema multiforme**

RESP: Asthmatic attack

SYST: **Angioedema, anaphylaxis**

Contraindications: Hypersensitivity, child <12 yr, intermittent porphyria

Precautions: Pregnancy **C,** renal disease, hepatic disease, addictive personality, elderly

Pharmacokinetics	
Absorption	Well absorbed
Distribution	Crosses placenta
Metabolism	Liver, partially
Excretion	Kidney, unchanged; breast milk
Half-life	8 hr

Pharmacodynamics	
Onset	½ hr
Peak	4 hr
Duration	4-6 hr

Interactions
Individual drugs
Alcohol: increased CNS depression
Drug classifications
Antidepressants (tricyclic), barbiturates, opioids, sedative/hypnotics: increased CNS depression
Drug/herb
Chamomile, kava, skullcap, valerian: increased CNS depression
Drug/lab test
Increased: AST, alkaline phosphatase, blood glucose

NURSING CONSIDERATIONS
Assessment
- Monitor ROM, atrophy, stiffness, and pain in muscles; assess throughout treatment
- Monitor ECG in seizure patients; poor seizure control has occurred with patients taking this drug
- Assess for idiosyncratic reaction within a few min or hr of administration (disorientation, restlessness, weakness, euphoria, blurred vision); patient should be reassured that reaction is temporary
- Check for allergic reactions: rash, fever

Nursing diagnoses
- Mobility, impaired (uses)
- Injury, risk for (adverse reactions)
- Knowledge, deficient (teaching)

Implementation
- Give with meals for GI symptoms
- Have patient use gum, frequent sips of water for dry mouth
- Store in tight container at room temp

Patient/family education
- Caution patient not to take with alcohol, other CNS depressants
- Advise patient to avoid altering activities while taking this drug
- Caution patient to avoid hazardous activities if drowsiness or dizziness occurs
- Caution patient to avoid using OTC medication such as cough preparations, antihistamines, unless directed by prescriber

Evaluation
Positive therapeutic outcome
- Decreased pain, spasticity

Treatment of overdose: Induce emesis of conscious patient, lavage, dialysis

! HIGH ALERT

carmustine (Rx)
(kar-mus'teen)

BiCNU, BCNU, Gliadel

Func. class.: Antineoplastic alkylating agent

Chem. class.: Nitrosourea

Pregnancy category D

Action: Alkylates DNA, RNA; inhibits enzymes that allow synthesis of amino acids in proteins; also responsible for cross-linking DNA strands; activity is not cell cycle phase specific

Therapeutic Outcome: Prevention of rapidly growing malignant cells

Uses: Brain tumors such as glioblastoma, medulloblastoma, astrocytoma, ependymoma, metastic brain tumors; multiple myeloma (with prednisone), Hodgkin's disease, other lymphomas; GI, breast, bronchogenic, and renal carcinomas, other lymphomas; wafer, as adjunct to surgery/radiation in newly diagnosed high-grade malignant glioma patients; in recurrent glioblastoma multiforme patients as adjunct to surgery

Investigational uses: Primary cutaneous T-cell lymphoma, malignant melanoma

Dosage and routes
Adult: **IV** 75-100 mg/m^2 over 1-2 hr × 2 days or 150-200 mg/m^2 × 1 dose q6-8 wk or 40 mg/m^2/day × 5 days q6 wk; if WBC 3000-3999/mm^3 give 50% of dose; if WBC is 2000-2999/mm^3 and platelet count is 25,000-75,000/mm^3 give 25% of dose; withhold dose if WBC <2000/mm^3 and platelets <25,000/mm^3

Adult: Intracavitary 8 wafers inserted into resection cavity

Available forms: Powder for inj 100 mg; wafer 7.7 mg intracavitary

Adverse effects
GI: *Nausea, vomiting, anorexia, stomatitis,* **hepatotoxicity**

GU: *Azotemia,* **renal failure**

HEMA: **Thrombocytopenia, leukopenia, myelosuppression, anemia**
INTEG: Burning, hyperpigmentation at inj site, alopecia
RESP: **Fibrosis, pulmonary infiltrate**

Contraindications: Pregnancy **D**, hypersensitivity, leukopenia, thrombocytopenia

Precautions: Lactation

Pharmacokinetics

Absorption	Completely absorbed
Distribution	Readily penetrates CSF
Metabolism	Liver, rapid
Excretion	Kidneys, breast milk
Half-life	Unknown

Pharmacodynamics

Unknown

Interactions
Individual drugs
Aspirin: increased risk of bleeding
Cimetidine, radiation: increased toxicity
Digoxin: decreased effects of digoxin
Phenytoin: decreased effects of phenytoin
Drug classifications
Anticoagulants: increased risk of bleeding
Antineoplastics: increased toxicity
Live vaccines: increased adverse reactions; decreased antibody reaction
Myelosuppressive agents: increased myelosuppression

NURSING CONSIDERATIONS
Assessment
- Assess buccal cavity q8h for dryness, sores or ulceration, white patches, pain, bleeding, dysphagia; obtain prescription for viscous lidocaine (Xylocaine)
- Assess symptoms indicating severe allergic reaction: rash, pruritus, urticaria, purpuric skin lesions, itching, flushing; drug should be discontinued
- Monitor CBC, differential, platelet count weekly; withhold drug if WBC $<4000/mm^3$ or platelet count is $<100,000/mm^3$; notify prescriber of results if WBC $<20,000/mm^3$, platelets $<150,000/mm^3$
- Monitor renal function studies: BUN, creatinine, urine CCr before and during therapy; I&O ratio; report fall in urine output to <30 ml/hr
- Monitor temp q4h (may indicate beginning of infection)
- Monitor liver function tests before and during therapy (bilirubin, AST, ALT, LDH) as needed or monthly; note yellowing of skin or sclera, dark urine, clay-colored stools, itchy skin, abdominal pain, fever, diarrhea; hepatotoxicity can be serious and fatal
- Assess for bleeding: hematuria, stool guaiac, bruising or petechiae, mucosa or orifices q8h; inflammation of mucosa, breaks in skin
- Monitor pulmonary function tests, chest x-ray films before, during therapy; chest film should be obtained q2 wk during treatment; monitor for dyspnea, cough, pulmonary fibrosis; infiltrate occurs after high doses or several low-dose courses
- Identify effects of alopecia on body image; discuss feelings about body changes

Nursing diagnoses
- Injury, risk for (adverse reactions)
- Body image, disturbed (adverse reactions)
- Infection, risk for (adverse reactions)
- Knowledge, deficient (teaching)

Implementation
- Blood transfusion or RBC colony-stimulating factors to counter anemia may be required
- Give fluids **IV** or PO before chemotherapy to hydrate patient
- Provide antiemetic 30-60 min before giving drug to prevent vomiting, and prn; antibiotics for prophylaxis of infection
- Provide liq diet (carbonated beverages); gelatin may be added if patient is not nauseated or vomiting
- Give all medications PO, if possible, avoid IM inj if platelets $<100,000/mm^3$

Wafer
- Foil pouches may be kept at room temp for 6 hr, if unopened
- If wafers are broken in several pieces, do not use

IV route
- Prepare in biologic cabinet wearing gown, gloves, mask; avoid contact with skin
- Administer after diluting 100 mg/3 ml ethyl alcohol (provided); then further dilute 27 ml sterile water for inj; then dilute with 100-500 ml 0.9% NaCl or D_5W; give over 1 hr or more; use only glass containers; reduce rate if discomfort is felt
- Flush **IV** line after carmustine with 10 ml 0.9% NaCl to prevent irritation at site
- Store reconstituted sol in refrigerator for 24 hr or room temp for 8 hr

Y-site compatibilities: Amifostine, aztreonam, cefepime, filgrastim, fludarabine, granisetron, melphalan, ondansetron, piperacillin/tazobactam, sargramostim, teniposide, thiotepa, vinorelbine

Additive incompatibilities: Sodium bicarbonate

Patient/family education
- Teach patient to avoid use of products containing aspirin or ibuprofen, razors, commercial mouthwash, since bleeding may occur; to report symptoms of bleeding (hematuria, tarry stools)
- Advise patient to avoid foods with citric acid, hot or rough texture if stomatitis is present
- Instruct patient to report signs of anemia (fatigue, headache, irritability, faintness, shortness of breath); avoid smoking
- Advise patient that hair may be lost during treatment; a wig or hairpiece may make patient feel better; new hair may be different in color, texture
- Caution patient not to have any vaccinations without the advice of the prescriber; serious reactions can occur
- Advise patient that contraception is needed during treatment and for several months after completion of therapy; drug has teratogenic properties

Evaluation
Positive therapeutic outcome
- Prevention of rapid division of malignant cells

carteolol (Rx)
(kar-tee'oe-lole)

Cartrol

Func.class.: Antihypertensive, antianginal

Chem. class.: Nonselective β-blocker

Pregnancy category C

Do Not Confuse:
carteolol/carvedilol

Action: Produces fall in B/P without reflex tachycardia or significant reduction in heart rate through mixture of α-blocking, β-blocking effects and intrinsic sympathomimetic activity; elevated plasma renins are reduced; decreased intraocular pressure in glaucoma and intraocular hypertension

Therapeutic Outcome: Decreased B/P, heart rate; decreased intraocular pressure

Uses: Mild to moderate hypertension; oph intraocular hypertension, open-angle glaucoma (see Appendix D)

Dosage and routes
Adult: PO 2.5 mg daily initially; may gradually increase to desired response, max 10 mg/day

Renal dose

Adult: PO CCr >60 ml/min give dose q24h, CCr 20-60 ml/min give dose q48h, CCr <20 ml/min give dose q72h

Available forms: Tabs 2.5, 5 mg

Adverse effects
CNS: Dizziness, mental changes, drowsiness, fatigue, headache, catatonia, depression, anxiety, nightmares, paresthesia, lethargy, insomnia, decreased concentration
CV: Orthostatic hypotension, **bradycardia, CHF, chest pain, ventricular dysrhythmias, AV block, peripheral vascular insufficency,** palpitations
EENT: Tinnitus, visual changes, sore throat, double vision, dry, burning eyes
GI: Nausea, vomiting, diarrhea, dry mouth, flatulence, constipation, anorexia
GU: Impotence, dysuria, ejaculatory failure, urinary retention
HEMA: **Agranulocytosis, thrombocytopenic purpura (rare)**
INTEG: Rash, alopecia, urticaria, pruritus, fever
MISC: Facial swelling, decreased exercise tolerance, weight change, Raynaud's disease, lupuslike syndrome
MS: Joint pain, arthralgia, muscle cramps, pain
RESP: **Bronchospasm,** dyspnea, wheezing, nasal stuffiness, pharyngitis

Contraindications: Hypersensitivity to β-blockers, cardiogenic shock, heart block (2nd or 3rd degree), sinus bradycardia, bronchial asthma

Precautions: Pregnancy **C,** major surgery, lactation, CHF, diabetes mellitus, renal disease, thyroid disease, COPD, well-compensated heart failure, nonallergic bronchospasm

Pharmacokinetics	
Absorption	80%-90%
Distribution	Unknown; protein binding 23%-30%
Metabolism	Liver to active metabolite
Excretion	Kidneys, unchanged (50%-75%)
Half-life	Carteolol (6-8 hr); metabolite (8-12 hr); increased renal disease

Pharmacodynamics	PO	OPHTH
Onset	Unknown	Unknown
Peak	1-3 hr	Unknown
Duration	Unknown	Unknown

Interactions

Individual drugs

Alcohol, clonidine: increased hypotension (large amounts)
DOBUTamine, dopamine: decreased CV effect
Insulin: increased hypoglycemia
Phenytoin (**IV**), verapamil: increased myocardial depression
Thyroid agents: decreased effectiveness of carteolol

Drug classifications

Amphetamines, MAOIs: increased hypertension
Antidiabetics, oral: increased hypoglycemia
Antihypertensives, general anesthetics, nitrates: increased hypotension
β_2-Agonists, theophyllines: decreased bronchodilatation
Cardiac glycosides: increased bradycardia
NSAIDs: decreased antihypertensive action

Drug/herb

Betel palm, butterbur, cola tree, figwort, fumitory, guarana, hawthorn, jaborandi tree, lily of the valley, motherwort, plantain: increased effect
Coenzyme Q10, yohimbe: decreased effect

Drug/lab test

Increased: ANA titer, blood glucose, BUN, uric acid, lipoprotein, triglyceride

NURSING CONSIDERATIONS

Assessment

- Monitor B/P during beginning treatment, periodically thereafter; pulse q4h; note rate, rhythm, quality: apical/radial pulse before administration; notify prescriber of any significant changes (pulse <50 bpm)
- Monitor blood glucose in those taking insulin, oral antidiabetics, dosage adjustment may be needed
- Check for baselines in renal, liver function tests before therapy begins
- Assess for edema in feet, legs daily; monitor I&O, daily weight; check for jugular vein distention and crackles bilaterally, dyspnea (CHF)
- Monitor skin turgor, dryness of mucous membranes for hydration status, especially elderly

Nursing diagnoses

- Cardiac output, decreased (uses)
- Injury, risk for (side effects)
- Knowledge, deficient (teaching)
- Noncompliance (teaching)

Implementation

- Give ac, at bedtime; tab may be crushed or swallowed whole; give with food to prevent GI upset
- Store protected from light, moisture; placed in cool environment

Patient/family education

- Teach patient not to discontinue drug abruptly; taper over 2 wk; may cause precipitate dysrhythmias, hypertension, myocardial ischemia if stopped abruptly
- Teach patient not to use OTC products containing α-adrenergic stimulants (such as nasal decongestants, cold preparations); to avoid alcohol, smoking and to limit sodium intake as prescribed
- Teach patient how to take pulse and B/P at home; advise when to notify prescriber
- Instruct patient to comply with weight control, dietary adjustments, modified exercise program
- Advise patient to carry/wear emergency ID to identify drug being taken, allergies; tell patient drug controls symptoms but does not cure
- Caution patient to avoid hazardous activities if dizziness, drowsiness present
- Teach patient to report symptoms of CHF; difficult breathing, especially on exertion or when lying down, night cough, swelling of extremities or bradycardia, dizziness, confusion, depression, fever
- Teach patient to take drug as prescribed, not to double doses, skip doses; take any missed doses as soon as remembered if at least 4 hr until next dose

Evaluation

Positive therapeutic outcome

- Decreased B/P in hypertension (after 1-2 wk)

Treatment of overdose: Lavage, **IV** atropine for bradycardia; **IV** theophylline for bronchospasm, digitalis, O_2, diuretic for cardiac failure; **IV** glucose for hypoglycemia; **IV** diazepam (or phenytoin) for seizures

carvedilol (Rx)

(kar-veh'dee-lol)

Coreg

Func. class.: Antihypertensive α/β-blocker

Pregnancy category C

Do Not Confuse:

Carvedilol/Captopril/Carteolol

Action: A mixture of nonselective β-blocking and α-blocking activity; decreases cardiac output, exercise-induced tachycardia, reflex orthostatic tachycardia; causes reduction in peripheral vascular resistance and vasodilatation

Therapeutic Outcome: Decreased B/P in hypertension

Uses: Essential hypertension alone or in combination with other antihypertensives, CHF

Investigational uses: Angina pectoris, idiopathic cardiomyopathy

Dosage and routes

Essential hypertension

Adult: PO 6.25 mg bid × 7-14 days if tolerated well, then increase to 12.5 mg bid × 7-14 days if tolerated well, may be increased if needed to 25 mg bid, max 50 mg daily

Congestive heart failure

Adult: PO 3.125 mg bid × 2 wk; if well tolerated, give 6.25 mg bid × 2 wk, then double q2wk to max dose 25 mg bid <85 kg or 80 mg bid >85 kg

Angina pectoris

Adult: PO 25-50 mg bid

Idiopathic cardiomyopathy

Adult: PO 6.25-25 mg bid

Available forms: Tabs 3.125, 6.25, 12.5, 25 mg

Adverse effects

CNS: *Dizziness,* somnolence, insomnia, ataxia, hyperesthesia, paresthesia, vertigo, depression, fatigue, weakness

CV: *Bradycardia, postural hypotension,* dependent edema, peripheral edema, **AV block, extrasystoles,** hypertension, hypotension, palpitations, peripheral ischemia, **CHF,** pulmonary edema

GI: *Diarrhea,* abdominal pain, increased alkaline phosphatase, increased ALT/AST

GU: Decreased libido, *impotence*

MISC: Fatigue, injury, back pain, UTI, viral infection, hypertriglyceridemia, **thrombocytopenia,** *hyperglycemia*

RESP: Rhinitis, pharyngitis, dyspnea

Contraindications: Hypersensitivity, bronchial asthma, class IV decompensated cardiac failure, 2nd- or 3rd-degree heart block, cardiogenic shock, severe bradycardia, pulmonary edema

Precautions: Pregnancy **C**, cardiac failure, hepatic injury, peripheral vascular disease, anesthesia, major surgery, diabetes mellitus, thyrotoxicosis, elderly, lactation, children, emphysema, chronic bronchitis, renal disease

Pharmacokinetics

Absorption	Readily and extensively absorbed
Distribution	>98% protein binding
Metabolism	Extensively liver
Excretion	Via bile into feces
Half-life	Terminal half-life 7-10 hr, increased in the elderly, hepatic disease

Pharmacodynamics

Unknown

Interactions

Individual drugs

Alcohol (acute ingestion), cimetidine: increased toxicity
Clonidine: decreased heart rate, B/P
Digoxin: increased concentrations of digoxin
Reserpine: increased hypotension, bradycardia
Rifampin: decreased levels of carvedilol

Drug classifications

Antihypertensives, nitrates: increased toxicity
Antidiabetic agents: increased hypoglycemia
Calcium channel blockers: increased conduction disturbance
MAOIs: increased bradycardia, hypotension
NSAIDs, thyroid hormones: decreased levels of carvedilol

Drug/herb

Aconite: increased toxicity, death
Astragalus, cola tree: increased or decreased antihypertensive effect
Barberry, betony, black catechu, black cohosh, bloodroot, broom, burdock, cat's claw, dandelion, goldenseal, Irish moss, Jamaican dogwood, kelp, khella, mistletoe, parsley: increased antihypertensive effect
Coltsfoot, guarana, khat, licorice: decreased antihypertensive effect

NURSING CONSIDERATIONS

Assessment

- Monitor renal studies including protein, BUN, creatinine; watch for increased levels that may indicate nephrotic syndrome; obtain baselines in renal and liver function studies before beginning treatment; if liver function studies are elevated, drug should be discontinued
- Monitor I&O, weight daily
- Monitor B/P during beginning treatment and periodically thereafter, pulse q4h, note rate, rhythm, quality
- Monitor apical/radial pulse before administration; notify prescriber of significant changes, pulse <50 bpm hold drug, notify prescriber
- Assess for edema in feet and legs daily, fluid

overload: dyspnea, weight gain, jugular vein distention, fatigue, crackles

Nursing diagnoses

- Cardiac output, decreased (uses)
- Injury, risk for (adverse reactions)
- Knowledge, deficient (teaching)
- Noncompliance (teaching)

Implementation

- Give PO ac, at bedtime; tablets may be crushed or swallowed whole, give with food to decrease orthostatic hypotension
- Administer reduced dosage in renal dysfunction

Patient/family education

- Tell patient to comply with dosage schedule even if feeling better, that improvement may take several weeks
- Teach patient to rise slowly to sitting or standing position to minimize orthostatic hypotension
- Encourage patient to report bradycardia, dizziness, confusion, depression, fever, weight gain, shortness of breath, cold extremities, rash, sore throat, bleeding, bruising
- Teach patient to take pulse at home; advise when to notify prescriber
- Encourage patient not to discontinue drug abruptly, taper over 1-2 wk
- Advise patient to avoid hazardous activities until stabilized on medication; dizziness may occur
- Advise patient to avoid all OTC medications unless approved by prescriber
- Advise patient to carry/wear emergency ID with drug name, prescriber at all times
- Advise patient to inform all health care providers of drugs, supplements taken

Evaluation

Positive therapeutic outcome

- Decreased B/P
- Decreased symptoms of CHF or angina

cascara sagrada/cascara sagrada aromatic fluid extract/cascara sagrada fluid extract (OTC)

(kas-kar'a)

Func. class.: Laxative
Chem. class.: Anthraquinone

Pregnancy category C

Action: Direct chemical irritation in colon; increases propulsion of stool; increases fluid in colon

Therapeutic Outcome: Decreased constipation; removal of bowel contents before surgery or diagnostic tests

Uses: Constipation; bowel or rectal preparation for surgery or examination

Dosage and routes

Adult: PO 325 mg at bedtime; fluid 1 ml daily; aromatic fluid 5 ml daily
Child 2-12 yr: PO/fluid/aromatic fluid ½ adult dose
Child <2 yr: PO/fluid/aromatic fluid ¼ adult dose

Available forms: Tabs 325 mg; fluid extract 1 g/ml; aromatic fluid extract 1 g/ml

Adverse effects

GI: *Nausea, vomiting, anorexia, cramps, diarrhea*
META: Hypocalcemia, enteropathy, alkalosis, hypokalemia, **tetany**

Contraindications: Hypersensitivity, GI bleeding, obstruction, CHF, lactation, abdominal pain, nausea/vomiting, appendicitis, acute surgical abdomen, alcoholics (aromatic fluid extract)

Precautions: Pregnancy **C**

Pharmacokinetics	
Absorption	Minimal
Distribution	Unknown
Metabolism	Liver, minimally
Excretion	Kidneys, feces, breast milk
Half-life	Not known

Pharmacodynamics	
Onset	Unknown
Peak	6-12 hr
Duration	Unknown

Interactions

Individual drugs

Digitalis, nitrofurantoin: decreased absorption

Drug classifications

Antibiotics, oral anticoagulants, salicylates, tetracyclines: decreased absorption

Drug/herb

Flax, lily of the valley, pheasant's eye, senna, squill: increased action, side effects

NURSING CONSIDERATIONS

Assessment

- Monitor blood, urine electrolytes if drug used often by patient; check I&O ratio to identify fluid loss
- Assess cramping, rectal bleeding, nausea, vomiting; if these symptoms occur, drug

should be discontinued; identify cause of constipation; identify whether fluids, bulk, or exercise is missing from lifestyle

Nursing diagnoses
- Constipation (uses)
- Diarrhea
- Knowledge, deficient (teaching)
- Noncompliance (teaching)

Implementation
- Swallow tabs whole; do not break, crush, or chew tabs
- Give alone with water only for better absorption; do not administer with food; do not take within 1 hr of antacids, milk, or cimetidine
- Give in AM or PM (oral dose); evacuation will occur 6-12 hr later

Patient/family education
- Discuss with the patient that adequate fluid consumption is necessary
- Teach patient that normal bowel movements do not always occur daily
- Teach patient not to use in presence of abdominal pain, nausea, vomiting; tell patient to notify prescriber if constipation unrelieved or if symptoms of electrolyte imbalance occur: muscle cramps, pain, weakness, dizziness, excessive thirst

Evaluation
Positive therapeutic outcome
- Decreased constipation in 6-12 hr
- Removal of bowel contents

cefaclor
See cephalosporins—2nd generation

cefadroxil
See cephalosporins—1st generation

cefazolin
See cephalosporins—1st generation

cefdinir
cefditoren pivoxil
See cephalosporins—3rd generation

cefepime
cefixime
See cephalosporins—3rd generation

cefmetazole
See cephalosporins—2nd generation

cefoperazone
cefotaxime
See cephalosporins—3rd generation

cefotetan
cefoxitin
See cephalosporins—2nd generation

cefpodoxime
See cephalosporins—3rd generation

cefprozil
See cephalosporins—2nd generation

ceftazidime
ceftibuten
ceftizoxime
ceftriaxone
See cephalosporins—3rd generation

cefuroxime
See cephalosporins—2nd generation

cephalexin
See cephalosporins—1st generation

! HIGH ALERT

celecoxib (Rx)
(cel-eh-cox'ib)

Celebrex

Func. class.: Nonsteroidal antiinflammatory, antirheumatic

Chem. class.: COX-2 inhibitor

Pregnancy category
C (1st/2nd trimesters),
D (3rd trimester)

Do Not Confuse:
Celebrex/Celexa/Cerebra/Cerebyx

Action: Inhibits prostaglandin synthesis by selectively inhibiting cyclooxygenase 2 (COX-2), an enzyme needed for biosynthesis

Therapeutic Outcome: Decreased pain, inflammation

Uses: Acute, chronic rheumatoid arthritis, osteoarthritis, familial adenomatous polyposis (FAP), acute pain, primary dysmenorrhea, ankylosing spondylitis

Investigational uses: Colorectal polyps

Dosage and routes

Do not exceed recommended dose, deaths have occurred

Acute pain/primary dysmenorrhea
Adult: PO 400 mg initially, then 200 mg on 1st day, then 200 mg bid prn on subsequent days, if needed

Osteoarthritis
Adult: PO 200 mg/day as a single dose or 100 mg bid

Rheumatoid arthritis
Adult: PO 100-200 mg bid

Ankylosing spondylitis
Adult: PO 200 mg daily or in divided dose (bid)

FAP
Adult: PO 400 mg bid

Colorectal polyps
Adult: PO 400 mg bid × 6 mo

Hepatic dose (Child-Pugh class II)
Adult: PO reduce dose by 50%

Available forms: Caps 100, 200 mg

Adverse effects

CNS: *Fatigue, anxiety, depression, nervousness, paresthesia,* dizziness, insomnia
CV: **Stroke, MI, tachycardia, CHF,** angina, palpitations, dysrhythmias, hypertension, fluid retention
EENT: Tinnitus, hearing loss, blurred vision, glaucoma, cataract, conjunctivitis, eye pain
GI: *Nausea, anorexia, vomiting, constipation, dry mouth,* diverticulitis, gastritis, gastroenteritis, hemorrhoids, hiatal hernia, stomatitis, **GI bleeding**
GU: **Nephrotoxicity: dysuria, hematuria, oliguria, azotemia, cystitis, UTI**
HEMA: *Blood dyscrasias,* epistaxis, bruising, anemia
INTEG: Purpura, rash, pruritus, sweating, erythema, petechiae, photosensitivity, alopecia, **serious sometimes fatal Stevens-Johnson syndrome, toxic epidermal necrolysis**
RESP: Pharyngitis, shortness of breath, pneumonia, coughing

Contraindications: Pregnancy **D** (3rd trimester), hypersensitivity to aspirin, iodides, other NSAIDs, sulfonamides, asthma, asthma triad

Precautions: Pregnancy **C** (1st/2nd trimester), renal, hepatic, hypertension, severe dehydration, children <18 yr, lactation, bleeding, GI, cardiac disorders, hypersensitivity to other antiinflammatories, glucocorticoids, anticoagulants, elderly

Pharmacokinetics	
Absorption	Well absorbed (PO)
Distribution	Crosses placenta, bound to plasma proteins
Metabolism	Liver
Excretion	Kidneys
Half-life	Unknown

Pharmacodynamics	
Onset	Unknown
Peak	3 hr
Duration	Unknown

Interactions

Individual drugs
Aspirin: decreased effectiveness; increased adverse reactions
Fluconazole: increased celecoxib level
Furosemide: decreased effect of furosemide
Lithium: increased toxicity
Warfarin: increased anticoagulant effects

Drug classifications
ACE inhibitors: may decrease effects of ACE inhibitors
Anticoagulants: increased risk of bleeding
Antineoplastics: increased risk of hematologic toxicity
Glucocorticoids, NSAIDs: increased adverse reactions
Thiazide diuretics: decreased effectiveness of diuretics

Drug/herb
Arginine, gossypol: increased gastric irritation
Bearberry, bilberry: increased celecoxib effect
Bogbean, saw palmetto, turmeric: increased bleeding risk
St. John's wort: severe photosensitivity

NURSING CONSIDERATIONS

Assessment

- Assess for pain of rheumatoid arthritis, osteoarthritis; check ROM, inflammation of joints, characteristics of pain
- Monitor blood counts during therapy; watch for decreasing platelets; if low, therapy may need to be discontinued, restarted after

hematologic recovery; and for blood dyscrasias (thrombocytopenia): bruising, fatigue, bleeding, poor healing
- Assess FAP patient for decreasing number of polyps

Nursing diagnoses
- Pain (uses)
- Mobility, physical, impaired (uses)
- Injury, risk for (side effects)
- Knowledge, deficient (teaching)

Implementation
- Do not break, crush, chew, or dissolve caps
- Administer with food or milk to decrease gastric symptoms
- Do not increase dose

Patient/family education
- ❗ Do not exceed recommended dose; notify prescriber immediately of chest pain, skin eruptions, stop drug
- Teach patient that drug must be continued for prescribed time to be effective; to avoid other NSAIDs, sulfonamides
- Caution patient to report bleeding, bruising, fatigue, malaise, since blood dyscrasias do occur; to report GI symptoms: black tarry stools, cramping
- Teach patient to take with a full glass of water to enhance absorption
- Teach patient to check with prescriber to determine when drug should be discontinued before surgery; advise patient to notify prescriber if pregnancy is planned or suspected

Evaluation
Positive therapeutic outcome
- Decreased pain in arthritic conditions
- Decreased inflammation in arthritic conditions
- Decreased number of polyps (FAP)

CEPHALOSPORINS—1ST GENERATION

cefadroxil (Rx)
(sef-a-drox'ill)
cefadroxil, Duricef

cefazolin (Rx)
(sef-a'zoe-lin)
Ancef, cefazolin

cephalexin (Rx)
(sef-a-lex'in)
Apo-Cephalex ✤, Biocef, cephalexin, Keflex, Keftab, Novo-Lexin ✤, Nu-Cephalex ✤

cephapirin (Rx)
(sef-a-pye'rin)
Cefadyl, cephapirin

cephradine (Rx)
(sef'ra-deen)
cephradine, Velosef

Func. class.: Antiinfective
Chem. class.: Cephalosporin (1st generation)

Pregnancy category B

Do Not Confuse:
cephalexin/cefaclor, cephapirin/cephradine, Kefzol/Cefzil

Action: Inhibits bacterial cell wall synthesis, rendering cell wall osmotically unstable, leading to cell death by binding to cell wall membrane

cefadroxil
Therapeutic Outcome: Bactericidal effects for the following: gram-negative bacilli *Escherichia coli, Proteus mirabilis, Klebsiella* (UTI only); gram-positive organisms *Streptococcus pneumoniae, Streptococcus pyogenes, Staphylococcus aureus*

Uses: Upper, lower respiratory tract, urinary tract, skin infections; otitis media; tonsillitis, pharyngitis; particularly for UTI

cefazolin
Therapeutic Outcome: Bactericidal effects for the following: gram-negative organisms *Enterobacter* sp., *Haemophilus influenzae, Escherichia coli, Proteus mirabilis, Klebsiella;* gram-positive organisms *Streptococcus pneumoniae, Streptococcus pyogenes, Staphylococcus aureus*

Uses: Upper, lower respiratory tract, urinary tract, skin infections; bone, joint, biliary, genital infections; endocarditis, surgical prophylaxis, septicemia

cephalexin
Therapeutic Outcome: Bactericidal effects for the following: gram-negative organisms *Haemophilus influenzae, Escherichia coli, Proteus mirabilis, Klebsiella;* gram-positive organisms *Streptococcus pneumoniae, Streptococcus pyogenes, Staphylococcus aureus*

Uses: Upper, lower respiratory tract, urinary tract, skin, bone infections; otitis media

cephapirin
Therapeutic Outcome: Bactericidal effects for the following: gram-negative bacilli *Haemophilus influenzae, Escherichia coli, Proteus mirabilis, Klebsiella;* gram-positive organisms *Streptococcus pneumoniae, Streptococcus viridans, Staphylococcus aureus*

Uses: Lower respiratory tract, urinary tract, skin infections; septicemia, endocarditis, bacterial peritonitis

cephradine
Therapeutic Outcome: Bactericidal effects for the following: gram-negative bacilli *Haemophilus influenzae, Escherichia coli, Proteus mirabilis, Klebsiella;* gram-positive organisms *Streptococcus pneumoniae, Streptococcus pyogenes, Staphylococcus aureus*

Uses: Serious respiratory tract, urinary tract, skin infections; otitis media

Dosage and routes

cefadroxil
Adult: PO 1-2 g daily or q12h in divided doses, give a loading dose of 1 g initially
Child: PO 30 mg/kg/day in divided doses bid

Renal dose
Adult: PO CCr 25-50 ml/min, 500 mg q12h; CCr 10-24 ml/min 500 mg q24h, CCr <10 ml/min 500 mg q36h

Available forms: Caps 500 mg; tabs 1 g; oral susp 125, 250, 500 mg/5 ml

cefazolin
Life-threatening infections
Adult: IM/**IV** 1-2 g q6h
Child >1 mo: IM/ 100 mg/kg in 3-4 divided doses

Mild/moderate infections
Adult: IM/**IV** 250 mg-1 g q8h
Child >1 mo: IM/ 25-50 mg/kg in 3-4 equal doses

Renal dose
CCr 35-54 ml/min 250-1000 mg q12h; CCr 10-34 ml/min 125-500 mg q12h; CCr <10 ml/min 125-500 mg q18-24h

Available forms: Inj 250, 500 mg, 1, 5, 10, 20 g; infusion 500 mg, 1 g/50 ml vial

cephalexin
Renal dose
CCr <40 ml/min q8-12h; CCr 5-10 ml/min q12h; CCr <5 ml/min q24h

Moderate infections
Adult: PO 250-500 mg q6h
Child: PO 25-50 mg/kg/day in 4 equal doses

Moderate skin infections
Adult: PO 500 mg q12h

Endocarditis prophylaxis: 2 g 1 hr before procedure

Severe infections
Adult: PO 500 mg-1 g q6h
Child: PO 50-100 mg/kg/day in 4 equal doses

Available forms: Caps 250, 500 mg; tabs 250, 500 mg, 1 g; oral susp 125, 250 mg/5 ml

cephapirin
Adult: IM/**IV** 500 mg-1 g q4-6h
Child: IM/ 40-80 mg/kg/day in divided doses q6h or 10-20 mg/kg q6h

Renal dose
CCr <10 ml/min give q12h

Available forms: Powder for inj 500 mg, 1, 2, 20 g; **IV** only 1, 2, 4 g

cephradine
Adult: PO 250 mg-1 g q6-12h
Child >1 yr: PO 6-12 mg/kg q6h

Renal dose
CCr >20 ml/min 500 mg q6h; CCr 5-20 ml/min 250 mg q6h

Available forms: Caps 250, 500 mg; oral susp 125, 250 mg/5 ml

Side effects/adverse reactions

CNS: Headache, dizziness, weakness, paresthesia, fever, chills, **seizures** (high doses)
GI: Nausea, vomiting, *diarrhea, anorexia,* pain, glossitis, bleeding; increased AST, ALT, bilirubin, LDH, alkaline phosphatase; abdominal pain, **pseudomembranous colitis**
GU: Proteinuria, vaginitis, pruritus, candidiasis, increased BUN, **nephrotoxicity, renal failure**
HEMA: **Leukopenia, thrombocytopenia, agranulocytosis,** anemia, **neutropenia, lymphocytosis, eosinophilia, pancytopenia, hemolytic anemia**
INTEG: Rash, urticaria, dermatitis
RESP: Dyspnea

SYST: **Anaphylaxis, serum sickness,** superinfection

Contraindications: Hypersensitivity to cephalosporins, infants <1 mo

Precautions: Pregnancy **B,** hypersensitivity to penicillins, lactation, renal disease

cefadroxil

Pharmacokinetics

Absorption	Well absorbed
Distribution	Widely distributed; crosses placenta
Metabolism	Not metabolized
Excretion	Unchanged by kidneys; enters breast milk
Half-life	1½-2 hr

Pharmacodynamics

	PO
Onset	Rapid
Peak	1½-2 hr
Duration	12-24 hr

cefazolin

Pharmacokinetics

Absorption	Well absorbed
Distribution	Widely distributed; crosses placenta
Metabolism	Not metabolized
Excretion	Unchanged by kidneys; enters breast milk
Half-life	1½-2½ hr

Pharmacodynamics

	IM	IV
Onset	Rapid	10 min
Peak	1-2 hr	Infusion's end
Duration	6-12 hr	

cephalexin

Pharmacokinetics

Absorption	Well absorbed
Distribution	Widely distributed; crosses placenta
Metabolism	Not metabolized
Excretion	Kidneys, unchanged; enters breast milk
Half-life	½-1 hr; increased in renal disease

Pharmacodynamics

Onset	15-30 min
Peak	1 hr
Duration	6-12 hr

cephapirin

Pharmacokinetics

Absorption	Well absorbed
Distribution	Widely distributed; crosses placenta
Metabolism	Not metabolized
Excretion	Kidneys, unchanged; enters breast milk
Half-life	½-1 hr

Pharmacodynamics

	IM	IV
Onset	Rapid	Immediate
Peak	½ hr	Infusion's end
Duration	4-6 hr	

cephradine

Pharmacokinetics

Absorption	Well absorbed
Distribution	Widely distributed; crosses placenta
Metabolism	Not metabolized
Excretion	Kidneys, unchanged; enters breast milk
Half-life	1-2 hr

Pharmacodynamics

	PO/IM	IV
Onset	Rapid	Immediate
Peak	1-2 hr	Infusion's end
Duration	6-12 hr	

Interactions
Individual drugs
Probenecid: increased toxicity
Drug classifications
Aminoglycosides, diuretics (loop): increased toxicity
Drug/herb
Acidophilus: do not use with antiinfectives
Drug/lab test
Increased: AST, ALT, alkaline phosphatase, LDH, BUN, creatinine, bilirubin

False positive: urinary protein, direct Coombs' test, urine glucose

Interference: cross-matching

NURSING CONSIDERATIONS
Assessment
- Assess patient for previous sensitivity reaction to penicillins or other cephalosporins;

cross-sensitivity between penicillins and cephalosporins is common
- Assess patient for signs and symptoms of infection including characteristics of wounds, sputum, urine, stool, WBC >10,000/mm^3, earache, fever; obtain baseline information and during treatment
- Obtain C&S before beginning drug therapy to identify if correct treatment has been initiated
- Assess for anaphylaxis: rash, urticaria, pruritus, chills, fever, joint pain; angioedema may occur a few days after therapy begins; epINEPHrine and resuscitation equipment should be available for anaphylactic reaction
- Identify urine output; if decreasing, notify prescriber (may indicate nephrotoxicity); also check for increased BUN, creatinine
- Monitor blood studies: AST, ALT, CBC, Hct, bilirubin, LDH, alkaline phosphatase, Coombs' test monthly if patient is on long-term therapy
- Monitor electrolytes: potassium, sodium, chloride monthly if patient is on long-term therapy
- Assess bowel pattern daily; if severe diarrhea occurs, drug should be discontinued; may indicate pseudomembranous colitis
- Monitor for bleeding: ecchymosis, bleeding gums, hematuria, stool guaiac daily if on long-term therapy
- Assess for superinfection: perineal itching, fever, malaise, redness, pain, swelling, drainage, rash, diarrhea, change in cough, sputum

Nursing diagnoses
- Infection, risk for (uses)
- Diarrhea (side effects)
- Fluid volume, deficient, risk for (side effects)
- Injury, risk for (side effects)
- Knowledge, deficient (teaching)
- Noncompliance (teaching)

cefadroxil
Implementation
- Give in even doses around the clock; if GI upset occurs, give with food; drug must be given for 10-14 days to ensure organism death and prevent superinfection
- Shake susp, refrigerate, discard after 2 wk

cefazolin
Implementation
IM route
- Reconstitute 250-500 mg of drug with 2 ml sterile or bacteriostatic water for inj, or 0.9% NaCl; reconstitute 1 g of drug with 2.5 ml; give deep in large muscle mass, massage

IV route
- Check for irritation, extravasation, phlebitis daily, change site q72h
- For direct **IV** dilute in 10 ml of sterile water for inj; give over 5 min
- For intermittent inf dilute reconstituted sol (500 mg or 1 mg) in 50-100 ml D_5W, $D_{10}W$, D_5/0.25% NaCl, D_5/0.45% NaCl, D_5/0.9% NaCl, D_5/LR, or LR, 0.9% NaCl; give over 30-60 min; may be refrigerated up to 96 hr or stored 24 hr at room temp

Syringe compatibilities: Heparin, vit B complex

Syringe incompatibilities: Ascorbic acid inj, cimetidine, lidocaine, vit B/C

Y-site compatibilities: Acyclovir, allopurinol, amifostine, atracurium, aztreonam, calcium gluconate, cyclophosphamide, diltiazem, enalaprilat, esmolol, famotidine, filgrastim, fluconazole, fludarabine, foscarnet, heparin, labetalol, lidocaine, magnesium sulfate, melphalan, meperidine, midazolam, morphine, multivitamins, ondansetron, perphenazine, pancuronium, regular insulin, sargramostim, tacrolimus, teniposide, theophylline, thiotepa, vecuronium, vit B/C

Y-site incompatibilities: Amiodarone, hetastarch, hydromorphone, idarubicin, vinorelbine tartrate

Additive compatibilities: Aztreonam, clindamycin, famotidine, fluconazole, metronidazole, verapamil

Additive incompatibilities: Amikacin, amobarbital, bleomycin, calcium gluceptate, calcium gluconate, colistimethate, erythromycin, kanamycin, oxytetracycline, pentobarbital, polymyxin B, tetracycline

cephalexin
Implementation
- Do not break, crush, or chew caps
- Give in even doses around the clock; if GI upset occurs, give with food; drug must be taken for 10-14 days to ensure organism death and prevent superinfection
- Shake susp, refrigerate, discard after 2 wk

cephapirin
Implementation
IM route
- Reconstitute 1-2 g/1-2 ml of sterile water for inj; give deep in large muscle mass and massage

IV route
- Check for irritation, extravasation, phlebitis daily; change site q72h
- For intermittent inf, reconstitute 250 mg/2.4 ml, 500 mg/4.8 ml, 1 g/9.6 ml, 2 g/19.2 ml sterile water for inj, D_5W, 0.9% NaCl; do not

use sol with benzyl alcohol for neonates; may be further diluted in 50-100 ml D_5W, $D_{10}W$, 0.9% NaCl, or LR; give over 30-60 min

- Store refrigerated 96 hr, room temp 24 hr

Y-site compatibilities: Acyclovir, cyclophosphamide, famotidine, heparin, hydrocortisone, hydromorphone, magnesium sulfate, meperidine, morphine, multivitamins, perphenazine, potassium chloride, vit B/C

Additive compatibilities: Bleomycin, calcium chloride, calcium gluconate, chloramphenicol, diphenhydrAMINE, ergonovine maleate, heparin, hydrocortisone, metaraminol, oxacillin, penicillin G potassium, pentobarbital, phenobarbital, phytonadione, potassium chloride, sodium bicarbonate, succinylcholine, verapamil, warfarin, vit B complex

Additive incompatibilities: Aminoglycosides, amikacin, ascorbic acid, epINEPHrine, gentamicin, kanamycin, mannitol, norepinephrine, oxytetracycline, phenytoin, tetracycline, thiopental

cephradine

Implementation

PO route

- May be given with food for GI symptoms
- When giving susp, shake well; refrigerate unused portion

IM route

- Reconstitute 250 mg/1.2 ml, 500 mg/ml, 1 g/4 ml sterile or bacteriostatic water for inj; give deep in large muscle mass, massage

IV route

- Check for irritation, extravasation, phlebitis daily; change site q72h
- For direct **IV** route, reconstitute 250-500 mg/5 ml sterile water, 0.9% NaCl, D_5W, or 1 g/10 ml, 2 g/20 ml; give over 3-5 min
- For intermittent inf, dilute 1 g/10 ml or more sterile water for inj, D_5W, $D_{10}W$, or D_5/0.9% NaCl; give over 30-60 min
- Store refrigerated 96 hr, room temp 24 hr

Additive incompatibilities: Other antibiotics, calcium salts, D_5W, epINEPHrine, lidocaine, Ringer's or LR sol, NormosolR, 0.9% NaCl, TPN #61, tetracycline

Patient/family education

- Teach patient to report sore throat, bruising, bleeding, joint pain; may indicate blood dyscrasias (rare)
- Advise patient to contact prescriber if vaginal itching, loose foul-smelling stools, furry tongue occur; may indicate superinfection
- Instruct patient to take all medication prescribed for the length of time ordered
- Advise patient to notify prescriber of diarrhea with blood, pus, mucus, which may indicate pseudomembranous colitis

Evaluation

Positive therapeutic outcome

- Absence of signs/symptoms of infection (WBC <10,000/mm^3, temp WNL, absence of red draining wounds, earache)
- Reported improvement in symptoms of infection
- Negative C&S

Treatment of anaphylaxis: EpINEPHrine, antihistamines, resuscitate if needed

CEPHALOSPORINS—2ND GENERATION

cefaclor (Rx)
(sef'a-klor)
Ceclor, Ceclor CD, Raniclor

cefmetazole (Rx)
(sef-met'a-zole)
Zefazone

cefotetan (Rx)
(sef'oh-tee-tan)
Cefotan

cefoxitin (Rx)
(se-fox'i-tin)
Mefoxin

cefprozil (Rx)
(sef-proe'zill)
Cefzil

cefuroxime (Rx)
(sef-yoor-ox'eem)
Ceftin, Cefuroxime, Zinacef

loracarbef (Rx)
(lor-a-kar'beff)
Lorabid

Func. class.: Antiinfective
Chem. class.: Cephalosporin (2nd generation)

Pregnancy category B

Do Not Confuse:
cefaclor/cephalexin, Cefotan/Ceftin, cefprozil/cefazolin, cefprozil/cefuroxime, Cefzil/Ceftin, Cefzil/Kefzol

Action: Inhibits bacterial cell wall synthesis, rendering cell wall osmotically unstable, leading to cell death by binding to cell wall membrane

cefaclor

Therapeutic Outcome: Bactericidal effects for the following: gram-negative bacilli *Haemophilus influenzae, Escherichia coli, Proteus mirabilis, Klebsiella;* gram-positive organisms *Streptococcus pneumoniae, Staphylococcus* β-hemolytic; streptococci, anaerobes, *Bacteroides* sp.

Uses: Upper and lower respiratory tract, urinary tract, skin infections; otitis media; increased bone, joint, gynecologic infections; septicemia

cefmetazole

Therapeutic Outcome: Bactericidal effects for the following: anaerobes, *Clostridium, Bacteroides* sp., *Fusobacterium* sp.; gram-negative organisms *Morganella morganii, Haemophilus influenzae, Escherichia coli, Proteus, Klebsiella, Bacteroides fragilis;* gram-positive organisms *Streptococcus pneumoniae, Streptococcus pyogenes, Staphylococcus aureus*

Uses: Infections of lower respiratory tract, urinary tract, skin, bone; intraabdominal infections

cefotetan

Therapeutic Outcome: Bactericidal effects for the following: gram-negative organisms *Haemophilus influenzae, Escherichia coli, Enterobacter aerogenes, Proteus mirabilis, Klebsiella, Morganella morganii, Proteus vulgaris, Providencia, Enterobacter, Salmonella, Shigella, Acinetobacter, Bacteroides fragilis, Neisseria, Serratia;* gram-positive organisms *Streptococcus pneumoniae, Streptococcus pyogenes, Staphylococcus aureus;* anaerobes *Bacteroides, Clostridium, Fusobacterium, Peptococcus, Peptostreptococcus*

Uses: Serious upper or lower respiratory tract, urinary tract, gynecologic, skin, bone, joint, gonococcal, intraabdominal infections

cefoxitin

Therapeutic Outcome: Bactericidal effects for the following: gram-negative bacilli *Haemophilus influenzae, Escherichia coli, Proteus, Klebsiella, Providencia, Neisseria gonorrhoeae;* gram-positive organisms *Streptococcus pneumoniae, Streptococcus pyogenes, Staphylococcus aureus;* anaerobes including *Clostridium, Bacteroides, Peptococcus, Peptostreptococcus*

Uses: Lower respiratory tract, urinary tract, skin, bone, gynecologic, gonococcal infections; septicemia, peritonitis

cefprozil

Therapeutic Outcome: Bactericidal effects for the following: gram-negative bacilli *Haemophilus influenzae, Escherichia coli;* gram-positive organisms *Streptococcus pneumoniae, Streptococcus pyogenes, Staphylococcus aureus*

Uses: Upper and lower respiratory tract, urinary tract, skin infections; otitis media

loracarbef

Therapeutic Outcome: Bactericidal effects for the following: gram-negative organisms *Haemophilus influenzae, Escherichia coli, Proteus mirabilis, Klebsiella;* gram-positive organisms *Streptococcus pneumoniae, Streptococcus pyogenes, Staphyloccus aureus*

Uses: Upper and lower respiratory tract, urinary tract, skin infections; otitis media, pharyngitis, tonsillitis

Dosage and routes

cefaclor

Adult: PO 250-500 mg q8h, not to exceed 4 g/day or 375-500 mg (ext rel) q12h × 7-10 days

Child >1 mo: PO 20-40 mg/kg daily in divided doses q8h, or total daily dose may be divided and given q12h, not to exceed 1 g/day

Acute bacterial exacerbations of chronic bronchitis or acute bronchitis

Adult: 500 mg/12 hr × 1 wk (ext rel)

Pharyngitis/tonsillitis

Adult: 375 mg/12 hr × 10 days (ext rel)

Available forms: Caps 250, 500 mg; oral susp 125, 187, 250, 375 mg/5 ml; ext rel tabs 375, 500 mg; chew tabs (Raniclor) 125, 187, 250, 375 mg

C

cefmetazole
Adult: **IV** 2 g divided q6-12h × 5-14 days

Renal dose
CCr <50 ml/min 1-2 g q12h; CCr 10-29 ml/min 1-2 g q24-48h; CCr <10 ml/min 1-2 g q48hr

Available forms: Powder for inj 1, 2 g/vial

cefotetan
Adult: **IV**/IM 1-2 g q12h × 5-10 days

Renal dose
CCr 10-30 ml/min q24h; CCr <10 ml/min q48h

Perioperative proplylaxis
Adult: **IV** 1-2 g ½-1 hr before surgery

Available forms: Inj 1, 2, 10 g

cefoxitin
Adult: IM/**IV** 1-2 g q6-8h

Renal dose
CCr <50 ml/min q8-12h; CCr 10-29 ml/min q24h; CCr <10 ml/min q24-48h
• Uncomplicated gonorrhea 2 g IM as single dose with 1 g PO probenecid at same time

Severe infections
Adult: IM/**IV** 2 g q4h
Child ≥3 mo: IM/**IV** 80-160 mg/kg/day divided q4-6h; max 12 g/day

Available forms: Powder for inj 1, 2, 10 g

cefprozil
Renal dose
CCr <30 ml/min 50% of dose

Upper respiratory infections
Adult: PO 500 mg q24h × 10 days

Otitis media
Child 6 mo-12 yr: PO 15 mg/kg q12h × 10 days

Lower respiratory infections
Adult: PO 500 mg q12h × 10 days

Skin/skin structure infections
Adult: PO 250-500 mg q12h × 10 days

Available forms: Tabs 250, 500 mg; susp 125, 250 mg/5 ml

cefuroxime
Adult and child: PO 250 mg q12h; may increase to 500 mg of q12h in serious infections
Adult: IM/**IV** 750 mg-1.5 g q8h for 5-10 days

Urinary tract infections
Adult: PO 125 mg q12h; may increase to 250 mg q12h if needed

Otitis media
Child <2 yr: PO 125 mg bid
Child >2 yr: PO 250 mg bid

Surgical prophylaxis
Adult: **IV** 1.5 g ½-1 hr preop

Severe infections
Adult: IM/**IV** 1.5 g q6h; may give up to 3 g q8h for bacterial meningitis
Child >3 mo: IM/**IV** 50-100 mg/kg/day; may give up to 200-240 mg/kg/day **IV** in divided doses for bacterial meningitis (not recommended)
• Dosage reduction indicated in severe renal impairment (CCr <20 ml/min)

Uncomplicated gonorrhea
Adult: 1.5 g IM as single dose with oral probenecid in 2 separate sites

Available forms: Tabs 125, 250, 500 mg: inj 150, 750 mg, 1.5, 7.5 g; inj 750 mg; 1.5 g powder, susp 125, 250 mg/5 ml

loracarbef
Adult and child >13 yr: PO 200-400 mg q12h
Child to 12 yr: PO 15-30 mg/kg/day in 2 divided doses q12h

Renal dose
CCr 10-49 ml/min 50% of dose; CCr <10 ml/min q3-5 days

Available forms: Caps 200, 400 mg; Oral susp 100, 200 mg/5 ml

Side effects/adverse reactions
CNS: Dizziness, headache, fatigue, paresthesia, fever, chills, confusion
GI: *Diarrhea,* nausea, vomiting, anorexia, dysgeusia, glossitis, bleeding; increased AST, ALT, bilirubin, LDH, alkaline phosphatase; abdominal pain, loose stools, flatulence, heartburn, stomach cramps, colitis, jaundice, **pseudomembranous colitis**
GU: Vaginitis, pruritus, candidiasis, increased BUN, **nephrotoxicity, renal failure,** pyuria, dysuria, reversible interstitial nephritis

HEMA: **Leukopenia, thrombocytopenia, agranulocytosis,** anemia, **neutropenia, lymphocytosis, eosinophilia, pancytopenia, hemolytic anemia, leukocytosis, granulocytopenia**
INTEG: Rash, urticaria, dermatitis, **Stevens-Johnson syndrome**
RESP: Dyspnea
SYST: **Anaphylaxis, serum sickness,** superinfection

Contraindications: Hypersensitivity to cephalosporins or related antibiotics, seizures

Precautions: Pregnancy **B**, lactation, children, renal disease

cefaclor

Pharmacokinetics	
Absorption	Well absorbed
Distribution	Widely distributed; crosses placenta
Metabolism	Not metabolized
Excretion	Unchanged by kidneys (60%-80%); enters breast milk
Half-life	36-54 min; increased in renal disease

Pharmacodynamics	
Onset	15 min
Peak	½-1 hr

cefmetazole

Pharmacokinetics	
Absorption	Complete
Distribution	Widely distributed; crosses placenta
Metabolism	Not metabolized
Excretion	Kidneys, unchanged (85%); enters breast milk
Half-life	½-2 hr; increased in renal disease

Pharmacodynamics	
Onset	Rapid
Peak	Infusion's end

cefotetan

Pharmacokinetics	
Absorption	Well absorbed (IM)
Distribution	Widely distributed; crosses placenta
Metabolism	Not metabolized
Excretion	Kidneys, unchanged; enters breast milk
Half-life	5 hr; increased in renal disease

Pharmacodynamics	IM	IV
Onset	Rapid	Immediate
Peak	1-3 hr	Infusion's end

cefoxitin

Pharmacokinetics	
Absorption	Well absorbed (IM)
Distribution	Widely distributed; crosses placenta
Metabolism	Not metabolized
Excretion	Kidneys, unchanged; enters breast milk
Half-life	½-1 hr; increased in renal disease

Pharmacodynamics	IM	IV
Onset	Rapid	Immediate
Peak	½ hr	Infusion's end

cefprozil

Pharmacokinetics	
Absorption	Well absorbed (PO)
Distribution	Widely distributed; crosses placenta
Metabolism	Not metabolized
Excretion	Kidneys, unchanged; enters breast milk
Half-life	1-1½ hr; increased in renal disease

Pharmacodynamics	PO
Onset	Unknown
Peak	Unknown

loracarbef

Pharmacokinetics

Absorption	Well absorbed
Distribution	Widely distributed; crosses placenta
Metabolism	Not metabolized
Excretion	Kidneys, unchanged; enters breast milk
Half-life	1 hr; increased in renal disease

Pharmacodynamics

Onset	Rapid
Peak	1 hr

Interactions

Individual drugs

Alcohol: disulfiram reaction if ingested within 48-72 hr of cephalosporin
Furosemide: increased toxicity
Plicamycin, valproic acid: increased bleeding
Probenecid: decreased excretion of drug and increased blood levels

Drug classifications

Aminoglycosides: increased toxicity
Anticoagulants, antiplatelets, NSAIDs, thrombolytics: increased bleeding (cefmetazole, cefotetan)

Drug/herb

(cefotetan, cefmetazole) Angelica, anise, arnica, bogbean, boldo, celery, chamomile, clove, fenugreek, feverfew, garlic, ginger, ginkgo, ginseng (*Panax*), horse chestnut, horseradish, licorice, meadowsweet, onion, papain, passion flower, prickly ash, red clover, turmeric, willow: increased bleeding risk
Acidophilus: do not use with antiinfectives

Drug/lab test

False: increased creatinine (serum urine), urinary 17-KS
False positive: urinary protein, direct Coombs' test, urine glucose (Clinitest)
Interference: cross-matching

NURSING CONSIDERATIONS

Assessment

- Assess patient for previous sensitivity reaction to penicillins or other cephalosporins; cross-sensitivity between penicillins and cephalosporins is common
- Assess patient for signs and symptoms of infection including characteristics of wounds, sputum, urine, stool, WBC >10,000/mm^3, earache, fever; obtain baseline information and during treatment
- Obtain C&S before beginning drug therapy to identify if correct treatment has been initiated
- Assess for anaphylaxis: rash, urticaria, pruritus, dyspnea, chills, fever, joint pain; angioedema may occur a few days after therapy begins; epINEPHrine and resuscitation equipment should be available for anaphylactic reaction
- Identify urine output; if decreasing, notify prescriber (may indicate nephrotoxicity); also check for increased BUN, creatinine
- Monitor blood studies: AST, ALT, CBC, Hct, bilirubin, LDH, alkaline phosphatase, Coombs' test monthly if patient is on long-term therapy
- Monitor electrolytes: potassium, sodium, chloride monthly if patient is on long-term therapy
- Assess bowel pattern daily; if severe diarrhea occurs, drug should be discontinued; may indicate pseudomembranous colitis
- Monitor for bleeding: ecchymosis, bleeding gums, hematuria, stool guaiac daily if on long-term therapy
- Assess for overgrowth of infection: perineal itching, fever, malaise, redness, pain, swelling, drainage, rash, diarrhea, change in cough, sputum

Nursing diagnoses

- Infection, risk for (uses)
- Diarrhea (side effects)
- Fluid volume, deficient, risk for (side effects)
- Injury, risk for (side effects)
- Knowledge, deficient (teaching)
- Noncompliance (teaching)

Implementation

cefaclor

- Do not break, crush, chew, or cut ext rel tabs
- Give in even doses around the clock; if GI upset occurs, give with food; drug must be given for 10-14 days to ensure organism death and prevent superinfection
- Shake susp, refrigerate, discard after 2 wk

cefmetazole

- Check for irritation, extravasation, phlebitis daily; change site q72h
- For intermittent inf, reconstitute with sterile, bacteriostatic water for inj or 0.9% NaCl; may be further diluted with 0.9% NaCl, LR, D_5W (1-20 mg/ml); give over 30-60 min; may be refrigerated for 1 wk or stored 24 hr at room temp

Additive compatibilities: Famotidine, clindamycin, KCI

cefotetan

IM route

- Reconstitute 1 g/2 ml or 2 g/3 ml of sterile or bacteriostatic water for inj; may be diluted with 0.5% of 1% lidocaine to prevent pain; give deep in large muscle mass, massage

IV route

- May be stored 96 hr refrigerated or 24 hr room temp
- Check for irritation, extravasation, phlebitis daily; change site q72h
- For direct **IV** dilute in 1 g/10 ml or more and give over 5 min
- For intermittent inf further dilute in 50-100 ml of 0.9% NaCl or D_5W; give over 3-5 min; discontinue primary line while running intermittent inf

Syringe incompatibilities: Doxapram
Y-site compatibilities: Allopurinol, amifostine, aztreonam, diltiazem, famotidine, filgrastim, fluconazole, fludarabine, heparin, regular insulin, melphalan, meperidine, morphine, paclitaxel, sargramostim, tacrolimus, teniposide, theophylline, thiotepa
Additive incompatibilities: Aminoglycosides, tetracyclines, heparin

cefoxitin

IM route

- Reconstitute 1 g/2 ml of sterile water for inj; may be diluted with 0.5% or 1% lidocaine to prevent pain; give deep in large muscle mass, massage

IV route

- Check for irritation, extravasation, phlebitis daily; change site q72h
- For direct **IV**, dilute 1 g/10 ml or 2 g/20 ml of sterile water for inj; shake, let stand until clear; give over 3-5 min
- For intermittent inf further dilute with 50-100 ml of D_5W, $D_{10}W$, D_5/0.25% NaCl, D_5/0.45% NaCl, D_5/0.9% NaCl, 0.9% NaCl D_5/LR, D_5/0.02%, sodium bicarbonate, Ringer's, or LR; give over 15-30 min; may store 96 hr refrigerated or 24 hr room temp
- For cont inf dilute in 500-1000 ml; give over prescribed rate

Syringe compatibilities: Heparin, insulin
Y-site compatibilities: Acyclovir, amifostine, aztreonam, cyclophosphamide, diltiazem, famotidine, fluconazole, foscarnet, hydromorphone, magnesium sulfate, meperidine, morphine, ondansetron, perphenazine, temiposide, thiotepa
Y-site incompatibilities: Hetastarch
Additive compatibilities: Amikacin, cimetidine, clindamycin, gentamicin, kanamycin, multivitamins, sodium bicarbonate, tobramycin, verapamil, vit B/C
Additive incompatibilities: Aztreonam

cefprozil

IM route

- Reconstitute with 1 g/2 ml or 2 g/3 ml of sterile or bacteriostatic water for inj; may be diluted with 0.5% or 1% lidocaine to prevent pain; give deep in large muscle mass, massage

IV route

- Check for irritation, extravasation, phlebitis daily; change site q72h
- For direct **IV**, dilute 1 g/10 ml or more and give over 5 min
- For intermittent inf further dilute with 50-100 ml of 0.9% NaCl or D_5W; give over 3-5 min; discontinue primary line while running intermittent infusion

Syringe incompatibilities: Doxapram
Y-site compatibilities: Famotidine, fluconazole, fludarabine, regular insulin, meperidine, morphine, sargramostim
Additive incompatibilities: Aminoglycosides, tetracyclines, heparin

loracarbef

- Do not break, crush, or chew caps
- Give on an empty stomach, 1 hr ac or 2 hr pc
- Oral susp should be shaken before administration; store for 2 wk at room temp, discard after 2 wk

Patient/family education

- Teach patient to report sore throat, bruising, bleeding, joint pain; may indicate blood dyscrasias (rare)
- Advise patient to contact prescriber if vaginal itching, loose foul-smelling stools, furry tongue occur; may indicate superinfection
- Instruct patient to take all medication prescribed for the length of time ordered; to use yogurt or buttermilk to maintain intestinal flora, decrease diarrhea
- Advise patient to notify prescriber of diarrhea with blood or pus, which may indicate pseudomembranous colitis

Evaluation

Positive therapeutic outcome

- Absence of signs/symptoms of infection (WBC <10,000/mm^3, temp WNL, absence of red draining wounds, earache)
- Reported improvement in symptoms of infection
- Negative C&S

Treatment of anaphylaxis: EpINEPHrine, antihistamines, resuscitate if needed

CEPHALOSPORINS—3RD GENERATION

cefdinir (Rx)
(sef'dih-ner)
Omnicef

cefditoren pivoxil (Rx)
(sef-dit'oh-ren pih-vox'il)
Spectracef

cefepime (Rx)
(sef'e-peem)
Maxipime

cefoperazone (Rx)
(sef-oh-per'a-zone)
Cefobid

cefotaxime (Rx)
(sef-oh-taks'eem)
Claforan

cefpodoxime (Rx)
(sef-poe-docks'eem)
Vantin

ceftazidime (Rx)
(sef'tay-zi-deem)
Ceptaz, Fortaz, Tazicef, Tazidime

ceftibuten (Rx)
(sef-ti-byoo'tin)
Cedax

ceftizoxime (Rx)
(sef-ti-zox'eem)
Cefizox

ceftriaxone (Rx)
(sef-try-ax'one)
Rocephin

Func. class.: Broad-spectrum antibiotic
Chem. class.: Cephalosporin (3rd generation)

Pregnancy category B

Do Not Confuse:
ceftazidime/ceftizoxime, Vantin/Ventolin

Action: Inhibits bacterial cell wall synthesis, rendering cell wall osmotically unstable, leading to cell death

cefdinir

Therapeutic Outcome: Bactericidal effects for the following: gram-negative organisms *Haemophilus influenzae, Serratia, Salmonella, Klebsiella, Citrobacter Shigella, Pseudomonas, Haemophilus parainfluenzae, Enterococcus faecalis,* gram-positive organisms *Streptococcus pneumoniae, Streptococcus pyogenes, Staphylococcus aureus*

Uses: Uncomplicated skin and skin structure infections, community-acquired pneumonia, acute exacerbations of chronic bronchitis, acute maxillary sinusitis, pharyngitis, tonsillitis, CNS infections, perioperative prophylaxis

cefditoren pivoxil

Therapeutic Outcome: Acute bacterial exacerbation of chronic bronchitis caused by *Haemophilus influenzae, Haemophilus parainfluenzae, Streptococcus pneumoniae, Moraxella catarrhalis;* pharyngitis/tonsillitus caused by *Streptococcus pyogenes;* uncomplicated skin, skin structure infections caused by *Staphylococcus aureus, S. pyogenes*

cefepime

Therapeutic Outcome: Bactericidal effects for the following: gram-negative bacilli, *Escherichia coli, Proteus, Klebsiella;* gram-positive organisms *Streptococcus pneumoniae, Streptococcus pyogenes, Staphylococcus aureus*

Uses: Lower respiratory tract, urinary tract, skin, bone, gonococcal infections; septicemia, peritonitis

cefoperazone

Therapeutic Outcome: Bactericidal effects for the following: gram-negative organisms *Acinetobacter, Morganella morganii, Neisseria gonorrhoeae, Proteus vulgaris;* gram-positive organisms *Staphylococci,* Streptococci, Streptococci (β-hemolytic), *Streptococcus pneumoniae, Haemophilus influenzae, Escherichia coli, Proteus mirabilis, Klebsiella, Enterobacter, Serratia, Citrobacter, Providencia, Pseudomonas aeruginosa;* anaerobes *Bacteroides, Clostridium, Eubacterium, Fusobacterium, Peptococcus, Peptostreptococcus*

Uses: Lower respiratory tract, urinary tract, skin, bone infections; bacterial septicemia, peritonitis, PID, endometritis

cefotaxime

Therapeutic Outcome: Bactericidal effects for the following: gram-negative organisms *Haemophilus influenzae, Escherichia coli, Neisseria meningitidis, Proteus mirabilis, Klebsiella, Citrobacter, Serratia, Salmonella, Shigella;* gram-positive organisms *Streptococcus pneumoniae, Streptococcus pyogenes, Staphylococcus aureus*

Uses: Lower serious respiratory tract, urinary tract, skin, bone, gonococcal infections; bacteremia, septicemia, meningitis

cefpodoxime

Therapeutic Outcome: Bactericidal effects for the following: gram-negative organisms *Neisseria gonorrhoeae, Haemophilus influenzae, Escherichia coli, Proteus mirabilis, Klebsiella;* gram-positive organisms *Streptococcus pneumoniae, Streptococcus pyogenes, Staphylococcus aureus*

Uses: Upper and lower respiratory tract, urinary tract, skin infections; otitis media, sexually transmitted diseases

ceftazidime

Therapeutic Outcome: Bactericidal effects for the following: gram-negative organisms *Haemophilus influenzae, Escherichia coli, Enterobacter aerogenes, Proteus mirabilis, Klebsiella, Citrobacter, Enterobacter, Pseudomonas aeruginosa, Shigella, Acinetobacter, Bacteroides fragilis, Neisseria;* gram-positive organisms *Streptococcus pneumoniae, Streptococcus pyogenes, Staphylococcus aureus*

Uses: Serious upper or lower respiratory tract, urinary tract, skin, gynecologic, bone, joint, intraabdominal infections; septicemia, meningitis

ceftibuten

Therapeutic Outcome: Bactericidal effects for the following: gram-negative bacilli *Haemophilus influenzae, Escherichia coli;* gram-positive organisms *Streptococcus pneumoniae, Streptococcus pyogenes, Staphylococcus aureus*

Uses: Upper and lower respiratory tract infections; otitis media

ceftizoxime

Therapeutic Outcome: Bactericidal effects for the following: gram-negative organisms *Haemophilus influenzae, Escherichia coli, Enterobacter aerogenes, Proteus mirabilis, Klebsiella, Acinetobacter, Neisseria gonorrhoeae, Providencia rettgeri, Pseudomonas aeruginosa, Serratia, Enterobacter;* gram-positive organisms *Streptococcus pneumoniae, Streptococcus pyogenes,*

Staphylococcus aureus; anaerobes *Bacteroides, Peptococcus, Peptostreptococcus*

Uses: Serious lower respiratory tract, urinary tract, skin, intraabdominalinfections; septicemia, meningitis; bone, joint infections; PID caused by *Neisseria gonorrhoeae*

ceftriaxone

Therapeutic Outcome: Bactericidal effects on the following: gram-negative organisms *Haemophilus influenzae, Escherichia coli, Enterobacter aerogenes, Proteus mirabilis, Klebsiella, Citrobacter, Enterobacter, Pseudomonas aeruginosa, Neisseria, Serratia;* gram-positive organisms *Streptococcus pneumoniae, Streptococcus pyogenes, Staphylococcus aureus;* anaerobes *Bacteroides*

Uses: Serious lower respiratory tract, urinary tract, skin, gonococcal, intraabdominal infections; septicemia, meningitis; bone, joint infections

Dosage and routes

cefdinir

Uncomplicated skin and skin structure infections/community-acquired pneumonia

Adult and child ≥13 yr: PO 300 mg q12h × 10 days

Child 6 mo-12 yr: PO 7 mg/kg q12h or 14 mg/kg q24h × 10 days; max 600 mg daily

Acute exacerbations of chronic bronchitis/acute maxillary sinusitis

Adult and child ≥13 yr: PO 300 mg q12h or 600 mg q24h × 10 days or 300 mg bid × 5 days in some infections

Pharyngitis/tonsillitis

Adult and child ≥13 yr: PO 300 mg q12h or 600 mg q24h × 10 days

Child 6 mo-12 yr: PO 7 mg/kg q12h × 5-10 days or 14 mg/kg q24h × 10 days

Renal dose

CCr <30 ml/min 300 mg daily (adult); 7 mg/kg daily (child)

Available forms: Caps 300 mg, oral susp 125 mg/5 ml

cefditoren pivoxil

Adult: PO 200-400 mg bid

Renal dose

Adult: PO CCr 30-50 ml/min, max 200 mg bid; CCr <30 ml/min, max 200 mg daily

Available forms: Tabs 200 mg

cefepime

Urinary tract infections (mild to moderate)

Adult: **IV**/IM 0.5-1 g q12h × 7-10 days

Urinary tract infections (severe)

Adult: **IV** 2 g q12h × 10 days

Pneumonia (moderate to severe)

Adult: **IV** 1-2 g q12h × 10 days

Dosage reduction indicated in renal impairment (CCr <50 ml/min)

Uncomplicated gonorrhea

- IM 2 g as a single dose with 1 g PO probenecid at the same time

Available forms: Powder for inj 500 mg, 1, 2 g

cefoperazone

Adult: IM/**IV** 1-2 g q12h

Severe infections

Adult: IM/**IV** 6-12 g/day divided in 2-4 equal doses

Hepatic dose: Give 50% of dose

Mild/moderate infections

Adult: IM/**IV** 1-2 g q12h

Available forms: Inj 1, 2 g

cefotaxime

Adult: IM/**IV** 1-2 g q12h as a single dose

Child 1 mo-12 yr: IM/**IV** 50-180 mg/kg/day in 4-6 divided doses

Severe infections

Adult: IM/**IV** 2 g q4h, not to exceed 12 g/day

Child 1 mo-12 yr: IM/**IV** 50 mg/kg q6h

Uncomplicated gonorrhea

Adult: IM 1 g; dosage reduction indicated for severe renal impairment (CCr <30 ml/min)

Available forms: Powder for inj 500 mg, 1, 2, 10 g; 1, 2 g premixed frozen

cefpodoxime

Adult >13 yr: *Pneumonia:* 200 mg q12h for 14 days; *uncomplicated gonorrhea:* 200

mg single dose; *skin and skin structure:* 400 mg q12h for 7-14 days; *pharyngitis and tonsillitis:* 100 mg q12h for 10 days; *uncomplicated UTI:* 100 mg q12h for 7 days; dosing interval increased in presence of severe renal impairment

Acute otitis media
Child 5 mo-12 yr: 5 mg/kg q12h for 10 days; *pharyngitis/tonsillitis:* 5 mg/kg q12h (max 100 mg/dose or 200 mg/day) × 5-10 days
Renal dose: Reduce dose in renal disease

Available forms: Tabs 100, 200 mg/ granules for susp 50, 100 mg/5 ml

ceftazidime
Adult: **IV**/IM 1-2 g q8-12h × 5-10 days
Child: **IV** 30-50 mg/kg q8h not to exceed 6 g/day
Neonate: **IV** 30-50 mg/kg q12h

Renal dose
Adult: **IV** CCr <50 ml/min q12h; CCr 10-30 ml/min q24h; CCr <10 ml/min q48h

Available forms: Inj 500 mg, 1, 2, 6 g

ceftibuten
Adult: PO 400 mg daily × 10 days
Child 6 mo-12 yr: PO 9 mg/kg daily × 10 days

Renal dose
Adult: PO CCr <50 ml/min 200 mg q24h; CCr 5-20 ml/min 100 mg q24h

Available forms: Caps 400 mg; susp 90, 180 mg/5 ml

ceftizoxime
Adult: IM/**IV** 1-2 g q8-12h, may give up to 4 g q8h in life-threatening infections
Child >6 mo: IM/**IV** 50 mg/kg q6-8h

Renal dose
Adult: IM/**IV** CCr <80 ml/min 500-1500 mg q8h; CCr 10-49 ml/min 250-1000 mg q12h

PID
Adult: **IV** 2 g q8h, may increase to 4 g q8h in severe infections

Available forms: Powder for inj 500 mg, 1, 2, 10 g; premixed 1 g, 2 g/50 ml

ceftriaxone
Reduce dosage in severe renal impairment (CCr <10 ml/min)
Adult: IM/**IV** 1-2 g daily, max 2 g q12h
Child: IM/**IV** 50-75 mg/kg/day in equal doses q12h

Uncomplicated gonorrhea
Adult: 250 mg IM as single dose

Meningitis
Adult and child: IM/**IV** 100 mg/kg/day in equal doses q12h, max 4 g/day

Surgical prophylaxis
Adult: **IV** 1 g ½-2 hr preop

Available forms: Inj 250, 500 mg, 1, 2, 10 g

Adverse effects
CNS: Headache, dizziness, weakness, paresthesia, fever, chills, **seizures**
GI: *Nausea, vomiting, diarrhea, anorexia,* pain, glossitis, **bleeding;** increased AST, ALT, bilirubin, LDH, alkaline phosphatase; abdominal pain, **pseudomembranous colitis**
GU: **Proteinuria,** vaginitis, pruritus, candidiasis, increased BUN, **nephrotoxicity, renal failure**
HEMA: **Leukopenia, thrombocytopenia, agranulocytosis,** anemia, **neutropenia, lymphocytosis, eosinophilia, pancytopenia, hemolytic anemia**
INTEG: Rash, urticaria, dermatitis
RESP: Dyspnea
SYST: **Anaphylaxis, serum sickness**

Contraindications: Hypersensitivity to cephalosporins, infants <1 mo

Precautions: Pregnancy **B,** hypersensitivity to penicillins, lactation, renal disease, children

cefdinir

Pharmacokinetics	
Absorption	Well absorbed
Distribution	Widely distributed; crosses placenta
Metabolism	Not metabolized
Excretion	Kidneys, unchanged; enters breast milk
Half-life	Unknown

Pharmacodynamics	PO
Onset	Unknown
Peak	Unknown

cefditoren pivoxil

Pharmacokinetics	
Absorption	Well absorbed after it is broken down (prodrug)
Distribution	Widely
Metabolism	Unknown
Excretion	Unknown
Half-life	100 mins

Pharmacodynamics

Onset	Rapid
Peak	0.5-3 hrs
Duration	12 hrs

cefepime

Pharmacokinetics

Absorption	Well absorbed (IM)
Distribution	Widely distributed; crosses placenta
Metabolism	Not metabolized
Excretion	Kidneys, unchanged; enters breast milk
Half-life	2 hr; increased in renal disease

Pharmacodynamics

	IM	IV
Onset	Rapid	Immediate
Peak	79 min	Infusion's end

cefoperazone

Pharmacokinetics

Absorption	Well absorbed (IM)
Distribution	Widely distributed; crosses placenta
Metabolism	Not metabolized
Excretion	Bile; enters breast milk
Half-life	2 hr

Pharmacodynamics

	IM	IV
Onset	Rapid	5 min
Peak	1-2 hr	Infusion's end

cefotaxime

Pharmacokinetics

Absorption	Widely distributed
Distribution	Breast milk, small amounts
Metabolism	Liver, active metabolites
Excretion	40%-65% unchanged, kidney
Half-life	1 hr

Pharmacodynamics

	IV	IM
Onset	5 min	30 min
Peak	Unknown	Unknown
Duration	Unknown	Unknown

cefpodoxime

Pharmacokinetics

Absorption	Well absorbed (PO)
Distribution	Widely distributed; crosses placenta
Metabolism	Not metabolized
Excretion	Kidneys, unchanged; enters breast milk
Half-life	2-3 hr, increased in renal disease

Pharmacodynamics

	PO
Onset	Unknown
Peak	Unknown

ceftazidime

Pharmacokinetics

Absorption	Well absorbed (IM)
Distribution	Widely distributed; crosses placenta
Metabolism	Not metabolized
Excretion	Kidneys, unchanged; enters breast milk
Half-life	½-1 hr; increased in renal disease

Pharmacodynamics

	IM	IV
Onset	Rapid	Immediate
Peak	1 hr	Infusion's end

ceftibuten

Pharmacokinetics

Absorption	Well absorbed
Distribution	Widely distributed; crosses placenta
Metabolism	Not metabolized
Excretion	Kidneys, unchanged; enters breast milk
Half-life	1-1½ hr; increased in renal disease

Pharmacodynamics

Onset	Unknown
Peak	Unknown

ceftizoxime

Pharmacokinetics

Absorption	Well absorbed (IM)
Distribution	Widely distributed; crosses placenta
Metabolism	Not metabolized
Excretion	Kidneys, unchanged; enters breast milk
Half-life	1½-2 hr; increased in renal disease

Pharmacodynamics

	IM	IV
Onset	Rapid	Immediate
Peak	1 hr	Infusion's end

ceftriaxone

Pharmacokinetics

Absorption	Well absorbed
Distribution	Widely distributed; crosses placenta; enters CSF
Metabolism	Liver
Excretion	Kidneys, partly
Half-life	5-8 hr

Pharmacodynamics

	IM	IV
Onset	Rapid	Immediate
Peak	1 hr	Infusion's end

Interactions

Individual drugs

Furosemide, probenecid: increased toxicity
Iron: decreased absorption of cefdinir
Plicamycin, valproic acid: increased bleeding

Drug classifications

Aminoglycosides: increased toxicity
Anticoagulants, NSAIDs, thrombolytics: increased bleeding

Drug/herb

Acidophilus: do not use with antiinfectives
Angelica, anise, arnica, bogbean, boldo, celery, chamomile, clove, fenugreek, feverfew, garlic, ginger, ginkgo, ginseng (*Panax*), horse chestnut, horseradish, licorice, meadowsweet, onion, papain, passion flower, poplar, prickly ash, red clover, turmeric, willow: increased risk of bleeding when used with cefoperazone

Drug/lab test

Increased: ALT, AST, alkaline phosphatase, LDH, bilirubin, BUN, creatinine
False increase: creatinine (serum urine), urinary 17-KS
False positive: urinary protein, direct Coombs' test, urine glucose
Interference: cross-matching

NURSING CONSIDERATIONS

Assessment

- Assess patient for previous sensitivity reaction to penicillins or other cephalosporins; cross-sensitivity between penicillins and cephalosporins is common
- Assess patient for signs and symptoms of infection including characteristics of wounds, sputum, urine, stool, WBC >10,000/mm^3, fever; obtain baseline information and during treatment
- Obtain C&S before beginning drug therapy to identify if correct treatment has been initiated
- Assess for anaphylaxis: rash, urticaria, pruritus, chills, fever, joint pain; angioedema may occur a few days after therapy begins; epINEPHrine and resuscitation equipment should be available for anaphylactic reaction
- Identify urine output; if decreasing, notify prescriber (may indicate nephrotoxicity); also check for increased BUN, creatinine
- Monitor blood studies: AST, ALT, CBC, Hct, bilirubin, LDH, alkaline phosphatase, Coombs' test monthly if patient is on long-term therapy
- Monitor electrolytes: potassium, sodium, chloride monthly if patient is on long-term therapy
- Assess bowel pattern daily; if severe diarrhea occurs, drug should be discontinued; may indicate pseudomembranous colitis
- Monitor for bleeding: ecchymosis, bleeding gums, hematuria, stool guaiac daily if on long-term therapy
- Assess for overgrowth of infection: perineal itching, fever, malaise, redness, pain, swelling, drainage, rash, diarrhea, change in cough, sputum

C

Nursing diagnoses
- Infection, risk for (uses)
- Injury, risk for (side effects)
- Diarrhea (side effects)
- Knowledge, deficient (teaching)

Implementation
cefdinir
PO route
- Give oral suspension after adding 39 ml water to the 60 ml bottle; 65 ml water to the 12.0 ml bottle; discard unused portion after 10 days

cefditoren pivoxil
- Give for 10 days to ensure organism death, prevent superinfection
- Give with food if needed for GI symptoms
- Give after C&S is completed

cefepime
IM route
- Reconstitute 1 g/2 ml of sterile water for inj; may be diluted with 0.5% or 1% lidocaine to prevent pain; give deep in large muscle mass, massage

IV route
- Check for irritation, extravasation, phlebitis daily; change site q72h
- For intermittent inf dilute with 50-100 ml of D_5W, give over 30 min

Solution compatibilities: 0.9% NaCl, D_5, 0.5, 1.0% lidocaine, bacteriostatic water for inj with parabens/benzyl alcohol

cefoperazone
IM route
- Reconstitute 1 g/2.8 ml of sterile or bacteriostatic water for inj, or 2 g/5.4 ml; may be diluted further with 1 ml or 1.8 ml of 2% lidocaine to prevent pain; give deep in large muscle mass, massage

IV route
- Check for irritation, extravasation, phlebitis daily; change site q72h
- For intermittent inf, reconstituted sol should be further diluted 1 g/20-40 ml of 0.9% NaCl, D_5W, D_5/0.9% NaCl, D_5/LR, or LR; give over 15-30 min; may be refrigerated up to 96 hr or stored 24 hr at room temp
- For cont inf, final concentration is 2-25 mg/ml, give at prescribed rate

Syringe compatibilities: Heparin

Syringe incompatibilities: Doxapram

Y-site compatibilities: Acyclovir, allopurinol, aztreonam, cyclophosphamide, enalaprilat, esmolol, famotidine, foscarnet, fludarabine, hydromorphone, magnesium sulfate, melphalan, morphine, teniposide, thiotepa

Y-site incompatibilities: Gentamicin, hetastarch, labetalol, meperidine, ondansetron, perphenazine, sargramostim, tobramycin, vinorelbine tartrate

Additive compatibilities: Cimetidine, clindamycin, furosemide

Additive incompatibilities: Aminoglycosides

cefotaxime
IV route
- Dilute 1 g/10 ml D_5W, NS, sterile H_2O for inj and give over 3-5 min by Y-tube or 3-way stopcock; may be diluted further with 50-100 ml of 0.9% NaCl or D_5W; run over ½-1 hr; discontinue primary inf during administration; or may be diluted in larger volume of sol and given as a cont inf over 6-24 hr
- Give for 10-14 days to ensure organism death, prevent superinfection
- Thaw frozen container at room temperature or refrigeration, do not force thaw by immersion or microwave; visually inspect container for leaks

Syringe compatibilities: Heparin, oflaxacin

Y-site compatibilities: Acyclovir, amifostine, aztreonam, cyclophosphamide, diltiazem, famotidine, fludarabine, hydromorphone, lorazepam, magnesium sulfate, melphalan, meperidine, midazolam, morphine, ondansetron, perphenazine, sargramostim, teniposide, thiotepa, tolazoline, vinorelbine

Additive compatibilities: Clindamycin, metronidazole, verapamil

cefpodoxime
IM route
- Reconstitute 1 g/2 ml or 2 g/3 ml of sterile or bacteriostatic water for inj; may be diluted with 0.5% of 1% lidocaine to prevent pain; give deep in large muscle mass, massage

IV route
- Check for irritation, extravasation, phlebitis daily; change site q72h
- For direct **IV** dilute in 1 g/10 ml or more and give over 5 min
- For intermittent inf further dilute in 50-100 ml of 0.9% NaCl or D_5W; give over 3-5 min; discontinue primary line while running intermittent inf

Syringe incompatibilities: Doxapram
Y-site compatibilities: Famotidine, fluconazole, fludarabine, regular insulin, meperidine, morphine, sargramostim
Additive incompatibilities: Aminoglycosides, heparin, tetracyclines

ceftazidime

IM route

- Reconstitute 500 mg/1.5 ml or 1 g/3 ml of sterile or bacteriostatic water for inj; may be diluted with 0.5% or 1% lidocaine to prevent pain; give deep in large muscle mass, massage

IV route

- Check for irritation, extravasation, phlebitis daily; change site q72h
- For direct **IV** dilute 500 mg/5 ml or 1 g/10 ml sterile water for inj; give over 3-5 min; do not use sol with benzyl alcohol for neonates
- For intermittent inf further dilute 1 g/10 ml or more 0.9% NaCl, D_5W, $D_{10}W$, D_5/0.25% NaCl, D_5/0.45% NaCl, D_5/0.9% NaCl, or LR; give over 30-60 min
- Store for 96 hr refrigerated, 24 hr room temp

Y-site compatibilities: Acyclovir, allopurinol, amifostine, aztreonam, ciprofloxacin, diltiazem, enalaprilat, esmolol, famotidine, filgrastim, fludarabine, foscarnet, granisetron, heparin, hydromorphone, labetalol, meperidine, melphalan, morphine, ondansetron, paclitaxel, rantidine, tacrolimus, teniposide, theophylline, thiotepa, vinorelbine tartrate, zidovudine
Y-site incompatibilities: Amsacrine, fluconazole, idarubicin, sargramostim
Additive compatibilities: Ciprofloxacin, clindamycin, fluconazole, metronidazole, ofloxacin
Additive incompatibilities: Aminoglycosides, sodium bicarbonate

ceftibuten

- Administer for 10 days to ensure organism death, prevent superimposed infection
- Administer after C&S

ceftizoxime

IM route

- Reconstitute 250 mg/0.9 ml, 500 mg/1.8 ml, 1 g/3.6 ml, 2 g/7.2 ml; may be diluted with 0.5% or 1% lidocaine to prevent pain; give deep in large muscle mass, massage

IV route

- Check for irritation, extravasation, phlebitis daily; change site q72h
- For intermittent inf reconstitute 250 mg/2.4 ml, 500 mg/4.8 ml, 1 g/9.6 mg/2 g/19.2 ml sterile water for inj, D_5W, or 0.9% NaCl; do not use sol with benzyl alcohol for neonates; may be further diluted in 50-100 ml of D_5W, $D_{10}W$, 0.9% NaCl, or LR; give over 30-60 min
- May store 96h refrigerated, 24h room temp

Y-site compatibilities: Acyclovir, allopurinol, amifostine, aztreonam, enalaprilat, esmolol, famotidine, fludarabine, foscarnet, hydromorphone, labetalol, melphalan, meperidine, morphine, ondansetron, sargramostim, teniposide, thiotepa, vinorelbine
Additive compatibilities: Clindamycin, metronidazole
Additive incompatibilities: Aminoglycosides

ceftriaxone

- Give for 10-14 days to ensure organism death, prevent superinfection
- Give IM inj deeply in large muscle mass

IV route

- Give **IV** after diluting 250 mg/2.4 ml of D_5W, H_2O for inj, 0.9% NaCl; may be further diluted with 50-100 ml of 0.9% NaCl, D_5W, $D_{10}W$, shake; run over ½-1 hr

Y-site compatibilities: Acyclovir, allopurinol, aztreonam, cisatracurium, diltiazem, DOXOrubicin liposome, fludarabine, foscarnet, heparin, melphalan, meperidine, methotrexate, morphine, paclitaxel, remifentanil, sargramostim, tacrolimus, teniposide, theophylline, vinorelbine, warfarin, zidovudine
Additive compatibilities: Amino acids or sodium bicarbonate, metronidazole

Patient/family education

- Teach patient to report sore throat, bruising, bleeding, joint pain; may indicate blood dyscrasias (rare)
- Advise patient to contact prescriber if vaginal itching, loose foul-smelling stools, furry tongue occur; may indicate superinfection
- Advise patient to notify prescriber of diarrhea with blood or pus, may indicate pseudomembranous colitis
- Cefditoren can be taken with oral contraceptives

Evaluation

Positive therapeutic outcome

- Absence of signs/symptoms of infection (WBC <10,000/mm^3, temp WNL, absence of red draining wounds, earache)
- Reported improvement in symptoms of infection
- Negative C&S

Treatment of anaphylaxis: EpINEPHrine, antihistamines, resuscitate if needed

C

cephapirin
cephradine
See cephalosporins—1st generation

cetirizine (Rx)

(se-tear'i-zeen)

Zyrtec

Func. class: Antihistamine, peripherally selective (2nd generation)

Chem. class.: Piperazine, H_1 histamine antagonist

Pregnancy category B

Do Not Confuse:
Zyrtec/Xanax/Zantac

Action: Acts on blood vessels, GI, respiratory system by competing with histamine for H_1-receptor site; decreases allergic response by blocking pharmacologic effects of histamine; less sedation rate than with other antihistamines; causes increased heart rate, vasodilatation, increased secretions

Therapeutic Outcome: Absence of allergy symptoms, rhinitis, and chronic idiopathic urticaria

Uses: Rhinitis, allergy symptoms, and chronic idiopathic urticaria

Dosage and routes

Adult and child ≥6 yr: PO 5-10 mg daily
Child 2-5 yr: PO 2.5 mg daily, may increase to 5 mg daily or 2.5 mg bid
Child 1-2 yr: PO 2.5 mg daily, may increase to 2.5 mg g12h
Child 6-11 mo: PO 2.5 mg daily
Elderly: PO 5 mg daily, may increase to 10 mg/day

Renal dose
Adult: PO CCr 11-31 ml/min 5 mg daily

Hepatic dose
Adult: PO 5 mg daily

Available forms: Tabs 5, 10 mg; syr 5 mg/5 ml

Adverse effects

CNS: *Headache,* stimulation, *drowsiness,* sedation, *fatigue,* confusion, blurred vision, tinnitus, restlessness, tremors, parodoxical excitation in children or elderly
GI: *Dry mouth,* increased liver function tests
INTEG: Rash, eczema, photosensitivity, urticaria
RESP: *Thickening of bronchial secretions;* dry nose, throat

Contraindications: Hypersensitivity to this drug or hydrOXYzine, newborn or premature infants, lactation, severe hepatic disease

Precautions: Pregnancy **B**, elderly, children, respiratory disease, narrow-angle glaucoma, prostatic hypertrophy, bladder neck obstruction, asthma

Pharmacokinetics	
Absorption	Well absorbed, rapid
Distribution	Protein binding 93%
Metabolism	Liver
Excretion	Kidneys
Half-life	8.3 hr, decreased in children, increased in hepatic/renal disease

Pharmacodynamics	
Onset	½ hr
Peak	1-2 hr
Duration	24 hr

Interactions

Individual drugs
Alcohol: increased CNS depression

Drug classifications
CNS depressants, opioids, sedative/hypnotics: increased CNS depression
MAOIs: increased anticholinergic effect

Drug/herb
Corkwood: increased anticholinergic effect
Hops, Jamaican dogwood, kava, senna, valerian: increased CNS depression

Drug/food
Prolongs absorption by 1.7 hr

Drug/lab test
False negative: skin allergy tests (discontinue antihistamine 3 days before testing)

NURSING CONSIDERATIONS

Assessment

- Assess respiratory status: rate, rhythm; increase in bronchial secretions, wheezing, chest tightness; provide fluids to 2 L/day to decrease secretion thickness
- Assess for allergy symptoms: pruritus, urticaria, watering eyes, baseline and during treatment

Nursing diagnoses

- Airway clearance, ineffective (uses)
- Injury, risk for (side effects)
- Knowledge, deficient (teaching)
- Noncompliance (teaching overuse)

Implementation

- Give without regard to meals
- Store in tight, light-resistant container

Patient/family education

- Teach all aspects of drug uses; to notify prescriber if confusion, sedation, hypotension occur; to avoid driving or other hazardous activity if drowsiness occurs; to avoid alcohol or other CNS depressants that may potentiate effect
- Instruct patient to take without regard to meals
- Instruct patient not to exceed recommended dose; dysrhythmias may occur
- Advise patient to avoid using if breast feeding
- Advise patient to avoid exposure to sunlight; burns may occur
- Advise patient to use sugarless gum, candy, frequent sips of water to minimize dry mouth

Evaluation

Positive therapeutic outcome

- Absence of runny or congested nose, rashes

Treatment of overdose:

Lavage, diazepam, vasopressors, barbiturates (short acting)

cetrorelix (Rx)

(set-roe-ree′lix)

Cetrotide

Func. class.: Gonadotropin-releasing hormone antagonist

Chem. class.: Synthetic decapeptide

Pregnancy category X

Action: Inhibitor of pituitary gonadotropin secretion; initially increases LH and FSH, induces a rapid suppression of gonadotropin secretion

Therapeutic Outcome: Pregnancy

Uses: For inhibition of premature LH surges in women undergoing controlled ovarian hyperstimulation

Dosage and routes

Single-dose regimen

Adult: SUBCUT 3 mg when serum estradiol level is at appropriate stimulation response, usually on stimulation day 7; if hCG has not been given within 4 days after inj of 3 mg cetrorelix, give 0.25 mg daily until day of hCG administration

Multiple-dose regimen

Adult: SUBCUT 0.25 mg is given on stimulation day 5 (either morning or evening) or 6 (morning) and continued daily until day hCG is given

Available forms: Inj 0.25, 3 mg

Adverse effects

CNS: Headache

ENDO: Ovarian hyperstimulation syndrome, abdominal pain (gyn)

GI: Nausea, vomiting, diarrhea

INTEG: Pain on inj; local site reactions

***SYST:* Fetal death**

Contraindications: Pregnancy **X**, hypersensitivity, latex allergy, lactation

Pharmacokinetics	
Absorption	Unknown
Distribution	Protein binding 86%
Metabolism	Liver to metabolites
Excretion	Feces/urine
Half-life	Depends on dosage

Pharmacodynamics

Unknown

Interactions: None known

NURSING CONSIDERATIONS

Assessment

- Assess for suspected pregnancy; drug should not be used
- Assess for latex allergy; drug should not be used
- Monitor ALT, AST, GGT, alkaline phosphatase

Nursing diagnoses

- Knowledge, deficient (teaching)

Implementation

- Give SUBCUT using abdomen, around navel or upper thigh, swab inj area with disinfectant, clean a 2 in circle and allow to dry, pinch up area between thumb and finger, insert needle at 45-90° to surface; if blood is drawn into the syringe, reposition needle without removing it
- Do not administer if patient is pregnant
- Protect from light

Patient/family education

- Instruct to report abdominal pain, vaginal bleeding, nausea, vomiting, diarthea, shortness of breath, peripheral edema
- Teach self-administration technique if needed

Evaluation

Positive therapeutic outcome

- Pregnancy

cetuximab (Rx)
(se-tux'i-mab)
Erbitux
Func. class.: Miscellaneous antineoplastic, monoclonal antibody
Chem. class.: Epidermal growth factor receptor inhibitor
Pregnancy category C

Action: Not fully understood. Binds to epidermal growth factor receptors (EGFR); inhibits phosphorylation and activation of receptor associated kinase resulting in inhibition of cell growth.

Therapeutic Outcome: Decrease in tumor size

Uses: Alone or in combination with irinotecan for EGFR expressing metastatic colorectal carcinoma

Dosage and routes
Adult: **IV** inf 400 mg/m^2 loading dose given over 120 min, max infusion rate 5 ml/min, weekly maintenance dose (all other infusions) is 250 mg/m^2 given over 60 min, max infusion rate 5 ml/min. Premedicate with an H_1 antagonist (diphenhydrAMINE 50 mg **IV**); dosage adjustments are made for infusion reactions or dermatologic toxicity

Available forms: Inj 50 ml, single use vial with 100 mg of cetuximab (2 mg/ml)

Adverse effects
CNS: *Headache, insomnia, depression*
GI: *Nausea, diarrhea, vomiting, anorexia, mouth ulceration, dehydration, constipation, abdominal pain*
HEMA: **Leukepenia, anemia**
INTEG: Rash, pruritus, acne, dry skin, **toxic epidermal neurolysis, angioedema,** *blepharitis, cheilitis, cellulitis, cysts, alopecia, skin/nail disorder*
MISC: *Conjunctivitis, asthma, malaise, fever,* **renal failure**
MS: *Back pain*
RESP: **Interstitial lung disease**, *cough, dyspnea,* **pulmonary embolus**, *peripheral edema*
SYST: **Anaphylaxis, sepsis, infection**

Contraindications: Hypersensitivity to this drug or murine proteins

Precautions: Pregnancy **C**, renal/hepatic disease, ocular, pulmonary disorders, lactation, children, elderly

Pharmacokinetics

Absorption	Unknown
Distribution	Unknown
Metabolism	Unknown
Excretion	Unknown
Half-life	114 hrs

Pharmacodynamics

Onset	Unknown
Peak	168-235 g/ml, trough 41-85 g/ml
Duration	Steady state by 3rd weekly infusion

Interactions: None known

NURSING CONSIDERATIONS
Assessment
- ⬥ Monitor pulmonary changes: lung sounds, cough, dyspnea; interstitial lung disease may occur, my be fatal; discontinue therapy if confirmed
- ⬥ Assess for toxic epidermal necrosis, angioedema, anaphylaxis
- Assess GI symptoms: frequency of stools, dehydration, abdominal pain, stomatitis

Nursing diagnoses
- Injury, risk for (adverse reactions)
- Body image, disturbed (adverse reactions)
- Infection, risk for (adverse reactions)
- Knowledge, deficient (teaching)

Implementation
IV infusion route
- Administer by **IV** infusion only, do not give by **IV** push or bolus
- Do not shake or dilute
- Infusion pump: draw up volume of a vial using appropriate syringe/needle (a vented spike or other appropriate transfer device); fill Erbitux into sterile evacuted container/bag, repeat until calculated volume has been put into the container. Use a new needle for each vial; give through in-line filter (low protein binding 0.22-micrometer); affix infusion line and prime before starting infusion, max rate 5 ml/min; flush line at end of infusion with 0.9% NaCl
- Syringe pump: Draw up volume of a vial using appropriate syringe/needle (a vented spike); place syringe into syringe driver of a syringe pump and set rate; use an in-line filter 0.22 micrometer (low protein binding); connect infusion line and start infusion after priming; repeat until calculated volume has been given.
- Use a new needle and filter for each vial,

max 5 ml/min rate; use 0.9% NaCl to flush line after infusion

- Do not piggyback to patient infusion line
- Observe patient for adverse reactions for 1 hr after infusion
- Infusion reactions: if mild (Grade 1 or 2) reduce all doses by 50%; if severe (Grade 3 or 4) permanently discontinue
- Store refrigerated 36-46° F, discard unused portions

Patient/family education

- Instruct patient to report adverse reactions immediately: SOB, severe abdominal pain, skin eruptions
- Explain reason for treatment, expected results
- Instruct patient to use contraception during treatment
- Advise patient to wear sunscreen and hats to limit sun exposure. Sun exposure can exacerbate any skin reactions

Evaluation

Positive therapeutic outcome

- Decrease growth, spread of EGFR expressing metastatic colorectal carcinoma

chloral hydrate (Rx)

(klor'al hye'drate)

Aquachloral, chloral hydrate, Novo-Chlorhydrate ✤, PMS-Chloral Hydrate

Func. class.: Sedative/hypnotic

Chem. class.: Chloral derivative

Pregnancy category C

Controlled substance schedule IV (USA), schedule F (Canada)

Action: Reduced to product trichloroethanol, which produces mild cerebral depression, causing sleep; generalized CNS depression

Therapeutic Outcome: Ability to sleep, sedation

Uses: Sedation, short-term treatment of insomnia, preoperative reduction of anxiety

Dosage and routes

Sedation

Adult: PO/rec 250 mg tid pc

Child: PO 25-50 mg/kg tid, not to exceed 500 mg tid

Procedure sedation

Child: PO/REC 25-50 mg/kg, not to exceed 100 mg/kg or 2 g

Insomnia

Adult: PO/REC 500 mg-1 g 30 min before bedtime

Child: PO/REC 50-75 mg/kg (one dose)

Renal dose

Adult: PO/REC CCr <50 ml/min avoid use

Available forms: Caps 250, 500, 650 mg; syr 250, 500 mg/5 ml; supp 325, 500 mg

Adverse effects

CNS: *Drowsiness,* dizziness, stimulation, nightmares, ataxia, hangover (rare), lightheadedness, headache, paranoia

CV: Hypotension, **dysrhythmias**

GI: *Nausea, vomiting, flatulence, diarrhea,* unpleasant taste, **gastric necrosis**

HEMA: **Eosinophilia, leukopenia**

INTEG: Rash, urticaria, **angioedema,** fever, purpura, eczema

RESP: **Depression**

Contraindications: Hypersensitivity to this drug or triclofos, severe renal disease, severe hepatic disease, GI disorders (oral forms), gastritis

Precautions: Pregnancy **C,** severe cardiac disease, depression, suicidal individuals, asthma, intermittent porphyria, lactation, elderly

Pharmacokinetics

Absorption	Well absorbed (PO, rec)
Distribution	Widely distributed; crosses placenta
Metabolism	Liver to trichloroethanol
Excretion	Kidneys (inactive metabolite), feces, breast milk
Half-life	8-10 hr; active metabolite

Pharmacodynamics

	PO	REC
Onset	½-1 hr	Slow
Peak	Unknown	Unknown
Duration	4-8 hr	4-8 hr

Interactions

Individual drugs

Alcohol: increased action of both drugs

Furosemide: increased action of furosemide

Phenytoin: decreased effect of phenytoin

Drug classifications

Anticoagulants (oral): increased action of anticoagulants

CNS depressants: increased action of both drugs

Drug/herb

Catnip, chamomile, clary, cowslip, kava, lavender, mistletoe, nettle, pokeweed, poppy,

Queen Anne's lace, senega, valerian: increased sedative effect
Black cohosh: increased hypotension

Drug/lab test
Interferences: urine catecholamines, urinary 17-OHCS

NURSING CONSIDERATIONS
Assessment
- Assess patient's sleep pattern and note physical (sleep apnea, obstructed airway, pain/discomfort, urinary frequency) and psychologic (fear, anxiety) circumstances that interrupt sleep
- Assess patient's bedtime routine, presleep cues/props
- Assess potential for abuse; this drug may lead to physical and psychologic dependency; amount of drug should be limited
- Monitor blood studies: Hct, Hgb, RBCs, serum folate (if on long-term therapy), protime in patients receiving anticoagulants since action of anticoagulant may be increased
- Monitor mental status: mood, sensorium, affect, memory (long, short)
- Monitor physical dependency: more frequent requests for medication, shakes, anxiety, pinpoint pupils
- Monitor respiratory dysfunction: respiratory depression, character, rate, rhythm; hold drug if respirations are <10/min or if pupils are dilated (rare)
- Assess for blood dyscrasias: fever, sore throat, bruising, rash, jaundice, epistaxis (rare)
- Assess previous history of substance abuse, cardiac disease, or gastritis

Nursing diagnoses
- Sleep patterns, disturbed (uses)
- Anxiety (uses)
- Knowledge, deficient (teaching)
- Noncompliance (teaching)

Implementation
- Regulate environmental stimuli (light, noise, temperature), remove foods and fluids that interfere with sleep
- Place side rails up after giving medication for hypnotic; remove cigarettes/matches from patient's environment to prevent fires

PO route
- Do not break, crush, or chew caps
- Give ½-1 hr before bedtime for sleeplessness; give on empty stomach with full glass of water or juice for best absorption and to decrease corrosion (do not chew); after meals to decrease GI symptoms if used for sedation; dilute syr in 4 oz water or juice
- (Alert) Check dose of syrup carefully, fatal overdoses have occurred

Rectal route
- Store supp in dark container, in refrigerator; remove outer wrapper before insertion

Patient/family education
- Caution patient to avoid driving and other activities requiring alertness; to avoid alcohol ingestion or CNS depressants; serious CNS depression may result plus tachycardia, flushing, headache, hypotension
- Instruct patient not to discontinue medication quickly after long-term use; drug should be tapered over 1-2 wk, delirium may occur; that benefits may take 2 nights to be noticed; withdrawal symptoms include tremors, anxiety, hallucinations, delirium
- Teach patient alternative measures to improve sleep (reading, exercise several hours before bedtime, warm bath, warm milk, TV, self-hypnosis, deep breathing)
- Instruct the patient about factors that contribute to sleep pattern disturbances (lifestyle, shift work, long work hours, environmental factors, frequent napping)
- Teach patient to take drug as prescribed, not to double doses
- Avoid breastfeeding

Evaluation
Positive therapeutic outcome
- Ability to sleep at night
- Decreased amount of early morning awakening if taking drug for insomnia
- Sedation

Treatment of overdose: Lavage, activated charcoal; monitor electrolytes, VS

chlorambucil (Rx)
(klor-am′byoo-sil)
Leukeran
Func. class.: Antineoplastic alkylating agent
Chem. class.: Nitrogen mustard
Pregnancy category D

Do Not Confuse:
Leukeran/leucovorin, Leukeran/Leukine

Action: Alkylates DNA, RNA; inhibits enzymes that allow synthesis of amino acids in proteins; activity is not cell cycle phase specific

Therapeutic Outcome: Prevention of rapidly growing malignant cells

Uses: Chronic lymphocytic leukemia, Hodgkin's disease, other lymphomas, macroglobulinemia, nephrotic syndrome, breast carcinoma, choreocarcinoma, ovarian carcinoma

Dosage and routes

Adult: PO 0.1-0.2 mg/kg/day × 3-6 wk initially, then 4-10 mg/day; maintenance 0.2 mg/kg × 2-4 wk; course may be repeated at 2-4 wk intervals or 0.4 mg/kg (12 mg/m^2) 2 ×/wk, may increase by 0.1 mg/kg (3 mg/m^2) q2 wk, adjust as needed

Elderly: PO initially ≤2-4 mg/day

Child: PO 0.1-0.2 mg/kg/day (4.5 mg/m^2/day) in divided doses or 4.5 mg/m^2/day as 1 dose or in divided doses

Macroglobulinemia (off-label)

Adult: PO 2-10 mg daily × 9 days, or 8 mg/m^2 daily with predniSONE × 10 days, repeat q6-8 wk as needed

Nephrotic syndrome

Child: PO 0.1-0.2 mg/kg daily with predniSONE × 8-12 wk

Intractable idiopathic uveitis, Behçet's syndrome

Adult: PO 6-12 mg or 0.1-0.2 mg/kg, × 1 yr or more

Available forms: Tabs 2 mg

Adverse effects

CNS: **Seizures,** tremors, confusion, agitation, ataxia

GI: *Nausea, vomiting, diarrhea, weight loss,* **hepatoxicity,** *jaundice*

GU: Hyperuremia

HEMA: **Thrombocytopenia, leukopenia, pancytopenia** (prolonged use), **permanent bone marrow suppression**

INTEG: Alopecia (rare), dermatitis, rash, **Stevens-Johnson syndrome**

RESP: **Fibrosis, pneumonitis**

Contraindications: Pregnancy **D**, radiation therapy within 1 mo, chemotherapy within 1 mo, thrombocytopenia, recent smallpox vaccination, lactation

Precautions: *Pneumococcus* vaccination, children

Pharmacokinetics	
Absorption	Rapidly, completely absorbed
Distribution	Crosses placenta
Metabolism	Liver, extensively
Excretion	Kidneys
Half-life	2 hr

Pharmacodynamics
Unknown

Interactions

Individual drugs

Radiation: increased toxicity, bone marrow suppression

Drug classifications

Anticoagulants, salicylates: increased risk of bleeding

Antineoplastics: increased toxicity

Antineoplastics: increased bone marrow suppression

Drug/lab test

Increased: uric acid

NURSING CONSIDERATIONS

Assessment

- Monitor CBC, differential, platelet count weekly; withhold drug if WBC is <2000/mm^3 or granulocyte count <1000/mm^3 notify prescriber of results if WBC <20,000/mm^3, platelets <50,000/mm^3
- Monitor pulmonary function tests, chest x-ray films before, during therapy; chest film should be obtained q2 wk during treatment; check for dyspnea, crackles, unproductive cough, chest pain, tachypnea
- Assess for increased uric acid levels, swelling, joint pain primarily in extremities; patient should be well hydrated to prevent urate deposits
- Monitor renal function studies: BUN, serum uric acid, urine CCr before, during therapy; I&O ratio; report fall in urine output of 30 ml/hr; monitor for decreased hyperuricemia
- Assess for jaundice of skin, sclera, dark urine, clay-colored stools, itchy skin, abdominal pain, fever, diarrhea
- Monitor for cold, fever, sore throat (may indicate beginning infection); identify edema in feet, joint, stomach pain, shaking; prescriber should be notified
- Assess for bleeding: hematuria, guaiac, bruising or petechiae, mucosa or orifices q8h, no rect temp

Nursing diagnoses

- Injury, risk for (adverse reactions)
- Body image, disturbed (adverse reactions)
- Infection, risk for (adverse reactions)
- Knowledge, deficient (teaching)

Implementation

- Give 1 hr ac or 2 hr pc to lessen nausea and vomiting or antacid before oral agent, give drug after evening meal, before bedtime or 1 hr before breakfast; antiemetic 30-60 min before giving drug to prevent vomiting

• Give allopurinol to maintain uric acid levels, alkalinization of urine; increase fluid intake to 2-3 L/day to prevent urate deposits, calculus formation
• Antibiotics for prophylaxis of infection may be prescribed, since infection potential is high
• Give all drugs PO if possible, avoid IM inj when platelets <100,000/mm^3
• Store in tight container

Patient/family education

• Teach patient to avoid use of products containing aspirin or ibuprofen, razors, commercial mouthwash, since bleeding may occur; to report symptoms of bleeding (hematuria, tarry stools)
• Instruct patient to report signs of anemia (fatigue, headache, irritability, faintness, shortness of breath)
• Instruct patient to report any changes in breathing or coughing even several mo after treatment; to avoid crowds and persons with respiratory tract or other infections
• Advise patient hair loss is common; discuss the use of wigs or hairpieces
• Instruct patient to drink 2-3 L of fluid daily unless contraindicated
• Caution patient not to have any vaccinations without the advice of the prescriber; serious reactions can occur
• Advise patient contraception is needed during treatment and for several months after the completion of therapy, may cause irreversible gonadal suppression

Evaluation

Positive therapeutic outcome

• Decreased size of tumor
• Decreased spread of malignancy
• Improved blood values
• Absence of sweating at night
• Increased appetite, increased weight

chloramphenicol (Rx)

(klor-am-fen'i-kole)

chloramphenicol, Chloromycetin, Pentamycetin ✤

Func. class.: Antiinfective, miscellaneous

Chem. class.: Dichloroacetic acid derivative

Pregnancy category C

Action: Binds to 50S ribosomal subunit, which interferes with or inhibits protein synthesis

Therapeutic Outcome: Bactericidal for *Haemophilus influenzae, Salmonella typhi, Rickettsia, Neisseria, Mycoplasma*

Uses: Meningitis, bacteremia, abdominal, skin, soft tissue infections; local infections of skin, ear, eye; not to be used if less-toxic drugs can be used

Dosage and routes

Adult/child: PO/**IV** 50-75 mg/kg/day in divided doses q6h, 100 mg/kg/day (for meningitis only) max 4 g/day

Premature infants and neonates: **IV**/PO 25 mg/kg/day in divided doses q12-24h

Adult and child: OPHTH 1-2 gtt of sol or ointment q3-6 mo; otic 2-3 gtt bid or tid; top 1% cream tid or qid

Available forms: Inj **IV** 1-g; caps 250 mg; ophth ointment 10 mg/g; ophth sol 25 mg/15 ml, 5 mg/ml; top cream 1%; otic sol 0.5%

Adverse effects

CNS: Headache, *depression,* confusion, peripheral neuritis

CV: **Gray syndrome in newborns: failure to feed, pallor, cyanosis, abdominal distention, irregular respiration, vasomotor collapse**

EENT: Optic neuritis, blindness

GI: *Nausea, vomiting, diarrhea,* abdominal pain, xerostomia, glossitis, colitis, pruritus ani

HEMA: **Anemia, thrombocytopenia, aplastic anemia, granulocytopenia, leukopenia** (rare)

INTEG: Itching, urticaria, contact dermatitis, rash

Contraindications: Hypersensitivity, severe renal disease, severe hepatic disease, minor infections

Precautions: Pregnancy **C,** hepatic disease, renal disease, infants, children, bone marrow depression (drug-induced), lactation

Pharmacokinetics	
Absorption	Well absorbed (PO), Completely absorbed (**IV**)
Distribution	Wide
Metabolism	Liver
Excretion	Kidneys, unchanged
Half-life	1½-4 hr

Pharmacodynamics	PO	IV	TOP	OPHTH	OTIC
Onset	15 min	Rapid	Unkn	Unkn	Unkn
Peak	1-2 hr	Inf end	Unkn	Unkn	Unkn

Interactions

Individual drugs

Folic acid: decreased action of folic acid
Hydantoins: increased action of hydantoins

Iron: increased action of iron
Rifampin: decreased action of rifampin
Vitamin B_{12}: decreased action of vit B_{12}

Drug classifications

Anticoagulants: increased prothrombin time
Antidiabetics: increased action of antidiabetics
Barbiturates: increased levels of barbiturates
Penicillins: decreased action of penicillins

Drug/herb

Acidophilus: do not use with antiinfectives

NURSING CONSIDERATIONS

Assessment

- Assess patient for previous sensitivity reaction to other antiinfectives; cross-sensitivity between penicillins and cephalosporins is common
- Assess patient for signs and symptoms of infection including characteristics of wounds, sputum, urine, stool, WBC >10,000/mm^3, fever; obtain baseline information and during treatment
- Perform C&S testing before starting drug therapy to identify if correct treatment has been initiated
- Monitor drug level in impaired hepatic, renal systems; peak 15-20 mg/ml 3 hr after dose, trough 5-10 mg/ml before next dose
- Monitor blood studies: platelets q2 days, CBC
- Assess bowel pattern daily; if severe diarrhea occurs, drug should be discontinued
- Monitor for bleeding: ecchymosis, bleeding gums, hematuria, stool guaiac daily if on long-term therapy
- Assess for overgrowth of infection: perineal itching, fever, malaise, redness, pain, swelling, drainage, rash, diarrhea, change in cough, sputum

Nursing diagnoses

- Infection, risk for (uses)
- Diarrhea (adverse reaction)
- Injury, risk for (side effects)
- Knowledge, deficient (teaching)
- Noncompliance (teaching)

Implementation

PO route

- Do not break, crush, or chew caps
- Give oral form on empty stomach with full glass of water
- Store cap in airtight container at room temp

Topical route

- Wash hands, clean area to be treated with soap and water before application

Ophthalmic route

- Apply a small amount of ointment in lower lid
- Have patient tilt head back before application

IV route

- Give after diluting 1 g/10 ml of sterile H_2O for inj or D_5W (10% sol); give >1 min
- May be further diluted in 50-100 ml of D_5W; give through Y-tube, 3-way stopcock, or additive infusion set; run over ½-1 hr; store reconstituted sol at room temp for up to 30 days

Syringe compatibilities: Ampicillin, cloxacillin, heparin, methicillin, penicillin G sodium

Y-site compatibilities: Acyclovir, cyclophosphamide, enalaprilat, esmolol, foscarnet, hydromorphone, labetalol, magnesium sulfate, meperidine, morphine, perphenazine, tacrolimus

Y-site incompatibilities: Fluconazole

Additive compatibilities: Amikacin, aminophylline, ascorbic acid, calcium chloride/gluconate, cephalothin, cephapirin, colistimethate, corticotropin, cyanocobalamin, dimenhyDRINATE, DOPamine, epHEDrine, heparin, hydrocortisone, kanamycin, lidocaine, magnesium sulfate, metaraminol, methicillin, methyldopate, methylPREDNISolone, metronidazole, nafcillin, oxacillin, oxytocin, penicillin G potassium, penicillin G sodium, pentobarbital, phenylephrine, phytonadione, plasma protein fraction, potassium chloride, promazine, ranitidine, sodium bicarbonate, thiopental, verapamil, vit B

Patient/family education

- Teach patient all aspects of drug therapy; need to complete entire course of medication to ensure organism death (10-14 days); culture may be taken after complete course of medication
- Advise patient to report sore throat, fever, fatigue, unusual bleeding, or bruising; could indicate bone marrow depression (may occur weeks or months after termination of drug)
- Tell patient that drug must be taken at regular intervals around the clock to maintain blood levels

Evaluation

Positive therapeutic outcome

- Decreased symptoms of infection

chlordiazepoxide (Rx)

(klor-dye-az-e-pox'ide)

Apo-Chlordiazepoxide ✦, chlordiazepoxide HCl, Librium, Novopoxide ✦

Func. class.: Antianxiety

Chem. class.: Benzodiazepine

Pregnancy category D

Controlled substance schedule IV

Do Not Confuse:

Librium/Librax

Action: Potentiates the actions of GABA, an inhibitory neurotransmitter, especially in the limbic system reticular formation, which depresses the CNS

Therapeutic Outcome: Decreased anxiety, successful alcohol withdrawal, relaxation

Uses: Short-term management of anxiety, acute alcohol withdrawal, preoperative relaxation

Dosage and routes

Mild anxiety

Adult: PO 5-10 mg tid-qid

Elderly: PO 5 mg bid-qid initially, increase as needed

Child >6 yr: PO 5 mg bid-qid, not to exceed 10 mg bid-tid

Severe anxiety

Adult: PO 20-25 mg tid-qid, IM/**IV** 50-100 mg initially, then 25-50 mg tid or 25-50 mg initially in elderly

Preoperatively

Adult: PO 5-10 mg tid-qid on day before surgery; IM 50-100 mg 1 hr before surgery

Alcohol withdrawal

Adult: PO/IM/**IV** 50-100 mg, not to exceed 300 mg/day

Available forms: Caps 5, 10, 25 mg; IM inj 100 mg ampule

Adverse effects

CNS: *Dizziness, drowsiness,* confusion, headache, anxiety, tremors, stimulation, fatigue, depression, insomnia, hallucinations

CV: *Orthostatic hypotension,* **ECG changes, tachycardia,** hypotension

EENT: *Blurred vision,* tinnitus, mydriasis

GI: Constipation, dry mouth, nausea, vomiting, anorexia, diarrhea

INTEG: Rash, dermatitis, itching

Contraindications: Pregnancy **D**, hypersensitivity to benzodiazepines, narrow-angle glaucoma, psychosis, child <6 yr

Precautions: Elderly, debilitated, hepatic disease, renal disease

Pharmacokinetics

Absorption	Well absorbed (PO); slow, erratic (IM)
Distribution	Widely distributed; crosses placenta, blood-brain barrier
Metabolism	Liver extensively
Excretion	Kidneys, breast milk
Half-life	5-30 hr (increased in elderly)

Pharmacodynamics

	PO	IM	IV
Onset	30 min	15-30 min	1-5 min
Peak	Within 2 hr	Unknown	Unknown
Duration	4-6 hr	Unknown	Up to 1 hr

Interactions

Individual drugs

Alcohol: increased CNS depression

Cimetidine, disulfiram, fluoxetine, isoniazid, ketoconazole, metoprolol, propranolol, valproic acid: increased action of chlordiazepoxide

Levodopa: decreased action of levodopa

Rifamycins: decreased action of chlordiazepoxide

Drug classifications

Barbiturates: decreased effect of chlordiazepoxide

CNS depressants: increased CNS depression

Contraceptives (oral): increased effect of chlordiazepoxide

Drug/herb

Cowslip, kava, Queen Anne's lace, valerian: increased effect

Drug/lab test

False increase: 17-OHCS

False positive: pregnancy test (some methods)

NURSING CONSIDERATIONS

Assessment

- Assess anxiety reaction: inability to sleep, apprehension, dread, foreboding, or uneasiness related to unidentified source of danger
- Assess for previous drug dependence or tolerance; if drug dependent or tolerant, amount of medication should be restricted
- Monitor B/P (with patient lying, standing), pulse; if systolic B/P drops 20 mm Hg, hold drug, notify prescriber

- Monitor blood studies: CBC during long-term therapy; blood dyscrasias have occurred rarely
- Monitor hepatic studies: AST, ALT, bilirubin, creatinine, LDH, alkaline phosphatase during long-term therapy
- Monitor mental status: mood, sensorium, affect, sleeping patterns, drowsiness, dizziness, suicidal tendencies

Nursing diagnoses
- Anxiety (uses)
- Knowledge, deficient (teaching)
- Noncompliance (teaching)

Implementation
PO route
- Give with food or milk for GI symptoms, crushed if patient unable to swallow medication whole; do not open capsules; provide sugarless gum, hard candy, frequent sips of water for dry mouth

IM route
- Reconstitute with diluent provided (2 ml); agitate slowly, do not shake; give deep in large muscle mass to prevent severe pain; do not use IM diluent for **IV** route

IV route
- Reconstitute 100 mg/5 ml sterile water for inj or 0.9% NaCl; give over at least 1 min to prevent cardiac arrest, apnea, bradycardia
- Keep powder from light; refrigerate, mix when ready to use

Y-site compatibilities: Heparin, hydrocortisone, potassium chloride, vit B with C

Solution compatibilities: D_5W, 0.9% NaCl

Patient/family education
- Instruct patient that drug may be taken with food; if dose is missed take as soon as remembered; do not double doses
- Tell patient to avoid OTC preparations unless approved by prescriber; to avoid alcohol ingestion or other psychotropic medications unless directed by a prescriber
- Caution patient to avoid driving and activities requiring alertness, since drowsiness may occur; until medication response is known, tell patient that drowsiness may worsen at beginning of treatment
- Instruct patient not to discontinue medication abruptly after long-term use, drug should be tapered over 1 wk
- Caution patient to rise slowly or fainting may occur, especially in elderly
- Advise patient that drug should be avoided during pregnancy

Evaluation
Positive therapeutic outcome
- Increased well being
- Decreased anxiety, restlessness, sleeplessness, dread
- Successful alcohol withdrawal

Treatment of overdose: Lavage, VS, supportive care

chloroquine (Rx)
(klor'oh-kwin)

Aralen HCl, Aralen Phosphate, chloroquine phosphate

Func. class.: Antimalarial

Chem. class.: Synthetic 4-aminoquinoline derivative

Pregnancy category C

Action: Inhibits parasite replications, transcription of DNA to RNA by forming complexes with DNA of parasite

Therapeutic Outcome: Decreased symptoms of malaria, amebiasis

Uses: Malaria caused by *Plasmodium vivax, Plasmodium malariae, Plasmodium ovale, Plasmodium falciparum* (some strains), amebiasis

Dosage and routes
Malaria suppression

Adult and child: PO 5 mg base/kg/wk on same day of week, not to exceed 300 mg base; treatment should begin 1-2 wk before exposure and for 8 wk after; if treatment begins after exposure, 600 mg base for adult and 10 mg base/kg for children in 2 divided doses 6 hr apart

Extraintestinal amebiasis

Adult: IM 160-200 mg base daily × 10-12 days or PO (HCl) 600 mg base daily × 2 days, then 300 mg base daily × 2-3 wk (phosphate)

Child: IM/PO 10 mg/kg daily (HCl) × 2-3 wk, not to exceed 300 mg/day

Available forms: Tabs 250 mg (150 mg base), 500 mg (300 mg base) phosphate; inj 50 mg (40 mg base)/ml HCl

Adverse effects
CNS: Headache, stimulation, fatigue, **seizure,** psychosis

CV: Hypotension, **heart block, asystole with syncope,** ECG changes

EENT: *Blurred vision, corneal changes, retinal changes, difficulty focusing,* tinnitus, vertigo, deafness, photophobia, corneal edema

GI: Nausea, vomiting, anorexia, diarrhea, cramps
***HEMA:* Thrombocytopenia, agranulocytosis, hemolytic anemia, leukopenia**
INTEG: Pruritus, pigmentary changes, skin eruptions, lichen planus–like eruptions, eczema, **exfoliative dermatitis**

Contraindications: Hypersensitivity, retinal field changes

Precautions: Pregnancy **C**, children, blood dyscrasias, severe GI disease, neurologic disease, alcoholism, hepatic disease, G6PD deficiency, psoriasis, eczema, lactation

Pharmacokinetics

Absorption	Well absorbed
Distribution	Widely
Metabolism	Liver
Excretion	Kidneys, feces
Half-life	3-5 days

Pharmacodynamics

	PO	IM
Onset	Rapid	Rapid
Peak	1-3 hr	30 min
Duration	6-8 hr	Unknown

Interactions
Individual drugs
Cimetidine: decreased oral clearance, metabolism
Kaolin: decreased absorption
Magnesium: decreased action of chloroquine
Drug classifications
Antacids (aluminum): decreased absorption

NURSING CONSIDERATIONS
Assessment
- Monitor liver studies weekly: ALT, AST, bilirubin; renal status: before exposure, monthly thereafter: BUN, creatinine, output, sp gr, urinalysis
- Assess mental status often: affect, mood, behavioral changes; psychosis may occur
- Assess hepatic status: decreased appetite, jaundice, dark urine, fatigue
- Assess for toxicity: blurring vision, difficulty focusing, headache, dizziness, decreased knee and ankle reflexes, drug should be discontinued immediately

Nursing diagnoses
- Infection, risk for (uses)
- Diarrhea (side effects)
- Knowledge, deficient (teaching)
- Noncompliance (teaching)
- Injury, risk for (side effects)

Implementation
PO route
- Give with meals to decrease GI symptoms; better to take on empty stomach 1 hr ac or 2 hr pc
- Give antiemetic if vomiting occurs
- Give after C&S is completed; monthly to detect resistance

IM route
- Give IM after aspirating to prevent inj into bloodstream

Additive compatibility: Promethazine

Patient/family education
- Advise patient that compliance with dosage schedule, duration is necessary
- Instruct patient that scheduled appointments must be kept or relapse may occur
- Caution patient to avoid alcohol while taking drug
- Instruct diabetic to use blood glucose monitor to obtain correct result
- Teach patient to report weakness, fatigue, loss of appetite, nausea, vomiting, yellowing of skin or eyes, tingling/numbness of hands/feet
- Advise patient that urine may turn rust brown color
- Instruct patient to use sunglasses in bright sunlight to prevent photophobia

Evaluation
Positive therapeutic outcome
- Decreased symptoms of malaria

Treatment of overdose: Induce vomiting, gastric lavage, administer barbiturate (ultrashort-acting), vasopressor; tracheostomy may be necessary

chlorothiazide (Rx)
(klor-oh-thye′a-zide)
Diuril
Func. class.: Diuretic, antihypertensive
Chem. class.: Thiazide; sulfonamide derivative

Pregnancy category B

Do Not Confuse:
chlorothiazide/chlorproMAZINE, chlorothiazide/chlorproPAMIDE, chlorothiazide/chlorthalidone

Action: Acts on the distal tubule and thick ascending limb of the loop of Henle in the kidney, increasing excretion of sodium, water, chloride, magnesium, potassium, and bicarbonate

Therapeutic Outcome: Decreased BP, decreased edema in tissues peripherally, diuresis

Uses: Edema in CHF, nephrotic syndrome; may be used alone or as adjunct with antihypertensives; also for edema in corticosteroids, estrogen therapy

Dosage and routes

Edema, hypertension

Adult: PO/**IV** 500 mg-2 g daily; may divide bid

Diuresis

Adult: **IV** 250 mg q6-12h

Child >6 mo: PO 10-20 mg/kg/day may divide bid

Child <6 mo: PO up to 40 mg/kg/day; may divide bid

Available forms: Tabs 250, 500 mg; oral susp 250 mg/5 ml; inj 500 mg

Adverse effects

CNS: Paresthesia, anxiety, depression, headache, *dizziness, fatigue, weakness, fever, insomnia*

CV: Irregular pulse, orthostatic hypotension, palpitations, volume depletion

EENT: Blurred vision

ELECT: *Hypokalemia,* hypercalcemia, hyponatremia, hypochloremia, hypophosphatemia, hypomagnesemia

GI: Nausea, vomiting, anorexia, constipation, diarrhea, cramps, pancreatitis, GI irritation, ***hepatitis***

GU: *Frequency,* polyuria, ***uremia,*** glucosuria, hematuria

HEMA: ***Aplastic anemia, hemolytic anemia, leukopenia, agranulocytosis, thrombocytopenia, neutropenia***

INTEG: Rash, urticaria, purpura, photosensitivity, alopecia

META: Hyperglycemia, *hyperuricemia,* increased creatinine, BUN

Contraindications: Hypersensitivity to thiazides or sulfonamides, anuria, renal decompensation, lactation, hepatic coma

Precautions: Pregnancy **B,** hypokalemia, renal disease, hepatic disease, gout, COPD, LE, diabetes mellitus, elderly, hyperlipidemia

Pharmacokinetics

	PO
Absorption	GI tract (10%-20%)
Distribution	Extracellular spaces; crosses placenta
Metabolism	Liver
Excretion	Urine, unchanged; breast milk
Half-life	1-2 hr

Pharmacodynamics

	PO	IV
Onset	2 hr	15 min
Peak	4 hr	½ hr
Duration	6-12 hr	2 hr

Interactions

Individual drugs

Alcohol: increased hypotension
Allopurinol, digitalis, lithium: increased toxicity
Amphotericin, mezlocillin, piperacillin, ticarcillin: increased hypokalemia
Cholestyramine, colestipol: decreased absorption of chlorothiazide

Drug classifications

Antihypertensives: increased antihypertensive effect
Glucocorticoids: increased hypokalemia
Nitrates: increased hypotension
NSAIDs: decreased diuretic action
Nondepolarizing skeletal muscle relaxants: increased toxicity

Drug/herb

Aloe, buckthorn, cascara sagrada, Chinese rhubarb, gossypol, licorice, nettle, senna: increased hypokalemia
Aloe, cucumber, dandelion, horsetail, pumpkin, Queen Anne's lace: increased diuretic effect
St. John's wort: increased severe photosensitivity

Drug/lab test

Increased: BSP retention, calcium, amylase, parathyroid test
Decreased: PBI, PSP
False negative: phentolamine and tyramine tests
Interference: urine steroid tests

NURSING CONSIDERATIONS

Assessment

- Assess glucose in urine if patient is diabetic
- Monitor improvement in CVP q8h
- Check for rashes, temp elevation daily
- Assess for confusion, especially in elderly; take safety precautions if needed

- Monitor manifestations of hypokalemia; *RENAL:* acidic urine, reduced urine osmolality, nocturia; *CV:* hypotension, broad T wave, U wave, ectopy, tachycardia, weak pulse; *NEURO:* muscle weakness, altered LOC, drowsiness, apathy, lethargy, confusion, depression; *GI:* anorexia, nausea, cramps, constipation, distention, paralytic ileus; *RESP:* hypoventilation, respiratory muscle weakness
- Monitor for manifestations of hypomagnesemia; *CNS:* agitation, muscle twitching, paresthesias, hyperactive reflexes, positive Babinski's reflex, dysphagia, nystagmus, seizures, tetany; *GI:* nausea, vomiting, diarrhea, anorexia, abdominal distention; *CV:* ectopy, tachycardia, broad, flat, or inverted T waves, depressed ST segment, prolonged QT interval, decreased cardiac output, hypotension
- Monitor for manifestations of hyponatremia: *CV:* increased B/P, cold, clammy skin, hypovolemia or hypervolemia; *GI:* anorexia, nausea, vomiting, diarrhea, abdominal cramps; *NEURO:* lethargy, increased ICP, confusion, headache, seizures, coma, fatigue, tremors, hyperreflexia
- Monitor for manifestations of hyperchloremia: *NEURO:* weakness, lethargy, coma; *RESP:* coma, deep rapid breathing
- Assess fluid volume status: I&O ratios and record, count or weigh diapers as appropriate, weight, distended red veins, crackles in lung, color, quality and sp gr of urine, skin turgor, adequacy of pulses, moist mucous membranes, bilateral lung sounds, peripheral pitting edema; dehydration symptoms of decreasing output, thirst, hypotension, dry mouth and mucous membranes should be reported
- Monitor electrolytes: potassium, sodium, calcium, magnesium; also include BUN, blood pH, ABGs, uric acid, CBC, blood glucose
- Assess B/P before and during therapy with patient lying, standing, and sitting as appropriate; orthostatic hypotension can occur rapidly

Nursing diagnoses

- Urinary elimination, impaired (adverse reactions)
- Fluid volume, deficient
- Fluid volume, excess (uses)
- Knowledge, deficient (teaching)

Implementation

- Give in AM to avoid interference with sleep
- Potassium replacement if potassium level is 3.0 mg/dl
- Give whole, or use oral sol; drug may be crushed if patient is unable to swallow

PO route

- Give with food; if nausea occurs, absorption may be increased

IV route

- Do not use sol that is yellow, has a precipitate, or crystals
- Administer **IV** after diluting 0.5 g/18 ml or more of sterile water for inj; may be diluted further with dextrose or NaCl: give over 5 min; sol is stable at room temp for 24 hr

Additive compatibilities: Cimetidine, lidocaine, nafcillin, sodium bicarbonate

Additive incompatibilities: Amikacin, blood, blood products, chlorproMAZINE, codeine, hydrALAZINE, insulin, levorphanol, methadone, morphine, multivitamins, norepinephrine, polymyxin B, procaine, prochlorperazine, promazine, promethazine, streptomycin, tetracycline, triflupromazine, vancomycin

Patient/family education

- Teach patient to take medication early in the day to prevent nocturia
- Instruct patient to take with food or milk if GI symptoms of nausea and anorexia occur
- Teach patient to maintain a weekly record of weight and notify prescriber of weight loss >5 lb
- Caution patient that this drug causes a loss of potassium, so food rich in potassium should be added to the diet; refer to a dietician for assistance in planning
- Caution patient not to exercise in hot weather or stand for prolonged periods, since orthostatic hypotension will be enhanced; to use sunscreen to prevent burning
- Teach patient not to use alcohol or any OTC medications without prescriber's approval; serious drug reactions may occur
- Emphasize the need to contact prescriber immediately if muscle cramps, weakness, nausea, dizziness, or numbness occurs
- Teach patient to take own B/P and pulse and record
- Caution patient that orthostatic hypotension may occur; patient should rise slowly from sitting or reclining positions and lie down if dizziness occurs
- Teach patient to continue taking medication even if feeling better; this drug controls symptoms but does not cure the condition
- Advise the patient with hypertension to continue other medical treatment (exercise, weight loss, relaxation techniques, cessation of smoking)

Evaluation

Positive therapeutic outcome

- Decreased edema
- Decreased B/P
- Increased diuresis

Treatment of overdose: Lavage if taken orally, monitor electrolytes; administer dextrose in saline; monitor hydration, CV, renal status

chlorpheniramine (OTC, Rx)

(klor-fen-ir'a-meen)

Aller-Chlor, Chlo-Amine, Chlorate, chlorpheniramine maleate, Chlor-Trimeton, Chlor-Tripolon ✱, Gen-Allerate, Novo-Pheniram ✱, PediaCare Allergy Formula, Phenetron, Teldrin

Func. class.: Antihistamine (1st generation, nonselective)

Chem. class.: Alkylamine, H_1-receptor antagonist

Pregnancy category B

Do Not Confuse:
Teldrin/Tedral

Action: Acts on blood vessels, GI, respiratory system by competing with histamine for H_1-receptor site; decreases allergic response by blocking histamine

Therapeutic Outcome: Absence of allergy symptoms and rhinitis

Uses: Allergy symptoms, rhinitis, allergic dermatoses, nasal allergies, hypersensitive reactions including blood transfusion reactions, anaphylaxis

Dosage and routes

Adult/child ≥12 yr: PO 2-4 mg tid-qid, not to exceed 24 mg/day; time rel 8-12 mg bid-tid, not to exceed 24 mg/day; IM/**IV**/SUBCUT 5-40 mg/day, max 40 mg/day

Child 6-12 yr: PO 2 mg q4-6h, not to exceed 12 mg/day; sus rel 8 mg at bedtime or daily; sus rel not recommended for child <6 yr; SUBCUT 87.5 mcg/kg or 2.5 mg/m^2 q6h

Child 2-5 yr: PO 1 mg q4-6h, not to exceed 4 mg/day

Available forms: Chewable tabs 2 mg; tabs 4, 8, 12 mg; time rel tabs 8, 12 mg; time rel caps 8, 12 mg; syr 1, 2, 2.5 mg/5 ml; inj 10, 100 mg/ml

Adverse effects

CNS: *Dizziness, drowsiness,* poor coordination, fatigue, anxiety, euphoria, confusion, paresthesia, neuritis

EENT: Blurred vision, dilated pupils, tinnitus, nasal stuffiness, dry nose, throat, mouth

GI: Nausea, anorexia, diarrhea

GU: *Retention,* dysuria, frequency

HEMA: **Thrombocytopenia, agranulocytosis, hemolytic anemia**

INTEG: Photosensitivity

RESP: Increased thick secretions, wheezing, chest tightness

Contraindications: Hypersensitivity to H_1-receptor antagonists, acute asthma attack, lower respiratory tract disease, stenosed peptic ulcers, bladder neck obstruction, angle-closure glaucoma, newborns/neonates

Precautions: Pregnancy **B**, increased intraocular pressure, renal disease, cardiac disease, hypertension, bronchial asthma, seizure disorder, hyperthyroidism, prostatic hypertrophy, lactation, elderly

Pharmacokinetics

Absorption	Well absorbed (PO, SUBCUT, IM, **IV**)
Distribution	Widely distributed; crosses blood-brain barrier
Metabolism	Liver, mostly
Excretion	Kidneys, metabolite; breast milk (minimal)
Half-life	12-15 hr

Pharmacodynamics

	PO	PO-ER	SUBCUT	IM	IV
Onset	15-30 min	Unknown	Unknown	Unknown	Immediate
Peak	1-2 hr	Unknown	Unknown	Unknown	Unknown
Duration	4-12 hr	8-24 hr	4-12 hr	4-12 hr	4-12 hr

Interactions

Individual drugs

Alcohol: increased CNS depression

Atropine, haloperidol, quinidine: increased anticholinergic reactions

Drug classifications

CNS depressants, opiates, sedative/hypnotics, tricyclics: increased CNS depression

Phenothiazines: increased anticholinergic reactions

MAOIs: increased effect of chlorpheniramine

Drug/herb

Corkwood, henbane leaf: increased anticholinergic effect

Hops, Jamaican dogwood, kava, khat, senega: increased sedative effect

Drug/lab test
False negative: skin allergy tests (discontinue antihistamines 3 days before testing)

NURSING CONSIDERATIONS
Assessment
- Assess respiratory status: rate, rhythm, increase in bronchial secretions, wheezing, chest tightness; provide fluids to 2 L/day to decrease secretion thickness
- Monitor I&O ratio: be alert for urinary retention, frequency, dysuria, especially elderly; drug should be discontinued if these occur
- **IV** administration may result in rapid drop in B/P, sweating, dizziness, especially in elderly

Nursing diagnoses
- Airway clearance, ineffective (uses)
- Injury, risk for (side effects)
- Knowledge, deficient (teaching)
- Noncompliance (teaching, overuse)

Implementation
PO route
- Swallow time rel tabs and caps whole
- Do not break, crush, chew, or open time rel tabs
- Chewable tabs should be chewed and not swallowed whole
- May give with food to decrease GI upset
- Store in tight, light-resistant container

IM/SUBCUT route
- Use only 20 and 100 mg/ml strengths; does not need to be reconstituted or diluted

IV route
Give undiluted by direct **IV** (10 mg/ml strength only); administer 10 mg over 1 min or more
Additive incompatibilities: Calcium chloride, kanamycin, norepinephrine, pentobarbital

Patient/family education
- Teach all aspects of drug use; to notify prescriber if confusion, sedation, hypotension, or difficulty voiding occurs; to avoid driving and other hazardous activity if drowsiness occurs; to avoid alcohol and other CNS depressants that may potentiate effect
- Teach patient not to exceed recommended dosage; dysrhythmias may occur
- Advise patient hard candy, gum, frequent rinsing of mouth may be used for dryness

Evaluation
Positive therapeutic outcome
- Absence of running or congested nose, rashes

Treatment of overdose: Administer lavage, diazepam, vasopressors, barbiturates (short acting)

chlorproMAZINE ⚷ (Rx)
(klor-proe'ma-zeen)
chlorproMAZINE HCl, Chlorpromanyl ♣, Largactil ♣, Novo-Chlorpromazine ♣, Thorazine, Thor-Prom
Func. class.: Antipsychotic/neuroleptic/antiemetic
Chem. class.: Phenothiazine, aliphatic
Pregnancy category C

Do Not Confuse:
chlorproMAZINE/chlorothiazide, chlorproMAZINE/chlorproPAMIDE, chlorproMAZINE/chlorthalidone, chlorproMAZINE/prochlorperazine

Action: Depresses cerebral cortex, hypothalamus, limbic system, which control activity aggression; blocks neurotransmission produced by dopamine at synapse; exhibits a strong α-adrenergic, anticholinergic blocking action; mechanism for antipsychotic effects is unclear

Therapeutic Outcome: Decreased signs and symptoms of psychosis; control of nausea, vomiting, intractable hiccups, decreased anxiety preoperatively

Uses: Psychotic disorders, Tourette's syndrome, mania, schizophrenia, anxiety, intractable hiccups (adults), nausea, vomiting, preoperative relaxation, acute intermittent porphyria, behavioral problems in children, nonpsychotic patients with dementia

Investigational uses: Vascular headache

Dosage and routes
Psychosis
Adult: PO 10-50 mg q1-4h initially, then increase up to 2 g/day if necessary; IM 10-50 mg q1-4h, usual dose 300-800 mg/day
Elderly: PO 10-25 mg daily-bid, increased by 10-25 mg/day q4-7 days, max 800 mg/day
Child >6 mo: PO 0.5 mg/kg q4-6h; IM 0.5 mg/kg q6-8h; REC 1 mg/kg q6-8h

Nausea and vomiting
Adult: PO 10-25 mg q4-6h prn; IM 25-50 mg q3h prn; rec 50-100 mg q6-8h prn, not to exceed 400 mg/day; **IV** 25-50 mg daily-qid
Child ≥6 mo: PO 0.55 mg/kg q4-6h; IM q6-8h; REC 1.1 mg/kg q6-8h, max IM ≤5 yr or ≤22.7 kg 40 mg; max IM 5-10 yr or 22.7-45.5 kg 75 mg

Intractable hiccups

Adult: PO 25-50 mg tid-qid; IM 25-50 mg (used only if PO dose does not work); **IV** 25-50 mg in 500-1000 ml saline (only for severe hiccups)

Available forms: Tabs 10, 25, 50, 100, 200 mg; sus rel caps 30, 75, 150, 200, 300 mg; syr 10, 25, 100 mg/5 ml; conc 30, 40, 100 mg/ml; supp 25, 100 mg; inj 25 mg/ml

Adverse effects

CNS: **Neuroleptic malignant syndrome,** dizziness, *extrapyramidal symptoms: pseudoparkinsonism, akathisia, dystonia, tardive dyskinesia,* **seizures,** *headache*

CV: *Orthostatic hypotension,* hypertension, **cardiac arrest,** ECG changes, **tachycardia**

EENT: Blurred vision, glaucoma, dry eyes

GI: *Dry mouth, nausea, vomiting, anorexia, constipation,* diarrhea, jaundice, weight gain

GU: Urinary retention, enuresis, impotence, amenorrhea, gynecomastia, breast engorgement

HEMA: Anemia, **leukopenia, leukocytosis, agranulocytosis**

INTEG: *Rash,* photosensitivity, dermatitis

RESP: **Laryngospasm,** dyspnea, **respiratory depression**

Contraindications: Hypersensitivity, circulatory collapse, liver damage, cerebral arteriosclerosis, coronary disease, severe hypertension/hypotension, blood dyscrasias, coma, child <6 mo, brain damage, bone marrow depression, alcohol and barbiturate withdrawal, narrow-angle glaucoma

Precautions: Pregnancy **C,** lactation, seizure disorders, hypertension, hepatic disease, cardiac disease, elderly, prostate enlargement

Pharmacokinetics

Absorption	Variable (PO); well absorbed (IM)
Distribution	Widely distributed; crosses placenta
Metabolism	Liver, GI mucosa extensively
Excretion	Kidneys
Half-life	30 hr

Pharmacodynamics

	PO	REC	IM	IV
Onset	½-1 hr	12 hr	Unknown	Rapid
Peak	Unknown	Unknown	Unknown	Unknown
Duration	4-6 hr*	3-4 hr	4-8 hr	Unknown

*Duration PO ext rel is 10-12 hr.

Interactions

Individual drugs

Alcohol: increased effects of both drugs, oversedation

Aluminum hydroxide, magnesium hydroxide: decreased absorption

Bromocriptine, levodopa: decreased antiparkinsonian activity

Epinephrine: increased toxicity

Lithium: decreased chlorproMAZINE levels

Valproic acid: increased valproic acid level

Warfarin: decreased anticoagulant effect

Drug classifications

Antacids: decreased absorption

Anticholinergics, antidepressants, antiparkinsonian agents: increased anticholinergic effects

Anticonvulsants: decreased seizure threshold

Antidepressants, antihistamines, barbiturate anesthetics, general anesthetics, MAOIs, opioids, sedative/hypnotics: increased CNS depression

Antithyroid agents: increased agranulocytosis

Barbiturates: decreased serum chlopro-MAZINE

β-Adrenergic blockers: increased effect of both drugs

Drug/herb

Cola tree, hops, nettle, nutmeg: increased action

Henbane leaf: increased anticholinergic effect

Betel palm, kava: increased EPS

Drug/lab test

Increased: liver function tests, cardiac enzymes, cholesterol, blood glucose, prolactin, bilirubin, PBI, cholinesterase I, alkaline phosphatase, leukocytes, granulocytes, platelets, ^{131}I

Decreased: hormones (blood and urine)

False positive: pregnancy tests, PKU, urine

False negative: urinary steroids, 17-OHCS

NURSING CONSIDERATIONS

Assessment

- Assess mental status: orientation, mood, behavior, presence of hallucinations, and type before initial administration and monthly; this drug should significantly reduce psychotic behavior
- Assess any potentially reversible cause of behavior problems in the elderly before and during therapy
- Check for swallowing of PO medication; check for hoarding or giving of medication to other patients
- Monitor I&O ratio; palpate bladder if low urinary output occurs, especially in elderly;

urinalysis recommended before, during prolonged therapy
- Monitor bilirubin, CBC, liver function studies monthly
- Assess affect, orientation, LOC, reflexes, gait, coordination, sleep pattern disturbances
- Monitor B/P with patient sitting, standing, and lying; take pulse and respirations q4h during initial treatment; establish baseline before starting treatment; report drops of 30 mm Hg; obtain baseline ECG, Q wave, and T wave changes
- Check for dizziness, faintness, palpitations, tachycardia on rising; severe orthostatic hypotension is common
- ❗ Identify for neuroleptic malignant syndrome: hyperpyrexia, muscle rigidity, increased CPK, altered mental status; drug should be discontinued
- Assess for EPS including akathisia (inability to sit still, no pattern to movements), tardive dyskinesia (bizarre movements of the jaw, mouth, tongue, extremities), pseudoparkinsonism (rigidity, tremors, pill rolling, shuffling gate); an antiparkinsonian drug should be prescribed
- Assess for constipation, urinary retention daily; if these occur, increase bulk, water in diet

Nursing diagnoses
- Thought processes, disturbed (uses)
- Coping, ineffective (uses)
- Knowledge, deficient (teaching)
- Noncompliance (teaching)

Implementation
PO route
- ❗ Do not break, crush, or chew time rel caps
- Give drug in liquid form mixed in glass of juice or cola if hoarding is suspected
- Periodically attempt dosage reduction in patients with behavioral problems
- Give with full glass of water, milk; or give with food to decrease GI upset
- Store in tight, light-resistant container, oral sol in amber bottle

IM route
- Inject in deep muscle mass; do not give SUBCUT; may be diluted with 0.9% NaCl, 2% procaine as prescribed; do not administer sol with a precipitate
- Remain lying down after IM inj for at least 30 min

Rectal route
- Give after placing in refrigerator for 30 min if too soft to insert; this route is used for nausea, vomiting, hiccups

IV route
- Give by direct **IV** by diluting with 0.9% NaCl to a concentration of 1 mg/1 ml; administer at a rate of 1 mg/2 min
- Give by cont inf after diluting 50 mg/500-1000 ml of D_5W, $D_{10}W$, 0.9% NaCl, 0.45% NaCl, LR, Ringer's or combinations (used for intractable hiccups)

Syringe compatibilities:
Atropine, benztropine, butorphanol, diphenhydrAMINE, doxapram, droperidol, fentanyl, glycopyrrolate, hydromorphone, hydrOXYzine, meperidine, metoclopramide, midazolam, morphine, pentazocine, perphenazine, prochlorperazine, promazine, promethazine, scopolamine

Syringe incompatibilities:
Cimetidine, dimenhyDRINATE, heparin, pentobarbital, thiopental

Y-site compatibilities:
Amsacrine, cisatracurium, cisplatin, cladribine, cyclophosphamide, cytarabine, DOXOrubicin, DOXOrubicin liposome, famotidine, filgrastim, fluconazole, granisetron, heparin, hydrocortisone, ondansetron, potassium chloride, propofol, teniposide, thiotepa, vinorelbine

Additive compatibilities:
Ascorbic acid, ethacrynate, netilmicin, theophylline, vit B/C

Additive incompatibilities:
Aminophylline, amphotericin B, ampicillin, chloramphenicol, chlorothiazide, methicillin, methohexital, penicillin G, phenobarbital

Patient/family education
- Teach patient to use good oral hygiene; frequent rinsing of mouth, sugarless gum, candy or ice chips for dry mouth
- Caution patient to avoid hazardous activities until drug response is determined; dizziness, blurred vision may occur
- Inform patient that orthostatic hypotension occurs often and to rise from sitting or lying position gradually, to remain lying down after IM inj for at least 30 min; tell patient to avoid hot tubs, hot showers, tub baths, since hypotension may occur; tell patient that in hot weather heat stroke may occur; take extra precautions to stay cool
- Advise patient to avoid abrupt withdrawal of this drug, or extrapyramidal symptoms may result; drug should be withdrawn slowly
- Teach patient to avoid OTC preparations (cough, hay fever, cold) unless approved by prescriber, since serious drug interactions may occur; avoid use with alcohol, CNS depressants, since increased drowsiness may occur

- Caution patient to use sunscreen and sunglasses to prevent burns
- Teach patient about extrapyramidal symptoms and necessity of meticulous oral hygiene, since oral candidiasis may occur
- Instruct patient to take antacids 2 hr before or after taking this drug
- Instruct patient to report sore throat, malaise, fever, bleeding, mouth sores; if these occur, CBC should be drawn and drug discontinued
- Teach that urine may turn pink or reddish-brown
- Teach patient to use contraceptive measures

Evaluation

Positive therapeutic outcome

- Decrease in emotional excitement, hallucinations, delusions, paranoia
- Reorganization of patterns of thought, speech
- Increase in target behaviors

Treatment of overdose: Lavage if orally ingested; provide airway, *do not induce vomiting or use epINEPHrine*

chlorthalidone (Rx)

(klor-tha'li-doan)

Apo-Chlorthalidone ✤, chlorthalidone, Hygroton, Thalitone, Uridon ✤

Func. class.: Diuretic, antihypertensive

Chem. class.: Thiazide-like phthalimindine derivative

Pregnancy category B

Do Not Confuse: chlorthalidone/chlorothiazide, chlorthalidone/chlorproMAZINE, chlorthalidone/chlorproPAMIDE, Hygroton/Regroton, Uridon ✤/Vicodin

Action: Acts on the distal tubule and thick ascending limb of the loop of Henle in the kidney, increasing excretion of sodium, water, chloride, magnesium, potassium, and bicarbonate, possible arteriolar dilatation

Therapeutic Outcome: Decreased B/P, decreased edema in lung tissues and peripherally, diuresis

Uses: Edema in congestive heart failure, nephrotic syndrome; may be used alone or as adjunct with antihypertensives; also for edema in corticosteroid, estrogen therapy

Dosage and routes

Adult: PO 25-200 mg/day or 100 mg every other day

Elderly: PO 12.5 mg daily, initially

Child: PO 2 mg/kg or 60 mg/m^2 3 ×/wk

Available forms: Tabs 25, 50, 100 mg

Adverse effects

CV: Irregular pulse, orthostatic hypotension, palpitations, volume depletion

CNS: Paresthesia, headache, *dizziness, fatigue, weakness,* fever

EENT: Blurred vision

ELECT: *Hypokalemia,* hypercalcemia, hyponatremia, hypochloremia, hypomagnesemia

GI: *Nausea, vomiting, anorexia,* constipation, diarrhea, cramps, pancreatitis, GI irritation, **hepatitis**

GU: *Frequency,* polyuria, **uremia,** glucosuria, impotence

HEMA: **Aplastic anemia, hemolytic anemia, leukopenia, agranulocytosis, thrombocytopenia, neutropenia**

INTEG: Rash, urticaria, purpura, photosensitivity

META: *Hyperglycemia, hyperuricemia,* increased creatinine, BUN, gout

Contraindications: Hypersensitivity to thiazides or sulfonamides, anuria, renal decompensation, lactation

Precautions: Pregnancy **B,** hypokalemia, renal disease, hepatic disease, gout, diabetes mellitus, elderly

Pharmacokinetics	
Absorption	Well absorbed
Distribution	Extracellular spaces; crosses placenta
Metabolism	Liver
Excretion	Urine, unchanged (30%-60%)
Half-life	40 hr

Pharmacodynamics	
Onset	2 hr
Peak	6 hr
Duration	24-72 hr

Interactions

Individual drugs

Alcohol: increased hypotensive effect
Allopurinol, lithium: increased toxicity
Amphotericin B: increased hypokalemia
Cholestyramine, colestipol: decreased absorption of chlorthalidone
Diazoxide: increased hyperglycemia, hypotension

Drug classifications

Nondepolarizing skeletal muscle relaxants: increased toxicity
Glucocorticoids: increased hypokalemia

Drug/herb
Buckthorn, cascara sagrada, Chinese rhubarb, gossypol, licorice, nettle, senna: increased hypokalemia
Cucumber, dandelion, horsetail, khella, pumpkin, Queen Anne's lace: increased hypotension
St. John's wort: severe photosensitivity

Drug/lab test
Increased: BSP retention, triglycerides, calcium, amylase, cholesterol
Decreased: PBI, PSP, parathyroid test

NURSING CONSIDERATIONS
Assessment
- Monitor manifestations of hypokalemia; *CV:* hypotension, broad T wave, U wave, ectopy, tachycardia, weak pulse; *GI:* anorexia, nausea, cramps, constipation, distention, paralytic ileus; *NEURO:* muscle weakness, altered LOC, drowsiness, apathy, lethargy, confusion, depression; *RENAL:* acidic urine, reduced urine, osmolality, nocturia; *RESP:* hypoventilation, respiratory muscle weakness
- Monitor for manifestations of hypomagnesemia; *CNS:* agitation, muscle twitching, paresthesias, hyperactive reflexes, positive Babinski's reflex, dysphagia, nystagmus seizures, tetany; *CV:* ectopy, tachycardia, broad, flat or inverted T waves, depressed ST segment, prolonged QT, decreased cardiac output, hypotension; *GI:* nausea, vomiting, diarrhea, anorexia, abdominal distention
- Monitor for manifestations of hyponatremia; *CV:* increased B/P, cold, clammy skin, hypovolemia or hypervolemia; *GI:* anorexia, nausea, vomiting, diarrhea, abdominal cramps; *NEURO:* lethargy, increased ICP, confusion, headache, seizures, coma, fatigue, tremors, hyperreflexia
- Monitor for manifestations of hyperchloremia; *NEURO:* weakness, lethargy, coma; *RESP:* coma, deep rapid breathing
- Assess fluid volume status: I&O ratios and record, count or weigh diapers as appropriate, weight, distended red veins, crackles in lung, color, quality and sp gr of urine, skin turgor, adequacy of pulses, moist mucous membranes, bilateral lung sounds, peripheral pitting edema; dehydration symptoms of decreasing output, thirst, hypotension, dry mouth, and mucous membranes should be reported
- Monitor electrolytes: potassium, sodium, calcium, magnesium; also include BUN, blood pH, ABGs, uric acid, CBC, blood glucose
- Assess B/P before and during therapy with patient lying, standing, and sitting as appropriate; orthostatic hypotension can occur rapidly

Nursing diagnoses
- Fluid volume, deficient (adverse reactions)
- Fluid volume, excess (uses)
- Knowledge, deficient (teaching)
- Urinary elimination, impaired (side effect)

Implementation
- Brand names Thalitone/Hygroton should not be used interchangeably
- Give in AM to avoid interference with sleep
- Provide potassium replacement if potassium level is 3.0 mg/dl; give whole, or use oral solutions lightly; drug may be crushed if patient is unable to swallow
- Give with food if nausea occurs; may crush tab and mix with fluids or applesauce for swallowing

Patient/family education
- Teach patient to take the medication early in the day to prevent nocturia
- Instruct patient to take with food or milk if GI symptoms of nausea and anorexia occur
- Teach patient to maintain weekly record of weight and notify prescriber of weight loss >5 lb
- Caution patient that this drug causes a loss of potassium, so foods rich in potassium should be added to the diet; refer to a dietician for assistance in planning
- Caution the patient not to exercise in hot weather or stand for prolonged periods, since orthostatic hypotension will be enhanced; to use sunscreen to prevent burns
- Teach patient not to use alcohol, or any OTC medications without prescriber's approval; serious drug reactions may occur
- Emphasize the need to contact prescriber immediately if muscle cramps, weakness, nausea, dizziness, or numbness occurs
- Teach patient to take own B/P and pulse and record
- Caution patient that orthostatic hypotension may occur; patient should rise slowly from sitting or reclining positions and lie down if dizziness occurs
- Teach patient to continue taking medication even if feeling better; this drug controls symptoms but does not cure the condition
- Advise patient with hypertension to continue other medical treatment (exercise, weight loss, relaxation techniques, cessation of smoking)

Evaluation
Positive therapeutic outcome
- Decreased edema
- Decreased B/P
- Increased diuresis

Treatment of overdose: Lavage if taken orally, monitor electrolytes; administer dextrose in saline; monitor hydration, CV, renal status

cholecalciferol
See vitamin D

cholestyramine (Rx)
(koe-less-tear'a-meen)
LoCHOLEST, LoCHOLEST Light, Prevalite, Questran, Questran Light
Func. class.: Antilipemic
Chem. class.: Bile acid sequestrant
Pregnancy category C

Action: Absorbs, combines with bile acids to form an insoluble complex that is excreted through feces; loss of bile acids lowers cholesterol levels

Therapeutic Outcome: Decreasing cholesterol levels and low-density lipoproteins, decreased pruritus

Uses: Primary hypercholesterolemia, pruritus associated with biliary obstruction, diarrhea caused by excess bile acid

Investigational uses: Diarrhea caused by excess bile acid

Dosage and routes
Adult: PO 4 g daily-bid, max 24 g/day
Child: PO 240 mg/kg/day in 3 divided doses; administer with food or drink, max 8 g/day

Available forms: Powder for susp 4 g/cholestyramine/packet or scoop

Adverse effects
CNS: Headache, dizziness, drowsiness, vertigo, tinnitus, anxiety
GI: *Constipation, abdominal pain, nausea,* fecal impaction, hemorrhoids, flatulence, vomiting, steatorrhea, peptic ulcer
HEMA: **Bleeding,** increased protime
INTEG: Rash, irritation of perianal area, tongue, skin
META: Decreased vit A, D, K, red cell folate content, **hyperchloremic acidosis**
MS: Muscle, joint pain

Contraindications: Hypersensitivity, biliary obstruction

Precautions: Pregnancy **C**, lactation, children

Pharmacokinetics
Absorption	Not absorbed
Distribution	Not distributed
Metabolism	Not metabolized; LDL lowered in 4-7 days, serum cholesterol lowered in 1 mo
Excretion	Binds with bile acids, feces
Half-life	Unknown

Pharmacodynamics
Onset	24-48 hr
Peak	1-3 wk
Duration	2-4 wk

Interactions
Individual drugs
Clindamycin, clofibrate, gemfibrozil, glipizide, penicillin G, phenytoin, propranolol, iron, thyroid hormones, warfarin: decreased absorption of each specific drug
Drug classifications
Anticoagulants (oral), β-adrenergic blockers, cardiac glycosides, corticosteroids, NSAIDs, tetracyclines, thiazides, vit A, D, E, K: decreased absorption
Drug/herb
Glucomannan: increased effect
Gotu kola: decreased effect
Drug/lab test
Increased: AST, ALT, alkaline phosphatase
Decreased: Na, K
Interference: cholecystography

NURSING CONSIDERATIONS
Assessment
- Assess nutrition: fat, protein, carbohydrates, nutritional analysis should be completed by dietician
- Assess skin integrity after patient has been receiving drug; itching, pruritus often occur from bile deposits on skin
- Monitor cardiac glycoside level if both drugs are being administered; cardiac glycoside levels will be decreased
- Monitor for signs of vit A, D, E, K deficiency; fasting LDL, HDL, total cholesterol, triglyceride levels, electrolytes if on extended therapy
- Monitor bowel pattern daily; increase bulk, water in diet if constipation develops

Nursing diagnoses
- Constipation (adverse reactions)
- Knowledge, deficient (teaching)
- Noncompliance (teaching)

Implementation

- Give drug daily-bid, at bedtime; give all other medications 1 hr before cholestyramine or 4-6 hr after cholestyramine to avoid poor absorption; do not take dry; mix drug with applesauce or stir into beverage (2-6 oz); let stand for 2 min; do not mix with carbonated beverages; avoid inhaling powder
- Provide supplemental doses of vit A, D, E, K, if levels are low

Patient/family education

- ❗ Teach patient symptoms of hypoprothrombinemia: bleeding mucous membranes, dark tarry stools, hematuria, petechiae; report immediately
- Teach patient importance of compliance
- Teach patient that risk factors should be decreased: high-fat diet, smoking, alcohol consumption, absence of exercise
- Have patient mix drug with 6 oz of milk, water, fruit juice; do not mix with carbonated beverages; rinse glass to make sure all medication is taken or may mix drug in applesauce; allow to stand for 2 min before mixing

Evaluation

Positive therapeutic outcome

- Decreased cholesterol level (hyperlipidemia)
- Decreased diarrhea, pruritus (excess bile acids)

choline salicylate (Rx)

(koe'leen sa-lis'ih-late)

Arthropan

choline/magnesium salicylates (Rx)

CMT, Tricosal, Trilisate

Func. class.: Nonopioid analgesic

Chem. class.: Salicylate

Pregnancy category C

Action: Blocks pain impulses in CNS that occur in response to inhibition of prostaglandin synthesis; antipyretic action results from inhibition of hypothalamic heat-regulating center to produce vasodilatation to allow heat dissipation

Therapeutic Outcome: Decreased pain, inflammation, fever

Uses: Mild to moderate pain or fever including arthritis, juvenile rheumatoid arthritis

Dosage and routes

Choline salicylate

Adult and child>12 yr: PO 870-1740 mg qid; max 6×/day

Pain/fever

Adult: PO 435-870 mg q3-4h prn

Choline/magnesium salicylates

Adult: PO 2-3 g salicylate/day divided bid-tid

Child>37 kg: PO 2.2 g of salicylate/day divided bid

Child<37 kg: PO 50 mg of salicylate/kg/day divided bid

Available forms: Choline salicylate liq 870 mg/5 ml; choline/magnesium salicylate tabs 500, 750, 1000 mg; liq 500 mg/5 ml

Adverse effects

CNS: Stimulation, drowsiness, dizziness, confusion, **seizure,** headache, flushing, hallucinations, **coma**

CV: Rapid pulse, pulmonary edema

EENT: Tinnitus, hearing loss

ENDO: Hypoglycemia, hyponatremia, hypokalemia

GI: *Nausea, vomiting, GI bleeding, diarrhea, heartburn,* anorexia, **hepatitis, hepatotoxicity**

HEMA: **Thrombocytopenia, agranulocytosis, leukopenia, neutropenia, hemolytic anemia,** increased protime

INTEG: *Rash,* urticaria, bruising, sweating

RESP: Wheezing, hyperpnea, hyperventilation

Contraindications: Hypersensitivity to salicylates, GI bleeding, bleeding disorders, children <3 yr, vit K deficiency, children with flulike symptoms

Precautions: Pregnancy **C,** anemia, hepatic disease, renal disease, Hodgkin's disease, lactation

Pharmacokinetics	
Absorption	Well absorbed
Distribution	Widely distributed; crosses placenta
Metabolism	Liver, extensively
Excretion	Kidney, active metabolites; breast milk
Half-life	2-3 hr (low doses); 15-30 hr (high doses)

Pharmacodynamics	
Onset	15-30 min
Peak	1-3 hr
Duration	3-6 hr

Interactions
Individual drugs
Alcohol, aspirin, cefamandole, heparin, plicamycin: increased bleeding
Ammonium chloride, nizatidine: increased salicylate levels
Insulin, methotrexate, penicillins, phenytoin, valproic acid, warfarin: increased effects
Probenecid, spironolactone, sulfinpyrazone: decreased effects
Drug classifications
Antacids, steroids, urinary alkalizers: decreased effects of choline salicylate
Anticoagulants, hypoglycemics (oral), thrombolytics: increased effects
Antiinflammatories, NSAIDs, steroids: increased gastric ulcers
β-Blockers, NSAIDS, sulfonamides: decreased effects
Corticosteroids: decreased salicylate effect
Urinary acidifiers: increased salicylate levels
Drug/herb
Bilberry, bogbean, chondroitin, Irish moss, kelpware, pansy: increased bleeding risk
Drug/lab test
Increased: coagulation studies, liver function studies, serum uric acid, amylase, CO_2, urinary protein
Decreased: serum potassium, PBI, cholesterol
Interference: urine catecholamines, pregnancy test

NURSING CONSIDERATIONS
Assessment
- Monitor pain: location, duration, type, intensity, before dose and 1 hr after
- Monitor musculoskeletal status: ROM before dose
- Identify fever, length of time and related symptoms
- Monitor liver function studies: AST, ALT, bilirubin, creatinine if patient is on long-term therapy
- Monitor renal function studies: BUN, urine creatinine if patient is on long-term therapy
- Monitor blood studies: CBC, Hct, Hgb, protime if patient is on long-term therapy
- Check I&O ratio; decreasing output may indicate renal failure (long-term therapy)
- Assess hepatotoxicity: dark urine, clay-colored stools, yellowing of the skin and sclera, itching, abdominal pain, fever, diarrhea if patient is on long-term therapy
- Assess for allergic reactions: rash, urticaria; if these occur, drug may have to be discontinued
- Assess for ototoxicity: tinnitus, ringing, roaring in ears; audiometric testing needed before, after long-term therapy
- Assess for visual changes: blurring, halos; corneal, retinal damage
- Check edema in feet, ankles, legs
- Identify prior drug history; there are many drug interactions

Nursing diagnoses
- Pain, acute (uses)
- Pain, chronic (uses)
- Mobility, physical, impaired (uses)
- Knowledge, deficient (teaching)
- Injury, risk for (side effects)

Implementation
- Administer to patient crushed or whole
- Give with food or milk to decrease gastric symptoms; give 30 min ac or 2 hr pc; absorption may be slowed; sit upright for 30 min after dose
- Give antacids 1-2 hr after enteric products

Patient/family education
- Teach patient to report any symptoms of hepatotoxicity, renal toxicity, visual changes, ototoxicity, allergic reactions, bleeding (long-term therapy)
- Advise patient to take with 8 oz of water
- Caution patient not to exceed recommended dosage; acute poisoning may result
- Caution patient to read label on other OTC drugs; many contain aspirin products
- Inform patient that the therapeutic response takes 2 wk (arthritis)
- Teach patient to report tinnitus, confusion, diarrhea, sweating, hyperventilation
- Caution patient to avoid alcohol ingestion; GI bleeding may occur
- Teach patient that patients who have allergies may develop allergic reactions
- Caution patient to avoid buffered or effervescent products
- Teach patient not to give to children; Reye's syndrome may develop

Evaluation
Positive therapeutic outcome
- Decreased pain
- Decreased inflammation
- Decreased fever
- Increased mobility

Treatment of overdose: Lavage, activated charcoal, monitor electrolytes, VS

cidofovir (Rx)

(si-doh-foh'veer)

Vistide

Func. class.: Antiviral

Chem. class.: Nucleotide analog

Pregnancy category C

Action: Suppresses cytomegalovirus (CMV) replication by selective inhibition of viral DNA synthesis

Therapeutic Outcome: Decreased symptoms of CMV

Uses: CMV retinitis in patients with HIV, used with probenecid

Dosage and routes

Dilute in 100 ml 0.9% NaCl sol before administration; probenecid must be given PO 2 g 3 hr before the cidofovir inf and 1 g at 2 and 8 hr after ending the cidofovir inf; give 1 L of 0.9% NaCl sol **IV** with each inf of cidofovir, give saline inf over 1-2 hr period immediately before cidofovir; patient should be given a second L if the patient can tolerate the fluid load; second L given at time of cidofovir or immediately afterward and should be given over a 1-3 hr period

Renal dose

Adult: **IV** CCr <50 ml/min reduce dose

Induction

Adult: **IV** inf initially 5 mg/kg given over 1 hr at a constant rate qwk × 2 consecutive wk; then **IV** inf 5 mg/kg given over 1 hr q2 wk

Available forms: Inj 75 mg/ml

Adverse effects

CNS: *Fever, chills,* **coma,** confusion, abnormal thought, *dizziness,* bizarre dreams, *headache,* psychosis, tremors, somnolence, paresthesia, *amnesia, anxiety, insomnia,* **seizures**

CV: **Dysrhythmias,** hypertension/hypotension

EENT: Retinal detachment in CMV retinitis

GI: Abnormal liver function tests, *nausea, vomiting, anorexia, diarrhea,* abdominal pain, **hemorrhage**

GU: **Hematuria,** increased creatinine, BUN, **nephrotoxicity**

HEMA: **Granulocytopenia, thrombocytopenia, irreversible neutropenia, anemia, eosinophilia**

INTEG: *Rash, alopecia, pruritus, acne,* urticaria, pain at inj site, phlebitis

RESP: Dyspnea

Contraindications: Hypersensitivity to this drug or probenecid, sulfa drugs

Precautions: Pregnancy **C,** preexisting cytopenias, renal function impairment, lactation, children <6 mo, elderly, platelet count <25,000/mm^3

Pharmacokinetics

Unknown

Pharmacodynamics

Unknown

Interactions

Individual drugs

Amphotericin B, foscarnet, pentamidine **IV**: increased nephrotoxicity; wait 7 days after use to begin cidofovir

Drug classifications

Aminoglycosides, NSAIDs: increased nephrotoxicity; wait 7 days after use to begin cidofovir

NURSING CONSIDERATIONS

Assessment

- Obtain culture before treatment is initiated; cultures of blood, urine, and throat may all be taken; CMV is not confirmed by this method; the diagnosis is made by an ophthalmic exam
- Monitor renal, liver function, increased hematopoietic studies and BUN; serum creatinine, AST, ALT, creatinine, CCr, A-G ratio, baseline and drip treatment, blood counts should be done q2 wk; watch for decreasing granulocytes, Hgb; if low, therapy may have to be discontinued and restarted after hematologic recovery; blood transfusions may be required
- Assess for GI symptoms: severe nausea, vomiting, diarrhea; severe symptoms may necessitate discontinuing drug
- Assess electrolytes and minerals: calcium, phosphorous, magnesium, sodium, potassium; watch closely for tetany during first administration
- Assess for symptoms of blood dyscrasias (anemia, granulocytopenia); bruising, fatigue, bleeding, poor healing
- Assess allergic reactions: flushing, rash, urticaria, pruritus
- Assess for leukopenia, neutropenia, thrombocytopenia: WBCs, platelets q2 days during 2×/day dosing and qwk thereafter; check for leukopenias, with daily WBC count in patients with prior leukopenia, with other nucleoside analogs, or for whom leukopenia counts are <1000 cells/mm^3 at start of treatment

- Monitor serum creatinine or CCr at least q2 wk; give only to those with creatinine levels ≤1.5 mg/dl, CCr >55 ml/min, urine protein <100 mg/dl

Nursing diagnoses
- Infection, risk for (uses)

Implementation
- Mix under strict aseptic conditions using gloves, gown, and mask, and using precautions for antineoplastics
- Administer after diluting in 100 ml of 0.9% NaCl
- Give slowly; do not give by bolus **IV**, **IV**, SUBCUT inj
- Use diluted sol within 12 hr, do not refrigerate or freeze; do not use sol with particulate matter or discoloration
- Refrigerate up to 24 hr; allow to warm to room temperature before using

Patient/family education
- Advise to notify prescriber if sore throat, swollen lymph nodes, malaise, fever occur, may indicate other infections
- Advise to report perioral tingling, numbness in extremities, and paresthesias
- Teach that serious drug interactions may occur if OTC products are ingested; check first with prescriber
- Teach that drug is not a cure, but will control symptoms
- Advise that regular ophthalmic exams must be continued
- Advise that major toxicities may necessitate discontinuing drug
- Advise to use contraception during treatment and that infertility may occur; men should use barrier contraception for 90 days after treatment

Evaluation
Positive therapeutic outcome
- Decreased symptoms of CMV

Treatment of overdose: Discontinue drug; use hemodialysis, and increase hydration

cilastatin
See imipenem/cilastatin

cilostazol
(sil-oo-stay′zole)
Pletal
Func. class.: Platelet aggregation inhibitor
Chem. class.: Quinolinone derivative

Pregnancy category C

Do Not Confuse:
Pletal/Plendil

Action: Reversibly inhibits cellular phosphodiesterase; inhibits platelet aggregation induced by thrombin, ADP, collagen, arachidonic acid, epINEPHrine, stress

Therapeutic Outcome: Increased walking distance

Uses: Intermittent claudication

Dosage and routes
Adult: PO 100 mg bid taken ≥30 min ac or 2 hr pc breakfast and dinner or 50 mg bid, if using drugs that inhibit CYP3A4 and CYP2C19; 12 wk of treatment may be needed

Available forms: Tabs 50, 100 mg

Adverse effects
CNS: Dizziness, headache
CV: Palpitations, tachycardia, **nodal dysrhythmia,** postural hypotension
EENT: Blindness, diplopia, ear pain, tinnitus, retinal hemorrhage
GI: Nausea, vomiting, diarrhea, GI disorder, colitis, cholelithiasis, ulcer, esophagitis, gastritis, anorexia, *flatulence, dyspepsia*
GU: Cystitis, frequency, vaginitis, **vaginal hemorrhage,** hematuria
HEMA: **Bleeding (epistaxis, hematuria, retinal hemorrhage, GI bleeding), thrombocytopenia,** anemia, polycythemia
INTEG: Rash, urticaria, dry skin
MISC: Back pain, infection, myalgia, peripheral edema, chills, fever, malaise, diabetes mellitus
RESP: Cough, pharyngitis, rhinitis, asthma, pneumonia

Contraindications: Hypersensitivity, CHF, acute MI

Precautions: Pregnancy **C,** past liver disease, renal disease, elderly, lactation, children, increased bleeding risk, low platelet count, platelet dysfunction, active bleeding

Pharmacokinetics

Absorption	Unknown
Distribution	95%-98% protein binding
Metabolism	Hepatic extensively by CYP450 enzymes
Excretion	Urine (74%), feces (20%)
Half-life	11-13 hr

Pharmacodynamics

Unknown

Interactions
Individual drugs
Diltiazem, erythromycin, omeprazole, verapamil: increased cilostazol levels
Fluconazole, fluoxetine, fluvoxamine, itraconazole, ketoconazole, nefazodone, voriconazole: may increase cilostazol levels; exercise caution when coadministering and reduce dose to 50 mg bid
Drug classifications
Anticoagulants, NSAIDs, thrombolytics: may increase bleeding tendencies
Protease inhibitors: increased cilostazol levels
Drug/herb
Agrimony, alfalfa, angelica, anise, bay, bilberry, black haw, bogbean, buchu, chondroitin, dong quai, fenugreek, feverfew, garlic, ginger, ginkgo, ginseng, green tea, horse chestnut, Irish moss, kelp, kelpware, khella, lovage, lungwort, meadowsweet, motherwort, mugwort, nettle, papaya, parsley (large amounts), pau d'arco, pineapple, poplar, prickly ash, safflower, saw palmetto, tonka bean, turmeric, wintergreen, yarrow: increased risk of bleeding
Chamomile, coenzyme Q10, flax, glucomannan, goldenseal: decreased anticoagulant effect
Drug/food
Do not use with grapefruit juice

NURSING CONSIDERATIONS
Assessment
- Assess for underlying CV disease since cardiovascular risk is great
- Assess for CV lesions with repeated oral administration
- Assess for CHF
- Monitor blood studies: CBC, Hct, Hgb, protime if patient is on long-term therapy; thrombocytopenia, neutropenia may occur

Nursing diagnoses
- Injury, risk for (uses)
- Knowledge, deficient (teaching)

Implementation
- Give bid ≥1 hr ac or 2 hr pc; do not give with grapefruit juice

Patient/family education
- Advise patient to report any unusual bleeding to prescriber
- Caution patient to report side effects such as diarrhea, skin rashes, subcutaneous bleeding
- Teach patient that effects may take 2-4 wk, treatment of up to 12 wk may be required for necessary effect
- Teach patients with CHF about potential risks
- Advise patient to take ≥1 hr ac or 2 hr pc
- Advise patient that reading patient package insert is necessary

Evaluation
Positive therapeutic outcome
- Increased walking distance and duration
- Decreased pain

cimetidine (Rx, OTC)
(sye-met'i-deen)
Apo-Cimetidine ✦, cimetidine, Novocimetine ✦, Peptol ✦ Tagamet, Tagamet HB
Func. class.: H_2-receptor antagonist
Chem. class.: Imidazole derivative
Pregnancy category B

Action: Inhibits histamine at H_2-receptor site in the gastric parietal cells, which inhibits gastric acid secretion

Therapeutic Outcome: Healing of duodenal or gastric ulcers; prevention of duodenal ulcers; decreases symptoms of gastroesophageal reflux disease (GERD) and Zollinger-Ellison syndrome

Uses: Short-term treatment of duodenal and gastric ulcers and maintenance; management of GERD and Zollinger-Ellison syndrome

Investigational uses: Prevention of aspiration pneumonitis, stress ulcers, upper GI bleeding, herpes infection, hirsutism, urticaria, cutaneous/nongenital warts, weight loss

Dosage and routes
Treatment of active ulcers
Adult and child: PO 300 mg qid with meals, at bedtime × 8 wk or 400 mg bid, 800 mg at bedtime; after 8 wk give at bedtime dose only; **IV** bol 300 mg/20 ml 0.9% NaCl over 1-2 min q6h; **IV** inf 300 mg/50 ml D_5W over 15-20 min; IM 300 mg q6h, not to exceed 2400 mg
Child: PO 20-40 mg/kg/day; IM/**IV** 5-10 mg/kg q6-8h

Prophylaxis of duodenal ulcer
Adult and child >16 yr: 400 mg at bedtime

GERD
Adult: PO 800-1600 mg/day in divided doses

Hypersecretory conditions (Zollinger-Ellison syndrome)
Adult: PO/IM/**IV** 300-600 mg q6h; may increase to 12 g/day if needed

Upper GI bleeding prophylaxis
Adult: **IV** 50 mg/hr; lowered in renal disease

Aspiration pneumonitis prophylaxis
Adult: IM/**IV** 300 mg IM 1 hr before anesthesia, then 300 mg **IV** q4h until patient is alert, max 2400 mg/day

Weight loss
Adult: PO 200-400 mg tid × 8-12 wk

Warts
Adult: PO 400-800 mg tid × 12 wk or 30-40 mg/kg/day given tid × 3 mo

Hirsutism
Adult: PO 300 mg qid × 5 day or 1600 mg daily up to 6 mo

Renal dose
Adult: PO CCr 20-40 ml/min 300 mg q8h; CCr <20 ml/min 300 mg q12h

Available forms: Tabs 100, 200, 300, 400, 800 mg; liq 200, 300 mg/5 ml; inj 300 mg/2 ml, 300 mg/50 ml 0.9% NaCl

Adverse effects
CNS: *Confusion, headache,* depression, dizziness, anxiety, weakness, psychosis, tremors, **seizures**
CV: Bradycardia, tachycardia, **dysrhythmias**
GI: *Diarrhea,* abdominal cramps, **paralytic ileus,** *jaundice*
GU: Gynecomastia, galactorrhea, impotence, increase in BUN, creatinine
HEMA: **Agranulocytosis, thrombocytopenia, neutropenia, aplastic anemia, increase in protime**
INTEG: Urticaria, rash, alopecia, sweating, flushing, **exfoliative dermatitis**

Contraindications: Hypersensitivity

Precautions: Pregnancy **B,** lactation, child <16 yr, organic brain syndrome, hepatic disease, renal disease, elderly

Pharmacokinetics

Absorption	Well absorbed (PO, IM); completely absorbed (**IV**)
Distribution	Widely distributed; crosses placenta
Metabolism	Liver (30%)
Excretion	Kidneys, unchanged (70%); breast milk
Half-life	1½-2 hr; increased in renal disease

Pharmacodynamics

	PO	IV/IM
Onset	½ hr	10 min
Peak	45-90 min	½ hr
Duration	4-5 hr	4-5 hr

Interactions
Individual drugs
Carbamazepine, chloroquine, lidocaine, metronidazole, moricizine, phenytoin, quinidine, quinine, valproic acid, warfarin: increased toxicity (CYP450 pathway)
Ketoconazole: decreased absorption of ketoconazole
Sucralfate: decreased cimetidine absorption
Drug classifications
Antacids: decreased absorption of cimetidine
Antidepressants (tricyclic), benzodiazepines, β-adrenergic blockers, calcium channel blockers, phenytoins, sulfonylureas, theophyllines: increased toxicity (CYP450 pathway)
Drug/lab test
Increased: alkaline phosphatase, AST, creatinine, prolactin
False positive: gastroccult, hemocult
False negative: TB skin tests

NURSING CONSIDERATIONS
Assessment
- Assess patient with ulcers or suspected ulcers: epigastric or abdominal pain, hematemesis, occult blood in stools, blood in gastric aspirate before and/or throughout treatment; monitor gastric pH (5 or > should be maintained)
- Monitor I&O ratio, BUN, creatinine, CBC with differential periodically

Nursing diagnoses
- Pain, acute (uses)
- Knowledge, deficient (teaching)

Implementation
PO route
- Give with meals for lengthened drug effect; antacids 1 hr before or 1 hr after cimetidine

IV route
- Give by direct **IV** after diluting 300 mg/20 ml of 0.9% NaCl for inj; give over 5 min or more

- Give intermittent **IV** by diluting 300 mg/50 ml of D_5W; run over 15-20 min
- Give by cont inf after using total daily dose (900 mg) diluted in 100-1000 ml D_5W given over 24 hr
- Store diluted sol at room temp up to 48 hr

Syringe compatibilities: Atropine, butorphanol, cephalothin, diazepam, diphenhydrAMINE, doxapram, droperidol, fentanyl, glycopyrrolate, heparin, hydromorphone, hydrOXYzine, lorazepam, meperidine, midazolam, morphine, nafcillin, nalbuphine, penicillin G sodium, pentazocine, perphenazine, prochlorperazine, promazine, promethazine, scopolamine

Syringe incompatibilities: Cefamandole, cefazolin, chlorproMAZINE, pentobarbital, secobarbital

Y-site compatibilities: Acyclovir, amifostine, aminophylline, inamrinone, atracurium, aztreonam, cisatracurium, cisplatin, cladribine, cyclosphosphamide, cytarabine, diltiazem, DOXOrubicin, DOXOrubicin liposome, enalaprilat, esmolol, filgrastim, fluconazole, fludarabine, foscarnet, gallium, granisetron, haloperidol, heparin, hetastarch, idarubicin, labetalol, melphalan, meropenem, methotrexate, midazolam, ondansetron, paclitaxel, pancuronium, piperacillin/tazobactam, propofol, sargramostim, tacrolimus, teniposide, theophylline, thiotepa, tolazoline, vecuronium, vinorelbine, zidovudine

Y-site incompatibilities: Amsacrine

Additive compatibilities: Acetazolamide, amikacin, aminophylline, atracurium, cefoperazone, cefoxitin, chlorothiazide, clindamycin, colistimethate, dexamethasone, digoxin, epINEPHrine, erythromycin, ethacrynate, floxacillin, flumazenil, furosemide, gentamicin, insulin, isoproterenol, lidocaine, lincomycin, meropenem, metaraminol, methylPREDNISolone, norepinephrine, penicillin G potassium, phytonadione, polymyxin B, potassium chloride, protamine, quinidine, tacrolimus, tetracycline, vancomycin, verapamil, vit B complex, vit B/C

Additive incompatibilities: Amphotericin B

Patient/family education

- Advise patient that any gynecomastia or impotence that develops is reversible after treatment is discontinued
- Caution patient to avoid driving, other hazardous activities until stabilized on this medication; drowsiness or dizziness may occur
- Advise patient to avoid black pepper, caffeine, alcohol, harsh spices, extremes in temp of food; tell patient to avoid OTC preparations: aspirin, cough, cold preparations; condition may worsen
- Advise patient that smoking decreases the effectiveness of the drug; smoking cessation should be considered
- Teach patient that drug must be continued for prescribed time to be effective and taken exactly as prescribed; doses are not to be doubled; to take missed dose when remembered up to 1 hr before next dose
- Instruct patient to report bruising, fatigue, malaise; blood dyscrasias may occur
- Have patient report to prescriber immediately any diarrhea, black tarry stools, sore throat, dizziness, confusion, or delirium

Evaluation

Positive therapeutic outcome

- Decreased pain in abdomen
- Healing of ulcers
- Absence of gastroesophageal reflux
- Gastric pH of ≥5

cinacalcet (Rx)

(sin-a-kal'set)

Sensipar

Func. class.: Calcium receptor agonist

Chem. class.: Polypeptide hormone

Pregnancy category C

Action: Directly lowers PTH levels by increasing sensitivity of calcium sensing receptors to extracellular calcium

Therapeutic Outcome: Decreased symptoms of hypercalcemia

Uses: Hypercalcemia in parathyroid carcinoma, secondary hyperparathyroidism in chronic kidney disease on dialysis

Dosage and routes

Parathyroid carcinoma

Adult: PO 30 mg bid, titrate q 2-4 wk, with sequential doses of 30 mg bid, 60 mg bid, 90 mg bid, 90 mg tid-qid to normalize calcium levels

Secondary hyperparathyroidism

Adult: PO 30 mg daily, titrate no more frequently than 2-4 wks with sequential doses of 30, 60, 90, 120, 180 mg daily

Available forms: Tabs 30, 60, 90 mg

Adverse effects

CNS: Dizziness

CV: Hypertension

GI: Nausea, diarrhea, vomiting, anorexia

MISC: Access infection, noncardiac chest pain, asthenia
MS: Myalgia

Contraindications: Hypersensitivity

Precautions: Pregnancy **C**, children, lactation, seizure disorders, hepatic disease

Pharmacokinetics

Absorption	93-97% bound to plasma
Distribution	Unknown
Metabolism	Proteins metabolized by CYP3A4, 2D6, 1A2
Excretion	Renal (80% renal, 15% feces)
Half-life	30-40 hr

Pharmacodynamics

Unknown

Interactions
Individual drugs
Ketoconazole, erythromycin, itraconazole (drugs metabolized by CYP3A4); flecainide, vinBLAStine, thioridazine, tricyclics (drugs metabolized by CYP2D6): adjustments may be necessary
Drug classifications
Tricyclics (metabolized by CYP2D6): adjustments may be necessary
Drug/food
High-fat meal: increased action

NURSING CONSIDERATIONS
Assessment
- Assess for hypocalcemia: cramping, seizures, tetany, myalgia, paresthesia
- Monitor calcium, phosphorous within 1 wk and iPTH 1-4 wk after initiation or dosage adjustment when maintenance is established; measure calcium, phosphorus monthly; iPTH q1-3 mo, target range 150-300 pg/ml for iPTH level
- If calcium < 8.4 mg/dl, do not start therapy

Nursing diagnoses
- Injury, risk for (uses)
- Knowledge, deficient (teaching)

Implementation
- Swallow tabs whole; do not break, crush, chew, or divide tabs
- Can be used alone or in combination with vit D sterols and/or phosphate binders
- Take with food or shortly after meal

Secondary hyperthyroidism
- Titrate q2-4 wk to target iPTH consistent with National Kidney Foundation-Kidney Disease Outcomes Quality Initiative (NKF-K/DOQI) for chronic kidney disease patient on dialysis of 150-300 pg/ml; if iPTH drops below 150-300 pg/ml, reduce dose of cinacalcet and/or vit D sterols or discontinue treatment
- Store at <77° F (25° C)

Patient/family education
- Instruct patient to take with food or shortly after a meal
- Instruct patient to immediately report cramping, seizures, muscle pain, tingling, tetany

Evaluation
Positive therapeutic outcome
- Calcium levels 9-10 mg/dl, decreasing symptoms of hypercalcemia

ciprofloxacin (Rx)
(sip-ro-floks'a-sin)
Cipro, Cipro IV, Cipro XR
Func. class.: Urinary antiinfectives, broad-spectrum
Chem. class.: Fluoroquinolone
Pregnancy category C

Do Not Confuse:
ciprofloxacin/cephalexin

Action: Interferes with conversion of intermediate DNA fragments into high-molecular-weight DNA in bacteria; DNA gyrase inhibitor

Therapeutic Outcome: Bactericidal action against the following: gram-positive organisms *Staphylococcus epidermidis,* methicillin-resistant strains of *Staphylococcus aureus, Streptococcus pyogenes, Streptococcus pneumoniae;* gram-negative organisms *Escherichia coli, Klebsiella* species, *Enterobacter, Salmonella, Shigella, Proteus vulgaris, Providencia stuartii, Providencia rettgeri, Morganella morganii, Pseudomonas aeruginosa, Serratia, Haemophilus, Acinetobacter, Neisseria gonorrhoeae, Neisseria meningitidis, Branhamella catarrhalis, Yersinia, Vibrio, Brucella, Campylobacter, Aeromonas*

Uses: Adult urinary tract infections (including complicated); chronic bacterial prostatitis; acute sinusitis; lower respiratory, skin, bone, joint infections; infectious diarrhea, exposure to inhalation anthrax; conjunctivitis, corneal ulcers (ophthalmic)

Dosage and routes

Uncomplicated urinary tract infections

Adult: PO 250 mg q12h × 3 days or 500 mg q24h × 3 days

Complicated/severe urinary tract infections

Adult: PO 500 mg q12h or 1000 mg q24h × 7-14 days; **IV** 400 mg q12h

Respiratory, bone, skin, joint infections

Adult: PO 500 mg q12h; **IV** 400 mg q12h

Corneal ulcers, conjunctivitis

Adult: Ophth 1-2 gtt q15-30 min until infection is controlled, then 1-2 gtt 4-6 times daily

Nosocomial pneumonia

Adult: **IV** 400 mg q8h × 10-14 days

Intraabdominal infections, complicated

Adult: PO 500 mg q12h × 7-14 days, **IV** 400 mg q12h × 7-14 days

Acute sinusitis, mild/moderate

Adult: PO 500 mg q12h × 10 days; **IV** 400 mg q12h × 10 days

Inhalational anthrax (postexposure)

Adult: PO 500 mg q12h × 60 days; **IV** 400 mg q12h × 60 days

Child: PO 15 mg/kg/dose, max 500 mg/dose; **IV** max 400 mg/dose × 60 days

Infectious diarrhea

Adult: PO 500 mg q12h × 5-7 days

Chronic bacterial prostatis

Adult: PO 500 mg q12h × 28 days; **IV** 400 mg q12h × 28 days

Pyelonephritis, acute uncomplicated

Adult: PO 1000 mg × q24h × 7-14 days

Renal dose

Adult: PO CCr 30-50 ml/min PO 250-500 mg q12h; CCr 5-29 ml/min PO 250-500 mg q18h; **IV** 200-400 mg q18-24h

Available forms: Tabs 100, 250, 500, 750 mg; ext rel tabs (XR) 500, 1000 mg; inj 200 mg/20 ml, 400 mg/40 ml, 200 mg/100 ml D_5, 400 mg/200 ml D_5; oral susp 250, 500 mg/5 ml

Adverse effects

CNS: *Headache,* dizziness, fatigue, insomnia, depression, *restlessness,* **seizures,** confusion

GI: *Nausea,* increased ALT, AST, flatulence, heartburn, *vomiting, diarrhea,* oral candidiasis, dysphagia, **pseudomembranous colitis,** dry mouth

INTEG: *Rash,* pruritus, urticaria, photosensitivity, flushing, fever, chills

MISC: **Anaphylaxis, Stevens-Johnson syndrome**

MS: Tremor, arthralgia, tendon rupture

Contraindications: Hypersensitivity to quinolones

Precautions: Pregnancy **C,** lactation, children, renal disease, epilepsy

Pharmacokinetics

Absorption	Well absorbed (75%) (PO)
Distribution	Widely distributed
Metabolism	Liver (15%)
Excretion	Kidneys (40%-50%)
Half-life	3-4 hr; increased in renal disease

Pharmacodynamics

	PO	IV
Onset	Rapid	Immediate
Peak	1 hr	Infusion's end

Interactions

Individual drugs

Calcium, enteral feeding, sucralfate, zinc sulfate, iron: decreased ciprofloxacin absorption

CycloSPORINE: increased nephrotoxicity

Probenecid: increased blood levels of ciprofloxacin, increased toxicity

Theophylline: increased theophylline levels, monitor blood levels

Warfarin: increased warfarin effect, monitor blood levels

Drug classifications

Antacids (containing magnesium, aluminum), iron salts: decreased absorption of ciprofloxacin

Drug/herb

Acidophilus: do not use with antiinfectives

Caffeine: increased caffeine levels

Fennel: decreased antiinfective effect

Yerba maté: increased toxicity

Drug/food

Dairy products, food: decreased absorption

Drug/lab test

Increased: AST, ALT, bilirubin, BUN, creatinine, alkaline phosphatase, LDH, glucose, proteinuria, albuminuria

Decreased: WBC, glucose

NURSING CONSIDERATIONS

Assessment

- Assess patient for previous sensitivity reaction
- Assess patient for signs and symptoms of infection including characteristics of wounds, sputum, urine, stool, WBC >10,000/mm^3, fever; obtain baseline information before and during treatment
- Obtain C&S before beginning drug therapy to identify if correct treatment has been initiated
- Assess for anaphylaxis: rash, urticaria, dyspnea, pruritus, chills, fever, joint pain; may occur a few days after therapy begins; epINEPHrine and resuscitation equipment should be available for anaphylactic reaction
- Identify urine output; if decreasing, notify prescriber (may indicate nephrotoxicity); also check for increased BUN, creatinine
- Monitor blood studies: AST, ALT, CBC, Hct, bilirubin, LDH, alkaline phosphatase, Coombs' test monthly if patient is on long-term therapy
- Monitor electrolytes: potassium, sodium, chloride monthly if patient is on long-term therapy
- Assess bowel pattern daily; if severe diarrhea occurs, drug should be discontinued
- Monitor for bleeding: ecchymosis, bleeding gums, hematuria, stool guaiac daily if on long-term therapy
- Assess for overgrowth of infection: perineal itching, fever, malaise, redness, pain, swelling, drainage, rash, diarrhea, change in cough, sputum

Nursing diagnoses

- Infection, risk for (uses)
- Diarrhea (side effects)
- Injury, risk for (side effects)
- Knowledge, deficient (teaching)
- Noncompliance (teaching)

Implementation

PO route

- Give around the clock to maintain proper blood levels
- Administer 2 hr before or 2 hr after antacids, zinc, iron, calcium

IV route

- Check for irritation, extravasation, phlebitis daily
- For intermittent inf, dilute to 1-2 mg/ml of D_5W, 0.9% NaCl; give over 60 min; it will remain stable under refrigeration for 2 wk

Y-site compatibilities: Amifostine, amino acids, aztreonam, calcium gluconate, ceftazidime, cisatracurium, digoxin, diltiazem, diphenhydrAMINE, DOBUTamine, DOPamine, DOXOrubicin liposome, gallium, gentamicin, granisetron, hydrOXYzine, lidocaine, lorazepam, metoclopramide, midazolam, midodrine, piperacillin, potassium acetate, potassium chloride, potassium phosphates, prednisoLONE, promethazine, propofol, ranitidine, remifentanil, Ringer's, sodium chloride, tacrolimus, teniposide, thiotepa, tobramycin, verapamil

Y-site incompatibilities: Heparin, mezlocillin

Additive compatibilities: Amikacin, aztreonam, ceftazidime, cycloSPORINE, gentamicin, metronidazole, netilmicin, piperacillin, potassium acetate, potassium chloride, potassium phosphates, prednisoLONE, promethazine, propofol, ranitidine, Ringer's, sodium chloride, tobramycin, vit B/C

Additive incompatibilities: Aminophylline, amoxicillin, clindamycin, floxacillin, mezlocillin

Patient/family education

- Teach patient to report sore throat, bruising, bleeding, joint pain; may indicate blood dyscrasias (rare)
- Teach patient to contact prescriber if adverse reaction occurs or if inflammation or pain in tendon occurs
- Advise patient to contact prescriber if vaginal itching, loose foul-smelling stools, furry tongue occur; may indicate superinfection; report itching, rash, pruritus, urticaria
- Instruct patient to take all medication prescribed for the length of time ordered; drug must be taken around the clock to maintain blood levels; do not give medication to others
- Advise patient to notify prescriber of diarrhea with blood or pus
- Advise patient to rinse mouth frequently, use sugarless candy or gum for dry mouth

Evaluation

Positive therapeutic outcome

- Absence of signs/symptoms of infection (WBC <10,000/mm^3, temp WNL, absence of red draining wounds)
- Reported improvement in symptoms of infection

C

cisatracurium (Rx)

(sis-a-tra-cyoor'ee-um)

Nimbex

Func. class.: Neuromuscular blocker (nondepolarizing)

Pregnancy category B

Action: Inhibits transmission of nerve impulses by binding with cholinergic receptor sites, antagonizing action of acetylcholine

Therapeutic Outcome: Paralysis of body for administration of anesthesia

Uses: Facilitation of endotracheal intubation, skeletal muscle relaxation during mechanical ventilation surgery, or general anesthesia

Dosage and routes

Adult: **IV** 0.15 and 0.2 mg/kg depending on desired time to intubate and length of surgery: use peripheral nerve stimulation to evaluate dosage

Child 2-12 yr: **IV** 0.1 mg/kg over 5-10 sec with halothane or opioid anesthesia

Available forms: Inj 2, 10 mg/ml

Adverse effects

CV: Bradycardia, tachycardia; increased, decreased B/P

EENT: Increased secretions

INTEG: Rash, flushing, pruritus, urticaria

RESP: **Prolonged apnea, bronchospasm, cyanosis, respiratory depression**

Contraindications: Hypersensitivity

Precautions: Pregnancy **B,** cardiac disease, lactation, children <2 yr electrolyte imbalances, dehydration, neuromuscular disease, respiratory disease

Pharmacokinetics

Unknown

Pharmacodynamics

Onset	1-3 min
Peak	2-5 min
Duration	30-40 min

Interactions

Individual drugs

Carbamazepine, phenytoin: decreased duration of neuromuscular blockade

Isoflurane, lithium: increased neuromuscular blockade

Succinylcholine: decreased neuromuscular blockade

Drug classifications

Aminoglycosides, antibiotics (polymix), β-Adrenergic blockers, opioids: increased neuromuscular blockade

NURSING CONSIDERATIONS

Assessment

- Assess for electrolyte imbalances (K, Mg), may lead to increased action of this drug
- Assess vital signs (B/P, pulse, respirations, airway) until fully recovered; rate, depth, pattern of respirations; strength of handgrip
- Assess I&O ratio: check for urinary retention, frequency, hesitancy
- Assess recovery: decreased paralysis of face, diaphragm, legs, arms, rest of body
- Assess allergic reactions: rash, fever, respiratory distress, pruritus; drug should be discontinued

Nursing diagnoses

- Breathing pattern, ineffective (uses)
- Communication, verbal, impaired (adverse reactions)
- Knowledge, deficient (teaching)

Implementation

IV route

- Use nerve stimulator by anesthesiologist to determine neuromuscular blockade
- Give anticholinesterase to reverse neuromuscular blockade
- Give by slow **IV** only by qualified person, do not administer IM
- Store in light-resistant area
- Reassure if communication is difficult during recovery from neuromuscular blockage

Evaluation

Positive therapeutic outcome

- Paralysis of jaw, eyelid, head, neck, rest of body

Treatment of overdose: Edrophonium or neostigmine, atropine, monitor VS; mechanical ventilation

! HIGH ALERT

cisplatin (Rx)

(sis'pla-tin)

Platinol, Platinol-AQ

Func. class.: Antineoplastic alkylating agent

Chem. class.: Inorganic heavy metal

Pregnancy category D

Do Not Confuse:

cisplatin/carboplatin

Platinol/Paraplatin

Action: Alkylates DNA, RNA; inhibits enzymes that allow synthesis of amino acids in proteins; activity is not cell cycle phase specific

Therapeutic Outcome: Prevention of rapidly growing malignant cells

Uses: Advanced bladder cancer; adjunctive in metastatic testicular cancer and metastatic ovarian cancer; head, neck, esophageal, prostatic, lung, and cervical cancer; lymphoma

Dosage and routes

Dosage protocols may vary

Metastatic testicular cancer

Adult: **IV** 20 mg/m^2 daily × 5 days, repeat q3 wk for 3 cycles or more, depending on response

Advanced bladder cancer

Adult: **IV** 50-70 mg/m^2 q3-4 wk

Metastatic ovarian cancer

Adult: **IV** 100 mg/m^2 q4 wk or 75 mg/m^2 q3 wk with cyclophosphamide therapy; mix with 2 L of NaCl and 37.5 g mannitol over 6 hr

Available forms: Inj 0.5 mg/ml 🍁, 1 mg/ml; powder for inj 10, 50 mg vials

Adverse effects

CNS: **Seizures,** peripheral neuropathy
CV: Cardiac abnormalities
EENT: *Tinnitus, hearing loss, vestibular toxicity,* blurred vision, altered color perception
GI: *Severe nausea, vomiting, diarrhea, weight loss*
GU: **Renal tubular damage,** renal insufficiency, impotence, sterility, amenorrhea, gynecomastia, hyperuremia
HEMA: **Thrombocytopenia, leukopenia, pancytopenia**
INTEG: *Alopecia,* dermatitis
META: Hypomagnesemia, hypocalcemia, hypokalemia, hypophosphatemia
RESP: **Fibrosis**
SYST: **Anaphylaxis**

Contraindications: Pregnancy **D,** radiation therapy within 1 mo, chemotherapy within 1 mo, thrombocytopenia, recent smallpox vaccination, aluminum products used to prepare or administer cisplatin

Precautions: Pneumococcal vaccination, lactation

Pharmacokinetics

Absorption	Complete
Distribution	Widely distributed, accumulates in body tissues for several months
Metabolism	Liver
Excretion	Kidneys
Half-life	30-100 hr

Pharmacodynamics

Unknown

Interactions

Individual drugs

Alcohol, aspirin: increased risk of bleeding
Bumetanide, ethacrynic acid, furosemide: ototoxicity
Phenytoin: decreased phenytoin effect

Drug classifications

Aminoglycosides, diuretics (loop): increased nephrotoxicity
Myelosuppressive agents, radiation: increased myelosuppression
NSAIDs: increased risk of bleeding
Vaccines, live virus: decreased antibody response

Drug/lab test

Increased: uric acid, BUN, creatinine
Decreased: CCr, calcium, phosphate, potassium, magnesium
Positive: Coombs' test

NURSING CONSIDERATIONS

Assessment

- Monitor for bone marrow depression: CBC, differential, platelet count weekly; withhold drug if WBC count is <4000/mm^3 or platelet count is <100,000/mm^3; notify prescriber of results if WBC <20,000/mm^3, platelets <150,000/mm^3
- Monitor renal function studies: BUN, creatinine, serum uric acid, urine CCr before and during therapy; I&O ratio; report fall in urine output to <30 ml/hr; dose should not be given if BUN <25 mg/dl; creatinine <1.5 mg/dl
- Assess for anaphylaxis: wheezing, tachycardia, facial swelling, fainting; discontinue drug and report to prescriber, resuscitation equipment should be nearby
- Monitor temp q4h (may indicate beginning of infection)
- Monitor liver function tests before and during therapy (bilirubin, AST, ALT, LDH) as needed or monthly; note yellowing of skin or sclera, dark urine, clay-colored stools, itchy skin, abdominal pain, fever, diarrhea
- Assess for increased uric acid levels, swelling, joint pain primarily in extremities; patient should be well hydrated to prevent urate deposits
- Assess for bleeding: hematuria, stool guaiac, bruising or petechiae, mucosa or orifices q8h; note inflammation of mucosa, breaks in skin
- Identify dyspnea, crackles, nonproductive cough, chest pain, tachypnea

- Identify effects of alopecia on body image; discuss feelings about body changes
- Identify edema in feet, joint pain, stomach pain, shaking; prescriber should be notified

Nursing diagnoses

- Injury, risk for (adverse reactions)
- Body image, disturbed (adverse reactions)
- Infection, risk for (adverse reactions)
- Knowledge, deficient (teaching)

Implementation

- Hydrate patient with 0.9% NaCl over 8-12 hr before treatment
- Give all medications PO, if possible; avoid IM inj when platelets <100,000/mm^3
- Give epINEPHrine, antihistamines, corticosteroids for hypersensitivity reaction; antiemetic 30-60 min before giving drug to prevent vomiting, and prn; allopurinol or sodium bicarbonate to maintain uric acid level, alkalinization of urine; antibiotics for prophylaxis of infection; diuretic (furosemide 40 mg **IV**) or mannitol after infusion
- After diluting 10 mg/10 ml or 50 mg/50 ml sterile water for inj; withdraw prescribed dose, dilute ½ dose with 1000 ml D_5 0.2 NaCl or D_5 0.45 NaCl with 37.5 g mannitol; **IV** inf is given over 3-4 hr; use a 0.45 μm filter; total dose 2000 ml over 6-8 hr; check site for irritation, phlebitis; do not use equipment containing aluminum
- Prepare in biologic cabinet using gown, gloves, mask; do not allow drug to come in contact with skin, use soap and water if contact occurs

Syringe compatibilities: Bleomycin, cyclophosphamide, doxapram, DOXOrubicin, droperidol, fluorouracil, furosemide, heparin, leucovorin, methotrexate, metoclopramide, mitomycin, vinBLAStine, vinCRIStine

Y-site compatibilities: Allopurinol, aztrenonam, bleomycin, chlorproMAZINE, cimetidine, cladribine, cyclophosphamide, dexamethasone, diphenhydrAMINE, doxapram, DOXOrubicin, DOXOrubicin liposome, droperidol, famotidine, filgrastim, fludarabine, fluorouracil, furosemide, ganciclovir, granisetron, heparin, hydromorphone, leucovorin, lorazepam, melphalan, methotrexate, methylPREDNISolone, metoclopramide, mitomycin, morphine, ondansetron, paclitaxel, prochlorperazine, promethazine, propofol, ranitidine, sargramostim, teniposide, vinBLAStine, vinCRIStine, vinorelbine

Additive compatibilities: Carboplatin, cyclophosphamide with etoposide, etoposide, etoposide with floxuridine, floxuridine, floxuridine with leucovorin, hydrOXYzine, ifosfamide, ifosfamide with etoposide, leucovorin, magnesium sulfate, mannitol, ondansetron

Additive incompatibilities: Fluorouracil, mesna, thiotepa

Solution compatibilities: D_5/0.225% NaCl, D_5/0.45% NaCl, D_5/0.9% NaCl, D_5/0.45% NaCl with mannitol 1.875%, D_5/0.33% NaCl with mannitol 1.875%, D_5/0.33% NaCl with KCl 20 mEq and mannitol 1.875%, 0.9% NaCl, 0.45% NaCl, 0.3% NaCl, 0.225% NaCl, water

Solution incompatibilities: Sodium bicarbonate 5%, 0.1% NaCl, water

Patient/family education

- Teach patient to avoid use of products containing aspirin or ibuprofen, NSAIDs, alcohol (may cause GI bleeding), razors, commercial mouthwash; to report symptoms of bleeding (hematuria, tarry stools, bruising, petechiae)
- Advise patient to report numbness, tingling in face or extremities, poor hearing or joint pain, swelling
- Instruct patient to report signs of anemia (fatigue, headache, irritability, faintness, shortness of breath)
- Instruct patient to report any changes in breathing or coughing even several months after treatment; to avoid crowds and persons with respiratory tract or other infections
- Advise patient that hair may be lost during treatment; a wig or hair piece may make patient feel better; new hair may be different in color, texture
- Tell patient not to have any vaccinations without the advice of the prescriber; serious reactions can occur
- Caution patient contraception is needed during treatment and for several months after the completion of therapy

Evaluation

Positive therapeutic outcome

- Prevention of rapid division of malignant cells

citalopram (Rx)

(sigh-tal′oh-pram)

Celexa

Func. class.: Antidepressant

Chem class.: Selective serotonin reuptake inhibitor (SSRI)

Pregnancy category C

Do Not Confuse:

Celexa/Celebrex/Cerebyx/Cerebra

Action: Inhibits CNS neuron uptake of

serotonin but not of norepinephrine; weak inhibitor of CYP450 enzyme system, making it more appealing than other drugs

Therapeutic Outcome: Decreased symptoms of depression after 2-3 wk

Uses: Major depressive disorder

Investigational uses: Fibromyalgia, premenstrual disorders, panic disorder, social phobia, impulsive aggression in children, obsessive-compulsive disorder in adolescents, treatment of psychotic symptoms in nondepressed, demented patients

Dosage and routes

Depression

Adult: PO 20 mg daily AM or PM, may increase if needed to 40 mg/day after 1 wk; maintenance: after 6-8 wk of initial treatment, continue for 24 wk (32 wk total), reevaluate long-term usefulness (max 60 mg/day)

Fibromyalgia

Adult: PO 20 mg daily × 4 wk, increase dose to 40 mg daily × 4 wk

Hepatic dose/elderly

Adult: PO 20 mg/day, may increase to 40 mg/day if no response

Panic disorder

Adult: PO 20-30 mg/day

Premenstrual dysphoria, social phobia, impulsive aggression in children

Adult: PO 20-40 mg/day used intermittently in premenstrual dysphoria

Available forms: Tabs 10, 20, 40 mg; oral sol 2 mg (as base)/ml

Adverse effects

CNS: *Headache, nervousness, insomnia, drowsiness, anxiety, tremor, dizziness, fatigue, sedation, poor concentration, abnormal dreams, agitation,* **seizures,** apathy, euphoria, hallucinations, delusions, psychosis, **suicidal attempts**

CV: *Hot flashes, palpitations,* angina pectoris, **hemorrhage,** hypertension, 1st-degree tachycardia, 1st-degree AV block, bradycardia, MI, thrombophlebitis

EENT: Visual changes, ear/eye pain, photophobia, tinnitus

GI: *Nausea, diarrhea, dry mouth, anorexia, dyspepsia, constipation, cramps, vomiting, taste changes, flatulence, decreased appetite*

GU: *Dysmenorrhea, decreased libido, urinary frequency, urinary tract infection,* amenorrhea, cystitis, impotence, urine retention

INTEG: *Sweating, rash, pruritus,* acne, alopecia, urticaria

MS: *Pain,* arthritis, twitching

RESP: *Infection, pharyngitis, nasal congestion, sinus headache, sinusitis, cough, dyspnea, bronchitis,* asthma, hyperventilation, pneumonia

SYST: *Asthenia, viral infection, fever, allergy, chills*

Contraindications: Hypersensitivity

Precautions: Pregnancy **C,** lactation, children, elderly

Pharmacokinetics	
Absorption	Well absorbed
Distribution	Unknown
Metabolism	Liver
Excretion	Kidneys, steady state 28-35 days
Half-life	Unknown

Pharmacodynamics	
Onset	Unknown
Peak	Unknown
Duration	Unknown

Interactions

Individual drugs

Alcohol: increased CNS depression
Carbamazepine: decreased citalopram levels
Lithium: increased serotonergic effects

Drug classifications

Antidepressants, tricyclics: increased effect, use cautiously
Antifungals (azole), macrolides: increased citalopram levels
Barbiturates, benzodiazepines, CNS depressants, sedative/hypnotics: increased CNS depression
β-Adrenergic blockers: increased plasma levels of β-blockers
MAOIs: hypertensive crisis, seizures, fatal reactions, do not use together

Drug/herb

SAM-e, St. John's wort: serotonin syndrome, do not use with citalopram, fatal reaction may occur
Yohimbe: increased CNS stimulation

Drug/lab test

Increased: serum bilirubin, blood glucose, alkaline phosphatase
Decreased: VMA, 5-HIAA
False increase: increased urinary catecholamines

NURSING CONSIDERATIONS

Assessment

- Monitor B/P (lying, standing), pulse q4h; if

systolic B/P drops 20 mm Hg, hold drug and notify prescriber; take vital signs q4h in patients with cardiovascular disease
- Monitor blood studies: CBC, leukocytes, differential, cardiac enzymes if patient is receiving long-term therapy; check platelets, bleeding can occur
- Monitor hepatic studies: AST, ALT, bilirubin
- Check weight qwk; appetite may increase with drug
- Assess ECG for flattening of T wave, bundle branch block, AV block, dysrhythmias in cardiac patients
- Assess extrapyramidial symptoms (EPS) primarily in elderly: rigidity, dystonia, akathisia
- Assess mental status: mood, sensorium, affect, suicidal tendencies; increase in psychiatric symptoms: depression, panic
- Monitor urinary retention, constipation; constipation is more likely to occur in children or elderly
- ❗ Assess for withdrawal symptoms: headache, nausea, vomiting, muscle pain, weakness; usually do not occur unless drug is discontinued abruptly
- Identify patient's alcohol consumption; if alcohol is consumed, hold dose until AM

Nursing diagnoses
- Coping, ineffective (uses)
- Injury, risk for (side effects)
- Knowledge, deficient (teaching)
- Noncompliance (teaching)

Implementation
- Give with food or milk for GI symptoms
- Give dosage at bedtime if oversedation occurs during day
- Store at room temp; do not freeze

Patient/family education
- Teach patient that therapeutic effects may take 2-3 wk
- Instruct patient to use caution in driving or other activities requiring alertness because of drowsiness, dizziness, blurred vision; to avoid rising quickly from sitting to standing, especially elderly
- Caution patient to avoid alcohol ingestion, other CNS depressants
- Advise patient not to discontinue medication quickly after long-term use: may cause nausea, headache, malaise
- Instruct patient to increase fluids, bulk in diet if constipation, urinary retention occur, especially elderly
- Advise patient to take gum, hard sugarless candy, or frequent sips of water for dry mouth

Evaluation
Positive therapeutic outcome
- Decreased in depression
- Absence of suicidal thoughts

clarithromycin (Rx)
(clare-i-thro-mye'sin)

Biaxin, Biaxin XL

Func. class.: Antiinfective

Chem. class.: Macrolide

Pregnancy category C

Action: Binds to 50S ribosomal subunits of susceptible bacteria and suppresses protein synthesis

Therapeutic Outcome: Bactericidal action against the following: *Streptococcus pneumoniae, Streptococcus pyogenes, Mycoplasma pneumoniae, Corynebacterium diphtheriae, Bordetella pertussis, Listeria monocytogenes, Haemophilus influenzae, Staphylococcus aureus, Mycobacterium avium (MAC), Mycobacterium intracellulare,* complex infections in AIDS patients, *Helicobacter pylori* in combination with omeprazole

Uses: Mild to moderate infections of the upper respiratory tract, lower respiratory tract; uncomplicated skin and skin structure infections

Dosage and routes
Acute exacerbation of chronic bronchitis

Adult: PO 250-500 mg q12h × 7-14 days or 1000 mg daily × 7 days (XL) bid-tid

Pharyngitis/tonsillitis

Adult: PO 250 mg q12h × 10 days

Renal dose

Adult: PO CCr <30 ml/min 250 mg daily × bid, may use an initial dose of 500 mg

Child: PO CCr <30 ml/min reduce dose by 50%

Community-acquired pneumonia

Adult: PO 250 mg q12h × 7-14 days or 1000 mg daily × 7 days (XL)

Endocarditis prophylaxis

Adult: PO 500 mg 1 hr before procedure

MAC prophylaxis/treatment

Adult: PO 500 mg bid, will require an additional antiinfective for active infection

H. pylori *infection*

Adult: PO 500 mg daily plus omeprazole 2 × 20 mg q AM (days 1-14), then omeprazole 20 mg q AM (days 15-28)

Acute maxillary sinusitis
Adult: PO 500 mg q12h × 14 days
Most infections
Child: PO 7.5 mg/kg q12h × 10 days, max 500 mg/dose for MAC

Available forms: Tabs 250, 500 mg; oral susp 125, 250 mg/5 ml; ext rel tab (XL) 500 mg

Adverse effects
CV: **Ventricular dysrhythmias**
GI: Nausea, vomiting, diarrhea, **hepatotoxicity,** abdominal pain, stomatitis, heartburn, anorexia, abnormal taste, **pseudomembranous colitis**
GU: Vaginitis, moniliasis
HEMA: Leukopenia, thrombocytopenia, increased INR
INTEG: Rash, urticaria, pruritus, **Stevens-Johnson syndrome**
MISC: Headache

Contraindications: Hypersensitivity to this drug or other macrolides

Precautions: Pregnancy **C,** lactation, hepatic/renal disease, elderly

Pharmacokinetics	
Absorption	50%
Distribution	Widely distributed
Metabolism	Liver
Excretion	Kidneys, unchanged (20%-30%)
Half-life	4-6 hr

Pharmacodynamics	
Onset	Unknown
Peak	2 hr

Interactions
Individual drugs
Alprazolam, busPIRone, carbamazepine, cycloSPORINE, digoxin, disopyramide, felodipine, fluconazole, omeprazole, tacrolimus, theophylline: increased levels, increased toxicity
Carbamazepine: increased toxicity, from increased levels of carbamazepine, increased oral anticoagulants effect
Cisapride, pimozide: increased effect, increased dysrhythmias
Digoxin: increased blood levels of digoxin, increased digoxin effects, increased oral anticoagulants effect
Fluconazole: increased clarithromycin levels
Rifabutin, rifampin: decreased levels
Theophylline: increased toxicity from increased levels of theophylline, increased oral anticoagulants effect
Zidovudine: increased or decreased action

Drug classifications
All drugs metabolized by CYP3A enzyme system: increased action, risk of toxicity
Ergots: increased levels, increased toxicity
HMG-CoA reductase inhibitors: increased levels
Oral anticoagulants: increased effects of oral anticoagulants

Drug/herb
Acidophilus: do not use with antiinfectives

Drug/lab test
Increased: 17-OHCS/17-KS, AST, ALT, BUN, creatinine, LDH, total bilirubin
Decreased: folate assay, WBC

NURSING CONSIDERATIONS
Assessment
- Assess patient for signs and symptoms of infection including characteristics of wounds, sputum, urine, stool, WBC >10,000/mm^3, earache, fever; obtain baseline information before and during treatment
- Obtain C&S before beginning drug therapy to identify if correct treatment has been initiated
- Monitor blood studies: AST, ALT, CBC, Hct, bilirubin, LDH, alkaline phosphatase, Coombs' test monthly if patient is on long-term therapy
- Assess bowel pattern daily; if severe diarrhea occurs, drug should be discontinued
- Assess for overgrowth of infection: perineal itching, fever, malaise, redness, pain, swelling, drainage, rash, diarrhea, change in cough, sputum

Nursing diagnoses
- Infection, risk for (uses)
- Diarrhea (side effects)
- Knowledge, deficient (teaching)
- Noncompliance (teaching)

Implementation
- Do not break, crush, or chew ext rel tab
- Ensure adequate fluid intake (2 L) during diarrhea episodes
- Give q12h to maintain serum level

Patient/family education
- Advise patient to contact physician if vaginal itching, loose foul-smelling stools, furry tongue occur; may indicate superinfection
- Instruct patient to take all medication prescribed for the length of time ordered
- Advise prescriber if pregnancy is planned or suspected

Evaluation
Positive therapeutic outcome
- Absence of signs/symptoms of infection (WBC <10,000/mm^3, temp WNL, absence of red draining wounds)

C

• Reported improvement in symptoms of infection

clavulanate

See amoxicillin/clavulanate, ticarcillin/clavulanate

clemastine (Rx)

(klem'as-teen)

Antihist-1, Contac Allergy 12 Hour, Tavist

Func. class.: Antihistamine

Chem. class.: Ethanolamine derivative, H_1-receptor antagonist

Pregnancy category B

Action: Acts on blood vessels, GI, respiratory system by competing with histamine for H_1-receptor site; decreases allergic response by blocking histamine

Therapeutic Outcome: Absence of allergy symptoms and rhinitis

Uses: Allergy symptoms, rhinitis, allergic dermatoses, nasal allergies, hypersensitive reactions including blood transfusion reactions, anaphylaxis

Dosage and routes

Adult and child >12 yr: PO 1.34-2.68 mg bid-tid, not to exceed 8.04 mg/day

Available forms: Tabs 1.34, 2.68 mg; syr 0.67 mg/ml

Adverse effects

CNS: *Dizziness, drowsiness,* poor coordination, fatigue, anxiety, euphoria, confusion, paresthesia, neuritis, paradoxic excitement (child)

CV: Hypotension, palpitations, tachycardia

EENT: *Blurred vision,* dilated pupils, tinnitus, nasal stuffiness, dry nose, throat, *mouth*

GI: *Constipation,* dry mouth, nausea, vomiting, anorexia, diarrhea

GU: *Retention,* dysuria, frequency

HEMA: **Thrombocytopenia, agranulocytosis, hemolytic anemia**

INTEG: Rash, urticaria, photosensitivity, sweating

RESP: Increased thick secretions, wheezing, chest tightness

Contraindications: Hypersensitivity to H_1-receptor antagonists, acute asthma attack, lower respiratory tract disease

Precautions: Pregnancy **B,** increased intraocular pressure, renal disease, cardiac disease, hypertension, bronchial asthma, seizure disorder, stenosed peptic ulcers, hyperthyroidism, prostatic hypertrophy, bladder neck obstruction, elderly

Pharmacokinetics

Absorption	Well absorbed
Distribution	Widely distributed
Metabolism	Liver, extensively
Excretion	Kidneys, breast milk (high)
Half-life	Unknown

Pharmacodynamics

Onset	15-60 min
Peak	1-2 hr
Duration	12 hr

Interactions

Individual drugs

Alcohol: increased CNS depression

Drug classifications

CNS depressants, opioids, sedative/hypnotics: increased CNS depression

MAOIs: increased anticholinergic effect

Drug/herb

Corkwood, henbane leaf: increased anticholinergic effect

Hops, Jamaican dogwood, kava, khat, senega: increased sedative effect

Drug/lab test

False negative: skin allergy tests (discontinue antihistamines 3 days before testing)

NURSING CONSIDERATIONS

Assessment

• Assess respiratory status: rate, rhythm, increase in bronchial secretions, wheezing, chest tightness; provide fluids to 2 L/day to decrease secretion thickness

• Monitor I&O ratio: be alert for urinary retention, frequency, dysuria, especially elderly; drug should be discontinued if these occur

Nursing diagnoses

• Airway clearance, ineffective (uses)
• Injury, risk for (side effects)
• Knowledge, deficient (teaching)
• Noncompliance (teaching, overuse)

Implementation

• Do not break, crush, or chew tabs
• May give with food to decrease GI upset
• Store in tight, light-resistant container

Patient/family education

• Teach all aspects of drug uses; to notify prescriber if confusion, sedation, hypotension occur; to avoid driving and other hazardous activity if drowsiness occurs; to avoid alcohol and other CNS depressants that may potentiate effect

- Instruct patient to take 1 hr ac or 2 hr pc to facilitate absorption
- Caution patient not to exceed recommended dosage; dysrhythmias may occur
- Teach patient hard candy, gum, frequent rinsing of mouth may be used for dryness
- Tell patient if EENT or CNS symptoms occur (blurred vision, severe dry mouth, dry throat, confusion, dizziness, poor coordination, euphoria), prescriber should be notified

Evaluation

Positive therapeutic outcome

- Absence of running or congested nose, rashes

Treatment of overdose: Administer lavage, diazepam, vasopressors, barbiturates (short acting)

clindamycin HCl (Rx)

(klin-dah-my'sin)

Cleocin HCl

clindamycin palmitate (Rx)

Cleocin Pediatric, Dalacin C Palmitate

clindamycin phosphate (Rx)

Cleocin Phosphate, Dalacin C, Dalacin C Phosphate

Func. class.: Antiinfective—miscellaneous

Chem. class.: Lincomycin derivative

Pregnancy category B

Action: Binds to 50S subunit of bacterial ribosomes; suppresses protein synthesis

Therapeutic Outcome: Absence of infection

Uses: Infections caused by staphylococci, streptococci, *Rickettsia, Fusobacterium, Actinomyces, Peptococcus, Clostridium*

Dosage and routes

Adults: PO 150-450 mg q6h, max 1.8 g/day; IM/**IV** 1.2-1.8 g/day in 2-4 divided doses q6-12h, not to exceed 4800 mg/day

Child <1 mo: 15-20 mg/kg/day divided q6-8h

Child >1 mo: PO 8-25 mg/kg/day in divided doses q6-8h; IM/**IV** 20-40 mg/kg/day in divided doses q6-8h in 3-4 equal doses

Vaginal route

Adult: 5 g applicatorful at bedtime × 1 wk

Topical route

Adult: Sol 1% apply bid

PID

Adult: **IV** 600 mg q6h plus gentamicin or 900 mg q8h

Bacterial endocarditis prophylaxis

Adult: 600 mg 1 hr before procedure

Available forms: Phosphate: inj 150, 300, 600 mg base/4 ml; 900 mg base/ml; inj inf in D_5 300, 600, 900 mg; HCl: caps 75, 150, 300 mg; palmitate: oral sol 75 mg/5 ml

Adverse effects

GI: *Nausea, vomiting, abdominal pain, diarrhea,* **pseudomembranous colitis,** *anorexia, weight loss,* increased AST, ALT, bilirubin, alkaline phosphatase, jaundice

GU: *Vaginitis,* urinary frequency

HEMA: **Leukopenia, eosinophilia, agranulocytosis, thrombocytopenia, polyarthritis**

INTEG: Rash, urticaria, pruritus, erythema, pain, abscess at inj site

Contraindications: Hypersensitivity to this drug or lincomycin, tartrazine dye, ulcerative colitis/enteritis

Precautions: Pregnancy **B,** renal disease, liver disease, GI disease, elderly, lactation, tartrazine sensitivity

Pharmacokinetics

Absorption	Well absorbed (PO, IM), minimal (top)
Distribution	Widely distributed; crosses placenta
Metabolism	Liver, extensively
Excretion	Kidneys, breast milk
Half-life	2½ hr

Pharmacodynamics

	PO	IM	IV	TOP	VAG
Onset	Rapid	Rapid	Rapid	Rapid	Rapid
Peak	½-1 hr	1½ hr	Infusion's end	Unknown	Unknown

Interactions

Individual drugs

Erythromycin: decreased action of clindamycin

Kaolin: decreased absorption

Drug classifications

Neuromuscular blockers: increased neuromuscular blockade

Drug/herb

Acidophilus: do not use with antiinfectives

Drug/lab test

Increased: alkaline phosphatase, bilirubin, CPK, AST, ALT

NURSING CONSIDERATIONS

Assessment

- Assess any patient with compromised renal system; drug is excreted slowly in poor renal system function; toxicity may occur rapidly
- Assess patient for signs and symptoms of infection including characteristics of wounds, sputum, urine, stool, WBC >10,000/mm^3, fever; obtain baseline information before and during treatment
- Complete C&S testing before beginning drug therapy; this will identify if correct treatment has been initiated
- Assess for allergic reactions: rash, urticaria, pruritus, chills, fever, joint pain; may occur a few days after therapy begins; epINEPHrine and resuscitation equipment should be available in case of an anaphylactic reaction
- Identify urine output; if decreasing, notify prescriber (may indicate nephrotoxicity); also look for increased BUN and creatinine levels
- Monitor blood studies: AST, ALT, CBC, Hct, bilirubin, LDH, alkaline phosphatase, Coombs' test monthly if patient is on long-term therapy
- Monitor electrolytes: potassium, sodium, chloride monthly if patient is on long-term therapy
- Assess bowel pattern daily; if severe diarrhea occurs, drug should be discontinued; may indicate pseudomembranous colitis
- Monitor for bleeding: ecchymosis, bleeding gums, hematuria, stool guaiac daily if on long-term therapy
- Assess for overgrowth of infection: perineal itching, fever, malaise, redness, pain, swelling, drainage, rash, diarrhea, change in cough, sputum

Nursing diagnoses

- Infection, risk for (uses)
- Diarrhea (adverse reactions)
- Injury, risk for (adverse reaction)
- Knowledge, deficient (teaching)
- Noncompliance (teaching)

Implementation

PO route

- Do not break, crush, or chew caps
- Give with 8 oz of water; give with meals for GI symptoms
- Shake liquids well
- Do not refrigerate oral preparations; stable at room temperature for 2 wk

IM route

- If more than 600 mg must be given, divide into 2 inj
- Give deeply in large muscle mass; rotate sites

Topical route

- Avoid contact with eyes, mucous membranes, and open cuts during topical application; if accidental contact occurs, rinse with cool water
- Wash affected areas with warm water and soap, rinse, pat dry before application

IV route

- Give by inf only; do not administer bolus dose; dilute 300 mg or more/50 ml or more of D_5W, 0.9% NaCl
- May be further diluted in greater amounts of D_5W, 0.9% NaCl and given as a cont inf in acute PID; give first dose 10 mg/min over ½ hr, then 0.75 mg/min; increased rates may be used to keep serum blood levels higher; run over >10 min; no more than 1200 mg in a 1 hr inf

Syringe compatibilities: Amikacin, aztreonam, gentamicin, heparin

Syringe incompatibilities: Tobramycin

Y-site compatibilities: Amifostine, amiodarone, amphotericin B cholesteryl, amsacrine, aztreonam, cisatracurium, cyclophosphamide, diltiazem, DOXOrubicin liposome, enalaprilat, esmolol, fludarabine, foscarnet, granisetron, heparin, hydromorphone, labetolol, magnesium sulfate, melphalan, meperidine, midazolam, morphine, multivitamins, odansetron, perphenazine, piperacillin/tazobactam, propofol, remifentanil, sargramostim, tacrolimus, teniposide, theophylline, thiotepa, vinorelbine, vit B/C, zidovudine

Y-site incompatibilities: Idarubicin

Additive compatibilities: Amikacin, ampicillin, aztreonam, cefamandole, cefazolin, cefepine, cefonicid, cefoperazone, cefotaxime, cefoxitin, ceftazidime, ceftizoxime, cefuroxime, cephalothin, cimetidine, fluconazole, heparin, hydrocortisone, kanamycin, methylPREDNISolone, metoclopramide, metronidazole, netilmicin, ofloxacin, penicillin G, pipercillin, potassium chloride, sodium bicarbonate, tobramycin, verapamil, vit B/C

Additive incompatibilities: Ciprofloxacin

Patient/family education

- Tell patient to take oral drug with full glass of water; may take with food if GI symptoms occur; antiperistaltic drugs may worsen diarrhea
- Teach patient aspects of drug therapy: need to complete entire course of medication to ensure organism death (10-14 days); culture may be taken after medication course has been completed

- Advise patient to report sore throat, fever, fatigue; may indicate superimposed infection
- Advise patient that drug must be taken at equal intervals around clock to maintain blood levels

Evaluation
Positive therapeutic outcome
- Decreased temperature, negative C&S

Treatment of hypersensitivity: Withdraw drug; maintain airway; administer epINEPHrine, aminophylline, O_2, **IV** corticosteroids

clomiPHENE (Rx)
(kloe'mi-feen)
Clomid, clomiPHENE citrate, Milophene, Serophene
Func. class.: Ovulation stimulant
Chem. class.: Nonsteroidal antiestrogenic
Pregnancy category X

Do Not Confuse:
clomiPHENE/clomiPRAMINE

Action: Increases LH, FSH release from the pituitary, which increases maturation of ovarian follicle, ovulation, development of corpus luteum

Therapeutic Outcome: Pregnancy

Uses: Female infertility (ovulatory failure)

Dosage and routes
Adult: PO 50-100 mg daily × 5 days or 50-100 mg daily beginning on day 5 of cycle; may be repeated until conception occurs or 3 cycles of therapy have been completed

Available forms: Tabs 50 mg

Adverse effects
CNS: *Headache, depression,* restlessness, anxiety, nervousness, fatigue, insomnia, dizziness, flushing
CV: Vasomotor flushing, phlebitis, **deep vein thrombosis**
EENT: Blurred vision, diplopia, photophobia
GI: *Nausea, vomiting, constipation,* abdominal pain, bloating
GU: Polyuria, frequency of urination, **birth defects, spontaneous abortions,** multiple ovulation, breast pain, oliguria, abnormal uterine bleeding
INTEG: *Rash, dermatitis,* urticaria, alopecia

Contraindications: Pregnancy **X,** hypersensitivity, hepatic disease, undiagnosed uterine bleeding, uncontrolled thyroid or adrenal dysfunction, intracranial lesion, ovarian cysts

Precautions: Hypertension, depression, seizures, diabetes mellitus

Pharmacokinetics
Absorption	Well distributed
Distribution	Unknown
Metabolism	Liver, extensively
Excretion	Feces
Half-life	5 days

Pharmacodynamics
Unknown

Interactions: None
Drug/lab test
Increased: FSH/LH, BSP, thyroxine, TBG

NURSING CONSIDERATIONS
Assessment
- Determine liver function tests before therapy: AST, ALT, alkaline phosphatase
- Monitor serum progesterone, urinary excretion of pregnanediol to identify occurrence of ovulation
- Pelvic examination should be done to determine ovarian size, cervical condition
- Endometrial biopsy may be done in women over 35 to rule out endometrial carcinoma

Nursing diagnoses
- Sexual dysfunction (uses)
- Knowledge, deficient (teaching)

Implementation
- Give after discontinuing estrogen therapy
- Give at same time daily to maintain drug level; begin on 5th day of menstrual cycle

Patient/family education
- Advise patient that multiple births are common after drug is taken
- Instruct patient to notify prescriber immediately if low abdominal pain occurs; may indicate ovarian cyst, cyst rupture
- Advise patient to notify prescriber of photophobia, blurred vision, diplopia, abnormal bleeding, hot flashes, nausea, vomiting, headache
- Teach patient if dose is missed, double at next time; if more than one dose is missed, call prescriber
- Instruct patient that response usually occurs 4-10 days after last day of treatment
- Teach patient method for taking, recording basal body temp to determine whether ovulation has occurred; if ovulation can be deter-

mined (there is a slight decrease in temp, then a sharp increase for ovulation), to attempt coitus 3 days before and every other day until after ovulation
- Teach patient if pregnancy is suspected, to notify prescriber immediately

Evaluation

Positive therapeutic outcome
- Fertility

clomiPRAMINE (Rx)

(klom-ip'ra-meen)

Anafranil

Func. class.: Tricyclic antidepressant

Chem. class.: Tertiary amine

Pregnancy category C

Do Not Confuse: clomiPRAMINE/clomiPHENE, clomiPRAMINE/desipramine/norpramin

Action: Potent inhibitor of serotonin and norepinephrine uptake; also increases dopamine metabolism

Therapeutic Outcome: Decreased signs and symptoms of obsessive-compulsive disorder, decreased depression

Uses: Obsessive-compulsive disorder, depression, dysphoria, anxiety, agoraphobia and other phobias

Dosage and routes

Obsessive-compulsive disorder

Adult: PO 25 mg at bedtime; increase gradually over 4 wk to a dosage of 75-250 mg/day in divided doses

Child 10-18 yr: PO 25-50 mg/day gradually increased or 3 mg/kg/day, whichever is smaller; not to exceed 200 mg/day

Depression

Adult: PO 50-150 mg/day in a single or divided dose

Anxiety/agoraphobia

Adult: PO 25-75 mg/day

Available forms: Caps 25, 50, 75 mg

Adverse effects

CNS: *Dizziness, tremors, mania,* **seizures,** aggressiveness, drowsiness, headache, extrapyramidal symptoms (EPS)

CV: Hypotension, tachycardia, **cardiac arrest**

EENT: Blurred vision

ENDO: Galactorrhea, hyperprolactinemia

GI: *Constipation, dry mouth, nausea, dyspepsia,* weight gain

GU: *Delayed ejaculation, anorgasmia,* retention, decreased libido

HEMA: **Agranulocytosis, neutropenia, pancytopenia**

INTEG: Diaphoresis, photosensitivity

META: Hyponatremia

Contraindications: Hypersensitivity, immediately after MI

Precautions: Pregnancy **C,** seizures, suicidal patients, elderly, cardiac disease, lactation

Pharmacokinetics

Absorption	Well absorbed
Distribution	Widely distributed
Metabolism	Liver, extensively
Excretion	Kidneys, breast milk
Half-life	19-37 hr; steady state 1-2 wk

Pharmacodynamics

Onset	≥2 wk
Peak	2-6 hr

Interactions

Individual drugs

Alcohol: increased CNS depression

Carbamazepine: decreased clomiPRAMINE action

Cimetidine, fluoxetine, fluvoxamine, sertraline: increased clomiPRAMINE level; do not use together

Clonidine, epINEPHrine, norepinephrine: severe hypertension; avoid use

Phenytoin: decreased clomiPRAMINE action

Drug classifications

Barbiturates: decreased clomiPRAMINE levels

CNS depressants: increased effects; do not use together

MAOIs: hypertensive crisis, seizures; do not use together

Drug/herb

SAM-e, St. John's wort: serotonin syndrome, do not use together

Belladonna, corkwood, henbane leaf, jimsonweed: increased anticholinergic effect

Hops, kava, lavender: increased sedative effect

Scopolia: increased clomiPRAMINE effect

Drug/lab test

Increased: prolactin, TBG, serum thyroid hormones

NURSING CONSIDERATIONS

Assessment

- Monitor B/P (with patient lying, standing), pulse q4h; if systolic B/P drops 20 mm Hg hold drug, notify prescriber; take VS q4h in patients with cardiovascular disease

- Monitor blood studies: CBC, leukocytes, differential, cardiac enzymes if patient is receiving long-term therapy
- Monitor hepatic studies: AST, ALT, bilirubin
- Check weight weekly; appetite may increase with drug
- Assess ECG for flattening of T wave, QTc prolongation bundle branch block, AV block, dysrhythmias in cardiac patients
- Assess for EPS primarily in elderly: rigidity, dystonia, akathisia
- Assess mental status: mood, sensorium, affect, suicidal tendencies; increase in psychiatric symptoms: depression, panic, frequency of obsessive-compulsive behaviors
- Monitor urinary retention, constipation; constipation is more likely to occur in children or elderly
- Assess for withdrawal symptoms: headache, nausea, vomiting, muscle pain, weakness; do not usually occur unless drug was discontinued abruptly
- Identify alcohol consumption; if alcohol is consumed, hold dose until morning

Nursing diagnoses
- Coping, ineffective (uses)
- Injury, risk for physical (side effects)
- Knowledge, deficient (teaching)
- Noncompliance (teaching)

Implementation
- Do not break, crush, or chew caps
- Give with food or milk for GI symptoms
- Store at room temp; do not freeze

Patient/family education
- Teach patient that therapeutic effects may take 2-3 wk
- Teach patient to use caution in driving or other activities requiring alertness because of drowsiness, dizziness, blurred vision; to avoid rising quickly from sitting to standing, especially elderly
- Teach patient to avoid alcohol ingestion, other CNS depressants
- Teach patient not to discontinue medication quickly after long-term use: may cause nausea, headache, malaise
- Teach patient to wear sunscreen or large hat, since photosensitivity occurs
- Teach patient to increase fluids, bulk in diet if constipation, urinary retention occur, especially elderly
- Teach patient to take gum, hard sugarless candy, or frequent sips of water for dry mouth
- Advise patient to notify prescriber if pregnancy is planned or suspected

Evaluation
Positive therapeutic outcome
- Decrease in depression
- Absence of suicidal thoughts

Treatment of overdose: ECG monitoring, induce emesis, lavage, activated charcoal, administer anticonvulsant

clonazepam (Rx)
(kloe-na'zi-pam)

Klonopin, Rivotril, Syn-Clonazepam ✦

Func. class.: Anticonvulsant

Chem. class.: Benzodiazepine derivative

Pregnancy category C

Controlled substance schedule IV

Do Not Confuse:
Klonopin/clonidine
clonazepam/lorazepam/clorazepate

Action: Inhibits spike, wave formation in absence seizures (petit mal), decreases amplitude, frequency, duration, spread of discharge in minor motor seizures

Therapeutic Outcome: Decreased frequency, severity of seizures

Uses: Absence, atypical absence, akinetic, myoclonic seizures, Lennox-Gastaut syndrome

Investigational uses: Parkinsonian dysarthrias, acute mania, adjunct in schizophrenia, neuralgias, multifocal tic disorders, restless legs syndrome, rectal administration

Dosage and routes
Adult: PO not to exceed 1.5 mg/day in 3 divided doses; may be increased 0.5-1 mg q3 days until desired response; not to exceed 20 mg/day; rec 0.02 mg/kg

Child<10 yr or 30 kg: PO 0.01-0.03 mg/kg/day in divided doses q8h, not to exceed 0.05 mg/kg/day; may be increased 0.25-0.5 mg q3 days until desired response; not to exceed 0.1-0.2 mg/kg/day; rec 0.05-0.1 mg/kg

Elderly: PO 0.25 daily bid initially, increase by 0.25 daily q7-14 days as needed

Available forms: Tabs 0.5, 1, 2 mg; oral susp; **IV** sol

Adverse effects
CNS: *Drowsiness,* dizziness, confusion, behavioral changes, tremors, insomnia, headache, **suicidal tendencies,** slurred speech

CV: Palpitations, bradycardia, tachycardia

EENT: *Increased salivation, nystagmus, diplopia,* abnormal eye movements

GI: *Nausea, constipation,* polyphagia, anorexia, xerostomia, diarrhea, gastritis, sore gums
GU: Dysuria, enuresis, nocturia, retention, libido changes
HEMA: **Thrombocytopenia, leukocytosis, eosinophilia**
INTEG: Rash, alopecia, hirsutism
RESP: **Respiratory depression,** dyspnea, congestion

Contraindications: Hypersensitivity to benzodiazepines, acute narrow-angle glaucoma, psychosis, severe liver disease

Precautions: Pregnancy **C,** open-angle glaucoma, chronic respiratory disease, renal/hepatic disease, elderly, lactation

Pharmacokinetics

Absorption	Well absorbed
Distribution	Crosses blood-brain barrier, placenta
Metabolism	Liver
Excretion	Kidneys
Half-life	18-50 hr

Pharmacodynamics

Onset	½-1 hr
Peak	1-2 hr
Duration	6-12 hr

Interactions
Individual drugs
Alcohol: increased CNS depression
Carbamazepine: decreased effectiveness
Phenobarbitol: decreased clonazepam effect
Phenytoin: decreased clonazepam levels

Drug classifications
Antidepressants, anticonvulsants, barbiturates, general anesthetics, opiates, sedative/hypnotics: increased CNS depression
Barbiturates: decreased effect of clonazepam

Drug/herb
Ginkgo: increased clonazepam effect
Ginseng, santonica: decreased clonazepam effect
Kava: increased sedative effect

Drug/lab test
Increased: AST, alkaline phosphatase

NURSING CONSIDERATIONS
Assessment
- Assess mental status: mood, sensorium, affect, memory (long, short), especially elderly
- Assess for blood dyscrasias: fever, sore throat, bruising, rash, jaundice, epistaxis (long-term treatment only)
- Assess seizure activity including type, location, duration, and character; provide seizure precaution
- Assess renal studies: urinalysis, BUN, urine creatinine
- Monitor blood studies: RBCs, Hct, Hgb, reticulocyte counts weekly for 4 wk then monthly
- Monitor hepatic studies: ALT, AST, bilirubin, creatinine
- Monitor drug levels during initial treatment
- Assess for signs of physical withdrawal if medication suddenly discontinued
- Assess eye problems: need for ophthalmic examinations before, during, after treatment (slit lamp, fundoscopy, tonometry)
- Assess allergic reaction: red raised rash; if this occurs, drug should be discontinued
- Monitor for toxicity: bone marrow depression, nausea, vomiting, ataxia, diplopia, cardiovascular collapse

Nursing diagnoses
- Injury, risk for (side effects)
- Knowledge, deficient (teaching)

Implementation
PO route
- Give on empty stomach for best absorption

Rectal route
- **IV** sol may be used rectally, 1 ml syringe inserted 3 cm into rectum
- Oral susp may be used rectally (1 mg/ml of drug with 1 ml of water), use plastic tube (volume 2.2-3.3 ml)

Patient/family education
- Teach patient to carry/wear emergency ID card stating patient's name, drugs taken, condition, physician's name, phone number
- Caution patient to avoid driving, other activities that require alertness
- Caution patient to avoid alcohol ingestion or CNS depressants; increased sedation may occur
- Teach patient not to discontinue medication quickly after long-term use; taper off over several weeks

Evaluation
Positive therapeutic outcome
- Decreased seizure activity

Treatment of overdose: Lavage, activated charcoal, VS, monitor electrolytes

clonidine (Rx)

(klon'i-deen)

Catapres, Catapres-TTS, clonidine HCl, Dixarit ✤, Duraclon

Func. class.: Antihypertensive, centrally acting analgesic

Chem. class.: Centrally acting α-adrenergic agonist

Pregnancy category C

Do Not Confuse:
Catapres/Cataflam/catarase
clonidine/Klonopin/clonazepam

Action: Inhibits sympathetic vasomotor center in CNS, which reduces impulses in sympathetic nervous system; B/P, pulse rate, cardiac output decreased; prevents pain signal transmission in CNS by α-adrenergic receptor stimulation of the spinal cord

Therapeutic Outcome: Decreased B/P in hypertension

Uses: Mild to moderate hypertension; used alone or in combination

Investigational uses: Opioid withdrawal, prevention of vascular headaches, treatment of menopausal symptoms, dysmenorrhea, attention deficit hyperactivity disorder (ADHD)

Dosage and routes

Hypertension

Adult: PO/trans 0.1 mg bid, then increase by 0.1-0.2 mg/day at weekly intervals, until desired response; range 0.2-0.6 mg/day in divided doses

Elderly: PO 0.1 mg at bedtime, may increase gradually

Child: PO 5-10 mcg/kg/day in divided doses q8-12h, max 0.9 mg/day

Opioid withdrawal (unlabeled use)

Adult: PO 0.3-1.2 mg/day; may decrease by 50% × 3 days then decrease by 0.1-0.2 mg/day or discontinue

Severe pain

Adult: Cont epidural inf 30 mcg/hr

Child: Cont epidural inf 0.5 mcg/kg/hr, then titrate to response

Menopausal symptoms (unlabeled use)

Adult: TD 0.1 mg patch q1 wk; PO 0.05-0.4 mg daily

ADHD (unlabeled use)

Child: PO 5 mcg/kg/day in 3-4 divided doses × 8 wk

Available forms: Tabs 0.025 ✤, 0.1, 0.2, 0.3 mg; trans sys 2.5, 5, 7.5 mg delivering 0.1, 0.2, 0.3 mg/24 hr, respectively; inj 100, 500 mcg/ml

Adverse effects

CNS: *Drowsiness, sedation, headache, fatigue,* nightmares, insomnia, mental changes, anxiety, depression, hallucinations, delirium

CV: *Orthostatic hypotension, palpitations,* **CHF**, ECG abnormalities

EENT: Taste change, parotid pain

ENDO: Hyperglycemia

GI: *Nausea, vomiting, malaise,* constipation, *dry mouth*

GU: Impotence, dysuria, *nocturia,* gynecomastia

INTEG: *Rash,* alopecia, facial pallor, pruritus, hives, edema, burning papules, excoriation (trans patches)

MISC: *Withdrawal symptoms*

MS: Muscle, joint pain, leg cramps

Contraindications: Hypersensitivity; (epidural) bleeding disorders, anticoagulants

Precautions: Pregnancy **C**, MI (recent), diabetes mellitus, chronic renal failure, Raynaud's disease, thyroid disease, depression, COPD, child<12 yr (transdermal), asthma, lactation, elderly, noncompliant patients

Pharmacokinetics

Absorption	Well absorbed (PO, trans)
Distribution	Widely distributed; crosses blood-brain barrier
Metabolism	Liver, extensively
Excretion	Kidneys, unchanged (30%)
Half-life	12-21 hr

Pharmacodynamics

	PO	TD
Onset	½-1 hr	3 days
Peak	2-4 hr	Unknown
Duration	8-12 hr	8 hr (after removal)

Interactions

Individual drugs

Alcohol: increased CNS depression
Levodopa: decreased levodopa effect
Prazosin: decreased hypotensive effects
Verapamil: AV block

Drug classifications

Amphetamines, appetite suppressants, MAOIs, tricyclics: decreased hypotensive effects
Anesthetics, opiates, sedatives/hypnotics: increased CNS depression

Antidepressants (tricyclic), β-adrenergic blockers: life-threatening increase in B/P
Diuretics, nitrates: increased hypotensive effects

Drug/herb

Aconite: increased toxicity, death
Astragalus, capsicum peppers, cola tree, coltsfoot, guarana, khat, licorice: decreased antihypertensive effect
Barberry, betony, black catechu, black cohosh, bloodroot, broom, burdock, cat's claw, dandelion, goldenseal, Irish moss, Jamaican dogwood, kelp, khella, mistletoe, parsley, Queen Anne's lace, rue: increased antihypertensive effect

Drug/lab test

Increased: blood glucose
Decreased: VMA, urinary catecholamines, aldosterone

NURSING CONSIDERATIONS

Assessment

- Assess pain: location, intensity, character, alleviating, aggravation factors, baseline and frequency
- Perform blood studies: neutrophils, decreased platelets
- Perform renal studies: protein, BUN, creatinine; watch for increased levels that may indicate nephrotic syndrome: polyuria, oliguria, frequency
- Monitor baselines for renal, liver function tests before therapy begins; check potassium levels, although hyperkalemia rarely occurs
- Monitor B/P, pulse if the drug is being used for hypertension; notify prescriber of changes
- Assess for opiate withdrawal in patients receiving the drug for opioid withdrawal, including fever, diarrhea, nausea, vomiting, cramps, insomnia, shivering, dilated pupils, weakness
- Check for edema in feet, legs daily; monitor I&O; check for decreasing output
- Note allergic reaction: rash, fever, pruritus, urticaria; drug should be discontinued if antihistamines fail to help
- Note allergic reaction from patches: rash, urticaria, angioedema; should not continue to use
- Assess for symptoms of CHF: edema, dyspnea, wet crackles, B/P, weight gain, report significant changes

Nursing diagnoses

- Injury, risk for physical (side effects)
- Knowledge, deficient (teaching)
- Noncompliance (teaching)

Implementation

PO route

- Give last dose at bedtime

Transdermal route

- Apply patch weekly; remove old patch and wash off residue; apply to site without hair; best absorption over chest or upper arm; rotate sites with each application; clean site before application; apply firmly, especially around edges
- Store patches in cool environment, tabs in tight container

Patient/family education

- Instruct patient not to discontinue drug abruptly, or withdrawal symptoms may occur: anxiety, increased B/P, headache, insomnia, increased pulse, tremors, nausea, sweating
- Caution patient not to use OTC (cough, cold, or allergy) products unless directed by prescriber
- Teach patient to comply with dosage schedule even if feeling better; drug controls symptoms, does not cure
- Caution patient to change position slowly, to rise slowly to sitting or standing position to minimize orthostatic hypotension, especially elderly
- Instruct patient to notify physician of mouth sores, sore throat, fever, swelling of hands or feet, irregular heartbeat, chest pain, signs of angioedema, increased weight
- Teach patient about excessive perspiration, dehydration, vomiting; diarrhea may lead to fall in B/P; consult prescriber if these occur
- Tell patient that drug may cause dizziness, fainting; light-headedness may occur during 1st few days of therapy; use hard candy, saliva product, or frequent rinsing of mouth for dry mouth
- Advise patient that compliance is necessary; not to skip or stop drug unless directed by prescriber
- Teach patient that drug may cause skin rash or impaired perspiration
- Teach patient that response may take 2-3 days if drug is given TD; instruct on administration of patch; return demonstration
- Teach patient to avoid hazardous activities, since drug may cause drowsiness, dizziness
- Teach patient to administer 1 hr ac

Evaluation

Positive therapeutic outcome

- Decrease in B/P in hypertension
- Decrease in withdrawal symptoms
- Decrease in pain
- Decrease in vascular headaches
- Decrease in dysmenorrhea
- Decrease in menopausal symptoms

Treatment of overdose: Supportive treatment; administer tolazoline, atropine, DOPamine prn

clopidogrel (Rx)
(klo-pid'oh-grel)
Plavix
Func. class.: Platelet aggregation inhibitor
Chem. class.: Thienopyridine derivative
Pregnancy category B

Action: Inhibits first and second phases of ADP-induced effects in platelet aggregation

Therapeutic Outcome: Decreased possibility of stroke, MI by decreasing platelet aggregation

Uses: Reducing the risk of stroke, MI, peripheral arterial disease in high-risk patients, acute coronary syndrome

Dosage and routes
Adult: PO 75 mg daily with or without food

Acute coronary syndrome
Adult: PO 300 mg then 75 mg daily

Available forms: Tabs 75 mg

Adverse effects
CNS: Headache, dizziness, depression, syncope, hyperesthesia, neuralgia
CV: Edema, hypertension
GI: Nausea, vomiting, diarrhea, GI discomfort, **GI bleeding**
HEMA: *Epistaxis,* purpura, **bleeding, neutropenia**
INTEG: Rash, pruritus
MISC: UTI, hypercholesterolemia, chest pain, fatigue, **intracranial hemorrhage**
MS: Arthralgia, back pain
RESP: Upper respiratory tract infection, dyspnea, rhinitis, bronchitis, cough

Contraindications: Hypersensitivity, active bleeding

Precautions: Pregnancy **B,** past liver disease, lactation, children, increased bleeding risk, neutropenia, agranulocytosis

Pharmacokinetics

Absorption	Rapidly absorbed
Distribution	Unknown
Metabolism	Liver, extensively, protein binding 95%
Excretion	Kidneys, unchanged drug
Half-life	8 hr

Pharmacodynamics

Onset	Unknown
Peak	1-3 hr
Duration	Unknown

Interactions
Individual drugs
Abciximab, aspirin, eptifibatide, ticlopidine, tirofiban: increased bleeding tendencies
Fluvastatin, phenytoin, tamoxifen, TOLBUTamide, torsemide, warfarin: increased action of each specific drug

Drug classifications
Anticoagulants, NSAIDs, thrombolytics: increased bleeding tendencies
NSAIDs: increased action of some NSAIDs

Drug/herb
Agrimony, alfalfa, angelica, anise, basil, bay, bilberry, black haw, bogbean, bromelain, buchu, chondroitin, cinchona bark, dong quai, fenugreek, feverfew, garlic, ginger, ginkgo, ginseng, horse chestnut, Irish moss, kelp, kelpware, khella, lovage, lungwort, meadowsweet, motherwort, mugwort, nettle, papaya, parsley (large amounts), pau d'arco, pineapple, poplar, prickly ash, safflower, saw palmetto, tonka bean, turmeric, wintergreen, yarrow: increased risk of bleeding
Chamomile, coenzyme Q10, flax, glucomannan, goldenseal, guar gum: decreased anticoagulant effect

NURSING CONSIDERATIONS
Assessment
- Assess for symptoms of stroke, MI during treatment
- Monitor liver function studies: AST, ALT, bilirubin, creatinine if patient is on long-term therapy (4 mo or more)
- Monitor blood studies: CBC, Hct, Hgb, protime, cholesterol if patient is on long-term therapy; thrombocytopenia, neutropenia may occur

Nursing diagnoses
- Injury, risk for (uses)
- Knowledge, deficient (teaching)

Implementation
- Give with food to decrease gastric symptoms

Patient/family education
- Advise patient that blood work will be necessary during treatment
- Advise patient to report any unusual bleeding to prescriber, that it may take longer to stop bleeding
- Instruct patient to take with food or just after eating to minimize GI discomfort

- Caution patient to report diarrhea, skin rashes, subcutaneous bleeding, chills, fever, sore throat
- Teach patient to tell all health care providers that clopidogrel is used

Evaluation

Positive therapeutic outcome

- Absence of stroke

clorazepate (Rx)

(klor-az′e-pate)

APO-Clorazepate ✤, clorazepate, Novo-Clopate ✤, Tranxene-SD, Tranxene-SD Half Strength, Tranxene T-tab

Func. class.: Antianxiety, anticonvulsant, sedative/hypnotic

Chem. class.: Benzodiazepine

Pregnancy category D

Controlled substance schedule IV

Do Not Confuse:

clorazapate/clonazepam

Action: Potentiates the actions of GABA; especially in limbic system, reticular formation has anticonvulsant effects

Therapeutic Outcome: Decreased anxiety, restlessness, insomnia

Uses: Anxiety, acute alcohol withdrawal, adjunct in seizure disorders

Dosage and routes

Anxiety

Adult: PO 15-60 mg/day or 7.5-15 mg 2-4×/day; ext rel 11.25-22.5 mg at bedtime, do not use ext rel to initiate therapy

Elderly: PO 7.5 mg daily bid

Alcohol withdrawal

Adult: PO 30 mg then day 1, 30-60 mg in divided doses; day 2, 45-90 mg in divided doses; day 3, 22.5-45 mg in divided doses; day 4, 15-30 mg in divided doses; then gradually reduce daily dose to 7.5-15 mg

Seizure disorders

Adult and child>12 yr: PO 7.5 mg tid; may increase by 7.5 mg/wk or less, not to exceed 90 mg/day

Child 9-12 yr: PO 3.75-7.5 mg bid; may increase by 3.75 mg/wk or less, not to exceed 60 mg/day

Available forms: Tabs 3.75, 7.5, 15 mg; ext rel tab (Tranxene SD Half Strength) 11.25 mg, (Tranxene SD) 22.5 mg

Adverse effects

CNS: *Dizziness, drowsiness,* confusion, headache, anxiety, tremors, stimulation, fatigue, depression, insomnia, hallucinations, lethargy

CV: *Orthostatic hypotension,* **ECG changes, tachycardia,** hypotension, chest pain

EENT: *Blurred vision,* tinnitus, mydriasis

GI: Constipation, dry mouth, nausea, vomiting, anorexia, diarrhea

INTEG: Rash, dermatitis, itching

Contraindications: Pregnancy **D,** hypersensitivity to benzodiazepines, narrow-angle glaucoma, psychosis, lactation, child<9 yr

Precautions: Elderly, debilitated, hepatic disease, renal disease

Pharmacokinetics	
Absorption	Well absorbed
Distribution	Widely distributed; crosses placenta
Metabolism	Liver
Excretion	Kidneys, breast milk
Half-life	30-100 hr

Pharmacodynamics	
Onset	1 hr
Peak	1-2 hr
Duration	Up to 24 hr

Interactions

Individual drugs

Alcohol: increased CNS depression

Cimetidine, disulfiram, fluoxetine, isoniazid, ketoconazole, propoxyphene, valproic acid: increased effects of clorazepate

Rifampin: decreased action of clorazepate

Drug classifications

Antidepressants, β-blockers (some), MAOIs, oral contraceptives: increased clorazepate action

Barbiturates: decreased clorazepate effect

CNS depressants: increased CNS depression

Drug/herb

Catnip, chamomile, clary, cowslip, kava, mistletoe, nettle, pokeweed, poppy, senega, Queen Anne's lace, valerian: increased CNS depression

Black cohosh: increased hypotension

Drug/lab test

Increased: AST/ALT

Decreased: HCT

NURSING CONSIDERATIONS

Assessment

- Assess seizures: duration, location, intensity, aura

• Monitor B/P (with patient lying, standing), pulse; if systolic B/P drops 20 mm Hg, hold drug, notify prescriber
• Monitor blood studies: CBC during long-term therapy; blood dyscrasias have occurred rarely
• Monitor hepatic studies: AST, ALT, bilirubin, creatinine, LDH, alkaline phosphatase
• Monitor I&O; may indicate renal dysfunction
• Monitor mental status: mood, sensorium, affect, sleeping pattern, drowsiness, dizziness, physical dependency; withdrawal symptoms: headache, nausea, vomiting, muscle pain, weakness after long-term use; suicidal tendencies

Nursing diagnoses
• Coping, ineffective (uses)
• Knowledge, deficient (teaching)
• Noncompliance (teaching)

Implementation
• Give with food or milk for GI symptoms
• Use sugarless gum, hard candy, frequent sips of water for dry mouth
• Check to see PO medication has been swallowed

Patient/family education
• Teach patient that drug may be taken with food
• Teach patient not to use for everyday stress or longer than 4 mo, unless directed by a prescriber; not to take more than prescribed amount; may be habit forming
• Caution patient to avoid OTC preparations unless approved by a prescriber
• Caution patient to avoid driving, activities that require alertness; drowsiness may occur, especially in elderly
• Advise patient to avoid alcohol ingestion or other psychotropic medications, unless prescribed
• Advise patient not to discontinue medication abruptly after long-term use; restlessness, insomnia, irritability may occur
• Advise patient to rise slowly or fainting may occur
• Teach patient that drowsiness may worsen at beginning of treatment

Evaluation
Positive therapeutic outcome
• Decreased anxiety, restlessness
• Decreased seizure activity

Treatment of overdose: Lavage, VS, supportive care, flumazenil

cloxacillin (Rx)
(klox-a-sill'in)

Apo-Cloxi ✤, cloxacillin, Cloxapen, Novo-cloxin ✤, Nu-Clox ✤, Orbenin ✤

Func. class.: Broad-spectrum antiinfective
Chem. class.: Penicillinase-resistant penicillin

Pregnancy category B

Action: Interferes with cell wall replication of susceptible organisms; the cell wall, rendered osmotically unstable, swells, bursts from osmotic pressure; resists the penicillinase action that inactivates penicillins

Therapeutic Outcome: Bactericidal effects for the following: gram-positive cocci *Staphylococcus aureus, Staphylococcus epidermidis,* penicillinase-producing staphylococci

Uses: Penicillinase-producing staphylococci, streptococci; respiratory tract, skin, skin structure infections; sinusitis

Dosage and routes
Adult: PO 1-4 g/day in divided doses q6h
Child: PO 50-100 mg/kg in divided doses q6h, max 4 g/day

Available forms: Caps 250, 500 mg; oral sol 125 mg/5 ml

Adverse effects
CNS: Lethargy, hallucinations, anxiety, depression, muscle twitching, **coma, seizures**
GI: *Nausea, vomiting, diarrhea,* increased AST, ALT, abdominal pain, glossitis, **pseudomembranous colitis,** colitis
GU: **Oliguria, proteinuria,** hematuria, *vaginitis, moniliasis,* **glomerulonephritis**
HEMA: Anemia, **increased bleeding time, bone marrow depression, granulocytopenia**
SYST: **Anaphylaxis, serum sickness**

Contraindications: Hypersensitivity to penicillins; neonates, severe renal, hepatic disease

Precautions: Pregnancy **B,** hypersensitivity to cephalosporins, lactation

Pharmacokinetics
Absorption	Moderate (35%-60%)
Distribution	Widely distributed; crosses placenta
Metabolism	Liver (up to 22%)
Excretion	Breast milk; kidneys, unchanged (30%-45%)
Half-life	0.5-1.1 hr, increased in hepatic/renal disease

Pharmacodynamics

Onset	½ hr
Peak	½-2 hr

Interactions

Individual drugs

Probenecid: increased cloxacillin concentrations; decreased renal excretion

Drug classifications

Anticoagulants (oral): increased anticoagulant effects

Drug/herb

Acidophilus: do not use with antiinfectives
Khat: decreased absorption, separate by ≥2 hr

Drug/food

Food, carbonated drinks, citrus fruit juices: decreased absorption

Drug/lab test

Decreased: uric acid
False positive: urine glucose, urine protein

NURSING CONSIDERATIONS

Assessment

- Assess patient for previous sensitivity reaction to penicillins or other cephalosporins; cross-sensitivity between penicillins and cephalosporins is common
- Assess patient for signs and symptoms of infection including characteristics of wounds, sputum, urine, stool, WBC >10,000/mm^3, fever; obtain baseline information and during treatment
- Obtain C&S before beginning drug therapy to identify if correct treatment has been initiated
- Assess for anaphylaxis: rash, urticaria, pruritus, chills, fever, joint pain may occur a few days after therapy begins; epINEPHrine and resuscitation equipment should be available for anaphylactic reaction
- (Alert) Identify urine output; if decreasing, notify prescriber (may indicate nephrotoxicity); also check for increased BUN, creatinine
- Monitor blood studies: AST, ALT, CBC, Hct, Hgb, bilirubin, LDH, alkaline phosphatase, Coombs' test monthly if patient is on long-term therapy
- Monitor electrolytes: potassium, sodium, chloride monthly if patient is on long-term therapy
- Assess bowel pattern daily; if severe diarrhea occurs, drug should be discontinued; may indicate pseudomembranous colitis
- Monitor for bleeding: ecchymosis, bleeding gums, hematuria, stool guaiac daily if on long-term therapy
- Assess for overgrowth of infection: perineal itching, fever, malaise, redness, pain, swelling, drainage, rash, diarrhea, change in cough, sputum

Nursing diagnoses

- Infection, risk for (uses)
- Diarrhea (side effects)
- Injury, risk for (side effects)
- Knowledge, deficient (teaching)
- Noncompliance (teaching)

Implementation

- Do not break, crush, or chew caps
- Give in even doses around the clock; if GI upset occurs, give with food; drug must be given for 10-14 days to ensure organism death and prevent superinfection; store in airtight container
- Shake susp well before each dose; store in refrigerator for 2 wk, 3 days at room temp

Patient/family education

- Teach patient to report sore throat, bruising, bleeding, joint pain; may indicate blood dyscrasias (rare)
- Advise patient to contact prescriber if vaginal itching, loose foul-smelling stools, furry tongue occur; may indicate superinfection
- Instruct patient to take all medications prescribed for the length of time ordered
- Advise patient to notify prescriber of diarrhea with blood or pus, which may indicate pseudomembranous colitis
- Advise patient to wear or carry emergency ID if allergic to penicillins

Evaluation

Positive therapeutic outcome

- Absence of signs/symptoms of infection (WBC <10,000/mm^3, temp WNL, absence of red, draining wounds)
- Reported improvement in symptoms of infection

Treatment of anaphylaxis: Withdraw drug, maintain airway, administer epINEPHrine, aminophylline, O_2, **IV** corticosteroids

clozapine (Rx)

(kloz'a-peen)

clozapine, Clozaril

Func. class.: Antipsychotic

Chem. class.: Tricyclic dibenzodiazepine derivative

Pregnancy category B

Do Not Confuse:

Clozaril/Clinoril/Colazal

Action: Interferes with dopamine receptor binding with lack of extrapyramidal symptoms and tardive dyskinesia; also acts as an adrenergic, cholinergic, histaminergic, serotonergic antagonist

Therapeutic Outcome: Decreased psychotic behavior

Uses: Management of psychotic symptoms in schizophrenic patients for whom other antipsychotics have failed

Dosage and routes

Adult: PO 12.5 mg daily or bid; may increase by 25-50 mg/day; normal range 300-450 mg/day after 2 wk; do not increase dosage more than 2 times/wk; do not exceed 900 mg/day; use lowest dosage to control symptoms

Available forms: Tabs 12.5, 25, 100 mg

Adverse effects

CNS: *Sedation, salivation, dizziness, headache, tremors, sleep problems, akinesia, fever,* **seizures,** *sweating, akathisia, confusion, fatigue, insomnia, depression, slurred speech, anxiety,* **neuroleptic malignant syndrome,** agitation

CV: *Tachycardia, hypotension, hypertension,* chest pain, ECG changes, orthostatic hypotension

EENT: Blurred vision

GI: *Drooling or excessive salivation, constipation, nausea, abdominal discomfort, vomiting, diarrhea,* anorexia, weight gain, dry mouth, heartburn, dyspepsia gastroesophageal reflux

GU: *Urinary abnormalities,* incontinence, ejaculation dysfunction, frequency, urgency, retention, dysuria

HEMA: **Leukopenia, neutropenia, agranulocytosis, eosinophilia**

MS: Weakness; pain in back, neck, legs; spasm; rigidity

RESP: Dyspnea, nasal congestion

OTHER: Diaphoresis

Contraindications: Hypersensitivity, myeloproliferative disorders, severe granulocytopenia (WBC <3500/mm^3 before therapy), CNS depression, coma, uncontrolled epilepsy

Precautions: Pregnancy **B,** lactation, children <16 yr, hepatic, renal, cardiac disease, seizures, prostatic enlargement, elderly, narrow-angle glaucoma

Pharmacokinetics	
Absorption	Well absorbed
Distribution	Widely distributed; crosses blood-brain barrier, placenta; 95% bound to plasma proteins
Metabolism	Liver
Excretion	Kidneys, feces (metabolites)
Half-life	8-12 hr

Pharmacodynamics	
Onset	Unknown
Peak	Steady state 2½ hr
Duration	4-12 hr

Interactions

Individual drugs

Alcohol: increased CNS depression
Carbamazepine, omeprazole, phenobarbitol, rifampin: decreased clozapine level
Caffeine, citalopram, erythromycin, fluoxetine, fluvoxamine, ketoconazole, risperidone, ritonaur, sertraline: increased clozapine levels
Digoxin: increased plasma concentration of digoxin
Warfarin: increased plasma concentrations

Drug classifications

Antihypertensives, nitrates: increased hypotension
Antineoplastics: increased bone marrow suppression
Benzodiazepines: increased hypotension, respiratory, cardiac arrest, collapse
CNS depressants, psychoactives: increased CNS depression
CYPIA2 inducers: decreased clozapine levels
CYP1A2 inhibiters, CYP3A4 inhibitors: increased clozapine level
Highly protein-bound drugs: increased plasma concentrations

Drug/herb

Kava, St. John's wort: increased CNS depression
Cola tree, hops, nettle, nutmeg: increased clozapine action
Betel palm, kava: increased extrapyramidal symptoms (EPS)

Drug/food

Caffeine: increased clozapine levels

Drug/lab test

Increased: liver function tests, cardiac enzymes, cholesterol, blood glucose, bilirubin, PBI, cholinesterase, ^{131}I
False positive: pregnancy tests, PKU
False negative: urinary steroids, 17-OHCS

NURSING CONSIDERATIONS

Assessment

- Assess mental status: orientation, mood, behavior, presence of hallucinations, and type before initial administration and monthly; this drug should significantly reduce psychotic behavior
- Check for swallowing of PO medication; check for hoarding or giving of medication to other patients
- Monitor I&O ratio, palpate bladder if low urinary output occurs, especially in elderly; urinalysis recommended before, during prolonged therapy
- Monitor bilirubin, CBC, liver function studies monthly; discontinue treatment if WBC $<3000/mm^3$ or if ANC $<1500/mm^3$; test qwk; may resume when normal; if WBC $<2000/mm^3$ or ANC $<1000/mm^3$, discontinue
- Assess affect, orientation, LOC, reflexes, gait, coordination, sleep pattern disturbances
- Monitor B/P with patient sitting, standing, and lying; take pulse and respirations q4h during initial treatment; establish baseline before starting treatment; report drops of 30 mm Hg
- Check for dizziness, faintness, palpitations, tachycardia on rising
- Assess for neuroleptic malignant syndrome: hyperpyrexia, muscle rigidity, increased CPK, altered mental status; drug should be discontinued
- Assess for EPS including akathisia (inability to sit still, no pattern to movements), tardive dyskinesia (bizarre movements of the jaw, mouth, tongue, extremities), pseudoparkinsonism (rigidity, tremors, pill rolling, shuffling gate)
- Assess for constipation, urinary retention daily; if these occur, increase bulk, water in diet

Nursing diagnoses

- Thought processes, disturbed (uses)
- Coping, ineffective (uses)
- Knowledge, deficient (teaching)
- Noncompliance (teaching)

Implementation

- Decrease dosage in elderly since metabolism is slowed
- Give with full glass of water, milk; or give with food to decrease GI upset
- Store in tight, light-resistant container; oral sol in amber bottle

Patient/family education

- Teach patient to use good oral hygiene; frequent rinsing of mouth, sugarless gum for dry mouth
- Caution patient to avoid hazardous activities until drug response is determined
- Inform patient that orthostatic hypotension occurs often and to rise from sitting or lying position gradually
- Caution patient to avoid hot tubs, hot showers, tub baths, since hypotension may occur
- Teach patient to avoid OTC preparations (cough, hay fever, cold) unless approved by prescriber, since serious drug interactions may occur; avoid use with alcohol, CNS depressants; increased drowsiness may occur
- Teach patient about EPS and necessity of meticulous oral hygiene, since oral candidiasis may occur
- Teach patient to report sore throat, malaise, fever, bleeding, mouth sores; if these occur, CBC should be performed and drug discontinued
- Advise patient that in hot weather, heat stroke may occur; take extra precautions to stay cool
- Teach patient symptoms of agranulocytosis and need for blood test qwk for 6 mo, then q2 wk; report flulike symptoms

Evaluation

Positive therapeutic outcome

- Decrease in emotional excitement, hallucinations, delusions, paranoia
- Reorganization of patterns of thought, speech

Treatment of anaphylaxis: Withdraw drug, maintain airway; if diabetic check blood glucose levels

! HIGH ALERT

coagulation factor VIIa, recombinant (Rx)

NovoSeven

Func. class.: Antihemophilic

Pregnancy category C

Action: Promotes hemostasis by activating the intrinsic pathway of coagulation

Uses: Bleeding in hemophilia A or B, with inhibitors to factor VIII or IX

Dosage and routes

Adult: **IV** bol 90 mcg/kg q2h until hemostasis occurs, or until therapy is deemed to be inadequate; posthemostatic doses q3-6h may be required

Available forms: Lyophilized powder 1.2 mg/vial (1200 mcg/vial); 4.8 mg/vial (4800

mcg/vial) recombinant human coagulation factor VIIa (rFVIIa)

Adverse effects

CNS: Fever, headache

INTEG: Pain, redness at inj site, pruritus, purpura, rash

SYST: **Hemorrhage not otherwise specified, hemarthrosis, fibrinogen plasma decreased,** hypertension, bradycardia, **DIC, coagulation disorder, thrombosis**

Contraindications: Hypersensitivity to this product or mouse, hamster, or bovine products

Precautions: Pregnancy **C,** lactation, children

Pharmacokinetics

Half-life	2-3 hr

Pharmacodynamics

Unknown

Interactions

Individual drugs

Activated prothrombin complex concentrate, prothrombin complex concentrate: do not use together

NURSING CONSIDERATIONS

Assessment

- Assess VS, B/P, pulse, respirations, neurologic signs, temp at least q4h, temperature 104° F (40° C) or indicators of internal bleeding, cardiac rhythm
- Monitor protime, APTT, plasma FVII clotting
- Monitor for thrombosis, dose should be reduced or stopped

Nursing diagnoses

- Tissue perfusion, ineffective (uses)
- Injury, risk for (uses, adverse reactions)

Implementation

IV route

- Bring to room temp; for 1.2 mg vial/2.2 ml sterile water for inj; 4.8 mg vial/8.5 ml sterile water for inj; remove caps from stopper, cleanse stopper with alcohol, allow to dry, draw back plunger of sterile syringe and allow air into syringe, insert needle of syringe into sterile water for inj, inject the air and withdraw amount required, insert syringe needle with diluent into drug vial, aim to side so liquid runs down vial wall, gently swirl until dissolved, use within 3 hr, give by bol over 3-5 min
- Do not admix, keep refrigerated until ready to use, avoid sunlight

Evaluation

Positive therapeutic outcome

- Therapeutic response: hemostasis

codeine (Rx)

(koe'deen)

Paveral ♣

Func. class.: Opiate, phenanthrene derivative

Pregnancy category C

Controlled substance schedule II, III, IV, V

(depends on route)

Do Not Confuse:

codeine/Lodine/Iodine/Cardene

Action: Depresses pain impulse transmission at the spinal cord level by interacting with opioid receptors; decreases cough reflex, GI motility

Therapeutic Outcome: Pain relief, decreased cough, decreased diarrhea depending on route

Uses: Moderate to severe pain, nonproductive cough

Investigational uses: Diarrhea

Dosage and routes

Pain

Adult: PO 15-60 mg q4h prn; IM/SUBCUT 15-60 mg q4h prn

Child: PO 3 mg/kg/day in divided doses q4h prn

Cough

Adult: PO 10-20 mg q4-6h, not to exceed 120 mg/day

Child: PO 1-1.5 mg/kg/day in 4 divided doses, not to exceed 60 mg/day

Diarrhea

Adult: PO 30 mg; may repeat qid prn

Renal dose

Adult: PO CCr 10-50 ml/min 75% of dose; CCr <10 ml/min 50% of dose

Available forms: Inj 30, 60 mg/ml; tabs 15, 30, 60 mg; oral sol 10 mg/5 ml, 15 mg/5 ml

Adverse effects

CNS: *Drowsiness, sedation,* dizziness, agitation, dependency, lethargy, restlessness, euphoria, **seizures**

CV: Bradycardia, palpitations, orthostatic hypotension, tachycardia, **circulatory collapse**

GI: *Nausea, vomiting, anorexia, constipation*
GU: Urinary retention
INTEG: Flushing, rash, urticaria, pruritus
RESP: **Respiratory depression, respiratory paralysis**
SYST: **Anaphylaxis**

Contraindications: Hypersensitivity to opiates, respiratory depression, increased intracranial pressure, seizure disorders, severe respiratory disorders

Precautions: Pregnancy **C**, elderly, cardiac dysrhythmias, prostatic hypertrophy, lactation

Pharmacokinetics

Absorption	Bioavailability 60%-90%
Distribution	Widely distributed; crosses placenta
Metabolism	Liver, extensively
Excretion	Kidneys (up to 15%), breast milk
Half-life	3-4 hr

Pharmacodynamics

	PO	IM	SUBCUT
Onset	30-45 min	15-30 min	15-30 min
Peak	1-2 hr	30-60 min	Unknown
Duration	4 hr	4 hr	4 hr

Interactions

Individual drugs
Alcohol: increased CNS, depression

Drug classifications
Antipsychotics, opiates, sedative/hypnotics, skeletal muscle relaxants: increased CNS depression
MAOIs: increased toxicity

Drug/herb
Corkwood: increased anticholinergic effects
Jamaican dogwood, kava, lavender, mistletoe, nettle, pokeweed, poppy, senega, valerian: increased CNS depression

Drug/lab test
Increased: amylase, lipase

NURSING CONSIDERATIONS

Assessment
- Assess pain: intensity, type, alleviating factors
- Assess GI function: nausea, vomiting, constipation
- Monitor VS after parenteral route; note muscle rigidity, drug history, liver, kidney function tests, respiratory dysfunction: respiratory depression, character, rate, rhythm; notify prescriber if respirations are <10/min
- Monitor CNS changes: dizziness, drowsiness, hallucinations, euphoria, LOC, pupil reaction
- Monitor allergic reactions: rash, urticaria

Nursing diagnoses
- Pain, acute (uses)
- Sensory perceptual, disturbed (adverse reactions)
- Breathing pattern, ineffective (adverse reactions)
- Knowledge, deficient (teaching)

Implementation
- Give with antiemetic if nausea, vomiting occur
- Administer when pain is beginning to return, determine dosage interval by patient response; continuous dosing of medication is more effective given prn; explain analgesic effect
- Medication should be slowly withdrawn after long-term use to prevent withdrawal symptoms
- Store in light-resistant container at room temp

PO route
- May be given with food or milk to lessen GI upset

IM/SUBCUT route
- Do not give if cloudy, or a precipitate has formed

IV route
- Give slowly by direct inj

Syringe compatibilities: Glycopyrrolate, hydrOXYzine
Y-site compatibilities: Cefmetazole
Additive incompatibilities: Aminophylline, amobarbital, chlorothiazide, heparin, methicillin, pentobarbital, phenobarbital, phenytoin, secobarbital, thiopental

Patient/family education
- Teach patient to report any symptoms of CNS changes, allergic reactions; to avoid CNS depressants: alcohol, sedative/hypnotics for at least 24 hr after taking this drug
- Discuss with patient that dizziness, drowsiness, and confusion are common
- Advise patient to avoid getting up without assistance
- Discuss in detail all aspects of the drug

Evaluation
Positive therapeutic outcome
- Decreased pain
- Decreased cough
- Decreased diarrhea

Treatment of overdose: Naloxone 0.2-0.8 **IV**, O_2, **IV** fluids, vasopressors

colchicine (Rx)

(kol'chi-seen)

Func. class.: Antigout agent
Chem. class.: Colchicum autumnale alkaloid

Pregnancy category
C (PO), D (IV)

Action: Inhibits microtubule formation of lactic acid in leukocytes, which decreases phagocytosis and inflammation in joints

Therapeutic Outcome: Decreased pain, inflammation of joints

Uses: Gout, gouty arthritis (prevention, treatment); to arrest progression of neurologic disability in multiple sclerosis

Investigational uses: Hepatic cirrhosis, familial Mediterranean fever, pericarditis

Dosage and routes

Prevention

Adult: PO 0.6-1.8 mg daily depending on severity; **IV** 0.5-1 mg daily-bid

Treatment

Adult: PO 0.6-1.2 mg, then 0.5-1.2 mg q1h, until pain decreases or side effects occur; **IV** 2 mg, then 0.5 mg q6h, not to exceed 4 mg/24 hr

Available forms: Tabs 0.6 mg; inj **IV** 0.5 mg/ml

Adverse effects

GI: *Nausea, vomiting, anorexia, malaise,* metallic taste, cramps, peptic ulcer, diarrhea
GU: Hematuria, **oliguria, renal damage**
HEMA: **Agranulocytosis, thrombocytopenia, aplastic anemia, pancytopenia**
INTEG: Chills, dermatitis, pruritus, purpura, erythema
MISC: Myopathy, alopecia, reversible azoospermia, peripheral neuritis

Contraindications: Pregnancy **D (IV)**, hypersensitivity; serious GI, renal, hepatic, cardiac disorders

Precautions: Pregnancy **C** (PO), severe renal disease, blood dyscrasias, hepatic disease, elderly, lactation, children

Pharmacokinetics

Absorption	Well absorbed
Distribution	WBCs
Metabolism	Deacetylates in liver
Excretion	Feces (metabolites/active drug)
Half-life	20 min

Pharmacodynamics

	PO
Onset	Unknown
Peak	½-2 hr
Duration	Unknown

Interactions

Individual drugs

CycloSPORINE, radiation: increased bone marrow depression
Clarithromycin, cycloSPORINE, erythromycin: toxicity
Ethanol: increased GI effects
Vitamin B_{12}: decreased action of vit B_{12}; may cause reversible malabsorption

Drug classifications

Bone marrow depressants: increased bone marrow depression
NSAIDs: increased GI effects

Drug/lab test

Increased: alkaline phosphatase, AST
False positive: urine, RBC, Hgb
Interference: urinary 17-hydroxycorticosteroids

NURSING CONSIDERATIONS

Assessment

- Assess pain and mobility of joints
- Monitor I&O ratio; observe for decrease in urinary output; CBC, platelets, reticulocytes before, during therapy (q3 mo), may cause aplastic anemia, agranulocytosis, decreased platelets
- Assess for toxicity: weakness, abdominal pain, nausea, vomiting, diarrhea

Nursing diagnoses

- Pain, chronic (uses)
- Mobility, impaired (uses)
- Knowledge, deficient (teaching)

Implementation

PO route

- Give with food for GI symptoms

IV route

- Give **IV** undiluted or diluted 1 mg/10-20 ml normal saline or sterile water for inj; give over 2-5 min
- Do not give IM or SUBCUT
- Do not dilute in D_5W or change in **IV** line that is running or contains D_5W
- Wait ≥1 wk after giving a full course of **IV** colchicine, before giving more doses

Patient/family education

- Caution patient to avoid alcohol, OTC preparations that contain alcohol

- Instruct patient to report any pain, redness, or hard area, usually in legs; rash, sore throat, fever, bleeding, bruising, weakness, numbness, tingling
- Teach patient importance of complying with medical regimen (diet, weight loss, drug therapy); bone marrow depression may occur

Evaluation
Positive therapeutic outcome
- Decreased stone formation on x-ray
- Decreased pain in kidney region
- Absence of hematuria
- Decreased pain in joints

Treatment of overdose: D/C medication, may need opioids to treat diarrhea

colesevelam (Rx)
(coal-see-vel′am)
Welchol
Func. class.: Antilipemic
Chem. class.: Bile acid sequestrant
Pregnancy category C

Action: Absorbs, combines with bile acids to form insoluble complex that is excreted through feces; loss of bile acids lowers cholesterol levels

Therapeutic Outcome: Decreasing LDL cholesterol

Uses: Elevated LDL cholesterol, alone or in combination with HMG-CoA reductase inhibitor

Dosage and routes
Adult: PO monotherapy: 3 625 mg tabs bid with meals or 6 tabs daily with a meal; may increase to 7 tabs if needed

Combination therapy
3 tabs bid with meals or 6 tabs daily with a meal given with an HMG-CoA reductase inhibitor

Available forms: Tabs 625 mg

Adverse effects
CNS: Headache, dizziness, drowsiness, vertigo, tinnitus
GI: *Constipation, abdominal pain, nausea,* fecal impaction, hemorrhoids, flatulence, vomiting, steatorrhea, peptic ulcer
HEMA: Decreased red cell folate content; **bleeding**, decreased protime
INTEG: Rash, irritation of perianal area, tongue, skin
META: Decreased vit A, D, K, **hyperchloremic acidosis**
MS: Muscle, joint pain

Contraindications: Hypersensitivity, biliary obstruction

Precautions: Pregnancy **C**, lactation, children

Pharmacokinetics	
Absorption	Unknown
Distribution	Unknown
Metabolism	Unknown
Excretion	Feces
Half-life	Unknown

Pharmacodynamics
LDL decreased in 4-7 days

Interactions
Individual drugs
Clindamycin, digitalis, gemfibrozil, glipiZIDE, iron, penicillin G, phenytoin, prepanolol, warfarin: decreased absorption of each specific drug
Corticosteroid: decreased corticosteroid action
Thyroid hormones: decreased absorption of thyroid
Drug classifications
Tetracyclines: decreased absorption of tetracyclines
Thiazides: decreased absorption of thiazides
Vitamins (fat-soluble): decreased absorption of fat-soluble vitamins
Drug/herb
Glucomannan: increased effect
Gotu kola: decreased effect
Drug/lab test
Increased: liver function studies, Cl, PO_4

NURSING CONSIDERATIONS
Assessment
- Assess cardiac glycoside level if both drugs are being administered
- Assess for signs of vit A, D, K deficiency
- Monitor fasting LDL, HDL, total cholesterol, triglyceride levels, electrolytes if on extended therapy
- Monitor bowel pattern daily; increase bulk, H_2O in diet for constipation

Nursing diagnoses
- Constipation (adverse reactions)
- Knowledge, deficient (teaching)
- Noncompliance (teaching)

Implementation
- Give drug daily, bid with meals; give all

other medications 1 hr before colesevelam or 4 hr after colesevelam to avoid poor absorption, take with liquid
- Give supplemental doses of vit A, D, K, if levels are low

Patient/family education
- Teach the symptoms of hypoprothrombinemia: bleeding mucous membranes, dark tarry stools, hematuria, petechiae; report immediately
- Teach the importance of compliance; toxicity may result if doses missed
- Teach that risk factors should be decreased: high-fat diet, smoking, alcohol consumption, absence of exercise
- Advise not to discontinue suddenly

Evaluation
Positive therapeutic outcome
- Decreased cholesterol level (hyperlipidemia); diarrhea, pruritus (excess bile acids)

colestipol (Rx)
(koe-les'ti-pole)
Colestid
Func. class.: Antilipemic
Chem. class.: Bile acid sequestrant
Pregnancy category B

Action: Absorbs, combines with bile acids to form an insoluble complex that is excreted through feces; loss of bile acids lowers cholesterol levels

Therapeutic Outcome: Decreasing cholesterol levels and low-density lipoproteins, decreased pruritus

Uses: Primary hypercholesterolemia, xanthomas

Investigational uses: Digitalis toxicity

Dosage and routes
Adult: PO tabs 2 g daily-bid, may increase by 1 g/mo, max 16 g/day; granules 5 g daily-bid, may increase qmo, max 30 g/day

Available forms: Granules 300, 450 g, 500 g bottles; 5 g colestipol/7.5 g powder; tabs 1 g

Adverse effects
GI: *Constipation, abdominal pain, nausea,* fecal impaction, hemorrhoids, flatulence, vomiting, steatorrhea, peptic ulcer
HEMA: **Bleeding, increased protime**
INTEG: *Rash,* irritation of perianal area, tongue, skin
META: *Decreased vit A, D, E, K,* red folate content; **hyperchloremic acidosis**

Contraindications: Hypersensitivity, biliary obstruction

Precautions: Pregnancy **B,** lactation, children, bleeding disorders

Pharmacokinetics	
Absorption	Not absorbed
Distribution	Not distributed
Metabolism	Not metabolized
Excretion	Binds with bile acids, feces
Half-life	Unknown

Pharmacodynamics	
Onset	24-48 hr
Peak	30 days
Duration	30 days

Interactions
Individual drugs
Clindamycin, digitalis, digoxin, folic acid, gemfibrozil, glipiZIDE, iron, penicillin G, propranolol, tetracycline, thyroid agents, warfarin: decreased action of each specific drug
Phenytoin, TOLBUTamide: decreased effect of each specific drug
Drug classifications
Diuretics (thiazide): decreased absorption
Corticosteroids: decreased corticosteroid action
Vitamins A, D, E, K: decreased absorption
Drug/herb
Glucomannan: increased effect
Gotu kola: decreased effect
Drug/lab test
Increased: Cl, PO_4, AST, ALT, alkaline phosphatase
Decreased: Na, K, Ca

NURSING CONSIDERATIONS
Assessment
- Assess nutrition: fat, protein, carbohydrates; nutritional analysis should be completed by dietician
- Assess skin integrity after patient has been receiving drug; itching, pruritus often occur from bile deposits on skin
- Monitor cardiac glycoside level, if both drugs are being administered; cardiac glycoside levels will be decreased
- Monitor for signs of vit A, D, E, K deficiency; check serum cholesterol, triglyceride levels, electrolytes if on extended therapy

• Monitor bowel pattern daily; increase bulk, water in diet if constipation develops

Nursing diagnoses

• Constipation (adverse reactions)
• Knowledge, deficient (teaching)
• Noncompliance (teaching)

Implementation

• Swallow tabs whole; do not break, crush, or chew
• Give drug daily or bid; give all other medications 1 hr before or 4 hr after colestipol to avoid poor absorption; give drug mixed with applesauce or stirred into beverage (2-6 oz), let stand for 2 min; rinse glass to make sure all medication is taken; do not take dry
• Provide supplemental doses of vit A, D, E, K, if levels are low

Patient/family education

◆ Teach patient symptoms of hypoprothrombinemia: bleeding mucous membranes, dark, tarry stools, hematuria, petechiae; report immediately
• Teach patient importance of compliance, not to miss or double doses
• Teach patient that risk factors should be decreased: high-fat diet, smoking, alcohol consumption, absence of exercise
• Tell patient to mix drug with 6 oz of milk, water, fruit juice; may be mixed with carbonated beverages; rinse glass to make sure all medication is taken or may mix drug in applesauce; allow to stand for 2 min before mixing

Evaluation

Positive therapeutic outcome

• Decreased cholesterol level (hyperlipidemia)

contraceptives (Rx)

Func. class.: Hormone
Chem. class.: Estrogen/progestin combinations

Pregnancy category X

Action: Prevents ovulation by suppressing FSH, LH; **monophasic:** estrogen/progestin (fixed dose) used during a 21-day cycle; ovulation is inhibited by suppression of FSH and LH; thickness of cervical mucus and endometrial lining prevents pregnancy; **biphasic:** ovulation is inhibited by suppression of FSH and LH; alteration of cervical mucus, endometrial lining prevents pregnancy; **triphasic:** ovulation is inhibited by suppression of FSH and LH; change of cervical mucus, endometrial lining prevents pregnancy; variable doses of estrogen/progestin combinations may be similar to natural hormonal fluctuations; **progestin-only pill and intrauterine implant:** change of cervical mucus and endometrial lining prevents pregnancy; ovulation may be suppressed

Therapeutic Outcome: Prevention of pregnancy, decreased severity of endometriosis, hypermenorrhea

Uses: To prevent pregnancy, emergency contraception, menstrual cycle regulation, and acne

Dosage and routes

Adult: PO 1 daily starting on day 5 of menstrual cycle; day 1 is 1st day of period

21-tablet packs

Adult: PO 1 daily starting on day 7 of menstrual cycle; day 1 is 1st day of period; then on 20 or 21 days, off 7 days

28-tablet packs

Adult: PO 1 daily continuously

Biphasic

Adult: 1 daily × 10 days, then next color 1 daily × 11 days

Triphasic

Adult: 1 daily; check package insert for each brand

Available forms: Check specific brand

Adverse effects

CNS: Depression, fatigue, dizziness, nervousness, anxiety, headache
CV: Increased B/P, **cerebral hemorrhage, thrombosis, pulmonary embolism,** fluid retention, edema
EENT: Optic neuritis, retinal thrombosis, cataracts
ENDO: Decreased glucose tolerance, increased TBG, PBI, T_4, T_3
GI: *Nausea,* vomiting, cramps, diarrhea, bloating, constipation, change in appetite, **cholestatic jaundice**
GU: Breakthrough bleeding, amenorrhea, spotting, dysmenorrhea, galactorrhea, endocervical hyperplasia, vaginitis, cystitis-like syndrome, breast change

HEMA: Increased fibrinogen, clotting factor
INTEG: *Chloasma, melasma,* acne, rash, urticaria, erythema, pruritus, hirsutism, alopecia, photosensitivity

Contraindications: Pregnancy **X,** lactation, reproductive cancer, thrombophlebitis, MI, hepatic tumors, hepatic disease, CAD, women 40 yr and over, CVA

Precautions: Depression, hypertension, renal disease, seizure disorders, lupus erythematosus, rheumatic disease, migraine headache, amenorrhea, irregular menses, breast cancer (fibrocystic), gallbladder disease, diabetes mellitus, heavy smoking, acute mononucleosis, sickle cell disease

Pharmacokinetics

Absorption	Well absorbed
Distribution	Unknown
Metabolism	Liver, extensively
Excretion	Kidneys
Half-life	Unknown

Pharmacodynamics

	PO	IM	IMPLANT
Onset	1 mo	1 mo	1 mo
Peak	1 mo	1 mo	1 mo
Duration	1 mo	3 mo	5 yr

Interactions

Individual drugs

Griseofulvin, rifampin: decreased effectiveness of oral contraceptive

Drug classifications

Analgesics, antibiotics, anticoagulants (oral), anticonvulsants, antihistamines: decreased action of oral contraceptives

Drug/herb

Alfalfa, black cohosh, chaste tree: altered action

Saw palmetto, St. John's wort: decreased oral contraceptive effect

Drug/food

Grapefruit juice: increased peak level

Drug/lab test

Increased: protime; clotting factors VII, VIII, IX, X; TBG, PBI, T_4, platelet aggregation, BSP, triglycerides, bilirubin, AST, ALT

Decreased: T_3, antithrombin III, folate, metyrapone test, GTT, 17-OHCS

NURSING CONSIDERATIONS

Assessment

- Assess for reproductive changes: change in breasts, tumors, positive Pap smear; drug should be discontinued if changes occur
- Monitor glucose, thyroid function, liver function tests, B/P

Nursing diagnoses

- Injury, risk for (adverse reactions)
- Body image, disturbed (adverse reactions)
- Knowledge, deficient (teaching)
- Noncompliance (teaching)

Implementation

PO route

- If GI symptoms occur, medication may be taken with food; take at same time each day

Implant route

- Inject 6 cap subdermally
- Implant is effective for 5 yr, should be removed after that

IM route

- Administer inj deep in large muscle mass after shaking susp well; ensure pregnancy has not occurred if inj are 2 wk or more apart

Patient/family education

- Teach patient about detection of clots using Homans' sign; teach monitoring technique for heat, redness, pain, swelling
- Teach patient to use sunscreen or to avoid sunlight; photosensitivity can occur
- Teach patient to take at same time each day to ensure equal drug level; to take another tab as soon as possible if one is missed
- Teach patient that after drug is discontinued, pregnancy may not occur for several mo
- Instruct patient to report GI symptoms that occur after 4 mo
- Advise patient to use another birth control method during first 3 wk of oral contraceptive use
- Teach patient to report abdominal pain, change in vision, shortness of breath, change in menstrual flow, spotting, breakthrough bleeding, breast lumps, swelling, headache, severe leg pain, mental changes; that continuing medical care is needed: Pap smear and gynecologic exam q6 mo
- Teach patient to notify physicians and dentist of oral contraceptive use

Evaluation

Positive therapeutic outcome

- Absence of pregnancy
- Decreased severity of endometriosis
- Decreased severity of hypermenorrhea

cortisone 🔑 (Rx)

(kor'ti-sone)

Cortone ✱, cortone acetate

Func. class.: Corticosteroid, synthetic

Chem. class.: Short-acting glucocorticoid

Pregnancy category D

Action: Decreases inflammation by suppression of migration of polymorphonuclear leukocytes, fibroblasts, reversal of increased capillary permeability, and lysosomal stabilization; suppresses adrenal function with long-term use

Therapeutic Outcome: Replacement of cortisol in adrenal insufficiency

Uses: Inflammation, severe allergy, adrenal insufficiency, collagen disorders, respiratory and dermatologic, rheumatic disorders

Dosage and routes

Adult: PO/IM 25-300 mg daily or q2 days, titrated to patient response

Child: PO 0.7-10 mg/kg/day; IM 0.2-5 mg/kg/day

Available forms: Tabs 5, 10, 25 mg; inj 50 mg/ml

Adverse effects

CNS: *Depression, flushing, sweating,* headache, mood changes

CV: *Hypertension,* **circulatory collapse, thrombophlebitis, embolism,** tachycardia, **necrotizing angiitis, CHF,** edema

EENT: Fungal infections, increased intraocular pressure, blurred vision

GI: *Diarrhea, nausea, abdominal distention,* **GI hemorrhage,** increased appetite, **pancreatitis**

HEMA: **Thrombocytopenia**

INTEG: Acne, poor wound healing, ecchymosis, bruising, petechiae

META: Sodium fluid retention; potassium loss

MS: Fractures, osteoporosis, weakness, loss of muscle mass

Contraindications: Pregnancy **D**, psychosis, hypersensitivity, idiopathic thrombocytopenia, acute glomerulonephritis, amebiasis, fungal infections, nonasthmatic bronchial disease, child <2 yr, AIDS, TB

Precautions: Diabetes mellitus, glaucoma, osteoporosis, seizure disorders, ulcerative colitis, CHF, myasthenia gravis, renal disease, esophagitis, peptic ulcer, lactation, hapatic disease

Pharmacokinetics

Absorption	Slowly IM
Distribution	Widely, crosses placenta
Metabolism	Liver
Excretion	Unknown
Half-life	8-12 hr

Pharmacodynamics

	PO	IM
Onset	Unknown	Unknown
Peak	2 hr	20-48 hr
Duration	1½ days	10 days

Interactions

Individual drugs

Alcohol: increased side effects

Indomethacin: increased GI symptoms, increased side effects, increased action of cortisone

Ketoconazole: increased cortisone action

Phenobarbital, phenytoin: decreased effectiveness of cortisone

Rifampin, theophylline: decreased cortisone action

Drug classifications

Anticoagulants: decreased anticoagulant effect

Antidiabetics: decreased antidiabetic effect

Antiinfectives (macrolide), estrogens: increased cortisone action

Acetylcholinesterases, barbiturates: decreased cortisone action

Contraceptives (oral): increased action of cortisone

Diuretics (potassium-wasting), salicylates: increased side effects

NSAIDs: increased GI symptoms

Salicylates: increased GI symptoms, increased cortisone effects, increased side effects; decreased salicylate effect

Toxoids: decreased toxoid effect

Vaccines: decreased vaccine effect

Drug/herb

Aloe, buckthorn bark/berry, cascara sagrada bark, Chinese rhubarb, rhubarb root, senna leaf/fruits: increased potassium deficiency

Aloe, licorice, perilla: increased steroid effect

Drug/lab test

Increased: cholesterol, sodium, blood glucose, uric acid, calcium, urine glucose

Decreased: calcium, potassium, T_4, T_3, thyroid ^{131}I uptake test, urine 17-OHCS, 17-KS, PBI

False negative: skin allergy tests

NURSING CONSIDERATIONS
Assessment
- Assess for adrenal insufficiency symptoms: weakness, nausea, vomiting, confusion, anxiety, restlessness, decreased B/P, weight loss; check before and during treatment
- Monitor potassium, blood/urine glucose for patient on long-term therapy; hypokalemia and hyperglycemia can occur
- Check B/P, pulse q4h; notify prescriber if chest pain occurs
- Monitor I&O ratio and weight daily; be alert for decreasing urinary output and increasing edema with bilateral crackles, dyspnea, weight gain
- Monitor plasma cortisol levels during long-term therapy (normal level: 138-635 nmol/L if checked at 8 AM)
- Assess for symptoms of infection: increased temp, WBC even after withdrawal of medication; drug masks symptoms of infection
- Monitor for potassium depletion: paresthesias, fatigue, nausea, vomiting, depression, polyuria, dysrhythmias, weakness, edema, hypertension, cardiac symptoms, weight daily; notify prescriber of weekly gain >5 lb
- Assess for mental changes: affect, mood, behavioral changes, aggression; depression, psychoses may occur

Nursing diagnoses
- Infection, risk for (adverse reactions)
- Injury, risk for (adverse reactions)
- Knowledge, deficient (teaching)

Implementation
PO route
- Administer in AM with food or milk to decrease GI symptoms

IM route
- Give after shaking susp (parenteral); titrate dose; use lowest effective dosage
- Give IM inj deep in large muscle mass; rotate sites; avoid deltoid; use a 21-G needle
- Administer in 1 dose in AM to prevent adrenal suppression; avoid SUBCUT administration; damage may be done to tissue; do not give **IV**

Patient/family education
- Advise patient to carry/wear emergency ID as steroid user at all times
- Instruct patient to notify prescriber if therapeutic response decreases; dosage adjustment may be needed; teach not to discontinue this medication abruptly or adrenal crisis can result; teach all aspects of drug usage, including cushingoid symptoms
- Caution patient to avoid OTC products: salicylates, potassium, alcohol in cough products, cold preparations unless directed by prescriber
- Teach patient symptoms of adrenal insufficiency: nausea, anorexia, fatigue, dizziness, dyspnea, weakness, joint pain, tarry stools, bruising, blurred vision
- Advise patient to avoid persons with known infections; report probable infection rapidly; drug masks infection
- Caution patient that diet modification is necessary if on long-term treatment: increased calcium, potassium, and protein; also low sodium and carbohydrates
- Advise the patient to avoid exposure to chickenpox, measles
- Advise the patient to take PO dose in AM with food or fluid (milk)

Evaluation
Positive therapeutic outcome
- Ease of respirations, decreased inflammation

cotrimoxazole
See trimethoprim/sulfamethoxazole

cyclobenzaprine (Rx)
(sye-kloe-ben′za-preen)

cyclobenzaprine HCl, Cycloflex, Flexeril

Func. class.: Skeletal muscle relaxant, central acting

Chem. class.: Tricyclic amine salt

Pregnancy category B

Do Not Confuse:
cyclobenzaprine/cyproheptadine

Action: Reduction of tonic muscle activity at the brain stem; may be related to antidepressant effects

Therapeutic Outcome: Relaxation of skeletal muscle

Uses: Adjunct for relief of muscle spasm and pain in musculoskeletal conditions

Dosage and routes
Musculoskeletal disorders

Adult: PO 10 mg tid × 1 wk, not to exceed 60 mg/day × 3 wk

Fibromyalgia

Adult: PO 5-40 mg at bedtime

Available forms: Tabs 10 mg

Adverse effects
CNS: *Dizziness, weakness, drowsiness,*

headache, tremor, depression, insomnia, confusion, paresthesia
CV: Postural hypotension, tachycardia, **dysrhythmias**
EENT: Diplopia, temporary loss of vision
GI: *Nausea,* vomiting, hiccups, dry mouth, constipation
GU: Urinary retention, frequency, change in libido
INTEG: Rash, pruritus, fever, facial flushing, sweating

Contraindications: Acute recovery phase of MI, dysrhythmias, heart block, CHF, hypersensitivity, child <12 yr, intermittent porphyria, thyroid disease

Precautions: Pregnancy **B,** renal disease, hepatic disease, addictive personality, elderly, lactation

Pharmacokinetics

Distribution	Well
Metabolism	Liver, partially
Excretion	Kidney (unchanged)
Half-life	1-3 days

Pharmacodynamics

Onset	1 hr
Peak	3-8 hr
Duration	12-24 hr

Interactions
Individual drugs
Alcohol: increased CNS depression
Tramadol: do not use within 14 days

Drug classifications
Antidepressants (tricyclic), barbiturates, opiates, sedative/hypnotics: increased CNS depression
MAOIs: do not use within 14 days

Drug/herb
Kava: increased CNS depression

NURSING CONSIDERATIONS
Assessment
- Assess pain periodically: location, duration, mobility, stiffness, baseline
- Monitor ECG in epileptic patients; poor seizure control has occurred in patients taking this drug
- Check for allergic reactions: rash, fever, respiratory distress
- Check for severe weakness, numbness, in extremities
- Assess for CNS depression: dizziness, drowsiness, psychiatric symptoms

Nursing diagnoses
- Mobility, physical, impaired
- Injury, risk for (adverse reactions)
- Knowledge, deficient (teaching)

Implementation
- Give without regard to meals
- Store in airtight container at room temp

Patient/family education
- Teach patient not to discontinue medication quickly; insomnia, nausea, headache, spasticity, tachycardia will occur; drug should be tapered off over 1-2 wk
- Caution patient not to take with alcohol, other CNS depressants
- Advise to avoid altering activities while taking this drug
- Caution patient to avoid hazardous activities if drowsiness/dizziness occurs
- Caution patient to avoid using OTC medication: cough preparations, antihistamines, unless directed by prescriber
- Teach patient to use gum, frequent sips of water for dry mouth

Evaluation
Positive therapeutic outcome
- Decreased pain, spasticity; muscle spasms of acute, painful musculoskeletal conditions are generally short term; long-term therapy is seldom warranted

Treatment of overdose: Empty stomach with emesis, gastric lavage, then administer activated charcoal; use anticonvulsants if indicated; monitor cardiac function

! HIGH ALERT

cyclophosphamide (Rx)
(sye-kloe-foss′fa-mide)
Cytoxan, Neosar, Procytox ♣
Func. class.: Antineoplastic alkylating agent
Chem. class.: Nitrogen mustard
Pregnancy category D

Do Not Confuse:
cyclophosphamide/cycloSPORINE, Cytoxan/Cytosar, Cytoxan/Cytotec/centoxin/Cytarabine

Action: Alkylates DNA, RNA; inhibits enzymes that allow synthesis of amino acids in proteins; is also responsible for cross-linking DNA strands; activity is not cell cycle phase specific

Therapeutic Outcome: Prevention of rapidly growing malignant cells

Uses: Hodgkin's disease, lymphomas, leukemia, multiple myeloma, neuroblastoma, retinoblastoma, Ewing's sarcoma, cancer of female reproductive tract, breast, lung, prostate

Dosage and routes

Adult: PO initially 1-5 mg/ kg over 2-5 days; maintenance 1-5 mg/kg; **IV** initially 40-50 mg/kg in divided doses over 2-5 days; maintenance 10-15 mg/kg q7-10 days, or 3-5 mg/kg q3 days

Child: PO/**IV** 2-8 mg/kg or 60-250 mg/m² in divided doses × 6 or more days; maintenance **IV** 10-15 mg/kg q7-10 days or 30 mg/kg q3-4 wk; dose should be reduced by half when bone marrow suppression occurs

Renal dose

Adult: PO/**IV** CCr 25-50 ml/min 50% of dose; CCr <25 ml/min avoid use

Available forms: Powder for inj **IV** 100, 200, 500 mg, 1, 2 g; tabs 25, 50 mg

Adverse effects

CNS: Headache, dizziness
CV: **Cardiotoxicity** (high doses)
ENDO: Syndrome of inappropriate antidiuretic hormone (SIADH), gonadal suppression
GI: *Nausea, vomiting, diarrhea, weight loss,* colitis, **hepatotoxicity**
GU: **Hemorrhagic cystitis,** hematuria, neoplasms, amenorrhea, azoospermia, sterility, ovarian fibrosis
HEMA: **Thrombocytopenia, leukopenia, pancytopenia, myelosuppression**
INTEG: *Alopecia,* dermatitis
META: Hyperuricemia
MISC: Secondary neoplasms, **anaphylaxis**
RESP: **Fibrosis**

Contraindications: Pregnancy **D,** lactation, severely depressed bone marrow function, hypersensitivity

Precautions: Radiation therapy

Pharmacokinetics

Absorption	Well absorbed (PO)
Distribution	Widely distributed; crosses placenta, blood-brain barrier (50%)
Metabolism	Liver to active drug
Excretion	Kidneys, unchanged (30%)
Half-life	4-6½ hr

Pharmacodynamics

Unknown

Interactions

Individual drugs

Allopurinol: increased bone marrow suppression
Chloramphenicol: decreased cyclophosphamide effect
Digoxin: decreased digoxin levels
Insulin: increased hypoglycemia
Succinylcholine: increased neuromuscular blockade
Warfarin: increased warfarin action

Drug classifications

Diuretics (thiazides): increased bone marrow suppression
Barbiturates: increased toxicity of cyclophosphamide
Corticosteroids: decreased cyclophosphamide effect
Live virus vaccines: decreased antibody reaction

Drug/lab test

Increased: uric acid
Decreased: pseudocholinesterase
False positive: Pap smear
False negative: PPD, mumps trichophytin, *Candida*

NURSING CONSIDERATIONS

Assessment

- Assess symptoms indicating severe allergic reaction: rash, pruritus, urticaria, purpuric skin lesions, itching, flushing
- Assess for tachypnea, ECG changes, dyspnea, edema, fatigue
- Monitor CBC, differential, platelet count weekly; withhold drug if WBC count is <2500/mm³ or platelet count is <75,000/mm³; notify prescriber of results
- Assess for hemorrhagic cystitis: renal function studies including BUN, creatinine, serum uric acid, urine CCr before and during therapy; I&O ratio; report fall in urine output to <30 ml/hr
- Monitor temp q4h (elevated temp may indicate beginning of infection)
- Monitor liver function tests before and during therapy (bilirubin, AST, ALT, LDH) as needed or monthly; note jaundice of skin or sclera, dark urine, clay-colored stools, itchy skin, abdominal pain, fever, diarrhea
- Assess for bleeding: hematuria, stool guaiac, bruising or petechiae, mucosa or orifices q8h
- Identify dyspnea, crackles, unproductive cough, chest pain, tachypnea
- Identify effects of alopecia on body image; discuss feelings about body changes

Nursing diagnoses

- Injury, risk for (adverse reactions)
- Body image, disturbed (adverse reactions)
- Infection, risk for (adverse reactions)
- Knowledge, deficient (teaching)

Implementation

- Give fluids **IV** or PO before chemotherapy to hydrate patient
- Give antacid before oral agent, pc PM, before bedtime; antiemetic 30-60 min before giving drug to prevent vomiting, and prn; antibiotics for prophylaxis of infection
- Give top or syst analgesics for pain; give in AM so drug can be eliminated before bedtime

IV route

- Give **IV** after diluting 100 mg/5 ml of sterile or bacteriostatic water; shake; let stand until clear; may be further diluted in up to 250 ml D_5 0.9% NaCl, 0.45% NaCl, LR, Ringer's; give 100 mg or less/min through 3-way stopcock of glucose or saline inf
- Use 21-, 23-, or 25-G needle; check site for irritation, phlebitis

Syringe compatibilities: Bleomycin, cisplatin, doxapram, DOXOrubicin, droperidol, fluorouracil, furosemide, heparin, leucovorin, methotrexate, metoclopramide, mitomycin, mitoxantrone, vinBLAStine, vinCRIStine

Y-site compatibilities: Amifostine, amikacin, ampicillin, azlocillin, aztreonam, bleomycin, cefamandole, cefazolin, cefepime, cefoperazone, cefotaxime, cefoxitin, cefuroxime, cephalothin, cephapirin, chloramphenicol, chlorproMAZINE, cimetidine, cisplatin, cladribine, clindamycin, dexamethasone, diphenhydrAMINE, DOXOrubicin, doxycycline, droperidol, erythromycin, famotidine, filgrastim, fludarabine, fluorouracil, furosemide, gallium, ganciclovir, gentamicin, granisetron, heparin, hydromorphone, idarubicin, kanamycin, leucovorin, lorazepam, melphalan, methotrexate, methylPREDNISolone, metoclopramide, metronidazole, mezlocillin, minocycline, mitomycin, moxalactam, nafcillin, ondansetron, oxacillin, paclitaxel, penicillin G potassium, piperacillin, piperacillin/tazobactam, prochlorperazine, promethazine, propofol, ranitidine, sargramostim, sodium bicarbonate, teniposide, tetracycline, thiotepa, ticarcillin, ticarcillin-clavulanate, tobramycin, trimethoprim-sulfamethoxazole, vancomycin, vinBLAStine, vinCRIStine, vinorelbine

Additive compatibilities: Cisplatin with etoposide, hydrOXYzine, methotrexate, methotrexate with fluorouracil, mitoxantrone, ondansetron

Solution compatibilities: Amino acids 4.25%/D_{25}, D_5/0.9% NaCl, D_5W, 0.9% NaCl

Patient/family education

- Teach patient to avoid use of products containing aspirin or ibuprofen, razors, commercial mouthwash, since bleeding may occur; to report symptoms of bleeding (hematuria, tarry stools, bruising)
- Instruct patient to report signs of anemia (fatigue, headache, irritability, faintness, shortness of breath)
- Teach patient to report any changes in breathing or coughing even several months after treatment
- Advise patient that hair may be lost during treatment; a wig or hairpiece may make patient feel better; new hair may be different in color, texture
- Teach patient not to have any vaccinations without the advice of the prescriber; serious reactions can occur
- Advise patient contraception is needed during treatment and for several months after the completion of therapy

Evaluation

Positive therapeutic outcome

- Prevention of rapid division of malignant cells
- Increased appetite, increased weight

cycloSPORINE (Rx)

(sye-kloe-spor'een)

Gengraf, Neoral, Sandimmune, SangCya

Func. class.: Immunosuppressant

Chem. class.: Fungus-derived peptide

Pregnancy category C

Do Not Confuse:

cycloSPORINE/CycloSERINE, cycloSPORINE/cyclophosphamide

Action: Produces immunosuppression by inhibiting T lymphocytes

Therapeutic Outcome: Absence of transplant rejection

Uses: Organ transplants (liver, kidney, heart) to prevent rejection, rheumatoid arthritis, psoriasis

Investigational uses: Recalcitrant ulcerative colitis

Dosage and routes

Prevention of transplant rejection

Adult and child: PO 15 mg/kg several hr before surgery, daily for 2 wk, reduce dosage by 2.5 mg/kg/wk to 5-10 mg/kg/day; **IV** 5-6

mg/kg several hr before surgery, daily, switch to PO form as soon as possible

Rheumatoid arthritis (Neoral/Gengraf)

Adult: PO 2.5 mg/kg/day divided bid, may increase 0.5-0.75 mg/kg/day after 8-12 wk, max 4 mg/kg/day

Psoriasis (Neoral/Gengraf)

Adult: PO 2.5 mg/kg/day divided bid × 4 wk, then increase by 0.5 mg/kg/day q2 wk, max 4 mg/kg/day

Available forms: Oral sol (Neoral) 100 mg/ml; soft gel cap 25, 100 mg; oral sol 100 mg/ml; inj 50 mg/ml

Adverse effects

CNS: *Tremors, headache,* **seizures**

GI: Nausea, vomiting, diarrhea, *oral Candida, gum hyperplasia,* **hepatotoxicity,** pancreatitis

GU: **Albuminuria, hematuria, proteinuria, renal failure**

INTEG: Rash, acne, *hirsutism*

META: Hyperkalemia, hypomagnesemia, hyperlipidemia, hyperuricemia

MISC: *Infection*

Contraindications: Hypersensitivity to polyxyethylated castor oil (inj only), psoriasis or rheumatoid arthrits in renal disease (Neoral/Gengraf), uncontrolled, malignant hypertension; Gengraf/Neoral used with PUVA/UVB; methotrexate, coal tar, radiation in psoriasis, lactation

Precautions: Pregnancy **C,** severe renal disease, severe hepatic disease, elderly

Pharmacokinetics	
Absorption	Poorly absorbed (PO)
Distribution	Crosses placenta
Metabolism	Liver to mercaptopurine
Excretion	Kidney, minimal
Half-life	Biphasic 1.2 hr, 25 hr

Pharmacodynamics	PO
Onset	Unknown
Peak	4 hr
Duration	Unknown

Interactions

Individual drugs

Allopurinol, amiodarone, amphotericin B, bromocriptine, carvedilol, cimetidine, colchicine, foscarnet, imipenem-cilastatin, ketoconazole, melphalan, metoclopramide: increased action, cycloSPORINE toxicity

Digoxin: increased digoxin level

Etoposide: increased etoposide level

Methotrexake: increased methotrexate level

Nafcillin, orlistat, phenobarbital, phenytoin, probucol terbinafine, ticlodipine, trimethoprim/sulfamethoxazole: decreased cycloSPORINE action

Sirolimus: increased sirolimus level

Tacrolimus: increased tacrolimus level

Drug classifications:

Androgens, antifungals (azole), beta-blockers, calcium channel blockers, contraceptives (oral), corticosteroids, fluoroquinolones, macrolides, NSAIDs: increased cycloSPORINE levels, toxicity

Anticonvulsants, rifamycins: decreased cycloSPORINE levels

Live virus vaccines: decreased antibody reaction

Drug/herb

Ginseng, maitake, mistletoe, schisandra, St. John's wort, turmeric: decreased effect

Safflower: increased effect

Drug/food

Grapefruit juice, food: increased slowed metabolism of drug

NURSING CONSIDERATIONS

Assessment

- Monitor renal studies: BUN, creatinine at least monthly during treatment, 3 mo after treatment
- Monitor liver function studies: alkaline phosphatase, AST, ALT, bilirubin
- Monitor drug blood levels during treatment
- Assess for hepatotoxicity: dark urine, jaundice, itching, light-colored stools; drug should be discontinued
- Assess for nephrotoxicity: 6 wk postop, CyA trough level >200 ng/ml, intracapsular pressure <40 mm Hg, rise in creatinine 0.15 mg/dl/day

Nursing diagnoses

- Mobility, impaired (uses)
- Infection, risk for (uses)
- Knowledge, deficient (teaching)

Implementation

PO route

- Do not break, crush, or chew caps
- Use pipette provided to draw up oral sol; may mix with milk or juice, wipe pipette, do not wash
- Give for several days before transplant surgery with corticosteroids
- Microemulsion products (Neoral) and other products are not interchangeable

- Give with meals for GI upset or drug placed in chocolate milk
- Give with oral antifungal for *Candida* infections

IV route

- Give **IV** after diluting each 50 mg/20-100 ml of 0.9% NaCl or D_5W; run over 2-6 hr; use an infusion pump, glass inf bottles only; may give as cont inf over 24 hr

Additive compatibilities: Ciprofloxacin

Y-site compatibility: Cefmetazole, propofol, sargramostim

Solution compatibilities: D_5W, NaCl 0.9%

- Give for several days before transplant surgery
- Give with corticosteroids

Patient/family education

- Advise patient to report fever, rash, severe diarrhea, chills, sore throat, fatigue, since serious infections may occur; also to report clay-colored stools, cramping (may indicate hepatotoxicity); tremors, bleeding gums, increased B/P
- Caution patient to use contraceptive measures during treatment and for 12 wk after ending therapy; drug is teratogenic
- Caution patient to avoid crowds and persons with known infections to reduce risk of infection

Evaluation

Positive therapeutic outcome

- Absence of graft rejection

cyproheptadine (Rx)

(si-proe-hep'ta-deen)

cyproheptadine HCl, Periactin, PMS-Cyproheptadine

Func. class.: Antihistamine, H_1-receptor antagonist

Chem. class.: Piperidine

Pregnancy category B

Do Not Confuse:
cyproheptadine/cyclobenzaprine

Action: Acts on blood vessels, GI, respiratory system by competing with histamine for H_1-receptor site; decreases allergic response by blocking histamine; blocks serotonin to increase appetite and relieve vascular headaches

Therapeutic Outcome: Absence of allergy symptoms and rhinitis

Uses: Allergy symptoms, rhinitis, pruritus, cold urticaria

Investigational uses: Appetite stimulant, management of vascular headache, nightmares, posttraumatic stress disorder

Dosage and routes

Adult: PO 4 mg tid-qid, not to exceed 0.5 mg/kg/day

Child 6-14 yr: PO 4 mg bid-tid, not to exceed 16 mg/day

Child 2-6 yr: PO 2 mg bid-tid, not to exceed 12 mg/day

Nightmares, posttraumatic stress disorder

Adult: PO 4-12 mg nightly, max 32 mg

Available forms: Tabs 4 mg; syr 2 mg/5 ml

Adverse effects

CNS: *Dizziness, drowsiness,* poor coordination, fatigue, anxiety, euphoria, confusion, paresthesia, neuritis

CV: Hypotension, palpitations, tachycardia

EENT: *Blurred vision,* dilated pupils; tinnitus; nasal stuffiness; dry nose, throat, mouth

GI: *Constipation, dry mouth,* nausea, vomiting, anorexia, diarrhea, weight gain, increased appetite

GU: *Urinary retention,* dysuria, urinary frequency

HEMA: **Hemolytic anemia, leukopenia, thrombocytosis, agranulocytosis**

INTEG: Rash, urticaria, photosensitivity

MISC: **Anaphylaxis**

RESP: Increased thick secretions, wheezing, chest tightness

Contraindications: Hypersensitivity to H_1-receptor antagonist, acute asthma attack, lower respiratory tract disease

Precautions: Pregnancy **B,** increased intraocular pressure, renal disease, cardiac disease, hypertension, bronchial asthma, seizure disorder, stenosed peptic ulcers, hyperthyroidism, prostatic hypertrophy, bladder neck obstruction, elderly, lactation

Pharmacokinetics	
Absorption	Well absorbed
Distribution	Unknown
Metabolism	Liver, complete
Excretion	Kidneys
Half-life	Unknown

Pharmacodynamics

Onset	15-60 min
Peak	1-2 hr
Duration	8 hr

Interactions

Individual drugs

Alcohol: increased CNS depression

Drug classifications

Antidepressants (tricyclics), barbiturates, CNS depressants, opiates, sedative/hypnotics: increased CNS depression

MAOIs: increased anticholinergic effect

Drug/herb

Corkwood, henbane leaf: increased anticholinergic effect

Hops, Jamaican dogwood, kava, khat, senega: increased CNS depression

Drug/lab test

False negative: skin allergy tests (discontinue antihistamine 3 days before testing)

NURSING CONSIDERATIONS

Assessment

- Assess respiratory status: rate, rhythm, increase in bronchial secretions, wheezing, chest tightness; provide fluids to 2 L/day to decrease secretion thickness
- Monitor I&O ratio: be alert for urinary retention, frequency, dysuria, especially elderly; drug should be discontinued if these occur; monitor food intake, weight if using as an appetite stimulant

Nursing diagnoses

- Airway clearance, ineffective (uses)
- Injury, risk for (side effects)
- Knowledge, deficient (teaching)
- Noncompliance (teaching, overuse)

Implementation

- May give with food to decrease GI upset
- Syrup may be used for patients with difficulty swallowing or children
- Store in tight, light-resistant container

Patient/family education

- Teach all aspects of drug uses; tell patient to notify prescriber if confusion, sedation, hypotension occur; to avoid driving and other hazardous activity if drowsiness occurs; to avoid alcohol and other CNS depressants that may potentiate effect
- Caution patient not to exceed recommended dosage; dysrhythmias may occur
- Teach patient hard candy, gum, frequent rinsing of mouth may be used for dryness

Evaluation

Positive therapeutic outcome

- Absence of runny or congested nose, rashes

Treatment of overdose: Administer lavage, diazepam, vasopressors, barbiturates (short acting)

C

! HIGH ALERT

cytarabine (Rx)

(sye-tare′a-been)

Ara-C, Cytosar ✦, Cytosar-U, cytosine arabinoside, Depo Cyt, Tarabine PFS

Func. class.: Antineoplastic, antimetabolite

Chem. class.: Pyrimidine nucleoside

Pregnancy category D

Do Not Confuse:

Cytosar/Cytovene, Cytosar/Cytoxan/Cytovene

Action: Competes with physiologic substrate of DNA synthesis, thus interfering with cell replication in the S phase of the cell cycle (before mitosis)

Therapeutic Outcome: Prevention of rapidly growing malignant cells

Uses: Acute myelocytic leukemia, acute lymphocytic leukemia, chronic myelocytic leukemia, lymphomatous meningitis (IT), and in combination for non-Hodgkin's lymphomas in children

Dosage and routes

Acute myelocytic leukemia

Adult: **IV** inf 200 mg/m^2/day × 5 days q2 wk as single agent or 2-6 mg/kg/day (100-200 mg/m^2/day) as single dose or 2-3 divided doses for 5-10 days until remission, used in combination; maintenance 70-200 mg/m^2/day for 2-5 days qmo; SUBCUT maintenance 1 mg/kg 1-2×/wk

Refractory acute leukemia/refractory non-Hodgkin's lymphoma

Adult: **IV** 3 g/m^2 over 1-3 hr q12h × 4-12 doses, repeat at 2-3 wk intervals, or when patient recovers from toxicities

Meningeal leukemia

Adult and child: IT 5-75 mg/m^2 variable daily × 4 days to q 2-7 days

Available forms: Powder for inj 100, 500 mg, 1, 2 g; sus rel (Depo Cyt) liposomal for IT use 10 mg/ml

Adverse effects

CNS: Neuritis, dizziness, headache, cerebellar syndrome, personality changes, ataxia, me-

chanical dysphasia, **coma; chemical arachnoiditis** (IT)
CV: Chest pain, **cardiopathy**
CYTARABINE SYNDROME: Fever, myalgia, bone pain, chest pain, rash, conjunctivitis, malaise (6-12 hr after administration)
EENT: Sore throat, conjunctivitis
GI: *Nausea, vomiting, anorexia, diarrhea, stomatitis,* **hepatotoxicity,** abdominal pain, hematemesis, **GI hemorrhage**
GU: Urinary retention, **renal failure, hyperuricemia**
HEMA: **Thrombophlebitis, bleeding, thrombocytopenia, leukopenia, myelosuppression, anemia**
INTEG: *Rash, fever,* freckling, cellulitis
META: Hyperuricemia
RESP: **Pneumonia,** dyspnea, **pulmonary edema** (high doses)
SYST: **Anaphylaxis**

Contraindications: Pregnancy **D,** hypersensitivity, infants

Precautions: Renal disease, hepatic disease, lactation

Pharmacokinetics

Absorption	Complete
Distribution	Widely distributed; crosses blood-brain barrier, placenta
Metabolism	Liver, extensively
Excretion	Kidneys
Half-life	1-3 hr; IT 100-236 hr

Pharmacodynamics

Unknown

Interactions

Individual drugs

Digoxin oral: decreased digoxin effects
Radiation: increased toxicity, bone marrow suppression

Drug classifications

Antineoplastics: increased toxicity, bone marrow suppression

NURSING CONSIDERATIONS

Assessment

- Assess buccal cavity q8h for dryness, sores or ulceration, white patches, pain, bleeding, dysphagia; obtain prescription for viscous lidocaine (Xylocaine)
- Assess symptoms indicating anaphylaxis: rash, pruritus, urticaria, purpuric skin lesions, itching, flushing, resuscitation equipment should be nearby
- (Alert) Assess for chemical arachnoiditis (IT): headache, nausea, vomiting, fever; neck rigidity/pain, meningism, CSF pleocytosis; may be decreased by dexamethasone
- Assess tachypnea, dyspnea, edema, fatigue; identify dyspnea, crackles, unproductive cough, chest pain, tachypnea; pulmonary edema may be fatal (rare)
- (Alert) Assess for cytarabine syndrome 6-12 hr after inf: fever, myalgia, bone pain, chest pain, rash, conjunctivitis, malaise; corticosteroid may be ordered
- Monitor CBC, differential, platelet count weekly; withhold drug if WBC count is <1000/mm^3 or platelet count is <50,000/mm^3
- Assess for increased uric acid levels, swelling, joint pain primarily in extremities; patient should be well hydrated to prevent urate deposits
- Monitor renal function studies: BUN, creatinine, serum uric acid, urine CCr before and during therapy; I&O ratio; report fall in urine output to <30 ml/hr
- Monitor temp q4h (may indicate beginning of infection)
- Monitor liver function tests before and during therapy (bilirubin, AST, ALT, LDH) as needed or monthly; note yellowing of skin or sclera, dark urine, clay-colored stools, pruritus, abdominal pain, fever, diarrhea; an antispasmodic may be used for GI symptoms
- Assess for bleeding: hematuria, stool guaiac, bruising or petechiae, mucosa or orifices q8h; identify inflammation of mucosa, breaks in skin

Nursing diagnoses

- Injury, risk for (adverse reactions)
- Body image, disturbed (adverse reactions)
- Infection, risk for (adverse reactions)
- Knowledge, deficient (teaching)

Implementation

- Avoid contact with skin; very irritating; wash completely to remove
- Give fluids **IV** or PO before chemotherapy to hydrate patient
- Give antiemetic 30-60 min before giving drug to prevent vomiting, and prn; antibiotics for prophylaxis of infection
- Increase fluids to 3 L/day
- Give top or syst analgesics for pain
- Give in AM so drug can be eliminated before bedtime
- Give **IV** direct after diluting 100 mg/5 ml of sterile water for inj; give by direct **IV** over 1-3 min through free-flowing tubing

IM/SUBCUT route

- Reconstitute 100 mg/5 ml or 500 mg/10 ml with bacteriostatic water for inj with benzyl alcohol 0.9%; do not use sol with precipitate; stable for 48 hr

Intrathecal route

- Liposomal: withdraw drug immediately before use; use within 4 hr, do not save unused portions, or use in-line filter; give directly into CSF by intraventricular reservoir or by direct inj into lumbar site
- Give slowly over 1-5 min, follow with lumbar puncture, instruct patient to lie flat, give dexamethasone 4 mg bid PO or **IV** × 5 days beginning on day of liposomal inj

IV infusion route

- May be further diluted in 50-100 ml 0.9% NaCl or D_5W and given over 30 min to 24 hr depending on dosage; may be given by cont inf also

Syringe compatibilities: Metoclopramide

Y-site compatibilities: Amifostine, amsacrine, aztreonam, cefepime, chlorproMAZINE, cimetidine, cladribine, dexamethasone, diphenhydrAMINE, droperidol, famotidine, filgrastim, fludarabine, gentamicin, granisetron, heparin, hydrocortisone, hydromorphone, idarubicin, lorazepam, melphalan, methotrexate, methylPREDNISolone, metoclopramide, morphine, ondansetron, paclitaxel, piperacillin/tazobactam, prochlorperazine, promethazine, propofol, ranitidine, sargramostim, sodium bicarbonate, teniposide, thiotepa, vinorelbine

Additive compatibilities: Corticotropin, DAUNOrubicin with etoposide, etoposide, hydrOXYzine, lincomycin, mitoxantrone, potassium chloride, prednisoLONE, ondansetron, sodium bicarbonate, vinCRIStine

Additive incompatibilities: Carbenicillin, fluorouracil, heparin, regular insulin, nafcillin, oxacillin, penicillin G sodium

Solution compatibilities: Amino acids, 4.25%/D_{25}, D_5/LR, D_5/0.2% NaCl, D_5/0.9% NaCl, D_{10}/0.9% NaCl, D_5W, invert glucose 10% in electrolyte #1, Ringer's LR, 0.9% NaCl, sodium lactate 1/6 mol/L, TPN #57

Patient/family education

- Advise patient that contraceptive measures are recommended during and 4 mo after therapy
- Teach patient to avoid use of products containing aspirin or ibuprofen, NSAIDs, razors, commercial mouthwash, since bleeding may occur; to report symptoms of bleeding (hematuria, tarry stools)
- Advise that fever, headache, nausea, vomiting are likely to occur, but to continue using dexamethasone with IT administration
- Provide liquid diet: carbonated beverages; gelatin may be added if patient is not nauseated or vomiting
- Provide rinsing of mouth tid-qid with water, club soda; brushing of teeth bid-qid with soft brush or cotton-tipped applicators for stomatitis; use unwaxed dental floss
- Advise patient to report signs of anemia (fatigue, headache, irritability, faintness, shortness of breath)
- Advise patient to avoid foods with citric acid, hot or rough texture if stomatitis is present, use sponge brush and rinse with water after each meal; to report stomatitis: any bleeding, white spots, ulcerations in mouth; tell patient to examine mouth daily, report any symptoms
- Instruct patient to report any changes in breathing or coughing even several months after treatment; to avoid crowds and persons with respiratory tract or other infections; neurotoxicity
- Caution patient not to have any vaccinations without the advice of the prescriber; serious reactions can occur
- Advise patient to take fluids 3 L/day to prevent renal damage

Evaluation

Positive therapeutic outcome

- Prevention of rapid division of malignant cells

! HIGH ALERT

dacarbazine (Rx)

(da-kar'ba-zeen)

dacarbazine, DTIC ✤, DTIC-Dome

Func. class.: Antineoplastic—miscellaneous agent

Chem. class.: Imidazole

Pregnancy category C

Action: Alkylates DNA, RNA; inhibits enzymes that allow synthesis of amino acids in proteins; also responsible for cross-linking DNA strands; activity is not cell cycle phase specific

Therapeutic Outcome: Prevention of rapidly growing malignant cells

Uses: Hodgkin's disease, sarcomas, neuroblastoma, malignant melanoma

Investigational uses: Metastatic sarcoma

Dosage and routes

Metastatic malignant melanoma

***Adult:* IV** 2-4.5 mg/kg daily × 10 days or 250 mg/m^2 daily × 5 days; repeat q3 wk depending on response

Hodgkin's disease

***Adult:* IV** 150 mg/m^2 daily × 5 days with other agents, repeat q4 wk or 375 mg/m^2 on day 1 when given in combination, repeat q15 days

Available forms: Inj 100, 200 mg

Adverse effects

CNS: Facial paresthesia, flushing, fever, malaise, confusion, headache, **seizures,** blurred vision (high doses)

GI: *Nausea, anorexia, vomiting,* **hepatotoxicity** (rare)

HEMA: **Thrombocytopenia, leukopenia,** anemia

INTEG: *Alopecia,* dermatitis, pain at inj site, photosensitivity; severe sun reactions (high doses)

MISC: Flulike symptoms, malaise, fever, myalgia

SYST: **Anaphylaxis**

Contraindications: Lactation

Precautions: Pregnancy **C** (1st trimester), radiation therapy

Pharmacokinetics

Absorption	Complete bioavailability (**IV**)
Distribution	Widely distributed; concentrates in liver
Metabolism	Liver (50%, 5% protein bound)
Excretion	Kidneys, unchanged (50%)
Half-life	Initial 35 min, terminal 5 hr

Pharmacodynamics

Unknown

Interactions

Individual drugs

Phenobarbital, phenytoin: increased metabolism; decreased effect

Radiation: bone marrow suppression, toxicity

Drug classifications

Aminoglycosides: increased nephrotoxicity

Anticoagulants, salicylates: increased risk of bleeding

Antineoplastics, bone marrow–suppressing drugs: increased toxicity, bone marrow suppression

Diuretics, loop: increased ototoxicity

Live virus vaccines: increased adverse reactions; decreased antibody reaction

NURSING CONSIDERATIONS

Assessment

- Assess symptoms indicating severe allergic reaction: rash, pruritus, urticaria, purpuric skin lesions, itching, flushing; drug should be discontinued
- Monitor CBC, differential, platelet count weekly; withhold drug if WBC is <4000/mm^3 or platelet count is <100,000/mm^3
- Monitor renal function studies: BUN, creatinine, urine CCr before and during therapy; I&O ratio; report fall in urine output to <30 ml/hr
- Monitor temp q4h (may indicate beginning of infection)
- Monitor liver function tests before and during therapy (bilirubin, AST, ALT, LDH) as needed or monthly; note jaundice of skin or sclera, dark urine, clay-colored stools, itchy skin, abdominal pain, fever, diarrhea; hepatotoxicity can be serious and fatal
- Assess for bleeding: hematuria, stool guaiac, bruising or petechiae, mucosa or orifices q8h; check for inflammation of mucosa, breaks in skin
- Identify effects of alopecia on body image; discuss feelings about body changes

Nursing diagnoses

- Injury, risk for (adverse reactions)
- Body image, disturbed (adverse reactions)
- Infection, risk for (adverse reactions)
- Knowledge, deficient (teaching)

Implementation

- Give fluids **IV** or PO before chemotherapy to hydrate patient
- Give antiemetic 30-60 min before giving drug to prevent vomiting, and prn; antibiotics for prophylaxis of infection
- Provide liquid diet: carbonated beverages; gelatin may be added if patient is not nauseated or vomiting
- After diluting 100 mg/9.9 ml of sterile water for inj (10 mg/ml), give by direct **IV** over 1 min through Y-tube or 3-way stopcock
- May be further diluted in 50-250 ml of D_5W or normal saline for inj and given over 30 min
- Watch for extravasation; give 3-5 ml of mixture of 4 ml sodium thiosulfate 10% plus 5 ml of sterile water SUBCUT as prescribed

Y-site compatibilities:

Amifostine, aztreonam, filgrastim, fludarabine, granisetron, melphalan, ondansetron, paclitaxel, sargramostim, teniposide, thiotepa, vinorelbine

Additive compatibilities:

Bleomycin, carmustine, cyclophosphamide, cytarabine, dactinomycin, DOXOrubicin, fluorouracil, mercaptopurine, methotrexate, ondansetron, vinBLAStine

Additive incompatibilities:
Hydrocortisone sodium succinate, cysteine

Patient/family education

- Teach patient to avoid use of products containing aspirin or ibuprofen, razors, commercial mouthwash, since bleeding may occur; to report symptoms of bleeding (hematuria, tarry stools)
- Instruct patient to report signs of anemia (fatigue, headache, irritability, faintness, shortness of breath)
- Advise patient that hair may be lost during treatment; a wig or hairpiece may make patient feel better; new hair may be different in color, texture
- Caution patient not to have any vaccinations without the advice of prescriber; serious reactions can occur
- Advise patient contraception is needed during treatment and for several months after the completion of therapy; drug has teratogenic properties

Evaluation

Positive therapeutic outcome

- Prevention of rapid division of malignant cells

! HIGH ALERT

daclizumab (Rx)

(dah-kliz'uh-mab)

Zenapax

Func. class.: Immunosuppressant

Chem class.: Humanized IgGl monoclonal antibody

Pregnancy category C

Action: Binds to the IL-2 receptor antagonist

Therapeutic Outcome: Prevention of graft rejection

Uses: Acute allograft rejection in renal transplant patients

Dosage and routes

Adult: **IV** 1 mg/kg as part of a regimen that includes cycloSPORINE and corticosteroids, mix calculated vol with 50 ml of 0.9% NaCl and give via peripheral/central vein over 15 min

Available forms: Inj 25 mg/ml

Adverse effects

CNS: *Chills, tremors, dizziness, insomnia,* headache, prickly sensation

CV: Hypertension, **tachycardia, thrombosis, bleeding**

GI: *Vomiting, nausea, diarrhea, constipation, abdominal pain, pyrosis*

GU: Oliguria, dysuria, **renal tubular necrosis, renal damage, hydronephrosis**

INTEG: Impaired wound healing, acne

RESP: *Dyspnea, wheezing,* **pulmonary edema,** coughing, atelectasis, congestion, hypoxia

Contraindications: Hypersensitivity

Precautions: Pregnancy **C**, child <2 yr, lactation, elderly

Pharmacokinetics

Unknown

Pharmacodynamics

Unknown

Interactions

Drug/herb

Ginseng, maitake, mistletoe, schisandra, St. John's wort, turmeric: decreased immunosuppressant effect

Safflower: increased immunosuppressant effect

NURSING CONSIDERATIONS

Assessment

- Monitor blood studies: Hgb, WBC, platelets during treatment qmo; if leukocytes are <3000/mm^3, drug should be discontinued
- Monitor liver function studies: alkaline phosphatase, AST, ALT, bilirubin
- Assess for hepatotoxicity: dark urine, jaundice, itching, light-colored stools; drug should be discontinued
- Assess for anaphylaxis: have corticosteroids, epINEPHrine available

Nursing diagnoses

- Injury, risk for (uses)
- Knowledge, deficient (teaching)

Implementation

- Give all other medications PO if possible; avoid IM inj, since infection may occur

IV route

- Solution compatibilities 0.9% NaCl
- Protect undiluted sol from direct light; should be used with drugs for immunosuppression

Patient/family education

- Teach patient to report fever, chills, sore throat, fatigue, since serious infection may occur
- Instruct patient to use contraception

(women), before, during, and for 4 mo after treatment

- Advise patient to avoid vaccinations during treatment
- Advise patient to drink fluids during treatment

Evaluation

Positive therapeutic outcome

- Absence of graft rejection

! HIGH ALERT

dactinomycin (Rx)

(dak-ti-noe-mye'sin)

Cosmegen

Func. class.: Antineoplastic, antibiotic

Pregnancy category C

Action: Inhibits DNA, RNA, protein synthesis; derived from *Streptomyces parvulus;* replication is decreased by binding to DNA, which causes strand splitting; cell cycle nonspecific; a vesicant

Therapeutic Outcome: Prevention of rapidly growing malignant cells, immunosuppression

Uses: Sarcomas, melanomas, trophoblastic tumors in women, testicular cancer, Wilms' tumor, rhabdomyosarcoma

Dosage and routes

Adult: **IV** 500 mcg/m^2/day × 5 days; stop drug for 2-4 wk; then repeat cycle

Child: **IV** 15 mcg/kg/day × 5 days, not to exceed 500 mcg/day; stop drug until bone marrow recovery, then repeat cycle

Available forms: Inj 0.5 mg/vial

Adverse effects

CNS: Malaise, fatigue, lethargy, fever

EENT: Cheilitis, dysphagia, esophagitis

GI: *Nausea, vomiting, anorexia, stomatitis,* **hepatotoxicity,** abdominal pain, diarrhea

HEMA: **Thrombocytopenia, leukopenia, aplastic anemia**

INTEG: *Rash,* alopecia, pain at inj site, folliculitis, acne, desquamation, *extravasation*

MS: Myalgia

Contraindications: Hypersensitivity, herpes infections, child <6 mo

Precautions: Pregnancy **C**, renal, hepatic disease, lactation, bone marrow suppression

Pharmacokinetics

Absorption	Complete bioavailability
Distribution	Widely distributed; crosses placenta
Metabolism	Unknown
Excretion	Bile; feces, unchanged (50%); kidneys (10%)
Half-life	36 hr

Pharmacodynamics

Unknown

Interactions

Individual drugs

Radiation: increased toxicity

Drug classifications

Antineoplastics: increased toxicity

Drug/lab test

Increased: uric acid

NURSING CONSIDERATIONS

Assessment

- Assess buccal cavity q8h for dryness, sores or ulceration, white patches, pain, bleeding, dysphagia; obtain prescription for viscous lidocaine (Xylocaine)
- (Alert) Assess symptoms indicating severe allergic reaction: rash, pruritus, urticaria, purpuric skin lesions, itching, flushing; drug should be discontinued
- Monitor CBC, differential, platelet count weekly; withhold drug if WBC is <4000/mm^3 or platelet count is <100,000/mm^3; notify prescriber of results if WBC <20,000/mm^3, platelets <150,000/mm^3
- Monitor renal function studies: BUN, creatinine, serum uric acid, urine CCr before and during therapy; I&O ratio; report fall in urine output to <30 ml/hr
- Monitor temp q4h (may indicate beginning of infection)
- Monitor liver function tests before and during therapy (bilirubin, AST, ALT, LDH) as needed or monthly; note jaundice of skin or sclera, dark urine, clay-colored stools, itchy skin, abdominal pain, fever, diarrhea
- Assess for bleeding: hematuria, stool guaiac, bruising or petechiae, mucosa or orifices q8h; check for inflammation of mucosa, breaks in skin
- Identify effects of alopecia on body image; discuss feelings about body changes

Nursing diagnoses

- Injury, risk for (adverse reactions)
- Body image, disturbed (adverse reactions)
- Oral mucous membranes, impaired (adverse reactions)

- Infection, risk for (adverse reactions)
- Knowledge, deficient (teaching)

Implementation

- Provide antacid before oral agent; give drug pc PM, before bedtime; antiemetic 30-60 min before giving drug to prevent vomiting, and prn; antibiotics for prophylaxis of infection
- Provide liquid diet: carbonated beverages; gelatin may be added if patient is not nauseated or vomiting
- Help patient rinse mouth tid-qid with water, club soda, brush teeth bid-qid with soft brush or cotton-tipped applicators for stomatitis, use unwaxed dental floss
- Drug should be prepared by experienced personnel using proper precautions
- Give after diluting 0.5 mg/1.1 ml of sterile water for inj without preservative; use 2.2 ml (0.25 mg/ml), give by direct **IV** at 0.5 mg or less/min through Y-tube or 3-way stopcock of inf in progress
- Increase fluids to 3 L/day

Intermittent IV infusion route

- May be further diluted in 50 ml of D_5W or 0.9% NaCl for inf; run over 10-15 min
- Give hydrocortisone, sodium thiosulfate to infiltration area, and ice compress after stopping inf
- Store in darkness in cool environment

Y-site compatibilities: Allopurinol, amifostine, aztreonam, cefepime, fludarabine, granisetron, melphalan, ondansetron, sargramostim, teniposide, thiotepa, vinorelbine

Patient/family education

- Teach patient to avoid use of products containing aspirin or ibuprofen, razors, commercial mouthwash, since bleeding may occur; to report symptoms of bleeding (hematuria, tarry stools)
- Instruct patient to report signs of anemia (fatigue, headache, irritability, faintness, shortness of breath)
- Advise patient that hair may be lost during treatment; a wig or hairpiece may make patient feel better; new hair may be different in color, texture
- Caution patient not to have any vaccinations without the advice of the prescriber, serious reactions can occur
- Advise patient that contraception is needed during treatment and for several months after the completion of therapy
- Advise patient to increase fluids to 3 L/day

Evaluation

Positive therapeutic outcome

- Prevention of rapid division of malignant cells

! HIGH ALERT

dalteparin (Rx)

(dahl'ta-pear-in)

Fragmin

Func. class.: Anticoagulant

Chem. class.: Low-molecular-weight heparin

Pregnancy category B

Action: Prevents conversion of fibrinogen to fibrin and prothrombin to thrombin by enhancing inhibitory effects of antithrombin III

Therapeutic Outcome: Absence of deep vein thrombosis

Uses: Unstable angina/non-Q-wave MI; prevention of deep vein thrombosis in abdominal surgery, hip replacement patients

Investigational uses: Systemic anticoagulation in venous/arterial thromboembolic complications

Dosage and routes

Hip replacement surgery/ DVT prophylaxis

Adult: SUBCUT 2500 international units 2 hr before surgery and 2nd dose in the evening the day of surgery, then 5000 international units SUBCUT 1st postop day and daily 5-10 days

Unstable angina/ non-Q-wave MI

Adult: SUBCUT 120 international units/kg, do not exceed 10,000 international units q12h with concurrent aspirin, continue until stable

Systemic anticoagulation

Adult: SUBCUT 200 international units/kg daily or 100 international units/kg bid

Deep vein thrombosis, prophylaxis for abdominal surgery

Adult: SUBCUT 2500 international units daily, 1-2 hr before abdominal surgery and repeat daily × 5-10 days; in high-risk patients 5000 international units may be used

Available forms: Prefilled syringes, 2500, 5000 international units/0.2 ml; 10,000 international units multidose vials; 7500 international units/0.3 ml, 10,000 international units/ml

Adverse effects

CNS: **Intracranial bleeding**

HEMA: **Thrombocytopenia**

INTEG: Pruritus, superficial wound infection

SYST: Hypersensitivity, **hemorrhage, anaphylaxis** possible

Contraindications: Hypersensitivity to this drug, heparin, pork products, benzyl alcohol; hemophilia, leukemia with bleeding, thrombocytopenic purpura, cerebrovascular hemorrhage, cerebral aneurysm, severe hypertension, other severe cardiac disease, those undergoing regional anesthesia for unstable angina, non-Q-wave MI

Precautions: Pregnancy **B,** elderly, hepatic disease, severe renal disease, blood dyscrasias, subacute bacterial endocarditis, acute nephritis, lactation, child, recent childbirth, peptic ulcer disease, pericarditis, pericardial effusion, recent lumbar puncture, vasculitis, other diseases where bleeding is possible

Pharmacokinetics	
Absorption	87%
Distribution	Unknown
Metabolism	Liver
Excretion	Kidney
Half-life	3-5 hr elimination

Pharmacodynamics	
Onset	Unknown
Peak	4 hr
Duration	Unknown

Interactions

Drug classifications

Anticoagulants, NSAIDs, platelet inhibitors, salicylates, thrombolytics: increased risk of bleeding

Drug/herb

Agrimony, alfalfa, angelica, anise, basil, bay, bilberry, black haw, bogbean, bromelain, buchu, chondroitin, cinchona bark, dong quai, fenugreek, feverfew, garlic, ginger, ginkgo, ginseng, horse chestnut, Irish moss, kelp, kelpware, khella, lovage, lungwort, meadowsweet, motherwort, mugwort, nettle, papaya, parsley (large amounts), pau d'arco, pineapple, poplar, prickly ash, safflower, saw palmetto, senega, tonka bean, turmeric, wintergreen, yarrow: increased risk of bleeding

Chamomile, coenzyme Q10, flax, glucomannan, goldenseal, guar gum: decreased anticoagulant effect

NURSING CONSIDERATIONS

Assessment

- Assess for bleeding (Hct, occult blood in stools) during treatment since bleeding can occur
- ◆ Assess for bleeding gums, petechiae, ecchymosis, black tarry stools, hematuria, epistaxis, decrease in Hct, B/P; may indicate bleeding, possible hemorrhage; notify prescriber immediately, drug should be discontinued
- Assess for hypersensitivity: fever, skin rash, urticaria; notify prescriber immediately
- Assess for needed dosage change q1-2 wk; dose may need to be decreased if bleeding occurs

Nursing diagnoses

- Injury, risk for (uses, adverse reactions)
- Tissue perfusion, ineffective (uses)
- Knowledge, deficient (teaching)

Implementation

SUBCUT route

- Cannot be used interchangeably (unit for unit with unfractionated heparin or LMWHs)
- Do not give IM or **IV** drug route; approved in SUBCUT only; do not mix with other inj or sol
- Give by SUBCUT only; have patient sit or lie down; SUBCUT inj may be 2 in from umbilicus in a U-shape, upper outer side of thigh, around navel, or upper outer quadrangle of the buttocks; rotate inj sites
- Changing needles is not recommended; change inj site daily, use at same time of day

Patient/family education

- Advise patient to avoid OTC preparations that contain aspirin, other anticoagulants; serious drug interaction may occur
- Advise patient to use soft-bristle toothbrush to avoid bleeding gums, avoid contact sports, use electric razor, avoid IM inj
- Instruct patient to report any signs of bleeding: gums, under skin, urine, stools; unusual bruising

Evaluation

Positive therapeutic outcome

- Absence of deep vein thrombosis

Treatment of overdose: Protamine sulfate 1% given **IV**; 1 mg protamine/100 anti-Xa international units of dalteparin given

danazol (Rx)

(da'na-zole)

Cyclomen ✚, danazol, Danocrine

Func. class.: Androgen, anabolic steroid

Chem. class.: α-Ethinyl testosterone derivative

Pregnancy category X

Do Not Confuse:
danazol/Dantrium

Action: Atrophy of endometrial tissue; decreases FSH, LH, which are controlled by pituitary; this leads to amenorrhea/anovulation; has weak androgen, anabolic activity

Therapeutic Outcome: Decreased pain and nodules/fibrocystic breast disease; correction in hereditary angioedema; atrophy of endometrial tissue (ectopic)

Uses: Endometriosis, prevention of hereditary angioedema, fibrocystic breast disease

Dosage and routes

Endometriosis

Adult: PO 100-500 mg bid, uninterrupted for 3-9 mo

Fibrocystic breast disease

Adult: PO 100-400 mg daily in 2 divided doses × 2-6 mo

Hereditary angioedema prevention

Adult: PO 200 mg bid-tid until desired response, then decrease dose to 100 mg at 1-3 mo intervals

Available forms: Caps 50, 100, 200 mg

Adverse effects

CNS: Dizziness, headache, fatigue, tremors, paresthesias, flushing, sweating, anxiety, *lability,* insomnia

CV: Increased B/P

EENT: Conjunctival edema, nasal congestion, voice weakness

ENDO: Abnormal GTT

GI: Nausea, vomiting, constipation, *weight gain,* **cholestatic jaundice**

GU: Hematuria, *amenorrhea,* atrophic vaginitis, decreased libido, *decreased breast size,* clitoral hypertrophy, testicular atrophy

INTEG: Rash, *acneiform lesions,* oily hair and skin, flushing, sweating, acne vulgaris, alopecia, *hirsutism,* pruritus

MS: Cramps, spasms, joint swelling

Contraindications: Pregnancy **X,** severe renal disease, severe cardiac disease, severe hepatic disease, hypersensitivity, genital bleeding (abnormal), children, lactation

Precautions: Migraine headaches, seizure disorders

Pharmacokinetics	
Absorption	GI absorption
Distribution	Unknown
Metabolism	Liver
Excretion	Kidneys
Half-life	4½ hr

Pharmacodynamics
Unknown

Interactions

Individual drugs

cycloSPORINE: increased risk of nephrotoxicity

Insulin: increased action

Drug classifications

Anticoagulants, antidiabetics, corticosteroids: increased action

Drug/lab test

Increased: cholesterol

Decreased: cholesterol, T_4, T_3, thyroid ^{131}I uptake test, 17-KS, PBI

Interferences: GTT

NURSING CONSIDERATIONS

Assessment

- Assess for pain before and after treatment in endometriosis, fibrocystic breast disease; tenderness, nodules in fibrocystic breast disease
- Monitor potassium, blood, urine glucose while patient is on long-term therapy; liver function tests, periodically; semen volume, sperm count, motility in hereditary angioedema
- Assess breast for fibrocystic nodules; check for pain, tenderness before therapy and throughout to identify if treatment is effective
- Monitor weight daily; notify prescriber if weekly weight gain is >5 lb; I&O ratio; be alert for decreasing urinary output, increasing edema, hypertension, cardiac symptoms, jaundice
- Assess for mental status: affect, mood, behavioral changes, aggression, sleep disorders, depression; change may be extreme
- Assess for signs of virilization: deepening of voice, decreased libido, facial hair (may not be reversible)

Nursing diagnoses

- Infection, risk for (adverse reactions)
- Injury, risk for (adverse reactions)
- Knowledge, deficient (teaching)

Implementation

- Do not break, crush, or chew caps
- Start treatment during menstruation in endometriosis, fibrocystic breast disease
- Store in airtight container at room temp
- Provide ROM exercise for patients who are immobile
- Give with food or milk to decrease GI symptoms

Patient/family education

- Teach patient to notify prescriber if therapeutic response decreases; advise that endometriosis tends to recur after drug is discontinued; not to discontinue medication abruptly but to taper over several weeks
- Advise patient that nonhormonal contraceptive measures are needed during treatment; amenorrhea may occur with higher dosages
- Teach patient to report menstrual irregularities; that amenorrhea usually occurs but menstruation resumes 2-3 mo after termination of therapy; that drug should induce anovulation; reversible within 60-90 days after drug is discontinued
- Teach patient about routine breast self-exam technique, to report any increase in nodule size
- Instruct patient to report masculinization: deepening voice, facial hair growth, body hair growth
- Advise patient to use sunscreen or stay out of the sun to prevent burns

Evaluation

Positive therapeutic outcome

- Decreased pain in endometriosis
- Decreased size, pain in fibrocystic breast disease
- Decreased signs of angioedema (hereditary)

dantrolene (Rx)

(dan'troe-leen)

Dantrium

Func. class.: Skeletal muscle relaxant, direct acting

Chem. class.: Hydantoin

Pregnancy category C

Do Not Confuse:

Dantrium/danazol

Action: Interferes with intracellular release from the sarcoplasmic reticulum of calcium necessary to initiate contraction; slows catabolism in malignant hyperthermia

Therapeutic Outcome: Decreased muscle spasticity; absence of malignant hyperthermia

Uses: Spasticity in multiple sclerosis, stroke, spinal cord injury, cerebral palsy, prevention and treatment of malignant hyperthermia

Dosage and routes

Spasticity

Adult: PO 25 mg/day; may increase by 25-100 mg bid-qid, not to exceed 400 mg/day × 1 wk

Child: PO 1 mg/kg/day given in divided doses bid; may increase gradually, not to exceed 100 mg daily

Malignant hyperthermia

Adult and child: **IV** 1 mg/kg; may repeat to total dose of 10 mg/kg; PO 4-8 mg/kg/day in 4 divided doses × 3 days to prevent further hyperthermia; postcrisis follow-up 4-8 mg/kg/day for 1-3 days

Prevention of malignant hyperthermia

Adult and child: PO 4-8 mg/kg/day in 3-4 divided doses × 1-2 days before procedures; give last dose 4 hr preoperatively; **IV** 2.5 mg/kg prior to anesthesia

Available forms: Caps 25, 50, 100 mg; powder for inj 20 mg/vial

Adverse effects

CNS: *Dizziness, weakness, fatigue, drowsiness,* headache, disorientation, insomnia, paresthesias, tremors, **seizures**

CV: Hypotension, chest pain, palpitations

EENT: Nasal congestion, blurred vision, mydriasis

GI: **Hepatic injury,** *nausea,* constipation, vomiting, increased AST and alkaline phosphatase, abdominal pain, dry mouth, anorexia, hepatitis, dyspepsia

GU: Urinary frequency, nocturia, impotence, crystalluria

HEMA: **Eosinophilia**

INTEG: Rash, pruritus, photosensitivity

RESP: Pleural effusion

Contraindications: Hypersensitivity, compromised pulmonary function, active hepatic disease, impaired myocardial function

Precautions: Pregnancy **C,** peptic ulcer disease, renal disease, hepatic disease, stroke, seizure disorder, diabetes mellitus, lactation, elderly

Pharmacokinetics

Absorption	PO (30%-35%), poor
Distribution	Unknown
Metabolism	Liver, extensively
Excretion	Kidney
Half-life	9 hr

Pharmacodynamics

	PO	IV
Onset	Unknown	Immediate
Peak	5 hr	5 hr
Duration	Dose related	Dose related

Interactions

Individual drugs

Alcohol: increased CNS depression
Verapamil: increased dysrhythmias

Drug classifications

Antidepressants (tricyclic), antihistamines, barbiturates, opiates, sedative/hypnotics: increased CNS depression
Estrogens, hepatotoxic agents: increased hepatotoxicity

NURSING CONSIDERATIONS

Assessment

- Monitor I&O ratio; check for urinary retention, frequency, hesitancy, especially elderly
- Monitor ECG in epileptic patients; poor seizure control has occurred with patients taking this drug; assess for increased seizure activity in epilepsy patient
- Monitor hepatic function by frequent determination of AST, ALT, bilirubin, alkaline phosphatase, GGTP, renal function studies, CBC
- Assess for allergic reactions: rash, fever, respiratory distress
- Monitor for severe weakness, numbness in extremities
- Assess for CNS depression: dizziness, drowsiness, psychiatric symptoms
- Assess for signs of hepatotoxicity: jaundice, yellow sclera, pain in abdomen, nausea, fever; drug should be discontinued if these signs and symptoms occur

Nursing diagnoses

- Pain, chronic (uses)
- Mobility, physical, impaired (uses)
- Injury, risk for (adverse reactions)
- Knowledge, deficient (teaching)

Implementation

PO route

- Do not crush or chew caps; caps may be opened and mixed with juice and swallowed; drink immediately after mixing
- Give with meals for GI symptoms
- Store in airtight container at room temp

IV route

- Administer **IV** after reconstituting 20 mg/60 ml sterile water for inj without bacteriostatic agent (333 mcg/ml); shake until clear; give by rapid **IV** push through Y-tube or 3-way stopcock; follow by prescribed doses immediately; may also give by intermittent inf over 1 hr before anesthesia; assess site for extravasation, phlebitis
- Protect diluted sol from light; use reconstituted sol within 6 hr
- Considered incompatible in sol or syringe, compatibility unknown

Patient/family education

- Notify prescriber of abdominal pain, jaundiced sclera, clay-colored stools, change in color of urine, rash, itching
- Caution patient not to take with alcohol, other CNS depressants; severe CNS depression can occur; avoid using OTC medication: cough preparations, antihistamines, unless directed by prescriber
- Tell patient that if improvement does not occur within 6 wk, prescriber may discontinue
- Caution patient to avoid hazardous activities if drowsiness, dizziness, blurred vision occurs; wait several days to identify patient response to medication
- Teach patient to use sunscreen, protective clothing for photosensitivity
- Instruct patient to take medication as prescribed; do not double doses; take missed dose within 1 hr of scheduled time

Evaluation

Positive therapeutic outcome

- Decreased pain, spasticity
- Absence or decreased symptoms of malignant hyperthermia

Treatment of overdose: Induce emesis of conscious patient; lavage, dialysis

daptomycin (Rx)

(dap′toe-mye-sin)
Cubicin
Func. class.: Antiinfective—miscellaneous
Chem. class.: Lipopeptides

Pregnancy category B

Action: New class of antiinfective; binds to the bacterial membrane and results in a rapid depolarization of the membrane potential, leading to inhibition of DNA, RNA, and protein synthesis

Therapeutic Outcome: Absence of infections

Uses: Complicated skin, skin structure infections caused by *Staphylococcus aureus,* including methicillin-resistant strains, *Streptococcus pyogenes, S. agalactiae, S. dysgalactiae, Enterococcus faecalis* (vancomycin-susceptible strains only)

Dosage and routes

Adult: **IV** INF 4 mg/kg over ½ hr diluted in 0.9% NaCl, give q24h ×7-14 days

Renal dose

Adult: **IV** INF CCr >30 ml/min 4 mg/kg q24h; CCr <30 ml/min; hemodialysis, CAPD 4 mg/kg q48h

Available forms: lyophilized powder for inj 250, 500 mg

Adverse effects

CNS: Headache, insomnia, dizziness

CV: Hypotension, hypertension, increased CPK

GI: Nausea, constipation, diarrhea, vomiting, dyspepsia, **pseudomembranous colitis**

GU: **Nephrotoxicity: increased BUN, creatinine, albumin**

INTEG: Rash, pruritus

MISC: Fungal infections, UTI, anemia

MS: Muscle pain or weakness, arthralgia, pain

Contraindications: Hypersensitivity

Precautions: Pregnancy **B**, renal disease, children, lactation, elderly

Pharmacokinetics	
Absorption	Unknown
Distribution	Protein binding 92%
Metabolism	Unknown
Excretion	Unknown
Half-life	Unknown

Pharmacodynamics	
Onset	Unknown
Peak	Unknown
Duration	Unknown

Interactions

Drug classifications

HMG-CoA reductase inhibitors: myopathy

NURSING CONSIDERATIONS

Assessment

- Monitor I&O ratio: report hematuria, oliguria; nephrotoxicity may occur
- (Alert) Monitor any patient with compromised renal system, toxicity may occur; BUN, creatinine
- Monitor blood studies: CBC
- Monitor C&S, drug may be given as soon as culture is taken
- Monitor B/P during administration; hypo/hypertension may occur
- Assess signs of infection
- Assess respiratory status: rate, character, wheezing
- Identify allergies before treatment, reaction of each medication

Nursing diagnoses

- Infection, risk for (uses)
- Knowledge, deficient (teaching)

Implementation

IV route

- Give after reconstitution with 5 ml 0.9% NaCl (250 mg/5 ml) or 10 ml 0.9% NaCl (500 mg/10 ml), further dilution is needed with 0.9% NaCl, infuse over ½ hr

Solution compatibilities: 0.9% NaCl, LR

Patient/family education

- Teach all aspects of drug therapy
- Advise to report sore throat, fever, fatigue; could indicate superinfection

Evaluation

Positive therapeutic outcome

- Negative culture

darbepoetin alfa (Rx)

(dar'bee-poh'-eh-tin al'fah)

Aranesp

Func. class.: Hematopoietic agent

Chem. class.: Recombinant human erythropoietin

Pregnancy category C

Action: Stimulates erythropoiesis by the same mechanism as endogenous erythropoietin; in response to hypoxia, erythropoietin is produced in the kidney and released into the bloodstream, where it interacts with progenitor stem cells to increase red cell production

Therapeutic Outcome: Decreased anemia with increased RBCs

Uses: Anemia associated with chronic renal failure in patients on and not on dialysis and anemic in nonmyeloid malignancies receiving coadministered chemotherapy

Dosage and routes

Correction of anemia

Adult: SUBCUT/**IV** 0.45 mcg/kg as a single inj, titrate not to exceed a target Hgb of 12 g/dl

Conversion from epoetin alfa to darbepoetin

Adult: SUBCUT/**IV** estimate starting dose based on weekly epoetin alfa dose; because of longer serum half-life, darbepoetin must be administered less frequently than epoetin alfa; if epoetin was given 2-3×/wk, give darbepoetin 1×/wk; if epoetin was given 1×/wk, give darbepoetin 1× q2 wk; do not increase doses more often than 1×/mo

Available forms: Sol for inj 25, 40, 60, 100, 150, 200, 300, 500 mcg/ml

Adverse effects

CNS: **Seizures**, sweating, headache, dizziness, **stroke**

CV: *Hypertension, hypotension,* **cardiac arrest,** *angina pectoris,* **thrombosis, CHF, acute MI, dysrhythmias,** chest pain, transient ischemic attacks

GI: *Diarrhea, vomiting, nausea, abdominal pain, constipation*

MISC: *Infection, fatigue, fever,* **death,** *fluid overload,* **vascular access hemorrhage**

MS: *Bone pain, myalgia, limb pain, back pain*

RESP: *Upper respiratory infection, dyspnea, cough, bronchitis*

SYST: Allergic reactions, **anaphylaxis**

Contraindications: Hypersensitivity to mammalian cell–derived products or human albumin, uncontrolled hypertension, red cell aplasia

Precautions: Pregnancy **C**, seizure disorder, porphyria, hypertension, lactation, children, sickle cell disease, vit B_{12} folate deficiency

Pharmacokinetics

Absorption	Slow, rate-limiting (SUBCUT)
Distribution	Vascular space
Metabolism	Metabolized in body (**IV**), extent unknown
Excretion	Unknown
Half-life	49 hr

Pharmacodynamics

Onset	Onset of increased reticulocyte count 1-6 wk
Peak	34 hr
Duration	Unknown

Interactions

Individual drugs

Do not use epoetin alfa with this drug

Drug classifications

Androgens: increased darbepoetin alfa effect

NURSING CONSIDERATIONS

Assessment

- Assess for serious allergic reactions: rash, urticaria; if anaphylaxis occurs, stop drug, administer emergency treatment (rare)
- Assess blood studies: ferritin, transferrin monthly; transferrin sat ≥20%, ferritin ≥100 ng/ml; Hgb 2×/wk until stabilized in target range (30%-33%) then at regular intervals; those with endogenous erythropoietin levels of <500 units/L respond to this agent
- Assess renal studies: urinalysis, protein, blood, BUN, creatinine
- Assess B/P, Hct; check for rising B/P as Hct rises, antihypertensives may be needed
- Assess CV status: hypertension may occur rapidly leading to hypertensive encephalopathy
- Assess I&O ratio; report drop in output to <50 ml/hr
- Assess for seizures if Hgb is increased within 2 wk by 4 pts
- Assess CNS symptoms: cold sensation, sweating, pain in long bones
- Assess dialysis patients for thrill, bruit of shunts; monitor for circulation impairment

Nursing diagnoses

- Fatigue (uses)
- Activity intolerance (uses)
- Knowledge, deficient (teaching)

Implementation

IV/SUBCUT

- Do not shake, do not dilute, do not mix with other drugs or solutions
- Check for discoloration, particulate matter; do not use if present, discard unused portion, do not pool unused portion

Patient/family education

- Caution patient to avoid driving or hazardous activity during beginning of treatment
- Advise patient to monitor B/P
- Advise patient to take iron supplements, vit B_{12}, folic acid as directed
- Advise patient to report side effects to prescriber, to comply with treatment regimen
- Teach home administration and review information for patients and caregivers if home administration is deemed appropriate

Evaluation

Positive therapeutic outcome

- Increased reticulocyte count, Hgb/Hct
- Increased appetite
- Enhanced sense of well-being

Treatment of overdose: If polycythemia occurs, discontinue drug temporarily; perform phlebotomy if clinically indicated

D

! HIGH ALERT

DAUNOrubicin (Rx)

(daw-noe-roo'bi-sin)

Cerubidine

DAUNOrubicin citrate liposome (Rx)

DaunoXome

Func. class.: Antineoplastic, antibiotic

Chem. class.: Anthracycline glycoside

Pregnancy category D

Do Not Confuse:
DAUNOrubicin/DOXOrubicin

Action: Inhibits DNA synthesis, primarily; derived from *Streptomyces coeruleorubidus;* replication is decreased by binding to DNA, which causes strand splitting; cell cycle specific (S phase); a vesicant

Therapeutic Outcome: Prevention of rapidly growing malignant cells; immunosuppression

Uses: Myelogenous, monocytic leukemia, acute nonlymphocytic leukemia, Ewing's sarcoma, Wilms' tumor, neuroblastoma, rhabdomyosarcoma; DAUNOrubicin citrate liposome: advanced Kaposi's sarcoma in HIV

Dosage and routes

Use decreased dose for those >60 yr

Single agent

Adult: **IV** 60 mg/m^2/day × 3-5 day q4 wk

In combination

Adult: **IV** 45 mg/m^2/day × 3 days, then 2 days of subsequent courses in combination

Child: **IV** 25-60 mg/m^2 depending on cycle

DAUNOrubicin citrate liposome

Adult: **IV** 40 mg/m^2 q2 wk

Renal dose

Adult: **IV** serum Cr >3 mg/dl reduce dose by 50%

Hepatic dose

Adult: **IV** serum bilirubin 1.2-3 mg/dl reduce dose by 25%; bilirubin >3 mg/dl reduce dose by 50%

Available forms: Inj 20 mg powder/vial, sol for inj 5 mg/ml; liposome: dispersion for inj 2 mg/ml

Adverse effects

DAUNOrubicin

CNS: Fever, chills

CV: **Dysrhythmias, CHF, pericarditis, myocarditis,** peripheral edema

GI: *Nausea, vomiting, anorexia, mucositis,* **hepatotoxicity**

GU: Impotence, sterility, amenorrhea, gynecomastia, hyperuricemia

HEMA: **Thrombocytopenia, leukopenia, anemia**

INTEG: *Rash, extravasation,* dermatitis, reversible alopecia, cellulitis, thrombophlebitis at inj site

MISC: **Anaphylaxis**

DAUNOrubicin citrate liposome

CNS: Fatigue, headache, depression, insomnia, dizziness, malaise, neuropathy

CV: Chest pain, edema

GI: Abdominal pain, nausea, vomiting, *diarrhea,* constipation, stomatitis

INTEG: *Alopecia,* sweating, *pruritus*

MS: *Rigors,* arthralgia, back pain

RESP: *Cough, dyspnea, rhinitis, sinusitis*

Contraindications: Pregnancy **D,** hypersensitivity, lactation, systemic infections, cardiac disease

Precautions: Renal, hepatic disease, gout, bone marrow suppression

Pharmacokinetics

Absorption	Complete
Distribution	Widely distributed; crosses placenta
Metabolism	Liver, extensively
Excretion	Biliary (40%-50%)
Half-life	18½ hr, liposome 55½ hr

Pharmacodynamics

Unknown

Interactions

Individual drugs

Cyclophosphamide, radiation: increased toxicity

Drug classifications

Antineoplastics: increased toxicity

Live virus vaccines: decreased antibody reaction

NSAIDs, salicylates: increased risk of bleeding

Drug/lab test

Increased: uric acid

NURSING CONSIDERATIONS

Assessment

- Assess buccal cavity q8h for dryness, sores or ulceration, white patches, pain, bleeding, dysphagia; obtain prescription for viscous lidocaine (Xylocaine)
- Assess symptoms indicating severe allergic reaction: rash, pruritus, urticaria, purpuric skin lesions, itching, flushing; drug should be discontinued

- Assess chest x-ray, echocardiography, radionuclide angiography, ECG; watch for ST-T wave changes, low QRS and T, possible dysrhythmias (sinus tachycardia, heart block, PVCs); watch for CHF (jugular vein distention, weight gain, edema, crackles), may occur after 2-6 mo of treatment
- Monitor CBC, differential, platelet count weekly, leukocyte nadir within 2 wk after administration, recovery within 3 wk; do not administer if absolute granulocyte count is <750/mm^3 (liposome)
- Assess for increased uric acid levels, swelling, joint pain primarily in extremities; patient should be well hydrated to prevent urate deposits
- Monitor renal function studies: BUN, creatinine, serum uric acid, urine CCr baseline and before each dose; I&O ratio; report fall in urine output to <30 ml/hr
- Monitor temp q4h (may indicate beginning of infection)
- Monitor liver function tests baseline and before each dose (bilirubin, AST, ALT, LDH) as needed or monthly; note jaundice of skin or sclera, dark urine, clay-colored stools, itchy skin, abdominal pain, fever, diarrhea; hepatotoxicity can be severe
- Assess for bleeding: hematuria, stool guaiac, bruising or petechiae, mucosa or orifices q8h; check for inflammation of mucosa, breaks in skin
- Identify effects of alopecia on body image; discuss feelings about body changes

Nursing diagnoses

- Injury, risk for (adverse reactions)
- Cardiac output, decreased (adverse reactions)
- Body image, disturbed (adverse reactions)
- Infection, risk for (adverse reactions)
- Knowledge, deficient (teaching)

Implementation

- Avoid contact with skin; very irritating; wash completely to remove
- Give fluids **IV** or PO before chemotherapy to hydrate patient; give antiemetic 30-60 min before giving drug to prevent vomiting, and prn; antibiotics for prophylaxis of infection
- Provide liquid diet: carbonated beverages; gelatin may be added if patient is not nauseated or vomiting
- Help patient rinse mouth tid-qid with water, club soda, brush teeth bid-qid with soft brush or cotton-tipped applicators for stomatitis, use unwaxed dental floss
- Drug should be prepared by experienced personnel using proper precautions

Cerubidine

IV route

- Give after diluting 20 mg/4 ml sterile water for inj (5 mg/ml); rotate; further dilute in 10-15 ml 0.9% NaCl; give over 3-5 min by direct **IV** through Y-tube or 3-way stopcock of inf of D_5W or 0.9% NaCl

Intermittent IV infusion route

- Dilute further in 50-100 ml 0.9% NaCl, LR, D_5W; give over 15 min (50 ml), 30 min (100 ml)

Y-site compatibilities: Amifostine, filgrastim, granisetron, melphalan, methotrexate, ondansetron, sodium bicarbonate, teniposide, thiotepa, vinorelbine

Y-site incompatibilities: Fludarabine

Additive compatibilities: Cytarabine with etoposide, hydrocortisone; not recommended for admixing

Additive incompatibilities: Dexamethasone, heparin

Solution compatibilities: $D_{3.3}$/0.3% NaCl, D_5W, Normosol-R, Ringer's, 0.9% NaCl

DaunoXome

IV route

- Dilute with D_5W (1 mg/ml), give over 60 min, do not use in-line filter, reconstituted sol may be stored ≤6 hr refrigerated; do not admix

Patient/family education

- Teach patient to avoid use of products containing aspirin or ibuprofen, razors, commercial mouthwash, since bleeding may occur; to report symptoms of bleeding (hematuria, tarry stools)
- Instruct patient to report signs of anemia (fatigue, headache, irritability, faintness, shortness of breath); signs of infection; bleeding, bruising, shortness of breath, swelling, change in heart rate; to avoid crowds, those with known infections
- Advise patient that hair may be lost during treatment; a wig or hairpiece may make patient feel better; new hair may be different in color, texture
- Caution patient not to have any vaccinations without the advice of the prescriber; serious reactions can occur
- Advise patient that contraception is needed during treatment and for 4 mo after the completion of therapy
- Advise patient to avoid alcohol, aspirin, NSAIDs

Evaluation
Positive therapeutic outcome
- Prevention of rapid division of malignant cells

delavirdine (Rx)
(de-la-veer'deen)
Rescriptor
Func. class.: Antiretroviral
Chem. class.: Nonnucleoside reverse transcriptase inhibitor (NNRII)
Pregnancy category C

Action: Binds directly to reverse transcriptase and blocks RNA, DNA causing a disruption of the enzyme's site

Therapeutic Outcome: Improvement of HIV-1 infection

Uses: HIV-1 in combination with other antiretrovirals

Dosage and routes
Adult and child ≥16 yr: 400 mg tid

Available forms: Tabs 100, 200 mg

Adverse effects
CNS: Headache, fatigue
GI: Diarrhea, anorexia, abdominal pain, nausea, vomiting, dyspepsia, **hepatotoxicity**
GU: **Nephrotoxicity**
HEMA: **Neutropenia, leukopenia, thrombocytopenia, anemia, granulocytopenia**
INTEG: Rash, pruritis
MS: Pain, myalgia
SYST: **Stevens-Johnson syndrome**

Contraindications: Hypersensitivity to this drug or atevirdine

Precautions: Pregnancy **C,** liver disease, lactation, children, renal disease, myelosuppression

Pharmacokinetics	
Absorption	Well
Distribution	98% protein bound
Metabolism	Liver, extensively
Excretion	Kidneys, feces
Half-life	2-11 hr

Pharmacodynamics	
Onset	Unknown
Peak	1 hr
Duration	8 hr

Interactions
Individual drugs
Alprazolam, amprenavir, atorvastatin, clarithromycin, dapsone, felodipine, indinavir, lovastatin, midazolam, nifidepine, saquinavir, simvastatin: increased level of each specific drug
Cisapride, pimozide, sildenafil: life-threatening reactions; do not combine
Clarithromycin, quinidine, warfarin: increased level of both drugs
Fluoxetine, ketoconazole: increased level of delavirdine

Drug classifications
Amphetamines, antidysrhythmics, benzodiazepines, calcium channel blockers, ergots: increased serious life-threatening adverse reaction
Antacids, anticonvulsants, protease inhibitors, rifamycins: decreased delavirdine levels
Antidysrhythmics, sedative/hypnotics: life-threatening reactions; do not combine
Contraceptives (oral): decreased action of oral contraceptives

NURSING CONSIDERATIONS
Assessment
- Assess signs of infection, anemia
- Assess liver studies: ALT, AST; renal studies
- Assess C&S before drug therapy; drug may be taken as soon as culture is taken; repeat C&S after treatment; determine the presence of other sexually transmitted disease
- Assess bowel pattern before, during teatment; if severe abdominal pain with bleeding occurs, drug should be discontinued; monitor hydration
- Assess skin eruptions; rash, urticaria, itching
- Assess allergies before treatment, reaction to each medication; place allergies on chart
- Assess plasma delavirdine concentrations (trough 10 μm)
- Assess CBC, blood chemistry, plasma HIV RNA, absolute $CD4^+/CD8^+$/cell counts/%, serum β_2 microglobulin, serum ICD+24 antigen levels
- Assess for signs of delavirdine toxicity: severe nausea, vomiting, maculopapular rash

Nursing diagnoses
- Infection, risk for (uses)
- Diarrhea (side effects)
- Knowledge, deficient (teaching)

Implementation
- Add 4 tabs/3-4 oz of water, let stand, stir, swallow, rinse glass, swallow; use only 100 mg tabs for dispersion

- Do not give within 1 hr of antacids or didanosine
- Take in equal intervals around the clock

Patient/family education

- Advise patient to take as prescribed; if dose is missed, take as soon as remembered up to 1 hr before next dose; do not double dose
- Advise patient that drug must be taken in equal intervals around the clock to maintain blood levels for duration of therapy
- Advise patient that tabs may be dissolved, drink right away, rinse cup with water, and drink that to get all medication
- Instruct patient to make sure health care provider knows of all the medications being taken
- Advise patient that if severe rash, mouth sores, swelling, aching muscles/joints, or eye redness occur, stop taking and notify health care provider
- Advise patient not to breastfeed if taking this drug

Evaluation

Positive therapeutic outcome

- Increased $CD4^+$ cell count
- Decreased viral load
- Improvement in symptoms of HIV

denileukin diftitox (Rx)

(den-ih-loo'kin dif'tih-tox)

Ontak

Func. class.: Antineoplastic miscellaneous agent

Pregnancy category C

Action: A recombinant DNA-derived cytotoxic protein; inhibits cellular protein synthesis

Therapeutic Outcome: Prevention of rapidly growing malignant cells

Uses: Cutaneous T-cell lymphoma that express CD25 component of the IL-2 receptor

Dosage and routes

Adult: **IV** 9-18 mcg/kg/day given for 5 days q21 days, give over ≥15 min

Available forms: Sol for inj, frozen 150 mcg/ml

Adverse effects

CNS: *Dizziness, paresthesia, nervousness, confusion, insomnia*

CV: *Hypotension, vasodilatation, tachycardia, thrombosis, hypertension, dysrhythmia*

GI: *Nausea, anorexia, vomiting, diarrhea, constipation, dyspepsia, dysphagia*

GU: *Hematuria,* albuminuria, pyuria, creatinine increase

HEMA: **Thrombocytopenia, leukopenia,** anemia

INTEG: *Rash, pruritus, sweating*

META: Hypoalbuminemia, edema, hypocalcemia, weight decrease, dehydration, hypokalemia

MISC: *Fever, chills, asthenia, infection, pain, headache, chest pain,* flulike symptoms

MS: Myalgia, arthralgia

RESP: *Dyspnea, cough, pharyngitis, rhinitis*

Contraindications: Hypersensitivity to denileukin, diphtheria toxin, interleukin-2

Precautions: Pregnancy **C**, radiation therapy, elderly, lactation, children

Pharmacokinetics

Absorption	Complete bioavailability (**IV**)
Distribution	Widely distributed; concentrates in liver/kidneys
Metabolism	Proteolytic degradation
Excretion	Unknown
Half-life	Unknown

Pharmacodynamics

Unknown

Interactions

Drug classifications

Antineoplastics, bone marrow-suppressing drugs, radiation: increased bone marrow suppression

Live virus vaccines: increased adverse reactions; decreased antibody reaction

NURSING CONSIDERATIONS

Assessment

- Assess symptoms indicating severe allergic reaction: rash, pruritus, urticaria, purpuric skin lesions, itching, flushing; drug should be discontinued
- Assess for vascular leak syndrome after 2 wk of treatment: hypotension, edema, hypoalbuminemia; monitor weight, B/P, serum albumin, edema
- Obtain CD25 expression on skin biopsy samples
- Monitor CBC, differential, platelet count weekly; withhold drug if WBC count is $<4000/mm^3$ or platelet count is $<100,000/mm^3$
- Monitor renal function studies: BUN, creatinine, urine CCr before and during therapy; I&O ratio; report fall in urine output to <30 ml/hr

• Monitor temp q4h (may indicate beginning of infection)
• Monitor liver function tests before and during therapy (bilirubin, AST, ALT, LDH) as needed or monthly; note jaundiced skin or sclera, dark urine, clay-colored stools, itchy skin, abdominal pain, fever, diarrhea; hepatotoxicity can be serious and fatal
• Assess for bleeding: hematuria, stool guaiac, bruising or petechiae, mucosa or orifices q8h; check for inflammation of mucosa, breaks in skin

Nursing diagnoses
• Injury, risk for (adverse reactions)
• Body image, disturbed (adverse reactions)
• Infection, risk for (adverse reactions)
• Knowledge, deficient (teaching)

Implementation
• Give fluids **IV** or PO before chemotherapy to hydrate patient
• Give antiemetic 30-60 min before giving drug to prevent vomiting, and prn; antibiotics for prophylaxis of infection
• Provide liquid diet: carbonated beverages; gelatin may be added if patient is not nauseated or vomiting
• Prepare and hold sol in plastic syringes or soft plastic **IV** bags only
• Draw calculated dose from vial, inject into empty **IV** infusion bag, for each 1 ml of drug removed from vial, no more than 9 ml of sterile saline without preservative should be added to **IV** bag; infuse over ≥15 min; do not give by bolus; do not admix with other drugs; do not use a filter
• Use within 6 hr, discard unused portions
• Watch for extravasation; give 3-5 ml of mixture of 4 ml sodium thiosulfate 10% plus 5 ml sterile water SUBCUT as prescribed

Patient/family education
• Teach patient to avoid use of products containing aspirin or NSAIDs, razors, commercial mouthwash, since bleeding may occur; to report symptoms of bleeding (hematuria, tarry stools)
• Instruct patient to report signs of anemia (fatigue, headache, irritability, faintness, shortness of breath)
• Caution patient not to have any vaccinations without the advice of prescriber; serious reactions can occur
• Advise patient contraception is needed during treatment and for several months after the completion of therapy; drug has teratogenic properties

Evaluation
Positive therapeutic outcome
• Prevention of rapid division of malignant cells

desipramine (Rx)
(dess-ip'ra-meen)
Apo-Desipramine ✤, desipramine HCl, Norpramin, Pertofrane ✤
Func. class.: Antidepressant, tricyclic
Chem. class.: Dibenzazepine, secondary amine
Pregnancy category C

Action: Blocks reuptake of norepinephrine, serotonin into nerve endings, increasing action of norepinephrine, serotonin in nerve cells

Therapeutic Outcome: Decreased depression

Uses: Depression

Investigational uses: Chronic pain

Dosage and routes
Adult: PO 100-200 mg/day in a single dose or in divided doses; max 300 mg/day
Elderly: PO 25-50 mg/day, may increase to 150 mg/day
Child >12 yr: PO 25-50 mg/day in divided doses, max 100 mg/day
Child 6-12 yr: PO 10-30 mg/day or 1-5 mg/kg/day in divided doses

Available forms: Tabs 10, 25, 50, 75, 100, 150 mg; caps 25, 50 mg

Adverse effects
CNS: *Dizziness, drowsiness,* confusion, headache, anxiety, tremors, stimulation, weakness, insomnia, nightmares, EPS (elderly), increased psychiatric symptoms, paresthenia
CV: *Orthostatic hypotension, ECG changes, tachycardia, hypertension,* palpitations
EENT: *Blurred vision,* tinnitus, mydriasis, ophthalmoplegia
GI: *Diarrhea, dry mouth,* nausea, vomiting, **paralytic ileus**, increased appetite, cramps, epigastric distress, jaundice, **hepatitis**, stomatitis, constipation
GU: *Retention,* **acute renal failure**
HEMA: **Agranulocytosis, thrombocytopenia, eosinophilia, leukopenia**
INTEG: Rash, urticaria, sweating, pruritus, photosensitivity

Contraindications: Hypersensitivity to tricyclic antidepressants, narrow-angle glaucoma

Precautions: Pregnancy **C**, suicidal patients, severe depression, increased intraocular pressure, elderly, lactation, seizure disorder, CV disease, prostatic hypertrophy

Pharmacokinetics

Absorption	Well
Distribution	Widely, protein binding 92%
Metabolism	Extensively, liver
Excretion	Unknown
Half-life	12-24 hr

Pharmacodynamics

Unknown

Interactions

Individual drugs

Alcohol, barbiturates, opioids, CNS depressants: increased CNS depression
Cimetidine, fluvoxamine, fluoxetine, paroxetine, sertraline: increased desipramine level
Clonidine: increased life-threatening B/P elevations, do not use concurrently
EpINEPHrine, norepinephrine: increased hypertension

Drug classifications

MAO inhibitors: increased hyperpyrexia, seizures, excitation, do not use within 14 days of MAOIs

Drug/herb

Evening primrose oil: may lower seizure threshold, do not use concurrently
Chamomile, hops, kavan, valerian: increased CNS depression
St. John's wort, SAM-e: may increase serotonin syndrome; avoid concurrent use

Drug/lab test

Increase: serum bilirubin, blood glucose, alkaline phosphatase

NURSING CONSIDERATIONS

Assessment

- Monitor B/P (lying, standing), pulse q4h; if systolic B/P drops 20 mm Hg, hold drug, notify prescriber; take vital signs q4h in patients with cardiovascular disease
- Monitor blood studies: CBC, leukocytes, differential, cardiac enzymes if patient is receiving long-term therapy
- Monitor hepatic studies: AST, ALT, bilirubin
- Check weight qwk; appetite may increase with this drug
- Monitor ECG for flattening T wave, bundle branch block, AV block, dysrhythmias in cardiac patients
- Assess for EPS primarily in elderly: rigidity, dystonia, akathisia
- Assess mental status: mood, sensorium, affect, suicidal tendencies, increase in psychiatric symptoms: depression, panic
- Assess for urinary retention, constipation; constipation most likely in children
- Assess for withdrawal symptoms: headache, nausea, vomiting, muscle pain, weakness; not usual unless drug discontinued abruptly
- Assess for alcohol consumption; if consumed, hold dose until morning

Nursing diagnoses

- Coping, ineffective (uses)
- Noncompliance (teaching)
- Knowledge, deficient (teaching)

Implementation

- Increase fluids, bulk in diet for constipation, especially in elderly
- Take with food or milk for GI symptoms
- Crush if patient is unable to swallow medication whole
- Give dosage at bedtime if oversedation occurs during day; may take entire dose at bedtime; elderly may not tolerate once a day dosing
- Give gum, hard candy, frequent sips of water for dry mouth
- Store at room temperature
- Provide assistance with ambulation during beginning of therapy for drowsiness/dizziness
- Provide safety measures, primarily in the elderly
- Check to see that PO medication is swallowed

Patient/family education

- Advise patient that therapeutic effects may take 2-3 wk
- Advise patient to use caution in driving, other activities requiring alertness because of drowsiness, dizziness, blurred vision
- Teach patient to avoid alcohol ingestion, other CNS depressants
- Teach patient not to discontinue medication quickly after long-term use; may cause nausea, headache, malaise
- Teach patient to wear sunscreen or large hat, since photosensitivity occurs

Evaluation

Positive therapeutic outcome

- Decreased depression

Treatment of overdose: ECG monitoring; induce emesis; lavage, activated charcoal; administer anticonvulsant

desirudin (Rx)

(des-i'rude'in)

Iprivask

Func. class.: Anticoagulant

Chem. class.: Thrombin inhibitor

Pregnancy category C

Action: Inhibits thrombin resulting in prolongation of clotting time

Therapeutic Outcome: Absence of deep vein thrombosis

Uses: Prophylaxis for deep vein thrombosis in those undergoing hip replacement

Dosage and routes

Adult: SUBCUT 15 mg, 1st dose 5-15 min before surgery, but after regional block anesthesia, then 15 mg q12h, up to 12 days

Available forms: Lyophilized powder 15 mg

Adverse effects

MISC: Inj site mass, nausea, deep thrombophlebitis, anemia, hypersensitivity

SYST: **Bleeding, hemorrhage**

Contraindications: Hypersensitivity to natural or synthetic hirudins, active bleeding, irreversible coagulation disorders

Precautions: Pregnancy **C**, lactation, children, elderly, hepatic and renal impairment, patients with increased risks of hemorrhage

Pharmacokinetics

Absorption	Unknown
Distribution	Unknown
Metabolism	Kidney (40%-50% unchanged)
Excretion	Kidney
Half-life	Unknown

Pharmacodynamics

Onset	Unknown
Peak	Unknown
Duration	Unknown

Interactions

Drug classifications

Anticoagulants: increased anticoagulant effect Antiplatelets (abciximab, clopidogrel, ketorolac, NSAIDs, salicylates, sulfinpyrazone, triclopidine): increased anticoagulant effect

Thrombolytics: increased anticoagulant effect

NURSING CONSIDERATIONS

Assessment

- Monitor APTT daily in those with increased risk for bleeding
- ◆ Assess for neurologic changes that may indicate intracranial bleeding
- ◆ Assess for retroperitoneal bleeding: back pain, leg weakness, diminished pulses
- Assess for bleeding: gums, petechiae, ecchymosis, black tarry stool, hematuria; notify prescriber

Nursing diagnoses

- Tissue perfusion, ineffective (uses)
- Injury, risk for (uses, adverse reactions)
- Knowledge, deficient (teaching)

Implementation

- Give alone, do not mix with other drugs or solutions
- Give for 9-12 days
- Give only after screening patient for bleeding disorders
- Give SUBCUT only, do not give IM
- Give with patient recumbent, rotate inj sites (left/right anterolateral, left/right posterolateral abdominal wall)
- Insert whole length of needle into skin fold held with thumb and forefinger
- Give at same time of day to maintain blood level
- Administer only this drug when ordered, not interchangeable with heparin
- Provide bed rest during entire course of treatment
- Avoid venous or arterial puncture, inj, rectal temp
- Treat fever with acetaminophen

Patient/family education

- Teach about drug use and expected results; to report adverse reactions; bleeding, bruising
- Advise to avoid all OTC drugs unless prescribed
- Instruct to use soft-bristle toothbrush to avoid bleeding gums, to use electric razor

Evaluation

Positive therapeutic outcome

- Absence of DVT

desloratadine (Rx)
(des-lor-at'ah-deen)

Clarinex, Clarinex Reditabs

Func. class.: Antihistamine, 2nd generation

Chem. class.: Selective histamine (H_1-) receptor antagonist

Pregnancy category C

Action: Binds to peripheral histamine receptors, providing antihistamine action without sedation

Therapeutic Outcome: Decreased nasal stuffiness, itching, swollen eyes

Uses: Seasonal allergic rhinitis, chronic idiopathic urticaria

Dosage and routes
Adult and child ≥12 yr: PO 5 mg daily

Child 6-11 yr: PO 2.5 mg daily

Child 1-5 yr: PO 1.25 mg daily

Child 6-11 mo: PO 1 mg daily

Hepatic/renal dose

Adult: PO 5 mg every other day

Available forms: Tabs 5 mg; orally disintegrating (Reditabs) 5 mg; syrup 0.5 mg/ml

Adverse effects
CNS: Sedation (more common with increased doses), headache

Contraindications: Hypersensitivity, acute asthma attacks, lower respiratory tract disease

Precautions: Pregnancy **C,** bronchial asthma, liver or renal impairment

Pharmacokinetics	
Absorption	Unknown
Distribution	Bound to plasma proteins (82%-87%)
Metabolism	Liver (active metabolites)
Excretion	Urine, feces (metabolites)
Half-life	8½-28 hr

Pharmacodynamics	
Onset	1 hr, relief in 1 day
Peak	1½ hr
Duration	24 hr

Interactions
Drug/food

Food may prolong time to peak with orally disintegrating tabs

NURSING CONSIDERATIONS
Assessment
- Assess for allergy: hives, rash, rhinitis; monitor respiratory status; test interaction, antigen skin test

Nursing diagnoses
- Airway clearance, ineffective (uses)
- Knowledge, deficient (teaching)
- Noncompliance (teaching, overuse)

Implementation
- May administer without regard to meals
- Store in airtight container at room temp

Patient/family education
- Advise patient to avoid driving, other hazardous activities if drowsiness occurs; to observe caution until drug's effects are known
- Advise patient that drug may cause photosensitivity; use sunscreen or stay out of the sun to prevent burns
- Caution patient to avoid use of other CNS depressants
- Teach not to remove Reditabs from blister until ready to use; to place Reditabs directly on tongue, may take with or without water

Evaluation
Positive therapeutic outcome
- Absence of running or congested nose, other allergy symptoms

desmopressin (Rx)
(des-moe-press'in)

DDAVP, Stimate

Func. class.: Pituitary hormone

Chem. class.: Synthetic antidiuretic hormone

Pregnancy category B

Action: Promotes reabsorption of water by action on renal tubular epithelium in the kidney; causes smooth muscle constriction and increase in plasma factor VIII levels, which increases platelet aggregation resulting in vasopressor effect; similar to vasopressor

Therapeutic Outcome: Prevention of nocturnal enuresis, decreased bleeding in hemophilia A, von Willebrand's disease type 1, control and stabilization of water in diabetes insipidus

Uses: Hemophilia A, von Willebrand's disease type 1, nonnephrogenic diabetes insipidus, symptoms of polyuria/polydipsia caused by pituitary dysfunction, nocturnal enuresis

Dosage and routes

Primary nocturnal enuresis

Adult and child ≥6 yr: Intranasal 20 mcg (10 mcg in each nostril) at bedtime; may increase to 40 mcg; PO 0.2 mg at bedtime, may be increased to max 0.6 mg at bedtime

Diabetes insipidus

Adult: Intranasal 0.1-0.4 ml daily in divided doses (1-4 sprays with pump); **IV**/SUBCUT 0.5-1 ml daily in divided doses

Child 3 mo-12 yr: Intranasal 0.05-0.3 ml daily in divided doses

Hemophilia/von Willebrand's disease

Adult and child >3 mo: **IV** 0.3 mcg/kg in NaCl over 15-30 min; may repeat if needed

Antihemorrhagic

Adult and child >3 mo: **IV** 0.3 mcg/kg

Adult and child <50 kg: Intranasal 1 spray in one nostril

Adult and child >50 kg: 1 spray each nostril

Available forms: Inj 4, 15 mcg/ml, Rhinal Tube del 2.5 mg/vial (0.1 mg/ml); tabs 0.1, 0.2 mg; nasal spray pump 10 mcg/spray (0.1 mg/ml); nasal sol 1.5 mg/ml (150 mcg/dose)

Adverse effects

CNS: Drowsiness, headache, lethargy, flushing

CV: Increased B/P

EENT: Nasal irritation, congestion, rhinitis

GI: Nausea, heartburn, cramps

GU: *Vulval pain*

SYST: **Anaphylaxis (IV)**

Contraindications: Hypersensitivity, nephrogenic diabetes insipidus

Precautions: Pregnancy **B**, CAD, lactation, hypertension

Pharmacokinetics

Absorption	Nasal (up to 20%)
Distribution	Unknown
Metabolism	Unknown
Excretion	Unknown; breast milk
Half-life	8 min (initial), 76 min (terminal)

Pharmacodynamics

	PO	INTRANASAL	IV/SUBCUT
Onset	1 hr	1 hr	Rapid
Peak	4-7 hr	1-4 hr	15-30 min
Duration	Unknown	8-20 hr	3 hr

Interactions

Individual drugs

Carbamazepine, chlorpropamide, clofibrate: increased antidiuretic action

Demeclocycline, epINEPHrine (large doses), alcohol, heparin, lithium: decreased antidiuretic action

NURSING CONSIDERATIONS

Assessment

- Monitor I&O ratio, urine osmolality, sp gr, weight daily; check for edema in extremities; if water retention is severe, diuretic may be prescribed; check pulse, B/P when giving drug **IV** or SUBCUT
- Assess for water intoxication: lethargy, behavioral changes, disorientation, neuromuscular excitability, dehydration, poor skin turgor, severe thirst, dry skin, tachycardia
- Assess intranasal use: nausea, congestion, cramps, headache; usually decreased with decreased dosage
- Monitor for enuresis during treatment (nocturnal enuresis)
- Assess for allergic reaction including anaphylaxis (**IV** route)
- Assess for nasal mucosa changes: congestion, edema, discharge, scarring (nasal route)
- Monitor urine volume osmolality and plasma osmolality (diabetes insipidus)
- Monitor factor VIII coagulant activity before using for hemostasis

Nursing diagnoses

- Fluid volume, deficient (uses)
- Fluid volume, excess (side effects)
- Knowledge, deficient (teaching)

Implementation

- Draw medication into tube, insert tube into nostril to instill drug and blow on other end to deliver sol into nasal cavity; rinse after use
- Store in refrigerator or cool environment

IV, direct route

- Give undiluted over 1 min in diabetes insipidus or **IV** for hemophilia

Intermittent IV infusion route

- Give single dose diluted in 50 ml of 0.9% NaCl (adult and child >10 kg); a single dose/10 ml as an **IV** inf over 15-30 min in von Willebrand's disease or hemophilia A

Patient/family education

- Use demonstration, return demonstration to teach technique for nasal instillation
- Teach patient to notify prescriber of dyspnea, vomiting, cramping, drowsiness, headache, nasal congestion
- Caution patient to avoid OTC products (cough, hay fever), since these preparations

may contain epINEPHrine and decrease drug response; do not use with alcohol
- Advise patient to carry/wear emergency ID or other identification specifying disease and medication used
- Advise patient if dose is missed, take when remembered up to 1 hr before next dose; do not double doses
- Teach patient to report upper respiratory infection, nasal congestion

Evaluation

Positive therapeutic outcome
- Absence of severe thirst
- Decreased urine output, osmolality
- Absence of bleeding (hemophilia)

desoxyribonuclease

See fibrinolysin/desoxyribonuclease

dexamethasone (Rx)

(dex-ah-meth'ah-sone)

Decadron, Deronil ✦, Dexasone ✦, Dexon, Hexadrol, Mymethasone

dexamethasone acetate (Rx)

Dalalone DP, Dalalone LA, Decadron-LA, Decaject-LA, Dexacen LA-8, Dexasone-LA, Dexone LA, Solurex-LA

dexamethasone sodium phosphate (Rx)

Dalalone, Decadron Phosphate, Decaject, Dexacen-4, Dexone, Hexadrol Phosphate, Solurex

Func. class.: Corticosteroid, synthetic
Chem. class.: Glucocorticoid, long-acting

Pregnancy category C

Do Not Confuse:
Decadron/Percodan

Action: Decreases inflammation by suppression of migration of polymorphonuclear leukocytes, fibroblasts, reversal of increased capillary permeability and lysosomal stabilization

Uses: Inflammation, allergies, neoplasms, cerebral edema, septic shock, collagen disorders

Dosage and routes

Inflammation

Adult: PO 0.75-9 mg/day, in divided doses q6-12h; or phosphate IM 0.5-9 mg/day divided q6-12h; or acetate IM 4-16 mg q1-3 wk

Child: PO 0.024-0.34 mg/kg/day in divided doses q6-12h

Shock

Adult: **IV** (phosphate) single dose 1-6 mg/kg or **IV** 40 mg q2-6h as needed up to 72 hr

Cerebral edema

Adult: **IV** (phosphate) 10 mg, then 4-6 mg IM q6h × 2-4 days, then taper over 1 wk

Child: PO/IM/**IV** loading dose 1-2 mg/kg, then 1-1.5 mg/kg/day, max 16 mg/day divided q4-6hr for 2-4 days, then taper down qwk

Adrenocortical insufficiency

Adult: PO 0.5-9 mg/day in divided doses

Child: PO 0.03-0.3 mg/kg/day divided in 2-4 doses

Suppression test

Adult: PO 1 mg at 11 PM or 0.5 mg q6h × 48 hr

Available forms: Dexamethasone: tabs 0.25, 0.5, 0.75, 1, 1.5, 2, 4, 6 mg; elix 0.5 mg/5 ml; oral sol 0.5 mg/5 ml, 1 mg/1 ml; inj acetate 8, 16 mg/ml; inj phosphate 4, 10, 20, 24 mg/ml

Adverse effects

CNS: *Depression, flushing, sweating,* headache, mood changes, euphoria, psychosis, **seizures**, insomnia

CV: *Hypertension,* **circulatory collapse, thrombophlebitis, embolism,** tachycardia, edema

EENT: Fungal infections, increased intraocular pressure, blurred vision

ENDO: Hypothalmic-pituitary-adrenal axis suppression, hyperglycemia, sodium, fluid retention

GI: *Diarrhea, nausea, abdominal distention,* **GI hemorrhage,** *increased appetite,* **pancreatitis**

HEMA: **Thrombocytopenia**

INTEG: Acne, poor wound healing, ecchymosis, petechiae, hirsutism

META: Hypokalemia

MS: Fractures, osteoporosis, weakness

Contraindications: Psychosis, hypersensitivity, idiopathic thrombocytopenia, acute glomerulonephritis, amebiasis, fungal infections, nonasthmatic bronchial disease, child <2 yr, AIDS, TB

Precautions: Pregnancy **C,** lactation, diabetes mellitus, glaucoma, osteoporosis, seizure disorders, ulcerative colitis, CHF, myasthenia gravis, renal disease, peptic ulcer, esophagitis

Pharmacokinetics

Absorption	Unknown
Distribution	Unknown
Metabolism	Liver
Excretion	Kidneys
Half-life	36-54 hr

Pharmacodynamics

	PO	IM
Onset	1 hr	Unknown
Peak	1-2 hr	8 hr
Duration	2½ days	6 days-3 wk

Interactions
Individual drugs
Alcohol, amphotericin B, cycloSPORINE, digitalis, indomethacin: increased side effects
Ambemonium, isoniazid, neostigmine, sometrem: decreased effects of each specific drug
Cholestyramine, colestipol, epHEDrine, phenytoin, rifampin, theophylline: decreased action of dexamethasone
Indomethacin, ketoconazole: increased action of dexamethasone
Drug classifications
Antacids, barbiturates: decreased action of dexamethasone
Antibiotics (macrolide), contraceptives (oral), estrogens, salicylates: increased action of dexamethasone
Anticholinesterases, anticoagulants, anticonvulsants, antidiabetics, salicylates, toxoids/vaccines: decreased effects of each specific drug
Diuretics, salicylates: increased side effects
Drug/herb
Aloe, buckthorn bark/berry, cascara sagrada, Chinese rhubarb, senna pod/leaf: increased hypokalemia
Aloe, licorice, perilla: increased corticosteroid effect
Drug/lab test
Increased: cholesterol, Na, blood glucose, uric acid, Ca, urine glucose
Decreased: Ca, K, T_4, T_3, thyroid ^{131}I uptake test, urine 17-OHCS, 17-KS, PBI
False negative: skin allergy tests

NURSING CONSIDERATIONS
Assessment
- Monitor K, blood, urine glucose while on long-term therapy; hypokalemia and hyperglycemia
- Monitor weight daily; notify prescriber of weekly gain >5 lb
- Monitor B/P q4h, pulse; notify prescriber of chest pain
- Monitor I&O ratio; be alert for decreasing urinary output, increasing edema
- Monitor plasma cortisol levels during long-term therapy (normal: 138-635 nmol/L SI units when assessed at 8 AM)
- Assess infection: fever, WBC even after withdrawal of medication; drug masks infection
- Assess potassium depletion: paresthesias, fatigue, nausea, vomiting, depression, polyuria, dysrhythmias, weakness
- Assess edema, hypertension, cardiac symptoms
- Assess mental status: affect, mood, behavioral changes, aggression

Nursing diagnoses
- Infection, risk for (adverse reaction)
- Knowledge, deficient (teaching)
- Mobility, impaired (uses)

Implementation
PO route
- Give with food or milk to decrease GI symptoms
- Provide assistance with ambulation in patient with bone tissue disease to prevent fractures

IM route
- IM inj deep in large muscle mass; rotate sites; avoid deltoid; use 21-G needle
- In one dose in AM to prevent adrenal suppression; avoid SUBCUT administration, may damage tissue

IV route
- **IV** undiluted direct over 1 min or less or diluted with 0.9% NaCl or D_5W and give as an **IV** inf at prescribed rate
- After shaking susp (parenteral); do not give susp **IV**
- Titrated dose; use lowest effective dose

Dexamethasone sodium phosphate
Syringe compatibilities: Granisetron, metoclopramide, ranitidine, sufentanil
Y-site compatibilities: Acyclovir, allopurinol, amifostine, amikacin, amphotericin B cholesteryl, amsacrine, aztreonam, cefepime, cisatracurium, cisplatin, cladribine, cyclophosphamide, cytarabine, DOXOrubicin, DOXOrubicin liposome, famotidine, filgrastim, fluconazole, fludarabine, foscarnet, heparin, melphalan, meperidine, meropenem, morphine, ondansetron, paclitaxel, piperacillin/tazobactam, potassium chloride, propofol, remifentanil, sargramostim, sodium bicarbon-

ate, sufentanil, tacrolimus, teniposide, theophylline, vinorelbine, vit B/C, zidovudine

Additive compatibilities: Aminophylline, bleomycin, cimetidine, floxacillin, furosemide, lidocaine, meropenem, nafcillin, netilmicin, ondansetron, prochlorperazine, ranitidine, verapamil

Patient/family education

- Advise that emergency ID as steroid user should be carried or worn
- Teach to notify prescriber if therapeutic response decreases; dosage adjustment may be needed
- Teach not to discontinue abruptly or adrenal crisis can result
- Teach to avoid OTC products: salicylates, alcohol in cough products, cold preparations unless directed by prescriber
- Instruct patient to contact prescriber if surgery, trauma, stress occurs, dose may need to be adjusted
- Teach patient all aspects of drug usage, including cushingoid symptoms
- Instruct patient to notify prescriber of infection
- Teach symptoms of adrenal insufficiency: nausea, anorexia, fatigue, dizziness, dyspnea, weakness, joint pain
- Advise patient to avoid exposure to chickenpox or measles, persons with infections

Evaluation

Positive therapeutic outcome

Ease of respirations, decreased inflammation

dexmedetomidine (Rx)

(deks-med-ee-tome'a-dine)

Precedex

Func. class.: Sedative, α_2-adrenoceptor agonist

Pregnancy category C

Action: Produces α_2 activity as seen at low and moderate doses; also, α_1 at high doses

Uses: Sedation in mechanically ventilated, intubated patients in ICU

Dosage and routes

Adult: **IV** Loading dose of 1 mcg/kg over 10 min, then 0.2-0.7 mcg/kg/hr, do not use for more than 24 hr

Available forms: Inj 100 mcg/ml

Adverse effects

CV: Bradycardia, hypotension, hypertension, **atrial fibrillation, infarction**

GI: Nausea, thirst

GU: Oliguria

HEMA: Leukocytosis, anemia

RESP: **Pulmonary edema, pleural effusion, hypoxia**

Contraindications: Hypersensitivity

Precautions: Pregnancy **C**, elderly, renal disease, respiratory depression, severe respiratory disorders, cardiac dysrhythmias, lactation, children

Pharmacokinetics	
Half-life	8 min

Interactions

Individual drugs

Alcohol: increased CNS depression

Drug classifications

Anesthetics, antipsychotics, opiates, sedative/hypnotics, skeletal muscle relaxants: increased CNS depression

NURSING CONSIDERATIONS

Assessment

- Assess inj site: phlebitis, burning, stinging
- Monitor ECG for changes: atrial fibrillation
- Assess CNS changes: movement, jerking, tremors, dizziness, LOC, pupil reaction
- Assess respiratory dysfunction: respiratory depression, character, rate, rhythm; notify prescriber if respirations are <10/min

Nursing diagnoses

- Injury, risk for (uses)

Implementation

IV route

- Give after diluting with D_5W, 0.9% NaCl, withdraw 2 ml of drug and add to 48 ml of 0.9% NaCl to a total of 50 ml, shake to mix well
- Give only with resuscitative equipment available
- Give only by qualified persons trained in management of ICU sedation

Solution compatibilities: LR, D_5W, 0.9% NaCl, 20% mannitol

Additive compatibilities: Atracurium, atropine, etomidate, fentanyl, glycopyrrolate, midazolam, mivacurium, morphine, pancuronium, phenylephrine, succinylcholine, thiopental, vecuronium

- Provide safety measures: side rails, nightlight, call bell within easy reach

Evaluation

Positive therapeutic outcome

- Induction of sedation

D

dexmethylphenidate (Rx)

(dex'meth-ul-fen'ih-dayt)

Focalin, Focalin XR

Func. class.: Central nervous system (CNS) stimulant

Pregnancy category C

Controlled substance schedule II

Action: Increases release of norepinephrine and dopamine into the extraneuronal space, also blocks reuptake of norepinephrine and dopamine into the presynaptic neuron; mode of action in treating attention deficit hyperactivity disorder (ADHD) is unknown

Therapeutic Outcome: Increased alertness, decreased fatigue, ability to stay awake (narcolepsy), increased attention span, decreased hyperactivity (ADHD)

Uses: ADHD, adjunctive treatment

Dosage and routes

Adult: PO ext rel 10 mg/day, may adjust to 20 mg/day in 10 mg increments

Child >6 yr: PO 2.5 mg bid with doses at least 4 hr apart, gradually increase to a maximum of 20 mg/day (10 mg bid); for those taking methylphenidate, use ½ of methylphenidate dose initially, then increase as needed to a maximum of 20 mg/day; ext rel 5 mg/day, may adjust to 20 mg/day in 5 mg increments

Available forms: Tabs 2.5, 5, 10 mg; ext rel caps (Focalin XR) 5, 10, 20 mg

Adverse effects

CNS: Dizziness, headache, drowsiness, **toxic psychosis, neuroleptic malignant syndrome (rare)**, Gilles de la Tourette's syndrome

CV: Palpitations, B/P changes, angina, **dysrhythmias**

GI: Nausea, anorexia, abnormal liver function, **hepatic coma**, *abdominal pain*

HEMA: **Leukopenia, anemia, thrombocytopenic purpura**

INTEG: **Exfoliative dermatitis**, urticaria, rash, erythema multiforme

MISC: Fever, arthralgia, scalp hair loss

Contraindications: Hypersensitivity to methylphenidate, anxiety, history of Gilles de la Tourette's syndrome; children <6 yr, glaucoma, concurrent treatment with MAOIs or within 14 days of discontinuing treatment with MAOIs, lactation

Precautions: Pregnancy **C**, hypertension, depression, seizures, drug abuse, cardiovascular disorders, alcoholism

Pharmacokinetics

Absorption	Readily absorbed
Distribution	Unknown
Metabolism	Liver
Excretion	Kidneys
Half-life	2.2 hr

Pharmacodynamics

	PO	EXT REL
Onset	½-1 hr	Unknown
Peak	1-1 ½ hr	4 hr
Duration	4 hr	8 hr

Interactions

Drug classifications

Anticoagulants (coumarin) (e.g., warfarin), anticonvulsants, SSRIs, tricyclics: increased effects

Antihypertensives: decreased effects

Decongestants, vasoconstrictors: increased sympathomimetic effect

MAOIs: hypertensive crisis if coadministered or given within 14 days

Vasopressors: hypertensive crisis

Drug/herb

Horsetail, yohimbe: increased stimulant effect

Melatonin: increased synergistic effect

NURSING CONSIDERATIONS

Assessment

- Assess VS, B/P; may reverse antihypertensives; check patients with cardiac disease more often for increased B/P
- Assess CBC, differential, platelet counts during long-term therapy, urinalysis; in diabetes: blood/urine glucose; insulin changes may have to be made, since eating will decrease
- Assess height, growth rate q3 mo in children; growth rate may be decreased
- Assess mental status: mood, sensorium, affect, stimulation, insomnia, aggressiveness
- ◆ Assess withdrawal symptoms: headache, nausea, vomiting, muscle pain, weakness
- Assess appetite, sleep, speech patterns
- Assess for attention span, decreased hyperactivity in persons with ADHD

Nursing diagnoses

- Thought processes, disturbed (uses, adverse reactions)
- Coping, ineffective (uses)
- Knowledge, deficient (teaching)
- Coping, family, disabled (uses)

Implementation

- Do not break, crush, or chew ext rel caps

- Twice daily at least 4 hr apart; ext rel once a day
- Without regard to meals

Patient/family education

- Advise patient to decrease caffeine consumption (coffee, tea, cola, chocolate); may increase irritability, stimulation
- Advise patient to avoid OTC preparations unless approved by prescriber
- Caution patient to taper off drug over several wk to avoid depression, increased sleeping, lethargy
- Caution patient to avoid alcohol ingestion
- Caution patient to avoid hazardous activities until stabilized on medication
- Advise patient to get needed rest; patients will feel more tired at end of day
- Notify all health providers including school nurse of medication and schedule
- Discuss information instructions provided in patient information section

Evaluation

Positive therapeutic outcome

- Decreased hyperactivity or ability to stay awake

Treatment of overdose: Administer fluids; hemodialysis or peritoneal dialysis; antihypertensive for increased B/P; administer short-acting barbiturate before lavage

dextroamphetamine (Rx)

(dex-troe-am-fet'a-meen)

Dexedrine, Dexedrine Spansule, dextroamphetamine, Dextrostat

Func. class.: Cerebral stimulant

Chem. class.: Amphetamine

Pregnancy category C

Controlled substance schedule II

Action: Increases release of norepinephrine, dopamine in cerebral cortex to reticular activating system

Therapeutic Outcome: Increased alertness, decreased fatigue, ability to stay awake (narcolepsy); increased attention span, decreased hyperactivity (ADHD)

Uses: Narcolepsy, attention deficit disorder with hyperactivity

Investigational use: Obesity

Dosage and routes

Narcolepsy

Adult: PO 5-60 mg daily in divided doses

Child >12 yr: PO 10 mg daily increasing by 10 mg/day at weekly intervals

Child 6-12 yr: PO 5 mg daily increasing by 5 mg/wk (max 60 mg/day)

ADHD

Adult: PO 5-60 mg/day in divided doses

Child >6 yr: PO 5 mg daily-bid increasing by 5 mg/day at weekly intervals

Child 3-6 yr: PO 2.5 mg daily increasing by 2.5 mg/day at weekly intervals

Available forms: Tabs 5, 10 mg; sus rel caps (Dexedrine Spansule) 5, 10, 15 mg

Adverse effects

CNS: *Hyperactivity, insomnia, restlessness, talkativeness,* dizziness, headache, chills, stimulation, dysphoria, irritability, aggressiveness, tremor, dependence, addiction

CV: *Palpitations,* **tachycardia,** hypertension, decrease in heart rate, **dysrhythmias**

GI: *Anorexia,* dry mouth, diarrhea, constipation, weight loss, metallic taste

GU: Impotence, change in libido

INTEG: Urticaria

Contraindications: Hypersensitivity to sympathomimetic amines, hyperthyroidism, hypertension, glaucoma, severe arteriosclerosis, drug abuse, cardiovascular disease, anxiety, anorexia nervosa, tartrazine dye hypersensitivity

Precautions: Pregnancy **C,** Gilles de la Tourette's disorder, lactation, child <3 yr, depression

Pharmacokinetics	
Absorption	Well absorbed
Distribution	Widely distributed; crosses placenta
Metabolism	Liver
Excretion	Kidneys, pH dependent: increased pH, increased reabsorption
Half-life	10-30 hr; increased when urine is alkaline

Pharmacodynamics	
Onset	½ hr
Peak	1-3 hr
Duration	4-10 hr

Interactions

Individual drugs

Acetazolamide, sodium bicarbonate: increased effect of dextroamphetamine

Ammonium chloride, ascorbic acid: decreased effect of dextroamphetamine

Haloperidol: increased CNS effect

Phenytoin: decreased absorption of phenytoin

Drug classifications
Adrenergic blockers: decreased adrenergic blocking effect
Antacids: increased effect of dextroamphetamine
Antidepressants (tricyclic), phenothiazines: increased CNS effect
Antidiabetics: decreased antidiabetic effect
Barbiturates: decreased absorption of barbiturate
MAOIs: hypertensive crisis if used within 14 days

Drug/herb
Eucalyptus: decreased stimulant effect
Khat: increased stimulant effect
St. John's wort: increased serotonin syndrome

Drug/food
Caffeine: increased amine effect

NURSING CONSIDERATIONS

Assessment
- Monitor VS, B/P, since this drug may reverse antihypertensives; check patients with cardiac disease more often for increased B/P
- Monitor CBC, urinalysis; for diabetic patients monitor blood, urine glucose; insulin changes may be required, since eating will decrease
- Monitor height and weight q3 mo since growth rate in children may be decreased; appetite is suppressed so weight loss is common during the first few months of treatment
- Monitor mental status: mood, sensorium, affect, stimulation, insomnia; aggressiveness may occur; depression with crying spells may occur after drug has worn off
- Assess for physical dependency; should not be used for extended time except in ADHD; dosage should be decreased gradually to prevent withdrawal symptoms
- Assess for narcoleptic symptoms before medication and after; ability to stay awake should increase significantly
- In children or adults with ADHD, monitor for improved organizational skills, attention span, attending to tasks, impulse control, socialization, and ability to get along better with others
- Assess for withdrawal symptoms: headache, nausea, vomiting, muscle pain, weakness; drug tolerance develops after long-term use; dosage should not be increased if tolerance develops; this medication has a high abuse potential

Nursing diagnoses
- Thought processes, disturbed (uses, adverse reactions)
- Coping, ineffective (uses)
- Coping, family, compromised (uses)
- Knowledge, deficient (teaching)

Implementation
- Do not break, crush, or chew sus rel caps
- Give at least 6 hr before bedtime to avoid sleeplessness; titrate to patient's response; lowest dosage should be used to control symptoms
- Give gum, hard candy, frequent sips of water for dry mouth at beginning of treatment; these symptoms tend to lessen with time

Patient/family education
- Advise patient to decrease caffeine consumption (coffee, tea, cola, chocolate), which may increase irritability and stimulation; to avoid OTC preparations unless approved by prescriber; to avoid alcohol ingestion; these may cause serious drug interactions
- Caution patient to taper off drug over several weeks, or depression, increased sleeping, lethargy may occur
- Caution patient to avoid hazardous activities until patient is stabilized on medication
- Instruct patient not to double doses if medication is missed; prescriber may suggest drug holidays (ADHD) during the school year to assess progress and determine continued drug necessity
- Instruct patient/family to notify prescriber if significant side effects occur: tremors, insomnia, palpitations, restlessness, drug changes may be needed
- Inform patient that if dry mouth occurs to use frequent sips of water, sugarless gum, hard candy during beginning therapy; dry mouth lessens with continued treatment
- Advise patient to get needed rest; patients will feel more tired at end of day; to give last dose at least 6 hr before bedtime to avoid insomnia

Evaluation
Positive therapeutic outcome
- Decreased activity in ADHD
- Absence of sleeping during day in narcolepsy

Treatment of overdose: Administer fluids, hemodialysis, peritoneal dialysis, antihypertensives for increased B/P; ammonium chloride for increased excretion

dextromethorphan (OTC)
(dex-troe-meth-or′fan)

Balminil DM ♣, Benylin DM, Broncho-Grippol-DM ♣, Children's Hold, Creo-Terpin, Delsym, dextromethorphan, Hold DM, Koffex ♣, Neo-DM ♣, Ornex-DM ♣, Pertussin, Pertussin ES, Robidex ♣, Robitussin Cough Calmers, Robitussin Pediatric, Sedatuss ♣, St. Joseph Cough Suppressant, Scot-Tussin DM, Sucrets Cough Control, Suppress, Vicks Formula 44

Func. class.: Antitussive, nonopioid
Chem. class.: Levorphanol derivative

Pregnancy category C

Action: Depresses cough center in medulla by direct effect related to levorphanol

Therapeutic Outcome: Absence of cough

Uses: Nonproductive cough carried by minor respiratory tract infections or irritants that might be inhaled

Investigational uses: Neuropathy

Dosage and routes
Adult and child ≥12 yr: PO 10-20 mg q4h, or 30 mg q6-8h, not to exceed 120 mg/day; sus rel liq 60 mg q12h, not to exceed 120 mg/day

Child 6-12 yr: PO 5-10 mg q4h; sus rel liq 30 mg bid, not to exceed 60 mg/day; lozenge 5-10 mg q1-4h, max 60 mg/day

Child 2-6 yr: PO 2.5-5 mg q4h, or 7.5 mg q6-8h, not to exceed 30 mg/day

Neuropathy

Adult: PO doses vary widely

Available forms: Loz 2.5, 5, 7.5, 15 mg; sol; liq 3.5 mg, 7.5, 15 mg/5 ml, 3.5, 5, 7.5, 10, 15 mg/5 ml; syr 15 mg/15 ml, 10 mg/5 ml; sus action liq equivalent to 30 mg/5 ml; caps 30 mg; ext rel susp 30 mg/5 ml; gel caps 15 mg

Adverse effects
CNS: *Dizziness,* sedation

GI: *Nausea*

Contraindications: Hypersensitivity, asthma/emphysema, productive cough

Precautions: Pregnancy **C**, nausea/vomiting, increased temp, persistent headache

Pharmacokinetics

Absorption	Rapid (PO); slow (sus rel)
Distribution	Unknown
Metabolism	Liver
Excretion	Kidneys
Half-life	Unknown

Pharmacodynamics

	PO	PO-SUS
Onset	15-30 min	Unknown
Peak	Unknown	Unknown
Duration	3-6 hr	12 hr

Interactions
Individual drugs

Alcohol: increased CNS depression
Amiodarone, fluoxetine, quinidine, sibutramine: increased adverse reactions

Drug classifications

Antihistamines, antidepressants, opiates, sedative/hypnotics: increased CNS depression
MAOIs: increased hypotension, hyperpyrexia, do not give within 2 wk of MAOI

NURSING CONSIDERATIONS
Assessment
- Assess cough: type, frequency, character including sputum; provide adequate hydration to 2 L/day to decrease viscosity of secretions

Nursing diagnoses
- Airway clearance, ineffective (uses)
- Knowledge, deficient (teaching)

Implementation
- Administer decreased dosage to elderly patients; their metabolism may be slowed; do not provide water within 30 min of administration because it dilutes drug
- Shake susp before administration

Patient/family education
- Caution patient to avoid driving or other hazardous activities until stabilized on this medication; may cause drowsiness, dizziness in some individuals
- Advise patient to avoid smoking, smoke-filled rooms, perfumes, dust, environmental pollutants, cleaners, which increase cough; may use gum, hard candy to prevent dry mouth
- Advise patient to avoid alcohol or other CNS depressants while taking this medication; drowsiness will be increased
- Caution patient that any cough lasting over a few days should be assessed by prescriber

Evaluation
Positive therapeutic outcome
- Absence of dry, irritating cough

D

dextrose (D-glucose) (Rx)

Glucose, Glutose, Insta-Glucose

Func. class.: Caloric agent

Action: Needed for adequate utilization of amino acids; decreases protein, nitrogen loss; prevents ketosis

Therapeutic Outcome: Provides calories, prevents severe hypoglycemia

Uses: Increases intake of calories; increases fluids in patients unable to take adequate fluids, calories orally; 2.5%-11.5% forms provide calories, increased hydration; 20%-70% forms used to treat severe hypoglycemia

Dosage and routes

Adult and child: **IV**, depends on individual requirements

Available forms: Inj **IV** 2.5%, 5%, 10%, 20%, 30%, 40%, 50%, 60%, 70%; oral gel 40%; chewable tabs 5 g

Adverse effects

CNS: Confusion, **loss of consciousness,** dizziness

CV: Hypertension, **CHF, pulmonary edema**

ENDO: Hyperglycemia, rebound hypoglycemia, hyperosmolar syndrome, hyperglycemic nonketolytic syndrome

GU: Glycosuria, osmotic diuresis

INTEG: Chills, flushing, warm feeling, rash, urticaria, extravasation necrosis

Contraindications: Hyperglycemia, delirium tremens, hemorrhage (cranial/spinal), CHF

Precautions: Renal, liver, cardiac disease, diabetes mellitus

Pharmacokinetics

Absorption	Well absorbed (PO); completely absorbed (**IV**)
Distribution	Widely distributed
Metabolism	Unknown
Excretion	Unknown
Half-life	Unknown

Pharmacodynamics

	IV	PO
Onset	Immediate	Rapid
Peak	Immediate	Rapid
Duration	Immediate	Rapid

Interactions

Individual drugs

Insulin: increased need for insulin

Drug classifications

Corticosteroids: increased fluid retention/electrolyte excretion

Hypoglycemics, oral: increased need for hypoglycemic

NURSING CONSIDERATIONS

Assessment

- Assess I&O, skin turgor, edema, electrolytes (potassium, sodium, calcium, chloride, magnesium), blood glucose, ammonia, phosphate
- Monitor inj site for extravasation: redness along vein, edema at site, necrosis, pain, hard tender area; site should be changed immediately
- Monitor temp q4h for increased fever, indicating infection; if infection suspected, inf is discontinued and tubing, bottle, catheter tip cultured
- Monitor serum glucose in patients receiving hypertonic glucose 5% and over
- Assess nutritional status: calorie count by dietician; GI system function

Nursing diagnoses

- Nutrition, less than body requirements, imbalanced (uses)
- Fluid volume, excess (adverse reactions)
- Knowledge, deficient (teaching)

Implementation

PO route

- Oral glucose preparations (gel, chewable tabs) are to be used for conscious patients only; serum blood glucose should be monitored after first oral dose; if glucose has not increased by 20 mg/100 ml in 20-30 min, dose should be repeated and serum glucose checked again

IV route

- Give only protein (4%) and dextrose (up to 12.5%) via peripheral vein; stronger sol requires central **IV** administration
- May be given undiluted via prepared sol; give 10% sol (5 ml/15 sec), 20% sol (1000 ml/3 hr or more), 50% sol (500 ml/30-60 min); too rapid **IV** administration may cause fluid overload and hyperglycemia
- After changing **IV** catheter, change dressing q24h with aseptic technique

Patient/family education

- Teach patient reason for dextrose infusion
- Provide literature and information on when and how to use oral products for hypoglycemia
- Review hypoglycemia/hyperglycemia symptoms
- Review blood glucose monitoring procedure

Evaluation

Positive therapeutic outcome

- Increased weight
- Blood glucose level at normal limits for patient
- Adequate hydration

diazepam (Rx)

(dye-az'e-pam)

Apo-Diazepam ✤, diazepam, Diazemuls ✤, Novo-Diapam ✤, PMS-Diazepam ✤, Valium, Vivol ✤

Func. class.: Antianxiety, anticonvulsant, skeletal muscle relaxant, central acting

Chem. class.: Benzodiazepine

Pregnancy category D

Controlled substance schedule IV

Do Not Confuse:
diazepam/Ditropan/lorazepam

Action: Potentiates the actions of GABA, especially in limbic system, reticular formation; enhances presympathetic inhibition, inhibits spinal polysynaptic afferent paths

Therapeutic Outcome: Decreased anxiety, restlessness, insomnia

Uses: Anxiety, acute alcohol withdrawal, adjunct in seizure disorders; preoperative skeletal muscle relaxation; rectally for acute repetitive seizures

Investigational uses: Panic attacks

Dosage and routes

Anxiety/convulsive disorders

Adult: PO 2-10 mg bid-qid

Elderly: PO 1-2 mg daily-bid, increase slowly as needed

Child >6 mo: PO 1-2.5 mg tid-qid

Precardioversion

Adult: **IV** 5-15 mg 5-10 min precardioversion

Preendoscopy

Adult: **IV** 2.5-20 mg, IM 5-10 mg ½ hr preendoscopy

Muscle relaxation

Adult: PO 2-10 mg tid-qid or ext rel 15-30 mg daily; **IV**/IM 5-10 mg repeat in 2-4 hr

Elderly: PO2-5 mg bid-qid; **IV**/IM 2-5 mg, may repeat in 2-4 hr

Tetanic muscle spasms

Child >5 yr: IM/**IV** 5-10 mg q3-4h prn

Infants >30 days: IM/**IV** 1-2 mg q3-4h prn

Status epilepticus

Adult: **IV**/IM 5-10 mg, 2 mg/min, may repeat q10-15 min, not to exceed 30 mg; may repeat in 2-4 hr if seizures reappear

Child >5 yr: **IV**/IM 1 mg q2-5 min, max 10 mg, may repeat in 2-4 hr

Child 1 mo-5 yr: **IV**/IM 0.2-0.5 mg slowly q2-5 min up to 5 mg

Adult: REC 0.2 mg/kg, may repeat 4-12 hr later

Child 6-11 yr: REC 0.3 mg/kg, may repeat 4-12 hr later

Child 2-5 yr: REC 0.5 mg/kg, may repeat 4-12 hr later

Alcohol withdrawal

Adult: PO 10 mg tid-qid in 1st 24 hr, then 5 mg tid-qid; IM/**IV** 10 mg, then 5-10 mg after 3 hr

Psychoneurotic reactions

Adult: **IV**/IM 2-10 mg; may repeat in 3-4h

Available forms: Tabs 2, 5, 10 mg; inj 5 mg/ml; oral sol 5 mg/5 ml; gel, rectal delivery system 2.5, 5, 10, 15, 20 mg, twin packs

Adverse effects

CNS: *Dizziness, drowsiness,* confusion, headache, anxiety, tremors, stimulation, fatigue, depression, insomnia, hallucinations

CV: *Orthostatic hypotension,* **ECG changes, tachycardia,** hypotension

EENT: *Blurred vision,* tinnitus, mydriasis, nystagmus

GI: Constipation, dry mouth, nausea, vomiting, anorexia, diarrhea

HEMA: **Neutropenia**

INTEG: Rash, dermatitis, itching

RESP: **Respiratory depression**

Contraindications: Pregnancy **D**, hypersensitivity to benzodiazepines, narrow-angle glaucoma, psychosis, coma, respiratory depression

Precautions: Elderly, debilitated, hepatic disease, renal disease, addiction, child <6 mo

Pharmacokinetics

Absorption	Rapid (PO); erratic (IM)
Distribution	Widely distributed; crosses blood-brain barrier, placenta
Metabolism	Liver, extensively
Excretion	Kidneys, breast milk
Half-life	20-80 hr

Pharmacodynamics

	PO	IM	IV
Onset	½ hr	15 min	Immediate
Peak	1-2 hr	½-1½ hr	15 min
Duration	2-3 hr	1-1½ hr	15 min-1 hr

Interactions

Individual drugs

Alcohol: increased CNS depression
Cimetidine, valproic acid: increased toxicity
Disulfiram, isoniazid, propranolol, valproic acid: decreased metabolism of diazepam

Drug classifications

Barbiturates, CNS depressants, SSRIs: increased toxicity
CNS depressants: increased CNS depression
Oral contraceptives: decreased metabolism of diazepam

Drug/herb

Cowslip, goldenseal, kava, melatonin, mistletoe, pokeweed, poppy, Queen Anne's lace, valerian: increased diazepam effect
Cola tree: decreased diazepam effect

Drug/lab test

Increased: AST/ALT, serum bilirubin
Decreased: radioactive iodine uptake
False increase: 17-OHCS

NURSING CONSIDERATIONS

Assessment

- Assess degree of anxiety; what precipitates anxiety and whether drug controls symptoms; other signs of anxiety: dilated pupils, inability to sleep, restlessness, inability to focus
- Assess for alcohol withdrawal symptoms, including hallucinations (visual, auditory), delirium, irritability, agitation, fine to coarse tremors
- Monitor B/P (with patient lying, standing), pulse, respiratory rate; if systolic B/P drops 20 mm Hg, hold drug, notify prescriber; monitor respirations q5-15 min if given **IV**
- Monitor blood studies: CBC during long-term therapy; blood dyscrasias have occurred (rarely)
- Monitor for seizure control; type, duration, and intensity of seizures; what precipitates seizures
- Monitor hepatic studies: AST, ALT, bilirubin, creatinine, LDH, alkaline phosphatase
- Assess mental status: mood, sensorium, affect, sleeping pattern, drowsiness, dizziness, suicidal tendencies, and ability of drug to control these symptoms; check for tolerance, withdrawal symptoms: headache, nausea, vomiting, muscle pain, weakness after long-term use

Nursing diagnoses

- Anxiety (uses)
- Injury, risk for (uses, adverse reactions)
- Coping, ineffective (uses)
- Knowledge, deficient (teaching)
- Noncompliance (teaching)

Implementation

PO route

- Give with food or milk for GI symptoms
- Crush tab if patient is unable to swallow medication whole
- Use sugarless gum, hard candy, frequent sips of water for dry mouth
- Reduce opioid dosage by ⅓ if given concomitantly with diazepam
- Check to see PO medication has been swallowed

Rectal route

- Do not use more than 5×/mo or for an episode q5 days

IV route

- Administer **IV** into large vein; do not dilute or mix with any other drug; give **IV** 5 mg or less/1 min or total dose over 3 min or more (children, infants); cont inf is not recommended
- Check **IV** site for thrombosis or phlebitis, which may occur rapidly

Sterile emulsion for injection route

- Use **IV** only, within 6 hr, flush line after use and after 6 hr

Syringe compatibilities: Cimetidine

Syringe incompatibilities: Benzquinamide, doxapram, glycopyrrolate, heparin, nalbuphine

Y-site compatibilities: Cefmetazole, DOBUTamine, nafcillin, quinidine, sufentanil

Y-site incompatibilities: Hydromorphone, fluconazole, foscarnet, heparin, pancuronium, potassium chloride, vecuronium, vit B with C

Additive compatibilities: Netilmicin, verapamil

Patient/family education

- Advise patient that drug may be taken with food; that drug is not to be used for everyday stress or used longer than 4 mo unless directed by prescriber; take no more than prescribed amount; may be habit forming
- Caution patient to avoid OTC preparations unless approved by a prescriber; to avoid alcohol, other psychotropic medications unless prescribed; that smoking may decrease diazepam effect by increasing diazepam metabolism; not to discontinue medication abruptly after long-term use
- Inform patient to avoid driving, activities that require alertness; drowsiness may occur; to rise slowly or fainting may occur, especially in elderly
- Advise patient not to become pregnant while using this drug

• Inform patient that drowsiness may worsen at beginning of treatment

Evaluation

Positive therapeutic outcome

• Decreased anxiety, restlessness, insomnia

Treatment of overdose: Lavage, VS, supportive care, flumazenil

diazoxide (Rx)

(dye-az-ox'ide)

Hyperstat IV, diazoxide parenteral

Func. class.: Antihypertensive

Chem. class.: Vasodilator

Pregnancy category C

Action: Decreases release of insulin from β-cells in pancreas, resulting in an increase in blood glucose; relaxes vascular smooth muscle (peripheral arterioles)

Therapeutic Outcome: Decreased B/P, increased blood glucose

Uses: Hypoglycemia caused by hyperinsulinism; emergency treatment of hypertension

Dosage and routes

Hypoglycemia

Adult and child: PO 3-8 mg/kg/day in 2-3 divided doses q8-12h

Infants and neonates: PO 8-15 mg/kg/day in 2-3 divided doses 8-12h

Hypertension

Adult: **IV** bol 1-3 mg/kg rapidly up to a max of 150 mg in a single inj; dose may be repeated until desired response is achieved; give **IV** in 30 sec or less

Child: **IV** bol 1-2 mg/kg rapidly: administration same as adult, not to exceed 150 mg

Available forms: Caps 50 mg; oral susp 50 mg/ml; inj 15 mg/ml, 300 mg/20 ml

Adverse effects

CNS: Headache, weakness, anxiety, dizziness, insomnia, paresthesia, **seizures, cerebral ischemia, paralysis,** sleepiness, euphoria, anxiety, extrapyramidial symptoms (EPS), confusion, tinnitus, blurred vision

CV: Palpitations, hypotension, **shock, MI,** T-wave changes, angina pectoris, **supraventricular tachycardia, edema,** rebound hypertension

ENDO: Hyperglycemia in diabetics, transient hyperglycemia in nondiabetics, increased uric acid

GI: Nausea, vomiting, dry mouth

GU: Breast tenderness, increased BUN, fluid, electrolyte imbalances, Na, water retention

HEMA: **Thrombocytopenia,** decreased Hgb, Hct

INTEG: Rash

Contraindications: Hypersensitivity to this drug or thiazides, sulfonamides, hypertension of aortic coarctation or AV shunt, pheochromocytoma, dissecting aortic aneurysm

Precautions: Pregnancy **C**, lactation, tachycardia, fluid/electrolyte imbalances, impaired cerebral or cardiac circulation, children

Pharmacokinetics

Absorption	Well absorbed (PO); completely absorbed (**IV**)
Distribution	Crosses blood-brain barrier, placenta, protein binding >90%
Metabolism	Liver (50%)
Excretion	Kidneys, unchanged (50%)
Half-life	20-36 hr

Pharmacodynamics

	PO	IV
Onset	1 hr	1-2 min
Peak	8-12 hr	5 min
Duration	8 hr	3-12 hr

Interactions

Drug classifications

Antihypertensives: severe hypotension

Diuretics (thiazides): increased hyperuricemic, antihypertensive effects of diazoxide

Hydantoins: decreased anticonvulsant effect

Sulfonylureas: increased hyperglycemia

Drug/herb

Aconite: increased toxicity, death

NURSING CONSIDERATIONS

Assessment

• Assess for allergies to sulfonamide; cross-sensitivity may occur

• Assess B/P q5 min until stabilized

• Monitor electrolytes, blood studies: potassium, sodium, chloride, carbon dioxide, CBC, serum glucose

• Monitor weight daily, I&O; edema in feet, legs daily; check skin turgor, dryness of mucous membranes for hydration status

• Assess for crackles, dyspnea, orthopnea; peripheral edema, fatigue, weight gain, jugular vein distention (CHF)

• Assess for signs of hyperglycemia: acetone breath, increased urinary output, severe thirst, lethargy, dizziness

Nursing diagnoses
- Cardiac output, decreased (adverse reactions)
- Injury, risk for (side effects)
- Knowledge, deficient (teaching)

Implementation
PO route
- Shake susp before using
- Store protected from light and heat

IV route
- Give by direct **IV** over 30 sec or less; may repeat q5-15 min until desired response; do not administer dark solution
- Give to patient in recumbent position; keep in that position for 1 hr after

Syringe compatibility: Heparin
Y-site incompatibilities: Hydralazine, propranolol

Evaluation
Positive therapeutic outcome
- Decreased B/P in hypertension

Treatment of overdose: Administer levarterenol, DOPamine, or norepinephrine for hypotension, dialysis

diclofenac potassium (Rx)
(dye-kloe'fen-ak)
Cataflam, Voltaren Rapide ✦
diclofenac sodium
Apo-Dilo ✦, Novo-Difenac ✦, Nu-Diclo, Voltaren, Voltaren XR
Func. class.: Nonsteroidal antiinflammatory (NSAIDs), nonopioid analgesic
Chem. class.: Phenylacetic acid

Pregnancy category B

Do Not Confuse:
Cataflam/Catapres

Action: Inhibits prostaglandin synthesis by decreasing enzyme needed for biosynthesis; analgesic, antiinflammatory, antipyretic properties

Therapeutic Outcome: Decreased pain, inflammation

Uses: Acute, chronic rheumatoid arthritis, osteoarthritis, ankylosing spondylitis, analgesia, primary dysmenorrhea

Dosage and routes
Osteoarthritis
Adult: PO 100-150 mg/day in 2-3 divided doses

Rheumatoid arthritis
Adult: PO 100-200 mg/day in 2-4 divided doses (potassium); 50 mg tid-qid, then reduce to lowest dose needed (25 mg tid) (sodium)

Ankylosing spondylitis
Adult: PO 100-125 mg/day in 4-5 divided doses; give 25 mg qid and 25 mg at bedtime if needed (potassium)

Postcataract surgery
Adult: Ophth 1 gtt of 0.1% sol qid × 2 wk postsurgery

Analgesia/primary dysmenorrhea
Adult: PO 50 mg tid, max 150 mg/day (potassium)

Available forms: Potassium: tabs 50, 75 mg; sodium: delayed rel tabs (enteric-coated) 25, 50, 75 mg; ext rel tabs 75, 100 mg; supp 50, 100 mg

Adverse effects
CNS: ***Dizziness, headache,*** drowsiness, fatigue, tremors, confusion, insomnia, anxiety, depression, nervousness, paresthesia, muscle weakness
CV: **CHF,** tachycardia, peripheral edema, palpitations, dysrhythmias, hypotension, hypertension, fluid retention
EENT: Tinnitus, hearing loss, blurred vision, **laryngeal edema**
GI: Nausea, anorexia, vomiting, diarrhea, jaundice, **cholestatic hepatitis,** constipation, flatulence, cramps, dry mouth, peptic ulcer, GI bleeding, **hepatotoxicity**
GU: **Nephrotoxicity: dysuria, hematuria, oliguria, azotemia, cystitis, UTI**
HEMA: **Blood dyscrasias,** epistaxis, bruising
INTEG: Purpura, rash, pruritus, sweating, erythema, petechiae, photosensitivity, alopecia
RESP: Dyspnea, hemoptysis, pharyngitis, **bronchospasm,** rhinitis, shortness of breath
SYST: **Anaphylaxis**

Contraindications: Pregnancy (3rd trimester), hypersensitivity to aspirin, iodides, other NSAIDs, asthma

Precautions: Pregnancy **B** (1st trimester), not recommended in 2nd half of pregnancy, lactation, children, bleeding disorders, GI disorders, cardiac disorders, hypersensitivity to other antiinflammatory agents, CCr <30 ml/min

Pharmacokinetics

Absorption	Well absorbed (PO, ophth)
Distribution	Crosses placenta; 90% bound to plasma proteins
Metabolism	Liver (50%)
Excretion	Breast milk
Half-life	1-2 hr

Pharmacodynamics

	PO	OPHTH
Onset	Unknown	Unknown
Peak	2-3 hr	Unknown
Duration	Unknown	Unknown

Interactions
Individual drugs
Aspirin: increased GI side effects
CycloSPORINE, lithium, methotrexate, phenytoin: increased toxicity
Drug classifications
Anticoagulants: increased risk of bleeding
Antidiabetics: increased need for dosage adjustment
β-blockers, diuretics: decreased antihypertensive effect
Diuretics (potassium-sparing): hyperkalemia
NSAIDs: increased GI side effects
Drug/herb
Arginine, gossypol: increased gastric irritation
Bearberry, bilberry: increased NSAIDs effect
Bogbean, chondroitin, saw palmetto, turmeric: increased bleeding risk
St. John's wort: increased severe photosensitivity

NURSING CONSIDERATIONS
Assessment
- Assess for pain of rheumatoid arthritis, osteoarthritis, ankylosing spondylitis; check ROM, inflammation of joints, characteristics of pain
- Assess ophth patients for pain, inflammation, redness, swelling
- ❗ Monitor blood counts during therapy; watch for decreasing platelets; if low, therapy may need to be discontinued, restarted after hematologic recovery
- Assess for asthma, aspirin hypersensitivity, nasal polyps; may develop hypersensitivity
- Monitor liver function tests (may be elevated) and uric acid (may be decreased—serum; increased—urine) periodically; also BUN, creatinine, electrolytes (may be elevated)
- ❗ Monitor for blood dyscrasias (thrombocytopenia): bruising, fatigue, bleeding, poor healing

Nursing diagnoses
- Pain, chronic (uses)
- Mobility, physical, impaired (uses)
- Injury, risk for (side effects)
- Knowledge, deficient (teaching)

Implementation
PO route
- Do not break, crush, chew or dissolve enteric-coated or ext rel tabs
- Administer with food or milk to decrease gastric symptoms
- Remain upright for ½ hr

Ophthalmic route
- Administer with patient recumbent or tilting head back; pull down on lower lid; when conjunctival sac is exposed, instill 1 drop; wait a few minutes before instilling other drops

Patient/family education
- Teach patient that drug must be continued for prescribed time to be effective; to avoid aspirin, NSAIDs, acetaminophen, or other OTC medications unless approved by prescriber, alcoholic beverages; to contact prescriber before surgery regarding when to discontinue this drug
- Caution patient to report bleeding, bruising, fatigue, malaise, since blood dyscrasias do occur
- Advise patient to report hepatotoxicity: flulike symptoms, nausea, vomiting, jaundice, pruritus, lethargy
- Instruct patient to use sunscreen to prevent photosensitivity
- Teach patient to avoid use in 3rd trimester of pregnancy
- Instruct patient to use caution when driving; drowsiness, dizziness may occur
- Teach patient to take with a full glass of water to enhance absorption; remain upright for ½ hr; if dose is missed, take as soon as remembered within 2 hr if taking 1-2 ×/day, do not double doses

Evaluation
Positive therapeutic outcome
- Decreased pain in arthritic conditions
- Decreased inflammation in arthritic conditions
- Decreased ocular irritation

dicloxacillin (Rx)
(dye-klox-a-sill′in)
dicloxacillin sodium, Dycill, Dynapen, Pathocil
Func. class.: Antiinfective
Chem. class.: Penicillinase-resistant penicillin

Pregnancy category B

Do Not Confuse:
Pathocil/Bactocil

Action: Interferes with cell wall replication of susceptible organisms; osmotically unstable cell wall swells, bursts from osmotic pressure

Therapeutic Outcome: Bactericidal effects for the following: gram-positive cocci *Staphylococcus aureus, Streptococcus pyogenes, Streptococcus viridans, Streptococcus faecalis, Streptococcus bovis, Streptococcus pneumoniae;* infections caused by penicillinase-producing *Staphylococcus* organisms

Uses: Penicillinase-producing staphylococci, streptococci; respiratory tract, skin, skin structure infections; sinusitis

Dosage and routes

Adult and child ≥40 kg: PO 0.5-4 g/day in divided doses q6h, max 4 g/day

Child ≤40 kg: PO 12.5-25 mg/kg in divided doses q6h, max 4 g/day

Available forms: Caps 250, 500 mg

Adverse effects

CNS: Lethargy, hallucinations, anxiety, depression, twitching, **coma, seizures**

GI: *Nausea, vomiting, diarrhea,* increased AST, ALT, abdominal pain, glossitis, **pseudomembranous colitis**

GU: **Oliguria, proteinuria, hematuria,** *vaginitis, moniliasis,* **glomerulonephritis**

HEMA: Anemia, increased bleeding time, **bone marrow depression, granulocytopenia**

SYST: **Anaphylaxis**

Contraindications: Hypersensitivity to penicillins; neonates

Precautions: Pregnancy **B,** hypersensitivity to cephalosporins, lactation, severe renal or hepatic disease

Pharmacokinetics	
Absorption	Rapid, incomplete (35%-75%)
Distribution	Widely distributed; crosses placenta
Metabolism	Liver (6%-10%)
Excretion	Kidneys, unchanged (60%); breast milk
Half-life	½-1 hr, increased in hepatic renal disease

Pharmacodynamics	
Onset	½ hr
Peak	½-2 hr

Interactions

Individual drugs

Probenecid: increased dicloxacillin levels

Drug classifications

Oral anticoagulants: decreased anticoagulant effects

Drug/herb

Acidophilus: do not use with antiinfectives

Khat: decreased absorption; separate by 2 hr

Drug/food

Food, citrus fruit juices: decreased absorption

Drug/lab test

False positive: urine glucose, urine protein

NURSING CONSIDERATIONS

Assessment

- Assess patient for previous sensitivity reaction to penicillins or other cephalosporins; cross-sensitivity between penicillins and cephalosporins is common
- Assess patient for signs and symptoms of infection including characteristics of wounds, sputum, urine, stool, WBC >10,000/mm^3, fever; obtain baseline information and during treatment
- Obtain C&S before beginning drug therapy to identify if correct treatment has been initiated
- Assess for anaphylaxis: rash, urticaria, pruritus, chills, fever, joint pain may occur a few days after therapy begins; epINEPHrine and resuscitation equipment should be available for anaphylactic reaction
- ❗ Identify urine output; if decreasing, notify prescriber (may indicate nephrotoxicity); check for increased BUN, creatinine
- Monitor blood studies: AST, ALT, CBC, Hct, bilirubin, LDH, alkaline phosphatase, Coombs' test monthly if patient is on long-term therapy
- Monitor electrolytes: potassium, sodium, chloride monthly if patient is on long-term therapy
- Assess bowel pattern daily; if severe diarrhea occurs, drug should be discontinued; may indicate pseudomembranous colitis
- Monitor for bleeding: ecchymosis, bleeding gums, hematuria, stool guaiac daily if on long-term therapy
- Assess for overgrowth of infection: perineal itching, fever, malaise, redness, pain, swelling, drainage, rash, diarrhea, change in cough, sputum

Nursing diagnoses

- Infection, risk for (uses)
- Diarrhea (side effects)
- Knowledge, deficient (teaching)
- Noncompliance (teaching)
- Injury, risk for (side effects)

Implementation

- Do not break, crush, or chew caps
- Give in even doses around the clock; if GI upset occurs, give with food; drug must be given for 10-14 days to ensure organism death

and prevent superinfection; store in airtight container
- Shake susp well before each dose; store in refrigerator for 2 wk or 1 wk at room temp

Patient/family education
- Teach patient to report sore throat, bruising, bleeding, joint pain; may indicate blood dyscrasias (rare)
- Advise patient to contact prescriber if vaginal itching, loose, foul-smelling stools, furry tongue occur; may indicate superinfection
- Instruct patient to take all medication prescribed for the length of time ordered, carry/wear emergency ID if allergic to penicillins
- Advise patient to notify prescriber of diarrhea with blood or pus, which may indicate pseudomembranous colitis

Evaluation
Positive therapeutic outcome
- Absence of signs/symptoms of infection (WBC <10,000/mm^3, temp WNL, absence of red draining wounds)
- Reported improvement in symptoms of infection

Treatment of anaphylaxis: Withdraw drug, maintain airway, administer epINEPHrine, aminophylline, O_2, **IV** corticosteroids

didanosine (Rx)
(dye-dan'oh-seen)
ddl, dideoxyinosine, Videx, Videx EC
Func. class.: Antiretroviral
Chem. class.: Synthetic purine nucleoside reverse transcriptase inhibitor
Pregnancy category B

Action: Nucleoside analog incorporating into cellular DNA by viral reverse transcriptase, thereby terminating the cellular DNA chain that prevents viral replication

Therapeutic Outcome: Antiviral against the retroviruses, primarily HIV-1

Uses: HIV-1 infection in combination with other antiretrovirals

Dosage and routes
Renal dose
Adult: PO reduce dosage CCr <60 ml/min
Adult: PO >60 kg, 200 mg bid tabs, or 250 mg bid buffered powder; caps, del rel 400 mg daily; <60 kg, 125 mg bid tabs, or 167 mg bid buffered powder; caps del rel 250 mg daily
Child: PO tabs 90-120 mg/m^2 q12h; buffered powder packets 112.5-150 mg/m^2 q12h; PO (child BSA 1.1-1.4 m^2) tab 100 mg q8-12h; reconstituted pediatric powder 125 mg q8-12h; PO (child BSA 0.8-1 m^2) tabs 75 mg q8-12h; reconstituted pediatric powder 94 mg q8-12h; PO (child BSA 0.5-0.7 m^2) tabs 50 mg q8-12h; reconstituted pediatric powder 62 mg q8-12h; PO (child BSA <0.4 m^2) tabs 25 mg q8-12h; reconstitutedpediatric powder 31 mg q8-12h

Available forms: Tabs, buffered, chewable/dispersible 25, 50, 100, 150, 200 mg; powder for oral sol, 10 mg/ml; del rel caps 125, 200, 250, 400

Adverse effects
CNS: **Peripheral neuropathy, seizures,** confusion, *anxiety,* hypertonia, abnormal thinking, asthenia, *insomnia, CNS depression,* pain, dizziness, chills, fever
CV: Hypertension, vasodilatation, **dysrhythmia,** syncope, **CHF,** palpitations
EENT: Ear pain, otitis, photophobia, visual impairment, retinal depigmentation
GI: **Pancreatitis,** *diarrhea, nausea,* vomiting, *abdominal pain,* constipation, stomatitis, dyspepsia, liver abnormalities, flatulence, taste perversion, dry mouth, oral thrush, melena, increased ALT, AST, alkaline phosphatase, amylase, **hepatic failure**
GU: Increased bilirubin, uric acid
HEMA: **Leukopenia, granulocytopenia, thrombocytopenia, anemia**
INTEG: *Rash, pruritus,* alopecia, ecchymosis, hemorrhage, petechiae, sweating
MS: Myalgia, arthritis, myopathy, muscular atrophy
RESP: Cough, pneumonia, dyspnea, asthma, epistaxis, hypoventilation, sinusitis
SYST: **Lactic acidosis, anaphylaxis**

Contraindications: Hypersensitivity, lactic acidosis, pancreatitis, phenylketonuria

Precautions: Pregnancy **B,** renal, hepatic disease, lactation, children, sodium-restricted diets, elevated amylase, preexistent peripheral neuropathy, hyperuricemia

Pharmacokinetics
Absorption	Rapidly absorbed (up to 40%)
Distribution	Unknown
Metabolism	Not metabolized
Excretion	Kidneys (55%)/feces
Half-life	0.8-1.6 hr, shorter in children

Pharmacodynamics	
Onset	Unknown
Peak	Up to 1 hr, del rel 2 hr
Duration	Unknown

Interactions

Individual drugs

Allopurinol, tenofovir: increased didanosine level
Dapsone, ketoconazole: decreased absorption of each specific drug
Itraconazole: decreased concentrations
Methadone: decreased didanosine level

Drug classifications

Antacids, magnesium, aluminum: increased side effects
Antiretrovirals, other: decreased concentration
Fluoroquinolones, tetracyclines: decreased concentrations of each specific drug

Drug/food

Do not use with acidic juices
Decreased: absorption

NURSING CONSIDERATIONS

Assessment

- Assess for peripheral neuropathy: tingling or pain in hands and feet, distal numbness; onset usually occurs 2-6 mo after beginning treatment, if these occur during therapy, drug may be decreased or discontinued
- Assess for pancreatitis: abdominal pain, nausea, vomiting, elevated liver enzymes; drug should be discontinued, since condition can be fatal
- Assess children by dilated retinal examination q6 mo to rule out retinal depigmentation
- Monitor CBC, differential, platelet count monthly; withhold drug if WBC is <4000/mm^3 or platelet count is <75,000 mm^3, viral load, CD4$^+$ count; notify prescriber of results
- Monitor renal function studies: BUN, serum uric acid, urine CCr before, during therapy; these may be elevated throughout treatment
- Assess for anaphylaxis, lactic acidosis
- Monitor temp q4h; may indicate beginning of infection
- Monitor liver function tests before, during therapy (bilirubin, AST, ALT, amylase, alkaline phosphatase) as needed or monthly

Nursing diagnoses

- Infection, risk for (uses)
- Injury, risk for (adverse reactions)
- Knowledge, deficient (teaching)

Implementation

- Give on empty stomach, 1 hr ac or 2 hr pc, q12h; food decreases effectiveness of drug; adjust dose in renal impairment
- Patient should chew tabs; may be crushed and mixed with water
- Pediatric powder for oral sol should be prepared in the pharmacy; shake before using
- Packets for oral sol must be mixed with ½ glass of water not fruit juice; stir until dissolved; drink immediately
- Store tabs, caps in tightly closed bottle at room temp; store oral sol after dissolving at room temp ≤4 hr
- Do not take dapsone at same time as ddl

Patient/family education

- Advise patient to take on empty stomach; not to mix powder with fruit juice; to chew tab or crush and dissolve in water; to drink powder immediately after mixing; to use exactly as prescribed
- Instruct patient to report signs of infection: increased temp, sore throat, flulike symptoms; to avoid crowds and those with known infections
- Instruct patient to report signs of anemia: fatigue, headache, faintness, shortness of breath, irritability
- Advise patient to report numbness/tingling in extremities
- Instruct patient to report bleeding; avoid use of razors and commercial mouthwash
- Advise patient that hair may be lost during therapy; a wig or hairpiece may make patient feel better
- Caution patient to avoid OTC products and other medications without approval of prescriber; to avoid alcohol
- Teach patient not to have any sexual contact without use of a condom; needles should not be shared; blood from infected individual should not come in contact with another's mucous membranes

Evaluation

Positive therapeutic outcome

- Absence of opportunistic infection, symptoms of HIV

difenoxin with atropine

See diphenoxylate with atropine

! HIGH ALERT

digoxin (Rx)

(di-jox'in)

digoxin, Lanoxicaps, Lanoxin

Func. class.: Inotropic antidysrhythmic, cardiac glycoside

Chem. class.: Digitalis preparation

Pregnancy category C

Do Not Confuse:
Lanoxin/Lasix/Lonox,
Lanoxin/Lomotil,
Lanoxin/Xanax/Levoxine

Action: Inhibits sodium-potassium ATPase, which makes more calcium available for contractile proteins, resulting in increased cardiac output; increases force of contraction (positive inotropic effect); decreases heart rate (chronotropic effect); decreases AV conduction speed

Therapeutic Outcome: Decreased edema, pulse, respiration, crackles

Uses: Rapid digitalization in acute and chronic CHF, atrial fibrillation, atrial flutter, atrial tachycardia; cardiogenic shock, paroxysmal atrial tachycardia

Dosage and routes

Adult: **IV** *digitalizing dose* 0.6-1.0 mg given as 50% of the dose initially, additional fractions given at 4-8 hr intervals; PO *digitalizing dose* 0.75-1.25 mg given as 50% of the dose initially, additional fractions given at 4-8 hr intervals; *maintenance* 0.063-0.5 mg/day (tabs), or 0.350-0.5 mg/day (gelatin cap)

Child >10 yr: **IV** *digitalizing dose* 8-12 mcg/kg given as 50% of the dose initially, additional fractions given at 4-8 hr intervals; PO *digitalizing dose* 0.01-0.015 mg/kg given as 50% of the dose initially, additional fractions given at 6-8 hr intervals; maintenance 25%-35% of the loading dose daily as a single dose

Child 5-10 yr: **IV** *digitalizing dose* 0.015-0.03 mg/kg given as 50% of the dose initially, additional fractions given at 4-8 hr intervals; PO *digitalizing dose* 0.02-0.035 mg/kg given as 50% of the dose initially, additional fractions given at 6-8 hr intervals; *maintenance* 25%-35% of the loading dose daily in 2 divided doses

Child 2-5 yr: **IV** *digitalizing dose* 0.025-0.035 mg/kg given as 50% of the dose initially, additional fractions given at 4-8 hr intervals; PO *digitalizing dose* 0.03-0.04 mg/kg given as 50% of the dose initially, additional fractions given at 6-8 hr intervals; *maintenance* 25%-35% of the loading dose daily in 2 divided doses

Child 1-2 yr: **IV** *digitalizing dose* 0.03-0.05 mg/kg given as 50% of the dose initially, additional fractions given at 4-8 hr intervals; PO *digitalizing dose* 0.035-0.06 mg/kg given as 50% of the dose initially, additional fractions given at 4-8 hr intervals; *maintenance* 25%-35% of the loading dose daily in 2 divided doses

Infants: **IV** *digitalizing dose* 0.02-0.03 mg/kg given as 50% of the dose initially, additional fractions given at 4-8 hr intervals; PO *digitalizing dose* 0.025-0.035 mg/kg given as 50% of the dose initially, additional fractions given at 6-8 hr intervals; *maintenance* 25%-35% of the loading dose daily in 2 divided doses

Infants, premature: **IV** *digitalizing dose* 0.015-0.025 mg/kg given as 50% of the dose initially, additional fractions given at 4-8 hr intervals; PO *digitalizing dose* 0.02-0.03 mg/kg given as 50% of the dose initially, additional fractions given at 6-8 hr intervals; *maintenance* 20%-30% of the loading dose daily in 2 divided doses

Available forms: Caps 0.05, 0.1, 0.2 mg; elix 0.05 mg/ml; tabs 0.125, 0.25, 0.5 mg; inj 0.5 🍁, 0.25 mg/ml; pediatric inj 0.1 mg/ml

Adverse effects

CNS: *Headache,* drowsiness, apathy, confusion, disorientation, fatigue, depression, hallucinations

CV: **Dysrhythmias,** hypotension, bradycardia, **AV block**

EENT: Blurred vision, yellow-green halos, photophobia, diplopia

GI: Nausea, vomiting, anorexia, abdominal pain, diarrhea

Contraindications: Hypersensitivity to digitalis, ventricular fibrillation, ventricular tachycardia, carotid sinus syndrome, 2nd- or 3rd-degree heart block

Precautions: Pregnancy **C,** renal disease, acute MI, AV block, severe respiratory disease, hypothyroidism, elderly, sinus nodal disease, lactation, hypokalemia

Pharmacokinetics

Absorption	Unknown
Distribution	Widely distributed; 20%-25% protein bound
Metabolism	Liver, small amount; also intestinal bacteria
Excretion	Urine
Half-life	1½ days

Pharmacodynamics

	PO	IV
Onset	½-1½ hr	5-30 min
Peak	2-6 hr	1-5 hr
Duration	After steady state	6-8 days

Interactions

Individual drugs

Amiodarone, diltiazem, NIFEdipine, propantheline, quinidine, verapamil: increased digoxin levels
Amphotericin B, carbenicillin, ticarcillin: increased hypokalemia, increased toxicity
Calcium IV: increased hypercalcemia, hypomagnesemia, digoxin toxicity
Cholestyramine, colestipol, metoclopramide, thyroid hormones: decreased digoxin levels
Diltiazem: increased blood levels
Kaolin/pectin: decreased absorption
Verapamil: decreased positive inotropic effect

Drug classifications

Antacids: decreased digoxin absorption
Anticholinergics: increased digoxin blood levels
Antidysrhythmics, β-adrenergic blockers: increased bradycardia
Diuretics (thiazide) corticosteroids: increased hypokalemia, hypercalcemia, hypomagnesemia, digitalis toxicity
Sympathomimetics: increased cardiac dysrhythmia risk

Drug/herb

Aconite, hawthorn, horsetail: increased toxicity
Aloe, betel palm, broom, buckthorn, cascara sagrada castor, Chinese rhubarb, figwort, fumitory, hawthorn, khat, kudzu, licorice, lily of the valley, Mayapple, mistletoe, motherwort, night blooming cereus, oleander, pheasant's eye, purple foxglove, Queen Anne's lace, rhubarb, rue, senna, Siberian ginseng, squill, yellow dock: increased digoxin action
Bethroot, goldenseal, St. John's wort: decreased digoxin effect
Blackroot: forms insoluble complex
Cocoa, coffee, cola, guarana, horsetail, licorice, yerba maté: increased hypokalemia
Indian snakeroot: increased bradycardia
Psyllium: decreased digoxin absorption

Drug/lab test

Increased: CPK

NURSING CONSIDERATIONS

Assessment

- Assess and document apical pulse for 1 min before giving drug; if pulse <60 in adult or <90 in an infant or is significantly different, take again in 1 hr; if <60 in adult, call prescriber; note rate, rhythm, character
- Monitor electrolytes: potassium, sodium, chloride, magnesium, calcium; renal function studies: BUN, creatinine; other blood studies: ALT, AST, bilirubin, Hct, Hgb, drug levels (therapeutic level 0.5-2 ng/ml) before initiating treatment and periodically thereafter
- Monitor I&O ratio, daily weights; monitor turgor, lung sounds, edema
- Monitor cardiac status: apical pulse, character, rate, rhythm; resolution of atrial dysrhythmias by ECG; if tachydysrhythmia develops, hold drug; delay cardioversion while drug levels are determined
- Monitor ECG continuously during parenteral loading doses and for patients with suspected toxicity; provide hemodynamic monitoring for patients with heart failure or administer multiple cardiac drugs

Nursing diagnoses

- Cardiac output, decreased (uses)
- Gas exchange, impaired (adverse reactions)
- Knowledge, deficient (teaching)

Implementation

- Do not give at same time as antacids or other drugs that decrease absorption

PO route

- Give PO with or without food; may crush tabs
- Take medication at same time each day
- Give potassium supplements if ordered for potassium levels <3, or give foods high in potassium: bananas, orange juice

IV route

- Give **IV** undiluted or 1 ml of drug/4 ml sterile water, D_5, or 0.9% NaCl; give over >5 min through Y-tube or 3-way stopcock; during digitalization close monitoring is necessary
- Store protected from light

Syringe compatibilities: Heparin, milrinone

Syringe incompatibility: Doxapram

Y-site compatibilities: Amrinone, cefmetazole, ciprofloxacin, cisatracurium, diltiazem, famotidine, meperidine, meropenem, midazolam, milrinone, morphine, potassium chloride, propofol, remifentanil, tacrolimus, vit B/C

Y-site incompatibilities: Fluconazole, foscarnet

Additive compatibilities: Bretylium, cimetidine, floxacillin, furosemide, lidocaine, ranitidine, verapamil

Additive incompatibility: DOBUTamine

Patient/family education

- Caution patient to avoid OTC medications including cough, cold, allergy preparations, antacids, since many adverse drug interactions may occur; do not take antacid at same time
- Instruct patient to notify prescriber of any loss of appetite, lower stomach pain, diarrhea, weakness, drowsiness, headache, blurred or yellow-green vision, rash, depression; teach toxic symptoms of this drug and when to notify prescriber
- Advise patient to maintain a sodium-restricted diet as ordered; to take potassium supplements as ordered to prevent toxicity
- Instruct patient to report shortness of breath, difficulty breathing, weight gain, edema, persistent cough
- Teach patient purpose of drug is to regulate the heart's functioning
- Teach patient as outpatient to check and record pulse for 1 min before taking dose; if there is a change of >15 bpm from usual pulse, prescriber should be notified
- Teach patient to take medication at the same time each day, take missed doses within 12 hr; do not double doses; notify prescriber if doses are missed for 2 days or more; how to monitor heart rate
- Advise patient to carry/wear emergency ID describing dosage and reason for digoxin

Evaluation

Positive therapeutic outcome

- Decreased weight, edema, pulse, respiration, crackles
- Increased urine output
- Serum digoxin level 0.5-2 ng/ml

Treatment of overdose: Discontinue drug, administer potassium, monitor ECG, administer an adrenergic blocking agent, digoxin immune Fab

digoxin immune Fab (ovine) (Rx)

(di-jox'in)

Digibind, DigiFab

Func. class.: Antidote, digoxin specific

Pregnancy category C

Action: Antibody fragments bind to free digoxin or to reverse toxicity by not allowing digoxin or digitoxin to bind to sites of action

Therapeutic Outcome: Correction of digoxin toxicity

Uses: Reversal of life-threatening digoxin or digitoxin toxicity, including severe bradycardia, ventricular tachycardia/fibrillation, severe hypertension

Dosage and routes

1 (38 mg) vial binds 0.5 mg digoxin

Digoxin toxicity (known amount) (tabs, oral sol, IM)

Adult/child: **IV** dose (mg) = dose ingested (mg) × 0.8/1000 × 38; if ingested amount is unknown, give 760 mg **IV**

Toxicity (known amount) (cap, IV)

Adult/child: **IV** dose = dose ingested (mg)/0.5 × 38

Toxicity (known amount) by serum digoxin concentrations (SDCs)

Adult/child: **IV** SDC (nanograms/ml) × kg of weight/100 × 38

Digoxin toxicity (unknown amount)

Adult/child >20 kg: **IV** 228 mg (6 vials)

Infant/child <20 kg: **IV** 38 mg (1 vial)

Skin test

Adult: ID 9.5 mcg

Available forms: Inj 38 mg/vial (binds 0.5 mg of digoxin), 40 mg/vial (binds 0.5 mg digoxin)

Adverse effects

CV: **CHF,** *ventricular rate increase,* **atrial fibrillation,** *low cardiac output*

INTEG: *Hypersensitivity,* allergic reactions, facial swelling, redness

META: *Hypokalemia*

MISC: **Anaphylaxis** (rare)

RESP: **Impaired respiratory function, rapid respiratory rate**

Contraindications: Mild digoxin toxicity, hypersensitivity to this product or papain

Precautions: Pregnancy **C,** children, lactation, cardiac disease, renal disease, allergy to ovine proteins, elderly

Pharmacokinetics	
Absorption	Complete
Distribution	Widely distributed into plasma, interstitial fluids
Metabolism	Unknown
Excretion	Kidneys
Half-life	Biphasic (14-20 hr); increased in renal disease

Pharmacodynamics

Onset	30 min (variable)
Peak	Unknown
Duration	Unknown

Interactions
Individual drugs
Considered incompatible with all drugs in syringe or sol
Drug/lab test
Interference: immunoassay (digoxin)

NURSING CONSIDERATIONS
Assessment
- Assess for hypokalemia: ST depression, flat T waves, presence of U wave, ventricular dysrhythmias
- Obtain information on previous allergies: previous exposure to sheep (ovine) proteins; scratch test may be performed before use of this product; hypersensitive reactions are more common in persons with previous exposure
- Monitor VS before, during, and after infusion
- Monitor heart rate, B/P q10 min during inf and after completion until stabilized; hemodynamic monitoring is used for unstable or hypotensive patients; check potassium levels until toxicity is resolved
- Assess for oxygen or perfusion deficit: hypotension, chest pain, dizziness, loss of consciousness
- Assess respiratory status: auscultate lung fields for bibasilar crackles in patients with advanced CHF

Nursing diagnoses
- Injury, risk for (uses)
- Knowledge, deficient (teaching)

Implementation
- Test doses have proven to be ineffective in the general population; only use test dose in those with known allergies or those previously treated with digoxin immune FAB
- For test dose dilute 0.1 ml or reconstituted drug (9.5 mg/ml) in 9.9 ml sterile isotonic saline, inj 0.1 ml (1:100 dilution) ID and observe for wheal with erythema; read in 20 min
- For scratch test place 1 gtt of sol on skin and make a scratch through the drop with a sterile needle; read in 20 min
- Give after diluting 40 mg/4 ml of sterile water (10 mg/ml), mix gently; may be further diluted with 0.9% NaCl; sol should be clear, colorless
- Give by bol if cardiac arrest is imminent or **IV** over 30 min using a 0.22-µm filter
- Store reconstituted sol for up to 4 hr in refrigerator; do not freeze DigiFab

Patient/family education
- Teach that purpose of medication is to bind excess digoxin and reduce high blood levels
- Instruct patients to report fever, chills, itching, sweating, dyspnea, delayed hypersensitivity
- Advise other prescribers that this medication has been used previously

Evaluation
Positive therapeutic outcome
- Correction of digoxin toxicity
- Digoxin blood level 0.5-2 ng/ml
- Digitoxin blood level 9-25 ng/ml

dihydroergotamine
See ergotamine

dihydrotachysterol (Rx)
(dye-hye-droh-tak-iss'ter-ole)

DHT Intensol ✤, Hytakerol

Func. class.: Parathyroid agent (calcium regulator)

Chem. class.: Vitamin D analog

Pregnancy category C

Action: Increases intestinal absorption of calcium, increases renal tubular absorption of phosphorus; is able to regulate calcium levels by regulation of calcitonin, parathyroid hormone

Therapeutic Outcome: Prevention of continued calcium loss in bones

Uses: Renal osteodystrophy, hypoparathyroidism, pseudohypoparathyroidism, familial hypophosphatemia, postoperative tetany

Investigational uses: Renal osteodystrophy

Dosage and routes
Hypophosphatemia
Adult and child: PO 0.5-2 mg daily, maintenance 0.2-1.5 mg daily

Hypoparathyroidism/pseudohypoparathyroidism
Adult: PO 0.8-2.4 mg daily × 4 days, maintenance 0.2-2 mg daily regulated by serum calcium levels

Neonates: PO 0.05-0.1 mg/day

Infants-young child: PO 0.1-0.5 mg/day

Older child: PO 0.5-1 mg/day

Renal osteodystrophy
Adult: PO 0.25-0.375 mg/day
Child: PO 0.125-0.5 mg/day

Rickets (vit D resistant)
Child: PO 0.25-1 mg/day

Available forms: Tabs 0.125, 0.2, 0.4 mg; caps 0.125 mg; oral sol 0.2, 0.25 mg/5 ml, 0.2 mg/ml ✦ (Intensol)

Adverse effects

CNS: Drowsiness, headache, vertigo, fever, lethargy, depression
CV: **Dysrhythmias,** hypertension
EENT: Tinnitus
GI: Nausea, diarrhea, vomiting, jaundice, anorexia, dry mouth, constipation, cramps, metallic taste, thirst
GU: **Polyuria,** hypercalciuria, hyperphosphatemia, **hematuria,** nocturia, renal calculi
MS: Myalgia, arthralgia, decreased bone development, weakness, ataxia

Contraindications: Hypersensitivity, renal disease, hyperphosphatemia, hypercalcemia

Precautions: Pregnancy **C,** renal calculi, lactation, CV disease

Pharmacokinetics

Absorption	Well absorbed from small intestine
Distribution	Liver, fat
Metabolism	Liver
Excretion	Feces (inactive, active metabolites)
Half-life	Unknown

Pharmacodynamics

Onset	2 wk
Peak	2 wk
Duration	2 wk

Interactions

Individual drugs

Cholestyramine, colestipol, mineral oil: decreased absorption of dihydrotachysterol
Phenytoin: decreased effect of dihydrotachysterol
Verapamil: increased dysrhythmias

Drug classifications

Barbiturates, corticosteroids: decreased effect of dihydrotachysterol
Calcium supplements, diuretics (thiazide): increased hypercalcemia
Cardiac glycosides: increased dysrhythmias

Drug/lab test

False increase: cholesterol

NURSING CONSIDERATIONS

Assessment

- Monitor BUN, urinary calcium, AST, ALT, cholesterol, alkaline phosphatase, creatinine, uric acid, chloride, magnesium, electrolytes, urine pH, phosphate; may increase calcium; should be kept at 9-10 mg/dl; keep vit D at 50-135 international units/dl, phosphate at 70 mg/dl; these tests should be checked before and throughout treatment
- Monitor for increased blood level, since toxic reaction may occur rapidly
- Monitor for dry mouth, metallic taste, polyuria, bone pain, muscle weakness, headache, fatigue, tinnitus, change in LOC, irregular pulse, dysrhythmias, increased respirations, anorexia, nausea, vomiting, cramps, diarrhea, constipation; may indicate hypercalcemia; if these occur, discontinue drug, give laxatives, low-calcium diet
- Monitor renal status: decreased urinary output (oliguria, anuria), edema in extremities, weight gain >5 lb, periorbital edema
- Assess nutritional status; check diet for sources of vit D (milk, some seafood), calcium (dairy products, dark green vegetables); phosphates (dairy products) must be avoided

Nursing diagnoses

- Nutrition: Less than body requirements, imbalanced (uses)
- Knowledge, deficient (teaching)

Implementation

- Do not break, crush, or chew caps
- May be increased q4 wk depending on blood level; give with meals for GI symptoms
- Store in tight, light-resistant containers at room temp
- Restrict sodium, potassium if required
- Restriction of fluids may be required for chronic renal failure

Patient/family education

- Teach symptoms of hypercalcemia and when to report symptoms to prescriber
- Teach patient about foods rich in calcium, vit D; provide list of calcium-rich foods; renal failure patients are given a renal diet
- Caution patient not to double doses, take exactly as prescribed

Evaluation

Positive therapeutic outcome

- Prevention of bone deficiencies
- Calcium, phosphorus at normal levels

D

! HIGH ALERT

diltiazem (Rx)

(dil-tye'a-zem)

Apo-Diltiaz ♣, Cardizem, Cardizem LA, Cardizem SR, Cardizem CD, diltiazem, Diltia XR, Dilacor-XR, Tiazac

Func. class.: Calcium channel blocker, antianginal

Chem. class.: Benzothiazepine

Pregnancy category C

Do Not Confuse:
Cardizem/Cardene, Cardizem CD/Cardizem SR, Cardizem SR/Cardene SR

Action: Inhibits calcium ion influx across cell membrane during cardiac depolarization, produces relaxation of coronary vascular smooth muscle, dilates coronary arteries, slows SA/AV node conduction times, dilates peripheral arteries

Therapeutic Outcome: Decreased angina pectoris, dysrhythmias, B/P

Uses
Oral: Angina pectoris due to coronary insufficiency, hypertension, coronary artery spasm
Parenteral: Atrial fibrillation, flutter

Investigational use: Raynaud's syndrome

Dosage and routes
Hypertension
Adult: PO 60-120 mg bid (sus rel) (Cardizem SR), max 540 mg/day, or 180-240 mg (ext rel) daily

Prinzmetal's or variant angina, chronic stable angina
Adult: PO 30 mg qid, increasing dose gradually to 180-360 mg/day in divided doses or 60-120 mg bid; may increase to 240-360 mg/day or 120 or 180 mg ext rel (LA, CD, XT, XR products) PO daily

Atrial fibrillation, flutter, paroxysmal supraventricular tachycardia
Adult: **IV** 0.25 mg/kg as bol over 2 min initially, then 0.35 mg/kg may be given after 15 min; if no response, may give cont inf 5-15 mg/hr for up to 24 hr

Available forms: Tabs 30, 60, 90, 120 mg; ext rel tab 120, 180, 240, 300, 360, 420 mg; ext rel caps 60, 90, 120, 180, 240, 300, 360, 420 mg; sus rel caps 60, 90, 120 mg; inj **IV** 5 mg/ml (5, 10 ml); inj 25 mg; inj for **IV** only 100 mg

Adverse effects
CNS: *Headache, fatigue, drowsiness,* dizziness, depression, weakness, insomnia, tremor, paresthesia
CV: **Dysrhythmia,** *edema,* **CHF,** bradycardia, hypotension, palpitations, **heart block**
GI: *Nausea,* vomiting, diarrhea, gastric upset, *constipation,* increased liver function studies
GU: Nocturia, polyuria, **acute renal failure**
INTEG: *Rash,* pruritus, flushing, photosensitivity, burning
RESP: Rhinitis, dyspnea, pharyngitis

Contraindications: Sick sinus syndrome, 2nd- or 3rd-degree heart block, hypotension less than 90 mm Hg systolic, acute MI, pulmonary congestion, intracranial surgery, bleeding aneurysms, severe hypotension (systolic <90 mm Hg or diastolic <60 mg Hg)

Precautions: Pregnancy **C,** CHF, hypotension, hepatic injury, lactation, children, renal disease

Pharmacokinetics

Absorption	Well absorbed
Distribution	Not known
Metabolism	Liver, extensively
Excretion	Metabolites (96%)
Half-life	3½-9 hr

Pharmacodynamics

	PO	PO-SUS REL	IV
Onset	½ hr	Unknown	Unknown
Peak	2-3 hr	Unknown	Unknown
Duration	6-8 hr	12 hr	Unknown

Interactions
Individual drugs
Carbamazepine, lithium, lovastatin: increased effects of each specific drug
Cimetidine: increased effects of diltiazem
CycloSPORINE: increased cycloSPORINE effect
Digoxin: increased digoxin effect
Theophylline: increased effect, toxicity
Drug classifications
Anesthetics: increased effects of anesthetics
Antihypertensives: increased hypotension
β-Adrenergic blockers: increased bradycardia, CHF, increased β-blocker effect
Benzodiazepines: increased effect of benzodiazepines
HMG-CoA reductase inhibitors: increased effects
Drug/herb
Barberry, betel palm, burdock, goldenseal, khat, khella, lily of the valley, plantain: increased diltiazem effect
Yohimbe: decreased diltiazem effect

Drug/food
Grapefruit juice: increased hypotension

NURSING CONSIDERATIONS
Assessment
- Assess fluid volume status: I&O ratio and record, weight, distended red veins, crackles in lung, color, quality, and sp gr of urine, skin turgor, adequacy of pulses, moist mucous membranes, bilateral lung sounds, peripheral pitting edema; dehydration symptoms of decreasing output, thirst, hypotension, dry mouth and mucous membranes should be reported
- Monitor B/P and pulse, respiration, ECG and intervals (PR, QRS, QT); PCWP, CVP often during infusion; if B/P drops 30 mm Hg, stop inf and call prescriber
- Monitor ALT, AST, bilirubin daily; if these are elevated, hepatotoxicity is suspected
- If platelets are $<150,000/mm^3$, drug is usually discontinued and another drug started
- Assess for extravasation: change site q48h

Nursing diagnoses
- Cardiac output, decreased (uses)
- Knowledge, deficient (teaching)

Implementation
PO route
- Do not break, crush, or chew sus rel caps
- Give with meals for GI symptoms; may be crushed and mixed with food/fluids for swallowing difficulty
- Store in airtight container at room temp

IV route
- Give direct **IV** undiluted over 2 min
- For continuous inf dilute 125 mg/100 ml (1.25 mg/ml) or 250 mg/250 ml (1 mg/ml) or 250 mg/500 ml (0.5 mg/ml) of D_5W, 0.9% NaCl, D_5/0.45% NaCl; give 10 mg/hr; may increase by 5 mg/hr to 15 mg/hr; may continue inf up to 24 hr

Y-site compatibilities: Albumin, amikacin, amphotericin B, aztreonam, bretylium, bumetanide, cefazolin, cefotaxime, cefotetan, cefoxitin, ceftazidime, ceftriaxone, cefuroxime, cimetidine, ciprofloxacin, clindamycin, digoxin, DOBUTamine, DOPamine, doxycycline, epINEPHrine, erythromycin, esmolol, fentanyl, fluconazole, gentamicin, hetastarch, hydromorphone, imipenem-cilastatin, labetalol, lidocaine, lorazepam, meperidine, metoclopramide, metronidazole, midazolam, milrinone, morphine, multivitamins, niCARdipine, nitroglycerin, norepinephrine, oxacillin, penicillin G potassium, pentamidine, piperacillin, potassium chloride, potassium phosphates, ranitidine, sodium nitroprusside, theophylline, ticarcillin, ticarcillin/clavulanate, tobramycin, trimethoprim-sulfamethoxazole, vancomycin, vecuronium

Patient/family education
- Caution patient to avoid hazardous activities until stabilized on drug and dizziness is no longer a problem
- Instruct patient to limit caffeine consumption; to avoid alcohol and OTC drugs unless directed by prescriber
- Tell patient to comply in all areas of medical regimen; diet, exercise, stress reduction, drug therapy; to notify prescriber of irregular heart beat, shortness of breath, swelling of feet and hands, pronounced dizziness, constipation, nausea, hypotension
- Teach patient to use as directed even if feeling better; may be taken with other cardiovascular drugs (nitrates, β-blockers)

Evaluation
Positive therapeutic outcome
- Decreased anginal pain
- Decreased B/P
- Absence of dysrhythmias

Treatment of overdose: Atropine for AV block, vasopressor for hypotension

dimenhyDRINATE (OTC, Rx)
(dye-men-hye'dri-nate)

Apo-Dimenhydrinate ♣, Calm-X, Children's Dramamine, dimenhyDRINATE, Dimentabs, Dinate, Dramamine, Dramanate, Dymenate, Gravol ♣, Gravol L/A ♣, Hydrate, Nauseatol ♣, Novo-Dimenate ♣, PMS-Dimenhydrinate ♣, Travamine ♣, Triptone Caplets

Func. class.: Antiemetic, antihistamine, anticholinergic

Chem. class.: H_1-receptor antagonist, ethanolamine derivative

Pregnancy category B

Do Not Confuse:
dimenhyDRINATE/diphenhydrAMINE

Action: Vestibular stimulator is decreased; anticholinergic, antiemetic, antihistamine response

Therapeutic Outcome: Absence of motion sickness

Uses: Motion sickness, nausea, vomiting

Dosage and routes
Adult: PO 50-100 mg q4h; IM/**IV** 50 mg q4h as needed

Child 6-12 yr: PO 25-50 mg q6-8hr prn, max 150 mg/day
Child 2-5 yr: PO 12.5-25 mg q6-8hr, max 75 mg/day

Available forms: Tab 50 mg; inj 50 mg/ml; elix 15 mg/5 ml ✦, chew tab 50 mg

Adverse effects
CNS: *Drowsiness,* restlessness, headache, dizziness, insomnia, confusion, nervousness, tingling, vertigo
CV: Hypertension, *hypotension,* palpitations
EENT: Dry mouth, blurred vision, diplopia, nasal congestion, photosensitivity
GI: Nausea, anorexia, vomiting, *constipation*
INTEG: Rash, urticaria, fever, chills, flushing
MISC: **Anaphylaxis**

Contraindications: Hypersensitivity to opioids, shock

Precautions: Pregnancy **B**, children, cardiac dysrhythmias, elderly, asthma, prostatic hypertrophy, bladder neck obstruction, narrow-angle glaucoma, stenosing peptic ulcer, pyloroduodenal obstruction

Pharmacokinetics

Absorption	Well absorbed (PO, IM)
Distribution	Unknown; crosses placenta
Metabolism	Liver
Excretion	Kidneys, breast milk
Half-life	Unknown

Pharmacodynamics

	PO	IM	IV
Onset	15-60 min	30 min	Immediate
Peak	1-2 hr	1-2 hr	Unknown
Duration	4-6 hr	4-6 hr	4-6 hr

Interactions
Individual drugs
Alcohol: increased CNS depression
Drug classifications
CNS depressants, opiates, sedative/hypnotics: increased CNS depression
Drug/herb
Corkwood, henbane leaf: increased anticholinergic effect
Hops, Jamaican dogwood, khat, senega: increased effect
Drug/lab test
False negative: skin allergy tests (discontinue antihistamines 3 days before testing)

NURSING CONSIDERATIONS

Assessment
- Assess for signs of toxicity to other drugs or masking of symptoms of disease (brain tumor, intestinal obstruction); monitor GI symptoms including nausea, vomiting, abdominal pain, increased bowel sounds
- Monitor VS, B/P; check patients with cardiac disease more often
- Monitor I&O; check for dehydration (poor skin turgor, increased sp gr, tachycardia, severe thirst) especially in the elderly

Nursing diagnoses
- Injury, risk for (side effects)
- Knowledge, deficient (teaching)

Implementation
PO route
- Tabs may be swallowed whole, chewed, or allowed to dissolve; give 1-2 hr before activity that may cause motion sickness; use measuring device for liq for correct dosing

IM route
- Give IM inj in large muscle mass; aspirate to avoid **IV** administration; massage

IV route
- Give **IV** directly after diluting 50 mg/10 ml or NaCl inj; give 50 mg or less over 2 min

Syringe compatibilities: Atropine, diphenhydrAMINE, droperidol, fentanyl, heparin, hydromorphone, meperidine, metoclopramide, morphine, pentazocine, perphenazine, ranitidine, scopolamine
Syringe incompatibilities: Butorphanol, chlorproMAZINE, glycopyrrolate, hydrOXYzine, midazolam, pentobarbital, prochlorperazine, promazine, promethazine, thiopental
Y-site compatibilities: Acyclovir
Y-site incompatibilities: Aminophylline, heparin, hydrocortisone sodium succinate, hydrOXYzine, phenobarbital, phenytoin, prednisoLONE, prochlorperazine, promazine, promethazine
Additive compatibilities: Amikacin, calcium gluconate, chloramphenicol, corticotropin, erythromycin, heparin, hydrOXYzine, methicillin, norepinephrine, penicillin G potassium, pentobarbital, phenobarbital, potassium chloride, prochlorperazine, vancomycin, vit B/C
Additive incompatibilities: Tetracycline, thiopental

Patient/family education
- Teach all aspects of drug uses; to notify prescriber if confusion, sedation, hypotension occur; to avoid driving and other hazardous activity if drowsiness occurs; to avoid alcohol and other CNS depressants that may potentiate effect

- Tell patient not to exceed recommended dosage
- Inform patient hard candy, gum, frequent rinsing of mouth may be used for dryness
- Advise patient that a false negative result may occur with skin testing; these procedures should not be scheduled until 4 days after discontinuing use
- Caution patient to avoid hazardous activities, activities requiring alertness; dizziness may occur; instruct patient to request assistance with ambulation

Evaluation

Positive therapeutic outcome

- Absence of motion sickness
- Absence of nausea, vomiting

dinoprostone (Rx)

(dye-noe-prost'one)

Cervidil Vaginal Insert, Prepidil, Endocervical Gel, Prostin E Vaginal Suppository

Func. class.: Oxytocic, abortifacient

Chem. class.: Prostaglandin E_2

Pregnancy category C

Do Not Confuse:

Prepidil/bepridil

Action: Stimulates uterine contractions similar to labor by myometrium stimulation, causing abortion; acts within 30 hr for complete abortion; GI smooth muscle stimulation, effacement, dilatation of the cervix

Therapeutic Outcome: Beginning of labor, fetal expulsion

Uses: Abortion during 2nd trimester, benign hydatidiform mole, expulsion of uterine contents in fetal deaths to 28 wk, missed abortion, cervical effacement and dilatation in term pregnancy when they have not occurred spontaneously

Dosage and routes

Abortifacient

Adult: VAG SUPP 20 mg; repeat q3-5h until abortion occurs; max dose is 240 mg

Cervical ripening

Adult: GEL; warm to room temperature; choose correct length shielded catheter (10 or 20 mm), fill catheter by pushing plunger; have patient recumbent for 15-30 min; insert one 10 mg insert

Available forms: Vag supp 20 mg; gel 0.5 mg/3 g (prefilled syringe); gel 0.5 mg; 10 mg insert

Adverse effects

CNS: *Headache,* dizziness, chills, fever
CV: Hypotension, **dysrhythmias**
EENT: Blurred vision
GI: *Nausea, vomiting, diarrhea*
GU: Vaginitis, vaginal pain, vulvitis, vaginismus
INTEG: Rash, skin color changes
MS: *Leg cramps, joint swelling,* weakness
Insert: Uterine hyperstimulation, fever, nausea, vomiting, diarrhea, abdominal pain
Gel: Uterine contractile abnormality, GI side effects, back pain, fever
Fetal: Bradycardia (i.e., deceleration)
Suppository: Uterine rupture, anaphylaxis

Contraindications: Hypersensitivity, uterine fibrosis, cervical stenosis, pelvic surgery, PID, respiratory disease

Precautions: Pregnancy **C**, hepatic, renal, cardiac disease, asthma, anemia, jaundice, diabetes mellitus, seizure disorders, hypertension, hypotension

Pharmacokinetics

Absorption	Rapidly absorbed
Distribution	Unknown
Metabolism	Enzymes
Excretion	Kidneys
Half-life	Unknown

Pharmacodynamics

	GEL	SUPP
Onset	Rapid	10 min
Peak	30-45 min	Unknown
Duration	Unknown	2-3 hr

Interactions

Individual drugs

Alcohol: decreased oxytoxic effect
Oxytocin: increased effect

NURSING CONSIDERATIONS

Assessment

- Assess dilatation and effacement of the cervix, uterine contractions, fetal heart tones; watch for contractions lasting over 1 min, hypertonus, fetal distress; drug should be slowed or discontinued
- Assess for fever that occurs approximately 30 min after supp insertion (abortion)
- Monitor for nausea, vomiting, diarrhea; these may require medication
- Assess for hypersensitivity reaction: dyspnea, rash, chest discomfort
- Assess respiratory rate, rhythm, depth; notify prescriber of abnormalities, in pulse, B/P

D

- Check vaginal discharge; itching, irritation indicates vaginal infection

Nursing diagnoses

- Injury, risk for (side effects)
- Knowledge, deficient (teaching)

Implementation

Suppository route

- Warm supp by running warm water over package; insert high in vagina, wear gloves to prevent absorption; have patient recumbent for at least 10 min

Gel route

- Do not allow to come in contact with skin; use soap and water to wash after use
- Gel should be at room temp
- Place patient in dorsal or lithotomy position to insert gel into cervical canal; remove catheter; discard all items after use; keep supine 15-30 min

Patient/family education

- Teach patient all aspects of treatment including purpose of medication and expected results
- Tell patient that gel may produce warmth in her vagina
- Caution patient that if contractions are longer than 1 min to notify nurse or prescriber
- Advise patient to notify prescriber of cramping, pain, increased bleeding, chills, increased temp, or foul-smelling discharge; these symptoms may indicate uterine infection
- Advise patient to remain supine 10-15 min after insertion of suppository; 2 hr after insert, 15-30 min after gel

Evaluation

Positive therapeutic outcome

- Progression of labor
- Abortion

diphenhydrAMINE ⊶

(OTC, Rx)

(dye-fen-hye′dra-meen)

Allerdryl ✤, AllerMax, Allermed, Banophen, Benadryl, Benadryl 25, Benadryl Kapseals, Benahist 10, Benahist 50, Ben-Allergin-50, Benoject-10, Benoject-50, Benylin Cough, Bydramine, Compoz, Diphenadryl, Diphen Cough, Diphenhist, diphenhydrAMINE HCl, Dormin, Genahist, Hydramine, Hydramyn, Hydril, Hyrexin-50, Insomnal ✤, Nidryl, Nighttime Sleep Aid, Nordryl, Nordryl Cough, Nytol, Phendry, Siladril, Sleep-Eze 3, Sominex 2, Tusstat, Twilite, Uni-Bent Cough, Wehdryl

Func. class.: Antihistamine (1st generation, nonselective), antitussive

Chem. class.: Ethanolamine derivative, H_1-receptor antagonist

Pregnancy category B

Do Not Confuse:

diphenhydrAMINE/dicyclomine

diphenhydrAMINE/dimenhyDRINATE

Action: Acts on blood vessels, GI, respiratory system by competing with histamine for H_1-receptor site; decreases allergic response by blocking histamine; causes increased heart rate, vasodilatation, secretions

Therapeutic Outcome: Absence of allergy symptoms and rhinitis, decreased dystonic symptoms, absence of motion sickness, absence of cough, ability to sleep

Uses: Allergy symptoms, rhinitis, motion sickness, antiparkinsonism, nighttime sedation, infant colic, nonproductive cough, anaphylaxis, nasal allergies, allergic dermatoses, dystonic reactions

Dosage and routes

Adult and child >12 yr: PO 25-50 mg q4-6h, not to exceed 400 mg/day; IM/**IV** 10-50 mg, not to exceed 400 mg/day

Child <12 yr: PO/IM/**IV** 5 mg/kg/day in 4 divided doses, not to exceed 300 mg/day

Nighttime sleep aid

Adult and child ≥12 yr: PO 25-50 mg at bedtime

Antitussive (syrup only)

Adult and child ≥12 yr: 25 mg q4h, max 100 mg/24 hr

Child 6-12 yr: 12.5 mg q4h, max 75 mg/24 hr

Child 2-6 yr: 6.25 mg q4h, max 37.5 mg/24 hr

Renal dose

Adult: PO CCr >50 ml/min give dose q6h; CCr 10-50 ml/min dose q6-12h; CCr <10 ml/min dose q12-18h

Available forms: Caps 25, 50 mg; tabs 25, 50 mg; chew tabs 12.5 mg; elix 12.5 mg/5 ml; syr 12.5 mg/5 ml; inj 10, 50 mg/ml; orally disintegrating tabs 12.5 mg

Adverse effects

CNS: *Dizziness, drowsiness,* poor coordination, fatigue, anxiety, euphoria, confusion, paresthesia, neuritis, **seizures**

EENT: Blurred vision, dilated pupils, tinnitus, nasal stuffiness, dry nose, throat, mouth

GI: Nausea, anorexia, diarrhea

GU: *Retention,* dysuria, frequency

HEMA: **Thrombocytopenia, agranulocytosis, hemolytic anemia**

INTEG: Photosensitivity

MISC: **Anaphylaxis**

RESP: Increased thick secretions, wheezing, chest tightness

Contraindications: Hypersensitivity to H_1-receptor antagonist, acute asthma attack, lower respiratory tract disease

Precautions: Pregnancy **B,** increased intraocular pressure, renal disease, cardiac disease, hypertension, bronchial asthma, seizure disorder, stenosed peptic ulcers, hyperthyroidism, prostatic hypertrophy, bladder neck obstruction, lactation

Pharmacokinetics

Absorption	Well absorbed (PO, IM); completely absorbed (**IV**)
Distribution	Widely distributed; crosses placenta
Metabolism	Liver (95%)
Excretion	Kidneys, breast milk
Half-life	2½-7 hr

Pharmacodynamics

	PO	IM	IV
Onset	15-60 min	30 min	Immediate
Peak	1-4 hr	1-4 hr	Unknown
Duration	4-8 hr	4-8 hr	4-8 hr

Interactions

Individual drugs

Alcohol: increased CNS depression

Drug classifications

Antidepressants (tricyclic), barbiturates, CNS depressants, opiates, sedative/hypnotics: increased CNS depression

MAOIs: increased effect of diphenhydrAMINE

Drug/herb

Corkwood, henbane leaf: increased anticholinergic effect

Hops, Jamaican dogwood, khat, senega: increased effect

Drug/lab test

False negative: skin allergy tests (discontinue antihistamines 3 days before testing)

D

NURSING CONSIDERATIONS

Assessment

- Assess respiratory status: rate, rhythm, increase in bronchial secretions, wheezing, chest tightness; provide fluids to 2 L/day to decrease secretion thickness
- Monitor I&O ratio: be alert for urinary retention, frequency, dysuria, especially elderly; drug should be discontinued if these occur
- Monitor CBC during long-term therapy; blood dyscrasias may occur but are rare
- If giving for dystonic reactions, assess type of involuntary movements and evaluate response to this medication
- Assess cough characteristics including type, frequency, thickness of secretions, and evaluate response to this medication if using for cough

Nursing diagnoses

- Injury, risk for (side effects)
- Sleep patterns, disturbed (uses)
- Knowledge, deficient (teaching)

Implementation

- Give 20 min before bedtime if using for sleep aid

PO route

- Give with meals if GI symptoms occur; absorption rate may be slightly decreased; cap may be opened and drug mixed with food/fluids for patients with swallowing difficulties

IM route

- Give IM inj in large muscle mass; aspirate to avoid **IV** administration; rotate sites

IV route

- Give **IV** undiluted 25 mg/min; may be diluted with 0.9% NaCl, D_5W, $D_{10}W$, 0.45% NaCl, D_5/0.9% NaCl, D_5/0.45% NaCl, D_5/0.25% NaCl, LR, Ringer's, give 25 mg/min or less

Syringe compatibilities: Atropine, butorphanol, chlorproMAZINE, cimetidine, cisatracurium, dimenhyDRINATE, DOXOrubicin liposome, droperidol, fentanyl, fluphenazine, glycopyrrolate, hydromorphone, hydrOXYzine, meperidine, metoclopramide, midazolam, morphine, nalbuphine, pentazocine, perphenazine, prochlorperazine, pro-

mazine, promethazine, ranitidine, remifentanil, scopolamine, sufentanil, thiothixene
Syringe incompatibilities: Pentobarbital, phenytoin, thiopental
Y-site compatibilities: Acyclovir, aldesleukin, amifostine, amsacrine, aztreonam, ciprofloxacin, cisplatin, cladribine, cyclophosphamide, cytarabine, DOXOrubicin, famotidine, filgrastim, fluconazole, fludarabine, gallium, granisetron, heparin, hydrocortisone, idarubicin, melphalan, meperidine, meropenem, methotrexate, ondansetron, paclitaxel, piperacillin/tazobactam, potassium chloride, propofol, sargramostim, sufentanil, tacrolimus, teniposide, thiotepa, vinorelbine, vit B/C
Y-site incompatibilities: Foscarnet
Additive compatibilities: Amikacin, aminophylline, ascorbic acid, bleomycin, cephapirin, erythromycin, hydrocortisone, lidocaine, methicillin, methyldopate, nafcillin, netilmicin, penicillin G potassium, penicillin G sodium, polymyxin B, vit B/C
Additive incompatibilities: Amobarbital, cephalothin, thiopental

Patient/family education

- Tell patient that a false-negative result may occur with skin testing; these procedures should not be scheduled until 3 days after discontinuing use
- Caution patient to avoid hazardous activities and activities requiring alertness, since dizziness may occur; instruct patient to request assistance with ambulation
- Teach patient to use sunscreen to prevent photosensitivity
- Advise patient to avoid alcohol, other depressants; may potentiate effect; CNS depression may occur
- Teach all aspects of drug uses; to notify prescriber if confusion, sedation, hypotension occur; to avoid driving and other hazardous activity if drowsiness occurs; to avoid alcohol or other CNS depressants that may potentiate effect

Evaluation

Positive therapeutic outcome

- Absence of motion sickness
- Absence of nausea, vomiting
- Ability to sleep
- Absence of cough
- Decrease in involuntary movements

Treatment of overdose:

- Administer lavage, diazepam, vasopressors, barbiturates (short acting)

diphenoxylate with atropine (Rx)

(dye-fen-ox'i-late)
Logen, Lomanate, Lomotil, Lonox

difenoxin/atropine

(dye-fen-ox'in/a'troe-peen)
Motofen
Func. class.: Antidiarrheal
Chem. class.: Phenylpiperidine derivative, opiate agonist

Pregnancy category C

Controlled substance schedule V **diphenoxylate/atropine; IV difenoxin/atropine (US)**

Do Not Confuse:

Diphenatol/diphenidol, Lomotil/Lamictal/Lamasil, Lomotil/Lanoxin, Lomotil/Lasix

Action: Inhibits gastric motility by acting on mucosal receptors responsible for peristalsis; related to opioid analgesics as adjunct

Therapeutic Outcome: Decreased loose stools

Uses: Diarrhea (cause undetermined)

Dosage and routes

diphenoxylate/atropine
Adult: 2.5-5 mg qid, titrated to patient response, not to exceed 8 tabs/24 hr
Child 2-12 yr: PO (liq only) 0.3-0.4 mg/kg/day in divided doses

difenoxin/atropine
Adult: initially 2 tabs, then 1 tab after each loose stool or q3-4hr PO max 8 tabs/day

Available forms: diphenoxylate/atropine: tab 2.5 mg diphenoxylate/0.025 mg atropine; liq 2.5 mg diphenoxylate/0.025 mg atropine/5 ml; difenoxin/atropine: tabs 1 mg difenoxin/0.025 atropine

Adverse effects

CNS: *Dizziness, drowsiness, lightheadedness, headache,* fatigue, nervousness, insomnia, confusion
EENT: Blurred vision, burning eyes
GI: *Nausea, vomiting, dry mouth, epigastric distress,* constipation, **paralytic ileus**
MISC: **Anaphylaxis, angioedema**
RESP: **Respiratory depression**

Contraindications: Hypersensitivity, pseudomembranous enterocolitis, jaundice, glaucoma, child <2 yr, severe electrolyte imbalances, diarrhea associated witih organisms that penetrate intestinal mucosa

Precautions: Pregnancy **C**, hepatic, renal disease, ulcerative colitis, lactation, severe liver disease

Pharmacokinetics

Absorption	Well absorbed
Distribution	Unknown
Metabolism	Liver, active metabolite
Excretion	Kidneys
Half-life	2½ hr

Pharmacodynamics

Onset	45-60 min
Peak	2 hr
Duration	3-4 hr

Interactions
Individual drugs
Alcohol: increased action of alcohol
Drug classifications
Anticholinergics: increased anticholinergic effect
Barbiturates: increased action of barbiturates
CNS depressants: increased action of CNS depressants
MAOIs: hypertensive crisis; do not use together
Opiates: increased action of opioids
Sedative/hypnotics: increased CNS depression
Drug/herb
Nutmeg: increased antidiarrheal effect

NURSING CONSIDERATIONS
Assessment
- Monitor electrolytes (potassium, sodium, chloride) if on long-term therapy; fluid status, skin turgor
- Assess bowel pattern before, during treatment; check for rebound constipation after termination of medication; check bowel sounds
- Check response after 48 hr; if no response, drug should be discontinued and other treatment initiated
- Assess for abdominal distention and toxic megacolon, which may occur in ulcerative colitis
- Assess hepatic function if on long-term therapy

Nursing diagnoses
- Diarrhea (uses)
- Constipation (adverse reactions)
- Knowledge, deficient (teaching)
- Noncompliance (teaching)

Implementation
- Give for 48 hr only; tabs may be given with food, crushed and mixed with fluids; liq should be measured accurately

Patient/family education
- Advise patient to avoid alcohol and OTC products unless directed by prescriber; may cause increased CNS depression
- Caution patient not to exceed recommended dosage; that drug may be habit forming
- Advise patient that drug may cause drowsiness; to avoid hazardous activities until response to drug is determined
- Teach patient that dry mouth can be decreased by frequent sips of water, hard candy, sugarless gum

Evaluation
Positive therapeutic outcome
- Decreased diarrhea

dipyridamole (Rx)
(dye-peer-id'a-mole)
Apo-Dipyridamole ✱, dipyridamole, Novo-Dipiradol ✱, Persantine, Persantine IV
Func. class.: Coronary vasodilator, antiplatelet agent
Chem. class.: Nonnitrate
Pregnancy category B

Action: Inhibits adenosine uptake, which produces coronary vasodilatation; increases oxygen saturation in coronary tissues, coronary blood flow; acts on small vessels with little effect on vascular resistance; may increase development of collateral circulation; decreased platelet aggregation by the inhibition of phosphodiesterases (enzymes)

Therapeutic Outcome: Inhibition of platelet aggregation; absence of ischemic attacks, reinfarction

Uses: Prevention of transient ischemic attacks, inhibition of platelet adhesion to prevent myocardial reinfarction, thromboembolism, with warfarin in prosthetic heart valves, prevention of coronary bypass graft occlusion with aspirin; **IV** form used to evaluate coronary artery disease; used as alternative to exercise in thallium myocardial perfusion imaging to evaluate coronary artery disease

Dosage and routes
Transient ischemic attacks
Adult: PO 50 mg tid, 1 hr ac, not to exceed 400 mg daily

Inhibition of platelet adhesion
Adult: PO 50-75 mg qid in combination with aspirin or warfarin

Thallium myocardial perfusion imaging
Adult: **IV** 570 mcg/kg

Available forms: Tabs 25, 50, 75 mg; inj 10 mg/2 ml

Adverse effects

CNS: *Headache, dizziness, weakness, fainting, syncope;* **IV**: transient cerebral ischemia, weakness
CV: *Postural hypotension;* **IV**: **MI**
GI: *Nausea, vomiting,* anorexia, diarrhea
INTEG: *Rash,* flushing
RESP: **IV: Bronchospasm**

Contraindications: Hypersensitivity

Precautions: Pregnancy **B,** hypotension

Pharmacokinetics

Absorption	30%-50% (PO)
Distribution	Widely distributed; crosses placenta
Metabolism	Liver
Excretion	Bile, undergoes enterohepatic recirculation; enters breast milk
Half-life	10 hr

Pharmacodynamics

	PO	IV
Onset	Unknown	Unknown
Peak	1.25 hr	6 min
Duration	6 hr	½ hr
Therapeutic effect	Several mo	

Interactions

Individual drugs
Aspirin, cefamandole, cefotetan, cefoperazone, plicamycin, sulfinpyrazone, valproic acid: increased risk of bleeding
Theophylline: decreased effects of disopyramide (thallium)

Drug classifications
Anticoagulants, NSAIDs, thrombolytics: increased risk of bleeding

Drug/herb
Arginine: increased gastric irritation
Bilberry, saw palmetto: decreased antiplatelet effect
Bogbean, dong quai, feverfew, ginger, ginkgo: increased antiplatelet effect

NURSING CONSIDERATIONS

Assessment

- Monitor B/P, pulse baseline and during treatment until stable; take B/P with patient lying, standing; orthostatic hypotension is common
- Assess cardiac status: chest pain, what aggravates or ameliorates condition
- If using by **IV** route, monitor VS before, during, and after infusion; monitor for chest pain, bronchospasm; use ECG for identifying dysrhythmias; use aminophylline up to 250 mg **IV** for bronchospasm and chest pain if chest pain is unrelieved with the 250 mg dose of aminophylline; give SL dose of nitroglycerin

Nursing diagnoses

- Cardiac output, decreased (uses)
- Pain, acute (uses)
- Knowledge, deficient (teaching)

Implementation

PO route
- Give with 8 oz of water; to improve absorption give on an empty stomach; if GI symptoms occur may give with meals
- Tabs may be crushed, mixed with food or fluids for swallowing difficulty or swallowed whole
- Store at room temp

Intermittent IV infusion route
- Give by **IV** after diluting to at least 1:2 ratio using D_5W, 0.45% NaCl, or 0.9% NaCl; 20-50 ml should be given; give over 4 min; do not give undiluted

Patient/family education

- Teach patient that this medication is not a cure; that drug may have to be taken continuously in evenly spaced doses only as directed; if a dose is missed, take one when remembered up to 4 hr; do not double doses
- Advise patient to rise slowly from sitting or lying down to prevent orthostatic hypotension
- Caution patient not to use alcohol or OTC medication unless approved by prescriber
- Caution patient to avoid hazardous activities until stabilized on medication; dizziness may occur

Evaluation

Positive therapeutic outcome
- Absence of reinfarction, ischemic attacks

Treatment of overdose: Administer **IV** phenylephrine

dirithromycin (Rx)

(die-rith-roe-mie'sin)

Dynabac

Func. class.: Antibacterial

Chem. class.: Macrolide

Pregnancy category C

Do Not Confuse:
Dynabac/DynaCirc

Action: Binds to 50S ribosomal subunits of susceptible bacteria; suppresses protein synthesis

Therapeutic Outcome: Bactericidal action against *Moraxella catarrhalis, Streptococcus pneumoniae, Streptococcus pyogenes, Streptococcus viridans, Legionella pneumophila, Mycoplasma pneumoniae, Staphylococcus aureus, Staphylococcus agalactiae, Bordetella pertussis*

Uses: Infections of upper and lower respiratory tract

Dosage and routes

Adult: PO 500 mg daily, given for 7-14 days depending on infections

Available forms: Enteric coated tab 250 mg

Adverse effects

CNS: *Headache, dizziness, insomnia*

GI: *Abdominal pain, nausea, diarrhea, vomiting, dyspepsia,* GI disorders, flatulence, abnormal stools, anorexia, constipation, **pseudomembranous colitis**

HEMA: Increased platelet count, increased eosinophils

INTEG: Pruritus, urticaria

RESP: Cough, dyspnea

Contraindications: Hypersensitivity to this drug or any other macrolide or to erythromycin, bacteremias

Precautions: Pregnancy **C,** lactation, children, hepatic, renal disease

Pharmacokinetics

Absorption	Rapidly absorbed
Distribution	Widely distributed
Metabolism	No hepatic metabolism
Excretion	Bile, feces (up to 97%)
Half-life	Plasma half-life 8 hr, terminal 44 hr

Pharmacodynamics

Unknown

Interactions

Drug classifications

Antacids, H_2 antagonists: slightly enhanced absorption of dirithromycin

Theophylline: may alter effect

Drug/herb

Acidophilus: do not use with antiinfectives

Drug/food

Increased: absorption

NURSING CONSIDERATIONS

Assessment

- Assess I&O ratio; report hematuria, oliguria in renal disease
- Monitor liver function studies: AST, ALT if on long-term therapy
- Monitor renal studies: urinalysis, protein, blood
- Monitor C&S before drug therapy; drug may be given as soon as culture is taken; C&S may be repeated after treatment
- Assess bowel pattern before, during treatment; pseudomembranous colitis may occur
- Assess for skin eruptions, itching
- Assess respiratory status: rate, character, wheezing, tightness in chest; discontinue drug

Nursing diagnoses

- Infection, risk for (uses)
- Diarrhea (side effects)
- Knowledge, deficient (teaching)
- Noncompliance (teaching)

Implementation

- Swallow tabs whole; do not break, crush, chew or cut
- Give adequate intake of fluids (2 L) during diarrhea episodes
- Give with food or within 1 hr of food at same time each day
- Store at room temp in tight container

Patient/family education

- Teach patient to take with full glass of water; give with food
- Instruct patient to report sore throat, fever, fatigue; may indicate superinfection
- Teach patient to notify nurse of diarrhea, dark urine, pale stools, yellow discoloration of eyes or skin, severe abdominal pain
- Instruct patient to take at evenly spaced intervals; complete dosage regimen

Evaluation

Positive therapeutic outcome

- C&S negative for infection

Treatment of hypersensitivity: Withdraw drug, maintain airway, administer epINEPHrine, aminophylline, O_2, **IV** corticosteroids

disopyramide (Rx)
(dye-soe-peer'a-mide)
disopyramide, Norpace, Norpace CR, Rhythmodan

Func. class.: Antidysrhythmic (class IA)
Chem. class.: Nonnitrate

Pregnancy category C

Action: Prolongs action potential duration and effective refractory period; reduces disparity in refractory period between normal and infarcted myocardium; prevents increased myocardial excitability and conduction contractility

Therapeutic Outcome: Suppression of supraventricular dysrhythmias

Uses: PVCs, ventricular tachycardia, supraventricular tachycardia, atrial flutter, fibrillation

Investigational uses: Supraventricular tachycardia (prevention, treatment)

Dosage and routes
Adult: PO 100-200 mg q6h; sus rel cap 200-400 mg q12h
Child 12-18 yr: PO 6-15 mg/kg/day, in divided doses q6h
Child 4-12 yr: PO 10-15 mg/kg/day in divided doses q6h
Child 1-4 yr: PO 10-20 mg/kg/day in divided doses q6h
Child <1 yr: PO 10-30 mg/kg/day, in divided doses q6h

Renal dose
Adult: PO CCr 30-40 ml/min dose q8h; CCr 15-30 ml/min dose q12h; CCr <15 ml/min dose q24h

Available forms: Caps 100, 150 mg; cont rel caps 100, 150 mg; sus rel tabs 250 mg ♣

Adverse effects
CNS: *Headache, dizziness,* psychosis, fatigue, depression, paresthesias, insomnia
CV: *Hypotension, bradycardia,* angina, PVCs, tachycardia, increases in QRS and QT segments, **cardiac arrest,** edema, weight gain, AV block, ***CHF,*** syncope, chest pain
EENT: *Blurred vision, dry nose, throat, eyes,* narrow-angle glaucoma
GI: *Dry mouth, constipation,* nausea, anorexia, flatulence, diarrhea, vomiting
GU: *Retention, hesitancy,* impotence
HEMA: **Thrombocytopenia, agranulocytosis,** anemia (rare), decreased Hgb, Hct
INTEG: Rash, pruritus, urticaria
META: Hypoglycemia, hypokalemia
MS: Weakness, pain in extremities

Contraindications: Hypersensitivity, 2nd- or 3rd-degree heart block, cardiogenic shock, CHF (uncompensated), sick sinus syndrome, QT prolongation

Precautions: Pregnancy **C,** lactation, diabetes mellitus, renal, hepatic disease, children, myasthenia gravis, narrow-angle glaucoma, cardiomyopathy, conduction abnormalities, potassium imbalance

Pharmacokinetics

Absorption	Well absorbed
Distribution	Widely distributed
Metabolism	Liver
Excretion	Kidneys
Half-life	4-10 hr

Pharmacodynamics

	PO	PO–SUS REL
Onset	½-3½ hr	Unknown
Peak	2 hr	Unknown
Duration	1½-8 hr	12 hr

Interactions
Individual drugs
Atenolol, erythromycin, lidocaine, procainamide, propranolol, quinidine: increased effects of disopyramide
Phenobarbital, phenytoin: decreased effects of disopyramide
Rifampin: decreased disopyramide levels

Drug classifications
Anticholinergics: increased side effects, urinary retention

Drug/herb
Aconite: increased toxicity, death
Aloe, broom, buckthorn (chronic use), cascara sagrada (chronic use), Chinese rhubarb, figwort, fumitory, goldenseal, kudzu, licorice, senna: increased effect
Coltsfoot: decreased effect
Horehound: increased serotonin effect

Drug/lab test
Increased: liver enzymes, lipids, BUN, creatinine
Decreased: Hgb/Hct, blood glucose

NURSING CONSIDERATIONS
Assessment
- Assess respiratory status: auscultate lung fields for bibasilar crackles in patients with advanced CHF
- Monitor I&O ratio and electrolytes: potas-

sium, sodium, chloride; watch for decreasing urinary output, possible retention
- Monitor liver function studies: AST, ALT, bilirubin, alkaline phosphatase
- Monitor ECG to determine drug effectiveness, measure PR, QRS, QT intervals; check for PVCs, other dysrhythmias; monitor B/P for hypotension; check for prolonged widening QT intervals, QRS complex; if QT or QRS increase by 50% or more, withhold next dose, notify prescriber
- Monitor for dehydration or hypovolemia
- Monitor for CNS symptoms: psychosis, numbness, depression; if these occur, drug should be discontinued

Nursing diagnoses
- Cardiac output, decreased (uses)
- Knowledge, deficient (teaching)

Implementation
- Do not break, crush, or chew sus rel tabs
- Give 1 hr ac or 2 hr pc
- If changing from regular release to sus rel cap, give sus rel 6 hr after last dose of regular release

Patient/family education
- Teach patient to report side effects immediately to prescriber; to take exactly as prescribed; if dose is missed take when remembered if within 3-4 hr of next dose; do not double doses
- Teach patient to complete follow-up appointment with prescriber including pulmonary function studies, chest x-ray
- Instruct patient that dry mouth may be relieved by frequent sips of water, hard candy, sugarless gum
- Caution patient to make position changes from lying to standing slowly to prevent orthostatic hypotension

Evaluation
Positive therapeutic outcome
- Decreased PVCs, ventricular tachycardia

Treatment of overdose: Administer O_2, artificial ventilation, ECG; administer DOPamine for circulatory depression; administer diazepam or thiopental for seizures, isoproterenol

divalproex sodium
See valproate

DOBUTamine (Rx)
(doe-byoo'ta-meen)
DOBUTamine, Dobutrex
Func. class.: Adrenergic direct-acting β_1-agonist, inotropic agent, cardiac stimulant
Chem. class.: Catecholamine
Pregnancy category B

Do Not Confuse:
DOBUTamine/DOPamine, Dobutrex/Diamox

Action: Causes increased contractility, increased cardiac output without marked increase in heart rate by acting on β_1-receptors in heart; minor α/β_2 effects

Therapeutic Outcome: Cardiac output increased with decreased fatigue and dyspnea

Uses: Cardiac decompensation due to organic heart disease or cardiac surgery

Investigational uses: Cardiogenic shock in children, congenital heart disease in children undergoing cardiac catherization

Dosage and routes
Adult: **IV** inf 2.5-10 mcg/kg/min; may increase to 40 mcg/kg/min if needed
Child: **IV** inf 5-20 mcg/kg/min over 10 min for cardiac cath

Available forms: Inj 12.5 mg/ml

Adverse effects
CNS: *Anxiety,* headache, dizziness
CV: Palpitations, tachycardia, hypertension, PVCs, angina, hypotension
GI: Heartburn, nausea, vomiting
MS: Muscle cramps (leg)

Contraindications: Hypersensitivity, idiopathic hypertrophic subaortic stenosis

Precautions: Pregnancy **B,** lactation, children, hypertension

Pharmacokinetics	
Absorption	Complete
Distribution	Unknown
Metabolism	Liver
Excretion	Kidneys
Half-life	2 min

Pharmacodynamics	
Onset	1-5 min
Peak	10 min
Duration	<10 min

Interactions

Individual drugs

Bretylium, oxytocin: increased dysrhythmias
Guanethidine: increased severe hypertension
Oxytocin: increased pressor effects

Drug classifications

Anesthetics, MAOIs: increased dysrhythmias
Antidepressants (tricyclic): increased pressor response, dysrhythmias
β-Blockers: decreased action of DOBUTamine
MAOIs: increased pressor effect

NURSING CONSIDERATIONS

Assessment

- Assess for hypovolemia; if present, correct before beginning treatment with DOBUTamine; avoid use in patients with atrial fibrillation before digitalization
- Monitor ECG for dysrhythmias, ischemia during treatment; some patients may not need continuous ECG monitoring; also monitor PCWP, CVP, CO_2, urinary output; notify prescriber if <30 ml/hr
- Assess for heart failure: bibasilar crackles, S_3 gallop, dyspnea, neck vein distention in patients with cardiomyopathy or CHF
- Assess for oxygenation or perfusion deficit: decreased B/P, chest pain, dizziness, loss of consciousness
- Monitor B/P and pulse q5 min during inf; if B/P drops 30 mm Hg, stop inf and call prescriber
- Monitor ALT, AST, bilirubin daily
- Monitor for sulfite sensitivity, which may be life threatening

Nursing diagnoses

- Cardiac output, decreased (uses)
- Knowledge, deficient (teaching)

Implementation

IV route

- Reconstitute 250 mg/10 ml of D_5W or sterile water for inj; may add another 10 ml to dissolve completely if needed, then dilute in 50 ml or more of D_5W, 0.9% NaCl, 0.45% NaCl, D_5/0.45% NaCl, D_5/0.9% NaCl, D_5/LR, LR; titrate to patient response; use infusion pump for correct dose
- Use a CVP catheter or large peripheral vein, use infusion pump, titrate to patient response
- Change **IV** site q48h

Syringe compatibilities: Heparin, ranitidine

Syringe incompatibility: Doxapram

Y-site compatibilities: Amifostine, inamrinone, atracurium, aztreonam, bretylium, calcium chloride, calcium gluconate, ciprofloxacin, cladribine, diazepam, diltiazem, DOPamine, enalaprilat, epINEPHrine, famotidine, fentanyl, fluconazole, granisetron, haloperidol, hydromorphone, regular insulin, labetalol, lidocaine, lorazepam, magnesium sulfate, meperidine, milrinone, morphine, niCARdipine, nitroglycerin, norepinephrine, pancuronium, potassium chloride, propofol, ranitidine, sodium nitroprusside, streptokinase, tacrolimus, theophylline, thiotepa, tolazoline, vecuronium, verapamil, zidovudine

Y-site incompatibilities: Acyclovir, alteplase, aminophylline, foscarnet, phytonadione

Additive compatibilities: Amiodarone, atracurium, atropine, DOPamine, enalaprilat, epINEPHrine, flumazenil, hydrALAZINE, isoproterenol, lidocaine, meperidine, meropenem, metaraminol, morphine, nitroglycerin, norepinephrine, phentolamine, phenylephrine, procainamide, propranolol, ranitidine, verapamil

Additive incompatibilities: Acyclovir, aminophylline, bumetanide, calcium gluconate, diazepam, digoxin, furosemide, insulin, magnesium sulfate, phenytoin, potassium phosphate, sodium bicarbonate

Patient/family education

- Teach patient reason for medication and expected results, reason for all monitoring and procedures
- Advise patient to report dyspnea, headache, **IV** site discomfort, chest pain, numbness of extremities

Evaluation

Positive therapeutic outcome

- Increased cardiac output
- Decreased PCWP, adequate CVP
- Decreased dyspnea, fatigue, edema, ECG
- Increased urine output

Treatment of overdose: Discontinue drug, support circulation

docetaxel (Rx)

(doe-se-tax'el)

Taxotere

Func. class.: Antineoplastic—miscellaneous

Pregnancy category D

Do Not Confuse:
Taxotere/Taxol

Action: Inhibits the reorganization of the microtubule network needed for interphase and mitotic cellular functions; also causes abnormal bundles of microtubules during cell cycle and multiple esters of microtubules during mitosis

Therapeutic Outcome: Prevention of rapidly growing malignant cells

Uses: Locally advanced or metastatic breast cancer, non–small-cell lung cancer, androgen independent metastatic prostate cancer, postsurgery operable node-positive breast cancer

Dosage and routes

Locally advanced or metastatic breast cancer after failure of other chemotherapy

Adult: **IV** 60-100 mg/m^2 given over 1 hr q3 wk; if neutrophil count is <500/mm^3 for >1 wk, reduce dose by 25%

Locally advanced or metastatic non–small-cell lung cancer after failure of cisplatin chemotherapy

Adult: **IV** 75 mg/m^2 over 1 hr q3 wk; if neutrophil count is <500/mm^3 for >1 wk, reduce dose to 55 mg/m^2; if patient develops grade 3 peripheral neuropathy, stop drug

Unresectable, locally advanced or metastatic non–small-cell lung cancer previously treated with chemotherapy

Adult: **IV** 75 mg/m^2 over 1 hr, then cisplatin 75 mg/m^2 **IV** given over 30-60 min q3 wk; reduce dose to 65 mg/m^2 in those with hematologic or non-hematologic toxicities

Androgen-independent metastatic prostate cancer

Adult: **IV** 75 mg/m^2 given over 1 hr q3 wk, with 5 mg predniSONE PO bid continuously; give dexamethasone 8 mg PO at 12 hr, 3 hr and 1 hr prior to docetaxel; if neutrophil count is <500 cells/mm^3 for more than 1 wk or other toxicities occur, reduce dose to 60 mg/m^2

Adjuvant postsurgery treatment of operable node-positive breast cancer

Adult: **IV** 75 mg/m^2 over 1 hr, given 1 hr after DOXOrubicin 50 mg/m^2, cyclophosphamide 500 mg/m^2 q3 wk × 6 cycles

Available forms: Inj 20, 80 mg in single dose vials

Adverse effects

CV: *Hypotension,* fluid retention, peripheral edema, flushing

GI: *Nausea, vomiting, diarrhea,* **hepatotoxicity**

HEMA: **Neutropenia, leukopenia, thrombocytopenia, anemia**, bleeding, infections, **myelosuppression**

INTEG: *Alopecia,* nail pain, rash, skin eruptions

MS: *Arthralgia, myalgia,* back pain

NEURO: *Peripheral neuropathy*

RESP: Dyspnea, **pulmonary edema**

❗ ***SYST:*** *Hypersensitivity reactions,* **death**

Contraindications: Pregnancy **D**, hypersensitivity to this drug or other drugs with polysorbate 80, neutropenia (neutrophils <1500/mm^3), severe hepatic disease, bilirubin exceeding upper normal limit, or severely elevated ALT, AST, alkaline phosphatase

Precautions: Children, lactation, CV disease

Pharmacokinetics

Absorption	Completely absorbed
Distribution	Unknown
Metabolism	Liver, extensively
Excretion	Fecal
Half-life	11.1 hr

Pharmacodynamics

Onset	Rapid
Peak	Unknown
Duration	Unknown

Interactions

Individual drugs

CycloSPORINE, erythromycin, ketoconazole, troleadomycin: altered metabolism of docetaxel

Drug classifications

Anineoplastics, radiation: increased myelosuppression

Live virus vaccines: decreased immune response

NURSING CONSIDERATIONS

Assessment

- Assess CNS changes: confusion, paresthesias, dysethenia, pain, weakness: if severe, drug should be discontinued
- Check buccal cavity q8h for dryness, sores or ulceration, white patches, oral pain, bleeding, dysphagia; obtain prescription for viscous lidocaine (Xylocaine) to use in mouth
- Assess symptoms indicating severe allergic reaction, anaphylaxis: rash, pruritus, urticaria, purpuric skin lesions, itching, flushing
- Monitor CBC, differential, platelet count weekly; withhold drug if WBC is <1500/mm^3 or platelet count is <100,000/mm^3, notify prescriber of results
- Monitor renal function studies: BUN, creatinine, serum uric acid, urine CCr before and during therapy; check I&O ratio; report fall in urine output to <30 ml/hr

- Monitor temp q4h (may indicate beginning of infection)
- Monitor liver function tests before and during therapy (bilirubin, AST, ALT, LDH) as needed or monthly; check for jaundice of skin and sclera, dark urine, clay-colored stools, itchy skin, abdominal pain, fever, diarrhea
- Assess for bleeding: hematuria, stool guaiac, bruising or petechiae, mucosa or orifices q8h; check for inflammation of mucosa, breaks in skin
- Assess effects of alopecia on body image; discuss feelings about body changes

Nursing diagnoses
- Injury, risk for (adverse reactions)
- Body image, disturbed (adverse reactions)
- Infection, risk for (adverse reactions)
- Knowledge, deficient (teaching)

Implementation
- Give top or systemic analgesics for pain to lessen effects of stomatitis
- Give liq diet: carbonated beverages; gelatin may be added if patient is not nauseated or vomiting

IV route
- Use gloves and cytotoxic handling precautions
- Allow vials to warm to room temperature, withdrawal all diluent and inject in vial of docetaxel, rotate gently to mix, allow to stand to decrease foaming, then withdraw the required amount (10 mg/ml) and inject in 250 ml of 0.9% NaCl or D_5W, mix gently, give over 1 hr

Y-site compatibilities: Acyclovir, amikacin, aminophylline, ampicillin/sulbactam, butorphanol, calcium gluconate, cefepime, cefotetan, ceftazidime, ceftriaxone, cimetidine, diphenhydrAMINE, droperidol, famotidine, fluconazole, furosemide, ganciclovir, gentamicin, granisetron, haloperidol, heparin, hydrocortisone, hydromorphone, lorazepam, magnesium sulfate, mannitol, meperidine, mesna, metoclopramide, morphine, ondansetron, potassium chloride, prochlorperazine, ranitidine, sodium bicarbonate, vancomycin, zidovudine

Patient/family education
- Inform patient that nonhormonal contraceptive measures are recommended during therapy and >4 mo after; teratogenic effects are possible
- Teach patient to avoid use of products containing aspirin or ibuprofen, razors, commercial mouthwash, since bleeding may occur; to report symptoms of bleeding (hematuria, tarry stools)
- Instruct patient to report signs of anemia (fatigue, headache, irritability, faintness, shortness of breath) and CNS reactions (confusion, psychosis nightmares, seizures, severe headaches)
- Inform patient that hair may be lost during treatment; a wig or hairpiece may make patient feel better; new hair may be different in color and texture
- Inform patient that receiving vaccinations during therapy may cause serious reactions
- Instruct patient to rinse mouth tid-qid with water, club soda; brush teeth bid-qid with soft brush or cotton-tipped applicators for stomatitis; use unwaxed dental floss

Evaluation
Positive therapeutic outcome
- Prevention of rapid division of malignant cells

docusate calcium (OTC)
(dok'yoo-sate)

DC Softgels, Pro-Cal-Sof, Sulfalax Calcium, Surfak

docusate sodium (OTC)
Colace, Correctol Extra Gentle, Dialose DOK, DOS, Diocto, Dioeze, Disonate, Di-Sosul, D-S-S, Ex-Lax, Modane, Regulax SS, Regulax ✦, Silace

Func. class.: Laxative, emollient

Chem. class.: Anionic surfactant

Pregnancy category C

Action: Increases water, fat penetration in intestine; allows for easier passage of stool; increases electrolyte, water secretion in colon

Therapeutic Outcome: Passage of softened stool, absence of constipation

Uses: To soften stools, prevent constipation, soften fecal impaction (rec route)

Dosage and routes
Adult: PO 50-300 mg daily (docusate sodium) or 240 mg (docusate calcium or docusate potassium) prn; enema 5 ml (docusate sodium)

Child >12 yr: Enema 2 ml (docusate sodium)

Child 6-12 yr: PO 40-150 mg daily (docusate sodium) in divided doses

Child 3-6 yr: PO 20-60 mg daily (docusate sodium) in divided doses

Child <3 yr: PO 10-40 mg daily (docusate sodium) in divided doses

Available forms

Docusate calcium: Caps 50, 240 mg
Docusate sodium: Caps 50, 100, 240, 250 mg; tabs 50, 100 mg; syr 16.75 mg/5 ml, 20 mg/5 ml, 50, 60 mg/15 ml; liq 150 mg/15 ml; oral sol 10, 50 mg/ml; enema 283 mg/3.9 g cap

Adverse effects

EENT: Bitter taste, throat irritation
GI: Nausea, anorexia, cramps, diarrhea
INTEG: Rash

Contraindications: Hypersensitivity, obstruction, fecal impaction, nausea/vomiting

Precautions: Pregnancy **C**

Pharmacokinetics

Absorption	Minimal (PO)
Distribution	Unknown
Metabolism	Not metabolized
Excretion	Bile
Half-life	Unknown

Pharmacodynamics

	PO	REC
Onset	24-72 hr	4-6 hr
Peak	Unknown	Unknown
Duration	Unknown	Unknown

Interactions

Individual drugs

Mineral oil: toxicity

Drug/herb

Flax, senna: increased laxative action

NURSING CONSIDERATIONS

Assessment

- Assess cramping, rectal bleeding, nausea, vomiting; if these symptoms occur, drug should be discontinued; identify cause of constipation; identify whether fluids, bulk, or exercise is missing from lifestyle

Nursing diagnoses

- Constipation (uses)
- Diarrhea (side effects)
- Knowledge, deficient (teaching)
- Noncompliance (teaching)

Implementation

PO route

- Dilute oral sol in juice or other fluid to disguise taste
- Give tabs or caps with 8 oz of liq; give on empty stomach for increased absorption, results

Patient/family education

- Discuss with patient that adequate fluid consumption is as necessary as bulk, exercise for adequate bowel function
- Teach patient that normal bowel movements do not always occur daily
- Advise patient not to use in presence of abdominal pain, nausea, vomiting; tell patient to notify prescriber if unrelieved constipation or if symptoms of electrolyte imbalance occur: muscle cramps, pain, weakness, dizziness, excessive thirst
- Advise patient that drug may take up to 3 days to soften stools
- Instruct patient to take oral preparation with a full glass of water and increase fluid intake unless on fluid restrictions
- Caution patients with heart disease to avoid using the Valsalva maneuver to expedite evacuation

Evaluation

Positive therapeutic outcome

- Decreased constipation within 3 days

dofetilide

(doff-ee-till′-lide)
Tikosyn
Func. class.: Antidysrhythmic (Class III)
Pregnancy category C

Action: Blocks cardiac ion channel carrying the rapid component of delayed potassium current, no effect on sodium channels

Therapeutic Outcome: Absence of atrial fibrillation

Uses: Atrial fibrillation, flutter, maintenance of normal sinus rhythm

Dosage and routes

Adult: PO 125-500 mcg bid depending on CCr, may be adjusted q2-3h to get appropriate increase in QTc

Renal dose: PO initial dose for CCr > 60 mg/ml 500 mcg bid; CCr 40-60 mg/min 250 mcg bid; CCr 20-39 mg/min 125 mcg bid; CCr <20 mg/min do not use

Available forms: Caps 125, 250, 500 mcg

Adverse effects

CNS: *Syncope, dizziness,* headache
CV: *Hypotension, postural hypotension, bradycardia,* angina, PVCs, substernal pressure, precipitation of angina transient hypertension
GI: *Nausea, vomiting,* severe diarrhea, anorexia

Contraindications: Hypersensitivity, digitalis toxicity, aortic stenosis, pulmonary hypertension, children, QT syndromes, severe renal disease

Precautions: Pregnancy **C**, renal disease, lactation

Pharmacokinetics

Absorption	>90%
Distribution	Steady state 2-3 days
Metabolism	Not metabolized
Excretion	Kidneys 80%
Half-life	10 hr

Pharmacodynamics

Unknown

Interactions

Individual drugs

Amiloride, cimetidine, ketoconazole, megestrol, metformin, prochlorperazine, triamterene, trimethoprim/sulfamethoxazole, verapamil: do not use together
Diuretics, potassium depletion: increased hypokalemia

NURSING CONSIDERATIONS

Assessment

- Monitor ECG continuously to determine drug effectiveness; measure PR, QRS, QT intervals; check for PVCs, other dysrhythmias; monitor B/P continuously; this drug is available only to facilities that have been educated in its administration; patient must be hospitalized
- Before administration, QTc must be determined using an average of 5-10 beats, if the QTc >440 msec or 500 msec in ventricular conduction abnormalities, do not use; do not use if heart rate <60 bpm
- Before dosing, identify CCr, using CCr to determine dosing

Nursing diagnoses

- Cardiac output, decreased (uses)
- Gas exchange, impaired (adverse reactions)
- Knowledge, deficient (teaching)

Implementation

- Give for 3 days with patient hospitalized
- Give dofetilide after withholding class I or III antidysrhythmic for 3 half-lives of dofetilide before starting dofetilide

Patient/family education

- Notify prescriber if fast heartbeats with fainting or dizziness occur
- Notify all prescribers of all medications and supplements taken
- Teach patient that if a dose is missed, do not double, take next dose at usual time

Evaluation

Positive therapeutic outcome

- Increased control in atrial fibrillation

dolasetron (Rx)

(do-la'se-tron)

Anzemet

Func. class.: Antiemetic

Chem. class.: 5-HT receptor antagonist

Pregnancy category B

Action: Prevents nausea, vomiting by blocking serotonin peripherally, centrally, and in the small intestine

Therapeutic Outcome: Control of nausea, vomiting

Uses: Prevention of nausea, vomiting associated with cancer chemotherapy and prevention of postoperative nausea, vomiting

Investigational uses: Radiotherapy-induced nausea/vomiting

Dosage and routes

Prevention of nausea/vomiting associated with cancer chemotherapy

Adult and child 2-16 yr: **IV** 1.8 mg/kg as a single dose ½ hr before chemotherapy

Adult: PO 100 mg 1 hr before chemotherapy

Child 2-16 yr: PO 1.8 mg/kg 1 hr before chemotherapy, max 100 mg

Prevention of postoperative nausea/vomiting

Adult: **IV** 12.5 mg as a single dose 15 min before cessation of anesthesia; PO 100 mg 2 hr before surgery (prevention only)

Child 2-16 yr: **IV** 0.35 mg/kg as a single dose 15 min before cessation of anesthesia; PO 1.2 mg/kg within 2 hr before surgery (prevention only)

Available forms: Tabs 50, 100 mg; inj 20 mg/ml (12.5 mg/0.625 ml)

Adverse effects

CNS: *Headache,* dizziness, fatigue, drowsiness

CV: **Dysrhythmias,** ECG changes, hypotension, tachycardia, hypertension, bradycardia

GI: *Diarrhea,* constipation, increased AST, ALT, abdominal pain, anorexia

GU: Urinary retention, oliguria
MISC: Rash, **bronchospasm**

Contraindications: Hypersensitivity

Precautions: Pregnancy **B,** lactation, children, elderly, hypokalemia, electrolyte imbalances, granisetron, ondansetron hypersensitivity

Pharmacokinetics

Absorption	Completely absorbed
Distribution	Unknown
Metabolism	Liver, extensively
Excretion	Kidneys
Half-life	Unknown

Pharmacodynamics

Unknown

Interactions

Individual drugs

Cimetidine: increased dolasetron levels
Rifampin: decreased dolasetron levels

Drug classifications

Antidysrhythmics: increased dysrhythmias
Thiazide, loop diuretics: increased QT prolongation

NURSING CONSIDERATIONS

Assessment

- Assess for absence of nausea, vomiting during chemotherapy
- Assess for hypersensitivity reaction: rash, bronchospasm
- Assess for cardiac conditions, electrolyte imbalances or dysrhythmias

Nursing diagnoses

- Knowledge, deficient (teaching)
- Noncompliance (teaching)

Implementation

IV route

- Administer by inj 100 mg/30 sec or less or diluted in 50 ml of compatible sol; give over 15 sec
- Store at room temp for 24 hr after dilution

Patient/family education

- Instruct patient to report diarrhea, constipation, rash, or changes in respirations; may cause headache, use analgesic
- Teach patient reason for medication and expected results

Evaluation

Positive therapeutic outcome

- Absence of nausea, vomiting during cancer chemotherapy

donepezil (Rx)

(don-ep-ee′zill)
Aricept
Func. class.: Reversible cholinesterase inhibitor

Pregnancy category C

D

Action: Elevates acetylcholine concentrations (cerebral cortex) by slowing degradation of acetylcholine released in cholinergic neurons; does not alter underlying dementia

Therapeutic Outcome: Decreased symptoms of Alzheimer's disease

Uses: Treatment of mild to moderate dementia in Alzheimer's disease

Dosage and routes

Adult: PO 5 mg daily at bedtime may increase to 10 mg daily after 4-6 wk

Available forms: Tabs 5, 10 mg

Adverse effects

CNS: Dizziness, insomnia, somnolence, headache, fatigue, abnormal dreams, syncope, **seizures**
CV: **Atrial fibrillation,** hypotension or hypertension
GI: Nausea, vomiting, anorexia, *diarrhea*
GU: Frequency, UTI, incontinence
INTEG: Rash, flushing
MS: Cramps, arthritis
RESP: Rhinitis, URI, cough, pharyngitis

Contraindications: Hypersensitivity to this drug or piperidine derivatives

Precautions: Pregnancy **C,** sick sinus syndrome, history of ulcers, GI bleeding, hepatic disease, bladder obstruction, asthma, lactation, children, seizures, asthma, COPD

Pharmacokinetics

Absorption	Well
Distribution	Unknown
Metabolism	Liver to metabolities
Excretion	Unknown
Half-life	10 hr (single dose)

Pharmacodynamics

Unknown

Interactions

Individual drugs

Carbamazepine, dexamethasone, phenobarbital, phenytoin, rifampin: decreased donepezil effect
Succinylcholine: synergistic effects

Drug classification
Anticholinergics: decreased activity
Cholinergic agonists, cholinesterase inhibitors: synergistic effects
NSAIDs: increased gastric acid secretions

NURSING CONSIDERATIONS
Assessment
- Monitor B/P: hypotension, hypertension
- Assess mental status: affect, mood, behavioral changes, depression, complete suicide assessment
- Assess GI status: nausea, vomiting, anorexia, diarrhea
- Assess GU status: urinary frequency, incontinence

Nursing diagnoses
- Confusion, chronic (uses)
- Memory, impaired (uses)

Implementation
- Give between meals; may be given with meals for GI symptoms
- Administer dosage adjusted to response no more than q6 wk
- Provide assistance with ambulation during beginning therapy; dizziness, ataxia may occur

Patient/family education
- Advise patient to report side effects: twitching, nausea, vomiting, sweating; indicates overdose
- Advise patient to use drug exactly as prescribed; at regular intervals, preferably between meals; may be taken with meals for GI upset
- Advise patient to notify prescriber of nausea, vomiting, diarrhea (dose increase or beginning treatment), or rash
- Advise patient not to increase or abruptly decrease dose, serious consequences may result
- Instruct patient that drug is not a cure

Evaluation
Positive therapeutic outcome
- Decrease in confusion; improved mood

Treatment of overdose:
Withdraw drug, administer tertiary anticholinergics, provide supportive care

! HIGH ALERT

DOPamine (Rx)
(doe'pa-meen)
DOPamine HCl, Intropin, Revimine ♣
Func. class.: Agonist, vasopressor, inotropic agent
Chem. class.: Catecholamine

Pregnancy category C

Do Not Confuse:
DOPamine/DOBUTamine

Action: Causes increased cardiac output; acts on β_1- and α-receptors, causing vasoconstriction in blood vessels; when low doses are administered, causes renal and mesenteric vasodilatation; β_1 stimulation produces inotropic effects with increased cardiac output

Therapeutic Outcome: Increased B/P, cardiac output

Uses: Shock; to increase perfusion; hypotension

Investigational uses: COPD, RDS in infants

Dosage and routes
Shock
Adult: **IV** inf 2-5 mcg/kg/min, not to exceed 50 mcg/kg/min; titrate to patient's response
Child: **IV** 5-20 mcg/kg/min adjust depending on response

COPD
Adult: **IV** 4 mcg/kg/min

CHF
Adult: **IV** 2-5 mcg/kg/min

RDS
Infants: **IV** 5 mcg/kg/min

Available forms: Inj 40, 80, 160 mg/ml; conc for **IV** inf 0.8, 1.6, 3.2 mg/ml in D_5W

Adverse effects
CNS: *Headache*
CV: *Palpitations,* **tachycardia,** *hypertension,* **ectopic beats,** *angina,* **wide QRS complex,** peripheral vasoconstriction
GI: *Nausea, vomiting, diarrhea*
INTEG: Necrosis, tissue sloughing with extravasation, **gangrene**
RESP: Dyspnea

Contraindications: Hypersensitivity, ventricular fibrillation, tachydysrhythmias, pheochromocytoma

Precautions: Pregnancy **C,** lactation, arterial embolism, peripheral vascular disease

Pharmacokinetics

Absorption	Complete
Distribution	Widely
Metabolism	Liver
Excretion	Kidney, plasma
Half-life	2 min

Pharmacodynamics

Onset	2-5 min
Peak	Unknown
Duration	<10 min

Interactions
Individual drugs
Phenytoin: bradycardia, hypotension
Drug classifications
α-Adrenergic blockers, β-adrenergic blockers: decreased action of dopamine
Anesthetics: increased dysrhythmias
Antidepressants (tricyclic): increased pressor response
Ergots: severe hypertension
MAOIs: increased hypertension (severe), do not use within 2 wk, increased pressor effect
Oxytocics: increased B/P
Drug/lab test
Increased: urinary catecholamine, serum glucose

NURSING CONSIDERATIONS
Assessment
- Monitor ECG for dysrhythmias, ischemia during treatment; some patients may not need continuous ECG monitoring; also monitor PCWP, CVP, CO_2, urinary output; notify prescriber if <30 ml/hr
- Assess for heart failure: bibasilar crackles, S_3 gallop, dyspnea, neck vein distention in patients with cardiomyopathy or CHF
- Assess for oxygenation or perfusion deficit: decreased B/P, chest pain, dizziness, loss of consciousness
- Monitor B/P and pulse q5 min during inf; if B/P drops 30 mm Hg, stop inf and call prescriber
- Check for extravasation: change site q48h

Nursing diagnoses
- Cardiac output, decreased (uses)
- Tissue perfusion, ineffective (uses)
- Fluid volume, excess (uses)
- Knowledge, deficient (teaching)

Implementation
Continuous infusion route
- Dilute 200-400 mg/250-500 ml of D_5W, 0.9% NaCl, D_5/LR, D_5/0.45% NaCl, D_5/0.9% NaCl, LR; do not use discolored sol; sol is stable for 24 hr; give 0.5-5 mcg/kg/min; may increase by 1-4 mcg/kg/min q15-30 min until desired patient response; use infusion pump

Syringe compatibilities: Doxapram, heparin, ranitidine

Y-site compatibilities: Aldesleukin, amifostine, amiodarone, inamrinone, atracurium, aztreonam, cefmetazole, cefpirome, ciprofloxacin, cladribine, diltiazem, DOBUTamine, enalaprilat, epINEPHrine, esmolol, famotidine, fentanyl, fluconazole, foscarnet, granisetron, haloperidol, heparin, hydrocortisone, hydromorphone, labetalol, lidocaine, lorazepam, meperidine, methylPREDNISolone, metronidazole, midazolam, milrinone, morphine, niCARdipine, nitroglycerin, norepinephrine, ondansetron, pancuronium, piperacillin/tazobactam, potassium chloride, propofol, ranitidine, sargramostim, sodium nitroprusside, streptokinase, tacrolimus, theophylline, thiotepa, tolazoline, vecuronium, verapamil, vit B/C, warfarin, zidovudine

Additive compatibilities: Aminophylline, atracurium, bretylium, calcium chloride, cephalothin, chloramphenicol, DOBUTamine, enalaprilat, flumazenil, heparin, hydrocortisone, kanamycin, lidocaine, meropenem, methylPREDNISolone, nitroglycerin, oxacillin, potassium chloride, ranitidine, verapamil

Patient/family education
- Teach patient reason for medication, expected results, reason for all monitoring, and procedures
- Advise patient to report all side effects

Evaluation
Positive therapeutic outcome
- Increased cardiac output

Treatment of overdose: Discontinue drug, support circulation; give a short-acting α-blocker

doxapram (Rx)
(dox'a-pram)
Dopram
Func. class.: Analeptic (respiratory/cerebral stimulant)

Pregnancy category B

Action: Respiratory stimulation through activation of peripheral carotid chemoreceptor in low dosages; with higher dosages medullary respiratory centers are stimulated, with progressive general CNS stimulation

Therapeutic Outcome: Ease of breathing, ABGs at normal limits

Uses: COPD, postanesthesia CNS and respiratory depression, prevention of acute hypercapnia, drug-induced CNS depression

Investigational uses: Treatment of apnea in premature infants when methylxanthines have failed

Dosage and routes

Postanesthesia stimulation

Adult: **IV** inj 0.5-1 mg/kg, not to exceed 1.5 mg/kg total as a single inj; **IV** inf 250 mg in 250 ml sol, not to exceed 4 mg/kg; run at 1-3 mg/min

Drug-induced CNS depression

Adult: **IV** priming dose of 2 mg/kg, repeated in 5 min; repeat q1-2h until patient awakens; **IV** inf priming dose 2 mg/kg at 1-3 mg/min, not to exceed 3 g/day

COPD (hypercapnia)

Adult: **IV** inf 1-2 mg/min, not to exceed 3 mg/min for no longer than 2 hr

Apnea of premature infant

Infant: **IV** 1-1.5 mg/kg/hr loading dose followed by inf of 0.5-2.5 mg/kg/hr

Available forms: Inj **IV** 20 mg/ml

Adverse effects

CNS: **Seizures** (clonus/generalized), *headache,* restlessness, dizziness, confusion, paresthesias, flushing, sweating, bilateral Babinski's sign, rigidity, depression

CV: *Chest pain, hypertension, change in heart rate,* lowered T waves, tachycardia, dysrhythmias

EENT: Pupil dilation, sneezing

GI: Nausea, vomiting, diarrhea, desire to defecate

GU: Retention, incontinence, elevation of BUN, albuminuria

INTEG: Pruritus, irritation at inj site

RESP: **Laryngospasm, bronchospasm,** rebound hypoventilation, dyspnea, cough, tachypnea, hiccups

Contraindications: Hypersensitivity, seizure disorders, severe hypertension, severe bronchial asthma, severe dyspnea, severe cardiac disorders, flail chest, pneumothorax, pulmonary embolism, severe respiratory disease

Precautions: Pregnancy **B**, bronchial asthma, pheochromocytoma, severe tachycardia, dysrhythmias, hypertension, lactation, children

Pharmacokinetics	
Absorption	Complete
Distribution	Unknown
Metabolism	Liver
Excretion	Kidneys, metabolites
Half-life	2.5-4 hr

Pharmacodynamics	
Onset	20-40 sec
Peak	1-2 min
Duration	5-10 min

Interactions

Individual drugs

Cyclopropane, enflurane, halothane: increased dysrhythmias; delay use of doxapram for 10 min

Drug classifications

MAOIs, sympathomimetics: synergistic pressor effect

NURSING CONSIDERATIONS

Assessment

- Monitor B/P, heart rate, deep tendon reflexes, level of consciousness, ABGs before administration q30 min; check for Po_2, Pco_2, O_2 saturation during treatment
- Monitor ECG; watch for hypertension, increased pulse, increased pulmonary artery pressures
- Monitor for hypertension: dysrhythmias, tachycardia, dyspnea, skeletal muscle hyperactivity; may indicate overdosage; discontinue if these occur
- Assess for respiratory stimulation: increased respiratory rate, depth, abnormal rhythm; check for patent airway; elevate head of bed to 45 degrees or higher, position patient on side
- Check for extravasation: redness, inflammation, pain; may cause phlebitis; change **IV** site q48h

Nursing diagnoses

- Breathing pattern, ineffective (uses)
- Gas exchange, impaired (uses)
- Knowledge, deficient (teaching)

Implementation

- May give **IV** diluted with equal parts of sterile water for inj; may be diluted 250 mg/250 ml (1 mg/ml) of D_5W, $D_{10}W$ (dilute 400 mg/180 ml of compatible **IV** sol [2 mg/ml] and run as inf over 2 hr)
- Give **IV** undiluted over 5 min; **IV** inf at 1-3 mg/min; adjust for desired respiratory response, using infusion pump **IV**; if an inf is used after initial dose, start at 1-3 mg/min; adjust for desired respiratory response, using infusion pump **IV**; if an inf is used after initial

dose, start at 1-3 mg/min depending on patient response; discontinue after 2 hr; wait 1-2 hr and repeat

- Give only after adequate airway is established; ensure O_2, **IV** barbiturates, resuscitative equipment available
- Discontinue inf if side effects occur; narrow margin of safety

Syringe compatibilities: Amikacin, bumetadine, chlorproMAZINE, cimetidine, cisplatin, cyclophosphamide, DOPamine, doxycycline, epINEPHrine, hydrOXYzine, imipramine, isoniazid, lincomycin, methotrexate, netilmicin, phytonadione, pyridoxine, terbutaline, thiamine, tobramycin, vinCRIStine

Syringe incompatibilities: Aminophylline, ascorbic acid, cefoperazone, cefotaxime, cefotetan, cefuroxime, dexamethasone, diazepam, digoxin, DOBUTamine, folic acid, furosemide, hydrocortisone, ketamine, methylPREDNISolone, minocycline, thiopental, ticarcillin

Patient/family education

- Teach all aspects of drug, purpose, expected reactions
- Caution patient if difficulty breathing or shortness of breath occurs to notify nurse or prescriber

Evaluation

Positive therapeutic outcome

- Increased breathing capacity
- ABGs WNL for patient

doxazosin (Rx)

(dox-ay'zoe-sin)

Cardura

Func. class.: Peripheral α-adrenergic blocker, antihypertensive

Chem. class.: Quinazoline

Pregnancy category C

Do Not Confuse:

Cardura/Coumadin/Cardene, Cardura/Ridaura

Action: Peripheral blood vessels are dilated, peripheral resistance lowered; reduction in B/P results from α-adrenergic receptors being blocked

Therapeutic Outcome: Decreased B/P, decreased symptoms of benign prostatic hypertrophy (BPH)

Uses: Hypertension alone or as an adjunct, urinary outflow obstruction, symptoms of benign prostatic hyperplasia

Investigational uses: CHF with digoxin and diuretics

Dosage and routes

BPH

Adult: PO 1 mg daily, increase in stepwise manner to 2, 4, 8 mg daily as needed at 1-2 wk intervals, max 8 mg

Hypertension

Adult: PO 1 mg daily, increasing up to 16 mg daily if required; usual range 4-16 mg/day

Elderly: PO 0.5 mg nightly, gradually increase

Available forms: Tabs 1, 2, 4, 8 mg

Adverse effects

CNS: *Dizziness,* headache, drowsiness, anxiety, depression, vertigo, weakness, fatigue, asthenia

CV: Palpitations, *orthostatic hypotension,* **tachycardia,** edema, **dysrhythmias,** chest pain

EENT: Epistaxis, tinnitus, dry mouth, red sclera, pharyngitis, rhinitis

GI: Nausea, vomiting, diarrhea, constipation, abdominal pain

GU: Incontinence, polyuria, priapism

Contraindications: Hypersensitivity to quinazolines

Precautions: Pregnancy **C,** children, lactation, hepatic disease

Pharmacokinetics	
Absorption	Well absorbed
Distribution	Not known; 98% plasma protein bound
Metabolism	Liver, extensively (<63%)
Excretion	Kidneys
Half-life	22 hr

Pharmacodynamics	
Onset	2 hr
Peak	2-6 hr
Duration	6-12 hr

Interactions

Individual drugs

Alcohol, sildenafil, vardenafil: increased hypotensive effects

Clonidine: decreased antihypertensive effect

Drug classifications

Other antihypertensives, nitrates: increased hypotensive effects

Drug/herb

Angelica: increased doxazosin effect

Butcher's broom, capsicum peppers: decreased doxazosin effect

Yohimbe: increased toxicity

NURSING CONSIDERATIONS
Assessment
- Monitor B/P (lying, standing) and pulse, syncope; check for edema in feet, legs daily; I&O; monitor for weight daily; notify prescriber of changes
- Assess skin turgor, dryness of mucous membranes for hydration status
- Assess for orthostatic hypotension; tell patient to rise slowly from sitting or lying position; assess pulse, jugular venous distention q4h, crackles, dyspnea, orthopnea with B/P

Nursing diagnoses
- Cardiac output, decreased (uses)
- Injury, risk for (side effects)
- Knowledge, deficient (teaching)
- Noncompliance (teaching)

Implementation
- Store in tight container at 86° F (30° C) or less
- May be used in combination with other antihypertensives
- May be given with food to prevent GI symptoms

Patient/family education
- Teach patient not to discontinue drug abruptly; emphasize the importance of complying with dosage schedule, even if feeling better; if dose is missed take as soon as remembered; take at same time each day
- Instruct patient to take 1st dose at bedtime to decrease orthostatic B/P changes
- Teach patient not to use OTC products (cough, cold, allergy) unless directed by prescriber; also to avoid large amounts of caffeine
- Emphasize the need to rise slowly to sitting or standing position to minimize orthostatic hypotension
- Teach patient to notify prescriber of mouth sores, sore throat, fever, swelling of hands or feet, irregular heartbeat, chest pain
- Caution patient to report excessive perspiration, dehydration, vomiting, diarrhea; may lead to fall in B/P
- Caution patient that drug may cause dizziness, fainting, lightheadedness; may occur during 1st few days of therapy; to avoid hazardous activities
- Teach patient how to take B/P, and normal readings for age-group; to take B/P q7 days

Evaluation
Positive therapeutic outcome
- Decreased B/P in hypertension
- Decreased symptoms of BPH

Treatment of overdose: Administer volume expanders or vasopressors; discontinue drug; place in supine position

doxepin (Rx)
(dox'e-pin)
doxepin HCl, Novo-Doxepin ✦, Sinequan, Sinequan Concentrate, Triadapin ✦, Zonolon Topical Cream
Func. class.: Antidepressant, tricyclic; antianxiety
Chem. class.: Dibenzoxepin, tertiary amine
Pregnancy category C

Do Not Confuse:
Sinequan/Serentil/Sarafem

Action: Blocks reuptake of norepinephrine, serotonin into nerve endings, increasing action of norepinephrine, serotonin in nerve cells; has anticholinergic effects

Therapeutic Outcome: Decreased symptoms of depression after 2-3 wk

Uses: Major depression, anxiety

Investigational uses: Chronic pain management; topical—pruritus

Dosage and routes
Depression/anxiety
Adult: PO 25-75 mg/day, may increase to 300 mg/day for severely ill
Elderly: PO 10-25 mg at bedtime, increase qwk by 10-25 mg to desired dose
Pruritus
Adult: PO 10 mg at bedtime, may increase to 25 mg at bedtime; top apply a thin film qid ≥3 hr apart

Available forms: Caps 10, 25, 50, 75, 100, 150 mg; oral conc 10 mg/ml; cream 5%

Adverse effects
CNS: *Dizziness, drowsiness,* confusion, headache, anxiety, tremors, stimulation, weakness, insomnia, nightmares, extrapyramidal symptoms (EPS) (elderly), increased psychiatric symptoms, paresthesia
CV: *Orthostatic hypotension, ECG changes,* **tachycardia,** *hypertension,* palpitations, **dysrhythmias**
EENT: *Blurred vision,* tinnitus, mydriasis, ophthalmoplegia, glossitis
GI: *Diarrhea, dry mouth,* nausea, vomiting, **paralytic ileus,** increased appetite, cramps, epigastric distress, jaundice, **hepatitis,** stomatitis, constipation
GU: *Retention,* **acute renal failure**

HEMA: **Agranulocytosis, thrombocytopenia, eosinophilia, leukopenia**
INTEG: Rash, urticaria, sweating, pruritus, photosensitivity

Contraindications: Hypersensitivity to tricyclic antidepressants, urinary retention, narrow-angle glaucoma, prostatic hypertrophy

Precautions: Pregnancy **C** (PO), suicidal patients, elderly, UK-PO lactation, seizures

Pharmacokinetics

Absorption	Well absorbed
Distribution	Widely distributed; crosses placenta
Metabolism	Liver, extensively
Excretion	Kidneys, breast milk
Half-life	8-24 hr

Pharmacodynamics

Unknown

Interactions

Individual drugs

Alcohol: increased CNS depression
Cimetidine, fluoxetine, sertraline: increased doxepin effect
Clonidine: severe hypotension; avoid use
EpINEPHrine, norepinephrine: increased hypertensive action

Drug classifications

Barbiturates, benzodiazepines, CNS depressants, sedative/hypnotics: increased CNS depression
MAOIs: hypertensive crisis, seizures, hyperpyretic crisis

Drug/herb

Belladonna, corkwood, henbane, jimsonweed: increased anticholinergic effect
Hops, kava, lavender, scopolia: increased action of doxepin
SAM-e, St. John's wort: increased serotonin syndrome
Yohimbe: increased hypertension

Drug/lab test

Increased: serum bilirubin, blood glucose, alkaline phosphatase

NURSING CONSIDERATIONS

Assessment

- Monitor B/P (with patient lying, standing), pulse q4h; if systolic B/P drops 20 mm Hg, hold drug, notify prescriber; take VS q4h in patients with CV disease
- Monitor blood studies: CBC, leukocytes, differential, cardiac enzymes if patient is receiving long-term therapy
- Monitor hepatic studies: AST, ALT, bilirubin
- Check weight weekly; appetite may increase with drug
- Assess ECG for flattening of T wave, bundle branch block, AV block, dysrhythmias in cardiac patients; drug should be discontinued gradually several days before surgery
- Assess for (EPS) primarily in elderly: rigidity, dystonia, akathisia
- Assess mental status: mood, sensorium, affect, suicidal tendencies; increase in psychiatric symptoms: depression, panic
- Monitor urinary retention, constipation; constipation is more likely to occur in children or elderly
- Assess for withdrawal symptoms: headache, nausea, vomiting, muscle pain, weakness; do not usually occur unless drug was discontinued abruptly
- Identify alcohol consumption; if alcohol is consumed, hold dose until AM

Nursing diagnoses

- Coping, ineffective (uses)
- Injury, risk for (side effects)
- Knowledge, deficient (teaching)

Implementation

- Oral conc should be diluted with 120 ml of water, milk, or orange, grapefruit, tomato, prune, pineapple juice; do not mix with grape juice
- Give with food or milk for GI symptoms; do not give with carbonated beverages
- Give dosage at bedtime if oversedation occurs during day; may take entire dose at bedtime; elderly may not tolerate once/day dosing
- Store at room temp; do not freeze
- Provide safety measures, primarily for elderly

Patient/family education

- Tell patient that therapeutic effects of decreased depression may take 2-3 wk, antianxiety effects sooner; to use caution in driving and other activities requiring alertness because of drowsiness, dizziness, blurred vision
- Advise patient to avoid rising quickly from sitting to standing, especially elderly
- Teach patient to avoid alcohol ingestion, other CNS depressants, may potentiate effects; not to discontinue medication quickly after long-term use: may cause nausea, headache, malaise
- Teach patient to wear sunscreen or large hat, since photosensitivity occurs
- Teach patient to increase fluids, bulk in diet if constipation occurs, especially elderly; to

D

take gum, hard sugarless candy, or frequent sips of water for dry mouth
• Teach patient to report urinary retention immediately

Evaluation

Positive therapeutic outcome
• Decrease in depression
• Absence of suicidal thoughts

Treatment of overdose: ECG monitoring, induce emesis, lavage, activated charcoal, administer anticonvulsant

doxercalciferol (Rx)

(dox-er-kal'-cif-er-ol)
Hectorol
Func. class.: Parathyroid agent (calcium regulator)
Chem. class.: Vitamin D hormone
Pregnancy category C

Therapeutic Outcome: Calcium at normal level

Uses: To lower high parathyroid hormone levels in patients undergoing chronic kidney dialysis, postmenopausal osteoporosis, prostate cancer

Dosage and routes

Adult: PO 10 mcg 3×/wk at dialysis
Adults: **IV** 4 mcg 3×/wk at end of dialysis, max 18 mcg/dose

Available forms: Caps 2.5 mcg; inj 2 mcg/ml

Adverse effects

CNS: Drowsiness, headache, lethargy
GI: Nausea, diarrhea, vomiting, anorexia, dry mouth, constipation, cramps, metallic taste
GU: Polyuria, hypercalciuria, hyperphosphatemia, hematuria
MS: Myalgia, arthralgia, decreased bone development
RESP: Shortness of breath

Contraindications: Hypersensitivity, hyperphosphatemia, hypercalcemia, vit D toxicity

Precautions: Pregnancy **C**, renal calculi, lactation, CV disease

Pharmacokinetics	
Absorption	Unknown
Distribution	Unknown
Metabolism	Liver
Excretion	Unknown
Half-life	96 hr, Terminal

Pharmacodynamics
Unknown

Interactions

Individual drugs
Cholestyramine, magnesium antacids, mineral oil: decreased doxercalciferol levels, do not use together

NURSING CONSIDERATIONS

Assessment

• Assess GI symptoms, polyuria, flushing, head swelling, tingling, headache; may indicate hypercalcemia
• Identify nutritional status; check diet for sources of vit D (milk, some seafood), calcium (dairy products, dark green vegetables), phosphates
• Monitor BUN, creatinine, uric acid, chloride electrolytes, urine pH, urinary calcium, magnesium, phosphate, urinalysis (calcium should be kept at 9-10 mg/dl; vit D 50-135 international units/dl), alkaline phosphatase baseline and q3-6 mo
(Alert) • Assess for increased drug level, since toxic reactions occur rapidly; have calcium chloride on hand if calcium level drops too low; check for tetany

Nursing diagnoses

• Injury, risk for (adverse reactions)
• Pain, chronic (uses)
• Knowledge, deficient (teaching)

Implementation

• Do not break, crush, or chew caps
• Give with meals for GI symptoms

Patient/family education

• Teach patient the symptoms of hypercalcemia and about foods rich in calcium
• Advise patient to avoid products with sodium: cured meats, dairy products, cold cuts, olives, beets, pickles, soups, meat tenderizers in chronic renal failure
• Advise patient to avoid products with potassium: oranges, bananas, dried fruit, peas, dark green leafy vegetables, milk, melons, beans in chronic renal failure
• Advise patient to avoid OTC products containing calcium, potassium, or sodium in chronic renal failure
• Instruct patient to avoid all preparations containing vit D
• Instruct patient to monitor weight weekly

Evaluation

Positive therapeutic outcome
• Calcium levels 9-10 mg/dl

! HIGH ALERT

DOXOrubicin (Rx)

(dox-oh-roo'bi-sin)

Adriamycin PFS, Adriamycin RDF, Rubex

DOXOrubicin liposome (Rx)

Doxil

Func. class.: Antineoplastic, antibiotic
Chem. class.: Anthracycline glycoside

Pregnancy category D

Do Not Confuse:
Adriamycin/Aredia, Adriamycin/Idamycin, DOXOrubicin/DAUNOrubicin, DOXOrubicin/idarubicin, DOXOrubicin/idamycin

Action: Inhibits DNA synthesis primarily; derived from *Streptomyces peucetius;* replication is decreased by binding to DNA, which causes strand splitting; active throughout entire cell cycle; a vesicant

Therapeutic Outcome: Prevention of rapidly growing malignant cells

Uses: Wilms' tumor; bladder, breast, cervical, head, neck, liver, lung, ovarian, prostatic, stomach, testicular, thyroid cancer; Hodgkin's disease; acute lymphoblastic leukemia; myeloblastic leukemia; neuroblastomas; lymphomas; sarcomas

Dosage and routes

DOXOrubicin

Adult: **IV** 60-75 mg/m^2 q3 wk, or 30 mg/m^2 on days 1-3 of 4-wk cycle, not to exceed 550 mg/m^2 cumulative dose

Child: **IV** 30 mg/m^2/day × 3 days, may repeat q4 wk

DOXOrubicin liposome

Adult: **IV** 20 mg/m^2 q3 wk

Ovarian cancer (DOXOrubicin liposomal)

Adult: **IV** 50 mg/m^2 (doxorubicin equivalent) given 1 mg/min if no adverse reactions, may increase to finish infusion in 1 hr

Available forms: Inj 10, 20, 50, 100, 150 mg; liposomal dispersion for inj (Doxil): 20 mg/ml, 50 mg /30 ml

Adverse effects

CV: Increased B/P, **sinus tachycardia, PVCs,** chest pain, **bradycardia, extrasystole**
GI: Nausea, vomiting, anorexia, mucositis, **hepatotoxicity**
GU: Impotence, sterility, amenorrhea, gynecomastia, hyperuricemia
***HEMA:* Thrombocytopenia, leukopenia, anemia**
INTEG: Rash, necrosis at inj site, dermatitis, reversible alopecia, cellulitis, thrombophlebitis at inj site

Contraindications: Pregnancy **D** (1st trimester), hypersensitivity, lactation, systemic infections, cardiac disorders

Precautions: Renal, hepatic, cardiac disease, gout, bone marrow suppression (severe)

D

Pharmacokinetics	
Absorption	Complete bioavailability
Distribution	Widely distributed; crosses placenta
Metabolism	Liver, extensively
Excretion	Bile (40%-50%)
Half-life	12 min; 3½ hr; 29⅔ hr

Pharmacodynamics

Unknown

Interactions

Individual drugs

Cyclophosphamide: increased cardiotoxicity, increased hemorrhagic cystitis risk
Mercaptopurine, radiation: increased toxicity, hypersensitivity
Radiation: increased bone marrow suppression, toxicity

Drug classifications

Antineoplastics: increased toxicity, bone marrow suppression
Live virus vaccines: decreased antibody response

Drug/lab test

Increased: uric acid

NURSING CONSIDERATIONS

Assessment

- Monitor ECG; watch for ST-T wave changes, low QRS and T; possible dysrhythmias (sinus tachycardia, heart block, PVCs); signs of irreversible cardiomyopathy
- Assess buccal cavity q8h for dryness, sores or ulceration, white patches, pain, bleeding, dysphagia; obtain prescription for viscous lidocaine (Xylocaine)
- Assess symptoms indicating severe allergic reaction: rash, pruritus, urticaria, purpuric skin lesions, itching, flushing; drug should be discontinued
- Assess tachypnea, ECG changes, dyspnea, edema, fatigue
- Monitor CBC, differential, platelet count weekly; withhold drug if WBC is <4000/mm^3 or platelet count is <100,000/mm^3; notify prescriber of results if WBC <20,000/mm^3, platelets <150,000/mm^3

- Assess for increased uric acid levels, swelling, joint pain, primarily extremities; patient should be well hydrated to prevent urate deposits
- Monitor renal function studies: BUN, creatinine, serum uric acid, urine CCr before and during therapy; I&O ratio; report fall in urine output to <30 ml/hr
- Monitor temp q4h (may indicate beginning of infection)
- Monitor liver function tests before and during therapy (bilirubin, AST, ALT, LDH) as needed or monthly; note jaundice of skin or sclera, dark urine, clay-colored stools, itchy skin, abdominal pain, fever, diarrhea
- Assess for bleeding: hematuria, stool guaiac, bruising or petechiae, mucosa or orifices q8h; inflammation of mucosa, breaks in skin
- Identify effects of alopecia on body image; discuss feelings about body changes

Nursing diagnoses

- Injury, risk for (adverse reactions)
- Body image, disturbed (adverse reactions)
- Infection, risk for (adverse reactions)
- Knowledge, deficient (teaching)

Implementation

- Avoid contact with skin; very irritating; wash completely to remove; give fluids **IV** or PO before chemotherapy to hydrate patient
- Give antiemetic 30-60 min before giving drug to prevent vomiting and prn; give antibiotics for prophylaxis of infection
- Provide liq diet: carbonated beverages; gelatin may be added if patient is not nauseated or vomiting
- Drug should be prepared by experienced personnel using proper precautions
- Do not interchange DOXOrubicin with DOXOrubicin liposome
- Give **IV** after diluting 10 mg/5 ml of NaCl for inj; another 5 ml of diluent/10 mg is recommended; shake; give over 3-5 min; give through Y-tube or 3-way stopcock through free-flowing D_5 inf or 0.9% NaCl
- **IV** liposome inj (Doxil): dilute dose up to 90 mg/250 ml of D_5W, give over ½ hr; do not admix with other solution medications
- Use hydrocortisone, dexamethasone, or sodium bicarbonate (1 mEq/1 ml) for extravasation: apply ice compress
- Dose modifications for HFS: Toxicity Grade 1, redose unless patient has experienced previous grade 3 or 4; Grade 2, delay dosing up to 2 wk, or until resolved to grades 0 or 1; Grade 3 delay dosing up to 2 wk or until resolved to grades 0 or 1; resume dose at 25% decrease, return to original dosing after interval; Grade 4 delay dosing up to 2 wk or until grades 0 or 1; resume dose at 25% decrease, then return to original dose; if after 2 wk there is no resolution, discontinue

Syringe compatibilities: Bleomycin, cisplatin, cyclophosphamide, droperidol, fluorouracil, leucovorin, methotrexate, metoclopramide, mitomycin, vinCRIStine

Syringe incompatibilities: Furosemide, heparin

Y-site compatibilities: Amifostine, aztreonam, bleomycin, chlorproMAZINE, cimetidine, cisplatin, cladribine, cyclophosphamide, dexamethasone, diphenhydrAMINE, droperidol, famotidine, filgrastim, fludarabine, fluorouracil, granisetron, hydromorphone, leucovorin calcium, lorazepam, melphalan, methotrexate, methylPREDNISolone, metoclopramide, mitomycin, morphine, ondansetron, paclitaxel, prochlorperazine, promethazine, propofol, ranitidine, sargramostim, sodium bicarbonate, teniposide, thiotepa, vinBLAStine, vinCRIStine, vinorelbine

Y-site incompatibilities: Furosemide, heparin

Additive compatibilities: Ondansetron

Additive incompatibilities: Aminophylline, cephalothin, dexamethasone, diazepam, fluorouracil, hydrocortisone

Patient/family education

- Help patient to rinse mouth tid-qid with water or club soda, brush teeth bid-qid with soft brush or cotton-tipped applicators for stomatitis, use unwaxed dental floss
- Advise patient to add 2-3 L of fluids unless contraindicated prior to and for 24-48 hr after, to decrease possible hemorrhagic cystitis
- Tell patient that urine and other body fluids may be red-orange for 48 hr; contraceptive measures are recommended during and 4 mo after therapy; drug is teratogenic to fetus
- Advise patient to avoid use of products containing aspirin or ibuprofen, razors, commercial mouthwash, since bleeding may occur; to report symptoms of bleeding (hematuria, tarry stools)
- Instruct patient to report signs of anemia (fatigue, headache, irritability, faintness, shortness of breath)
- Inform patient that hair may be lost during treatment; a wig or hairpiece may make patient feel better; new hair may be different in color, texture
- Caution patient not to have any vaccinations without the advice of the prescriber; serious reactions can occur

Evaluation

Positive therapeutic outcome

- Prevention of rapid division of malignant cells

doxycycline (Rx)

(dox-i-sye'kleen)

Apo-Doxy ✤, Doryx, Doxy, Doxycin ✤, doxycycline, Monodox, Novodoxyclin ✤, Periostat, Vibramycin, Vibra-Tabs

Func. class.: Antiinfective

Chem. class.: Tetracycline

Pregnancy category D

Do Not Confuse:
doxycycline/doxepin

Action: Inhibits protein synthesis, phosphorylation in microorganisms by binding to 30S ribosomal subunits, reversibly binding to 50S ribosomal subunits; bacteriostatic

Therapeutic Outcome: Bactericidal action against the following: gram-positive pathogens *Bacillus anthracis, Clostridium perfringens, Clostridium tetani, Listeria monocytogenes, Nocardia, Propionibacterium acnes, Actinomyces israelii;* gram-negative pathogens *Haemophilus influenzae, Legionella pneumophila, Versinia enterocolitica, Versinia pestis, Neisseria gonorrhoeae, Neisseria meningitidis, Mycoplasma, Chlamydia, Rickettsia*

Uses: Syphilis, gonorrhea, *Chlamydia,* lymphogranuloma venereum, uncommon gram-negative or -positive organisms, malaria prophylaxis, acne, anthrax

Investigational uses: Traveler's diarrhea, Lyme disease, prevention of chronic bronchitis

Dosage and routes

Adult: PO/**IV** 100 mg q12h on day 1, then 100 mg/day; **IV** 200 mg in 1-2 inf on day 1, then 100-200 mg/day

Child >8 yr (>45 kg): PO/**IV** 2.2-4.4 mg/kg/day in divided doses q12h

Gonorrhea (uncomplicated) (patients allergic to penicillin)

Adult: PO 100 mg q12h × 7 days, or 300 mg followed 1 hr later by another 300 mg

Malaria prophylaxis

Adult: 100 mg daily 1-2 days prior to travel and daily during travel

Chlamydia trachomatis

Adult: PO 100 mg bid × 7days

Syphilis

Adult: PO 300 mg/day in divided doses × 10 days

Periodontitis

Adult: 20 mg bid after sealing and root planing for ≤9 mo; give ≥1 hr before meal AM or PM

Available forms: Tabs 100 mg; caps 50, 100 mg; syr 50 mg/5 ml; powder for inj 100, 200 mg; powder for oral susp 25 mg/5 ml; mouth products: tabs 20 mg; inj 42.5 mg

Adverse effects

CNS: Fever

CV: Pericarditis

EENT: Dysphagia, glossitis, decreased calcification of deciduous teeth, oral candidiasis

GI: *Nausea, abdominal pain, vomiting, diarrhea,* anorexia, enterocolitis, **hepatotoxicity,** flatulence, abdominal cramps, gastric burning, stomatitis

GU: *Increased BUN*

HEMA: **Eosinophilia, neutropenia, thrombocytopenia, hemolytic anemia**

INTEG: Rash, urticaria, photosensitivity, increased pigmentation, **exfoliative dermatitis,** pruritus, **angioedema**

Contraindications: Pregnancy **D**, hypersensitivity to tetracyclines, children <8 yr

Precautions: Hepatic disease, lactation

Pharmacokinetics

Absorption	Well absorbed
Distribution	Widely distributed, crosses placenta
Metabolism	Some hepatic recycling
Excretion	Bile, feces; kidneys unchanged (20%-40%), enters breast milk
Half-life	14-17 hr; increased in severe renal disease

Pharmacodynamics

	PO	IV
Onset	1½-4 hr	Immediate
Peak	1½-4 hr	Infusion's end

Interactions

Individual drugs

Bismuth, carbamazepine, cimetidine, cholestyramine, colestipol, kaolin/pectin, $NaHCO_3$, phenytoin, rifampin, sucralfate: decreased effect of doxycycline

Digoxin: decreased effect of digoxin

Iron: forms chelates, decreased absorption

Penicillins: decreased effects of penicillins

Warfarin: increased effect of warfarin

Drug classifications
Alkali products, antacids, barbiturates: decreased effect of doxycycline
Anticoagulants (oral): increased effect of anticoagulants
Contraceptives (oral): decreased effect of oral contraceptive

Drug/herb
Bromelain: increased action
Acidophilus: do not use with antiinfectives

Drug/food
Decreased: absorption with dairy products

Drug/lab test
False increase: urinary catecholamines, ALT, AST

NURSING CONSIDERATIONS

Assessment

- Assess patient for previous sensitivity reaction
- Assess patient for signs and symptoms of infection including characteristics of wounds, sputum, urine, stool, WBC >10,000/mm^3, fever; obtain baseline information before and during treatment
- Obtain C&S before beginning drug therapy to identify if correct treatment has been initiated
- Assess for allergic reactions: rash, urticaria, pruritus, chills, fever, joint pain; angioedema may occur a few days after therapy begins
- Assess bowel pattern daily; if severe diarrhea occurs, drug should be discontinued
- Monitor for bleeding: ecchymosis, bleeding gums, hematuria, stool guaiac daily if on long-term therapy; blood dyscrasias may occur
- Assess for overgrowth of infection: perineal itching, fever, malaise, redness, pain, swelling, drainage, rash, diarrhea, change in cough, sputum

Nursing diagnoses

- Infection, risk for (uses)
- Diarrhea (side effects)
- Injury, risk for (side effects)
- Knowledge, deficient (teaching)
- Noncompliance (teaching)

Implementation

PO route

- Do not break, crush, or chew caps
- Give around the clock to maintain proper blood levels; give with food to increase absorption of drug; do not give within 3 hr of other agents; drug reactions may occur
- Give with 8 oz of water, 1 hr before bedtime to prevent ulceration
- Shake liq preparation well before giving; use calibrated device for proper dosing
- Do not give with iron, calcium, magnesium products or antacids, which decrease absorption and form insoluble chelate

IV route

- Check for irritation, extravasation, phlebitis daily; change site q72h
- For intermittent inf, dilute each 100 mg/10 ml of 0.9% NaCl, sterile water for inj; further dilute in at least 100 ml of 0.9% NaCl, D_5W, Ringer's, LR, D_5/LR; protect from direct light; keep at room temp; give over 1-4 hr; **IV** sol stable for 12 hr at room temp, 72 hr refrigerated, discard if precipitate forms

Syringe compatibilities: Doxapram

Y-site compatibilities: Acyclovir, amifostine, amiodarone, aztreonam, cyclophosphamide, diltiazem, filgrastim, fludarabine, granisetron, hydromorphone, magnesium sulfate, melphalan, meperidine, morphine, ondansetron, perphenazine, propofol, sargramostim, tacrolimus, teniposide, theophylline, thiotepa, vinorelbine

Y-site incompatibilities: Hetastarch

Additive compatibilities: Ranitidine

Patient/family education

- Teach patient to report sore throat, bruising, bleeding, joint pain; may indicate blood dyscrasias (rare)
- Advise patient to contact prescriber if vaginal itching, loose foul-smelling stools, furry tongue occur; may indicate superinfection; report itching, rash, pruritus, urticaria
- Instruct patient to take all medication prescribed for the length of time ordered; drug must be taken around the clock to maintain blood levels; do not give medication to others
- Advise patient to notify prescriber of diarrhea with blood or pus

Evaluation

Positive therapeutic outcome

- Absence of signs/symptoms of infection (WBC <10,000/mm^3, temp WNL, absence of red draining wounds)
- Reported improvement in symptoms of infection

! HIGH ALERT

droperidol (Rx)

(droe-per'i-dole)

droperidol, Inapsine

Func. class.: Neuroleptic, tranquilizer, antiemetic

Chem. class.: Butyrophenone derivative

Pregnancy category C

Action: Acts on CNS at subcortical levels, producing tranquilization, sleep; antiemetic; mild α-blockade

Therapeutic Outcome: Maintenance of anesthesia

Uses: Premedication for surgery; induction, maintenance in general anesthesia; postoperatively for nausea and vomiting

Dosage and routes

Induction, adjunct

Adult: **IV**/IM 1.25-2.5 mg, may give additional 1.25 mg

Child 2-12 yr: **IV** 0.05-0.1 mg/kg titrate to response

Premedication

Adult: IM 2.5-10 mg ½-1 hr before surgery, may give 1.25-2.5 mg additionally

Child 2-12 yr: IM 0.05-0.1 mg/kg

Maintaining general anesthesia

Adult: **IV** 1.25-2.5 mg

Available forms: Inj 2.5 mg/ml

Adverse effects

CNS: EPS: Dystonia, akathisia, flexion of arms, fine tremors; dizziness, anxiety, drowsiness, restlessness, hallucinations, depression, **seizures,** extrapyramidal symptoms, **neuroleptic malignant syndrome**

CV: **Tachycardia,** *hypotension,* prolonged QT

EENT: Upward rotation of eyes, oculogyric crisis

INTEG: *Chills, facial sweating, shivering*

RESP: **Laryngospasm, bronchospasm**

Contraindications: Hypersensitivity, child <2 yr, lactation

Precautions: Pregnancy **C**, elderly, CV disease (hypotension, bradydysrhythmias), renal, liver disease, Parkinson's disease, pheochromocytoma

Pharmacokinetics

Absorption	Well absorbed (IM)
Distribution	Crosses blood-brain barrier, placenta
Metabolism	Liver
Excretion	Kidneys, unchanged (10%)
Half-life	2-3 hr

Pharmacodynamics

	IM/IV
Onset	3-10 min
Peak	30 min
Duration	3-6 hr

Interactions

Individual drugs

Alcohol: increased CNS depression

Lithium: increased side effects of lithium

Drug classifications

Antihistamines, antipsychotics, barbiturates, CNS depressants, opiates: increased CNS depression

Antihypertensives, nitrates: increased hypotension

Drug/herb

Kava: increased action

NURSING CONSIDERATIONS

Assessment

- Check VS q10 min during **IV** administration, q30 min after IM dose; for increasing heart rate or decreasing B/P, notify prescriber at once; do not place patient in Trendelenburg's position, sympathetic blockade may occur, causing respiratory arrest
- Assess extrapyramidal reactions: dystonia, akathisia, extended neck, restlessness, tremors; if these occur, an anticholinergic should be given
- If given for nausea or vomiting, monitor for significant loss of fluids, bowel sounds before and during administration
- EKG prior to and 2-3 hr after administration for serious arrhythmias

Nursing diagnoses

- Injury, risk for (adverse reactions)
- Knowledge, deficient (teaching)

Implementation

- Protect from light

IM route

- Give deeply in large muscle mass

IV route

- Give direct **IV** undiluted; give through Y-tube or 3-way stopcock at 10 mg or less/min; titrate to patient response
- Intermittent inf may be given by adding dose

to 250 ml of LR, D_5W, 0.9% NaCl; give slowly, titrate to patient response

- Give anticholinergics (benztropine, diphenhydrAMINE) for extrapyramidal reaction
- Give only with resuscitative equipment nearby

Syringe compatibilities: Atropine, bleomycin, butorphanol, chlorproMAZINE, cimetidine, cisplatin, cyclophosphamide, dimenhyDRINATE, diphenhydrAMINE, DOXOrubicin, fentanyl, glycopyrrolate, hydrOXYzine, meperidine, metoclopramide, midazolam, mitomycin, morphine, nalbuphine, pentazocine, perphenazine, prochlorperazine, promazine, promethazine, scopolamine, vinBLAStine, vinCRIStine

Syringe incompatibilities: Fluorouracil, furosemide, heparin, leucovorin, methotrexate, pentobarbital

Y-site compatibilities: Amifostine, aztrenonam, bleomycin, cisatracurium, cisplatin, cladribine, cyclophosphamide, cytarabine, DOXOrubicin, DOXOrubicin liposome, famotidine, filgrastim, fluconazole, fludarabine, granisetron, hydrocortisone sodium succinate, idarubicin, melphalen, meperidine, metoclopramide, mitomycin, ondansetron, paclitaxel, potassium chloride, propofol, remifentanil, sargramostim, teniposide, thiotepa, vinBLAStine, vinCRIStine, vinorelbine, vit B/C

Y-site incompatibilities: Fluorouracil, foscarnet, furosemide, leucovorin, methotrexate, nafcillin

Additive incompatibilities: Barbiturates

Patient/family education

- Advise patient that orthostatic hypotension is common; to rise from lying or sitting position slowly; to avoid ambulation without assistance
- Caution patient that drowsiness may occur; to call for assistance for ambulation

Evaluation

Positive therapeutic outcome

- Decreased anxiety
- Absence of vomiting during and after surgery

drotrecogin alfa (Rx)

(droh'treh-koh-jin al'fah)

Xigris

Func. class.: Thrombolytic agent

Chem. class.: Recombinant human activated protein C

Pregnancy category C

Action: Activated protein C exerts an antithrombotic effect by inhibiting factor Va/VIIIa

Therapeutic Outcome: Reduction of mortality in adult patients with severe sepsis who have a high risk of death

Uses: Severe sepsis (sepsis associated with acute organ dysfunction)

Dosage and routes

Adult: **IV** inf 24 mcg/kg/hr × 96 hr

Available forms: Powder for inj, lyophilized, 5 mg, 20 mg

Adverse effects

HEMA: Decreased Hct, **bleeding**

SYST: **GI, GU, intracranial, intraabdominal, intrathoracic, retroperitoneal bleeding; surface bleeding**

Contraindications: Hypersensitivity, internal active bleeding, intraspinal surgery, CNS neoplasms, ulcerative colitis, enteritis, hepatic disease, hypocoagulation, hemorrhagic stroke, epidural catheter in place, cerebral embolism/thrombosis/hemorrhage, recent major surgery, trauma

Precautions: Pregnancy **C,** recent GI bleeding, prothrombin time –INR >3, lactation, children, use >96 hr

Pharmacokinetics	
Absorption	Rapid
Distribution	Plasma
Metabolism	Unknown
Excretion	Unknown
Half-life	Unknown

Pharmacodynamics	
Onset	Within 2 hr of beginning infusion
Peak	96 hr
Duration	2 hr postinfusion

Interactions

Individual drugs

Asprin, indomethacin, phenylbutazone: increased bleeding risk

Drug classifications

Anticoagulants, glycoprotein IIb/IIIa inhibitors,

salicylates, thrombolytics: increased bleeding risk

Drug/herb

Agrimony, alfalfa, angelica, anise, basil, bay, bilberry, black haw, bogbean, bromelain, buchu, chondroitin, cinchona bark, dong quai, fenugreek, feverfew, garlic, ginger, ginkgo, ginseng, horse chestnut, Irish moss, kelp, kelpware, khella, lovage, lungwort, meadowsweet, motherwort, mugwort, nettle, papaya, parsley (large amounts), pau d'arco, pineapple, poplar, prickly ash, safflower, saw palmetto, tonka bean, turmeric, wintergreen, yarrow: increased risk of bleeding

Chamomile, coenzyme Q10, flax, glucomannan, goldenseal, guar gum: decreased anticoagulant effect

Drug/lab test

Possible variably prolonged APTT, possible altered one-stage coagulation assays based on APTT (factor VIII, IX, XI assays)

NURSING CONSIDERATIONS

Assessment

- Assess for bleeding during treatment; hematuria, hematemesis, bleeding from mucous membranes, epistaxis, ecchymosis; may require transfusion (rare), continue to assess for bleeding
- Assess blood studies (Hct, platelets, PTT, PT, TT, APTT) before starting therapy; PT or APTT must be less than 2× control before starting therapy; PTT or PT q3-4h during treatment
- Assess VS, B/P, pulse, respirations, neurologic signs, temp at least q4h; temp >104° F (40° C) indicates internal bleeding; systolic pressure increase >25 mm Hg should be reported to prescriber
- Assess for neurologic changes that may indicate intracranial bleeding
- Assess for retroperitoneal bleeding: back pain, leg weakness, diminished pulses

Nursing diagnoses

- Knowledge, deficient (teaching)

Implementation

- Store in refrigerator at 2°-8° C (36°-46° F); do not freeze
- Protect unreconstituted vials from light; keep in carton until time of use

IV route

- Reconstitute 5 mg vial/2.5 ml; 20 mg vial/10 ml sterile water for inj to a concentration of 2 mg/ml; slowly add sterile water for inj; do not shake or invert, gently swirl until dissolved
- Further dilute with 0.9% NaCl, slowly withdraw prescribed amount and add to bag of 0.9% NaCl, direct stream to side of bag, gently invert bag; do not transport infusion bag between locations using mechanical delivery systems
- Use immediately after reconstituting, may be held for only 3 hr at controlled room temp 59°-86° F and must complete inf within 12 hr after preparation
- Do not use if discolored or if particulate is present
- If using an infusion pump, usual concentration is 100-200 mcg/ml; if using a syringe pump, usual concentration is 100-1000 mcg/ml
- Use a dedicated **IV** line, or dedicated lumen of central venous catheter, may use only 0.9% NaCl, LR, dextrose, or dextrose/saline mixtures through same line
- Do not expose to heat or direct sunlight
- Discontinue 2 hr prior to invasive surgery or procedures introducing risk of bleeding

Evaluation

Positive therapeutic outcome

- Decreasing symptoms of sepsis, lack of mortality

D

duloxetine (Rx)

(du-lox'uh-teen)

Cymbalta

Func. class.: Miscellaneous antidepressant

Chem. class: Serotonin, norepinephrine reuptake inhibitor

Pregnancy category C

Action: Unknown, may potentiate serotonergic, nonadrenergic activity in the CNS. In studies duloxetine is a potent inhibitor of neuronal serotonin and norepinephrine reuptake

Therapeutic Outcome: Decreased depression, decreased neuropathic pain

Uses: Major depressive disorder (MDD), neuropathic pain associated with diabetic neuropathy

Dosage and routes

Depression

Adult: PO 20 mg bid, may increase to 30 mg bid if needed

Diabetic neuropathy

Adult: PO 60 mg q day

Available forms: Caps 20, 30, 60 mg

Adverse effects

CNS: Insomnia, anxiety, dizziness, tremor, fatigue, decreased appetite, decreased weight

CV: Thrombophlebitis, peripheral edema
EENT: Abnormal vision
GI: Constipation, diarrhea, dysphagia, nausea, vomiting, anorexia, dry mouth, colitis, gastritis
GU: Abnormal ejaculation, urinary hesitation, ejaculation delayed, erectile dysfunction
INTEG: Photosensitivity, bruising, sweating

Contraindications: Hypersensitivity, narrow-angle glaucoma

Precautions: Pregnancy **C**, mania, lactation, children, elderly, hypertension, cardiac disease, narrow-angle glaucoma, renal disease, hepatic disease, seizures

Pharmacokinetics

Absorption	Well absorbed
Distribution	90% protein binding
Metabolism	Extensively metabolized (CYP 2D6, CYP 1A2) in the liver to an active metabolite
Excretion	70% of drug recovered in urine, 20% in feces
Half-life	12 hr

Pharmacodynamics

Unknown

Interactions

Individual drugs

Alcohol: increased ALT, bilirubin

Drug classifications

⚠ MAOIs: coadministration is contraindicated or within 14 days of MAOIs use: hyperthermia, rigidity, rapid fluctuations of vital signs, mental status changes, neuroleptic malignant syndrome
Opioids, antihistamines, sedative/hypnotics: increased CNS depression
CYP 1A2 inhibitors (fluvoxamine, quinolone antiinfectives); CYP 2D6 (fluoxetine, quinidine, paroxetine): increased action of duloxetine
CYP 2D6 extensively metabolized drugs (flecainide, phenothiazines, propafenone, tricyclics, thioridazine): narrow therapeutic index

Drug/herb

Chamomile, hops, kava, lavender, skullcap, valerian: increased CNS depression
Corkwood, jimsonweed: increased anticholinergic effect
SAM-e, St. John's wort: serotonin syndrome
Yohimbe: increased hypertension

NURSING CONSIDERATIONS

Assessment

- Assess B/P lying, standing; pulse q4h; if systolic B/P drops 20 mm Hg, hold drug, notify prescriber; take VS q4h in patients with cardiovascular disease
- Monitor hepatic studies: AST, ALT, bilirubin
- Monitor weight qwk; weight loss or gain; appetite may increase; peripheral edema may occur
- Offer sugarless gum, hard candy, frequent sips of water for dry mouth
- Assess mental status: mood, sensorium, affect, suicidal tendencies, increase in psychiatric symptoms; depression, panic
- Assess for withdrawal symptoms: headache, nausea, vomiting, muscle pain, weakness; not usual unless drug is discontinued abruptly

Nursing diagnoses

- Injury, risk for (uses)
- Knowledge, deficient (teaching)
- Noncompliance (teaching)

Implementation

- Swallow caps whole; do not break, crush, or chew; do not sprinkle on food or mix with liquid
- Store in tight container at room temperature; do not freeze
- Provide assistance with ambulation during beginning therapy, since drowsiness, dizziness occur
- Check to see if PO medication was swallowed

Patient/family education

- Advise that drug is dispensed in small amounts because of suicide potential, especially in the beginning of therapy
- Teach patient/family to use caution when driving or other activities requiring alertness because of drowsiness, dizziness, blurred vision
- Advise patient to avoid alcohol ingestion, MAOIs, other CNS depressants
- Advise patient not to discontinue medication quickly after long-term use; may cause nausea, headache, malaise
- Advise patient to wear sunscreen or large hat, since photosensitivity may occur
- Advise patient to notify prescriber if pregnancy is planned or suspected, or if breastfeeding
- Tell patient that improvement may occur in 1-4 wk

Evaluation

Positive therapeutic outcome

- Decreased depression

dutasteride (Rx)
(doo-tass'ter-ide)
Duagen
Func. class.: Sex hormone, 5α-reductase inhibitor
Chem. class.: Synthetic 4-azasteroid compound
Pregnancy category X

Action: Inhibits both types 1 and 2 forms of a steroid enzyme that converts testosterone to 5 µ-dihydrotestosterone (DHT), which is responsible for the initial growth of prostatic tissue

Therapeutic Outcome: Decreased symptoms of benign prostatic hyperplasia (BPH)

Uses: Treatment of symptomatic BPH in men with an enlarged prostate gland

Dosage and routes
Adult: PO 0.5 mg daily

Available forms: Caps 0.5 mg

Adverse effects
GU: Decreased libido, impotence, gynecomastia, ejaculation disorders (rare), mastalgia, teratogenesis

Contraindications: Pregnancy **X,** hypersensitivity, lactation, women, children

Precautions: Hepatic disease

Pharmacokinetics	
Absorption	Absolute bioavailability ~60%
Distribution	Protein binding 99%
Metabolism	Liver (CYP3A4)
Excretion	Feces
Half-life	5 wk at steady state

Pharmacodynamics	
Onset	Rapid
Peak	2-3 hr
Duration	Levels detectable 4-6 mo posttreatment

Interactions
Individual drugs
Cimetidine, ciprofloxacin, diltiazem, ketoconazole, ritonavir, verapamil: increased dutasteride concentrations
Drug classifications
Antiretroviral protease inhibitors or other CYP3A4-metabolized drugs: increased dutasteride concentrations
Drug/lab test
Increased: TSH
Decreased: prostate-specific antigen (PSA)

NURSING CONSIDERATIONS
Assessment
- Assess for decreasing symptoms in BPH: decreasing urinary retention, frequency, urgency, nocturia
- Assess PSA levels, digital rectal exam, urinary obstruction; determine the absence of urinary cancer before starting treatment
- Assess liver function studies: ALT, AST, bilirubin

Nursing diagnoses
- Knowledge, deficient (teaching)
- Body image, disturbed (adverse reactions)

Implementation
- Swallow caps whole: do not break, crush, chew, or open
- May be given without regard to meals

Patient/family education
- Advise patient to notify prescriber if therapeutic response decreases, if edema occurs
- Caution patient not to discontinue drug abruptly
- Inform patient about changes in sex characteristics
- Caution patient not to donate blood for at least 6 mo after last dose to prevent possible blood administration to pregnant female
- Advise patient and family that caps should not be handled by pregnant women since this drug can be absorbed through the skin
- Inform patient that ejaculate volume may decrease during treatment, that drug rarely interferes with sexual function
- Advise patient to read patient information leaflet before starting therapy and reread it upon prescription renewal

Evaluation
Positive therapeutic outcome
- Decreased levels of DHT (5 α-dihydrotestosterone)
- Decreased urinary frequency
- Decreased urinary retention
- Decreased urinary urgency
- Decreased nocturia

D

dyphylline (Rx)

(dye'fi-lin)

Dilor, Dyflex-200, Dylline, dyphylline, Lufyllin, Neothylline

Func. class.: Bronchodilator, phosphodiesterase inhibitor

Chem. class.: Xanthine, theophylline derivative

Pregnancy category C

Action: Relaxes smooth muscle of respiratory system by blocking phosphodiesterase, which increases cyclic AMP; cyclic AMP results in positive inotropic, chronotropic effects, bronchodilatation, stimulation of CNS

Therapeutic Outcome: Bronchodilatation with ease of breathing

Uses: Bronchial asthma, bronchospasm in chronic bronchitis and emphysema, COPD

Dosage and routes

Adult: PO 200-800 mg q6h; IM 250-500 mg q6h injected slowly, max 15 mg/kg/q6h

Child > 6 yr: PO 4-7 mg/kg/day in 4 divided doses

Available forms: Tabs 200, 400 mg; elix 33.3, 53.3 mg/5 ml; inj 250 mg/ml

Adverse effects

CNS: *Anxiety, restlessness, insomnia, dizziness,* **seizures,** headache, lightheadedness, muscle twitching

CV: *Palpitations, sinus tachycardia,* hypotension, flushing, **dysrhythmias, circulatory failure**

GI: *Nausea,* diarrhea, *vomiting, anorexia,* dyspepsia, epigastric pain, rectal irritation, bleeding, reflux

INTEG: Flushing, urticaria

OTHER: Fever, dehydration, **albuminuria,** hyperglycemia, increased diuresis

RESP: Tachypnea, **respiratory arrest**

Contraindications: Hypersensitivity to xanthines, active peptic ulcer disease, seizure disorder

Precautions: Pregnancy **C,** elderly, CHF, cor pulmonale, hepatic disease, diabetes mellitus, hypertension, children, renal disease, glaucoma, hyperthyroidism

Pharmacokinetics

Absorption	Well absorbed (PO)
Distribution	Unknown
Metabolism	Liver
Excretion	Kidneys (85%), breast milk
Half-life	2 hr; increased in renal disease

Pharmacodynamics

	PO	IM
Onset	Unknown	Unknown
Peak	1 hr	Unknown
Duration	6 hr	Unknown

Interactions

Individual drugs

Cimetidine, erythromycin, propranolol, probenecid: increased action of dyphylline

Phenytoin: decreased levels of phenytoin, increased metabolism of dyphylline

Drug classifications

Barbiturates: increased metabolism of dyphilline

β-Adrenergic blockers: increased cardiotoxicity

Uricosurics: decreased elimination of dyphylline

NURSING CONSIDERATIONS

Assessment

- Monitor dyphylline blood levels (therapeutic level is <20 mcg/ml); toxicity (dysrhythmias, seizures, diuresis, flushing, headache) may occur with small increase above 20 mcg/ml, especially elderly; determine whether theophylline was given recently (24 hr)
- Monitor I&O; an increase in diuresis occurs; dehydration may result in elderly or children
- Assess respiratory rate, rhythm, depth; before and during treatment auscultate lung fields bilaterally; notify prescriber of abnormalities
- Assess for allergic reactions: rash, urticaria; if these occur, drug should be discontinued
- Assess for drug toxicity: nausea, vomiting, anorexia, cramping, diarrhea, confusion

Nursing diagnoses

- Injury, risk for (uses, adverse reactions)
- Airway clearance, ineffective (uses)
- Activity intolerance (uses)
- Knowledge, deficient (teaching)

Implementation

PO route

- Give around the clock to maintain blood levels, daily dose each AM
- Give 1 hr ac and 2 hr pc to increase absorption; elix should be measured accurately
- Take with 8 oz of water and food if GI upset occurs
- Increased fluids to 2 L/day

IM route

- Inject slowly; do not give by **IV** route; do not administer if cloudy or a precipitate occurs, avoid this route, do not give **IV**

Patient/family education

- Teach patient to take doses as prescribed, not to skip doses or double dose; patient should check OTC medications and current prescription medications for epHEDrine, which increases CNS stimulation; tell patient not to drink alcohol or caffeine products (tea, coffee, chocolate, colas) or CV effects may occur, not to change brands
- Advise patient to avoid hazardous activities; dizziness may occur
- Caution patient if GI upset occurs, to take drug with 8 oz of water and food
- Teach patient to notify prescriber of change in smoking habit; a change in dosage may be required
- Instruct patient to report nausea, vomiting, insomnia, tachycardia, dysrhythmias, seizures, or restlessness; can indicate toxicity
- Teach patient to increase fluids to 2 L/day to decrease viscosity of secretions
- Advise patient to obtain drug level q6-12 mo

Evaluation

Positive therapeutic outcome

- Decreased dyspnea
- Clear lung fields bilaterally

edrophonium (Rx)

(ed-roe-fone'ee-yum)

Enlon, Reversol, Tensilon

Func. class.: Cholinergics, anticholinesterase

Chem. class.: Quaternary ammonium compound

Pregnancy category C

Action: Inhibits destruction of acetylcholine, which increases concentration at sites where acetylcholine is released; this facilitates transmission of impulses across myoneural junction

Therapeutic Outcome: Reversal of nondepolarizing neuromuscular blockers; absence of difficulty with muscular function in myasthenia gravis

Uses: Diagnosis of myasthenia gravis; curare antagonist; differentiation of myasthenic crisis from cholinergic crisis; reversal of nondepolarizing neuromuscular blockers

Dosage and routes

Tensilon test (myasthenia gravis diagnosis)

Adult: **IV** 1-2 mg over 15-30 sec, then 8 mg if no response; IM 10 mg; if cholinergic reaction occurs, retest after ½ hr with 2 mg IM

Child >34 kg: **IV** 2 mg; if no response in 45 sec, then 1 mg q45 sec, not to exceed 10 mg; IM 5 mg

Child <34 kg: **IV** 1 mg; if no response in 45 sec, then 1 mg q45 sec, not to exceed 5 mg; IM 2 mg

Infant: **IV** 0.5 mg

Reversal of nondepolarizing neuromuscular blockers

Adult: **IV** 10 mg over 30-45 sec, may repeat, not to exceed 40 mg

Differentiation of myasthenic crisis from cholinergic crisis

Adult: **IV** 1 mg, if no response in 1 min, may repeat

Available forms: Inj 10 mg/ml

Adverse effects

CNS: Dizziness, headache, sweating, weakness, **seizures**, uncoordination, **paralysis**, drowsiness, **loss of consciousness**

CV: Dysrhythmias, bradycardia, hypotension, **AV block**, ECG changes, **cardiac arrest**, syncope

EENT: Miosis, blurred vision, lacrimation, visual changes

GI: *Nausea, diarrhea, vomiting, cramps, increased salivary and gastric secretions, dysphagia, increased peristalsis*

GU: Frequency, incontinence, urgency

INTEG: Rash, urticaria

RESP: **Respiratory depression, bronchospasm, constriction, laryngospasm, respiratory arrest**, dyspnea, increased bronchial secretions

Contraindications: Obstruction of intestine, renal system, hypersensitivity

Precautions: Pregnancy **C**, seizure disorders, bronchial asthma, coronary occlusion, hyperthyroidism, dysrhythmias, peptic ulcer, megacolon, poor GI motility, bradycardia, hypotension

Pharmacokinetics	
Absorption	Unknown
Distribution	Unknown
Metabolism	Unknown
Excretion	Unknown
Half-life	Unknown

Pharmacodynamics

	IM	IV
Onset	2-10 min	30-60 sec
Peak	Unknown	Unknown
Duration	12-45 min	6-25 min

Interactions

Individual drugs

Atropine, haloperidol, magnesium, procainamide, quinidine: decreased action of edrophonium

Digitalis: increased bradycardia

Drug classifications

Anesthetics, antidysrhythmics, antihistamines, corticosteroids, phenothiazines: decreased action of edrophonium

Muscle relaxants, depolarizing: increased action of muscle relaxant

NURSING CONSIDERATIONS

Assessment

- Assess vital signs, respiration during test
- Monitor diabetic patient carefully, this drug lowers blood glucose

Nursing diagnoses

- Breathing pattern, ineffective (uses)
- Knowledge, deficient (teaching)

Implementation

IV route

- Administer undiluted 2 mg or less over 15-30 sec, or give as continuous inf in myasthenia crisis
- ◆ Give only after ensuring that atropine sulfate is available for cholinergic crisis
- Give only after all other cholinergics have been discontinued
- Store at room temp

Y-site compatibilities: Heparin, hydrocortisone, potassium chloride, vit B/C

Patient/family education

- Instruct patient to carry/wear emergency ID specifying myasthenia gravis and drugs taken

Evaluation

Positive therapeutic outcome

- Increased muscle strength, hand grasp; improved gait; absence of labored breathing (if severe)

Treatment of overdose: Respiratory support, atropine 1-4 mg (**IV**)

efavirenz (Rx)

(ef-ah-veer'enz)

Sustiva

Func. class.: Antiretroviral

Chem. class.: Nonnucleoside reverse transcriptase inhibitor (NNRTI)

Pregnancy category D

Action: Binds directly to reverse transcriptase and blocks RNA, DNA causing a disruption of the enzyme's site

Therapeutic Outcome: Improvement of HIV-1 infection

Uses: HIV-1 in combination with other antiretrovirals

Dosage and routes

Given in combination with protease inhibitor or nucleoside analog reverse transcriptase inhibitors (NRTIs)

Adult and child >40 kg: PO 600 mg daily at bedtime

Child:

10-15 kg: PO 200 mg daily at bedtime
15-20 kg: PO 250 mg daily at bedtime
20-25 kg: PO 300 mg daily at bedtime
25-32.5 kg: PO 350 mg daily at bedtime
32.5-40 kg: PO 400 mg daily at bedtime

Available forms: Caps 50, 100, 200, 600 mg

Adverse effects

CNS: Headache, dizziness, fatigue, impaired concentration, insomnia, abnormal dreams, depression, anxiety, drowsiness

GI: *Diarrhea,* abdominal pain, *nausea,* hyperlipidemia

GU: Hematuria, kidney stones

INTEG: *Rash,* **erythema multiforme, Stevens-Johnson syndrome, toxic epidermal necrolysis**

Contraindications: Pregnancy **D**, hypersensitivity

Precautions: Liver disease, lactation, children <3 yr, renal disease, myelosuppression, depression, seizures

Pharmacokinetics

Absorption	Well
Distribution	Highly protein bound (99%)
Metabolism	Liver
Excretion	Kidneys, feces
Half-life	Terminal 52-76 hr

Pharmacodynamics	
Peak	3-5 hr

Interactions

Individual drugs

Alcohol: increased CNS depression
Clarithromycin, indinavir, methadone, saquinavir: decreased level of each specific drug
Midazolam, triazolam, warfarin: increased level of each specific drug
Cisapride, midazolam, triazolam: do not give together
Ritonavir: increased levels of both drugs

Drug classifications

Anticonvulsants, ergots, statins (except pravastatin, fluvastatin): increased levels of each specific drug
Antidepressants, antihistamines, opioids: increased CNS depression
Benzodiazepines, ergots: do not give together
Estrogens: increased level of both drugs
Rifamycins: decreased efavirenz action

Drug/herb

St. John's wort: do not use together

Drug/food

Increased: absorption of high-fat foods

Drug/lab test

Increased: ALT
False positive: cannabinoids

NURSING CONSIDERATIONS

Assessment

- Assess signs of infection, anemia
- Assess liver studies: ALT, AST; renal studies
- Assess bowel pattern before, during treatment; if severe abdominal pain with bleeding occurs, drug should be discontinued; monitor hydration
- Assess skin eruptions; rash, urticaria, itching
- Assess allergies before treatment, reaction to each medication
- Assess CBC, blood chemistry, plasma HIV RNA, absolute $CD4^+/CD8^+$/cell counts/%, serum β_2 microglobulin, serum ICD+24 antigen levels, cholesterol, hepatic enzymes
- Assess for signs of toxicity: severe nausea/vomiting, maculopapular rash

Nursing diagnoses

- Infection, risk for (uses)
- Diarrhea (side effects)
- Knowledge, deficient (teaching)

Implementation

- Give at bedtime to decrease CNS side effects, give on empty stomach

Patient/family education

- Inform patient that drug does not cure disease but controls symptoms, HIV still can be transmitted to others
- Advise patient to take as prescribed; if dose is missed, take as soon as remembered; do not double dose, take on empty stomach with water/juice
- Instruct patient to make sure health care provider knows of all the medications being taken, supplements, herbs, OTC drugs
- Advise patient that if severe rash occurs, stop taking and notify health care provider
- Advise patient not to breastfeed or become pregnant (serious birth defects have occured) if taking this drug
- Advise patient that adverse reactions: rash, dizziness, abnormal dreams, insomnia, lessen after a month
- Teach patient to avoid hazardous activities if dizziness, drowsiness occurs

Evaluation

Positive therapeutic outcome

- Increased CD4, cell counts
- Decreased viral load
- Improvement in symptoms and progression of HIV-1 infection

eletriptan (Rx)

(el-ee-trip'tan)
Relpax
Func. class.: Antimigraine agent
Pregnancy category C

Action: Binds selectively to the vascular 5-HT_1-receptor subtype, exerts antimigraine effect; causes vasoconstriction in cranial arteries

Therapeutic Outcome: Decreased severity of migraine

Uses: Acute treatment of migraine with or without aura

Dosage and routes

Adult: **PO** 20 mg, may increase if needed, max 40 mg (single dose); may repeat in 2 hr if headache improves but returns, max 80 mg/day

Available forms: Tabs 20, 40 mg

Adverse effects

CNS: *Dizziness,* headache, anxiety, paresthesia, asthenia, somnolence, flushing, fatigue, hot/cold sensation
CV: Chest pain, palpitations, hypertension

GI: Nausea, dry mouth
MS: Weakness
RESP: Chest tightness, pressure

Contraindications: Concurrent use of ergotamine-containing preparations, uncontrolled hypertension, hypersensitivity, basilar or hemiplegic migraine; ischemic bowel disease; severe hepatic disease; coronary artery vasospasm; peripheral vascular disease; heart disease

Precautions: Postmenopausal women, men >40 yr, risk factors of CAD, MI, or other cardiac disease, hypercholesterolemia, obesity, diabetes, impaired hepatic or renal function, pregnancy **C**, lactation, children, elderly

Pharmacokinetics

Absorption	Unknown
Distribution	Unknown
Metabolism	Liver
Excretion	Urine, feces
Half-life	Unknown

Pharmacodynamics

Onset	Of pain relief 2 hr
Peak	Unknown
Duration	Unknown

Interactions

Individual drugs

Clarithromycin, erythromycin, itraconazole, ketoconazole, nelfinavir, propanolol, ritonavir: increased plasma concentration of eletriptan

Drug classifications

CYP3A4 inhibitors: increased concentration of eletriptan

Drug/herb

Butterbur: increased effect

NURSING CONSIDERATIONS

Assessment

- Monitor B/P; signs/symptoms of coronary vasospasms
- Assess for tingling, hot sensation, burning, feeling of pressure, numbness, flushing
- Assess stress level, activity, recreation, coping mechanisms
- Assess neurologic status: LOC, blurring vision, nausea, vomiting, tingling in extremities preceding headache
- Identify ingestion of tyramine foods (pickled products, beer, wine, aged cheese), food additives, preservatives, colorings, artificial sweeteners, chocolate, caffeine, which may precipitate these types of headaches

Nursing diagnoses

- Pain, acute (uses)
- Knowledge, deficient (teaching)

Implementation

- Swallow tabs whole; do not break, crush, or chew
- Provide quiet, calm environment with decreased stimulation from noise, bright light, excessive talking

Patient/family education

- Have patient report any side effects to prescriber
- Teach patient to use contraception while taking drug
- Teach patient to have dark, quiet environment
- Teach patient that drug does not prevent or reduce number of migraine attacks

Evaluation

Positive therapeutic outcome

- Decreased in severity of migraine

emtricitabine (Rx)

(em-tri-sit′uh-bean)

Emtriva

Func. class.: Antiretroviral

Chem. class.: Nucleoside reverse transcriptase inhibitor (NRTI)

Pregnancy category B

Action: Synthetic nucleoside analog of cytosine; inhibits replication of HIV virus by competing with the natural substrate and then becoming incorporated into cellular DNA by viral reverse transcriptase, thereby terminating cellular DNA chain

Therapeutic Outcome: Decreasing symptoms of HIV

Uses: HIV-1 infection with other antiretrovirals.

Dosage and routes

Adult: PO 200 mg daily

Renal dose

Adult: PO CCr 30-49 ml/min 200 mg q48h; 15-29 ml/min 200 mg q72h; <15 ml/min 200 mg q96h

Available forms: Caps 200 mg

Adverse effects

CNS: Headache, abnormal dreams, depression, dizziness, insomnia, neuropathy, paresthesia
GI: Nausea, vomiting, diarrhea, anorexia, abdominal pain, dyspepsia

INTEG: Rash, skin discoloration
MS: Arthralgia, myalgia
RESP: Cough
SYST: Change in body fat distribution

Contraindications: Hypersensitivity

Precautions: Pregnancy **B**, lactation, children, elderly, renal disease, hepatic insufficiency, chronic hepatitis B

Pharmacokinetics	
Absorption	Rapidly, extensively absorbed
Distribution	Protein binding <4%
Metabolism	Unknown
Excretion	Excreted unchanged in urine (86%), feces (14%)
Half-life	10 hr

Pharmacodynamics	
Onset	Unknown
Peak	1-2 hr
Duration	Unknown

Interactions: None known

NURSING CONSIDERATIONS

Assessment

- Monitor liver, renal function tests: AST, ALT, bilirubin, amylase, lipase, triglycerides periodically during treatment
- Assess for lactic acidosis, severe hepatomegaly with steatosis; if lab reports confirm these conditions, discontinue treatment

Nursing diagnoses

- Infection, risk for (uses)
- Injury, risk for (adverse reactions)
- Knowledge, deficient (teaching)

Implementation

- Give without regard to meals
- Store at 25° C (77° F)
- Take at same time every day

Patient/family education

- Teach that GI complaints resolve after 3-4 wk of treatment
- Advise not to breastfeed while taking this drug
- Instruct that drug must be taken at same time of day to maintain blood level
- Advise that drug will control symptoms, but is not a cure for HIV; patient is still infectious, may pass HIV virus on to others
- Instruct that other drugs may be necessary to prevent other infections
- Advise that changes in body fat distribution may occur

Evaluation

Positive therapeutic outcome

- Decrease in signs/symptoms of HIV

enalapril/enalaprilat (Rx)

(e-nal'april/e-nal'a-pril-at)

Vasotec, Vasotec IV

Func. class.: Antihypertensive

Chem. class.: Angiotensin-converting enzyme (ACE) inhibitor

Pregnancy category
C (1st trimester),
D (2nd/3rd trimesters)

Do Not Confuse:
enalapril/Eldepryl, enalapril/ramipril/Anafranil

Action: Selectively suppresses renin-angiotensin-aldosterone system; inhibits ACE; prevents conversion of angiotensin I to angiotensin II, resulting in dilatation of arterial and venous vessels

Therapeutic Outcome: Decreased B/P in hypertension; decreased preload, afterload in CHF

Uses: Hypertension, CHF, left ventricular dysfunction

Dosage and routes

Hypertension

Adult: PO 5 mg/day, may increase or decrease to desired response; range 10-40 mg/day

Adult: **IV** 1.25 mg q6h over 5 min

Child: PO 0.08 mg/kg/day in 1-2 divided doses, max 0.58 mg/kg/day

Child: **IV** 5-10 mcg/kg/dose q8-24h

Patients on diuretics

Adult: **IV** 0.625 mg over 5 min, may give additional doses of 1.25 mg q6h

Renal dose

Adult: PO 2.5 mg daily (CCr <30 ml/min) increase gradually; **IV** CCr >30 ml/min 1.25 mg q6h; CCr <30 ml/min 0.625 mg as one-time dose, increase as per B/P

CHF

Adult: PO 2.5-20 mg/day in 2 divided doses, max 40 mg daily in divided doses

Available forms: Enalapril: tabs 2.5, 5, 10, 20 mg; enalaprilat: inj 1.25 mg/ml

Adverse effects

CNS: *Insomnia, dizziness,* paresthesias, headache, fatigue, anxiety

CV: *Hypotension,* chest pain, tachycardia, **dysrhythmias**, syncope, angina, **MI**, orthostatic hypotension
EENT: *Tinnitus,* visual changes, sore throat, double vision, dry burning eyes
GI: Nausea, vomiting, colitis, cramps, diarrhea, constipation, flatulence, dry mouth, loss of taste
GU: **Proteinuria, renal failure,** increased frequency of polyuria or oliguria
HEMA: **Agranulocytosis, neutropenia**
INTEG: Rash, purpura, alopecia, hyperhidrosis, photosensitivity
META: Hyperkalemia
RESP: Dyspnea, dry cough, crackles, angioedema

Contraindications: Pregnancy **D** (2nd/3rd trimesters), hypersensitivity, history of angioedema

Precautions: Pregnancy **C** (1st trimester), renal disease, hyperkalemia, hepatic failure, dehydration, bilateral renal artery stenosis, lactation

Pharmacokinetics

Absorption	Well absorbed (PO), complete (**IV**)
Distribution	Unknown
Metabolism	Liver (active metabolite—enalaprilat)
Excretion	Kidneys (60%—enalaprilat, 20%—enalapril)
Half-life	Enalaprilat 11 hr, increased in renal disease

Pharmacodynamics

	PO	IV
Onset	1 hr	15 min
Peak	4-6 hr	1-4 hr
Duration	24 hr	6 hr

Interactions
Individual drugs
Alcohol: increased hypotension (large amounts)
Allopurinol: increased hypersensitivity
CycloSPORINE, indomethacin: increased potassium levels
Digoxin, lithium: increased serum levels
Rifampin: decreased effects of enalapril
Drug classifications
α-Adrenergic blockers, diuretics, general anesthesia, nitrates, other antihypertensives, phenothiazines: increased hypotension
Antacids: decreased absorption
Diuretics (potassium-sparing), potassium supplements, salt substitutes: increased potassium levels
Drug/herb
Arginine: fatal hypokalemia
Pill-bearing spurge: increased effect
Pineapple, yobimbe: decreased effect
St. John's wort: severe photosensitivity
Drug/lab test
Increased: ALT, AST, bilirubin, alkaline phosphatase, glucose, uric acid
False positive: ANA titer

NURSING CONSIDERATIONS
Assessment
- Monitor blood studies: neutrophils, decreased platelets with differential baseline and q3 mo if neutrophils <1000/mm^3, discontinue treatment
- Monitor B/P, orthostatic hypotension, syncope; if changes occur dosage change may be required; obtain peak/trough levels
- Monitor electrolytes: K, Na, Cl during 1st 2 wk of therapy
- Monitor renal studies: protein, BUN, creatinine; increased levels may indicate nephrotic syndrome and renal failure
- Monitor renal symptoms: polyuria, oliguria, frequency, dysuria
- Establish baselines in renal, liver function tests before therapy begins and 1 wk into therapy
- Check potassium levels throughout treatment, although hyperkalemia rarely occurs
- Check for edema in feet, legs daily
- Assess for allergic reactions: rash, fever, pruritus, urticaria; drug should be discontinued if antihistamines fail to help

Nursing diagnoses
- Cardiac output, decreased (uses)
- Injury, risk for (adverse reactions)
- Knowledge, deficient (teaching)
- Noncompliance (teaching)

Implementation
PO route
- Store in air-tight container at 86° F (30° C) or less
- Severe hypotension may occur after 1st dose of this medication; decreased hypotension may be prevented by reducing or discontinuing diuretic therapy 3 days before beginning benazepril therapy
- Give by **IV** inf of 0.9% NaCl (as ordered) to expand fluid volume if severe hypotension occurs

IV route
- Give **IV** direct over 5 min

- Dilute in 50 ml of 0.9% NaCl, D_5W, D_5/0.9% NaCl, D_5/LR; diluted solution may be used for 24 hr

Y-site compatibilities: Allopurinol, amifostine, amikacin, aminophylline, ampicillin, ampicillin/sulbactam, aztreonam, butorphanol, calcium gluconate, cefazolin, cefoperazone, ceftazidime, ceftizoxime, chloramphenicol, cimetidine, cladribine, clindamycin, dextran 40, DOBUTamine, DOPamine, erythromycin lactobionate, esmolol, famotidine, fentanyl, filgrastim, ganciclovir, gentamicin, granisetron, heparin, hetastarch, hydrocortisone, labetalol, lidocaine, magnesium sulfate, melphalan, meropenem, methylPREDNISolone, metronidazole, morphine, nafcillin, niCARdipine, penicillin G potassium, phenobarbital, piperacillin, piperacillin/tazobactam, potassium chloride, potassium phosphate, propofol, ranitidine, teniposide, thiotepa, tobramycin, trimethoprim/sulfamethoxazole, vancomycin, vinorelbine

Y-site incompatibilities: Amphotericin B, phenytoin

Additive compatibilities: DOBUTamine, DOPamine, heparin, meropenem, nitroglycerin, nitroprusside, potassium chloride

Patient/family education

- Advise patient not to discontinue drug abruptly; advise patient to tell all persons associated with health care that drug is being taken
- Teach patient not to use OTC products (cough, cold, allergy medications) unless directed by physician, to avoid potassium, salt substitutes; serious side effects can occur; xanthines, such as coffee, tea, chocolate, cola can prevent action of drug
- Instruct patient on the importance of complying with dosage schedule, even if feeling better; to continue with medical regimen to decrease B/P: exercise, cessation of smoking, decreasing stress, diet modifications
- Emphasize the need to rise slowly to sitting or standing position to minimize orthostatic hypotension; not to exercise in hot weather, which can cause increased hypotension
- Advise patient to notify prescriber of mouth sores, sore throat, fever, swelling of hands or feet, irregular heartbeat, chest pain, coughing, shortness of breath
- Caution patient to report excessive perspiration, dehydration, vomiting, diarrhea; may lead to fall in B/P
- Caution patient that drug may cause skin rash or impaired perspiration; that angioedema may occur and to discontinue if it occurs
- Caution patient that drug may cause dizziness, fainting, light-headedness; may occur during 1st few days of therapy; to avoid activities that may be hazardous
- Teach patient how to take B/P, and normal readings for age-group

Evaluation

Positive therapeutic outcome

- Decreased B/P in hypertension

Treatment of overdose: Lavage, **IV** atropine for bradycardia; **IV** theophylline for bronchospasm, digitalis, O_2; diuretic for cardiac failure, hemodialysis

enfuvirtide (Rx)

(en-fyoo'vir-tide)

Fuzeon

Func. class.: Antiretroviral

Chem. class.: Fusion inhibitor

Pregnancy category B

Action: Inhibitor of the fusion of HIV-1 with CD4+ cells

Therapeutic Outcome: Decreasing symptoms of HIV

Uses: Treatment of HIV-1 infection in combination with other antiretrovirals

Dosage and routes

Adult: SUBCUT 90 mg (1 ml) bid

Child 6-16 yr: SUBCUT 2 mg/kg bid, max 90 mg bid

Available forms: Powder for inj, lyophilized 108 mg (90 mg/ml when reconstituted)

Adverse effects

CNS: Anxiety, peripheral neuropathy, taste disturbance, **Guillain-Barré syndrome,** insomnia, depression

GI: Abdominal pain, anorexia, constipation, pancreatitis

GU: **Glomerulonephritis, renal failure**

HEMA: **Thrombocytopenia, neutropenia**

INTEG: Inj site reactions

MISC: Influenza, cough, conjunctivitis, lymphadenopathy, myalgias, hyperglycemia, pneumonia, rhinitis, fatigue

Contraindications: Hypersensitivity

Precautions: Pregnancy **B**, liver disease, lactation, children <6 yr, myelosuppression, infections

Pharmacokinetics

Absorption	Well
Distribution	92% protein binding
Metabolism	Undergoes catabolism
Excretion	Unknown
Half-life	Terminal 3.8 hr

Pharmacodynamics

Onset	Unknown
Peak	8 hrs
Duration	Unknown

Interactions: None known

NURSING CONSIDERATIONS
Assessment
- Assess for signs of infection, inj site reactions
- Monitor renal studies: BUN, creatinine, renal failure may occur
- Monitor bowel pattern before, during treatment; if severe abdominal pain or constipation occurs, notify prescriber; monitor hydration
- Assess skin eruptions, rash, urticaria, itching
- Identify allergies before treatment, reaction to each medication
- CBC, blood chemistry, plasma HIV RNA, absolute CD4+/CD8+ cell counts/%, serum β_2 microglobulin, serum ICD+24 antigen levels, cholesterol

Nursing diagnoses
- Infection, risk for (uses)
- Injury, risk for (adverse reactions)
- Knowledge, deficient (teaching)

Implementation
- Give SUBCUT, bid, rotate sites

Patient/family education
- Instruct to notify prescriber if pregnancy is suspected, or if breastfeeding
- Advise that pneumonia may occur, to contact prescriber if cough, fever occur
- Teach that hypersensitive reactions may occur, rash, pruritus; stop drug, contact prescriber
- Teach that this drug is not a cure for HIV-1 infection but controls symptoms, HIV-1 can still be transmitted to others
- Teach that this drug is to be used in combination only with other antiretrovirals

Evaluation
Positive therapeutic outcome
- Increased CD4 cell counts; decreased viral load; slowing progression of HIV-1 infection

enoxacin (Rx)
(en-ox'a-sin)

Penetrex

Func. class.: Antiinfective

Chem. class.: Fluoroquinolone

Pregnancy category C

Do Not Confuse:
enoxacin/enoxaparin

Action: Interferes with conversion of intermediate DNA fragments into high molecular weight DNA in bacteria; DNA gyrase inhibitor

Therapeutic Outcome: Bactericidal against the following organisms: staphylococci, *Enterobacter* sp, *Escherichia coli, Klebsiella* sp, *Neisseria gonorrhoeae, Pseudomonas aeruginosa*

Uses: Uncomplicated urethral or cervical gonorrhea, uncomplicated and complicated UTI

Dosage and routes
Gonorrhea

Adult: PO 400 mg as a single dose

Uncomplicated UTI

Adult: PO 200 mg q12h × 7 days

Complicated UTI

Adult: PO 400 mg q12h × 14 days

Renal dose

Adult: PO CCr <30 ml/min give initial dose, then give 50% of dose q12h

Available forms: Tabs 200, 400 mg

Adverse effects
CNS: *Dizziness, headache,* fatigue, somnolence, depression, insomnia, anxiety, **seizures**

EENT: Visual disturbances, dizziness

GI: *Diarrhea, nausea, vomiting,* anorexia, flatulence, heartburn, abdominal pain, dry mouth, increased AST, ALT, **pseudomembranous colitis**

INTEG: Rash, pruritus, photosensitivity

SYST: **Anaphylaxis, Stevens-Johnson syndrome**

Contraindications: Hypersensitivity to quinolones

Precautions: Pregnancy **C,** lactation, children, elderly, renal disease, seizure disorders

Pharmacokinetics

Absorption	Well absorbed
Distribution	Widely
Metabolism	Liver 20%
Excretion	Kidneys 50%-80%
Half-life	3-6 hr, increased in renal disease

Pharmacodynamics

Onset	Unknown
Peak	Unknown

Interactions

Individual drugs

Aluminum, iron salts, sucralfate: decreased enoxacin absorption
Aminophylline: increased level of aminophylline
Bismuth subsalicylate: decreased enoxacin level, decreased effects of enoxacin
Cimetidine: increased levels of cimetidine
CycloSPORINE: increased levels of cycloSPORINE
Digoxin: increased digoxin levels, monitor for toxicity
Theophylline: increased toxicity, do not use together
Warfarin: increased levels of warfarin

Drug classifications

Antacids, magnesium: decreased enoxacin absorption
Oral anticoagulants: increased anticoagulation

Drug/herb

Acidophilus: do not use with antiinfectives

Drug/food

Decreased: absorption, dairy products

NURSING CONSIDERATIONS

Assessment

- Assess patient for previous sensitivity reaction to quinolones
- Assess patient for signs and symptoms of infection including WBC >10,000/mm^3, hematuria, foul-smelling urine; obtain baseline information before and during treatment
- Complete C&S testing before beginning drug therapy; this will identify if correct treatment has been initiated
- Assess for anaphylaxis: rash, urticaria, pruritus; may occur a few days after therapy begins, emergency equipment should be available
- Identify urine output; also monitor increases in BUN, creatinine
- Monitor blood studies: AST, ALT, alkaline phosphatase

Nursing diagnoses

- Infection, risk for (uses)
- Diarrhea (adverse reactions)
- Knowledge, deficient (teaching)
- Noncompliance (teaching)

Implementation

- Give 1 hr ac or 2 hr pc to maintain proper blood levels
- Give with 8 oz of water, 1 hr before bedtime to prevent ulceration
- Do not give 4 hr before or 2 hr after medication
- Give 2 hr before or 2 hr after antacids, zinc, iron, or calcium
- Increase fluids to 2 L/day

Patient/family education

- Instruct patient to increase fluids to 2 L/day to prevent crystallization in the kidney
- Instruct patient to report itching, rash, pruritus, urticaria
- Instruct patient to contact prescriber if adverse reactions occur or if inflammation or pain of tendon occurs
- Instruct patient to take all medication prescribed for the length of time ordered; drug must be taken as ordered
- Advise patient to limit intake of alkaline foods and drugs: milk, dairy products, peanuts, vegetables, alkaline antacids, sodium bicarbonate, not to double or miss doses
- Advise patient to ambulate, perform activities with assistance, do not perform hazardous activities
- Advise to avoid OTC medications unless approved by prescriber

Evaluation

Positive therapeutic outcome

- Reported improvement in symptoms of infection
- Negative C&S test results

! HIGH ALERT

enoxaparin (Rx)

(ee-nox'a-par-in)

Lovenox

Func. class.: Anticoagulant, antithrombotic
Chem. class.: Unfractionated porcine heparin (low-molecular-weight heparin)

Pregnancy category B

Do Not Confuse:

enoxaparin/enoxacin
Lovenox/Lotronex

E

Action: Prevents conversion of fibrinogen to fibrin and prothrombin to thrombin by enhancing inhibitory effects of antithrombin III; produces higher ratio of anti-factor Xa to anti-factor IIa

Therapeutic Outcome: Prevention of deep vein thrombosis

Uses: Prevention of deep vein thrombosis, pulmonary emboli in hip and knee replacement, abdominal surgery at risk for thrombosis; unstable angina/non–Q-wave MI

Dosage and routes

DVT prevention before hip/knee surgery

Adult: SUBCUT 30 mg bid given 12-24 hr postoperatively for 7-10 days, provided that hemostasis has been established

DVT prevention before hip replacement

Adult: SUBCUT 40 mg daily started 12 hr preop or 30 mg q12h started 12-24 hr postop

DVT prophylaxis before abdominal surgery

Adult: SUBCUT 40 mg daily × 7-10 days to prevent thromboembolic complications, start 2 hr before surgery

DVT/PE

Adult: SUBCUT (outpatient without PE) 1 mg/kg q12h or 1.5 mg/kg daily (outpatient/inpatient)

Prevention of ischemic complications in unstable angina/non–Q-wave MI with aspirin

Adult: SUBCUT 1 mg/kg q12h until stable with aspirin 100-325 mg daily

Available forms: Inj 30 mg/0.3 ml, 40 mg/0.4 ml, 60 mg/0.6 ml, 80 mg/0.8 ml, 100 mg/1 ml, 120 mg/0.8 ml, 150 mg/ml, 300 mg/3 ml

Adverse effects

CNS: Fever, confusion

GI: Nausea

HEMA: **Hemorrhage, hypochromic anemia, thrombocytopenia,** bleeding

INTEG: Ecchymosis, inj site hematoma

SYST: Edema, peripheral edema

Contraindications: Hypersensitivity to this drug, heparin, or pork; hemophilia; leukemia with bleeding; peptic ulcer disease; thrombocytopenic purpura, heparin-induced thrombocytoparia, increased risk of bleeding

Precautions: Pregnancy **B,** alcoholism, elderly, hepatic disease (severe), renal disease (severe), blood dyscrasias, severe hypertension, subacute bacterial endocarditis, acute nephritis, lactation, children, recent burn, spinal surgery

Pharmacokinetics

Absorption	Well absorbed (90%)
Distribution	Unknown
Metabolism	Unknown
Excretion	Kidneys
Half-life	4½ hr

Pharmacodynamics

Onset	Unknown
Peak	3-5 hr
Duration	Unknown

Interactions

Drug classifications

Anticoagulants, antiplatelets, NSAIDs, salicylates, thrombolytics: increased bleeding

Drug/herb

Agrimony, alfalfa, angelica, anise, basil, bay, bilberry, black haw, bogbean, bromelain, buchu, chondroitin, cinchona bark, dong quai, fenugreek, feverfew, garlic, ginger, ginkgo, ginseng, horse chestnut, Irish moss, kelp, kelpware, khella, lovage, lungwort, meadowsweet, motherwort, mugwort, nettle, papaya, parsley (large amounts), pau d'arco, pineapple, poplar, prickly ash, safflower, saw palmetto, tonka bean, turmeric, wintergreen, yarrow: increased risk of bleeding

Chamomile, coenzyme Q10, flax, glucomannan, goldenseal, guar gum: decreased anticoagulant effect

Drug/lab test

Increased: AST/ALT

Decreased: platelets

NURSING CONSIDERATIONS

Assessment

- Monitor blood studies (Hct, CBC, coagulation studies, occult blood in stools), anti-Xa levels q3 mo; platelet count q2-3 days; thrombocytopenia may occur
- Assess patient for bleeding gums, petechiae, ecchymosis, black tarry stools, hematuria, epistaxis, decrease in B/P; indicate bleeding and possible hemorrhage; notify prescriber immediately
- Assess for neurosymptoms in patients that have received spinal anesthesia

Nursing diagnoses

- Injury, risk for (uses, adverse reactions)
- Tissue perfusion, ineffective (uses)
- Knowledge, deficient (teaching)

Implementation
- Give at same time each day to maintain steady blood levels
- Administer SUBCUT deeply; do not give IM, begin 2 hr before surgery, do not aspirate, do not expel bubble from syringe before administration; sol is clear to yellow; do not use sol with precipitate; apply gentle pressure for 1 min
- Leave vascular access sheath in place for 6 hr after dose, then give next dose, 6 hr after sheath removed
- Do not mix with other drugs or infusion fluids
- Give to recumbent patient, rotate sites (left/right anterolateral, left/right posterolateral abdominal wall)
- Only this drug when ordered; not interchangeable with heparin or LMWHs

Patient/family education
- Warn patient to avoid OTC preparations unless directed by prescriber because they could cause serious drug interactions
- Instruct patient to use soft-bristled toothbrush to avoid bleeding gums; to avoid contact sports; to use electric razor; to avoid IM inj
- Advise patient to report any signs of bleeding, bruising: gums, under skin, urine, stools

Evaluation
Positive therapeutic outcome
- Absence of deep vein thrombosis

entacapone (Rx)
(en-ta'-ka-pone)
Comtan
Func. class.: Antiparkinsonian agent
Chem. class.: COMT
Pregnancy category C

Action: Inhibits COMT (catechol *O*-methyltransferase) and alters the plasma pharmacokinetics of levodopa; given with levodopa/carbidopa

Therapeutic Outcome: Decreased symptoms of Parkinson's disease (involuntary movements)

Uses: Parkinsonism in those experiencing end of dose, decreased effect as an adjunct to levodopa/carbidopa

Dosage and routes
Adult: PO 200 mg given with carbidopa/levodopa, max 1600 mg/day

Available forms: Tabs 200 mg film coated

Adverse effects
CNS: *Involuntary choreiform movements, dyskinesia, hypokinesia, hyperkinesia, hand tremors, fatigue, headache, anxiety, twitching, numbness, weakness, confusion, agitation, nightmares,* psychosis, hallucinations, hypomania, severe depression, dizziness, **neuroleptic malignant syndrome**
CV: *Orthostatic hypotension*
GI: *Nausea, vomiting, anorexia, abdominal distress, dry mouth, flatulence, dyspepsia,* gastritis, GI disorder, *diarrhea, constipation,* bitter taste
INTEG: Rash, sweating, alopecia
MISC: Dark urine and other body fluids, back pain, dyspnea, purpura, fatigue, asthenia, infection-bacterial, **rhabdomyolysis**

Contraindications: Hypersensitivity

Precautions: Pregnancy **C**, renal, hepatic disease, affective disorders, psychosis, lactation, children

Pharmacokinetics	
Absorption	Well absorbed
Distribution	Protein binding 98%
Metabolism	Liver extensively
Excretion	Kidneys, feces; breast milk
Half-life	0.5 hr initial, 2.5 hr second

Pharmacodynamics	
Onset	Unknown
Peak	Unknown
Duration	≤8 hr

Interactions
Individual drugs
Ampicillin, chloramphenicol, erythromycin, rifampin: decreased excretion of entacapone
Apomorphine, bitolterol, DOBUTamine, DOPamine, epINEPHrine, isoetharine, methyldopa, norepinephrine: increased CV reactions, avoid use
Cholestyramine: decreased excretion
Probenecid: may decrease excretion of entacapone
Drug classifications
MAOIs: prevents catecholamine metabolism, do not use together
Drug/herb
Kava: decreased effect

NURSING CONSIDERATIONS

Assessment

- Assess for neuroleptic malignant syndrome: high temp, increased CPK, rigidity, change in consciousness
- Monitor B/P, respiration during initial treatment; hypotension should be reported
- Assess mental status: affect, mood, behavioral changes, depression; complete suicide assessment
- Monitor liver function enzymes: AST, ALT, alkaline phosphatase; also check LDH, bilirubin, CBC
- Assess for involuntary movements in parkinsonism: akinesia, tremors, staggering gait, muscle rigidity, drooling; these symptoms should improve with therapy when given with levodopa/carbidopa

Nursing diagnoses

- Mobility, impaired (uses)
- Injury, risk for (uses)
- Knowledge, deficient (teaching)
- Noncompliance (teaching)

Implementation

- Adjust dosage to patient response
- Give with meals to decrease GI upset; limit protein taken with drug
- Give only after MAOIs have been discontinued for 2 wk

Patient/family education

- Advise patient that hallucinations, mental changes, nausea, dyskinesia can occur
- Caution patient to change positions slowly to prevent orthostatic hypotension; not to drive or operate machinery until stabilized on medication and mental performance is not affected
- Instruct patient to use drug exactly as prescribed
- Inform patient that urine, sweat may darken
- Inform patient to notify prescriber if pregnancy is suspected; if lactating, drug is excreted in breast milk

Evaluation

Positive therapeutic outcome

- Decreased akathisia, other involuntary movements when used with levodopa/carbidopa
- Increased mood when used with levodopa/carbidopa

entecavir

Baraclude

See Appendix A, Selected New Drugs

! HIGH ALERT

epHEDrine (Rx, OTC)

(e-fed′rin)

epHEDrine sulfate, Pretz-D

Func. class.: Bronchodilator, nonselective, adrenergic, mixed direct and indirect effects; bronchodilator, nasal decongestant, vasopressor

Chem. class.: Phenylisopropylamine

Pregnancy category C

Do Not Confuse:
epHEDrine/epINEPHrine

Action: Increases contractility and heart rate by acting on β-receptors in the heart; also acts on α-receptors, causing vasoconstriction in blood vessels

Therapeutic Outcome: Decreased nasal congestion, bronchodilatation, stimulation, increased B/P

Uses: Shock; increased perfusion; hypotension, bronchodilatation; nasal congestion; orthostatic hypotension, depression, narcolepsy; vasopressor

Dosage and routes

Bronchodilator

Adult and child >12 yr: PO 12.5-50 mg q3-4h prn, max 150 mg/24 hr; NASAL 2-3 sprays in each nostril q4h

Child 2-12 yr: PO 2-3 mg/kg or 100 mg/m^2/day in 4-6 divided doses

Child 6-12 yr: PO 6.25-12.5 mg q4h, max 75 mg/24 hr; NASAL 1-2 sprays in each nostril q4h

Nasal decongestant

Adult: Fill dropper to the level marked, then use in each nostril q4h or less

Adult and child >6 yr: Nasal 1-2 sprays in each nostril prn q4h for <3-4 days

Child: PO 3 mg/kg/day or 100 mg/m^2/day in 4-6 divided doses

Hypotension

Adult: PO 25 mg daily-qid; IM/SUBCUT 25-50 mg; **IV** 10-25 mg max 150 mg/24 hr

Child: SUBCUT/**IV** 25-100 mg/m^2/day in 4-6 divided doses

Available forms: Inj 25, 30, 50 mg/ml; caps 25, 50 mg

Adverse effects

CNS: *Tremors, anxiety,* insomnia, sweating, headache, dizziness, confusion, hallucinations, **seizures, CNS depression, cerebral hemorrhage**

CV: Palpitations, tachycardia, hypertension, chest pain, **dysrhythmias**
EENT: Rebound congestion (nasal)
GI: *Anorexia, nausea, vomiting*
GU: Dysuria, urinary retention
RESP: *Dyspnea*

Contraindications: Hypersensitivity to sympathomimetics, narrow-angle glaucoma, nonanaphylactic shock during general anesthesia

Precautions: Pregnancy **C**, cardiac disorders, hyperthyroidism, diabetes mellitus, prostatic hypertrophy, hypertension

Pharmacokinetics

Absorption	Well absorbed (PO/IM/SC) complete (**IV**)
Distribution	Unknown
Metabolism	Liver
Excretion	Kidneys—unchanged
Half-life	3-5 hr

Pharmacodynamics

	PO	SUBCUT	IM	IV	NASAL
Onset	¼-1 hr	Unkn	15-30 min	5 min	Unkn
Peak	Unkn	Unkn	Unkn	Unkn	Unkn
Duration	2-4 hr	1 hr	1 hr	2 hr	6 hr

Interactions
Drug classifications
α-Adrenergic blockers, antidepressants (tricyclic), diuretics, methyldopa, rauwolfia alkaloids, urinary acidifiers: decreased effect of epHEDrine
Anesthetics (halothane), cardiac glycosides, levodopa: increased dysrhythmias
Guanethidine: decreased effect of guanethedine
MAOIs: increased chance of hypertensive crisis, do not use together
Oxytoxics: increased severe hypertension
Sympathomimetics: increased adrenergic side effects
Urinary alkalizers: increased effect of epHEDrine

NURSING CONSIDERATIONS
Assessment
- Monitor respiratory function: vital capacity, forced expiratory volume, ABGs, lung sounds, heart rate, baseline rhythm (bronchodilator)
- Monitor for evidence of allergic reactions; paradoxical bronchospasm; withhold dose; notify prescriber
- Monitor ECG, B/P, pulse, q5 min when using **IV** route (shock)
- Assess for paresthesias and coldness of extremities; peripheral blood flow may decrease; long-term use may produce pseudo anxiety state requiring sedatives, increased lactic acid with severe metabolic acidosis
- Assess nasal congestion to identify factors contributing to ongoing congestion (nasal use)
- Assess mental status and sleeping patterns; mood, sensorium, ability to stay awake

Nursing diagnoses
- Airway clearance, ineffective (uses)
- Gas exchange, impaired (uses)
- Sleep pattern, disturbed (uses)
- Knowledge, deficient (teaching)

Implementation
PO route
- Administer several hr (up to 6 hr) before bedtime to prevent sleeplessness

IV route
- Give **IV** directly undiluted using 3-way stopcock or Y-site; give 10-25 mg slowly, may repeat in 5-10 min
- Use clear sol without precipitate; unused sol should be discarded, protect from light

Syringe compatibilities: Pentobarbital
Y-site compatibilities: Etomidate, propofol
Additive compatibilities: Chloramphenicol, lidocaine, metaraminol, nafcillin, penicillin G potassium
Solution compatibilities: 0.9% NaCl, 0.45% NaCl, D_5W, $D_{10}W$, Ringer's, LR

Patient/family education
- Advise patient to avoid use of OTC medications; extra stimulation may occur, and not to use alcohol

Evaluation
Positive therapeutic outcome
- Increased B/P (vasopressor)
- Ability to stay awake (absence of narcolepsy) or improved mood (absence of depression)
- Absence of bronchospasm
- Decreased nasal congestion

E

! HIGH ALERT

epINEPHrine (Rx, OTC)

(ep-i-nef'rin)

Adrenalin, Ana-Guard, AsthmaHaler Mist, AsthmaNefrin (racepinephrine), Bronitin Mist, Bronkaid Mist, epINEPHrine, Epinal, Epitrate, Eppy/N, Epinephrine Pediatric, EpiPen, EpiPen Jr., Medihaler, microNefrin, Nephron, Primatene Mist, S-2, Sus-Phrine, Vaponefrin (racepinephrine)

Func. class.: Bronchodilator, nonselective adrenergic agonist, cardiac stimulant, vasopressor

Chem. class.: Catecholamine

Pregnancy category C

Do Not Confuse:
epINEPHrine/epHEDrine

Action: β_1- and β_2-agonist causing increased levels of cyclic AMP producing bronchodilatation, cardiac and CNS stimulation; large doses cause vasoconstriction via α-receptors; small doses can cause vasodilatation via β_2-vascular receptors

Therapeutic Outcome: Vasoconstrictor, cardiac stimulator, bronchodilator, decreased aqueous humor

Uses: Acute asthmatic attacks, hemostasis, bronchospasm, anaphylaxis, allergic reactions, cardiac arrest, adjunct in anesthesia, shock

Dosage and routes

Asthma

Adult and child: INH 1-2 puffs of 1:100 or 2.25% racemic q15 min

Bronchodilator

Adult: SUBCUT/IM 0.1-0.5 mg (1:1000 sol) q10-15 min-4 hr, max 1 mg/dose

Anaphylactic reaction/asthma

Adult: SUBCUT/IM 0.1-0.5 mg, repeat q10-15 min, not to exceed 1 mg/dose; epINEPHrine susp 0.5 mg SUBCUT, may repeat 0.5-1.5 mg q6h

Child: SUBCUT 0.01 mg/kg, repeat q15 min × 2 doses, then q4h as needed, up to 0.5 mg/dose; epINEPHrine susp 0.025 mg/kg SUBCUT, may repeat q6h, max 0.75 mg in child ≤30 kg

Cardiac arrest

Adult: **IV** 1 mg q3-5 min, ENDOTRACHEAL 2-25 mg IC 0.3-0.5 mg

Symptomatic bradycardia/pulseless arrest (PALS)

Child: **IV** 0.01 mg/kg, may repeat q3-5 min; endotracheal give 2-10 × **IV** dose diluted to a volume of 3-5 mg of 0.9% NaCl, followed by positive pressure ventilation

Available forms: Aerosol 0.16, 0.2, 0.25 mg/spray, inj 1:1000 (1 mg/ml), 1:200 (5 mg/ml), 0.01 mg/ml (1:100,000), 0.1 mg/ml (1:10,000), 0.5 mg/ml (1:2,000); sol for nebulization 1:100, 1.25% 2.25% (base)

Adverse effects

CNS: *Tremors, anxiety,* insomnia, headache, dizziness, weakness, drowsiness, confusion, hallucinations, **cerebral hemorrhage**

CV: *Palpitations, tachycardia,* hypertension, *dysrhythmias,* increased T-wave

GI: *Anorexia, nausea, vomiting*

RESP: *Dyspnea*

Contraindications: Hypersensitivity to sympathomimetics, narrow-angle glaucoma, nonanaphylactic shock during general anesthesia, organic brain syndrome, local anesthesia of certain areas, labor, cardiac dilation, coronary insufficiency, cerebral arteriosclerosis, organic heart disease

Precautions: Pregnancy **C**, cardiac disorders, hyperthyroidism, diabetes mellitus, prostatic hypertrophy, elderly, lactation, hypertension

Pharmacokinetics

Absorption	Well absorbed (PO), complete (**IV**)
Distribution	Unknown, crosses placenta
Metabolism	Liver
Excretion	Breast milk
Half-life	Unknown

Pharmacodynamics

	SUBCUT	IM	IV	INH
Onset	3-5 min	5-10 min	Immediate	1 min
Peak	Unknown	Unknown	Unknown	Unknown
Duration	1-4 hr	1-4 hr	Unknown	1-4 hr

Interactions

Drug classifications

α-Adrenergic blockers: decreased hypertensive effects

Antidepressants, tricyclic: increased chance of hypertensive crisis; do not use together

MAOIs: increased chance of hypertensive crisis, do not use together
Other sympathomimetics: toxicity

NURSING CONSIDERATIONS

Assessment

- Monitor respiratory function: vital capacity, forced expiratory volume, ABGs, lung sounds, heart rate, rhythm (baseline); amount, color of sputum
- Monitor ECG during administration continuously; if B/P increases, drug should be decreased; check B/P, pulse q5 min after parenteral route; CVP, PCWP, SVR; inadvertent high arterial B/P can result in angina, aortic rupture, cerebral hemorrhage
- Check inj site for tissue sloughing; if this occurs, administer phentolamine mixed with 0.9% NaCl
- Monitor for evidence of allergic reactions, paradoxical bronchospasm, withhold dose, notify prescriber; sulfite sensitivity, which may be life threatening

Nursing diagnoses

- Airway clearance, ineffective (uses)
- Gas exchange, impaired (uses)
- Cardiac output, decreased (uses)
- Sensory perception, disturbed, visual (uses) (ophth)
- Knowledge, deficient (teaching)

Implementation

- Check for correct concentration, route, dosage before administration
- Use this medication before other medications and allow at least 5 min between each to prevent overstimulation

IM/SUBCUT route

- Rotate inj sites, massage well, do not use gluteal (IM) site
- Shake susp before using

Inhalation route

- Use 2.25% sol diluted in nebulizer/respirator
- Rinse mouth after inh
- 10 gtt of a 1% sol should be placed in nebulizer
- Dilute racepinephrine 2.25% sol

Endotracheal route

- Only used in intubated patient; use **IV** dose that should be injected by endotracheal tube into bronchi

IV route

- Give after diluting 1 mg of 1:1000 sol/10 ml or more; 0.9% NaCl yields 1:10,000 sol, give 1 mg/min
- Give by continuous inf after further diluting in 0.9% NaCl, D_5W, $D_{10}W$, D_5/LR, LR via 3-way stopcock; for Y-site, use infusion pump, protect from light; increase dose of insulin in diabetic patients

Syringe compatibilities: Doxapram, heparin, milrinone

Y-site compatibilities: Amrinone, atracurium, calcium chloride, calcium gluconate, diltiazem, DOBUTamine, DOPamine, famotidine, fentanyl, furosemide, heparin, hydrocortisone sodium succinate, hydromorphone, labetalol, lorazepam, midazolam, milrinone, morphine, niCARdipine, nitroglycerin, norepinephrine, pancuronium, phytonadione, potassium chloride, propofol, ranitidine, vecuronium, vit B/C

Y-site incompatibilities: Ampicillin

Additive compatibilities: Amikacin, cimetidine, DOBUTamine, floxacillin, furosemide, metaraminol, ranitidine, verapamil

Additive incompatibilities: Aminophylline, mephentermine, sodium bicarbonate, warfarin

Patient/family education

- Tell patient not to use OTC medications; extra stimulation may occur; to use this medication before other medications and allow at least 5 min between each, to prevent overstimulation
- Teach patient that paradoxical bronchospasm may occur and to stop drug immediately and notify prescriber; to limit caffeine products such as chocolate, coffee, tea, and colas
- Patient should rinse mouth after inh
- Patient should report blurred vision, irritation with ophth preparations

Evaluation

Positive therapeutic outcome

- Absence of dyspnea, wheezing
- Improved airway exchange, improved ABGs
- Decreased aqueous humor
- Stabilization of heart rate and cardiac output

Treatment of overdose: Administer a β_2-adrenergic blocker, vasodilators, α-blocker

! HIGH ALERT

epirubicin (Rx)

(ep-i-roo′-bi-sin)

Ellence

Func. class.: Antineoplastic, antibiotic
Chem. class.: Anthracycline

Pregnancy category D

Action: Inhibits DNA synthesis primarily; replication is decreased by binding to DNA, which causes strand splitting; maximum cytotoxic effects at S and G_2 phases; a vesicant

Therapeutic Outcome: Prevention of rapidly growing malignant cells

Uses: Breast cancer as an adjuvant therapy, with axillary node involvement, after resection

Dosage and routes

Adult: **IV** inf 100-120 mg/m^2 initially given with other antineoplastics (cyclophosphamide, 5-fluorouracil); given in repeated cycles; 3-4 wk cycles

Epirubicin dosage adjustments

Adult: **IV** 100 mg/m^2 on day 1 of each cycle; toxicity nadir platelet counts <50,000 mm^3, ANC 250 mm^3, neutropenic fever or grade 3 or 4 nonhematologic toxicity; next cycle give 75% of day 1 dose; delay next cycle until platelets are ≥100,000 m^3, ANC >1500 mm^3, and nonhematologic toxicities have recovered to < grade 1

Hepatic dose

Adult: **IV**, bilirubin 1.2-3 mg/dl or AST 2-4 × normal upper limit, 50% of starting dose; bilirubin >3 mg/dl or AST >4 × normal upper limit, 25% of starting dose

Available forms: Inj 2 mg/ml

Adverse effects

CV: Increased B/P, **sinus tachycardia, PVCs,** chest pain, **bradycardia, extrasystole, CHF; confirm for doses >900 mg/m^2**

GI: Nausea, vomiting, diarrhea, anorexia, mucositis

GU: *Hot flashes, amenorrhea, hyperuricemia*

HEMA: **Thrombocytopenia, leukopenia, anemia, neutropenia, secondary AML**

INTEG: *Rash, necrosis at inj site, reversible alopecia*

MISC: Infection, febrile neutropenia, lethargy, fever, conjunctivitis

Contraindications: Pregnancy **D,** hypersensitivity to this drug, anthracyclines, anthracenediones, lactation, systemic infections, severe hepatic disease, baseline neutrophil count <1500 cell/mm^3, severe myocardial insufficiency, recent MI

Precautions: Renal, hepatic, cardiac disease, gout, bone marrow suppression (severe), elderly, children

Pharmacokinetics

Absorption	Complete bioavailability
Distribution	Widely distributed, crosses placenta
Metabolism	Liver, extensively
Excretion	Bile (60%)
Half-life	3 min; 2.5 hr; 33 hr

Pharmacodynamics

Unknown

Interactions

Individual drugs

Cimetidine, radiation: increased toxicity

Drug classifications

Antineoplastics: increased toxicity

Live virus vaccines: decreased antibody response

NURSING CONSIDERATIONS

Assessment

- Monitor left ventricular ejection fraction, multigated acquisition scan or echocardiogram, ECG; watch for ST-T wave changes, low QRS and T; possible dysrhythmias (sinus tachycardia, heart block, PVCs) may occur; assess tachypnea, ECG changes, dyspnea, edema, fatigue; cardiac status: B/P, pulse, character, rhythm, rate, ABGs
- Assess for bone marrow depression, infection
- Assess symptoms indicating severe allergic reaction: rash, pruritus, urticaria, purpuric skin lesions, itching, flushing; drug should be discontinued
- Monitor CBC, differential, platelet count weekly; withhold drug if baseline neutrophil count is <1500/mm^3; notify prescriber of results if WBC <20,000/mm^3, platelets <150,000/mm^3; leukocyte nadir occurs 10-14 days after administration, recovery by 21st day
- Assess for increased uric acid levels, swelling, joint pain, primarily extremities; patient should be well hydrated to prevent urate deposits
- Monitor renal function studies: BUN, creatinine, serum uric acid, urine CCr before and during therapy; I&O ratio; report fall in urine output to <30 ml/hr; dosage adjustment is needed if serum creatinine >5 mg/dl
- Monitor liver function tests before and during therapy (bilirubin, AST, ALT, LDH) as needed or monthly; note jaundice of skin or sclera, dark urine, clay-colored stools, itchy skin, abdominal pain, fever, diarrhea
- Assess for bleeding: hematuria, stool guaiac,

bruising or petechiae, mucosa or orifices q8h; inflammation of mucosa, breaks in skin
- Identify effects of alopecia on body image; discuss feeling about body changes

Nursing diagnoses
- Injury, risk for (adverse reactions)
- Body image, disturbed (adverse reactions)
- Infection, risk for (adverse reactions)
- Knowledge, deficient (teaching)

Implementation
- Avoid contact with skin; very irritating; wash completely to remove; give fluids **IV** or PO before chemotherapy to hydrate patient
- Give antiemetic 30-60 min before giving drug to prevent vomiting and prn
- Administer prophylactic antibiotic with a fluoroquinolone or trimethoprim/sulfamethoxazole if dose of epirubicin is 120 mg/m^2
- Provide liq diet: carbonated beverages; gelatin may be added if patient is not nauseated or vomiting
- Drug should be prepared by experienced personnel using proper precautions
- Give into tubing of free-flowing **IV** inf 0.9% NaCl or D_5 over 3-5 min; do not admix with other drugs in syringe
- Use hydrocortisone, dexamethasone, or sodium bicarbonate (1 mEq/1 ml) for extravasation: apply ice compress

Patient/family education
- Advise patient to avoid use of products containing aspirin or NSAIDs, razors, commercial mouthwash, since bleeding may occur; to report symptoms of bleeding (hematuria, tarry stools)
- Instruct patient to report signs of anemia (fatigue, headache, irritability, faintness, shortness of breath)
- Inform patient that hair may be lost during treatment; a wig or hairpiece may make patient feel better; new hair may be different in color, texture
- Caution patient not to have any vaccinations without the advice of the prescriber; serious reactions can occur
- Advise patient to use contraception during treatment and 4 mo afterward
- Advise patient that urine may appear red for 2 days
- Instruct patient to avoid crowds, persons with known infection
- Caution patient to avoid OTC medications, supplements unless approved by prescriber

Evaluation
Positive therapeutic outcome
- Prevention of rapid division of malignant cells

eplerenone (Rx)
(ep-ler-ee'known)
Inspra
Func. class.: Antihypertensive
Pregnancy category B

Action: Binds to mineralocorticoid receptor and blocks the binding of aldosterone, a component of the renin-angiotensin-aldosterone system (RAAS)

Therapeutic Outcome: Absence of hypertension

Uses: Hypertension, alone or in combination with thiazide diuretics

Dosage and routes
Adult: **PO** 50 mg daily initially, may increase to 50 mg bid after 4 wk; start dose at 25 mg daily if patient is taking CYP3A4 inhibitors

Available forms: Tabs 25, 50, 100 mg

Adverse effects
CNS: Headache, dizziness, fatigue
CV: Angina, **MI**
GI: Increased GGT diarrhea, abdominal pain, increased ALT
GU: Increased BUN, creatinine, gynecomastia, mastodynia (males), abnormal vaginal bleeding
META: Hyperkalemia, hyponatremia, hypercholesteremia, hypertriglyceridemia, increased uric acid
RESP: Cough

Contraindications: Hypersensitivity, lactation, children, increased serum creatinine >2 mg/dl (male) or >1.8 mg/dl (female), potassium >5.5 mEq/L, type 2 diabetes with microalbuminuria, hepatic disease, CCr >50 ml/min, <50 ml/min in hypertension

Precautions: Pregnancy **B;** impaired renal, liver function; elderly; hyperkalemia; lactation

Pharmacokinetics

Absorption	Unknown
Distribution	Protein binding 50%
Metabolism	Liver (CYP3A4 inhibitor)
Excretion	Urine
Half-life	4-6 hr

Pharmacodynamics

Onset	Unknown
Peak	1½ hr
Duration	Unknown

Interactions

Individual drugs

Erythromycin, fluconazole, itraconazole, ketoconazole, saquinavir, verapamil: increased levels of eplerenone
Lithium: increased serum lithium levels

Drug classifications

ACE inhibitors, angiotensin II antagonists, NSAIDs, potassium supplements: increased hyperkalemia
CYP3A4 inhibitors: increased levels of eplerenone
NSAIDs: decreased antihypertensive effect

Drug/herb

Aconite: increased toxicity, death
Astragalus, cola tree: increased or decreased antihypertensive effect
Barberry, betony, black catechu, black cohosh, bloodroot, broom, burdock, cat's claw, dandelion, goldenseal, Irish moss, Jamaican dogwood, kelp, khella, mistletoe, parsley: increased antihypertensive effect
Coltsfoot, guarana, khat, licorice: decreased antihypertensive effect
St. John's wort: decreased levels of eplerenone

Drug/food

Grapefruit juice: increased drug level by 25%

NURSING CONSIDERATIONS

Assessment

- Monitor B/P at peak/trough level of drug, orthostatic hypotension, syncope when used with diuretic
- Monitor renal studies: protein, BUN, creatinine; increased liver function tests; uric acid may be increased
- Monitor potassium levels, hyperkalemia may occur

Nursing diagnoses

- Tissue perfusion, ineffective (uses)
- Cardiac output, decreased (uses)
- Diarrhea (side effects)
- Knowledge, deficient (teaching)
- Noncompliance (teaching)

Implementation

- Store in tight container at 86° F (30° C) or less

Patient/family education

- Advise not to discontinue drug abruptly
- Advise not to use OTC products (cough, cold, allergy) unless directed by prescriber; do not use salt substitutes containing potassium without consulting prescriber
- Teach the importance of complying with dosage schedule, even if feeling better
- Teach that drug may cause dizziness, fainting, light-headedness; may occur during first few days of therapy
- Teach how to take B/P, and normal readings for age-group

Evaluation

Positive therapeutic outcome

- Decreased in B/P

epoetin (Rx)

(ee-poe'e-tin)

Epogen, EPO, Eprex ✱, Procrit

Func. class.: Antianemic, biologic modifier, hormone

Chem. class.: Amino acid polypeptide

Pregnancy category C

Action: Erythropoietin is one factor controlling rate of red cell production; drug is developed by recombinant DNA technology

Therapeutic Outcome: Decreased anemia with increased RBCs

Uses: Anemia caused by reduced endogenous erythropoietin production, primarily end-stage renal disease; to correct hemostatic defect in uremia; anemia caused by AZT (zidovudine) treatment in HIV-positive patients; anemia caused by chemotherapy; reduction of allogeneic blood transfusion in surgery patients

Investigational uses: Pruritus, anemia in premature preterm infants, anemia in myelodysplastic syndrome, anemia in chronic inflammatory disorders

Dosage and routes

Anemia secondary to chemotherapy

Adult: SUBCUT 150 units/kg 3×/wk, may increase after 2 mo up to 300 units/kg 3×/wk

Anemia in chronic renal failure

Adult: SUBCUT/**IV** 50-100 units/kg 3×/wk, then adjust to maintain the target Hct of 30%-36%
Child: **IV**/SUBCUT 50 units/kg 3×/wk

Anemia secondary to zidovudine treatment

Adult: SUBCUT/**IV** 100 units/kg 3×/wk × 2 mo; may increase by 50-100 units/kg q1-2 mo, up to 300 units/kg 3×/wk

Surgery
Adult: SUBCUT 300 units/kg/day × 10 days before surgery, the day of surgery and for 4 days postsurgery or 600 units/kg 3, 2, 1 wk before and on day of surgery

Available forms: Inj 2000, 3000, 4000, 10,000, 20,000, 40,000 units/ml

Adverse effects

CNS: **Seizures,** coldness, sweating, headache
CV: *Hypertension,* **hypertensive encephalopathy**
MS: Bone pain

Contraindications: Hypersensitivity to mammalian cell-derived products, or human albumin, uncontrolled hypertension

Precautions: Pregnancy **C**, seizure disorder, porphyria, children <1 mo, lactation, multidose preserved formulation contains benzyl alcohol and should not be used in premature infants

Pharmacokinetics

Absorption	Well absorbed (SUBCUT), completely absorbed (**IV**)
Distribution	Unknown
Metabolism	Unknown
Excretion	Unknown
Half-life	5-14 hr

Pharmacodynamics

	SUBCUT/IV
Onset	Unknown
Peak	Immediate
Duration	Unknown
Increased RBC count	2-6 wk

Interactions

Drug classifications

Anticoagulants: need for increased anticoagulants during hemodialysis

NURSING CONSIDERATIONS

Assessment

- Monitor renal studies: urinalysis, protein, blood, BUN, creatinine; I&O; report drop in output to <50 ml/hr
- Monitor blood studies: ferritin, transferrin monthly, transferrin sat ≥20%; ferritin ≥100 ng/ml; Hct 2×/wk until stabilized in target range (30%-36%) then at regular intervals; those with endogenous erythropoietin levels of <500 units/L respond to this agent; check for symptoms of anemia: fatigue, pallor, dyspnea; monitor Hct 2×/wk in chronic renal failure; those being treated with zidovudine or cancer patients should be monitored weekly, then periodically after stabilization
- Assess for CNS symptoms: coldness, sweating, pain in long bones
- Assess CV status: B/P before and during treatment; hypertension may occur rapidly leading to hypertension encephalopathy, antihypertensives may be needed
- Assess patient during hemodialysis for bruits, thrills, or shunts; drug prevents severe anemia in chronic renal failure; clotting may need to be treated with increased anticoagulant
- Assess for seizures if Hct is increased within 2 wk by 4 pts
- Monitor serum iron levels, ferritin, transferrin levels; iron therapy may be needed to prevent recurring anemia
- Monitor B/P, check for rising B/P as Hct rises
- Monitor blood studies: BUN, creatinine, uric acid, platelets, WBC, phosphorus, potassium, bleeding time; Hct, Hgb, RBCs, reticulocytes should be checked in chronic renal failure
- For hypersensitivity reactions: Skin rashes, urticaria (rare), antibody development does not occur
- ❗ For pure cell aplasia (PRCA) in absence of other causes, evaluate by testing sera for recombinant erythropoietin antibodies; any loss of response to epoetin should be evaluated

Nursing diagnoses

- Fatigue (uses)
- Activity intolerance (uses)
- Knowledge, deficient (teaching)

Implementation

SUBCUT route

- Before injecting, preservative-free, single dose formulation may be admixed by using 0.9% NaCl, USP, with benzyl alcohol 0.9% at a 1:1 ratio to reduce injection site discomfort

IV route

- Administer by direct route at end of dialysis by venous line, do not shake vial
- If Hct increases by 4% in 2 wk, decrease dose by 25 units/kg; increase dose if Hct does not increase by 5-6 pts after 8 wk of therapy, suggested target Hct range 30%-36%
- Give additional heparin to lower chance of clots

Solution compatibilities: Do not dilute or administer with other solutions

Patient/family education

- Teach patient how to take B/P

- Advise patients to take iron supplements, vit B_{12}, folic acid as directed
- Teach patient to avoid driving or hazardous activity during treatment
- Teach patients with renal disease to include high-iron and low-potassium foods in their diets (meat, dark green leafy vegetables, eggs, enriched breads)
- Teach patient the reason for treatment, expected results
- Advise patient to use contraception

Evaluation

Positive therapeutic outcome

- Increased appetite
- Enhanced sense of well-being
- Increased in reticulocyte count in 2-6 wk, Hgb, Hct

eprosartan (Rx)

(ep-roh-sar'tan)

Teveten

Func. class.: Antihypertensive

Chem. class.: Angiotensin II receptor antagonist (Subtype AT_1)

Pregnancy category C (1st trimester), D (2nd/3rd trimesters)

Action: Blocks the vasoconstrictor and aldosterone-secreting effects of angiotensin II; selectively blocks the binding of angiotensin II to the AT_1 receptor found in tissues

Therapeutic Outcome: Decreased B/P

Uses: Hypertension, alone or in combination with other antihypertensives

Dosage and routes

Adult: PO 600 mg daily; dose may be divided and given bid with total daily doses ranging from 400-800 mg

Available forms: Tabs 400, 600 mg

Adverse effects

CNS: *Dizziness*, depression, fatigue, headache
CV: Chest pain
EENT: Sinusitis
GI: *Diarrhea, dyspepsia,* abdominal pain
GU: UTI
META: Hypertriglyceridemia
MS: Myalgia, arthralgia
RESP: *Cough, upper respiratory infection,* rhinitis, pharyngitis, viral infection

Contraindications: Pregnancy **D** (2nd/3rd trimesters), hypersensitivity

Precautions: Pregnancy **C** (1st trimester), hypersensitivity to ACE inhibitors; lactation, children, elderly; renal, hepatic disease

Pharmacokinetics	
Absorption	Absolute bioavailability ~13%; food delays absorption
Distribution	Protein binding 98%
Metabolism	Moderate renal impairment increases drug levels by 30%, hepatic impairment increases levels by 40%
Excretion	Urine, feces
Half-life	5-9 hr

Pharmacodynamics	
Onset	Unknown
Peak	1-2 hr
Duration	Unknown

Interactions

Drug/herb

Aconite: increased toxicity, death
Astragalus, cola tree: increased or decreased antihypertensive effect
Barberry, betony, black catechu, black cohosh, bloodroot, broom, burdock, cat's claw, dandelion, goldenseal, Irish moss, Jamaican dogwood, kelp, khella, mistletoe, parsley: increased antihypertensive effect
Coltsfoot, guarana, khat, licorice: decreased antihypertensive effect

Drug/lab test

Increased: ALT, AST, alkaline phosphatase
Decreased: Hgb

NURSING CONSIDERATIONS

Assessment

- Assess B/P with position changes, pulse q4h; note rate, rhythm, quality
- Assess electrolytes: K, Na, Cl
- Assess baselines in renal, liver function tests before therapy begins
- Assess for edema in feet, legs daily
- Assess skin turgor, dryness of mucous membranes for hydration status

Nursing diagnoses

- Fluid volume, deficient (adverse reactions)
- Noncompliance (teaching)
- Knowledge, deficient (teaching)
- Injury, risk for (adverse reactions)

Implementation

- May be given without regard to meals

Patient/family education

- Advise patient to comply with dosage schedule, even if feeling better

- Advise patient to notify prescriber of fever, swelling of hands or feet, chest pain
- Inform patient that excessive perspiration, dehydration, diarrhea may lead to fall in blood pressure; consult prescriber if these occur
- Inform patient that drug may cause dizziness; advise to avoid hazardous activities until effect is known
- Advise patient not to take this medication if pregnant or breastfeeding, or if allergic reaction to this drug has occurred
- Advise patient to take missed dose as soon as possible, unless within 1 hr of next dose

Evaluation

Positive therapeutic outcome

- Decreased B/P

! HIGH ALERT

eptifibatide (Rx)

(ep-tih-fib'ah-tide)

Integrilin

Func. class.: Antiplatelet agent

Chem. class.: Glycoprotein IIb/IIIa inhibitor

Pregnancy category B

Action: Platelet glycoprotein antagonist; reversibly prevents fibrinogen, von Willebrand's factor from binding to the glycoprotein IIb/IIIa receptor, inhibiting platelet aggregation

Therapeutic Outcome: Decreased platelets

Uses: Acute coronary syndrome including those undergoing percutaneous coronary intervention (PCI)

Dosage and routes

Acute coronary syndrome

Adult: **IV** BOL 180 mcg/kg as soon as diagnosed, max 22.6 mg; then **IV** cont inf 2 mcg/kg/min until discharge or coronary artery bypass graft (CABG) up to 72 hr, max 15 mg/hr

PCI in patients without acute coronary syndrome

Adult: **IV** BOL 180 mcg/kg given immediately before PCI; then 2 mcg/kg/min × 18 hr and a second 180 mcg/kg bolus, 10 min after 1st bolus; continue inf for up to 18-24 hr

Renal dose

CCr <50 ml/min 2-4 mg/dl same loading dose, then ½ usual inf dose

Available forms: Sol for inj 2 mg/ml (10 ml), 0.75 mg/ml (100 ml)

Adverse effects

CV: **Stroke,** hypotension

GU: Hematuria

HEMA: **Thrombocytopenia**

SYST: **Bleeding, anaphylaxis**

Contraindications: Hypersensitivity, active internal bleeding; history of bleeding, stroke within 1 mo; major surgery with severe trauma, severe hypertension, history of intracranial bleeding, current or planned use of another parenteral GPIIb/IIIa inhibitor, dependence on renal dialysis, coagulopathy

Precautions: Pregnancy **B,** bleeding, lactation, children, elderly, renal function impairment

Pharmacokinetics	
Absorption	Unknown
Distribution	Unknown
Metabolism	Limited
Excretion	Kidneys
Half-life	2.5 hr

Pharmacodynamics	
Onset	Unknown
Peak	Unknown
Duration	Unknown

Interactions

Individual drugs

Abciximab, aspirin, clopidogrel, dipyridamole, heparin, ticlopidine, valproate: increased bleeding

Drug classifications

Anticoagulants, NSAIDs, thrombolytics: increased bleeding

Platelet receptor inhibitors IIb, IIIa: do not give together

NURSING CONSIDERATIONS

Assessment

- Monitor platelets, Hgb, Hct, creatinine, PT/APTT baseline, INR, within 6 hr of loading dose and daily thereafter; patients undergoing PCI should have ACT monitored; maintain APTT 50-70 sec unless PCI is to be performed; during PCI, ACT should be 200-300 sec; if platelets drop <100,000/mm^3, obtain additional platelet counts; if thrombocytopenia is confirmed, discontinue drug; also draw Hct, Hgb, serum creatinine
- Assess for bleeding: gums, bruising, ecchymosis, petechiae; from GI, GU tract, cardiac catheter sites, IM inj sites

Nursing diagnoses
- Tissue perfusion, ineffective (uses)
- Knowledge, deficient (teaching)

Implementation
- Aspirin and heparin may be given with this drug
- Discontinue heparin before removing femoral artery sheath after PCI

IV route
- After withdrawing the bolus dose from 10-ml vial, give **IV** push over 1-2 min; follow bolus dose with cont inf using infusion pump, give drug undiluted directly from the 100-ml vial, spike the 100-ml vial with a vented infusion set, use caution when centering the spike on the circle of the stopper top
- Do not use discolored sol or those with particulate

Y-site compatibilities: Alteplase, atropine, DOBUTamine, heparin, lidocaine, meperidine, metoprolol, midazolam, morphine, nitroglycerin, verapamil

Solution compatibilities: 0.9% NaCl, D_5/0.9% NaCl
- Discontinuing drug before CABG
- Give all medications PO if possible, avoid IM inj and catheters

Patient/family education
- Teach patient to report bruising, bleeding, chest pain immediately
- Inform patient of reason for medication and expected results

Evaluation
Positive therapeutic outcome
- Decreased platelets

ergocalciferol
See vitamin D

ergonovine (Rx)
(er-goe-noe'veen)

Ergometrine, ergotrate

Func. class.: Oxytocic

Chem. class.: Ergot alkaloid

Pregnancy category UK

Action: Stimulates uterine and vascular smooth muscle contractions, decreases bleeding

Therapeutic Outcome: Uterine contraction, decreases bleeding

Uses: Treatment of postpartum or postabortion hemorrhage

Investigational uses: To induce a coronary artery spasm for diagnostic purposes

Dosage and routes
Oxytoxic

Adult: PO/SL 0.2-0.4 mg q6-12h; IM 0.2 mg q2-4h, not to exceed 5 doses; **IV** 0.2 mg given over 1 min

Induced coronary artery spasm

Adult: **IV** 50 mg q5 min up to 400 mcg or until chest pain occurs

Available forms: Inj 0.2, 0.25 mg/ml; tab 0.2 mg

Adverse effects
CNS: *Headache, dizziness,* fainting

CV: Hypertension, chest pain

EENT: Tinnitus

GI: *Nausea, vomiting,* diarrhea

GU: Cramping

INTEG: Sweating

RESP: Dyspnea

Contraindications: Hypersensitivity to ergot medication, augmentation of labor, before delivery of placenta, spontaneous abortion (threatened), PID

Precautions: Hepatic, renal, cardiac disease, asthma, anemia, seizure disorders, hypertension, glaucoma, obliterative vascular disease

Pharmacokinetics	
Absorption	Well absorbed (IM), completely absorbed (**IV**)
Distribution	Unknown
Metabolism	Liver
Excretion	Kidneys
Half-life	Unknown

Pharmacodynamics	IM	IV
Onset	2-5 min	Immediate
Peak	Unknown	Unknown
Duration	3 hr	45 min

Interactions
Drug classifications

Ergots, sympathomimetics: increased hypertension

Drug/herb

Horehound: increased serotonin effect

NURSING CONSIDERATIONS

Assessment

- Monitor B/P, pulse; watch for change that may indicate hemorrhage; check respiratory rate, rhythm, depth; notify prescriber of abnormalities
- Assess fundal tone, nonphasic contractions; check for relaxation or severe cramping
- Assess for ergotism or overdose: nausea, vomiting, weakness, muscular pain, insensitivity to cold, paresthesia of extremities; drug should be decreased or inf discontinued
- Before administering ergonovine, calcium levels should be checked; if hypocalcemia is present, correction should be made to increase effectiveness of this drug
- Monitor prolactin levels and decreased breast milk production

Nursing diagnoses

- Tissue perfusion, ineffective (uses)
- Injury, risk for (adverse reactions)
- Knowledge, deficient (teaching)

Implementation

IM route

- Contractions begin in 2-5 min, drug is given q2-4h for contractions to continue; give deeply in large muscle mass; rotate inj sites if additional doses are given

IV route

- Give **IV** directly after dilution with 5 ml of 0.9% NaCl, give over >1 min through Y-site of free-running **IV** of 0.9% NaCl or D_5W

Additive compatibilities: Amikacin, cephapirin, sodium bicarbonate

Patient/family education

- Advise patient to report increased blood loss, increased temp or foul-smelling lochia; need for pad count
- Inform patient that cramping is normal; pad count should be done to determine amount of bleeding
- Tell patient not to smoke during treatment to prevent excessive vasoconstriction

Evaluation

Positive therapeutic outcome

- Absence of severe bleeding

Treatment of overdose: Stop drug; give vasodilators, heparin, dextran

ergotamine (Rx)

(er-got'a-meen)

Ergostat, Ergomar ✦, Gynergen

dihydroergotamine

(dy-hy'droh-er-got'ah-meen)

DHE 45, Dihydroergotamine Sandoz ✦, Migranal

Func. class.: α-Adrenergic blocker, vascular headache suppressant

Chem. class.: Ergot alkaloid–amino acid

Pregnancy category X

Action: Constricts smooth muscle in peripheral, cranial blood vessels; relaxes uterine muscle; blocks serotonin release

Therapeutic Outcome: Absence of headache

Uses: Vascular headache (migraine, histamine, cluster)

Dosage and routes

Ergotamine

Adult: SL 1 tab (2 mg), may use q30 min, max 3 tabs (6 mg)/24 hr or 10 mg/wk

Dihydroergotamine

Adult: SUBCUT/IM 1 mg, may repeat in 1 hr to 3 mg, max 3 mg/day or 6 mg/ wk; **IV** 0.5 mg, may repeat in 1 hr, max 2 mg/day or 6 mg/wk; INTRANASAL: 1 spray in each nostril, repeat in 15 min, max 3 mg/24 hr, 4 mg/wk

Child ≥6 yr: SUBCUT/IM 0.5 mg, may repeat in 1 hr; **IV** 0.25 mg, may repeat in 1 hr

Severe acute migraine

Child 12-16 yr: **IV** 0.25-0.5 mg, may repeat q20 min for 1-2 doses

Available forms: Ergotamine: SL tab 2 mg; tabs 1 mg; dihydroergotamine: inj 1 mg/ml; nasal spray 4 mg/ml

Adverse effects

CNS: *Numbness in fingers, toes,* headache, weakness

CV: Transient tachycardia, chest pain, bradycardia, edema, claudication, increase or decrease in B/P, **MI,** peripheral vascular ischemia

GI: Nausea, vomiting, diarrhea, abdominal cramps

MS: Muscle pain

Contraindications: Pregnancy **X,** hypersensitivity to ergot preparations, occlusion (peripheral, vascular), CAD, hepatic, renal disease, peptic ulcer, hypertension, Raynaud's disease, peripheral vascular disease, intermittent claudication, glaucoma, angina

Precautions: Lactation, elderly, children, anemia, basilar/hemiplagic migraine

Pharmacokinetics

Absorption	Erratic (PO), poor (SL), rapidly (SUBCUT, IM)
Distribution	Crosses blood-brain barrier
Metabolism	Liver—extensively
Excretion	Kidneys (metabolites)
Half-life	Biphasic 2.7 hr, 21 hr

Pharmacodynamics

	PO	SL	IM/SUBCUT	IV
Onset	1-2 hr	Unknown	Unknown	Unknown
Peak	½-3 hr	Unknown	Unknown	¼-2 hr
Duration	Unknown	Unknown	8 hr	8 hr

Interactions
Individual drugs
Nicotine: increased vasoconstriction
Drug classifications
CYP450384 inhibitors (protease inhibitors, some macrolides, azole antifungals): increased ergot toxicity, do not use together
β-Blockers, contraceptives (oral vasoconstrictors, other migraine agents): increased vasoconstriction
Drug/herb
Horehound: increased serotonin effect

NURSING CONSIDERATIONS
Assessment
- Assess characteristics of pain: duration, intensity, location, frequency, alleviating factors; also identify if halos, nausea, vomiting, blurred vision occur with headache; assess before and during treatment
- Assess for ergotism or overdose: nausea, vomiting, weakness, muscular pain, insensitivity to cold, paresthesia of extremities; drug should be decreased or infusion discontinued
- Check for hypertension: B/P, pulse, monitor all peripheral pulses; if hypertension occurs, notify prescriber; also check for tachycardia or bradycardia

Nursing diagnoses
- Pain, acute (uses)
- Injury, risk for (adverse reactions)
- Knowledge, deficient (teaching)

Implementation
SL route
- Do not break, crush, chew or swallow SL tab
- Place tab under tongue, do not drink, eat, or smoke until tab has dissolved

Inhalation route
- Teach patient how to use inhaler, protect ampules from heat/light

IV route
- Give dihydroergotamine undiluted over 1 min

Patient/family education
- Caution patient not to smoke during treatment to prevent excessive vasoconstriction
- Advise patient to avoid alcohol or OTC medications unless approved by prescriber
- Tell patient to inform prescriber if pregnancy occurs

Evaluation
Positive therapeutic outcome
- Decreasing headache

Treatment of overdose: Stop drug, give vasodilators, heparin, dextran

erlotinib (Rx)
(er-loe'tye-nib)
Tarceva
Func. class.: Misc. antineoplastic
Chem. class.: Epidermal growth factor receptor inhibitor

Pregnancy category D

Action: Not fully understood. Inhibits intracellular phosphorylation of cell surface receptors associated with epidermal growth factor receptors.

Therapeutic Outcome: Decrease in tumor size

Uses: Nonsmall cell lung cancer (NSCLC)

Dosage and routes
Adult: PO 150 mg daily taken at least 1 hr before or 2 hr after food

CYP3A4 inducers concurrently (such as rifampin or phenytoin)
Dosage increase is advised

CYP3A4 inhibitors (atazanavir, clarithromycin, indinavir, itraconazole, ketoconazole, telithromycin, ritonavir, saquinavir, troleandomycin, nelfinavir)
Dosage reduction may be needed.

Available forms: Tabs 25, 100, 150 mg

Adverse effects

GI: *Nausea, diarrhea, vomiting, anorexia, mouth ulceration*
INTEG: *Rash*
MISC: *Conjunctivitis, eye pain, fatigue, infection*
RESP: **Interstitial lung disease**, *cough, dyspnea*

Contraindications: Pregnancy **D**, hypersensitivity

Precautions: Renal, hepatic, ocular, pulmonary disorders, lactation, children, elderly

Pharmacokinetics	
Absorption	Slowly absorbed
Distribution	Unknown
Metabolism	Metabolized by CYP3A4
Excretion	Feces (86%), urine (<4%)
Half-life	36 hr

Pharmacodynamics	
Onset	Unknown
Peak	3-7 hr
Duration	Unknown

Interactions

Individual drugs

Warfarin, metoprolol: increased plasma concentrations

Drug classifications

CYP3A4 inhibitors (atazanavir, clarithromycin, indinavir, itraconazole, ketoconazole, telithromycin, ritonavir, saquinavir, troleandomycin, nelfinavir): increased erlotinib concentrations
CYP3A4 inducers (phenytoin, rifampin, carbamazepine, phenobarbital): decreased erlotinib levels

Drug/herb

St. John's wort: decreased erlotinib levels

NURSING CONSIDERATIONS

Assessment

- ⚠ Assess for pulmonary changes: lung sounds, cough, dyspnea; interstitial lung disease may occur, may be fatal; discontinue therapy if confirmed
- Assess for ocular changes: eye irritation, corneal erosion/ulcer, aberrant eyelash growth
- Assess for GI symptoms: frequency of stools, if diarrhea is poorly tolerated, therapy may be discontinued for up to 14 days

Nursing diagnoses

- Injury, risk for (adverse reactions)
- Body image, disturbed (adverse reactions)
- Infection, risk for (adverse reactions)
- Knowledge, deficient (teaching)

Implementation

- Administer 1 hr before or 2 hr after food

Patient/family education

- ⚠ Teach patient to report adverse reactions immediately: SOB, severe abdominal pain, persistent diarrhea or vomiting, ocular changes, skin eruptions
- Explain reason for treatment, expected results
- Advise patient to use contraception during treatment

Evaluation

Positive therapeutic outcome

- Decrease non–small cell lung cancer cells

ertapenem (Rx)

(er-tah-pen′em)

Invanz

Func. class.: Antiinfective—miscellaneous
Chem. class.: Carbapenem

Pregnancy category B

Do Not Confuse:
Invanz/Aninza

Action: Interferes with cell wall replication of susceptible organisms; osmotically unstable cell wall swells, bursts from osmotic pressure

Therapeutic Outcome: Bactericidal action against the following organisms: *Bacteroides fragilis, Bacteroides distasonis, Bacteroides ovatus, Bacteroides thetaiotaomicron, Bacteroides uniformis; Clostridium clostridioforme, Escherichia coli, Eubacterium lentum, Haemophilus influenzae* (beta-lactamase-negative), *Klebsiella pneumoniae, Moraxella catarrhalis, Peptostreptococcus* sp., *Porphyromonas asaccharolytica, Prevotella bivia, Staphylococcus aureus* (methicillin-susceptible); *Streptococcus agalactiae, Streptococcus pneumoniae* (penicillin-susceptible), *Streptococcus pyogenes*

Uses: Adult patients with moderate to severe intraabdominal infections, complicated skin/skin structure infections, community-acquired pneumonia, complicated UTI, acute pelvic infections

Dosage and routes

Complicated intraabdominal infections

Adult: **IV**/IM 1 g daily × 5-14 days

Complicated skin/skin structure infections

Adult: **IV**/IM 1 g daily × 7-14 days

Community-acquired pneumonia

Adult: **IV**/IM 1 g daily × 10-14 days

Complicated UTI

Adult: **IV**/IM 1 g daily × 10-14 days

Acute pelvic infections

Adult: **IV**/IM 1 g daily × 3-10 days

Available forms: Powder, lyophilized, 1 g

Adverse effects

CNS: Insomnia, **seizures**, dizziness, *headache*
GI: *Diarrhea, nausea, vomiting,* **pseudomembranous colitis**
GU: *Vaginitis*
INTEG: *Rash,* urticaria, *pruritus,* pain at inj site, *infused vein complication, phlebitis/thrombophlebitis*, erythema at inj site
RESP: Dyspnea, cough, pharyngitis, crackles, respiratory distress
SYST: **Anaphylaxis**

Contraindications: Hypersensitivity to this drug or its components, to amide-type local anesthetics (IM only); anaphylactic reactions to beta-lactams

Precautions: Pregnancy **B,** lactation, elderly, children, renal disease

Pharmacokinetics

Absorption	Almost completely absorbed (IM); completely (**IV**)
Distribution	85%-95% plasma protein bound
Metabolism	Liver (IM, **IV**)
Excretion	Urine (80%), feces (10%), breast milk (IM, **IV**)
Half-life	4 hr (**IV**)

Pharmacodynamics

	IM	IV
Onset	Unknown	Immediate
Peak	2.3 hr	Dose-dependent
Duration	Unknown	Unknown

Interactions

Individual drugs

Probenecid: increased ertapenem plasma levels; do not coadminister

Drug/herb

Acidophilus: do not use with antiinfectives

NURSING CONSIDERATIONS

Assessment

- Assess for sensitivity to carbapenem antibiotics, other beta-lactam antibiotics, penicillins
- Assess for renal disease: lower dose may be required
- Assess bowel pattern daily: if severe diarrhea occurs, drug should be discontinued; may indicate pseudomembranous colitis
- Assess for infection: temp, sputum, characteristics of wound before, during, after treatment
- (Alert) Assess for allergic reactions, anaphylaxis: rash, urticaria, pruritus; may occur a few days after therapy begins
- Assess for overgrowth of infection: perineal itching, fever, malaise, redness, pain, swelling, drainage, rash, diarrhea, change in cough or sputum

Nursing diagnoses

- Infection, risk for (uses)
- Diarrhea (adverse reaction)
- Injury, risk for (adverse reactions)
- Knowledge, deficient (teaching)
- Noncompliance (teaching)

Implementation

- Administer by **IV** or IM
- Give after C&S is taken

IM route

- Reconstitute 1 g vial of ertapenem with 3.2 ml of 1% lidocaine HCl without epINEPHrine, shake well
- Withdraw contents, administer deep IM in large muscle mass, use within 1 hr

IV route

- Do not co-infuse or mix with other medications; do not use diluents containing dextrose
- Reconstitute 1 g vial of ertapenem with either 10 ml of water for inj, 0.9% NaCl, or bacteriostatic water for inj
- Shake well to dissolve, transfer contents of reconstituted vial to 50 ml 0.9% NaCl inj
- Complete inf within 6 hr

Patient/family education

- Advise patient to report severe diarrhea; may indicate pseudomembranous colitis
- Advise patient to report overgrowth of infection: black, furry tongue, vaginal itching, foul-smelling stools
- Caution patient to avoid breastfeeding; drug is excreted in breast milk

Evaluation

Positive therapeutic outcome

- Negative C&S, absence of signs and symptoms of infection

Treatment of overdose: Administer epINEPHrine, antihistamines; resuscitate if needed (anaphylaxis)

erythromycin base (Rx)

(eh-rith-roh-my'sin)

Apo Erythro ♣, E-base, E-Mycin, Eramycin, Erybid ♣, Eryc, Ery-Tab, Erythromid ♣, Erythromycin Base Filmtab, Erythromycin Delayed-Release, Novo-Rythro Encap ♣, PCE

erythromycin estolate (Rx)

Ilosone, Novo-Rythro ♣

erythromycin ethylsuccinate (Rx)

Apo-Erythro-ES ♣, EES, Ery Ped, Novo-Rythro ♣

erythromycin gluceptate (Rx)

erythromycin lactobionate (Rx)

Erythrocin

erythromycin stearate (Rx)

Apo-Erythro-s ♣, Novo-Rythro ♣

Func. class.: Antiinfective

Chem. class.: Macrolide

Pregnancy category B

Action: Binds to 50S ribosomal subunits of susceptible bacteria and suppresses protein synthesis

Therapeutic Outcome: Bactericidal action against the following organisms: *Neisseria gonorrhoeae, Streptococcus pneumoniae, Mycoplasma pneumoniae, Corynebacterium diphtheriae, Bordetella pertussis, Borrelia burgdorferi, Listeria monocytogenes;* syphilis, Legionnaire's disease; streptococci, staphylocci; gram-positive bacilli: *Clostridium, Corynebacterium;* gram-negative pathogens: *Neisseria, Haemophilus influenzae, Legionella pneumophila, Mycoplasma, Chlamydia trachomatis, Entamoeba histolytica*

Uses: Mild to moderate respiratory tract, skin, soft tissue infections

Dosage and routes

Soft tissue infections

Adult: PO 250-500 mg q6-12h (base, estolate, stearate); PO 400-800 mg q6-12h (ethylsuccinate); **IV** inf 15-20 mg/kg/day (lactobionate) divided q6h

Child: PO 30-50 mg/kg/day in divided doses q6h (salts); **IV** 20-40 mg/kg/day in divided doses q6h (lactobionate), max adult dose

N. gonorrhoeae/*PID*

Adult: **IV** 500 mg q6h × 3 days (gluceptate, lactobionate), then PO 250 mg (base, estolate, stearate) or 400 mg (ethylsuccinate) q6h × 1 wk

Syphilis

Adult: PO 20-40 g in divided doses over 15 days (base, estolate, stearate)

Chlamydia

Adult: PO 500 mg q6h × 1 wk or 250 mg qid × 2 wk

Infant: PO 50 mg/kg/day in 4 divided doses × 3 wk or more

Newborn: PO 50 mg/kg/day in 4 divided doses × 2 wk or more

Intestinal amebiasis

Adult: PO 250 mg q6h × 10-14 days (base, estolate, stearate)

Child: PO 30-50 mg/kg/day in divided doses q6h × 10-14 days (base, estolate, stearate)

Available forms: Base: enteric-coated tab 250, 333, 500 mg; film-coated tab 250, 500 mg; enteric-coated caps, 250, 333 mg; estolate: tabs 500 mg; caps 125, 250 mg; drops 100 mg/ml; susp 125, 250 mg/5 ml; stearate: film-coated tabs, 250 mg; ethylsuccinate: chewable tabs 200 mg; susp 100 mg/2.5 ml, 200, 400 mg/5 ml; susp 200, 400 mg; powder for susp 100 mg/2.5 ml, 200, 400 mg/ 5 ml; powder for inj 500 mg, 1 g (lactobionate); 1 g (as gluceptate)

Adverse effects

CV: **Dysrhythmias**

EENT: Hearing loss, tinnitus

GI: Nausea, vomiting, diarrhea, **hepatotoxicity,** abdominal pain, stomatitis, heartburn, anorexia, pruritus ani

GU: Vaginitis, moniliasis

INTEG: Rash, urticaria, pruritus, thrombophlebitis (**IV** site)

SYST: **Anaphylaxis**

Contraindications: Hypersensitivity, preexisting liver disease (estolate), hepatic disease

Precautions: Pregnancy **B,** lactation

Pharmacokinetics

Absorption	Well absorbed (PO)
Distribution	Widely distributed; minimally distributed (CSF); crosses placenta
Metabolism	Liver, partially
Excretion	Bile, unchanged; kidneys (minimal), unchanged
Half-life	1-3 hr

Pharmacodynamics

	PO	IV
Onset	1 hr	Rapid
Peak	4 hr	Infusion's end

Interactions
Individual drugs
Bromocriptine, clindamycin, cycloSPORINE, diazepam, digoxin, dihydropyridine, disopyramide, lovastatin, methylPREDNISolone, midazolam, simvastatin, theophylline, triazolam, warfarin: increased toxicity, increased action
Clindamycin, digoxin, dihydropyridine, disopyramide, lovastatin, midazolam, simvastatin: increased action of each specific drug
Digoxin: increased blood levels of digoxin
Pimozide, sparfloxacin: increased serious dysrhythmias, do not use together
Triazolam: increased effects of triazolam
Drug classifications
Calcium antagonists: increased action of calcium antagonists
Calcium antagonists, ergots: increased toxicity
Ergots: increased action
HMG-CoA reductase inhibitors: increased action, toxicity
Oral anticoagulants: increased effects of oral anticoagulants
Drug/herb
Acidophilus: do not use with antiinfectives
Drug/lab test
Increased: AST/ALT
Decreased: folate assay
False increase: 17-OHCS/17-KS

NURSING CONSIDERATIONS
Assessment
- Assess patient for previous sensitivity reaction
- Assess patient for signs and symptoms of infection including characteristics of wounds, sputum, urine, stool, WBC >10,000/mm^3, earache, fever; obtain baseline information before and during treatment
- Obtain C&S test results before beginning drug therapy to identify if correct treatment has been initiated
- Assess for allergic reactions: rash, urticaria may occur a few days after therapy begins
- Identify urine output; if decreasing, notify prescriber (may indicate nephrotoxicity); also monitor increases in BUN, creatinine
- Monitor blood studies: AST, ALT, CBC, Hct, bilirubin, LDH, alkaline phosphatase, Coombs' test monthly if patient is on long-term therapy
- Monitor electrolytes: potassium, sodium, chloride monthly if patient is on long-term therapy
- Assess bowel pattern daily; if severe diarrhea occurs, drug should be discontinued
- Assess for overgrowth of infection: perineal itching, fever, malaise, redness, pain, swelling, drainage, rash, diarrhea, change in cough, sputum

Nursing diagnoses
- Infection, risk for (uses)
- Diarrhea (adverse reactions)
- Knowledge, deficient (teaching)
- Noncompliance (teaching)
- Injury, risk for (adverse reactions)

Implementation
PO route
- Give around the clock on an empty stomach, at least 1 hr ac or 2 hr pc; may be taken with food if GI upset occurs; do not take with juices; take dose with a full glass of water: use calibrated measuring device for drops or susp; shake well
- Store susp in refrigerator
- Chewable tab may be crushed or chewed, not swallowed whole
- Do not crush or chew enteric-coated tab

IV route
- Add 10 ml of sterile water for inj without preservatives to 250- or 500-mg vials and 20 ml to 1-g vial; sol is stable for 1 wk after reconstitution if refrigerated

Intermittent IV infusion
- Dilute further in 100-250 ml of 0.9% NaCl or D_5W
- Give over 20-60 min to avoid phlebitis; assess for pain along vein; slow inf if pain occurs; apply ice to site and notify prescriber if unable to relieve pain

Continuous infusion
- May also be administered as an infusion in a dilution of 1 g/L of 0.9% NaCl, D_5W, over 4 hr

Syringe incompatibilities: Heparin
Additive compatibilities: Calcium gluconate, hydrocortisone, lidocaine, methicil-

lin, penicillin G potassium, potassium chloride, sodium bicarbonate
Additive incompatibilities: Aminophylline, cephapirin, pentobarbital, secobarbital, streptomycin, tetracycline

Erythromycin lactobionate
Syringe compatibilities: Methicillin
Syringe incompatibilities: Ampicillin, heparin
Y-site compatibilities: Acyclovir, amiodarone, cyclophosphamide, enalapri-lat,esmolol, famotidine, foscarnet, hydromorphone, idarubicin, labetalol, lorazepam, magnesium sulfate, merperidine, midazolam, morphine, multivitamins, perphenazine, vit B/C, zidovudine
Y-site incompatibilities: Fluconazole
Additive compatibilities: Aminophylline, ampicillin, cimetidine, diphenhydrAMINE, hydrocortisone, lidocaine, methicillin, penicillin G potassium, penicillin G sodium, pentobarbital, polymyxin B, potassium chloride, prednisoLONE, prochlorperazine, promazine, ranitidine, sodium bicarbonate, verapamil
Additive incompatibilities: Cephalothin, colistimethate, floxacillin, furosemide, heparin, metaraminol, metoclopramide, tetracycline, vit B/C

Patient/family education

- Teach patient to report sore throat, bruising, bleeding, joint pain; may indicate blood dyscrasias (rare)
- Advise patient to contact prescriber if vaginal itching, loose foul-smelling stools, furry tongue occur; may indicate superimposed infection
- Instruct patient to take all medication prescribed for the length of time ordered

Evaluation

Positive therapeutic outcome

- Absence of signs/symptoms of infection (WBC <10,000/mm^3, temp WNL, absence of red, draining wounds, earache)
- Reported improvement in symptoms of infection

Treatment of overdose: Withdraw drug, maintain airway, administer epINEPHrine, aminophylline, O_2, **IV** corticosteroids

escitalopram (Rx)

(es-sit-tal'oh-pram)
Lexapro
Func. class.: Antidepressant, SSRI (selective serotonin reuptake inhibitor)
Pregnancy category C

Action: Inhibits CNS neuron uptake of serotonin but not of norepinephrine

Therapeutic Outcome: Decreased symptoms of depression

Uses: Major depressive disorder

Dosage and routes

Adult: PO 10 mg daily in AM or PM; after 1 wk if no clinical improvement is noted, dose may be increased to 20 mg daily PM; maintenance 10-20 mg/day, reassess to determine need for treatment
Elderly/hepatic dose: PO 10 mg/day

Available forms: Tabs 10, 20 mg; oral sol 5 mg (as base)/5 ml

Adverse effects

CNS: *Headache, nervousness, insomnia, drowsiness, anxiety, tremor, dizziness, fatigue, sedation, poor concentration, abnormal dreams, agitation,* **seizures,** apathy, euphoria, hallucinations, delusions, psychosis
CV: *Hot flashes, palpitations,* angina pectoris, **hemorrhage,** hypertension, **tachycardia,** 1st-degree AV block, **bradycardia, MI, thrombophlebitis,** postural hypotension
EENT: Visual changes, ear/eye pain, photophobia, tinnitus
GI: *Nausea, diarrhea, dry mouth, anorexia, dyspepsia, constipation, cramps, vomiting, taste changes, flatulence, decreased appetite*
GU: *Dysmenorrhea, decreased libido, urinary frequency, UTI,* amenorrhea, cystitis, impotence, urine retention
INTEG: *Sweating, rash, pruritus,* acne, alopecia, urticaria, photosensitivity
MS: *Pain,* arthritis, twitching
RESP: *Infection, pharyngitis, nasal congestion, sinus headache, sinusitis, cough, dyspnea, bronchitis,* asthma, hyperventilation, pneumonia
SYST: *Asthenia, viral infection, fever, allergy, chills*

Contraindications: Hypersensitivity

Precautions: Pregnancy **C**, lactation, children, elderly, renal disease, history of seizures

Pharmacokinetics

Absorption	Unknown
Distribution	Unknown
Metabolism	Liver
Excretion	Urine
Half-life	Unknown

Pharmacodynamics

Unknown

Interactions

Individual drugs

Alcohol: increased CNS depression
Amantadine, bromocriptine, buspirone, lithium, tryptophan: increased serotonin syndrome
Buspirone: increased symptoms of OCD
Carbamazepine, lithium, phenytoin, warfarin: increased levels or toxicity of each specific drug
Cyproheptadine: decreased escitalopram effect
Diazepam: increased half-life of diazepam
Haloperidol: increased effect of haloperidol

Drug classifications

Antidepressants, amphetamines: increased serotonin syndrome
Highly protein-bound drugs: increased side effects of escitalopram
MAOIs: do not use with or 14 days before escitalopram
Opioids, sedatives: increased CNS depression
Phenothiazines: increased levels of phenothiazines
Tricyclics: increased levels of tricyclics

Drug/herb

Corkwood, jimsonweed: increased anticholinergic effect
Hops, kava, lavender: increased CNS effect
SAM-e, St. John's wort: do not use together
Yohimbe: increased hypertension

NURSING CONSIDERATIONS

Assessment

- Assess mental status: mood, sensorium, affect, suicidal tendencies, increase in psychiatric symptoms, depression, panic
- Assess appetite in bulimia nervosa, weight daily, increase nutritious foods in diet, watch for bingeing and vomiting
- Assess allergic reactions: itching, rash, urticaria; drug should be discontinued, may need to give antihistamine
- Monitor B/P (lying/standing), pulse q4h; if systolic B/P drops 20 mm Hg, hold drug, notify prescriber; take VS q4h in patients with cardiovascular disease
- Monitor blood studies: CBC, leukocytes, differential, cardiac enzymes if patient is receiving long-term therapy; check platelets; bleeding can occur
- Montior liver function tests: AST, ALT, bilirubin, creatinine
- Monitor weight qwk; appetite may decrease with drug
- Monitor ECG for flattening of T wave, bundle branch, AV block, dysrhythmias in cardiac patients
- Monitor alcohol consumption; if alcohol is consumed, hold dose until AM

Nursing diagnoses

- Coping, ineffective (uses)
- Injury, risk for (uses/adverse reactions)
- Knowledge, deficient (teaching)

Implementation

- Give with food or milk for GI symptoms
- Give crushed if patient is unable to swallow medication whole
- Give dosage at bedtime if oversedation occurs during the day
- Give gum, hard candy, frequent sips of water for dry mouth
- Store at room temperature; do not freeze
- Provide assistance with ambulation during therapy, because drowsiness, dizziness occur
- Provide safety measures primarily in elderly
- Check to see if PO medication swallowed

Patient/family education

- Teach that therapeutic effect may take 1-4 wk
- Advise to use caution in driving, other activities requiring alertness because of drowsiness, dizziness, blurred vision
- Advise to use sunscreen to prevent photosensitivity
- Advise to avoid alcohol ingestion, other CNS depressants
- Advise patient to notify prescriber if pregnant or plan to become pregnant or breastfeed
- Advise patient to change positions slowly, orthostatic hypotension may occur
- Teach to avoid all OTC drugs unless approved by prescriber
- To report immediately signs of urinary retention

Evaluation

Positive therapeutic outcome

- Decreased depression

esmolol (Rx)
(ez'moe-lole)

Brevibloc

Func. class.: β-Adrenergic blocker (antidysrhythmic II)

Pregnancy category C

Do Not Confuse:
Brevibloc/Brevital
esmolol/Osmitrol

Action: Competitively blocks stimulation of β_1-adrenergic receptors in the myocardium; produces negative chronotropic, inotropic activity (decreases rate of SA node discharge, increases recovery time), slows conduction of AV node, decreases heart rate, decreases O_2 consumption in myocardium; also decreases renin-aldosterone-angiotensin system at high doses; inhibits β_2-receptors in bronchial system at higher doses

Therapeutic Outcome: Decreased supraventricular tachycardia

Uses: Supraventricular tachycardias, noncompensatory sinus tachycardia, hypertensive crisis, intraoperative and postoperative tachycardia, hypertension

Dosage and routes
Adult: **IV** loading dose 500 mcg/kg/min over 1 min; maintenance 50 mcg/kg/min for 4 min; if no response in 5 min, give 2nd loading dose; then increase inf to 100 mcg/kg/min for 4 min; if no response, repeat loading dose, then increase maintenance inf by 50 mcg/kg/min (max of 200 mcg/kg/min); titrate to patient response

Child: **IV** 50 mcg/kg/min, may increase q10 min, max 300 mcg/kg/min

Available forms: Inj 10 mg, 250 mg/ml

Adverse effects
CNS: Confusion, light-headedness, paresthesia, somnolence, fever, dizziness, fatigue, headache, depression, anxiety, **seizures**

CV: Hypotension, bradycardia, chest pain, peripheral ischemia, shortness of breath, CHF, conduction disturbances 1st-, 2nd-, 3rd-degree heart block

GI: *Nausea,* vomiting, anorexia, gastric pain, flatulence, constipation, heartburn, bloating

GU: Urinary retention, impotence, dysuria

INTEG: *Induration, inflammation at inj site,* discoloration, edema, erythema, burning pallor, flushing, rash, pruritus, dry skin, alopecia

RESP: **Bronchospasm,** dyspnea, cough, wheezing, nasal stuffiness

Contraindications: Heart block (2nd- or 3rd-degree), cardiogenic shock, CHF, cardiac failure, hypersensitivity

Precautions: Pregnancy **C,** hypotension, peripheral vascular disease, diabetes, hypoglycemia, thyrotoxicosis, renal disease, lactation

Pharmacokinetics	
Absorption	Complete
Distribution	Unknown
Metabolism	Liver
Excretion	Kidneys
Half-life	9 min

Pharmacodynamics	
Onset	Rapid
Peak	Unknown
Duration	1-2 min

Interactions
Individual drugs
Amphetamine, epHEDrine, epINEPHrine, norepinephrine, phenylephrine, pseudoephedrine: increased α-adrenergic stimulation

Digoxin: increased digoxin levels

Thyroid hormones: decreased effect of esmolol, decreased action of thyroid hormone

Drug classifications
MAOIs: avoid use

Drug/herb
Aloe, buckthorn, cascara sagrada, senna: increased hypokalemia

Betel palm, butterbur, cola tree, figwort, fumitory, guarana, hawthorn, lily of the valley, motherwort, plantain: increased β-blocking effect

Coenzyme Q10, yohimbe: decreased β-blocking effect

Jamborandi tree: increased CV reactions

Drug/lab test
Interference: glucose/insulin tolerance test

NURSING CONSIDERATIONS
Assessment
- Monitor B/P during beginning treatment, periodically thereafter; pulse q4h; note rate, rhythm, quality; apical/radial pulse before administration; notify prescriber of any significant changes (pulse <50 bpm)
- Check for baselines in renal, liver function tests before therapy begins
- Assess for edema in feet, legs daily, monitor I&O, daily weight; check for jugular vein

E

distention, crackles bilaterally, dyspnea (CHF)
- Monitor skin turgor, dryness of mucous membranes for hydration status, especially elderly

Nursing diagnoses
- Cardiac output, decreased (uses)
- Injury, risk for (adverse reactions)
- Knowledge, deficient (teaching)
- Noncompliance (teaching)

Implementation
- Give by intermittent inf after diluting 5 g/500 ml of D_5W, 0.9% NaCl, D_5/0.45% NaCl, D_5/LR, D_5/0.9% NaCl, 0.45% NaCl, LR (10 mg/ml)
- Give loading dose over 1 min, then maintenance dose over 4 min, may repeat loading dose q5 min with increased maintenance dose; maintenance dose should not be >200 mcg/kg/min and be administered up to 48 hr; dosage should be tapered at a rate of 25 mcg/kg/min
- Store at room temp for 24 hr; sol should be clear

Y-site compatibilities: Amikacin, aminophylline, ampicillin, amiodarone, atracurium, butorphanol, calcium chloride, cefazolin, cefmetazole, cefoperazone, ceftazidime, ceftizoxime, chloramphenicol, cimetidine, cisatracurium, clindamycin, diltiazem, DOPamine, enalaprilat, erythromycin, famotidine, fentanyl, gentamicin, heparin, hydrocortisone, regular insulin, labetalol, magnesium sulfate, methyldopate, metronidazole, midazolam, morphine, nafcillin, nitroglycerin, norepinephrine, nitroprusside, pancuronium, penicillin G potassium, phenytoin, piperacillin, polymyxin B, potassium chloride, potassium phosphate, propofol, ranitidine, remifentanil, streptomycin, tacrolimus, tobramycin, trimethoprim/sulfamethoxazole, vancomycin, vecuronium

Y-site incompatibilities: Furosemide

Additive compatibilities: Aminophylline, atracurium, bretylium, heparin

Additive incompatibilities: Diazepam, procainamide, sodium bicarbonate, thiopental

Patient/family education
- Teach patient need for medication and expected results
- Caution patient to rise slowly to prevent orthostatic hypotension
- Advise patient to notify if pain, swelling occurs at **IV** site

Evaluation
Positive therapeutic outcome
- Absence of dysrhythmias

Treatment of overdose: Defibrillation, vasopressor for hypotension

esomeprazole (Rx)
(es'oh-mep'rah-zohl)

Nexium

Func. class.: Anti-ulcer, proton pump inhibitor

Chem. class.: Benzimidazole

Pregnancy category B

Action: Suppresses gastric secretion by inhibiting hydrogen/potassium ATPase enzyme system in the gastric parietal cell; characterized as gastric acid pump inhibitor, since it blocks final step of acid production

Therapeutic Outcome: Absence of duodenal ulcers; decreased gastroesophageal reflux

Uses: Gastroesophageal reflux disease (GERD), severe erosive esophagitis; treatment of active duodenal ulcers in combination with antiinfectives for *Helicobacter pylori* infection

Dosage and routes
Active duodenal ulcers associated with H. pylori

Adult: PO 40 mg daily × 10 days in combination with clarithromycin 500 mg bid × 10 days and amoxicillin 1000 mg bid × 10 days

GERD

Adult: PO 20 or 40 mg daily × 4-8 wk, no adjustment needed in renal, liver failure, elderly

Available forms: Caps 20, 40 mg

Adverse effects
CNS: *Headache, dizziness*

GI: *Diarrhea, flatulence,* abdominal pain, constipation, dry mouth

GU: UTI, urinary frequency

INTEG: *Rash,* dry skin

RESP: *Cough*

Contraindications: Hypersensitivity

Precautions: Pregnancy **B,** lactation, children, elderly

Pharmacokinetics

Absorption	Unknown
Distribution	97% plasma protein bound
Metabolism	Liver (metabolites)
Excretion	Urine (metabolites), feces (metabolites); in elderly, elimination rate decreased, bioavailability increased
Half-life	1-1½ hr

Pharmacodynamics

Onset	Unknown
Peak	1½ hr
Duration	Unknown

Interactions
Individual drugs
Diazepam, digoxin, penicillins: increased effect, toxicity
Dapsone, iron, itraconazole, ketoconazole: decreased effect

NURSING CONSIDERATIONS
Assessment
- Assess GI system: bowel sounds q8h, abdomen for pain, swelling, anorexia
- Assess hepatic enzymes: AST, ALT, alkaline phosphatase during treatment

Nursing diagnoses
- Pain, acute (uses)
- Pain, chronic (uses)
- Knowledge, deficient (teaching)

Implementation
- Swallow caps whole; do not break, crush, or chew
- Administer at least 1 hr before eating

Patient/family education
- Instruct patient to report severe diarrhea; drug may have to be discontinued
- Advise diabetic patients that hypoglycemia may occur
- Advise patient to avoid hazardous activities; dizziness may occur
- Advise patient to avoid alcohol, salicylates, ibuprofen; may cause GI irritation

Evaluation
Positive therapeutic outcome
- Absence of epigastric pain, swelling, fullness

estradiol (Rx)
(ess-tra-dye'ole)
Estrace
estradiol cypionate
depGynogen, Depo-Estradiol, Depogen, Dura-Estrin, E-Cypionate, Estragyn LAS, Estro-Cyp, Estrofem, Estroject-LA, Estro-L.A.
estradiol topical emulsion
Estrasorb
estradiol valerate
Clinagen LA, Delestrogen, Dioval, Duragan, Estra-L, Estro-span, Femogex ♣, Gynogen LA, Menaval, Valergen
estradiol transdermal system
Alora, Climara, Esclim, Estraderm, FemPatch, Vivelle
estradiol vaginal tablet
Vagifem
estradiol vaginal ring
Estring

Func. class.: Estrogen, progestin
Chem. class.: Nonsteroidal synthetic estrogen

Pregnancy category X

Action: Needed for adequate functioning of female reproductive system; affects release of pituitary gonadatropins, inhibits ovulation, promotes adequate calcium use in bone structure

Therapeutic Outcome: Decreased tumor size in prostatic cancer; increased estrogen levels in menopause, female hypogonadism

Uses: Symptoms associated with menopause, breast cancer, prostatic cancer, atrophic vaginitis, kraurosis vulvae, hypogonadism, castration, primary ovarian failure, prevention of osteoporosis

Dosage and routes
Hormone replacement
Adult: TD 0.05-0.1 mg/24 hr apply 2×/wk

Menopause/hypogonadism/castration/ovarian failure
Adult: PO 1-2 mg daily 3 wk on, 1 wk off or 5 days on, 2 days off; IM 1-5 mg q3-4 wk (cypionate), 10-20 mg q4 wk (valerate); top Estraderm 0.05 mg/24 hr applied 2×/wk, Climara 0.05 mg/hr applied 1×/wk in a cyclic regimen, women with hysterectomy may use continuously

Prostatic cancer
Adult: IM 30 mg q1-2wk (valerate); PO 1-2 mg tid (oral estradiol)
Breast cancer
Adult: PO 10 mg tid × 3 mo or longer
Atropic vaginitis/kraurosis vulvae
Adult: Vag cream 2-4 g daily × 1-2 wk, then 1 g 1-3 ×/wk cycled; vag tab 1 daily × 2 wk, maintenance 1 tab 2×/wk; vag ring inserted and left in place continuously for 3 mo
Vasomotor symptoms
Adult: TOP after cleaning and drying skin on left thigh, calf, rub in contents of pouch using both hands until completely absorbed, wash hands

Available forms: Estradiol: tabs 0.5, 1, 2 mg; valerate: inj 10, 20, 40 mg/ml; TD: 0.025, 0.0375, 0.05, 0.075, 0.1 mg/24-hr release rate; vag cream: 100 mcg/g; vag ring: 2 mg/90 days; vag tab: 25 mcg

Adverse effects
CNS: Dizziness, headache, migraine, depression, **seizures**
CV: Hypotension, thrombophlebitis, edema, **thromboembolism, stroke, pulmonary embolism, MI**
EENT: Contact lens intolerance, increased myopia, astigmatism
GI: *Nausea,* vomiting, diarrhea, anorexia, pancreatitis, cramps, constipation, increased appetite, increased weight, **cholestatic jaundice, hepatic adenoma**
GU: Amenorrhea, cervical erosion, breakthrough bleeding, dysmenorrhea, vaginal candidiasis, breast changes, *gynecomastia, testicular atrophy, impotence,* **increased risk of breast, endometrial cancer,** changes in libido
INTEG: Rash, urticaria, acne, hirsutism, alopecia, oily skin, seborrhea, purpura, melasma
META: Folic acid deficiency, hypercalcemia, hyperglycemia

Contraindications: Pregnancy **X**, breast cancer, thromboembolic disorders, reproductive cancer, genital bleeding (abnormal, undiagnosed), lactation

Precautions: Hypertension, asthma, blood dyscrasias, gallbladder disease, CHF, diabetes mellitus, bone disease, depression, migraine headache, seizure disorders, hepatic, renal disease, family history of cancer of breast or reproductive tract, smoking

Pharmacokinetics

Absorption	Well absorbed
Distribution	Widely distributed, crosses placenta
Metabolism	Unknown
Excretion	Unknown
Half-life	Unknown

Pharmacodynamics

	PO	IM	IV
Onset	Rapid	Slow	Rapid
Peak	Unknown	Unknown	Unknown
Duration	Unknown	Unknown	Unknown

Interactions
Individual drugs
Calcium, phenylbutazone, rifampin: decreased estradiol action
CycloSPORINE, dantrolene: increased toxicity
Tamoxifen: decreased tamoxifen action
Drug classifications
Anticoagulants: decreased action of anticoagulants
Anticonvulsants, barbiturates: decreased estradiol action
Corticosteroids: increased action of corticosteroids
Hypoglycemics (oral): decreased action of hypoglycemics
Drug/herb
Alfalfa, hops: increased estrogen effect
Saw palmetto: decreased estrogen effect
Black cohosh, DHEA: altered estrogen effect
Drug/food
Grapefruit juice: increased estrogen level
Drug/lab test
Increased: BSP retention test; PBI; T_4; serum sodium; platelet aggregation; thyroxine-binding globulin (TBS); prothrombin; factors VII, VIII, IX, X; triglycerides
Decreased: serum folate, serum triglyceride, T_3 resin uptake test, glucose tolerance test, antithrombin III, pregnanediol, metyrapone test
False positive: LE prep, ANA titer

NURSING CONSIDERATIONS
Assessment
- Monitor blood glucose in patient with diabetes; hyperglycemia may occur
- Monitor B/P q4h; watch for increase caused by water and sodium retention
- Monitor I&O ratio; be alert for decreasing urinary output and increasing edema; monitor weight daily; notify prescriber if weekly weight

gain is >5 lb; if increased, diuretic may be ordered
- Obtain liver function studies baseline, periodically, including AST, ALT, bilirubin, alkaline phosphatase
- Assess edema, hypertension, cardiac symptoms, jaundice
- Assess mental status: affect, mood, behavioral changes, aggression; depression may occur, drug may need to be discontinued
- Assess female patient for intact uterus, if so, progesterone should be added to estrogen therapy to decrease risk of endometrial cancer

Nursing diagnoses
- Sexual dysfunction (uses)
- Injury, risk for (adverse reactions)

Implementation
PO route
- Give titrated dose, use lowest effective dose
- Give with food or milk to decrease GI symptoms

IM route
- Administer deeply in large muscle mass; drug is painful
- Rotate syringe to mix oil and medication

TD route
- Apply to area free of hair to ensure adhesion on trunk of body 2×/wk; press firmly and hold in place for 10 sec to ensure good contact
- Start TD dose 7 days before last PO dose if routes are to be changed

Vaginal route
- Place cream in applicator by attaching tube to applicator; squeeze cream into tube to mark; insert with patient reclining
- Applicator should be washed after each use

Patient/family education
- Tell patient to take exactly as prescribed; do not double doses
- Advise patient that increased weight gain and symptoms of fluid retention should be reported to prescriber: edema of feet, ankles, sacral area; abnormal vaginal bleeding; breast lumps; hepatic disease (dark urine, clay-colored stools, jaundice of skin, sclera, pruritus)
- Caution patient that thromboembolic symptoms should be reported: tenderness in legs, chest pain, dyspnea, headaches, blurred vision
- Inform patient to use sunscreen and protective clothing because sunburns may occur
- Advise patient to stop smoking; smokers have a greater chance of thromboembolic disorder
- Tell patient to use nonhormonal birth control, and to notify prescriber if pregnancy is suspected

Evaluation
Positive therapeutic outcome
- Reversal of menopausal symptoms
- Decreased in tumor size in prostatic or breast cancer
- Decreased in itching, inflammation of vagina
- Absence of symptoms of osteoporosis

estrogens, conjugated (Rx)
Cenestin, C.E.S ♣, Congest ♣, conjugated estrogens, Premarin, Premarin Intravenous

estrogens, conjugated synthetic B
Enjuvia

Pregnancy category X

Do Not Confuse:
Premarin/Provera

Action: Needed for adequate functioning of female reproductive system; affects release of pituitary gonadotropins; inhibits ovulation; promotes adequate calcium use in bone structures

Therapeutic Outcome: Decreased tumor size in prostatic cancer; increased estrogen levels in menopause, female hypogonadism

Uses: Symptoms associated with menopause, breast cancer, prostatic cancer, abnormal uterine bleeding, hypogonadism, castration, primary ovarian failure, prevention of osteoporosis

Dosage and routes
Menopause
Adult: PO 0.3-1.25 mg daily 3 wk on, 1 wk off

Prevention of osteoporosis
Adult: PO 0.625 mg daily or in a cycle

Atrophic vaginitis
Adult: Vag 2-4 g cream daily × 21 days, off 7 days, repeat

Prostatic cancer
Adult: PO 1.25-2.5 mg tid

Advanced inoperable breast cancer
Adult: PO 10 mg tid × 3 mo or longer

Abnormal uterine bleeding
Adult: **IV**/IM 25 mg, repeat in 6-12 hr
Ovariectomy/primary ovarian failure/castration
Adult: PO 1.25 mg daily 3 wk on, 1 wk off
Hypogonadism
Adult: PO 2.5 mg bid-tid × 20 days/mo
Estrogens conjugated synthetic B menopause
Adult: PO 0.625 mg daily initially, may increase based on response

Available forms: Tabs 0.3, 0.625, 0.9, 1.25, 2.5 mg; inj 25 mg/vial; vag cream 0.625 mg/g; synthetic B: tabs 0.625, 1.25 mg

Adverse effects
CNS: Dizziness, headache, migraine, depression, **seizures**
CV: Hypotension, thrombophlebitis, edema, **thromboembolism, stroke, pulmonary embolism, MI**
EENT: Contact lens intolerance, increased myopia, astigmatism
GI: *Nausea,* vomiting, diarrhea, anorexia, pancreatitis, cramps, constipation, increased appetite, increased weight, **cholestatic jaundice, hepatic adenoma**
GU: Amenorrhea, cervical erosion, breakthrough bleeding, dysmenorrhea, vaginal candidiasis, breast changes, *gynecomastia, testicular atrophy, impotence,* **increased risk of breast, endometrial cancer,** libido changes
INTEG: Rash, urticaria, acne, hirsutism, alopecia, oily skin, seborrhea, purpura, melasma
META: Folic acid deficiency, hypercalcemia, hyperglycemia

Contraindications: Pregnancy **X,** thromboembolic disorders, reproductive cancer, genital bleeding (abnormal, undiagnosed), lactation

Precautions: Hypertension, asthma, blood dyscrasias, gallbladder disease, CHF, diabetes mellitus, bone disease, depression, migraine headache, seizure disorders, hepatic, renal disease, family history of cancer of breast or reproductive tract, smoking

Pharmacokinetics

Absorption	Well absorbed (PO), completely absorbed **(IV)**
Distribution	Widely distributed, crosses placenta
Metabolism	Liver—exclusively; hepatic recirculation
Excretion	Kidney
Half-life	Unknown

Pharmacodynamics

	PO	IM	IV
Onset	Rapid	Slow	Immediate
Peak	Unknown	Unknown	Unknown
Duration	Unknown	Unknown	Unknown

Interactions
Individual drugs
Cyclosporine, dantrolene: increased toxicity
Phenylbutazone, rifampin: decreased action of estrogens
Tamoxifen: decreased tamoxifen action
Drug classifications
Anticoagulants: decreased action of anticoagulants
Anticonvulsants, barbiturates: decreased action of estrogens
Corticosteroids: increased action of corticosteroids
Oral hypoglycemics: decreased action of hypoglycemics
Drug/herb
Alfalfa, hops: increased estrogen level
Black cohosh, DHEA: altered estrogen effect
Saw palmetto: decreased estrogen level
Drug/food
Grapefruit juice: increased estrogen level
Drug/lab test
Increased: BSP retention test; PBI, T_4; serum sodium; platelet aggregation; thyroxine-binding globulin (TBG); prothrombin; factors VII, VIII, IX, X; triglycerides
Decreased: serum folate, serum triglyceride, T_3 resin uptake test, glucose tolerance test, antithrombin III, pregnanediol, metyrapone test
False positive: LE prep, ANA titer

NURSING CONSIDERATIONS
Assessment
- Monitor blood glucose in patient with diabetes; hyperglycemia may occur
- Monitor B/P q4h; watch for increase caused by water and sodium retention
- Monitor I&O ratio; be alert for decreasing urinary output and increasing edema; monitor

weight daily; notify prescriber if weekly weight gain is >5 lb; if increased, diuretic may be ordered
- Obtain liver function studies, including AST, ALT, bilirubin, alkaline phosphatase
- Assess edema, hypertension, cardiac symptoms, jaundice
- Assess mental status: affect, mood, behavioral changes, aggression; depression may occur, drug may need to be discontinued
- Assess female patient for intact uterus; if so, progesterone should be added to estrogen therapy to decrease risk of endometrial cancer

Nursing diagnoses
- Sexual dysfunction (uses)
- Injury, risk for (adverse reactions)

Implementation
PO route
- Give titrated dose, use lowest effective dose
- Give in 1 dose in AM for prostatic cancer, vaginitis, hypogonadism
- Give with food or milk to decrease GI symptoms

IM route
- Reconstitute after withdrawing at least 5 ml of air from container and inject sterile diluent on vial side, rotate to dissolve
- Give IM inj deeply in large muscle

Vaginal route
- Place cream in applicator by attaching tube to applicator, squeeze cream into tube to mark, insert with patient recumbent
- Applicator should be washed after each use

IV route
- Direct **IV**: reconstitute as for IM, inject into distal port of running **IV** line of D_5W, 0.9% NaCl, LR, at a rate of 5 mg/min or less

Y-site compatibilities: Heparin/hydrocortisone, potassium chloride, vit B/C

Patient/family education
- Caution patient to take exactly as prescribed and not to double doses
- Advise patient that increased weight gain and symptoms of fluid retention should be reported to prescriber: edema of feet, ankles, sacral area; abnormal vaginal bleeding; breast lumps; hepatic disease (dark urine, clay-colored stools, jaundice of skin, sclera, pruritus)
- Caution patient that thromboembolic symptoms should be reported: pain, redness, tenderness in legs; chest pain, dyspnea, headaches, blurred vision
- Inform patient that sunburns may occur and to use sunscreen and protective clothing
- Advise patient to stop smoking; smokers have a greater chance of thromboembolic disorder
- Tell patient to use nonhormonal birth control, and to notify prescriber if pregnancy is suspected

Evaluation
Positive therapeutic outcome
- Reversal of menopause symptoms
- Decrease in tumor size in prostatic, breast cancer
- Decrease in itching, inflammation of vagina
- Absence of symptoms of osteoporosis

etanercept (Rx)
(eh-tan'er-sept)

Enbrel

Func. class.: Antirheumatic agent (disease-modifying)

Pregnancy category B

Action: Binds to tumor necrosis factor (TNF), which decreases inflammation and immune response

Therapeutic Outcome: Decreased pain, inflammation

Uses: Acute, chronic rheumatoid arthritis that has not responded to other disease-modifying agents; polyarticular course juvenile rheumatoid arthritis (JRA)

Investigational uses: CHF, psoriasis/psoriatic arthritis

Dosage and routes
Osteoarthritis

Adult: SUBCUT 25 mg 2×/wk, may be given with other drugs for rheumatoid arthritis

Child 4-17 yr: SUBCUT 0.4 mg/kg 2×/wk, max 25 mg/dose

CHF

Adult: SUBCUT 5-12 mg/m^2 2×/wk × 3 mo

Psoriasis/psoriatic arthritis

Adult: SUBCUT 25 mg 2×/wk × 12 wk

Available forms: Powder for inj: 25 mg

Adverse effects
CNS: Headache, asthenia, dizziness
GI: Abdominal pain, dyspepsia
INTEG: Rash, *inj site reaction*
RESP: Pharyngitis, rhinitis, *cough, URI,* non-URI sinusitis

Contraindications: Hypersensitivity, sepsis

Precautions: Pregnancy **B**, lactation, children <4 yr, elderly

Pharmacokinetics

Absorption	Rapidly (60%)
Distribution	Unknown
Metabolism	Unknown
Excretion	Unknown
Half-life	115 hr

Pharmacodynamics

Onset	Unknown
Peak	Unknown
Duration	Unknown

Interactions
Drug classifications
Immunizations: should be brought up to date before treatment
Immunizations, vaccines: do not give concurrently

NURSING CONSIDERATIONS
Assessment
- Assess for pain of rheumatoid arthritis; check ROM, inflammation of joints, characteristics of pain
- Assess inj site for pain, swelling, usually occurs after 2 inj (4-5 days)

Nursing diagnoses
- Pain, chronic (uses)
- Mobility, physical, impaired (uses)
- Injury, risk for (side effects)
- Knowledge, deficient (teaching)

Implementation
- Administer after reconstituting 1 ml of supplied diluent, slowly inject diluent into vial, swirl contents, do not shake, sol should be clear/colorless, do not use if cloudy or discolored
- Do not admix with other sol or medications; do not use filter
- May be injected SUBCUT into upper arm, abdomen, thigh; rotate inj sites

Patient/family education
- Teach patient that drug must be continued for prescribed time to be effective; to avoid aspirin, alcoholic beverages
- Instruct patient to use caution when driving; dizziness may occur
- Teach patient about self-administration, if appropriate: inj should be made in thigh, abdomen, upper arm; rotate sites at least 1 in from old site

Evaluation
Positive therapeutic outcome
- Decreased pain in arthritic conditions
- Decreased inflammation in arthritic conditions

ethambutol (Rx)
(e-tham'byoo-tole)
Etibi ✤, Myambutol
Func. class.: Antitubercular
Chem. class.: Diisopropylethylene diamide derivative

Pregnancy category B

Do Not Confuse:
ethambutol/Ethmozine

Action: Inhibits RNA synthesis, decreases tubercle bacilli replication

Therapeutic Outcome: Resolution of TB infection

Uses: Pulmonary TB, as an adjunct, other mycobacterial infections

Dosage and routes
Adult and child >13 yr: PO 15-25 mg/kg/day as a single dose or 50 mg/kg 2×/wk or 25-30 mg/kg 3×/wk

Renal dose
Adult: PO CCr 10-50 ml/min dose q24-36h; CCr <10 ml/min dose q48h

Retreatment
Adult: PO 25 mg/kg/day as single dose × 2 mo with at least 1 other drug, then decrease to 15 mg/kg/day as single dose, max 2.5 g/day
Child: PO 15 mg/kg/day

Available forms: Tabs 100, 400 mg

Adverse effects
CNS: *Headache, confusion,* fever, malaise, dizziness, *disorientation,* hallucinations
EENT: Blurred vision, optic neuritis, photophobia, decreased visual acuity
GI: *Abdominal distress, anorexia, nausea, vomiting*
INTEG: Dermatitis, pruritus, **toxic epidermal necrolysis**
META: *Elevated uric acid, acute gout,* liver function impairment
MISC: **Thrombocytopenia,** joint pain, bloody sputum, **anaphylaxis**

Contraindications: Hypersensitivity, optic neuritis, child <13 yr

Precautions: Pregnancy **B,** renal disease, diabetic retinopathy, cataracts, ocular defects, hepatic and hematopoietic disorders, lactation

Pharmacokinetics	
Absorption	Rapidly absorbed
Distribution	Widely distributed, crosses blood-brain barrier, placenta
Metabolism	Liver
Excretion	Kidneys—unchanged
Half-life	3 hr, increased in liver, kidney disease

Pharmacodynamics	
Onset	Rapid
Peak	2-4 hr

Interactions

Drug classifications

Antacids, aluminum: decreased absorption
Neurotoxic agents, other: increased neurotoxicity

NURSING CONSIDERATIONS

Assessment

- Obtain C&S tests including sputum tests before initiating treatment; monitor qmo to detect resistance
- Monitor liver function studies qwk × 2 wk, then q2 mo: ALT, AST, bilirubin; renal studies: before, qmo: BUN, creatinine, output, sp gr, urinalysis, uric acid
- Assess patient's mental status often: affect, mood, behavioral changes; psychosis may occur with hallucinations, confusion
- Assess patient's hepatic status: decreased appetite, jaundice, dark urine, fatigue
- Assess patient for visual disturbance that may indicate optic neuritis: blurred vision, change in color perception; may lead to blindness

Nursing diagnoses

- Infection, risk for (uses)
- Diarrhea (adverse reactions)
- Sensory perception, disturbed (adverse reactions)
- Knowledge, deficient (teaching)
- Noncompliance (teaching)

Implementation

- Give with meals to decrease GI symptoms, at same time each day to maintain blood level
- Give 2 hr before antacids
- Give antiemetic if vomiting occurs

Patient/family education

- Advise patient that compliance with dosage schedule and duration is necessary to eradicate disease; to keep scheduled appointments including ophthalmic appointments or relapse may occur
- Caution patient to report weakness, fatigue, loss of appetite, nausea, vomiting, yellowing of skin or eyes, tingling/numbness of hands/feet, weight gain, or decreased urine output
- Instruct patient to report any visual changes; rash; hot, swollen, painful joints; numbness or tingling of extremities to physician
- Caution patient to inform prescriber if pregnancy is suspected

Evaluation

Positive therapeutic outcome

- Decreased symptoms of TB
- Decrease in acid-fast bacteria

E

etidronate (Rx)

(eh-tih-droe'nate)

Didronel, Didronel IV

Func. class.: Bone resorption inhibitor

Chem. class.: Bisphosphonate

Pregnancy category C

Do Not Confuse:
etidronate/etomidate, etidronate/etretinate

Action: Decreases bone resorption and new bone development (accretion)

Therapeutic Outcome: Decreased bone reabsorption, calcium levels WNL

Uses: Paget's disease, heterotopic ossification, hypercalcemia of malignancy

Dosage and routes

Paget's disease

Adult: PO 5-10 mg/kg/day, 2 hr ac with water, not to exceed 20 mg/kg/day, max 6 mo or 11-20 mg/kg/day for max of 3 mo

Heterotopic ossification

Adult: PO 20 mg/kg daily × 2 wk, then 10 mg/kg/day for 10 wk, total 12 wk

Hypercalcemia

Adult: **IV** 7.5 mg/kg/day × 3 days, then 20 mg/kg/day (PO)

Heterotopic ossification/hip replacement

Adult: PO 20 mg/kg/day × 4 wk before and 3 mo after surgery (4 months total)

Available forms: Tabs 200, 400 mg; inj 50 mg/ml

Adverse effects
GI: *Nausea,* constipation, metallic taste, diarrhea(**IV**)
GU: **Nephrotoxicity**
MISC: Dyspnea; low magnesium, phosphorous, alopecia
MS: *Bone pain,* hypocalcemia, decreased mineralization of nonaffected bones

Contraindications: Pathologic fractures, clinically overt osteomalacia, severe renal disease with creatinine >5 mg/dl

Precautions: Pregnancy **C,** renal disease, lactation, restricted vit D/Ca, children, enterocolitis

Pharmacokinetics

Absorption	Poorly absorbed (PO), completely absorbed (**IV**)
Distribution	50% bond to crystals in osteogenesis
Metabolism	None
Excretion	Feces (unabsorbed), kidney (unchanged)
Half-life	5-7 hr; in bone >3 mo

Pharmacodynamics

	PO	IV
Onset	4 wk	24 hr
Peak	Unknown	3-4 days
Duration	Up to 1 yr	10-12 days

Interactions
Individual drugs
Warfarin: increased protime
Drug classifications
Antacids, mineral supplements with magnesium, calcium, iron products, or aluminum: decreased absorption of etidronate
Drug/food
Dairy products: decreased absorption of etidronate

NURSING CONSIDERATIONS
Assessment
- Assess for GI symptoms, polyuria, flushing, head swelling, tingling, headache, may indicate hypercalcemia; nervousness, irritability, twitching, seizures, spasm, paresthesia indicates hypocalcemia at start of treatment
- Identify nutritional status; evaluate diet for sources of vit D (milk, some seafood), calcium (dairy products, dark green vegetables), phosphates
- Monitor BUN, creatinine, uric acid, chloride, electrolytes, urine pH, urinary calcium, magnesium, phosphate, urinalysis (calcium-should be kept at 9-10 mg/dl), albumin, alkaline phosphatase baseline and q3-6 mo; check urine sediment for casts throughout treatment
- Assess for increased drug level; toxic reactions occur rapidly; have calcium chloride or gluconate on hand if calcium level drops too low; check for tetany

Nursing diagnoses
- Injury, risk for (adverse reactions)
- Pain, chronic (uses)
- Knowledge, deficient (teaching)

Implementation
PO route
- Administer on empty stomach to improve absorption (2 hr ac)

IV route
- Used in hypercalcemias; give by intermittent inf after diluting 300 mg/250 ml or more 0.9% NaCl; run over 2-3 hr, therapy should not last >6 mo

Patient/family education
- Teach method of inj if patient will be responsible for self-medication
- Caution patient to notify prescriber if hypercalcemia recurs: renal calculi, nausea, vomiting, thirst, lethargy, deep bone or flank pain, heat over bone, restricted mobility
- Teach patient that warmth and flushing occur and last 1 hr
- Teach patient to follow a low-calcium diet as prescribed (Paget's disease, hypercalcemia)
- Advise patient to notify prescriber of diarrhea, nausea; dose may be divided to lessen these symptoms
- Inform patient that metallic taste may occur with **IV** dosing

Evaluation
Positive therapeutic outcome
- Calcium levels 9-10 mg/dl
- Decreasing symptoms of Paget's disease including pain
- Decreased bone loss in osteoporosis

etodolac (Rx)
(ee-toe-doe'lak)
Lodine, Lodine XL
Func. class.: Nonsteroidal antiinflammatory, nonopioid analgesic
Pregnancy category C

Do Not Confuse:
Lodine/codeine/iodine

Action: Inhibits prostaglandin synthesis by decreasing enzyme needed for biosynthesis; analgesic, antiinflammatory properties

Therapeutic Outcome: Decreased pain, inflammation

Uses: Mild to moderate pain, osteoarthritis

Dosage and routes

Osteoarthritis

Adult: PO 800-1200 mg/day in divided doses q6-8h initially, then adjust to 600-1200 mg/day in divided doses; do not exceed 1200 mg/day; patients <60 kg not to exceed 20 mg/kg

Analgesia

Adult: PO 200-400 mg q6-8h prn for acute pain; do not exceed 1200 mg/day; patients <60 kg not to exceed 20 mg/kg

Available forms: Caps 200, 300 mg; tabs 400, 500 mg; ext rel tabs 400, 600 mg

Adverse effects

CNS: Dizziness, headache, drowsiness, fatigue, tremors, confusion, insomnia, anxiety, depression, light-headedness, vertigo
CV: Tachycardia, peripheral edema, fluid retention, palpitations, dysrhythmias, CHF
EENT: Tinnitus, hearing loss, blurred vision, photophobia
GI: *Nausea, anorexia,* vomiting, diarrhea, jaundice, **cholestatic hepatitis,** constipation, flatulence, cramps, dry mouth, peptic ulcer, dyspepsia, **GI bleeding**
GU: **Nephrotoxicity, dysuria, hematuria, oliguria, azotemia, cystitis, UTI**
HEMA: **Blood dyscrasias**
INTEG: Erythema, urticaria, purpura, rash, pruritus, sweating, **Stevens-Johnson syndrome**
SYST: **Angioedema, anaphylaxis**

Contraindications: Hypersensitivity; patients in whom aspirin, iodides, or other NSAIDs have produced asthma, rhinitis, urticaria, nasal polyps, angioedema, bronchospasm; avoid in 2nd half of pregnancy

Precautions: Pregnancy **C,** lactation, children, bleeding, GI, cardiac disorders, elderly; renal, hepatic disorders

Pharmacokinetics	
Absorption	Well absorbed
Distribution	Highly bound to plasma protein
Metabolism	Unknown
Excretion	Unknown
Half-life	7 hr

Pharmacodynamics	
Onset	½ hr
Peak	1-2 hr
Duration	4-12 hr

Interactions

Individual drugs

Aspirin: may increase GI toxicity
CycloSPORINE, digoxin, lithium, methotrexate, phenytoin: increased toxicity

Drug classifications

Antacids: delayed etodolac effect
β-Adrenergic blockers: decreased effect
Diuretics: decreased effectiveness of diuretics

Drug/herb

Arginine, gossypol: increased gastric irritation
Bearberry, bilberry: increased NSAIDs action
Bogbean, chondroitin, saw palmetto, turmeric: increased bleeding risk
St. John's wort: severe photosensitivity

NURSING CONSIDERATIONS

Assessment

- Assess pain: location, frequency, characteristics; relief after medication
- Assess for GI bleeding: black stools, hematemesis
- Assess for asthma, aspirin hypersensitivity, nasal polyps that may be hypersensitive to etodolac
- Monitor blood counts during therapy; watch for decreasing platelets; if low, therapy may need to be discontinued, then restarted after hematologic recovery; watch for blood dyscrasia (thrombocytopenia): bruising, fatigue, bleeding, poor healing

Nursing diagnoses

- Pain, acute (uses)
- Pain, chronic (uses)
- Mobility, physical, impaired (uses)
- Knowledge, deficient (teaching)
- Injury, risk for (adverse reactions)

Implementation

- Do not break, crush, or chew ext rel tabs
- Administer with full glass of water to enhance absorption
- Administer with food or milk to decrease gastric symptoms; food will slow absorption slightly, will not decrease absorption

Patient/family education

- Inform patient that drug must be continued for prescribed time to be effective; to avoid aspirin, alcoholic beverages, NSAIDs
- Caution patient to report bleeding, bruising, fatigue, malaise because blood dyscrasias can occur

- Instruct patient to use caution when driving; drowsiness, dizziness may occur
- Teach patient to take with a full glass of water to enhance absorption

Evaluation

Positive therapeutic outcome

- Decreased pain
- Decreased inflammation
- Increased mobility

! HIGH ALERT

etoposide (Rx)

(e-toe'poe-side)

VePesid, VP-16

Func. class.: Antineoplastic—miscellaneous

Chem. class.: Semisynthetic podophyllotoxin

Pregnancy category D

Do Not Confuse:

VePesid/Versed

Action: Inhibits mitotic activity through metaphase to mitosis; also inhibits cells from entering mitosis, depresses DNA, RNA synthesis, cell cycle specific S and G_2

Therapeutic Outcome: Prevention of rapid growth of malignant cells

Uses: Leukemias, lung, testicular cancer, lymphomas, neuroblastoma, melanoma, ovarian cancer; being investigated for use in leukemia, lymphoma

Dosage and routes

Testicular cancer

Adult: **IV** 50-100 mg/m^2/day × 3-5 days given q3-5 wk or 200-250 mg/m^2/wk, or 125-140 mg/m^2/day 3 × wk, q5 wk

Small cell carcinoma of the lung

Adult: PO 70 mg/m^2/day × 4 days, repeated q3-4 wk; **IV** 35 mg/m^2/day × 4 days, up to 50 mg/m^2 daily × 5 day q3-4 wk

Available forms: Inj 20 mg/ml, caps 50 mg

Adverse effects

CNS: Headache, *fever,* peripheral neuropathy, paresthesia, confusion

CV: *Hypotension,* **MI,** dysrhythmia

GI: *Nausea, vomiting, anorexia,* **hepatotoxicity,** dyspepsia, diarrhea, constipation

GU: **Nephrotoxicity**

HEMA: **Thrombocytopenia, leukopenia, myelosuppression, anemia**

INTEG: *Rash, alopecia,* phlebitis at **IV** site, radiation recall

RESP: **Bronchospasm,** pleural effusion

SYST: **Anaphylaxis**

Contraindications: Pregnancy **D,** hypersensitivity, bone marrow depression, severe hepatic disease, severe renal disease, bacterial infection, viral infection

Precautions: Renal, hepatic disease; lactation, children, gout

Pharmacokinetics

Absorption	Variably absorbed
Distribution	Rapidly absorbed, 97% protein binding, crosses placenta
Metabolism	Liver—some
Excretion	Kidneys, unchanged 50%, breast milk
Half-life	3 hr initially, 15 hr terminally

Pharmacodynamics

Unknown

Interactions

Individual drugs

Radiation: increased bone marrow depression

Drug classifications

Antineoplastics: increased bone marrow depression

Live virus vaccines: increased adverse reactions

NURSING CONSIDERATIONS

Assessment

- Monitor B/P (baseline and q15 min) during administration
- Monitor CBC, differential, platelet count weekly; withhold drug if WBC is <4000/mm^3 or platelet count is <75,000/mm^3; notify prescriber of results; recovery will take 3 wk
- Monitor renal function studies: BUN, urine CCr before, during therapy; I&O ratio; report fall in urine output of 30 ml/hr; for decreased hyperuricemia
- Monitor for cold, fever, sore throat (may indicate beginning of infection); notify prescriber if these occur
- Assess for bleeding: hematuria, guaiac, bruising or petechiae, mucosa or orifices q8h: no rectal temp; avoid IM inj; use pressure to venipuncture sites
- Identify nutritional status: an antiemetic may need to be prescribed
- (Alert) Assess for symptoms indicating severe allergic reactions: rash, pruritus, urticaria,

itching, flushing, bronchospasm, hypotension; epINEPHrine and crash cart should be nearby

Nursing diagnoses

- Injury, risk for (adverse reactions)
- Body image, disturbed (adverse reactions)
- Infection, risk for (adverse reactions)
- Knowledge, deficient (teaching)

Implementation

PO route

- Caps need to be refrigerated

IV route

- Give by intermittent inf
- Sol should be prepared by qualified personnel and only under controlled conditions
- Use Luer-Lok tubing to prevent leakage; do not let sol come in contact with skin; if contact occurs, wash well with soap and water
- Give after diluting 100 mg/250 ml or more D_5W or NaCl to a concentration of 0.2-0.4 mg/ml; infuse over 30-60 min; phosphate may be given over 5 min-3½ hr; may dilute further to 0.1 mg/ml in 0.9% NaCl, D_5W
- Give hyaluronidase 150 units/ml to 1 ml NaCl to infiltration area; ice compress for treatment of vesicant activity

Y-site compatibilities: Allopurinol, amifostine, aztreonam, cladribine, fludarabine, granisetron, melphalan, ondansetron, paclitaxel, piperacillin/tazobactam, sargramostim, sodium bicarbonate, teniposide, thiotepa, vinorelbine

Y-site incompatibility: Idarubicin

Additive compatibilities: Carboplatin, cisplatin, cytarabine, floxuridine, fluorouracil, hydrOXYzine, ifosfamide, ondansetron

Patient/family education

- Teach patient to avoid use of products containing aspirin or ibuprofen, razors, commercial mouthwash because bleeding may occur; to report symptoms of bleeding (hematuria, tarry stools)
- Instruct patient to report signs of anemia (fatigue, headache, irritability, faintness, shortness of breath)
- Teach patient to report any changes in breathing or coughing even several months after treatment
- Advise patient that contraception will be necessary during treatment because teratogenesis may occur
- Caution patient that hair loss may occur during treatment; a wig or hairpiece may make patient feel better; new hair will be different in color, texture
- Advise patient to avoid vaccinations during treatment because serious reactions may occur
- Teach patient to report signs/symptoms ofinfection; fever, chills, sore throat; patient should avoid crowds and persons with known infections

Evaluation

Positive therapeutic outcome

- Decreased spread of malignant, leukemic cells

exemestane (Rx)

(x-ee-mes'-tane)

Aromasin

Func. class.: Antineoplastic

Chem. class.: Aromatase inhibitor

Pregnancy category D

Action: Lowers serum estradiol concentrations; many breast cancers have strong estrogen receptors

Therapeutic Outcome: Prevention of rapidly growing malignant cells

Uses: Advanced breast carcinoma that has not responded to other therapy in estrogen receptor–positive patients (postmenopausal)

Dosage and routes

Adult: PO 25 mg daily pc

Available forms: Tabs 25 mg

Adverse effects

CNS: Hot flashes, headache, fatigue, depression, insomnia, anxiety

CV: Hypertension

GI: Nausea, vomiting, increased appetite, diarrhea, constipation, abdominal pain

HEMA: *Lymphopenia*

RESP: Cough, dyspnea

Contraindications: Pregnancy **D**, hypersensitivity, premenopausal women

Precautions: Lactation, children, elderly, hepatic, renal disease

Pharmacokinetics

Absorption	Rapidly absorbed
Distribution	Unknown
Metabolism	Liver
Excretion	Feces, urine
Half-life	24 hr

Pharmacodynamics

Unknown

Interactions
Drug classifications
CYP3A4 inducers, estrogens: decreased exemestane action

NURSING CONSIDERATIONS
Assessment
- Assess B/P, hypertension may occur

Nursing diagnoses
- Injury, risk for (adverse reactions)
- Knowledge, deficient (teaching)

Implementation
- Give with food or fluids for GI upset
- Store in light-resistant container at room temp

Patient/family education
- Instruct patient to report any complaints, side effects to prescriber; if dose is missed, do not double next dose
- Advise patient that hot flashes can occur, and are reversible after discontinuing treatment
- Inform patient about who should be told about therapy

Evaluation
Positive therapeutic outcome
- Decreased spread of malignant cells in breast cancer

exenatide
Byetta
See Appendix A, Selected New Drugs

ezetimibe (Rx)
(ehz-eh-tim′bee)
Zetia
Func. class.: Antilipemic
Pregnancy category C

Action: Inhibits absorption of cholesterol by the small intestine

Therapeutic Outcome: Decreased cholesterol levels

Uses: Hypercholesterolemia, homozygous familial hypercholesterolemia (HoFH), homozygous sitosterolemia

Dosage and routes
Adult: **PO** 10 mg daily; may be given with HMG-CoA reductase inhibitor at same time; may be given with bile acid sequestrant; give ezetimibe 2 hr before or 4 hr after the bile acid sequestrant

Available forms: Tabs 10 mg

Adverse effects
CNS: Fatigue, dizziness, headache
GI: Diarrhea, abdominal pain
MISC: Chest pain
MS: *Myalgias, arthralgias,* back pain
RESP: Pharyngitis, sinusitis, cough, URI

Contraindications: Hypersensitivity, severe hepatic disease

Precautions: Pregnancy **C,** lactation, children, hepatic disease

Pharmacokinetics

Absorption	Unknown
Distribution	Unknown
Metabolism	Small intestine, liver
Excretion	Urine (11%), feces (78%)
Half-life	Unknown

Pharmacodynamics
Unknown

Interactions
Individual drugs
Cholestyramine: decreased ezetimibe action
CycloSPORINE: increased action of ezetimibe
Drug classifications
Antacids: decreased action of ezetimibe
Fibric acid derivatives: increased ezetimibe action
Drug/herb
Glucomannan: increased effect
Gotu kola: decreased effect

NURSING CONSIDERATIONS
Assessment
- Monitor lipid levels, liver function tests baseline and periodically during treatment

Nursing diagnoses
- Knowledge, deficient (teaching)
- Noncompliance (teaching)

Implementation
- Give without regard to meals

Patient/family education
- Teach patient that compliance is needed
- Advise that risk factors should be decreased: high-fat diet, smoking, alcohol consumption, absence of exercise
- Advise patient to notify prescriber if pregnancy is suspected or planned

Evaluation
Positive therapeutic outcome
- Decreased cholesterol

! HIGH ALERT

factor IX complex (human)/ factor IV (Rx)

Benefix, Konyne 80, Profilnine/Alpha Nine, Proplex T, Proplex SX-T, Alpha Nine SD, Mononine

Func. class.: Hemostatic

Chem. class.: Factors II, VII, IX, X

Pregnancy category C

Action: Causes an increase in blood levels of clotting factors II, VII, IX, X; factor IX (human) has IX activity only

Therapeutic Outcome: Replacement of factors II, VII, IX, X

Uses: Hemophilia B (Christmas disease), factor IX deficiency, anticoagulant reversal, control of bleeding in patients with factor VIII inhibitors; reversal of overdose of anticoagulants in emergencies

Dosage and routes

Bleeding in hemophilia A and inhibitors of factor VIII (Proplex T, Konyne 80)

Adult and child: 75 units/kg, repeat in 12 hr

Bleeding in hemophilia B

Adult and child: **IV** establish 25% of normal factor IX activity or 60-75 units/kg then 10-20 units/kg/day × 1-2 wk

Prophylaxis of bleeding in hemophilia B

Adult and child: 10-20 units/kg 1-2 × wk

Reversal of oral anticoagulant

Adult and child: 15 units/kg

Factor VII deficiency (use Proplex T only)

Adult and child: 0.5 units/kg × body weight (kg) × desired factor IX increase (in % of normal); repeat q4-6h if needed

Factor IX, (human) minor to moderate hemorrhage

Use only Alpha Nine, Alpha Nine SD

Adult and child: **IV** dose to increase plasma factor IX level to 20%-30% in one dose

Serious hemorrhage

Adult and child: **IV** dose to increase plasma factor IX level to 30%-50% given as daily inf

Minor hemorrhage (Mononine only)

Adult and child: **IV** dose to increase plasma factor IX level to 15%-25% (20-30 units/kg), may repeat in 24 hr if needed

Major hemorrhage

Adult and child: **IV** dose to increase plasma factor IX level to 25%-50% (75 units/kg) q18-30h for up to 10 days

Available forms: Inj (number of units noted on label)

Adverse effects

CNS: *Headache, dizziness,* malaise, paresthesia, *lethargy, chills, fever, flushing*

CV: *Hypotension,* tachycardia, **MI, venous thrombosis, pulmonary embolism**

GI: Nausea, vomiting, abdominal cramps, jaundice, **viral hepatitis**

HEMA: **Thrombosis, hemolysis, AIDS, disseminated intravascular coagulation (DIC)**

INTEG: Rash, flushing, *urticaria*

RESP: **Bronchospasm**

Contraindications: Hypersensitivity to mouse protein, hepatic disease, DIC, elective surgery, mild factor IX deficiency

Precautions: Pregnancy **C**, neonates/infants

Pharmacokinetics

Absorption	40% (PO), complete (**IV**)
Distribution	Unknown
Metabolism	Rapidly cleared from plasma, liver 30%
Excretion	Kidneys—70% unchanged
Half-life	24 hr

Pharmacodynamics

Unknown

Interactions

Individual drugs

Aminocaproic acid: increased risk of thrombosis; do not use together

Warfarin: decreased effect of warfarin

Drug classifications

Incompatible with protein products

NURSING CONSIDERATIONS

Assesment

- Monitor blood studies (coagulation factor assays by % normal: 5% prevents spontaneous hemorrhage, 30%-50% for surgery, 80%-100% for severe hemorrhage); check for bleeding q15-30 min, immobilize and apply ice to affected joints

F

- Monitor for increased B/P, pulse
- Monitor I&O; if urine becomes orange or red, notify prescriber
- Assess for allergic or pyrogenic reaction: fever, chills, rash, itching; slow inf rate if not severe
- ❗ Assess for DIC: bleeding, ecchymosis, hypersensitivity, changes in coagulation tests

Nursing diagnoses
- Injury, risk for (uses)
- Tissue perfusion, ineffective (uses)
- Knowledge, deficient (teaching)

Implementation
IV route
- Give hepatitis B vaccine before administration
- Give **IV** after warming to room temp 3 ml/min or less, with plastic syringe only; do not admix
- Give after dilution with provided diluent, 50 or 25 units/ml; give so as not to exceed 10 ml/min; decrease rate if fever, headache, flushing, tingling occur
- Give after crossmatch is completed if patient has blood type A, B, AB, to determine incompatibility with factor
- Store reconstituted sol for 3 hr at room temp or up to 2 yr if refrigerated (powder); check expiration date
- Incompatible with protein products

Patient/family education
- Advise patient to report any signs of bleeding: gums, under skin, urine, stools, emesis
- Caution patient about risk of viral hepatitis, AIDS; that immunization for hepatitis B may be given first; to be tested q2-3 mo for HIV, even though the risk is low
- Tell patient to carry/wear emergency ID identifying disease and treatment; avoid salicylates, NSAIDs, to inform other health professionals about condition

Evaluation
Positive therapeutic outcome
- Prevention of hemorrhage

famciclovir (Rx)
(fam-sye-klo'vir)
Famvir
Func. class.: Antiviral
Chem. class.: Guanosine nucleoside
Pregnancy category B

Action: Inhibits DNA polymerase and viral DNA synthesis by the conversion of this guanosine nucleoside to penciclovir

Therapeutic Outcome: Decreasing size and number of lesions

Uses: Treatment of acute herpes zoster (shingles), genital herpes, recurrent mucocutaneous herpes simplex virus (HSV) in HIV patients

Investigational uses: Initial episodes of herpes genitalis

Dosage and routes
Herpes zoster
Adult: PO 500 mg q8h × 7 days

Renal dose
Adult: PO CCr ≥ 60 ml/min 500 mg q8h; 40-59 ml/min 500 mg q12h; 20-39 ml/min 500 mg q24h

Recurrent mucocutaneous herpes simplex
Adult: PO 500 mg q12h × 1 wk

Recurrent HSV
Adult: PO 125 mg q12h × 5 days

Suppression of recurrent HSV
Adult: PO 250 mg q12h up to 1 yr

Genital herpes (recurrent)
Adult: PO 125 mg bid × 5 days; begin treatment at first sign of recurrence

Suppression of recurrent genital herpes
Adult: PO 250 mg bid for up to a year

Herpes genitalis
Initial episodes (off-label)
Adult: PO 25 mg tid × 7-10 days

Available forms: Tabs 125, 250, 500 mg

Adverse effects
CNS: *Headache, fatigue, dizziness,* paresthesia, somnolence, fever
GI: Nausea, vomiting, diarrhea, constipation, abdominal pain, anorexia
GU: Decreased sperm count
INTEG: *Pruritus*
MS: Back pain, arthralgia
RESP: Pharyngitis, sinusitis

Contraindications: Hypersensitivity to this drug or penciclovir

Precautions: Pregnancy **B**, renal disease, hypersensitivity to acyclovir, ganciclovir, lactation

Pharmacokinetics	
Absorption	Well absorbed
Distribution	Unknown
Metabolism	Intestinal tissue, blood, liver
Excretion	Breast milk, kidney, bile
Half-life	3 hr

Pharmacodynamics	
Onset	Unknown
Peak	1 hr
Duration	8 hr

Interactions

Individual drugs

Cimetidine: decreased metabolism

Digoxin, probenecid, theophylline: decreased renal excretion

NURSING CONSIDERATIONS

Assessment

- Assess amount and distribution of lesions; also burning, itching, or pain (early symptoms of herpes infection); neuralgia during and after treatment
- Monitor renal function studies: urine CCr, BUN before and during treatment if patient has decreased renal function; dose may need to be lowered
- Monitor bowel pattern before, during treatment; diarrhea may occur

Nursing diagnoses

- Infection, risk for (uses)
- Knowledge, deficient (teaching)

Implementation

- Give with or without meals; absorption does not appear to be lowered when taken with food
- Give within 72 hr of the appearance of rash in herpes zoster

Patient/family education

- Teach patient how to recognize signs of beginning of infection
- Teach patient how to prevent the spread of infection to others
- Teach patient reason for medication and expected results
- Advise patient that this medication does not prevent spread of disease to others, that condoms should be used
- Advise women with genital herpes to have yearly Pap smears, cervical cancer is more likely

Evaluation

Positive therapeutic outcome

- Decreased size and spread of lesions

famotidine (Rx, OTC)

(fa-moe'to-deen)

Mylanta AR, Pepcid AC, Pepcid, Pepcid IV, Pepcid RPD ♣

Func. class.: H_2-histamine receptor antagonist, antiulcer agent

Pregnancy category B

Action: Inhibits histamine at H_2-receptor site in gastric parietal cells, which inhibits gastric acid secretion

Therapeutic Outcome: Healing of duodenal ulcers or gastric ulcers; prevention of duodenal ulcers; decreases symptoms of gastroesophageal reflux disease or Zollinger-Ellison syndrome, heartburn

Uses: Short-term treatment of active duodenal ulcer, maintenance therapy for duodenal ulcer, Zollinger-Ellison syndrome, multiple endocrine adenomas, gastric ulcers, heartburn

Investigational uses: GI disorders in those taking NSAIDs, urticaria, prevention of stress ulcers, aspiration pneumonitis, inactivation of oral pancreatic enzymes in pancreatic disorders, prevention of paclitaxel hypersensitivity reactions

Dosage and routes

Active ulcer

Adult: PO 40 mg daily at bedtime × 4-8 wk, then 20 mg daily at bedtime if needed (maintenance); **IV** 20 mg q12h if unable to take PO

Child 1-16 yr: PO 0.5 mg/kg/day at bedtime or divided bid, max 40 mg daily

Hypersecretory conditions

Adult: PO 20 mg q6h; may give 160 mg q6h if needed; **IV** 20 mg q12h if unable to take PO

Child 1-16 yr: PO 1 mg/kg/day divided bid, max 40 mg bid

Paclitaxel hypersensitivity reactions

Adult: **IV** 20 mg ½ hr before inf

Heartburn relief/prevention

Adult: PO 10 mg with water or 1 hr before eating

F

Renal dose

Adult: PO CCr <10 ml/min 20 mg at bedtime or dose q36-48h

Available forms: Tabs 10, 20, 40 mg; powder for oral susp 40 mg/5 ml; inj 10 mg/ml, 20 mg/50 ml 0.9% NaCl; orally disintegrating tabs (RPD) 20, 40 mg; chew tabs 10 mg

Adverse effects

CNS: *Headache, dizziness,* paresthesia, depression, anxiety, somnolence, insomnia, fever

CV: **Dysrhythmias**

EENT: Taste change, tinnitus, orbital edema

GI: *Constipation,* nausea, vomiting, anorexia, cramps, abnormal liver enzymes, diarrhea

HEMA: **Thrombocytopenia, aplastic anemia**

INTEG: Rash

MS: Myalgia, arthralgia

Contraindications: Hypersensitivity

Precautions: Pregnancy **B,** lactation, children <12 yr, severe renal disease, severe hepatic disease, elderly

Pharmacokinetics

Absorption	50% absorbed (PO)
Distribution	Plasma, protein binding (15%-20%)
Metabolism	Liver (30% active metabolizing)
Excretion	Kidneys (70%)
Half-life	2½-3½ hr

Pharmacodynamics

	PO	IV
Onset	30-60 min	Immediate
Peak	1-3 hr	½-3 hr
Duration	6-12 hr	8-15 hr

Interactions

Individual drugs

Ketoconazole: decreased absorption of ketoconazole

Drug classifications

Antacids: decreased absorption of famotidine

NURSING CONSIDERATIONS

Assessment

- Assess patient with ulcers or suspected ulcers: epigastric, abdominal pain, hematemesis, occult blood in stools, blood in gastric, aspirate before treatment; throughout treatment, monitor gastric pH (5 should be maintained)
- Monitor I&O ratio, BUN, creatinine, CBC with differential monthly

Nursing diagnoses

- Pain, acute (uses)
- Knowledge, deficient (teaching)

Implementation

PO route

- Give antacids 1 hr before or 2 hr after famotidine; may be given with foods or liq
- Administer oral susp after shaking well; discard unused sol after 1 mo

IV route

- Give **IV** direct after diluting 2 ml of drug (10 mg/ml) in 0.9% NaCl to total volume of 5-10 ml; inject over 2 min to prevent hypotension
- Administer **IV** intermittent inf after diluting 20 mg of drug in 100 ml of LR, 0.9% NaCl, D_5W, $D_{10}W$; run over 15-30 min
- Store in cool environment (oral); **IV** solution is stable for 48 hr at room temp; do not use discolored sol

Y-site compatibilities: Acyclovir, allopurinol, amifostine, aminophylline, amphotericin, ampicillin, ampicillin/sulbactam, inamrinone, amsacrine, atropine, aztreonam, bretylium, calcium gluconate, cefazolin, cefoperazone, cefotaxime, cefotetan, cefoxitin, ceftazidime, ceftizoxime, ceftriaxone, cefuroxime, cephalothin, cephapirin, chlorproMAZINE, cisplatin, cladribine, cyclophosphamide, cytarabine, dexamethasone, dextran 40, digoxin, diphenhydrAMINE, DOBUTamine, DOPamine, DOXOrubicin, droperidol, enalaprilat, epINEPHrine, erythromycin lactobionate, esmolol, filgrastim, fluconazole, fludarabine, folic acid, gentamicin, granisetron, haloperidol, heparin, hydrocortisone, hydromorphone, hydrOXYzine, imipenem/cilastatin, regular insulin, isoproterenol, labetalol, lidocaine, lorazepam, magnesium sulfate, melphalan, meperidine, methotrexate, methylPREDNISolone, metoclopramide, mezlocillin, midazolam, morphine, nafcillin, nitroglycerin, nitroprusside, norepinephrine, ondansetron, oxacillin, paclitaxel, perphenazine, phenylephrine, phenytoin, phytonadione, piperacillin, potassium chloride, potassium phosphate, procainamide, propofol, sargramostim, sodium bicarbonate, teniposide, theophylline, thiamine, thiotepa, ticarcillin, ticarcillin/clavulanate, verapamil, vinorelbine

Additive compatibilities: Cefazolin, cefmetazole, flumazenil

Patient/family education

- Caution patient to avoid driving, other hazardous activities until stabilized on this medication; dizziness may occur
- Advise patient to avoid black pepper, caf-

feine, alcohol, harsh spices, extremes in temp of food; tell patient to avoid OTC preparations: aspirin, cough, cold preparations; condition may worsen

- Advise patient to avoid taking the OTC and the prescription preparations of this drug concurrently
- Tell patient that smoking decreases the effectiveness of the drug; that smoking cessation should be considered
- Instruct patient that drug must be continued for prescribed time to be effective and taken exactly as prescribed; doses are not to be doubled; take missed dose when remembered up to 1 hr before next dose
- Tell patient to report bruising, fatigue, malaise; blood dyscrasias may occur
- Tell patient to report diarrhea, black tarry stools, sore throat, rash, dizziness, confusion, or delirium to prescriber immediately

Evaluation

Positive therapeutic outcome

- Decreased pain in abdomen
- Healing of ulcers

fat emulsions (Rx)

(fat ee-mul'shuns)

Intralipid 10%, Intralipid 20%, Liposyn II 10%, Liposyn II 20%, Liposyn III 10%, Liposyn III 20%, Soyacal 20%

Func. class.: Caloric

Chem. class.: Fatty acid, long chain

Pregnancy category C

Action: Needed for energy, heat production; consists of neutral triglycerides, primarily unsaturated fatty acids

Therapeutic Outcome: Increased available calories and fatty acids

Uses: Increase calorie intake, prevent fatty acid deficiency

Dosage and routes

Deficiency

Adult and child: **IV** 8%-10% of required calorie intake (intralipid)

Adjunct to TPN

Adult: **IV** 1 ml/min over 15-30 min (10%) or 0.5 ml/min over 15-30 min (20%); may increase to 500 ml over 4-8 hr if no adverse reactions occur; not to exceed 2.5 g/kg

Child: **IV** 0.1 ml/min over 10-15 min (10%) or 0.05 ml/ min over 10-15 min (20%); may increase to 1 g/kg over 4 hr if no adverse reactions occur; not to exceed 4 g/kg

Prevention of deficiency

Adult: **IV** 500 ml 2 × wk (10%), given 1 ml/min for 30 min, not to exceed 500 ml over 6 hr

Child: **IV** 5-10 ml/kg/day (10%), given 0.1 ml/min for 30 min, not to exceed 100 ml/hr

Available forms: Inj 10% (50, 100, 200, 250, 500 ml), 20% (50, 100, 200, 250, 500 ml)

Adverse effects

CNS: Dizziness, headache, drowsiness, **focal seizures**

CV: **Shock**

GI: Nausea, vomiting, **hepatomegaly**

HEMA: **Hyperlipemia, hypercoagulation, thrombocytopenia, leukopenia, leukocytosis**

RESP: Dyspnea, **fat in lung tissue**

Contraindications: Hypersensitivity, hyperlipemia, lipid necrosis, acute pancreatitis accompanied by hyperlipemia, hyperbilirubinemia of the newborn

Precautions: Pregnancy **C,** severe liver disease, diabetes mellitus, thrombocytopenia, gastric ulcers, premature, term newborns, sepsis

Pharmacokinetics

Absorption	Completely absorbed
Distribution	Intravascular space
Metabolism	Conversion to triglycerides, to free fatty acids
Excretion	Unknown
Half-life	Unknown

Pharmacodynamics

Unknown

Interactions: None known

NURSING CONSIDERATIONS

Assessment

- Monitor triglycerides, free fatty acid levels, platelet counts daily to prevent fat overload, thrombocytopenia
- Monitor liver function studies: AST, ALT, Hct, Hgb; notify prescriber if abnormal
- Assess nutritional status: calorie count by dietitian; monitor weight daily

Nursing diagnoses

- Nutrition: less than body requirements, imbalanced (uses)
- Knowledge, deficient (teaching)

Implementation

- Administer using infusion pump at prescribed rate; do not use in-line filter sized for lipid emulsion; clogging will occur

- Do not use mixed sol that looks oily or is not separated; discard unused sol
- Change **IV** tubing at each inf: infection may occur with old tubing
- Give by intermittent inf at a rate of 10% sol (1 ml/min); 20% sol (0.5 ml/min) initially for 15-30 min; may be increased to 10% sol (120 ml/hr) or 20% sol (62.5 ml/hr) if no adverse reactions occur; do not give more than 500 ml during the first day; children should be given 10% (0.1 mg/ ml) or 20% (0.05 ml/min) initially for 15-30 min, may be increased 1 g/kg/4 hr, do not give more than 10% (100 ml/hr) or 20% (50 ml/hr)

Y-site compatibilities: Ampicillin, cefamandole, cefazolin, cefoxitin, cephapirin, clindamycin, digoxin, DOPamine, erythromycin, furosemide, gentamicin, IL-2, isoproterenol, lidocaine, kanamycin, norepinephrine, oxacillin, penicillin G potassium, ticarcillin, tobramycin

Y-site incompatibilities: Amikacin, tetracycline

Additive compatibilities: Cefamandole, chloramphenicol, cimetidine, cycloSPORINE, diphenhydrAMINE, famotidine, heparin, hydrocortisone, multivitamins, nizatidine, penicillin G potassium

Patient/family education

- Teach patient reason for use of lipids and expected results

Evaluation

Positive therapeutic outcome

- Increased weight
- Fatty acids at adequate levels

felodipine (Rx)

(feh-loh'dih-peen)

Plendil, Renedil ✤

Func. class.: Calcium-channel blocker, antihypertensive, antianginal

Chem. class.: Dihydropyridine

Pregnancy category C

Do Not Confuse:

Plendil/pindolol, Plendil/Prinivil, Plendil/Prilosec, Plendil/Pletal

Action: Inhibits calcium ion influx across cell membrane, resulting in inhibition of excitation/contraction

Therapeutic Outcome: Decreased B/P in hypertension

Uses: Essential hypertension, alone or with other antihypertensives, angina pectoris, Prinzmetal's angina (vasospastic)

Dosage and routes

Adult: PO 5 mg daily initially, usual range 5-10 mg daily; max 10 mg daily; do not adjust dosage at intervals of <2 wk

Elderly: PO 2.5 mg daily

Hepatic dose

Adult: PO 2.5-5 mg daily, max 10 mg/day

Available forms: Ext rel tabs 2.5, 5, 10 mg

Adverse effects

CNS: Headache, fatigue, drowsiness, dizziness, anxiety, depression, nervousness, insomnia, light-headedness, paresthesia, tinnitus, psychosis, somnolence

CV: **Dysrhythmias**, edema, **CHF**, hypotension, palpitations, **MI, pulmonary edema,** tachycardia, syncope, AV block, angina

GI: Nausea, vomiting, diarrhea, gastric upset, constipation, increased liver function studies, dry mouth

GU: Nocturia, polyuria

HEMA: Anemia

INTEG: Rash, pruritus

MISC: Flushing, sexual difficulties, cough, nasal congestion, shortness of breath, wheezing, epistaxis, respiratory infection, chest pain, **Stevens-Johnson syndrome,** gingival hyperplasia

Contraindications: Hypersensitivity, sick sinus syndrome, 2nd- or 3rd-degree heart block, hypotension <90 mm Hg systolic

Precautions: Pregnancy **C**, CHF, hepatic injury, lactation, children, renal disease, elderly

Pharmacokinetics	
Absorption	Well absorbed
Distribution	Unknown; protein binding >99%
Metabolism	Liver, extensively
Excretion	Kidneys
Half-life	11-16 hr

Pharmacodynamics	
Onset	2-3 hr
Peak	2½-5 hr
Duration	<24 hr

Interactions

Individual drugs

Alcohol, fentanyl, quinidine: increased hypotension

Digoxin: increased digoxin levels

Digoxin, disopyramide, phenytoin: increased bradycardia, increased CHF
Erythromycin, ketoconazole, itraconazole, propanolol: increased toxicity

Drug classifications

Antihypertensives, nitrates: increased hypotension
β-Adrenergic blockers: increased bradycardia, CHF
NSAIDs: decreased antihypertensive effects

Drug/herb

Aconite: increased toxicity, death
Astragalus, cola tree: increased or decreased antihypertensive effect
Barberry, betony, black catechu, black cohosh, bloodroot, broom, burdock, cat's claw, dandelion, goldenseal, Irish moss, Jamaican dogwood, kelp, khella, mistletoe, parsley: increased antihypertensive effect
Coltsfoot, guarana, khat, licorice: decreased antihypertensive effect

Drug/food

Grapefruit juice: increased felodipine level

NURSING CONSIDERATIONS

Assessment

- Assess fluid volume status: I&O ratio and record; weight; skin turgor; adequacy of pulses; moist mucous membranes; bilateral lung sounds; peripheral pitting edema; dehydration symptoms of decreasing output, thirst, hypotension, dry mouth, and mucous membranes should be reported; for CHF: weight gain, crackles, dyspnea, edema, jugular venous distention
- Monitor ALT, AST, bilirubin daily if these are elevated
- Monitor cardiac status: B/P, pulse, respiration, ECG, periodically
- Assess for anginal pain: duration, intensity, ameliorating, aggravating factors

Nursing diagnoses

- Cardiac output, decreased (uses)
- Knowledge, deficient (teaching)

Implementation

- Do not break, crush, or chew ext rel tabs
- Give once a day with food for GI symptoms

Patient/family education

- Caution patient to avoid hazardous activities until stabilized on drug, and dizziness is no longer a problem
- Instruct patient to limit caffeine consumption; to avoid alcohol and OTC drugs unless directed by prescriber
- Urge patient to comply in all areas of medical regimen: diet, exercise, stress reduction, drug therapy; to notify prescriber of irregular heartbeat, shortness of breath, swelling of feet and hands, pronounced dizziness, constipation, nausea, hypotension
- Advise patient to use protective clothing, sunscreen to prevent photosensitivity
- Teach patient to change positions slowly to prevent orthostatic hypotension
- Advise patient to obtain correct pulse, to contact prescriber if pulse is <50 bpm
- Teach patient to use as directed even if feeling better; may be taken with other CV drugs (nitrates, β-blockers), that capsules may appear in stools but are insignificant

Evaluation

Positive therapeutic outcome

- Decreased B/P
- Decreased anginal attacks
- Increase in activity tolerance

fenofibrate (Rx)

(fen-oh-fee' brate)
Tricor
Func. class.: Antilipemic
Chem. class.: Fibric acid derivative
Pregnancy category C

Action: Increases lipolysis and elimination of triglyceride-rich particles from plasma by activating lipoprotein lipase, resulting in triglyceride change in size and composition of LDL, leading to rapid breakdown of LDL; mobilizes triglycerides from tissue; increases excretion of neutral sterols

Therapeutic Outcome: Decreasing cholesterol levels and low-density lipoproteins, decreased pruritus

Uses: Patients with types IV, V hyperlipidemia who do not respond to other treatment and who are at risk for pancreatitis Fredrickson type IIa, IIb, hypertriglyceridemia

Investigational uses: Polymetabolic syndrome X

Dosage and routes

Hypertriglyceridemia

Adult: PO 54-160 mg/day, may increase q4-8 wk, max 160 mg/day

Primary hypercholesterolemia/ mixed hyperlipidemia

Adult: PO 160 mg/day

Renal dose/elderly

Adult: PO 54 mg/day (CCr <50 ml/min)

Available forms: Tabs 54, 160 mg

F

Adverse effects

CNS: Fatigue, weakness, drowsiness, dizziness, insomnia, depression, vertigo
CV: Angina, **dysrhythmias,** hypertension
GI: Nausea, vomiting, dyspepsia, increased liver enzymes, flatulence, hepatomegaly, gastritis
GU: Dysuria, proteinuria, oliguria, urinary frequency
HEMA: Anemia, leukopenia, ecchymosis
INTEG: *Rash,* urticaria, pruritus
MISC: Polyphagia, weight gain
MS: Myalgias, arthralgias, myopathy
RESP: Pharyngitis, bronchitis, cough

Contraindications: Hypersensitivity, severe hepatic disease, severe renal disease, primary biliary cirrhosis, preexisting gallbladder disease

Precautions: Pregnancy **C,** peptic ulcer, lactation, pancreatitis, renal, hepatic disease, elderly

Pharmacokinetics

Absorption	Unknown
Distribution	Protein binding 99%
Metabolism	Liver
Excretion	Urine 60%
Half-life	20 hr

Pharmacodynamics

Peak	6-8 hr

Interactions

Drug classifications

Anticoagulants (oral): increased effect of anticoagulants
Bile acid sequestrants: decreased absorption
CycloSPORINE: increased nephrotoxicity
HMG-CoA reductase inhibitors: do not use together, rhabdomyolysis may occur

Drug/herb

Glucomannan: increased effect
Gotu kola: decreased effect

Drug/food

Increased absorption

NURSING CONSIDERATIONS

Assessment

- Assess lipid levels, liver function tests, baseline and periodically during treatment; CPK if muscle pain occurs, CBC, Hct, Hgh, protime with anticoagulant therapy
- Assess for pancreatitis, cholelithiasis, renal failure, rhabdomyolysis, (when combined with HMG-CoA reductase inhibitors) myositis, drug should be discontinued
- Assess nutrition: fat, protein, carbohydrates, nutritional analysis should be completed by dietician
- Assess skin integrity after patient has been receiving drug; itching, pruritus often occur from bile deposits on skin
- Monitor cardiac glycoside level if both drugs are being administered; cardiac glycoside levels will be decreased
- Monitor for signs of vit A, D, K deficiency; serum cholesterol, triglyceride levels, electrolytes if on extended therapy
- Monitor bowel pattern daily; increase bulk, water in diet if constipation develops

Nursing diagnoses

- Knowledge, deficient (teaching)
- Noncompliance (teaching)

Implementation

- Do not break, crush, or chew tabs
- Give with evening meal; if dose is increased, take with breakfast and evening meal
- Store in cool environment in tight, light-resistant container

Patient/family education

- Inform patient that compliance is needed
- Teach patient that risk factors—high-fat diet, smoking, alcohol consumption, absence of exercise—should be decreased
- Caution patient to notify prescriber if pregnancy is planned or suspected
- Teach patient to notify prescriber if the GI symptoms of diarrhea, abdominal or epigastric pain, nausea, or vomiting occur
- Instruct patient to report GU symptoms: dysuria, proteinuria, oliguria, decreased libido, impotence
- Advise patient to notify prescriber of muscle pain, weakness, fever, fatigue, epigastric pain

Evaluation

Positive therapeutic outcome

- Decrease in cholesterol to desired level after 8 wk

fenoldopam (Rx)

(fen-nahl'doh-pam)
Corlopam
Func. class.: Antihypertensive, vasodilator
Pregnancy category B

Action: Agonist at D_1-like dopamine receptors; binds to α_2-adrenoreceptors; increases renal blood flow

Therapeutic Outcome: B/P, decreased

Uses: Hypertensive crisis, malignant hypertension

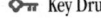

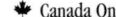

Dosage and routes
Adult: **IV** 0.01-1.6 mcg/kg/min

Available forms: Inj conc 10 mg/ml in single-use ampules

Adverse effects
CNS: *Headache,* anxiety, dizziness
CV: *Hypotension,* ST-T-wave changes, angina pectoris, palpitations, **MI, ischemic heart disease,** *flushing*
GI: Nausea, vomiting, constipation, diarrhea
HEMA: **Leukocytosis, bleeding**
META: Increased BUN, glucose, LDH, creatinine, hypokalemia

Contraindications: Hypersensitivity, sulfite sensitivity

Precautions: Pregnancy **B,** tachycardia, lactation, children, intraocular pressure, hypokalemia

Pharmacokinetics	
Absorption	Unknown
Distribution	Steady state 20 min
Metabolism	Unknown
Excretion	Unknown
Half-life	5 min (elimination)

Pharmacodynamics	
Onset	Unknown
Peak	Unknown
Duration	Unknown

Interactions
Drug classifications
β-Adrenergic blockers: increased hypotension
Drug/herb
Aconite: increased toxicity, death
Astragalus, cola tree: increased or decreased antihypertensive effect
Barberry, betony, black catechu, black cohosh, bloodroot, broom, burdock, cat's claw, dandelion, goldenseal, Irish moss, Jamaican dogwood, kelp, khella, mistletoe, parsley: increased antihypertensive effect
Coltsfoot, guarana, khat, licorice: decreased antihypertensive effect

NURSING CONSIDERATIONS
Assessment
- Monitor B/P q5 min until stabilized, then q1h × 2 hr, then q4h; pulse, jugular venous distention q4h
- Monitor electrolytes, blood studies: K, Na, Cl, CO_2, CBC, serum glucose
- Assess skin turgor, dryness of mucous membranes for hydration status
- Assess **IV** site for extravasation, rate

Nursing diagnoses
- Tissue perfusion, ineffective (uses)
- Knowledge, deficient (teaching)
- Noncompliance (teaching)

Implementation
IV route
- Administer after diluting contents of ampules in 0.9% NaCl, or 5% dextrose inj (40 mcg/ml); then add 4 ml of conc (40 mg of drug/1000 ml); 2 ml of conc (20 mg of drug/500 ml); 1 ml of conc (10 mg of drug/250 ml); do not admix
- Give to patient in recumbent position; keep in that position for 1 hr after administration
- Diluted sol is stable in normal light/temp for 24 hr

Patient/family education
- Teach patient reason for medication and expected results
- Instruct patient to report dyspnea, chest pain, bleeding

Evaluation
Positive therapeutic outcome
- Decreased B/P

! HIGH ALERT

fentanyl (Rx)
(fen'ta-nill)
fentanyl, Sublimaze, Fentanyl Oralet, Actiq
Func. class.: Opioid analgesic
Chem. class.: Synthetic phenylpiperidine derivative

Pregnancy category C

Controlled substance schedule II

Do Not Confuse:
fentanyl/Sufenta

Action: Inhibits ascending pain pathways in CNS, increases pain threshold, alters pain perception by binding to opiate receptors

Therapeutic Outcome: Relief of pain, supplement to anesthesia

Uses: Preoperatively, postoperatively; adjunct to general anesthetic, adjunct to regional anesthesia; Fentanyl Oralet for anesthesia as premedication, conscious sedation; Actiq for breakthrough cancer pain

Dosage and routes
Anesthetic
Adult: **IV** 25-100 mcg (0.7-2 mcg/kg) q2-3 min prn

Anesthesia supplement
Adult: **IV** 2-20 mcg/kg **IV** INF 0.025-0.25 mcg/kg/min

Induction and maintenance
Adult: **IV** Bol 5-40 mcg/kg
Child 2-12 yr: **IV** 2-3 mcg/kg

Preoperatively
Adult: IM 0.05-0.1 mg q30-60 min before surgery

Postoperatively
Adult: IM 0.05-0.1 mg q1-2hr prn

Fentanyl Oralet
Adult: Transmucosal: 5 mcg/kg = fentanyl IM 0.75-1.25 mcg/kg, do not exceed 5 mcg/kg
Child: Transmucosal may need doses of 5-15 mcg/kg; must be watched continuously for hypoventilation

Actiq
Adult: Transmucosal 200 mcg, redose if needed 15 min after completion of 1st dose, do not give more than 2 doses during titration period

Available forms: Inj 0.05 mg/ml; lozenges 100, 200, 300, 400 mcg; lozenges on a stick 200, 400, 600, 800, 1200, 1600 mcg

Adverse effects
CNS: Dizziness, delirium, euphoria
CV: **Bradycardia, cardiac arrest,** hypotension or hypertension
EENT: Blurred vision, miosis
GI: Nausea, vomiting
GU: Urinary retention
INTEG: Rash, diaphoresis
MS: Muscle rigidity
RESP: **Respiratory depression, arrest, laryngospasm**

Contraindications: Hypersensitivity to opiates, myasthenia gravis

Precautions: Pregnancy **C**, elderly, respiratory depression, increased ICP, seizure disorders, severe respiratory disorders, cardiac dysrhythmias, lactation

Pharmacokinetics

Absorption	Well absorbed (IM), completely absorbed (**IV**)
Distribution	Unknown, crosses placenta
Metabolism	Extensively—liver, 80% bound to plasma proteins
Excretion	Kidneys—up to 25% unchanged, breast milk
Half-life	1½-6 hr

Pharmacodynamics

	IM	IV
Onset	7-8 min	Rapid
Peak	30 min	3-5 min
Duration	1-2 hr	½-1 hr

Interactions
Individual drugs
Alcohol: increased respiratory depression, hypotension, increased sedation
Drug classifications
CNS depressants, sedative/hypnotics: increased respiratory depression, hypotension
Opioids, skeletal muscle relaxants: effects increased
Drug/herb
Corkwood: increased anticholinergic effect
Jamaican dogwood, kava, lavender, mistletoe, nettle, pokeweed, poppy, senaga, valerian: increased fentanyl action
Drug/lab test
Increased: amylase, lipase

NURSING CONSIDERATIONS
Assessment
- Monitor VS after parenteral route (B/P, pulse, respiration); note muscle rigidity; take drug history before administering drug; check liver, kidney function tests; assess for respiratory dysfunction: respiratory depression, character, rate, rhythm; notify prescriber if respirations are <10/min
- Monitor CNS changes: dizziness, drowsiness, hallucinations, euphoria, LOC, pupil reaction
- Monitor allergic reactions: rash, urticaria; drug should be discontinued
- Assess for pain: intensity, location, duration, type, before and 15 min after IM route or 3-5 min after **IV** route

Nursing diagnoses
- Pain, acute (uses)
- Sensory perception, disturbed: visual, auditory (adverse reactions)
- Breathing pattern, ineffective (adverse reactions)
- Knowledge, deficient (teaching)

Implementation
- Give by inj (IM, **IV**), only with resuscitative equipment available; give slowly to prevent rigidity
- Give **IV** undiluted by anesthesiologist or diluted with 5 ml or more sterile water or 0.9% NaCl given through Y-tube or 3-way stopcock given at 0.1 mg or less/1.2 min
- Store in light-resistant area at room temp

Transmucosal route

- Remove foil just before administration, instruct patient to place under tongue and suck, not chew (Oralet); place between cheek and lower gum, moving it back and forth and suck, not chew (Actiq); all products not used or partially used should be flushed down the toilet

Syringe compatibilities: Atracurium, atropine, bupivacaine/ketamine, butorphanol, chlorproMAZINE, cimetidine, clonidine/lidocaine, dimenhyDRINATE, diphenhydrAMINE, droperidol, heparin, hydromorphone, hydrOXYzine, meperidine, metoclopramide, midazolam, morphine, pentazocine, perphenazine, prochlorperazine, promazine, promethazine, ranitidine, scopolamine

Syringe incompatibilities: Pentobarbital

Y-site compatibilities: Amphotericin B cholesteryl, atracurium, cisatracurium, diltiazem, dobutamine, DOPamine, enalaprilat, epINEPHrine, esmolol, etomidate, furosemide, heparin, hydrocortisone, hydromorphone, labetalol, lorazepam, midazolam, milrinone, morphine, nafcillin, niCARdipine, nitroglycerin, norepinephrine, pancuronium, potassium chloride, propofol, ranitidine, remifentanil, sargramostim, thiopental, vecuronium, vit B/C

Additive compatibilities: Bupivacaine, sodium bicarbonate

Additive incompatibilities: Methohexital, pentobarbital, thiopental

Solution compatibilities: D_5W, 0.9% NaCl

Patient/family education

- Advise patient to report any symptoms of CNS changes, allergic reactions
- Instruct patient to avoid CNS depressants: alcohol, sedative/hypnotics for at least 24 hr after taking this drug
- Teach patient that dizziness, drowsiness, confusion are common, and to avoid getting up without assistance
- Discuss in detail with patient all aspects of the drug

Evaluation

Positive therapeutic outcome

- Maintenance of anesthesia
- Decreased pain

Treatment of overdose: Naloxone 0.2-0.8 **IV**, O_2, **IV** fluids, vasopressors

fentanyl transdermal (Rx)

(fen'ta-nill)

Duragesic

Func. class.: Opioid, analgesic

Chem. class.: Synthetic phenylpiperidine

Pregnancy category C

Controlled substance schedule II

Action: Inhibits ascending pain pathways in CNS, increases pain threshold, alters pain perception by binding to opiate receptors

Therapeutic Outcome: Relief of chronic pain

Uses: Management of chronic pain for those requiring opioid analgesia

Dosage and routes

Adult: TD 25 mcg/hr; may increase until pain relief occurs; apply patch to flat surface on upper torso and wear for 72 hr; apply new patch on different site for continued relief

Available forms: Patches 12, 25, 50, 75, 100 mcg/hr

Adverse effects

CNS: Dizziness, delirium, euphoria, lightheadedness, sedation, dysphoria, agitation, anxiety, confusion, headache, depression

CV: Bradycardia, **cardiac arrest,** hypotension or hypertension, facial flushing, chills, chest pain, dysrhythmia

EENT: Blurred vision, miosis

GI: Nausea, vomiting, diarrhea, cramps, anorexia, constipation, dyspepsia

GU: Urinary retention, urgency, dysuria, frequency, oliguria

INTEG: Sweating, pruritus, rash, erythema, papules

MS: Asthenia

RESP: **Respiratory depression, laryngospasm, bronchospasm;** depresses cough; hypoventilation, dyspnea, hiccups, **apnea**

Contraindications: Hypersensitivity to opiates, myasthenia gravis, children <12 yr, patient <18 yr with weight <110 lb

Precautions: Pregnancy **C,** elderly, respiratory depression, increased ICP, seizure disorders, severe respiratory disorders, cardiac dysrhythmias, fever

Pharmacokinetics

Absorption	92% (skin), continuously for 72 hr
Distribution	Crosses placenta
Metabolism	Extensively—liver
Excretion	Up to 25%—kidneys unchanged
Half-life	17 hr after removal of patch

Pharmacodynamics

Onset	6 hr
Peak	12-24 hr
Duration	72 hr

Interactions

Individual drugs

Alcohol: increased respiratory depression, hypotension, increased sedation

Drug classifications

Antihistamines, CNS depressants, phenothiazines, sedative/hypnotics: increased respiratory depression, hypotension

Opioids, skeletal muscle relaxants: effects may be increased

Drug/herb

Corkwood: increased anticholinergic effect

Jamaican dogwood, kava, lavender, mistletoe, nettle, pokeweed, poppy, senega, valerian: increased fentanyl level

NURSING CONSIDERATIONS

Assessment

- Assess for respiratory dysfunction: respiratory depression, character, rate, rhythm; notify prescriber if respirations are <10/min
- Monitor CNS changes: dizziness, drowsiness, hallucinations, euphoria, LOC, pupil reaction
- Monitor allergic reactions: rash, urticaria; drug should be discontinued
- Assess for pain: intensity, location, duration, type, before and after administration

Nursing diagnoses

- Pain, chronic (uses)
- Sensory perception, disturbed: visual, auditory (adverse reactions)
- Breathing pattern, ineffective (adverse reactions)
- Knowledge, deficient (teaching)

Implementation

- Opioids should be used to control pain until relief is obtained with TD patch; patients may continue to require other opioids for breakthrough pain; if >100 mcg/hr is required, use multiple systems
- Apply patch to chest on a flat area with skin intact; for skin preparation, use clear water with no soap; clip hair, skin should be dry before applying patch; apply immediately after removing from package and press firmly in place with palm of hand; flush old patch down toilet immediately upon removal

Use pain dosing

- Dosage is titrated based on patient's report of pain; dosage is determined by calculating the previous 24-hr requirement and converting to equianalgesic morphine dose
- To convert to another opioid analgesic, remove TD patch and begin treatment with half the equal pain-controlling dose of the new analgesic in 12-18 hr
- Medication should be tapered gradually after long-term use to prevent withdrawal symptoms

Patient/family education

- Advise patient to report any symptoms of CNS changes, allergic reactions
- Instruct patients to avoid CNS depressants: alcohol, sedative/hypnotics for at least 24 hr after this drug
- Discuss with patient that dizziness, drowsiness, and confusion are common and to avoid getting up without assistance
- Discuss with patient that excessive heat may increase absorption; excessive perspiration may alter adhesiveness

Evaluation

Positive therapeutic outcome

- Decreased pain

Treatment of overdose: Naloxone 0.2-0.8 mg **IV**, O_2, **IV** fluids, vasopressors

ferrous fumarate (Rx, OTC)

(fer'us fyu'-muh-rāt)

Femiron, Feostat, Feostat Drops, Hemocyte, Ircon, Nephro-Fer, Novofumar ✱, Palafer ✱, Span-FF

ferrous gluconate (Rx, OTC)

Fergon, Fertinic ✱, Novoferrogluc ✱

ferric gluconate complex (Rx, OTC)

Ferrlecit

ferrous sulfate (Rx, OTC)

Apo-Ferrous Sulfate ✱, ED-INSOL, Feosol, Fer-gen-sol, Fer-Iron Drops, Fero-Grad, Mol-Iron

ferrous sulfate, dried (Rx, OTC)

Fe^{50}, Feosol, Feratab, Novoferrosulfa ✱, PMS-Ferrous Sulfate, Slow Fe

iron, carbonyl (OTC)

(kar'boh-nil)

Feosol, Icar

iron polysaccharide (OTC)

(pah-lee-sack'ah-ride)

Hytinic, Niferex, Nu-Iron, Nu-Iron 150

Func. class.: Hematinic

Chem. class.: Iron preparation

Pregnancy category B, C

Action: Replaces iron stores needed for red blood cell development, energy and O_2 transport, utilization; fumarate contains 33% elemental iron; gluconate, 12%; sulfate, 20%; iron, 30%; ferrous sulfate exsiccated

Therapeutic Outcome: Prevention and correction of iron deficiency

Uses: Iron deficiency anemia, prophylaxis for iron deficiency in pregnancy

Dosage and routes

Fumarate

Adult: PO 200 mg daily-qid

Child 2-12 yr: PO 3 mg/kg/day (elemental iron) tid-qid

Child 6 mo-2 yr: PO up to 6 mg/kg/day (elemental iron) tid-qid

Infants: PO 10-25 mg/day (elemental iron) in 3-4 divided doses, max 15 mg/day

Gluconate

Adult: PO 200-600 mg daily-tid

Child 6-12 yr: PO 300-900 mg daily

Child <6 yr: PO 100-300 mg daily

Sulfate

Adult: PO 0.750-1.5 g/day in divided doses tid

Child 6-12 yr: 600 mg/day in divided doses

Pregnancy

Adult: PO 300-600 mg/day in divided doses

Complex

Adult: **IV** inf (125 mg) 10 ml/100 ml of NaCl for inj given over 1 hr

Iron polysaccharide

Adult: 100-200 mg tid

Child: PO 4-6 mg/kg/day in 3 divided doses

Available forms

Fumarate: Tabs 63, 195, 200, 324, 325 mg; chewable tabs 100 mg; controlled-release tabs 300 mg; oral susp 100 mg/5 ml, 45 mg/0.6 ml

Gluconate: Tabs 300, 320, 325 mg; caps 86, 325, 435 mg; film-coated tabs 300 mg; elix 300 mg/5 ml

Sulfate: Tabs 195, 300, 325 mg; enteric-coated tabs 325 mg; ext rel tabs, time-rel caps 525 mg

Dried: Tabs 200 mg; ext rel tabs 160 mg; ext rel caps 160 mg

Complex: Inj 62.5 mg/5 ml (12.5 mg/ml)

Iron polysaccharide: Tabs 50 mg; caps 150 mg; sol 100 mg/5 ml

Adverse effects

GI: *Nausea, constipation, epigastric pain, black and red tarry stools,* vomiting, diarrhea

INTEG: Temporarily discolored tooth enamel and eyes

Contraindications: Hypersensitivity, ulcerative colitis/regional enteritis, hemosiderosis/hemochromatosis, peptic ulcer disease, hemolytic anemia, cirrhosis

Precautions: Pregnancy **B** (ferric gluconate complex), **C** (iron dextran, oral products), anemia (long-term)

Pharmacokinetics

Absorption	Up to 30%
Distribution	Bound to transferrin, crosses placenta
Metabolism	Recycled
Excretion	Feces, urine, skin, breast milk
Half-life	Unknown

Pharmacodynamics

Unknown

Interactions

Individual drugs

Chloramphenicol, vit C: increased absorption of iron products

Cholestyramine: decreased absorption of iron

L-Thyroxine: decreased L-thyroxine absorption

Levodopa: decreased absorption of levodopa

Methyldopa: decreased absorption of methyldopa

Penicillamine: decreased absorption of penicillamine

Tetracycline: decreased absorption of tetracycline

Vit E: decreased absorption of iron preparations

Drug classifications

Antacids, H_2 antagonists, proton pump inhibitors: decreased absorption of iron preparations

Fluoroquinolones: decreased absorption of fluoroquinolone

Drug/herb

Allspice, bilberry, condurango, elderberry, eye bright (PO), gentian, ground ivy, marshmallow, meadowsweet, mistletoe, motherwort, nettle, raspberry, valerian, tea made with artichoke, hawthorn, horse chestnut, lady mantle, lemon balm, oak bark, plantain, poplar, prickly ash, sage: decreased iron absorption

Anise: increased iron effect

Black catechu: forms insoluble complex

Drug/food

Caffeine, dairy products, eggs: decreased absorption

Drug/lab test

False positive: occult blood

NURSING CONSIDERATIONS

Assessment

- Monitor blood studies: Hct, Hgb, reticulocytes, bilirubin before treatment, at least monthly; iron studies (Fe, TIBC, ferritin)

- Assess for toxicity: nausea, vomiting, diarrhea (green, then tarry stools,) hematemesis, pallor, cyanosis, shock, coma
- Assess bowel elimination; if constipation occurs, increase water, bulk, activity before laxatives are required
- Assess nutrition: amount of iron in diet (meat, dark green leafy vegetables, dried beans, dried fruits, eggs); provide referral to dietitian if indicated
- Identify cause of iron loss or anemia, including salicylates, sulfonamides, antimalarials, quinidine

Nursing diagnoses

- Nutrition, less than body requirements, imbalanced (uses)
- Fatigue (uses)
- Knowledge, deficient (teaching)

Implementation

- Swallow all tabs whole; do not break, crush, or chew
- Give between meals for best absorption; may give with juice; do not give with antacids or milk, delay at least 1 hr; if GI symptoms occur, give pc even if absorption is decreased; eggs, milk products, chocolate, caffeine interfere with absorption; ferrous gluconate is less GI irritating than ferrous sulfate
- Give liq preparations through plastic straw to avoid discoloration of tooth enamel; dilute thoroughly
- Give at least 1 hr before bedtime because corrosion may occur in stomach
- Give for <6 mo for anemia
- Store in airtight, light-resistant container

Patient/family education

- Advise patient that iron will make stools black or dark green; that iron poisoning may occur if increased beyond recommended level
- Keep out of reach of children
- Caution patient not to substitute one iron salt for another; elemental iron content differs (e.g., 300 mg ferrous fumarate contains about 100 mg elemental iron, whereas 300 mg ferrous gluconate contains only about 30 mg elemental iron)
- Caution patient to avoid reclining position for 15-30 min after taking drug to avoid esophageal corrosion; to follow diet high in iron

Evaluation

Positive therapeutic outcome

- Decreased fatigue, weakness
- Improvement in Hct, Hgb, reticulocytes

Treatment of overdose: Induce vomiting; give eggs, milk until lavage can be done

fexofenadine (Rx)

(fex-oh-fin'a-deen)

Allegra

Func. class.: H_1-histamine antagonist

Chem. class: Piperidine, peripherally selective

Pregnancy category C

Do Not Confuse:

Allegra/Viagra

Action: Acts on blood vessels, GI, respiratory system by competing with histamine for H_1-receptor site; decreases allergic response by blocking pharmacologic effects of histamine; less sedation rate than with other antihistamines; causes increased heart rate, vasodilatation, increased secretions

Therapeutic Outcome: Absence of allergy symptoms and rhinitis

Uses: Rhinitis, allergy symptoms, chronic idiopathic urticaria

Dosage and routes

Adult and child >12 yr: 60 mg bid

Child 6-11 yr: PO 30 mg bid

Renal dose

Adult and child ≥12 yr: PO CCr <80 ml/min 60 mg daily

Available forms: Caps 60 mg; ext rel tabs 180 mg; tabs 30, 60, 180 mg

Adverse effects

CNS: Headache, stimulation, drowsiness, sedation, fatigue, confusion, blurred vision, tinnitus, restlessness, tremors, paradoxical excitation in children or elderly

CV: Hypotension, palpitations, bradycardia, tachycardia, **dysrhythmias (rare)**

GI: Nausea, diarrhea, abdominal pain, vomiting, constipation

GU: Frequency, dysuria, urinary retention, impotence

HEMA: **Hemolytic anemia, thrombocytopenia, leukopenia, agranulocytosis, pancytopenia**

INTEG: Rash, eczema, photosensitivity, urticaria

RESP: Thickening of bronchial secretions; dry nose, throat

Contraindications: Hypersensitivity, newborn or premature infants, lactation, severe hepatic disease

Precautions: Pregnancy **C**, elderly, children, respiratory disease, narrow-angle glaucoma, prostatic hypertrophy, bladder neck obstruction, asthma

Pharmacokinetics	
Absorption	Well absorbed
Distribution	Unknown
Metabolism	Liver
Excretion	Kidneys

Pharmacodynamics	
Onset	1 hr
Peak	2-3 hr
Duration	12-24 hr

Interactions
Individual drugs
Alcohol: increased sedation
Drug classifications
Aluminum, antacids, magnesium: decreased fexofenadine effect
CNS depressants, opiates, sedative/hypnotics: increased sedation
Drug/herb
Corkwood, henbane leaf: increased anticholinergic effect
Hops, Jamaican dogwood, khat, senega: increased sedation
Drug/food
Apple, orange, grapefruit juice: decreased absorption
Drug/lab test
False negative: skin allergy tests (discontinue antihistamine 3 days before testing)

NURSING CONSIDERATIONS
Assessment
- Assess respiratory status: rate, rhythm, increase in bronchial secretions, wheezing, chest tightness; provide fluids to 2 L/day to decrease secretion thickness
- Monitor I&O ratio: be alert for urinary retention, frequency, dysuria, especially elderly; drug should be discontinued if these occur

Nursing diagnoses
- Airway clearance, ineffective (uses)
- Injury, risk for (side effects)
- Knowledge, deficient (teaching)
- Noncompliance (teaching, overuse)

Implementation
- Give on an empty stomach 1 hr before or 2 hr pc to facilitate absorption, with food or milk for GI symptoms, do not take with juice
- Store in tight, light-resistant container

Patient/family education
- Teach all aspects of drug uses; to notify prescriber if confusion, sedation, hypotension occur; to avoid driving or other hazardous activity if drowsiness occurs; to avoid alcohol or other CNS depressants that may potentiate effect
- Instruct patient to take 1 hr before or 2 hr pc to facilitate absorption
- Instruct patient not to exceed recommended dose; dysrhythmias may occur
- Teach patient that hard candy, gum, frequent rinsing of mouth may be used for dryness

Evaluation
Positive therapeutic outcome
- Absence of running or congested nose, rashes

Treatment of overdose:
Administer lavage, diazepam, vasopressors, barbiturates (short acting)

F

fibrinolysin/desoxyribonuclease (Rx)
(fye-brin-oe-lye'sin/dez-ox-ee-rye-boe-nuke'lee-ase)
Elase
Func. class.: Enzyme
Chem. class.: Proteolytic, bovine
Pregnancy category C

Action: Dissolves fibrin in clots and fibrinous exudates, attacks DNA in areas of disintegrating cells

Therapeutic Outcome: A clean wound

Uses: Debridement of wounds, vaginitis, cervicitis, ulcerative colitis, 2nd-, 3rd-degree burns; irrigating wounds, topically

Dosage and routes
Debridement/intravaginally
Adult: Oint 5 g × 5 applications
Irrigating
Adult: Irrigating dilution depends on type of wound

Available forms: Fibrinolysin with desoxyribonuclease 666.6 units/g; powder for reconstitution fibrinolysin 25 units/desoxyribonuclease 15,000 units

Adverse effects
INTEG: Hyperemia

Contraindications: Hypersensitivity to bovine or mercury products, hematoma

Precautions: Pregnancy **C**

Pharmacokinetics

Absorption	Not absorbed
Distribution	Unknown
Metabolism	Unknown
Excretion	Unknown
Half-life	Unknown

Pharmacodynamics

Unknown

Interactions: None known

NURSING CONSIDERATIONS

Assessment

- Assess for signs of irritation and inflammation around wound; drug should be discontinued
- Assess wound for drainage, color, odor, size, depth before and during therapy

Nursing diagnoses

- Skin integrity, impaired (uses)
- Knowledge, deficient (teaching)

Implementation

TOP route

- Apply after reconstituting top sol with 10-50 ml of sterile NaCl sol; use only fresh sol; reconstituted sol is stable for 24 hr; remove necrotic debris, dry eschar
- Saturate gauze with sol; pack area; remove in 6-8 hr and clean; repeat tid-qid
- Apply top oint after flushing wound with saline, water, or let dry or pat dry, then apply a small amount of oint to area and cover with a nonadhesive dressing; change daily or bid

Vaginal route

- Place 5 ml in applicator, apply with patient recumbent

Patient/family education

- Teach patient reason for treatment and expected results

Evaluation

Positive therapeutic outcome

- Decrease in wound scarring, tissue necrosis

filgrastim (Rx)

(fill-gras'stim)

G-CSF, granulocyte colony stimulator, Neupogen

Func. class.: Biologic modifier

Chem. class.: Granulocyte colony-stimulating factor

Pregnancy category C

Action: Stimulates proliferation and differentiation of neutrophils; a glycoprotein

Therapeutic Outcome: Absence of infection

Uses: To decrease infection in patients receiving antineoplastics that are myelosuppressive; to increase WBC in patients with drug-induced neutropenia

Investigational uses: Neutropenia in HIV infection

Dosage and routes

After myelosuppressive chemotherapy

Adult and child: **IV**/SUBCUT 5 mcg/kg/day in a single dose × 14 days; may increase by 5 mcg/kg in each chemotherapy cycle; give daily for up to 2 wk until ANC has reached 10,000/mm^3; response to G-CSF is much greater with SUBCUT than **IV** therapy

After bone marrow transplantation

Adult: **IV**/SUBCUT 10 mcg/kg as an inf (**IV**) over 4 or 24 hr, begin 24 hr after chemotherapy and 24 hr after bone marrow transplantation

Peripheral blood progenitor cell collection/therapy

Adult: 10 mcg/kg/day as a bol or cont inf × 4 days or more before leukapheresis, continue to last leukapheresis, may alter dose if WBC >100,000/mm^3

Severe neutropenia (chronic)

Adult: SUBCUT 5 mcg/kg daily-bid

Available forms: Inj 300 mcg/ml

Adverse effects

CNS: Fever

GI: Nausea, vomiting, diarrhea, mucositis, anorexia

HEMA: **Thrombocytopenia**

INTEG: Alopecia, exacerbation of skin conditions

MS: Osteoporosis, skeletal pain

OTHER: Chest pain

RESP: **Respiratory distress syndrome**

Contraindications: Hypersensitivity to proteins of *Escherichia coli*

Precautions: Pregnancy **C**, lactation, cardiac conditions, children, myeloid malignancies, radiation therapy, sepsis, sickle cell disease

Pharmacokinetics

Absorption	Well absorbed (SUBCUT), completely absorbed (**IV**)
Distribution	Unknown
Metabolism	Unknown
Excretion	Unknown
Half-life	Unknown

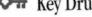

Pharmacodynamics

	IV	SUBCUT
Onset	5-60 min	5-60 min
Peak	24 hr	2-8 hr
Duration	up to 1 wk	up to 1 wk

Interactions
Drug classifications
Antineoplastics: increased neutrophils, do not use together 24 hr before or after antineoplastics
Drug/lab test
Increased: uric acid, lactate dehydrogenase, alkaline phosphatase

NURSING CONSIDERATIONS
Assessment
- Monitor blood studies: CBC, platelet count before treatment and twice weekly; neutrophilcounts (ANC) may be increased for 2 days after therapy, but treatment should continue until ANC >10,000/mm^3
- Assess for bone pain: frequency, intensity, duration; analgesics may be given; opiates should not be used
- Check B/P, heart rate, respiration, baseline and during treatment

Nursing diagnoses
- Infection, risk for (uses)
- Pain, acute (adverse reaction)
- Knowledge, deficient (teaching)

Implementation
IV route
- Give 300 mcg/ml or 480 mcg/1.6 ml; allow to warm to room temp; give single dose over 1 min or less through Y-tube or medport
- Use single-use vials; after dose is withdrawn, do not reenter vial
- Give for 2 wk or until ANC = 10,000/mm^3 after the expected chemotherapy neutrophil nadir
- Store in refrigerator; do not freeze; may store at room temp for up to 6 hr; avoid shaking

Y-site compatibilities: Acyclovir, allopurinol, amikacin, aminophylline, ampicillin, ampicillin/sulbactam, aztreonam, bleomycin, bumetanide, buprenorphine, butorphanol, calcium gluconate, carboplatin, carmustine, cefazolin, cefotetan, ceftazidime, chlorproMAZINE, cimetidine, cisplatin, cyclophosphamide, cytarabine, dacarbazine, DAUNOrubicin, dexamethasone, diphenhydrAMINE, DOXOrubicin, doxycycline, droperidol, enalaprilat, famotidine, floxuridine, fluconazole, fludarabine, gallium, ganciclovir, granisetron, haloperidol, hydrocortisone, hydromorphone, hydrOXYzine, idarubicin, ifosfamide, leucovorin, lorazepam, mechlorethamine, melphalan, meperidine, mesna, methotrexate, metoclopramide, miconazole, minocycline, mitoxantrone, morphine, nalbuphine, netilmicin, ondansetron, plicamycin, potassium chloride, promethazine, ranitidine, sodium bicarbonate, streptozocin, ticarcillin, ticarcillin/clavulanate, tobramycin, trimethoprim-sulfamethoxazole, vancomycin, vinBLAStine, vinCRIStine, vinorelbine, zidovudine

Patient/family education
- Teach patient technique for self-administration: dose, side effects, disposal of containers and needles; provide instruction sheet

Evaluation
Positive therapeutic outcome
- Absence of infection

F

finasteride (Rx)
(fin-ass'te-ride)

Propecia, Proscar

Func. class.: Androgen hormone inhibitor, hair stimulant

Chem. class.: 5-α-Reductase inhibitor

Pregnancy category X

Do Not Confuse:
Proscar/Prosom, Proscar/Prozac

Action: Inhibits 5-α-reductase and reduction in dihydrotestosterone (DHT); DHT induces androgenic effects by binding to androgen receptors in the cell nuclei of the prostate gland, liver, skin; prevents development of benign prostatic hypertrophy (BPH)

Therapeutic Outcome: Reduced prostate size

Uses: Symptomatic BPH; male-pattern baldness (Propecia)

Dosage and routes
BPH
Adult: PO 5 mg daily × 6-12 mo

Male pattern baldness
Adult: PO 1 mg daily

Available forms: Tabs 1, 5 mg

Adverse effects
GU: Impotence, decreased libido, decreased volume of ejaculate

Contraindications: Pregnancy **X**, hypersensitivity, children, women who are pregnant or may become pregnant should not handle tabs

Precautions: Large residual urinary volume, severely diminished urinary flow, liver function abnormalities

Pharmacokinetics

Absorption	63%, readily
Distribution	Plasma protein binding, crosses blood-brain barrier
Metabolism	Liver
Excretion	Kidneys—metabolites (39%), feces (57%)
Half-life	6-15 hr

Pharmacodynamics

Onset	Immediate
Peak	1-2 hr
Duration	14 days

Interactions
Drug classifications

Anticholinergics, bronchodilators (adrenergic), theophylline: decreased effect of finasteride

NURSING CONSIDERATIONS
Assessment
- Assess urinary patterns, residual urinary volume, severely diminished urinary flow; prostate-specific antigen (PSA) levels and digital rectal exam results before initiating therapy and periodically thereafter
- Monitor liver function studies before initiating treatment; extensively metabolized in liver

Nursing diagnoses
- Urinary elimination, impaired (uses)
- Knowledge, deficient (teaching)

Implementation
- Administer without regard to meals; give for a minimum of 6 mo; not all patients will respond
- Store at temp <86° F (30° C); protect from light; keep container tightly closed

Patient/family education
- Advise patient that pregnant women or women who may become pregnant should not touch crushed tab or come into contact with semen of a patient taking this drug; may adversely affect development of male fetus
- Inform patient that volume of ejaculate may be decreased during treatment; impotence and decreased libido may also occur
- Inform patient that Propecia results may not occur for 3 mo
- Inform patient that Proscar results may not occur for 6-12 mo

Evaluation
Positive therapeutic outcome
- Decreased postvoiding dribbling, frequency, nocturia
- Increased urinary flow
- Hair growth within 3-6 mo

flavocoxid (Rx)
(flav-uh-kox'id)

Limbrel

Func. class.: Oral nutritional supplement

Pregnancy category UK

Action: Exhibits anti-inflammatory, analgesic properties, thought to be due to inhibition of prostaglandin synthesis via inhibition of cyclooxygenase

Therapeutic Outcome: Decreased pain, inflammation in osteoarthritis

Uses: For dietary management of osteoarthritis

Dosage and routes
Adult: PO 250 mg q12hr

Available forms: Caps 250 mg

Adverse effects
MISC: Hypertension, increase in varicose veins, psoriasis

MS: Fluid accumulation in the knees

Contraindications: Hypersensitivity

Precautions: Pregnancy **UK,** lactation, children <18 yrs, history of stomach ulcers

Pharmacokinetics

Absorption	Unknown
Distribution	Unknown
Metabolism	Primarily via glucuronidation and sulfation
Excretion	Unknown
Half-life	Unknown

Pharmacodynamics

Unknown

Interactions: None known

NURSING CONSIDERATIONS
Assessment
- Assess for pain of rheumatoid arthritis, osteoarthritis; check ROM, inflammation of joints, characteristics of pain

Nursing diagnoses
- Injury, risk for (uses)
- Knowledge, deficient (teaching)

Implementation
- Administer 1 hr before or after meals

Patient/family education
- Teach patient that drug does not take the place of other drugs including corticosteroids for osteoarthritis
- Advise patient to notify prescriber if pregnancy is planned or suspected

Evaluation
Positive therapeutic outcome
- Decreased pain, inflammation in arthritic conditions

flecainide (Rx)
(flek'a-nide)
Tambocor
Func. class.: Antidysrhythmic (Class IC)
Pregnancy category C

Action: Decreases conduction in all parts of the heart, with greatest effect on the His-Purkinje system, which stabilizes the cardiac membrane

Therapeutic Outcome: Absence of dysrhythmias

Uses: Life-threatening ventricular dysrhythmias, sustained ventricular tachycardia; supraventricular tachydysrhythmias, paroxysmal atrial fibrillation/flutter associated with disabling symptoms

Dosage and routes
PSVTT/PAT
Adult: PO 50-100 mg q12h; may increase every 4 days by 50 mg q12h to desired response, not to exceed 300 mg/day

Life-threatening ventricular dysrhythmias
Adult: PO 100 mg q12h, may increase by 50 mg q12h q4d, max 400 mg/day

Renal dose
Adult: PO CCr <35 ml/min dose 50%-75%

Available forms: Tabs 50, 100, 150 mg

Adverse effects
CNS: *Headache, dizziness,* involuntary movement, confusion, psychosis, restlessness, irritability, paresthesias, ataxia, flushing, somnolence, depression, anxiety, malaise, fatigue, asthenia, tremors
CV: *Hypotension,* **bradycardia,** angina, PVCs, **heart block, cardiovascular collapse, arrest, dysrhythmias, CHF, fatal ventricular tachycardia**
EENT: Tinnitus, *blurred vision,* hearing loss
GI: Nausea, vomiting, anorexia, constipation, abdominal pain, flatulence, change in taste
GU: Impotence, decreased libido, polyuria, urinary retention
HEMA: **Leukopenia, thrombocytopenia**
INTEG: Rash, urticaria, edema, swelling
RESP: Dyspnea, **respiratory depression**

Contraindications: Hypersensitivity, severe heart block, cardiogenic shock, nonsustained ventricular dysrhythmias, frequent PVCs, non–life-threatening dysrhythmias

Precautions: Pregnancy **C,** lactation, children, renal disease, liver disease, CHF, respiratory depression, myasthenia gravis

F

Pharmacokinetics	
Absorption	Well absorbed
Distribution	Widely distributed
Metabolism	Liver
Excretion	30% kidneys, unchanged
Half-life	14 hr

Pharmacodynamics	
Onset	Unknown
Peak	3 hr
Duration	Unknown

Interactions
Individual drugs
Amiodarone, cimetidine, ritonavir: increased level of flecainide
Digoxin: increased digoxin levels
Disopyramide, verapamil: increased CV depressant action
Propanolol: increased both drugs

Drug classifications
Acidifying agents, alkalizing agents: increased or decreased effect
β-Adrenergic blockers: increased CV depressant action

Drug/herb
Aconite: increased toxicity, death
Aloe, broom, buckthorn (chronic use), cascara sagrada (chronic use), Chinese rhubarb, figwort, fumitory, goldenseal, kudzu, licorice: increased effect
Coltsfoot: decreased effect
Horehound: increased serotonin effect

NURSING CONSIDERATIONS
Assessment
- Monitor ECG continuously to determine drug effectiveness; measure PR, QRS, QT intervals; check for PVCs, other dysrhythmias; monitor B/P continuously for hypotension, hypertension, and rebound hypertension (after 1-2 hr); check for dehydration or hypovolemia

• Monitor I&O ratio; electrolytes: (K [potassium], Na [sodium]), Cl (chloride); check weight daily and for signs of CHF or pulmonary toxicity: dyspnea, fatigue, cough, fever, chest pain, jugular vein distention, crackles; if these occur, drug should be discontinued
• Monitor liver function studies: AST, ALT, bilirubin, alkaline phosphatase
• Assess patient for CNS symptoms: confusion, psychosis, numbness, depression, involuntary movements; if these occur, drug should be discontinued
• Monitor cardiac rate, respiration: rate, rhythm, character, chest pain; watch for ventricular tachycardia, supraventricular tachycardia, or fibrillation

Nursing diagnoses

• Cardiac output, decreased (uses)
• Knowledge, deficient (teaching)

Implementation

• Give reduced dosage slowly with ECG monitoring; do not increase dose fewer than 4 days apart
• Give with meals if GI upset occurs

Patient/family education

• Instruct patient to report side effects immediately to prescriber
• Instruct patient to complete follow-up appointment with health care provider including pulmonary function studies, chest x-ray
• Teach patient to change position slowly from lying or sitting to standing to minimize orthostatic hypotension
• Advise patient not to skip or double doses
• Advise patient to carry/wear emergency ID with disorder, medications taken
• Advise patient to avoid hazardous activities that require alertness until response is known

Evaluation

Positive therapeutic outcome

• Absence of dysrhythmias

fluconazole (Rx)

(floo-kon'a-zole)

Diflucan

Func. class.: Antifungal

Pregnancy category B

Do Not Confuse:

Diflucan/Diprivan

Action: Inhibits ergosterol biosynthesis, causes direct damage to membrane phospholipids in the cell wall of fungi

Therapeutic Outcome: Fungistatic fungicidal against the following susceptible organisms: *Candida, Cryptococcus neoformans*

Uses: Oropharyngeal esophageal candidiasis in AIDS patients, chronic mucocutaneous candidiasis, urinary candidiasis, cryptococcal meningitis, peritonitis

Dosage and routes

Renal dose

Adult: PO CCr 11-50 ml/min dose 50%

Vaginal candidiasis

Adult: PO 150 mg as a single dose

Serious fungal infections

Adult: PO/**IV** 50-400 mg initially, then 200 mg once daily for 4 wk

Child: 6-12 mg/kg/day

Oropharyngeal candidiasis

Adult: PO 200 mg initially, then 100 mg daily for at least 2 wk

Child: 3 mg/kg/day

Available forms: Tabs 50, 100, 150, 200 mg; inj 2 mg/ml; powder for oral susp 50, 200 mg/ml

Adverse effects

CNS: Headache

GI: Nausea, vomiting, diarrhea, cramping, flatus, increased AST, ALT, **hepatotoxicity**

INTEG: **Stevens-Johnson syndrome**

Contraindications: Hypersensitivity to azoles

Precautions: Pregnancy **B,** renal disease, lactation, hepatic disease

Pharmacokinetics

Absorption	Well absorbed (PO)
Distribution	Widely distributed (peritoneum, CSF)
Metabolism	<10%—liver
Excretion	80% kidneys (unchanged)
Half-life	30 hr, increased in renal disease

Pharmacodynamics

	PO	IV
Onset	Unknown	Immediate
Peak	2-4 hr	Infusion's end
Duration	Unknown	Unknown

Interactions

Individual drugs

CycloSPORINE, phenytoin, rifabutin, tacrolimus, theophylline: increased plasma concentrations
Warfarin: increased anticoagulation
Zidovudine: increased effect

Drug classification
Contraceptives (oral): decreased effect
Oral antidiabetics: hypoglycemia
Drug/herb
Gossypol: increased nephrotoxicity

NURSING CONSIDERATIONS
Assessment
- Assess for signs and symptoms of infection: clearing of CSF culture during treatment, obtain C&S baseline and during treatment, drug may be started as soon as culture is taken
- Monitor for hepatotoxicity: increased AST, ALT, alkaline phosphatase, bilirubin; drug will be discontinued if hepatotoxicity occurs

Nursing diagnoses
- Infection, risk for (uses)
- Injury, risk for (adverse reactions)
- Knowledge, deficient (teaching)

Implementation
- Take with food to reduce GI effects

PO route
- Shake oral susp before each use

IV route
- Give after diluting according to package directions; run at 200 mg/hr or less; do not use plastic containers in connections
- Do not admix
- Administer **IV** using an in-line filter, using distal veins; check for extravasation and necrosis q2h
- Give drug only after C&S confirms organism, drug needed to treat condition
- Store protected from moisture and light, diluted sol is stable for 24 hr

Y-site compatibilities: Acyclovir, aldesleukin, allopurinol, amifostine, amikacin, aminophylline, ampicillin/sulbactam, aztreonam, benztropine, cefazolin, cefepime, cefotetan, cefoxitin, chlorproMAZINE, cimetidine, dexamethasone, diphenhydrAMINE, DOBUTamine, DOPamine, droperidol, famotidine, filgrastim, fludarabine, foscarnet, gallium, ganciclovir, gentamicin, granisetron, heparin, hydrocortisone, immune globulin, leucovorin, lorazepam, melphalan, meperidine, meropenem, metoclopramide, metronidazole, midazolam, morphine, nafcillin, nitroglycerin, ondansetron, oxacillin, paclitaxel, pancuronium, penicillin G, potassium, phenytoin, piperacillin/tazobactam, prochlorperazine, promethazine, propofol, ranitidine, sargramostim, sulfamethoxazole, tacrolimus, teniposide, theophylline, thiotepa, ticarcillin/clavulanate, tobramycin, vancomycin, vecuronium, vinorelbine, zidovudine

Y-site incompatibilities: Amphotericin B, ampicillin, calcium gluconate, cefotaxime, ceftriaxone, ceftazidime, cefuroxime, chloramphenicol, clindamycin, diazepam, digoxin, erythromycin lactobionate, furosemide, haloperidol, hydrOXYzine, imipenem/cilastatin, pentamidine, ticarcillin, trimethoprim/sulfamethoxazole

Additive compatibilities: Acyclovir, amikacin, amphotericin B, cefazolin, ceftazidime, clindamycin, gentamicin, heparin, meropenem, metronidazole, morphine, piperacillin, potassium chloride, theophylline

Patient/family education
- Caution patient that long-term therapy may be needed to clear infection; to take entire course of medication; take in equal intervals (PO)
- Teach patient the signs and symptoms of hepatotoxicity: nausea, vomiting, clay-colored stools, dark urine, anorexia, fatigue, jaundice; prescriber should be notified immediately
- Inform patient that medication may be taken with food to reduce GI effects
- Advise patient to consider using alternative contraception if using oral contraceptives

Evaluation
Positive therapeutic outcome
- Decreasing oral candidiasis, fever, malaise, rash
- Negative C&S for infecting organism

F

fludrocortisone (Rx)
(floo-droe-kor′ti-sone)
Florinef
Func. class.: Corticosteroid, synthetic
Chem. class.: Mineralocorticoid
Pregnancy category C

Action: Promotes increased reabsorption of sodium and loss of potassium, water, hydrogen from the distal renal tubules

Therapeutic Outcome: Treatment of adrenal insufficiency symptoms

Uses: Adrenal insufficiency, salt-losing adrenogenital syndrome

Investigational uses: Renal tubular acidosis (type IV), idiopathic orthostatic hypertension

Dosage and routes
Adult: PO 0.1-0.2 mg daily
Child: PO 0.05-0.1 mg/day

Available forms: Tabs 0.1 mg

Adverse effects

CNS: *Flushing, sweating,* headache, paralysis, dizziness
CV: *Hypertension,* **circulatory collapse, thrombophlebitis, embolism,** tachycardia, **CHF,** edema
ENDO: Weight gain, adrenal suppression
META: *Hypokalemia*
MISC: Hypersensitivity
MS: Fractures, osteoporosis, weakness

Contraindications: Hypersensitivity, acute glomerulonephritis, amebiasis, psychoses, Cushing's syndrome, fungal infections, child <2 yr

Precautions: Pregnancy **C**, osteoporosis, CHF, lactation, child >2 yr, hypertension, diabetes

Pharmacokinetics

Absorption	Well absorbed
Distribution	Widely
Metabolism	Liver
Excretion	Kidneys, breast milk
Half-life	3½ hr

Pharmacodynamics

Peak	1.5 hr

Interactions

Individual drugs

Amphotericin B, mezlocillin, piperacillin: increased hypokalemia
Phenytoin: decreased action of fludrocortisone
Rifampin: decreased effect of fludrocortisone

Drug classifications

Barbiturates: decreased action of fludrocortisone
Diuretics (loop), thiazides, potassium-wasting drugs: decreased potassium levels

Drug/herb

Aloe, buckthorn, cascara sagrada, Chinese rhubarb, senna: increased hypokalemia
Aloe, licorice, perilla: increased corticosteroid effect

Drug/food

Increased salt/sodium ingestion: increased B/P

Drug/lab test

Increased: potassium, sodium
Decreased: hematocrit

NURSING CONSIDERATIONS

Assessment

- Monitor patient for fluid retention: weigh daily, notify prescriber of weekly gain >5 lb; B/P q4h, pulse; notify prescriber if chest pain occurs; I&O ratio; be alert for decreasing urinary output and increasing edema
- Check for potassium depletion: paresthesias, fatigue, nausea, vomiting, depression, polyuria, dysrhythmias, weakness; also sodium, chloride

Nursing diagnoses

- Fluid volume, deficient (uses)
- Fluid volume, excess (adverse reactions)
- Knowledge, deficient (teaching)

Implementation

- Administer titrated dose; use lowest effective dose; scored tab may be broken if lower dose is necessary
- Give with food or milk to decrease GI symptoms

Patient/family education

- Advise patient to carry/wear emergency ID as steroid user at all times during diagnosis and treatment
- Caution patient not to discontinue this medication abruptly; Addisonian crisis may occur
- Counsel patient to follow dietary regimen recommended by prescriber; should include high potassium and, possibly, low sodium
- Advise patient to report weight gain >5 lb; edema in legs, hands; abdominal cramping; muscle cramps; nausea; vomiting; anorexia; dizziness or weakness, infection, trauma stress
- Advise patient not to breastfeed

Evaluation

Positive therapeutic outcome

- Correction of adrenal insufficiency
- Electrolytes and fluids in normal range

flumazenil (Rx)

(flu-maz'e-nil)

Anexate ✤, Romazicon

Func. class.: Benzodiazepine receptor antagonist
Chem. class.: Imidazobenzodiazepine derivative

Pregnancy category C

Do Not Confuse:
Mazicon/Mivacron

Action: Antagonizes the actions of benzodiazepines on the CNS, competitively inhibits the activity at the benzodiazepine receptor complex

Therapeutic Outcome: Reversed benzodiazepine toxic effects

Uses: Reversal of the sedative effects of benzodiazepines

Dosage and routes

Reversal of conscious sedation or in general anesthesia

Adult: **IV** 0.2 mg (2 ml) given over 15 sec; wait 45 sec, then give 0.2 mg (2 ml) if consciousness does not occur; may be repeated at 60-sec intervals as needed (max 3 mg/hr)

Child: **IV** 10 mcg (0.01 mg)/kg; cumulative dose of 1 mg or less

Management of suspected benzodiazepine overdose

Adult: **IV** 0.2 mg (2 ml) given over 30 sec; wait 30 sec, then give 0.3 mg (3 ml) over 30 sec if consciousness does not occur; further doses of 0.5 mg (5 ml) can be given over 30 sec at intervals of 1 min up to cumulative dose of 3 mg

Child: **IV** 100 mcg (0.1 mg)/kg; cumulative dose of 1 mg or less

Available forms: Inj 0.1 mg/ml

Adverse effects

CNS: Dizziness, agitation, emotional lability, confusion, **seizures,** somnolence

CV: Hypertension, palpitations, cutaneous vasodilatation, **dysrhythmias,** bradycardia, tachycardia, chest pain

EENT: Abnormal vision, blurred vision, tinnitus

GI: Nausea, vomiting, hiccups

SYST: Headache, inj site pain, increased sweating, fatigue, rigors

Contraindications: Hypersensitivity to this drug or benzodiazepines, serous tricyclic antidepressant overdose, patients given benzodiazepine for control of life-threatening condition

Precautions: Pregnancy **C,** lactation, children, elderly, renal disease, status epilepticus, head injury, labor and delivery, hepatic disease, hypoventilation, panic disorder, drug and alcohol dependency, ambulatory patients

Pharmacokinetics	
Absorption	Complete
Distribution	Unknown
Metabolism	Liver
Excretion	Unknown
Half-life	41-79 min

Pharmacodynamics	
Onset	1 min
Peak	10 min
Duration	Unknown

Interactions

Individual drugs

Zaleplon, zolpidem: antagonize action

Drug classifications

Benzodiazepines: antagonize action

Toxicity: mixed drug overdosage

NURSING CONSIDERATIONS

Assessment

- Assess cardiac status using continuous monitoring
- Assess for seizures, protect patient from injury; most likely in those who usually experience withdrawal from sedatives
- Assess for GI symptoms: nausea, vomiting; place in side-lying position to prevent aspiration
- Assess for allergic reactions: flushing, rash, urticaria, pruritus

Nursing diagnoses

- Injury, risk for (uses)
- Poisoning, risk for (uses)

Implementation

- Give directly undiluted or diluted in 0.9% NaCl, D_5W, or LR; give over 15 sec into running **IV**
- Check airway and **IV** access before administration

Additive compatibilities: Aminophylline, cimetidine, DOBUTamine, DOPamine, famotidine, heparin, lidocaine, procainamide, ranitidine

Patient/family education

- Caution patient that amnesia may continue
- Instruct patient to avoid any hazardous activities for 18-24 hr after discharge
- Inform patient not to take any alcohol or nonprescription drugs for 18-24 hr; serious reactions may occur

Evaluation

Positive therapeutic outcome

- Decreased sedation, respiratory depression
- Absence of toxicity

! HIGH ALERT

fluorouracil (Rx)

(flure-oh-yoor′a-sil)

Adrucil, Efudex, 5-FU

Func. class.: Antineoplastic, antimetabolite

Chem. class.: Pyrimidine antagonist

Pregnancy category D

Do Not Confuse:

fluorouracil/flucytosine

F

Action: Inhibits DNA, RNA synthesis; interferes with cell replication by competitively inhibiting thymidylate synthesis, cell cycle–specific (S phase), a vesicant

Therapeutic Outcome: Prevention of rapidly growing malignant cells

Uses: *Systemic:* cancer of breast, colon, rectum, stomach, pancreas; multiple active keratoses; *Topical:* basal cell carcinoma

Dosage and routes

Adult: **IV** 12 mg/kg/day × 4 days, not to exceed 800 mg/day; may repeat with 6 mg/kg on day 6, 8, 10, 12; maintenance is 10-15 mg/kg/wk as a single dose, not to exceed 1 g/wk

Actinic/solar keratoses

Adult: TOP 1% cream/sol 1-2×/day

Superficial basal cell carcinoma

Adult: TOP 5% sol 2×/day × 3-12 wk

Available forms: Inj 50 mg/ml; cream 1, 5%; sol 1, 2, 5%

Adverse effects

Systemic use

CNS: Lethargy, malaise, weakness, acute cerebellar dysfunction
CV: Myocardial ischemia, angina
EENT: Epistaxis
GI: *Anorexia, stomatitis,* diarrhea, nausea, vomiting, **hemorrhage, enteritis glossitis**
HEMA: **Thrombocytopenia, leukopenia, myelosuppression, anemia, agranulocytosis**
INTEG: *Rash,* fever, photosensitivity

Contraindications: Pregnancy **D,** hypersensitivity, myelosuppression, poor nutritional status, serious infections, major surgery within 1 mo

Precautions: Renal disease, hepatic disease, bone marrow depression, angina, lactation, children

Pharmacokinetics

Absorption	Completely bioavailable (**IV**), minimal (top)
Distribution	Widely distributed, concentration in tumor
Metabolism	Liver—converted to active metabolite
Excretion	Lungs (60%-80%), kidneys (up to 15%)
Half-life	20 hr terminal

Pharmacodynamics

Unknown

Interactions

Individual drugs

Irinotecan: increased toxicity
Radiation: increased toxicity, bone marrow suppression

Drug classifications

Antineoplastics: increased toxicity, bone marrow depression
Live virus vaccines: decreased antibody response

Drug/lab test

Increased: liver function studies, 5-HIAA
Decreased: albumin

NURSING CONSIDERATIONS

Assessment

- Monitor ECG; watch for ST-T wave changes, low QRS and T, possible dysrhythmias (sinus tachycardia, heart block, PVCs)
- Assess buccal cavity q8h for dryness, sores or ulceration, white patches, oral pain, bleeding, dysphagia; obtain prescription for viscous lidocaine (Xylocaine)
- Assess tachypnea, ECG changes, dyspnea, edema, fatigue; identify dyspnea, crackles, unproductive cough, chest pain, tachypnea
- Monitor CBC, differential, platelet count daily (**IV**); withhold drug if WBC is <4000/mm^3 or platelet count is <100,000/mm^3; notify prescriber of results if WBC <20,000/mm^3, platelets <50,000/mm^3; nadir of leukopenia within 2 wk, recovery 1 mo
- Monitor renal function studies: BUN, creatinine, serum uric acid, urine CCr before and during therapy; I&O ratio; report fall in urine output to <30 ml/hr
- Monitor temp q4h (may indicate beginning of infection)
- Monitor liver function tests before and during therapy (bilirubin, AST, ALT, LDH) as needed or monthly; jaundice of skin, sclera, dark urine, clay-colored stools, itchy skin, abdominal pain, fever, diarrhea
- Assess for bleeding: hematuria, stool guaiac, bruising or petechiae, mucosa or orifices q8h; inflammation of mucosa, breaks in skin

Nursing diagnoses

- Injury, risk for (adverse reactions)
- Body image, disturbed (adverse reactions)
- Infection, risk for (adverse reactions)
- Knowledge, deficient (teaching)

Implementation

- Avoid contact with skin (very irritating); wash completely to remove
- Give fluids **IV** or PO before chemotherapy to hydrate patient
- Give antiemetic 30-60 min before giving

drug to prevent vomiting, and prn for several days thereafter; antibiotics for prophylaxis of infection

- Provide liq diet: carbonated beverages; gelatin may be added if patient is not nauseated or vomiting
- Provide rinsing of mouth tid-qid with water, club soda; brushing of teeth bid-qid with soft brush or cotton-tipped applicators for stomatitis; use unwaxed dental floss

Topical route

- Wear gloves when applying; may use with a loose dressing, use a plastic or wooden applicator

IV route

- Prepare in biologic cabinet using gloves, gown, mask
- **IV** undiluted; may inject through Y-tube or 3-way stopcock; give over 1-3 min
- May be diluted in 0.9% NaCl, D_5W, given over 2-8 hr as an **IV** inf

Syringe compatibilities: Bleomycin, cisplatin, cyclophosphamide, furosemide, heparin, leucovorin, methotrexate, metoclopramide, mitomycin, vinBLAStine, vinCRIStine

Syringe incompatibilities: Droperidol

Y-site compatibilities: Allopurinol, amifostine, aztreonam, bleomycin, cefepime, cisplatin, cyclophosphamide, DOXOrubicin, fludarabine, furosemide, granisetron, heparin, hydrocortisone, leucovorin, mannitol, melphalan, methotrexate, metoclopramide, mitomycin, paclitaxel, piperacillin/tazobactam, potassium chloride, propofol, sargramostin, thiotepa, thiposide, vinBLAStine, vinCRIStine, vit B/C

Y-site incompatibilities: Droperidol, vinorelbine

Additive compatibilities: Bleomycin, cephalothin, cyclophosphamide, etoposides, floxuridine, hydromorphone, ifosfamide, leucovorin, methotrexate, mitoxantrone, prednisoLONE, vinCRIStine

Additive incompatibilities: Carboplatin, cisplatin, cytarabine, diazepam, DOXOrubicin

Solution compatibilities: Amino acids 4.25%/D_{25}, D_5/LR, $D_{3.3}$/0.3% NaCl, D_5W, 0.9% NaCl, TPN #23

Patient/family education

- Caution patient that contraceptive measures are recommended during therapy
- Teach patient to avoid using aspirin, NSAIDs, or ibuprofen-containing products, razors, commercial mouthwash because bleeding may occur; to report symptoms of bleeding (hematuria, tarry stools)
- Instruct patient to report signs of anemia (fatigue, headache, irritability, faintness, shortness of breath)
- Instruct patient to report signs of stomatitis (bleeding, white spots, ulcerations in the mouth); tell patient to examine mouth daily, to report symptoms; viscous lidocaine (Xylocaine) may be used
- Teach patient to avoid crowds, persons with known infections
- Advise patient to avoid vaccinations during therapy, to use sunscreen or stay out of the sun to prevent burns; about hair loss, explore use of wigs or other products until hair regrowth occurs

Evaluation

Positive therapeutic outcome

- Prevention of rapid division of malignant cells

F

fluoxetine (Rx)

(floo-ox'uh-teen)

Prozac, Prozac Weekly, Sarafem

Func. class.: Antidepressant, SSRI (selective serotonin reuptake inhibitor)

Pregnancy category B

Do Not Confuse:

Prozac/Proscar, Prozac/Prilosec, Prozac/Prosom

Sarafem/Serophene

Action: Inhibits CNS neuron uptake of serotonin, but not of norepINEPHrine

Therapeutic Outcome: Decreased symptoms of depression after 2-3 wk

Uses: Major depressive disorder, obsessive-compulsive disorder (OCD), bulimia nervosa; sarafem: premenstrual dysphoric disorder (PMDD)

Investigational uses: Alcoholism, anorexia nervosa, attention deficit hyperactivity disorder, bipolar II affective disorder, borderline personality disorder, cataplexy, narcolepsy, kleptomania, migraine, obesity, posttraumatic stress disorder, schizophrenia, Gilles de la Tourette's syndrome, trichotillomania, levodopa-induced dyskinesia, social phobia

Dosage and routes

Depression/OCD

Adult: PO 20 mg daily AM; after 4 wk if no clinical improvement is noted, dose may be increased to 20 mg bid in AM, afternoon, not to exceed 80 mg/day; PO weekly

Elderly: PO 5-10 mg/day, increase as needed

Child 5-18 yr: PO 5-10 mg/day, max 20 mg/day

Bulimia nervosa
Adult: PO 60 mg/day in AM

ADHD (unlabeled)
Adult: PO 20-60 mg/day

Alcoholism (unlabeled)
Adult: PO 20-80 mg/day

Anorexia nervosa (unlabeled)
Adult: PO 10 mg every other day-20 mg/day

Bipolar II affective disorder (unlabeled)
Adult: PO 10 mg every other day-20 mg/day

Borderline personality disorder (unlabeled)
Adult: PO 20 mg/day

Kleptomania (unlabeled)
Adult: PO 60-80 mg/day

Migraine, chronic daily headaches (unlabeled)
Adult: PO 10-80 mg/day

Narcolepsy (unlabeled)
Adult: PO 20-40 mg/day

Posttraumatic stress disorder (unlabeled)
Adult: PO 10-80 mg/day

Premenstrual dysphoric disorder (Sarafem)
Adult: PO 20 mg daily, may be taken daily week before menses

Schizophrenia (unlabeled)
Adult: PO 20-60 mg/day

Available forms: Caps 10, 20, 40 mg; tabs 10, 20 mg; oral sol 20 mg/5 ml; del rel caps (Prozac Weekly) 90 mg

Adverse effects

CNS: *Headache, nervousness, insomnia, drowsiness, anxiety, tremor, dizziness, fatigue, sedation, poor concentration, abnormal dreams, agitation,* **seizures,** apathy, euphoria, hallucinations, delusions, psychosis

CV: *Hot flashes, palpitations,* angina pectoris, **hemorrhage,** hypertension, **tachycardia,** 1st-degree AV block, **bradycardia, MI, thrombophlebitis**

EENT: Visual changes, ear/eye pain, photophobia, tinnitus

GI: *Nausea, diarrhea, dry mouth, anorexia, dyspepsia, constipation, cramps, vomiting, taste changes, flatulence, decreased appetite*

GU: *Dysmenorrhea, decreased libido, urinary frequency, urinary tract infection,* amenorrhea, cystitis, impotence, urine retention

INTEG: *Sweating, rash, pruritus,* acne, alopecia, urticaria

MS: *Pain,* arthritis, twitching

RESP: *Infection, pharyngitis, nasal congestion, sinus headache, sinusitis, cough, dyspnea, bronchitis,* asthma, hyperventilation, pneumonia

SYST: *Asthenia, viral infection, fever, allergy, chills*

Contraindications: Hypersensitivity

Precautions: Pregnancy **B,** lactation, children, elderly, diabetes mellitus

Pharmacokinetics

Absorption	Well absorbed
Distribution	Crosses blood-brain barrier
Metabolism	Liver, extensively to norfluoxetine
Excretion	Kidneys, unchanged (12%), metabolite (7%); steady state 28-35 days, protein binding 94%
Half-life	1-3 days metabolite up to 1 wk

Pharmacodynamics

Onset	Unknown
Peak	6-8 hr
Duration	Unknown

Interactions

Individual drugs

Alcohol: increased CNS depression
Buspirone: increased worsening of OCD
Carbamazepine, digoxin, lithium, phenytoin, warfarin: increased toxicity
Cyproheptadine: decreased fluoxetine effect
Diazepam: increased half-life of diazepam
Haloperidol: increased haloperidol effect
Thioridazine: do not use, or use within 5 wk of discontinuing fluoxetine

Drug classifications

Antidepressants, barbiturates, benzodiazepines, CNS depressants, opioids, sedative/hypnotics: increased CNS depression
Highly protein-bound drugs: increased side effects
MAOIs: hypertensive crisis, seizures; do not use with or 14 days prior to fluoxetine
Phenothiazines, tricyclic antidepressants: increased levels

Drug/herb

Corkwood, jimsonweed: increased anticholinergic effect
Hops, kava, lavender: increased CNS effect
St. John's wort, SAM-e: do not use together; increased risk of serotonin syndrome

Drug/lab test
Increased: serum bilirubin, blood glucose, alkaline phosphatase
Decreased: VMA, 5-HIAA
False increase: urinary catecholamines

NURSING CONSIDERATIONS
Assessment
- Monitor B/P (lying, standing), pulse q4h; if systolic B/P drops 20 mm hg, hold drug and notify prescriber; take VS q4h in patients with CV disease
- Monitor blood studies: CBC, leukocytes, differential, cardiac enzymes if patient is receiving long-term therapy; check platelets, bleeding can occur
- Monitor hepatic studies: AST, ALT, bilirubin
- Check weight qwk; appetite may increase with drug
- Assess ECG for flattening of T wave, bundle branch block, AV block, dysrhythmias in cardiac patients
- Assess mental status: mood, sensorium, affect, suicidal tendencies; increase in psychiatric symptoms: depression, panic; monitor for seizures; seizure potential is increased
- Monitor urinary retention, constipation; constipation is more likely to occur in children or elderly
- Identify patient's alcohol consumption; if alcohol is consumed, hold dose until AM
- Assess appetite in bulimia nervosa, weight daily, increase nutritious foods in diet, watch for bingeing and vomiting
- Assess allergic reactions: itching, rash, urticaria, drug should be discontinued; may need to give antihistamine

Nursing diagnoses
- Coping, ineffective (uses)
- Injury, risk for (side effects)
- Knowledge, deficient (teaching)
- Noncompliance (teaching)

Implementation
- Give with food or milk for GI symptoms
- Give dosage at bedtime if oversedation occurs during day; may take entire dose at bedtime; elderly may not tolerate once/day dosing, crushed if patient unable to swallow whole (tabs only)
- Prozac weekly: Give on same day each week
- Store at room temp; do not freeze

Patient/family education
- Teach patient that therapeutic effects may take 1-4 wk
- Instruct patient to use caution in driving or other activities requiring alertness because of drowsiness, dizziness, blurred vision; to avoid rising quickly from sitting to standing, especially elderly; to use sunscreen to prevent photosensitivity
- Caution patient to avoid alcohol ingestion, other CNS depressants
- Advise patient not to discontinue medication quickly after long-term use: may cause nausea, headache, malaise
- Instruct patient to increase fluids, bulk in diet if constipation, urinary retention occur, especially elderly
- Advise patient to take gum, hard sugarless candy, or frequent sips of water for dry mouth
- Teach patient to avoid all OTC drugs unless approved by prescriber
- Advise patient to change positions slowly, orthostatic hypotension may occur

Evaluation
Positive therapeutic outcome
- Decrease in depression
- Absence of suicidal thoughts
- Decreased symptoms of OCD

fluphenazine decanoate (Rx)
(floo-fen'ah-zeen)
Modecate ✦, Modecate Concentrate, Prolixin Decanoate

fluphenazine hydrochloride (Rx)
Apo-Fluphenazine ✦, Moditen HCL ✦, Moditen HCl-H.P. ✦, Permitil ✦, Prolixin
Func. class.: Antipsychotic/neuroleptic
Chem. class.: Phenothiazine, piperazine

Pregnancy category C

Do Not Confuse:
Prolixin/Proloid

Action: Depresses cerebral cortex, hypothalamus, limbic system, which control activity and aggression; blocks neurotransmission produced by dopamine at synapse; exhibits strong α-adrenergic and anticholinergic blocking action; mechanism for antipsychotic effects is unclear

Therapeutic Outcome: Decreased signs and symptoms of psychosis

Uses: Psychotic disorders, schizophrenia

Dosage and routes
Decanoate
Adult and child >16 yr: IM/SUBCUT 12.5-25 mg q1-3 wk, may increase slowly
Child 12-16 yr: IM/SUBCUT 6.25-18.75

mg, then repeat q1-3 wk, then increase slowly, max 25 mg
Child 5-12 yr: IM/SUBCUT 3.125-12.5 mg, then repeat q1-3 wk, increase slowly

HCl
Adult: PO 2.5-10 mg, in divided doses q6-8h, not to exceed 20 mg daily; IM initially 1.25 mg then 2.5-10 mg in divided doses q6-8h
Child: PO 0.25-3.5 mg daily in divided doses q4-6h, max 10 mg/daily

Available forms: HCl tabs 1, 2.5, 5, 10 mg; elixir 2.5 mg/5 ml; inj 2.5 mg/ml; decanoate: inj 25 mg/ml

Adverse effects
CNS: Extrapyramidal symptoms (EPS), pseudoparkinsonism, akathisia, dystonia, tardive dyskinesia, drowsiness, headache, **seizures, neuroleptic malignant syndrome**
CV: Orthostatic hypotension, hypertension, **cardiac arrest,** ECG changes, **tachycardia**
EENT: Blurred vision, glaucoma, dry eyes
GI: Dry mouth, nausea, vomiting, anorexia, constipation, diarrhea, jaundice, weight gain, **paralytic ileus, hepatitis,** cholecystic jaundice
GU: Urinary retention, urinary frequency, enuresis, impotence, amenorrhea, gynecomastia
HEMA: Anemia, **leukopenia, leukocytosis, agranulocytosis, aplastic anemia, thrombocytopenia**
INTEG: Rash, photosensitivity, dermatitis
RESP: **Laryngospasm,** dyspnea, **respiratory depression**

Contraindications: Hypersensitivity, circulatory collapse, liver damage, cerebral arteriosclerosis, coronary disease, severe hypertension/hypotension, blood dyscrasias, coma, brain damage, bone marrow depression, alcohol and barbiturate withdrawal, narrow-angle glaucoma

Precautions: Pregnancy **C,** lactation, seizure disorders, hypertension, hepatic disease, cardiac disease, elderly, child <12 yr

Pharmacokinetics

Absorption	Well absorbed (PO, IM)
Distribution	Widely absorbed, crosses blood-brain barrier, placenta
Metabolism	Liver, extensively
Excretion	Kidneys (metabolites)
Half-life	HCl-4.7-15.3 hr, enanthate 3½-4 days, decanoate 6.8-14.3 days

Pharmacodynamics

	PO/IM HCl	IM Enanthate	IM Decanoate
Onset	1 hr	1-2 days	1-3 days
Peak	1½-2 hr	2-3 days	1-2 days
Duration	6-8 hr	1-3 wk	>4 wk

Interactions
Individual drugs
Alcohol: increased effects of both drugs, oversedation
Epinephrine: increased toxicity
Levodopa: decreased antiparkinson activity
Lithium: decreased effects of lithium
Drug classifications
Anticholinergics: increased anticholinergic effects
Barbiturates: decreased effect of fluphenazine, oversedation
CNS depressants: oversedation
Smoking: decreased effects of fluphenazine
Drug/herb
Betel palm, kava: increased EPS
Cola tree, hops, kava, nettle, nutmeg: possible increased action
Henbane leaf: increased anticholinergic effect
Drug/lab test
Increased: liver function tests, cardiac enzymes, cholesterol, blood glucose, prolactin, bilirubin, PBI, cholinesterase
Decreased: hormones (blood and urine)
False positive: pregnancy tests, PKU, urinary steroids, 17-OHCS

NURSING CONSIDERATIONS
Assessment
- Assess mental status: orientation, mood, behavior, presence of hallucinations, and type before initial administration and monthly; this drug should significantly reduce psychotic behavior
- Check for swallowing of PO medication; check for hoarding or giving of medication to other patients
- Monitor I&O ratio, palpate bladder if low urinary output occurs, especially in elderly; urinalysis recommended before, during prolonged therapy
- Monitor bilirubin, CBC, liver function studies monthly
- Assess affect, orientation, LOC, reflexes, gait, coordination, sleep pattern disturbances
- Monitor B/P with patient sitting, standing, and lying down; take pulse and respirations q4h during initial treatment; establish baseline before starting treatment; report drops of 30

mm Hg; obtain baseline ECG, Q-wave and T-wave changes
- Check for dizziness, faintness, palpitations, tachycardia on rising; severe orthostatic hypotension is common
- Assess for neuroleptic malignant syndrome: hyperpyrexia, musclerigidity, increased CPK, altered mental status; drug should be discontinued
- Assess for EPS including akathisia (inability to sit still, no pattern to movements), tardive dyskinesia (bizarre movements of the jaw, mouth, tongue, extremities), pseudoparkinsonism (rigidity, tremors, pill rolling, shuffling gate), an antiparkinson drug should be prescribed
- Assess for constipation, urinary retention daily; if these occur, increase bulk, water in diet

Nursing diagnoses
- Thought processes, disturbed (uses)
- Coping, ineffective (uses)
- Knowledge, deficient (teaching)
- Noncompliance (teaching)

Implementation
PO route
- Give drug in liq form mixed in glass of juice or cola if hoarding is suspected; do not mix in caffeine drinks, tannics, or pectinates; decrease dose in elderly
- Give PO with full glass of water, milk; or give with food to decrease GI upset
- Take antacids 2 hr before or after this drug
- Store in tight, light-resistant container, oral sol in amber bottle

SUBCUT route
- May be given by this route; however, it is painful

IM route
- Inject in deep muscle mass, use a 21G needle into dorsal gluteal site, keep patient recumbent for ½ hr to prevent orthostatic hypotension
- Patient should remain lying down after IM inj for at least 30 min

Syringe compatibilities: Benztropine, diphenhydrAMINE, hydrOXYzine

Patient/family education
- Teach patient to use good oral hygiene; frequent rinsing of mouth, sugarless gum for dry mouth
- Caution patient to avoid hazardous activities until drug response is determined; dizziness, blurred vision may occur
- Inform patient that orthostatic hypotension occurs often and to rise from sitting or lying position gradually; tell patient to avoid hot tubs, hot showers, tub baths because hypotension may occur; tell patient that in hot weather, heat stroke may occur; extra precautions are necessary to stay cool
- Instruct patient to avoid abrupt withdrawal of this drug, or EPS may result; drug should be withdrawn slowly
- Teach patient to avoid OTC preparations (cough, hay fever, cold) unless approved by physician because serious drug interactions may occur; avoid use with alcohol, CNS depressants; increased drowsiness may occur
- Instruct patient to use a sunscreen and sunglasses to prevent burns
- Teach patient about EPS and necessity of meticulous oral hygiene because oral candidiasis may occur
- Instruct patient to take antacids 2 hr before or after this drug
- Advise patient to report sore throat, malaise, fever, bleeding, mouth sores; if these occur, CBC should be performed and drug discontinued

Evaluation
Positive therapeutic outcome
- Decrease in emotional excitement, hallucinations, delusions, paranoia
- Reorganization of patterns of thought, speech

Treatment of overdose: Lavage if orally ingested; provide airway; *do not induce vomiting or use epiNEPHrine*

flurazepam (Rx)
(flure-az'e-pam)

Apo-flurazepam ✤, Dalmane, flurazepam, Novoflupam ✤, Somnol ✤

Func. class.: Sedative-hypnotic
Chem. class.: Benzodiazepine derivative

Pregnancy category UK

Controlled substance schedule IV (USA), schedule F (Canada)

Do Not Confuse:
flurazepam/temazepam

Action: Produces CNS depression at the limbic, thalamic, hypothalamic levels of CNS; may be mediated by neurotransmitter γ-aminobutyric acid (GABA); results are sedation, hypnosis, skeletal muscle relaxation, anticonvulsant activity, anxiolytic action

Therapeutic Outcome: Ability to sleep, relaxation

Uses: Insomnia

Dosage and routes

Adult: PO 15-30 mg at bedtime; may repeat dose once if needed

Elderly: PO 15 mg at bedtime; may increase if needed

Available forms: Caps 15, 30 mg

Adverse effects

CNS: *Lethargy, drowsiness, daytime sedation,* dizziness, confusion, light-headedness, headache, anxiety, irritability

CV: Chest pain, pulse changes, palpitations

GI: Nausea, vomiting, diarrhea, heartburn, abdominal pain, constipation

HEMA: **Leukopenia, granulocytopenia (rare)**

MISC: Physical, psychologic dependence

Contraindications: Hypersensitivity to this drug or benzodiazepines, lactation, intermittent porphyria, uncontrolled pain

Precautions: Pregnancy **UK,** anemia, hepatic disease, renal disease, suicidal individuals, drug abuse, elderly, psychosis, child <15 yr

Pharmacokinetics

Absorption	Well absorbed
Distribution	Widely absorbed, crosses blood-brain barrier, crosses placenta
Metabolism	Liver to active, inactive metabolites
Excretion	Kidneys, breast milk
Half-life	2½ hr, 30-200 hr active metabolites

Pharmacodynamics

Onset	15-30 min
Peak	½-1 hr
Duration	7-8 hr

Interactions

Individual drugs

Alcohol: increased CNS depression
Cimetidine, disulfiram, fluoxetine, isoniazid, ketoconazole, propranolol, valproic acid: increased action of flurazepam
Probenecid: increased effects of flurazepam
Rifampin: decreased action of flurazepam
Theophylline: decreased effect of flurazepam

Drug classifications

Barbiturates: decreased effect of flurazepam
CNS depressants: increased CNS depression
Oral contraceptives: increased effect of flurazepam

Drug/herb

Black cohosh: increased hypotension
Catnip, chamomile, clary, cowslip, kava, lavender, mistletoe, nettle, pokeweed, poppy, Queen Anne's lace, senega, valerian: increased effect

Drug/lab test

Increased: AST, ALT, serum bilirubin
Decreased: radioactive iodine uptake
False increase: urinary 17-OHCS

NURSING CONSIDERATIONS

Assessment

- Assess anxiety reaction: inability to sleep, apprehension, dread, foreboding, or uneasiness related to unidentified source of danger
- Assess for previous drug dependence or tolerance; if drug dependent or tolerant, amount of medication should be restricted
- Monitor B/P (lying, standing), pulse; if systolic B/P drops 20 mm Hg, hold drug, notify prescriber; I&O, may indicate renal dysfunction
- Monitor blood studies: CBC during long-term therapy; blood dyscrasias have occurred rarely
- Monitor hepatic studies: AST, ALT, bilirubin, creatinine, LDH, alkaline phosphatase
- Monitor patient's mental status: mood, sensorium, affect, sleeping patterns, drowsiness, dizziness, suicidal tendencies

Nursing diagnoses

- Sleep pattern, disturbed (uses)
- Knowledge, deficient (teaching)
- Noncompliance (teaching)

Implementation

- Give after removing cigarettes to prevent fires
- Give after trying conservative measures for insomnia
- Give ½-1 hr before bedtime for sleeplessness; caps may be opened and mixed with food; give pc to decrease GI symptoms if used for sedation
- Provide assistance with ambulation after receiving dose
- Provide safety measures: nightlight, call bell within easy reach
- Check to see if PO medication has been swallowed
- Store in tight container in cool environment

Patient/family education

- Inform patient that drug may be taken with food; if dose is missed take as soon as remembered; do not double doses
- Advise patient to avoid OTC preparations unless approved by a physician, to avoid alcohol ingestion or other psychotropic medications unless approved by prescriber,

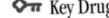

that 1-2 wk of therapy may be required before therapeutic effects occur

- Caution patient to avoid driving, activities requiring alertness, drowsiness may occur; until medication response is known, tell patient that drowsiness may worsen at beginning of treatment
- Instruct patient not to discontinue medication abruptly after long-term use
- Caution patient to rise slowly or fainting may occur, especially in elderly
- Inform patient that hangover is common in elderly

Evaluation

Positive therapeutic outcome

- Increased well-being
- Decreased anxiety, restlessness, sleeplessness, dread

Treatment of overdose: Lavage, activated charcoal; monitor electrolytes, VS

flutamide (Rx)

(floo'ta-mide)

Eulexin

Func. class.: Antineoplastic hormone

Chem. class.: Antiandrogen

Pregnancy category D

Do Not Confuse:
Eulexin/Edecrin

Action: Interferes with testosterone uptake in the nucleus or testosterone activity in target tissues; arrests tumor growth in androgen-sensitive tissue (i.e., prostate gland)

Therapeutic Outcome: Prevention of rapidly growing malignant cells

Uses: Metastatic prostatic carcinoma, stage D_2 in combination with LHRH agonistic analogs (leuprolide)

Dosage and routes

Adult: PO 250 mg q8h tid, for a daily dosage of 750 mg

Available forms: Caps 125, 250 mg

Adverse effects

CNS: *Hot flashes,* drowsiness, confusion, depression, anxiety, paresthesia

GI: *Diarrhea, nausea, vomiting,* increased liver function studies, **hepatitis,** anorexia, **hepatotoxicity**

GU: *Decreased libido, impotence, gynecomastia*

HEMA: Leukopenia, thrombocytopenia, hemolytic anemia

INTEG: Irritation at site, rash, photosensitivity

MISC: Edema, neuromuscular and pulmonary symptoms, hypertension

Contraindications: Pregnancy **D,** hypersensitivity

Pharmacokinetics

Absorption	Well absorbed
Distribution	Unknown
Metabolism	Liver
Excretion	Unknown
Half-life	6 hr

Pharmacodynamics

Unknown

Interactions

Individual drugs

Leuprolide: decreased flutamide action

Warfarin: increased PT

NURSING CONSIDERATIONS

Assessment

- Monitor CBC, bilirubin, creatinine, AST, ALT, alkaline phosphatase, which may be elevated, drug may need to be discontinued
- Identify CNS symptoms: drowsiness, confusion, depression, anxiety

Nursing diagnoses

- Injury, risk for (adverse reactions)
- Sexual dysfunction (adverse reactions)
- Body image, disturbed (adverse reactions)
- Infection, risk for (adverse reactions)
- Knowledge, deficient (teaching)

Implementation

- Used in combination with LHRH agonist (leuprolide)
- May be given with food or fluids

Patient/family education

- Tell the patient to report side effects: decreased libido, impotence, breast enlargement, hot flashes, diarrhea, which occur when the two drugs are given together; also nausea, vomiting; jaundice in eyes, skin; dark urine, clay-colored stools, hepatotoxicity may occur
- Inform patient that this drug is taken with leuprolide for medical castration, do not change dosing

Evaluation

Positive therapeutic outcome

- Prevention of rapid division of malignant cells

fluvastatin (Rx)
(flu'vah-stay-tin)
Lescol
Func. class.: Antilipidemic
Chem. class.: HMG-CoA reductase inhibitor
Pregnancy category X

Action: Inhibits HMG-CoA reductase enzyme, which reduces cholesterol synthesis

Therapeutic Outcome: Decreased cholesterol levels and LDLs, increased HDLs

Uses: As an adjunct in primary hypercholesterolemia (types Ia, Iib), coronary atherosclerosis in CAD

Dosage and routes
Adult: PO 20-40 mg daily in PM initially, usual range 20-80, not to exceed 80 mg; may be given in 2 doses (40 mg AM, 40 mg PM); dosage adjustments may be made in 4-wk intervals or more

Available forms: Caps 20, 40 mg; ext rel tab 80 mg

Adverse effects
CNS: Headache, dizziness, insomnia
EENT: Lens opacities
GI: *Nausea, constipation, diarrhea, abdominal pain, cramps, dyspepsia, flatus,* liver dysfunction, pancreatitis
***HEMA:* Thrombocytopenia, hemolytic anemia, leukopenia**
INTEG: Rash, pruritus
MISC: Fatigue, influenza, photosensitivity
MS: Myalgia, *arthritis, arthralgia,* myositis, **rhabdomyolysis**
RESP: Upper respiratory infection, rhinitis, cough, pharyngitis, sinusitis

Contraindications: Pregnancy **X,** hypersensitivity, lactation, active liver disease

Precautions: Past liver disease, alcoholism, severe acute infections, trauma, hypotension, uncontrolled seizure disorders, severe metabolic disorders, electrolyte imbalance

Pharmacokinetics

Absorption	Unknown
Distribution	Unknown
Metabolism	Liver
Excretion	Feces, kidneys
Half-life	14 hr

Pharmacodynamics
Unknown

Interactions
Individual drugs
Alcohol, cimetidine, ranitidine, omeprazole, saquinavir: increased fluvastatin effect
Rifampin: decreased action of fluvastatin
Clofibrate, cycloSPORINE, erythromycin, gemfibrozil, niacin: increased myalgia, myositis
Digoxin, warfarin: increased action
Drug classifications:
Azole antiinfectives given with clofibrate: increased myalgia, increased myositis
Drug/herb
Glucomannan: increased effect
Gotu kola: decreased effect
Drug/food
Grapefruit juice: possible increased fluvastatin toxicity

NURSING CONSIDERATIONS
Assessment
- Assess nutrition: fat, protein, carbohydrates; nutritional analysis should be completed by dietitian before treatment
- Monitor bowel pattern daily; diarrhea may be a problem
- Assess fasting lipid profile (cholesterol, LDL, HDL, triglycerides) q8 wk, then q3-6 mo when stable
- Monitor liver function studies q1-2 mo during the first 1½ yr of treatment; AST, ALT, liver function test results may be increased
- Monitor renal studies in patients with compromised renal system: BUN, I&O ratio, creatinine
- Obtain ophth exam before, 1 mo after treatment begins, annually; lens opacities may occur

Nursing diagnoses
- Diarrhea (adverse reactions)
- Knowledge, deficient (teaching)
- Noncompliance (teaching)

Implementation
- Give with evening meal; if dosage is increased, take with breakfast and evening meal
- Store in cool environment in airtight, light-resistant container

Patient/family education
- Inform patient that compliance is needed for positive results to occur, not to double doses
- Advise patient to notify prescriber if GI symptoms of diarrhea, abdominal or epigastric pain, nausea, vomiting, or if chills, fever, sore throat occur; also muscle pain, weakness, tenderness

- Advise patient that treatment is chronic
- Advise patient that blood studies and eye exam will be necessary during treatment
- Instruct patient to report suspected pregnancy, not to use during pregnancy
- Advise patient that previously prescribed regimen will continue, including diet, exercise, smoking cessation
- Advise patient to use sunscreen or stay out of the sun to prevent burns
- Instruct patient to notify all health care providers of drugs taken

Evaluation

Positive therapeutic outcome

- Decreased LDL, VLDL, total cholesterol levels
- Improved ratio of HDLs

folic acid (vitamin B_9) (PO, OTC; IM/IV, Ph)

(foe-lik a'sid)

Apo-Folic ✤, Folate, Folvite, Novofolacid ✤, Vitamin B_9

Func. class.: Vitamin B-complex group

Chem. class.: Supplement

Pregnancy category A

Action: Needed for erythropoiesis; increases RBC, WBC, and platelet formation in megaloblastic anemias

Therapeutic Outcome: Absence of macrocytic, megaloblastic anemias

Uses: Megaloblastic or macrocytic anemia caused by folic acid deficiency; liver disease; alcoholism; hemolysis; intestinal obstruction; pregnancy

Dosage and routes

RDA

Adult/child ≥14 yr: 400 mcg
Child 9-13 yr: 300 mcg
Child 4-8 yr: 200 mcg
Child 1-3 yr: 150 mcg
Infant 6 mo-1 yr: 80 mcg
Neonates/infants <6 mo: 65 mcg
Pregnancy: 600 mcg
Lactating: 500 mcg

Megaloblastic/macrocytic anemia due to folic acid or nutritional deficiency

Therapeutic dose

Adult and child: PO/IM/SUBCUT/**IV** up to 1 mg daily

Maintenance dose

Adult and child >4 yr: PO/IM/**IV**/SUBCUT 0.4 mg/day
Child <4 yr: PO/IM/**IV**/SUBCUT up to 0.3 mg/day
Infants: PO/IM/**IV**/SUBCUT up to 0.1 mg/day

Pregnant and/or lactating: PO/IM/**IV**/SUBCUT 0.8 mg/day

Prevention of neural tube defects during pregnancy

Adult: PO 0.4 mg daily

Prevention of megaloblastic anemia during pregnancy

Adult: PO/IM/SUBCUT up to 1 mg/day

Tropical sprue

Adult: PO 3-15 mg daily

Available forms: Tabs 0.1, 0.4, 0.8, 1, 5 mg; inj 5, 10 mg/ml

Adverse effects

INTEG: *Flushing*
RESP: **Bronchospasm**

Contraindications: Hypersensitivity, anemias other than megaloblastic/macrocytic anemia, vit B_{12} deficiency anemia, uncorrected pernicious anemia

Precautions: Pregnancy **A**

Pharmacokinetics	
Absorption	Well absorbed
Distribution	Liver, crosses placenta
Metabolism	Liver (converted to active metabolite)
Excretion	Kidneys (unchanged)
Half-life	Unknown

Pharmacodynamics	
Onset	Unknown
Peak	½-1 hr
Duration	Unknown

Interactions

Individual drugs

Carbamazepine: increased need for folic acid
Fosphenytoin: decreased fosphenytoin levels, may increase seizures
Methotrexate, sulfasalazine: decreased action of folic acid
Phenytoin: decreased phenytoin levels, may increase seizures

Drug classifications

Estrogens, glucocorticoids, hydantoins: increased need for folic acid
Sulfonamides: decreased action of folic acid

F

NURSING CONSIDERATIONS

Assessment

- Assess patient for fatigue, dyspnea, weakness, shortness of breath, activity intolerance (signs of megaloblastic anemia)
- Monitor Hgb, Hct, and reticulocyte count; folate levels: 6-15 mcg/ml baseline and throughout treatment
- Assess nutritional status: bran, yeast, dried beans, nuts, fruits, fresh vegetables, asparagus; if high folic acid foods are missing from the diet, a referral to a dietitian may be indicated
- Identify drugs currently taken: alcohol, oral contraceptives, estrogens, glucocorticoids, carbamazepine, hydantoins, trimethoprim; these drugs may cause increased folic acid use by the body and contribute to deficiency

Nursing diagnoses

- Nutrition: less than body requirements, imbalanced (uses)
- Fatigue (uses)
- Activity intolerance (uses)
- Knowledge, deficient (teaching)

Implementation

IV route

- Give **IV** directly, undiluted 5 mg or less over 1 min or more, or may be added to most **IV** sol or TPN
- Store in light-resistant container

Y-site compatibilities: Famotidine
Solution compatibilities: $D_{20}W$
Solution incompatibilities: $D_{40}W$, $D_{50}W$, calcium gluconate

Patient/family education

- Advise patient to take drug exactly as prescribed; not to double doses, toxicity may occur
- Instruct patient to notify prescriber of side effects; rash or fever may indicate hypersensitivity
- Advise patient that urine may become more yellow
- Instruct patient to increase intake of foods rich in folic acid in diet as recommended by dietitian or health care provider

Evaluation

Positive therapeutic outcome

- Absence of fatigue, weakness, dyspnea
- Absence of symptoms of megaloblastic anemia
- Increase in reticulocyte count within 5 days

fondaparinux (Rx)

(fon-dah-pair'ih-nux)
Arixtra
Func. class.: Anticoagulant, antithrombotic
Chem. class.: Synthetic, selective factor Xa inhibitor

Pregnancy category B

Do Not Confuse:
Arixtra/Anti-Xa

Action: Acts by antithrombin III (ATIII)-mediated selective inhibition of factor Xa; neutralization of factor Xa interrupts blood coagulation and inhibits thrombin formation; does not inactivate thrombin (activated factor II) or affect platelets

Therapeutic Outcome: Prevention of deep vein thrombosis

Uses: Prevention of deep vein thrombosis, pulmonary emboli in hip and knee replacement, hip fracture surgery

Dosage and routes

Adult: SUBCUT 2.5 mg daily; after hemostasis established, initial dose is given 6-8 hr after surgery, usual duration 5-9 days

Available forms: Inj 2.5 mg/0.5 ml single-dose syringe

Adverse effects

CNS: *Fever*, confusion, headache, dizziness, *insomnia*
GI: *Nausea, vomiting*, diarrhea, dyspepsia, *constipation*, increased AST, ALT
GU: UTI, urinary retention
HEMA: *Anemia*, minor bleeding, purpura, hematoma, **thrombocytopenia, major bleeding (intracranial, cerebral, retroperitoneal hemorrhage), postoperative hemorrhage**
INTEG: Local reaction—*rash*, pruritus, inj site bleeding, increased wound drainage, bullous eruption
META: Hypokalemia
MISC: Hypotension, pain, *edema*

Contraindications: Hypersensitivity to this drug; hemophilia, leukemia with bleeding, peptic ulcer disease, hemorrhagic stroke, surgery, thrombocytopenic purpura, weight <50 kg, severe renal disease (CCr <30 ml/min)

Precautions: Pregnancy **B**, alcoholism, hepatic disease (severe), blood dyscrasias, heparin-induced thrombocytopenia, severe hypertension, subacute bacterial endocarditis, acute nephritis, lactation, elderly, children, mild-moderate renal disease

Pharmacokinetics

Absorption	Rapidly, completely absorbed
Distribution	Blood; does not bind to plasma proteins except 94% to ATIII
Metabolism	Unknown
Excretion	Eliminated unchanged in 72 hr in normal renal function
Half-life	17-21 hr

Pharmacodynamics

Onset	Unknown
Peak	3 hr
Duration	Unknown

Interactions

Before starting fondaparinux, discontinue use of other drugs that may increase the risk of hemorrhage; monitor closely if coadministration is essential

Drug/herb

Agrimony, alfalfa, angelica, anise, basil, bay, bilberry, black haw, bogbean, bromelain, buchu, chondroitin, cinchona bark, dong quai, fenugreek, feverfew, garlic, ginger, ginkgo, ginseng, horse chestnut, Irish moss, kelp, kelpware, khella, lovage, lungwort, meadowsweet, motherwort, mugwort, nettle, papaya, parsley (large amounts), paud'arco, pineapple, poplar, prickly ash, safflower, saw palmetto, tonka bean, turmeric, wintergreen, yarrow: increased risk of bleeding

Chamomile, coenzyme Q10, flax, glucomannan, goldenseal, guar gum: decreased anticoagulant effect

NURSING CONSIDERATIONS

Assessment

- Assess blood studies (Hct, CBC, coagulation studies, platelets, occult blood in stools), anti-Xa; thrombocytopenia may occur
- Assess for bleeding: gums, petechiae, ecchymosis, black tarry stools, hematuria; notify prescriber
- Assess for neurologic symptoms in patients who have received spinal anesthesia

Nursing diagnoses

- Injury, risk for (uses, adverse reactions)
- Tissue perfusion, ineffective (uses)
- Knowledge, deficient (teaching)

Implementation

- Do not mix with other drugs or solutions; cannot be used interchangeably (unit to unit) with other anticoagulants
- Administer for 5-9 days
- Give only after screening patient for bleeding disorders
- Administer SUBCUT only; do not give IM
- Store at 77° F (25° C); do not freeze

SUBCUT route

- Check for discolored sol or sol with particulate; if present, do not give
- Begin 2 hr prior to surgery
- Administer to recumbent patient, rotate inj sites (left/right anterolateral, left/right posterolateral abdominal wall)
- Wipe surface of inj site with alcohol swab, twist plunger cap and remove, remove rigid needle guard by pulling straight off needle, do not aspirate, do not expel air bubble from surface
- Insert whole length of needle into skin fold held with thumb and forefinger
- When drug is injected, a soft click may be felt or heard
- Give at same time each day to maintain steady blood levels
- Avoid all IM inj that may cause bleeding
- ❗ Administer only this drug when ordered; not interchangeable with heparin

Patient/family education

- Advise patient to use soft-bristle toothbrush to avoid bleeding gums, to use electric razor
- Advise patient to report any signs of bleeding: gums, under skin, urine, stools
- Caution patient to avoid OTC drugs containing aspirin

Evaluation

Positive therapeutic outcome

- Absence of deep vein thrombosis

formoterol (Rx)

(for-moh'ter-ahl)

Foradil Aerolizer

Func. class.: β-Adrenergic agonist

Chem. class.: Sympathomimetic catecholamine

Pregnancy category C

Do Not Confuse:

Foradil/Toradol

Action: Has β_1 and β_2 action; relaxes bronchial smooth muscle and dilates the trachea and main bronchi by increasing levels of cAMP, which relaxes smooth muscles; causes increased contractility and heart rate by acting on β-receptors in the heart

Therapeutic Outcome: Bronchodilation, increased heart rate and cardiac output from action on β-receptors in heart

Uses: Maintenance, treatment of asthma, COPD, prevention of exercise-induced bronchospasm

Dosage and routes

Maintenance, treatment of asthma

Adult/child ≥5 yr: INH AM and PM long-term, 1 cap q12h using aerolizer inhaler

Maintenance of COPD

Adult: INH 12 mcg q12h

Prevention of exercise-induced bronchospasm

Adult/child ≥12 yr: prn occasionally 1 cap (12 mcg) at least 15 min before exercise

Available forms: INH powder in cap 12 mcg

Adverse effects

CNS: Tremors, *anxiety*, insomnia, headache, dizziness, stimulation

CV: Palpitations, tachycardia, hypertension

GI: Nausea, vomiting

RESP: Bronchial irritation, dryness of oropharynx, **bronchospasms** (overuse)

Contraindications: Hypersensitivity to sympathomimetics, narrow-angle glaucoma

Precautions: Pregnancy **C**, cardiac disorders, hyperthyroidism, diabetes mellitus, prostatic hypertrophy, elderly

Pharmacokinetics	
Absorption	Rapid (INH)
Distribution	Plasma protein binding 61%-64% at concentrations of 0.1-100 ng/mL; 31%-38% at concentrations of 5-500 ng/mL
Metabolism	Liver, lungs, GI tract
Excretion	Urine, feces
Half-life	10 hr mean terminal elimination half-life

Pharmacodynamics	
Onset	Unknown
Peak	5 min (INH)
Duration	Unknown

Interactions

Drug classifications

β-Blockers: decreased action of formoterol
MAOIs, antidepressants (tricyclics): serious dysrhythmias
Sympathomimetics: increased action of both drugs

NURSING CONSIDERATIONS

Assessment

- Assess respiratory function: B/P, pulse, lung sounds
- Assess I&O ratio; check for urinary retention, frequency, hesitancy
- Assess for paresthesias and coldness of extremities; peripheral blood flow may decrease

Nursing diagnoses

- Airway clearance, ineffective (uses)
- Gas exchange, impaired (uses)
- Knowledge, deficient (teaching)

Implementation

- Store at room temp, protect from heat, moisture
- Do not use discolored solution
- Rinse mouth after use

Patient/family education

- Review package insert with patient and inform about all aspects of drug
- Teach correct use of inhaler
- Teach use of spacer device in elderly or children
- Advise patient to avoid getting aerosol in eyes
- Instruct patient to rinse mouth after use
- Advise patient to wash inhaler in warm water and dry daily
- Advise patient to avoid smoking, smoke-filled rooms, persons with respiratory infections

Evaluation

Positive therapeutic outcome

- Absence of dyspnea, wheezing
- Improved airway exchange
- Improved ABGs

Treatment of overdose: Administer β-blocker

foscarnet (Rx)

(foss-kar′net)

Foscavir

Func. class.: Antiviral

Chem. class.: Inorganic pyrophosphate organic analog

Pregnancy category C

Action: Antiviral activity is produced by selective inhibition at the pyrophosphate binding site on virus-specific DNA polymerases and reverse transcriptases at concentrations that do not affect cellular DNA polymerases

Therapeutic Outcome: Virostatic agents against cytomegalovirus (CMV) retinitis

Uses: Treatment of CMV, retinitis, herpes simplex virus (HSV) infections; used with ganciclovir for relapsing patients

Dosage and routes

CMV retinitis

Adult: **IV** inf 60 mg/kg given over at least 1 hr, q8h × 2-3 wk initially, then 90-120 mg/kg/day over 2 hr, usually give with at least 750-1000 ml of 0.9% NaCl daily

HSV

Adult: **IV** 40 mg/kg q8-12h × 2-3 wk

Renal dose

Adult: **IV**

Male:

$$\frac{140 - \text{age}}{72 \times \text{serum creatinine (mg/dl)}} = \text{CCr}$$

Female: 0.85 × above value; dose based on table provided in package insert

Available forms: Inj 24 mg/ml

Adverse effects

CNS: *Fever,* dizziness, *headache,* **seizures,** *fatigue,* neuropathy, tremor, ataxia, dementia, stupor, EEG abnormalities, vertigo, **coma,** abnormal gait, hypertonia, extrapyramidal disorders, hemiparesis, **paralysis,** hyperreflexia, paraplegia, **tetany,** hyporeflexia, neuralgia, neuritis, celebral edema, *paresthesia,* depression, *confusion, anxiety,* insomnia, somnolence, amnesia, hallucinations, agitation

CV: Hypertension, palpitations, ECG abnormalities, 1st-degree AV block, nonspecific ST-T segment changes, hypotension, cerebrovascular disorder, cardiomyopathy, **cardiac arrest,** bradycardia, **dysrhythmias**

EENT: Visual field defects, vocal cord paralysis, speech disorders, taste perversion, eye pain, conjunctivitis, tinnitus, otitis

GI: *Nausea, vomiting, diarrhea, anorexia,* abdominal pain, constipation, dysphagia, rectal hemorrhage, dry mouth, melena, flatulence, ulcerative stomatitis, pancreatitis, enteritis, enterocolitis, glossitis, proctitis, stomatitis, increased amylases, gastroenteritis, **pseudomembranous colitis,** duodenal ulcer, **paralytic ileus, esophageal ulceration,** abnormal A-G ratio, increased AST, ALT, cholecystitis, **hepatitis,** dyspepsia, tenesmus, hepatosplenomegaly, jaundice

GU: **Acute renal failure,** decreased CCr and increased serum creatinine, **glomerulonephritis, toxic nephropathy, nephrosis, renal tubular disorders, pyelonephritis, uremia, hematuria, albuminuria,** dysuria, polyuria

HEMA: Anemia, **granulocytopenia, leukopenia, thrombocytopenia, platelet abnormalities, thrombosis, pulmonary embolism, coagulation disorders, decreased prothrombin, hypochromic anemia, pancytopenia, hemolysis, leukocytosis,** lymphadenopathy, epistaxis, lymphopenia

INTEG: *Rash,* sweating, pruritus, skin ulceration, seborrhea, SKIN discoloration, alopecia, acne, dermatitis, pain/inflammation at injection site, facial edema, dry skin, urticaria

MS: Arthralgia, myalgia

RESP: *Coughing, dyspnea,* pneumonia, sinusitis, pharyngitis, **pulmonary infiltration,** stridor, **pneumothorax, hemoptysis, bronchospasm,** bronchitis, **respiratory depression, pleural effusion, pulmonary hemorrhage,** rhinitis

SYST: *Hypokalemia, hypocalcemia, hypomagnesemia,* increased alkaline phosphatase, LDH, BUN, acidosis, hypophosphatemia, hyperphosphatemia, dehydration, glycosuria, increased creatine phosphokinase, hypervolemia, infection, **sepsis, death, ascites,** hyponatremia, hypochloremia, hypercalcemia

Contraindications: Hypersensitivity, CCr <0.4 ml/min/kg

Precautions: Pregnancy **C,** lactation, children, elderly, renal disease, seizure disorders, electrolyte/mineral imbalances, severe anemia

Pharmacokinetics	
Absorption	Complete (**IV**)
Distribution	14%-17% plasma protein binding
Metabolism	Not metabolized
Excretion	Kidneys (90%) unchanged, breast milk
Half-life	2-8 hr; increased in renal disease

Pharmacodynamics	
Onset	48 hr
Peak	2 wk
Duration	Unknown

Interactions

Individual drugs

Amphotericin B: increased nephrotoxicity
Pentamide: increased hypocalcemia

Drug classification

Aminoglycosides: increased nephrotoxicity

NURSING CONSIDERATIONS

Assessment

- Culture should be done before treatment with foscarnet is begun; cultures of blood, urine, and throat may all be taken; CMV is not confirmed by this method; the diagnosis is made by an ophth exam

- Assess kidney and liver function; increased hemopoietic studies: BUN, serum creatinine, creatinine clearance, if CCr <0.4 ml/min/kg, discontinue drug; AST, ALT, A-G ratio, baseline and during treatment; blood counts should be done q2wk; watch for decreasing granulocytes, Hgb; if low, therapy may have to be discontinued and restarted after hematologic recovery; blood transfusions may be required
- Assess for GI symptoms: severe nausea, vomiting, diarrhea; severe symptoms may necessitate discontinuing drug
- Monitor electrolytes and minerals: calcium, phosphorous, magnesium, sodium, potassium; watch closely for tetany during first administration
- ❗ Assess for symptoms of blood dyscrasias (anemia, granulocytopenia); bruising, fatigue, bleeding, poor healing
- Assess for symptoms of allergic reactions: flushing, rash, urticaria, pruritus

Nursing diagnoses

- Infection, risk for (uses)
- Injury, risk for (adverse reactions)
- Knowledge, deficient (teaching)

Implementation

IV route

- Administer increased fluids before and during drug administration to induce diuresis and minimize renal toxicity
- Administer via infusion pump, at no more than 1 mg/kg/min; do not give by rapid or bolus **IV**; give by central venous line or peripheral vein; standard 24 mg/ml sol may be used without dilution if using by central line; dilute the 24 mg/ml sol to 12 mg/ml with D_5W or 0.9% NaCl if using peripheral vein
- Monitor patient closely during therapy; if tingling, numbness, paresthesias occur, stop inf and obtain lab sample for electrolytes

Y-site compatibilities: Aldesleukin, aminophylline, amikacin, ampicillin, aztreonam, benzquinamide, cefazolin, cefoperazone, cefoxitin, ceftazidime, ceftizoxime, ceftriaxone, cefuroxime, chloramphenicol, cimetidine, clindamycin, dexamethasone, DOPamine, erythromycin, fluconazole, flucytosine, furosemide, gentamicin, heparin, hydrocortisone, hydromorphone, hydrOXYzine, imipenem-cilastatin, metoclopramide, metronidazole, miconazole, morphine, nafcillin, oxacillin, penicillin G potassium, phenytoin, piperacillin, ranitidine, ticarcillin/clavulanate, tobramycin

Y-site incompatibilities: Acyclovir, amphotericin B, calcium, cotrimoxazole, diazepam, digoxin, gancyclovir, haloperidol, leucovorin, midazolam, pentamidine, phenytoin, prochlorperazine, vancomycin

Patient/family education

- Advise patient to notify prescriber if sore throat, swollen lymph nodes, malaise, fever occur, may indicate presence of other infections
- Advise patient to report perioral tingling, numbness in extremities, and paresthesias; inf should be stopped and electrolytes should be requested
- Caution patient that serious drug interactions may occur if OTC products are ingested; check first with prescriber
- Inform patient that drug is not a cure, but will control symptoms
- Advise patient that ophth exams must be continued

Evaluation

Positive therapeutic outcome

- Improvement in CMV retinitis

fosamprenavir (Rx)

(fos-am-pren′a-veer)

Lexiva

Func. class.: Antiretroviral

Chem. class.: Protease inhibitor

Pregnancy category C

Action: Prodrug of amprenavir; inhibits human immunodeficiency virus (HIV) protease, which prevents maturation of the infectious virus

Therapeutic Outcome: Decreasing symptoms of HIV

Uses: HIV-1 infection in combination with antiretrovirals

Dosage and routes

Therapy-naïve patients

Adult: PO 1400 mg bid without ritonavir, or fosamprenavir 1400 mg daily and ritonavir 200 mg daily, or fosamprenavir 700 mg bid and ritonavir 100 mg bid

Protease experienced patients (PI)

Adult: PO 700 mg bid and ritonavir 100 mg bid

Combination with efavirenz

Adult: PO add another 100 mg/day of ritonavir for a total of 300 mg/day when all three drugs are given

Hepatic dose
Adult (Child-Pugh 5-8): PO 700 mg bid; do not use in Child-Pugh 9-12

Available forms: Tabs 700 mg (equivalent to 600 mg amprenavir)

Adverse effects
CNS: Headache, fatigue, depression, oral paresthesia
GI: *Nausea, diarrhea, vomiting, abdominal pain*
INTEG: Rash, pruritus
MISC: Redistribution or accumulation of body fat, hyperglycemia

Contraindications: Hypersensitivity to protease inhibitors

Precautions: Pregnancy **C,** liver disease, hemolytic anemia, diabetes, sulfa sensitivity, lactation, elderly

Pharmacokinetics	
Absorption	Unknown
Distribution	90% protein binding
Metabolism	In the liver by CYP4503AY (CYP3A4)
Excretion	Excretion of unchanged drug is minimal
Half-life	Unknown

Pharmacodynamics	
Onset	Unknown
Peak	1½-4 hr
Duration	Unknown

Interactions
Individual drugs
Amiodarone, antacids, lidocaine: serious dysrhythmias
Carbamazepine, efavirenz, nevirapine, phenytoin, ranitidine, saquinavir: decreased fosamprenavir levels
Itraconazole, ketoconazole, rifbutin, sildenafil, vardenafil: increased effect
Avoid use with rifampin, delavirdine, carbamazepine, phenobarbital, phenytoin because may lose virologic response and possibly lead to resistance to fosamprenavir
Warfarin: may affect coagulation
Drug classifications
Calcium channel blockers: serious dysrhythmias
HMG-CoA reductase inhibitors: increased toxicity; do not use with pimozide, ergots, midazolam, triazolam, flecainide, propafenone
Contraceptives (oral): decreased effect
Avoid use with H_2 receptor antagonists, proton pump inhibitors because may lose virologic response and possibly lead to resistance of fosamprenavir
Drug/herb
Avoid use with St. John's wort because may lose virologic response and possibly lead to resistance of fosamprenavir

NURSING CONSIDERATIONS
Assessment
- Assess bowel pattern before, during treatment; monitor hydration
- Assess skin eruptions, rash, urticaria, itching
- Monitor viral load, CD4 cell counts baseline and throughout treatment

Nursing diagnoses
- Infection, risk for (uses)
- Injury, risk for (adverse reactions)
- Knowledge, deficient (teaching)

Implementation
- Administer without regard to food
- Patients receiving phosphodiesterase type 5 inhibitors may be at increased risk for PDE5 inhibitor adverse effects

Patient/family education
- Advise to avoid taking with other medications unless directed by provider
- Teach that drug does not cure, but does manage symptoms; that drug does not prevent transmission of HIV to others
- Advise to use nonhormonal form of birth control while taking this drug
- Instruct if dose is missed, take as soon as remembered up to 1 hr before next dose; do not double dose
- Instruct not to alter dose or stop therapy without talking to physician
- Advise physician if patient has a sulfa allergy
- Advise to report all medications, including herbal supplements, to physician

Evaluation
Positive therapeutic outcome
- Decreasing symptoms of HIV

fosinopril (Rx)
(foss-in-o'pril)
Monopril
Func. class.: Antihypertensive
Chem. class.: Angiotensin-converting enzyme (ACE) inhibitor

Pregnancy category
C (1st trimester),
D (2nd/3rd trimesters)

Do Not Confuse:
Monopril/minoxidil/Accupril/Monoket

Action: Selectively suppresses renin-angiotensin-aldosterone system; inhibits ACE; prevents conversion of angiotensin I to angiotensin II; results in dilatation of arterial, venous vessels

Therapeutic Outcome: Decreased B/P in hypertension

Uses: Hypertension, alone or in combination with thiazide diuretics, systolic CHF

Dosage and routes

Hypertension

Adult: PO 10 mg daily initially, then 20-40 mg/day divided bid or daily, max 80 mg/day

CHF

Adult: PO 10 mg daily, then up to 40 mg/day, increased over several weeks, use lower dose in those undergoing diuresis before fosinopril

Available forms: Tabs 10, 20, 40 mg

Adverse effects

CNS: *Insomnia, paresthesia, headache, dizziness,* fatigue, memory disturbance, tremor, mood change

CV: *Hypotension,* chest pain, palpitations, angina, orthostatic hypotension, dysrhythmias, tachycardia

GI: *Nausea,* constipation, vomiting, diarrhea

GU: **Proteinuria,** increased BUN, creatinine, decreased libido

HEMA: Decreased Hct, Hgb, **eosinophilia, leukopenia, neutropenia**

INTEG: **Angioedema,** rash, flushing, sweating, photosensitivity, pruritus

META: Hyperkalemia

MS: Arthralgia, myalgia

RESP: Cough, sinusitis, dyspnea, **bronchospasm**

Contraindications: Pregnancy **D** (2nd/3rd trimesters), hypersensitivity to ACE inhibitors, lactation, children

Precautions: Pregnancy **C** (1st trimester), impaired liver function, hypovolemia, blood dyscrasias, CHF, COPD, asthma, elderly

Pharmacokinetics	
Absorption	30%
Distribution	Crosses placenta
Metabolism	Liver—converted to fosinoprilate
Excretion	50% kidneys (metabolites), 50% feces
Half-life	12 hr—fosinoprilat

Pharmacodynamics	
Onset	1 hr
Peak	2-6 hr
Duration	24 hr

Interactions

Individual drugs

Alcohol (acute ingestion): increased hypotension (large amounts)
Allopurinol: increased hypersensitivity
Digoxin, hydralazine, lithium, prazosin: increased toxicity
Indomethacin: decreased antihypertensive effect

Drug classifications

Adrenergic blockers, antihypertensives, diuretics, ganglionic blockers, nitrates, phenothiazines: increased hypotension
Antacids: decreased absorption
Diuretics (potassium-sparing), sympathomimetics, vasodilators: increased toxicity

Drug/herb

Arginine: fatal hypokalemia
Pill-bearing spurge: increased antihypertensive effect
Pineapple, yohimbe: decreased antihypertensive effect
St. John's wort: severe photosensitivity

Drug/lab test

Increased: AST, ALT, alkaline phosphatase, glucose, bilirubin, uric acid
Positive: ANA titer
False positive: urine acetone

NURSING CONSIDERATIONS

Assessment

- Monitor blood studies: neutrophils, decreased platelets; obtain WBC with differential baseline and qmo × 6 mo, then q2-3 mo × 1 yr; if neutrophils <1000/mm^3, discontinue
- Monitor B/P, check for orthostatic hypotension, syncope; if changes occur, dosage change may be required
- Monitor renal studies: protein, BUN, creatinine; watch for increased levels that may indicate nephrotic syndrome and renal failure; monitor urine daily for protein; monitor renal symptoms: polyuria, oliguria, frequency, dysuria
- Establish baselines in renal, liver function tests before therapy begins
- Check potassium levels throughout treatment although hyperkalemia rarely occurs
- Check for edema in feet, legs daily, monitor weight daily
- Assess for allergic reactions: rash, fever, pruritus, urticaria; drug should be discontinued if antihistamines fail to help

Nursing diagnoses

- Cardiac output, decreased (uses)
- Injury, risk for (side effects)
- Knowledge, deficient (teaching)
- Noncompliance (teaching)

Implementation

- Store in airtight container at 86° F (30° C) or less
- Severe hypotension may occur after 1st dose of this medication; hypotension may be prevented by reducing or discontinuing diuretic therapy 3 days before beginning benzapril therapy

Patient/family education

- Advise patient not to discontinue drug abruptly; warn patient to tell all persons associated with his or her care
- Teach patient not to use OTC products (cough, cold, allergy) unless directed by prescriber because serious side effects can occur; xanthines such as coffee, tea, chocolate, cola can prevent action of drug
- Teach patient the importance of complying with dosage schedule, even if feeling better; to continue with medical regimen to decrease B/P: exercise, smoking cessation, decreasing stress, diet modifications
- Emphasize the need to rise slowly to sitting or standing position to minimize orthostatic hypotension; not to exercise in hot weather or increased hypotension can occur
- Teach patient to notify prescriber of mouth sores, sore throat, fever, swelling of hands or feet, irregular heartbeat, chest pain, coughing, shortness of breath
- Instruct patient to report excessive perspiration, dehydration, vomiting, diarrhea; may lead to fall in B/P
- Caution patient that drug may cause dizziness, fainting, light-headedness; may occur during 1st few days of therapy; to avoid activities that may be hazardous
- Teach patient how to take B/P, and normal readings for age-group
- Advise patient to notify prescriber if pregnancy is planned or suspected

Evaluation

Positive therapeutic outcome

- Decreased B/P in hypertension

Treatment of overdose: 0.9% NaCl **IV** inf, hemodialysis

fosphenytoin (Rx)

(foss-fen'i-toy-in)

Cerebyx

Func. class.: Anticonvulsant

Chem. class.: Hydantoin

Pregnancy category D

Action: Inhibits spread of seizure activity in motor cortex by altering ion transport; increases AV conduction

Therapeutic Outcome: Decreased seizures, absence of dysrhythmias

Uses: Generalized tonic-clonic seizures, status epilepticus

Dosage and routes

PE = Phenytoin equivalent

Status epilepticus

Adult and child: **IV**/IM loading dose 15-20 mg PE/kg given at 100-150 mg PE/min

Nonemergency/maintenance dosing

Adult and child: **IV**/IM loading dose 10-20 mg PE/kg; maintenance dosing 4-6 mg PE/kg/day given at a rate of <150 mg PE/min

Available forms: Inj 150 mg (100 mg PE) 750 mg (500 mg PE)

Adverse effects

CNS: Drowsiness, dizziness, insomnia, paresthesias, depression, suicidal tendencies, aggression, headache, confusion

CV: Hypotension, **ventricular fibrillation**

EENT: Nystagmus, diplopia, blurred vision

GI: Nausea, vomiting, diarrhea, constipation, anorexia, weight loss, **hepatitis,** jaundice, gingival hyperplasia

HEMA: **Agranulocytosis, leukopenia, aplastic anemia, thrombocytopenia, megaloblastic anemia**

INTEG: Rash, lupus erythematosus, **Stevens-Johnson syndrome,** hirsutism

SYST: Hyperglycemia

Contraindications: Pregnancy **D**, hypersensitivity, psychiatric conditions, bradycardia, SA and AV block, Stokes-Adams syndrome

Precautions: Allergies, hepatic disease, renal disease, lactation, myocardial insufficiency

Pharmacokinetics

Absorption	Unknown
Distribution	Unknown
Metabolism	Liver
Excretion	Kidneys
Half-life	Unknown

Pharmacodynamics

Unknown

Interactions

Individual drugs

Alcohol: decreased effects of fosphenytoin (chronic use)

Amiodarone, chloramphenicol, cimetidine, methylphenidate, trazodone: increased fosphenytoin level

Carbamazepine: decreased effectiveness

Folic acid, reserpine, rifampin, theophylline: decreased effects of fosphenytoin

Isoniazid: decreased metabolism; increased action

Drug classifications

Antacids, antineoplastics, antihistamines, barbiturates: decreased effects of fosphenytoin

Antidepressants (tricyclics), estrogens, H_2-receptor antagonists, phenothiazines, sulfonamides: increased fosphenytoin level

Antihistamines, barbiturates, general anesthetics, hypnotics, opiates, sedatives: increased CNS depression

Salicylates: increased fosphenytoin level

Drug/herb

Ginseng, santonica, valerian: decreased anticonvulsant effect

Ginkgo: increased anticonvulsant effect

Drug/food

Decreased folic acid absorption

Drug/lab test

Increased: glucose, alkaline phosphatase

Decreased: dexamethasone, metyrapone test serum, PBI, urinary steroids

NURSING CONSIDERATIONS

Assessment

- Assess drug level: toxic level 30-50 mcg/ml, wait at least 2 hr after dose before testing
- Assess seizure activity including type, location, duration, and character; provide seizure precaution
- Assess renal studies: urinalysis, BUN, urine creatinine
- Monitor hepatic studies: ALT, AST, bilirubin, creatinine
- Assess allergic reaction: red raised rash; if this occurs, drug should be discontinued
- Monitor for toxicity: bone marrow depression, nausea, vomiting, ataxia, diplopia, cardiovascular collapse, slurred speech, confusion
- Assess drug level: toxic level 30-50 mcg/ml

❗ Assess for rash, discontinue as soon as rash develops, serious adverse reactions such as Stevens-Johnson syndrome can occur

- Assess mental status: mood, sensorium, affect, memory (long, short), especially elderly
- Assess for blood dyscrasias: fever, sore throat, bruising, rash, jaundice, epistaxis (long-term treatment only)
- Monitor blood studies: RBC, Hct, Hgb, reticulocyte counts weekly for 4 wk then monthly; also check thyroid function tests, serum calcium, albumin, phosphorus

Nursing diagnoses

- Injury, risk for (uses, adverse reactions)
- Knowledge, deficient (teaching)
- Noncompliance (teaching)

Implementation

IV route

- Administer by direct **IV** after diluting with D_5 or 0.9% NaCl to 1.5-25 mg PE/ml

Solution compatibilities: D_5W, $D_{10}W$, amino acid inj 10%, D_5LR, D_5/0.9% NaCl, Plasmalyte A, LR, per sterile water for inj

Additive compatibilities: Potassium chloride

Patient/family education

- Teach patient the reason for and expected outcome of treatment
- Instruct patient not to use machinery or engage in hazardous activity; drowsiness, dizziness may occur
- Advise patient to carry/wear emergency ID identifying drug used, name of prescriber
- Advise patient to notify prescriber of rash, bleeding, bruising, slurred speech, jaundice of skin or eyes, joint pain, nausea, vomiting, severe headache
- Advise patient to keep all medical appointments, including lab work, physical assessment
- Advise patient to notify prescriber if pregnancy is planned or suspected; to use contraception with this product

Evaluation

Positive therapeutic outcome

- Decreased seizure activity

frovatriptan (Rx)

(froh-vah-trip'tan)

Frova

Func. class.: Antimigraine agent

Chem. class.: 5-HT_1 receptor agonist

Pregnancy category C

Action: Binds selectively to the vascular 5-HT_{1B}, 5-HT_{1D} receptor subtypes, exerts antimigraine effect; binds to benzodiazepine receptor sites

Therapeutic Outcome: Absence of migraines

Uses: Acute treatment of migraine with or without aura

Dosage and routes

Adult: PO 2.5 mg, a 2nd dose may be taken after ≥2 hr; max 3 tabs/day (7.5 mg)

Available forms: Tabs 2.5 mg

Adverse effects

CNS: *Hot sensation*, paresthesia, *dizziness,* headache, fatigue, cold sensation
CV: *Flushing,* chest pain, palpitation
GI: Dry mouth, dyspepsia, abdominal pain
INTEG: Photosensitivity
MS: Skeletal pain

Contraindications: Angina pectoris, history of MI, documented silent ischemia, Prinzmetal's angina, ischemic heart disease, concurrent ergotamine-containing preparations, uncontrolled hypertension, hypersensitivity, basilar or hemiplegic migraine; ischemic bowel disease; peripheral vascular disease, severe hepatic disease, prophylactic migraine treatment

Precautions: Pregnancy **C**, postmenopausal women, men >40 yr, risk factors for CAD, hypercholesterolemia, obesity, diabetes, impaired hepatic function, lactation, children, elderly, seizure disorder

Pharmacokinetics

Absorption	Absolute bioavailability of PO dose ~20% in males, 30% in females
Distribution	Protein binding 15%; reversibly bound to blood cells at equilibrium 60%
Metabolism	Liver
Excretion	Urine (32%), feces (62%)
Half-life	25-29 hr

Pharmacodynamics

Onset	10 min-2 hr
Peak	2-4 hr
Duration	Unknown

Interactions

Individual drugs

Estrogen, propranolol: increased effects of frovatriptan

Drug classifications

CYP1A2 inhibitors (cimetidine, ciprofloxacin, erythromycin): increased frovatriptan levels
SSRIs, other serotonin agonists (dextromethorphan, tramadol, antidepressants): increased toxicity

Drug/herb

Butterbur: increased effect

NURSING CONSIDERATIONS

Assessment

- Assess B/P; signs/symptoms of coronary vasospasms
- Assess for stress level, activity, recreation, coping mechanisms
- Assess neurologic status: LOC, paresthesia, hot/cold sensations, dizziness, headache, fatigue
- Assess for ingestion of tyramine-containing foods (pickled products, beer, wine, aged cheese), food additives, preservatives, colorings, artificial sweeteners, chocolate, caffeine, which may precipitate these types of headaches

Nursing diagnoses

- Pain, acute (uses)
- Knowledge, deficient (teaching)

Implementation

- Ensure that tablets are swallowed whole
- Provide quiet, calm environment with decreased stimulation from noise, bright light, excessive talking

Patient/family education

- Instruct patient to report any side effects to prescriber
- Advise patient to use contraception while taking drug
- Advise patient that photosensitivity may occur, to use sunscreen and wear protective clothing when outdoors
- Advise patient to have dark, quiet environment available

Evaluation

Positive therapeutic outcome

- Decrease in frequency, severity of migraine

Treatment of overdose: No specific antidote; monitor patient closely for ≥48 hr, treat any symptoms as necessary

fulvestrant (Rx)

(full-ves'trant)

Faslodex

Func. class.: Antineoplastic

Pregnancy category D

Action: Inhibits cell division by binding to cytoplasmic estrogen receptors; resembles normal cell complex but inhibits DNA synthesis and estrogen response of target tissue

Therapeutic Outcome: Decreased tumor size, spread of malignancy

Uses: Advanced breast carcinoma in estrogen-receptor–positive patients (usually postmenopausal)

Dosage and routes

Adult: **IM** 250 mg qmo

Available forms: Inj 50 mg/ml

Adverse effects

CNS: ***Headache,*** depression, dizziness, insomnia, paresthesia, anxiety

GI: ***Nausea, vomiting,*** anorexia, constipation, diarrhea, abdominal pain

INTEG: ***Rash,*** sweating, hot flashes, inj site pain

MS: Bone pain, arthritis, back pain

RESP: Pharyngitis, dyspnea, cough

Contraindications: Pregnancy **D,** hypersensitivity

Precautions: Lactation, children, hepatic disease

Pharmacokinetics

Absorption	Unknown
Distribution	Unknown
Metabolism	CYP3A4
Excretion	Feces 90%
Half-life	40 days

Pharmacodynamics

Unknown

NURSING CONSIDERATIONS

Assessment

Monitor for side effects, report to prescriber

Nursing diagnoses

- Infection, risk for (adverse reactions)
- Nutrition: less than body requirements, imbalanced (adverse reactions)
- Knowledge, deficient (teaching)

Implementation

- Give IM 5 ml as a single inj or 2, 2.5 ml inj; give slowly in buttock
- Give antacid before oral agent; give drug after evening meal, before bedtime
- Give antiemetic 30-60 min before giving drug to prevent vomiting
- Provide liquid diet, if needed, including cola, Jell-O; dry toast or crackers may be added if patient is not nauseated or vomiting
- Provide nutritious diet with iron, vitamin supplements as ordered
- Increase fluids to 2 L/day unless contraindicated
- Store in refrigerator

Patient/family education

- Advise patient to report any complaints, side effects to prescriber
- Teach patient to increase fluids to 2 L/day unless contraindicated
- Advise patient to report vaginal bleeding immediately
- Teach patient that tumor flare—increase in size of tumor, increased bone pain—may occur and will subside rapidly; may take analgesics for pain
- Teach that premenopausal women must use mechanical birth control because ovulation may be induced

Evaluation

Positive therapeutic outcome

- Decreased tumor size, spread of malignancy

furosemide (Rx)

(fur-oh'se-mide)

Apo-Furosemide ♣, Furoside ♣, Lasix, Lasix Special ♣, Myrosemide, Novosemide ♣, Uritol ♣

Func. class.: Loop diuretic

Chem. class.: Sulfonamide derivative

Pregnancy category C

Do Not Confuse:

furosemide/torsemide, Lasix/Lanoxin, Lasix/Lomotil, Lasix/Luvox

Action: Acts on the ascending loop of Henle in the kidney, inhibiting reabsorption of electrolytes sodium and chloride, causing excretion of sodium, calcium, magnesium, chloride, water, and some potassium; decreases reabsorption of sodium and chloride and increases excretion of potassium in the distal tubule of the kidney; responsible for slight antihypertensive effect and peripheral vasodilatation

Therapeutic Outcome: Decreased edema in lung tissue, peripherally; decreased B/P

Uses: Edema in CHF, nephrotic syndrome, ascites, caused by hepatic disease, hepatic cirrhosis; may be used alone or as adjunct with antihypertensives such as spironolactone, triamterene; should not be used with ethacrynic acid

Investigational uses: Hypercalcemia in malignancy

Dosage and routes

Adult: PO 20-80 mg/day in AM, may give another dose in 6 hr, up to 600 mg/day; IM/**IV**

20-40 mg, increased by 20 mg q2h until desired response

Child: PO/IM/**IV** 2 mg/kg, may increase by 1-2 mg/kg/q6-8h up to 6 mg/kg

Pulmonary edema

Adult: **IV** 40 mg given over several min, repeated in 1 hr; increase to 80 mg if needed

Hypertensive crisis/acute renal failure

Adult: **IV** 100-200 mg over 1-2 min

Antihypercalcemia

Adult: IM/**IV** 80-100 mg q1-4h or PO 120 mg daily or divided bid

Child: IM/**IV** 25-50 mg, repeat q4h if needed

Available forms: Tabs 20, 40, 80 mg; oral sol 10 mg/ml, 40 mg/5 ml; inj IM, **IV** 10 mg/ml

Adverse effects

CNS: Headache, fatigue, weakness, vertigo, paresthesias

CV: Orthostatic hypotension, chest pain, ECG changes, **circulatory collapse**

EENT: *Loss of hearing,* ear pain, tinnitus, blurred vision

ELECT: *Hypokalemia, hypochloremic alkalosis, hypomagnesemia, hyperuricemia, hypocalcemia, hyponatremia,* metabolic alkalosis

ENDO: *Hyperglycemia*

GI: *Nausea,* diarrhea, dry mouth, vomiting, anorexia, cramps, oral or gastric irritations, pancreatitis

GU: *Polyuria,* **renal failure,** *glycosuria*

HEMA: **Thrombocytopenia, agranulocytosis, leukopenia, neutropenia, anemia**

INTEG: *Rash, pruritus, purpura,* **Stevens-Johnson syndrome,** sweating, photosensitivity, urticaria

MS: Cramps, stiffness

Contraindications: Hypersensitivity to sulfonamides, anuria, hypovolemia, infants, lactation, electrolyte depletion

Precautions: Pregnancy **C,** diabetes mellitus, dehydration, severe renal disease, cirrhosis, ascites

Pharmacokinetics

	PO
Absorption	GI tract (60%-70%)
	PO/IM/**IV**
Distribution	Crosses placenta
Metabolism	Liver (30%-40%)
Excretion	Breast milk, urine, feces
Half-life	½-1 hr

Pharmacodynamics

	PO	IM	IV
Onset	1 hr	½ hr	5 min
Peak	1-2 hrs	Unknown	½ hr
Duration	6-8 hr	4-8 hr	2 hr

Interactions

Individual drugs

Cisplatin, vancomycin: increased risk of ototoxicity

Clofibrate: increased furosemide effects

Digitalis: increased toxicity

Lithium: decreased renal clearance, causing increased toxicity

Drug classifications

Aminoglycosides: increased ototoxicity

Antihypertensives: increased antihypertensive effect

Nitrates: increased hypotensive action

Nondepolarizing skeletal muscle relaxants: increased toxicity

Drug/herb

Aloe, cucumber, dandelion, horsetail, khella, pumpkin, Queen Anne's lace: increased diuretic effect

St. John's wort: severe photosensitivity

Drug/lab test

Interference: GTT

NURSING CONSIDERATIONS

Assessment

- Assess patient for tinnitus, hearing loss, ear pain; periodic testing of hearing is needed when high doses of this drug are given by **IV** route
- Monitor for renal, cardiac, neurologic, GI, pulmonary manifestations of hypokalemia: acidic urine, reduced urine osmolality, nocturia, polyuria and polydipsia; hypotension, broad T-wave, U-wave, ectopy, tachycardia, weak pulse; muscle weakness, altered LOC, drowsiness, apathy, lethargy, confusion, depression; anorexia, nausea, cramps, constipation, distention, paralytic ileus; hypoventilation, respiratory muscle weakness
- Monitor for CNS, GI, cardiovascular, integumentary, neurologic manifestations of hypocalcemia: personality changes, anxiety, disturbances, depression and psychosis; nausea, vomiting, constipation, abdominal pain from muscle spasm; decreased contractility, decreased cardiac output, hypotension, lengthened ST segment, prolonged QT interval; scaling eczema, alopecia, hyperpigmentation; tetany, muscle twitching, cramping grimacing, seizure, altered deep tendon reflexes, spasm
- Monitor for CNS, neuromuscular, GI,

cardiac manifestations of hypomagnesemia, agitation; muscle twitching, paresthesias, hyperactive reflexes, positive Babinski reflex, dysphagia, nystagmus seizures, tetnany; nausea, vomiting, diarrhea, anorexia, abdominal distention; ectopy, tachycardia, broad, flat or inverted T-waves, depressed ST segment, prolonged QT, decreased cardiac output, hypotension

- Monitor for CV, GI, neurologic manifestations of hyponatremia: increased B/P, cold, clammy skin, hypovolemia or hypervolemia; anorexia, nausea, vomiting, diarrhea, abdominal cramps; lethargy, increased ICP, confusion, headache, seizures, coma, fatigue, tremors, hyperreflexia
- Monitor for neurologic, respiratory manifestations of hyperchloremia: weakness, lethargy, coma; deep rapid breathing
- Assess fluid volume status: I&O ratios and record, count or weigh diapers as appropriate, weight, distended red veins, crackles in lung, color, quality and sp gr of urine, skin turgor, adequacy of pulses, moist mucous membranes, bilateral lung sounds, peripheral pitting edema; dehydration symptoms of decreasing output, thirst, hypotension, dry mouth and mucous membranes should be reported
- Monitor electrolytes: potassium, sodium, calcium, magnesium; also include BUN, blood pH, ABGs, uric acid, CBC, blood glucose
- Assess B/P before and during therapy lying, standing and sitting as appropriate; orthostatic hypotension can occur rapidly

Nursing diagnoses

- Fluid volume, deficient (side effects)
- Fluid volume, excess (uses)
- Knowledge, deficient (teaching)

Implementation

- Give in AM to avoid interference with sleep
- Potassium replacement if potassium level is <3.0 mg/dl, or use oral sol slightly, drug may be crushed if patient is unable to swallow

PO route

- With food or milk if nausea occurs, absorption may be reduced

IV route

- Do not use sol that is yellow, has a precipitate, or crystals

IV, direct route

- Give undiluted through Y-tube on 3-way stopcock; give 20 mg or less/min

Intermittent IV infusion route

- May be added to 0.9% NaCl, D_5W, $D_{10}W$, $D_{20}W$; invert sugar 10% in electrolyte #1, LR, use within 24 hr to ensure compatibility; give through Y-tube or 3-way stopcock; give at 4 mg/min or less, use infusion pump

Syringe compatibilities: Bleomycin, cisplatin, cyclophosphamide, fluorouracil, heparin, leucovorin, methotrexate, mitomycin

Syringe incompatibilities: Doxapram, DOXOrubicin, droperidol, metaclopramide, milrinone

Y-site compatibilities: Allopurinol, amifostine, amikacin, aztreonam, bleomycin, cefepime, cefmetazole, cisplatin, cladribine, cyclophosphamide, cytarabine, dexamethasone, epINEPHrine, fentanyl, fludarabine, fluorouracil, foscarnet, gallium, granisetron, heparin, hydrocortisone, hydromorphone, indomethacin, kanamycin, leucovorin, lorazepam, melphalan, meropenem, methotrexate, mitomycin, morphine, nitroglycerin, norepinephrine, paclitaxel, piperacillin/tazobactam, potassium chloride, propofol, ranitidine, sargramostim, tacrolimus, teniposide, thiotepa, tobramycin, tolazoline, vit B complex with C

Y-site incompatibilities: Amsacrine, bleomycin, DOXOrubicin, droperidol, esmolol, fluconazole, gentamicin, idarubicin, metoclopramide, milrinone, netilmicin, ondansetron, quinidine, vinBLAStine, vinCRIStine

Additive compatibilities: Amikacin, aminophylline, ampicillin, atropine, bumetanide, calcium gluconate, cefamandole, cefoperazone, cefuroxime, cimetidine, cloxacillin, dexamethasone, diamorphine, digoxin, epINEPHrine, heparin, isosorbide, kanamycin, lidocaine, meropenem, morphine, nitroglycerin, penicillin G, potassium chloride, ranitidine, scopolamine, sodium bicarbonate, theophylline, tobramycin, verapamil

Additive incompatibilities: Bleomycin, DOBUTamine, gentamicin, chlorproMAZINE, diazepam, erythromycin, isoproterenol, meperidine, metoclopramide, netilmicin, opium alkaloids, prochlorperazine, tetracycline

Patient/family education

- Teach patient to take the medication early in the day to prevent nocturia
- Instruct the patient to take with food or milk if GI symptoms of nausea and anorexia occur
- Teach patient to maintain a record of weight on a weekly basis and notify physician of weight loss of >5 lb
- Caution the patient that this drug causes a loss of potassium, that food rich in potassium should be added to the diet; refer to a dietitian for assistance in planning
- Caution the patient to rise slowly from sitting

or reclining positions, not to exercise in hot weather or stand for prolonged periods of time because orthostatic hypotension will be enhanced; lie down if dizziness occurs

- Advise patient to wear protective clothing and sunscreen to prevent photosensitivity
- Teach patient not to use alcohol or any OTC medications without physician's approval, serious drug reactions may occur
- Emphasize the need to contact physician immediately if muscle cramps, weakness, nausea, dizziness, or numbness occurs
- Teach patient to take and record own B/P and pulse
- Teach patient to continue taking medication even if feeling better, this drug controls symptoms but does not cure the condition
- Advise the patient with hypertension to continue other medical treatment (exercise, weight loss, relaxation techniques, cessation of smoking)

Evaluation

Positive therapeutic outcome

- Decreased edema
- Decreased B/P
- Lowered calcium level in malignancy
- Increased diuresis

gabapentin (Rx)

(gab'a-pen-tin)

Neurontin

Func. class.: Anticonvulsant

Pregnancy category C

Do Not Confuse:

Neurontin/Noroxin/Neoral

Action: Mechanism unknown; may increase seizure threshold; structurally similar to GABA; gabapentin binding sites in neocortex, hippocampus

Therapeutic Outcome: Decreased seizure activity

Uses: Adjunct treatment of partial seizures, with or without generalization in patients >12 yr; adjunct in partial seizures in children 3-12 yr, postherpetic neuralgia

Investigational uses: Tremors in multiple sclerosis, neuropathic pain, bipolar disorder, migraine prophylaxis, diabetic neuropathy

Dosage and routes

Adult and child >12 yr: PO 900-1800 mg/day in 3 divided doses; may titrate by giving 300 mg on the first day, 300 mg bid on second day, 300 mg tid on third day; may increase to 1800 mg/day by adding 300 mg on subsequent days

Child 5-12 yr: PO 10-15 mg/kg/day in 3 divided doses, initially titrate dose upward over approximately 3 days; 25-35 mg/kg/day; all given in 3 divided doses; rec 200 mg as a single dose

Child 3-4 yr: PO 10-15 mg/kg/day in 3 divided doses, initially titrate dose upward over approximately 3 days, 40 mg/kg/day; all given in 3 divided doses, rect 200 mg as a single dose

Postherpetic neuralgia

Adult: PO 300 mg on day 1, 600 mg/day divided bid on day 2, 900 mg/day divided tid, may titrate to 1800 mg divided tid if needed

Renal dose

Adult and child >12 yr: CCr 30-60 ml/min 300 mg bid; CCr 15-30 ml/min 300 mg daily; CCr <15 ml/min 125 mg daily

Available forms: Caps 100, 300, 400 mg; tabs 600, 800 mg; oral sol 250 mg/5 ml

Adverse effects

CNS: Dizziness, fatigue, anxiety, somnolence, ataxia, amnesia, abnormal thinking, unsteady gait, depression; 3-12 yr old, emotional lability, aggression, thought disorder, hyperkinesia

CV: Vasodilatation, peripheral edema, hypotension

EENT: Dry mouth, blurred vision, diplopia, nystagmus

GI: Constipation, increased appetite, dental abnormalities, nausea, vomiting

GU: Impotence, bleeding, *UTI*

HEMA: **Leukopenia,** decreased WBC

INTEG: Pruritus, abrasion

MS: Myalgia

RESP: Rhinitis, pharyngitis, coughing

Contraindications: Hypersensitivity to this drug

Precautions: Pregnancy **C,** renal disease, lactation, child <12 yr, elderly, hemodialysis

Pharmacokinetics	
Absorption	Unknown
Distribution	Unknown
Metabolism	None
Excretion	Urine unchanged
Half-life	5-7 hr, 130 hr in ESRD

Pharmacodynamics	
Onset	Unknown
Peak	Unknown
Duration	Unknown

Interactions

Individual drugs

Alcohol: increased CNS depression

Drug classifications

Antacids: decreased gabapentin levels

Antihistamines, CNS depressants (other sedatives): increased CNS depression

Drug/herb

Chamomille, hops, kava, skullcap, valerian: increased CNS depression

Drug/lab test

False positive: urinary protein using Ames N-multistix SG

NURSING CONSIDERATIONS

Assessment

- Assess seizures: aura, location, duration, activity at onset
- Assess renal studies: urinalysis, BUN, urine creatinine q3 mo
- Assess mental status: mood, sensorium, affect, behavioral changes; if mental status changes, notify prescriber
- Assess eye problems, need for ophth exam before, during, after treatment (slit lamp, fundoscopy, tonometry)

Nursing diagnoses

- Knowledge, deficient (teaching)
- Noncompliance (teaching)

Implementation

- Do not break, crush, or chew caps
- Give at least 2 hr pc with antacids, give without regard to meals
- Store at room temp away from heat and light
- Provide assistance with ambulation during early part of treatment; dizziness occurs
- Provide seizure precautions: padded side rails; move objects that may harm patient

Patient/family education

- Advise patient to carry/wear emergency ID stating patient's name, drugs taken, condition, prescriber's name and phone number
- Teach patient to avoid driving, other activities that require alertness
- Teach patient not to discontinue medication quickly after long-term use, withdrawal-precipitated seizures may occur, not to double dose; if dose is missed, take if 2 hr or more before next dose
- Teach patient to gradually withdraw over 7 days; abrupt withdrawal may precipitate seizures
- Teach patient to use hard candy, gum, and frequent rinsing of mouth for dry mouth
- Teach patient to increase fluids, bulk in diet for constipation
- Advise patient to notify prescriber if pregnancy is planned or suspected, avoid breast feeding

Evaluation

Positive therapeutic outcome

- Decreased seizure activity; document on patient's chart

Treatment of overdose: Lavage, VS

galantamine (Rx)

(gah-lan'tah-meen)

Razadyne

Func. class.: Anti-Alzheimer's agent, cholinesterase inhibitor

Pregnancy category B

Action: May enhance cholinergic functioning by increasing acetylcholine

Therapeutic Outcome: Decreased signs and symptoms of Alzheimer's dementia

Uses: Mild to moderate dementia of Alzheimer's type

Dosage and routes

Adult: PO 4 mg bid with morning and evening meals; after 4 wk or more may increase to 8 mg bid; after another 4 wk may increase to 12 mg bid; usual dose 16-24 mg/day in 2 divided doses

Hepatic dose

Child-Pugh 7-9: Max 16 mg/day

Child-Pugh 10-15: Avoid use

Renal dose/moderate renal impairment: Max 16 mg/day

CCr <9 ml/min: Avoid use

Available forms: Tabs 4, 8, 12 mg; oral sol 4 mg/ml

Adverse effects

CNS: *Tremors, insomnia,* depression, dizziness, headache, somnolence, fatigue

CV: Bradycardia, chest pain

GI: *Nausea, vomiting, anorexia, abdominal distress, flatulence,* diarrhea

GU: Urinary incontinence, bladder outflow obstruction, hematuria

META: Weight decrease

MISC: Anemia, hematuria

MS: Asthenia, anemia

RESP: URI, rhinitis

Contraindications: Hypersensitivity to this drug

Precautions: Pregnancy **B,** renal disease, hepatic disease, respiratory disease, seizure disorder, peptic ulcer, asthma, lactation, children

Pharmacokinetics

Absorption	Rapidly and completely absorbed
Distribution	Unknown
Metabolism	P450 enzyme
Excretion	Kidneys; clearance decreased in the elderly, hepatic disease, females (20% lower)
Half-life	Elimination 7 hr

Pharmacodynamics

Onset	Unknown
Peak	Unknown
Duration	Unknown

Interactions

Individual drugs

Amitriptyline, cimetidine, erythromycin, fluvoxamine, ketoconazole, paroxetine, quinidine: increased galantamine bioavailability

Drug classifications

Cholinesterase inhibitors, cholinomimetics: synergistic effect

Drug/herb

Jimsonweed, scopolia: cholinergic antagonism
Pill-bearing spurge: increased effect

NURSING CONSIDERATIONS

Assessment

- Assess liver function enzymes: AST, ALT, alkaline phosphatase, LDH, bilirubin, CBC
- Assess for severe GI effects: nausea, vomiting, anorexia, weight loss
- Assess B/P, respiration during initial treatment
- Assess mental status: affect, mood, behavioral changes, depression

Nursing diagnoses

- Knowledge, deficient (teaching)
- Thought processes, disturbed

Implementation

- Give with meals, morning and evening
- Dose increase after minimum of 4 wk at prior dose
- Provide assistance with ambulation during beginning therapy
- Perform complete suicide assessment

Patient/family education

- Teach patient or caregiver correct procedure for giving oral solution, using instruction sheet provided
- Instruct patient or caregiver to notify prescriber of severe GI effects
- Instruct patient or caregiver to report hypo/hypertension

Evaluation

Positive therapeutic outcome

- Decreased symptoms of dementia
- Increased coherence
- Improved cognitive performance (memory, orientation, attention, reasoning, language, praxis)

Treatment of overdose: Administer **IV** atropine titrated to effect at an initial dose of 0.5-1 mg, with subsequent doses based on clinical response; provide general supportive measures

G

gallium (Rx)

(gal'ee-yum)

Ganite

Func. class.: Electrolyte modifier
Chem. class.: Hypocalcemic drug

Pregnancy category C

Action: Lowers serum calcium levels by inhibiting calcium resorption from bone

Therapeutic Outcome: Decrease calcium level to 5-9 mg/dl

Uses: Cancer-related hypercalcemia

Dosage and routes

Adult: **IV** 100-200 mg/m^2 daily × 5 days; inf over 24 hr, rest period of 2-4 wk between courses

Available forms: Inj 25 mg/ml

Adverse effects

CV: Tachycardia, hypotension
EENT: Blurred vision, optic neuritis, hearing loss
GI: Nausea, vomiting, diarrhea, constipation, mucositis, metallic taste
GU: **Nephrotoxicity,** increased BUN, creatinine
HEMA: **Anemia, leukopenia, thrombocytopenia**
META: *Hypophosphatemia,* hypocalcemia, decreased serum bicarbonate

Contraindications: Hypersensitivity, hypocalcemia, renal failure, severe renal disease (specific gravity >2.5 mg/dl)

Precautions: Pregnancy **C,** lactation, children, mild renal disease, dehydration

Pharmacokinetics

Absorption	Completely absorbed
Distribution	Unknown
Metabolism	Unknown
Excretion	Kidneys (unchanged)
Half-life	Unknown

Pharmacodynamics

Onset	12-48 hr
Peak	Unknown
Duration	4-14 days

Interactions

Individual drugs

Amphotericin B, cisplatin, foscarnet, ganciclovir, vancomycin: increased nephrotoxicity

Drug classifications

Aminoglycosides: increased nephrotoxicity

NURSING CONSIDERATIONS

Assessment

- Renal status: BUN, creatinine, urine output; if creatinine level is 2.5 mg/dl or more, drug should be discontinued
- Monitor calcium, phosphate, bicarbonate; all levels may be decreased and supplements of phosphate may be needed; calcium daily, phosphate 2-3 ×/wk
- Assess for hypercalcemia: nausea, vomiting, fatigue, weakness, thirst, dehydration, dysrhythmias, headache, confusion, coma, decreased reflexes
- For hypocalcemia: dysrhythmias, hypotension, paresthesia; twitching, colic, laryngospasm; hypercalcemia: poor coordination, myalgia, hypotonia, shortened ST segment and QT interval, prolonged PR interval, cone-shaped T wave, sinus bradycardia; Trousseau's, Chvostek's sign: tremors, tetany, cramping, grimacing, seizures, altered deep tendon reflexes and spasms, personality changes including irritability, depression, psychosis
- Monitor for indications of hypophosphatemia: weakness, malaise, tremors, memory loss, inattention, confusion, decreased reflexes, aching bone pain, joint stiffness, rapid, shallow respiration, decreased tidal volume, nausea, vomiting, anorexia, portal hypertension

Nursing diagnoses

- Injury, risk for (uses)
- Knowledge, deficient (teaching)

Implementation

- Provide adequate hydration with **IV** saline, 2 L/day during treatment; saline increases the extracellular calcium
- Give by cont **IV** inf after dilution of dose/1 L of 0.9% NaCl or D_5W, run over 24 hr, use infusion pump
- Store solution for 48 hr at room temp or 1 wk in refrigerator

Y-site compatibilities: Acyclovir, allopurinol, aminophylline, ampicillin/sulbactam, amifostine, aztreonam, cefazolin, ceftazidime, ceftriaxone, cimetidine, ciprofloxacin, cladribine, cyclophosphamide, dexamethasone, diphenhydrAMINE, filgrastim, fluconazole, furosemide, granisetron, heparin, hydrocortisone, fosfamide, magnesium sulfate, mannitol, melphalan, meperidine, mesna, methotrexate, metoclopramide, ondansetron, piperacillin, piperacillin/tazobactam, potassium chloride, ranitidine, sodium bicarbonate, teniposide, thiotepa, ticarcillin/clavulanate, trimethoprim, sulfamethoxazole, vancomycin, vinorelbine

Patient/family education

- Instruct patient to follow dietary guidelines given by prescriber, including avoiding calcium (dietary products, broccoli) and vit D (fortified milk, grain products, fish oil)
- Explain purpose of drug and expected results

Evaluation

Positive therapeutic outcome

- Decreased serum calcium levels to 5-9 mg/dl

galsulfase

Naglazyme

See Appendix A, Selected New Drugs

ganciclovir (Rx)

(gan-sye'kloe-vir)

Cytovene, Vitrasert

Func. class.: Antiviral

Chem. class.: Synthetic nucleoside analog

Pregnancy category C

Do Not Confuse:

Cytovene/Cytosar

Action: Inhibits replication of herpes viruses in vitro, competitively inhibits human cytomegalovirus (CMV) DNA polymerase and is incorporated, resulting in termination of DNA elongation

Therapeutic Outcome: Decreased proliferation of virus responsible for CMV retinitis

Uses: CMV retinitis in immunocompromised persons, including those with AIDS, after indirect ophthalmoscopy confirms diagnosis, prophylaxis of CMV in transplantation

Investigational uses: CMV pneumonia in organ transplant patients, CMV gastroenteritis in patients with irritable bowel syndrome, CMV pneumonitis

Dosage and routes

Induction treatment

Adult: **IV** 5 mg/kg/dose given over 1 hr q12h × 2-3 wk

Maintenance treatment

Adult: **IV** inf 5 mg/kg daily given over 1 hr, daily × 7 days/wk; or 6 mg/kg daily × 5 days/wk; PO 1000 mg tid with food or 500 mg q3h while awake; intravitreal: 4.5-mg implant for 6 doses

Prevention of CMV infection

Adult: **IV** 5 mg/kg/dose over 1 hr q12h × 1-2 wk, then 5 mg/kg/day × 7 days/wk then 6 mg/kg/day × 5 days/wk; PO 1000 mg tid

Renal dose

CCr <70 ml/min reduce dose

Available forms: Powder for inj 500 mg/vial, caps 250, 500 mg; implant, intravitreal 4.5 mg

Adverse effects

CNS: *Fever,* chills, **coma,** *confusion,* abnormal thoughts, dizziness, bizarre dreams, *headache,* psychosis, tremors, somnolence, *paresthesia, weakness,* **seizures**
CV: Dysrhythmia, hypertension/hypotension
EENT: Retinal detachment in CMV retinitis
GI: *Abnormal liver function tests, nausea, vomiting, anorexia, diarrhea, abdominal pain,* **hemorrhage**
GU: **Hematuria,** *increased creatinine,* BUN
HEMA: **Granulocytopenia, thrombocytopenia, irreversible neutropenia, anemia, eosinophilia**
INTEG: *Rash,* alopecia, *pruritus,* urticaria, pain at inj site, phlebitis, **Stevens-Johnson syndrome**
RESP: Dyspnea

Contraindications: Hypersensitivity to acyclovir or ganciclovir, ANC <500/mm^3, platelet count <25,000/mm^3

Precautions: Pregnancy **C,** preexisting cytopenias, renal function impairment, lactation, children <6 mo, elderly

Pharmacokinetics

Absorption	Completely absorbed
Distribution	Crosses blood-brain barrier, CSF
Metabolism	Not metabolized
Excretion	Kidneys (90%) unchanged, breast milk
Half-life	3 hr

Pharmacodynamics

Unknown

Interactions

Individual drugs

Amphotericin B, adriamycin, cycloSPORINE, dapsone, DOXOrubicin, flucytosine, pentamidine, probenecid, trimethoprim/sulfa combinations, vinBLAStine, vinCRIStine: increased ganciclovir toxicity
Didanosine: decreased effect
Imipenem with cilastatin: increased chance of seizures
Probenecid: decreased renal clearance of ganciclovir
Radiation, zidovudine: severe granulocytopenia; do not give together

Drug classifications

Antineoplastics: severe granulocytopenia; do not give together
Nucleoside analogs: increased toxicity

NURSING CONSIDERATIONS

Assessment

- Culture should be done before treatment with ganciclovir is initiated; cultures of blood, urine, and throat may all be taken; CMV is not confirmed by this method; the diagnosis is made by an ophth exam
- Assess kidney, liver function; increases in hemopoietic studies: BUN, serum creatinine, AST creatinine clearance, ALT, A-G ratio, baseline, and drip treatment; blood counts should be done q2 wk; watch for decreasing granulocytes, Hgb; if low, therapy may have to be discontinued and restarted after hematologic recovery; blood transfusions may be required
- Assess for GI symptoms: severe nausea, vomiting, diarrhea; severe symptoms may necessitate discontinuing drug
- Monitor electrolytes and minerals: calcium, phosphorus, magnesium, sodium, potassium; watch closely for tetany during 1st administration
- Assess for symptoms of blood dyscrasias (anemia, granulocytopenia); bruising, fatigue, bleeding, poor healing
- Assess for symptoms of allergic reactions: flushing, rash, urticaria, pruritus
- Monitor for leukopenia/neutropenia/thrombocytopenia: WBCs, platelets q2 days during 2 ×/day dosing and q1 wk thereafter; check for leukopenia with daily WBC count in patients with prior leukopenia with other nucleoside analogs or for whom leukopenia

G

counts are <1000 cells/mm^3 at start of treatment
- Monitor serum creatinine or creatinine clearance at least q2 wk

Nursing diagnoses
- Infection, risk for (uses)
- Injury, risk for (uses, adverse reactions)
- Knowledge, deficient (teaching)

Implementation
PO route
- Give with food

IV route
- Medicine should be mixed under strict aseptic conditions using gloves, gown, and mask, and using precautions for antineoplastics

Intermittent IV infusion route
- Administer **IV** after diluting 500 mg/10 ml of sterile water for inj (50 mg/ml); shake; further dilute in 100 ml of D_5W, 0.9% NaCl, LR, Ringer's and run over 1 hr; use infusion pump, in-line filter
- Give slowly; do not give by bolus **IV**, IM, SUBCUT inj
- Use reconstituted sol within 12 hr, do not refrigerate or freeze; infusion solution is stable for 14 days when refrigerated; do not use sol with particulate matter or discoloration, fludarabine, sargramostim

Y-site compatibilities: Allopurinol, cisplatin, cyclophosphamide, enalaprilat, etoposide, filgrastim, fluconazole, gatifloxacin, granisetron, linezolid, melphalan, methotrexate, paclitaxel, propofol, tacrolimus, teniposide, thiotepa

Y-site incompatibilities: Amsacrine, fludarabine, foscarnet, ondansetron, sargramostim, vinorelbine

Patient/family education
- Advise patient to notify prescriber if sore throat, swollen lymph nodes, malaise, fever occur; may indicate other infections
- Advise patient to report perioral tingling, numbness in extremities, and paresthesias
- Caution patient that serious drug interactions may occur if OTC products are ingested; check first with prescriber
- Inform patient that drug is not a cure, but will control symptoms
- Advise patient that regular blood tests, ophth exams must be continued
- Inform patient that major toxicities may necessitate discontinuing drug
- Instruct patient to use contraception during treatment and that infertility may occur; men should use barrier contraception for 90 days after treatment
- Teach patient to take PO with food
- Teach patient to report infection: fever, chills, sore throat; blood dyscrasias: bruising, bleeding, petechiae
- Tell patient to avoid crowds, persons with respiratory infection
- Advise patient to use sunscreen to prevent burns

Evaluation
Positive therapeutic outcome
- Decreased symptoms of CMV infection

ganirelix (Rx)
(gan-i-rell′-ex)
Antagon
Func. class.: Gonadotropin-releasing hormone antagonist
Chem. class.: Synthetic decapeptide

Pregnancy category X

Action: Inhibitor of pituitary gonadotropin secretion; initially increases LH and FSH, induces a rapid suppression of gonadotropin secretion

Therapeutic Outcome: Pregnancy

Uses: For inhibition of premature LH surges in women undergoing controlled ovarian hyperstimulation

Dosage and routes
Adult: SUBCUT 250 mcg daily during early to mid follicular phase, continue until day of hCG administration

Available forms: Inj 250 mcg/0.5 ml

Adverse effects
CNS: Headache
ENDO: Ovarian hyperstimulation syndrome, abdominal pain (gynecologic)
GI: Nausea
GU: *Spotting, breakthrough bleeding*
INTEG: Pain on inj
SYST: **Fetal death**

Contraindications: Pregnancy **X,** hypersensitivity, latex allergy, lactation

Pharmacokinetics

Absorption	Unknown
Distribution	Unknown
Metabolism	To metabolites
Excretion	Unknown
Half-life	13-16 hr

Pharmacodynamics	
Onset	Unknown
Peak	Unknown
Duration	Treatment length

Interactions: None known

NURSING CONSIDERATIONS

Assessment

- Assess for suspected pregnancy, drug should not be used
- Assess for latex allergy, drug should not be used

Nursing diagnoses

- Sexual dysfunction (uses)
- Knowledge, deficient (teaching)

Implementation

- Administer SUBCUT using abdomen, around navel or upper thigh, swab inj area with disinfectant, clean a 2-in circle and allow to dry, pinch up area between thumb and finger, insert needle at 45-90 degrees to surface, if positioned correctly, no blood will be drawn back into syringe, if blood is drawn into syringe, reposition needle without removing it
- Protect from light

Patient/family education

- Teach patient to report abdominal pain, vaginal bleeding

Evaluation

Positive therapeutic outcome

- Pregnancy

gatifloxacin (Rx)

(gat-i-floks'-a-sin)

Tequin

Func. class.: Urinary antiinfective

Chem. class.: Fluoroquinolone

Pregnancy category C

Action: Interferes with conversion of intermediate DNA fragments into high-molecular-weight DNA in bacteria; DNA gyrase inhibitor

Therapeutic Outcome: Bactericidal action against the following: gram-positive organisms methicillin-resistant strains of *Staphylococcus aureus, Streptococcus pneumoniae;* gram-negative organisms *Escherichia coli, Haemophilus influenzae, Haemophilus parainfluenzae, Klebsiella pneumoniae, Moraxella catarrhalis, Neisseria gonorrhoeae, Proteus mirabilis;* and other microorganisms: *Chlamydia pneumoniae, Legionella pneumophilia, Mycoplasma pneumoniae*

Uses: Adult urinary tract infections (including complicated); lower respiratory, skin, bone, joint infections, acute bacterial exacerbation of chronic bronchitis, acute sinusitis, community-acquired respiratory tract infections, gonorrhea

Investigational uses: Multidrug-resistant *S. pneumoniae;* in children with acute otitis media; sinusitis; *Mycobacterium leprae,* atypical pneumonia, uncomplicated skin, soft tissue infections, chronic prostatitis

Dosage and routes

Renal dose

CCr ≥40 ml/min 400 mg daily; CCr <40 ml/min 200 mg daily after 400 mg initially; hemodialysis 200 mg daily after 400 mg initially

Uncomplicated urinary tract infections

Adult: PO/**IV** 400 mg single dose

Complicated/severe urinary tract infections

Adult: PO/**IV** 400 mg × 7-10 days

Chronic bronchitis

Adult: PO/**IV** 400 mg × 5 days

Acute sinusitis

Adult: PO/**IV** 400 mg × 10 days

Community-acquired pneumonia

Adult: PO/**IV** 400 mg × 7-14 days

Gonorrhea

Adult: PO/**IV** 400 mg single dose

Available forms: Tabs 200, 400; inj 20 ml (200 mg), 40 ml (400 mg), inj premix 200, 400 mg

Adverse effects

CNS: Headache, dizziness, insomnia, paresthesia, tremor, vasodilatation

ENDO: Increased blood glucose

GI: Nausea, increased ALT, AST, diarrhea, **pseudomembranous colitis, hepatotoxicity**

INTEG: Rash, pruritus, urticaria, photosensitivity, flushing, fever, chills

RESP: Dyspnea, pharyngitis

SYST: **Anaphylaxis, Stevens-Johnson syndrome**

Contraindications: Hypersensitivity to quinolones, severe hepatic disease

Precautions: Pregnancy **C,** lactation, children, renal disease

Pharmacokinetics

Absorption	Well absorbed (PO); complete (**IV**)
Distribution	Protein binding 20%
Metabolism	Liver
Excretion	Kidneys unchanged (70%)
Half-life	1 hr

Pharmacodynamics

	PO	IV
Onset	Rapid	Immediate
Peak	1-2 hr	Infusion's end
Duration	24 hr	

Interactions

Individual drugs

Aluminum hydroxide, calcium, sucralfate: decreased absorption of gatifloxacin

Cimetidine: increased serum levels of gatifloxacin

CycloSPORINE: increased nephrotoxicity

Probenecid: increased blood levels of gatifloxacin

Warfarin: increased warfarin level

Drug classifications

Antacids (magnesium): decreased absorption of gatifloxacin

NURSING CONSIDERATIONS

Assessment

- Assess patient for previous sensitivity reaction
- Assess patient for signs and symptoms of infection including characteristics of wounds, sputum, urine, stool, WBC >10,000/mm^3, fever; obtain baseline information before and during treatment
- Obtain C&S before beginning drug therapy to identify if correct treatment has been initiated
- Assess for allergic reactions and anaphylaxis: rash, urticaria, pruritus, chills, fever, joint pain; may occur a few days after therapy begins; epiNEPHrine and resuscitation equipment should be available for anaphylactic reaction
- Identify urine output; if decreasing, notify prescriber (may indicate nephrotoxicity); also check for increased BUN, creatinine
- Monitor blood studies: AST, ALT, CBC, Hct, bilirubin, LDH, alkaline phosphatase, blood glucose, Coombs' test monthly if patient is on long-term therapy
- Monitor electrolytes: potassium, sodium, chloride monthly if patient is on long-term therapy
- Assess bowel pattern daily; if severe diarrhea occurs, drug should be discontinued
- Monitor for bleeding: ecchymosis, bleeding gums, hematuria, stool guaiac daily if on long-term therapy
- Assess for overgrowth of infection: perineal itching, fever, malaise, redness, pain, swelling, drainage, rash, diarrhea, change in cough, sputum

Nursing diagnoses

- Infection, risk for (uses)
- Diarrhea (side effects)
- Injury, risk for (side effects)
- Knowledge, deficient (teaching)
- Noncompliance (teaching)

Implementation

PO route

- Give 2 hr before or 2 hr after antacids, zinc, iron, calcium
- Give around clock to maintain blood levels
- Check to see if patient is taking theophylline

IV route

- Check for irritation, extravasation, phlebitis daily
- Do not use flexible containers in series connections, air embolism may occur
- Do not use if particulate matter is present
- Do not admix with other drugs
- Dilute with compatible sol to 2 mg/ml before administration; give over 1 hr; do not give by bolus or rapid **IV**

Solution compatibilities: D_5, 0.9% NaCl, D_5/0.9% NaCl LR/D_5, water for inj

Patient/family education

- Teach patient to report sore throat, bruising, bleeding, joint pain; may indicate blood dyscrasias (rare)
- Instruct patient to increase fluid intake to 2 L/day to prevent crystalluria
- Advise patient to contact prescriber if vaginal itching; loose, foul-smelling stools; furry tongue occur; may indicate superinfection; report itching, rash, pruritus, urticaria
- Instruct patient to take all medication prescribed for the length of time ordered; drug must be taken around the clock to maintain blood levels: do not give medication to others
- Advise patient to notify prescriber of diarrhea with blood or pus
- Advise patient to notify prescriber if theophylline is also being taken

Evaluation

Positive therapeutic outcome

- Absence of signs/symptoms of infection

(WBC <10,000/mm^3, temp WNL, absence of pain on urination, urgency)
- Reported improvement in symptoms of infection

gefitinib (Rx)
(ge-fi'tye-nib)
Iressa
Func. class.: Antineoplastic—miscellaneous
Chem. class.: Epidermal growth factor receptor inhibitor
Pregnancy category D

Action: Not fully understood; inhibits intracellular phosphorylation of cell surface receptors associated with epidermal growth factor receptors

Therapeutic Outcome: Decreased growth and spread of malignant cells

Uses: Non–small cell lung cancer (NSCLC)

Dosage and routes
Adult: PO 250 mg daily
CYP3A4 inducers concurrently (such as rifampin or phenytoin)
Adult: PO 500 mg daily

Available forms: Tabs 250 mg

Adverse effects
EENT: Amblyopia, conjunctivitis, eye pain, corneal erosion/ulcer
GI: Nausea, diarrhea, vomiting, anorexia, **pancreatitis,** mouth ulceration
INTEG: Rash, pruritus, acne, dry skin, **toxic epidermal neurolysis, angioedema**
MISC: Peripheral edema
RESP: **Interstitial lung disease,** cough, dyspnea

Contraindications: Pregnancy **D,** hypersensitivity

Precautions: Renal, hepatic, ocular, pulmonary disorders, lactation, children, elderly

Pharmacokinetics	
Absorption	Slowly
Distribution	Unknown
Metabolism	Unknown
Excretion	In feces (86%), urine (<4%)
Half-life	Unknown

Pharmacodynamics	
Onset	Unknown
Peak	3-7 hr
Duration	Unknown

Interactions
Individual drugs
Cimetidine, phenytoin, ranitidine, rifampin, sodium bicarbonate: decreased levels
Clarithromycin, erythromycin, itraconazole, ketoconazole: increased concentration
Metoprolol, warfarin: increased plasma concentration

NURSING CONSIDERATIONS
Assessment
- Assess pulmonary changes: lung sounds, cough, dyspnea; interstitial lung disease may occur, may be fatal; discontinue therapy if confirmed
- Assess ocular changes: eye irritation, corneal erosion/ulcer, aberrant eyelash growth
- Assess for pancreatitis: abdominal pain, levels of amylase, lipase
- Assess for toxic epidermal necrosis, angioedema
- Monitor GI symptoms: frequency of stools; if diarrhea is poorly tolerated, therapy may be discontinued for up to 14 days

Nursing diagnoses
- Injury, risk for (adverse reactions)
- Body image, disturbed (adverse reactions)
- Infection, risk for (adverse reactions)
- Knowledge, deficient (teaching)

Implementation
- Give without regard to food

Patient/family education
- Teach to report adverse reactions immediately: SOB, severe abdominal pain, occular changes, skin eruptions
- Advise of reason for treatment, expected results
- Advise to use contraception during treatment

Evaluation
Positive therapeutic outcome
- Decreased non–small cell lung cancer cells

gemcitabine (Rx)
(gem-sit'a-been)
Gemzar
Func. class.: Antineoplastic—miscellaneous
Chem. class.: Nucleoside analog
Pregnancy category D

Do Not Confuse:
Gemzar/Zinecard

Action: Exhibits antitumor activity by killing

cells undergoing DNA synthesis (S phase) and blocking G_1/S-phase boundary

Therapeutic Outcome: Prevention of growth of tumor

Uses: Adenocarcinoma of the pancreas: nonresectable stage II, III, or metastatic stage IV; in combination with cisplatin for inoperable, advanced, or metastatic non–small cell lung cancer

Dosage and routes

Pancreatic carcinoma

Adult: **IV** 1000 mg/m^2 given over ½ hr qwk × 7 wk, then 1 wk rest period; subsequent cycles should be infused once qwk × 3 wk out of every 4 wk

Non–small cell lung cancer

4 wk schedule

Adult: **IV** 1000 mg/m^2 given over ½ hr on days 1, 8, 15 of each 28-day cycle; give cisplatin **IV** 100 mg/m^2 on day 1 after gemcitabine

3 wk schedule

Adult: **IV** 1250 mg/m^2 given over ½ hr on days 1, 8 of each 21-day cycle; give cisplatin 100 mg/m^2 after the inf of gemcitabine on day 1

Available forms: Lyophilized powder for inj 20 mg/ml

Adverse effects

GI: Diarrhea, nausea, vomiting, anorexia, constipation, stomatitis

GU: Proteinuria, hematuria

HEMA: **Leukopenia, anemia, neutropenia, thrombocytopenia**

INTEG: Irritation at site, rash, alopecia

MISC: Dyspnea, fever, ***hemorrhage***, infection, flulike syndrome, paresthesia

Contraindications: Pregnancy **D**, hypersensitivity, lactation

Precautions: Children, elderly, myelosuppression, irradiation, renal/hepatic disease

Pharmacokinetics

Absorption	Unknown
Distribution	Crosses placenta
Metabolism	Unknown
Excretion	Unknown
Half-life	42-79 min

Pharmacodynamics

Unknown

Interactions

Individual drug

Alcohol: increased bleeding

Drug classifications

Antineoplastics, radiation: increased myelosuppression, diarrhea

Live virus vaccines: decreased antibody response

NSAIDs, salicylates: increased bleeding

NURSING CONSIDERATIONS

Assessment

- Monitor CBC, differential, platelet count before each dose; absolute granulocyte count >1000/mm^3, platelets >100,000/mm^3, give complete dose; absolute granulocyte count 500-1000/mm^3, platelets 50,000-100,000/mm^3, give 75%; absolute granulocyte count <500/mm^3, platelets <50,000/mm^3, do not give
- Assess for blood dyscrasias: bruising, bleeding, petechiae
- Monitor I&O, nutritional intake
- Monitor hepatic/renal studies before and during treatment, may increase AST, ALT, alkaline phosphatase, bilirubin, BUN, creatinine
- Assess food preferences: list likes, dislikes
- Assess buccal cavity q8h for dryness, sores or ulceration, white patches, oral pain, bleeding, dysphagia
- Assess GI symptoms: frequency of stools; cramping
- Assess signs of dehydration: rapid respirations, poor skin turgor, decreased urine output, dry skin, restlessness, weakness

Nursing diagnoses

- Infection, risk for (adverse reactions)
- Nutrition: less than body requirements, imbalanced (adverse reaction)

Implementation

- Give nutritious diet with iron, vitamin supplement, low fiber, few dairy products
- Give increased fluid intake to 2-3 L/day to prevent dehydration, unless contraindicated

IV route

- Prepare in biologic cabinet using gown, mask, gloves
- After reconstituting with 0.9% NaCl 5 ml/200 mg vial of drug or 25 ml/1 g of drug, shake (40 mg/ml); may be further diluted with 0.9% NaCl to concentrate as low as 0.1 mg/ml; discard unused portion, give over ½ hr, do not admix
- Change **IV** site q48h

Patient/family education

- Teach patient to rinse mouth tid-qid with water, club soda; brush teeth bid-tid with soft brush or cotton-tipped applicator for stomatitis; use unwaxed dental floss
- Advise patient to avoid foods with citric acid or hot or rough texture if stomatitis is present; to drink adequate fluids
- Advise patient to report stomatitis; any bleeding, white spots, ulcerations in mouth; tell patient to examine mouth daily, report symptoms
- Advise patient to report signs of anemia: fatigue, headache, faintness, shortness of breath, irritability; hematuria, dysuria
- Advise patient to use contraception during therapy and for 4 mo after
- Instruct patient to avoid use with NSAIDs, salicylates, alcohol; not to receive vaccinations during treatment

Evaluation

Positive therapeutic outcome

- Decrease in tumor size, decrease in spread of cancer

Treatment of overdose:

Induce vomiting, provide supportive care

gemfibrozil (Rx)

(gem-fye'broe-zil)

gemfibrozil, Lopid

Func. class.: Antilipemic

Chem. class.: Fibric acid derivative

Pregnancy category C

Do Not Confuse: Lopid/Levbid/Slo-bid

Action: Inhibits biosynthesis of VLDL, decreases triglycerides, increases HDLs

Therapeutic Outcome: Decreased hepatic triglyceride production, VLDL; accelerates removal of cholesterol from liver

Uses: Type IIb, IV, V hyperlipidemia as adjunct with diet therapy

Dosage and routes

Adult: PO 1200 mg in divided doses bid 30 min ac

Available forms: Tabs 600 mg

Adverse effects

CNS: Fatigue, vertigo, headache, paresthesia, dizziness, somnolence

GI: Nausea, vomiting, *dyspepsia, diarrhea, abdominal pain*

HEMA: **Leukopenia, anemia, eosinophilia, thrombocytopenia**

INTEG: Rash, urticaria, pruritus

MISC: Task perversion

Contraindications: Severe hepatic disease, preexisting gallbladder disease, severe renal disease, primary biliary cirrhosis, hypersensitivity

Precautions: Pregnancy **C,** monitor hematologic and hepatic function, lactation

Pharmacokinetics	
Absorption	Well absorbed
Distribution	Unknown, plasma protein binding >90%
Metabolism	Liver—minimal
Excretion	Kidney—unchanged (70%), feces (6%)
Half-life	1½ hr

Pharmacodynamics	
Onset	1-2 hr
Peak	1-2 hr
Duration	2-4 months

Interactions

Individual drugs

CycloSPORINE: decreased cycloSPORINE effect

Drug classifications

Anticoagulants (oral): increased effect of anticoagulants

HMG-CoA reductase inhibitors: increased risk of myositis, myalgia

Sulfonylureas: increased hypoglycemic effect

Drug/herb

Glucomannan: increased effect

Gotu kola: decreased effect

Drug/lab test

Increased: liver function studies, CPK, BSP, thymol turbidity, glucose

Decreased: Hgb, Hct, WBC

NURSING CONSIDERATIONS

Assessment

- Assess nutrition: fat, protein, carbohydrates; nutritional analysis should be performed by dietitian before treatment is initiated
- Assess renal function studies, liver function tests, CBC, blood glucose if patient is on long-term therapy; if liver function test results increase, drug should be discontinued
- Monitor bowel pattern daily; diarrhea may be a problem
- Monitor triglycerides, cholesterol, lipids baseline and during treatment; LDL and VLDL

G

should be watched closely and if increased, drug should be discontinued

Nursing diagnoses

- Diarrhea (adverse reactions)
- Knowledge, deficient (teaching)
- Noncompliance (teaching)

Implementation

- Give 30 min before AM and PM meals

Patient/family education

- Inform patient that compliance is needed for positive results to occur; not to double doses; that drug may be discontinued if no improvement in 3 mo
- Caution patient to decrease risk factors: high-fat diet, smoking, alcohol consumption, lack of exercise
- Advise patient to notify prescriber if GI symptoms of diarrhea, abdominal or epigastric pain, nausea, vomiting occur; or if chills, fever, sore throat occur; also occurrence of muscle cramps, abdominal cramps, severe flatulence

Evaluation

Positive therapeutic outcome

- Decreased cholesterol levels, serum triglyceride and improved ratio with HDLs

gemifloxacin (Rx)

(gem-ah-flox'a-sin)

Factive

Func. class.: Antiinfective

Chem. class.: Fluoroquinolone

Pregnancy category C

Action: Inhibits DNA gyrase, which is an enzyme involved in replication, transcription, and repair of bacterial DNA

Therapeutic Outcome: Negative C&S, decreasing symptoms of infection

Uses: Acute bacterial exacerbation of chronic bronchitis caused by *Streptococcus pneumoniae, Haemophilus influenzae, H. parainfluenzae, Moraxella catarrhalis;* community-acquired pneumonia caused by *Streptococcus pneumoniae* including multidrug-resistant strains, *H. influenzae, M. catarrhalis, Mycoplasma pneumoniae, Chlamydia pneumoniae, Klebsiella pneumoniae*

Dosage and routes

Adult: PO 320 mg/day × 5-7 days depending on type of infection

Renal dose

Adult: PO CCr ≤40 ml/min 160 mg q24hr

Available forms: Tabs 320 mg

Adverse effects

CNS: *Dizziness, headache,* somnolence, depression, insomnia, nervousness, confusion, agitation, **seizures**

EENT: Visual disturbances

GI: Diarrhea, *nausea,* vomiting, anorexia, flatulence, heartburn, dry mouth; increased AST, ALT; constipation, abdominal pain, oral thrush, glossitis, stomatitis, pseudomembranous colitis

INTEG: Rash, pruritus, urticaria, *photosensitivity*

SYST: **Anaphylaxis, Stevens-Johnson syndrome**

Contraindications: Hypersensitivity to quinolones

Precautions: Pregnancy **C**, hypokalemia, hypomagnesemia, lactation, children, elderly, renal disease, seizure disorders, excessive exposure to sunlight, psychosis, increased intracranial pressure, history of dysrhythmias, history of QT interval prolongation

Pharmacokinetics	
Absorption	Unknown
Distribution	Unknown
Metabolism	Unknown
Excretion	In urine as active drug, metabolites
Half-life	6-8 hr

Pharmacodynamics	
Onset	Unknown
Peak	1-2 hr
Duration	Unknown

Interactions

Individual drugs

Probenecid: may increase toxicity

Drug classifications

Antacids containing aluminum, iron, magnesium, sucralfate, zinc: decreased absorption, give 4 hr ac or 2 hr pc

Antiarrhythmics (amiodarone, disopyramide, procainamide, quinidine, sotalol): may decrease effect, resulting in life-threatening dysrhythmias

NURSING CONSIDERATIONS

Assessment

- Monitor kidney, liver function tests: BUN, creatinine, AST, ALT
- Monitor I&O ratio; urine pH, <5.5 is ideal
- Assess CNS symptoms: insomnia, vertigo, headache, agitation, confusion
- ❗ Assess allergic reactions and anaphylaxis: rash, flushing, urticaria, pruritus, chills, fever, joint pain; may occur a few days after therapy

begins; epINEPHrine and resuscitation equipment should be available for anaphylactic reaction
- Monitor bowel pattern daily, if severe diarrhea occurs, drug should be discontinued
- Assess for overgrowth of infection: perineal itching, fever, malaise, redness, pain, swelling, drainage, rash, diarrhea, change in cough, sputum

Nursing diagnoses
- Infection, risk for (uses)
- Knowledge, deficient (teaching)
- Noncompliance (teaching)

Implementation
- Give with or without food
- Theophylline should not be used with this product, toxicity may result
- Administer 4 hr before or 2 hr after antacids, iron, calcium, zinc products

Patient/family education
- Advise that fluids must be increased to 2 L/day to avoid crystallization in kidneys
- Instruct that if dizziness or light-headedness occurs, to ambulate, perform activities with assistance
- Instruct to complete full course of drug therapy
- Teach to contact prescriber if adverse reactions occur
- Teach to avoid iron- or mineral-containing supplements or antacids within 4 hr before and 2 hr after dosing
- Advise that photosensitivity may occur and sunscreen should be used
- Advise to use frequent rinsing of mouth, sugarless candy or gum for dry mouth
- Teach to avoid other medication unless approved by prescriber

Evaluation
Positive therapeutic outcome
- Negative C&S, absence of signs/symptoms of infection

! HIGH ALERT

gemtuzumab (Rx)
(gem-tue-zue′mab)

Mylotarg

Func. class.: Antineoplastic—miscellaneous
Chem. class.: Monoclonal antibody

Pregnancy category D

Action: Composed of recombinant humanized IgG_4 κ antibody, binds to CD33 antigen that is released in myeloid cells

Therapeutic Outcome: Decreasing signs/symptoms of leukemia

Uses: Acute myeloid leukemia (AML) in patients with first relapse who are 60 yrs or older

Dosage and routes
Adult: **IV** 9 m/m^2 as a 2 hr inf; before giving inf, give diphenhydrAMINE 50 mg PO, acetaminophen 650-1000 mg PO 1 hr before inf; then use acetaminophen 650-1000 mg q1-4h prn

Available forms: Powder for inj, lyophilized 5 mg

Adverse effects
CNS: *Dizziness,* insomnia, depression
CV: Hypertension, **hemorrhage,** tachycardia, hypotension
INTEG: *Rash,* herpes simplex, local reaction, petechiae
GI: Anorexia, diarrhea, constipation, nausea, stomatitis, vomiting
GU: Hematuria, **vaginal hemorrhage**
META: Hypokalemia, hypomagnesemia
MISC: *Fever, myalgias, headache, chills*
RESP: Cough, pneumonia, epistaxis, rhinitis

Contraindications: Pregnancy **D,** hypersensitivity, severe myelosuppression, lactation

Precautions: Children, severe renal or hepatic disease

Pharmacokinetics	
Absorption	Unknown
Distribution	Unknown
Metabolism	Unknown
Excretion	Unknown
Half-life	45, 100 hr, respectively

Pharmacodynamics

Unknown

Interactions: None known

NURSING CONSIDERATIONS
Assessment
- Assess for symptoms of infection; chills, fever, headache, may be masked by drug
- Assess CNS reaction: LOC, mental status, dizziness, confusion
- Assess cardiac status: lung sounds; ECG before and during treatment, especially in those with cardiac disease
- Assess bone marrow depression: bruising, bleeding, blood in stools, urine, sputum, emesis

Nursing diagnoses
- Infection, risk for (adverse reactions)
- Nutrition: less than body requirements, imbalanced (adverse reactions)
- Oral mucous membrane, impaired (adverse reactions)

Implementation
- Do not give **IV** push or bolus
- Protect from light, use biologic safety hood, allow to come to room temp
- Reconstitute each vial with 5 ml of sterile water for inj using sterile syringes, swirl each vial, check for discoloration or particulate matter, give over 2 hr, use a separate line with 1.2 micron terminal filter
- Store reconstituted sol for ≤8 hr in refrigerator

Patient/family education
- Advise patient to take acetaminophen for fever
- Instruct patient to avoid hazardous tasks, since confusion, dizziness may occur; avoid prolonged sunlight, use sunscreen
- Instruct patient to report signs of infection: sore throat, fever, diarrhea, vomiting
- Teach patient to avoid immunizations, crowds, people with known infections

Evaluation
Positive therapeutic outcome
- Decrease in size, number of lesions

gentamicin (Rx)
(jen-ta-mye'sin)

Cidomycin ✤, G-mycin, Garamycin, Gentamicin Sulfate, Jenamicin

Func. class.: Antiinfective

Chem. class.: Aminoglycoside

Pregnancy category C

Do Not Confuse:
Garamycin/kanamycin

Action: Interferes with protein synthesis in bacterial cell by binding to ribosomal subunit, causing misreading of genetic code; inaccurate peptide sequence forms in protein chain, causing bacterial death

Therapeutic Outcome: Bactericidal effects for the following organisms: *Pseudomonas aeruginosa, Proteus, Klebsiella, Serratia, Escherichia coli, Enterobacter, Citrobacter, Staphylococcus, Shigella, Salmonella, Acinetobacter*

Uses: Severe systemic infections of CNS; respiratory, GI, and urinary tracts; bone; skin; soft tissues; acute PID caused by susceptible strains

Dosage and routes
Severe systemic infections

Adult: **IV** inf 3-5 mg/kg/day in 3 divided doses q8h; dilute in 50-200 ml 0.9% NaCl or D_5W given over 30 min-1 hr; IM 3 mg/kg/day in divided doses q8h

Child: **IV**/IM 2-2.5 mg/ kg q8h

Neonates and infants: **IV**/IM 2.5 mg/kg q8-12h

Neonates <1 wk: 2.5 mg/kg q12-24h

Once-daily dosing/extended interval dosing (unlabeled)

Adult: **IV** 4-7 mg/kg q24h adjust according to levels

Renal dose

Adult: IM/**IV** 1-1.7 mg/kg initially, then adjust according to CCr levels

Available forms: Inj 10, 40 mg/ml; premixed inj 40, 60, 70, 80, 100 mg/50 ml; 40, 60, 80, 90, 100, 120, 160, 180 mg/ml

Adverse effects
CNS: Confusion, depression, numbness, tremors, **seizures,** muscle twitching, **neurotoxicity,** dizziness, vertigo

CV: Hypotension, hypertension, palpitations

EENT: Ototoxicity, deafness, visual disturbances, tinnitus

GI: Nausea, vomiting, anorexia, increased ALT, AST, bilirubin, hepatomegaly, **hepatic necrosis,** splenomegaly

GU: **Oliguria, hematuria, renal damage, azotemia, renal failure, nephrotoxicity**

HEMA: **Agranulocytosis, thrombocytopenia, leukopenia, eosinophilia,** anemia

INTEG: Rash, burning, urticaria, dermatitis, alopecia

Contraindications: Severe renal disease, hypersensitivity

Precautions: Pregnancy **C,** neonates, mild renal disease, hearing deficits, myasthenia gravis, lactation, elderly, Parkinson's disease

Pharmacokinetics	
Absorption	Well absorbed (IM)
Distribution	Distributed in extracellular fluids, poorly distributed in CSF; crosses placenta
Metabolism	Liver, minimal
Excretion	Mostly unchanged (79%) kidneys
Half-life	1-2 hr, infants 6-7 hr, increased in renal disease

Pharmacodynamics

	IM	IV
Onset	Rapid	Rapid
Peak	½-1½ hr	Infusion's end

Interactions
Individual drugs
Amphotericin B, cisplatin, ethacrynic acid, furosemide, mannitol, methoxyflurane, polymyxin, vancomycin: increased ototoxicity, neurotoxicity, nephrotoxicity
Drug classifications
Aminoglycosides, cephalosporins, penicillins: increased otoxicity, neurotoxicity, nephrotoxicity
Nondepolarizing neuromuscular blockers: increased neuromuscular blockade, respiratory depression

NURSING CONSIDERATIONS
Assessment
- Assess patient for previous sensitivity reaction
- Assess patient for signs and symptoms of infection including characteristics of wounds, sputum, urine, stool, WBC >10,000/mm^3, fever; obtain baseline information and during treatment
- Complete culture and sensitivity before beginning drug therapy; this will ensure that correct treatment has been initiated
- Assess for allergic reactions: rash, urticaria, pruritus, chills, fever, joint pain may occur a few days after therapy begins
- Identify urine output; if decreasing, notify prescriber (may indicate nephrotoxicity); also, increased BUN, creatinine, urine CCr <80 ml/min
- Monitor blood studies: AST, ALT, CBC, Hct, bilirubin, LDH, alkaline phosphatase, Coombs' test monthly if patient is on long-term therapy
- Monitor electrolytes: potassium, sodium, chloride, magnesium monthly if patient is on long-term therapy
- Monitor for bleeding: ecchymosis, bleeding gums, hematuria; assess stool guaiac daily if on long-term therapy
- Assess for overgrowth of infection: perineal itching, fever, malaise, redness, pain, swelling, drainage, rash, diarrhea, change in cough, sputum
- Obtain weight before treatment; calculation of dosage is usually based on ideal body weight but may be calculated on actual body weight
- Monitor I&O ratio; urinalysis daily for proteinuria, cells, casts; report sudden change in urine output
- Monitor VS during inf, watch for hypotension, change in pulse
- Assess **IV** site for thrombophlebitis including pain, redness, swelling q30 min, change site if needed; apply warm compresses to discontinued site
- Obtain serum peak, measured at 30-60 min after **IV** inf or 60 min after IM inj, trough level measured just before next dose; blood level should be 2-4 times bacteriostatic level
- Assess urine pH if drug is used for UTI; urine should be kept alkaline
- Assess for deafness by audiometric testing, ringing, roaring in ears, vertigo; assess hearing before, during, after treatment
- Assess for dehydration: high specific gravity, decrease in skin turgor, dry mucous membranes, dark urine

Nursing diagnoses
- Infection, risk for (uses)
- Diarrhea (side effects)
- Knowledge, deficient (teaching)
- Noncompliance (teaching)
- Injury, risk for (side effects)

Implementation
IM route
- Give inj deeply in large muscle mass; rotate sites

Topical route
- Wash hands, wear gloves, clean skin before applying

IV route
- Give in even doses around the clock; drug must be given for 10-14 days to ensure organism death and prevent superimposed infection
- Give by intermittent inf over ½-1 hr, flush with 0.9% NaCl or D_5W after inf
- Separate aminoglycosides and penicillins by ≥1 hr
- Store in tight container

Syringe compatibilities: Clindamycin, methicillin, penicillin G sodium
Y-site compatibilities: Acyclovir, amifostine, amiodarone, amsacrine, atracurium, aztreonam, cefpirome, ciprofloxacin, cyclophosphamide, cytarabine, diltiazem, enalaprilat, esmolol, famotidine, fluconazole, fludarabine, foscarnet, granisetron, hydromorphone, IL-2, insulin, labetalol, lorazepam, magnesium sulfate, melphalan, meperidine, meropenem, midazolam, morphine, multivitamins, ondansetron, paclitaxel, pancuronium, perphenazine, sargramostim, tacrolimus, teniposide, theophylline, thiotepa, tolazine,

G

vecuronium, vinorelbine, vit B with C, zidovudine

Y-site incompatibilities: Idarubicin, indomethacin, zidovudine

Additive compatibilities: Atracurium, aztreonam, bleomycin, cefoxitin, cimetidine, ciprofloxacin, fluconazole, meropenem, methicillin, metronidazole, ofloxacin, penicillin G sodium, ranitidine, verapamil

Patient/family education

- Teach patient to report sore throat, bruising, bleeding, joint pain; may indicate blood dyscrasias (rare)
- Advise patient to contact prescriber if vaginal itching, loose foul-smelling stools, furry tongue occur; may indicate superimposed infection

Evaluation

Positive therapeutic outcome

- Absence of signs/symptoms of infection (WBC <10,000/mm^3, temp WNL, absence of red, draining wounds)
- Reported improvement in symptoms of infection

Treatment of overdose: Withdraw drug, hemodialysis

glatiramer (Rx)

(glah-teer'a-mer)

Copaxone

Func. class.: Multiple sclerosis agent

Pregnancy category B

Action: Unknown; may modify the immune responses responsible for multiple sclerosis

Therapeutic outcome: Decreased symptoms of multiple sclerosis

Uses: Reduction of the frequency of relapses in patients with relapsing-remitting multiple sclerosis

Dosage and routes

Adult: SUBCUT 20 mg/day

Available forms: Inj premixed 20 mg/ml

Adverse effects

CNS: Anxiety, hypertonia, tremor, vertigo, speech disorder, agitation, confusion

CV: Migraine, palpitations, syncope, tachycardia, vasodilatation, chest pain

EENT: Ear pain, blurred vision

GI: Nausea, vomiting, diarrhea, anorexia, gastroenteritis

GU: Urgency, dysmenorrhea, vaginal moniliasis

HEMA: Ecchymosis, lymphadenopathy

INTEG: Pruritus, rash, sweating, urticaria, erythema

META: Edema, weight gain

MS: Arthralgia, back pain, neck pain

RESP: Bronchitis, dyspnea, laryngismus, rhinitis

Contraindications: Hypersensitivity to this drug or mannitol

Precautions: Pregnancy **B,** immune disorders, renal disease, lactation, child <18 yr

Pharmacokinetics	
Absorption	Unknown
Distribution	Unknown
Metabolism	Unknown
Excretion	Unknown
Half-life	Unknown

Pharmacodynamics

Unknown

NURSING CONSIDERATIONS

Assessment

- Monitor blood, renal, hepatic studies; before treatment
- Assess for CNS symptoms: anxiety, confusion, vertigo
- Assess GI status: diarrhea, vomiting, abdominal pain, gastroenteritis
- Assess cardiac status: tachycardia, palpitations, vasodilatation, chest pain

Nursing diagnoses

- Knowledge, deficient (teaching)
- Noncompliance (teaching)

Implementation

SUBCUT route

- Use a sterile syringe/needle to transfer the supplied diluent into the vial, rotate vial gently, do not shake; withdraw medication using a syringe with 27G needle; administer SUBCUT into hip, thigh, arm; discard unused portion
- Use SUBCUT route only; do not give IM or

IV

- Do not use sol that contains precipitate or is discolored

Patient/family education

- Give written, detailed instructions about the drug; provide initial and return demonstrations on inj procedure; give information on use and disposal of drug
- Advise patient that blurred vision, sweating may occur
- Advise patient that irregular menses, dysmenorrhea, or metorrhagia, as well as breast

pain may occur; use contraception during treatment
- Advise patient that if pregnancy is suspected or if nursing to notify prescriber
- Advise patient not to change dosing or to stop taking drug without advice of prescriber

Evaluation
Positive therapeutic outcome
- Decreased symptoms of multiple sclerosis

glimepiride (Rx)
(gly-meh'pih-ride)
Amaride
glipiZIDE (Rx)
(glip-i'zide)
Glucotrol, Glucotrol **XL**
Func. class.: Antidiabetic
Chem. class.: Sulfonylurea (2nd generation)
Pregnancy category C

Do Not Confuse:
glipiZIDE/glucotrol/glyBURIDE

Action: Causes functioning β-cells in pancreas to release insulin, leading to drop in blood glucose levels; may improve insulin binding to insulin receptors or increase the number of insulin receptors with prolonged administration; may also reduce basal hepatic glucose secretion; not effective if patient lacks functioning β-cells

Therapeutic Outcome: Decrease in polyuria, polydipsia, polyphagia, clear sensorium, absence of dizziness, stable gait

Uses: Type 2 diabetes mellitus

Dosage and routes
Glimepiride
Adult: PO 1-2 mg daily, then increase q1-2 wk up to 8 mg/day

Renal dose
Adult: CCr <20 ml/min; PO 1 mg daily with breakfast, may titrate upward as needed

GlipiZIDE
Adult: PO 5 mg initially, then increase to desired response; max 40 mg/day in divided doses or 15 mg/dose
Elderly/hepatic dose: PO 2.5 mg initially, then increase to desired response; max 40 mg/day in divided doses or 15 mg/dose

Available forms: Glimepiride: tabs 1, 2, 4 mg; glipiZIDE: tabs 5, 10 mg scored; ext rel tabs 5, 10 mg

Adverse effects
CNS: *Headache, weakness, dizziness, drowsiness,* tinnitus, fatigue, vertigo
ENDO: **Hypoglycemia**
GI: **Hepatotoxicity, cholestatic jaundice,** nausea, vomiting, diarrhea, heartburn
HEMA: **Leukopenia, thrombocytopenia, agranulocytosis, aplastic anemia,** increased AST, ALT, alkaline phosphatase, **pancytopenia, hemolytic anemia**
INTEG: Rash, allergic reactions, pruritus, urticaria, eczema, photosensitivity, erythema

Contraindications: Hypersensitivity to sulfonylureas, type 1/juvenile diabetes, diabetic ketoacidosis

Precautions: Pregnancy **C,** elderly, cardiac disease, severe renal disease, severe hepatic disease, thyroid disease

Pharmacokinetics	
Absorption	Completely absorbed GI tract
Distribution	Unknown
Metabolism	Liver
Excretion	Via kidneys
Half-life	2-4 hr

Pharmacodynamics	
Onset	1-1½ hr
Peak	1-3 hr
Duration	10-24 hr

Interactions
Individual drugs
Charcoal, cholestyramine, isoniazid, rifampin: possible decreased action of glipiZIDE
Chloramphenicol, cimetidine, clofibrate, fenfluramine, gemfibrozil, methyldopa, phenylbutazone, probenecid, sulfinpyrizine: increased hypoglycemia
Digitalis: increased action of digitalis
Drug classifications
Androgens, anticoagulants, H_2-antagonists, magnesium salts, MAOIs, NSAIDs, salicylates, sulfonamides, tricyclics, urinary acidifiers: increased hypoglycemia
β-Blockers: may mask symptoms of hypoglycemia
Diuretics (thiazide), hydantoins, urinary alkalinizers: possible decreased action of glipiZIDE
Glycosides: increased action of glycosides
Drug/herb
Alfalfa, aloe, basil, bay, bilberry, bitter melon, black catechu, buchu, burdock, coriander, dandelion, eyebright (po), garlic, glucomannan, glucosamine, goat's rue, gymnema,

G

horehound, horse chestnut, jambul, myrrh, myrtle: increased antidiabetic effect
Bee pollen, blue cohosh, broom, chromium, elecampane, eucalyptus, gotu kola: decreased antidiabetic effect
Broom, buchu, dandelion, glucosamine, juniper: decreased hypoglycemic effect
Chromium, coenzyme Q10, fenugreek, ginseng: increased or decreased hypoglycemic effect
Karela: increased glucose tolerance

NURSING CONSIDERATIONS

Assessment

- Assess for hypoglycemic/hyperglycemic reactions that can occur soon pc; hypoglycemic reactions (sweating, weakness, dizziness, anxiety, tremors, hunger); hyperglycemic reactions
- Monitor CBC, A1c (baseline, q3 mo) during treatment; check liver function tests periodically: AST, LDH, and renal studies: BUN, creatinine during treatment

Nursing diagnoses

- Nutrition: more than body requirements, imbalanced (uses)
- Nutrition: less than body requirements, imbalanced (adverse reactions)
- Injury, risk for (adverse reactions)
- Knowledge, deficient (teaching)
- Noncompliance (teaching)

Implementation

- Do not break, crush, or chew ext rel tabs
- Convert from other oral hypoglycemic agents or insulin dosage of <40 units/day; change may be made without gradual dosage change.
- Patients taking >40 units/day of insulin convert gradually by receiving oral hypoglycemic agents and 50% of previous insulin dosage for 3-5 days
- Monitor serum or urine glucose and ketones 3 ×/day during conversion
- Give drug 30 min before breakfast; if large dose is required, may be divided into 2 doses; give with meals to decrease GI upset and provide best absorption; if patient is NPO, may need to hold dose to prevent hypoglycemia
- Give tab crushed and mixed with meal or fluids for patients with difficulty swallowing
- For severe hypoglycemia give **IV** $D_{50}W$, then **IV** dextrose solution
- Store in tight container in cool environment

Patient/family education

- Teach patient to check for symptoms of cholestatic jaundice: dark urine, pruritus, yellow sclera; if these occur, prescriber should be notified
- Teach patient to use capillary blood glucose test
- Teach patient symptoms of hypo/hyperglycemia, what to do about each
- Instruct patient that drug must be continued on daily basis; explain consequence of discontinuing drug abruptly
- Teach patient to take drug in AM to prevent hypoglycemic reactions at night
- Caution patient to avoid OTC medications unless approved by a prescriber
- Teach patient that diabetes is a lifelong illness; that this drug is not a cure
- Teach patient to avoid alcohol; inform about disulfiram reaction (nausea, headache, cramps, flushing, hypoglycemia)
- Instruct patient that all food included in diet plan must be eaten to prevent hypoglycemia
- Advise patient to use sunscreen or stay out of the sun to prevent burns
- Advise patient to carry/wear emergency ID and carry a glucagon emergency kit for emergency purposes; also prescriber name, phone number, and medications taken
- Teach patient ext rel tab may appear in stool

Evaluation

Positive therapeutic outcome

- Decrease in polyuria, polydipsia, polyphagia, clear sensorium, absence of dizziness, stable gait

glyBURIDE (Rx)

(glye'byoor-ide)

Apo-Glyburide ✤, DiaBeta ✤, Euglucon ✤, Gen-Glyben ✤, Glynase PresTab, Micronase, novo-Glyburide ✤, nu-Glyburide ✤

Func. class.: Antidiabetic

Chem. class.: Sulfonylurea (2nd generation)

Pregnancy category B

Do Not Confuse:
DiaBeta/Zebeta, glyBURIDE/Glucotrol/glipiZIDE

Action: Causes functioning β-cells in pancreas to release insulin, leading to drop in blood glucose levels; may improve insulin binding to insulin receptors and increase number of insulin receptors with prolonged administration; may also reduce basal hepatic glucose secretion; not effective if patient lacks functioning β-cells

Therapeutic Outcome: Decrease in polyuria, polydipsia, polyphagia, clear sensorium, absence of dizziness, stable gait

Uses: Type 2 diabetes mellitus

Dosage and routes

DiaBeta/Micronase

Adult: PO 1.25-5 mg initially, then increased to desired response at weekly intervals up to 20 mg/day

Elderly: PO 1.25 mg initially, then increased to desired response; max 20 mg/day, maintenance 1.25-20 mg/daily

Glynase PresTab (micronized)

Adult: PO 1.5-3 mg/day initially, may increase by 1.5 mg/wk, max 12 mg/day

Elderly: PO 0.75-3 mg/day, may increase by 1.5 mg/wk

Available forms: Tabs (Diabeta) 1.25, 2.5, 5 mg; tabs micronized (Glynase PresTab) 1.5, 3, 6 mg

Adverse effects

CNS: *Headache, weakness,* paresthesia, tinnitus, fatigue, vertigo

ENDO: **Hypoglycemia**

GI: Nausea, fullness, heartburn, **hepatoxicity, cholestatic jaundice,** vomiting, diarrhea

HEMA: **Leukopenia, thrombocytopenia, agranulocytosis, aplastic anemia,** increased AST, ALT, alkaline phosphatase

INTEG: Rash, allergic reactions, pruritus, urticaria, eczema, photosensitivity, erythema

MS: Joint pains

Contraindications: Hypersensitivity to sulfonylureas, juvenile or type 1 diabetes, diabetic ketoacidosis

Precautions: Pregnancy **B,** elderly, cardiac disease, severe renal disease, severe hepatic disease, thyroid disease, severe hypoglycemic reactions

Pharmacokinetics	
Absorption	Completely absorbed GI tract
Distribution	99% plasma protein binding
Metabolism	Liver
Excretion	Urine, feces (metabolites), crosses placenta
Half-life	10 hr

Pharmacodynamics	
Onset	2-4 hr
Peak	4 hr
Duration	24 hr

Interactions

Individual drugs

Charcoal, cholestyramine, isoniazid, rifampin: decreased action of glyBURIDE

Chloramphenicol, fenfluramine, fluconazole, gemfibrozil, guanethidine, insulin, methyldopa, phenylbutazone, probenecid, sulfinpyrazone: increased hypoglycemia

Diazoxide: both drugs may have action decreased

Digoxin: increased level

Drug classifications

Androgens, anticoagulants, antidepressants (tricyclics), H_2-antagonists, magnesium salts, MAOIs, NSAIDs, salicylates, sulfonamides, urinary acidifiers: increased hypoglycemia

β-Adrenergic blockers: increased masking of symptoms of hypoglycemia

Diuretics (thiazide), hydantoins, urinary alkalinizers: decreased action of glyBURIDE

Drug/herb

Alfalfa, aloe, basil, bay, bilberry, bitter melon, black catechu, buchu, burdock, coriander, dandelion, eyebright (po), garlic, glucomannan, glucosamine, goat's rue, gymnema, horehound, horse chestnut, jambul, myrrh, myrtle: increased antidiabetic effect

Bee pollen, blue cohosh, broom, chromium, elecampane, eucalyptus, gotu kola: decreased antidiabetic effect

Broom, buchu, dandelion, juniper: decreased hypoglycemic effect

Chromium, coenzyme Q10, fenugreek, ginseng: increased or decreased hypoglycemic effect

Karela: increased glucose tolerance

NURSING CONSIDERATIONS

Assessment

- Assess for hypo/hyperglycemic reactions that can occur soon pc; hypoglycemic reactions (sweating, weakness, dizziness, anxiety, tremors, hunger); hyperglycemic reactions
- Monitor CBC, A1c (baseline, q3 mo) during treatment; check liver function tests periodically, AST, LDH, and renal studies: BUN, creatinine during treatment

Nursing diagnoses

- Nutrition: more than body requirements, imbalanced (uses)
- Nutrition: less than body requirements, imbalanced (adverse reactions)
- Injury, risk for (adverse reactions)
- Knowledge, deficient (teaching)
- Noncompliance (teaching)

Implementation

- Conversion from other oral hypoglycemic agents or insulin dosage of <40 units/day; change may be made without gradual dosage change
- Patients taking >40 units/day of insulin

G

convert gradually by receiving oral hypoglycemic agents and 50% of previous insulin dosage for 3-5 days

- Monitor serum or urine glucose and ketones 3 ×/day during conversion
- Give drug 30 min before breakfast; if large dose is required, may be divided into two; give with meals to decrease GI upset and provide best absorption, if patient is NPO, may need to hold dose to avoid hypoglycemia
- Give tab crushed and mixed with meal or fluids for patients with difficulty swallowing
- For severe hypoglycemia, give **IV** $D_{50}W$, then **IV** dextrose sol
- Store in tight container in cool environment

Patient/family education

- Teach patient to check for symptoms of cholestatic jaundice: dark urine, pruritus, yellow sclera; if these occur, prescriber should be notified
- Teach patient to use capillary blood glucose test
- Teach patient symptoms of hypo/hyperglycemia, what to do about each
- Instruct patient that drug must be continued on daily basis; explain consequence of discontinuing drug abruptly
- Teach patient to take drug in AM to prevent hypoglycemic reactions at night
- Caution patient to avoid OTC medications unless approved by a prescriber
- Teach patient that diabetes is a lifelong illness; that this drug is not a cure
- Instruct patient that all food included in diet plan must be eaten to prevent hypoglycemia
- Advise patient to carry/wear emergency ID and carry a glucagon emergency kit for emergency purposes: have sugar packets available; also prescriber name, phone number, and medications
- Advise patient to use sunscreen or stay out of the sun to prevent burns

Evaluation

Positive therapeutic outcome

- Decrease in polyuria, polydipsia, polyphagia, clear sensorium, absence of dizziness, stable gait

glycopyrrolate (Rx)

(glye-koe-pye'roe-late)

glycopyrrolate, Robinul, Robinul-Forte

Func. class.: Cholinergic blocker

Chem. class.: Quaternary ammonium compound

Pregnancy category B

Action: Inhibits action of acetylcholine at receptor sites in autonomic nervous system, which controls secretions, free acids in stomach

Therapeutic Outcome: Decreased secretions in the respiratory tract, GI system

Uses: Decreased secretions before surgery, reversal of neuromuscular blockade, peptic ulcer disease, irritable bowel syndrome

Investigational uses: Drooling, hypersalivation

Dosage and routes

Preoperatively

Adult: IM 4.4 mcg/kg ½-1 hr before surgery, max 0.1 mg

Child: IM 4.4-8.8 mcg/kg ½-1 hr before surgery

Reversal of neuromuscular blockage

Adult and child: **IV** 200 mcg for each 1 mg of neostigmine or 5 mg **IV** of pyridostigmine simultaneously

Drooling

Adult: PO doses vary widely

GI disorders

Adult: PO 1-2 mg bid-tid; IM/**IV** 100-200 mcg tid-qid, titrated to patient response

Antidysrhythmic

Adult: **IV** 100 mcg, may repeat q2 min

Child: **IV** 4.4 mcg/kg, may repeat q2 min, max 100 mcg

Available forms: Tabs 1, 2 mg; inj 200 mcg 0.2 mg/ml

Adverse effects

CNS: Confusion, anxiety, restlessness, irritability, delusions, hallucinations, headache, sedation, depression, incoherence, dizziness, lethargy, flushing, weakness

CV: Palpitations, tachycardia, postural hypotension, paradoxical bradycardia

EENT: Blurred vision, photophobia, dilated pupils, difficulty swallowing, increased intraocular pressure, mydriasis, cycloplegia

GI: *Dryness of mouth, constipation,* nausea, vomiting, abdominal distress, paralytic ileus, altered taste perception
GU: Hesitancy, retention, impotence
INTEG: Urticaria, allergic reactions
MISC: Suppression of lactation, nasal congestion, decreased sweating
SYST: **Anaphylaxis**

Contraindications: Hypersensitivity, narrow-angle glaucoma, myasthenia gravis, GI/GU obstruction, child <3 yr, tachycardia, myocardial ischemia, hepatic disease, ulcerative colitis, toxic megacolon, prostatic hypertrophy

Precautions: Pregnancy **B,** elderly, lactation, renal disease, CHF, pulmonary disease, hyperthyroidism

Pharmacokinetics

Absorption	Well absorbed (PO, SUBCUT, IM)
Distribution	Unknown
Metabolism	Not metabolized
Excretion	Unchanged feces
Half-life	2 hr

Pharmacodynamics

	PO	IM	IV
Onset	Unknown	15-30 min	Immediate
Peak	1 hr	30-45 min	10-15 min
Duration	8-12 hr	2-7 hr	2-7 hr

Interactions
Individual drugs
Alcohol, amantadine: increased anticholinergic effect
Drug classifications
Antacids: decreased absorption of glycopyrrolate
Antidepressants (tricyclic), antihistamines, phenothiazines: increased anticholinergic effect
Antidiarrheals: decreased absorption of glycopyrrolate

NURSING CONSIDERATIONS
Assessment
- Monitor I&O ratio; retention commonly causes decreased urinary output; check for urinary hesitation; palpate bladder if retention occurs
- Monitor ECG for ectopic ventricular beats, PVC, tachycardia
- Monitor for bowel sounds; check for constipation; increase fluids, bulk, exercise if constipation occurs
- Assess mental status: affect, mood, CNS depression, worsening of psychiatric symptoms during early therapy

Nursing diagnoses
- Knowledge, deficient (teaching)

Implementation
PO route
- Give PO with or after meals to prevent GI upset; may give with fluids other than water

IM route
- Give IM inj deeply in large muscle mass

IV route
- Administer **IV** undiluted, give at a rate of 0.2 mg or less over 5-15 min through Y-tube or 3-way stopcock; do not add to **IV** sol
- Administer parenteral dose with patient recumbent to prevent postural hypotension

Syringe compatibilities: Atropine, benzquinamide, chlorproMAZINE, cimetidine, codeine, diphenhydrAMINE, droperidol, droperidol/fentanyl, hydromorphone, hydrOXYzine, levorphanol, lidocaine, meperidine, meperidine/promethazine, midazolam, morphine, nalbuphine, neostigmine, oxymorphone, procaine, prochlorperazine, promazine, promethazine, pyridostigmine, ranitidine, scopolamine, triflupromazine, trimethobenzamide
Y-site compatibilities: Propofol
Solution compatibilities: D_5W, 0.9% NaCl, Ringer's D_5/0.45% NaCl

Patient/family education
- Caution patient not to operate machinery or engage in hazardous activities if drowsiness, blurred vision occurs
- Advise patient not to take OTC products, cough, cold preparations with alcohol, antihistamines without approval of prescriber
- Teach patient to avoid hot temp; since sweating is decreased, heat stroke is possible
- Advise patient to notify prescriber of eye pain, blurred vision, light sensitivity
- Caution patient not to discontinue this drug abruptly; tapering should be done over 1 wk

Evaluation
Positive therapeutic outcome
- Decreased secretions, bronchial, GI
- Decreased pain in GI disorders
- Reversal of neuromuscular blockade

G

goserelin (Rx)

(goe'se-rel-lin)

Zoladex

Func. class.: Gonadotropin-releasing hormone, antineoplastic

Chem. class.: Synthetic decapeptide analog of LHRH

Pregnancy category D, X

Action: Inhibitor of pituitary gonadotropin secretion; initially increases LH and FSH, with increases in testosterone, reduction in sex steroid levels (substitute serum testosterone levels)

Therapeutic Outcome: Decrease in tumor size and spread of malignant cells

Uses: Advanced prostate cancer (10.8 mg); endometriosis, advanced breast cancer, endometrial thinning (3.6 mg)

Dosage and routes

Adult: SUBCUT 3.6 mg q4 wk (implant) or 10.8 mg q12 wk

Endometrial thinning

Adult: SUBCUT 1-2 depot inj; usually 1 depot, surgery performed at 4 wk; if 2 depots, surgery performed 2-4 wk after 2nd depot

Available forms: Depot inj 3.6, 10.8 mg

Adverse effects

CNS: Headaches, **spinal cord compression,** anxiety, depression, dizziness, insomnia, lethargy

CV: **Dysrhythmia, cerebrovascular accident,** hypertension, **MI,** chest pain, CHF

ENDO: Gynecomastia, breast tenderness, hot flashes

GI: Nausea, vomiting, constipation, diarrhea, ulcer

GU: *Spotting, breakthrough bleeding, decreased libido,* renal insufficiency, urinary obstruction, urinary tract infection, impotence

INTEG: Rash, pain on inj

MS: Osteoneuralgia

RESP: *COPD, URI*

Contraindications: Pregnancy **D** (breast cancer), pregnancy **X** (endometriosis, lactation, nondiagnosed vaginal bleeding), hypersensitivity to LHRH, LHRH-agonist analogs

Pharmacokinetics	
Absorption	Well absorbed
Distribution	Unknown
Metabolism	Unknown
Excretion	Unknown
Half-life	4½ hr

Pharmacodynamics	
Onset	Unknown
Peak	14-28 days
Duration	Treatment length

Interactions: None known

Drug/lab test

Increased: alkaline phosphatase, estradiol, FSH, LH, testosterone levels

Decreased: testosterone levels, progesterone

NURSING CONSIDERATIONS

Assessment

- Assess for relief of bone pain (back pain), change in motor function
- Monitor I&O ratios, palpate bladder for distention (urinary obstruction) at beginning of treatment; renal insufficiency and obstruction may occur
- Monitor acid phosphatase, PSA baseline and periodically

Nursing diagnoses

- Sexual dysfunction (uses)
- Knowledge, deficient (teaching)

Implementation

- Administer via implant inserted by qualified persons into upper subcutaneous tissue in abdominal wall q28 days or q12 wk (10.8 mg)

Patient/family education

- Caution patient that gynecomastia and postmenopausal symptoms may occur but will decrease after treatment is discontinued; that bone pain may increase, then decrease
- Teach patient to contact prescriber if difficulty urinating, hot flashes occur during treatment
- Advise patient not to breastfeed while taking drug; use effective nonhormonal contraception

Evaluation

Positive therapeutic outcome

- More normal levels of PSA, acid phosphatase, alkaline phosphatase; testosterone level of <25 mg/dl

granisetron (Rx)

(grane-iss'e-tron)

Kytril

Func. class.: Antiemetic

Chem. class.: 5-HT_3 receptor antagonist

Pregnancy category B

Action: Prevents nausea, vomiting by blocking serotonin peripherally, centrally, and in the small intestine

Therapeutic Outcome: Absence of nausea and vomiting

Uses: Prevention of nausea, vomiting associated with cancer chemotherapy including high-dose cisplatin

Investigational uses: Acute nausea, vomiting after surgery

Dosage and routes

Nausea, vomiting in chemotherapy

Adult and child ≥2 yr: **IV** 10 mcg/kg over 5 min, 30 min before the start of cancer chemotherapy

Adult: PO 1 mg bid, give 1st dose 1 hr before chemotherapy and next dose 12 hr after 1st

Nausea, vomiting in radiation therapy

Adult: PO 2 mg daily 1 hr prior to radiation

Available forms: Inj 1 mg/ml; tabs 1 mg

Adverse effects

CNS: *Headache, asthenia,* anxiety, dizziness

CV: Hypertension

GI: Diarrhea, *constipation,* increased AST, ALT, *nausea*

HEMA: **Leukopenia,** anemia, **thrombocytopenia**

MISC: Rash, **bronchospasm**

Contraindications: Hypersensitivity

Precautions: Pregnancy **B,** lactation, children, elderly, ondansetron hypersensitivity

Pharmacokinetics

Absorption	Unknown
Distribution	Unknown
Metabolism	Liver
Excretion	Unknown
Half-life	10-12 hr

Pharmacodynamics

Unknown

Interactions: None known

NURSING CONSIDERATIONS

Assessment

- Assess patient for absence of nausea, vomiting during chemotherapy
- Assess patient for hypersensitive reaction: rash, bronchospasm

Nursing diagnoses

- Fluid volume, deficient (uses)
- Knowledge, deficient (teaching)

Implementation

- Administer **IV**
- Dilute in 0.9% NaCl for inj or D_5W (20-50 ml), give over 5-15 min
- Store at room temp for 24-hr dilution

Y-site compatibilities: Acyclovir, allopurinol, amifostine, amikacin, aminophylline, amphotericin B cholesteryl, ampicillin, ampicillin/sulbactam, amsacrine, aztreonam, bleomycin, bumetanide, buprenorphine, butorphanol, calcium gluconate, carboplatin, carmustine, cefazolin, cefepime, cefonicid, cefoperazone, cefotaxime, cefotetan, cefoxitin, ceftazidime, ceftizoxime, ceftriaxone, cefuroxime, chlorproMAZINE, cimetidine, ciprofloxacin, cisplatin, cladribine, clindamycin, cyclophosphamide, cytarabine, dacarbazine, dactinomycin, DAUNOrubicin, dexamethasone, diphenhydrAMINE, DOBUTamine, DOPamine, DOXOrubicin, DOXOrubicin liposome, doxycycline, droperidol, enalaprilat, etoposide, famotidine, filgrastim, floxuridine, fluconazole, fluorouracil, fludarabine, furosemide, gallium, ganciclovir, gentamicin, haloperidol, heparin, hydrocortisone, hydromorphone, hydrOXYzine, idarubicin, ifosfamide, imipenem-cilastatin, leucovorin, lorazepam, magnesium sulfate, melphalan, meperidine, mesna, methotrexate, methylPREDNISolone, metoclopramide, metronidazole, mezlocillin, miconazole, minocycline, mitomycin, mitoxantrone, morphine, nalbuphine, netilmicin, ofloxacin, paclitaxel, piperacillin, piperacillin/tazobactam, plicamycin, potassium chloride, prochlorperazine, promethazine, propofol, ranitidine, sargramostim, sodium bicarbonate, streptozocin, teniposide, thiotepa, ticarcillin, ticarcillin/clavulanate, tobramycin, trimethoprim/sulfamethoxazole, vancomycin, vinBLAStine, vinCRIStine, vinorelbine, zidovudine

Y-site incompatibilities: Fluorouracil, furosemide, sodium bicarbonate

Additive compatibilities: Dexamethasone, methylPREDNISolone

Solution compatibilities: D_5W, 0.9% NaCl

Patient/family education

- Advise patient to report diarrhea, constipation, rash, or changes in respirations

Evaluation

Positive therapeutic outcome

- Absence of nausea, vomiting during cancer chemotherapy

guaifenesin (Rx, OTC)

(gwye-fen'e-sin)

Altarussin, Anti-tuss, Benylin-E ✤, Calmylin Expectorant ✤, Diabetic Tussin EX, Ganidin NR, guaifenesin, Guaifenesin NR, Guaifenex LA, Guiatuss, Hytuss, Hytuss 2X, Liquibid, Monafed, Mucine X, Naldecon Senior EX, Organidin NR, Pneumomist, Respa-GF, Resyl ✤, Robitussin, Scot-Tussin Expectorant, Siltussin DAS, Siltussin SA

Func. class.: Expectorant

Pregnancy category C

Action: Acts as an expectorant by stimulating a gastric mucosal reflex to increase the production of lung mucus

Therapeutic Outcome: Decreased cough

Uses: Productive and nonproductive cough

Dosage and routes

Adult: PO 200-400 mg q4h, or 600-1200 mg q12h (ext rel); not to exceed 2.4 g/day

Child 6-12 yr: PO 100-200 mg q4h or 600 mg q12h (ext rel); not to exceed 1.2 g/day

Child 2-6 yr: PO: 50-100 mg q4h; not to exceed 600 mg/day

Available forms: Tabs 100, 200 mg; ext rel tabs 600, 1200 mg; caps 200 mg; syr 100 mg, 200/5 ml; ext rel caps 300 mg

Adverse effects

CNS: Drowsiness, headache, dizziness

GI: Nausea, anorexia, vomiting

Contraindications: Hypersensitivity, chronic persistent cough

Precautions: Pregnancy **C**

Pharmacokinetics

Absorption	Well absorbed
Distribution	Unknown
Metabolism	Unknown
Excretion	Unknown
Half-life	1 hr

Pharmacodynamics

	PO	PO–EXT–REL
Onset	½ hr	Unknown
Peak	Unknown	Unknown
Duration	4-6 hr	12 hr

Interactions: None known

NURSING CONSIDERATIONS

Assessment

- Assess cough: type, frequency, character, including characteristics of sputum; lung sounds bilaterally; fluids should be increased to 2 L/day to decrease secretion viscosity (thickness)

Nursing diagnoses

- Airway clearance, ineffective (uses)
- Knowledge, deficient (teaching)

Implementation

- Store at room temp; provide room humidification to assist with liquefying secretions
- Avoid fluids for ½ hr after administration

Patient/family education

- Caution patient to avoid driving, other hazardous activities if drowsiness occurs (rare)
- Advise patient to avoid smoking, smoke-filled rooms, perfumes, dust, environmental pollutants, cleansers
- Instruct patient to notify prescriber if dry, nonproductive cough lasts over 7 days

Evaluation

Positive therapeutic outcome

- Absence of dry cough
- Thinner, more productive cough that raises secretions

guanfacine (Rx)

(gwahn'fa-seen)

Tenex

Func. class.: Antihypertensive

Chem. class.: Central α_2-adrenergic agonist

Pregnancy category B

Action: Stimulates central α_2-adrenergic receptors in the CNS, resulting in decreased sympathetic outflow from brain with decreased peripheral resistance

Therapeutic Outcome: Decreased B/P in hypertension

Uses: Hypertension in individual using a thiazide diuretic

Dosage and routes

Adult: PO 1 mg/day at bedtime; may increase dose in 2-3 wk to 2-3 mg/day

Available forms: Tabs 1, 2 mg

Adverse effects

CNS: *Somnolence, dizziness, headache, fatigue*
CV: Bradycardia, chest pain, rebound hypertension, palpitations
EENT: Taste change, tinnitus, vision change, rhinitis, nasal congestion
GI: *Dry mouth, constipation,* cramps, nausea
GU: *Impotence*, urinary incontinence
INTEG: Dermatitis, pruritus, purpura
MS: Leg cramps
RESP: Dyspnea

Contraindications: Hypersensitivity

Precautions: Pregnancy **B,** lactation, children <12 yr, severe coronary insufficiency, recent MI, renal or hepatic disease, CVA

Pharmacokinetics	
Absorption	Well absorbed (80%)
Distribution	Widely distributed
Metabolism	Liver (50%)
Excretion	Kidneys—unchanged (50%)
Half-life	17 hr

Pharmacodynamics	
Onset	Unknown
Peak	8-12 hr
Duration	24 hr

Interactions

Individual drugs

Alcohol: increased hypotension, increased sedation

Drug classifications

Analgesics, opioids: increased sedation
Antidepressants, tricyclic: decreased effect of guanfacine
Antihypertensives: increased hypotension
β-Adrenergic blockers: increased bradycardia, CHF
MAOI: decreased effectiveness of guanabenz
Nitrates: increased nitrates
Sedatives/hypnotics: increased sedation

NURSING CONSIDERATIONS

Assessment

- Monitor blood studies: neutrophils, decreased platelets
- Monitor renal studies: protein, BUN, creatinine; watch for increased levels that may indicate nephrotic syndrome; polyuria, oliguria, frequency
- Obtain baselines in renal, liver function tests before therapy begins; potassium levels, although hyperkalemia rarely occurs
- Monitor B/P, pulse if the drug is being used for hypertension; notify prescriber of changes
- Assess for edema in feet, legs daily; monitor I/O; check weight for decreasing output
- Assess for allergic reaction: rash, fever, pruritus, urticaria, drug should be discontinued if antihistamines fail to help
- Assess for symptoms of CHF: edema, dyspnea, wet crackles, BP, weight gain

Nursing diagnoses

- Cardiac output, decreased (uses)
- Injury, risk for (adverse reactions)
- Knowledge, deficient (teaching)
- Noncompliance (teaching)

Implementation

- Give at bedtime
- Store in air-tight container at room temp

Patient/family education

- Instruct patient not to discontinue drug abruptly, or withdrawal symptoms may occur: anxiety, increased B/P, headache, insomnia, increased pulse, tremors, nausea, sweating
- Caution patient not to use OTC (cough, cold, or allergy) products unless directed by prescriber
- Teach patient to comply with dosage schedule even if feeling better; drug controls symptoms, does not cure
- Caution patient (especially the elderly) to change position slowly; to rise slowly to sitting or standing position to minimize orthostatic hypotension
- Instruct patient to notify prescriber of sore throat, fever, swelling of hands or feet, irregular heartbeat, chest pain, increased weight
- Inform patient that drug may cause dizziness, fainting; light-headedness may occur during 1st few days of therapy; drug may cause dry mouth—use hard candy or saliva product, or rinse mouth frequently
- Teach patient that compliance is necessary; not to skip or stop drug unless directed by prescriber
- Caution patient that drug may cause skin rash
- Teach patient to avoid hazardous activities—drug may cause drowsiness; dizziness

Evaluation

Positive therapeutic outcome

- Decreased B/P

G

haloperidol (Rx)
(hal-oh-pehr'ih-dol)

Apo-Haloperidol ✦, Haldol, Novo-Peridol ✦, Peridol ✦

haloperidol decanoate (Rx)
Haldol Decanoate, Haldol LA ✦

haloperidol lactate (Rx)
Haldol, Haldol Concentrate, Haloperidol Intensol

Func. class.: Antipsychotic/neuroleptic
Chem. class.: Butyrophenone

Pregnancy category C

Do Not Confuse:
Haldol/Stadol, haloperidol/Halotestin

Action: Depresses cerebral cortex, hypothalamus, limbic system, which control activity and aggression; blocks neurotransmission produced by dopamine at synapse; exhibits strong α-adrenergic, anticholinergic blocking action; mechanism for antipsychotic effects unclear

Therapeutic Outcome: Decreased signs and symptoms of psychosis

Uses: Psychotic disorders, control of tics, vocal utterances in Gilles de la Tourette syndrome, short-term treatment of hyperactive children showing excessive motor activity, prolonged parenteral therapy in chronic schizophrenia, control of severe nausea and vomiting in chemotherapy, organic mental syndrome with psychotic features, hiccups (short-term), emergency sedation of severely agitated or delirious patients

Investigational uses: Nausea, vomiting in chemotherapy, surgery

Dosage and routes

Psychosis

Adult: PO 0.5-5 mg bid or tid initially depending on severity of condition; increase to desired dosage, max 100 mg/day; IM (lactate) 2-5 mg q4-8h or bid-tid

Elderly: 0.25-0.5 mg daily-bid, titrate q3-4 days by 0.25-0.5 mg/dose

Child 3-12 yr: PO/IM (lactate) 0.05-0.15 mg/kg/day

Decanoate

Adult: Initial dose IM is 10-15 mg × daily oral dose at 4-wk interval; do not administer **IV**; not to exceed 100 mg

Chronic schizophrenia

Adult: IM 50-100 mg q4 wk (decanoate)

Child 3-12 yr: PO/IM 0.05-0.15 mg/kg/day

Tics/vocal utterances

Adult: PO 0.5-5 mg bid or tid, increased until desired response occurs

Child 3-12 yr: PO 0.05-0.075 mg/kg/day

Hyperactive children

Child 3-12 yr: PO 0.05-0.075 mg/kg/day

Available forms: Tabs 0.5, 1, 2, 5, 10, 20 mg; lactate: conc 2 mg/ml; inj 5 mg/ml; decanoate: 50, 100 mg base/ml

Adverse effects

CNS: *Extrapyramidal symptoms (EPS), pseudoparkinsonism, akathisia, dystonia, tardive dyskinesia, drowsiness, headache,* **seizures, neuroleptic malignant syndrome,** confusion

CV: *Orthostatic hypotension,* hypertension, **cardiac arrest,** ECG changes, **tachycardia**

EENT: Blurred vision, glaucoma, dry eyes

GI: *Dry mouth, nausea, vomiting, anorexia, constipation,* diarrhea, jaundice, weight gain, **ileus, hepatitis**

GU: Urinary retention, urinary frequency, dysuria, enuresis, impotence, amenorrhea, gynecomastia

INTEG: *Rash,* photosensitivity, dermatitis

RESP: **Laryngospasm,** dyspnea, **respiratory depression**

Contraindications: Hypersensitivity, blood dyscrasias, coma, child <3 yr, brain damage, bone marrow depression, alcohol and barbiturate withdrawal states, Parkinson's disease, angina, epilepsy, urinary retention, narrow-angle glaucoma

Precautions: Pregnancy **C,** lactation, seizure disorders, hypertension, hepatic disease, cardiac disease, elderly,

Pharmacokinetics

Absorption	Well absorbed (PO, IM); decanoate (IM) absorbed slowly
Distribution	High concentrations in liver, crosses placenta
Metabolism	Liver, extensively
Excretion	Kidneys, breast milk
Half-life	21-24 hr

Pharmacodynamics

	PO	IM	IM (decanoate)
Onset	Erratic	½ hr	3-9 days
Peak	2-6 hr	30-45 min	4-11 days
Duration	8-12 hr	4-8 hr	3 wk

Interactions

Individual drugs

Alcohol: increased effects of both drugs, oversedation
Carbamazepine: decreased effects of haloperidol
EpINEPHrine: increased toxicity
Levodopa: decreased effects of levodopa
Lithium: increased toxicity; decreased effects of lithium
Phenobarbital: decreased effects of haloperidol

Drug classifications

Anticholinergics: increased anticholinergic effects
Barbiturate anesthetics: oversedation
β-Adrenergic blockers: increased effects of both drugs
CNS depressants: oversedation

Drug/herb

Chamomile, cola tree, hops, kava, nettle, nutmeg, skullcap, valerian: increased action
Betel palm, kava: increased extrapyramidal symptoms
Jimsonweed, scopolia: antagonist action

Drug/lab test

Increased: liver function tests, cardiac enzymes, cholesterol, blood glucose, prolactin, bilirubin, PBI, cholinesterase, alkaline phosphatase
Decreased: hormones (blood and urine), protime
False positive: pregnancy tests, PKU
False negative: urinary steroids

NURSING CONSIDERATIONS

Assessment

- Assess mental status: orientation, mood, behavior, presence and type of hallucinations before initial administration and monthly; this drug should significantly reduce psychotic behavior
- Check for swallowing of PO medication; check for hoarding or giving of medication to other patients
- Monitor I&O ratio; palpate bladder if low urinary output occurs, especially in elderly; urinalysis is recommended before, during prolonged therapy
- Monitor bilirubin, CBC, liver function studies monthly
- Assess affect, orientation, LOC, reflexes, gait, coordination, sleep pattern disturbances
- Monitor B/P with patient sitting, standing, and lying; take pulse and respirations q4h during initial treatment; establish baseline before starting treatment; report drops of 30 mm Hg; obtain baseline ECG, Q-wave and T-wave changes
- Check for dizziness, faintness, palpitations, tachycardia on rising; severe orthostatic hypotension is common
- Assess for neuroleptic malignant syndrome: hyperpyrexia, muscle rigidity, increased CPK, altered mental status; drug should be discontinued immediately; if seizures, hyper/hypotension, tachycardia occur, notify prescriber immediately
- Assess for EPS including akathisia (inability to sit still, no pattern to movements), tardive dyskinesia (bizarre movements of the jaw, mouth, tongue, extremities), pseudoparkinsonism (ragged tremors, pill rolling, shuffling gate); an antiparkinsonian drug should be prescribed
- Assess for constipation and urinary retention daily; if these occur, increase bulk, water in diet

H

Nursing diagnoses

- Thought processes, disturbed (uses)
- Coping, ineffective (uses)
- Knowledge, deficient (teaching)
- Noncompliance (teaching)

Implementation

PO route

- Give drug in liquid form mixed in glass of juice or caffeine-free cola if hoarding is suspected; do not mix in caffeine drinks, tannics, pectins
- Give decreased dosage in elderly because of slower metabolism
- Give PO with full glass of water, milk; or give with food to decrease GI upset
- Give antacids 2 hr before or after this drug
- Store in tight, light-resistant container, oral sol in amber bottle

IM route

- Inject in deep muscle mass, do not give SUBCUT; use 21G 2-in needle; do not administer sol with a precipitate; give <3 ml per inj site; give slowly, may be painful
- Patient should remain lying down after IM inj for at least 30 min

IV route

- Give undiluted for psychotic episode at 5 mg/min
- Give by intermittent inf after dilution in 30-50 ml of D_5W, run over ½ hr

Syringe compatibilities: Hydromorphone, sufentanil

Y-site compatibilities: Amifostine, amsacrine, aztreonam, cimetidine, cisatracurium, cladribine, DOBUTamine, DOPamine, DOXOrubicin liposome, famotidine, filgrastim, fludarabine, granisetron, lidocaine, lorazepam, melphalan, midazolam, nitroglycerin, norepinephrine, ondansetron, paclitaxel, phenylephrine, propofol, remifentanil, sufentanil, tacrolimus, teniposide, theophylline, thiotepa, vinorelbine

Y-site incompatibilities: Fluconazole, foscarnet, heparin, sargramostim

Patient/family education

- Teach patient to use good oral hygiene; use frequent rinsing of mouth, sugarless gum for dry mouth, oral candidiasis may occur
- Advise patient to avoid hazardous activities until drug response is determined; dizziness, blurred vision are common
- Inform patient that orthostatic hypotension occurs often and to rise from sitting or lying position gradually; tell patient to avoid hot tubs, hot showers, tub baths, since hypotension may occur; tell patient that in hot weather heat stroke may occur; take extra precautions to stay cool
- Instruct patient to avoid abrupt withdrawal of this drug, or EPS may result; drug should be withdrawn slowly
- Caution patient to avoid OTC preparations (cough, hay fever, cold) unless approved by prescriber, since serious drug interactions may occur; avoid use with alcohol, CNS depressants since increased drowsiness may occur
- Advise patient to use a sunscreen and sunglasses to prevent burns
- Instruct patient to take antacids 2 hr before or after this drug
- Tell patient to report sore throat, malaise, fever, bleeding, mouth sores; if these occur, CBC should be obtained and drug discontinued

Evaluation

Positive therapeutic outcome

- Decrease in emotional excitement, hallucinations, delusions, paranoia, reorganization of patterns of thought, speech; improvement in specific behaviors

Treatment of overdose: Lavage if orally ingested; provide airway; *do not induce vomiting*

! HIGH ALERT

heparin (Rx)

(hep'a-rin)

Calcilean ✤, Calciparine, Hepalean ✤, heparin sodium, Heparin Leo ✤, Hep-Lock, Hep-Lock U/P

Func. class.: Anticoagulant, antithrombotic

Pregnancy category C

Do Not Confuse:

heparin/Hespan

Action: Prevents conversion of fibrinogen to fibrin and prothrombin to thrombin by enhancing inhibitory effects of antithrombin III

Therapeutic Outcome: Prevention of thrombi

Uses: Prevention of deep vein thrombosis (DVT) and pulmonary emboli (PE) (treatment and prevention), MI, open heart surgery, disseminated intravascular clotting syndrome, atrial fibrillation with embolization, as an anticoagulant in transfusion and dialysis procedures, prevention of DVT/PE, to maintain patency of indwelling venipuncture devices, diagnosis, treatment of disseminated intravascular coagulation (DIC)

Dosage and routes

DVT/MI

Adult: **IV** bol 5000-7000 units q4h then titrated to PTT or activated coagulation time (ACT) level; **IV** inf after bol dose, then 1000 units/hr titrated to PTT or ACT level

Child: **IV** inf 50 units/kg, maintenance 100 units/kg q4h or 20,000 units/m^2 daily

Anticoagulation

Adult: SUBCUT 500 units **IV** then 10,000-20,000 units, then 8,000-10,000 units 8qh or 15,000-20,000 units q12h

Pulmonary embolism

Adult: **IV** bol 7500-10,000 units q4h then titrated to PTT or ACT level; **IV** inf after bol dose, then 1000 units/hr titrated to PTT or ACT level

Child: **IV** inf 50 units/kg; maintenance 100 units/kg q4h or 20,000 units/m^2 daily

CV surgery

Adult: **IV** inf 150-300 units/kg

Prophylaxis for DVT/PE

Adult: SUBCUT 5000 units q8-12h

Heparin flush

Adult/child: **IV** 10-100 units

Available forms: Carpuject (sodium) 5000 units/ml; disposable inj 1000, 2500,

5000, 7500, 10,000, 15,000, 20,000, 40,000 units/ml; unit dose 1000, 5000, 10,000, 20,000, 40,000 units/ml; vials 1000, 2000, 2500, 5000, 7500, 10,000, 20,000, 40,000 units/ml; flush, disposable syringes 10, 100 units/ml; vials, 100 units/ml; ca inj: 5000 units/0.2 ml; ampules 12,500 units/0.5 ml; 20,000 units/0.8 ml

Adverse effects

CNS: *Fever,* chills
GU: **Hematuria**
HEMA: **Hemorrhage, thrombocytopenia, anemia**
INTEG: *Rash,* dermatitis, urticaria, pruritus, delayed transient alopecia, hematoma, cutaneous necrosis (SUBCUT)
SYST: **Anaphylaxis**

Contraindications: Hypersensitivity, hemophilia, leukemia with bleeding, peptic ulcer disease, severe thrombocytopenic purpura, hepatic disease (severe), renal disease (severe), blood dyscrasias, severe hypertension, subacute bacterial endocarditis, acute nephritis

Precautions: Pregnancy **C**, alcoholism, elderly, children, hyperlipidemia, diabetes, renal disease

Pharmacokinetics

Absorption	Well absorbed (SUBCUT)
Distribution	Unknown
Metabolism	Partially in kidney, liver
Excretion	Lymph, spleen, in urine (<50% unchanged)
Half-life	1½ hr

Pharmacodynamics

	SUBCUT	IV
Onset	½-1 hr	5 min
Peak	2 hr	10 min
Duration	8-12 hr	2-6 hr

Interactions

Individual drugs

Dextran, dipyridole, ticlopidine: increased action of heparin
Diazepam: increased action of diazepam
Digitalis: decreased action of heparin
Streptokinase: resistance to heparin

Drug classifications

Anticoagulants (oral), cephalosporins, NSAIDs, penicillins, platelet inhibitors, salicylates: increased action of heparin
Antihistamines, tetracyclines: decreased action of heparin
Corticosteroids: decreased action of corticosteroids

Drug/herb

Agrimony, alfalfa, angelica, anise, basil, bay, bilberry, black haw, bogbean, bromelain, buchu, chondroitin, cinchona bark, dong quai, fenugreek, feverfew, garlic, ginger, ginkgo, ginseng, horse chestnut, Irish moss, kelp, kelpware, khella, lovage, lungwort, meadowsweet, motherwort, mugwort, nettle, papaya, parsley (large amounts), pau d'arco, pineapple, poplar, prickly ash, safflower, saw palmetto, tonka bean, turmeric, wintergreen, yarrow: increased risk of bleeding
Chamomile, coenzyme Q10, flax, glucomannan, goldenseal, guar gum: decreased anticoagulant effect

Drug/lab test

Increased: ALT, AST, INR, PT, PTT
Decreased: platelets

H

NURSING CONSIDERATIONS

Assessment

- Assess for blood studies (Hct, occult blood in stools) q3 mo if patient is on long-term therapy
- Monitor PPT, which should be 1½-2 × control, PTT; often done daily, APTT, ACT
- Monitor platelet count q2-3 days; thrombocytopenia may occur on 4th day of treatment and resolve, or continue to 8th day of treatment
- ❗ Assess for bleeding gums, petechiae, ecchymosis, black tarry stools, hematuria, epistaxis, decrease in Hct, B/P; may indicate bleeding and possible hemorrhage; notify prescriber immediately
- Monitor for hypersensitivity: fever, skin rash, urticaria; notify prescriber immediately

Nursing diagnoses

- Injury, risk for (uses, adverse reactions)
- Tissue perfusion, ineffective (uses)
- Knowledge, deficient (teaching)

Implementation

SUBCUT route

- Give SUBCUT with at least 25-G ⅜-in needle; do not massage area or aspirate fluid when giving SUBCUT inj; give in abdomen between pelvic bones, rotate sites; do not pull back on plunger, leave in for 10 sec; apply gentle pressure for 1 min
- Give at same time each day to maintain steady blood levels
- Changing needles is not recommended

Heparin lock route

- Inject 10-100 units/0.5-1 ml after each inf or q8-12h

IV route

- Cannot be used interchangeably (unit for unit) with LMWHs or heparinoids
- Give directly; **IV** loading dose over 1 min
- Give **IV** diluted in 0.9% NaCl, dextrose, Ringer's and by intermittent or cont inf; inf may run from 4-24 hr; use infusion pump
- When drug is added to inf sol for cont **IV**, invert container at least 6× to ensure adequate mixing

Syringe compatibilities: Aminophylline, amphotericin B, ampicillin, atropine, azlocillin, bleomycin, cefamandole, cefazolin, cefoperazone, cefotaxime, cefoxitin, chloramphenicol, cimetidine, cisplatin, clindamycin, cyclophosphamide, diazoxide, digoxin, dimenhyDRINATE, DOBUTamine, DOPamine, epINEPHrine, fentanyl, fluorouracil, furosemide, leucovorin, lidocaine, lincomycin, methotrexate, metoclopramide, mezlocillin, mitomycin, moxalactam, nafcillin, naloxone, neostigmine, nitroglycerin, norepinephrine, pancuronium, penicillin G, phenobarbital, piperacillin, sodium nitroprusside, succinylcholine, trimethoprim-sulfamethoxazole, verapamil, vinCRIStine

Y-site compatibilities: Acyclovir, aldesleukin, allopurinol, amifostine, aminophylline, ampicillin, ampicillin/sulbactam, atracurium, atropine, aztreonam, betamethasone, bleomycin, calcium gluconate, cefazolin, cefotetan, ceftazidime, ceftriaxone, cephalothin, cephapirin, chlordiazepoxide, chlorproMAZINE, cimetidine, cisplatin, cladribine, clindamycin, conjugated estrogens, cyanocobalamin, cyclophosphamide, cytarabine, dexamethasone, digoxin, diphenhydrAMINE, DOPamine, DOXOrubicin liposome, edrophonium, enalaprilat, epINEPHrine, erythromycin, esmolol, ethacrynate, famotidine, fentanyl, fluconazole, fludarabine, fluorouracil, foscarnet, furosemide, gallium, granisetron, hydrALAZINE, hydrocortisone, hydromorphone, regular insulin, isoproterenol, kanamycin, leucovorin, lidocaine, lorazepam, magnesium sulfate, melphalan, menadiol sodium, meperidine, meropenem, methicillin, methotrexate, methoxamine, methyldopate, methylergonovine, metoclopramide, metronidazole, midazolam, milrinone, minocycline, mitomycin, morphine, nafcillin, neostigmine, nitroglycerin, nitroprusside, norepinephrine, ondansetron, oxacillin, oxytocin, paclitaxel, pancuronium, penicillin G potassium, pentazocine, phytonadione, piperacillin, piperacillin/tazobactam, propofol, potassium chloride, prednisoLONE, procainamide, prochlorperazine, propofol, propranolol, pyridostigmine, ranitidine, remifentanil, sargramostim, scopolamine, sodium bicarbonate, streptokinase, succinylcholine, tacrolimus, teniposide, theophylline, thiopental, thiotepa, ticarcillin, ticarcillin/clavulanate, trimethobenzamide, vecuronium, vinBLAStine, vinorelbine, warfarin, zidovudine

Y-site incompatibilities: Alteplase, ciprofloxacin, dacarbazine, diazepam, DOBUTamine, DOXOrubicin, ergotamine, gentamicin, haloperidol, idarubicin, methotrimeprazine, phenytoin, promethazine, tobramycin, triflupromazine

Additive compatibilities: Aminophylline, amphotericin, ascorbic acid, bleomycin, calcium gluconate, cefepime, cephapirin, chloramphenicol, clindamycin, colistimethate, dimenhyDRINATE, doxacillin, DOPamine, enalaprilat, erythromycin, esmolol, floxacillin, fluconazole, flumazenil, furosemide, hydrocortisone, isoproterenol, lidocaine, lincomycin, magnesium sulfate, meropenem, methyldopate, methylPREDNISolone, metronidazole/sodium bicarbonate, nafcillin, norepinephrine, octreotide, penicillin G, potassium chloride, prednisoLONE, promazine, ranitidine, sodium bicarbonate, verapamil, vit B complex, vit B complex with C

Additive incompatibilities: Amikacin, erythromycin lactobionate, gentamicin, kanamycin, meperidine, methadone, morphine, polymyxin B, streptomycin

Patient/family education

- Advise patient to avoid OTC preparations that may cause serious drug interactions unless directed by prescriber; may contain aspirin or other anticoagulants
- Tell patient that drug may be held during active bleeding (menstruation), depending on condition
- Caution patient to use soft-bristle toothbrush to avoid bleeding gums; avoid contact sports; use electric razor; avoid IM inj
- Instruct patient to carry/wear emergency ID or other identification identifying drug taken and condition treated
- Advise patient to report any signs of bleeding: gums, under skin, urine, stools; or unusual bruising

Evaluation

Positive therapeutic outcome

- Decrease of DVT
- PTT of 1.5-2.5 × control
- Free-flowing **IV**

Treatment of overdose: Withdraw drug, give protamine sulfate 1 mg protamine/100 units heparin

hepatitis B immune globulin (Rx)

(hep-a-tite'iss)

BayHep B, Nabi-HB

Func. class.: Immune globulin

Pregnancy category C

Action: Provides passive immunity to hepatitis B

Therapeutic Outcome: Passive immunity to hepatitis B

Uses: Prevention of hepatitis B virus in exposed patients, including passive immunity in neonates born to HBsAg-positive mothers

Dosage and routes

Acute exposure to blood with HBsAg

Adult: 2 doses, given after exposure and 1 mo later

Perinatal exposure of infants born to HBsAg-positive mothers

Infant: 1 dose at birth, then start hepatitis B vaccine series soon after birth

Sexual exposure to HBsAg

Adult: Administer 1 dose within 2 wk of exposure

Available forms: Sol for inj (Bay Hep B): 15%-18% protein; sol for inj (Nabi-HB): 5% ± 1% protein

Adverse effects

CNS: Headache, dizziness, fever

INTEG: Soreness at inj site, urticaria, erythema, swelling

SYST: Induration, **anaphylaxis, angioedema**

Contraindications: Hypersensitivity to immune globulins, coagulation disorders

Precautions: Pregnancy **C,** hemophilia, elderly, lactation, children, active infection, IgA deficiency

Pharmacokinetics

Absorption	Slowly absorbed
Distribution	Unknown
Metabolism	Unknown
Excretion	Unknown
Half-life	3 wk

Pharmacodynamics

Onset	1-7 days
Peak	3-10 days
Duration	2-6 mo

Interactions

Drug classifications

MMR, varicella, rotavirus vaccines: do not use within 3 mo of hepatitis B immune globulin

NURSING CONSIDERATIONS

Assessment

- Assess for history of allergies, skin conditions (eczema, psoriasis, dermatitis), reactions to vaccinations
- Assess for skin reactions: rash, induration, urticaria
- Assess for sneezing, pruritus, angioedema, dysphagia, vomiting, abdominal pain
- Assess for anaphylaxis: inability to breathe, bronchospasm, hypotension, wheezing, diaphoresis, fever, flushing; epINEPHrine and emergency equipment should be available

Nursing diagnoses

- Infection, risk for (uses)
- Knowledge, deficient (teaching)

Implementation

- Give after rotating vial; do not shake
- Give in deltoid (adult) or anterolateral thigh for better protection; give 2-ml dose in two different sites; do not give **IV**
- Refrigerate unused portion; sol should be clear, light amber, and thick

Patient/family education

- Teach patient purpose of medication and expected results
- Give patient a list of adverse reactions that need to be reported immediately: wheezing, vomiting, sneezing, abdominal pain, sweating, tightness in chest
- Advise patient that pain, rash, swelling at inj site can be expected
- Give patient written record of immunization

Evaluation

Positive therapeutic outcome

- Prevention of hepatitis B

hetastarch (Rx)

(het'a-starch)

Hespan

Func. class.: Plasma expander

Chem. class.: Synthetic polymer

Pregnancy category C

Do Not Confuse:
Hespan/heparin

Action: Similar to human albumin, which expands plasma volume by colloidal osmotic pressure

Therapeutic Outcome: Increased plasma volume

Uses: Plasma volume expander for sepsis, trauma, burns, leukapheresis

Dosage and routes

Adult: **IV** inf 500-1000 ml (30-60 g); total dose not to exceed 1500 ml/day, not to exceed 20 ml/kg/hr (hemorrhagic shock)

Leukapheresis

Adult: **IV** inf 250-700 ml infused at 1:8 ratio with whole blood; may be repeated twice weekly up to 10 treatments

Renal dose

Adult: CCr <10 ml/min give initial dose, but reduce subsequent doses by 25%-50%

Available forms: 6% hetastarch/0.9% NaCl (6 g/100 ml)

Adverse effects

CNS: Headache
EENT: Periorbital edema
GI: Nausea, vomiting
HEMA: Decreased hematocrit, platelet function, increased bleeding/coagulation times, increased erythrocyte sedimentation rate
INTEG: Rash, urticaria, pruritus, chills, fever, flushing, peripheral edema
RESP: Wheezing, dyspnea, **bronchospasm, pulmonary edema**
SYST: **Anaphylaxis, angioedema**

Contraindications: Hypersensitivity, severe bleeding disorders, renal failure, CHF (severe), anuria, oliguria, intracranial bleeding

Precautions: Pregnancy **C**, liver disease, pulmonary edema

Pharmacokinetics	
Absorption	Completely absorbed
Distribution	Unknown
Metabolism	Degraded
Excretion	Kidneys, unchanged
Half-life	17 days (90%); 48 days (10%)

Pharmacodynamics	
Onset	Immediate
Peak	Infusion's end
Duration	Over 24 hr

Interactions

Individual drugs

Fludrocortisone: increased sodium, water retention

Drug/lab test

False increase: bilirubin

NURSING CONSIDERATIONS

Assessment

- Monitor VS q5 min for 30 min; CVP during inf (5-10 cm H_2O normal range); PCWP; urine output q1h: watch for increase, which is common; if output does not increase, inf should be decreased or discontinued
- Monitor CBC with differential, Hgb, Hct, protime, PTT, platelet count, clotting time during treatment; treatment may increase clotting time, PTT, protime, sedimentary rates, Hct may drop due to increased volume and hemodilution; do not allow Hct to be <30% by volume
- Monitor I&O ratio and specific gravity, urine osmolarity; if sp gr is very low, renal clearance is low; drug should be discontinued
- Assess for allergy: rash, urticaria, pruritus, wheezing, dyspnea, bronchospasm; drug should be discontinued immediately
- (Alert) Assess for circulatory overload: increased pulse, respirations, dyspnea, wheezing, chest tightness, chest pain, increased CVP, jugular vein distention
- Assess for dehydration after inf; decreased output, increased temp, poor skin turgor, increased sp gr, dry skin

Nursing diagnoses

- Fluid volume, deficient (uses)
- Tissue perfusion, ineffective (uses)
- Fluid volume, excess (adverse reactions)
- Knowledge, deficient (teaching)

Implementation

- Give by **IV** cont inf, undiluted, run at 20 ml/kg/hr; reduced rate in septic shock, burns; rate is calculated by blood volume and response of patient
- Give up to 20 ml kg (1.2 g/ kg)/hr
- Store at room temp; discard unused portions; do not freeze; do not use if turbid or deep brown or precipitate forms

Y-site compatibilities: Cimetidine, diltiazem, doxycycline, enalaprilat
Y-site incompatibilities: Amikacin, cefamandole, cefoperazone, cefotaxime, cefoxitin, gentamicin, theophylline, tobramycin
Additive compatibilities: Cloxacillin, fosphenytoin

Patient/family education

- Teach patient the reason for administration and expected results
- Advise patient to notify prescriber if flulike symptoms or allergic symptoms occur

Evaluation

Positive therapeutic outcome

- Increased plasma volume as evidenced by higher B/P, blood volume, output

hydrALAZINE (Rx)

(hye-dral'a-zeen)

Alazine, Apresoline, Novo-Hylazin ♣, hydrALAZINE HCl, Pralzine, Rolzine, Supres ♣

Func. class.: Antihypertensive, direct-acting peripheral vasodilator

Chem. class.: Phthalazine

Pregnancy category C

Do Not Confuse:

Apresoline/allopurinol

hydrALAZINE/hydrOXYzine

Action: Vasodilates arterioles in smooth muscle by direct relaxation; reduces B/P with reflex increases in heart rate, stroke volume, cardiac output

Therapeutic Outcome: Decreased B/P in hypertension, decreased afterload in CHF

Uses: Essential hypertension, severe essential hypertension, CHF

Investigational uses: CHF

Dosage and routes

Hypertension

Adult: PO 10 mg qid 2-4 days, then 25 mg for rest of 1st wk, then 50 mg qid individualized to desired response, not to exceed 300 mg daily

Child: PO 0.75-3 mg/kg/day in 4 divided doses; max 7.5 mg/kg/24 hr

Hypertensive crisis

Adult: **IV**/IM bol 20-40 mg q4-6h; administer PO as soon as possible; IM 20-40 mg q4-6h

Child: **IV** bol 0.1-0.2 mg/kg q4-6h; IM 0.1-0.2 mg/kg q4-6h

CHF

Adult: PO 10-25 mg bid, max 75 mg tid

Available forms: Inj 20 mg/ml; tabs 10, 25, 50, 100 mg

Adverse effects

CNS: *Headache, tremors, dizziness, anxiety,* peripheral neuritis, depression, fever, chills

CV: *Palpitations, reflex tachycardia, angina,* **shock,** rebound hypertension

GI: *Nausea, vomiting, anorexia, diarrhea,* constipation, paralytic ileus

GU: Urinary retention

HEMA: **Leukopenia, agranulocytosis,** anemia, **thrombocytopenia**

INTEG: Rash, pruritus, urticaria

MISC: Nasal congestion, muscle cramps, *lupuslike symptoms,* flushing, edema, dyspnea

Contraindications: Hypersensitivity to hydrALAZINEs, CAD, mitral valvular rheumatic heart disease

Precautions: Pregnancy **C,** CVA, advanced renal disease, elderly, lactation

Pharmacokinetics

Absorption	Rapidly absorbed (PO); well absorbed (IM); completely absorbed (**IV**)
Distribution	Widely distributed; crosses placenta
Metabolism	GI mucosa, liver extensively
Excretion	Kidneys, urine (12%-14%)
Half-life	2-8 hr

Pharmacodynamics

	PO	IM	IV
Onset	½ hr	10-30 min	5-20 min
Peak	1-2 hr	1 hr	10-80 min
Duration	6-12 hr	4-6 hr	4-6 hr

Interactions

Individual drugs

Indomethacin: decreased effects of hydrALAZINE

Drug classifications

MAOIs: severe hypotension

β-Adrenergic blockers: increased effects

Sympathomimetics (epinephrine, norepinephrine): increased tachycardia, angina

Drug/herb

Aconite: increased toxicity, death

Astragalus, cola tree: increased or decreased antihypertensive effect

Barberry, betony, black catechu, black cohosh, bloodroot, broom, burdock, cat's claw, dandelion, goldenseal, Irish moss, Jamaican dogwood, kelp, khella, mistletoe, parsley: increased antihypertensive effect

Coltsfoot, guarana, khat, licorice: decreased antihypertensive effect

NURSING CONSIDERATIONS

Assessment

- Assess B/P q5 min for 2 hr, then q1h for 2 hr, then q4h; pulse, jugular venous distention q4h
- Monitor electrolytes, blood studies: potassium, sodium, chloride, carbon dioxide, CBC,

serum glucose; LE prep, ANA titer before starting treatment
- Monitor weight daily, I&O; edema in feet, legs daily; check skin turgor, dryness of mucous membranes for hydration status
- Assess for crackles, dyspnea, orthopnea; peripheral edema, fatigue, weight gain, jugular vein distention (CHF)
- For fever, joint pain, rash, sore throat (lupuslike symptoms), notify prescriber

Nursing diagnoses
- Cardiac output, decreased (adverse reactions)
- Injury, risk for (side effects)
- Knowledge, deficient (teaching)

Implementation
PO route
- Give with meals to enhance absorption
- Store protected from light and heat

IV route
- Give by **IV** undiluted through Y-tube or 3-way stopcock, give ≤10 mg/min
- Administer with patient in recumbent position; keep in that position for 1 hr after administration

Y-site compatibilities: Heparin, hydrocortisone, potassium chloride, verapamil, vit B/C

Y-site incompatibilities: Aminophylline, ampicillin, diazoxide, furosemide, paclitaxel

Additive incompatibilities: Aminophylline, ampicillin, chlorothiazide, edetate calcium disodium, ethacrynate, hydrocortisone, melphalan, mephentermine, methohexital, nitroglycerin, phenobarbital, verapamil, vinorelbine

Additive compatibilities: DOBUTamine

Patient/family education
- Teach patient to take with food to increase bioavailability (PO)
- Teach patient to avoid OTC preparations unless directed by prescriber
- Advise patient to notify prescriber if chest pain, severe fatigue, fever, muscle or joint pain occur
- Advise patient to rise slowly to prevent orthostatic hypertension
- Advise patient to notify prescriber if pregnancy is suspected

Evaluation
Positive therapeutic outcome
- Decreased B/P in hypertension

Treatment of overdose: Administer vasopressors, volume expanders for shock; if PO, lavage or give activated charcoal, digitalization

hydrochlorothiazide
🔑 (Rx)

(hye-droe-klor-oh-thye′a-zide)

Apo-Hydrol ✤, HCTZ, Esidrix, Hydro-Chlor, hydrochlorothiazide, HydroDIURIL, Microzide, Neo-Codema ✤, Novohydrazide ✤, Oretic, Urozide ✤

Func. class: Diuretic, antihypertensive

Chem. class: Thiazide, sulfonamide derivative

Pregnancy category B

Action: Acts on the distal tubule in the kidney, increasing excretion of sodium, water, chloride, magnesium, potassium, and bicarbonate

Therapeutic Outcome: Decreased B/P, decreased edema in lung tissues peripherally

Uses: Edema in CHF, nephrotic syndrome; edema in corticosteroid, NSAID therapy; idiopathic lower extremity edema; may be used alone or as adjunct with antihypertensives

Dosage and routes
Adult: PO 25-200 mg/day

Elderly: PO 12.5 mg/day, initially

Child >6 mo: PO 2 mg/kg/day

Child <6 mo: PO up to 4 mg/kg/day in divided doses

Available forms: Tabs 25, 50, 100 mg; caps 12.5 mg; oral sol 10 mg/5 ml, 100 mg/ml

Adverse effects
CNS: Drowsiness, paresthesia, depression, headache, *dizziness, fatigue, weakness,* fever

CV: Irregular pulse, orthostatic hypotension, palpitations, volume depletion, allergic myocarditis

EENT: Blurred vision

ELECT: *Hypokalemia,* hypercalcemia, hyponatremia, hypochloremia, hypomagnesemia

GI: *Nausea, vomiting, anorexia,* constipation, diarrhea, cramps, pancreatitis, GI irritation, **hepatitis**

GU: *Frequency,* polyuria, **uremia,** glucosuria, hyperuricemia

HEMA: **Aplastic anemia, hemolytic anemia, leukopenia, agranulocytosis, thrombocytopenia, neutropenia**

INTEG: *Rash,* urticaria, purpura, photosensitivity, alopecia, erythema multiforme

META: *Hyperglycemia, hyperuricemia,* increased creatinine, BUN

Contraindications: Hypersensitivity to thiazides or sulfonamides, anuria, renal decompensation, hypomagnesemia

Precautions: Pregnancy **B,** hypokalemia, renal disease, hepatic disease, gout, COPD, lupus erythematosus, diabetes mellitus, hyperlipidemia, CCr <25 ml/min, lactation

Pharmacokinetics

	PO
Absorption	Variable
Distribution	Extracellular spaces; crosses placenta
Metabolism	Excreted unchanged in urine
Excretion	Breast milk
Half-life	6-15 hr

Pharmacodynamics

Onset	2 hr
Peak	4 hr
Duration	6-12 hr

Interactions

Individual drugs

Amphotericin B: increased hypokalemia
Cholestyramine, colestipol: decreased absorption of hydrochlorothiazide
Diazoxide: increased hyperglycemia, hyperuricemia, hypotension
Lithium: increased toxicity

Drug classifications

Antidiabetics: decreased effect of antidiabetic agent
Cardiac glycosides, nondepolarizing skeletal muscle relaxants: increased toxicity
Diuretics (loop): increased effects of diuretic
Glucocorticoids: increased hypokalemia
NSAIDs: increased risk of renal failure

Drug/herb

Aloe, buckthorn, cascara sagrada, Chinese rhubarb, gossypol, licorice, nettle, senna: increased hypokalemia
Cucumber, dandelion, ginkgo, horsetail, khella, licorice, nettle, pumpkin, Queen Anne's lace: increased effect
St. John's wort: severe photosensitivity

Drug/lab test

Increased: BSP retention, amylase, parathyroid test
Decreased: PBI, PSP

NURSING CONSIDERATIONS

Assessment

- Monitor glucose in urine if patient is diabetic
- Assess improvement in CVP q8h
- Check for rashes, temp elevation daily
- Assess for confusion, especially in elderly; take safety precautions if needed
- Monitor manifestations of hypokalemia: acidic urine, reduced urine, osmolality, nocturia; hypotension, broad T wave, U wave, ectopy, tachycardia, weak pulse; muscle weakness, altered LOC, drowsiness, apathy, lethargy, confusion, depression; anorexia, nausea, cramps, constipation, distention, paralytic ileus; hypoventilation, respiratory muscle weakness
- Monitor for manifestations of hypomagnesemia: agitation, muscle twitching, paresthesias, hyperactive reflexes, positive Babinski reflex, dysphagia, nystagmus seizures, tetany; nausea, vomiting, diarrhea, anorexia, abdominal distention; ectopy, tachycardia, broad, flat, or inverted T waves, depressed ST segment, prolonged QT interval, decreased cardiac output, hypotension
- Monitor for manifestations of hyponatremia: increased B/P, cold, clammy skin, hypovolemia or hypervolemia; anorexia, nausea, vomiting, diarrhea, abdominal cramps; lethargy, increased ICP, confusion, headache, seizures, coma, fatigue, tremors, hyperreflexia
- Monitor for manifestations of hyperchloremia: weakness, lethargy, coma, deep rapid breathing
- Assess fluid volume status: I&O ratios, record, count, or weigh diapers as appropriate, weight, distended red veins, crackles in lungs, color, quality, and sp gr of urine, skin turgor, adequacy of pulses, moist mucous membranes, bilateral lung sounds, peripheral pitting edema; assess for dehydration: symptoms of decreasing output, thirst, hypotension; dry mouth and mucous membranes should be reported
- Monitor electrolytes: potassium, sodium, calcium, magnesium; also include BUN, blood pH, ABGs, uric acid, CBC, blood glucose, renal function
- Assess B/P before and during therapy with patient lying, standing, and sitting as appropriate; orthostatic hypotension can occur rapidly

Nursing diagnoses

- Urinary elimination, impaired (side effect)
- Fluid volume, deficient (side effects)
- Fluid volume, excess (uses)
- Knowledge, deficient (teaching)

Implementation

- Give in AM to avoid interference with sleep
- Provide potassium replacement if potassium level is ≤3.0 mg/dl; give whole tab or use oral

H

sol lightly; drug may be crushed if patient is unable to swallow
- Administer with food; if nausea occurs, absorption may be increased

Patient/family education
- Teach patient to take the medication early in the day to prevent nocturia
- Instruct patient to take with food or milk if GI symptoms of nausea and anorexia occur
- Teach patient to maintain a weekly record of weight and notify prescriber of weight loss >5 lb
- Caution patient that this drug causes a loss of potassium and that food rich in potassium should be added to the diet; refer to a dietitian for assistance in planning
- Caution patient to rise slowly from sitting or reclining positions, not to exercise in hot weather or stand for prolonged periods since orthostatic hypotension will be enhanced; lie down if dizziness occurs
- Teach patient not to use alcohol or any OTC medications without prescriber's approval; serious drug reactions may occur
- Emphasize the need to contact prescriber immediately if muscle cramps, weakness, nausea, dizziness, or numbness occurs
- Teach patient to take own B/P and pulse and record findings
- Teach patient to continue taking medication even if feeling better; this drug controls symptoms but does not cure the condition
- Advise patient with hypertension to continue other medical treatment (exercise, weight loss, relaxation techniques, cessation of smoking)

Evaluation
Positive therapeutic outcome
- Decreased edema
- Decreased B/P
- Increased diuresis

Treatment of overdose: Lavage if taken orally, monitor electrolytes, administer dextrose in saline, monitor hydration, CV, renal status

hydrocodone (Rx)
(hye-droe-koe'done)
Hycodan ✤, Robidone ✤, Tussigon

hydrocodone/ acetaminophen
Allay, Anexsia, Anolor DH, Bancap HC, Co-Gesic, Dolacet, Dolagesic, Duocet, Hycomed, Hyco-Pap, Hydracet, Hydrogesic, Lorcet, Lortab, Onset, Pancet, Panlor, Polygesic, Stagesic, T-Gesic, Ugesic, Vanacet, Vandone, Vicodin, Zydone

hydrocodone/aspirin
Azdone, Damason-P, Lortab ASA, Panasol

hyprocodone/ibuprofen
Vicoprofen

Func. class.: Antitussive opioid analgesic, nonopioid analgesic

Pregnancy category C

Controlled substance schedule III

Do Not Confuse:
Hycodan/Vicodin, hydrocodone/ hydrocortisone

Action: Acts directly on cough center in medulla to suppress cough; binds to opiate receptors in the CNS to reduce pain

Therapeutic Outcome: Pain relief, decreased cough, decreased diarrhea

Uses: Hyperactive and nonproductive cough, mild pain

Dosages and routes
Analgesic
Adult: PO 2.5-10 mg q3-6h prn
Child: PO 0.15-0.2 mg/kg q3-6h prn

Antitussive
Adult: PO 5 mg q4-6h prn

Available forms: Hydrocodone: tabs 5 mg (Hycodan); syr 5 mg/ml (Hycodan, Robidone ✤; hydrocodone/acetaminophen: tabs 2.5 mg hydrocodone/500 mg acetaminophen (Lortabs 2.5/500), 5 mg hydrocodone/ 400 mg acetaminophen (Zydone), 5 mg hydrocodone/500 mg acetaminophen (Anexsia 5/500, Co-Gesic, Dolacet, Hydrocet, Hydrogesic, Hy-Phen, Loracet, Loratab 5/500, Maragesic-H, Panacet 5/500, Stagesic, T-Gesic, Vicodin); 7.5 mg hydrocodone/400 mg acetaminophen (Zydone), 7.5 mg hydrocodone/ 500 mg acetaminophen (Loratab 7.5/500, 7.5 mg hydrocodone/650 mg acetaminophen (Anexsia 7.5/650, Loracet Plus), 7.5 mg hydrocodone/750 mg acetaminophen (Vicodin ES), 10 mg hydrocodone/325 mg acetaminophen (Norco), 10 mg hydrocodone/500 mg acetaminophen (Lortab 10/500), 10 mg hydrocodone/650 mg acetaminophen (Loracet 10/650, Vicodin HP), 10 mg hydrocodone/660 acetaminophen (Anexia 10/660); caps 5 mg hydrocodone/500 mg acetaminophen (Bancap-HC, Dolacet, Hydrocet, Hydrogesic, Loracet-HD, Maragesic-H, Stragesic, T-Gesic, Zydone); elixir or oral solution 2.5 mg hydrocodone/167 mg acetaminophen/5 ml; hydrocodone/aspirin: tabs 5 mg hydrocodone/500 mg aspirin (Alor 5/500, Azdone, Damason-P, Loratab ASA, Panasal 5/500); hydrocodone/ibuprofen: tabs 7.5 mg hydrocodone/200 mg ibuprofen (Vicoprofen)

Adverse effects

CNS: *Drowsiness,* dizziness, lightheadedness, confusion, headache, sedation, euphoria, dysphoria, weakness, hallucinations, disorientation, mood changes, dependence, **seizures**
CV: Palpitations, tachycardia, bradycardia, change in B/P, **circulatory depression,** syncope
EENT: Tinnitus, blurred vision, miosis, diplopia
GI: *Nausea, vomiting, anorexia, constipation,* cramps, dry mouth
GU: Increased urinary output, dysuria, urinary retention
INTEG: Rash, urticaria, flushing, pruritus
RESP: **Respiratory depression**

Contraindications: Hypersensitivity, addiction (opioid)

Precautions: Pregnancy **C**, addictive personality, lactation, increased ICP, MI (acute), severe heart disease, respiratory depression, hepatic disease, renal disease

Pharmacokinetics

Absorption	Well absorbed
Distribution	Unknown; crosses placenta
Metabolism	Liver, extensively
Excretion	Kidneys
Half-life	3½-4½ hr

Pharmacodynamics

	PO **(analgesic)**	PO **(antitussive)**
Onset	10-20 min	Unknown
Peak	30-60 min	Unknown
Duration	4-6 hr	4-6 hr

Interactions

Individual drugs

Alcohol: increased CNS depression

Drug classifications

Antidepressants (tricyclic), CNS depressants, general anesthetics, opioids, phenothiazines, sedative/hypnotics, skeletal muscle relaxants: increased CNS depression
Tricyclics: increased CNS depression

Drug/herb

Corkwood: increased anticholinergic effect
Jamacian dogwood, lavender, mistletoe, nettle, pokeweed, poppy, senega, valerian: increased CNS depression

Drug/lab test

Increased: amylase, lipase

NURSING CONSIDERATIONS

Assessment

- Assess pain: intensity, type, location, duration, precipitating factor
- Monitor VS after parenteral route; note muscle rigidity, drug history, liver, kidney function tests, cough, and respiratory dysfunction: respiratory depression, character, rate, rhythm; notify prescriber if respirations are <10/min
- Monitor CNS changes: dizziness, drowsiness, hallucinations, euphoria, LOC, pupil reaction
- Monitor allergic reactions: rash, urticaria

Nursing diagnoses

- Pain, acute (uses)
- Sensory perception, disturbed: visual, auditory (adverse reactions)
- Breathing pattern, ineffective (adverse reactions)
- Knowledge, deficient (teaching)

Implementation

- Do not break, crush, or chew tabs; only scored tabs can be broken
- Give with antiemetic if nausea, vomiting occur
- Give when pain is beginning to return; determine dosage interval by patient response; continuous dosing of medication is more effective given prn
- Medication should be slowly withdrawn after long-term use to prevent withdrawal symptoms
- Store in light-resistant container at room temp
- May be given with food or milk to lessen GI upset

Patient/family education

- Instruct patient to report any symptoms of CNS changes, allergic reactions; to avoid CNS depressants: alcohol, sedative/hypnotics for at least 24 hr after taking this drug
- Teach patient that dizziness, drowsiness, and confusion are common and to avoid getting up without assistance, driving, or other hazardous activities
- Discuss in detail all aspects of the drug

H

Evaluation
Positive therapeutic outcome
- Decreased pain
- Decreased cough

Treatment of overdose: Naloxone HCl (Narcan) 0.2-0.8 **IV**, O_2, **IV** fluids, vasopressors

hydrocortisone (Rx)
(hy-droh-kor'tih-sone)
Cortef, Cortenema, Hydrocortone
hydrocortisone acetate (Rx)
Cortifoam, Hydrocortone Acetate
hydrocortisone cypionate (Rx)
Cortef
hydrocortisone sodium phosphate (Rx)
Hydrocortone Phosphate
hydrocortisone sodium succinate (Rx)
A-hydroCort, Solu-Cortef

Func. class.: Short-acting glucocorticoid
Chem. class.: Natural nonfluorinated, group IV potency (valerate), group VI potency (acetate and plain)

Pregnancy category C

Do Not Confuse:
hydrocortisone/hydrocodone

Action: Decreases inflammation by suppressing migration of polymorphonuclear leukocytes and fibroblasts and reversing increased capillary permeability and lysosomal stabilization (systemic); antipruritic, antiinflammatory (top)

Therapeutic Outcome: Decreased inflammation

Uses: Severe inflammation, septic shock, adrenal insufficiency, ulcerative colitis, collagen disorders (systemic), psoriasis, eczema, contact dermatitis, pruritus (top)

Dosage and routes
Adrenal insufficiency/inflammation
Adult: PO 5-30 mg bid-qid; IM/**IV** 100-250 mg (succinate), then 50-100 mg IM as needed; IM/**IV** 15-240 mg q12h (phosphate)

Shock
Adult: 500 mg-2 g q2-6h (succinate)
Child: IM/**IV** 0.186-1 mg/kg bid-tid (succinate)

Colitis
Adult: Enema 100 mg nightly for 21 days

Topical route
Adult and child >2 yr: Apply to affected area daily-qid

Available forms: Tabs 5, 10, 20 mg; inj 25, 50 mg/ml; enema 100 mg/60 ml; acetate: inj 25 ♣, 50 mg/ml ♣, enema 10% aerosol foam, supp 25 mg; cypionate: oral susp 10 mg/5 ml; phosphate: inj 50 mg/ml; succinate: inj 100 mg ♣, 250 mg ♣, 500 mg ♣, 1000 mg/vial ♣

Adverse effects
CNS: Depression, flushing, sweating, headache, mood changes
CV: Hypertension, **circulatory collapse, thrombophlebitis, embolism,** tachycardia, edema
EENT: Fungal infections, increased intraocular pressure, blurred vision
GI: Diarrhea, nausea, abdominal distention, **GI hemorrhage,** increased appetite, pancreatitis
HEMA: **Thrombocytopenia**
INTEG: Acne, poor wound healing, ecchymosis, petechiae
MS: Fractures, osteoporosis, weakness

Contraindications: Psychosis, hypersensitivity, idiopathic thrombocytopenia (IM), acute glomerulonephritis, amebiasis, fungal infections, nonasthmatic bronchial disease, child <2 yr, AIDS, TB

Precautions: Pregnancy **C,** diabetes mellitus, glaucoma, osteoporosis, seizure disorders, ulcerative colitis, CHF, myasthenia gravis, renal disease, esophagitis, peptic ulcer, lactation

Pharmacokinetics
Absorption	Well absorbed (PO); systemic (top)
Distribution	Crosses placenta
Metabolism	Liver, extensively
Excretion	Kidney
Half-life	3-5 hr, adrenal suppression 3-4 days

Pharmacodynamics
	PO	IM	IV	TOP
Onset	1-2 hr	20 min	Rapid	Min to hr
Peak	1 hr	4-8 hr	Unkn	Hr to days
Duration	1½ days	1½ days	1½ days	Hr to days

Interactions
Individual drugs
Alcohol, amphotericin B, cycloSPORINE, digitalis: increased side effects
Cholestyramine, colestipol, ePHEDrine,

phenytoin, rifampin, theophylline: decreased action of hydrocortisone

Drug classifications

Anticoagulants, toxoids, vaccines: decreased action of anticoagulant
Anticonvulsants: decreased effects of anticonvulsant
Antidiabetics: decreased effects of antidiabetics
Barbiturates: decreased action of hydrocortisone
Diuretics: increased side effects
NSAIDs, salicylates: increased risk of GI bleeding

Drug/herb

Aloe, buckthorn, cascara sagrada, Chinese rhubarb, senna: increased hyokalemia
Aloe, licorice, perilla: increased corticosteroid effect

Drug/lab test

Increased: cholesterol, sodium, blood glucose, uric acid, calcium, urine glucose
Decreased: calcium, potassium, T_4, T_3, thyroid ^{131}I uptake test, urine 17-OHCS, 17-KS
False negative: skin allergy tests

NURSING CONSIDERATIONS

Assessment

- Monitor potassium, blood glucose, urine glucose while patient is on long-term therapy; hypokalemia and hyperglycemia may occur
- Monitor I&O ratio; be alert for decreasing urinary output and increasing edema; weigh daily; notify prescriber of weekly gain >5 lb or edema, hypertension, cardiac symptoms
- Monitor plasma cortisol levels during long-term therapy (normal level is 138-635 nmol/L when obtained at 8 AM); check adrenal function periodically for hypothalamic-pituitary-adrenal axis suppression
- Assess for infection: increased temp, WBC even after withdrawal of medication; drug masks infection symptoms; if fever develops, drug should be discontinued
- Check for potassium depletion: paresthesias, fatigue, nausea, vomiting, depression, polyuria, dysrhythmias, weakness
- Assess mental status: affect, mood, behavioral changes, aggression
- Check nasal passages during long-term treatment for changes in mucus (nasal)
- Assess for systemic absorption: increased temp, inflammation, irritation (top)

Nursing diagnoses

- Infection, risk for (adverse reactions)
- Knowledge, deficient (teaching)
- Noncompliance (teaching) (top/nasal preparation)

Implementation

PO route

- Give with food or milk to decrease GI symptoms

Rectal route

- Use applicator provided
- Clean applicator after each use

Topical route

- Apply only to affected areas; do not get in eyes
- Cleanse and dry area before applying medication, then cover with occlusive dressing (only if prescribed); seal to normal skin; change q12h; systemic absorption may occur; use only on dermatoses; do not use on weeping, denuded, or infected area
- Use for a few days after area has cleared
- Store at room temp

Nasal route

- Patient should clear nasal passages before administration; use decongestant if needed; shake inhaler, invert, tilt head backward, insert nozzle into nostril, away from septum; hold other nostril closed and depress activator, inhale through nose, exhale through mouth

IV route

- Give only sodium phosphate product **IV**; reconstitute with sol provided; give 100 mg over >1 min
- May be given by intermittent inf in compatible sol
- Give titrated dose; use lowest effective dosage

Sodium phosphate preparations

Syringe compatibilities: Fluconazole, fludarabine, metoclopramide

Additive compatibilities: Amikacin, amphotericin B, bleomycin, cephapirin, metaraminol, sodium bicarbonate, verapamil

Y-site compatibilities: Allopurinol, amifostine, aztreonam, cefepime, cladribine, famotidine, filgrastim, fluconazole, fludarabine, granisetron, melphalan, ondansetron, paclitaxel, piperacillin/tazobactam, teniposide, thiotepa, vinorelbine

Sodium succinate preparations

Syringe compatibilities: Metoclopramide, thiopental

Y-site compatibilities: Acyclovir, allopurinol, amifostine, aminophylline, ampicillin, amphotericin B cholesteryl, inamrinone, amsacrine, atracurium, atropine, aztreonam, betamethasone, calcium gluconate, cefepime, cefmetazole, cephalothin, cephapirin, chlordiazepoxide, chlorproMAZINE, cisatracurium, cladribine, cyanocobalamin, cytarabine, dexamethasone, digoxin, diphenhydrAMINE, DOPamine, DOXOrubicin liposome, droperidol, edrophonium, enalaprilat, epINEPHrine, esmolol, conjugated estrogens, ethacrynate, famotidine, fentanyl, fentanyl/droperidol, filgrastim, fludarabine, fluorouracil, foscarnet, furosemide, gallium, granisetron, heparin, hydrALAZINE, regular insulin, isoproterenol, kanamycin, lidocaine, lorazepam, magnesium sulfate, melphalan, menadiol, meperidine, methicillin, methoxamine, methylergonovine, minocycline, morphine, neostigmine, norepinephrine, ondansetron, oxacillin, oxytocin, paclitaxel, pancuronium, penicillin G potassium, pentazocine, phytonadione, piperacillin/tazobactam, prednisoLONE, procainamide, prochlorperazine, propofol, propranolol, pyridostigmine, remifentanil, scopolamine, sodium bicarbonate, succinylcholine, tacrolimus, teniposide, theophylline, thiotepa, trimethaphan, trimethobenzamide, vecuronium, vinorelbine

Y-site incompatibilities: Diazepam, ergotamine tartrate, idarubicin, phenytoin, sargramostim

Additive compatibilities: Amikacin, aminophylline, amphotericin B, calcium chloride, calcium gluconate, cephalothin, cephapirin, chloramphenicol, clindamycin, cloxacillin, corticotropin, DAUNOrubicin, diphenhydrAMINE, DOPamine, erythromycin, floxacillin, lidocaine, magnesium sulfate, mephentermine, metronidazole/sodium bicarbonate, mitomycin, mitoxantrone, netilmicin, netilmicin/potassium chloride, norepinephrine, penicillin G potassium/sodium, piperacillin, polymyxin B, potassium chloride, sodium bicarbonate, theophylline, thiopental, vancomycin, verapamil, vit B/C

Additive incompatibilities: Bleomycin, DOXOrubicin

Patient/family education

- Teach patient all aspects of drug usage, including cushingoid symptoms
- Advise patient to carry/wear emergency ID as steroid user; not to discontinue abruptly; adrenal crisis can result
- Instruct patient to notify prescriber if therapeutic response decreases; dosage adjustment may be needed
- Instruct patient to notify prescriber of signs of infection
- Caution patient to avoid OTC products unless directed by perscriber: salicylates, alcohol in cough products, cold preparations
- Teach patient symptoms of adrenal insufficiency: nausea, anorexia, fatigue, dizziness, dyspnea, weakness, joint pain, and when to notify prescriber
- Advise patient that long-term therapy may be needed to resolve infection (1-2 mo depending on type of infection)

Nasal route

- Instruct patient to clear nasal passages if sneezing attack occurs, then repeat dose; to continue using product even if mild nasal bleeding occurs; bleeding is usually transient
- Teach method of instillation after providing written instruction from manufacturer on instillation

Evaluation

Positive therapeutic outcome

- Decrease in runny nose (nasal)
- Ease of respirations, decreased inflammation
- Absence of severe itching, patches on skin, flaking (top)

! HIGH ALERT

hydromorphone (Rx)

(hye-droe-mor′fone)

Dilaudid, Dilaudid-HP, Hydromorphone HCl, Hydrostat IR, PMS Hydromorphone

Func. class.: Antitussive, opioid analgesic agonist

Chem. class.: Phenanthrene derivative, guaifenesin

Pregnancy category C

Controlled substance schedule II

Do Not Confuse:
Dilaudid/Demerol, hydromorphone/meperidine, hydromorphone/morphine

Action: Depresses pain impulse transmission at the spinal cord level by interacting with opioid receptors; increases respiratory tract fluid by decreasing surface tension and adhesiveness, which increases removal of mucus; analgesic, antitussive

Therapeutic Outcome: Decreased cough, decreased pain

Uses: As an antitussive to suppress cough; moderate to severe pain

Dosage and routes

Antitussive

Adult: PO 1 mg q3-4h prn

Analgesic

Adult: PO 1-6 mg q4-6h prn; SUBCUT/IM/**IV** 1.5 mg q3-4h prn, may be increased; rec 3 mg q4-6h prn

Geriatric: PO 1-2 mg q4-6h
Child: 0.03-0.08 mg/kg q4-6h, max 5 mg/dose

Available forms: Inj 1, 2, 3, 4, 10 mg/ml; tabs 1, 2, 3, 4, 8 mg; oral sol 5 mg/5 ml; syr 1 mg/5 ml supp 3 mg

Adverse effects

CNS: Dizziness, drowsiness, *sedation, confusion,* headache, euphoria, mood changes, **seizures**
CV: *Hypotension, bradycardia,* palpitations, change in B/P, tachycardia
EENT: Miosis, diplopia, blurred vision, tinnitus
GI: *Nausea, constipation, vomiting, anorexia,* dry mouth, cramps
GU: Increased urinary output, dysuria, urinary retention
INTEG: Urticaria, rash, flushing, bruising, diaphoresis, pruritus
RESP: **Respiratory depression**

Contraindications: Hypersensitivity, opiate addiction

Precautions: Pregnancy **C,** increased ICP, addictive personality, hepatic disease, renal disease, lactation, MI (acute), severe heart disease, respiratory depression, child <18 yr

Pharmacokinetics

Absorption	Well absorbed (PO), complete (**IV**)
Distribution	Unknown; crosses placenta
Metabolism	Liver, extensively
Excretion	Kidneys
Half-life	2-3 hr

Pharmacodynamics

	PO/IM/SUBCUT	IV	REC
Onset	15-30 min	10-15 min	15-30 min
Peak	30-60 min	15-30 min	30-90 min
Duration	4-5 hr	2-3 hr	4-5 hr

Interactions

Individual drugs

Alcohol: increased respiratory depression, hypotension, sedation
Nalbuphine, pentazocine: decreased analgesia

Drug classifications

Antipsychotics, opiates, sedative/hypnotics, skeletal muscle relaxants: increased effects

Drug/herb

Chamomile, hops, Jamaican dogwood, lavender, kava, mistletoe, nettle, pokeweed, poppy, senega, skullcap, valerian: increased action
Corkwood: increased anticholinergic effect

Drug/lab test

Increased: amylase

NURSING CONSIDERATIONS

Assessment

- Assess pain control, sedation by scoring on 0-10 scale, around-the-clock dosing is best for pain control
- Monitor VS after parenteral route; note muscle rigidity, drug history, liver, kidney function tests, respiratory dysfunction: respiratory depression, character, rate, rhythm; notify prescriber if respirations are <10/min
- Monitor CNS changes: dizziness, drowsiness, hallucinations, euphoria, LOC, pupil reaction
- Monitor allergic reactions: rash, urticaria; bowel function, constipation

Nursing diagnoses

- Pain, acute (uses)
- Sensory perception, disturbed: visual, auditory (adverse reactions)
- Breathing pattern, ineffective (adverse reactions)
- Knowledge, deficient (teaching)

Implementation

- Give with antiemetic if nausea, vomiting occur
- Give when pain is beginning to return; determine dosage interval by patient response; continuous dosing of medication is more effective given prn; explain analgesic effect
- Withdraw medication slowly after long-term use to prevent withdrawal symptoms
- Store in light-resistant container at room temp

PO route

- May be given with food or milk to lessen GI upset

IM/SUBCUT route

- Do not give if sol is cloudy or a precipitate has formed; rotate inj sites

IV route

- Give by direct **IV** after diluting with 5 ml or more of sterile water or 0.9% NaCl for inj
- Give slowly at 2 mg over 3-5 min or less through Y-connector or 3-way stopcock

Syringe compatibilities: Atropine, bupivacaine, ceftazidime, chlorproMAZINE, cimetidine, dimenhyDRINATE, diphenhydrAMINE, fentanyl, glycopyrrolate, haloperidol, hydrOXYzine, lorazepam, midazolam, pentazocaine, pentobarbital, prochlorperazine, promethazine, ranitidine, scopolamine, tetracaine, thiethylperazine, trimethobenzamide

H

Y-site compatibilities: Acyclovir, allopurinol, amifostine, amikacin, amsacrine, aztreonam, cefamandole, cefepime, cefmetazole, cefoperazone, cefotaxime, cefoxitin, ceftazidime, ceftizoxime, cefuroxime, cephalothin, cephapirin, chloramphenicol, cisplatin, cladribine, clindamycin, cyclophosphamide, cytarabine, diltiazem, DOBUTamine, DOPamine, DOXOrubicin, doxycycline, epINEPHrine, erythromycin lactobionate, famotidine, fentanyl, filgrastim, fludarabine, foscarnet, furosemide, gentamicin, granisetron, heparin, kanamycin, labetalol, lorazepam, magnesium sulfate, melphalan, methotrexate, metronidazole, mezlocillin, midazolam, milrinone, morphine, moxalactam, nafcillin, niCARdipine, nitroglycerin, norepinephrine, ondansetron, oxacillin, paclitaxel, penicillin G potassium, piperacillin, piperacillin/tazobactam, propofol, ranitidine, teniposide, thiotepa, ticarcillin, tobramycin, trimethoprim/sulfamethoxazole, vancomycin, vecuronium, vinorelbine
Y-site incompatibilities: Ampicillin, diazepam, minocycline, phenobarbital, phenytoin, sargramostim
Additive compatibilities: Bupivacaine, fluorouracil, midazolam, ondansetron, promethazine, verapamil
Additive incompatibilities: Sodium bicarbonate, thiopental
Solution compatibilities: D_5W, D_5/0.45% NaCl, D_5/0.9% NaCl, D_5/LR, D_5/Ringer's, 0.45% NaCl, 0.9% NaCl, Ringer's and lactated Ringer's

Patient/family education

- Instruct patient to report any symptoms of CNS changes, allergic reactions; to avoid CNS depressants: alcohol, sedative/hypnotics for at least 24 hr after taking this drug
- Advise patient that dizziness, drowsiness, and confusion are common and to avoid getting up without assistance, driving, or other hazardous activities
- Discuss in detail all aspects of the drug

Evaluation

Positive therapeutic outcome

- Decreased pain
- Decreased cough

Treatment of overdose: Naloxone HCl (Narcan) 0.2-0.8 **IV**, O_2, **IV** fluids, vasopressors

hydroxychloroquine (Rx)

(hye-drox-ee-klor'oh-kwin)

Plaquenil

Func. class.: Antimalarial, antirheumatic (DMARDs)

Chem. class.: 4-Aminoquinoline derivative

Pregnancy category C

Action: Inhibits parasite replications, transcription of DNA to RNA by forming complexes with DNA in parasite

Therapeutic Outcome: Resolution of infection

Uses: Malaria caused by *Plasmodium vivax, P. malariae, P. ovale, P. falciparum* (some strains): LE, rheumatoid arthritis

Dosage and routes

Malaria

Adult: PO suppression or prevention 200 mg qwk, begin 1-2 wk before travel, continue 4 wk after returning; treatment 400 mg, then 200 mg at 6, 24, 48 hr after 1st dose
Child: PO suppression or prevention 5 mg/kg qwk, begin 1-2 wk before travel, continue 4 wk after returning; treatment 10 mg/kg, then 5 mg/kg at 6, 24, 48 hr after 1st dose

Lupus erythematosus

Adult: PO 400 mg daily-bid; length depends on patient response; maintenance 200-400 mg daily

Rheumatoid arthritis

Adult: PO 400-600 mg daily for 4-12 wk; then 200-300 mg daily after good response

Available forms: Tabs 200 mg

Adverse effects

CNS: Headache, stimulation, fatigue, irritability, **seizures**, bad dreams, dizziness, confusion, psychosis, decreased reflexes
CV: Hypotension, heart block, **asystole with syncope**
EENT: *Blurred vision, corneal changes, retinal changes, difficulty focusing*, tinnitus, vertigo, deafness, photophobia, corneal edema
GI: *Nausea, vomiting, anorexia,* diarrhea, cramps
HEMA: **Thrombocytopenia, agranulocytosis, leukopenia, aplastic anemia**
INTEG: Pruritus, pigmentation changes, skin eruptions, lichen planus-like eruptions, eczema, **exfoliative dermatitis**, alopecia

Contraindications: Hypersensitivity, retinal field changes, children (long-term)

Precautions: Pregnancy **C,** blood dyscrasias, severe GI disease, neurologic disease, alcoholism, hepatic disease, G6PD deficiency, psoriasis, eczema, lactation

Pharmacokinetics	
Absorption	Well absorbed
Distribution	Widely distributed, crosses placenta
Metabolism	Liver
Excretion	Urine/feces
Half-life	3-5 day

Pharmacodynamics	
Onset	Rapid
Peak	1-2 hr
Duration	Days-weeks

Interactions
Individual drugs
Magnesium, aluminum products: decreased malarial action
Digoxin: increased levels
Rabies vaccine: increased antibody titer

NURSING CONSIDERATIONS
Assessment
- Assess for lupus erythematosus, malaria symptoms
- Assess for rheumatoid arthritis: pain, swelling, ROM, temperature of joints
- Assess ophthalmic exam baseline and q6mo if long-term treatment or drug dosage >150 mg/day
- Assess hepatic studies qwk: AST, ALT, bilirubin
- Assess blood studies: CBC, platelets; WBC, RBC, platelets may be decreased; if severe, drug should be discontinued
- Assess for decreased reflexes: knee, ankle
- Assess ECG during therapy
- Assess for depression of T waves, widening of QRS complex
- Assess allergic reactions: pruritus, rash, urticaria
- Assess blood dyscrasias: malaise, fever, bruising, bleeding (rare)
- Assess for ototoxicity (tinnitus, vertigo, change in hearing); audiometric testing should be done before, after treatment
- ❗ Assess for toxicity: blurring vision, difficulty focusing, headache, dizziness, knee, ankle reflexes; drug should be discontinued immediately

Nursing diagnoses
- Infection, risk for (uses)
- Pain, chronic (uses)
- Knowledge, deficient (teaching)

Implementation
- Give before or after meals with milk, at same time each day to maintain drug level
- Tabs may be crushed and mixed with food, fluids
- Malaria prophylaxis should be started 2 wk prior to exposure and 4-6 wk after leaving exposure area
- Store in tight, light-resistant container at room temperature

Patient/family education
- Teach patient to use sunglasses in bright sunlight to decrease photophobia
- Teach patient that urine may turn rust or brown
- Teach patient to report hearing, visual problems, fever, fatigue, bruising, bleeding, which may indicate blood dyscrasias

Evaluation
Positive therapeutic outcome
- Decreased symptoms of malaria, LE, rheumatoid arthritis

Treatment of overdose: Induce vomiting; gastric lavage; administer barbiturate (ultra–short-acting), vasopressor, ammonium chloride; tracheostomy may be necessary

hydroxyurea (Rx)
(hye-drox-ee-yoo-ree′ah)
Droxia, Hydrea
Func. class.: Antineoplastic, antimetabolite
Chem. class.: Synthetic urea analog
Pregnancy category D

Action: Acts by inhibiting DNA synthesis without interfering with RNA or protein synthesis; incorporates thymidine into DNA, causing direct damage to DNA strands; cell cycle specific (S phase)

Therapeutic Outcome: Prevention of rapidly growing malignant cells

Uses: Melanoma, chronic myelocytic leukemia, recurrent or metastatic ovarian cancer, squamous cell carcinoma of the head and neck, sickle cell anemia, psoriasis

Dosage and routes
Solid tumors
Adult: PO 80 mg/kg as a single dose q3 days or 20-30 mg/kg as a single dose daily

In combination with radiation
Adult: PO 80 mg/kg as a single dose q3 days; should be started 7 days before irradiation

Resistant chronic myelocytic leukemia
Adult: PO 20-30 mg/kg/day as a single daily dose

Sickle cell anemia
Adult: PO 15 mg/kg/day, may increase by 5 mg/kg/day, max 35 mg/kg/day

Renal dose
Adult: CCr 10-50 ml/min dose 50%; CCr <10 ml/min PO dose 20%

Available forms: Caps 200, 300, 400, 500 mg

Adverse effects
CNS: Headache, confusion, hallucinations, dizziness, **seizures**
CV: Angina, ischemia
GI: Nausea, vomiting, anorexia, diarrhea, stomatitis, constipation
GU: Increased BUN, uric acid, creatinine, temporary renal function impairment
HEMA: **Leukopenia, anemia, thrombocytopenia, megaloblastic erythropoiesis**
INTEG: *Rash,* urticaria, pruritus, dry skin, facial erythema
MISC: Fever, chills, malaise

Contraindications: Pregnancy **D,** hypersensitivity, leukopenia (<2500/mm^3), thrombocytopenia (<100,000/mm^3), anemia (severe), lactation

Precautions: Renal disease (severe)

Pharmacokinetics	
Absorption	Well absorbed
Distribution	Crosses blood-brain barrier
Metabolism	Liver (50%)
Excretion	Kidneys, unchanged (50%), eliminated as CO_2
Half-life	4 hr

Pharmacodynamics	
Onset	Unknown
Peak	2 hr
Duration	Unknown

Interactions
Individual drugs
Radiation: increased toxicity
Drug classifications
Antineoplastics: increased toxicity
Drug/lab test
Increased: renal function studies

NURSING CONSIDERATIONS

Assessment
- Assess buccal cavity q8h for dryness, sores or ulceration, white patches, oral pain, bleeding, dysphagia; obtain prescription for viscous lidocaine (Xylocaine)
- Assess symptoms indicating severe allergic reaction: rash, pruritus, urticaria, purpuric skin lesions, itching, flushing
- Monitor CBC, differential, platelet count weekly; withhold drug if WBC is <2500/mm^3 or platelet count is <100,000/mm^3; notify prescriber of results if WBC <20,000/mm^3, platelets <150,000/mm^3
- Assess for increased uric acid levels, swelling, joint pain primarily in extremities; patient should be well hydrated to prevent urate deposits
- Monitor renal function studies: BUN, creatinine, serum uric acid, urine CCr before and during therapy; I&O ratio; report fall in urine output to <30 ml/hr
- Monitor temp q4h (may indicate beginning of infection)
- Monitor liver function tests before and during therapy (bilirubin, AST, ALT, LDH) as needed or monthly
- Assess for bleeding: hematuria, stool guaiac, bruising or petechiae, mucosa or orifices q8h; check for inflammation of mucosa, breaks in skin

Nursing diagnoses
- Injury, risk for (adverse reactions)
- Body image, disturbed (adverse reactions)
- Infection, risk for (adverse reactions)
- Knowledge, deficient (teaching)

Implementation
- Do not crush or chew caps; for difficulty swallowing, caps can be opened and contents mixed with water
- Avoid contact with skin, very irritating; wash completely to remove
- Give fluids **IV** or PO before chemotherapy to hydrate patient
- Give antiemetic 30-60 min before giving drug and prn to prevent vomiting; antibiotics for prophylaxis of infection
- Provide liq diet: carbonated beverages; gelatin may be added if patient is not nauseated or vomiting

Patient/family education
- Advise patient that contraceptive measures are recommended during therapy
- Teach patient to avoid use of products containing aspirin or ibuprofen, razors, commercial mouthwash, since bleeding may

occur; instruct patient to report symptoms of bleeding (hematuria, tarry stools)

- Teach patient to rinse mouth tid-qid with water, club soda; brush teeth bid-qid with soft brush or cotton-tipped applicators for stomatitis; use unwaxed dental floss
- Instruct patient to report signs of anemia (fatigue, headache, irritability, faintness, shortness of breath)
- Advise patient to report any changes in breathing or coughing even several mo after treatment; to avoid crowds and persons with respiratory tract or other infections
- Caution patient not to have any vaccinations without the advice of the prescriber, serious reactions can occur

Evaluation

Positive therapeutic outcome

- Prevention of rapid division of malignant cells

hydrOXYzine (Rx)

(hye-drox'i-zeen)

Apo-hydroxyzine ✤, Atarax, Multipax ✤, Novohydroxyzine ✤, Vistaril

Func. class.: Antianxiety, sedative, hypnotic, antihistamine, antiemetic

Chem. class.: Piperazine derivative

Pregnancy category C

Do Not Confuse:

Atarax/amoxicillin/Ativan
Vistaril/Versed
hydrOXYzine/hydrALAZINE

Action: Depresses subcortical levels of CNS, including limbic system, reticular formation; anticholinergic, antiemetic, antihistaminic responses; competes with H_1-receptor sites

Therapeutic Outcome: Absence of allergy symptoms, rhinitis, pruritus, absence of nausea/vomiting, sedation, absence of anxiety

Uses: Anxiety preoperatively, postoperatively to prevent nausea, vomiting; to potentiate opioid analgesics; sedation; pruritus; prevention of alcohol, drug withdrawal

Dosage and routes

Adult: PO 25-100 mg tid-qid, max 600 mg/day
Elderly: PO 10 mg tid-qid (pruritus)
Child >6 yr: PO 50-100 mg/day in divided doses
Child <6 yr: PO 50 mg/day in divided doses

Preoperatively/postoperatively
Adult: IM 25-100 mg q4-6h
Child: IM 0.5-1.1 mg/kg q4-6h

Pruritus
Adult: PO 25 mg tid-qid

Antiemetic
Adult: IM 25-100 mg/dose q4-6h prn

Available forms: Tabs 10, 25, 50, 100 mg; caps 10, 25, 50, 100 mg; oral susp 25 mg/5 ml; inj 25, 50 mg/ml

Adverse effects

CNS: *Dizziness, drowsiness,* confusion, headache, tremors, fatigue, depression, **seizures**
CV: Hypotension
GI: Dry mouth, nausea, diarrhea, increased appetite, weight gain

Contraindications: Pregnancy (1st trimester), hypersensitivity to this drug or cetirizine, lactation, acute asthma

Precautions: Pregnancy **C** (2nd/3rd trimesters), elderly, debilitated patients, hepatic disease, renal disease, narrow-angle glaucoma, COPD, prostatic hypertrophy

Pharmacokinetics

Absorption	Well absorbed
Distribution	Not known
Metabolism	Liver, completely
Excretion	Feces, urine, bile
Half-life	3 hr

Pharmacodynamics

	PO/IM
Onset	15-30 min
Peak	2-4 hr
Duration	4-6 hr

Interactions

Individual drugs
Alcohol: increased CNS depression
Atropine, disopyramide, haloperidol, quinidine: increased anticholinergic reactions

Drug classifications
Analgesics, barbiturates, CNS depressants, opiates, sedative/hypnotics: increased CNS depression
Antidepressants, antihistamines, phenothiazines: increased anticholinergic reactions

Drug/herb
Corkwood, henbane leaf, jimsonweed, scopolia: increased anticholinergic effect
Chamomile, cowslip, hops, Jamaican dogwood, khat, kava, Queen Anne's lace, senega, skullcap, valerian: increased sedative action

H

Drug/lab test

False increase: 17-OHCS

NURSING CONSIDERATIONS

Assessment

- Assess mental status: mood, sensorium, affect, behavior, increased sedation
- Assess respiratory status: rate, rhythm, increase in bronchial secretions, wheezing, chest tightness; provide fluids to 2 L/day to decrease secretion thickness
- Monitor I&O ratio: be alert for urinary retention, frequency, dysuria, especially in the elderly; drug should be discontinued if these occur
- Observe for drowsiness, dizziness
- Assess cough characteristics including type, frequency, thickness of secretions; evaluate response to this medication if using for cough

Nursing diagnoses

- Injury, risk for (side effects)
- Anxiety (uses)
- Knowledge, deficient (teaching)

Implementation

PO route

- Take 1 hr pc or 2 hr ac to facilitate absorption
- May crush tab if patient unable to swallow whole
- Give with meals if GI symptoms occur; absorption may be slightly decreased
- Caps may be opened and drug mixed with food/fluids for patients with swallowing difficulties

IM route

- Give IM inj in large muscle mass; aspirate to prevent **IV** administration; use Z-track method; severe necrosis can result with improper technique; never give **IV**/SUBCUT

Syringe compatibilities: Atropine, atropine/meperidine, benzquinamide, bupivacaine, butorphanol, chlorproMAZINE, cimetidine, codeine, diphenhydrAMINE, doxapram, droperidol, fentanyl, fluphenazine, glycopyrrolate, hydromorphone, lidocaine, meperidine, meperidine/atropine, methotrimeprazine, metoclopramide, midazolam, morphine, nalbuphine, oxymorphone, pentazocine, perphenazine, procaine, prochlorperazine, promazine, promethazine, remifentanil, scopolamine, sufentanil, thiothixene

Syringe incompatibilities: Aminophylline, chloramphenicol, dimenhyDRINATE, heparin, penicillin G potassium, pentobarbital, phenobarbital, phenytoin

Additive compatibilities: Cisplatin, cyclophosphamide, cytarabine, dimenhyDRINATE, etoposide, lidocaine, mesna, methotrexate, nafcillin

Patient/family education

- Caution patient to avoid hazardous activities and activities requiring alertness, since dizziness may occur; instruct patient to request assistance with ambulation
- Advise patient to avoid alcohol, other CNS depressants including cough, cold preparations; CNS depression may occur
- Teach all aspects of drug use; to notify prescriber if confusion, sedation, hypotension occur; to avoid driving and other hazardous activity if drowsiness occurs
- Caution patient not to exceed recommended dosage; dysrhythmias may occur
- Tell patient hard candy, gum, frequent rinsing of mouth may be used for dryness

Evaluation

Positive therapeutic outcome

- Absence of nausea, vomiting
- Decreased anxiety

Treatment of overdose: Lavage if orally ingested, VS, supportive care, **IV** norepINEPHrine for hypotension

hyoscyamine (Rx)

(hye-oh-sye′a-meen)

Anaspaz, A-Spas S/L, Cystospaz, Cystospaz-M, Donnamar, ED-SPAZ, Gastrosed, Levsin, Levsinex, NuLev Timecaps

Func. class.: Anticholinergic/antispasmodics

Chem. class.: Belladonna alkaloid

Pregnancy category C

Action: Inhibits muscarinic actions of acetylcholine at postganglionic parasympathetic neuroeffector sites, reduces rigidity, tremors, hyperhidrosis of parkinsonism

Therapeutic Outcome: Absence of peptic ulcer after treatment

Uses: Treatment of peptic ulcer disease in combination with other drugs; other GI disorders, other spastic disorders, IBS, urinary incontinence

Dosage and routes

Adult: PO/SL 0.125-0.25 mg tid-qid ac, at bedtime; time rel 0.375 q12h; IM/SUBCUT/**IV** 0.25-0.5 mg q6h

Child 2-12 yr: PO (orally disintegrating tabs) 0.0625-0.125 mg (½-1 tab) q4h, max 6×/day

Child 34-36 kg: PO 125-187 mcg q4h prn

Child 22.7-33 kg: PO 94-125 mcg q4h prn
Child 13.6-22.6 kg: PO 63 mcg q4h prn
Child 9.1-13.5 kg: PO 31.3 mcg q4h prn
Child 6.8-9 kg: PO 25 mcg q4h prn
Child 4.5-6.7 kg: PO 18.8 mcg q4h prn
Child 3.4-4.4 kg: PO 15.6 mcg q4h prn
Child 2.3-3.3 kg: PO 12.5 mcg q4h prn

Available forms: Tabs 0.125, 0.13, 0.15 mg; time rel caps 0.375 mg; sol 0.125 mg/ml; elix 0.125 mg/ml; inj 0.5 mg/ml

Adverse effects

CNS: *Confusion, stimulation in elderly,* headache, insomnia, dizziness, drowsiness, anxiety, weakness, hallucination
CV: *Palpitations*, tachycardia
EENT: *Blurred vision*, photophobia, mydriasis, cycloplegia, increased ocular tension
GI: *Dry mouth, constipation, paralytic ileus*, heartburn, nausea, vomiting, dysphagia, absence of taste
GU: *Urinary hesitancy, retention*, impotence
INTEG: Urticaria, rash, pruritus, anhidrosis, fever, allergic reactions

Contraindications: Hypersensitivity to anticholinergics, narrow-angle glaucoma, GI obstruction, myasthenia gravis, paralytic ileus, GI atony, toxic megacolon, prostatic hypertrophy

Precautions: Pregnancy **C**, hyperhydroidism, coronary artery disease, dysrhythmias, CHF, ulcerative colitis, hypertension, hiatal hernia, hepatic disease, renal disease, urinary retention, elderly

Pharmacokinetics

Absorption	Well
Distribution	Cross blood-brain barrier, placenta
Metabolism	Liver
Excretion	Urine
Half-life	3½ hr

Pharmacodynamics

	PO	IM/IV/SUBCUT
Onset	30 min	2-3 min
Peak	Unknown	Unknown
Duration	4-6 hr	4-6 hr

Interactions

Individual drugs

Amantidine: increased anticholinergic effect
Levodopa, ketoconazole: decreased effects

Drug classifications

Antacids: decreased hyoscyamine effect
Antihistamines, H_1, antidepressants, tricyclics, MAOIs: increased anticholinergic effect
Phenothiazines: decreased effect of phenothiazines

Drug/herb

Black catechu: increased constipation
Butterbur, jimsonweed: increased anticholinergic effect
Jaborandi tree, pill-bearing spurge: decreased anticholinergic effect

NURSING CONSIDERATIONS

Assessment

- Monitor VS, cardiac status: checking for dysrhythmias, increased rate, palpitations
- Monitor I/O ratio; check for urinary retention or hesitancy
- Monitor GI complaints: pain, bleeding (frank or occult), nausea, vomiting, anorexia

H

Nursing diagnoses

- Constipation (adverse reactions)
- Injury, risk for (adverse reactions)
- Knowledge, deficient (teaching)

Implementation

- Do not break, crush, or chew time rel caps
- Give ½ hour ac for better absorption
- Give decreased dose to elderly patients; metabolism may be slowed
- Store in tight container protected from light

Patient/family education

- Teach patient to avoid driving, other hazardous activities until stabilized on medication
- Teach patient to avoid alcohol or other CNS depressants; will enhance sedating properties of this drug
- Teach patient to avoid hot environments; heat stroke may occur; drug suppresses perspiration
- Teach patient to use sunglasses when outside to prevent photophobia; may cause blurred vision
- Teach patient to use gum, hard candy, frequent rinsing of mouth for dryness of oral cavity
- Teach patient to increase fluids, bulk, exercise to decrease constipation

Evaluation

Positive therapeutic outcome

- Absence of epigastric pain, bleeding, nausea, vomiting

ibritumomab tiuxetan (Rx)
(ee-brit-u-moe'mab)
Zevalin
Func. class.: Antineoplastic—miscellaneous
Pregnancy category D

Action: High affinity for indium-111, yttrium-90; induces CD20+ B-cell lines

Therapeutic Outcome: Decrease in tumor size, spread of malignancy

Uses: Non-Hodgkin's lymphoma, B-cell NHL

Dosage and routes
Adult: **IV INF** 250 mg/m^2 at a rate of 50 mg/hr; if hypersensitivity does not occur, increase rate by 50 mg/hr q½h, max 400 mg/hr; slow/interrupt inf if hypersensitivity occurs

Available forms: Inj 3.2 mg/2 ml

Adverse effects
CV: **Cardiac dysrhythmias**
GI: *Nausea, vomiting, anorexia,* abdominal pain, diarrhea
GU: **Renal failure**
HEMA: **Leukopenia, neutropenia, thrombocytopenia,** anemia
INTEG: *Irritation at site, rash,* **fatal mucocutaneous infections (rare)**
OTHER: Fever, chills, asthenia, headache, angioedema, hypotension, myalgia, **bronchospasm, hemorrhage,** infections, cough, dyspnea, dizziness, anxiety
SYST: **Stevens-Johnson syndrome**

Contraindications: Pregnancy **D**, hypersensitivity to this agent or murine proteins

Precautions: Lactation, children, elderly, cardiac conditions, immunizations after therapy

Pharmacokinetics

Absorption	Unknown
Distribution	Unknown
Metabolism	Unknown
Excretion	Unknown
Half-life	30 hr

Pharmacodynamics
Unknown

NURSING CONSIDERATIONS
Assessment
- ⚠ Assess for signs of fatal infusion reaction: hypoxia, pulmonary infiltrates, ARDS, MI, ventricular fibrillation, cardiogenic shock; most fatal infusion reactions occur with first infusion; potentially fatal
- Assess biodistribution: 1st image 2-24 hr, 2nd image 48-72 hr, 3rd image 90-120 hr (optimal)
- Assess for signs of severe mucocutaneous reactions: Stevens-Johnson syndrome, lichenoid dermatitis, toxic epidermal lysis; occur 1-13 wk after drug was given
- ⚠ Assess for tumor lysis syndrome: acute renal failure requiring hemodialysis, hyperkalemia, hypocalcemia, hyperuricemia, hyperphosphatemia
- Monitor CBC, differential, platelet count weekly; withhold drug if WBC is <3500/mm^3 or platelet count <100,000/mm^3; notify prescriber of these results; drug should be discontinued
- Monitor GI symptoms: frequency of stools
- Assess for signs of dehydration: rapid respirations, poor skin turgor, decreased urine output, dry skin, restlessness, weakness

Nursing diagnoses
- Infection, risk for (adverse reactions)
- Nutrition: less than body requirements, imbalanced (adverse reactions)
- Knowledge, deficient (teaching)

Implementation
- Do not use as bolus or **IV** direct
- Provide increased fluid intake to 2-3 L/day to prevent dehydration, unless contraindicated
- Provide nutritious diet with iron, vitamin supplement, low fiber, few dairy products

IV infusion route
- See manufacturer's product labeling for preparation
- Have emergency equipment nearby with epinephrine, antihistamines, corticosteroids
- Change **IV** site q48h
- Store vials at 36°-46° F (2°-7° C), do not freeze

Patient/family education
- Advise patient to report adverse reactions
- Advise patient to use contraception during and for 12 mo after therapy

Evaluation
Positive therapeutic outcome
- Decrease in tumor size, decrease in spread of cancer

ibuprofen (OTC)

(eye-byoo-proe'fen)

Actiprofen ♣, Advil, Advil Migraine, Apo-Ibuprofen ♣, Bayer Select Ibuprofen Pain Relief, Children's Advil, Children's Motrin, Excedrin IB, Genpril, Haltran, ibuprofen, Medipren, Menadol, Midol Maximum Strength Cramp Formula, Motrin, Motrin IB, Motrin Junior Strength, Motrin Migraine Pain, Nu-Ibuprofen, Novoprofen ♣, Nuprin, PediaCare Children's Fever

Func. class.: Nonsteroidal antiinflammatory; nonopiate analgesic, antipyretic

Chem. class.: Propionic acid derivative

Pregnancy category B

Do Not Confuse:
Nuprin/Lupron

Action: Inhibits prostaglandin synthesis by decreasing enzyme needed for biosynthesis; analgesic, antiinflammatory, antipyretic

Therapeutic Outcome: Decreased pain, inflammation, fever

Uses: Rheumatoid arthritis, osteoarthritis, primary dysmenorrhea, gout, dental pain, musculoskeletal disorders, fever

Dosage and routes

Analgesia

Adult: PO 200-400 mg q4-6h, not to exceed 3.2 g/day

Child: PO 4-10 mg/kg/dose q6-8h

Antipyretic

Child 6 mo-12 yr: PO 5 mg/kg (temp <102.5° F or 39.2° C), 10 mg/kg (temp >102.5° F), may repeat q4-6h; max 40 mg/kg/day

Antiinflammatory

Adult: PO 300-800 mg tid-qid; max 3.2 g/day

Child: PO 30-40 mg/kg/day in 3-4 divided doses; max 50 mg/kg/day

Available forms: Tabs 100, 200, 300, 400, 600, 800 mg; liqui-gel caps 200 mg; oral susp 100 mg/2.5 ml, 100 mg/5 ml; liq 100 mg/5 ml; chew tabs 50, 100 mg; drops 50 mg/1.25 ml

Adverse effects

CNS: *Headache,* dizziness, drowsiness, fatigue, tremors, confusion, insomnia, anxiety, depression

CV: Tachycardia, peripheral edema, palpitations, dysrhythmias

EENT: Tinnitus, hearing loss, blurred vision

GI: *Nausea, anorexia,* vomiting, diarrhea, jaundice, **hepatitis,** constipation, flatulence, cramps, dry mouth, peptic ulcer, **GI bleeding**

GU: **Nephrotoxicity,** dysuria, hematuria, oliguria, azotemia

HEMA: **Blood dyscrasias,** increased bleeding time

INTEG: Purpura, rash, pruritus, sweating, urticaria, **necrotizing fasciitis**

SYST: **Anaphylaxis, Stevens-Johnson syndrome**

Contraindications: Avoid in 2nd/3rd trimester of pregnancy, hypersensitivity, asthma, severe renal disease, severe hepatic disease

Precautions: Pregnancy **B** (1st trimester), lactation, children, bleeding disorders, GI disorders, cardiac disorders, hypersensitivity to other antiinflammatory agents, elderly, CHF, CCr <25 ml/min

Pharmacokinetics	
Absorption	Well absorbed
Distribution	Not known; crosses placenta
Metabolism	Liver, extensively
Excretion	Kidneys, unchanged (10%)
Half-life	3½ hr

Pharmacodynamics	
Onset	½ hr
Peak	1-2 hr
Duration	4-6 hr

Interactions

Individual drugs

Alcohol, aspirin: increased GI reactions
Aspirin: decreased ibuprofen action
Cefamandole, cefotetan, cefoperazone, valproic acid, warfarin: increased risk of bleeding
CycloSPORINE, digoxin, lithium, probenecid: increased toxicity
Furosemide: decreased effect of furosemide
Insulin: increased hypoglycemia
Radiation: increased risk of blood dyscrasias

Drug classifications

Anticoagulants, antiplatelet agents, thrombolytics: increased risk of bleeding
Anticoagulants (oral): increased toxicity
Antidiabetics (oral): increased hypoglycemia
Antihypertensives: decreased effect of antihypertensives
Antineoplastics: increased risk of blood dyscrasias
Corticosteroids, NSAIDs: increased GI reactions
Diuretics: decreased effectiveness of diuretics (thiazides)

Drug/herb
Arginine, gossypol: increased gastric irritation
Arnica, bogbean, chamomile, chondroitin, clove, dong quai, fenugreek, feverfew, garlic, ginger, ginkgo, ginseng *(Panax)*: increased risk of bleeding
Bearberry, bilberry: increased NSAIDs effect

Drug/lab test
Increased: bleeding time

NURSING CONSIDERATIONS

Assessment
- Assess pain: location, duration, type, intensity before dose and 1 hr after
- Assess musculoskeletal status: ROM before dose and 1 hr after
- Monitor liver function studies: AST, ALT, bilirubin, creatinine if patient is on long-term therapy
- Monitor renal function studies: BUN, urine creatinine if patient is on long-term therapy
- Assess cardiac status: edema (peripheral), tachycardia, palpitations; monitor B/P, pulse for character, quality, rhythm
- Monitor blood studies: CBC, Hct, Hgb, protime if patient is on long-term therapy
- Check I&O ratio; decreasing output may indicate renal failure if patient is on long-term therapy
- Assess hepatotoxicity: dark urine, clay-colored stools, jaundice of skin and sclera, itching, abdominal pain, fever, diarrhea if patient is on long-term therapy
- Assess for history of peptic ulcer disorder; asthma, aspirin, hypersensitivity, check closely for hypersensitivity reactions
- Assess for allergic reactions: rash, urticaria; if these occur, drug may have to be discontinued
- Assess for ototoxicity: tinnitus, ringing, roaring in ears; audiometric testing needed before, after long-term therapy
- Assess for visual changes: blurring, halos; may indicate corneal, retinal damage
- Identify prior drug history; there are many drug interactions
- Identify fever: length of time in evidence and related symptoms

Nursing diagnoses
- Pain, acute (uses)
- Pain, chronic (uses)
- Mobility, physical, impaired (uses)
- Injury, risk for (side effects)
- Knowledge, deficient (teaching)

Implementation
- Administer to patient crushed or whole; 800-mg tab may be dissolved in water
- Give with food or milk to decrease gastric symptoms; give 30 min pc or 2 hr ac; absorption may be slowed

Patient/family education
- Teach patient to report any symptoms of hepatotoxicity, renal toxicity, visual changes, ototoxicity, allergic reactions, bleeding if patient is on long-term therapy
- Caution patient not to exceed recommended dosage; acute poisoning may result
- Advise patient to read label on other OTC drugs
- Inform patient that the therapeutic response takes 1 mo (arthritis)
- Caution patient to avoid alcohol ingestion, salicylates, NSAIDs; GI bleeding may occur
- Advise patient with allergies that allergic reactions may develop
- Advise patient to use sunscreen to prevent photosensitivity

Evaluation
Positive therapeutic outcome
- Decreased pain
- Decreased inflammation
- Decreased fever
- Increased mobility

! HIGH ALERT

ibutilide (Rx)
(eye-byoo′te-lide)
Corvert
Func. class.: Antidysrhythmic (Class III)

Pregnancy category C

Action: Prolongs duration of action potential and effective refractory period

Uses: For rapid conversion of atrial fibrillation/flutter occurring within 1 wk of coronary artery bypass or valve surgery

Dosage and routes
Adult: **IV** inf (≥60 kg) 1 vial (1 mg) given over 10 min, may repeat same dose in 10 min; **IV** inf (<60 kg) 0.01 mg/kg given over 10 min, may repeat same dose in 10 min

Available forms: Inj 0.1 mg/ml

Adverse effects
CNS: *Headache*
CV: *Hypotension, bradycardia,* **sinus arrest, CHF, dysrhythmias,** hypertension, extrasystoles, ventricular tachycardia, bundle branch block, AV block, palpitations, supraventricular extrasystoles, syncope
GI: Nausea

Contraindications: Hypersensitivity

Precautions: Pregnancy **C,** sinus node dysfunction, 2nd- or 3rd-degree AV block, electrolyte imbalances, bradycardia, lactation, children <18 yr, renal/hepatic disease, elderly

Pharmacokinetics	
Absorption	Unknown
Distribution	Unknown
Metabolism	Liver
Excretion	Kidney
Half-life	6 hr

Interactions
Individual drugs
Digoxin: masking of cardiotoxicity
Drug classifications
Antidepressants (tricyclic/tetracyclic): prodysrhythmia
Antihistamines, H_2-receptor antagonists, phenothiazines: increased prodysrhythmia
Class Ia antidysrhythmics (disopyramide, quinidine, procainamide), class III agents (amiodarone, sotalol): do not use within 4 hr of ibutilide
Drug/herb
Aconite: increased toxicity, death
Aloe, broom, buckthorn (chronic use), cascara sagrada (chronic use), Chinese rhubarb, figwort, fumitory, goldenseal, kudzu, licorice: increased effect
Coltsfoot: decreased effect
Horehound: increased serotonin effect

NURSING CONSIDERATIONS
Assessment
- Monitor I&O ratio; monitor electrolytes: potassium, sodium, chloride
- Monitor liver function studies: AST, ALT, bilirubin, alkaline phosphatase
- Monitor ECG continuously to determine drug effectiveness; measure PR, QRS, QT intervals; check for PVCs, other dysrhythmias; monitor B/P continuously for hypotension, hypertension; check for rebound hypertension after 1-2 hr; discontinue drug when atrial fibrillation/flutter ceases
- Monitor for dehydration or hypovolemia
- Assess for CNS symptoms: confusion, psychosis, numbness, depression, involuntary movements; if these occur drug should be discontinued
- Monitor cardiac rate, respiration; rate, rhythm, character, chest pain, ventricular tachycardia, supraventricular tachycardia or fibrillation

Nursing diagnoses
- Cardiac output, decreased (uses)
- Gas exchange, impaired (adverse reactions)
- Knowledge, deficient (teaching)

Implementation
IV route
- Give reduced dosage slowly with ECG monitoring only
- Give undiluted or diluted in 50 ml of 0.9% NaCl or D_5W (0.017 mg/ml), give over 10 min
- Solution is stable for 48 hr refrigerated or 24 hr at room temp
- Do not admix with other solution, drugs

Patient/family education
- Instruct patient to report side effects immediately to prescriber

Evaluation
Positive therapeutic outcome
- Decrease in atrial fibrillation/flutter

I

! HIGH ALERT

idarubicin (Rx)
(eye-da-roo'bi-sin)
Idamycin, Idamycin PFS
Func. class.: Antineoplastic, antibiotic
Chem. class.: Anthracycline glycoside

Pregnancy category D

Do Not Confuse:
Idamycin/Adriamycin, idarubicin/DOXOrubicin

Action: Inhibits DNA synthesis derived from DAUNOrubicin by binding to DNA, which causes strand splitting; cell cycle specific (Sphase); a vesicant

Therapeutic Outcome: Prevention of rapidly growing malignant cells

Uses: Used in combination with other antineoplastics for acute myelocytic leukemia in adults

Investigational uses: Breast cancer, solid tumors

Dosage and routes
Adult: **IV** 12 mg/m²/day × 3 days in combination with cytosine (induction)

Renal/hepatic dose
Adult: **IV** reduce dose; if bilirubin is 75 mg/dl, do not administer

Available forms: Inj 1 mg/ml

Adverse effects
CNS: Fever, chills, headache
CV: **Dysrhythmias, CHF, pericarditis, myocarditis,** peripheral edema, angina, **MI**

GI: Nausea, vomiting, abdominal pain, mucositis, diarrhea, **hepatotoxicity**
GU: **Nephrotoxicity**
HEMA: **Thrombocytopenia, leukopenia, anemia**
INTEG: Rash, extravasation, dermatitis, reversible alopecia, urticaria, thrombophlebitis, tissue necrosis at inj site

Contraindications: Pregnancy **D**, hypersensitivity, lactation, myelosuppression

Precautions: Renal and hepatic disease, gout, bone marrow depression, children, preexisting CV disease

Pharmacokinetics

Absorption	Complete bioavailability
Distribution	Rapidly distributed; high tissue binding
Metabolism	Liver, extensively
Excretion	Bile
Half-life	22 hr

Pharmacodynamics

Unknown

Interactions
Individual drugs
Radiation: increased toxicity
Drug classifications
Antineoplastics: increased toxicity
Live virus vaccines: decreased antibody response
Drug/lab test
Increased: uric acid

NURSING CONSIDERATIONS
Assessment
- Assess symptoms indicating severe allergic reaction: rash, pruritus, urticaria, purpuric skin lesions, itching, flushing; drug should be discontinued
- Assess for tachypnea, ECG changes, dyspnea, edema, fatigue
- Assess for cardiac toxicity: CHF, dysrhythmias, cardiomyopathy; cardiac studies should be done before and periodically during treatment; ECG, chest x-ray
- Monitor CBC, differential, platelet count weekly; withhold drug if WBC is $<4000/mm^3$ or platelet count is $<100,000/mm^3$; notify prescriber of results if WBC $<20,000/mm^3$, platelets $<150,000/mm^3$
- Monitor renal function studies: BUN, uric acid, urine CCr, electrolytes, before, during therapy
- Monitor temp q4h (may indicate beginning of infection)
- Monitor liver function tests before and during therapy (bilirubin, AST, ALT, LDH) as needed or monthly; note jaundice of skin and sclera, dark urine, clay-colored stools, itchy skin, abdominal pain, fever, diarrhea; hepatoxicity can be severe
- Assess for bleeding: hematuria, stool guaiac, bruising or petechiae, mucosa or orifices q8h; assess for inflammation of mucosa, breaks in skin
- Identify effects of alopecia on body image; discuss feelings about body changes

Nursing diagnoses
- Injury, risk for (adverse reactions)
- Cardiac output, decreased (adverse reactions)
- Body image, disturbed (adverse reactions)
- Infection, risk for (adverse reactions)
- Knowledge, deficient (teaching)

Implementation
- Avoid contact with skin; very irritating; wash completely to remove
- Give fluids **IV** or PO before chemotherapy to hydrate patient
- Administer antiemetic 30-60 min before giving drug and prn to prevent vomiting; administer antibiotics for prophylaxis of infection
- Give a liq diet: carbonated beverages; gelatin may be added if patient is not nauseated or vomiting
- Drug should be prepared by experienced personnel using proper precautions (biologic cabinet, wearing gown, gloves, mask)
- Give after reconstituting 5-mg vial with 5 ml of 0.9% NaCl (1 mg/1 ml); give over 10-15 min through Y-tube or 3-way stopcock of inf of D_5 or 0.9% NaCl; discard unused portion
- Inject hydrocortisone for extravasation; apply ice compress after stopping inf
- Store at room temp for 3 days after reconstituting or 7 days refrigerated

Y-site compatibilities: Amifostine, amikacin, aztreonam, cimetidine, cladribine, cyclophosphamide, cytarabine, diphenhydrAMINE, droperidol, erythromycin, filgrastim, granisetron, imipenem/cilastatin, magnesium sulfate, mannitol, melphalan, metoclopromide, potassium chloride, ranitidine, sargramostim, thiotepa, vinorelbine

Y-site incompatibilities: Acyclovir, ampicillin/sulbactam, cefazolin, ceftazidine, clindamycin, dexamethasone, etoposide, furosemide, gentamicin, hydrocortisone, lorazepam, meperidine, methotrexate, mezlocillin, sargramostim, sodium bicarbonate, vancomycin, vinCRIStine

Solution compatibilities: $D_{3.3}$/0.3% NaCl, D_5/0.9% NaCl, D_5W, Ringer's, 0.9% NaCl, LR

Patient/family education
- Teach patient to avoid use of products containing aspirin or ibuprofen, razors, commercial mouthwash, since bleeding may occur; to report symptoms of bleeding (hematuria, tarry stools)
- Instruct patient to report signs of anemia (fatigue, headache, irritability, faintness, shortness of breath)
- Advise patient that hair may be lost during treatment; a wig or hairpiece may make patient feel better; new hair may be different in color, texture
- Teach patient to rinse mouth tid-qid with water, club soda; brush teeth bid-qid with soft brush or cotton-tipped applicators for stomatitis; use unwaxed dental floss
- Tell patient not to have any vaccinations without the advice of the prescriber; serious reactions can occur
- Advise patient that contraception is needed during treatment and for several mo after the completion of therapy

Evaluation
Positive therapeutic outcome
- Prevention of rapid division of malignant cells

! HIGH ALERT

ifosfamide (Rx)
(i-foss'fa-mide)
Ifex
Func. class.: Antineoplastic alkylating agent
Chem. class.: Nitrogen mustard
Pregnancy category D

Action: Alkylates DNA, RNA; inhibits enzymes that allow synthesis of amino acids in proteins; also responsible for cross-linking DNA strands; activity is not cell cycle stage specific

Therapeutic Outcome: Prevention of rapidly growing malignant cells

Uses: Testicular cancer, soft-tissue sarcoma, Ewing's sarcoma, non-Hodgkin's lymphoma, lung, pancreatic cancer, sarcoma

Dosage and routes
Adult: **IV** 1.2 g/m²/day × 5 days; repeat course q3 wk; give with mesna

Available forms: Inj 1, 3 g

Adverse effects
CNS: Facial paresthesia, fever, malaise, somnolence, confusion, depression, hallucinations, dizziness, disorientation, **seizures, coma,** cranial nerve dysfunction
GI: Nausea, vomiting, anorexia, **hepatotoxicity,** stomatitis, constipation, diarrhea
GU: **Hematuria, nephrotoxicity, hemorrhagic cystitis,** dysuria, urinary frequency
HEMA: **Thrombocytopenia, leukopenia, anemia**
INTEG: Dermatitis, alopecia, pain at inj site

Contraindications: Pregnancy **D,** hypersensitivity, bone marrow suppression

Precautions: Renal disease, lactation, children

Pharmacokinetics

Absorption	Complete bioavailability
Distribution	Saturation at high dosages
Metabolism	Liver
Excretion	Breast milk
Half-life	15 hr

Pharmacodynamics
Unknown

Interactions
Individual drugs
Allopurinol: increased toxicity
Radiation: increased bone marrow suppression
Drug classifications
Antineoplastics: increased bone marrow suppression
Barbiturates: increased toxicity
Live virus vaccines: decreased antibody response

NURSING CONSIDERATIONS
Assessment
- Monitor CBC, differential, platelet count weekly; withhold drug if WBC is <2000 or platelet count is <50,000; notify prescriber of results if WBC <10,000/mm³, platelets <100,000/mm³
- Monitor renal function studies: BUN, serum uric acid, urine CCr before, during therapy; I&O ratio; report fall in urine output of 30 ml/hr
- Monitor for cold, fever, sore throat (may indicate beginning of infection); identify edema in feet and joints, stomach pain, shaking; prescriber should be notified
- Assess for bleeding: hematuria, guaiac, bruising or petechiae, mucosa or orifices q8h; no rec temp

• Monitor liver function studies before and during therapy (ALT, AST, LDH); jaundice of skin, sclera, dark urine, clay-colored stools, itching, abdominal pain, fever, diarrhea that may indicate liver involvement

Nursing diagnoses

- Injury, risk for (adverse reactions)
- Body image, disturbed (adverse reactions)
- Infection, risk for (adverse reactions)
- Knowledge, deficient (teaching)

Implementation

- Give fluids **IV** or PO before chemotherapy to hydrate patient
- Give antiemetic 30-60 min before giving drug and prn to prevent vomiting
- Provide liq diet: carbonated beverages; gelatin may be added if patient is not nauseated or vomiting
- Give **IV** after diluting 1 g/20 ml of sterile or bacteriostatic water for inj with parabens or benzyl only; shake
- Give by intermittent inf after further diluting with D_5W, LR, 0.9% NaCl, sterile water for inj (1 g/20 ml = 50 mg/ml; 1 g/50 ml = 20 mg/ml; 1 g/200 ml = 5 mg/ml); give over ≥30 min; may also give as a cont inf over 72 hr
- Store powder at room temp; always give with mesna, increase fluids to 3 L/day to prevent ifosfamide-induced hemorrhagic cystitis

Syringe compatibilities: Mesna
Y-site compatibilities: Allopurinol, amifostine, aztreonam, filgrastim, fludarabine, gallium, granisetron, melphalan, ondansetron, paclitaxel, piperacillin/tazobactam, propofol, sargramostim, teniposide, thiotepa, vinorelbine
Additive compatibilities: Carboplatin, cisplatin, etoposide, fluorouracil, mesna

Patient/family education

- Teach patient to avoid use of products containing aspirin or NSAIDs, razors, commercial mouthwash, since bleeding may occur; to report symptoms of bleeding (hematuria, tarry stools)
- Instruct patient to report signs of anemia (fatigue, headache, irritability, faintness, shortness of breath)
- Advise patient to report any changes in breathing or coughing even several mo after treatment; to avoid crowds and persons with respiratory tract or other infections
- Teach patient that hair loss is common; discuss the use of wigs or hairpieces; that hair may be a different texture when regrowth occurs
- Caution patient not to have any vaccinations without the advice of the prescriber; serious reactions can occur
- Advise patient that contraception is needed during treatment and for several mo after completion of therapy
- Advise patient to report confusion, hallucinations, extreme drowsiness, numbness, tingling; avoid use of alcohol for ≥4 months after treatment

Evaluation

Positive therapeutic outcome

- Prevention of rapid division of malignant cells
- Absence of swelling at night
- Increased appetite, increased weight

imatinib (Rx)

(im-ah-tin′ib)

Gleevec

Func. class.: Antineoplastic—miscellaneous
Chem. class.: Protein-tyrosine kinase inhibitor

Pregnancy category D

Action: Inhibits Bcr-Abl tyrosine kinase created in chronic myeloid leukemia (CML)

Therapeutic Outcome: Decreased tumor size, prevention of spread of cancer

Uses: Treatment of chronic myeloid leukemia (CML) in blast cell crisis or chronic failure after treatment failure with interferon alfa, gastrointestinal stromal tumors (GIST)

Investigational uses: Polycythemia vera, medullary thyroid carcinoma, recurrent extraabdominal desmoid tumors

Dosage and routes

CML, chronic phase
Adult: PO 400 mg/day
Child: PO 260 mg/m^2/day

CML, accelerated phase/blast crisis
Adult: PO 600 mg/day GIST
Adult: PO 400 or 600 mg/day

Available forms: Tabs 100, 400 mg

Adverse effects

CNS: **CNS hemorrhage**, headache, dizziness, insomnia
CV: Hemorrhage
GI: *Nausea,* **hepatotoxicity**, *vomiting, dyspepsia,* **GI hemorrhage**, *anorexia,* abdominal pain
HEMA: **Neutropenia, thrombocytopenia, bleeding**
INTEG: *Rash, pruritus*
META: Edema, fluid retention, hypokalemia,

MISC: Fatigue, epistaxis, pyrexia, night sweats, increased weight
MS: Cramps, pain, arthralgia, myalgia
RESP: Cough, dyspnea, nasopharyngitis, pneumonia, URI

Contraindications: Pregnancy **D**, hypersensitivity

Precautions: Lactation, children, elderly

Pharmacokinetics	
Absorption	Well absorbed; bound to plasma protein (98%)
Distribution	Unknown
Metabolism	Liver (metabolites)
Excretion	Feces, primarily (metabolites)
Half-life	18-40 hr

Pharmacodynamics	
Onset	Unknown
Peak	2-4 hr
Duration	24 hr (imatinib) 40 hr (metabolite)

Interactions

Individual drugs

Acetaminophen: increased hepatotoxicity
Carbamazepine, dexamethasone, phenobarbital, phenytoin, rifampin: decreased imatinib concentrations
Clarithromycin, erythromycin, ketoconazole, itraconazole: increased imatinib concentrations
Simvastatin: increased plasma concentrations
Warfarin: increased plasma concentration of warfarin; avoid coadministration; use low-molecular-weight anticoagulants instead

Drug classifications

Calcium channel blockers: increased plasma concentrations

Drug/herb

St. John's wort: decreased imatinib concentration

NURSING CONSIDERATIONS

Assessment

- Assess ANC and platelets; in chronic phase if ANC $<1 \times 10^9$/L and/or platelets $<50 \times 10^9$/L, stop until ANC $>1.5 \times 10^9$/L and platelets $>75 \times 10^9$/L; in accelerated phase/blast crisis if ANC $<0.5 \times 10^9$/L and/or platelets $<10 \times 10^9$/L, determine whether cytopenia is related to biopsy/aspirate, if not, reduce dose by 200 mg, if cytopenia continues, reduce dose by another 100 mg; if cytopenia continues for 4 wk, stop drug until ANC $\geq 1 \times 10^9$/L
- Assess for hepatotoxicity: monitor liver function tests, before treatment and qmo
- Assess CBC, differential, platelet count weekly; withhold drug if WBC is $<3500/mm^3$, or platelet count $<100,000/mm^3$; notify prescriber of these results; drug should be discontinued
- Assess food preferences: list likes, dislikes
- Assess GI symptoms: frequency of stools
- Assess signs of fluid retention, edema: weigh, monitor lung sounds, assess for edema, 50-ml fluid retention is dose dependent

Nursing diagnoses

- Injury, risk for (side effects)
- Knowledge, deficient (teaching)

Implementation

- Give with meal and large glass of water to decrease GI symptoms
- Store at 25° C (77° F)

Patient/family education

- Instruct patient to report adverse reactions immediately: shortness of breath, swelling of extremities, bleeding
- Teach patient reason for treatment, expected result
- Instruct patient to eat a nutritious diet with iron, vit supplement, low fiber, few dairy products

Evaluation

Positive therapeutic outcome

- Decrease in leukemic cells, size of tumors

imipenem/ cilastatin (Rx)

(i-me-pen'em sye-la-stat'in)
Primaxin IM, Primaxin IV
Func. class.: Antiinfective—misc. penicillin
Chem. class.: Carbapenem

Pregnancy category C

Do Not Confuse:
imipenem/Omnipen, Primaxin/Premarin

Action: Interferes with cell wall replication of susceptible organisms; osmotically unstable cell wall swells and bursts from osmotic pressure; addition of cilastatin prevents renal inactivation that occurs with high urinary concentrations of imipenem

Therapeutic Outcome: Bactericidal action against the following: *Streptococcus pneumoniae,* group A β-hemolytic streptococci, *Staphylococcus aureus,* enterococcus; gram-negative organisms: *Klebsiella, Proteus, Escherichia coli, Acinetobacter, Serratia, Pseudomonas aeruginosa; Salmonella, Shigella*

Uses: Serious infections caused by gram-positive or gram-negative organisms

Dosage and routes

Adult: **IV** 250-500 mg q6-8h; severe infections may require 1 g q8h; may give IM q12h (total daily IM dose >1500 mg not recommended); mild to moderate infections

Child: **IV** 60-100 mg/kg/day in divided doses max 4 g/day

Renal dose

Adult: **IV** CCr 30-70 ml/min give 50% dose q6-8h; CCr 20-30 ml/min give 40% of dose q8-12h; CCr 5-20 ml/min give 25% of dose q12h

Available forms: IV inj 250, 500; IM inj 500, 750 mg

Adverse effects

CNS: Fever, somnolence, **seizures,** confusion, dizziness, weakness, myoclonia

CV: Hypotension, palpitations

GI: *Diarrhea, nausea, vomiting,* **pseudomembranous colitis, hepatitis,** glossitis

HEMA: **Eosinophilia, neutropenia,** decreased Hgb, Hct

INTEG: Rash, urticaria, pruritus, pain at inj site, phlebitis, erythema at inj site

RESP: Chest discomfort, dyspnea, hyperventilation

SYST: **Anaphylaxis**

Contraindications: Hypersensitivity, IM hypersensitivity to local anesthetics of the amide type

Precautions: Pregnancy **C,** lactation, elderly, hypersensitivity to penicillins, seizure disorders, renal disease, children

Pharmacokinetics

Absorption	Complete bioavailability (**IV**)
Distribution	Widely distributed; crosses placenta
Metabolism	Liver
Excretion	Kidneys, unchanged (70%-80%); breast milk
Half-life	1 hr; increased in renal disease

Pharmacodynamics

	IV	IM
Onset	Rapid	Unknown
Peak	½-1 hr	Unknown

Interactions

Individual drugs

Ganciclovir: increased risk of seizures

Probenecid: increased imipenem plasma levels

Drug classifications

β-Lactam antibiotics: increased antagonistic effect

Drug/lab test

Increased: AST, ALT, LDH, BUN, alkaline phosphatase, bilirubin, creatinine

False positive: direct Coombs' test

NURSING CONSIDERATIONS

Assessment

- Assess patient for previous penicillin sensitivity reaction, may have sensitivity to this drug
- Assess patient for signs and symptoms of infection, including characteristics of wounds, sputum, urine, stool, WBC >10,000/mm^3, fever; obtain baseline information before and during treatment
- Complete C&S tests before beginning drug therapy to identify if correct treatment has been initiated
- Assess for allergic reactions, anaphylaxis: rash, urticaria, pruritus, chills, wheezing, laryngeal edema, fever, joint pain; angioedema may occur a few days after therapy begins; epiNEPHrine, resuscitation equipment should be available for anaphylactic reaction
- Identify urine output; if decreasing, notify prescriber (may indicate nephrotoxicity); also check for increased BUN, creatinine
- Monitor blood studies: AST, ALT, CBC, Hct, bilirubin, LDH, alkaline phosphatase, Coombs' test monthly if patient is on long-term therapy
- Monitor electrolytes: potassium, sodium, chloride monthly if patient is on long-term therapy
- Assess bowel pattern daily; if severe diarrhea occurs, drug should be discontinued; may indicate pseudomembranous colitis
- Monitor for bleeding: ecchymosis, bleeding gums, hematuria, stool guaiac daily if patient is on long-term therapy
- Assess for overgrowth of infection: perineal itching, fever, malaise, redness, pain, swelling, drainage, rash, diarrhea, change in cough, sputum

Nursing diagnoses

- Infection, risk for (uses)
- Diarrhea (adverse reactions)
- Injury, risk for (adverse reactions)
- Knowledge, deficient (teaching)
- Noncompliance (teaching)

Implementation

IM route

- Reconstitute 500 mg/2 ml or 750 mg/3 ml lidocaine without epiNEPHrine; shake well, withdraw and administer entire vial; give inj deep in large muscle mass, massage

IV route

- Reconstitute each 250 or 500 mg/10 ml of compatible diluent; shake well; transfer the resulting susp to not less than 100 ml of compatible diluent; add 10 ml to each previously reconstituted vial and shake to ensure all medication is used; transfer the remaining contents of the vial to the infusion container; do not administer susp by direct inj; reconstitute 120-ml infusion bottles/100 ml of a compatible diluent; shake until clear; may use 0.9% NaCl, D_5W, $D_{10}W$, D_5/0.2% sodium bicarbonate, D_5/0.9% NaCl, D_5/0.45% NaCl, D_5/0.225% NaCl, mannitol 2.5%, 5%, or 10%
- Give by intermittent inf: each 250- or 500-mg dose over 20-30 min, and each 1-g dose over 40-60 min; administer over 15-20 min for pediatric patients; do not administer direct **IV**; do not admix with other antibiotics

Y-site compatibilities: Acyclovir, amifostine, aztreonam, cefepime, diltiazem, famotidine, fludarabine, foscarnet, granisetron, idarubicin, regular insulin, melphalan, methotrexate, ondansetron, propofol, tacrolimus, teniposide, thiotepa, vinorelbine, zidovudine

Y-site incompatibilities: Fluconazole, meperidine, sargramostim

Additive incompatibilities: Fluconazole, meperidine, sargramostim

Patient/family education

- Teach patient to report sore throat, bruising, bleeding, joint pain; may indicate blood dyscrasias (rare)
- Advise patient to contact prescriber if vaginal itching, loose foul-smelling stools, furry tongue occur; may indicate superinfection
- Advise patient to notify prescriber of diarrhea with blood or pus; may indicate pseudomembranous colitis

Evaluation

Positive therapeutic outcome

- Absence of signs/symptoms of infection (WBC <10,000/mm^3, temp WNL, absence of red, draining wounds)
- Reported improvement in symptoms of infection

Treatment of anaphylaxis: EpINEPHrine, antihistamines, resuscitate if needed

imipramine (Rx)

(im-ip'ra-meen)

Apo-Imipramine ✦, Imipramine HCl, Impril ✦, Norfranil, Novo Pramine ✦, Tofranil, Tofranil PM, Tipramine

Func. class.: Antidepressant, tricyclic

Chem. class.: Dibenzazepine, tertiary amine

Pregnancy category C

Do Not Confuse:
imipramine/desipramine

Action: Blocks reuptake of norepinephrine and serotonin into nerve endings, increasing action of norepinephrine and serotonin in nerve cells; has anticholinergic effects

Therapeutic Outcome: Decreased symptoms of depression after 2-3 wk; decreased bedwetting in children

Uses: Depression, enuresis in children

Investigational uses: Chronic pain, migraine headaches, cluster headaches as adjunct, incontinence

Dosage and routes

Adult: PO/IM 75-100 mg/day in divided doses; may increase by 25-50 mg up to 200 mg, not to exceed 300 mg/day; may give daily dose at bedtime

Elderly: PO 25 mg at bedtime, may increase to 100 mg/day in divided doses

Child: PO 25-75 mg/day

Enuresis

Child 6-12 yr: PO 10 mg at bedtime, max 50 mg

Available forms: Tabs 10, 25, 50, 75 mg; inj 25 mg/2 ml; caps 75, 100, 125, 150 mg

Adverse effects

CNS: *Dizziness, drowsiness,* confusion, headache, anxiety, tremors, stimulation, weakness, insomnia, nightmares, extrapyramidal symptoms (EPS) (elderly), increased psychiatric symptoms, paresthesia, **seizures**

CV: *Orthostatic hypotension, ECG changes, tachycardia,* hypertension, palpitations, **dysrhythmias**

EENT: Blurred vision, tinnitus, mydriasis

GI: *Diarrhea, dry mouth,* nausea, vomiting, **paralytic ileus,** increased appetite, cramps, epigastric distress, jaundice, **hepatitis,** stomatitis, constipation, taste change

GU: *Retention,* **acute renal failure**

HEMA: **Agranulocytosis, thrombocytopenia, eosinophilia, leukopenia**

INTEG: Rash, urticaria, sweating, pruritus, photosensitivity

Contraindications: Hypersensitivity to tricyclic antidepressants, recovery phase of MI, seizure disorders, prostatic hypertrophy

Precautions: Pregnancy **C**, suicidal patients, severe depression, increased intraocular pressure, narrow-angle glaucoma, urinary retention, cardiac disease, hepatic disease, hyperthyroidism, electroshock therapy, elective surgery, elderly, lactation

Pharmacokinetics

Absorption	Well absorbed
Distribution	Widely distributed; crosses placenta
Metabolism	Liver, extensively
Excretion	Kidneys, breast milk
Half-life	6-20 hr

Pharmacodynamics

	PO	IM
Onset	1 hr	1 hr
Peak	Unknown	Unknown
Duration	Unknown	Unknown

Interactions
Individual drugs
Alcohol: increased effects
Clonidine: hyperpyretic crisis, seizures, hypertensive episode
Clonidine, guanethidine: decreased effects
Drug classifications
Barbiturates, benzodiazepines, CNS depressants: increased effects
MAOIs: hyperpyretic crisis, hypertensive episode, seizures
Selective serotonin reuptake inhibitors: increased toxicity, avoid concurrent use
Sympathomimetics (direct acting): increased effects
Sympathomimetics (indirect acting): decreased effects
Drug/herb
Belladonna, corkwood, henbane, jimsonweed, scopolia: increased anticholinergic effect
Chamomile, hops, kava, lavender, skullcap, valerian: increased imipramine effect
SAM-e, St. John's wort: serotonin syndrome
Yohimbe: increased hypertension
Drug/lab test
Increased: serum bilirubin, blood glucose, alkaline phosphatase
Decreased: VMA, 5-HIAA, urinary catecholamines

NURSING CONSIDERATIONS
Assessment
- Monitor B/P (with patient lying, standing), pulse q4h; if systolic B/P drops 20 mm Hg, hold drug, notify prescriber; take vital signs q4h in patients with CV disease
- Monitor blood studies: CBC, leukocytes, differential, cardiac enzymes if patient is receiving long-term therapy
- Monitor hepatic studies: AST, ALT, bilirubin
- Check weight weekly; appetite may increase with drug
- Assess ECG for flattening of T wave, bundle branch block, AV block, dysrhythmias in cardiac patients
- Assess for EPS primarily in elderly: rigidity, dystonia, akathisia
- Assess mental status: mood, sensorium, affect, suicidal tendencies; increase in psychiatric symptoms: depression, panic
- Monitor urinary retention, constipation; constipation is more likely to occur in children or elderly
- (Alert) Assess for withdrawal symptoms: headache, nausea, vomiting, muscle pain, weakness, diarrhea, insomnia, restlessness; do not usually occur unless drug was discontinued abruptly
- Identify alcohol consumption; if alcohol is consumed, hold dose until AM

Nursing diagnoses
- Coping, ineffective (uses)
- Injury, risk for (side effects)
- Knowledge, deficient (teaching)
- Noncompliance (teaching)

Implementation
PO route
- Do not break, crush, or chew caps
- Give with food or milk
- Store at room temp; do not freeze

IM route
- Put ampule under warm running water for 1 min to dissolve crystals; sol may be yellow or red

Syringe compatibilities: Doxapram
Y-site compatibilities: Cladribine

Patient/family education
- Teach patient that therapeutic effects may take 2-3 wk
- Teach patient to use caution in driving and other activities requiring alertness because of drowsiness, dizziness, blurred vision; to avoid rising quickly from sitting position, especially elderly; orthostatic hypotension may occur
- Teach patient to avoid alcohol ingestion, other CNS depressants during treatment
- Teach patient not to discontinue medication quickly after long-term use: may cause nausea, headache, malaise
- Teach patient to wear sunscreen or large hat, since photosensitivity occurs

- Teach patient to increase fluids, bulk in diet if constipation, urinary retention occur, especially elderly
- Teach patient to take gum, hard sugarless candy, or frequent sips of water for dry mouth

Evaluation

Positive therapeutic outcome

- Decreased depression
- Absence of suicidal thoughts
- Decreased enuresis in children
- Decreased pain

Treatment of overdose: ECG monitoring, induce emesis, lavage, activated charcoal, administer anticonvulsant

immune globulin (Rx)

gamma globulin, IG, IGIM, Bay Gam

immune globulin IV (IGIV) (Rx)

Carimune NF, Flebogamma 5%, Gamimune N, Gamma-Gard S/D, gamma globulin, Gammar-PIV, Gamunex, Iveegam, Octagam, Panglobulin NF, Polygam, Polygam SD, Sandoglobulin, Venoglobulin-I, Venoglobulin-S

Func. class.: Immune serum

Chem. class.: IgG

Pregnancy category C

Action: Provides passive immunity to hepatitis A, measles, varicella, rubella, immune globulin deficiency; contains γ-globulin antibodies (IgG)

Therapeutic Outcome: Absence of infection

Uses: Immunodeficiency syndrome, B-cell chronic lymphocytic leukemia, Kawasaki syndrome, bone marrow transplantation, pediatric HIV infection, agammaglobulinemia, hepatitis A, B exposure, measles exposure, measles vaccine complications, purpura, rubella exposure, chickenpox exposure

Dosage and routes

Primary immunodeficiency

Adult and child: **IV** (Carimune, Panglobulin NF) 200 mg/kg qmo, max 300 mg/kg qmo or give more frequently if needed; **IV** (Gamimune N) 100-200 mg/kg qmo, max 400 mg/kg; **IV** (Gammagard S/D) 200-400 mg qmo, minimum 100 mg/kg qmo

Hepatitis A exposure

Adult and child: IM 0.02-0.04 ml/kg or 0.1 mg/kg if treatment is delayed

Hepatitis B exposure

Adult and child: IM 0.06 ml/kg within 1 wk, qmo

Rubella exposure in pregnancy (1st trimester)

Women: IM 0.55 ml/kg as soon as possible, within 72 hr

Chickenpox exposure

Adult and child: IM 0.6-1.2 ml/kg as soon as exposed

Measles (postexposure)

Child: IM 0.25 ml/kg within 6 days

B-cell chronic lymphocytic leukemia (CLL) (Gammagard S/D, Polygam S/D)

Adult: **IV** 400 mg/kg q3-4 wk

Immunoglobulin deficiency

Adult and child: IM 1.3 ml/kg, then 0.66 ml/kg after 2-4 wk and q2-4 wk thereafter

Idiopathic thrombocytopenic purpura

Adult and child: **IV** 0.4 g/kg/day × 5 days or 1 g/kg/day × 1-2 days

Kawasaki syndrome (Iveegam, Venoglobulin-S, Gammagard S/D, Polygam S/D)

Adult and child: **IV** (Iveegam, Venglobulin-S 5% or 10%) 2000 mg/kg over 10-12 hr, may repeat; **IV** (Gammagard S/D, Polygam S/D) 1 g/kg as single dose

Bone marrow transplantation (BMT) (Gamimune N)

Adult >20 yr: **IV** 500 mg/kg 5% or 10% sol on days 2, 7 before transplant then qwk for 90 days thereafter

Pediatric HIV (Gamimune N)

Child: **IV** 400 mg/kg 5% or 10% sol q28days

Available forms: IM (Bay Gam) inj 2, 10 ml vial; **IV** (Gamimune N, Venoglobulin-S) 5%, 10% sol; powder for inj (Carimune NF) 1-, 3-, 6-, 12-g vials; (Gammagard S/D) 50 mg protein/ml in 2.5-, 5-, 10-g vials; (Gammar-P IV) 1-, 2.5-, 5-, 10-g vials; (Iveegam) 500 mg, 1-, 2.5-, 5-g vials; (Panglobulin) 6-, 12-g vials; (Polygam S/D) 2.5-, 5-, 10-g vials; sol for inj (Gamunex) 1-, 2.5-, 5-, 10-, 20-g vials

Adverse effects

CNS: Headache, fatigue, malaise

GI: Abdominal pain

INTEG: Pain at inj site, rash, pruritus, chills

MS: Arthralgia, chest pain

SYST: Lymphadenopathy, **anaphylaxis**

Contraindications: Hypersensitivity

Precautions: Pregnancy **C**

Pharmacokinetics

Absorption	Well absorbed (IM); completely absorbed (**IV**)
Distribution	Rapidly
Metabolism	Liver, catabolism
Excretion	Kidneys
Half-life	3-4 wk

Pharmacodynamics

	IM	IV
Onset	Unknown	Rapid
Peak	Unknown	Unknown
Duration	Unknown	Unknown

Interactions

Live virus vaccines: do not give within 3 mo

NURSING CONSIDERATIONS

Assessment

- Assess for exposure date: this drug should be given within 6 days of measles, 1 wk of hepatitis B, 14 days of hepatitis A; if the date of exposure is outside these limits, immune globulin will not be effective
- Monitor blood studies in leukemia, idiopathic thrombocytopenic purpura: WBCs (leukemia), platelets
- Identify the number of inj of this drug patient has received; multiple inj may lead to sensitization (diaphoresis, fever, chills, malaise)
- Assess for anaphylaxis in patient receiving **IV** immune globulin: diaphoresis, flushing, nausea, vomiting, wheezing, difficulty breathing, hypotension, chest tightness, fever, weakness, sneezing, abdominal pain; VS should be monitored during inf and 1 hr after beginning inf; emergency equipment should be available with epINEPHrine and antihistamines to treat anaphylaxis

Nursing diagnoses

- Infection, risk for (uses)
- Knowledge, deficient (teaching)

Implementation

IM route

- Give IM (IGIM) inj in deltoid or anterolateral thigh in adults or anterolateral thigh in young children; if large amounts are given, several inj may be needed
- Do not give the IM preparation **IV**, SUBCUT, or intradermally
- Sol should be transparent and clear or slightly colored

IV route

- Warm to room temp before administration (diluent, powder for inj)
- A transfer device is provided by manufacturer; this drug should not be agitated or shaken
- Do not give the **IV** preparation SUBCUT, IM, or intradermally
- Check for adverse reaction during inf; stop inf if adverse reactions are present

Y-site compatibilities: Fluconazole, sargramostim

Gamimune N: Dilute **IV** with D_5; give 0.01 ml/kg/min; may increase to 0.02-0.04 ml/kg/min if no adverse reactions are present; may increase to 0.08 ml/kg/hr; sol should be refrigerated; do not freeze

Gammagard S/D: Reconstitute with sterile water for inj (50 mg protein/ml); give within 2 hr of reconstitution; give 0.5 ml/kg/hr; may increase to 4 ml/kg/hr if no adverse reactions occur; use inf set provided

Gammar-P IV: Give 0.01 ml/kg/min (50 mg/ml sol) over 15-30 min; may increase to 0.02 ml/kg/min; if adverse reactions are not present, may increase to 0.03-0.06 ml/kg/min; do not freeze; store at room temp

Iveegam (5%): Give 1-2 ml/min; refrigerate, do not freeze

Sandoglobulin: IV diluted with provided diluent; give 0.5-1 ml/min over 15-30 min; may increase to 1.5-2.5 ml/min; other inf may be given 2-2.5 ml/min; store at room temp

Venoglobulin-I: Give 50 mg/ml sol 0.01-0.02 ml/kg/min over 30 min if no adverse reactions; increase 0.04 ml/kg/min; store at room temp

Patient/family education

- Advise patient that passive immunity is temporary; explain reason for and expected results of this drug
- Advise patient that pain and tenderness may occur at inj site

Evaluation

Positive therapeutic outcome

- Prevention of infection
- Increased platelets

Treatment of anaphylaxis: EpINEPHrine, diphenhydrAMINE, O_2, vasopressors, corticosteroids

! HIGH ALERT

inamrinone (Rx)

(in-am'rih-nohn)

Inocor

Func. class.: Inotropic agent

Chem. class.: Bipyrimidine derivative

Pregnancy category C

Do Not Confuse:
inamrinone/amiodarone

Action: Positive inotropic agent with vasodilator properties; reduces preload and afterload by direct relaxation of vascular smooth muscle; increases myocardial contractility

Therapeutic Outcome: Increased inotropic effect resulting in increased cardiac output

Uses: Short-term management of CHF that has not responded to other medication; can be used with digitalis products

Dosage and routes

Adult and child: **IV** bol 0.75 mg/kg given over 2-3 min; start inf of 5-10 mcg/kg/min; may give another bol 30 min after start of therapy, max 10 mg/kg total daily dose

Infants: **IV** 3-4.5 mg/kg in divided doses, then give by inf 10 mcg/kg/min

Neonates: **IV** 3-4.5 mg/kg in divided doses, then give by inf 3-5 mcg/kg/min

Available forms: Inj 5 mg/ml

Adverse effects

CV: *Dysrhythmias, hypotension,* chest pain

GI: *Nausea, vomiting, anorexia,* abdominal pain, **hepatotoxicity (rare), ascites,** jaundice, hiccups

HEMA: **Thrombocytopenia**

INTEG: Allergic reactions, burning at inj site

RESP: Pleuritis, **pulmonary densities, hypoxemia**

Contraindications: Hypersensitivity to this drug or bisulfites, severe aortic disease, severe pulmonic valvular disease, acute MI

Precautions: Pregnancy **C**, lactation, children, renal disease, hepatic disease, atrial flutter/fibrillation, elderly, asthma

Pharmacokinetics

Absorption	Complete bioavailability
Distribution	Unknown
Metabolism	Liver, 50%
Excretion	Kidney, metabolites (60%-90%)
Half-life	4-6 hr, increased in CHF

Pharmacodynamics

Onset	2-5 min
Peak	10 min
Duration	Variable

Interactions

Individual drugs

Disopyramide: increased hypotension

Drug classifications

Antihypertensives: increased hypotension

Cardiac glycosides: increased additive effect

Drug/herb

Aloe, buckthorn, cascara sagrada, senna: increased inamrinone action

Drug/lab test

Increased: hepatic enzymes

Decreased: potassium

NURSING CONSIDERATIONS

Assessment

- Monitor manifestations of hypokalemia: *RENAL:* acidic urine, reduced urine, osmolality, nocturia; *CV:* hypotension, broad T wave, U wave, ectopy, tachycardia, weak pulse; *NEURO:* muscle weakness, altered LOC, drowsiness, apathy, lethargy, confusion, depression; *GI:* anorexia, nausea, cramps, constipation, distention, paralytic ileus; *RESP:* hypoventilation, respiratory muscle weakness
- Assess fluid volume status: CVP in elderly, I&O ratio and record, weight, distended red veins, crackles in lung, color, quality, and sp gr of urine, skin turgor, adequacy of pulses, moist mucous membranes, bilateral lung sounds, peripheral pitting edema; dehydration symptoms of decreasing output, thirst, hypotension, dry mouth, and mucous membranes should be reported
- Monitor electrolytes: potassium, sodium, calcium, magnesium; also include BUN, blood pH, ABGs
- Monitor B/P and pulse, PCWP, CVP, index, often during inf; if B/P drops 30 mm Hg, stop infusion and call prescriber
- Monitor ALT, AST, bilirubin daily; if these are elevated, hepatotoxicity is suspected
- If platelets are <150,000/mm^3, drug is usually discontinued and another drug started
- Assess for extravasation: change site q48h

Nursing diagnoses

- Cardiac output, decreased (uses)
- Fluid volume, excess (uses)
- Knowledge, deficient (teaching)

Implementation

- Patients with low potassium levels (hypokalemia) should receive potassium supplements before inamrinone administration

I

- Administer potassium supplements if ordered for potassium levels <3.0 mg/dl, correct before using inamrinone

IV route

- Do not mix directly with dextrose sol; chemical reaction occurs over 24 hr; precipitate forms if inamrinone and furosemide come in contact

IV, direct route

- May inject into running dextrose inf through Y-connector or directly into tubing; may give undiluted over 2-3 min or dilute with 0.9%, 0.45% NaCl to concentration of 1-3 mg/ml; run at prescribed rate by cont inf; another loading dose may be given in 30 min

Continous IV route

- Give after diluting with 0.9% or 0.45% NaCl (1-3 mg/ml); do not dilute with dextrose sol; decomposition of drug will occur; use infusion pump; use sol within 24 hr of dilution; titrate to patient response

Syringe compatibilities: Propranolol, verapamil

Y-site compatibilities: Aminophylline, atropine, bretylium, calcium chloride, cimetidine, cisatracurium, digoxin, DOBUTamine, DOPamine, epINEPHrine, famotidine, hydrocortisone, isoproterenol, lidocaine, metaraminol, methylPREDNISolone, nitroglycerin, nitroprusside, norepinephrine, phenylephrine, potassium chloride, procainamide, propranolol, remifentanil, verapamil

Y-site incompatibilities: Furosemide, inamrinone, sodium bicarbonate

Patient/family education

- Teach patient reason for medication and expected results
- Instruct patient to make position changes slowly; orthostatic hypotension may occur
- Teach patient signs and symptoms of hypersensitivity reactions and hypokalemia
- Advise patient that burning may occur at **IV** site

Evaluation

Positive therapeutic outcome

- Increased cardiac output
- Decreased PCWP, adequate CVP
- Decreased dyspnea, fatigue, edema, ECG

Treatment of overdose: Discontinue drug, support circulation

indapamide (Rx)

(in-dap'a-mide)

indapamide, Lozide ✦, Lozol

Func. class.: Diuretic, thiazide-like, antihypertensive

Chem. class.: Thiazide-like sulfonamide derivative

Pregnancy category B

Action: Acts on the distal tubule and thick ascending loop of Henle in the kidney, increasing excretion of sodium, water, chloride, magnesium, potassium, and bicarbonate

Therapeutic Outcome: Decreased B/P, decreased edema in lung tissues, peripherally

Uses: May be used alone or as adjunct with antihypertensives (mild to moderate)

Dosage and routes

Edema

Adult: PO 2.5 mg daily in AM; may be increased to 5 mg daily if needed

Antihypertensive

Adult: PO 1.25-5 mg daily; may increase to 5 mg/day over 8 wks

Available forms: Tabs 1.25, 2.5 mg

Adverse effects

CNS: Depression, *headache, dizziness, fatigue, weakness, nervousness, agitation,* extremity numbness

CV: Orthostatic hypotension, palpitations, volume depletion, PVCs, dysrhythmias

EENT: Blurred vision, nasal congestion, increased intraocular pressure

ELECT: *Hypokalemia, hypercalcemia, hyponatremia, hypochloremic alkalosis, hypomagnesemia*, hyperuricemia, hyperglycemia

GI: *Nausea,* vomiting, anorexia, constipation, diarrhea, cramps, abdominal pain, dry mouth

GU: *Frequency, polyuria, nocturia*, impotence

INTEG: Rash, *pruritus,*

MS: Cramps

Contraindications: Hypersensitivity, anuria, hepatic coma

Precautions: Pregnancy **B**, hypokalemia, severe renal disease, hepatic disease, ascites, dehydration, lactation, CCr <25 ml/min (not effective)

Pharmacokinetics	
Absorption	Well absorbed
Distribution	Widely distributed
Metabolism	Liver; 7%
Excretion	Unchanged (urine)
Half-life	14-18 hr

Pharmacodynamics	
Onset	1-2 hr
Peak	2 hr
Duration	Up to 36 hr

Interactions
Individual drugs
Amphotericin B: decreased potassium
Cholestyramine, colestipol: decreased absorption
Diazoxide: hyperglycemia
Digitalis, lithium: increased toxicity
Indomethacin: decreased hypotensive effect
Drug classifications
Anticoagulants, antidiabetics, antigout agents: decreased effects
Diuretics (other), steroids: decreased potassium
Muscle relaxants, steroids: increased toxicity
NSAIDs: decreased hypotensive effects
Drug/herb
Aloe, buckthorn, cascara sagrada, Chinese cucumber, licorice, senna: increased hypokalemia
Aloe, cucumber, dandelion, horsetail, pumpkin, Queen Anne's lace: increased diuretic effect
St. John's wort: severe photosensitivity
Drug/lab test
Increased: calcium, parathyroid test, glucose, uric acid

NURSING CONSIDERATIONS
Assessment
- Check for rashes, temp elevation daily
- Monitor patients that receive cardiac glycosides for increased hypokalemia, toxicity
- Monitor manifestations of hypokalemia: acidic or reduced urine, osmolality, nocturia; hypotension, broad T-wave, U-wave, ectopy, tachycardia, weak pulse; muscle weakness, altered LOC, drowsiness, apathy, lethargy, confusion, depression; anorexia, nausea, cramps, constipation, distention, paralytic ileus; hypoventilation, respiratory muscle weakness
- Monitor for manifestations of hypomagnesemia: agitation, muscle twitching, paresthesias, hyperactive reflexes, positive Babinski reflex, dysphagia, nystagmus, seizures, tetany; nausea, vomiting, diarrhea, anorexia, abdominal distention; ectopy, tachycardia, broad, flat- or inverted T-waves, depressed ST segment, prolonged QT interval, decreased cardiac output, hypotension
- Monitor for manifestations of hyponatremia: increased B/P, cold, clammy skin, hypo/hypervolemia; anorexia, nausea, vomiting, diarrhea, abdominal cramps; lethargy, increased ICP, confusion, headache, seizures, coma, fatigue, tremors, hyperreflexia
- Monitor for manifestations of hyperchloremia: weakness, lethargy, coma, deep rapid breathing
- Assess fluid volume status: I&O ratios and record, weight, distended red veins, crackles in lung, color, quality and sp gr of urine, skin turgor, adequacy of pulses, moist mucous membranes, bilateral lung sounds, peripheral pitting edema; dehydration symptoms of decreasing output, thirst, hypotension, dry mouth and mucous membranes should be reported
- Monitor electrolytes: potassium, sodium, calcium, magnesium; also include BUN, blood pH, ABGs, uric acid, CBC, blood glucose
- Assess B/P before and during therapy with patient lying, standing, and sitting as appropriate; orthostatic hypotension can occur rapidly

Nursing diagnoses
- Urinary elimination, impaired (side effect)
- Fluid volume, deficient (side effects)
- Fluid volume, excess (uses)
- Knowledge, deficient (teaching)

Implementation
- Give in AM to avoid interference with sleep
- Provide potassium replacement if potassium level is <3.0 mg/dl; give whole
- Give with food and milk if nausea occurs, absorption may be increased

Patient/family education
- Teach patient to take the medication early in the day to prevent nocturia
- Instruct the patient to take with food or milk if GI symptoms of nausea and anorexia occur
- Teach patient to maintain weekly record of weight and notify prescriber of weight loss >5 lb
- Caution the patient that this drug causes a loss of potassium, so food rich in potassium should be added to the diet; refer to a dietitian for assistance in planning
- Caution the patient to rise slowly from sitting or reclining positions, not to exercise in hot weather or stand for prolonged periods, since orthostatic hypotension will be enhanced; lie down if dizziness occurs
- Teach patient not to use alcohol or any OTC medications without prescriber's approval; serious drug reactions may occur
- Emphasize the need to contact prescriber immediately if muscle cramps, weakness, nausea, dizziness, or numbness occurs

I

- Teach patient to take own B/P and pulse and record findings
- Teach patient to continue taking medication even if feeling better; this drug controls symptoms but does not cure the condition
- Advise the patient with hypertension to continue other medical treatment (exercise, weight loss, relaxation techniques, cessation of smoking)

Evaluation

Positive therapeutic outcome

- Decreased edema
- Decreased B/P
- Increased diuresis

Treatment of overdose: Lavage, monitor electrolytes, administer **IV** fluids, monitor hydration, CV, renal status

indinavir (Rx)

(en-den′a-veer)

Crixivan

Func. class.: Antiretroviral

Chem. class.: Protease inhibitor

Pregnancy category C

Do Not Confuse:
idinavir/Denavir

Action: Inhibits HIV-1 protease; this prevents maturation of the infectious virus

Therapeutic Outcome: Decreased signs/symptoms of HIV-1 infection

Uses: HIV-1 in combination with other antiretrovirals

Investigational uses: Prevention of HIV after exposure

Dosage and routes

Reduce dose in mild/moderate hepatic impairment and ketoconazole coadministration

Adult: PO 800 mg q8h; if given with didanosine, give 1 hr apart on empty stomach

Available forms: Caps 100, 200, 333, 400 mg

Adverse effects

CNS: *Headache, insomnia,* dizziness, somnolence

GI: *Diarrhea, abdominal pain, nausea, vomiting,* anorexia, dry mouth

GU: Nephrolithiasis

INTEG: Rash

MISC: Asthenia, **insulin-resistant hyperglycemia,** hyperlipidemia, **ketoacidosis**, lipodystrophy

MS: Pain

Contraindications: Hypersensitivity

Precautions: Pregnancy **C,** liver disease, lactation, children, renal disease, history of renal stones, diabetes, hypercholesterolemia

Pharmacokinetics

Absorption	Unknown
Distribution	Unknown
Metabolism	60% protein binding; liver
Excretion	20% unchanged, urine
Half-life	Terminal 1-2 hr

Pharmacodynamics

Unknown

Interactions

Individual drugs

Atorvastatin, lovastatin, simvastatin: increased myopathy
Clarithromycin, zidovudine: increased levels of both drugs
Delavirdine, itraconazole, ketoconazole: increased indinavir level
Efavirenz, fluconazole, nevirapine: decreased indinavir level
Isoniazid: increased isoniazid level
Midazolam, rifampin, triazolam: increased life-threatening dysrhythmias

Drug classifications

Anticonvulsants: decreased effect of both drugs
Ergots: increased life-threatening dysrhythmias
Oral contraceptives: decreased levels of oral contraceptives
Rifamycins: decreased indinavir levels

Drug/herb

St. John's wort: decreased indinavir level, avoid use

Drug/food

High fat, high protein, grapefruit juice: decreased absorption

NURSING CONSIDERATIONS

Assessment

- Assess for lower back, flank pain, indicates kidney stones
- Monitor signs of infection, anemia
- Monitor liver studies: ALT, AST; total bilirubin, amylase; all may be elevated
- Determine the presence of other sexually transmitted diseases
- Assess bowel pattern before, during treatment; if severe abdominal pain with bleeding occurs, drug should be discontinued; monitor hydration
- Assess skin eruptions; rash, urticaria, itching
- Assess allergies before treatment, reaction of each medication; place allergies on chart
- Monitor viral load CD4 during treatment

Nursing diagnoses
- Infection, risk for (uses)
- Knowledge, deficient (teaching)

Implementation
- Do not break, crush, or chew caps
- Give with water, 1 hr ac or 2 hr pc; may be given with other liquids or small meal; do not give with high-fat, high-protein meals
- Give in equal intervals around the clock
- Dosage adjustment will need to be considered when given with efavirenz
- Give water to 1.5 L/day minimum, to prevent nephrolithiasis

Patient/family education
- Advise to take as prescribed; if dose is missed, take as soon as remembered up to 1 hr before next dose; do not double dose
- Advise that drug must be taken in equal intervals around the clock to maintain blood levels for duration of therapy
- Instruct patient to increase fluids to prevent kidney stones, if stone formation occurs, treatment may need to be interrupted
- Inform patient that drug does not cure AIDS, controls symptoms only; not to donate blood
- Advise patient that hyperglycemia may occur, watch for symptoms (thirst, hunger, dry, itchy skin); notify prescriber

Evaluation
Positive therapeutic outcome
- Decreased signs/symptoms of infection, HIV

indomethacin (Rx)
(in-doe-meth′a-sin)

Apo-Indomethacin ✤, Indameth ✤, Indochron E-R, Indocid ✤, Indocin, Indocin IV, Indocin PDA ✤, Indocin SR, indomethacin, Novomethacin ✤, Nu-Indo ✤

Func. class.: NSAID (nonsteroidal antiinflammatory), antirheumatic

Chem. class.: Propionic acid derivative

Pregnancy category B (1st trimester), X (2nd/3rd trimesters)

Action: Inhibits prostaglandin synthesis by decreasing enzyme needed for biosynthesis; analgesic, antiinflammatory, antipyretic

Therapeutic Outcome: Decreased pain, inflammation; or closure of patent ductus arteriosus (premature infants)

Uses: Rheumatoid arthritis, ankylosing rheumatoid spondylitis, acute gouty arthritis; closure of patent ductus arteriosus in premature infants (**IV**)

Dosage and routes
Arthritis/antiinflammatory
Adult: PO/REC 25-50 mg bid; may increase by 25 mg/day qwk, not to exceed 200 mg/day; sus rel 75 mg daily; may increase to 75 mg bid

Acute arthritis
Adult: PO/REC 100 mg initially, then 50 mg tid; use only for acute attack, then reduce dosage

Patent ductus arteriosus
Longer or repeated treatment courses may be necessary for very premature infants

Infant <2 days: **IV** 0.2 mg/kg, then 0.1 mg/kg × 2 doses after 12, 24 hr

Infant 2-7 days: **IV** 0.2 mg/kg, then 0.2 mg/kg × 2 doses after 12, 24 hr

Infant >7 days: **IV** 0.2 mg/kg, then 0.25 mg/kg × 2 doses after 12, 24 hr

Available forms: Caps 25, 50 mg; sus rel caps 75 mg; oral susp 25 mg/5 ml; rec supp 50, 100 mg; inj 1-mg vials

Adverse effects
CNS: Dizziness, drowsiness, fatigue, tremors, confusion, insomnia, anxiety, depression, headache

CV: Tachycardia, peripheral edema, palpitations, dysrhythmias, hypertension

EENT: Tinnitus, hearing loss, blurred vision

GI: *Nausea,* anorexia, *vomiting,* diarrhea, jaundice, **cholestatic hepatitis,** *constipation,* flatulence, cramps, dry mouth, peptic ulcer, **ulceration, perforation, GI bleeding**

GU: **Nephrotoxicity (dysuria, hematuria, oliguria, azotemia)**

HEMA: **Blood dyscrasias,** prolonged bleeding

INTEG: Purpura, rash, pruritus, sweating

Contraindications: Pregnancy **X** (2nd/3rd trimesters) hypersensitivity, asthma, severe renal disease, severe hepatic disease, ulcer disease

Precautions: Pregnancy **B** (1st trimester), lactation, children, bleeding disorders, GI disorders, cardiac disorders, hypersensitivity to other antiinflammatory agents, depression

Pharmacokinetics

Absorption	Well absorbed (PO); erratic (rec); complete (**IV**)
Distribution	Crosses blood-brain barrier; placenta, 99% plasma protein binding
Metabolism	Liver, extensively
Excretion	Breast milk
Half-life	2.6-11 hr

Pharmacodynamics

	IV	PO	PO–EXT REL
Onset	2 day	1-2 hr	½ hr
Peak	Unknown	3 hr	Unknown
Duration	Unknown	4-6 hr	4-6 hr

Interactions

Individual drugs

Abciximab, cefamandole cefoperazone, cefotetan, clopidogrel, eptifibatide, plicamycin, ticlodipine, tirofiban, valproic acid: increased bleeding risk
CycloSPORINE: increased nephrotoxicity
Lithium, methotrexate, zidovudine: increased toxicity

Drug classifications

Aminoglycosides: increased effects of aminoglycosides
Anticoagulants, cephalosporins, thrombolytics: increased risk of bleeding
Antihypertensives: decreased effect of antihypertensives
Digoxin, penicillamine, phenyton: increased effect of each specific drug
Diuretics (potassium sparing): increased hyperkalemia

Drug/herb

Anise, arnica, bogbean, chamomile, chondroitin, clove, dong quai, feverfew, garlic, ginger, ginkgo, ginseng (*Panax*): increased bleeding risk
Arginine, gossypol: increased gastric irritation
Bearberry, bilberry: increased NSAIDs effect

NURSING CONSIDERATIONS

Assessment

- Assess for patent ductus arteriosus: respiratory rate, character, heart sounds
- Assess for joint pain (duration, intensity, ROM), baseline and during treatment
- Assess for confusion, mood changes, hallucinations, especially in elderly
- Assess renal, liver, blood studies: BUN, creatinine, AST, ALT, Hgb before treatment and periodically thereafter; if renal function decreases, do not give subsequent doses

Nursing diagnoses

- Pain, acute (uses)
- Pain, chronic (uses)
- Mobility, impaired (uses)
- Knowledge, deficient (teaching)

Implementation

PO route

- Swallow sus rel cap whole; do not break, crush, or chew sus rel cap
- Give with food or milk to decrease gastric symptoms, and prevent ulceration
- Shake susp, do not mix with other liquids

Rectal route

- Have patient retain rec supp for 1 hr after insertion

IV route

- Give after diluting 1-2 mg/ml or more normal saline or sterile water for inj without preservative; give over 5-10 sec to avoid dramatic shift in cerebral blood flow; avoid extravasation

Y-site compatibilities: Furosemide, insulin (regular), potassium chloride, sodium bicarbonate, sodium nitroprusside

Patient/family education

- Advise patient to report change in vision, blurring, rash, tinnitus, black stools
- Tell patient not to use for any other condition than prescribed
- Advise patient to avoid use with OTC medications for pain unless approved by prescriber
- Advise patient to avoid hazardous activities, since dizziness or drowsiness can occur
- Instruct patient to use sunscreen to prevent photosensitivity

Evaluation

Positive therapeutic outcome

- Decreased stiffness
- Increased joint mobility
- Decreased pain

infliximab (Rx)

(in-fliks'ih-mab)
Remicade
Func. class.: Monoclonal antibody
Pregnancy category B

Action: Monoclonal antibody that neutralizes the activity of tumor necrosis factor α (TNFα) that has been found in Crohn's disease; decreased infiltration of inflammatory cells

Therapeutic Outcome: Decreased cramping and blood in stools

Uses: Crohn's disease, fistulizing, moderate-severe; rheumatoid arthritis given with methotrexate

Investigational uses: Plaque psoriasis, ankylosing spondylitis, ulcerative colitis, psoriatic arthritis, psoriasis, Behçet syndrome, uveitis, juvenile arthritis

Dosage and routes

Crohn's disease (moderate-severe)

Adult: **IV** inf 5 mg/kg × 1

Crohn's disease (fistulizing)
Adult: **IV** inf 5 mg/kg initially, then repeat dose 2, 6 wk after 1st dose

Rheumatoid arthritis
Adult: **IV** 3 mg/kg initially, and 2, 6 wk and q8 wk thereafter, given with methotrexate

Available forms: Powder for inj 100 mg

Adverse effects

CNS: *Headache, dizziness, depression, vertigo, fatigue, anxiety, fever,* **seizures**
CV: Chest pain, hypertension and hypotension, tachycardia
GI: *Nausea, vomiting, abdominal pain, stomatitis, constipation, dyspepsia, flatulence*
GU: Dysuria, frequency
HEMA: **Anemia**
INTEG: *Rash, dermatitis, urticaria,* dry skin, sweating, flushing, hematoma, pruritus
MS: Myalgia, back pain, arthralgia
RESP: URI, pharyngitis, bronchitis, cough, dyspnea, sinusitis
SYST: **Anaphylaxis, fatal infections, sepsis, malignancies, immunogenicity**

Contraindications: Hypersensitivity to murines, moderate to severe CHF (NYHA class III/IV)

Precautions: Pregnancy **B,** lactation, children, elderly

Pharmacokinetics

Absorption	Unknown
Distribution	Vascular compartment
Metabolism	Unknown
Excretion	Unknown
Half-life	9½ days

Pharmacodynamics

Onset	Unknown
Peak	Unknown
Duration	Unknown

Interactions

Drug classifications
Live virus vaccines: do not administer live vaccines concurrently

NURSING CONSIDERATIONS

Assessment

- Assess GI symptoms: nausea, vomiting, abdominal pain
- Take periodic blood counts: CBC
- Assess CV status: B/P, pulse, chest pain
- Assess for allergic reaction, anaphylaxis: rash, dermatitis, urticaria, fever, chills, dyspnea, hypotension; discontinue if severe, administer epINEPHrine, corticosteroids; antihistamines; assess for allergy to murine proteins before starting therapy
- Fatal infections: discontinue if infection occurs, do not administer to patients with active infections
- Identify TB before beginning treatment; a TB test should be obtained; if present, TB should be treated prior to receiving infliximab

Nursing diagnoses

- Injury, risk for (uses)
- Diarrhea (uses)
- Knowledge, deficient (teaching)

Implementation

IV infusion route

- Administer immediately after reconstitution; reconstitute each vial with 10 ml of sterile water for inj, further dilute total dose/250 ml of 0.9% NaCl inj to a total conc of between 0.4 and 4 mg/ml; use 21G or smaller needle for reconstitution, direct sterile water at glass wall of vial, gently swirl
- Give over ≥2 hr, use polyethylene-lined infusion with in-line, sterile, low-protein-bind filter
- Do not admix
- Provide refrigerated storage, do not freeze

Patient/family education

- Teach patient not to breastfeed while taking this drug
- Advise patient to notify prescriber of GI symptoms, hypersensitivity reactions
- Advise patient not to operate machinery or drive if dizziness, vertigo occurs

Evaluation

Positive therapeutic outcome

- Absence of blood in stool
- Reported improvement in comfort
- Weight gain

insulin, inhaled

Exubera

See Appendix A, Selected New Drugs

! HIGH ALERT

insulins

RAPID ACTING

insulin glulisine (Rx)
Apidra
insulin aspart (Rx)
Novolog
insulin lispro (Rx)
Humalog

SHORT ACTING

insulin, regular ⚷ (OTC)
Humulin R ✦, Novolin ge Toronto ✦, Novolin R
insulin, regular concentrated (Rx)
regular (concentrated), Iletin II U-500

INTERMEDIATE ACTING

insulin, isophane suspension (NPH) ⚷ (OTC)
Humulin N, Novolin N
insulin, zinc suspension (Lente) (OTC)
Novolin ge Lente ✦, Novolin L

LONG ACTING

insulin, zinc suspension extended (Ultralente) (OTC)
insulin detemir (Rx)
Levemir
insulin glargine (Rx)
Lantus

MIXTURES

insulin, isophane suspension and regular insulin (Rx)
Humulin 70/30, Humalin 30/70 ✦, Novolin 70/30, Novolin 70/30 PenFill, Novolin 70/30 Prefilled, Novolin ge 30/70 ✦
isophane insulin suspension (NPH) and insulin mixtures (Rx)
Humulin 50/50, Novolin 50/50

Func. class.: Antidiabetic, pancreatic hormone

Chem. class.: Exogenous unmodified insulin

Pregnancy category B, C

Do Not Confuse:
Novolin 70/30 Penfill/Novolin 70/30 Prefilled, Lantus/Lente

Action: Decreases blood glucose; by transport of glucose into cells and the conversion of glucose to glycogen indirectly increases blood pyruvate and lactate, decreases phosphate and potassium; insulin may be pork or human (processed by recombinant DNA technologies)

Therapeutic Outcome: Decreased blood glucose levels in diabetes mellitus

Uses: Type 1 diabetes mellitus, type 2 diabetes mellitus, gestational diabetes, insulin lispro may be used in combination with sulfonylureas in children >3 yr

Dosage and routes

Insulin glulisine

Adult: SUBCUT dosage individualized, give within 15 min before or 20 minutes after starting a meal

Insulin aspart

Adult/child ≥6 yr: 0.5-1 unit/kg/day divided in treatment, meal-related, highly individualized

Insulin lispro

Adult: SUBCUT 15 min ac

Human regular

Adult: SUBCUT ½-1 ac

Insulin, isophane suspension

Adult: SUBCUT dosage individualized by blood, urine glucose; usual dose 7-26 units; may increase by 2-10 units/day if needed

Insulin detemir

Adult: SUBCUT 1 or 2 times daily; if 1 time give with evening meal

Insulin glargine

Adult and child ≥ 6 yr: SUBCUT 10 international units daily, range 2-100 international units/day

Regular insulin

Ketoacidosis

Adult: **IV** 5-10 units, then 5-10 units/hr until desired response, then switch to SUBCUT dose; **IV**/ inf 2-12 units (50 units/500 ml of normal saline)

Child: **IV** 0.1 unit/kg

Replacement

Adult and child: SUBCUT 0.5-1 units/kg/day qid given 30 min ac

Adolescents: SUBCUT 0.8-1.2 mg/kg/day; this dosage is used during rapid growth

Available forms: NPH: inj 100 units/ml; regular inj 100 units/ml, cartridges 100 units/ml; insulin analog inj 100 units/ml; insulin zinc susp ext (ultralente): 100 units/ml; isophane insulin susp inj 100 units/ml, cartridges 100 units/ml; zinc susp 100 units/ml; insulin lispro: 100 units/ml, 1.5 ml cartridges; insulin glulisine: inj 100 units/ml;

insulin detemir: 100 units/ml in 10 vials, 3 ml cartridges; insulin glargine: inj 100 units/ml; insulin detemir: inj 100 units/ml

Adverse effects

EENT: Blurred vision, dry mouth
INTEG: Flushing, rash, urticaria, warmth, *lipodystrophy,* lipohypertrophy, swelling, redness
META: *Hypoglycemia,* rebound hyperglycemia (Somogyi effect 12-72 hr or longer)
SYST: **Anaphylaxis**

Contraindications: Hypersensitivity to protamine

Precautions: Pregnancy **C** (glargine); **B** (lispro); **C** (all others)

Pharmacokinetics	
Absorption	Rapidly absorbed (SUBCUT)
Distribution	Widely distributed
Metabolism	Liver, muscle, kidney
Excretion	Kidneys
Half-life	Regular 3-5 min; NPH 10 min

Interactions

Individual drugs

Alcohol: increased hypoglycemia
Dobutamine: increased insulin need
EpINEPHrine: decreased hypoglycemia
Fenfluramine, guanethedine, phenylbutazone, sulfinpyrazone, tetracycline: decreased insulin need
Smoking: increased insulin need

Drug classifications

Anabolic steroids, β-adrenergic blockers, hypoglycemics (oral), salicylates: increased hypoglycemia
Contraceptives (oral), corticosteroids, diuretics (thiazide), thyroid hormones: decreased hypoglycemia
Estrogens: increased insulin need
MAOIs: decreased insulin need

Drug/herb

Aceitilla, adiantam, agrimony, aloe gel, banana flowers/roots, banyan stem bark, bilberry, bitter melon, broom, bugleweed, burdock, carob, cumin, damiana, dandelion, eucalyptus, fenugreek, fo-ti, garlic, goat's rue, guar gum, horse chestnut, jambul, juniper, konjac, maitake, onion, psyllium, reishi: increased hypoglycemia
Alfalfa, aloe, basil, bay, bilberry, bitter melon, black catechu, buchu, burdock, coriander, dandelion, eyebright (po), fenugreek, garlic, ginseng, glucomannan, glucosamine, goat's rue, gymnema, horehound, horse chestnut, jambul, myrrh, myrtle: increased antidiabetic effect
Annato, cocoa seeds, coffee beans, cola seeds, guarana, ma huang, rosemary, yerba maté: decreased hypoglycemic effect
Bee pollen, blue cohosh, broom, chromium, elecampane, eucalyptus, gotu kola: decreased antidiabetic effect
Chromium: increased or decreased hypoglycemia
Karela: increased glucose tolerance

Pharmacokinetics	
Rapid acting	
Insulin glulisine	Onset 15-30 min, peak ½-1½ hr, duration 3-4 hr
Insulin aspart	Onset 15-30 min, peak ½-1½ hr, duration 3-4 hr
Insulin lispro	Onset 15-30 min, peak ½-1½ hr, duration 3-4 hr
Short acting	
Insulin, regular	Onset ½-1 hr, peak 2-3 hr, duration 3-6 hrs
Intermediate acting	
Insulin, isophane suspension (NPH)	Onset 2-4 hr, peak 6-10 hr, duration 10-16 hr
Insulin, zinc suspension (Lente)	Onset 3-4 hr, peak 6-12 hr, duration 12-18 hr
Long acting	
Insulin, zinc suspension extended (Ultralente)	Onset 6-10 hr, peak 10-16 hr, duration 18-20 hr
Insulin glargine	Onset 5 hrs, no peak identified, duration ≥24 hr
Mixtures	
Insulin, isophane suspension and regular insulin (70/30)	Onset ½-1 hr, peak dual, duration 10-16 hr
Isophane insulin suspension (NPH) and insulin mixtures (50/50)	Onset ½-1 hr, peak dual, duration 10-16 hr

Drug/lab test
Increased: VMA
Decreased: potassium, calcium
Interference: liver function studies, thyroid function studies

NURSING CONSIDERATIONS
Assessment
- Monitor fasting blood glucose, 2 hr pc (80-150 mg/dl, normal fasting level; 70-130 mg/dl, normal 2-hr level); also A1c may be measured to identify treatment effectiveness
- Monitor urine ketones during illness; insulin requirements may increase during stress, illness, surgery
- Assess for hypoglycemic reaction that can occur during peak time (sweating, weakness, dizziness, chills, confusion, headache, nausea, rapid weak pulse, fatigue, tachycardia, memory lapses, slurred speech, staggering gait, anxiety, tremors, hunger)
- Assess for hyperglycemia: acetone breath, polyuria, fatigue, polydipsia, flushed, dry skin, lethargy

Nursing diagnoses
- Injury, risk for (adverse reactions)
- Knowledge, deficient (teaching)
- Noncompliance (teaching)

Implementation
SUBCUT route
- Give after warming to room temp by rotating in palms to prevent injecting cold insulin; use only insulin syringes with markings or syringe matching units/ml; rotate inj sites within one area: abdomen, upper back, thighs, upper arm, buttocks; keep record of sites
- Give increased dosages if tolerance occurs; give human insulin to those allergic to pork
- Give lispro 15 min ac
- Premixed insulins and NPH are cloudy suspensions
- Regular human insulin, rapid-acting analogs, and long-acting analogs are clear; do not use if cloudy, thick, or discolored
- Store at room temp for <1 mo; keep away from heat and sunlight; refrigerate all other supply; do not freeze

IV route, regular only
- Do not use if cloudy, thick, or discolored
- Give **IV** direct, undiluted via vein, Y-site, 3-way stopcock; give at 50 units/min or less
- Give by cont inf after diluting with **IV** sol and run at prescribed rate; use **IV** infusion pump for correct dosing; give reduced dose at serum glucose level of 250 mg/100 ml

Syringe compatibilities: Metoclopramide
Y-site compatibilities: Amiodarone, ampicillin, ampicillin/sulbactam, aztreonam, cefazolin, cefotetan, DOBUTamine, esmolol, famotidine, gentamicin, heparin, heparin/hydrocortisone, imipenen/cilastatin, indomethacin sodium trihydrate, magnesium sulfate, meperidine, meropenem, midazolam, morphine, nitroglycerin, nitroprusside, oxytocin, pentobarbital, potassium chloride, propofol, ritodrine, sodium bicarbonate, tacrolimus, terbutaline, ticarcillin, ticarcillin/clavulanate, tobramycin, vancomycin, vit B/C
Y-site incompatibilities: Nafcillin
Additive compatibilities: Bretylium, cimetidine, lidocaine, meropenem, ranitidine, verapamil
Additive incompatibilities: Aminophylline, amobarbital, chlorothiazide, cytarabine, DOBUTamine, pentobarbital, phenobarbital, phenytoin, secobarbital, sodium bicarbonate, thiopental

Patient/family education
- Advise patient that blurred vision occurs; not to change corrective lenses until vision is stabilized after 1-2 mo of therapy
- Advise patient to keep insulin and equipment available at all times; carry a glucagon kit, candy or lump sugar to treat hypoglycemia
- Advise patient to carry/wear emergency ID as diabetic
- Teach patient dosage, route, mixing instructions, disease process; tell patient to continue to use the same brand of insulin and to rotate inj sites
- Instruct patient to recognize hyperglycemia reaction: frequent urination, thirst, fatigue, hunger
- Teach patient symptoms of ketoacidosis: nausea, thirst, polyuria, dry mouth, decreased B/P, dry, flushed skin, acetone breath, drowsiness, Kussmaul respirations
- Advise patient that a plan is necessary for diet, exercise; all food on diet should be eaten, exercise routine should not vary
- Teach patient to avoid OTC drugs and alcohol unless approved by a prescriber
- Instruct patient to notify prescriber if pregnancy is planned
- Caution patient that treatment is lifelong; insulin does not cure condition

Evaluation
Positive therapeutic outcome
- Decrease in polyuria, polydipsia, polyphagia; clear sensorium, absence of dizziness, stable gait
- Blood glucose level under control

Treatment of overdose: Glucose 25 g **IV**, via dextrose 50% sol, 50 ml or glucagon 1 mg

interferon alfa-2a/ interferon alfa-2b (Rx)

(in-ter-feer'on)

Roferon-A/Intron-A

Func. class.: Antineoplastic—miscellaneous

Chem. class.: Protein product

Pregnancy category C

Do Not Confuse:
Roferon-A/Imferon

Action: Antiviral action inhibits viral replication by reprogramming virus; antitumor action suppresses cell proliferation; immunomodulating action phagocytizes target cells; may also inhibit virus replication

Therapeutic Outcome: Prevention of rapid growth of malignant cells; treatment of hepatitis non-A, non-B (liver function improvement)

Uses: Hairy cell leukemia in persons >18 yr, condylomata acuminata (alfa 2b), malignant melanoma, AIDS-related Kaposi's sarcoma, chronic hepatitis non-A, non-B (alfa 2b), chronic hepatitis B, C (alfa 2b)

Investigational uses: Bladder tumors, carcinoid tumors, non-Hodgkin's lymphoma, essential thrombocytopenia, cytomegaloviruses, herpes simplex, human papilloma virus–associated diseases

Dosage and routes

Hairy cell leukemia (2a)

Adult: SUBCUT/IM 3 million international units/day × 16-24 wk, then 3 million international units 3 ×/wk maintenance

Hairy cell leukemia (2b)

2 million international units/m^2 3 ×/wk; if severe adverse reactions occur, dose should be skipped or reduced by half

Kaposi's sarcoma (2b)

Adult: SUBCUT/IM 30 million international units m^2 3 ×/wk

Condylomata acuminata (2a)

1 million international units/lesion 3 ×/wk × 3 wk

Chronic hepatitis B (2b)

Adult: SUBCUT/IM 3 million international units 3 ×/wk × 18-24 mo or 5 million international units/day or 10 million international units 3 ×/wk × 16 wk

Available forms: Alfa-2a: inj 3, 6, 36 million international units/ml; alfa-2b: inj 3, 5, 10, 18, 25 million units/vial, powder for inj 5, 10, 18, 25, 50 million units/vial

Adverse effects

CNS: *Dizziness, confusion, numbness, paresthesia,* hallucinations, **seizures, coma,** amnesia, anxiety, mood changes, depression, somnolence, paranoia, irritability

CV: *Edema, hypotension,* hypertension, chest pain, palpitations, dysrhythmias, **CHF, MI, CVA,** tachycardia, syncope

GI: *Weight loss, taste changes,* nausea, anorexia, diarrhea, xerostomia

GU: *Impotence*

HEMA: **Neutropenia, thrombocytopenia**

INTEG: *Rash, dry skin, itching, alopecia,* flushing, photosensitivity

MISC: *Flulike symptoms: fever, fatigue, myalgias, headache, chills*

Contraindications: Hypersensitivity

Precautions: Pregnancy **C,** severe hypotension, dysrhythmia, tachycardia, lactation, children, severe renal or hepatic disease, seizure disorder

Pharmacokinetics	
Absorption	80%-90% (SC/IM)
Distribution	Unknown
Metabolism	Renal tubular (degraded)
Excretion	Kidneys
Half-life	3.7-8.5 hr (2a); 2-7 hr (2b)

Pharmacodynamics	
Onset	Unknown
Peak	3-8 hr
Duration	Unknown

Interactions

Individual drugs

Aminophylline: increased toxicity, blood levels

Zidovudine: increased neutropenia

Drug/lab test

Interference: AST, ALT, LDH, alkaline phosphatase, WBC, platelets, granulocytes, creatinine

NURSING CONSIDERATIONS

Assessment

- Assess cardiac status: lung sounds, ECG before and during treatment, especially in those with cardiac disease
- Assess bone marrow depression: bruising, bleeding, blood in stools, urine, sputum, emesis
- Assess mental status: depression, suicidal thoughts, hallucinations, amnesia
- Assess for symptoms of infection; may be masked by drug fever; fever, chills, headache, sore throat may occur 6 hr after dose; give acetaminophen for symptoms

I

- In AIDS patients with Kaposi's sarcoma, assess characteristics of lesions during therapy; symptoms should decrease
- Assess for bleeding: hematuria, stool guaiac, bruising or petechiae, mucosa or orifices q8h; check for inflammation of mucosa, breaks in skin; avoid IM inj, rec temp, or any other procedures that break the skin
- Assess for CNS reaction: LOC, mental status, dizziness, confusion, poor coordination, difficulty speaking, behavior changes; notify prescriber (alfa-2b)

Nursing diagnoses

- Injury, risk for (adverse reactions)
- Body image, disturbed (adverse reactions)
- Infection, risk for (adverse reactions)
- Knowledge, deficient (teaching)

Implementation

- Sol should be prepared by qualified personnel only under controlled conditions in biologic cabinet using gown, gloves, and mask
- Use Luer-Lok tubing to prevent leakage; do not let sol come in contact with skin; if contact occurs, wash well with soap and water
- Give at bedtime to minimize side effects
- Give acetaminophen as ordered to alleviate fever and headache
- Give by IM/SUBCUT after reconstituting 3-5 million international units/1 ml, 10 million international units/2 ml, 25 million international units/5 ml, of diluent provided; mix gently

Alfa-2a

- SUBCUT/IM after reconstituting 18 million units/3 ml of diluent provided (6 million units/ml)
- 36 million units/ml is used for Kaposi's sarcoma only
- Store reconstituted sol; must be used within 30 days

Intralesional route (2b)

- Give by intralesional route after reconstituting 10 million international units/1 ml of bacteriostatic water for inj; no more than 5 lesions can safely be treated at a time; using a 25G needle inject 0.1 ml into base at center

Patient/family education

- Caution patient to avoid hazardous tasks, since confusion, dizziness may occur; fatigue is common; activity may have to be altered; to take at bedtime to minimize flulike symptoms; to take acetaminophen for fever; avoid prolonged sunlight
- Advise patient that brands of this drug should not be changed; each form is different, with different dosages
- Caution patient not to become pregnant while taking drug; possible mutagenic effects; impotence may occur during treatment but is temporary
- Advise patient to report signs of infection: sore throat, fever, diarrhea, vomiting; sores or white patches in mouth
- Advise patient that emotional lability is common; notify prescriber if severe or incapacitating

Evaluation

Positive therapeutic outcome

- Leukocytes, Hgb, platelets, WNL
- Decreased amount of lesions in AIDS patients with Kaposi's sarcoma
- Decreased amount of genital warts

interferon alfa-n 1 lymphoblastoid (Rx)

(in-ter-feer′on)

Wellferon

Func. class.: Recombinant type I interferon

Pregnancy category UK

Action: Induces biologic responses and has antiviral, antiproliferative, and immunomodulatory effects; mixture of α-interferons isolated from human cells after induction with parainfluenza virus

Uses: Chronic hepatitis C infections

Dosage and routes

Adult: SUBCUT/IM 3 million units × 3 ×/wk × 6-12 mo

Available forms: Sol 3 million units/ml

Adverse effects

CNS: *Headache, fever, insomnia, dizziness, anxiety, hostility, lability, nervousness, depression, confusion, abnormal thinking, amnesia*

GI: *Abdominal pain, nausea, diarrhea, anorexia, vomiting*

HEMA: **Granulocytopenia, thrombocytopenia, leukopenia, ecchymosis**

INTEG: *Alopecia, pruritus, rash, erythema, dry skin*

MS: *Back pain*

PSYCH: *Nervousness, depression, anxiety, lability, abnormal thinking*

RESP: *Pharyngitis, upper respiratory infection, cough, dyspnea, bronchitis,* epistaxis

Contraindications: Hypersensitivity to α interferons, history of anaphylactic reaction to bovine or ovine immunoglobulins, egg protein, polymyxin B, neomycin sulfate

Precautions: Pregnancy **UK,** thyroid disorders, myelosuppression, hepatic, cardiac disease, lactation, children <18 yr, depression/suicidal tendencies

Pharmacokinetics	
Peak	24-36 hr

Interactions

Individual drugs

Theophylline: use cautiously

Drug classifications

Myelosuppressive agents: use together cautiously

NURSING CONSIDERATIONS

Assessment

- Monitor ALT, hepatitis C viral load, patients who show no reduction in ALT, hepatitis C viral load are unlikely to show benefit from treatment after 6 mo
- Monitor platelet counts, heme concentration, ANC, serum creatinine concentration, albumin, bilirubin, TSH, T_4, AFP
- Monitor for myelosuppression, hold dose if neutrophil count is $<500 \times 10^6$/L or if platelets are $<50 \times 10^9$/L
- Assess for hypersensitivity: discontinue immediately if hypersensitivity occurs

Nursing diagnoses

- Infection, risk for (uses)
- Knowledge, deficient (teaching)

Implementation

- Give the same brand of product during the course of treatment

Patient/family education

- Provide patient or family member with written, detailed information about drug
- Teach patient instructions for home use if appropriate
- Advise patient to take in evening to reduce discomfort, sleep through some side effects

Evaluation

Positive therapeutic outcome

- Decrease chronic hepatitis C signs/symptoms
- Undetectable viral load

interferon alfacon-1 (Rx)

(in-ter-feer'on al'fa-kon)

Infergen

Func. class.: Recombinant type I interferon

Pregnancy category C

Action: Induces biologic responses and has antiviral, antiproliferative, and immunomodulatory effects

Therapeutic Outcome: Decreased signs/symptoms of hepatitis C

Uses: Chronic hepatitis C infections

Investigational uses: Hairy cell leukemia when used with G-CSF

Dosage and routes

Adult: SUBCUT 9 mcg as a single inj 3×/wk × 24 wk

Available forms: Inj 9 mg/0.3 ml, 15 mg/0.5 ml

Adverse effects

CNS: Headache, fatigue, fever, rigors, insomnia, dizziness

CV: Hypertension, palpitation

EENT: Tinnitus, earache, conjunctivitis, eye pain

GI: Abdominal pain, nausea, diarrhea, anorexia, dyspepsia, vomiting, constipation, flatulence, hemorrhoids, decreased salivation

GU: Dysmenorrhea, vaginitis, menstrual disorders

HEMA: **Granulocytopenia, thrombocytopenia, leukopenia,** ecchymosis

INTEG: Alopecia, pruritus, rash, erythema, dry skin

MS: Back, limb, neck, skeletal pain

PSYCH: Nervousness, depression, anxiety, lability, abnormal thinking

RESP: Pharyngitis, upper respiratory infection, cough, sinusitis, rhinitis, respiratory tract congestion, epistaxis, dyspnea, bronchitis

Contraindications: Hypersensitivity to α-interferons, or products from *Escherichia coli*

Precautions: Pregnancy **C,** thyroid disorders, myelosuppression, hepatic, cardiac disease, lactation, children <18 yr

Pharmacokinetics	
Absorption	Unknown
Distribution	Unknown
Metabolism	Unknown
Excretion	Unknown
Half-life	Unknown

Pharmacodynamics

Onset	Unknown
Peak	24-36 hr
Duration	Unknown

Interactions: None known

NURSING CONSIDERATIONS

Assessment

- Assess platelet counts, heme concentration, ANC, serum creatinine concentration, albumin, bilirubin, TSH, T_4
- Assess for myelosuppression, low dose if neutrophil count is <500 × 10-6/L or if platelets are <50 × 10-9/L
- Assess for hypersensitivity; discontinue immediately if hypersensitivity occurs

Nursing diagnoses

- Infection, risk for (uses)
- Knowledge, deficient (teaching)

Patient/family education

- Provide patient or family member with written, detailed instructions about the drug
- Caution patient to use contraception during treatment

Evaluation

Positive therapeutic outcome

- Decreased hepatitis C signs/symptoms

interferon β-1a (Rx)

(in-ter-feer′on)

Avonex

interferon β-1b (Rx)

Betaseron

Func. class.: Multiple sclerosis agent, immune modifier

Chem. class.: Interferon, *Escherichia coli* derivative

Pregnancy category C

Action: Antiviral, immunoregulatory; action not clearly understood; biologic response-modifying properties mediated through specific receptors on cells, inducing expression of interferon-induced gene products

Therapeutic Outcome: Decreased symptoms of multiple sclerosis

Uses: Ambulatory patients with relapsing or remitting multiple sclerosis

Investigational uses: May be useful in treatment of AIDS, AIDS-related Kaposi's sarcoma, malignant melanoma, metastatic renal cell carcinoma, cutaneous T-cell lymphoma, acute non-A, non-B hepatitis

Dosage and routes

Interferon-β-1a

Adult: IM 30 mcg qwk

Interferon-β-1b

Relapsing/remitting multiple sclerosis

Adult: SUBCUT 0.25 mg (8 international units) every other day

Available forms: β-1a: 33 mcg (6.6 million international units/vial); β-1b: powder for inj 0.3 mg (9.6 milli-international units)

Adverse effects

CNS: *Headache, fever, pain, chills, mental changes,* hypertonia, **suicide attempts, seizures**

CV: *Migraine, palpitations, hypertension,* tachycardia, peripheral vascular disorders

EENT: Conjunctivitis, blurred vision

GI: *Diarrhea, constipation, vomiting, abdominal pain*

GU: *Dysmenorrhea, irregular menses, metorrhagia,* cystitis, breast pain

HEMA: **Decreased lymphocytes,** ANC, WBC; *lymphadenopathy*

INTEG: *Sweating, inj site reaction,*

MS: *Myalgia,* **myasthenia**

RESP: *Sinusitis,* dyspnea

Contraindications: Hypersensitivity to natural or recombinant interferon-β or human albumin, hamster protein

Precautions: Pregnancy **C**, lactation, children <18 yr, chronic progressive multiple sclerosis, depression, mental disorders, seizure disorders, latex allergy

Pharmacokinetics

Absorption	50% is absorbed
Distribution	Unknown
Metabolism	Unknown
Excretion	Unknown
Half- ife	8 min-4½ hr (β-1b), 8.6 hr (β-1a) β-1a up to 12 hr, 48 hr, 4 days, β-1b

Pharmacodynamics

Onset	Rapid
Peak	2-8 hr
Duration	Unknown

Interactions

Individual drugs

Zidovudine: decreased clearance

NURSING CONSIDERATIONS

Assessment

- Monitor blood, renal, hepatic studies: CBC, differential, platelet counts, BUN, creatinine, ALT, urinalysis; if neutrophil count is <750/mm^3, or if AST, ALT, is 10 × greater than upper normal limit, or if bilirubin is 5 × greater than upper normal limit; when neutrophil count exceeds 750/mm^3 and liver function or renal studies return to normal, treatment may resume at 50% original dosage
- Assess for CNS symptoms: headache, fatigue, depression; if depression occurs and is severe, drug should be discontinued
- Assess for multiple sclerosis symptoms
- Assess mental status: depression, depersonalization, suicidal thoughts, insomnia
- Monitor GI status: diarrhea or constipation, vomiting, abdominal pain
- Monitor cardiac status: increased B/P, tachycardia

Nursing diagnoses

- Mobility, physical, (uses) impaired
- Knowledge, deficient (teaching)

Implementation

- Reconstitute 0.3 mg (9.6 million international units)/1.2 ml of supplied diluent (0.2 mg or 8 million international units concentration); rotate vial gently, do not shake; withdraw 1 ml using a syringe with 27G needle; administer SUBCUT only into hip, thigh, arm; discard unused portion
- Products are not interchangeable

Interferon β-1a

- Reconstitute with 1.1 ml of diluent, swirl, give within 6 hr

Interferon β-1b

- Reconstitute by injecting diluent provided (1.2 ml) into vial, swirl (8 milli-international units/ml), use 27-G needle for inj
- Give acetaminophen for fever, headache; use SUBCUT route only; do not give IM or **IV**
- Store reconstituted sol in refrigerator; do not freeze; do not use sol that contains precipitate or is discolored

Patient/family education

- Provide patient or family member with written, detailed instructions about the drug; provide initial and return demonstrations on inj procedure; give information on use and disposal of drug
- Inform patient that blurred vision, sweating may occur
- Advise women patients that irregular menses, dysmenorrhea, or metorrhagia as well as breast pain may occur; use contraception during treatment; drug may cause spontaneous abortion
- Teach patient to use sunscreen to prevent photosensitivity
- Instruct patient to notify prescriber if pregnancy is suspected
- Teach patient inj technique and care of equipment
- Instruct patient to notify prescriber of increased temp, chills, muscle soreness, fatigue

Evaluation

Positive therapeutic outcome

- Decreased symptoms of multiple sclerosis

interferon gamma-1b (Rx)

(in-ter-feer'on)

Actimmune

Func. class.: Biologic response modifier

Chem. class.: Lymphokine, interleukin type

Pregnancy category C

Action: Species-specific protein synthesized in response to viruses; potent phagocyte-activating effects; capable of mediating the killing of *Staphylococcus aureus, Toxoplasma gondii, Leishmania donovani, Listeria monocytogenes, Mycobacterium avium-intracellulare;* enhances oxidative metabolism of macrophages; enhances antibody-dependent cellular cytotoxicity

Therapeutic Outcome: Decreased signs/symptoms of infection (serious) in chronic granulomatous disease

Uses: Serious infections associated with chronic granulomatous disease, osteoporosis

Dosage and routes

Adult: SUBCUT 50 mcg/m^2 (1.5 million units/m^2) for patients with a surface area of >0.5 m^2; 1.5 mcg/kg/dose for patient with a surface area of <0.5/m^2; give on Monday, Wednesday, Friday for 3 ×/wk dosing

Available forms: Inj 100 mcg (3 million units)/single-dose vial

Adverse effects

CNS: *Headache, fatigue,* depression, fever, chills

GI: *Nausea, anorexia,* abdominal pain, weight loss, diarrhea, vomiting

INTEG: Rash, pain at inj site

MS: Myalgia, arthralgia

Contraindications: Hypersensitivity to

interferon γ, *Escherichia coli*–derived products

Precautions: Pregnancy **C,** cardiac disease, seizure disorders, CNS disorders, myelosuppression, lactation, children

Pharmacokinetics

Absorption	Slowly absorbed; 89%
Distribution	Unknown
Metabolism	Unknown
Excretion	Unknown
Half-life	5.9 hr

Pharmacodynamics

Onset	Unknown
Peak	7 hr
Duration	Unknown

Interactions
Individual drugs
Aminophylline, theophylline: increased levels
Fosphenyton, phenyton, warfarin: increased interference
Drug classifications
Myelosuppressive agents: increased myelosuppression

NURSING CONSIDERATIONS
Assessment
- Monitor blood, renal, hepatic studies: CBC with differential, platelet count, BUN, creatinine, ALT, urinalysis before and q3 mo during treatment
- Assess for infection: headache, fever, chills, fatigue; these are common adverse reactions
- Monitor CNS symptoms: headache, fatigue, depression

Nursing diagnoses
- Infection, risk for (uses)
- Knowledge, deficient (teaching)

Implementation
- Give at bedtime to minimize adverse reactions; administer acetaminophen for fever, headache; use 50% of the dosage prescribed if severe reactions occur or discontinue treatment until reactions subside
- Give in right or left deltoid and anterior thigh; warm to room temp before use; do not leave at room temp over 12 hr (unopened vial); does not contain preservatives
- Store in refrigerator upon receipt; do not freeze; do not shake

Patient/family education
- Provide patient or family member with written, detailed instructions about the drug; provide initial and return demonstrations on inj procedure; give information on use and disposal of drug
- Caution patient to use contraception during treatment

Evaluation
Positive therapeutic outcome
- Decreased serious infections
- Improvement in existing infections and inflammatory conditions

ipratropium (Rx)
(i-pra-troe'pee-um)
Atrovent
Func. class.: Anticholinergic, bronchodilator
Chem. class.: Synthetic quaternary ammonium compound
Pregnancy category B

Do Not Confuse:
Atrovent/Alupent

Action: Inhibits interaction of acetylcholine at receptor sites on the bronchial smooth muscle, resulting in decreased cyclic guanosine monophosphate (cGMP) and bronchodilatation

Therapeutic Outcome: Bronchodilatation

Uses: Bronchodilatation during bronchospasm for patients with COPD; rhinorrhea in children 6-11 yr (nasal spray)

Dosage and routes
Adult: INH 2 puffs qid, not to exceed 12 puffs/24 hr; sol 500 mcg (1 unit dose) given 3-4 ×1 day
Child 6-11 yr: Nasal, 1 spray in each nostril

Available forms: Aerosol 18 mcg/actuation; nasal spray 0.03%, 0.06%; sol for inh 0.02%

Adverse effects
CNS: *Anxiety, dizziness, headache,* nervousness
CV: Palpitations
EENT: Dry mouth, blurred vision
GI: *Nausea, vomiting, cramps*
INTEG: Rash
RESP: *Cough, worsening of symptoms,* **bronchospasm**

Contraindications: Hypersensitivity to this drug, atropine, soya lecithin

Precautions: Pregnancy **B,** lactation, children <12 yr, narrow-angle glaucoma, prostatic hypertrophy, bladder neck obstruction

Pharmacokinetics

Absorption	Minimal
Distribution	Does not cross blood-brain barrier
Metabolism	Liver, minimal
Excretion	Unknown
Half-life	2 hr

Pharmacodynamics

Onset	5-15 min
Peak	1-1½ hr
Duration	3-6 hr

Interactions
Drug/herb
Black catechu: increased constipation
Butterbur, jimsonweed: increased anticholinergic effect
Green tea (large amounts), guarana: increased bronchodilator effect
Jamborandi tree, pill-bearing spurge: decreased anticholinergic effect

NURSING CONSIDERATIONS
Assessment
- Monitor respiratory function: vital capacity, FEV, ABGs, lung sounds, heart rate, rhythm (baseline and during treatment); if severe bronchospasm is present, a more rapid medication is required
- Monitor for evidence of allergic reactions, paradoxic bronchospasm; withhold dose and notify prescriber; identify if patient is allergic to belladonna products or atropine; allergy to this drug may occur

Nursing diagnoses
- Airway clearance, ineffective (uses)
- Gas exchange, impaired (uses)
- Knowledge, deficient (teaching)

Implementation
- Give after shaking container; have patient exhale, place mouthpiece in mouth, inhale slowly, hold breath, remove, exhale slowly; allow at least 1 min between inhalations
- Give this medication before other medications and allow at least 5 min between each

Nebulizer route
- Use solution in nebulizer with a mouthpiece rather than a face mask

Nasal route
- Prime pump, initially requires 7 actuations of the pump, priming again is not necessary if used regularly
- Store in light-resistant container; do not expose to temp over 86° F (30° C)

Patient/family education
- Advise patient not to use OTC medications unless approved by prescriber; extra stimulation may occur; to use this medication before other medications and allow at least 5 min between each to prevent overstimulation
- Teach patient that compliance is necessary with number of inhalations/24 hr, or overdose may occur
- Instruct patient to use spacer device if elderly
- Teach patient the proper use of the inhaler; review package insert with patient; to avoid getting aerosol in eyes; blurring may result; to wash inhaler in warm water daily and dry; to avoid smoking, smoke-filled rooms, persons with respiratory tract infections
- Teach patient if paradoxic bronchospasm occurs to stop drug immediately and notify prescriber; to limit caffeine products such as chocolate, coffee, tea, and colas
- Instruct patient on administration of dose, not to use more than prescribed; serious side effects may occur; if dose is missed, take when remembered; space other doses on new time schedule; do not double doses

Evaluation
Positive therapeutic outcome
- Absence of dyspnea, wheezing after 1 hr
- Improved airway exchange
- Improved ABGs

irbesartan (Rx)
(er-be-sar'tan)

Avapro

Func. class.: Antihypertensive

Chem. class.: Angiotensin II receptor (Type AT_1)

Pregnancy category
C (1st trimester),
D (2nd/3rd trimesters)

Do Not Confuse:
Avapro/Anaprox

Action: Blocks the vasoconstrictor and aldosterone-secreting effects of angiotensin II; selectively blocks the binding of angiotensin II to the AT_1 receptor found in tissues

Therapeutic Outcome: Decreased B/P

Uses: Hypertension, alone or in combination, nephropathy in type 2 diabetic patients

I

Investigational uses: Heart failure, hypertensive patients with diabetic nephropathy caused by type 2 diabetes

Dosage and routes

Hypertension

Adult: PO 150 mg daily; may be increased to 300 mg daily

Nephropathy in type 2 diabetic patients

Adult: PO maintenance dose 300 mg daily

Child 13-16 yr: PO 150 mg daily, may increase to 300 mg daily

Child 6-12 yr: PO 75 mg daily may increase to 150 mg daily

Volume and salt depleted patients

Adult: PO 75 mg daily

Available forms: Tabs 75, 150, 300 mg

Adverse effects

CNS: Dizziness, anxiety, headache, fatigue

GI: *Diarrhea, dyspepsia*

MISC: Edema, chest pain, rash, tachycardia, UTI, **angioedema,** hyperkalemia

RESP: *Cough, upper respiratory infection,* rhinitis, pharyngitis, sinus disorder

Contraindications: Pregnancy **D** (2nd/3rd trimesters), hypersensitivity

Precautions: Pregnancy **C** (1st trimester), hypersensitivity to ACE inhibitors; lactation, children, elderly, renal disease

Pharmacokinetics

Absorption	Well
Distribution	Bound to plasma proteins (90%)
Metabolism	Liver (minimal)
Excretion	Feces, urine
Half-life	11-15 hr

Pharmacodynamics

Unknown

Interactions

Drug classifications

NSAIDs: decreased antihypertensive effect

Diuretics (potassium sparing), potassium salt substitutes: increased hyperkalemia

Drug/herb

Aconite: increased toxicity, death

Astragalus, cola tree: increased or decreased antihypertensive effect

Barberry, betony, black catechu, black cohosh, bloodroot, broom, burdock, cat's claw, dandelion, goldenseal, Irish moss, Jamaican dogwood, kelp, khella, mistletoe, parsley: increased antihypertensive effect

Coltsfoot, guarana, khat, licorice: decreased antihypertensive effect

NURSING CONSIDERATIONS

Assessment

- Assess B/P, pulse q4h; note rate, rhythm, quality
- Monitor electrolytes: potassium, sodium, chloride
- Obtain baselines for renal liver function tests before therapy begins
- Monitor for edema in feet, legs daily
- Assess for skin turgor, dryness of mucous membranes for hydration status

Nursing diagnoses

- Fluid volume, deficient (side effects)
- Noncompliance (teaching)
- Knowledge, deficient (teaching)

Implementation

- Administer without regard to meals

Patient/family education

- Advise patient to comply with dosage schedule, even if feeling better
- Inform patient that drug may cause dizziness, fainting; lightheadedness may occur
- Caution patient to rise slowly to sitting or standing position to minimize orthostatic hypotension
- Advise patient to notify prescriber if pregnancy is suspected

Evaluation

Positive therapeutic outcome

- Decreased B/P

! HIGH ALERT

irinotecan (Rx)

(ear-een-oh-tee'kan)

Camptosar

Func. class.: Antineoplastic hormone

Chem. class.: Topoisomerase inhibitor

Pregnancy category D

Action: Cytotoxic by producing damage to double-strand DNA during DNA synthesis

Therapeutic Outcome: Prevention in growth of tumor size

Uses: Metastatic carcinoma of colon or rectum, or 1st line treatment in combination with fluorouracil (5-FU) and leucovorin for metastatic carcinoma of colon or rectum

Dosage and routes

Single agent

Adult: **IV** 125 mg/m^2 given over 1½ hr qwk × 4 wk, then 2 wk rest period, may be repeated; 4 wk or 2 wk off, dosage adjustments may be made to 150 mg/m^2 (high) or 50 mg/m^2 (low); adjustments should be made in increments of 25-50 mg/m^2 depending on patient's tolerance

Combination dosage schedule

Regimen 1: Irinotecan 75-125 mg/m^2, leucovorin 20 mg/m^2, 5-FU 300-500 mg/m^2, depending on dosing levels

Regimen 2: Irinotecan 120-180 mg/m^2, leucovorin 200 mg/m^2, 5 FU-BOL 240-400 mg/m^2, 5 FU infusion 360-600 mg/m^2

Hepatic impairment

Adult: 100 mg/m^2 qwk × 4 wk, then 2 wk rest; may repeat cycle or 300 mg/m^2 q3wk, dose may be adjusted up or down

Available forms: Inj 20 mg/ml

Adverse effects

CNS: Fever, headache, chills, dizziness
CV: Vasodilation
GI: **Severe diarrhea,** nausea, vomiting, anorexia, constipation, cramps, flatus, stomatitis, dyspepsia, **hepatotoxicity**
HEMA: **Leukopenia,** anemia, **neutropenia**
INTEG: Irritation at site, rash, sweating, alopecia
MISC: Edema, asthenia, weight loss
RESP: Dyspnea, increased cough, rhinitis

Contraindications: Pregnancy **D,** hypersensitivity

Precautions: Lactation, children, elderly, myelosuppression, irradiation

Pharmacokinetics

Absorption	Complete
Distribution	Widely, 30%-68% bond to plasma proteins
Metabolism	Unknown
Excretion	Urine/bile
Half-life	Unknown

Pharmacodynamics

Unknown

Interactions

Individual drugs

Dexamethasone: increased lymphocytopenia
Prochlorperazine: increased akathisia
Radiation: increased myelosuppression, diarrhea

Drug classifications

Antineoplastics: increased myelosuppression, diarrhea
Diuretics: increased dehydration

NURSING CONSIDERATIONS

Assessment

- Assess for CNS symptoms: fever, headache, chills, dizziness
- Assess CBC, differential, platelet count weekly; withhold drug if WBC is <2000/mm^3, or platelet count is <100,000/mm^3, Hgb ≤ g/dl, neutrophils ≤1000/mm^3; notify prescriber of these results, drug should be discontinued and colony-stimulating factor given
- Assess buccal cavity q8h for dryness, sores or ulceration, white patches, oral pain, bleeding, dysphagia
- Assess GI symptoms: frequency of stools; cramping; severe life-threatening diarrhea may occur with fluid and electrolyte imbalances
- Assess early diarrhea and other cholinergic symptoms, treat with atropine; late diarrhea must be treated promptly with loperimide, late diarrhea can be life threatening
- Assess signs of dehydration: rapid respirations, poor skin turgor, decreased urine output; dry skin, restlessness, weakness
- Assess for bone marrow depression: bruising, bleeding, blood in stools, urine, sputum, emesis

Nursing diagnoses

- Infection, risk for (adverse reactions)
- Knowledge, deficient (teaching)

Implementation

- Give antiemetics and dexamethasone 10 mg at least ½ hr before antineoplastics
- Give after preparing in biologic cabinet using gloves, mask, gown

IV route

- Give by intermittent inf after diluting with 0.9% NaCl or D_5W (0.12-1.1 mg/ml); give over 1½ hr
- Do not admix with other solutions or medications
- Provide increased fluid intake to 2-3 L/day to prevent dehydration, unless contraindicated
- Change **IV** site q48h
- Provide rinsing of mouth tid-qid with water, club soda; brushing of teeth bid-tid with soft brush or cotton-tipped applicator for stomatitis; use unwaxed dental floss
- Provide nutritious diet with iron, vitamin supplement, low fiber, few dairy products
- Stable for 24 hr at room temp, 48 hr if refrigerated

I

Patient/family education

- Advise patient to avoid foods with citric acid or hot or rough texture if stomatitis is present; to drink adequate fluids
- Advise patient to report stomatitis; any bleeding, white spots, ulcerations in mouth; tell patient to examine mouth daily, report symptoms
- Advise patient to report signs of anemia: fatigue, headache, faintness, shortness of breath, irritability
- Advise patient to use contraception during therapy
- Advise patient to avoid vaccinations while taking this drug
- Instruct patient to report diarrhea that occurs 24 hr after administration; severe dehydration can occur rapidly
- Teach patient to avoid salicylates, NSAIDs, alcohol; bleeding may occur

Evaluation

Positive therapeutic outcome

- Decrease in tumor size, decrease in spread of cancer

Treatment of overdose: Induce vomiting, provide supportive care, prevent dehydration

iron, carbonyl

See ferrous fumarate

iron dextran (Rx)

DexFerrum, Imferon, InFed

Func. class.: Hematinic

Chem. class.: Ferric hydroxide complex with dextran

Pregnancy category C

Do Not Confuse:

Imferon/Imuran, Imferon/Roferon-A

Action: Iron is carried by transferrin to the bone marrow, where it is incorporated into hemoglobin

Therapeutic Outcome: Prevention and resolution of iron-deficiency anemia

Uses: Iron-deficiency anemia in patients who cannot take oral preparations

Dosage and routes

Adult and child: IM 0.5 ml as a test dose by Z-track, then no more than the following per day:

Adult <50 kg: IM 100 mg

Adult >50 kg: IM 250 mg

Infant <5 kg: IM 25 mg

Child 5-9 kg: IM 50 mg

Adult: **IV** 0.5 ml (25 mg) test dose, then 100 mg daily after 2-3 days; give 25 mg test dose, wait 5 min, then inf over 6-12 hr or follow equation:

$$\frac{0.3 \times \text{weight (lb)} \times 100\ \text{Hgb (g/dl)} \times 100}{14.8} = \text{mg iron}$$

Patients <30 lb (66 kg) should be given 80% of above formula dose

Available forms: Inj IM/**IV** 50 mg/ml; inj IM only 50 mg/ml (2 ml, 10 ml vials)

Adverse effects

CNS: Headache, paresthesia, dizziness, shivering, weakness, **seizures**

CV: Chest pain, **shock,** hypotension, tachycardia

GI: *Nausea,* vomiting, metallic taste, abdominal pain

HEMA: **Leukocytosis**

INTEG: Rash, pruritus, urticaria, fever, sweating, chills, brown skin discoloration, pain at inj site, necrosis, sterile abscesses, phlebitis

MISC: **Anaphylaxis**

RESP: Dyspnea

Contraindications: Hypersensitivity, all anemias excluding iron-deficiency anemia, hepatic disease

Precautions: Pregnancy **C,** acute renal disease, children, asthma, lactation, rheumatoid arthritis (**IV**), infants <4 mo

Pharmacokinetics	
Absorption	Well absorbed; lymphatics over wk or mo
Distribution	Crosses placenta
Metabolism	Slow; blood loss, desquamation
Excretion	Breast milk, feces, urine, bile
Half-life	6 hr

Pharmacodynamics

Unknown

Interactions

Individual drugs

Chloramphenicol: decreased reticulocyte response

Oral iron: do not use together, increased toxicity

Penicillamine: decreased absorption of penicillamine

Drug/lab test

False increase: serum bilirubin
False decrease: serum calcium
False positive: ^{99m}Tc diphosphate bone scan, iron test (large doses >2 ml)

NURSING CONSIDERATIONS

Assessment

- Observe for 1 hr after test dose
- Monitor blood studies: Hct, Hgb, reticulocytes, transferrin, plasma iron concentrations, ferritin, total iron-binding bilirubin before treatment, at least monthly
- Assess for allergic reaction and anaphylaxis; rash, pruritus, fever, chills, wheezing, notify prescriber immediately, keep emergency equipment available
- Assess cardiac status: anginal pain, hypotension, tachycardia
- Assess for nutrition: amount of iron in diet (meat, dark green leafy vegetables, dried fruits, eggs); cause of iron loss or anemia, including salicylates, sulfonamides
- Monitor pulse, B/P during **IV** administration
- Assess for toxicity: nausea, vomiting, diarrhea, fever, abdominal pain (early symptoms); cyanotic lips, nailbeds, seizures, CV collapse (late symptoms)

Nursing diagnoses

- Fatigue (uses)
- Activity intolerance (uses)
- Knowledge, deficient (teaching)

Implementation

IM route

- Discontinue oral iron before parenteral; give only after test dose of 25 mg by preferred route; wait at least 1 hr before giving remaining portion
- Give IM inj deep in large muscle mass; use Z-track method and 19G, 20G 2-, 3-inch needle; ensure needle is long enough to place drug deep in muscle; change needles after withdrawing medication and injecting to prevent skin and tissue staining

IV route

- Give **IV** after flushing tubing with 10 ml of 0.9% NaCl; give undiluted; give 1 ml (50 mg) or less over 1 min or more; flush line after use with 10 ml of 0.9% NaCl; patient should remain recumbent for 30-60 min to prevent orthostatic hypotension
- **IV** inj requires single-dose vial without preservative; verify on label **IV** use is approved
- Give by cont inf after diluting in 50-250 ml of 0.9% NaCl for inf; administer over 4-5 hr
- Give only with epINEPHrine available in case of anaphylactic reaction during dose
- Store at room temp in cool environment

Additive compatibilities: Netilmicin

Patient/family education

- Caution patient that iron poisoning may occur if increased beyond recommended level; to not take oral iron preparation unless approved by prescriber
- Advise patient that delayed reaction may occur 1-2 days after administration and last 3-4 days (**IV**) or 3-7 days (IM); report fever, chills, malaise, muscle, joint aches, nausea, vomiting, backache

Evaluation

Positive therapeutic outcome

- Increased serum iron levels, Hct, Hgb

Treatment of overdose:

- Discontinue drug, treat allergic reaction, give diphenhydrAMINE or epINEPHrine as needed for anaphylaxis; give iron-chelating drug in acute poisoning

I

iron polysaccharide

See ferrous fumarate

iron sucrose (Rx)

Venofer
Func. class.: Hematinic
Chem. class.: Ferric hydroxide complex with dextran

Pregnancy category B

Action: Iron is carried by transferrin to the bone marrow, where it is incorporated into hemoglobin

Therapeutic Outcome: Improved signs/symptoms of iron deficiency anemia; iron levels improved

Uses: Iron deficiency anemia

Investigational uses: Dystrophic epidermolysis bullosa (DEB)

Dosage and routes

Adult: **IV** 5 ml (100 mg of elemental iron) given during dialysis, most will need 1000 mg of elemental iron over 10 dialysis sessions

Available forms: Inj 20 mg/ml

Adverse effects

CNS: Headache, dizziness
CV: Chest pain, hypo/hypertension, hypervolemia

GI: *Nausea, vomiting, abdominal pain*
INTEG: Rash, pruritus, urticaria, fever, sweating, chills
MISC: **Anaphylaxis**
RESP: Dyspnea, pneumonia, cough

Contraindications: Hypersensitivity, all anemias excluding iron deficiency anemia, iron overload

Precautions: Pregnancy **B**, lactation (**IV**), elderly, children

Pharmacokinetics

Absorption	Unknown
Distribution	Unknown
Metabolism	Unknown
Excretion	Urine
Half-life	6 hr

Pharmacodynamics

Unknown

Interactions
Individual drugs
Iron (oral): increased toxicity, do not use together

NURSING CONSIDERATIONS
Assessment
- Monitor blood studies: Hct, Hgb, reticulocytes, transferrin, plasma iron concentrations, ferritin, total iron binding, bilirubin before treatment, at least monthly
- Assess for allergy: anaphylaxis, rash, pruritus, fever, chills, wheezing; notify prescriber immediately, keep emergency equipment available
- Assess cardiac status: hypotension, hypertension, hypervolemia
- Assess for toxicity: nausea, vomiting, diarrhea, fever, abdominal pain (early symptoms), cyanotic-looking lips and nailbeds, seizures, CV collapse (late symptoms)

Nursing diagnoses
- Nutrition, less than body requirements, imbalanced (uses)
- Knowledge, deficient (teaching)

Implementation
- ◆ Give only with epINEPHrine available in case of anaphylactic reaction during dose

IV route
- Give directly in dialysis line by slow inj or inf; give by slow inj at 1 ml/min (5 min/vial); inf dilute each vial exclusively in a maximum of 100 ml of 0.9% NaCl, give at rate of 100 mg of iron/15 min, discard unused portions
- Store at room temp in cool environment, do not freeze

Patient/family education
- Teach patient that iron poisoning may occur if increased beyond recommended level; not to take oral iron preparations

Evaluation
Positive therapeutic outcome
- Increased serum iron levels, Hct, Hgb

Treatment of overdose: Discontinue drug, treat allergic reaction, give diphenhydrAMINE or epINEPHrine as needed, give iron-chelating drug in acute poisoning

isoniazid 🔑 (Rx)
(eye-soe-nye'a-zid)
INH, isoniazid, Isotamine ✤, Laniazid, Nydrazid, PMS-Isoniazid ✤
Func. class.: Antitubercular
Chem. class.: Isonicotinic acid hydrazide

Pregnancy category C

Action: Inhibits RNA synthesis, decreases tubercle bacilli replication

Therapeutic Outcome: Resolution of TB infection

Uses: Pulmonary TB as an adjunct; other infections caused by mycobacteria

Dosage and routes
Treatment
Adult: PO/IM 300 mg/day or 15 mg/kg 2-3 ×/wk, max 900 mg 2-3 ×/wk
Child and infant: PO/IM 10-20 mg/kg daily in 1-2 divided doses; max 300 mg/day or 20-40 mg/kg, max 900 mg 2-3 ×/wk

Available forms: Tabs 50, 100, 300 mg; inj 100 mg/ml; powder 50 mg/5 ml; syr 50 mg/5 ml

Adverse effects
Hypersensitivity: Fever, skin eruptions, lymphadenopathy, vasculitis
CNS: *Peripheral neuropathy, dizziness,* memory impairment, **toxic encephalopathy, convulsions,** psychosis, **seizures,** slurred speech
EENT: Blurred vision, optic neuritis
GI: *Nausea, vomiting,* epigastric distress, **jaundice, fatal hepatitis**
HEMA: **Agranulocytosis, hemolytic anemia, aplastic anemia, thrombocytopenia, eosinophilia, methemoglobinemia**

MISC: Dyspnea, vit B_6 deficiency, pellagra, hyperglycemia, metabolic acidosis, gynecomastia, rheumatic syndrome, systemic lupus erythematosus–like syndrome

Contraindications: Hypersensitivity, acute liver disease

Precautions: Pregnancy **C**, renal disease, diabetic retinopathy, cataracts, ocular defects, hepatic disease, child <13 yr

Pharmacokinetics

Absorption	Well
Distribution	Widely
Metabolism	Liver
Excretion	Kidneys
Half-life	1-4 hr

Pharmacodynamics

	PO	IM
Onset	Rapid	Rapid
Peak	1-2 hr	45-60 min
Duration	6-8 hr	6-8 hr

Interactions

Individual drugs

Alcohol, carbamazepine, cycloSERINE, ethionamide, meperidine, phenytoin, rifampin, warfarin: increased toxicity
BCG vaccine, ketoconazole: decreased effectiveness

Drug classifications

Antacids, aluminum: decreased absorption
Benzodiazepines: increased toxicity

Drug/food

Tyramine foods: increased toxicity

NURSING CONSIDERATIONS

Assessment

- Obtain C&S tests, including sputum tests, before treatment; monitor every mo to detect resistance
- Monitor liver studies weekly: ALT, AST, bilirubin, increased results may indicate hepatitis; renal studies during treatment and monthly: BUN, creatinine, output, sp gr, urinalysis, uric acid
- Assess mental status often: affect, mood, behavioral changes; psychosis may occur with hallucinations, confusion
- Assess hepatic status: decreased appetite, jaundice, dark urine, fatigue
- Assess for visual disturbance that may indicate optic neuritis: blurred vision, change in color perception; may lead to blindness

Nursing diagnoses

- Infection, risk for (uses)
- Diarrhea (adverse reactions)
- Injury, risk for (adverse reactions)
- Knowledge, deficient (teaching)
- Noncompliance (teaching)

Implementation

- Give antiemetic for vomiting
- Provide a list of foods to avoid while taking this drug

PO route

- Give with meals to decrease GI symptoms; absorption is better when taken on empty stomach, 1 hr ac or 2 hr pc

IM route

- Give inj deep in large muscle mass, massage; rotate inj sites, warm inj to room temp to dissolve crystals

Patient/family education

!

- Instruct patient that compliance with dosage schedule for duration is necessary; not to skip or double doses; that scheduled appointments must be kept or relapse may occur
- Caution patient to avoid alcohol while taking drug or hepatoxicity may result; to avoid ingestion of aged cheeses, fish or hypertensive crisis may result; give patient written directions on which foods to avoid while taking this medication
- Tell patient to report peripheral neuritis: weakness, tingling/numbness of hands/feet, fatigue; hepatoxicity: loss of appetite, nausea, vomiting, jaundice of skin or eyes

Evaluation

Positive therapeutic outcome

- Decreased symptoms of TB
- Culture negative for TB

Treatment of overdose: Pyridoxine

isosorbide dinitrate (Rx)

(eye-soe-sor'bide)

Apo-ISDN ✦, Cedocard-SR ✦, Coronex ✦, Dilatrate-SR, ISDN, Iso-Bid, Isonate, Isorbid, Isordil, Isosorbide dinitrate, Isotrate, Novasorbide ✦, Sorbitrate

isosorbide mononitrate (Rx)

Imdur, ISMO, Isotrate ER, Monoket

Func. class.: Antianginal, vasodilator

Chem. class.: Nitrate

Pregnancy category C

Do Not Confuse: Monoket/Monopril, Imdur/Imuran/Inderal/K-Dur

Action: Relaxation of vascular smooth muscle, which leads to decreased preload, afterload, thus decreasing left ventricular end-diastolic pressure, systemic vascular resistance, and reducing cardiac O_2 demand

Therapeutic Outcome: Relief and prevention of angina pectoris

Uses: Treatment, prevention of chronic stable angina pectoris

Dosage and routes

Dinitrate

Adult: PO 5-40 mg qid; SL, buccal tab 2.5-5 mg; may repeat q5-10min × 3 doses; chew tab 5-10 mg prn or q2-3h as prophylaxis; sus rel cap 40-80 mg q8-12h

Mononitrate

Adult: PO (ISMO, Monoket) 10-20 mg bid, 7 hr apart; (Imdur) initiate at 30-60 mg/day as a single dose, increase q3d as needed, may increase to 120 mg daily, max 240 mg/day

Available forms: Dinitrate: sus rel caps 40 mg; tabs 5, 10, 20, 30, 40 mg; SL tabs 2.5, 5, 10 mg; chew tabs 5, 10 mg; mononitrate: tabs (Monoket, ISMO) 10, 20 mg; ext rel tabs (Imdur, ER) 30, 60, 120 mg

Adverse effects

CNS: ***Vascular headache, flushing, dizziness,*** weakness, faintness

CV: ***Postural hypotension,*** tachycardia, **collapse,** syncope, palpitations

GI: Nausea, vomiting, diarrhea

INTEG: Pallor, sweating, rash

MISC: Twitching, hemolytic anemia, **methemoglobinemia**

Contraindications: Hypersensitivity to this drug or nitrates, severe anemia, increased ICP, cerebral hemorrhage, acute MI

Precautions: Pregnancy **C,** postural hypotension, lactation, children, MI, CHF, severe renal, hepatic disease

Pharmacokinetics

Absorption	Well
Distribution	Unknown
Metabolism	Liver
Excretion	Urine, metabolites
Half-life	Dinitrate 1 hr, mononitrate 5 hr

Pharmacodynamics

	SUS REL	SL	PO
Onset	Up to 4 hr	2-5 min	15-30 min
Peak	Unknown	Unknown	Unknown
Duration	6-8 hr	1-4 hr	4-6 hr

Interactions

Individual drugs

Alcohol: increased hypotension

Drug classifications

Antihypertensives, β-adrenergic blockers, calcium channel blockers, diuretics, phenothiazines: increased hypotension

Sildenafil, tadalofil, vardenafil: fatal hypotension

Drug/herb

Blue cohosh: decreased antianginal effect

NURSING CONSIDERATIONS

Assessment

- Assess for pain: duration, time started, activity being performed, character, intensity
- Monitor for orthostatic B/P, pulse at baseline and during treatment

Nursing diagnoses

- Cardiac output, decreased (uses)
- Tissue perfusion, ineffective (uses)
- Knowledge, deficient (teaching)

Implementation

PO route

- Swallow sus rel tab and ext rel tab whole; do not break, crush, or chew
- Do not swallow SL tab; tab should be dissolved under tongue
- Chew tab should be chewed thoroughly
- Give 1 hr ac or 2 hr pc with 8 oz of water

SL route

- Hold SL tab under tongue until dissolved (a few min); do not take anything PO when SL tab is in place

Patient/family education

- Instruct patient to not skip or double doses; if dose is missed take when remembered if 2 hr before next dose (dinitrate), 6 hr before next dose (sus rel), or 8 hr before next dose (mononitrate)

- Caution patient to avoid alcohol and OTC medications unless approved by prescriber
- Inform patient that drug may be taken before stressful activity: exercise, sexual activity
- Advise patient that SL tab may sting mucous membranes
- Caution patient to avoid driving and hazardous activities if dizziness occurs
- Advise patient to comply with complete medical regimen
- Caution patient to make position changes slowly to prevent orthostatic hypotension

Evaluation

Positive therapeutic outcome

- Decrease in, prevention of anginal pain

isradipine (Rx)

(is-ra′di-peen)

DynaCirc, DynaCirc CR

Func. class.: Calcium channel blocker, antihypertensive, antianginal

Chem. class.: Dihydropyridine

Pregnancy category C

Do Not Confuse:

DynaCirc/Dynabac/Dynacin

Action: Inhibits calcium ion influx across cell membrane during cardiac depolarization; produces relaxation of coronary vascular smooth muscle and peripheral vascular smooth muscle; dilates coronary vascular arteries

Therapeutic Outcome: Decreased B/P

Uses: Hypertension, pectoris, vasospastic angina

Dosage and routes

Adult: PO 2.5 mg bid; increase at 2-4 wk intervals up to 10 mg bid or 5 mg daily; cont rel, may be increased q2-4wk, max 20 mg/day

Available forms: Caps 2.5, 5 mg; cont rel tabs 5, 10 mg

Adverse effects

CNS: Headache, fatigue, dizziness, fainting, sleep disturbances, weakness, depression, drowsiness

CV: Peripheral edema, tachycardia, hypotension, chest pain, **dysrhythmias**, syncope

GI: Nausea, vomiting, diarrhea, gastric upset, constipation, **hepatitis,** abdominal pain, distention, dry mouth

GU: Nocturia, urinary frequency

HEMA: **Leukopenia**

INTEG: Rash, pruritus, urticaria

MISC: Flushing

Contraindications: Sick sinus syndrome, 2nd- or 3rd-degree heart block, hypotension less than 90 mm Hg systolic, hypersensitivity

Precautions: Pregnancy **C,** CHF, hypotension, hepatic disease, lactation, children, renal disease, elderly

Pharmacokinetics

Absorption	Well absorbed
Distribution	High plasma protein binding (95%)
Metabolism	Liver, extensively and rapidly
Excretion	Kidney
Half-life	8 hr

Pharmacodynamics

Onset	1-2 hr
Peak	1.5 hr (immediate rel), 7-18 hr (cont rel)
Duration	12 hr

Interactions

Individual drugs

Cimetidine, ranitidine: increased serum concentration of isradipine

Disopyramide: increased bradycardia, conduction effects

Fentanyl: increased hypotension

Flovastatin: decreased flovastatin concentration

Lovastatin: decreased lovastatin concentration

Rifampin: decreased serum concentration of isradipine

Drug classifications

Antihypertensives, nitrates: increased hypotension

β-Adrenergic blockers: increased synergistic effect

Drug/herb

Aconite: increased toxicity, death

Astragalus, cola tree: increased or decreased antihypertensive effect

Barberry, betony, black catechu, black cohosh, bloodroot, broom, burdock, cat's claw, dandelion, goldenseal, Irish moss, Jamaican dogwood, kelp, khella, mistletoe, parsley: increased antihypertensive effect

Coltsfoot, guarana, khat, licorice: decreased antihypertensive effect

NURSING CONSIDERATIONS

Assessment

- Assess fluid volume status: I&O ratio and record, weight, distended red veins, crackles in lung, color, quality, and sp gr of urine, skin turgor, adequacy of pulses, moist mucous membranes, bilateral lung sounds, peripheral pitting edema; dehydration symptoms of decreasing output, thirst, hypotension, dry mouth and mucous membranes should be reported
- Monitor ALT, AST, bilirubin; if these are elevated, hepatotoxicity is suspected
- Assess renal, hepatic status, electrolytes before and during treatment
- Monitor cardiac status: B/P, pulse, respiration, ECG; assess anginal pain, precipitating, ameliorating factors

Nursing diagnoses

- Cardiac output, decreased (uses)
- Knowledge, deficient (teaching)

Implementation

- Do not break, crush, or chew caps, cont rel tabs
- Give once a day with full glass of water; with food for GI symptoms

Patient/family education

- Instruct patient to avoid hazardous activities until stabilized on drug and dizziness is no longer a problem
- Instruct patient to limit caffeine consumption; to avoid alcohol and OTC drugs unless directed by prescriber
- Advise patient to comply in all areas of medical regimen: diet, exercise, stress reduction, drug therapy; to notify prescriber of irregular heartbeat, shortness of breath, swelling of feet and hands, pronounced dizziness, constipation, nausea, hypotension
- Teach patient to use as directed even if feeling better
- Teach patient to take with a full glass of water

Evaluation

Positive therapeutic outcome

- Decreased B/P

Treatment of overdose: Defibrillation, atropine for AV block, vasopressor for hypotension

itraconazole (Rx)

(it-tra-kon′a-zol)

Sporanox

Func. class.: Antifungal (systemic)

Chem. class.: Triazole derivative

Pregnancy category C

Action: Increases cell membrane permeability in susceptible organisms by binding sterols in fungal cell membrane; decreases potassium, sodium, and nutrients in cell

Therapeutic Outcome: Fungistatic against *Histoplasma capsulatum, Blastomyces dermatitis, Cryptococcus neoformans, Aspergillus fumigatus, Candida*

Uses: Systemic candidiasis, chronic mucocandidiasis, oral thrush, candiduria, coccidioidomycosis, histoplasmosis, chromomycosis, paracoccidioidomycosis, blastomycosis (pulmonary and extrapulmonary)

Investigational uses: Dermatophytoses, pityriasis versicolor, sebopsoriasis, vaginal candidiasis, cryptococcal, subcutaneous mycoses, dimorphic infections, leishmaniasis, fungal keratitis, alternariosis, zygomycosis

Dosage and routes

Dose varies with type of infection

Adult: PO 200 mg daily with food; may increase to 400 mg daily if needed; life-threatening infections may require a loading dose of 200 mg tid × 3 days; **IV** 200 mg bid × 4 doses, then 200 mg daily; give each dose over 1 hr, maintenance PO 100 mg/day

Child: PO 3-5 mg/kg/day

Available forms: Caps 100 mg; oral sol 10 mg/ml; inj 10 mg/ml

Adverse effects

CNS: Headache, dizziness, insomnia, somnolence, depression

GI: Nausea, vomiting, anorexia, diarrhea, cramps, abdominal pain, flatulence, **GI bleeding, hepatotoxicity**

GU: Gynecomastia, impotence, decreased libido

INTEG: Pruritus, fever, rash, **toxic epidermal necrolysis**

MISC: Edema, fatigue, malaise, hypertension, hypokalemia, tinnitus, **rhabdomyolysis**

Contraindications: Hypersensitivity, fungal meningitis, onychomycosis, or dermatomycosis in cardiac dysfunction

Precautions: Pregnancy **C**, hepatic disease, achlorhydria or hypochlorhydria (drug-induced), children, lactation

Pharmacokinetics

Absorption	Variable
Distribution	Tissue, plasma, CSF, highly protein bound
Metabolism	Liver, extensively, inhibits CYP4503A enzyme
Excretion	Feces, breast milk
Half-life	20-21 hr

Pharmacodynamics

Onset	Unknown
Peak	4 hr
Duration	Unknown

Interactions
Individual drugs
Busulfan, clarithromycin, cycloSPORINE, diazepam, digoxin, felodipine, indinavir, isradipine, niCARdipine, NIFEdipine, nimoldipine, phenytoin, ritonavir, saquinavir, tacrolimus, warfarin: increased toxicity
BusPIRone: increased busPIRone levels, toxicity
Didanosine: decreased antifungal action
Dofetilide, pimozide, quinidine: life-threatening CV reaction
Midazolam: increased sedation
Quinidine: increased tinnitus, hearing loss, increased toxicity
Rifamycins: decreased action of itraconazole
Triazolam: increased sedation
Drug classifications
Antacids, H_2-receptor antagonists: decreased action of itraconazole
Calcium channel blockers: increased edema
Contraceptives (oral): decreased effect
Hepatotoxic drugs: hepatotoxicity
Oral hypoglycemics: increased effects of oral hypoglycemics
Drug/herb
Gossypol: nephrotoxicity
Drug/food
Increased: absorption

NURSING CONSIDERATIONS
Assessment
- Assess for infection: WBC, sputum baseline and periodically, may start treatment before obtaining results
- Monitor for hepatotoxicity: increasing AST, ALT, alkaline phosphatase, bilirubin
- Monitor for allergic reaction: dermatitis, rash; drug should be discontinued, antihistamines (mild reaction) or epINEPHrine (severe reaction) administered; check inj site for thrombophlebitis
- Monitor for hypokalemia, check potassium level: anorexia, drowsiness, weakness, decreased reflexes, dizziness, increased urinary output, increased thirst, paresthesias; if these occur, drug should be decreased or discontinued and potassium administered

Nursing diagnoses
- Infection, risk for (uses)
- Injury, risk for (adverse reaction)
- Knowledge, deficient (teaching)

Implementation
PO route
- Swallow caps whole; do not break, crush, or chew
- Give caps after full meal to ensure absorption
- Give with food or milk to prevent nausea and vomiting
- Take 2 hr before administration of other drugs that increase gastric pH
- Store in tight container at room temp
- Oral sol and caps are not interchangeable on a mg/mg basis
- Oral sol: patient should swish in mouth vigorously

IV route
- **IV** after adding full contents 25 ml to 50 ml of NaCl, mix gently, use flow control device, give over 1 hr; use separate line, flush after use

Patient/family education
- Advise patient that long-term therapy may be needed to clear infection (1 wk-6 mo depending on type of infection)
- Teach patient side effects and when to notify prescriber
- Instruct patient to avoid hazardous activities if dizziness occurs
- Instruct patient to take 2 hr before administration of other drugs that increase gastric pH (antacids, H_2-blockers, omeprazole, sucralfate, anticholinergics)
- Teach patient importance of compliance with drug regimen
- Instruct patient to notify prescriber of GI symptoms, signs of liver dysfunction (fatigue, nausea, anorexia, vomiting, dark urine, pale stools)

Evaluation
Positive therapeutic outcome
- Decreased fever, malaise, rash
- Negative C&S for infectious organism

ketoconazole (Rx)

(kee-toe-koe'na-zole)

Nizoral

Func. class.: Antifungal

Chem. class.: Imidazole derivative

Pregnancy category C

Do Not Confuse:
Nizoral/Nasarel/Neoral

Action: Alters cell membrane and inhibits several fungal enzymes; prevents production of adrenal sterols; prevents fungal metabolism

Therapeutic Outcome: Fungistatic/ fungicidal against susceptible organisms: *Blastomycoses, Candida, Coccidioides, Cryptococcus, Histoplasma;* top route: tinea cruris, tinea corporis, tinea versicolor, *Pityrosporum ovale*

Uses: Systemic candidiasis, chronic mucocandidiasis, oral thrush, candiduria, coccidioidomycosis, histoplasmosis, chromomycosis, paracoccidioidomycosis, blastomycosis

Investigational uses: Cushing's syndrome, advanced prostatic cancer

Dosage and routes

Adult: PO 200-400 mg once daily for 1-2 wk (candidiasis), 6 wk (other infections); 400 mg tid (prostate cancer, unlabeled)

Children >2 yr: 3.3-6.6 mg/kg/day as single daily dose

Available forms: Tabs 200 mg; oral susp ♣ 100 mg/5 ml topical (see Appendix D)

Adverse effects

CNS: Headache, dizziness, somnolence

GI: Nausea, vomiting, anorexia, diarrhea, abdominal pain, **hepatotoxicity**

GU: Gynecomastia, impotence

HEMA: **Thrombocytopenia, leukopenia, hemolytic anemia**

INTEG: Pruritus, fever, chills, photophobia, rash, dermatitis, purpura, urticaria

SYST: **Anaphylaxis**

Contraindications: Hypersensitivity, lactation, fungal meningitis; coadministration with terfenadine or drugs that prolong QTc interval

Precautions: Pregnancy **C,** renal, hepatic disease, achlorhydria (drug induced), children <2 yr, other hepatotoxic agents including terfenadine, other drugs metabolized by CYP450

Pharmacokinetics

Absorption	pH dependent; decreased pH increased absorption
Distribution	Widely distributed; crosses placenta
Metabolism	Liver, partially
Excretion	Feces, bile, breast milk
Half-life	Biphasic: 2 hr, 8 hr

Pharmacodynamics

Onset	Unknown
Peak	1-3 hr
Duration	Unknown

Interactions

Individual drugs

Alcohol: increased hepatotoxicity

Alfentanil, alprazolam, amprenavir, atorvastatin, carbamazepine, cerivastatin, clarithromycin, cyclophosphamide, cycloSPORINE, donepezil, erythromycin, fentanyl, ifosfamide, indinavir, lovastatin, midazolam, nelfinavir, nisoldipine, quinidine, ritonavir, saquinavir, sildenafil, simvastatin, sufentanil, tamoxifen, triazolam, vinBLAStine, vinCRIStine, zolpidem: increased toxicity, inhibition of CYP450 3A4 pathway

Isoniazid, phenytoin, rifampin: decreased effect of ketoconazole

Paclitaxel: inhibited metabolism

Theophylline: decreased effectiveness

Warfarin: increased effects of warfarin

Drug classifications

Antacids, anticholinergics, gastric pump inhibitors, H_2-receptor agonists: decreased ketoconazole action

Anticoagulants (oral): increased effects of oral anticoagulants

Calcium channel blockers, corticosteroids, vinca alkaloids: increased toxicity

Contraceptives (oral): decreased effect of oral contraceptives

Hepatotoxic agents: increased hepatotoxicity

Drug/herb

Gossypol: nephrotoxicity

Yew: decreased ketoconazole action

NURSING CONSIDERATIONS

Assessment

- Assess for signs and symptoms of infection: drainage, sore throat, urinary pain, hematuria, fever
- Obtain cultures for C&S before beginning treatment; therapy may be started after culture is taken
- ❗ Monitor for hepatotoxicity: increased AST,

ALT, alkaline phosphatase, bilirubin; drug is discontinued if hepatotoxicity occurs

Nursing diagnoses
- Infection, risk for (uses)
- Injury, risk for (adverse reactions)
- Knowledge, deficient (teaching)

Implementation
PO route
- Give in the presence of acid products only; do not use alkaline products, proton pump inhibitors, H_2-antagonists, or antacids within 2 hr of drug; may give coffee, tea, acidic fruit juices, cola; give with food to decrease GI symptoms; dissolve tab/4 ml of aqueous sol 0.2 N HCl, use straw to avoid contact with, rinse with water afterward and swallow
- Give with HCI if achlorhydria is present
- Store in tight container at room temp

Topical route
- Use enough medication to cover fungally infected and surrounding area; rub in; do not use occlusive dressing; do not get in eyes

Shampoo
- Hair should be wet; apply shampoo, lather, rub gently into scalp and hair for 1 min; rinse; reapply × 3 min; continue treatment 2 ×/wk for 1 mo, no more than once q3 days

Patient/family education
- Advise patient that long-term therapy may be needed to clear infection (1 wk-6 mo depending on infection)
- Advise patient to avoid hazardous activities if dizziness occurs
- Instruct patient to take 2 hr before administration of other drugs that increase gastric pH (antacids, H_2-blockers, omeprazole, sucralfate, anticholinergics)
- Stress the importance of compliance with drug regimen
- Advise patient to notify prescriber of GI symptoms, signs of liver dysfunction (fatigue, nausea, anorexia, vomiting, dark urine, pale stools)
- Teach patient proper hygiene: hand washing, nail care, use of concomitant topical agents if prescribed
- Caution patient to avoid alcohol, since nausea, vomiting, hypertension may occur
- Advise patient to use sunscreen or avoid direct sunlight to prevent photosensitivity
- Advise patient to notify prescriber of sore throat, fever, skin rash, which may indicate superinfection
- Advise patient to use sunglasses to prevent photophobia

Evaluation
Positive therapeutic outcome
- Decreased oral candidiasis, fever, malaise, rash
- Negative C&S for infectious organism
- Absence of dandruff, scaling

ketoprofen (OTC, Rx)
(ke-to-proe'fen)

Actron, Apo-Keto ✤, Apo-Keto-E ✤, Ketoprofen, Orudis, Orudis-E ✤, Orudis-KT, Orudis-SR ✤, Oruvail, Rhodis ✤

Func. class.: NSAID; nonopioid analgesic, antirheumatic

Chem. class.: Propionic acid derivative

Pregnancy category B

Do Not Confuse:
Oruvail/Clinoril, Oruvail/Elavil

Action: Inhibits prostaglandin synthesis by decreasing enzyme needed for biosynthesis; analgesic, antiinflammatory

Therapeutic Outcome: Decreased pain, inflammation

Uses: Mild to moderate pain, osteoarthritis, rheumatoid arthritis, dysmenorrhea

Dosage and routes
Antiinflammatory

Adult: PO 150-300 mg in divided doses tid-qid, not to exceed 300 mg/day or ext rel 150-200 mg daily

Analgesic

Adult: PO 25-50 mg q6-8h

Available forms: Caps 25, 50, 75 mg; ext rel caps 100, 150, 200 mg; tabs 12.5 mg

Adverse effects
CNS: Dizziness, drowsiness, fatigue, tremors, confusion, insomnia, anxiety, depression, headache

CV: Tachycardia, peripheral edema, palpitations, dysrhythmias, hypertension

EENT: Tinnitus, hearing loss, blurred vision

GI: *Nausea, anorexia, vomiting, diarrhea,* jaundice, **hepatitis,** constipation, flatulence, cramps, dry mouth, peptic ulcer, **GI bleeding**

GU: **Nephrotoxicity: dysuria, hematuria, oliguria, azotemia**

HEMA: **Blood dyscrasias**

INTEG: Purpura, rash, pruritus, sweating

SYST: **Anaphylaxis**

Contraindications: Avoid in 2nd/3rd trimesters of pregnancy; hypersensitivity,

K

asthma, severe renal disease, severe hepatic disease, ulcer disease

Precautions: Pregnancy **B** (1st trimester), lactation, children, bleeding disorders, GI disorders, cardiac disorders, hypersensitivity to other antiinflammatory agents, elderly

Pharmacokinetics

Absorption	Well absorbed
Distribution	Not known
Metabolism	Liver
Excretion	Kidneys
Half-life	2-4 hr

Pharmacodynamics

Onset	Unknown
Peak	2 hr
Duration	Unknown

Interactions
Individual drugs
Alcohol: increased adverse GI reactions, toxicity
Aspirin: increased ketoprofen levels, increased adverse GI reactions
Cefamandole, cefaperazone, cefotetan, clopidogrel, eptifibatide, plicamycin, ticlopidine, tirofiban, valproic acid: increased risk of bleeding
CycloSPORINE, digoxin, lithium, methotrexate, phenytoin: increased ketoprofen levels, increased toxicity
Insulin: increased hypoglycemia
Radiation: increased risk of hematologic toxicity
Warfarin: increased anticoagulant effect
Drug classifications
Anticoagulants, thrombolytics: increased risk of bleeding
Antihypertensives: decreased effect of antihypertensives
Corticosteroids: increased adverse GI reactions
Diuretics: decreased effectiveness of diuretics
Sulfonylureas: increased hypoglycemia
NSAIDs: increased adverse GI reactions
Drug/herb
Anise, arnica, bogbean, chamomile, chondroitin, clove, dong quai, feverfew, garlic, ginger, ginkgo, ginseng (*Panax*): increased risk of bleeding
Arginine, gossypol: increased gastric irritation
Bearberry, bilberry: increased NSAIDs effect
Drug/lab test
Increased: bleeding time, potassium, BUN, alkaline phosphatase, AST, ALT, creatinine, LDH
Decreased: blood glucose, Hct, Hgb, CCr, platelets, leukocytes
Interference: urine albumin, 17 KS, 17 hydroxycorticosteroids, bilirubin

NURSING CONSIDERATIONS
Assessment
- Assess for pain: type, location, intensity; ROM before and 1-2 hr after treatment
- Monitor liver function, renal function, studies: AST, ALT, bilirubin, creatinine, BUN, urine creatinine, CBC Hct, Hgb, protime if patient is on long-term therapy
- Check I&O ratio; decreasing output may indicate renal failure (long-term therapy)
- Assess hepatotoxicity: dark urine, clay-colored stools, jaundice of skin and sclera, itching, abdominal pain, fever, diarrhea if patient is on long-term therapy
- Assess for allergic reactions: rash, urticaria; if these occur, drug may have to be discontinued
- Assess for ototoxicity: tinnitus, ringing, roaring in ears; audiometric testing needed before, after long-term therapy
- Assess for visual changes: blurring, halos; may indicate corneal, retinal damage
- Assess for GI bleeding: blood in sputum, emesis, stools
- Check edema in feet, ankles, legs
- Identify prior drug history; there are many drug interactions
- Monitor pain: location, duration, type, intensity, before dose and 1 hr after; ROM before dose and after

Nursing diagnoses
- Pain, acute (uses)
- Pain, chronic (uses)
- Mobility, physical, (uses) impaired
- Injury, risk for (adverse reactions)
- Knowledge, deficient (teaching)

Implementation
- Swallow whole; do not break, crush, chew, or open cap
- Give with 8 oz of water and sit upright for 30 min after dose to prevent ulceration
- Give with food or milk to decrease gastric symptoms; give 30 min ac or 2 hr pc; absorption may be slowed

Patient/family education
- Teach patient to report any symptoms of hepatotoxicity, renal toxicity, visual changes, ototoxicity, allergic reactions, bleeding (long-term therapy)
- Advise patient to take with 8 oz of water and sit upright for 30 min after dose to prevent ulceration
- Caution patient not to exceed recommended

dosage; acute poisoning may result; to take as prescribed; do not double dose

- Advise patient to read label on other OTC drugs; many contain other antiinflammatories
- Advise patient to use sunscreen to prevent photosensitivity
- Inform patient that the therapeutic response takes 2 wk (arthritis)
- Teach patient to report tinnitus, confusion, diarrhea, sweating, hyperventilation, blurred vision, fever, joint aches
- Caution patient to avoid alcohol ingestion; GI bleeding may occur

Evaluation

Positive therapeutic outcome

- Decreased pain
- Decreased inflammation
- Increased mobility
- Decreased fever

ketorolac (Rx)

(kee'toe-role-ak)

Acular, Toradol

Func. class.: NSAID, nonopioid analgesic

Chem. class.: Acetic acid

Pregnancy category C

Do Not Confuse:

Toradol/Tegretol/Foradil, Toradol/Inderal, Toradol/Torecan, Toradol/tramadol

Action: Inhibits prostaglandin synthesis by decreasing an enzyme needed for biosynthesis; analgesic, antiinflammatory, antipyretic effects

Therapeutic Outcome: Decreased pain, inflammation, ocular itching

Uses: Mild to moderate pain (short term); decreased ocular itching in seasonal allergic conjunctivitis

Dosage and routes

Adult <65 yr: PO 20 mg, then 10 mg q4-6h prn, max 40 mg/day; (single dose) IM 60 mg; **IV** 30 mg; (multiple dosing) IM/**IV** 15 mg q6h, max 60 mg/day × 5 days combined either PO/IM/**IV**

Adult ≥65 yr, renal disease, <50 kg: PO 10 mg q4-6h prn, max 40 mg/day; (single dose) IM 30 mg; **IV** 15 mg; (multiple dosing) IM/**IV** 15 mg q6h, max 60 mg/day × 5 days combined either PO/IM/**IV**

Ophthalmic route

See Appendix D

Adult: 1 gtt (0.25 mg) qid × 7 days

Child: **IV** 1 mg/kg then 0.5 mg/kg q6h

Available forms: Inj 15, 30 mg/ml (prefilled syringes); ophth 0.5% sol; tabs 10 mg

Adverse effects

CNS: Dizziness, *drowsiness,* tremors

CV: Hypertension, flushing, syncope, pallor, edema, vasodilation

EENT: Tinnitus, hearing loss, blurred vision

GI: Nausea, anorexia, vomiting, diarrhea, constipation, flatulence, cramps, dry mouth, peptic ulcer, **GI bleeding, perforation,** taste change

GU: **Nephrotoxicity: dysuria, hematuria, oliguria, azotemia**

HEMA: **Blood dyscrasias,** prolonged bleeding

INTEG: Purpura, rash, pruritus, sweating

Contraindications: Hypersensitivity, asthma, severe renal disease, severe hepatic disease, peptic ulcer disease, labor and delivery, lactation, CV bleeding

Precautions: Pregnancy **C,** lactation, children, bleeding disorders, GI disorders, cardiac disorders, hypersensitivity to other antiinflammatory agents, elderly, CCr <25 ml/min

Pharmacokinetics

Absorption	Rapidly, completely absorbed
Distribution	Bound to plasma proteins (99%)
Metabolism	Liver (<50%)
Excretion	Kidney, metabolites (92%); breast milk (6%); feces
Half-life	6 hr (IM); increased in renal disease

Pharmacodynamics

	IM	OPHTH/PO
Onset	Up to 10 min	Unknown
Peak	50 min IM; 2-3 hr PO	Unknown
Duration	4-6 hr PO	Unknown

Interactions

Individual drugs

Alcohol, aspirin: increased GI effects

Aspirin, probenecid: increased ketorolac levels

Cefamandole, cefoperazone, cefotetan, clopidogrel, eptifibatide, plicamycin, ticlopidine, tirofiban, valproic acid: increased risk of bleeding

Cyclosporine, lithium, methotrexate: increased toxicity

Heparin: increased bleeding

Drug classifications

ACE inhibitors: increased renal impairment

K

Anticoagulants: increased effects
Antihypertensives: decreased antihypertensive effect
Cephalosporins (some), salicylates, thrombolytics: increased risk of bleeding
Corticosteroids, NSAIDs, potassium products, steroids: increased GI effects
Diuretics: decreased diuretic effect

Drug/herb

Anise, arnica, bogbean, chamomile, chondroitin, clove, dong quai, feverfew, garlic, ginger, ginkgo, ginseng *(Panax)*: increased risk of bleeding
Arginine, gossypol: increased gastric irritation
Bearberry, bilberry: increased NSAIDs effect

Drug/lab test

Increased: liver function studies, bleeding time, BUN, creatinine, potassium

NURSING CONSIDERATIONS

Assessment

- ❗ Monitor blood counts during therapy; watch for decreasing platelets; if low, therapy may need to be discontinued and restarted after hematologic recovery; assess for blood dyscrasia (thrombocytopenia): bruising, fatigue, bleeding, poor healing
- Monitor for aspirin sensitivity, asthma; these patients may be more likely to develop hypersensitivity to NSAIDs
- Assess patient's eyes: redness swelling, tearing, itching
- Monitor for pain: type, location, intensity, ROM before and 1 hr after treatment
- Assess for GI bleeding: blood in sputum, emesis, stools

Nursing diagnoses

- Pain, acute (uses)
- Mobility, physical, impaired (uses)
- Injury, risk for (adverse reactions)
- Knowledge, deficient (teaching)

Implementation

PO route

- Administer to patient crushed or whole
- Give with full glass of water; give with food or milk to decrease gastric symptoms; give 30 min ac or 2 hr pc; absorption may be slowed

IM/IV route

- **IV** give undiluted ≥15 sec
- Give IM/**IV** for 5 days or less, continue with PO
- Give IM inj deeply in large muscle mass

Y-site compatibilities: Cisatracurium, remifentanil, sufentanil

Syringe incompatibilities: Morphine, meperidine, promethazine, hydrOXYzine

Solution compatibilities: D_5W, 0.9% NaCl, LR, D_5, plasmalate

Patient/family education

- Teach patient that drug must be continued for prescribed time to be effective; to avoid aspirin, alcoholic beverages, other NSAIDs, acetaminophen
- Caution patient to report bleeding, bruising, fatigue, malaise, since blood dyscrasias do occur
- Instruct patient to use caution when driving; drowsiness, dizziness may occur
- Teach patient to take with a full glass of water to enhance absorption
- Caution patient that this drug may cause eye redness, burning if soft contact lenses are worn

Evaluation

Positive therapeutic outcome

- Decreased pain
- Decreased inflammatory response
- Increased mobility
- Decreased ocular itching

labetalol (Rx)

(la-bet'a-lole)

Normodyne, Trandate

Func. class.: Antihypertensive, antianginal

Chem. class.: α- and β-blocker

Pregnancy category C

Do Not Confuse:

Trandate/Tridate

Action: Competitively blocks stimulation of β-adrenergic receptor within vascular smooth muscle; produces chronotropic, inotropic activity (decreases rate of SA node discharge, increases recovery time), slows conduction of AV node, decreases heart rate, which decreases O_2 consumption in myocardium; also has α-adrenergic blocking activity

Therapeutic Outcome: Decreased B/P

Uses: Mild to moderate hypertension; treatment of severe hypertension (**IV**)

Investigational uses: Hypertension in patients with pheochromocytoma, hypertension in clonidine withdrawal

Dosage and routes

Hypertension

Adult: PO 100 mg bid; may be given with a diuretic; may increase to 200 mg bid after 2

days; may continue to increase q1-3 days; max 2400 mg/day in divided doses

Hypertensive crisis

Adult: **IV** inf 200 mg/160 ml D_5W, run at 2 ml/min; stop inf after desired response obtained; repeat q6-8h as needed; **IV** bol 20 mg over 2 min; may repeat 40-80 mg q10 min, not to exceed 300 mg

Available forms: Tabs 100, 200, 300 mg; inj 5 mg/ml in 20-ml ampules

Adverse effects

CNS: Dizziness, mental changes, drowsiness, fatigue, headache, catatonia, depression, anxiety, nightmares, paresthesias, lethargy
CV: *Orthostatic hypotension,* **bradycardia, CHF,** chest pain, **ventricular dysrhythmias,** AV block, scalp tingling
EENT: *Tinnitus,* visual changes, sore throat, double vision, dry burning eyes
GI: *Nausea, vomiting, diarrhea,* dyspepsia, taste distortion
GU: Impotence, dysuria, ejaculatory failure
HEMA: **Agranulocytosis, thrombocytopenia, purpura** (rare)
INTEG: Rash, alopecia, urticaria, pruritus, fever
RESP: **Bronchospasm,** dyspnea, wheezing

Contraindications: Hypersensitivity to β-blockers, cardiogenic shock, heart block (2nd or 3rd degree), sinus bradycardia, CHF, bronchial asthma

Precautions: Pregnancy **C,** major surgery, lactation, diabetes mellitus, renal disease, thyroid disease, COPD, well-compensated heart failure, CAD, nonallergic bronchospasm, elderly, hepatic disease

Pharmacokinetics

Absorption	Bioavailability 25% (PO); complete (**IV**)
Distribution	Crosses placenta, CNS
Metabolism	Liver, extensively
Excretion	Breast milk, kidneys, bile
Half-life	6-8 hr

Pharmacodynamics

	PO	IV
Onset	1-2 hr	5 min
Peak	2-4 hr	15 min
Duration	8-12 hr	2-4 hr

Interactions

Individual drugs

Alcohol (large amounts), cimetidine, nitroglycerin: increased hypotension
Glutethimide: decreased effect of labetalol
Indomethacin, lidocaine: decreased effect of each specific drug
Verapamil: increased myocardial depression

Drug classifications

Antihypertensives: increased hypotension
β-Blockers, bronchodilators, sympathomimetics, xanthines: decreased effects
Diuretics: increased hypotension
General anesthetics, hydantoins: increased myocardial depression
MAOIs: do not use within 2 wk
Theophyllines: decreased bronchodilation

Drug/herb

Aconite: increased toxicity, death
Astragalus, cola tree: increased or decreased antihypertensive effect
Barberry, betony, black catechu, black cohosh, bloodroot, broom, burdock, cat's claw, dandelion, goldenseal, Irish moss, Jamaican dogwood, kelp, khella, mistletoe, parsley: increased antihypertensive effect
Coltsfoot, guarana, khat, licorice: decreased antihypertensive effect

Drug/lab test

Increased: ANA titer, blood glucose, alkaline phosphatase, LDH, AST, ALT, BUN, potassium, triglycerides, uric acid
False increase: urinary catecholamines

L

NURSING CONSIDERATIONS

Assessment

- Monitor B/P at beginning of treatment, periodically thereafter; pulse q4h; note rate, rhythm, quality: apical/radial pulse before administration; notify prescriber of any significant changes (pulse <50 bpm)
- Check for baselines in renal, liver function tests before therapy begins
- Assess for edema in feet, legs daily, monitor I&O, daily weight; check for jugular vein distention, crackles bilaterally, dyspnea (CHF)
- Monitor skin turgor, dryness of mucous membranes for hydration status, especially elderly

Nursing diagnoses

- Cardiac output, decreased (uses)
- Injury, risk for (side effects)
- Knowledge, deficient (teaching)
- Noncompliance (teaching)

Implementation

PO route

- Given ac, at bedtime, tab may be crushed or swallowed whole; give with food to prevent GI upset, increase absorption; reduce dosage in renal dysfunction
- Store protected from light, moisture; place in cool environment

IV route

- Give **IV** undiluted 20 mg/2 min; may increase q10 min 40-80 mg until desired effect
- Give **IV** cont inf by diluting in LR, D_5W, D_5 in 0.2%, 0.9%, 0.33% NaCl or Ringer's; inf is titrated to patient response; 200 mg of drug/160 ml sol (1 mg/ml); 300 mg of drug/240 ml sol (1 mg/ml); 200 mg of drug/250 ml sol (2 mg/3ml); use infusion pump
- Keep patient recumbent during and for 3 hr after inf, monitor VS q5-15 min

Y-site compatibilities: Amikacin, aminophylline, amiodarone, ampicillin, butorphanol, calcium gluconate, cefazolin, ceftazidime, ceftizoxime, chloramphenicol, cimetidine, clindamycin, diltiazem, DOBUTamine, DOPamine, enalaprilat, epINEPHrine, erythromycin, esmolol, famotidine, fentanyl, gentamicin, hydromorphone, lidocaine, lorazepam, magnesium sulfate, meperidine, metronidazole, midazolam, milrinone, morphine, niCARdipine, nitroglycerin, nitroprusside, norepinephrine, oxacillin, penicillin G potassium, piperacillin, potassium chloride, potassium phosphate, propofol, ranitidine, sodium acetate, tobramycin, trimethoprim/sulfamethoxazole, vancomycin, vecuronium

Y-site incompatibilities: Cefoperazone, nafcillin

Solution compatibilities: D_5R, D_5LR, $D_{2\frac{1}{2}}$/0.45% NaCl, D_5/0.2% NaCl, D_5/0.33% NaCl, D_5/0.9% NaCl, D_5W, Ringer's, LR

Solution incompatibilities: Sodium bicarbonate 5%

Patient/family education

- Teach patient not to discontinue drug abruptly, or precipitate angina might occur; taper over 2 wk
- Teach patient not to use OTC products containing α-adrenergic stimulants (such as nasal decongestants, cold preparations); to avoid alcohol, smoking and to limit sodium intake as prescribed
- Teach patient how to take pulse and B/P at home; advise when to notify prescriber
- Instruct patient to comply with weight control, dietary adjustments, modified exercise program
- Advise patient to carry/wear emergency ID to identify drugs being taken, allergies; that drug controls symptoms but does not cure the condition
- Caution patient to avoid hazardous activities if dizziness, drowsiness are present
- Teach patient to report symptoms of CHF: difficult breathing, especially on exertion or when lying down, night cough, swelling of extremities, bradycardia, dizziness, confusion, depression, fever
- Teach patient to take drug as prescribed, not to double or skip doses; take any missed doses as soon as remembered if at least 4 hr until next dose

Evaluation

Positive therapeutic outcome

- Decreased B/P in hypertension (after 1-2 wk)
- Absence of dysrhythmias

Treatment of overdose: Lavage, **IV** atropine for bradycardia, **IV** theophylline for bronchospasm, digitalis, O_2, diuretic for cardiac failure, hemodialysis, **IV** glucose for hyperglycemia, **IV** diazepam (or phenytoin) for seizures

lactulose (Rx)

(lak'tyoo-lose)

Cephulac, Cholac, Chronulac, Constilac, Constulose, Duphalac, Enulose, Evalose, Heptalac, Kristalose, Lactulax ✦, Lactulose PSE, Portalac

Func. class.: Laxative (hyperosmotic/ammonia detoxicant)

Chem. class.: Lactose synthetic derivative

Pregnancy category B

Action: Increases osmotic pressure; draws fluid into colon; prevents absorption of ammonia in colon; increases water in stool

Therapeutic Outcome: Decreased constipation, decreased blood ammonia level

Uses: Chronic constipation, portal-systemic encephalopathy in patients with hepatic disease

Dosage and routes

Constipation

Adult: PO 15-60 ml daily or 10-20 g powder for oral sol daily

Child (unlabeled): PO 7.5 ml daily

Encephalopathy

Adult: PO 30-45 ml tid or qid until stools are soft; retention enema 300 ml diluted

Infant (unlabeled): PO 2.5-10 ml/day in divided doses

Child (unlabeled): PO 40-90 ml/day in divided doses given 2-4 ×/day

Available forms: Syr 10 g/15 ml, single-use packets (Kristalose) 10, 20 g

Adverse effects

GI: *Nausea, vomiting, anorexia, abdominal cramps, diarrhea,* flatulence, *distention, belching*

Contraindications: Hypersensitivity, low-galactose diet

Precautions: Pregnancy **B,** lactation, diabetes mellitus, elderly and debilitated patient

Pharmacokinetics

Absorption	Poorly absorbed
Distribution	Not known
Metabolism	Colonic bacteria to acids
Excretion	Kidneys, unchanged
Half-life	Unknown

Pharmacodynamics

Unknown

Interactions

Individual drugs

Neomycin: decreased effectiveness (portal-systemic encephalopathy)

Drug classifications

Antiinfectives (oral): decreased lactulose effect

Laxatives: do not use together

Drug/herb

Flax, senna: increased laxative effect

NURSING CONSIDERATIONS

Assessment

- Monitor glucose levels in diabetic patients (increases)
- Monitor blood, urine, electrolytes if used often by patient; may cause diarrhea, hypokalemia, hypernatremia; check I&O ratio to identify fluid loss
- Assess cramping, rectal bleeding, nausea, vomiting; if these symptoms occur, drug should be discontinued; identify cause of constipation; identify whether fluids, bulk, or exercise is missing from lifestyle
- Monitor blood ammonia level (30-70 mg/100 ml); monitor for clearing of confusion, lethargy, restlessness, irritability (hepatic encephalopathy); may decrease ammonia level by 50%

Nursing diagnoses

- Constipation (uses)
- Diarrhea (adverse reactions)
- Knowledge, deficient (teaching)
- Noncompliance (teaching)

Implementation

PO route

- Give with full glass of fruit juice, water, milk to increase palatability of oral form; increase fluids by 2 L/day; do not give with other laxatives; if diarrhea occurs, reduce dosage

Rectal route

- Administer retention enema by diluting 300 ml of lactulose/700 ml of water or of 0.9% NaCl; administer by rec balloon catheter; retain for 30-60 min; repeat if evacuated too quickly

Patient/family education

- Discuss with patient that adequate fluid consumption is necessary
- Teach patient that normal bowel movements do not always occur daily
- Teach patient not to use in presence of abdominal pain, nausea, vomiting; tell patient to notify prescriber if constipation unrelieved or if symptoms of electrolyte imbalance occur: muscle cramps, pain, weakness, dizziness, excessive thirst
- Teach patient not to use laxatives for long-term therapy; bowel tone will be lost
- Do not give at bedtime as a laxative; may interfere with sleep
- Notify prescriber if diarrhea occurs; may indicate overdosage

Evaluation

Positive therapeutic outcome

- Decreased constipation
- Decreased blood ammonia level
- Clearing of mental state

L

lamivudine (3TC) (Rx)

(lam-i'vue-dine)

Epivir, Epivir-HBV

Func. class.: Antiretroviral

Chem. class.: Nucleoside reverse transcriptase inhibitor

Pregnancy category C

Do Not Confuse:
lamivudine/Lamotrigine

Action: Inhibits replication of HIV virus by incorporating into cellular DNA by viral reverse transcriptase, thereby terminating the cellular DNA chain

Therapeutic Outcome: Improved symptoms of HIV infection

Uses: HIV infection in combination with other antiretrovirals; chronic hepatitis B (Epivir-HBV)

Investigational uses: Prophylaxis of HIV postexposure with indinavir and zidovudine

Dosage and routes

HIV infection

Adult/child >16 yr: PO 150 mg bid or 300 mg daily

Child 3 mo-16 yr: PO 4 mg/kg bid; max 150 mg bid

Renal dose

Adult: PO CCr 30-49 ml/min 150 mg daily; CCr 15-29 ml/min 150 mg 1st dose, then 100 mg daily; CCr 5-14 ml/min 150 mg daily, then 50 mg daily; CCr <5 ml/min 50 mg 1st dose, then 25 mg daily

Chronic hepatitis B

Adult: PO 100 mg daily

Renal dose

Adult: PO CCr 30-49 ml/min 150 mg daily; CCr 15-29 ml/min 150 mg 1st dose, then 100 mg daily; CCr 5-14 ml/min 150 mg daily; CCr <5 ml/min 50 mg 1st dose, then 25 mg daily

Available forms: Oral sol (Epivir) 10 mg/ml, tabs 150, 300/mg; oral sol (Epivir-HBV) 5 mg/ml, tabs 100 mg

Adverse effects

CNS: *Fever, headache, malaise, dizziness, insomnia, depression, fatigue, chills,* **seizures**

EENT: Taste change, hearing loss, photophobia

GI: *Nausea, vomiting, diarrhea,* anorexia, cramps, dyspepsia, **hepatomegaly with steatosis, pancreatitis**

HEMA: **Neutropenia,** anemia, **thrombocytopenia**

INTEG: *Rash*

MS: *Myalgia, arthralgia, pain*

RESP: *Cough*

SYST: **Lactic acidosis, anaphylaxis, Stevens-Johnson syndrome**

Contraindications: Hypersensitivity

Precautions: Pregnancy **C,** granulocyte count <1000/mm^3 or Hgb <9.5 g/dl, lactation, children, renal disease, severe hepatic dysfunction, pancreatitis, elderly

Pharmacokinetics

Absorption	Rapidly absorbed
Distribution	Extravascular space
Metabolism	Protein binding <36%
Excretion	Unchanged in urine
Half-life	Terminal half-life 5-7 hr

Pharmacodynamics

Unknown

Interactions

Individual drugs

Trimethoprim/sulfamethoxazole: increased level of lamivudine

Zalcitabine: decreased both drugs

Zidovudine: increased level

Drug/lab test

Increased: ALT, bilirubin

Decreased: Hgb, neutrophil, platelet count

NURSING CONSIDERATIONS

Assessment

- Monitor blood counts q2 wk; watch for neutropenia, thrombocytopenia, Hgb, CD4, viral load, lipase, triglycerides periodically during treatment; if low, therapy may have to be discontinued and restarted after hematologic recovery; blood transfusions may be required
- Monitor liver function studies: AST, ALT, bilirubin; amylase
- Monitor children for pancreatitis: abdominal pain, nausea, vomiting
- Assess for lactic acidosis, severe hepatomegaly with steatosis: obtain baseline liver function tests; if elevated, discontinue treatment; discontinue even if liver function tests are normal and symptoms of lactic acidosis, severe hepatomegaly develop

Nursing diagnoses

- Infection, risk for (uses)
- Injury, risk for (adverse reactions)
- Knowledge, deficient (teaching)

Implementation

- Administer PO daily, bid without regard to meals
- Give with other antiretrovirals only
- Store in cool environment; protect from light

Patient/family education

- Teach patient that GI complaints and insomnia resolve after 3-4 wk of treatment
- Tell patient that drug is not a cure for AIDS but will control symptoms
- Teach patient to notify prescriber of sore throat, swollen lymph nodes, malaise, fever; other infections may occur
- Teach patient that virus is still infective, may pass AIDS virus to others
- Encourage patient to continue follow-up visits since serious toxicity may occur; blood counts must be done q2 wk
- Teach patient that drug must be taken as prescribed, even if feeling better
- Tell patient that other drugs may be necessary to prevent other infections

• Teach patient that drug may cause fainting or dizziness

Evaluation

Positive therapeutic outcome

• Absence of infection, symptoms of HIV infection

lamotrigine (Rx)

(lam-o-trye'geen)

Lamictal, Lamictal Chewable Dispersible

Func. class.: Anticonvulsant—miscellaneous

Chem. class.: Phenyltriazine

Pregnancy category C

Do Not Confuse:

Lamictal/Lamisil, Lamictal/Lomotil, Lamotrigine/Lamivudine

Action: Unknown; may inhibit voltage-sensitive sodium channels

Therapeutic Outcome: Decrease in intensity and amount of seizures

Uses: Adjunct in the treatment of partial seizures; children with Lennox-Gastaut syndrome

Investigational uses: Refractory bipolar disorder, generalized tonic-clonic, absence, atypical absence and myoclonic seizures

Dosage and routes

Monotherapy

Adult: PO 50 mg/day for wk 1 and 2, then increase to 100 mg divided bid for wk 3 and 4; maintenance 300-500 mg/day

Child: 2 mg/kg/day in 2 divided doses × 2 wk, then 10 mg/kg/day, max 15 mg/kg/day or 400 mg/day

Multiple therapy

Adult: PO 25 mg every other day, wk 1 through 4, then 150 mg/day in divided doses

Child: 0.1-0.2 mg/kg/day initially, then increase q2 wk as needed to 2 mg/kg/day or 150 mg/day

Hepatic dose

Adult (Child-Pugh grade B): PO reduce by 50%

Adult (Child-Pugh grade C): PO reduce by 75%

Bipolar disorder

Adult: PO wk 1-2 25 mg daily; wk 3-4 50 mg daily; wk 5 100 mg daily; wk 6-7 200 mg daily; for patients taking valproic acid: wk 1-2 25 mg every other day; wk 3-4 25 mg daily; wk 5 50 mg daily; wk 6 100 mg daily; wk 7 100 mg daily

Available forms: Tabs 25, 100, 150, 200 mg; chew tabs 2, 5, 25 mg

Adverse effects

CNS: Fever, insomnia, tremor, depression, anxiety, *dizziness,* ataxia, *headache*

EENT: Nystagmus, **diplopia,** *blurred vision*

GI: *Nausea, vomiting, anorexia,* abdominal pain, **hepatotoxicity**

GU: *Dysmenorrhea*

INTEG: **Rash (potentially life-threatening),** alopecia, photosensitivity

SYST: **Stevens-Johnson syndrome**

Contraindications: Hypersensitivity

Precautions: Pregnancy **C,** lactation, children <16 yr, renal, hepatic disease, elderly, cardiac disease, severe depression, suicidal, blood dyscrasias

Pharmacokinetics

Absorption	Well absorbed, rapid
Distribution	Unknown
Metabolism	Glucuronic acid
Excretion	Unknown
Half-life	Varies, depending on dose

Pharmacodynamics

Unknown

Interactions

Individual drugs

Acetaminophen, carbamazepine, oxcarbazepine, phenobarbital, phenytoin, primidone: decreased lamotrigine serum concentration

Valproic acid: decreased metabolic clearance of lamotrigine

Drug classifications

Contraceptives (oral), succinimides, rifamycins: decreased lamotrigine serium concentration

Drug/herb

Ginkgo: increased anticonvulsant effect

Ginseng, santonica: decreased anticonvulsant effect

NURSING CONSIDERATIONS

Assessment

• Assess for rash (Stevens-Johnson syndrome or toxic epidermal necrolysis) in pediatric patients, drug should be discontinued at first sign of rash

• Assess for seizure activity: duration, type, intensity, halo before seizure

• Assess for hypersensitive reactions

Nursing diagnoses

• Injury, risk for (uses)

• Knowledge, deficient (teaching)

Implementation

- Give in divided doses with or after meals to decrease adverse effects
- May be given with food or fluids
- Dispersible tabs should be swallowed whole, chewed, dispersed in water or diluted fruit juice; if chewed, a small amount of water should be taken

Patient/family education

- Caution patient not to discontinue drug abruptly; seizures may occur
- Caution patient to avoid hazardous activities until stabilized on drug
- Advise patient to notify prescriber of skin rash or increased seizure activity
- Instruct patient to report to prescriber if pregnancy is suspected or planned
- Teach patient to use sunscreen and protective clothing, photosensitivity occurs
- Advise patient to carry/wear emergency ID stating drug use

Evaluation

Positive therapeutic outcome

- Decrease in severity of seizures

lansoprazole (Rx)

(lan-soe'prah-zole)

Prevacid

Func. class.: Anti-ulcer–proton pump inhibitor

Chem. class.: Benzimidazole

Pregnancy category B

Do Not Confuse:
Prevacid/Pravachol/Prinivil

Action: Suppresses gastric secretion by inhibiting hydrogen/potassium ATPase enzyme system in gastric parietal cell; characterized as gastric acid pump inhibitor since it blocks final step of acid production

Therapeutic Outcome: Reduction in gastric pain, swelling, fullness

Uses: Gastroesophageal reflux disease (GERD), severe erosive esophagitis, poorly responsive systemic GERD, pathologic hypersecretory conditions (Zollinger-Ellison syndrome, systemic mastocytosis, multiple endocrine adenomas); possibly effective for treatment of duodenal, gastric ulcers, maintenance of healed duodenal ulcers

Dosage and routes

NG tube

Adult: Use intact granules mixed in 40 ml of apple juice injected through NG tube, then flush with apple juice

Duodenal ulcer

Adult: PO 15 mg daily ac for 4 wk, then 15 mg daily to maintain healing of ulcers; ulcers associated with *Helicobacter:* 30 mg lansoprazole, 500 mg clarithromycin, 1 g amoxicillin bid × 14 days or 30 mg lansoprazole, 1 g amoxicillin tid × 14 days

Erosive esophagitis

Adult: PO 30 mg daily ac for up to 8 wk, may use another 8-wk course if needed

Pathologic hypersecretory conditions

Adult: PO 60 mg daily, may give up to 90 mg bid, administer doses of >120 mg/day in divided doses

GERD/esophagitis

Child 1-11 yr (>30 kg): PO 30 mg daily ≤12 wk

Child 1-11 yr (≤30 kg): 15 mg daily ≤12 wk

Available forms: Del rel caps 15, 30 mg; granules for oral susp 15, 30 mg/packet

Adverse effects

CNS: Headache, dizziness, confusion, agitation, amnesia, depression

CV: Chest pain, angina, tachycardia, bradycardia, palpitations, **CVA,** hypertension/hypotension, **MI,** shock, vasodilation

EENT: Tinnitus, taste perversion, deafness, eye pain, otitis media

GI: Diarrhea, abdominal pain, vomiting, nausea, constipation, flatulence, acid regurgitation, anorexia, irritable colon

GU: Hematuria, glycosuria, impotence, kidney calculus, breast enlargement

HEMA: **Hemolysis,** anemia

INTEG: Rash, urticaria, pruritus, alopecia

META: Weight gain/loss, gout

RESP: Upper respiratory infections, cough, epistaxis, asthma, bronchitis, dyspnea

Contraindications: Hypersensitivity

Precautions: Pregnancy **B,** lactation, children

Pharmacokinetics	
Absorption	Rapid after granules leave stomach
Distribution	Protein binding 97%
Metabolism	Liver extensively
Excretion	Urine, feces; clearance decreased in elderly, renal, hepatic disease
Half-life	Plasma 1.5 hr

Pharmacodynamics

Unknown

Interactions
Individual drugs

Ampicillin, digoxin, iron, itraconazole, ketoconazole, theophylline: decreased absorption of each specific drug

Sucralfate: delayed absorption of lansoprazole

NURSING CONSIDERATIONS
Assessment
- Assess GI system; bowel sounds q8h, abdomen for pain, swelling, anorexia
- Monitor hepatic enzymes (AST, ALT, alkaline phosphatase) during treatment

Nursing diagnoses
- Pain, chronic (uses)
- Knowledge, deficient (teaching)

Implementation
- Swallow del rel cap whole; do not break, crush, chew, or open
- Administer before eating

Patient/family education
- Instruct patient to report severe diarrhea; drug may have to be discontinued
- Inform diabetic patient that hypoglycemia may occur
- Encourage patient to avoid hazardous activities; dizziness may occur
- Tell patient to avoid alcohol, salicylates, ibuprofen; may cause GI irritation

Evaluation
Positive therapeutic outcome
- Absence of gastric pain, swelling, fullness

leflunomide (Rx)
(leh-floo′noh-mide)

Arava

Func. class.: Antirheumatic (DMARDs)

Chem. class.: Immune modulator, pyrimidine synthesis inhibitor

Pregnancy category X

Action: Inhibits an enzyme involved in pyrimidine synthesis and has antiproliferative, antiinflammatory effect

Therapeutic Outcome: Decreased pain, joint swelling, increased mobility

Uses: Rheumatoid arthritis, to reduce disease process as well as symptoms

Dosage and routes
Adult: **PO** loading dose 100 mg/day × 3 days maintenance 20 mg/day, may be decreased to 10 mg/day if not well tolerated

Juvenile rheumatoid arthritis (off-label)

Adolescents and child: PO 10 mg (10-19.9 kg); 15 mg (20-40 kg); 20 mg (>40 kg)

Available forms: Tabs 10, 20, 100 mg

Adverse effects
CNS: Dizziness, insomnia, depression, paresthesia, anxiety, migraine, neuralgia, headache

CV: Palpitations, hypertension, chest pain, angina pectoris, peripheral edema

EENT: Pharyngitis, oral candidiasis, stomatitis, dry mouth, blurred vision

GI: *Nausea, anorexia, vomiting, constipation, flatulence, diarrhea, increased liver function tests,* **hepatotoxicity**

HEMA: Anemia, ecchymosis, hyperlipidemia

INTEG: Rash, pruritus, alopecia, acne, hematoma, herpes infections

RESP: Pharyngitis, rhinitis, bronchitis, cough, respiratory infection, pneumonia, sinusitis

Contraindications: Pregnancy **X,** hypersensitivity, lactation, jaundice, lactase deficiency, hepatic disease

Precautions: Renal disorders, vaccinations, infection, alcoholism, children, immunosuppression

Pharmacokinetics

Absorption	Unknown
Distribution	Unknown
Metabolism	Liver
Excretion	Kidneys
Half-life	Unknown

Pharmacodynamics

Onset	Unknown
Peak	Unknown
Duration	Unknown

Interactions
Individual drugs

Activated charcoal, cholestyramine: decreased effect of leflunomide

Methotrexate: increased leflunomide side effects

Rifampin: increased rifampin levels

Drug classifications

Live virus vaccines: decreased antibody reaction

NSAIDs: increased NSAID effect

Hepatotoxic agents: increased side effects of leflunomide

L

NURSING CONSIDERATIONS

Assessment

- Monitor liver function studies: if ALT elevations are >2 times baseline, reduce dose to 10 mg/day
- Assess arthritic symptoms: ROM, mobility, swelling of joints, baseline and during treatment

Nursing diagnoses

- Mobility, impaired (uses)
- Pain, chronic (uses)
- Knowledge, deficient (teaching)

Implementation

- Give with full glass of water to enhance absorption
- Give PO with food, milk, or antacids for GI upset
- To eliminate drug give cholestyramine 8 g tid × 11 days, check levels

Patient/family education

- Teach patient that drug must be continued for prescribed time to be effective
- Instruct patient to take with food, milk, or antacids to avoid GI upset
- Advise patient to use caution when driving; drowsiness, dizziness may occur
- Advise patient to take with a full glass of water to enhance absorption
- Advise patient to avoid pregnancy while taking this drug
- Inform patient that hair may be lost, review alternatives
- Advise patient to avoid live virus vaccinations during treatment

Evaluation

Positive therapeutic outcome

- Increased joint mobility without pain
- Decreased joint swelling

! HIGH ALERT

lepirudin (Rx)

(lep-ih-roo'din)

Refludan

Func. class.: Anticoagulant

Chem. class.: Thrombin inhibitor, hirudin

Pregnancy category B

Action Direct inhibitor of thrombin that is highly specific

Therapeutic Outcome: Absence of thrombocytopenia, stroke, MI, or other thromboembolic conditions

Uses: Heparin-induced thrombocytopenia and other thromboembolic conditions

Investigational uses: Adjunct therapy in unstable angina, acute MI without ST elevation, prevention of deep vein thrombosis, percutaneous coronary intervention

Dosage and routes

Adult: **IV** 0.4 mg/kg (≤110 kg) over 15-20 sec; then 0.15 mg/kg (≤110 kg/hr) as a cont inf for 2-10 days or longer

Renal dose

Adult: **IV** bol 0.2 mg/kg over 15-20 sec; CCr 45-60 ml/min 0.075 mg/kg/hr; CCr 30-44 ml/min 0.045 mg/kg/hr; CCr 15-29 ml/min 0.0225 mg/kg/hr

Concomitant use with thrombolytic therapy

Adult: **IV** bol 0.2 mg/kg initially

Adult: Cont **IV** inf 0.1 mg/kg/hr

Available forms: Powder for inj 50 mg

Adverse effects

CNS: *Fever*, **intracranial bleeding**

CV: **Heart failure, pericardial effusion, ventricular fibrillation**

GI: GI bleeding, abnormal liver function tests

GU: **Hematuria,** abnormal kidney function, vaginal bleeding

HEMA: **Hemorrhage, thrombocytopenia**

INTEG: Allergic skin reactions

RESP: Pneumonia

SYST: **Multiorgan failure, sepsis, anaphylaxis**

Contraindications: Hypersensitivity to hirudins

Precautions: Pregnancy **B,** intracranial bleeding, lactation, children, hepatic disease, recent major surgery, hemorrhagic diathesis, bacterial endocarditis, severe uncontrolled hypertension, advanced renal disease, recent active peptic ulcer, recent CVA, stroke, intracerebral surgery, elderly, women

Pharmacokinetics	
Absorption	Unknown
Distribution	Unknown
Metabolism	Possibly by the release of amino acids during catabolism
Excretion	50% unchanged in urine
Half-life	Unknown

Pharmacodynamics	
Onset	Unknown
Peak	Unknown
Duration	Unknown

Interactions
Individual drugs
Aspirin, cefamandole, cefoperazone, cefotetan, clopidogrel, dipyridamole, eptifibatide, plicamycin, ticlopidine, tirofiban, valproic acid: increased bleeding risk
Drug classifications
NSAIDs, thrombolytics, warfarin derivatives: increased bleeding risk
Drug/herb
Agrimony, alfalfa, angelica, anise, basil, bay, bilberry, black haw, bogbean, bromelain, buchu, chondroitin, cinchona bark, dong quai, fenugreek, feverfew, garlic, ginger, ginkgo, ginseng, horse chestnut, Irish moss, kelp, kelpware, khella, lovage, lungwort, meadowsweet, motherwort, mugwort, nettle, papaya, parsley (large amounts), paud'arco, pineapple, poplar, prickly ash, safflower, saw palmetto, tonka bean, turmeric, wintergreen, yarrow: increased risk of bleeding
Chamomile, coenzyme Q10, flax, glucomannan, goldenseal, guar gum: decreased anticoagulant effect

NURSING CONSIDERATIONS
Assessment
- Obtain baseline APTT before treatment; do not start treatment if APTT ratio is ≥2.5, then APTT 4 hr after initiation of treatment and at least daily thereafter; if APTT is above target, stop infusion for 2 hr, then restart at 50%, take APTT in 4 hr; if below target, increase inf rate by 20%, take APTT in 4 hr, do not exceed inf rate of 0.21 mg/kg/hr without checking for coagulation abnormalities
- Monitor APTT, which should be 1.5-2.5 × control
- ◆ Assess bleeding gums, petechiae, ecchymosis, black tarry stools, hematuria/epistaxis, B/P, vaginal bleeding, puncture sites; may indicate bleeding and possible hemorrhage
- Assess fever, skin rash, urticaria

Nursing diagnoses
- Tissue perfusion, ineffective (uses)
- Injury, risk for (side effects)
- Knowledge, deficient (teaching)

Implementation
- Administer after reconstitution and further dilution under sterile conditions; use water for inj or 0.9% NaCl; for further dilution 0.9% NaCl or D_5; for rapid and complete reconstitution, inject 1 ml of diluent into vial and shake gently, use immediately, warm to room temp before use
- Avoid all IM inj that may cause bleeding

IV route
- Administer **IV** bol: use sol with conc of 5 mg/ml, reconstitute 5 mg (1 vial)/1 ml of water for inj or 0.9% NaCl, use body weight for correct weight calculation
- Administer **IV** inf: use sol with a conc of 0.2 or 0.4 mg/ml; reconstitute 100 mg (2 vials) with 1 ml each (2 ml) water for inj or 0.9% NaCl, transfer to infusion bag with either 500 or 250 ml of 0.9% NaCl or D_5W

Patient/family education
- Teach patient to use soft bristle toothbrush to avoid bleeding gums, avoid contact sports, use electric razor, avoid IM inj
- Teach patient to report any signs of bleeding: gums, under skin, urine, stools

Evaluation
Positive therapeutic outcome
- Absence of thrombocytopenia without significant bleeding

letrozole (Rx)
(let'tro-zohl)
Femara
Func. class.: Antineoplastic, nonsteroidal aromatase inhibitor

Pregnancy category D

Action: Binds to the heme group of aromatase; inhibits conversion of androgens to estrogens to reduce plasma estrogen levels; 30% of breast cancers decrease in size when deprived of estrogen

Therapeutic Outcome: Decreased spread of malignancy

Uses: Metastatic breast cancer in postmenopausal women

Dosage and routes
Adult: PO 2.5 mg daily

Available forms: Tabs 2.5 mg

Adverse effects
CNS: Somnolence, dizziness, depression, anxiety, *headache, lethargy*
CV: Hypertension
GI: *Nausea, vomiting, anorexia,* **hepatotoxicity,** constipation, heartburn, diarrhea
INTEG: *Rash, pruritus,* alopecia, sweating, hot flashes
RESP: Dyspnea, cough

Contraindications: Pregnancy **D,** hypersensitivity

Precautions: Hepatic disease, respiratory disease

Pharmacokinetics

Absorption	Well absorbed
Distribution	Widely
Metabolism	Liver
Excretion	Kidneys
Half-life	Unknown

Pharmacodynamics

Unknown

NURSING CONSIDERATIONS

Assessment

- Monitor temperature q4h; may indicate beginning of infection
- Monitor liver function tests before, during therapy (bilirubin, AST, ALT, LDH) as needed or monthly
- Monitor inflammation of mucosa, breaks in skin, yellowing of skin and sclera, dark urine, clay-colored stools, itchy skin, abdominal pain, fever, diarrhea

Nursing diagnoses

- Injury, risk for (adverse reactions)
- Body image, disturbed (adverse reactions)
- Infection, risk for (adverse reactions)
- Knowledge, deficient (teaching)

Implementation

- Give with food or fluids for GI upset
- Give in equal intervals q6h

Patient/family education

- Instruct patient to report side effects
- Advise patient to avoid use of alcohol, which potentiates this drug
- Tell patient that drug may be taken without regard to meals

Evaluation

Positive therapeutic outcome

- Prevention of rapid division of malignant cells, postmenopausal cancer, prostate cancer

Treatment of overdose:

Induce vomiting, provide supportive care

leucovorin (Rx)

(loo-koe-vor′in)

Citrovorum Factor, Folinic Acid, leucovorin calcium, Wellcovorin

Func. class.: Vitamin/folic acid antagonist antidote

Chem. class.: Tetrahydrofolic acid derivative

Pregnancy category C

Do Not Confuse:

leucovorin/Leukeran, leucovorin/Leukine

Action: Needed for normal growth patterns; prevents toxicity during antineoplastic therapy by protecting normal cells

Therapeutic Outcome: Reversal of severe toxic effects of folic acid antagonists

Uses: Megaloblastic or macrocytic anemia caused by folic acid deficiency, overdose of folic acid antagonist, methotrexate toxicity, toxicity caused by pyrimethamine or trimethoprim, pneumocystosis, toxoplasmosis

Dosage and routes

Megaloblastic anemia caused by enzyme deficiency

Adult and child: PO/IM/**IV** up to 6 mg/day

Megaloblastic anemia caused by deficiency of folate

Adult and child: IM 1 mg or less daily until adequate response

Advanced colorectal cancer

Adult: **IV** 200 mg/m^2, then 5-fluorouracil 370 mg/m^2; or leucovorin 20 mg/m^2, then 5-fluorouracil 425 mg/m^2; give daily × 5 days q4-5 wk

Methotrexate toxicity

Adult and child: PO/IM/**IV** (normal elimination) given 6-36 hr after dose of methotrexate 10 mg/m^2 until methotrexate is $<10^{-8}$ M, CCr has increased 50% above prior level or methotrexate level is 5 × 10 at 24 hr, or at 48 hr level is >9 × 10 M, give leucovorin 100 mg/m^2 q3h until level drops to <10 M

Pyrimethamine toxicity

Adult and child: PO/IM 5-15 mg daily

Trimethoprim toxicity

Adult and child: PO/IM 400 mcg daily

Available forms: Tabs 5, 10, 15, 25 mg; inj 3, 5 mg/ml; powder for inj 10 mg/ml

Adverse effects

HEMA: Thrombocytosis (intraarterial)

INTEG: Rash, pruritus, erythema, thrombocytosis, urticaria

RESP: Wheezing

Contraindications: Hypersensitivity, anemias other than megaloblastic not associated with vit B_{12} deficiency

Precautions: Pregnancy **C**

Pharmacokinetics

Absorption	Rapidly absorbed (PO); completely absorbed (**IV**)
Distribution	Widely distributed
Metabolism	Liver
Excretion	Kidney
Half-life	3½ hr

Pharmacodynamics

	PO/IM/IV
Onset	Up to 5 min
Peak	Unknown
Duration	4-6 hr

Interactions

Individual drugs

Chloramphenicol: decreased folate levels
Phenobarbital: increased metabolism of phenobarbital

Drug classifications

Hydantoins: increased metabolism of hydantoins

NURSING CONSIDERATIONS

Assessment

- Obtain CCr before leucovorin rescue and daily to detect nephrotoxicity, methotrexate level
- Monitor I&O; watch for nausea and vomiting; if vomiting occurs IM or **IV** route may be necessary
- Assess drugs currently taken: alcohol, hydantoins, trimethoprim may cause increased folic acid use by body
- Assess for allergic reactions: rash, dyspnea, wheezing

Nursing diagnoses

- Injury, risk for (uses)
- Nutrition: less than body requirements, imbalanced (uses)
- Knowledge, deficient (teaching)

Implementation

- Instruct patient about leucovorin rescue; have patient drink 3 L of fluid each day of rescue

PO route

- Use PO route only if patient is not vomiting

IM route

- Treatment of megaloblastic anemia uses IM dosing
- Give within 1 hr of folic acid antagonist, no reconstitution needed
- Give increased fluid intake if used to treat folic acid inhibitor overdose
- Provide protection from light and heat when storing ampules

IV route

- Reconstitute 50 mg/5 ml of bacteriostatic water or sterile water for inj (10 mg/ml) or 100 mg/10 ml; use immediately if sterile water for inj is used to reconstitute
- Give by direct **IV** over 160 mg/min or less (16 ml of 10 mg/ml sol/min)
- Give by intermittent inf after diluting in 100-500 ml of 0.9% NaCl, D_5W, $D_{10}W$, LR, Ringer's

Syringe compatibilities: Bleomycin, cisplatin, cyclophosphamide, DOXOrubicin, fluorouracil, furosemide, heparin, methotrexate, metoclopramide, mitomycin, vinBLAStine, vinCRIStine

Y-site compatibilities: Amifostine, aztreonam, bleomycin, cefepime, cisplatin, cladribine, cyclophosphamide, DOXOrubicin, filgrastim, fluconazole, fluorouracil, furosemide, granisetron, heparin, methotrexate, metoclopramide, mitomycin, piperacillin/tazobactam, tacrolimus, teniposide, thiotepa, vinBLAStine, vinCRIStine

Additive compatibilities: Cisplatin, cisplatin/floxuridine, floxuridine

Patient/family education

- Advise patient to take drug exactly as prescribed; to notify prescriber of side effects immediately
- Advise patient to report signs of hypersensitivity reaction immediately
- Advise patient with folic acid deficiency to eat folic acid–rich foods: bran, yeast, dried beans, nuts, fruits, fresh green leafy vegetables, asparagus

Evaluation

Positive therapeutic outcome

- Increased weight
- Improved orientation, well-being
- Absence of fatigue
- Reversal of toxicity: methotrexate, folic acid antagonist overdose

! HIGH ALERT

leuprolide (Rx)

(loo-proe'lide)

Leupron Depo PED, Lupron Depot, Lupron, Lupron Depot-3 month, Viadur

Func. class.: Antineoplastic hormone
Chem. class.: Gonadotropin-releasing hormone

Pregnancy category X (depot)

Do Not Confuse:

Lupron/Lopurin, Lupron/Nuprin

Action: Causes initial increase in circulating levels of LH, FSH; continuous administration results in decreased LH, FSH; in men testosterone is reduced to castration levels; in premenopausal women estrogen is reduced to menopausal levels

Therapeutic Outcome: Prevention of rapidly growing malignant cells in prostate cancer, decreased pain in endometriosis, resolution of cenral precocious puberty (CPP)

Uses: Metastatic prostate cancer, management of endometriosis (depot), CPP

Dosage and routes

Prostate cancer

Adult: SUBCUT 1 mg/day; Depot IM 7.5 mg/dose qmo; or IM 22.5 mg q3 mo; or IM 30 mg q4mo; or implant 1 implant q12 mo Viadur implant 72 mg qyr

Endometriosis/fibroids

Adult: IM 3.75 mg once a month or 11.25 mg q3 mo; or IM 30 mg q4 mo

Central precocious puberty

Child: SUBCUT 50 mcg/kg/day; increase as needed by 10 mcg/kg/day

Child: >37.5 kg: IM 15 mg q4 wk
25-37.5 kg: IM 11.25 mg q4 wk
≤25 kg: 7.5 mg q4 wk

Available forms: Inj (Depot) 3.75, 7.5 mg single-dose, multiple-dose vials (5 mg/ml); single-use kit 11.25 mg vial; pediatric (Depot) 7.5, 11.25, 15 mg; (3 mo Depot) 22.5 mg single use; (Viadur) once/yr implant

Adverse effects

CV: **MI, pulmonary emboli, dysrhythmias**

GI: Anorexia, diarrhea, **GI bleeding**

GU: Edema, hot flashes, impotence, decreased libido, amenorrhea, vaginal dryness, gynecomastia

Contraindications: Pregnancy **X**, hypersensitivity to GnRH or analogs, thromboembolic disorders, lactation, undiagnosed vaginal bleeding

Precautions: Edema, hepatic disease, CVA, MI, seizures, hypertension, diabetes mellitus

Pharmacokinetics

Absorption	Rapidly absorbed (SC); slowly absorbed (IM depot)
Distribution	Unknown
Metabolism	Unknown
Excretion	Unknown
Half-life	3-4 hr

Pharmacodynamics

Unknown

Interactions

Individual drugs

Flutamide, megestrol: increased antineoplastic action

NURSING CONSIDERATIONS

Assessment

- Assess for symptoms of endometriosis/fibroids including lower abdominal pain, excessive vaginal bleeding, bloating if drug is given for the diagnosis of endometriosis
- If giving this drug for CPP, the diagnosis should have been confirmed by development of secondary sex characteristics in child <9 yr; also included to confirm the diagnosis of CPP is estradiol/testosterone, GnRH test, tomography of head, adrenal steroid, chorionic gonadotropin, wrist x-ray, height, weight; patients diagnosed with CPP display the signs of testicular growth, facial, body hair (males), breast development, menses (females)
- Monitor liver function tests before, during therapy (bilirubin, AST, ALT, LDH) as needed or monthly; prostate-specific antigen in prostate cancer
- Monitor pituitary gonadotropic and gonadal function during therapy and 4-8 wk after therapy is decreased; check LH, FSH, acid phosphate at beginning of treatment
- Monitor worsening of signs and symptoms (normal during beginning therapy): fatigue, increased pulse, pallor, lethargy, edema in feet, joints, stomach pain, shaking
- Monitor renal status: I&O ratio, check for bladder distention daily during beginning therapy (renal obstruction)

Nursing diagnoses

- Sexual dysfunction (adverse reactions)
- Injury, risk for (adverse reactions)
- Knowledge, deficient (teaching)

Implementation

- Use syringe and drug packaged together; give deep in large muscle mass; rotate sites
- Use depot only IM; never give SUBCUT
- Unused vials may be stored at room temp
- Give monthly: reconstitute single use vial with 1 ml of diluent, if multiple vials are used, withdraw 0.5 ml and inject into each vial (1 ml) withdraw all and inject
- Give 3 month: reconstitute microspheres using 1.5 ml of diluent and inject in vial, shake, withdraw and inject; 12-month: inserted into upper arm at the end of 12 months, implant must be removed

Patient/family education

- Advise patient to notify prescriber if menstruation continues; menstruation should stop; to use a nonhormonal method of contraception during therapy
- Instruct patient to report any complaints, side effects to nurse or prescriber; hot flashes may occur; record weight, report gain of 2 lb/day
- Teach patient how to prepare, administer; to rotate sites for SUBCUT inj; to keep accurate records of dosing (prostate cancer)
- Instruct patient that tumor flare may occur: increase in size of tumor, increased bone pain; tell patient that bone pain disappears after 1 wk; may take analgesics for pain; premenopausal women must use mechanical birth control; ovulation may be induced
- Advise the patient not to breastfeed while taking this drug
- Inform patient that voiding problems may increase in beginning of therapy, but will decrease in several weeks

Evaluation

Positive therapeutic outcome

- Decreased size, spread of malignancy
- Decreased pain in endometriosis, fibroids
- Decreased signs of CPP

levalbuterol (Rx)

(lev-al-bute'er-ole)

Xopenex

Func. class.: Bronchodilator

Chem. class.: Adrenergic β_2-agonist

Pregnancy category C

Action: Causes bronchodilatation by action on β_2 (pulmonary) receptors by increasing levels of cyclic adenosine monophosphate (cAMP), which relaxes smooth muscle; produces bronchodilatation; CNS, cardiac stimulation, increased diuresis, and increased gastric acid secretion; longer acting than isoproterenol

Therapeutic Outcome: Increased ability to breathe because of bronchodilatation

Uses: Treatment or prevention of bronchospasm (reversible obstructive airway disease)

Dosage and routes

Adult and child ≥12 yr: INH 0.63 mg tid, q6-8h by nebulization; may increase to 1.25 mg q8h

Child 6-11 yr: INH 0.31 mg tid via neb, max 0.63 mg tid

Available forms: Sol, inh 0.63, 1.25 mg/3 ml

Adverse effects

CNS: *Tremors, anxiety,* insomnia, headache, dizziness, stimulation, *restlessness,* hallucinations, flushing, irritability

CV: Palpitations, tachycardia, hypertension, angina, hypotension, dysrhythmias

EENT: Dry nose, irritation of nose and throat

GI: Heartburn, nausea, vomiting

MS: Muscle cramps

Contraindications: Hypersensitivity to sympathomimetics, tachydysrhythmias, severe cardiac disease

Precautions: Pregnancy **C,** lactation, cardiac disorders, hyperthyroidism, diabetes mellitus, hypertension, prostatic hypertrophy, narrow-angle glaucoma, seizures

Pharmacokinetics	
Absorption	Unknown
Distribution	Unknown
Metabolism	Liver extensively, tissues
Excretion	Unknown, breast milk
Half-life	Unknown

Pharmacodynamics	INH
Onset	5-15 min
Peak	1-1½ hr
Duration	6-8 hr

Interactions

Drug classifications

Adrenergics: increased levalbuterol action

Antidepressants (tricyclics): increased levalbuterol action

β-Adrenergic blockers: decreased levabuterol action

Bronchodilators (aerosol): increased action of bronchodilator

MAOIs: increased levalbuterol action

Drug/herb

Cola nut, guarana, tea (black/green), yerba maté: increased stimulation

NURSING CONSIDERATIONS

Assessment

- Assess respiratory function: vital capacity, forced expiratory volume, ABGs, lung sounds, heart rate, rhythm (baseline and during therapy); character of sputum: color, consistency, amount
- Determine that patient has not received theophylline therapy before giving dose, to

L

prevent additive effect; client's ability to self-medicate
- Monitor for evidence of allergic reactions; paradoxic bronchospasm; withhold dose; notify prescriber

Nursing diagnoses
- Airway clearance, ineffective (uses)
- Gas exchange, impaired (uses)
- Knowledge, deficient (teaching)

Implementation
- Give by nebulization q6-8h; wait at least 1 min between inhalation of aerosols
- Use this medication before other medications and allow 5 min between each to prevent overstimulation

Patient/family education
- Tell patient not to use OTC medications before consulting prescriber; extra stimulation may occur; instruct patient to use this medication before other medications and allow at least 5 min between each to prevent overstimulation; to limit caffeine products such as chocolate, coffee, tea, and cola or herbs such as cola nut, guarana, yerba maté
- ◆ Teach patient that if paradoxic bronchospasm occurs to stop drug immediately and notify prescriber

Evaluation
Positive therapeutic outcome
- Absence of dyspnea and wheezing after 1 hr
- Improved airway exchange
- Improved ABGs

Treatment of overdose: Administer a β_1-adrenergic blocker

levetiracetam (Rx)
(lev-ee-tye′ra-see-tam)

Keppra

Func. class.: Anticonvulsant

Pregnancy category C

Action: Unknown; may inhibit nerve impulses by limiting influx of sodium ions across cell membrane in motor cortex

Therapeutic Outcome: Absence of seizures

Uses: Adjunctive therapy in partial onset seizures

Dosage and routes
Adult: PO 500 mg bid, may increase by 1000 mg/day q2 wk, max 3000 mg/day

Available forms: Tabs 250, 500, 750 mg; oral sol 100 mg/ml

Adverse effects
CNS: Dizziness, somnolence, asthenia
HEMA: Decreased Hct, Hgb, RBC, infection
MISC: Abdominal pain, pharyngitis, infection

Contraindications: Hypersensitivity

Precautions: Pregnancy **C**, renal disease, cardiac disease, lactation, children, psychosis

Pharmacokinetics

Absorption	Rapidly absorbed
Distribution	Widely distributed, not protein bound
Metabolism	Small amount liver
Excretion	Kidneys (66%) unchanged
Half-life	6-8 hr or more in elderly

Pharmacodynamics
Unknown

Interactions: None known

NURSING CONSIDERATIONS
Assessment
- Monitor urine function tests (BUN, urine protein) periodically during treatments
- Assess seizure activity including type, location, duration, and character; provide seizure precautions

Nursing diagnoses
- Injury, risk for (side effects)
- Knowledge, deficient (teaching)

Implementation
- Give with food, milk to decrease GI symptoms (rare)

Patient/family education
- Teach patient to carry/wear emergency ID stating patient's name, drugs taken, condition, prescriber's name, phone number
- Caution patient to avoid driving, other activities that require alertness until stabilized on medication
- Teach patient not to discontinue medication quickly after long-term use
- Teach patient to use a nonhormonal type of contraception to prevent harm to the fetus
- Teach patient to take exactly as prescribed, do not double or omit doses

Evaluation
Positive therapeutic outcome
- Decreased seizure activity

levodopa (Rx)

(lee'voe-doe-pa)

Dopar, Larodopa, L-Dopa

Func. class.: Antiparkinsonian agent

Chem. class.: Catecholamine, dopamine agonist

Pregnancy category C

Do Not Confuse:
L-dopa/methyldopa

Action: Decarboxylation to dopamine, which increases dopamine levels in brain

Therapeutic Outcome: Decreased symptoms of Parkinson's disease (involuntary movements)

Uses: Parkinsonism

Dosage and routes

Adult: PO 0.5-1 g daily divided bid-qid with meals; may increase by up to 0.75 g q3-7 days, max 8 g/day unless closely supervised

Available forms: Caps 100, 250, 500 mg; tabs 100, 250, 500 mg

Adverse effects

CNS: *Involuntary choreiform movements, hand tremors, fatigue, headache, anxiety, twitching, numbness, weakness, confusion, agitation, insomnia, nightmares,* psychosis, hallucinations, hypomania, severe depression, dizziness

CV: *Orthostatic hypotension,* tachycardia, hypertension, palpitations

EENT: Blurred vision, diplopia, dilated pupils

GI: *Nausea, vomiting, anorexia, abdominal distress, dry mouth, flatulence, dysphagia,* bitter taste, diarrhea, constipation

HEMA: **Hemolytic anemia, leukopenia, agranulocytosis**

INTEG: Rash, sweating, alopecia

MISC: Urinary retention, incontinence, weight change, dark urine

Contraindications: Hypersensitivity, narrow-angle glaucoma, undiagnosed skin lesions

Precautions: Pregnancy **C,** renal disease, cardiac disease, hepatic disease, respiratory disease, MI with dysrhythmias, seizures, peptic ulcer, asthma, endocrine disease, affective disorders, psychosis, lactation, children <12 yr

Pharmacokinetics

Absorption	Well absorbed
Distribution	Widely distributed
Metabolism	Liver, GI tract, extensively
Excretion	Kidneys to metabolites; breast milk
Half-life	1 hr

Pharmacodynamics

Onset	10-15 min
Peak	1-3 hr
Duration	Up to 24 hr

Interactions

Individual drugs

Papaverine, pyridoxine: decreased effects of levodopa

Drug classifications

Antacids: increased levodopa effects

Anticholinergics, hydantoins: decreased effects of levodopa

MAOIs: hypertensive crisis

Drug/herb

Kava: increased Parkinson's symptoms

Indian snakeroot: increased extrapyramidal symptoms (EPS); decreased levodopa effect

Drug/food

Increased: protein food will decrease absorption

Drug/lab test

Decreased: VMA

False positive: urine ketones, urine glucose, Coombs' test

False negative: urine glucose (glucose oxidase)

False increase: uric acid, urine protein

NURSING CONSIDERATIONS

Assessment

- Monitor B/P, respiration during initial treatment; hypotension or hypertension should be reported
- Assess mental status: affect, mood, behavioral changes, depression; complete suicide assessment
- Monitor liver function, renal function studies: AST, ALT, alkaline phosphatase; also check LDH, bilirubin, CBC, BUN, PBI
- Assess for involuntary movements in parkinsonism: akinesia, tremors, staggering gait, muscle rigidity, drooling; these symptoms should improve with levodopa therapy
- Assess for levodopa toxicity: mental, personality changes, increased twitching, grimacing, tongue protrusion; these should be reported to prescriber

Nursing diagnoses
- Mobility, impaired (uses)
- Injury, risk for (uses)
- Knowledge, deficient (teaching)
- Noncompliance (teaching)

Implementation
- Levodopa/carbidopa should not be started until levodopa is withheld for 8 hr; toxicity may result if the two drugs are taken close together
- Give levodopa until NPO before surgery
- Adjust dosage to patient response
- Give with meals to decrease GI upset; limit protein taken with drug
- Give only after MAOIs have been discontinued for 2 wk

Patient/family education
- Advise patient that therapeutic effects may take several wk to a few months
- Caution patient to change positions slowly to prevent orthostatic hypotension
- Instruct patient to report side effects: twitching, eye spasms; indicate overdose
- Instruct patient to use drug exactly as prescribed; if drug is discontinued abruptly, parkinsonian crisis may occur
- Inform patient that urine, sweat may darken
- Advise patient to avoid vit B_6 preparations, vitamin-fortified foods containing B_6; these foods can reverse effects of levodopa; also OTC preparations should be avoided unless approved by prescriber

Evaluation
Positive therapeutic outcome
- Decreased akathisia, other involuntary movements
- Improved mood

levofloxacin (Rx)
(lev-o-floks'a-sin)

Levaquin

Func. class.: Antiinfective

Chem. class.: Fluoroquinolone antibacterial

Pregnancy category C

Action: Interferes with conversion of intermediate DNA fragments into high molecular weight DNA in bacteria; DNA gyrase inhibitor

Therapeutic Outcome: Bacterial action against the following: *Streptococcus pneumoniae, Haemophilus influenzae, Haemophilus parainfluenzae, Moraxella catarrhalis, Staphylococcus aureus, Klebsiella pneumoniae, Mycoplasma pneumoniae*

Uses: Adult urinary tract infections (including complicated); lower respiratory, skin infection

Dosage and routes
Adult: **IV** inf 500 mg by slow inf over 1 hr q24h × 7-14 days depending on infection; PO 500 mg q24h × 7-14 days depending on infection

Renal dose
Adult: PO/**IV** CCr 20-49 ml/min initial 500 mg, then 250 mg q24h; CCr 10-19 ml/min 250 or 500 mg, depending on condition, then 250 mg q48h

Available forms: Single-use vials (500, 750 mg), premixed flexible container; 250 mg/50 ml D_5W, 500 mg/100 ml D_5W, 750 mg/150 ml D_5W; tabs 250, 500, 750 mg

Adverse effects:
CNS: *Headache,* dizziness, *insomnia,* anxiety, **seizures,** encephalopathy, paresthesia

CV: Chest pain, palpitations, vasodilatation

EENT: Dry mouth

GI: *Nausea,* flatulence, *vomiting,* diarrhea, abdominal pain, **pseudomembranous colitis**

GU: Vaginitis, crystalluria

HEMA: Eosinophilia, **hemolytic anemia,** lymphophemia

INTEG: Rash, pruritus, photosensitivity

MISC: Hypoglycemia, hypersensitivity

RESP: Pneumonitis

SYST: **Anaphylaxis, multisystem organ failure, Stevens-Johnson syndrome**

Contraindications: Hypersensitivity to quinolones, photosensitivity

Precautions: Pregnancy **C,** lactation, children

Pharmacokinetics

Absorption	Unknown
Distribution	Unknown
Metabolism	Liver
Excretion	Kidneys unchanged
Half-life	6-8 hr

Pharmacodynamics

Onset	Immediate
Peak	Infusion's end

Interactions
Individual drugs
Calcium, iron, sucralfate, zinc: decreased absorption of levofloxacin

Foscarnet: increased CNS stimulation, seizures

Magnesium: decreased levofloxacin absorption; do not use in same **IV** line

Theophylline: decreased theophylline clearance, toxicity may result
Warfarin: increased bleeding

Drug classifications

Antacids (magnesium, aluminum): decreased absorption of levofloxacin
Antidiabetics: altered blood glucose levels
NSAIDs: increased CNS stimulation, seizures

Drug/herb

Cola tree: increased antiinfective effect

Drug/lab test

Decreased: glucose, lymphocytes

NURSING CONSIDERATIONS

Assessment

- Assess patient for previous sensitivity reaction
- Assess patient for signs and symptoms of infection including characteristics of wounds, sputum, urine, stool, WBC >10,000/mm^3, fever; baseline and during treatment
- Obtain C&S before beginning drug therapy to identify if correct treatment has been initiated
- Assess for allergic reactions and anaphylaxis: rash, urticaria, pruritus, chills, fever, joint pain; may occur a few days after therapy begins; epINEPHrine and resuscitation equipment should be available for anaphylactic reaction
- Determine urine output; if decreasing, notify prescriber (may indicate nephrotoxicity); also check for increased BUN, creatinine
- Monitor blood studies: AST, ALT, CBC, Hct, bilirubin, LDH, alkaline phosphatase, Coombs' test monthly if patient is on long-term therapy
- Monitor electrolytes: potassium, sodium, chloride monthly if patient is on long-term therapy
- Assess bowel pattern daily; if severe diarrhea occurs, drug should be discontinued
- Monitor for bleeding: ecchymosis, bleeding gums, hematuria, stool guaiac daily if on long-term therapy
- Assess for overgrowth of infection: perineal itching, fever, malaise, redness, pain, swelling, drainage, rash, diarrhea, change in cough, sputum

Nursing diagnoses

- Infection, risk for (uses)
- Diarrhea (side effects)
- Injury, risk for (side effects)
- Knowledge, deficient (teaching)
- Noncompliance (teaching)

Implementation

- Give PO 4 hr before or 2 hr after antacids, iron, calcium, zinc
- Check for irritation, extravasation, phlebitis daily
- Give drug around the clock to maintain blood levels
- Do not use theophylline with this product

Patient/family education

- Teach patient to report sore throat, bruising, bleeding, joint pain; may indicate blood dyscrasias (rare)
- Advise patient to contact prescriber if vaginal itching, loose foul-smelling stools, furry tongue occur, may indicate superinfection; report itching, rash, pruritus, urticaria
- Instruct patient to take all medication prescribed for the length of time ordered; drug must be taken around the clock to maintain blood levels; do not give medication to others
- Advise patient to notify prescriber of diarrhea with blood or pus
- Instruct patient to take 4 hr before antacids, iron, calcium, zinc products
- Tell patient to complete full course of therapy; to increase fluid intake to 2 L/day to prevent crystalluria
- Advise patient to avoid hazardous activities until response to drug is known
- Instruct patient to rinse mouth frequently and use sugarless candy or gum for dry mouth
- Instruct patient to avoid taking other medications unless approved by prescriber
- Advise patient to avoid sun exposure or use sunscreen to prevent phototoxicity

Evaluation

Positive therapeutic outcome

- Absence of signs/symptoms of infection (WBC <10,000/mm^3, temp WNL)
- Reported improvement in symptoms of infection

levothyroxine 🗝 (Rx)

(lee-voe-thye-rox'een)

Eltroxin ✦, Levo-T, Levothroid, levothyroxine sodium, Levoxyl, PMS-Levothyroxine Sodium ✦, Synthroid, T_4

Func. class.: Thyroid hormone
Chem. class.: Levoisomer of thyroxine

Pregnancy category A

Do Not Confuse:
Synthroid/Symmetrel

Action: Controls protein synthesis; increases metabolic rate, cardiac output, renal blood flow, O_2 consumption, body temp, blood

L

volume, growth, development at cellular level, exact mechanism unknown

Therapeutic Outcome: Correction of lack of thyroid hormone

Uses: Hypothyroidism, myxedema coma, thyroid hormone replacement, cretinism, thyrotoxicosis, congenital hypothyroidism, some types of thyroid cancer

Dosage and routes

Severe hypothyroidism

Adult: PO 50 mcg daily, increase by 25 mcg q2-3 wk, average dose 100-200 mcg daily, max 200 mcg daily; IM/**IV** 50-100 mcg/day as a single dose or 50% of usual oral dosage

Child >12 yr: PO 2-3 mcg/kg/day given as a single dose AM

Child 6-12 yr: PO 4-5 mcg/kg/day given as a single dose AM

Child 1-5 yr: PO 5-6 mcg/kg/day given as a single dose AM

Child 6-12 mo: PO 6-8 mcg/kg/day given as a single dose AM

Child to 6 mo: PO 8-10 mcg/kg/day given as a single dose AM

Myxedema coma

Adult: **IV** 200-500 mcg; may increase by 100-300 mcg after 24 hr; give oral medication as soon as possible

Available forms: Powder for inj 200, 500 mcg/vial; tabs 0.025, 0.05, 0.075, 0.088, 0.1, 0.112, 0.125, 0.137, 0.15, 0.175, 0.2, 0.3 mg

Adverse effects

CNS: *Anxiety, insomnia, tremors,* headache, **thyroid storm**

CV: *Tachycardia, palpitations, angina, dysrhythmias,* hypertension, **cardiac arrest**

GI: Nausea, diarrhea, increased or decreased appetite, cramps

MISC: Menstrual irregularities, weight loss, sweating, heat intolerance, fever, alopecia

Contraindications: Adrenal insufficiency, recent MI, thyrotoxicosis, hypersensitivity to beef, alcohol intolerance (inj only)

Precautions: Pregnancy **A,** elderly, angina pectoris, hypertension, ischemia, cardiac disease, lactation, diabetes

Pharmacokinetics

Absorption	Erratic (PO); complete (**IV**)
Distribution	Widely distributed
Metabolism	Liver; enterohepatic recirculation
Excretion	Feces via bile; breast milk (small amounts)
Half-life	6-7 days

Pharmacodynamics

	PO	IV
Onset	3-5 days	6-8 hr
Peak	12-48 hr	12-48 hr
Duration	Unknown	Unknown

Interactions

Individual drugs

Cholestyramine, colestipol, ferrous sulfate: decreased absorption of levothyroxine

Digitalis: decreased effect of digitalis

Insulin: increased requirement for insulin

Drug classifications

Anticoagulants (oral): increased anticoagulant effect

Antidepressants (tricyclics): increased tricyclic effect

epINEPHrine products: increased cardiac insufficiency risk

Estrogens: decreased thyroid hormone effects

Hypoglycemics: decreased hypoglycemic effect

SSRIs: decreased levothyroxine effects

Sympathomimetics: increased sympathomimetic effect

Drug/herb

Agar, bugleweed, carnitine, kelpware, soy, spirulina: decreased thyroid hormone effect

Drug/lab test

Increased: CPK, LDH, AST, PBI, blood glucose

Decreased: thyroid function tests

NURSING CONSIDERATIONS

Assessment

- Determine if the patient is taking anticoagulants, antidiabetic agents; document on chart
- Take B/P, pulse before each dose; monitor I&O ratio and weight every day in same clothing, using same scale, at same time of day
- Monitor height, weight, psychomotor development and growth rate if given to a child
- Monitor T_3, T_4, which are decreased; radioimmunoassay of TSH, which is increased; radioactive iodine uptake (RAIU), which is increased if patient is on too low a dosage of medication
- Monitor protime (may require decreased anticoagulant); check for bleeding, bruising
- Assess for increased nervousness, excitability, irritability, which may indicate too high a dosage of medication, usually after 1-3 wk of treatment
- Assess cardiac status: angina, palpitations, chest pain, change in VS; the elderly patient may have undetected cardiac problems and baseline ECG should be completed before treatment

Nursing diagnoses
- Knowledge, deficient (teaching)
- Noncompliance (teaching)

Implementation
PO route
- Give in AM if possible as a single dose to decrease sleeplessness; give at same time each day to maintain drug level
- Give crushed and mixed with water, non-soy formula, or breast milk for infants/children
- Give only for hormone imbalances; not to be used for obesity, male infertility, menstrual conditions, lethargy; give lowest dosage that relieves symptoms; lower dosage for the elderly and in cardiac diseases
- Store in tight, light-resistant container
- Remove medication 4 wk before RAIU test

IV route
- Give **IV** after diluting with provided diluent (0.9% NaCl), 0.5 mg/5 ml; shake well; give through Y-tube or 3-way stopcock; give 0.1 mg or less over 1 min; do not add to **IV** inf; 0.1 mg = 1 ml; discard any unused portion

Patient/family education
- Teach patient that drug is not a cure but controls symptoms and treatment is long term
- Instruct patient to report excitability, irritability, anxiety, sweating, heat intolerance, chest pain, palpitations, which indicate overdose
- Advise patient not to switch brands unless approved by prescriber; bioavailability may differ; do not take with food; absorption will be decreased
- Teach patient that drug may be discontinued after giving birth; thyroid panel will be evaluated after 1-2 mo
- Teach patient or parent that hyperthyroid child will show almost immediate behavior/ personality change; that hair loss will occur in child but is temporary
- Caution patient that drug is not to be taken to reduce weight
- Caution patient to avoid OTC preparations with iodine; read labels; other medications should not be used unless approved by prescriber
- Teach patient to avoid iodine-rich food: iodized salt, soybeans, tofu, turnips, high iodine seafood, some bread

Evaluation
Positive therapeutic outcome
- Absence of depression
- Weight loss, increased diuresis, pulse, appetite
- Absence of constipation, peripheral edema, cold intolerance, pale, cool dry skin, brittle nails, alopecia, coarse hair, menorrhagia, night blindness, paresthesias, syncope, stupor, coma, rosy cheeks
- Improved levels of T_3, T_4 by laboratory tests
- Child: age-appropriate weight, height and psychomotor development

Treatment of overdose: Withhold dose for up to 1 wk: acute overdose: gastric lavage or induced emesis, activated charcoal; provide supportive treatment to control symptoms

! HIGH ALERT

lidocaine, parenteral
(Rx)

(lye'doe-kane)

Lidopen Auto-Injector, Xylocard ♣, Xylocaine

Func. class.: Antidysrhythmic (class IB)

Chem. class.: Aminoacyl amide

Pregnancy category B

Action: Increases electrical stimulation threshold of ventricle and His-Purkinje system, which stabilizes cardiac membrane and decreases automaticity; locally produces anesthesia by preventing initiation and conduction of nerve impulses

Therapeutic Outcome: Decreased ventricular dysrhythmia; produces anesthesia locally

Uses: Ventricular tachycardia, ventricular dysrhythmias during cardiac surgery, MI, digitalis toxicity, cardiac catheterization; anesthesia locally

Dosage and routes
Adult: **IV** bol 50-100 mg (1 mg/kg) over 2-3 min; repeat q3-5 min, max 300 mg in 1 hr; begin **IV** inf 20-50 mcg/kg/min; IM 200-300 mg (4.3 mg/kg) in deltoid muscle, may repeat in 1-1½ hr if needed

Elderly with CHF, reduced liver function: **IV** bol ½ adult dose

Child: **IV** bol 1 mg/kg, then **IV** inf 30 mcg/kg/min

Available forms: **IV** inf 0.2% (2 mg/ml), 0.4% (4 mg/ml), 0.8% (8 mg/ml); **IV** admixture 4% (40 mg/ml), 10% (100 mg/ml), 20% (200 mg/ml); **IV** direct 1% (10 mg/ml), 2% (20 mg/ml); IM 300 mg/3 ml

Adverse effects
CNS: *Headache, dizziness,* involuntary movement, confusion, tremor, *drowsiness,* euphoria, **seizures**

L

CV: *Hypotension, bradycardia,* **heart block, cardiovascular collapse, arrest**
EENT: Tinnitus, blurred vision
GI: Nausea, vomiting, anorexia
INTEG: Rash, urticaria, edema, swelling
MISC: Febrile response, phlebitis at inj site
RESP: Dyspnea, **respiratory depression**

Contraindications: Hypersensitivity to amides, severe heart block, supraventricular dysrhythmias, Adams-Stokes syndrome, Wolff-Parkinson-White syndrome

Precautions: Pregnancy **B**, lactation, children, renal disease, liver disease, CHF, respiratory depression, malignant hyperthermia, elderly, myasthenia gravis, weight <50 kg

Pharmacokinetics

Absorption	Complete bioavailability (**IV**)
Distribution	Erythrocytes, cardiovascular endothelium
Metabolism	Liver
Excretion	Kidneys
Half-life	Biphasic 8 min, 1-2 hr

Pharmacodynamics

	IV	IM	TOP
Onset	2 min	5-15 min	Unknown
Peak	Unknown	½ hr	5 min
Duration	20 min	1½ hr	½-1 hr

Interactions
Individual drugs
Cimetidine, metoprolol, phenytoin, propranolol: increased lidocaine effects
Tubocurarine: increased neuromuscular blockade
Drug classifications
Barbiturates: decreased lidocaine effects
Neuromuscular blockers: increased neuromuscular blockade
Drug/herb
Aconite: increased toxicity, death
Aloe, broom, buckthorn (chronic use), cascara sagrada (chronic use), Chinese rhubarb, figwort, fumitory, goldenseal, kudzu, licorice: increased effect
Coltsfoot: decreased effect
Horehound: increased serotonin effect
Drug/lab test
Increased: CPR

NURSING CONSIDERATIONS
Assessment
- Assess for oxygenation or perfusion deficit: decreased B/P, chest pain, dizziness, loss of consciousness
- Assess respiratory status: auscultate lung fields for bibasilar crackles in patients with advanced CHF
- Assess for urinary retention: check for pain, abdominal absorption, palpate bladder; check males with benign prostatic hypertrophy; anticholinergic reaction may cause retention
- Monitor I&O ratio, electrolytes (potassium, sodium, chloride); watch for decreasing urinary output, possible retention
- Monitor liver function studies: AST, ALT, bilirubin, alkaline phosphatase
- Monitor ECG continuously to determine drug effectiveness, measure PR, QRS, QT intervals, check for PVCs, other dysrhythmias; monitor B/P continuously for hypotension, hypertension; check for rebound hypertension after 1-2 hr, prolonged PR/QT intervals, QRS complex; if QT or QRS increases by 50% or more, withhold next dose, notify prescriber
- Monitor for CNS symptoms: confusion, numbness, depression, involuntary movements; if these occur, drug should be discontinued
- Monitor blood levels (therapeutic level 1.5-5 mcg/ml), notify prescriber of abnormal results

Nursing diagnoses
- Cardiac output, decreased (uses)
- Gas exchange, impaired (adverse reactions)
- Knowledge, deficient (teaching)

Implementation
IM route
- Administer in deltoid, aspirate to prevent **IV** administration
- Check site daily for extravasation

IV route
- Give **IV** bolus undiluted (1%, 2% only); give 6 mg or less over 1 min; if using an **IV** line, use port near insertion site, flush with 0.9% NaCl (50 ml)
- Store at room temp; sol should be clear
- Give by cont inf after adding 1 g/250-1000 ml of D_5W; give 1-4 mg/min; use infusion pump for correct dosage; pediatric inf is 120 mg of lidocaine/100 ml of D_5W; 1-2.5 ml/kg/hr = 20-50 mcg/kg/min; use only 1%, 2% sol

Solution compatibilities: D_5W, D_5/0.9% NaCl, D_5/0.45% NaCl, D_5/LR, LR, 0.9% NaCl, 0.45% NaCl

Syringe compatibilities: Cloxacillin, glycopyrrolate, heparin, hydrOXYzine, methicillin, metoclopramide, milrinone, moxalactam, nalbuphine

Syringe incompatibilities: Cefazolin

Y-site compatibilities: Alteplase, amiodarone, inamrinone, cefazolin, ciprofloxacin, diltiazem, DOBUTamine, DOPamine, enalaprilat, etomidate, famotidine, haloperidol, heparin, heparin with hydrocortisone, labetalol, meperidine, morphine, nitroglycerin, nitroprusside, potassium chloride, propofol, streptokinase, theophylline, vit B/C, warfarin

Additive compatibilities: Alteplase, aminophylline, amiodarone, atracurium, bretylium, calcium chloride, calcium gluceptate, calcium gluconate, chloramphenicol, chlorothiazide, cimetidine, dexamethasone, digoxin, diphenhydrAMINE, DOBUTamine, DOPamine, epHEDrine, erythromycin, floxacillin, flumazenil, furosemide, heparin, hydrocortisone, nafcillin, hydrOXYzine, regular insulin, mephentermine, metaraminol, nafcillin, nitroglycerin, penicillin G potassium, pentobarbital, phenylephrine, potassium chloride, procainamide, prochlorperazine, promazine, ranitidine, sodium bicarbonate, sodium lactate, theophylline, verapamil, vit B/C

Additive incompatibilities: Methohexital, phenytoin; do not admix with blood transfusions

Infiltration

Physician may order lidocaine with epINEPHrine to minimize systemic absorption and prolong local anesthesia

Patient/family education

- Teach patient or family reason for use of medication and expected results
- Instruct patient in at-home use of Lidopen Auto-Injector; patient should call prescriber before use if heart attack is imminent

Evaluation

Positive therapeutic outcome

- Decreased B/P, dysrhythmias
- Decreased heart rate
- Normal sinus rhythm

Treatment of overdose: Oxygen, artificial ventilation, ECG, administer DOPamine for circulatory depression, diazepam or thiopental for seizures, decreased drug or discontinuation may be required

lindane (OTC)

(lin-dane)

GBH ✤, G-Well, Hexit ✤, Kwell, lindane, PMS Lindane ✤, Scabene

Func. class.: Scabicide/pediculicide

Chem. class.: Chlorinated hydrocarbon (synthetic)

Pregnancy category B

Action: Stimulates nervous system of arthropods, resulting in seizures, death of organism

Therapeutic Outcome: Resolution of infestation

Uses: Scabies, lice (head/pubic/body), nits

Dosage and routes

Lice

Adult and child: Top/cream/lotion: wash area with soap and water, remove visible crusts; apply to skin surfaces; remove with soap, water 8-12 hr after application; may reapply in 1 wk if needed; shampoo using 30 ml: work into lather, rub for 5 min, rinse, dry with towel; use fine-toothed comb to remove nits

Scabies

Adult and child: Top apply 1% cream/lotion to skin from neck to bottom of feet, toes; repeat in 1 wk if necessary

Available forms: Lotion, shampoo, cream (1%)

Adverse effects

CNS: Tremors, **seizures,** stimulation, dizziness (chronic inhalation of vapors), **CNS toxicity**

CV: **Ventricular fibrillation** (chronic inhalation of vapors)

GI: *Nausea, vomiting, diarrhea,* liver damage (inhalation of vapors)

GU: **Kidney damage** (chronic inhalation of vapors)

HEMA: **Aplastic anemia** (chronic inhalation of vapors)

INTEG: *Pruritus, rash, irritation, contact dermatitis*

Contraindications: Hypersensitivity, premature neonate, patients with known seizure disorders, inflammation of skin, abrasions, or breaks in skin

Precautions: Pregnancy **B,** children <10 yr, infants, lactation; avoid contact with eyes

Pharmacokinetics	
Absorption	20%
Distribution	Fat
Metabolism	Liver
Excretion	Kidneys
Half-life	18 hr

Pharmacodynamics	
Onset	Rapid
Peak	Rapid
Duration	3 hr

Interactions

Oil-based hair dressing: increased absorption; wash, rinse, and dry hair before using lindane

NURSING CONSIDERATIONS

Assessment

- Assess head, hair for lice and nits before and after treatment; if scabies are present, check all skin surfaces
- Identify source of infection: school, family members, sexual contacts

Nursing diagnoses

- Skin integrity, impaired (uses)
- Knowledge, deficient (teaching)

Implementation

- Apply to body areas, scalp only; do not apply to face, lips, mouth, eyes, any mucous membrane, anus, or meatus
- Give top corticosteroids as ordered to decrease contact dermatitis; provide antihistamines
- Apply menthol or phenol lotions to control itching
- Give top antibiotics for infection
- Provide isolation until areas on skin, scalp have cleared and treatment is completed
- Remove nits by using a fine-toothed comb rinsed in vinegar after treatment; use gloves

Patient/family education

- Advise patient to wash all inhabitants' clothing, using insecticide; preventive treatment may be required for all persons living in same house, using lotion or shampoo to decrease spread of infection; use rubber gloves when applying drug
- Instruct patient that itching may continue for 4-6 wk; that drug must be reapplied if accidently washed off, or treatment will be ineffective; remove after specified time to prevent toxicity
- Advise patient not to apply to face; if accidental contact with eyes occurs, flush with water
- Advise patient that sexual contacts should be treated simultaneously
- Inform the patient of CNS toxicity: dizziness, cramps, anxiety, nausea, vomiting, seizures

Evaluation

Positive therapeutic outcome

- Decreased crusts, nits, brownish trails on skin, itching papules in skinfolds
- Decreased itching after several wk

Treatment of ingestion: Gastric lavage, saline laxatives, **IV** diazepam (Valium) for seizures (if taken orally)

linezolid (Rx)

(lih-nee'zoh-lid)

Zyvox

Func. class.: Broad-spectrum antiinfective

Chem. class.: Oxazolidinone

Pregnancy category C

Action: Binds to bacterial 23S ribosomal RNA of the 50S subunit preventing formation of the bacterial translation process

Therapeutic Outcome: Negative blood cultures, absence of signs/symptoms of infection

Uses: Vancomycin-resistant *Enterococcus faecium* infections, nosocomial pneumonia, uncomplicated or complicated skin and skin structure infections, community-acquired pneumonia

Dosage and routes

Vancomycin-resistant* E. faecium *infections

Adult: **IV** 600 mg q12h × 14-28 days PO

Nosocomial pneumonia/complicated skin infections/community-acquired pneumonia/concurrent bacterial infection

Adult: **IV**/PO 600 mg q12h × 10-14 days

Uncomplicated skin infections

Adult: **IV**/PO 400 mg q12h × 10-14 days; *Adolescents:* PO 600 mg q12h × 10-14 days

Available forms: Tabs 400, 600 mg; oral susp 100 mg/5 ml; inj 2 mg/ml

Adverse effects

CNS: *Headache,* dizziness

GI: *Nausea, diarrhea,* increased ALT, AST, *vomiting,* taste change, tongue color change

HEMA: **Myelosuppression**

MISC: Vaginal moniliasis, fungal infection, oral moniliasis

Contraindications: Hypersensitivity

Precautions: Pregnancy **C**, lactation, children, thrombocytopenia

Pharmacokinetics

Absorption	Rapidly, excessively
Distribution	Protein binding 31%
Metabolism	Oxidation of the morpholine ring
Excretion	Unknown
Half-life	Unknown

Pharmacodynamics

Unknown

Interactions
Drug classifications
Adrenergic blockers: increased effects of adrenergics
Serotonergic agents: increased effect

NURSING CONSIDERATIONS
Assessment
- Assess CNS symptoms: headache, dizziness
- Monitor liver function studies: AST, ALT
- Monitor allergic reactions: fever, flushing, rash, urticaria, pruritus
- Assess for pseudomembranous colitis: severe diarrhea, cramping
- Monitor CBC weekly, assess for myelosuppression (anemia, leukopenia, pancytopenia, thrombocytopenia)

Nursing diagnoses
- Infection, risk for (uses)
- Knowledge, deficient (teaching)

Implementation
PO route
- Store reconstituted oral suspension at room temperature, use within 3 wk

IV route
- Give over 30-120 min; do not use **IV** infusion bag in series connections, do not use with additives in sol, do not use with another drug, administer separately

Y-site compatibilities: Acyclovir, alfentanil, amikacin, aminophylline, ampicillin, aztreonam, bretylium, buprenorphine, butorphanol, calcium gluconate, carboplatin, cefazolin, cefoperazone, cefotetan, cefoxitin, ceftazidine, ceftizoxime, ceftriaxone, cefuroxime, cimetidine, ciprofloxacin, cisatracurium, cisplatin, clindamycin, cyclophosphamide, cycloSPORINE, cytarabine, hydromorphone, ifosfamide, labetalol, leucovorin, levofloxacin, lidocaine, lorazepam, magnesium sulfate, mannitol, meperidine, meropenem, mesna, methotrexate, methylPREDNISolone, metoclopramide, metronidazole, midazolam, minocycline, mitoxantrone, morphine, nalbuphine, naloxone, nitroglycerin, ofloxacin, ondansetron, paclitaxel, pentobarbital, piperacillin, potassium chloride, prochlorperazine, promethazine, propranolol, ranitidine, remifentanil, theophylline, ticarcillin, tobramycin, vancomycin, vecuronium, verapamil, vinCRIStine, zidovudine

Solution compatibilities: D_5, 0.9% NaCl, LR

Patient/family education
- Advise patient if dizziness occurs, to ambulate, perform activities with assistance
- Advise patient to complete full course of drug therapy
- Advise patient to contact prescriber if adverse reaction occurs
- Advise patient to avoid large amounts of tyramine-containing foods (give list)

Evaluation
Positive therapeutic outcome
- Decreased symptoms of infection, blood cultures negative

liothyronine (T_3) (Rx)
(lye-oh-thye′roe-neen)
Cytomel, l-Triiodothyronine, liothyronine sodium, Triostat, T_3
Func. class.: Thyroid hormone
Chem. class.: Synthetic T_3

Pregnancy category A

Action: Controls protein synthesis; increases metabolic rates, cardiac output, renal blood flow, O_2 consumption, body temp, blood volume, growth, development at cellular level, exact mechanism unknown

Therapeutic Outcome: Correction of lack of thyroid hormone

Uses: Hypothyroidism, myxedema coma, thyroid hormone replacement, nontoxic goiter, T_3 suppression test, congenital hypothyroidism

Dosage and routes
Adult: PO 25 mcg daily, increased by 12.5-25 mcg q1-2 wk until desired response, maintenance dosage 25-75 mcg daily
Elderly: PO 5 mcg/day, increase by 5 mcg/day q1-2 wk, maintenance 25-75 mcg/day

Congenital hypothyroidism
Child >3 yr: PO 50-100 mcg daily
Child <3 yr: PO 5 mcg daily, increased by 5 mcg q3-4 days titrated to response, maintenance 20 mcg/day

Myxedema, severe hypothyroidism
Adult: PO 25-50 mcg then may increase by 5-10 mcg q1-2 wk; maintenance dosage 50-100 mcg daily

Myxedema coma/precoma
Adult: **IV** 25-50 mcg initially; 5 mcg in elderly; 10-20 mcg in cardiac disease; give doses q4-12h

Nontoxic goiter
Adult: PO 5 mcg daily, increased by 12.5-25 mcg q1-2 wk; maintenance dosage 75 mcg daily

L

Suppression test (T_3)
Adult: PO 75-100 mcg daily × 1 wk; ^{131}I is given before and after 1st wk dose

Available forms: Tabs 5, 25, 50 mcg; inj 10 mcg/ml

Adverse effects
CNS: *Insomnia, tremors,* headache, **thyroid storm**
CV: *Tachycardia, palpitations, angina, dysrhythmias,* hypertension, **cardiac arrest**
GI: Nausea, diarrhea, increased or decreased appetite, cramps
MISC: Menstrual irregularities, weight loss, sweating, heat intolerance, fever, alopecia

Contraindications: Adrenal insufficiency, MI, thyrotoxicosis

Precautions: Pregnancy **A,** elderly, angina pectoris, hypertension, ischemia, cardiac disease, lactation, diabetes

Pharmacokinetics

Absorption	Well (PO); complete (**IV**)
Distribution	Widely distributed; does not cross placenta
Metabolism	Liver
Excretion	Feces via bile, breast milk
Half-life	1-2 days

Pharmacodynamics

	PO/IV
Onset	Unknown
Peak	12-24 hr
Duration	72 hr

Interactions
Individual drugs
Cholestyramine, colestipol: decreased absorption of thyroid hormone
Insulin: increased requirement for insulin
Drug classifications
Amphetamines, anticoagulants (oral), antidepressants (tricyclics), decongestants, sympathomimetics, tricyclics, vasopressors: increased effect of each specific drug
Digoxin: decreased effects of digoxin
Estrogens: decreased effects of liothyronine
Hypoglycemics: decreased effect of each specific drug
Drug/herb
Agar, bugleweed, carnitine, kelpware, soy, spirulina: decreased thyroid hormone effect
Drug/lab test
Increased: CPK, LDH, AST, PBI, blood glucose
Decreased: thyroid function tests

NURSING CONSIDERATIONS
Assessment
- Determine if the patient is taking anticoagulants, antidiabetic agents; document on patient record
- Take B/P, pulse before each dose; monitor I&O ratio and weight every day in same clothing, using same scale, at same time of day
- Monitor height, weight, psychomotor development, and growth rate if given to a child
- Monitor T_3, T_4, FTIs, which are decreased; radioimmunoassay of TSH, which is increased; radioactive iodine uptake, which is increased if medication dose is too low
- Monitor protime; may require decreased anticoagulant; check for bleeding, bruising
- Assess for increased nervousness, excitability, irritability, which may indicate too high a dose, usually after 1-3 wk of treatment
- Assess cardiac status: angina, palpitations, chest pain, change in VS; elderly patients may have undetected cardiac problems, and baseline ECG should be completed before treatment

Nursing diagnoses
- Knowledge, deficient (teaching)
- Noncompliance (teaching)

Implementation
PO route
- Give in AM if possible as a single dose to decrease sleeplessness; give at same time each day to maintain drug level
- Do not take with food or absorption will be decreased
- Give only for hormone imbalances; not to be used for obesity, male infertility, menstrual conditions, lethargy; give lowest dose that relieves symptoms; give lower dose to the elderly and those with cardiac diseases
- Store in airtight, light-resistant container

IV route
- Administer **IV** for myxedema coma and precoma; do not give IM or SUBCUT; give q4-12h; use PO dose as soon as feasible

Patient/family education
- Teach patient that drug is not a cure but controls symptoms, and treatment is long term
- Instruct patient to report excitability, irritability, anxiety, sweating, heat intolerance, chest pain, palpitations, which indicate overdose
- Advise patient not to switch brands unless approved by prescriber; bioavailability may differ
- Teach patient that drug may be discontinued after giving birth; thyroid panel will be evaluated after 1-2 mo

- Teach patient that hyperthyroid child will show almost immediate behavior/personality change; that hair loss will occur in child but is temporary
- Caution patient that drug is not to be taken to reduce weight
- Caution patient to avoid OTC preparations with iodine; read labels; other medications should not be used unless approved by prescriber
- Teach patient to avoid iodine-rich food: iodized salt, soybeans, tofu, turnips, high iodine seafood, some bread

Evaluation

Positive therapeutic outcome

- Absence of depression
- Weight loss
- Increased diuresis, pulse, appetite
- Absence of constipation, peripheral edema, cold intolerance, pale, cool dry skin, brittle nails, alopecia, coarse hair, menorrhagia, night blindness, paresthesias, syncope, stupor, coma, rosy cheeks
- Improved levels of T_3, T_4 by laboratory tests
- Child:age-appropriate weight, height, and psychomotor development

Treatment of overdose: Withhold dose for up to 1 wk; for acute overdose: gastric lavage or induce emesis, then activated charcoal; provide supportive treatment to control symptoms

liotrix (Rx)

(lye'oh-trix)

T_3/T_4, Thyrolar

Func. class.: Thyroid hormone

Chem. class.: Levothyroxine/liothyronine (synthetic T_4, T_3)

Pregnancy category A

Do Not Confuse:

Thyrolar/Thyrar

Action: Controls protein synthesis; increases metabolic rates, cardiac output, renal blood flow, O_2 consumption, body temp, blood volume, growth, development at cellular level, exact mechanism unknown

Therapeutic Outcome: Correction of lack of thyroid hormone

Uses: Hypothyroidism, thyroid hormone replacement

Dosage and routes

Adult and child: PO 50 mcg levothyroxine/12.5 mcg liothyronine daily, increased by 50 mcg levothyroxine/12.5 mcg liothyronine q2-3 wk until desired response; may increase by 15-30 mg q2 wk in child

Elderly: PO 12.5-25 mcg levothyroxine/3.1-6.2 mcg liothyronine, may increase by 12.5-25 mcg levothyroxine/3.1-6.2 mcg liothyronine q6-8 wk until adequate response

Available forms: Tabs 12.5/3.1, 25/6.25, 50/12.5, 100/25, 150 mcg levothyroxine/37.5 mcg liothyronine

Adverse effects

CNS: *Insomnia, tremors,* headache, **thyroid storm**

CV: *Tachycardia, palpitations, angina, dysrhythmias,* hypertension, **cardiac arrest**

GI: Nausea, diarrhea, increased or decreased appetite, cramps

MISC: Menstrual irregularities, weight loss, sweating, heat intolerance, fever

Contraindications: Adrenal insufficiency, MI, thyrotoxicosis

Precautions: Pregnancy **A,** elderly, angina pectoris, hypertension, ischemia, cardiac disease, lactation, diabetes

Pharmacokinetics

Absorption	50%-80% (T_4); 95% (T_3)
Distribution	Widely distributed; does not cross placenta
Metabolism	Liver, tissues
Excretion	Feces via bile; breast milk
Half-life	6-7 days (T_4); 2 days (T_3)

Pharmacodynamics

	PO (T_4)	PO (T_3)
Onset	Unknown	Unknown
Peak	Unknown	24-72 hr
Duration	Unknown	72 hr

Interactions

Individual drugs

Cholestyramine: decreased absorption of thyroid hormone
Colestipol: decreased absorption of liotrix
Insulin: increased requirement for insulin

Drug classifications

Amphetamines, decongestants, vasopressors: increased effect of each specific drug
Anticoagulants (oral): increased effect of anticoagulants
Antidepressants (tricyclics): increased tricyclic effect
Catecholamines: increased catecholamine effect
Digoxin: decreased effect of digoxin
Estrogens: decreased liotrix effect

Hypoglycemics: decreased hypoglycemic effect
Sympathomimetics: increased sympathomimetic effect

Drug/herb

Agar, bugleweed, carnitine, kelpware, soy, spirulina: decreased thyroid hormone effect

Drug/lab test

Increased: CPK, LDH, AST, PBI, blood glucose
Decreased: thyroid function tests

NURSING CONSIDERATIONS

Assessment

- Determine if the patient is taking anticoagulants, antidiabetic agents; document on chart
- Take B/P, pulse before each dose; monitor I&O ratio and weight every day in same clothing, using same scale, at same time of day
- Monitor height, weight, psychomotor development, and growth rate if given to a child
- Monitor T_3, T_4, FTIs, which are decreased; radioimmunoassay of TSH, which is increased; radioactive iodine uptake (RA international units), which is increased if medication dose is too low
- Monitor protime; may require decreased anticoagulant; check for bleeding, bruising
- Assess for increased nervousness, excitability, irritability, which may indicate too high a dose of medication, usually after 1-3 wk of treatment
- Assess cardiac status: angina, palpitations, chest pain, change in VS; the elderly patient may have undetected cardiac problems, and baseline ECG should be completed before treatment

Nursing diagnoses

- Knowledge, deficient (teaching)
- Noncompliance (teaching)

Implementation

- Give in AM if possible as a single dose to decrease sleeplessness; give at same time each day to maintain drug level
- Do not take with food or absorption will be decreased
- Give only for hormone imbalances; not to be used for obesity, male infertility, menstrual conditions, lethargy; give lowest dose that relieves symptoms; give lower dose to the elderly and those with cardiac diseases
- Store in airtight, light-resistant container
- Remove medication 4 wk before RAIU test

Patient/family education

- Teach patient that drug is not a cure but controls symptoms, and treatment is long term
- Instruct patient to report excitability, irritability, anxiety, sweating, heat intolerance, chest pain, palpitations, which indicate overdose
- Advise patient not to switch brands unless approved by prescriber; bioavailability may differ
- Teach patient that drug may be discontinued after giving birth; thyroid panel will be evaluated after 1-2 mo
- Teach patient that hyperthyroid child will show almost immediate behavior/personality change; that hair loss will occur in child but is temporary
- Caution patient that drug is not to be taken to reduce weight
- Caution patient to avoid OTC preparations with iodine; read labels; other medications should not be used unless approved by prescriber
- Teach patient to avoid iodine-rich food: iodized salt, soybeans, tofu, turnips, high iodine seafood, some bread

Evaluation

Positive therapeutic outcome

- Absence of depression
- Weight loss
- Increased diuresis, pulse, appetite
- Absence of constipation, peripheral edema, cold intolerance, pale, cool dry skin, brittle nails, alopecia, coarse hair, menorrhagia, night blindness, paresthesias, syncope, stupor, coma, rosy cheeks
- Improved levels of T_3, T_4 by laboratory tests
- Child: age-appropriate weight, height, and psychomotor development

Treatment of overdose: Withhold dose for up to 1 wk; acute overdose: gastric lavage or induce emesis, then activated charcoal; provide supportive treatment to control symptoms

lisinopril (Rx)

(lyse-in′oh-pril)
Prinivil, Zestril
Func. class.: Antihypertensive, angiotensin converting enzyme (ACE) inhibitor
Chem. class.: Enalaprilat lysine analog

Pregnancy category
C (1st trimester),
D (2nd/3rd trimesters)

Do Not Confuse:

Prinivil/Plendil, Prinivil/Prilosec, Prinivil/Proventil
lisinopril/Risperdal

Action: Selectively suppresses renin-angiotensin-aldosterone system; inhibits ACE; prevents conversion of angiotensin I to angiotensin II; results in dilatation of arterial, venous vessels

Therapeutic Outcome: Decreased B/P in hypertension, decreased preload, afterload in CHF

Uses: Mild to moderate hypertension, adjunctive therapy of systolic CHF, acute MI

Dosage and routes

Hypertension

Adult: PO 10-40 mg daily; may increase to 80 mg daily if required

Elderly: PO 2.5-5 mg/day, increase q7 days

CHF

Adult: PO 5 mg initially with diuretics/digitalis, range 5-20 mg

Available forms: Tabs 2.5, 5, 10, 20, 30 40 mg

Adverse effects

CNS: *Vertigo,* depression, **stroke,** insomnia, paresthesias, *headache,* fatigue, asthenia, dizziness

CV: Chest pain, hypotension

EENT: Blurred vision, nasal congestion

GI: Nausea, vomiting, anorexia, constipation, flatulence, GI irritation, diarrhea

GU: **Proteinuria, renal insufficiency,** sexual dysfunction, impotence

INTEG: Rash, pruritus

MISC: Muscle cramps

RESP: Dry cough, dyspnea

SYST: **Angioedema**

Contraindications: Pregnancy **D** (2nd/3rd trimesters), hypersensitivity

Precautions: Pregnancy **C** (1st trimester), lactation, renal disease, hyperkalemia, renal artery stenosis

Pharmacokinetics	
Absorption	Variable
Distribution	Unknown
Metabolism	Not metabolized
Excretion	Kidneys, unchanged
Half-life	12 hr

Pharmacodynamics	
Onset	1 hr
Peak	6-8 hr
Duration	24 hr

Interactions

Individual drugs

Alcohol (large amounts), probenecid: increased hypotension
Allopurinol: increased hypersensitivity
Aspirin: decreased lisinopril effect
CycloSPORINE: increased hyperkalemia
Digoxin: increased serum levels, toxicity
Indomethacin: decreased antihypertensive effect
Lithium: increased levels of lithium, toxicity

Drug classifications

Antihypertensives, diuretics, nitrates, phenothiazines: increased hypotension
Diuretics, potassium-sparing, potassium salt substitutes, potassium supplements: increased hyperkalemia
NSAIDs: decreased lisinopril effect

Drug/herb

Aconite: increased toxicity, death
Astragalus, cola tree: increased or decreased antihypertensive effect
Barberry, betony, black catechu, black cohosh, bloodroot, broom, burdock, cat's claw, dandelion, goldenseal, Irish moss, Jamaican dogwood, kelp, khella, mistletoe, parsley: increased antihypertensive effect
Coltsfoot, guarana, khat, licorice: decreased antihypertensive effect

Drug/food

High-potassium diet (bananas, orange juice, avocados, broccoli, nuts, spinach) should be avoided; hyperkalemia may occur

Drug/lab test

Interference: glucose/insulin tolerance tests, ANA titer

NURSING CONSIDERATIONS

Assessment

- Assess blood studies: platelets, WBC with differential, baseline and periodically q3 mo; if neutrophils <1000/mm^3, discontinue treatment
- Monitor B/P, check for orthostatic hypotension, syncope; if changes occur, dosage change may be required
- Establish baselines in renal, liver function tests before therapy begins
- Monitor renal, liver studies: protein, BUN, creatinine; watch for increased levels that may indicate nephrotic syndrome and renal failure; monitor renal symptoms: polyuria, oliguria, frequency, dysuria; liver function tests
- Check potassium levels throughout treatment, although hyperkalemia rarely occurs
- Check for edema in feet, legs daily
- Assess for allergic reactions: rash, fever,

pruritus, urticaria; drug should be discontinued if antihistamines fail to help

Nursing diagnoses

- Cardiac output, decreased (uses)
- Injury, risk for (side effects)
- Knowledge, deficient (teaching)
- Noncompliance (teaching)

Implementation

- Store in airtight container at 86° F (30° C) or less
- Severe hypotension may occur after 1st dose of this medication; may be prevented by reducing or discontinuing diuretic therapy 3 days before beginning lisinopril therapy

Patient/family education

- Caution patient not to discontinue drug abruptly; advise patient to inform all health care providers about taking this drug
- Teach patient not to use OTC products (cough, cold, allergy) unless directed by prescriber; serious side effects can occur
- Teach patient the importance of complying with dosage schedule, even if feeling better; to continue with medical regimen to decrease B/P: exercise, cessation of smoking, decreasing stress, diet modifications
- Teach patient to notify prescriber of mouth sores, sore throat, fever, swelling of hands or feet, irregular heartbeat, chest pain, coughing, shortness of breath
- Caution patient to report excessive perspiration, dehydration, vomiting, diarrhea; may lead to fall in B/P
- Emphasize the need to rise slowly to sitting or standing position to minimize orthostatic hypotension; not to exercise in hot weather or increased hypotension can occur
- Caution patient that drug may cause dizziness, fainting, light-headedness; may occur during 1st few days of therapy; to avoid activities that may be hazardous
- Teach patient how to take B/P, and normal readings for age group; advise patient to take B/P regularly
- Instruct patient to avoid increasing potassium in the diet

Evaluation

Positive therapeutic outcome

- Decreased B/P in hypertension
- Decreased CHF symptoms

Treatment of overdose: 0.9% NaCl **IV** inf, hemodialysis

lithium (Rx)

(li'thee-um)

Carbolith ♣, Duralith ♣, Eskalith, Eskalith CR, lithium carbonate, Lithizine ♣, Lithonate, Lithotabs

Func. class.: Antimanic, antipsychotic

Chem. class.: Alkali metal ion salt

Pregnancy category D

Action: May alter sodium, potassium ion transport across cell membrane in nerve, muscle cells; may balance biogenic amines of norepinephrine, serotonin in CNS areas involved in emotional responses

Therapeutic Outcome: Stable mood

Uses: Bipolar disorders (manic phase), prevention of bipolar manic-depressive psychosis

Dosage and routes

Adult: PO 300-600 mg tid; maintenance 300 mg tid or qid; slow rel tab 300 mg bid; dosage should be individualized to maintain blood levels at 0.5-1.5 mEq/L

Elderly: PO 300 mg bid, increase q7 days by 300 mg to desired dose

Child: PO 15-20 mg (0.4-0.5 mEq)/kg/day in 2-3 divided doses, increase as needed, do not exceed adult doses

Renal dose

Adult: PO CCr 10-50 ml/min 50-75% of dose; CCr <10 ml/min 25%-50% of dose

Available forms: Caps 150, 300, 600 mg; tabs 300 mg; ext rel tabs 300, 450 mg; syr 300 mg/5 ml (8 mEq/5 ml); slow rel caps 150, 300 mg ♣

Adverse effects

CNS: *Headache, drowsiness, dizziness, tremors,* twitching, ataxia, **seizures,** slurred speech, restlessness, *confusion,* stupor, memory loss, clonic movements, *fatigue*

CV: *Hypotension,* ECG changes, **dysrhythmias, circulatory collapse, edema**

EENT: Tinnitus, blurred vision

ENDO: Hypothyroidism, goiter, hyperglycemia, hyperthyroidism, hypernatremia

GI: *Dry mouth, anorexia, nausea, vomiting, diarrhea,* incontinence, abdominal pain, metallic taste

GU: **Polyuria, glycosuria, proteinuria, albuminuria,** urinary incontinence, polydipsia

HEMA: **Leukocytosis**

INTEG: Drying of hair, alopecia, rash, pruritus, hyperkeratosis, *acneiform rash, folliculitis*

MS: *Muscle weakness,* rigidity

Contraindications: Pregnancy **D**, hepatic disease, renal disease, brain trauma, OBS, lactation, schizophrenia, severe cardiac disease, severe renal disease, severe dehydration, children <12 yr

Precautions: Elderly, thyroid disease, seizure disorders, diabetes mellitus, systemic infection, urinary retention

Pharmacokinetics

Absorption	Completely absorbed
Distribution	Reabsorbed by renal tubules (80%); crosses blood-brain barrier; crosses placenta
Metabolism	Unknown
Excretion	Urine, unchanged
Half-life	18-36 hr depending on age

Pharmacodynamics

Onset	Rapid
Peak	½-4 hr
Duration	Unknown

Interactions
Individual drugs
Acetazolamide, aminophylline, mannitol, sodium bicarbonate: increased renal clearance
Calcium iodide, iodinated glycerol, iodide, potassium: increased hypothyroid effect
Carbamazepine, fluoxetine, methyldopa, probenecid: increased lithium toxicity
Haloperidol: increased neurotoxicity
Indomethacin, losartan, urea: increased toxicity
Thioridazine: brain damage
Drug classifications
Antithyroid agents: increased hypothyroid effects
Neuromuscular blocking agents: increased effect of neuromuscular blocking effects
NSAIDs, thiazides: increased lithium toxicity
Phenothiazines: increased effect of phenothiazines
Theophyllines, urinary alkalinizers: decreased effect of lithium
Drug/herb
Broom, buchu, dandelion, goldenrod, horsetail, juniper, nettle, parsley: increased lithium effect
Cola nut, guarana, plantain, tea (black/green), yerba maté: decreased lithium effect
Drug/food
Significant changes in sodium intake will alter lithium excretion
Drug/lab test
Increased: potassium excretion, urine glucose, blood glucose, protein, BUN
Decreased: VMA, T_3, T_4, PBI, ^{131}I

NURSING CONSIDERATIONS
Assessment
- Assess for minor lithium toxicity: vomiting, diarrhea, poor coordination, fine motor tremors, weakness, lassitude; major toxicity: coarse tremors, severe thirst, tinnitus, dilute urine
- Assess weight daily; check for edema in legs, ankles, wrists; report if present; check skin turgor at least daily
- Monitor sodium intake; decreased sodium intake with decreased fluid intake may lead to lithium retention; increased sodium and fluids may decrease lithium retention
- Monitor urine for albuminuria, glycosuria, uric acid during beginning treatment, q2 mo thereafter
- Assess neurologic status: LOC, gait, motor reflexes, hand tremors
- Monitor serum lithium levels weekly initially, then q2 mo (therapeutic level: 0.5-1.5 mEq/L); toxicity and therapeutic levels are very close; toxicity may occur rapidly; blood levels are measured before the AM dose

Nursing diagnoses
- Coping, ineffective (uses)
- Thought processes, disturbed (uses)
- Knowledge, deficient (teaching)
- Noncompliance (teaching)

Implementation
- Do not break, crush, or chew caps
- Administer reduced dosage to elderly; give with meals to avoid GI upset
- Provide adequate fluids (2-3 L/day) to prevent dehydration during initial treatment, 1-2 L/day during maintenance
- Give list of drugs that interact with lithium

Patient/family education
- Provide patient with written information on symptoms of minor toxicity: vomiting, diarrhea, poor coordination, fine motor tremors, weakness, lassitude; major toxicity: coarse tremors, severe thirst, tinnitus, dilute urine
- Advise patient to monitor urine sp gr; emphasize need for follow-up care to determine lithium effects
- Advise patient that contraception is necessary, since lithium may harm fetus
- Caution patient not to operate machinery until lithium levels are stable and response determined; that beneficial effects may take 1-3 wk
- Provide to the patient a list of drugs that interact with lithium and discuss need for adequate, stable intake of salt and fluid
- Advise to have lithium levels monitored to ensure effectiveness

L

Evaluation

Positive therapeutic outcome

- Decrease in excitement, poor judgment, insomnia (manic phase)
- Decreased mood swings and lability

Treatment of overdose: Induce emesis or lavage, maintain airway, respiratory function; dialysis for severe intoxication

lomefloxacin (Rx)

(lome-flocks'a-sin)

Maxaquin

Func. class.: Antiinfective

Chem. class.: Fluoroquinolone

Pregnancy category C

Action: Interferes with conversion of intermediate DNA fragments into high molecular weight DNA in bacteria; DNA gyrase inhibitor

Therapeutic Outcome: Bactericidal for gram-negative organisms *Aeromonas, Citrobacter, Enterobacter, Escherichia coli, Haemophilus influenzae, Klebsiella, Legionella, Moraxella catarrhalis, Morganella morganii, Proteus vulgaris, Proteus mirabilis, Providencia alcalifaciens, Providencia rettgeri, Pseudomonas aeruginosa, Serratia;* gram-positive organisms *Staphylococcus aureus, Staphylococcus epidermidis, Staphylococcus saprophyticus* (methicillin-resistant strains also)

Uses: Treatment of lower respiratory tract infections (pneumonia, bronchitis), genitourinary tract infections (prostatitis, UTIs), preoperatively to reduce UTIs in transurethral surgical procedures

Dosage and routes

Lower respiratory tract infection/ uncomplicated cystitis

Adult: PO 400 mg × 10 days

Complicated UTI

Adult: PO 400 mg × 14 days depending on type of infection

Renal dose

Adult: PO CCr ≤40 ml/min 400 mg, then 200 mg/day

Surgical prophylaxis of UTI

Adult: PO 400 mg 2-6 hr before surgery

Available forms: Tabs 400 mg

Adverse effects

CNS: *Dizziness, headache,* somnolence, depression, insomnia, nervousness, confusion, agitation, **seizures**

EENT: Visual disturbances

GI: Diarrhea, *nausea,* vomiting, anorexia, flatulence, heartburn, dry mouth, increased AST, ALT, constipation, abdominal pain, oral thrush, glossitis, stomatitis, **pseudomembranous colitis**

INTEG: Rash, pruritus, urticaria, *photosensitivity*

SYST: **Anaphylaxis, Stevens-Johnson syndrome**

Contraindications: Hypersensitivity to quinolones

Precautions: Pregnancy **C**, lactation, children, elderly, renal disease, seizure disorders, excessive exposure to sunlight, psychosis, ICP

Pharmacokinetics	
Absorption	Well absorbed
Distribution	Widely distributed
Metabolism	Unknown
Excretion	Kidney, unchanged
Half-life	6-8 hr; increased in renal disease

Pharmacodynamics	
Onset	Unknown
Peak	1-2 hr

Interactions

Individual drugs

Cimetidine, probenecid: increased lomefloxacin levels, toxicity

CycloSPORINE: increased levels of cycloSPORINE, toxicity

Sucralfate: decreased lomefloxacin levels

Warfarin: increased levels of warfarin, toxicity

Drug classifications

Antacids (aluminum, magnesium), iron sulfate, zinc sulfate: decreased levels of lomefloxacin

NSAIDs: increased CNS stimulation, seizures

Drug/herb

Cola tree: increased antiinfective effect

NURSING CONSIDERATIONS

Assessment

- Assess patient for previous sensitivity reaction
- Assess patient for signs and symptoms of infection: characteristics of wounds, sputum, urine, stool, WBC >10,000/mm^3, fever; baseline and during treatment
- Obtain C&S before beginning drug therapy to identify if correct treatment has been initiated
- Assess for allergic reactions and anaphylaxis: rash, urticaria, pruritus, chills,

fever, joint pain; may occur a few days after therapy begins; epINEPHrine and resuscitation equipment should be available for anaphylactic reaction

- Monitor blood studies: AST, ALT, CBC, Hct, bilirubin, LDH, alkaline phosphatase, Coombs' test monthly if patient is on long-term therapy
- Assess bowel pattern daily; if severe diarrhea occurs, drug should be discontinued
- Assess for overgrowth of infection: perineal itching, fever, malaise, redness, pain, swelling, drainage, rash, diarrhea, change in cough, sputum
- Assess for CNS symptoms: insomnia, vertigo, headaches, agitation, confusion

Nursing diagnoses
- Infection, risk for (uses)
- Diarrhea (adverse reactions)
- Injury, risk for (adverse reactions)
- Knowledge, deficient (teaching)
- Noncompliance (teaching)

Implementation
- Give with food for GI symptoms; give with 8 oz of water
- Give 2 hr before or 2 hr after iron, calcium, zinc, magnesium products, or antacids, which decrease absorption

Patient/family education
- Instruct patient to take all medication prescribed for the length of time ordered; drug must be taken around the clock to maintain blood levels; do not give medication to others
- Teach patient to use sunscreen when outdoors to decrease phototoxicity
- Advise patient to increase fluids to 2 L/day to prevent crystalluria
- Caution patient to avoid driving and other hazardous activities until response is known; dizziness, confusion, drowsiness may occur
- Advise patient to rinse mouth frequently, use sugarless candy or gum for dry mouth
- Instruct patient to avoid other medications unless approved by prescriber

Evaluation
Positive therapeutic outcome
- Negative C&S, absence of signs/symptoms of infection (WBC <10,000/mm^3, temp WNL)
- Reported improvement in symptoms of infection

lomustine (Rx)
(loe-mus'teen)
CCNU, CeeNU
Func. class.: Antineoplastic alkylating agent
Chem. class.: Nitrosourea
Pregnancy category D

Action: Changes essential cellular ions to covalent bonding with resultant alkylation; this interferes with normal biologic function of DNA; activity is not phase specific; action is due to myelosuppression

Therapeutic Outcome: Prevention of rapid growth of malignant cells in chronic myelocytic leukemia

Uses: Hodgkin's disease, lymphomas, multiple myeloma

Investigational uses: Brain, breast, renal, GI tract, bronchogenic carcinoma; melanomas

Dosage and routes
Adult: PO 100, 130 mg/m^2 as a single dose q6 wk; titrate dosage to WBC level; do not give repeat dose unless WBCs are >4000/mm^3, platelet count >100,000/mm^3

Available forms: Caps 10, 40, 100 mg

Adverse effects
GI: Nausea, vomiting, anorexia, stomatitis, **hepatotoxicity**
GU: **Azotemia, renal failure**
HEMA: **Thrombocytopenia, leukopenia, myelosuppression, anemia**
RESP: **Fibrosis, pulmonary infiltrate**

Contraindications: Pregnancy **D**, lactation, "blastic" phase of chronic myelocytic leukemia, hypersensitivity, leukopenia, thrombocytopenia

Precautions: Radiation therapy

Pharmacokinetics
Absorption	Rapidly absorbed
Distribution	Widely
Metabolism	Liver
Excretion	Kidneys, breast milk
Half-life	16-48 hr

Pharmacodynamics
Unknown

Interactions
Individual drugs
Allopurinol: increased bone marrow suppression
Aspirin: increased bleeding

L

Chloral hydrate, phenytoin: increased toxicity
Phenobarbital: increased lomustine metabolism
Succinylcholine: increased lomustine effect

Drug classifications
Anticoagulants: increased bleeding
Barbiturates: increased toxicity

Drug/lab test
False positive: cytology tests for breast, bladder, cervix, lung

NURSING CONSIDERATIONS

Assessment

- ⚠ Monitor CBC, differential, platelet count weekly; withhold drug if WBC is <4000/mm^3 or platelet count is <100,000/mm^3; notify prescriber of results if WBC <20,000/mm^3, platelets <150,000/mm^3
- Monitor pulmonary function tests, chest x-ray films before, during therapy; chest film should be obtained q2 wk during treatment; assess for dyspnea, crackles, unproductive cough, chest pain, tachypnea
- Monitor renal function studies: BUN, serum uric acid, urine CCr before, during therapy; I&O ratio; report fall in urine output of 30 ml/hr; check for decreased hyperuricemia
- Monitor for cold, fever, sore throat (may indicate beginning of infection); identify edema in feet, joint and stomach pain, shaking; prescriber should be notified
- Assess for bleeding: hematuria, guaiac, bruising or petechiae, mucosa or orifices q8h, no rec temp

Nursing diagnoses

- Injury, risk for (adverse reactions)
- Body image, disturbed (adverse reactions)
- Infection, risk for (adverse reactions)
- Knowledge, deficient (teaching)

Implementation

- Give drug after evening meal, before bedtime; administer antiemetic 30-60 min before giving drug to prevent vomiting
- Antiinfectives for prophylaxis of infection may be prescribed since infection potential is high
- Store in tight container

Patient/family education

- Teach patient to avoid use of products containing aspirin or ibuprofen, razors, commercial mouthwash, since bleeding may occur; to report symptoms of bleeding (hematuria, tarry stools)
- Advise patient to report signs of anemia (fatigue, headache, irritability, faintness, shortness of breath)
- Caution patient to report any changes in breathing or coughing even several mo after treatment; to avoid crowds and persons with respiratory tract or other infections
- Caution patient not to have any vaccinations without the advice of prescriber; serious reactions can occur
- Tell patient contraception is needed during treatment and for several mo after the completion of therapy, avoid breastfeeding

Evaluation

Positive therapeutic outcome

- Decreased tumor sizes
- Decreased spread of malignancy

loperamide (OTC, Rx)

(loe-per'a-mide)

loperamide solution, Imodium, Imodium A-D, Imodium A-D Caplet, Loperamide, Kaopectate II Caplets, Maalox Antidiarrheal Caplets, Neo-Diaral, Pepto Diarrhea Control

Func. class.: Antidiarrheal
Chem. class.: Piperidine derivative

Pregnancy category B

Action: Direct action on intestinal muscles to decrease GI peristalsis; reduces volume, increases bulk; electrolytes are not lost

Therapeutic Outcome: Absence of diarrhea

Uses: Diarrhea (cause undetermined), chronic diarrhea, to decrease amount of ileostomy discharge, traveler's diarrhea

Dosage and routes

Adult: PO 4 mg, then 2 mg after each loose stool, max 16 mg/day
Child 9-11 yr: PO 2 mg, then 1 mg after each loose stool, max 6 mg/24 hr
Child 2-5 yr: PO 1 mg, then 0.1 mg/kg after each loose stool, max 4 mg/24 hr

Available forms: Caps 2 mg; liq 1 mg/5 ml; tabs 2 mg

Adverse effects

CNS: Dizziness, drowsiness, fatigue, fever
GI: *Nausea, dry mouth, vomiting, constipation,* abdominal pain, anorexia, **toxic megacolon**
INTEG: Rash

Contraindications: Hypersensitivity, severe ulcerative colitis, pseudomembranous colitis, acute diarrhea associated with *Escherichia coli*

Precautions: Pregnancy **B,** lactation, children <2 yr, liver disease, dehydration, bacterial disease

Pharmacokinetics

Absorption	Poor
Distribution	Unknown
Metabolism	Liver
Excretion	Feces, unchanged; small amount in urine
Half-life	7-14 hr

Pharmacodynamics

Onset	½-1 hr
Peak	Unknown
Duration	4-5 hr

Interaction
Individual drugs
Alcohol: increased CNS depression
Drug classifications
Antihistamines, analgesics (opioids), sedative/hypnotics: increased CNS depression
Solutions: do not mix with other oral sol
Drug/herb
Chamomile, hops, kava, skullcap, valerian: increased CNS depression
Nutmeg: increased antidiarrheal effect

NURSING CONSIDERATIONS
Assessment
- Monitor electrolytes (potassium, sodium, chloride) if patient is on long-term therapy; check fluid status, skin turgor
- Assess bowel pattern before, during treatment; check for rebound constipation after termination of medication; check bowel sounds
- Check response after 48 hr; if no response, drug should be discontinued and other treatment initiated
- Assess for abdominal distention, toxic megacolon, which may occur in ulcerative colitis
- Assess for dehydration, CNS symptoms in children

Nursing diagnoses
- Diarrhea (uses)
- Constipation (adverse reactions)
- Knowledge, deficient (teaching)
- Noncompliance (teaching)

Implementation
- Do not break, crush, or chew caps
- Store in airtight containers

Patient/family education
- Caution patient to avoid alcohol and OTC products unless directed by prescriber; may cause increased CNS depression
- Advise patient not to exceed recommended dosage; drug may be habit forming; ileostomy patient may take this drug for extended time
- Advise patient that drug may cause drowsiness and to avoid hazardous activities until response to drug is determined
- Teach patient that dry mouth can be decreased by frequent sips of water, hard candy, sugarless gum

Evaluation
Positive therapeutic outcome
- Decreased diarrhea

loracarbef
See cephalosporins—2nd generation

loratadine (Rx, OTC)
(lor-a′ti-deen)
Alavert, Claritin, Claritin Non-Drowsy Allergy, Claritin Reditabs, Tavist ND
Func. class.: Antihistamine (2nd generation)
Chem. class.: Selective histamine (H_1) receptor antagonist

Pregnancy category B

Action: Binds to peripheral histamine receptors, which provides antihistamine action without sedation

Therapeutic Outcome: Decreased nasal stuffiness, itching, swollen eyes

Uses: Seasonal rhinitis, chronic idiopathic urticaria for those ≥2 yr

Dosage and routes
Adult and child ≥6 yr: PO 10 mg daily
Child 2-5 yr: PO 5 mg daily

Renal dose
Adult: (CCr <30 ml/min) PO 10 mg every other day

Hepatic dose
Adult: PO 10 mg every other day

Available forms: Tabs 10 mg; rapid-disintegrating tabs 10 mg; orally disintegrating tabs 10 mg; syr 1 mg/ml, susp 5 mg/ml

Adverse effects
CNS: Sedation (more common with increased dosages), headache

Contraindications: Hypersensitivity, acute asthma attacks, lower respiratory tract disease

L

Precautions: Pregnancy **B,** increased intraocular pressure, bronchial asthma

Pharmacokinetics

Absorption	Well absorbed
Distribution	Unknown
Metabolism	Liver, extensively, to active metabolite desloratadine
Excretion	Kidneys
Half-life	17-28 hr

Pharmacodynamics

Onset	1-3 hr
Peak	8-12 hr
Duration	> 24 hr

Interactions

Individual drugs

Alcohol: increased CNS depression
Cimetidine, ketoconazole: increased loratadine level

Drug classifications

CNS depressants, antihistamines (other), opiates, sedative/hypnotics: increased CNS depression
Macrolides (clarithromycin, erythromycin): increased loratadine level
MAOIs: increased antihistamine effects

Drug/herb

Chamomile, hops, Jamaican dogwood, kava, khat, senega, skullcap, valerian: increased CNS depression
Corkwood, henbane: increased anticholinergic effect

Drug/food

Increased: absorption

NURSING CONSIDERATIONS

Assessment

- Assess allergy: hives, rash, rhinitis
- Assess respiratory status: rate, rhythm, increase in bronchial secretions, wheezing, chest tightness; provide fluids to 2 L/day to decrease secretion thickness

Nursing diagnoses

- Airway clearance, ineffective (uses)
- Knowledge, deficient (teaching)
- Noncompliance (teaching, overuse)

Implementation

- Give on an empty stomach, 1 hr ac or 2 hr pc to facilitate absorption
- Place rapidly disintegrating tabs on tongue, then swallow after disintegrated with or without water
- Use within 6 mo of opening pouch; immediately after opening blister pack
- Store in airtight, light-resistant container

Patient/family education

- Teach all aspects of drug uses; to notify prescriber if confusion, sedation, hypotension occur; to avoid driving and other hazardous activity if drowsiness occurs; to avoid alcohol and other CNS depressants that may potentiate effect
- Teach patient to take 1 hr ac or 2 hr pc to facilitate absorption
- Advise patient to use sunscreen or stay out of the sun to prevent burns
- Caution patient not to exceed recommended dosage; dysrhythmias may occur
- Teach patient that hard candy, gum, frequent rinsing of mouth may be used for dryness

Evaluation

Positive therapeutic outcome

- Absence of runny or congested nose, other allergy symptoms

lorazepam (Rx)

(lor-az′e-pam)

Apo-Lorazepam ♣, Ativan, lorazepam, Novo-Lorazem ♣, Nu-Loraz ♣

Func. class.: Sedative/hypnotic, antianxiety agent

Chem. class.: Benzodiazepine

Pregnancy category D

Controlled substance schedule IV

Do Not Confuse:
lorazepam/alprazolam/clonazepam

Action: Potentiates the actions of GABA, an inhibitory neurotransmitter, especially in the limbic system and reticular formation, which depresses the CNS

Therapeutic Outcome: Decreased anxiety, relaxation

Uses: Anxiety, irritability in psychiatric or organic disorders, preoperatively, insomnia

Investigational uses: Antiemetic before chemotherapy, status epilepticus, rectal use

Dosage and routes

Anxiety

Adult: PO 2-6 mg/day in divided doses, not to exceed 10 mg/day

Elderly: PO 0.5-1 mg/day in divided doses; or 0.5-1 mg at bedtime

Child: PO 0.05 mg/kg/dose, q4-8 hr

Insomnia

Adult: PO 2-4 mg at bedtime; only minimally effective after 2 wk continuous therapy
Elderly: PO 1-2 mg initially

Preoperatively

Adult: IM 50 mcg/kg 2 hr before surgery; **IV** 44 mcg/kg 15-20 min before surgery, max 2 mg 15-20 min prior to surgery
Child: 0.05 mg/kg

Status epilepticus

Neonate: 0.05 mg/kg
Child: 0.1 mg/kg up to 4 mg/dose; rec (off label) 0.05-0.1 mg × 2; wait 7 min before giving 2nd dose

Available forms: Tabs 0.5, 1, 2 mg; inj 2, 4 mg/ml; conc sol 2 mg/ml

Adverse effects

CNS: *Dizziness, drowsiness,* confusion, headache, anxiety, tremors, stimulation, fatigue, depression, insomnia, hallucinations, weakness, unsteadiness
CV: *Orthostatic hypotension,* **ECG changes, tachycardia,** hypotension; **apnea, cardiac arrest (IV, rapid)**
EENT: *Blurred vision,* tinnitus, mydriasis
GI: Constipation, dry mouth, nausea, vomiting, anorexia, diarrhea
INTEG: Rash, dermatitis, itching

Contraindications: Pregnancy **D,** hypersensitivity to benzodiazepines, narrow-angle glaucoma, psychosis, lactation

Precautions: Elderly, debilitated patients, history of drug abuse, COPD, child <12 yr, hepatic disease, renal disease

Pharmacokinetics

Absorption	Well absorbed (PO); completely absorbed (IM)
Distribution	Widely distributed; crosses placenta, blood-brain barrier
Metabolism	Liver, extensively
Excretion	Kidneys, breast milk
Half-life	14 hr

Pharmacodynamics

	PO	IM	IV
Onset	½ hr	15-30 min	5-15 min
Peak	1-3 hr	1-1½ hr	Unknown
Duration	3-6 hr	3-6 hr	3-6 hr

Interactions

Individual drugs

Alcohol: increased CNS depression

Drug classifications

CNS depressants, oral contraceptives: increased lorazepam effects
Disulfiram: increased lorazepam effects
Smoking: increased metabolism, decreased effect
Valproic acid: decreased lorazepam effects

Smoking

Increased metabolism, decreased effect

Drug/herb

Black cohosh: increased hypotension
Catnip, chamomile, clary, cowslip, hops, kava lavender, mistletoe, nettle, pokeweed, poppy, Queen Anne's lace, senega, skullcap, valerian: increased CNS depression

Drug/lab test

Increased: AST, ALT, serum bilirubin
False: increased 17-OHCS
Decreased: radioactive iodine uptake

NURSING CONSIDERATIONS

Assessment

- Assess degree of anxiety; what precipitates anxiety and whether drug controls symptoms; other signs of anxiety: dilated pupils, inability to sleep, restlessness, inability to focus
- Assess for alcohol withdrawal symptoms, including hallucinations (visual, auditory), delirium, irritability, agitation, fine to coarse tremors
- Monitor B/P (with patient lying/standing), pulse, check respiratory rate; if systolic B/P drops 20 mm Hg, hold drug, notify prescriber; respirations q5-15 min if given **IV**
- Monitor CBC during long-term therapy; blood dyscrasias have occurred (rarely)
- Monitor for seizure control; type, duration, and intensity of seizures; what precipitates seizures
- Monitor hepatic studies: AST, ALT, bilirubin, creatinine, LDH, alkaline phosphatase
- Assess mental status: mood, sensorium, affect, sleeping pattern, drowsiness, dizziness, suicidal tendencies, and ability of drug to control these symptoms; check for tolerance, withdrawal symptoms: headache, nausea, vomiting, muscle pain, weakness after long-term use

Nursing diagnoses

- Sleep pattern, disturbed (uses)
- Coping, ineffective (uses)
- Knowledge, deficient (teaching)
- Noncompliance (teaching)

Implementation

PO route

- Give with food or milk for GI symptoms; crush tab if patient is unable to swallow medication whole; provide sugarless gum, hard candy, frequent sips of water for dry mouth
- Use by SL route for rapid response (investigational use)

L

IM route

- Give deep in muscle mass; if using for preoperative sedation, give 2 hr or more before surgical procedure

IV route

- Prepare immediately before use, short stability time
- Dilute with sterile water for inj, 0.9% NaCl, or D_5W just before using; give by Y-site or 3-way stopcock at 2 mg/min
- Do not use sol that is discolored or contains a precipitate

Syringe compatibilities: Cimetidine, hydromorphone

Y-site compatibilities: Acyclovir, albumin, allopurinol, amifostine, amikacin, amoxicillin, amoxicillin/clavulanate, amsacrine, atracurium, bumetanide, cefepime, cefmetazole, cefotaxime, ciprofloxacin, cisatracurium, cisplatin, cladribine, clonidine, cyclophosphamide, cytarabine, dexamethasone, diltiazem, DOBUTamine, DOPamine, DOXOrubicin, epINEPHrine, erythromycin, etomidate, famotidine, fentanyl, filgrastim, fluconazole, fludarabine, furosemide, gentamicin, granisetron, haloperidol, heparin, hydrocortisone, hydromorphone, ketanserin, labetalol, melphalan, methotrexate, metronidazole, midazolam, milrinone, morphine, niCARdipine, nitroglycerin, norepinephrine, paclitaxel, pancuronium, piperacillin, piperacillin/tazobactam, potassium chloride, propofol, ranitidine, tacrolimus, teniposide, thiotepa, trimethoprim/sulfamethoxazole, vancomycin, vecuronium, vinorelbine, zidovudine

Y-site incompatibilities: Idarubicin, ondansetron, sargramostim

Patient/family education

- Advise patient that drug may be taken with food; that drug is not to be used for everyday stress or used longer than 4 mo unless directed by a prescriber; to take no more than prescribed amount; may be habit forming
- Caution patient to avoid OTC preparations unless approved by prescriber; to avoid alcohol, other psychotropic medications unless prescribed by physician; not to discontinue medication abruptly after long-term use
- Inform patient to avoid driving and activities that require alertness; drowsiness may occur; to rise slowly or fainting may occur, especially in elderly
- Inform patient that drowsiness may worsen at beginning of treatment

Evaluation

Positive therapeutic outcome

- Decreased anxiety, restlessness, insomnia

Treatment of overdose: Lavage, VS, supportive care

losartan (Rx)

(low-sar'tan)

Cozaar

Func. class.: Antihypertensive

Chem. class.: Angiotensin II receptor (type AT_1)

Pregnancy category
C (1st trimester),
D (2nd/3rd trimesters)

Do Not Confuse:
Cozaar/Zocor
losartan/valsartan

Action: Blocks the vasoconstrictor and aldosterone-secreting effects of angiotensin II; selectively blocks the binding of angiotensin II to the AT_1 receptor found in tissues

Therapeutic Outcome: Decreased B/P

Uses: Hypertension, alone or in combination; nephropathy in type 2 diabetes, hypertension with left ventricular hypertrophy

Dosage and routes

Hypertension

Adult: PO 50 mg daily alone or 25 mg daily when used in combination with diuretic

Nephropathy in type 2 diabetes

Adult: PO 50 mg daily, may increase to 100 mg daily

Hepatic dose

Adult: PO 25 mg daily as starting dose

Hypertension with left ventricular hypertrophy

Adult: PO 50 mg daily, add hydrochlorothiazide 12.5 mg/day and/or increase losartan to 100 mg daily, then increase hydrochlorothiazide to 25 mg daily

Available forms: Tabs 25, 50, 100 mg

Adverse effects

CNS: *Dizziness, insomnia,* anxiety, confusion, abnormal dreams, migraine, tremor, vertigo, headache

CV: Angina pectoris, 2nd- degree AV block, **CVA,** hypotension, **MI, dysrhythmias**

EENT: Blurred vision, burning eyes, conjunctivitis

GI: *Diarrhea, dyspepsia,* anorexia, constipation, dry mouth, flatulence, gastritis, vomiting

GU: Impotence, nocturia, urinary frequency, urinary tract infection, **renal failure**

HEMA: Anemia

INTEG: Alopecia, dermatitis, dry skin, flushing, photosensitivity, rash, pruritus, sweating **angioedema**
META: Gout
MS: Cramps, myalgia, pain, stiffness
RESP: *Cough, upper respiratory infection,* congestion, dyspnea, bronchitis

Contraindications: Pregnancy **D** (2nd/3rd trimesters), hypersensitivity

Precautions: Pregnancy **C** (1st trimester); hypersensitivity to ACE inhibitors; lactation, children, elderly

Pharmacokinetics

Absorption	Well
Distribution	Bound to plasma proteins
Metabolism	Extensive
Excretion	Feces, urine
Half-life	Biphasic, 2 hr, 6-9 hr

Pharmacodynamics

Unknown

Interactions

Individual drugs

Fluconazole: increased antihypertensive effect
Lithium: increased toxicity
Phenobarbital, rifamycin: decreased antihypertensive effect

Drug/herb

Aconite: increased toxicity, death
Astragalus, cola tree: increased or decreased antihypertensive effect
Barberry, betony, black catechu, black cohosh, bloodroot, broom, burdock, cat's claw, dandelion, goldenseal, Irish moss, Jamaican dogwood, kelp, khella, mistletoe, parsley: increased antihypertensive effect
Coltsfoot, guarana, khat, licorice: decreased antihypertensive effect

NURSING CONSIDERATIONS

Assessment

- Assess B/P with position changes, pulse q4h; note rate, rhythm, quality
- Monitor electrolytes: potassium, sodium, chloride
- Obtain baselines for renal, liver function tests before therapy begins
- Monitor for edema in feet, legs daily
- Assess for skin turgor, dryness of mucous membranes for hydratio status

Nursing diagnoses

- Fluid volume, deficient (side effects)
- Noncompliance (teaching)
- Knowledge, deficient (teaching)

Implementation

- Administer without regard to meals

Patient/family education

- Teach patient to avoid sunlight or wear sunscreen if in sunlight; photosensitivity may occur
- Advise patient to comply with dosage schedule, even if feeling better
- Teach patient to notify prescriber of mouth sores, fever, swelling of hands or feet, irregular heartbeat, chest pain
- Advise patient that excessive perspiration, dehydration, vomiting, diarrhea may lead to fall in blood pressure, consult prescriber if these occur
- Inform patient that drug may cause dizziness, fainting; light-headedness may occur
- Caution patient to rise slowly to sitting or standing position to minimize orthostatic hypotension
- Advise patient to use contraception while taking this product

Evaluation

Positive therapeutic outcome

- Decreased B/P

L

lovastatin (Rx)

(loe'va-sta-tin)
Altocor, Mevacor
Func. class.: Antilipemic
Chem. class.: HMG-CoA reductase inhibitor
Pregnancy category X

Do Not Confuse:
lovastatin/Lotensin

Action: By inhibiting HMG-CoA reductase, inhibits biosynthesis of VLDL and LDL, which are responsible for cholesterol development

Therapeutic Outcome: Decreased cholesterol levels and LDLs, increased HDLs

Uses: As an adjunct in primary hypercholesterolemia (types IIa, IIb), atherosclerosis, primary and secondary prevention of coronary events

Dosage and routes

(Patient should first be consuming a cholesterol-lowering diet)
Adult: PO 20 mg daily with evening meal; may increase to 20-80 mg/day in single or divided doses; not to exceed 80 mg/day; dosage adjustments should be made monthly; reduce dose in renal disease; ext rel 20-60 mg daily at bedtime

Available forms: Tabs 10, 20, 40 mg; ext rel tab (Altocor) 10, 20, 40, 60 mg

Adverse effects

CNS: Dizziness, headache, tremor, insomnia, paresthesia
EENT: Blurred vision, lens opacities
GI: Nausea, constipation, diarrhea, dyspepsia, *flatus,* abdominal pain, heartburn, **liver dysfunction,** vomiting, acid regurgitation, dry mouth, dysgeusia
HEMA: **Thrombocytopenia, hemolytic anemia, leukopenia**
INTEG: Rash, pruritus, photosensitivity
MS: Muscle cramps, myalgia, **myositis, rhabdomyolysis,** leg, shoulder or localized pain

Contraindications: Pregnancy **X,** hypersensitivity, lactation, active liver disease

Precautions: Past liver disease, alcoholism, severe acute infections, trauma, hypotension, uncontrolled seizure disorders, severe metabolic disorders, electrolyte imbalances, visual condition, children

Pharmacokinetics

Absorption	Poorly absorbed, erratic
Distribution	Crosses placenta, blood-brain barrier
Metabolism	Liver, extensively
Excretion	Feces (83%); kidneys, urine (10%)
Half-life	3-4 hr

Pharmacodynamics

Onset	Unknown
Peak	2-4 hr
Duration	Unknown

Interactions

Individual drugs

Cholestyramine: decreased action of lovastatin
Clofibrate, cycloSPORINE, erythromycin, gemfibrozil, niacin: increased myalgia, myositis
Digoxin: increased digoxin effect
Warfarin: increased bleeding

Drug classifications

Azole antifungals: increased myositis, myalgia
Bile acid sequestrants: increased lovastatin effects

Drug/herb

Glucomannan: increased effect
Gotu kola: decreased effect

Drug/food

Increased levels of lovastatin with food, must be taken with food
Grapefruit juice: increased toxicity

Drug/lab test

Increased: CPK, liver function tests

NURSING CONSIDERATIONS

Assessment

- Assess nutrition: fat, protein, carbohydrates; nutritional analysis should be completed by dietitian before treatment
- Monitor bowel pattern daily; diarrhea may be a problem
- Monitor triglycerides, fasting cholesterol LDL, HDL at baseline and throughout treatment; watch LDL and VLDL closely; if increased, drug should be discontinued
- Assess for muscle pain, tenderness, obtain CPK; if these occur, drug may need to be discontinued

Nursing diagnoses

- Diarrhea (adverse reactions)
- Knowledge, deficient (teaching)
- Noncompliance (teaching)

Implementation

- Give with evening meal; if dosage is increased, take with breakfast and evening meal
- Store in cool environment in airtight, light-resistant container

Patient/family education

- Inform patient that compliance is needed for positive results to occur; not to double doses
- Inform patient that blood work and ophthalmic exam will be necessary during treatment
- Teach patient that risk factors should be decreased: high-fat diet, smoking, alcohol consumption, absence of exercise
- Advise patient to report if pregnancy is suspected
- Advise patient to notify prescriber if the GI symptoms of diarrhea, abdominal or epigastric pain, nausea, vomiting occur; or if chills, fever, sore throat, blurred vision, dizziness, headache, muscle pain, weakness occur
- Advise patient to stay out of the sun or use sunscreen to prevent burns

Evaluation

Positive therapeutic outcome

- Decreased cholesterol, serum triglyceride levels
- Improved ratio of HDLs

loxapine (Rx)

(lox′a-peen)

Loxapac ✤, loxapine succinate ✤, Loxitane IM, Loxitane, Loxitane-C

Func. class.: Antipsychotic/neuroleptic

Chem. class.: Dibenzoxazepine

Pregnancy category C

Do Not Confuse:
Loxitane/Soriatane

Action: Depresses cerebral cortex, hypothalamus, limbic system, which control activity and aggression; blocks neurotransmission produced by DOPamine at synapse; exhibits strong α-adrenergic, anticholinergic blocking action; mechanism for antipsychotic effects is unclear

Therapeutic Outcome: Decreased psychotic behavior

Uses: Psychotic disorders, nonpsychotic symptoms associated with dementia

Investigational uses: Depression, anxiety

Dosage and routes

Adult: PO 10 mg bid-qid initially; may be rapidly increased depending on severity of condition; maintenance 60-100 mg/day; IM 12.5-50 mg q4-6h or more until desired response, then start PO form

Elderly: PO 5-10 mg daily bid, increase q4-7 days by 5-10 mg, max 125 mg

Available forms: Caps 5, 10, 25, 50 mg; conc 25 mg/ml; inj 50 mg/ml; tabs 5, 10, 25, 50 mg

Adverse effects

CNS: *Extrapyramidal symptoms (EPS): pseudoparkinsonism, akathisia, dystonia, tardive dyskinesia, drowsiness, headache,* **seizures,** confusion, **neuroleptic malignant syndrome**

CV: *Orthostatic hypotension,* **cardiac arrest,** ECG changes, tachycardia

EENT: Blurred vision, glaucoma

GI: *Dry mouth, nausea, vomiting, anorexia, constipation,* diarrhea, jaundice, weight gain

GU: Urinary retention, urinary frequency, enuresis, impotence, amenorrhea, gynecomastia

HEMA: **Anemia, leukopenia, leukocytosis, agranulocytosis**

INTEG: *Rash,* photosensitivity, dermatitis

RESP: **Laryngospasm,** dyspnea, **respiratory depression**

Contraindications: Hypersensitivity, blood dyscrasias, coma, severe CNS depression, brain damage, bone marrow depression, alcohol and barbiturate withdrawal states, narrow-angle glaucoma

Precautions: Pregnancy **C,** lactation, seizure disorders, hepatic disease, cardiac disease, prostatic hypertrophy, cardiac conditions, child <16 yr, elderly

Pharmacokinetics

Absorption	Well absorbed (PO)
Distribution	Unknown
Metabolism	Liver, extensively
Excretion	Kidneys
Half-life	Biphasic 5 hr, 19 hr

Pharmacodynamics

	PO	IM
Onset	½ hr	15-30 min
Peak	2-4 hr	15-20 min
Duration	12 hr	12 hr

Interactions

Individual drugs

Alcohol: increased CNS depression
EpINEPHrine: increased toxicity
Guanadrel, guanethidine: decreased effects

Drug classifications

Anticholinergics: increased anticholinergic effects
Antidepressants, MAOIs: increased CNS depression
Antipsychotics: increased EPS

Drug/herb

Betel palm, kava: increased EPS
Chamomile, cola tree, hops, nettle, nutmeg, skullcap, valerian: increased CNS depression

NURSING CONSIDERATIONS

Assessment

- Assess mental status: orientation, mood, behavior, presence and type of hallucinations before initial administration and monthly; this drug should significantly reduce psychotic behavior
- Check for swallowing of PO medication; check for hoarding or giving of medication to other patients
- Monitor I&O ratio; palpate bladder if low urinary output occurs, especially in elderly; urinalysis recommended before, during prolonged therapy, urinary retention may be cause
- Monitor bilirubin, CBC, liver function studies monthly
- Assess affect, orientation, LOC, reflexes, gait, coordination, sleep pattern disturbances
- Monitor B/P with patient sitting, standing,

L

and lying; take pulse and respirations q4h during initial treatment; establish baseline before starting treatment; report drops of 30 mm Hg
- Check for dizziness, faintness, palpitations, tachycardia on rising; severe orthostatic hypotension is common
- Identify for neuroleptic malignant syndrome: hyperpyrexia, muscle rigidity, increased CPK, altered mental status; drug should be discontinued
- Assess for EPS including akathisia (inability to sit still, no pattern to movements), tardive dyskinesia (bizarre movements of the jaw, mouth, tongue, extremities), pseudoparkinsonism (ragged tremors, pill rolling, shuffling gait); an antiparkinsonian drug should be prescribed
- Assess for constipation, urinary retention daily; if these occur, increase bulk, water in diet

Nursing diagnoses
- Thought processes, disturbed (uses)
- Coping, ineffective (uses)
- Knowledge, deficient (teaching)
- Noncompliance (teaching)

Implementation
PO route
- Administer drug in liq form mixed in glass of juice or cola if hoarding is suspected; do not mix in caffeine drinks, tannics, pectins
- Administer lowered dose in elderly, since metabolism is slowed
- Administer with full glass of water or milk; or give with food to decrease GI upset
- Give antacids 2 hr before or after taking this drug
- Store in airtight, light-resistant container, oral sol in amber bottle

IM route
- Inject deep in muscle mass; do not give SUBCUT; do not administer sol with a precipitate; amber-colored sol can be used
- Patient should remain lying down after IM inj for at least 30 min

Patient/family education
- Teach patient to use good oral hygiene; suggest frequent rinsing of mouth, sugarless gum for dry mouth; oral candidiasis can occur
- Caution patient to avoid hazardous activities until drug response is determined; dizziness, blurred vision may occur
- Inform patient that orthostatic hypotension occurs often and to rise from sitting or lying position gradually; caution patient to avoid hot tubs, hot showers, tub baths, since hypotension may occur; tell patient that in hot weather heat stroke may occur; take extra precautions to stay cool
- Advise patient to avoid abrupt withdrawal of this drug, or EPS may result; drug should be withdrawn slowly
- Advise patient to avoid use with alcohol, CNS depressants; increased drowsiness may occur
- Advise patient to use a sunscreen and sunglasses to prevent burns
- Suggest patient take antacids 2 hr before or after taking this drug
- Instruct patient to report sore throat, malaise, fever, bleeding, mouth sores; if these occur, CBC should be performed and drug discontinued

Evaluation
Positive therapeutic outcome
- Decrease in emotional excitement, hallucinations, delusions, paranoia
- Reorganization of patterns of thought, speech

Treatment of overdose: Lavage if orally ingested; barbiturates; provide airway, **IV** fluids; do not use epINEPHrine, which may increase hypotension

lymphocyte immune globulin (anti-thymocyte) (Rx)
Atgam

Func. class.: Immune globulin immunosuppressant

Pregnancy category C

Action: Produces immunosuppression by inhibiting the function of T-lymphocytes

Therapeutic Outcome: Absence of transplant rejection; hematologic remission (aplastic anemia)

Uses: Organ transplants to prevent rejection, aplastic anemia

Investigational uses: Multiple sclerosis, myasthenia gravis, immunosuppressant in liver, bone marrow, heart and other organ transplants, pure red cell aplasia, scleroderma

Dosage and routes
Renal allograft

Adult: **IV** 10-30 mg/kg/day

Child: **IV** 5-25 mg/kg/day

Delay of renal allograft rejection

Adult: **IV** 15 mg/kg/day × 14 days, then every other day × 14 days for a total of 21 doses in 28 days

Aplastic anemia
Adult: **IV** 10-20 mg/kg/day × 8-14 days

Available forms: Inj 50 mg horse gamma globulin/ml

Adverse effects
Renal transplant
CNS: *Fever, chills, headache, dizziness, weakness, faintness, seizures*
CV: *Chest pain, hypertension, tachycardia*
GI: *Diarrhea, nausea, vomiting, epigastric pain*
INTEG: *Rash, pruritus, urticaria, wheal*
SYST: **Anaphylaxis**
Aplastic anemia
CNS: Fever, chills, headache, **seizures,** light-headedness, encephalitis, postviral encephalopathy
CV: Bradycardia, myocarditis, irregularity
GI: Nausea, liver function test abnormality

Contraindications: Hypersensitivity

Precautions: Pregnancy **C,** severe renal disease, severe hepatic disease, lactation, children

Pharmacokinetics	
Absorption	Unknown
Distribution	Unknown
Metabolism	Unknown
Excretion	Unknown
Half-life	5.7 days

Pharmacodynamics	
Onset	Rapid
Peak	Unknown
Duration	Unknown

Interactions: None known

NURSING CONSIDERATIONS
Assessment
- Assess for infection, if infection occurs evaluation will be needed to continue treatment
- Monitor renal studies: BUN, creatinine at least monthly during treatment, 3 mo after treatment
- Monitor liver function studies: alkaline phosphatase, AST, ALT, bilirubin

Nursing diagnoses
- Mobility, impaired (uses)
- Infection, risk for (uses)
- Knowledge, deficient (teaching)

Implementation
IV route
- Do not infuse <4 hr
- Keep emergency equipment nearby for severe allergic reactions
- Skin testing must be completed before treatment; use intradermal inj of 0.1 ml of a 1:1000 dilution (5 mcg of horse IgG) in 0.9% NaCl, if a wheal or rash >10 mm or both, use caution during inf
- Dilute in saline sol before inf; invert **IV** bag, so undiluted drug does not contact the air inside, concentration should not be >1 mg/ml

Patient/family education
- Advise patient to report fever, rash, chills, sore throat, fatigue, since serious infections may occur
- Caution patient to use contraceptive measures during treatment and for 12 wk after ending therapy; drug is teratogenic
- Caution patient to avoid crowds and persons with known infections to reduce risk of infection

Evaluation
Positive therapeutic outcome
- Absence of graft rejection
- Hematologic recovery (aplastic anemia)

M

magaldrate (OTC)
(mag′al-drate)
Losapan ✤, Lowsium, Riopan, Riopan Extra Strength ✤
Func. class.: Antacid
Chem. class.: Aluminum/magnesium hydroxide

Pregnancy category C

Action: Neutralizes gastric acidity; drug is dissolved in gastric contents; this drug is a combination of aluminum and magnesium

Therapeutic Outcome: Decreased pain of ulcers

Uses: Antacid, peptic ulcer disease (adjunct), indigestion/heartburn, duodenal and gastric ulcers, reflex esophagitis, hyperacidity

Dosage and routes
Adult: SUSP 5-10 ml (400-800 mg) with water between meals, at bedtime, not to exceed 100 ml/day

Available forms: Susp 540 mg/5 ml; liq 540 mg/5 ml

Adverse effects

GI: Constipation, diarrhea
META: Hypermagnesemia, hypophosphatemia

Contraindications: Hypersensitivity to this drug or aluminum products

Precautions: Pregnancy **C**, elderly, fluid restriction, decreased GI motility, GI obstruction, dehydration, renal disease, sodium-restricted diets

Pharmacokinetics

Absorption	Not absorbed
Distribution	Not distributed
Metabolism	Not metabolized
Excretion	Kidneys
Half-life	Unknown

Pharmacodynamics

Onset	Unknown
Peak	½ hr
Duration	1 hr

Interactions

Individual drugs

Chlordiazepoxide, cimetidine, isoniazid, ketoconazole, phenytoin, tetracycline: decreased absorption of each specific drug
Flecainide, quinidine: increased action when taken in large amounts

Drug classifications

Amphetamines: increased action when taken in large amounts
Anticholinergics, corticosteroids, fluoroquinolones, iron salts, phenothiazines: decreased absorption of each specific drug
Salicylates: decreased action when taken in large amounts

NURSING CONSIDERATIONS

Assessment

- Assess GI status: location of pain, intensity, characteristics, what aggravates, ameliorates pain; heartburn/indigestion; hematemesis
- Monitor serum magnesium, calcium, phosphate, potassium if using long term or with impaired renal function
- Assess for constipation: increase bulk in diet if needed or obtain order for stool softener

Nursing diagnoses

- Pain, acute (uses)
- Knowledge, deficient (teaching)

Implementation

- Take antacids 2 hr before or 2 hr after taking enteric-coated drugs
- Give laxatives or stool softeners if constipation occurs
- Give susp after shaking; give between meals and at bedtime
- Give when stomach is empty pc and at bedtime

Patient/family education

- Advise patient to separate ingestion of enteric-coated drugs and antacid by 2 hr
- Advise patient to use 2 wk or less; drug should not be used for long periods
- Teach patient to notify prescriber immediately if coffee-ground emesis, emesis with frank blood, or black tarry stools occur

Evaluation

Positive therapeutic outcome

- Absence of abdominal pain
- Decreased acidity

magnesium salts (OTC)

(mag-neez′ee-um)

magnesium chloride (OTC)
Chloromag, Slo-Mag

magnesium citrate (OTC)
Citrate of Magnesia, Citroma, Citromag ✤

magnesium gluconate (OTC)
Almoate Magonate, magtrate

magnesium hydroxide (OTC)
Phillips Magnesia Tablets, Phillips Milk of Magnesia, MOM

magnesium oxide (OTC)
Mag-Ox 400, Maox, Uro-Mag

magnesium sulfate (OTC, Rx)
epsom salt, magnesium sulfate (**IV**)

HIGH ALERT

Func. class.: Electrolyte; anticonvulsant, laxative, saline; antacid

Pregnancy category A, B

Action: Increases osmotic pressure, draws fluid into colon, neutralizes HCl

Therapeutic Outcome: Magnesium levels WNL, absence of constipation

Uses: Constipation, bowel preparation before surgery or exam, electrolyte, anticonvulsant, in preeclampsia, eclampsia (magnesium sulfate)

Dosage and routes

Laxative

Adult: PO 30-60 ml at bedtime (Milk of Magnesia), 300 mg
Adult and child >6 yr: PO 15 g in 8 oz of H_2O (magnesium sulfate); PO 10-20 ml

(Concentrated Milk of Magnesia); PO 5-10 oz at bedtime (magnesium citrate)
Child 2-6 yr: 5-15 ml/day (Milk of Magnesia)

Prevention of magnesium deficiency
Adult and child ≥10 yr: PO male: 350-400 mg/day; female: 280-300 mg/day; lactation: 335-350 mg/day; pregnancy 320 mg/day
Child 8-10 yr: PO 170 mg/day
Child 4-7 yr: PO 120 mg/day
Infant to 4 yr: 40-80 mg/day

Magnesium sulfate deficiency
Adult: PO 200-400 mg in divided doses tid-qid; IM 1 g q6h × 4 doses; **IV** 5 g (severe)
Child 6-12 yr: 3-6 mg/kg/day in divided doses tid-qid

Preeclampsia/eclampsia magnesium sulfate
Adult: IM/**IV** 4-5 g **IV** inf; with 5 g IM in each gluteus, then 5 g q4h or 4 g **IV** inf, then 1-2 g/hr cont inf, max 40 g/day or 20 g/48 hr in severe renal disease

Available forms: Chloride: sus rel tabs 535 mg (64 mg Mg); enteric tabs 833 mg (100 mg Mg); hydroxide: liq 400 mg/5 ml (164 mg Mg/5 ml); conc liq 800 mg/5 ml (328 mg Mg/5 ml); chew tabs 300, 600 mg; oxide: tabs 400 mg (241.3 mg Mg); caps 140 mg (84.5 mg Mg); sulfate: powder for oral; bulk packages; (epsom salts) bulk packages; inj 10, 12.5, 25, 50%; citrate: oral sol 240, 296, 300 ml bottles (77 mEq/100 ml)

Adverse effects

CNS: Muscle weakness, flushing, sweating, confusion, sedation, depressed reflexes, **flaccid paralysis, hypothermia**
CV: Hypotension, heart block, **circulatory collapse**
GI: *Nausea, vomiting, anorexia, cramps*
META: Electrolyte, fluid imbalances
RESP: Respiratory depression

Contraindications: Hypersensitivity, abdominal pain, nausea/vomiting, obstruction, acute surgical abdomen, rectal bleeding

Precautions: Pregnancy **A, B** (magnesium sulfate), renal disease, cardiac disease

Pharmacokinetics

PO	Onset 3-6 hr
IM	Onset 1 hr, duration 4 hr
IV	Duration ½ hr

Pharmacodynamics

Onset	Unknown
Distribution	Unknown
Metabolized	Unknown
Excreted	Kidneys
Half-life	Unknown effective anticonvulsant levels 2.5-7.5 mEq/L

Interactions

Individual drugs
Nitrofurantoin: decreased absorption

Drug classifications
Antiinfectives (aminoquinolones), tetracyclines: decreased absorption
Neuromuscular blockers: increased effect

NURSING CONSIDERATIONS

Assessment

- Assess I&O ratio; check for decrease in urinary output
- Assess cause of constipation; lack of fluids, bulk, exercise
- Assess cramping, rectal bleeding, nausea, vomiting; drug should be discontinued
- Assess Mg toxicity: thirst, confusion, decrease in reflexes
- Assess visual changes: blurring, halos, corneal and retinal damage
- Assess edema in feet, ankles, legs
- Assess prior drug history; there are many drug interactions

Nursing diagnoses

- Constipation (uses)
- Injury, risk for, physical
- Knowledge, deficient (teaching)

Implementation

PO route

- Administer with 8 oz of H_2O
- Refrigerate magnesium citrate before administration
- Shake susp before using
- Give as antacid at least 2 hr pc
- Administer to patient crushed or whole; chewable tablets may be chewed
- Administer with food or milk to decrease gastric symptoms; give 30 min before or 2 hr after antacids

IV route

- Administer only when calcium gluconate available for magnesium toxicity
- Administer **IV** undiluted 1.5 ml of 10% sol over 1 min; may dilute to 20% sol, infuse over 3 hr
- Administer **IV** at less than 150 mg/min; circulatory collapse may occur

M

Y-site compatibilities: Acyclovir, aldesleukin, amifostine, amikacin, ampicillin, aztreonam, cefamandole, cefazolin, cefmetazole, cefoperazone, cefotaxime, cefoxitin, cephalothin, cephapirin, chloramphenicol, cisatracurium, DOBUTamine, doxycycline, DOXOrubicin liposome, enalaprilat, erythromycin, esmolol, famotidine, fludarabine, gallium, gentamicin, granisetron, heparin, hydromorphone, idarubicin, insulin, kanamycin, labetalol, meperidine, metronidazole, minocycline, morphine, moxalactam, nafcillin, ondansetron, oxacillin, paclitaxel, penicillin G potassium, piperacillin, piperacillin/tazobactam, potassium chloride, propofol, remifentanil, sargramostim, thiotepa, ticarcillin, tobramycin, trimethoprim/sulfamethoxazole, vancomycin, vit B complex/C

Additive compatibilities: Cephalothin, chloramphenicol, cisplatin, heparin, hydrocortisone, isoproterenol, meropenem, methyldopate, norepinephrine, penicillin G potassium, potassium phosphate, verapamil

Patient/family education

- Inform patient to report any symptoms of hepatotoxicity, renal toxicity, visual changes, ototoxicity, allergic reactions, bleeding (long-term therapy)
- Inform patient not to exceed recommended dosage; acute poisoning may result
- Inform patient to read label on other OTC drugs; many contain aspirin
- Inform patient that therapeutic response takes 2 wk (arthritis)
- Inform patient to avoid alcohol ingestion; GI bleeding may occur
- Inform patient that if anticoagulants are given with this drug, both should be discontinued 2 wk before surgery

Evaluation

Positive therapeutic outcome

- Decreased pain, fever

Treatment of overdose: Lavage, activated charcoal, monitor electrolytes, VS

mannitol (Rx)

(man'i-tole)

mannitol, Osmitrol, Resectisol

Func. class.: Diuretic-osmotic

Chem. class.: Hexahydric alcohol

Pregnancy category C

Action: Increases osmolarity of glomerular filtrate, which raises osmotic pressure of fluid in renal tubules; there is a decrease in reabsorption of water, electrolytes; increases in urinary output, sodium, chloride, potassium, calcium, phosphorus, uric acid, urea, magnesium

Uses: Edema; promote systemic diuresis in cerebral edema, decrease intraocular pressure, improve renal function in acute renal failure, chemical poisoning

Dosage and routes

Oliguria, prevention

Adult: **IV** 50-100 g of a 5%-25% sol, may use test dose 0.2 g/kg over 3-5 min

Oliguria, treatment

Adult: **IV** 300-400 mg/kg of a 20%-25% sol up to 100 g of a 15%-20% sol over 30-60 min

Child: **IV** 0.25-2 g/kg as a 15%-20% sol, run over 2-6 hr

Intraocular pressure/ICP

Adult: **IV** 1.5-2 g/kg of a 15%-25% sol over 30-60 min

Child: **IV** 1-2 g/kg (30-60 g/m^2) as a 15%-20% sol run over 30-60 min

Renal failure

Adult: **IV** 50-200 g/24 hr, adjusting to maintain output of 30-50 mg/hr

Diuresis in drug intoxication

Adult and child >12 yr: 5%-10% sol continuously up to 200 g **IV**, while maintaining 100-500 ml urine output/hr

Available forms: Inj 5%, 10%, 15%, 20%, 25%; GU irrigation 5%

Adverse effects

CNS: Dizziness, headache, **seizures, rebound increased ICP,** confusion

CV: Edema, hypotension, hypertension, **tachycardia, CHF,** thrombophlebitis, angina-like chest pains, fever, chills

EENT: Loss of hearing, blurred vision, nasal congestion, decreased intraocular pressure

ELECT: Fluid, electrolyte imbalances, **acidosis,** electrolyte loss, dehydration

GI: *Nausea, vomiting,* dry mouth, diarrhea

GU: Marked diuresis, urinary retention, thirst

RESP: Pulmonary congestion

Contraindications: Active intracranial bleeding, hypersensitivity, anuria, severe pulmonary congestion, edema, severe dehydration, progressive heart disease, renal failure

Precautions: Pregnancy **C,** dehydration, severe renal disease, CHF, lactation

Pharmacokinetics

Absorption	Complete
Distribution	Extracellular spaces
Metabolism	Minimal
Excretion	Renal
Half-life	100 min

Pharmacodynamics

Onset	½-1 hr
Peak	1 hr
Duration	6-8 hr

Interactions

Individual drugs

Lithium: decreased action; increased excretion

Drug/food

Potassium foods: increased hyperkalemia

Drug/lab test

Interference: inorganic phosphorus, ethylene glycol

NURSING CONSIDERATIONS

Assessment

- Assess neurologic status: LOC, ICP reading, pupil size and reaction when drug is given for increased ICP
- Assess for visual changes or eye discomfort or pain before and during treatment; (increases intraocular pressure); neurologic checks, ICP during treatment (increased ICP)
- Assess patient for tinnitus, hearing loss, ear pain; periodic testing of hearing is needed when high doses of this drug are given by **IV** route
- Monitor manifestations of hypokalemia: acidic urine, reduced urine osmolality, nocturia, polyuria, polydipsia; hypotension, broad T wave, U wave, ectopy, tachycardia, weak pulse; muscle weakness, altered LOC, drowsiness, apathy, lethargy, confusion, depression; anorexia, nausea, cramps, constipation, distention, paralytic ileus; hypoventilation, respiratory muscle weakness
- Monitor for manifestations of hyponatremia: increased B/P, cold, clammy skin, hypovolemia or hypervolemia; anorexia, nausea, vomiting, diarrhea, abdominal cramps; lethargy, increased ICP, confusion, headache, seizures, coma, fatigue, tremors, hyperreflexia
- Assess fluid volume status: check I&O ratios and record hourly urine values, CVP, breath sounds, weight, distended red veins, crackles in lung, color, quality and sp gr of urine, skin turgor, adequacy of pulses, moist mucous membranes, bilateral lung sounds, peripheral pitting edema
- Assess for dehydration; symptoms of decreasing output, thirst, hypotension, dry mouth and mucous membranes should be reported
- Monitor electrolytes: potassium, sodium, calcium, magnesium; also include BUN, ABGs, CVP, PAP, CBC; regularly monitor serum and urine levels of sodium and potassium
- Assess B/P before and during therapy with patient lying, standing, and sitting as appropriate; orthostatic hypotension can occur rapidly
- Monitor for rebound ICP: headache, confusion

Nursing diagnoses

- Urinary elimination, impaired (adverse reactions)
- Fluid volume, deficient (adverse reactions)
- Fluid volume, excess (uses)
- Knowledge, deficient (teaching)

Implementation

- Administer potassium replacement if potassium level is less than 3 mg/ml
- Use an in-line filter for 15%, 20%, 25% give with infusion pump; check **IV** patency at infusion site before and during administration; do not use sol that is yellow or has a precipitate or crystals; to redissolve, run bottle under hot water and shake vigorously; cool to body temp before giving
- Run at 30-50 ml/hr in oliguria
- Run over 30-60 min in increased ICP
- Run over 30 min for intraocular pressure; 60-90 min after surgery

Irrigation

- Use 100 ml of 25%/900 ml of sterile water for inj (2.5% sol)

Y-site compatibilities: Allopurinol, amifostine, aztreonam, cladribine, fludarabine, fluorouracil, gallium, idarubicin, melphalan, ondansetron, paclitaxel, piperacillin, propofol, sargramostim, teniposide, thiotepa, vinorelbine

Y-site incompatibilities: Amsacrine, bleomycin, DOXOrubicin, fluconazole, gentamicin, quinidine, vinBLAStine, vinCRIStine

Additive compatibilities: Amikacin, bretylium, cefamandole, cefoxitin, cimetidine, cisplatin, DOPamine, fosphenytoin, furosemide, gentamicin, metoclopramide, netilmicin, nizatidine, ofloxacin, ondansetron, sodium bicarbonate, tobramycin, verapamil

Additive incompatibilities: Blood, blood products, imipenem-cilastatin, potassium chloride, sodium chloride

Patient/family education

- Teach patient reason for and method of treatment

M

Evaluation

Positive therapeutic outcome

- Decreased intraocular pressure
- Prevention of hypokalemia (diuretic use)
- Decreased edema
- Decreased ICP
- Increased diuresis of >30 ml/hr
- Increased excretion of toxic substances

Treatment of overdose: Discontinue inf, correct fluid, electrolyte imbalances, hemodialysis, monitor hydration, CV, renal function

mebendazole (Rx)

(me-ben′da-zole)

Vermox

Func. class.: Anthelmintic

Chem. class.: Carbamate

Pregnancy category C

Action: Inhibits glucose uptake, degeneration of cytoplasmic microtubules in the cell; interferes with absorption, secretory function

Therapeutic Outcome: Parasite, cyst, egg death

Uses: Infestation with pinworms, roundworms, hookworms, whipworms, threadworms, pork tapeworms, dwarf tapeworms, beef tapeworms; hydatid cyst

Dosage and routes

Adult and child >2 yr: PO 100 mg as a single dose (pinworms) or bid × 3 days (whip-, round-, or hookworms); course may be repeated in 3 wk if needed

Available forms: Chew tabs 100 mg

Adverse effects

CNS: Dizziness, fever, headache

GI: Transient diarrhea, abdominal pain, nausea, vomiting

Contraindication: Hypersensitivity

Precautions: Pregnancy **C** (1st trimester), child <2 yr, lactation, Crohn's disease, hepatic disease, IBD, ulcerative colitis

Pharmacokinetics	
Absorption	Minimal
Distribution	Highly bound to plasma proteins
Metabolism	Liver
Excretion	Feces in metabolites (>95%); urine, unchanged
Half-life	2½-9 hr; increased in hepatic disease

Pharmacodynamics	
Onset	Unknown
Peak	½-7 hr
Duration	Unknown

Interactions

Individual drugs

Carbamazepine: decreased effect of mebendazole

Drug classifications

Hydantoins: decreased effect of mebendazole

Drug/food

High-fat foods: increased absorption

NURSING CONSIDERATIONS

Assessment

- Assess stools during entire treatment, also 1-3 wk after treatment is completed; specimens must be sent to lab while still warm; monitor for diarrhea during expulsion of worms; avoid self-contamination with patient's feces
- Assess for allergic reaction: rash (rare)
- Identify infestation in other family members, since transmission from person to person is common
- If pinworms are suspected, place a piece of cellophane tape over the anal area at night for 1 wk after treatment at night to identify ova; negative perianal swabs taken every AM for 3 days confirm that the patient is no longer infested
- Monitor blood studies: AST, ALT, alkaline phosphatase, BUN, CBC during treatment

Nursing diagnoses

- Infection, risk for (uses)
- Knowledge, deficient (teaching)

Implementation

- Tabs may be chewed or crushed and mixed with food if patient is unable to swallow whole
- Give PO after meals to avoid GI symptoms, since absorption is not decreased by food
- Give second course after 3 wk if needed; usually recommended (pinworms)
- Store in airtight container

Patient/family education

- Teach patient proper hygiene after bowel movements, including hand-washing technique; tell patient to avoid putting fingers in mouth; clean fingernails
- Advise patient that infested person should sleep alone; do not shake bed linen; wash bed linen daily in hot water; change and wash undergarments daily; that all members of the family should be treated (pinworms)

- Advise patient to clean toilet daily with disinfectant (green soap sol)
- Inform patient that compliance is needed with dosage schedule, duration of treatment
- Tell patient to wear shoes, wash all fruits and vegetables well before eating, use commercial fruit and vegetable cleaner solution

Evaluation

Positive therapeutic outcome
- Expulsion of worms
- Three negative stool cultures after completion of treatment

mechlorethamine (Rx)

(me-klor-eth'a-meen)

Mustargen, nitrogen mustard

Func. class.: Antineoplastic alkylating agent

Chem. class.: Nitrogen mustard

Pregnancy category D

Action: Alkylates DNA, RNA; inhibits enzymes that allow synthesis of amino acids in proteins; activity is not cell cycle phase specific; a vesicant

Therapeutic Outcome: Prevention of rapidly growing malignant cells

Uses: Hodgkin's disease, lymphomas, leukemias, lymphosarcoma; ovarian, breast, lung carcinoma; neoplastic effusions

Dosage and routes

Adult: **IV** 0.4 mg/kg or 10 mg/m^2 as 1 dose or 2-4 divided doses over 2-4 days; second course after 3 wk depending on blood cell count

Neoplastic effusions

Adult: Intracavity 0.4 mg/kg, may be 200-400 mcg/kg

Available forms: Inj 10 mg/vial

Adverse effects

CNS: *Headache, dizziness, drowsiness, paresthesia,* peripheral neuropathy, **coma**

EENT: Tinnitus, hearing loss

GI: *Nausea, vomiting, diarrhea, stomatitis, weight loss,* colitis, **hepatotoxicity**

HEMA: **Thrombocytopenia, leukopenia, agranulocytosis,** anemia

INTEG: *Alopecia,* pruritus, herpes zoster, extravasation

Contraindications: Pregnancy **D**, lactation, myelosuppression, acute herpes zoster

Precautions: Radiation therapy, chronic lymphocytic leukopenia

Pharmacokinetics

Absorption	Complete (**IV**)
Distribution	Unknown
Metabolism	Tissues/fluids
Excretion	Kidneys
Half-life	Unknown

Pharmacodynamics

	IV
Onset	1 day
Peak	1-2 wk
Duration	1-3 wk

Interactions

Individual drugs

Amphotericin B: increased blood dyscrasia
Aspirin: increased bleeding
Radiation: increased toxicity

Drug classifications

Anticoagulants: increased bleeding
Antineoplastics: increased toxicity
Live virus vaccines: decreased antibody reaction

Drug/lab test

Increased: uric acid

NURSING CONSIDERATIONS

Assessment

- Monitor CBC, differential, platelet count weekly; withhold drug if WBC is <1000/mm^3 or platelet count is <75,000/mm^3; notify prescriber of results if WBC <20,000/mm^3, platelets <150,000/mm^3; recovery of WBC platelets within 20 days
- Monitor pulmonary function tests, chest x-ray films before, during therapy; chest film should be obtained q2 wk during treatment; assess for dyspnea, crackles, unproductive cough, chest pain, tachypnea
- Assess for increased uric acid levels, swelling, joint pain primarily in extremities; patient should be well hydrated to prevent urate deposits
- Monitor renal function studies: BUN, serum uric acid, urine CCr before, during therapy; I&O ratio; report fall in urine output of 30 ml/hr; for decreased hyperuricemia
- Monitor for cold, fever, sore throat (may indicate beginning of infection); identify edema in feet, joint and stomach pain, shaking; prescriber should be notified
- Assess for bleeding: hematuria, guaiac, bruising or petechiae, mucosa or orifices q8h; no rec temp

Nursing diagnoses

- Injury, risk for (adverse reactions)
- Body image, disturbed (adverse reactions)

M

- Infection, risk for (adverse reactions)
- Knowledge, deficient (teaching)

Implementation

- Give fluids **IV** or PO before chemotherapy to hydrate patient
- Give antacid before oral agent; give drug after evening meal, before bedtime; administer antiemetic 30-60 min before giving drug and prn to prevent vomiting; give antibiotics for prophylaxis of infection
- Give top or systemic analgesics for pain
- Give in AM so drug can be eliminated before bedtime
- Use a liq diet: carbonated beverages; gelatin may be added if patient is not nauseated or vomiting

Intracavity route

- Further dilute in 100 ml of 0.9% NaCl; administration is completed by prescriber
- Watch for infiltration; if infiltration occurs, infiltrate area with isotonic sodium thiosulfate or 1% lidocaine; apply ice for 6-12 hr

IV route

- Give **IV** after diluting 10 mg/10 ml sterile water or 0.9% NaCl; leave needle in vial, shake, withdraw dose, give through Y-tube or 3-way stopcock or directly over 3-5 min into running **IV** of 0.9% NaCl

Y-site compatibilities: Amifostine, aztreonam, filgrastim, fludarabine, granisetron, melphalan, ondansetron, sargramostim, teniposide, vinorelbine

Additive incompatibilities: Methohexital

Solution incompatibilities: D_5W, 0.9% NaCl (**IV** only)

Patient/family education

- Teach patient to avoid use of products containing aspirin or ibuprofen, razors, commercial mouthwash, since bleeding may occur; to report symptoms of bleeding (hematuria, tarry stools)
- Teach patient to report signs of anemia (fatigue, headache, irritability, faintness, shortness of breath)
- Advise patient to report any changes in breathing or coughing even several mo after treatment; to avoid crowds and persons with respiratory tract or other infections
- Tell patient hair loss is common; discuss the use of wigs or hairpieces
- Caution patient not to have any vaccinations without the advice of the prescriber, serious reactions can occur
- Advise patient that contraception is needed during treatment and for several mo after the completion of therapy
- Have patient rinse mouth tid-qid with water, club soda; brush teeth bid-qid with soft brush or cotton-tipped applicators for stomatitis; use unwaxed dental floss

Evaluation

Positive therapeutic outcome

- Decreased size of tumor
- Decreased spread of malignancy
- Improved blood values
- Absence of sweating at night
- Increased appetite, increased weight

meclizine (OTC, Rx)

(mek'li-zeen)

Antivert, Antrizine, Bonamine ✤, Bonine, Dramamine Less Drowsy Formula, meclizine HCl, Meni-D, Vergan

Func. class.: Antiemetic, antihistamine, anticholinergic

Chem. class.: H_1-Receptor antagonist, piperazine derivative

Pregnancy category B

Action: Acts centrally by blocking chemoreceptor trigger zone, which in turn acts on vomiting center

Therapeutic Outcome: Decreased nausea in motion sickness; decreased vertigo

Uses: Vertigo, motion sickness

Dosage and routes

Vertigo

Adult: PO 25-100 mg daily in divided doses

Motion sickness

Adult: PO 12.5-25 mg 1 hr before traveling; repeat dose q12-24 hr prn

Available forms: Tabs 12.5, 25, 50 mg; chew tabs 25 mg; caps 25, 30 mg

Adverse effects

CNS: *Drowsiness,* fatigue, restlessness, headache, insomnia

CV: Hypotension

EENT: Dry mouth, blurred vision

GI: Nausea, anorexia, constipation, increased appetite

GU: Urinary retention

Contraindications: Hypersensitivity to cyclizines, shock

Precautions: Pregnancy **B**, children, narrow-angle glaucoma, glaucoma, urinary retention, lactation, prostatic hypertrophy, elderly, CV disease, hypertension, seizure disease

Pharmacokinetics

Absorption	Well
Distribution	Unknown
Metabolism	Unknown
Excretion	Unknown
Half-life	6 hr

Pharmacodynamics

Onset	1 hr
Peak	Unknown
Duration	8-24 hr

Interactions

Drug classifications

CNS depressants: increased CNS depression
Anticholinergics: increased anticholinergic effect

Drug/herb

Corkwood, henbane leaf: increased anticholinergic effect
Hops, Jamaican dogwood, khat, senega: increased sedative effect

Drug/lab test

False negative: allergy skin testing

NURSING CONSIDERATIONS

Assessment

- Monitor VS, B/P
- Assess for signs of toxicity of other drugs or masking of symptoms of disease: brain tumor, intestinal obstruction
- Observe for drowsiness, dizziness, level of consciousness

Nursing diagnoses

- Injury, risk for (adverse reactions)
- Knowledge, deficient (teaching)

Implementation

- Tablets may be swallowed whole, chewed, or allowed to dissolve; give with food to decrease GI upset
- Give lowest possible dose in elderly, anticholinergic effects

Patient/family education

- Teach patient that a false-negative result may occur with skin testing for allergies; these procedures should not be scheduled for 4 days after discontinuing use
- Teach patient to avoid hazardous activities, activities requiring alertness; dizziness may occur; instruct patient to request assistance with ambulation
- Teach patient to avoid alcohol, other depressants

Evaluation

Positive therapeutic outcome

- Absence of dizziness, vomiting

medroxyPROGESTERone (Rx)

(me-drox-ee-proe-jess'te-rone)
Amen, Curretab, Cycrin, Depo-Provera, medroxyPROGESTERone, Provera
Func. class.: Hormone—progestogen; contraceptive; antineoplastic
Chem. class.: Progesterone derivative

Pregnancy category X

Do Not Confuse:
Amen/Ambien, medroxyPROGESTERone/methylPREDNISolone, Provera/Premarin

Action: Inhibits secretion of pituitary gonadotropins, which prevents follicular maturation and ovulation; stimulates growth of mammary tissue; antineoplastic action against endometrial cancer

Therapeutic Outcome: Decreased abnormal uterine bleeding, absence of amenorrhea

Uses: Uterine bleeding (abnormal), secondary amenorrhea, endometrial cancer, renal cancer, contraceptive, prevention of endometrial changes associated with estrogen replacement therapy (ERT)

Investigational uses: Pickwickian syndrome, sleep apnea, hypersomnolence

Dosage and routes

Secondary amenorrhea

Adult: PO 5-10 mg daily × 5-10 days

Uterine bleeding

Adult: PO 5-10 mg daily × 5-10 days starting on 16th or 21st day of menstrual cycle

With ERT

Adult: PO monophasic 2.5 mg daily; biphasic 5 mg days 15-28 of cycle

Available forms: Tabs 2.5, 5, 10 mg; inj susp 50, 100, 150, 400 mg/ml

Adverse effects

CNS: Dizziness, headache, migraines, depression, fatigue
CV: Hypotension, thrombophlebitis, edema, **thromboembolism, stroke, pulmonary embolism, MI**
EENT: Diplopia
GI: *Nausea,* vomiting, anorexia, cramps, increased weight, **cholestatic jaundice**
GU: Amenorrhea, cervical erosion, breakthrough bleeding, dysmenorrhea, vaginal candidiasis, breast changes, *gynecomastia, testicular atrophy, impotence,* endometriosis, **spontaneous abortion**

M

INTEG: Rash, urticaria, acne, hirsutism, alopecia, oily skin, seborrhea, purpura, melasma, photosensitivity
META: Hyperglycemia
***SYST:* Angioedema, anaphylaxis**

Contraindications: Pregnancy **X,** breast cancer, hypersensitivity, thromboembolic disorders, reproductive cancer, genital bleeding (abnormal, undiagnosed)

Precautions: Lactation, hypertension, asthma, blood dyscrasias, gallbladder disease, CHF, diabetes mellitus, bone disease, depression, migraine headache, seizure disorders, hepatic disease, renal disease, family history of cancer of breast or reproductive tract

Pharmacokinetics

Absorption	Unknown
Distribution	Unknown
Metabolism	Unknown
Excretion	Unknown
Half-life	Unknown

Pharmacodynamics

	PO	IM
Onset	Unknown	Unknown
Peak	Unknown	Unknown
Duration	2-4 hr	Unknown

Interactions
Individual drugs
Aminoglutethimide: decreased contraceptive effect
Drug/lab test
Increased: alkaline phosphatase, pregnanediol, amino acids, sodium
Decreased: GTT, HDL

NURSING CONSIDERATIONS
Assessment
- Assess for symptoms indicating severe allergic reaction, angioedema; have epINEPHrine and resuscitative equipment available
- Monitor B/P at beginning of treatment and periodically; check weight daily; notify prescriber of weekly weight gain >5 lb
- Monitor I&O ratio: be alert for decreasing urinary output, increasing edema, hypertension
- Assess liver function studies: ALT, AST, bilirubin, periodically during long-term therapy
- Assess for edema, hypertension, cardiac symptoms, jaundice
- Assess mental status: affect, mood, behavioral changes, depression

Nursing diagnoses
- Sexual dysfunction (uses)
- Tissue perfusion, ineffective (adverse reactions)
- Injury, risk for (adverse reactions)
- Knowledge, deficient (teaching)

Implementation
PO route
- Give with food or milk to decrease GI symptoms

IM route
- Store in dark area
- Give titrated dosage; use lowest effective dosage; give oil sol deep in large muscle mass (IM); rotate sites; use after warming to dissolve crystals

Patient/family education
- Advise patients to avoid sunlight or use sunscreen; photosensitivity and melasma (brown patches on the face) can occur
- Teach patient about cushingoid symptoms: weight gain, moon face, buffalo hump, acne
- Teach women patients to report breast lumps, vaginal bleeding, edema, jaundice, dark urine, clay-colored stools, dyspnea, headache, blurred vision, abdominal pain, numbness or stiffness in legs, chest pain; men to report impotence or gynecomastia
- Teach patient to report suspected pregnancy immediately

Evaluation
Positive therapeutic outcome
- Decreased abnormal uterine bleeding
- Absence of amenorrhea
- Prevention of pregnancy
- Arrested spread of malignant cells

megestrol (Rx)
(me-jess'trole)
Megace, megestrol
Func. class.: Antineoplastic hormone
Chem. class.: Progestin

Pregnancy category
D (tabs),
X (susp)

Do Not Confuse:
Megace/Reglan

Action: Affects endometrium by antiluteinizing effect; this is thought to bring about cell death

Therapeutic Outcome: Prevention of rapidly growing malignant cells; weight gain, increased appetite in AIDS

Uses: Breast, endometrial, renal cell cancer; increase weight, decrease cachexia and anorexia associated with AIDS

Investigational uses: Hot flashes

Dosage and routes

Endometrial/ovarian carcinoma

Adult: PO 40-320 mg/day in divided doses

Breast carcinoma

Adult: PO 40 mg qid or 160 mg daily

Anorexia (AIDS)

Adult: PO 800 mg daily (oral susp)

Hot flashes (off-label)

Adult: PO 20 mg daily

Available forms: Tabs 20, 40 mg; oral susp 40 mg/ml

Adverse effects

CNS: Mood swings

CV: **Thrombophlebitis, thromboembolism**

GI: Nausea, vomiting, diarrhea, abdominal cramps, weight gain

GU: Gynecomastia, fluid retention, hypercalcemia, vaginal bleeding, discharge, impotence, decreased libido

INTEG: Alopecia, rash, pruritus, purpura, itching

Contraindications: Hypersensitivity, pregnancy **X** (susp), **D** (tabs)

Pharmacokinetics	
Absorption	Well absorbed
Distribution	Unknown
Metabolism	Liver, completely
Excretion	Unknown
Half-life	1 hr

Pharmacodynamics	
Onset	Several wk-mo
Peak	Unknown
Duration	1-3 days

Interactions: None known

Drug/lab test

Increased: alkaline phosphatase, urinary pregnanediol, plasma amino acids, urinary sodium

Decreased: HDL, GTT

False positive: urine glucose

NURSING CONSIDERATIONS

Assessment

- Monitor effects of alopecia on body image; discuss feelings about body changes
- In AIDS patients monitor calorie counts, weight, appetite
- Assess for thrombophlebitis: pain, redness, swelling in legs; notify prescriber immediately if these occur

Nursing diagnoses

- Knowledge, deficient (teaching)

Implementation

- Administer with meals for GI symptoms
- Oral susp is usually used for AIDS patients, shake well
- Give tablets for carcinoma

Patient/family education

- Teach patient to report any complaints or side effects to prescriber
- Advise patient that contraceptive measures must be used during and several mo after treatment; drug is teratogenic
- Explore with patient the need for wig or a hairpiece for hair loss
- Caution patient to report vaginal bleeding to prescriber
- Review with patient the need to comply with dosage schedule, not to miss or double doses; missed doses may be taken up to 1 hr before next dose
- Teach patient how to recognize signs of fluid retention, thromboembolism and report immediately

Evaluation

Positive therapeutic outcome

- Decreased spread of malignant cells
- Weight gain, increased appetite in AIDS patients

M

meloxicam (Rx)

(mel-ox′i-kam)

Mobic

Func. class.: Nonsteroidal antiinflammatory/nonopioid analgesic (NSAIDs)

Chem. class.: Oxicam

Pregnancy category

C (1st trimester),

D (2nd/3rd trimesters)

Action: Inhibits prostaglandin synthesis by decreasing an enzyme needed for biosynthesis; analgesic, antiinflammatory, antipyretic effects

Therapeutic Outcome: Decreased pain, swelling of joints; improved mobility

Uses: Osteoarthritis, rheumatoid arthritis, juvenile arthritis

Dosage and routes

Adult: PO 7.5 mg daily, may increase to 15 mg daily

Available forms: Tabs 7.5 mg; susp 7.5 mg/ml

Adverse effects

CNS: Dizziness, drowsiness, tremors, headache, nervousness, malaise, fatigue, insomnia, depression, **seizures**
CV: Hypertension, angina, **cardiac failure, MI,** hypotension, palpitations, **dysrhythmias,** tachycardia
EENT: Tinnitus, hearing loss
GI: Pancreatitis, nausea, colitis, GERD, vomiting, diarrhea, constipation, flatulence, cramps, dry mouth, peptic ulcer, **GI bleeding, perforation**
GU: **Nephrotoxicity: dysuria, hematuria, oliguria, azotemia**
HEMA: **Blood dyscrasias,** anemia, prolonged bleeding
INTEG: Rash, urticaria, photosensitivity
SYST: **Angioedema, anaphylaxis**

Contraindications: Pregnancy D (2nd/3rd trimesters), hypersensitivity, asthma, severe renal disease, severe hepatic disease, peptic ulcer disease, labor and delivery, lactation, CV bleeding

Precautions: Pregnancy **C** (1st trimester), children, bleeding disorders, GI disorders, cardiac disorders, hypersensitivity to other antiinflammatory agents, elderly, CCr <25 ml/min

Pharmacokinetics

Absorption	Unknown
Distribution	Unknown
Metabolism	Liver <50%
Excretion	Breast milk, kidneys
Half-life	6 hr

Pharmacodynamics

	PO	IM
Onset	Unknown	Unknown
Peak	4-5 hr	50 min
Duration	Unknown	Unknown

Interactions

Individual drugs

Cholestyramine: decreased action of meloxicam
CycloSPORINE: increased nephrotoxicity
Phenytoin: increased action of meloxicam

Drug classifications

Aminoglycosides, anticoagulants, diuretics, hydantoins: increased action of each specific drug
β-Adrenergic blockers: decreased action of β-blockers
Salicylates, sulfonamides: increased action of meloxicam

Drug/herb

Arginine, gossypol: increased gastric irritation
Bearberry, bilberry: increased NSAIDs effect
Bogbean, chondroitin: increased bleeding risk

NURSING CONSIDERATIONS

Assessment

- Monitor renal, liver, blood studies: BUN, creatinine, AST, ALT, Hgb before treatment, periodically thereafter
- Assess for bleeding times; check for bruising, bleeding; test for occult blood in urine
- ◆ Assess for anaphylaxis and angioedema; emergency equipment should be nearby
- ◆ Assess for hepatic dysfunction: jaundice, yellow sclera and skin, clay-colored stools
- Assess for audiometric, ophth exam before, during, after treatment
- Assess for GI condition, hypertension, cardiac conditions

Nursing diagnoses

- Mobility, physical, impaired (uses)
- Pain, chronic (uses)
- Knowledge, deficient (teaching)

Implementation

- May take without regard to meals, take with food for GI upset
- Take with full glass of water and sit upright for ½ hr
- Store at room temp

Patient/family education

- Advise patient to report blurred vision or ringing, roaring in ears (may indicate toxicity)
- Advise patient to avoid driving, other hazardous activities if dizziness or drowsiness occurs
- Teach patient to report change in urine pattern, weight increase, edema, pain increase in joints, fever, blood in urine (indicates nephrotoxicity); to report rash, black stools, or continuing headache
- Teach patient to not use alcohol, aspirin, acetaminophen without consulting prescriber

Evaluation

Positive therapeutic outcome

- Decreased pain, stiffness, swelling in joints, able to move more easily

! HIGH ALERT

melphalan (Rx)

(mel'fa-lan)

Alkeran, L-Pam, phenylalanine mustard

Func. class.: Antineoplastic, alkylating agent

Chem. class.: Nitrogen mustard

Pregnancy category D

Do Not Confuse:
melphalan/myleran

Action: Alkylates DNA, RNA; inhibits enzymes that allow synthesis of amino acids in proteins; activity is not cell cycle phase specific

Therapeutic Outcome: Prevention of rapidly growing malignant cells

Uses: Multiple myeloma, malignant melanoma, advanced ovarian cancer

Investigational uses: Breast, testicular, prostate carcinoma; osteogenic sarcoma, chronic myelogenous leukemia

Dosage and routes

Multiple myeloma

Adult: PO 150 mcg/kg/day × 1 wk, then 21 days off, then 50 mcg/kg/day or 100-150 mcg/kg/day or 250 mcg/kg/day × 4 days for 2-3 wk, then 2-4 wk off, then 2-4 mg/day or 7 mg/m^2 × 5 days q5-6 wk

Adult: **IV** inf 16 mg/m^2; reduce in renal insufficiency; give over 15-20 min; give at 2-wk intervals × 4 doses, then at 4-wk intervals

Ovarian carcinoma

Adult: PO 200 mcg/kg/day × 5 days q4-5 wk

Available forms: Tabs 2 mg; inj 50 mg

Adverse effects

GI: *Nausea, vomiting,* stomatitis, diarrhea

GU: Amenorrhea, hyperuricemia, gonadal suppression

HEMA: **Thrombocytopenia, neutropenia, leukopenia,** anemia

INTEG: Rash, urticaria, alopecia, pruritus

RESP: **Fibrosis, dysplasia**

SYST: **Anaphylaxis,** allergic reaction

Contraindications: Pregnancy **D**, lactation, hypersensitivity to this drug or other nitrogen mustards

Precautions: Radiation therapy, bone marrow depression, infection, renal disease, children

Pharmacokinetics

Absorption	Variable; incompletely absorbed
Distribution	Rapidly distributed
Metabolism	Bloodstream
Excretion	Kidneys, unchanged (10%)
Half-life	1½ hr

Pharmacodynamics

Unknown

Interactions

Individual drugs

Carmustine: increased pulmonary toxicity
CycloSPORINE: increased renal failure risk
Nalidixic acid: increased enterocolitis risk
Radiation: increased toxicity

Drug classifications

Antineoplastics: increased toxicity
Live virus vaccines: increased adverse reactions; decreased antibody reaction

Drug/lab test

Increased: uric acid

NURSING CONSIDERATIONS

Assessment

- Monitor CBC, differential, platelet count weekly; withhold drug if WBC is <3000/mm^3 or platelet count is <100,000/mm^3; notify prescriber of results if WBC <20,000/mm^3, platelets <100,000/mm^3; recovery usually occurs in 6 wk
- Monitor pulmonary function tests, chest x-ray films before, during therapy; chest film should be obtained q2 wk during treatment; check for dyspnea, crackles, unproductive cough, chest pain, tachypnea
- Assess for increased uric acid levels, swelling, joint pain primarily in extremities; patient should be well hydrated to prevent urate deposits
- Monitor renal function studies: BUN, serum uric acid, urine CCr before, during therapy; check I&O ratio; report fall in urine output of 30 ml/hr; check for decreased hyperuricemia; monitor AST, ALT
- Monitor for cold, fever, sore throat (may indicate beginning of infection); identify edema in feet, joint and stomach pain, shaking; prescriber should be notified
- Assess for bleeding: hematuria, guaiac, bruising or petechiae, from mucosa or orifices q8h; no rec temp
- Assess for symptoms indicating severe allergic reaction: rash, pruritus, urticaria, purpuric skin lesions, itching, flushing; assess allergy to chlorambucil, cross-sensitivity may occur

M

Nursing diagnoses
- Injury, risk for (adverse reactions)
- Body image, disturbed (adverse reactions)
- Infection, risk for (adverse reactions)
- Knowledge, deficient (teaching)

Implementation
- Give fluids **IV** or PO before chemotherapy to hydrate patient
- Give antacid before oral agent; give drug after evening meal, before bedtime; provide antiemetic 30-60 min before giving drug and prn to prevent vomiting; give antibiotics for prophylaxis of infection
- Give in AM so drug can be eliminated before bedtime
- Use a liq diet: carbonated beverages; gelatin may be added if patient is not nauseated or vomiting

PO route
- Give 1 hr ac or 2 hr pc to prevent nausea/ vomiting

IV route
- Give as intermittent inf: reconstitute with provided diluent (10 ml) to 5 mg/ml; shake until clear; further dilute with 0.9% NaCl to <0.45 mg/ml; give over 15 min, give within 1 hr

Y-site compatibilities: Acyclovir, amikacin, aminophylline, ampicillin, aztreonam, bleomycin, bumetanide, buprenorphine, butorphanol, calcium gluconate, carboplatin, carmustine, cefazolin, cefepime, cefoperazone, cefotaxime, cefotetan, ceftazidime, ceftizoxime, ceftriaxone, cefuroxime, cimetidine, cisplatin, clindamycin, cyclophosphamide, cytarabine, dacarbazine, dactinomycin, DAUNOrubicin, dexamethasone, diphenhydrAMINE, DOXOrubicin, doxycycline, droperidol, enalaprilat, etoposide, famotidine, floxuridine, fluconazole, fludarabine, fluorouracil, furosemide, gallium, ganciclovir, gentamicin, granisetron, haloperidol, heparin, hydrocortisone sodium phosphate, hydromorphone, hydrOXYzine, idarubicin, ifosfamide, imipenem-cilastatin, lorazepam, mannitol, mechlorethamine, meperidine, mesna, methylPREDNISolone, metoclopramide, methotrexate, metronidazole, miconazole, minocycline, mitomycin, mitoxantrone, morphine, nalbuphine, netilmicin, ondansetron, pentostatin, piperacillin, plicamycin, potassium chloride, prochlorperazine, promethazine, ranitidine, sodium bicarbonate, streptozocin, teniposide, thiotepa, ticarcillin, ticarcillin/clavulanate, tobramycin, trimethoprim/sulfamethoxazole, vancomycin, vinBLAStine, vinCRIStine, vinorelbine, zidovudine

Patient/family education
- Teach patient to avoid use of products containing aspirin or ibuprofen, razors, commercial mouthwash, since bleeding may occur; to report symptoms of bleeding (hematuria, tarry stools)
- Instruct patient to report signs of anemia (fatigue, headache, irritability, faintness, shortness of breath)
- Instruct patient to report any changes in breathing or coughing even several mo after treatment; to avoid crowds and persons with respiratory tract or other infections
- Tell patient hair loss is common; discuss the use of wigs or hairpieces
- Caution patient not to have any vaccinations without the advice of the prescriber, serious reactions can occur
- Advise patient that contraception is needed during treatment and for several mo after the completion of therapy
- Teach patient to rinse mouth tid-qid with water, club soda; brush teeth bid-qid with soft brush or cotton-tipped applicators for stomatitis; use unwaxed dental floss

Evaluation
Positive therapeutic outcome
- Decreased size of tumor
- Decreased spread of malignancy

memantine (Rx)
(me-man'teen)
Namenda
Func. class.: Anti-Alzheimer's disease agent
Chem. class.: NMDA receptor antagonist
Pregnancy category B

Action: Antagonist action of CNS NMDA receptors that may contribute to the symptoms of Alzheimer's disease

Therapeutic Outcome: Improved mood, orientation, decreasing confusion

Uses: Treatment of moderate to severe dementia in Alzheimer's disease

Investigational uses: Vascular dementia

Dosage and routes
Adult: PO 5 mg daily, may increase dose in 5-mg increments ≥1-wk intervals; recommended target dose 20 mg/day

Available forms: Tabs 5, 10 mg

Adverse effects
CNS: *Dizziness, confusion,* somnolence, headache, hallucinations
CV: Hypertension

GI: Vomiting, constipation
INTEG: Rash
MISC: Back pain, fatigue, pain
RESP: Coughing, dyspnea

Contraindications: Hypersensitivity

Precautions: Pregnancy **B**, renal disease, GU conditions, which raise urine pH; lactation, children

Pharmacokinetics

Absorption	Rapidly absorbed PO
Distribution	44% protein binding
Metabolism	Very little
Excretion	57%-82% excreted unchanged in urine
Half-life	Terminal elimination half-life 60-80 hr

Pharmacodynamics

Onset	Unknown
Peak	Unknown
Duration	Unknown

Interactions
Individual drugs
Cimetidine, hydrochlorothiazide, nicotine, quinidine, ranitidine, triamterene: may alter levels of both drugs
Drug classifications
Drugs that make the urine alkaline (sodium bicarbonate, carbonic anhydrase inhibitors): decreased clearance

NURSING CONSIDERATIONS
Assessment
- Monitor B/P: hypertension
- Assess mental status: affect, mood, behavioral changes; hallucinations, confusion
- Assess GI status: vomiting, constipation, add bulk, increase fluids for constipation
- Assess GU status: urinary frequency

Nursing diagnoses
- Thought processes, disturbed (uses)
- Injury, risk for (uses)
- Knowledge, deficient (teaching)
- Noncompliance (teaching)

Implementation
- Can be taken without regard to meals
- Give twice a day if dose >5 mg
- Dosage is adjusted to response no more than q1 wk
- Provide assistance with ambulation during beginning therapy; dizziness may occur

Patient/family education
- Advise to report side effects: restlessness, psychosis, visual hallucinations, stupor, loss of consciousness; indicate overdose
- Advise to use drug exactly as prescribed; drug is not a cure

Evaluation
Positive therapeutic outcome
- Decrease in confusion, improved mood

menotropins (Rx)
(men-oh-troe'pinz)
Humegon, Pergonal, Repronex
Func. class.: Gonadotropin
Chem. class.: Exogenous gonadotropin
Pregnancy category X

Action: In women, increases follicular growth, maturation; in men, when given with hCG, stimulates spermatogenesis; contains FSH and LH

Therapeutic Outcome: Pregnancy, ovulation

Uses: Infertility, anovulation in women; stimulates spermatogenesis in men; usually used with hCG

Dosage and routes
Infertility
Adult (men): IM 1 ampule 3 times a wk with hCG 2000 units 2 times a wk × 4 mo
Adult (women): IM 75 international units of FSH, LH daily × 9-12 days, then 10,000 units of hCG 1 day after these drugs; repeat × 2 menstrual cycles, then increase to 150 international units of FSH, LH daily × 9-12 days, then 10,000 units of hCG 1 day after these drugs × 2 menstrual cycles

Anovulation
Adult (women): IM 75 international units FSH, LH daily × 9-12 days, then 10,000 units hCG 1 day after last dose of these drugs: repeat × 1-3 menstrual cycles

Available forms: Powder for inj lyophilized 75, 150 international units FSH, LH activity

Adverse effects
CNS: Fever
CV: **Hypovolemia**
GI: *Nausea,* vomiting, diarrhea, anorexia
GU: **Ovarian enlargement,** multiple births, abdominal distention, pain, ovarian hyperstimulation, sudden ovarian enlargement, ascites with or without pain, gynecomastia in men

M

HEMA: **Hemoperitoneum, arterial thromboembolism**
OTHER: **Anaphylaxis**
RESP: **ARDS, pulmonary embolism, pulmonary infarction, pleural effusion**

Contraindications: Pregnancy **X**, primary ovarian failure, abnormal bleeding, thyroid/adrenal dysfunction, organic intracranial lesion, ovarian cysts, primary testicular failure

Pharmacokinetics

Absorption	Well absorbed
Distribution	Unknown
Metabolism	Unknown
Excretion	Kidneys, unchanged (8%)
Half-life	70 hr (FSH); 4 hr (LH)

Pharmacodynamics

Unknown

Interactions: None known

NURSING CONSIDERATIONS

Assessment

- Monitor weight daily; notify prescriber if weight gain increases rapidly
- Monitor estrogen excretion level; if >100 mcg/24 hr, drug is withheld; hyperstimulation syndrome may occur
- Monitor I&O ratio; be alert for decreasing urinary output
- Assess for ovarian enlargement, abdominal distention/pain; report symptoms immediately

Nursing diagnoses

- Sexual dysfunction (uses)
- Knowledge, deficient (teaching)

Implementation

- Give after reconstituting with 1-2 ml of sterile saline inj; use immediately

Patient/family education

- Advise patient that multiple births are possible; if pregnancy occurs, it is usually 4-6 wk after start of treatment
- Instruct patient to keep daily appointment for 2 wk during treatment

Evaluation

Positive therapeutic outcome

- Pregnancy

! HIGH ALERT

meperidine (Rx)

(me-per'i-deen)

Demerol, meperidine HCl, Pethidine

Func. class.: Opioid analgesic

Chem. class.: Phenylpiperidine derivative

Pregnancy category B

Controlled substance schedule II

Do Not Confuse:
Demerol/Dilaudid, meperidine/hydromorphone, meprobamate/morphine

Action: Depresses pain impulse transmission at the spinal cord level by interacting with opioid receptors; produces CNS depression

Therapeutic Outcome: Relief of pain

Uses: Moderate to severe pain, preoperatively, during labor

Investigational uses: Rigors

Dosage and routes

Pain

Adult: PO/SUBCUT/IM 50-150 mg q3-4h prn; **IV** 15-35 mg/hr as a cont inf; PCA 10 mg, then 1-5 mg incremental dose; lockout interval 6-10 min

Child: PO/SUBCUT/IM 1 mg/kg q3-4h prn, not to exceed 100 mg q4h

Preoperatively

Adult: IM/SUBCUT 50-100 mg q30-90 min before surgery; dosage should be reduced if given **IV**

Child: IM/SUBCUT 1-2.2 mg/kg 30-90 min before surgery

Renal dose

Adult: CCr 10-50 ml/min 75% of dose; CCr <10 ml/min 50% of dose

Labor analgesia

Adult: SUBCUT/IM 50-100 mg given when contractions are regulary spaced, repeat q1-3h prn

Available forms: Inj 10, 25, 50, 75, 100 mg/ml; tabs 50, 100 mg; syr 50 mg/5 ml

Adverse effects

CNS: Drowsiness, dizziness, confusion, headache, sedation, euphoria, **increased ICP, seizures**
CV: Palpitations, bradycardia, change in B/P, tachycardia (**IV**)
EENT: Tinnitus, blurred vision, miosis, diplopia, depressed corneal reflex
GI: Nausea, vomiting, anorexia, constipation, cramps

GU: Urinary retention, dysuria
INTEG: Rash, urticaria, bruising, flushing, diaphoresis, pruritus
***RESP:* Respiratory depression**

Contraindications: Hypersensitivity, addiction (opiate)

Precautions: Pregnancy **B**, addictive personality, lactation, increased ICP, MI (acute), severe heart disease, respiratory depression, hepatic disease, renal disease, child <18 yr, elderly

Pharmacokinetics

Absorption	Well absorbed (IM, SUBCUT); 50% (PO)
Distribution	Widely distributed; crosses placenta
Metabolism	Liver, extensively
Excretion	Kidneys; breast milk
Half-life	3-4 hr

Pharmacodynamics

	PO	IM/ SUBCUT	IV
Onset	15 min	10 min	Rapid
Peak	½-1 hr	½-1 hr	5-7 min
Duration	2-4 hr	2-4 hr	2-4 hr

Interactions
Individual drugs
Alcohol: increased respiratory depression, hypotension, sedation
Phenytoin: decreased meperidine effect
Procarbazine: fatal reaction, do not use together
Drug classifications
CNS depressants, opioids, sedative/hypnotics, antipsychotics, skeletal muscle relaxants: increased effects
MAOIs: do not use for 2 wk before taking meperidine; may cause fatal reaction
Protease inhibitor antiretrovirals: increased adverse reactions
Drug/herb
Chamomile, hops, Jamaican dogwood, kava, lavender, mistletoe, nettle, pokeweed, poppy, senega, skullcap, valerian: increased CNS depression
Parsley: may promote serotonin syndrome, avoid concurrent medicinal use
Drug/lab test
Increased: amylase, lipase

NURSING CONSIDERATIONS
Assessment
- Assess pain: location, duration, intensity before and 1 hr (IM, SUBCUT, PO) and 5-10 min (**IV**) after administration
- Assess renal function before initiating therapy; poor renal function can lead to accumulation of toxic metabolite and seizures
- Monitor VS after parenteral route; note muscle rigidity, drug history, liver, kidney function tests, respiratory dysfunction: respiratory depression, character, rate, rhythm; notify prescriber if respirations are <10/min
- Monitor CNS changes: dizziness, drowsiness, hallucinations, euphoria, LOC, pupil reaction; these are due to metabolite produced, CNS stimulation occurs with chronic or high doses
- Monitor allergic reactions: rash, urticaria

Nursing diagnoses
- Pain, acute (uses)
- Sensory perception, disturbed: visual, auditory (adverse reactions)
- Breathing pattern, ineffective (adverse reactions)
- Injury, risk for (adverse reactions)
- Knowledge, deficient (teaching)

Implementation
- Give with antiemetic if nausea, vomiting occur
- Administer when pain is beginning to return; determine dosage interval by patient response; continuous dosing of medication is more effective given prn
- Medication should be slowly withdrawn after long-term use to prevent withdrawal symptoms
- Store in light-resistant container at room temp

PO route
- May be given with food or milk to lessen GI upset
- Syr should be mixed with 4 oz of water

IM/SUBCUT route
- Do not give if cloudy or a precipitate has formed
- Patient should remain recumbent for 1 hr after administration

IV route
- Give by direct **IV** after diluting to 10 mg/ml with sterile water, 0.9% NaCl for inj; give slowly at 25 mg/1 min; rapid administration may cause respiratory depression, hypotension, circulatory collapse
- Give cont inf after diluting to 1 mg/ml with D_5W, $D_{10}W$, dextrose/saline combinations, dextrose/Ringer's, inj combinations, 0.45% NaCl, 0.9% NaCl, Ringer's, LR; give by infusion pump; titrate according to response

Syringe compatibilities: Atropine, benzquinamide, butorphanol, chlorproMAZINE, cimetidine, dimenhyDRINATE, diphenhydrAMINE, droperidol, fentanyl, glycopyrrolate,

M

hydrOXYzine, ketamine, metoclopramide, midazolam, pentazocine, perphenazine, prochlorperazine, promazine, promethazine, ranitidine, scopolamine

Syringe incompatibilities: Heparin, morphine, pentobarbital

Y-site compatibilities: Amifostine, amikacin, ampicillin, atenolol, aztreonam, bumetanide, cefamandole, cefazolin, cefmetazole, cefotaxime, cefotetan, cefoxitin, ceftazidime, ceftizoxime, ceftriaxone, cefuroxime, cephalothin, cephapirin, chloramphenicol, cladribine, clindamycin, dexamethasone, diltiazem, diphenhydrAMINE, DOBUTamine, DOPamine, doxycycline, droperidol, erythromycin lactobionate, famotidine, filgrastim, fluconazole, fludarabine, gallium, gentamicin, granisetron, heparin, hydrocortisone, regular insulin, kanamycin, labetalol, lidocaine, magnesium sulfate, melphalan, methyldopate, methylPREDNISolone, metoclopramide, metoprolol, metronidazole, moxalactam, ondansetron, oxacillin, oxytocin, paclitaxel, penicillin G potassium, piperacillin, potassium chloride, propofol, propranolol, ranitidine, sargramostim, teniposide, thiotepa, ticarcillin, ticarcillin/clavulanate, tobramycin, trimethoprim/sulfamethoxazole, vancomycin, verapamil, vinorelbine

Y-site incompatibilities: Cefoperazone, idarubicin, imipenem/cilastatin, mezlocillin, minocycline

Additive compatibilities: Cefazolin, DOBUTamine, ondansetron, scopolamine, succinylcholine, triflupromazine, verapamil

Patient/family education

- Advise patients to avoid CNS depressants (alcohol, sedative/hypnotics) for at least 24 hr after taking this drug
- Discuss with patient that dizziness, drowsiness, and confusion are common; to avoid getting up without assistance
- Discuss in detail with patient all aspects of the drug, including its purpose and what to expect
- Caution patient to make position changes carefully to lessen orthostatic hypotension

Evaluation

Positive therapeutic outcome

- Decreased pain

Treatment of overdose: Naloxone 0.2-0.8 mg **IV**, O_2, **IV** fluids, vasopressors

mercaptopurine (Rx)
(mer-kap-toe-pyoor′een)
6-MP, Purinethol
Func. class.: Antineoplastic, antimetabolite
Chem. class.: Purine analog
Pregnancy category D

Action: Inhibits purine metabolism at multiple sites, which inhibits DNA and RNA synthesis S phase of cell cycle

Therapeutic Outcome: Prevention of rapidly growing malignant cells

Uses: Chronic myelocytic leukemia, acute lymphoblastic leukemia in children, acute myelogenous leukemia

Investigational uses: Polycythemia vera, psoriatic arthritis, colitis, lymphoma

Dosage and routes

Adult: PO 80-100 mg/m^2 daily, max 5 mg/kg/day; maintenance 1.5-2.5 mg/kg/day
Child: PO 75 mg/m^2/day (2.5 mg/kg/day); maintenance 1.5-2.5 mg/kg/day

Available forms: Tabs 50 mg

Adverse effects

CNS: Fever, headache, weakness
GI: *Nausea, vomiting, anorexia, diarrhea, stomatitis,* **hepatotoxicity** (with high doses), jaundice, gastritis
GU: **Renal failure,** hyperuricemia, **oliguria,** crystalluria, **hematuria**
HEMA: **Thrombocytopenia, leukopenia, myelosuppression, anemia**
INTEG: *Rash,* dry skin, urticaria

Contraindications: Pregnancy **D,** patients with prior drug resistance, leukopenia (<2500/mm^3), thrombocytopenia (<100,000/mm^3), anemia, lactation

Precautions: Renal disease

Pharmacokinetics	
Absorption	Variable
Distribution	Widely—body water
Metabolism	Liver—extensively
Excretion	Kidneys unchanged (small amounts)
Half-life	Unknown

Pharmacodynamics

Unknown

Interactions

Individual drugs

Allopurinol, cotrimoxazole: increased bone marrow depression

Radiation: increased toxicity
Warfarin: increased or decreased effect of warfarin

Drug classifications
Antineoplastics: increased toxicity
Live virus vaccines: decreased antibodies
Nondepolarizing muscle relaxants: reversal of neuromuscular blockade

NURSING CONSIDERATIONS

Assessment

- Assess buccal cavity q8h for dryness, sores or ulceration, white patches, oral pain, bleeding, dysphagia; obtain prescription for viscous lidocaine (Xylocaine)
- ! Assess symptoms indicating severe allergic reaction: rash, pruritus, urticaria, purpuric skin lesions, itching, flushing
- Monitor CBC, differential, platelet count weekly; withhold drug if WBC is <4000/mm^3 or platelet count is <100,000/mm^3; notify prescriber of results if WBC <20,000/mm^3, platelets <150,000/mm^3
- Assess for increased uric acid levels, swelling, joint pain primarily in extremities; patient should be well hydrated to prevent urate deposits
- Monitor renal function studies: BUN, creatinine, serum uric acid, urine CCr before and during therapy; check I&O ratio; report fall in urine output to <30 ml/hr
- Monitor temp q4h (may indicate beginning of infection)
- Monitor liver function tests before and during therapy (bilirubin, AST, ALT, LDH) as needed or monthly; check for yellowing of skin or sclera, dark urine, clay-colored stools, itchy skin, abdominal pain, fever, diarrhea
- Assess for bleeding: hematuria, stool guaiac, bruising or petechiae, mucosa or orifices q8h; check for inflammation of mucosa, breaks in skin

Nursing diagnoses

- Injury, risk for (adverse reactions)
- Body image, disturbed (adverse reactions)
- Infection, risk for (adverse reactions)
- Knowledge, deficient (teaching)

Implementation

- Give fluids **IV** or PO before chemotherapy to hydrate patient
- Give antiemetic 30-60 min before giving drug and prn to prevent vomiting; give antibiotics for prophylaxis of infection
- Give in AM so drug can be eliminated before bedtime
- Give entire dose at one time
- Provide liq diet: carbonated beverages; gelatin may be added if patient is not nauseated or vomiting
- Tab may be crushed and added to fluids or food to facilitate swallowing

Patient/family education

- Encourage patient to rinse mouth tid-qid with water, club soda; brush teeth bid-qid with soft brush or cotton-tipped applicators for stomatitis; use unwaxed dental floss
- Advise patient that contraceptive measures are recommended during therapy; serious teratogenic effects may occur, to avoid breastfeeding
- Teach patient to avoid use of products containing aspirin or NSAIDs, razors, commercial mouthwash, since bleeding may occur; to report symptoms of bleeding (hematuria, tarry stools)
- Instruct patient to report signs of anemia (fatigue, headache, irritability, faintness, shortness of breath)
- Instruct patient to report any changes in breathing or coughing even several mo after treatment; to avoid crowds and persons with respiratory tract or other infections
- Caution patient not to have any vaccinations without the advice of the prescriber; serious reactions can occur
- Advise patient to take entire dose at one time

Evaluation

Positive therapeutic outcome

- Prevention of rapid division of malignant cells

meropenem (Rx)

(mer-oh-pen′em)
Merrem **IV**
Func. class.: Antiinfective—miscellaneous
Pregnancy category B

Action: Interferes with cell wall replication of susceptible organisms; osmotically unstable cell wall swells and bursts from osmotic pressure

Therapeutic Outcome: Bactericidal action against the following: *Streptococcus pneumoniae,* group A β-hemolytic streptococci, *viridans* group streptococci, enterococcus; gram-negative organisms *Klebsiella, Proteus, Escherichia coli, Pseudomonas aeruginosa, Bacteroides fragilis, Bacteroides thetaiotamicron,* bacterial meningitis (>3 mo old)

M

Uses: Serious infections caused by gram-positive or gram-negative organisms (appendicitis, peritonitis)

Dosage and routes

Adult: **IV** 1 g q8h, given over 15-30 min or as an **IV** bolus 5-20 ml given over 3-5 min

Renal dose

Adult: **IV** CCr 26-50 ml/min 1 g q12h; CCr 10-25 ml/min 500 mg q12h; CCr <10 ml/min 500 mg q24h

Child ≥ 3 mo: **IV** 20-40 mg/kg q8h (max 2 g q8h meningitis)

Child >50 kg: **IV** 1 g q8h (intraabdominal infection) or 2 g q8h (meningitis) given over 15-30 min or as an **IV** bolus 5-20 ml over 3-5 min

Available forms: Inj 500 mg, 1 g

Adverse effects

CNS: Fever, somnolence, ***seizures,*** dizziness, weakness, *headache,* myoclonia

CV: Hypotension, palpitations

GI: Diarrhea, nausea, vomiting, **pseudomembranous colitis, hepatitis,** glossitis

HEMA: **Eosinophilia, neutropenia,** decreased Hgb, Hct

INTEG: *Rash,* urticaria, *pruritus,* pain at inj site, phlebitis, erythema at inj site

RESP: Chest discomfort, dyspnea, hyperventilation

SYST: **Anaphylaxis**

Contraindications: Hypersensitivity to meropenem or imipenem

Precautions: Pregnancy **B**, lactation, elderly, renal disease

Pharmacokinetics

Absorption	Complete bioavailability
Distribution	Widely distributed
Metabolism	Liver
Excretion	Kidneys
Half-life	1 hr; increased in renal disease

Pharmacodynamics

Onset	Rapid
Peak	Dose dependent

Interactions

Individual drugs

Probenecid: increased meropenem levels

Drug/lab test

Increased: AST, ALT, LDH, BUN, alkaline phosphatase, bilirubin, creatinine

False positive: direct Coombs' test

NURSING CONSIDERATIONS

Assessment

- Assess patient for previous sensitivity reaction to carbapenem antiinfectives, penicillins
- Assess patient for signs and symptoms of infection, including characteristics of wounds, sputum, urine, stool, WBC >10,000/100 mm^3, fever; obtain baseline information before and during treatment
- Complete C&S tests before beginning drug therapy to identify if correct treatment has been initiated
- Assess for allergic reactions, anaphylaxis: rash, urticaria, pruritus, chills, fever, joint pain; angioedema may occur a few days after therapy begins; epINEPHrine and resuscitation equipment should be available for anaphylactic reaction
- Identify urine output; if decreasing, notify prescriber (may indicate nephrotoxicity); also check for increased BUN, creatinine
- Monitor blood studies: AST, ALT, CBC, Hct, bilirubin, LDH, alkaline phosphatase, Coombs' test monthly if patient is on long-term therapy
- Monitor electrolytes: potassium, sodium, chloride monthly if patient is on long-term therapy
- Assess bowel pattern daily; if severe diarrhea occurs, drug should be discontinued; may indicate pseudomembranous colitis
- Monitor for bleeding: ecchymosis, bleeding gums, hematuria, stool guaiac daily if on long-term therapy
- Assess for overgrowth of infection: perineal itching, fever, malaise, redness, pain, swelling, drainage, rash, diarrhea, change in cough, sputum

Nursing diagnoses

- Infection, risk for (uses)
- Diarrhea (adverse reactions)
- Injury, risk for (adverse reactions)
- Knowledge, deficient (teaching)
- Noncompliance (teaching)

Implementation

IV route

- Reconstitute with 0.9% NaCl, D_5W, LR, dilute in 5-20 ml of compatible sol; give by direct **IV** over 3-5 min
- Give by intermittent inf, dilute in 5-20 ml of compatible sol, give over 15-30 min

Y-site compatibilities: Aminophylline, atenolol, atropine, cimetidine, dexamethasone, digoxin, diphenhydrAMINE, enalaprilat, fluconazole, furosemide, gentamicin, heparin, insulin (regular), metoclopramide, morphine, norepinephrine, phenobarbital, vancomycin

Additive compatibilities: Aminophylline, atropine, cimetidine, dexamethasone, DOBUTamine, DOPamine, enalaprilat, fluconazole, furosemide, gentamicin, heparin, insulin (regular), magnesium sulfate, metoclopramide, morphine, norepinephrine, phenobarbital, ranitidine, vancomycin

Patient/family education
- Teach patient to report sore throat, bruising, bleeding, joint pain; may indicate blood dyscrasias (rare)
- Advise patient to contact prescriber if vaginal itching, loose foul-smelling stools, furry tongue occur; may indicate superinfection
- Advise patient to avoid breastfeeding, drug is excreted in breast milk
- Advise patient to notify prescriber of diarrhea with blood or pus, may indicate pseudomembranous colitis

Evaluation
Positive therapeutic outcome
- Absence of signs/symptoms of infection (WBC <10,000/mm^3, temp WNL, absence of red draining wounds)
- Reported improvement in symptoms of infection

Treatment of anaphylaxis: EpINEPHrine, antihistamines, resuscitate if needed

mesalamine (Rx)
(mez-al'a-meen)
Asacol, Canasa, Mesasal, Pentasa, Rowasa, Salofulk ✤
Func class.: GI antiinflammatory
Chem class.: 5-Aminosalicylic acid
Pregnancy category B

Do Not Confuse:
Asacol/Ansaid

Action: May diminish inflammation by blocking cyclooxygenase, inhibiting prostaglandin production in colon, local action only

Therapeutic Outcome: Decreased cramping, pain in GI conditions

Uses: Mild to moderate active distal ulcerative colitis, proctosigmoiditis, proctitis

Dosage and routes
Adult: Rec 60 ml (4 g) at bedtime, retained for 8 hr × 3-6 wk; PO 800 mg tid for 6 wk; supp 500 mg bid for 3-6 wk, retain 1-3 hr

Available forms: Rec susp 4 g/60 ml; supp 500 mg; del rel tabs 400 mg; cont rel caps (Pentasa) 250 mg

Adverse effects
CNS: *Headache, fever, dizziness,* insomnia, asthenia, weakness, fatigue
CV: Pericarditis, myocarditis
EENT: Sore throat, cough, pharyngitis, rhinitis
GI: *Cramps, gas, nausea, diarrhea,* rectal pain, constipation
INTEG: *Rash, itching,* acne
SYST: *Flulike symptoms, malaise,* back pain, peripheral edema, leg and joint pain, arthralgia, dysmenorrhea, **anaphylaxis,** acute intolerance syndrome

Contraindications: Hypersensitivity to this drug or salicylates

Precautions: Pregnancy **B,** renal disease, lactation, children, sulfite sensitivity, elderly, pyloric stenosis

Pharmacokinetics	
Absorption	20%-30% (PO), 10%-25% (rec)
Distribution	Unknown
Metabolism	Unknown
Excretion	Feces
Half-life	1 hr; metabolite 5-10 hr

Pharmacodynamics
Unknown

Interactions
Individual drugs
Azathioprine: increased azathioprine action
Digoxin: decreased digoxin level
Lactulose: decreased mesalamine absorption
Omeprazole: increased mesalamine absorption
Drug/lab test
Increased: AST, ALT, alkaline phosphatase, LDH, GGTP, amylase, lipase

NURSING CONSIDERATIONS
Assessment
- Assess for GI symptoms: cramping, gas, nausea, diarrhea, rectal pain, abdominal pain; if severe, the drug should be discontinued
- Assess for allergy to salicylates, sulfonamides; if allergic reactions occur, discontinue drug
- Assess renal function before and during treatment: BUN, creatinine
- Monitor I & O ratios, increase fluids to 1500 ml daily to prevent crystalluria

Nursing diagnoses
- Pain, chronic (uses)
- Diarrhea (uses)
- Knowledge, deficient (teaching)

M

Implementation

PO route
- Do not break, crush, or chew del rel tabs
- May give orally

Rectal route (susp)
- Give at bedtime, retained until AM; empty bowel before insertion
- Store at room temp
- Usual course of therapy is 3-6 wk
- Give after shaking bottle well

Patient/family education
- Advise patient to notify prescriber if abdominal pain, cramping, diarrhea with blood, headache, fever, rash, chest pain occur; drug should be discontinued
- Teach correct administration for PO, or enema

Evaluation

Positive therapeutic outcome
- Absence of pain, bleeding from GI tract

mescasermin

Increlex

See Appendix A, Selected New Drugs

metaproterenol (Rx)

(met-a-proe-ter'e-nole)

Alupent, Arm-a-Med, Dey-Lute

Func. class.: Selective β_2-agonist, bronchodilator

Pregnancy category C

Do Not Confuse:
Alupent/Atrovent

Action: Relaxes bronchial smooth muscle by direct action on β_2-adrenergic receptors, with increased levels of cAMP and increased bronchodilatation, diuresis, and cardiac and CNS stimulation

Therapeutic Outcome: Bronchodilatation with ease of breathing

Uses: Bronchial asthma, bronchospasm

Dosage and routes

Adult and child >12 yr: INH 2-3 puffs; may repeat q3-4h, not to exceed 12 puffs/day; IPPB or NEB 0.2-0.3 ml of 5% sol diluted in 2.5 ml of ½ NS or NS; or 2.5 mil of 0.4, 0.6% sol q4h prn

Child 6-12 yr: IPPB/NEB 0.1-0.2 ml of a 5% sol diluted in NS to a final volume of 3 ml q4h prn

Adult: PO 20 mg q6-8h

Elderly: PO 10 mg tid-qid, initially

Child >9 yr or >27 kg: PO 20 mg q6-8h or 0.4-0.9 mg/kg tid

Child 6-9 yr or <27 kg: PO 10 mg q6-8h or 0.4-0.9 mg/kg tid

Child 2-6 yr: PO 1.3-2.6 mg/kg divided q6-8h

Available forms: Tabs 10, 20 mg; aerosol 0.65 mg/dose; syr 10 mg/5 ml; sol for inh 0.4%, 0.6%, 5%

Adverse effects

CNS: *Tremors,* anxiety, insomnia, headache, dizziness, stimulation

CV: Palpitations, tachycardia, hypertension, **dysrhythmias, cardiac arrest** (high dose)

GI: Nausea, vomiting, dry mouth

RESP: **Paradoxical bronchospasm**

Contraindications: Hypersensitivity to sympathomimetics, narrow-angle glaucoma, cardiac dysrhythmias with tachycardia

Precautions: Pregnancy **C**, cardiac disorders, hyperthyroidism, diabetes mellitus, prostatic hypertrophy, seizure disorder, elderly, child <6 yr (PO)

Pharmacokinetics

Absorption	Well absorbed (PO)
Distribution	Unknown
Metabolism	Liver, tissues
Excretion	Unknown
Half-life	2-4 hr

Pharmacodynamics

	PO	INH
Onset	15 min	5 min
Peak	1 hr	1 hr
Duration	4 hr	1-6 hr

Interactions

Drug classifications

β-Adrenergic blockers: block therapeutic effect

Bronchodilators, aerosol: increased action of both drugs

MAOIs: increased chance of hypertensive crisis

Sympathomimetics: increased effects of both drugs

Drug/herb

Coffee, cola nut, guarana, tea (black/green): increased effect

Drug/lab test

Decreased: potassium

NURSING CONSIDERATIONS

Assessment

- Monitor respiratory function: vital capacity, FEV, ABGs, lung sounds, heart rate, rhythm (baseline)
- Determine that patient has not received theophylline therapy before giving dose; identify client's ability to self-medicate
- Monitor for evidence of allergic reactions; paradoxic bronchospasm; withhold dose; notify prescriber

Nursing diagnoses

- Airway clearance, ineffective (uses)
- Gas exchange, impaired (uses)
- Knowledge, deficient (teaching)

Implementation

- Give this medication before other medications and allow 5 min between each to prevent overstimulation

PO route

- Give PO with meals to decrease gastric irritation; syr to children (no alcohol, sugar)

Aerosol route

- Give after shaking, exhale, place mouthpiece in mouth, inhale slowly, hold breath, remove, exhale slowly; allow at least 1 min between inhalations
- Store in light-resistant container, do not expose to temp over 86° F (30° C)
- Provide spacer device for elderly

Patient/family education

- Advise patient not to use OTC medications; excess stimulation may occur; to use this medication before other medications and allow at least 5 min between each to prevent overstimulation
- Teach patient use of inhaler; review package insert with patient; teach patient to avoid getting aerosol in eyes, since blurring may result; to wash inhaler in warm water daily and dry; to avoid smoking, smoke-filled rooms, persons with respiratory tract infections
- Advise patient that paradoxic bronchospasm may occur and to stop drug immediately and notify prescriber; to limit caffeine products such as chocolate, coffee, tea, and colas
- Instruct patient on administration of dose; not to use more than prescribed; serious side effects may occur

Evaluation

Positive therapeutic outcome

- Absence of dyspnea, wheezing after 1 hr
- Improved airway exchange
- Improved ABGs

Treatment of overdose: Administer a β_1-adrenergic blocker

metformin (Rx)

(met-for′min)

Fortamet, Glucophage, Glucophage XR, Novo-Metformin ✦, Riomet

Func. class.: Antidiabetic, oral

Chem. class.: Biguanide

Pregnancy category B

Action: Inhibits hepatic glucose production and increases sensitivity of peripheral tissue to insulin

Therapeutic Outcome: Blood glucose at normal levels

Uses: Type 2 diabetes mellitus

Dosage and routes

Adult: PO 500 mg bid initially, then increase to desired response 1-2 g; dosage adjustment q2-3 wk or 850 mg daily with morning meal with dosage increased every other week, max 2500 mg/day; ext rel max 2000 mg/day

Elderly: PO use lowest effective dose

Available forms: Tabs 500, 850, 1000 mg; ext rel tabs 500 mg; oral sol (Riomet) 500 mg/5 ml

Adverse effects:

CNS: *Headache, weakness, dizziness, drowsiness,* tinnitus, fatigue, vertigo, *agitation*

ENDO: **Lactic acidosis,** hypoglycemia

GI: Nausea, vomiting, diarrhea, heartburn, anorexia, metallic taste

HEMA: **Thrombocytopenia,** decreased vit B_{12} levels

INTEG: Rash

Contraindications: Hypersensitivity, hepatic disease, creatinine >1.5 mg/ml (males) ≥1.4 (females), CHF, alcoholism, cardiopulmonary disease, history of lactic acidosis

Precautions: Pregnancy **B,** elderly, thyroid disease, previous hypersensitivity

Pharmacokinetics	
Absorption	Unknown
Distribution	Unknown
Metabolism	Unknown
Excretion	Kidneys, unchanged (35%-50%)
Half-life	1½-5, Terminal 6-20 hr

Pharmacodynamics	
Onset	Unknown
Peak	1-3 hr
Duration	Unknown

M

Interactions

Individual drugs

Acetazolamide: increased blood glucose levels
Cimetidine, digoxin, morphine, procainamide, ranitidine, triamterone, vancomycin: increased metformin level
Cimetidine, phenytoin: increased hypoglycemia
Ethanol: increased risk of lactic acidosis
Radiologic contrast media: do not give together, may cause renal failure

Drug classifications

Calcium channel blockers, contraceptives (oral), corticosteroids, diuretics, estrogens, phenothiazines, sympathomimetics: increased hypoglycemia

Drug/herb

Alfalfa, aloe, basil, bay, bilberry, bitter melon, black catechu, buchu, burdock, coriander, dandelion, eyebright (po), fenugreek, garlic, ginseng, glucomannan, glucosamine, goat's, gymnema, horehound, horse chestnut, jambul, myrrh, myrtle, rue: increased antidiabetic effect
Bee pollen, blue cohosh, broom, chromium, elecampane, eucalyptus, gotu kola: decreased antidiabetic effect
Chromium, coenzyme Q10, fenugreek: increased hypoglycemia
Glucosamine: increased hyperglycemia
Quinine: increased metformin level

NURSING CONSIDERATIONS

Assessment

- Assess for hypoglycemic reactions (sweating, weakness, dizziness, anxiety, tremors, hunger), hyperglycemic reactions soon after meals
- Monitor CBC (baseline, q3 mo) during treatment; check liver function tests (AST, LDH) and renal studies (BUN, creatinine) periodically during treatment; glucose, A1c
- (Alert) Monitor for lactic acidosis: malaise, myalgia, abdominal distress; risk increases with age, poor renal function; monitor electrolytes, lactate, pyruvate, blood pH, ketones, glucose

Nursing diagnoses

- Knowledge, deficient (teaching)

Implementation

- Do not break, crush, or chew ext rel tabs
- Conversion from other oral hypoglycemic agents; change may be made without gradual dosage change; monitor serum or urine glucose and ketones tid during conversion
- Give twice a day with meals to decrease GI upset and provide best absorption, may also be taken as a single dose
- Give in AM to prevent hypoglycemic reactions in PM
- Give tabs crushed and mixed with meal or fluids for patients with difficulty swallowing
- Store in tight container in cool environment

Patient/family education

- Teach patient to regularly self-monitor blood glucose using blood glucose meter
- Teach patient symptoms of hypo/hyperglycemia, what to do about each
- Advise patient that drug must be continued on daily basis; explain consequence of discontinuing drug abruptly
- Advise patient to take drug in morning to prevent hypoglycemic reactions at night
- Advise patient to avoid OTC medications unless approved by the prescriber
- Teach patient that diabetes is a lifelong illness; that this drug controls symptoms, but does not cure the condition
- Teach patient symptoms of lactic acidosis: hyperventilation, fatigue, malaise, myalgia, chills, somnolence to notify prescriber immediately
- Teach patient that all food included in diet plan must be eaten to prevent hypoglycemia
- Teach patient to carry/wear emergency ID and glucagon emergency kit for emergencies
- Advise patient that glucophage XR tab may appear in stool

Evaluation

Positive therapeutic outcome

- Decrease in polyuria, polydipsia, polyphagia; clear sensorium; absence of dizziness; stable gait, blood glucose at normal level

Treatment of overdose: Glucose 25 g **IV** via dextrose 50% sol, 50 ml or 1 mg glucagon

! HIGH ALERT

methadone (Rx)

(meth'a-done)

Dolophine, methadone, Methadose

Func. class.: Opioid analgesic

Chem. class.: Synthetic diphenylheptane derivative

Pregnancy category C

Controlled substance schedule II

Do Not Confuse:
methadone/methylphenidate

Action: Depresses pain impulse transmission at the spinal cord level by interacting with opioid receptors; produces CNS depression

Therapeutic Outcome: Relief of pain; successful opioid withdrawal

Uses: Severe pain, opiate withdrawal

Dosage and routes

Severe pain

Adult: PO/SUBCUT/IM 2.5-10 mg q3-4h prn

Opiate withdrawal

Adult: PO 15-40 mg/day individualized initially, then 20-120 mg/day titrated to patient response

Child: 0.05-0.1 mg/kg/dose q6-12h

Renal dose

Adult: PO CCr 10-50 ml/min dose q8h; CCr <10 ml/min dose q8-12h

Available forms: Inj 10 mg/ml; tabs 5, 10 mg; oral sol 5, 10 mg/5 ml; dispersible tabs 40 mg; oral conc 10 mg/ml; oral sol 5, 10 mg/5 ml, 10 mg/10 ml

Adverse effects

CNS: *Drowsiness, dizziness, confusion, headache, sedation,* euphoria, **seizures**

CV: Palpitations, bradycardia, change in B/P, **cardiac arrest, shock**

EENT: Tinnitus, blurred vision, miosis, diplopia

GI: *Nausea, vomiting, anorexia, constipation, cramps,* biliary tract spasm

GU: Increased urinary output, dysuria, urinary retention

INTEG: *Rash,* urticaria, bruising, flushing, diaphoresis, pruritus

RESP: **Respiratory depression, respiratory arrest**

Contraindications: Hypersensitivity to this drug, or hypersensitivity to chlorobutanol (inj route), addiction (opiate)

Precautions: Pregnancy **C**, addictive personality, lactation, increased ICP, MI (acute), severe heart disease, respiratory depression, hepatic disease, renal disease, child <18 yr, elderly

Pharmacokinetics

Absorption	Well absorbed (PO, SUBCUT, IM)
Distribution	Widely distributed; crosses placenta, half as active PO, as Inj
Metabolism	Liver, extensively
Excretion	Kidneys, breast milk
Half-life	15-30 hr; extended interval with continued dosing

Pharmacodynamics

	PO	IM/SUBCUT
Onset	½-1hr	20 min
Peak	1½-2 hr	1½-2 hr
Duration	4-12 hr	4-6 hr

Interactions

Individual drugs

Alcohol: increased respiratory depression, hypotension, sedation

Nalbuphine, pentazine, phenytoin, rifampin: decreased analgesia

Drug classifications

Antipsychotics, CNS depressants, opiates, phenothiazines, sedative/hypnotics, skeletal muscle relaxants: increased respiratory depression, hypotension

MAOIs: do not use for 2 wk before taking methadone, unpredictable reactions

Drug/herb

Chamomile, hops, Jamaican dogwood, kava, lavender, mistletoe, nettle, pokeweed, poppy, senega, skullcap, valerian: increased CNS depression

Corkwood: increased anticholinergic effect

Drug/lab test

Increased: amylase, lipase

NURSING CONSIDERATIONS

Assessment

- Assess for pain: type, location, intensity, grimacing before and 1½-2 hr after administration; use pain scoring
- Monitor VS after parenteral route; note muscle rigidity, drug history, liver, kidney function tests, respiratory dysfunction: respiratory depression, character, rate, rhythm; notify prescriber if respirations are <10/min
- Monitor CNS changes: dizziness, drowsiness, hallucinations, euphoria, LOC, pupil reaction
- Monitor allergic reactions: rash, urticaria
- Monitor opioid detoxification: no analgesia occurs, only prevention of withdrawal symptoms
- Monitor B/P, pulse
- Monitor bowel changes, bulk, fluids, laxatives should be used for constipation

Nursing diagnoses

- Pain, acute (uses)
- Sensory perception, disturbed: visual, auditory (adverse reactions)
- Breathing pattern, ineffective (adverse reactions)
- Knowledge, deficient (teaching)

Implementation

- Medication should be slowly withdrawn after long-term use to prevent withdrawal symptoms

PO route

- May be given with food or milk to lessen GI upset
- Store in light-resistant container at room temp

M

IM/SUBCUT route

- Do not give if cloudy or a precipitate has formed
- Give deeply in large muscle mass; rotate inj sites

Patient/family education

- Instruct patient to report any symptoms of CNS changes, allergic reactions; to avoid CNS depressants: alcohol, sedative/hypnotics for at least 24 hr after taking this drug
- Discuss with patient that dizziness, drowsiness, and confusion are common; to avoid getting up without assistance
- Discuss in detail with patient all aspects of the drug
- Caution patient to make position changes slowly to prevent orthostatic hypotension

Evaluation

Positive therapeutic outcome

- Decreased pain
- Successful opioid withdrawal

Treatment of overdose: Naloxone (Narcan) 0.2-0.8 mg **IV**, O_2, **IV** fluids, vasopressors

methimazole (Rx)

(meth-im′a-zole)

Tapazole

Func. class.: Thyroid hormone antagonist (antithyroid)

Chem. class.: Thioamide

Pregnancy category D

Action: Inhibits synthesis of thyroid hormones by decreasing iodine use in the manufacture of thyroglobin and iodothyronine; does not affect already formed hormones

Therapeutic Outcome: Decreased T_4 levels, hyperthyroid symptoms

Uses: Hyperthyroidism, preparation for thyroidectomy, thyrotoxic crisis, thyroid storm

Dosage and routes

Hyperthyroidism

Adult: PO 15 mg/day (mild hyperthyroidism); 30-40 mg/day (moderate-severe); 60 mg/day (severe); maintenance dosage 5-15 mg daily

Child: PO 0.4 mg/kg/day in divided doses q8h; continue until euthyroid; maintenance dosage 0.2 mg/kg/day in divided doses q8h, max 30 mg/24 hr

Preparation for thyroidectomy

Adult and child: PO same as above; iodine may be added for 10 days before surgery

Thyrotoxic crisis

Adult and child: PO same as hyperthyroidism with iodine and propranolol

Available forms: Tabs 5, 10 mg

Adverse effects

CNS: *Drowsiness, headache, vertigo, fever,* paresthesias, neuritis

ENDO: *Enlarged thyroid*

GI: *Nausea, diarrhea, vomiting, jaundice,* **hepatitis,** loss of taste

GU: **Nephritis**

HEMA: **Agranulocytosis, leukopenia, thrombocytopenia, hypothrombinemia, lymphadenopathy,** bleeding, vasculitis

INTEG: *Rash, urticaria, pruritus, alopecia, hyperpigmentation,* lupus-like syndrome

MS: Myalgia, arthralgia, nocturnal muscle cramps

Contraindications: Pregnancy **D,** hypersensitivity, lactation

Precautions: Infection, bone marrow depression, hepatic disease

Pharmacokinetics	
Absorption	Rapidly absorbed
Distribution	Crosses placenta
Metabolism	Liver, extensively
Excretion	Kidneys, unchanged; breast milk
Half-life	5-13 hr

Pharmacodynamics	
Onset	½ hr
Peak	Unknown
Duration	2-4 hr

Interactions

Individual drugs

Amiodarone, potassium iodide: decreased effectiveness

Digitalis, warfarin: increased response

Radiation: increased bone marrow depression

Drug classifications

Antineoplastics: increased bone marrow depression

Phenothiazines: increased agranulocytosis

Drug/lab test

Increased: protime, AST, ALT, alkaline phosphatase

NURSING CONSIDERATIONS
Assessment
- Monitor pulse, B/P, temp; check I&O ratio; check for edema (puffy hands, feet, periorbititis); indicates hypothyroidism
- Check weight daily; same clothing, scale, time of day
- Monitor T_3, T_4, which are increased; serum TSH, which is decreased; free thyroxine index, which is increased if dosage is too low; discontinue drug 3-4 wk before radioactive iodine uptake
- ⚠ Monitor blood studies: CBC for blood dyscrasias (leukopenia, thrombocytopenia, agranulocytosis), if these occur, drug should be discontinued and other treatment initiated; liver function tests
- Assess for hypersensitivity (rash, enlarged cervical lymph nodes); drug may have to be discontinued
- Assess for hypoprothrombinemia (bleeding, petechiae, ecchymosis)
- Monitor clinical response: after 3 wk should include increased weight, pulse, decreased T_4
- ⚠ Assess for bone marrow depression: sore throat, fever, fatigue

Nursing diagnoses
- Knowledge, deficient (teaching)
- Noncompliance (teaching)

Implementation
- Give with meals to decrease GI upset; give at same time each day to maintain drug level
- Give lowest dosage that relieves symptoms
- Store in light-resistant container
- Increase fluids to 3-4 L/day, unless contraindicated

Patient/family education
- Advise patient to abstain from breastfeeding after delivery; drug appears in breast milk
- Instruct patient to take pulse daily; to keep graph of weight, pulse, mood
- Advise patient to report redness, swelling, sore throat, mouth lesions, which indicate blood dyscrasias
- Caution patient to avoid OTC products that contain iodine; that seafood and other iodine-containing products may be restricted by prescriber
- Caution patient not to discontinue this medication abruptly; thyroid crisis may occur; stress patient compliance
- Advise patient that response may take several mo if thyroid is large
- Teach patient symptoms/signs of overdose: periorbital edema, cold intolerance, mental depression; notify prescriber at once
- Teach patient symptoms of inadequate dosage: tachycardia, diarrhea, fever, irritability; prescriber should be notified to adjust
- Teach patient to take medication exactly as prescribed, not to skip or double doses; missed doses should be taken when remembered up to 1 hr before next dose
- Instruct patient to carry ID describing medication taken and condition being treated

Evaluation
Positive therapeutic outcome
- Decreased weight gain
- Decreased pulse
- Decreased T_4
- Decreased B/P

methocarbamol (Rx)
(meth-oh-kar'ba-mole)

Carbacot, methocarbamol, Robaxin

Func. class.: Skeletal muscle relaxant, central acting

Chem. class.: Carbamate derivative

Pregnancy category C

Action: Depresses multisynaptic pathways in the spinal cord, causing skeletal muscle relaxation

Therapeutic Outcome: Decreased pain, spasm, resolution of tetanic spasms

Uses: Adjunct for relief of spasm and pain in musculoskeletal conditions

Dosage and routes
Pain of muscle spasm

Adult: PO 1.5 g qid × 2-3 days, then 1 g qid; IM 500 mg in each gluteal region; may repeat q8h; **IV** bol 1-3 g/day max at 3 ml/min; **IV** inf 1 g/250 ml D_5W or 0.9% NaCl, not to exceed 3 g/day

Elderly: PO 500 mg qid, titrate to needed dose

Tetanus management

Adult: **IV** direct 1-2 g or **IV** inf 1-3 g q6h

Child: **IV** 15 mg/kg q6h prn

Available forms: Tabs 500, 750 mg; inj 100 mg/ml

Adverse effects
CNS: *Dizziness, weakness, drowsiness,* headache, tremor, depression, insomnia; **seizures** (**IV**, IM only)

CV: Postural hypotension, *bradycardia*

EENT: Diplopia, temporary loss of vision, blurred vision, nystagmus

GI: *Nausea,* vomiting, hiccups, anorexia, metallic taste

M

GU: Brown, black, green urine
HEMA: Hemolysis, increased hemoglobin (**IV** only)
INTEG: Rash, pruritus, fever, facial flushing, urticaria, phlebitis
MISC: **Anaphylaxis** (IM, **IV**)

Contraindications: Hypersensitivity, child <12 yr, intermittent porphyria

Precautions: Pregnancy **C**, renal disease, hepatic disease, addictive personalities, myasthenia gravis, epilepsy

Pharmacokinetics

Absorption	Rapidly absorbed (PO)
Distribution	Widely distributed; crosses placenta
Metabolism	Liver, partially
Excretion	Kidney, unchanged
Half-life	1-2 hr

Pharmacodynamics

	PO	IM	IV
Onset	½ hr	Rapid	Rapid
Peak	1-2 hr	Unknown	Inf end
Duration	>8 hr	Unknown	Unknown

Interactions
Individual drugs
Alcohol: increased CNS depression
Drug classifications
Antidepressants, barbiturates, opioids, sedative/hypnotics, tricyclic: increased CNS depression
Drug/herb
Chamomile, hops, kava, skullcap, valerian: increased CNS depression
Drug/lab test
False increase: VMA, urinary 5-HIAA

NURSING CONSIDERATIONS
Assessment
- Assess for pain and spasm: location, duration, intensity, range of motion
- Monitor during and after inj: CNS effects, rash, conjunctivitis, and nasal congestion may occur
- Monitor ECG in epileptic patients; poor seizure control has occurred in patients taking this drug
- Assess allergic reactions: rash, fever, respiratory distress; check for severe weakness, numbness in extremities
- Assess for tolerance: increased need for medication, more frequent requests for medication, increased pain
- Assess for CNS depression: dizziness, drowsiness, psychiatric symptoms

Nursing diagnoses
- Mobility, physical, impaired (uses)
- Injury, risk for (adverse reactions)
- Knowledge, deficient (teaching)

Implementation
- Methocarbamol incompatible with any drug in sol or syringe

PO route
- Give with meals if GI symptoms occur
- Store in airtight container at room temp

IM route
- Give inj deep in large muscle mass; rotate sites
- Do not give SUBCUT

IV route
- Give **IV** undiluted over 1 min or more; give 300 mg or less/1 min or longer; may be diluted in 250 ml or less D_5 or isotonic NaCl sol for slow **IV** infusion
- Give by slow **IV** to prevent phlebitis; keep recumbent during and for 15 min after to prevent orthostatic hypotension; check for extravasation

Patient/family education
- Advise patient not to discontinue medication quickly; insomnia, nausea, headache, spasticity, tachycardia will occur; drug should be tapered off over 1-2 wk
- Inform patient that urine may turn green, black, or brown
- Caution patient not to take with alcohol, other CNS depressants; increased CNS depression can occur
- Advise patient to avoid altering activities while taking this drug
- Caution patient to avoid hazardous activities if drowsiness, dizziness occur; driving should be avoided until drug response is known
- Advise patient to avoid using OTC medications that are CNS depressants (cough preparations, antihistamines) unless directed by prescriber; CNS depression can occur

Evaluation
Positive therapeutic outcome
- Decreased pain, spasticity

Treatment of overdose: Induce emesis in conscious patient; lavage, dialysis; have epINEPHrine, antihistamines, and corticosteroids available, enhance elimination with osmotic diureses, **IV** fluids for hypotension

! HIGH ALERT

methotrexate, (amethopterin, MTX)

(Rx)

(meth-oh-trex'ate)

Methotrexate, Rheumatrex, Dose Pack, Trexall

Func. class.: Antineoplastic, antimetabolite

Chem. class.: Folic acid antagonist

Pregnancy category X

Do Not Confuse: methotrexate/metolazone

Action: Inhibits an enzyme that reduces folic acid, which is needed for nucleic acid synthesis in all cells; cell cycle specific (S phase); immunosuppressive

Therapeutic Outcome: Prevention of rapidly growing malignant cells; immunosuppression

Uses: Acute lymphocytic leukemia, in combination for breast, lung, head, neck carcinoma, lymphosarcoma, gestational choriocarcinoma, hydatidiform mole, psoriasis, rheumatoid arthritis, mycosis fungoides

Dosage and routes

Acute lymphocytic leukemia

Adult and child: PO/IM/**IV** 3.3 mg/m^2/day × 4-6 wk until remission, then 20-30 mg/m^2 PO/IM qwk in 2 divided doses or 2.5 mg/kg **IV** × 2 wk

Burkitt's lymphoma (stages I, II, III)

Adult: PO 10-25 mg daily × 4-8 days with 7-day rest period

Lymphosarcoma (stage III)

Adult: PO/IM/**IV**, 0.625-2.5 mg/kg/day

Meningeal leukemia

Adult and child: 12 mg/m^2 IT q2-5 days until CSF is normal, then one additional dose, max 15 mg

Choriocarcinoma

Adult and child: PO/IM 15-30 mg/m^2 daily × 5 days, then off 1 wk; may repeat

Breast cancer

Adult: **IV** 40 mg/m^2 on days 1 and 8 with other antineoplastics

Rheumatoid arthritis

Adult: PO 7.5 mg/wk or divided doses of 2.5 mg q12h × 3 given qwk, max 20 mg/wk

Polyarticular-course juvenile RA

Child: PO 10 mg/m^2 qwk

Osteosarcoma

Adult and child: **IV** 12 g/m^2 given over 4 hr, then leucovorin rescue is given

Mycosis fungoides

Adult: PO 2.5-10 mg/day until cleared (may be many mo); IM 50 mg qwk or 25 mg 2 ×/wk

Psoriasis

Adult: PO/IM/**IV** 10-25 mg qwk or 2.5 mg PO q12hr × 3 doses; may increase to 25 mg qwk

Available forms: Tabs 2.5, 5, 7.5, 10, 15 mg; inj 25 mg/ml; powder for inj 20 mg, 1 g

Adverse effects

CNS: Dizziness, **seizures,** headache, confusion, hemiparesis, malaise, fatigue, chills, fever, **leukoencephalopathy; arachnoiditis** (intrathecal)

GI: *Nausea, vomiting, anorexia, diarrhea, ulcerative stomatitis,* **hepatotoxicity,** cramps, ulcer, gastritis, **GI hemorrhage,** abdominal pain, hematemesis, **hepatic fibrosis, acute toxicity**

GU: Urinary retention, **renal failure,** menstrual irregularities, defective spermatogenesis, **hematuria, azotemia, uric acid nephropathy**

HEMA: **Leukopenia, thrombocytopenia, myelosuppression, anemia**

INTEG: *Rash, alopecia,* dry skin, urticaria, photosensitivity, folliculitis, vasculitis, petechiae, ecchymosis, acne, alopecia, **severe fatal skin reactions**

RESP: **Methotrexate-induced lung disease**

SYST: **Sudden death, *pneumocystis jiroveci* pneumonia**

Contraindications: Pregnancy **X**, hypersensitivity, leukopenia (<3500/mm^3), thrombocytopenia (<100,000/mm^3), anemia, psoriatic patients with severe renal/hepatic disease, alcoholism, HIV infection

Precautions: Renal disease, lactation, children

Pharmacokinetics

Absorption	Well absorbed (GI)
Distribution	Widely distributed; crosses placenta
Metabolism	Not metabolized
Excretion	Kidneys, unchanged; breast milk (minimal)
Half-life	2-4 hr; increased in renal disease

M

Pharmacodynamics

	PO	IM/IV	IT
Onset	Unknown	Unknown	Unknown
Peak	1-4 hr	½-2 hr	Unknown
Duration	Unknown	Unknown	Unknown

Interactions
Individual drugs
Alcohol, phenylbutazone, probenecid, radiation, theophylline: increased toxicity
Digoxin (PO), fosphenytoin, phenytoin: decreased effect of each specific drug
Folic acid: decreased effect of methotrexate
Radiation: increased bone marrow suppression
Drug classifications
Anticoagulants (oral): increased hypoprothrombinemia
Antineoplastics, NSAIDs, penicillins, salicylates, sulfa drugs: increased toxicity
Live virus vaccines: decreased antibodies

NURSING CONSIDERATIONS
Assessment
- Assess buccal cavity q8h for dryness, sores or ulceration, white patches, oral pain, bleeding, dysphagia; obtain prescription for viscous lidocaine (Xylocaine)
- Assess symptoms indicating severe allergic reaction: rash, pruritus, urticaria, purpuric skin lesions, itching, flushing
- Assess tachypnea, ECG changes, dyspnea, edema, fatigue; identify dyspnea, crackles, unproductive cough, chest pain, tachypnea
- Monitor CBC, differential, platelet count weekly; withhold drug if WBC is <3500/mm^3 or platelet count is <100,000/mm^3; notify prescriber of results if WBC <20,000/mm^3, platelets <150,000/mm^3; WBC, platelet nadirs occur on day 7
- Assess for increased uric acid levels, swelling, joint pain primarily in extremities; patient should be well hydrated to prevent urate deposits
- Monitor renal function studies: BUN, creatinine, serum uric acid, urine CCr before and during therapy; check I&O ratio; report fall in urine output to <30 ml/hr
- Monitor temp q4h (may indicate beginning of infection)
- Monitor liver function tests before and during therapy (bilirubin, AST, ALT, LDH) as needed or monthly; check for jaundice of skin and sclera, dark urine, clay-colored stools, itchy skin, abdominal pain, fever, diarrhea (hepatotoxicity)
- Assess for bleeding: hematuria, stool guaiac, bruising or petechiae, mucosa or orifices q8h; check for inflammation of mucosa, breaks in skin
- Identify effects of alopecia on body image; discuss feelings about body changes
- Identify edema in feet, joint and stomach pain, shaking; prescriber should be notified
- Monitor methotrexate levels, adjust leucovorin dose based on the level

Nursing diagnoses
- Injury, risk for (adverse reactions)
- Body image, disturbed (adverse reactions)
- Infection, risk for (adverse reactions)
- Knowledge, deficient (teaching)

Implementation
- Avoid contact with skin, since drug is very irritating; wash completely to remove
- (Alert) Administer leucovorin calcium within 24 hr of giving this drug to prevent tissue damage; check agency policy; continue until methotrexate level <10^{-8}m
- Give fluids **IV** or PO before chemotherapy to hydrate patient
- Give antacid before oral agent; give drug after evening meal, before bedtime; give antiemetic 30-60 min before giving drug and prn to prevent vomiting; administer antibiotics for infection prophylaxis
- Give in AM so drug can be eliminated before bedtime
- Provide liq diet: carbonated beverages; gelatin may be added if patient is not nauseated or vomiting

PO route
- Give 1 hr ac or 2 hr pc to prevent vomiting
- Make sure drug is taken weekly in RA, JRA

IM route
- Give deeply in large muscle mass

IV route
- Give **IV** after diluting 5 mg/2 ml of sterile water for inj; give through Y-tube or 3-way stopcock at 10 mg or less/min
- Give **IV** inf after diluting in 0.9% NaCl, D_5W, D_5/0.9% NaCl and give as prescribed
- (Alert) Give sodium bicarbonate tabs or **IV** fluids to prevent precipitation of drug at high doses, urine pH should be >7; may need to reduce dose if BUN is 20-30 mg/dl or creatinine is 1.2-2 mg/dl; stop drug if BUN >30 mg/dl or creatitine is >2 mg/dl

Syringe compatibilities: Bleomycin, cisplatin, cyclophosphamide, doxapram, DOXOrubicin, fluorouracil, furosemide, heparin, leucovorin, mitomycin, vinBLAStine, vinCRIStine

Syringe incompatibilities: Droperidol, ranitidine

Y-site compatibilities: Allopurinol, amifostine, asparaginase, aztreonam, bleomycin, cefepime, ceftriaxone, cimetidine, cisplatin, cyclophosphamide, cytarabine, DAUNOrubicin, dexchlorpheniramine, diphenhydrAMINE, DOXOrubicin, etoposide, famotidine, filgrastim, fludarabine, fluorouracil, furosemide, gallium, ganciclovir, granisetron, heparin, hydromorphone, imipenem-cilastatin, leucovorin, lorazepam, melphalan, mesna, methylPREDNISolone, metoclopramide, mitomycin, morphine, ondansetron, oxacillin, paclitaxel, piperacillin/tazobactam, prochlorperazine, ranitidine, sargramostim, teniposide, thiotepa, vinBLAStine, vinCRIStine, vinorelbine
Y-site incompatibilities: Droperidol, idarubicin
Additive compatibilities: Cephalothin, cyclophosphamide, cytarabine, fluorouracil, hydrOXYzine, mercaptopurine, ondansetron, sodium bicarbonate, vinCRIStine
Additive incompatibilities: Bleomycin, prednisoLONE
Solution compatibilities: Amino acids, 4.25%/D_{25}, D_5W, sodium bicarbonate 0.05 mol/L, sodium chloride 0.9%

Patient/family education

- Encourage patient to rinse mouth tid-qid with water, club soda; brush teeth bid-qid with soft brush or cotton-tipped applicators for stomatitis; use unwaxed dental floss
- Advise patient that contraceptive measures are recommended during therapy; drug is teratogenic; contraception should be used for 3 mo (male) and 4-6 wk (female); to discontinue breastfeeding; toxicity to infant may occur
- Teach patient to avoid use of products containing aspirin or NSAIDs, razors, commercial mouthwash, since bleeding may occur; to report symptoms of bleeding (hematuria, tarry stools)
- Caution patient to report signs of anemia (fatigue, headache, irritability, faintness, shortness of breath)
- Advise patient to report any changes in breathing or coughing even several mo after treatment; to avoid crowds and persons with respiratory tract or other infections
- Advise patient to report stomatitis: any bleeding, white spots, ulcerations in mouth to prescriber; tell patient to examine mouth daily, report symptoms, use good oral hygiene
- Teach patient that hair may be lost during treatment; a wig or hairpiece may make patient feel better; new hair may be different in color, texture
- Caution patient not to have any vaccinations without the advice of the prescriber; serious reactions can occur
- Advise patient to use sunblock or protective clothing to prevent burns

Evaluation

Positive therapeutic outcome

- Prevention of rapid division of malignant cells

methyldopa/ methyldopate (Rx)

(meth-ill-doe'pa)

Aldomet, Apo-methyldopa ♣, Dopamet ♣, methyldopa/methyldopate, Novamedopa, Nu-Medopa ♣

Func. class.: Antihypertensive

Chem. class.: Centrally acting α-adrenergic inhibitor

Pregnancy category B (PO), C (IV)

Do Not Confuse:
methyldopa/L-dopa (levodopa)

Action: Stimulates central α_2-adrenergic receptors in the CNS, resulting in decreased sympathetic outflow from the brain with decreased peripheral resistance

Therapeutic Outcome: Decreased B/P in hypertension

Uses: Hypertension, hypertensive crisis

Dosage and routes

Adult: PO 250-500 mg bid or tid, then adjusted q2 days prn, 0.5-2 g daily in 2-4 divided doses (maintenance), max 3 g/day; **IV** 250-500 mg in 100 ml D_5W q6h, run over 30-60 min, not to exceed 1 g q6h, switch to PO as soon as possible
Elderly: PO 125 mg bid tid, increase q2 days as needed, max 3 g/day
Child: PO 10 mg/kg/day in 2-4 divided doses, max 65 mg/kg or 3 g/day, whichever is less; **IV** 20-40 mg/kg/day in 4 divided doses, max 65 mg/kg or 3 g, whichever is less

Available forms: Methyldopa: tabs 125, 250, 500 mg; oral susp 50 mg/ml; methydopate: inj 50 mg/ml (250 mg/5 ml)

Adverse effects

CNS: *Drowsiness, weakness, dizziness, sedation, headache,* depression, psychosis, paresthesias, parkinsonism, Bell's palsy, nightmares

M

CV: Bradycardia, **myocarditis,** orthostatic hypotension, angina, edema, weight gain, **CHF,** paradoxical pressor response (**IV** use)
EENT: Nasal congestion, eczema
ENDO: Breast enlargement, gynecomastia, lactation, amenorrhea
GI: Nausea, vomiting, diarrhea, constipation, **hepatic dysfunction,** sore or "black" tongue, **pancreatitis,** colitis, flatulence
GU: Impotence, failure to ejaculate
HEMA: **Leukopenia, thrombocytopenia, hemolytic anemia, granulocytopenia,** positive Coombs' test
INTEG: Lupus-like syndrome, rash, **toxic epidural necrolysis**

Contraindications: Active hepatic disease, hypersensitivity

Precautions: Pregnancy **B** (PO), **C** (**IV**) liver disease, eclampsia, severe cardiac disease, renal disease

Pharmacokinetics

Absorption	50% (PO)
Distribution	Crosses placenta, blood-brain barrier
Metabolism	Liver, moderately
Excretion	Kidneys, unchanged (partially)
Half-life	1½ hr

Pharmacodynamics

	PO	IV
Onset	Unknown	Unknown
Peak	2-4 hr	2 hr
Duration	12-24 hr	10-16 hr

Interactions

Individual drugs

Alcohol: CNS depression
Alcohol, levodopa: increased hypotension
Haloperidol: increased psychosis
Levodopa: increased CNS toxicity
Lithium: increased lithium toxicity
Tolbutamide: increased hypoglycemia

Drug classifications

Amphetamines, antidepressants (tricyclic), barbiturates, NSAIDs: decreased antihypertensive effect
Analgesics, antidepressants, antihistamines, sedative/hypnotics: increased CNS depression
Antihypertensives, diuretics: increased hypotension
β-Adrenergic blockers: increased B/P
MAOIs: increased pressor effect
Sympathomimetic amines: increased pressor effect

Drug/herb

Aconite: increased toxicity, death
Astragalus, cola tree: increased or decreased antihypertensive effect
Barberry, betony, black catechu, black cohosh, bloodroot, broom, burdock, cat's claw, dandelion, goldenseal, Irish moss, Jamaican dogwood, kelp, khella, mistletoe, parsley: increased antihypertensive effect
Coltsfoot, guarana, khat, licorice: decreased antihypertensive effect

Drug/lab test

Interference: urinary uric acid, serum creatinine, AST
False increase: urinary catecholamines

NURSING CONSIDERATIONS

Assessment

- Monitor blood studies: neutrophils, decreased platelets; direct Coombs' test before and after 6, 12 mo of therapy
- Monitor renal studies: protein, BUN, creatinine; watch for increased levels that may indicate nephrotic syndrome: polyuria, oliguria, frequency; report weight gain >5 lb
- Obtain baselines in renal, liver function tests before therapy begins; check potassium levels, although hyperkalemia rarely occurs
- Monitor B/P, pulse if the drug is being used for hypertension; notify prescriber of changes
- Monitor edema in feet, legs daily; monitor I&O; check weight for decreasing output
- Assess for allergic reaction: rash, fever, pruritus, urticaria; drug should be discontinued if antihistamines fail to help
- Monitor CNS symptoms, especially in the elderly, depression, change in mental status

Nursing diagnoses

- Cardiac output, decreased (uses)
- Injury, risk for (side effects)
- Knowledge, deficient (teaching)
- Noncompliance (teaching)

Implementation

PO route

- Give ac
- Shake susp before using
- Store in airtight container at room temp

IV route

- Give by intermittent inf after diluting in 100 ml of 0.9% NaCl, D_5W, $D_5/0.9\%$ NaCl, 5% sodium bicarbonate, Ringer's; administer over 30-60 min

Y-site compatibilities: Esmolol, heparin, meperidine, morphine, theophylline

Additive compatibilities: Aminophylline, ascorbic acid, chloramphenicol, diphenhydrAMINE, heparin, magnesium sulfate, multivitamins, netilmicin, potassium chloride, promazine, sodium bicarbonate, succinylcholine, verapamil, vit B/C

Additive incompatibilities: Amphotericin B, barbiturates, methohexital, sulfonamides

Solution compatibilities: D_5W, D_5/0.9% NaCl, Ringer's, sodium bicarbonate 5%, 0.9% NaCl, amino acids 4.25%/D_{25}, Dextran$_6$/0.9% NaCl, Normosol R, Normosol M/D_5W

Patient/family education

- Instruct patient not to discontinue drug abruptly, or withdrawal symptoms may occur: anxiety, increased B/P, headache, insomnia, increased pulse, tremors, nausea, sweating
- Caution patient not to use OTC (cough, cold, or allergy) products unless directed by prescriber
- Teach patient to comply with dosage schedule even if feeling better; drug controls symptoms, does not cure
- Caution patient to change position slowly, to rise slowly to sitting or standing position to minimize orthostatic hypotension, especially elderly
- Teach patient about excessive perspiration, dehydration, vomiting, diarrhea, may lead to fall in B/P; consult prescriber if these occur
- Advise patient that drug may cause dizziness, fainting; lightheadedness may occur during 1st few days of therapy; that drug may cause dry mouth; use hard candy, saliva product, or frequent rinsing of mouth
- Caution patient that compliance is necessary; not to skip or stop drug unless directed by prescriber
- Teach patient that drug may cause skin rash
- Teach patient to avoid hazardous activities, since drug may cause drowsiness, dizziness

Evaluation

Positive therapeutic outcome

- Decreased B/P

Treatment of overdose: Gastric evacuation, sympathomimetics, may be indicated if severe; hemodialysis

methylergonovine (Rx)

(meth-ill-er-goe-noe'veen)

Methergine, methylergonovine

Func. class.: Oxytocic

Chem. class.: Ergot alkaloid

Pregnancy category C

Action: Stimulates uterine and vascular smooth muscle, causing contractions, decreased bleeding

Therapeutic Outcome: Absence of hemorrhage

Uses: Treatment of hemorrhage postpartum or after abortion

Dosage and routes

Adult: PO 200-400 mcg q6-12h × 2-7 days IM/**IV** 200 mcg q2-4hr for 1-5 doses

Available forms: Inj 200 mcg/ml; tabs 200 mcg

Adverse effects

CNS: *Headache, dizziness,* **seizures**

CV: **Hypotension,** chest pain, palpitations, *hypertension,* **dysrhythmias; CVA (IV)**

EENT: Tinnitus

GI: *Nausea, vomiting*

GU: Cramping

INTEG: Sweating, rash, allergic reactions

RESP: *Dyspnea*

Contraindications: Hypersensitivity to ergot preparations, indication of labor, before delivery of placenta, hypertension, pelvic inflammatory disease, respiratory disease, cardiac disease, peripheral vascular disease

Precautions: Pregnancy **C,** severe hepatic disease, severe renal disease, jaundice, diabetes mellitus, convulsive disorders, sepsis

M

Pharmacokinetics

Absorption	Well absorbed (PO, IM)
Distribution	Unknown
Metabolism	Liver, possibly
Excretion	Unknown
Half-life	½-2 hr

Pharmacodynamics

	PO	IM	IV
Onset	5-15 min	5 min	Immediate
Peak	Unknown	Unknown	Unknown
Duration	3 hr	3 hr	Unknown

Interactions

Drug classifications

Vasopressors: increased vasoconstriction

Smoking: increased vasoconstriction

NURSING CONSIDERATIONS

Assessment

- Monitor B/P, pulse; watch for change that may indicate hemorrhage; check respiratory rate, rhythm, depth; notify prescriber of abnormalities
- Assess fundal tone, nonphasic contractions; check for relaxation or severe cramping

- Assess for ergotism or overdose: nausea, vomiting, weakness, muscular pain, insensitivity to cold, paresthesia of extremities; drug should be decreased or inf discontinued
- Before administering ergonovine, check calcium levels; if hypocalcemia is present, correction should be made to increase effectiveness of this drug
- Monitor prolactin levels and for decreased breast milk production

Nursing diagnoses

- Tissue perfusion, ineffective (uses)
- Injury, risk for (adverse reactions)
- Knowledge, deficient (teaching)

Implementation

PO route

- PO is the preferred route

IM route

- Give inj deeply in large muscle mass

IV route

- Give by this route for severe, life-threatening hemorrhage
- Give directly undiluted or diluted with 5 ml of 0.9% NaCl given through Y-site or 3-way stopcock; give 0.2 mg/min; use clear, colorless sol
- Store up to 2 mo if unused

Y-site compatibilities: Heparin, hydrocortisone sodium succinate, potassium chloride, vit B/C

Patient/family education

- Advise patient to stop smoking, since increased vasoconstriction will result
- Inform patient that abdominal cramps are a side effect of this medication
- Instruct patient to notify prescriber if chest pain, nausea, vomiting, headache, muscle pain, weakness or cold, numb extremities occur

Evaluation

Positive therapeutic outcome

- Prevention of hemorrhage

methylphenidate (Key Drug) (Rx)

(meth-ill-fen'i-date)

Concerta, Metadate CD, Metadate ER, Methidate, Methylin, Methylin ER, PMS-Methylphenidate, Riphenidate (Canada Only), Ritalin, Ritalin SR, Ritalin LA

Func. class.: Cerebral stimulant

Chem. class.: Piperidine derivative

Pregnancy category C

Controlled substance schedule II

Do Not Confuse:
methylphenidate/methadone

Action: Increases release of norepinephrine and dopamine in cerebral cortex to reticular activating system; exact action not known

Therapeutic Outcome: Increased alertness, decreased fatigue, ability to stay awake (narcolepsy), increased attention span, decreased hyperactivity (ADHD)

Uses: Attention deficit disorder with hyperactivity (ADHD), narcolepsy (except Concerta, Metadate CD, Ritalin LA), attention deficit disorder (ADD)

Investigational uses: Depression in the elderly, cancer, poststroke, HIV, brain injury, improvement of pain control, sedation in patients receiving opiates

Dosage and routes

ADHD

Child >6 yr: PO (immediate release tab, chew tabs, oral sol) 5 mg before breakfast and lunch, increasing by 5-10 mg/wk, not to exceed 60 mg/day; ext rel 20 mg daily-tid

Narcolepsy

Adult: PO 10 mg bid-tid, 30-45 min ac; may increase up to 40-60 mg/day

Depression

Elderly: PO 2.5 mg q AM, increase q 3rd day by 2.5 mg to desired dose, max 20 mg/day

Available forms: Tabs 5, 10, 20 mg; ext rel tabs 10, 20 mg; ext rel tabs (Concerta) 18, 27, 36, 54 mg; chew tabs (Methylin) 2.5, 5, 10 mg; ext rel cap 10, 20, 30, 40 mg; oral sol 5 mg, 10 mg/ml

Adverse effects

CNS: *Hyperactivity, insomnia, restlessness, talkativeness,* dizziness, headache, akathisia, dyskinesia, masking or worsening of Gilles de la Tourette's syndrome, **seizures,** drowsiness, toxic psychosis

CV: *Palpitations, tachycardia,* B/P changes, angina, **dysrhythmias**

ENDO: Growth retardation

GI: Nausea, anorexia, dry mouth, weight loss, abdominal pain
HEMA: **Leukopenia,** anemia, **thrombocytopenic purpura**
INTEG: **Exfoliative dermatitis,** urticaria, rash, erythema multiforme
MISC: Fever, arthralgia, scalp hair loss

Contraindications: Hypersensitivity, anxiety, history of Gilles de la Tourette's syndrome; children <6 yr, glaucoma, anorexia nervosa, tartrazine dye hypersensitivity

Precautions: Pregnancy **C,** hypertension, depression, seizures, lactation, drug abuse

Pharmacokinetics

Absorption	Well absorbed (PO); delayed (ext rel)
Distribution	Widely distributed; crosses placenta
Metabolism	Liver
Excretion	Kidneys
Half-life	1-3 hr

Pharmacodynamics

	PO	PO–EXT-REL
Onset	½-1 hr	2 hr
Peak	1-3 hr	4 hr
Duration	4-6 hr	6-8 hr

Interactions
Drug classifications
Anticonvulsants, antidepressants (tricyclics), SSRIs: increased effects
MAOIs (or within 14 days of MAOIs), vasopressors: hypertensive crisis
Drug/herb
Cola nut, guarana, horsetail, yerba maté, yohimbe: increased CNS stimulation
Melatonin: synergistic effect
Drug/food
Caffeine: increased stimulation

NURSING CONSIDERATIONS
Assessment
- Monitor VS, B/P, since this drug may reverse antihypertensives; check patients with cardiac disease more often for increased B/P
- Perform CBC, urinalysis; for diabetic patients monitor blood glucose, urine glucose; insulin changes may be required, since eating will decrease
- Monitor height and weight q3 mo since growth rate in children may be decreased; appetite is suppressed, weight loss is common during the first few mo of treatment
- Monitor mental status: mood sensorium, affect, stimulation, insomnia; aggressiveness may occur; depression with crying spells may occur after drug has worn off
- Assess for tolerance; should not be used for extended time except in ADHD; dosage should be discontinued gradually to prevent withdrawal symptoms
- Assess for narcoleptic symptoms before medication and after; ability to stay awake should increase significantly
- In children or adults with ADHD, monitor for improved organizational skills, attention span, attending to tasks, impulse control, socialization, and ability to get along better with others
- Assess for withdrawal symptoms: headache, nausea, vomiting, muscle pain, weakness; drug tolerance will develop after long-term use; dosage should not be increased if tolerance develops
- Assess appetite, sleep, speech patterns

Nursing diagnoses
- Thought processes, disturbed (uses, adverse reactions)
- Coping, ineffective (uses)
- Knowledge, deficient (teaching)
- Coping, family, compromised (uses)

Implementation
- Do not chew, crush time rel tabs; caps may be opened and beads sprinkled over spoonful of applesauce
- Give at least 6 hr before bedtime (regular release); at least 10 hr (ext rel) to avoid sleeplessness; titrate to patient's response; lowest dosage should be used to control symptoms
- Give gum, hard candy, frequent sips of water for dry mouth at beginning of treatment; these symptoms tend to lessen with time

Patient/family education
- Teach patient to decrease caffeine consumption (coffee, tea, cola, chocolate); not to use guarana, cola nut, yerba maté, which may increase irritability and stimulation; to avoid OTC preparations unless approved by prescriber; to avoid alcohol ingestion; these may cause serious drug interactions
- Advise patient to taper off drug over several wk, or depression, increased sleeping, lethargy may occur
- Caution patient to avoid hazardous activities until stabilized on medication
- Instruct patient not to double doses if medication is missed; prescriber may suggest drug holidays (ADHD) during the school year to assess progress and determine continued drug necessity

- Instruct patient/family to notify presciber if significant side effects occur: tremors, insomnia, palpitations, restlessness; drug changes may be needed
- Inform patient that if dry mouth occurs to use frequent sips of water, sugarless gum, hard candy during beginning therapy; dry mouth lessens with continued treatment
- Encourage patient to get needed rest; patient will feel more tired at end of day; to take last dose at least 6 hr before bedtime to avoid insomnia
- Advise patient that shell of Concerta tab may appear in stools

Evaluation

Positive therapeutic outcome

- Decreased hyperactivity in ADHD
- Improved attention span in ADHD
- Absence of sleeping during day in narcolepsy

Treatment of overdose: Administer fluids, hemodialysis, peritoneal dialysis, antihypertensives for increased B/P

methylPREDNISolone (Rx)

(meth-ill-pred-niss'oh-lone)

A-Methapred, dep Medalone, Depoject, Depo-Medrol, Depopred, Depo-Predate, Duralone, Medralone, Medrol, Rep-Pred, Solu-Medrol

Func. class.: Corticosteroid, synthetic

Chem. class.: Glucocorticoid, immediate acting

Pregnancy category C

Do Not Confuse:
methylPREDNISolone/medroxyPROGESTERone, methylPREDNISolone/predniSONE, methylPREDNISolone/methylTESTOSTERone

Action: Decreases inflammation by suppression of migration of polymorphonuclear leukocytes, fibroblasts; reverses increased capillary permeability and lysosomal stabilization; antipruritic, antiinflammatory (top)

Therapeutic Outcome: Decreased inflammation

Uses: Severe inflammation, shock, adrenal insufficiency, collagen disorders, management of acute spinal cord injury, multiple sclerosis

Dosage and routes

Adrenal insufficiency/inflammation

Adult: PO 2-60 mg in 4 divided doses; IM 10-80 mg (acetate); IM/**IV** 10-250 mg (succinate); intraarticular 4-30 mg (acetate); Rec 40 mg 3-7 × wk for ≥2 wk

Child: **IV** 117 mcg-1.66 mg/kg in 3-4 divided doses (succinate); Rec 0.5-1 mg/kg (15-30 mg/m^2) daily or every other day × 1 wk or more

Shock

Adult: **IV** 100-250 mg q2-6h or 30 mg/kg, then q4-6h prn × 2-3 days (succinate)

Multiple sclerosis

Adult: PO 160 mg/day × 1 wk, then 64 mg every other day × 30 days

Available forms: Tabs 2, 4, 6, 8, 16, 24, 32 mg; inj 20, 40, 80 mg/ml acetate; inj 40, 125, 500, 1000, 2000 mg/vial succinate, dose pack 4 mg tabs; susp for inj 20, 40, 80 mg/ml; enema 40 mg

Adverse effects

CNS: Depression, flushing, sweating, headache, mood changes

CV: Hypertension, **circulatory collapse, thrombophlebitis, embolism,** tachycardia

EENT: Fungal infections, increased intraocular pressure, blurred vision, cataracts

GI: Diarrhea, nausea, abdominal distention, **GI hemorrhage,** increased appetite, **pancreatitis**

HEMA: **Thrombocytopenia**

INTEG: Acne, poor wound healing, ecchymosis, petechiae

MS: Fractures, osteoporosis, weakness

Contraindications: Hypersensitivity to corticosteroids, fungal infections, psychosis, idiopathic thrombocytopenia, acute glomerulonephritis, amebiasis, nonasthmatic bronchial disease, child <2 yr, AIDS, TB

Precautions: Pregnancy **C,** lactation, diabetes mellitus, glaucoma, osteoporosis, seizure disorders, ulcerative colitis, CHF, myasthenia gravis, renal disease, esophagitis, peptic ulcer

Pharmacokinetics

Absorption	Well absorbed (PO); systemic (top)
Distribution	Crosses placenta
Metabolism	Liver, extensively
Excretion	Kidney
Half-life	3-5 hr (plasma) 18-36 hr (tissue); adrenal suppression 3-4 days

Pharmacodynamics

	PO	IM	IV	TOP
Onset	Unknown	Unknown	Rapid	Min to hr
Peak	2 hr	4-8 days	Unknown	Hr to days
Duration	1½ days	1-4 wk	Unknown	Hr to days

Interactions

Individual drugs

Amphotericin B: increased side effects
Insulin: increased need for insulin
Phenytoin, rifampin, theophylline: decreased action; increased metabolism
Somatrem: decreased effect

Drug classifications

Contraceptives, oral: increased methylPREDNISolone action
Diuretics: increased side effects
Hypoglycemic agents: increased need for hypoglycemic agents
NSAIDs: increased GI reactions

Drug/herb

Aloe, buckthorn, cascara sagrada, Chinese rhubarb, rhubarb root, senna: increased hypokalemia
Aloe, licorice, perilla: increased corticosteroid effect

Drug/food

Grapefruit juice: increased methylPREDNISolone level, do not use concurrently

Drug/lab test

Increased: cholesterol, sodium, blood glucose, uric acid, calcium, urine glucose
Decreased: calcium, potassium, T_4, T_3, thyroid radioactive iodine uptake test, urine 17-OHCS, 17-KS
False negative: skin allergy tests

NURSING CONSIDERATIONS

Assessment

- Monitor potassium, blood glucose, urine glucose while patient is on long-term therapy; hypokalemia and hyperglycemia
- Monitor weight daily; notify prescriber of weekly gain >5 lb
- Monitor B/P q4h, pulse; notify prescriber if chest pain occurs
- Monitor I&O ratio; be alert for decreasing urinary output and increasing edema
- Monitor plasma cortisol levels during long-term therapy (normal level 138-635 nmol/L when drawn at 8 AM)
- Monitor adrenal function periodically for hypothalamic-pituitary-adrenal axis suppression
- Assess for infection: increased temp, WBC even after withdrawal of medication; drug masks infection symptoms
- Assess for potassium depletion: paresthesias, fatigue, nausea, vomiting, depression, polyuria, dysrhythmias, weakness
- Assess for edema, hypertension, cardiac symptoms
- Assess mental status: affect, mood, behavioral changes, aggression
- Check temp; if fever develops, drug should be discontinued
- Assess for systemic absorption: increased temp, inflammation, irritation (top)

Nursing diagnoses

- Infection, risk for (adverse reactions)
- Knowledge, deficient (teaching)
- Noncompliance (teaching)

Implementation

PO route

- Give with food or milk to decrease GI symptoms

IM route

- Give IM inj deep in large muscle mass; rotate sites; avoid deltoid; use 21-G needle
- Give in one dose in AM to prevent adrenal suppression; avoid SUBCUT administration; may damage tissue

Inhalation route

- Give inh with water to decrease possibility of fungal infections
- Give titrated dosage; use lowest effective dosage
- Clean aerosol top daily with warm water; dry thoroughly
- Store in cool environment; do not puncture or incinerate container

Topical route

- Cleanse area before applying drug
- Apply only to affected areas; do not get in eyes
- Apply medication, then cover with occlusive dressing (only if prescribed); seal to normal skin; change q12h; systemic absorption may occur
- Apply only to dermatoses; do not use on weeping, denuded, or infected area
- Apply treatment for a few days after area has cleared
- Store at room temp

IV route

- Give **IV**, use only sodium phosphate product; give >1 min; may be given by **IV** inf in compatible sol
- Give after shaking susp (parenteral)
- Give titrated dosage; use lowest effective dosage

M

Syringe compatibilities: Granisetron, metoclopramide

Y-site compatibilities: Acyclovir, amifostine, aztreonam, cefepime, cisplatin, cladribine, cyclophosphamide, cytarabine, DOPamine, DOXOrubicin, enalaprilat, famotidine, fludarabine, granisetron, heparin, inamrinone, melphalan, meperidine, methotrexate, metronidazole, midazolam, morphine, piperacillin/tazobactam, sodium bicarbonate, tacrolimus, teniposide, theophylline, thiotepa, vit B with C

Y-site incompatibilities: Ondansetron, paclitaxel, sargramostim, vinorelbine

Additive compatibilities: Chloramphenicol, cimetidine, clindamycin, DOPamine, granisetron, heparin, norepinephrine, penicillin G potassium, ranitidine, theophylline, verapamil

Patient/family education

- Teach patient that emergency ID as steroid user should be carried/worn
- Advise patient to notify prescriber if therapeutic response decreases; dosage adjustment may be needed
- Caution patient not to discontinue abruptly; adrenal crisis can result
- Caution patient to avoid OTC products: salicylates, alcohol in cough products, cold preparations unless directed by prescriber
- Teach patient all aspects of drug usage including cushingoid symptoms
- Teach patient symptoms of adrenal insufficiency: nausea, anorexia, fatigue, dizziness, dyspnea, weakness, joint pain
- Inform patient that long-term therapy may be needed to clear infection (1-2 mo depending on type of infection)

Nasal route

- Advise patient to clear nasal passages if sneezing attack occurs; repeat dose
- Advise patient to continue using product even if mild nasal bleeding occurs; is usually transient
- Teach patient method of instillation after providing written instructions from manufacturer

Topical route

- Advise patient to avoid sunlight on affected area; burns may occur

Evaluation

Positive therapeutic outcome

- Ease of respirations, decreased inflammation
- Absence of severe itching, patches on skin, flaking (top)

methysergide (Rx)

(meth-i-ser'jide)

Sansert

Func. class.: Adrenergic blocker, serotonin antagonist

Chem. class.: Ergot derivative

Pregnancy category X

Action: Competitively blocks serotonin (hydroxytryptamine) receptors in CNS and periphery; potent vasoconstrictor

Therapeutic Outcome: Absence of migraines and other vascular headaches

Uses: Prophylaxis for migraine and other vascular headaches; if no improvement is noted in 3 wk, drug is unlikely to be beneficial

Dosage and routes

Adult: PO 2-4 mg bid with meals; 3-4 wk rest period after each 6-mo treatment

Available forms: Tabs 2 mg

Adverse effects

CNS: *Tremors, anxiety,* insomnia, headache, dizziness, euphoria, confusion, depersonalization, hallucinations, paresthesias, drowsiness

CV: **Retroperitoneal fibrosis,** valvular thickening, palpitations, tachycardia, postural hypertension, angina, thrombophlebitis, ECG changes, **cardiac fibrosis**

GI: Nausea, vomiting, weight gain

HEMA: **Blood dyscrasias**

INTEG: Flushing, rash, alopecia

MS: Arthralgia, myalgia

Contraindications: Pregnancy **X**, hypersensitivity to ergot, tartrazine, peripheral vascular occlusion, CAD, hepatic disease, renal disease, peptic ulcer, hypertension, connective tissue disease, fibrotic pulmonary disease

Precautions: Lactation, children

Pharmacokinetics	
Absorption	Rapidly absorbed
Distribution	Widely distributed
Metabolism	Liver
Excretion	Kidneys, breast milk
Half-life	10 hr

Pharmacodynamics

Unknown

Interactions

Drug classifications

β-Adrenergic blockers: increased vasoconstriction

Opiates: decreased effect of opiates
Smoking: increased vasoconstriction

NURSING CONSIDERATIONS
Assessment
- Monitor stress level, activity, reaction, coping mechanisms of patient
- Assess neurologic status: LOC, blurring vision, nausea, vomiting, tingling in extremities preceding headache
- Assess for ingestion of tyramine-containing foods (pickled products, beer, wine, aged cheese), food additives, preservatives, colorings, artificial sweeteners, chocolate, caffeine, which may precipitate these types of headaches

Nursing diagnoses
- Pain, chronic (uses)
- Injury, risk for (adverse reactions)
- Knowledge, deficient (teaching)

Implementation
- Provide quiet, calm environment with decreased stimulation; no noise, bright lights, or excessive talking
- Give with or pc to avoid GI symptoms
- Store in dark area

Patient/family education
- Caution patient to avoid OTC medications and alcohol; serious drug interactions may occur
- Caution patient to maintain dosage at approved level; not to increase even if drug does not relieve headache
- Advise patient that an increase in headaches may occur when this drug is discontinued after long-term use
- Caution patient to keep drug out of the reach of children; death may occur
- Caution patient to use drug for less than 6 mo continuously; a 3-4 wk drug-free period must follow each 6-mo period

Evaluation
Positive therapeutic outcome
- Decrease in frequency, severity of headache

metoclopramide (Rx)
(met-oh-kloe-pra′mide)

Apo-Metoclop ♣, Emex ♣, Maxeran ♣, metoclopramide, Octamide, Reclomide, Reglan, Sensamide IV

Func. class.: Cholinergic, antiemetic
Chem. class.: Central dopamine receptor antagonist

Pregnancy category B

Do Not Confuse:
metoclopramide/metolazone, Reglan/Megace

Action: Enhances response to acetylcholine of tissue in upper GI tract, which causes contraction of gastric muscle, relaxes pyloric, duodenal segments, increases peristalsis without stimulating secretions, blocks dopamine in chemoreceptor trigger zone of CNS

Therapeutic Outcome: Decreased symptoms of delayed gastric emptying, decreased nausea, vomiting

Uses: Prevention of nausea, vomiting induced by chemotherapy, radiation; delayed gastric emptying, gastroesophageal reflux

Investigational uses: Hiccups, migraines, lactation induction, lung cancer

Dosage and routes
Nausea/vomiting
Adult: **IV** 1-2 mg/kg 30 min before administration of chemotherapy, then q2h × 2 doses, then q3h × 3 doses
Child: **IV** 0.1-0.2 mg/kg/dose

Facilitation of small bowel intubation in radiologic exams
Adult and child >14 yr: **IV** 10 mg over 1-2 min
Child 6-14 yr: **IV** 2.5-5 mg
Child <6 yr: **IV** 0.1 mg/kg

Diabetic gastroparesis
Adult: PO 10 mg 30 min ac, at bedtime × 2-8 wk
Elderly: PO 5 mg ½ hr ac, at bedtime, increase to 10 mg if needed

Hiccups (off-label)
Adult: PO/IM/**IV** 10 mg q6h

Gastroesophageal reflux
Adult: PO 10-15 mg qid 30 min ac
Child: PO 0.4-0.8 mg/kg/day divided in 4 doses

Lactation induction (off-label)
Adult: PO 10 mg bid-tid, may increase to 20-45 mg/day in divided doses

M

Non–small cell lung cancer (NSCLC) radiation sensitizer (off-label) (Sensamide IV)
Adult: **IV** 2 mg/kg given 1 hr prior to radiation therapy 3 ×/wk

Renal dose
Adult: **IV** CCr <40 ml/min 50% of dose

Available forms: Tabs 5, 10 mg; syr 5 mg/5 ml; inj 5 mg/ml, conc sol 10 mg/ml

Adverse effects
CNS: *Sedation, fatigue, restlessness, headache, sleeplessness, dystonia,* dizziness, drowsiness, **suicide ideation, seizures,** extrapyramidal symptoms (EPS)
CV: Hypotension, **supraventricular tachycardia**
GI: Dry mouth, constipation, nausea, anorexia, vomiting, diarrhea
GU: Decreased libido, prolactin secretion, amenorrhea, galactorrhea
HEMA: **Neutropenia, leukopenia, agranulocytosis**
INTEG: Urticaria, rash

Contraindications: Hypersensitivity to this drug or procaine or procainamide, seizure disorder, pheochromocytoma, breast cancer (prolactin dependent), GI obstruction

Precautions: Pregnancy **B,** lactation, GI hemorrhage, CHF, Parkinson's disease, tardive dyskinesia

Pharmacokinetics

Absorption	Well absorbed (PO)
Distribution	Widely distributed; crosses blood-brain barrier, placenta
Metabolism	Liver, minimally
Excretion	Kidneys, breast milk
Half-life	4 hr

Pharmacodynamics

	PO	IM	IV
Onset	½-1 hr	10-15 min	1-3 min
Peak	Unknown	Unknown	Unknown
Duration	1-2 hr	1-2 hr	1-2 hr

Interactions
Individual drugs
Alcohol: increased sedation
Haloperidol: increased extrapyramidal reaction
Drug classifications
Anticholinergics, opiates: decreased action of metoclopramide
CNS depressants: increased sedation
MAOIs: avoid use
Phenothiazines: increased extrapyramidal reaction
Drug/lab test
Increased: prolactin, aldosterone, thyrotropin

NURSING CONSIDERATIONS
Assessment
- Assess GI complaints: nausea, vomiting, anorexia, constipation, abdominal distention before and after administration
- Assess for extrapyramidal symptoms and tardive dyskinesia, more likely to occur in elderly patient: rigidity, grimacing, shuffling gait, tremors, rhythmic involuntary movements of tongue, mouth, jaw, feet, hands; these side effects should be reported to prescriber immediately; some effects may be irreversible
- Assess mental status: depression, anxiety, irritability during treatment

Nursing diagnoses
- Injury, risk for (adverse reactions)
- Knowledge, deficient (teaching)

Implementation
PO route
- Use gum, hard candy, frequent rinsing of mouth for dryness of oral cavity
- Give ½-1 hr before meals for better absorption

IV route
- Give **IV** undiluted if dose is ≤10 mg; give over 2 min
- Dilute more than 10 mg in 50 ml or more D_5W, NaCl, Ringer's, LR and give over 15 min or more
- Give diphenhydrAMINE **IV** for EPS
- Discard open ampules

Syringe compatibilities: Aminophylline, ascorbic acid, atropine, benztropine, bleomycin, butorphanol, chlorproMAZINE, cisplatin, cyclophosphamide, cytarabine, dexamethasone, dimenhyDRINATE, diphenhydrAMINE, DOXOrubicin, droperidol, fentanyl, fluorouracil, heparin, hydrocortisone, hydrOXYzine, regular insulin, leucovorin, lidocaine, magnesium sulfate, meperidine, methotrimeprazine, methylPREDNISolone, midazolam, mitomycin, morphine, pentazocine, perphenazine, prochlorperazine, promazine, promethazine, ranitidine, scopolamine, sufentanil, vinBLAStine, vinCRIStine, vit B/C

Syringe incompatibilities: Ampicillin, calcium gluconate, cephalothin, chloramphenicol, furosemide, penicillin G potassium, sodium bicarbonate

Y-site compatibilities: Acyclovir, aldesleukin, amifostine, aztreonam, bleomycin, ciprofloxacin, cisplatin, cladribine, cyclophosphamide, cytarabine, diltiazem, DOXOrubicin, droperidol, famotidine, filgrastim, fluconazole, fludarabine, fluorouracil, foscarnet, gallium, granisetron, heparin, idarubicin, leucovorin, melphalan, meperidine, meropenem, methotrexate, mitomycin, morphine, ondansetron, paclitaxel, piperacillin/tazobactam, propofol, sargramostim, sufentanil, tacrolimus, teniposide, thiotepa, vinBLAStine, vinCRIStine, vinorelbine, zidovudine

Y-site incompatibilities: Furosemide

Additive compatibilities: Clindamycin, meropenem, morphine, multivitamins, potassium acetate/chloride/phosphate, verapamil

Additive incompatibilities: Cisplatin, erythromycin, tetracycline

Patient/family education

- Instruct patient to avoid driving, other hazardous activities until stabilized on this medication
- Advise patient to avoid alcohol and other CNS depressants that enhance sedating properties of this drug
- Advise patient to notify prescriber if involuntary movements occur

Evaluation

Positive therapeutic outcome

- Absence of nausea, vomiting, anorexia, fullness

metolazone (Rx)

(me-tole'a-zone)

Mykrox, Zaroxolyn

Func. class.: Diuretic, antihypertensive

Chem. class.: Thiazide-like quinazoline derivative

Pregnancy category B

Do Not Confuse:

metolazone/methotrexate, metolazone/metoclopramide

Action: Acts on the distal tubule and cortical thick ascending limb of the loop of Henle in the kidney, increasing excretion of sodium, water, chloride, magnesium, potassium, and bicarbonate

Therapeutic Outcome: Decreased B/P, decreased edema in lung tissue and peripherally

Uses: Edema in CHF, nephrotic syndrome; may be used alone or as adjunct with antihypertensives for mild to moderate hypertension

Dosage and routes

Edema

Adult: PO 5-20 mg/day

Hypertension

Adult: PO 2.5-5 mg/day (Zaroxolyn)

Child: PO 0.2-0.4 mg/kg/day divided q12-24h

Adult: PO 0.5 mg (Mykrox) daily in AM: may increase to 1 mg

Available forms: Tabs (Mykrox) 0.5; tabs (Zaroxolyn) 2.5, 5, 10 mg

Adverse effects

CNS: Drowsiness, paresthesia, anxiety, depression, headache, *dizziness, fatigue, weakness*

CV: Irregular pulse, orthostatic hypotension, palpitations, volume depletion

EENT: Blurred vision

ELECT: *Hypokalemia,* hypercalcemia, hyponatremia, hypochloremia, hypomagnesemia, hypophosphatemia

GI: *Nausea, vomiting, anorexia,* constipation, diarrhea, cramps, **pancreatitis,** GI irritation, **hepatitis**

GU: *Frequency,* polyuria, **uremia,** glucosuria

HEMA: **Aplastic anemia, hemolytic anemia, leukopenia, agranulocytosis, neutropenia**

INTEG: *Rash,* urticaria, purpura, photosensitivity, fever

META: *Hyperglycemia,* increased creatinine, BUN

Contraindications: Hypersensitivity to thiazides or sulfonamides, anuria, lactation

Precautions: Pregnancy **B,** hypokalemia, renal disease, hepatic disease, gout, COPD, lupus erythematosus, diabetes mellitus, elderly

Pharmacokinetics	
Absorption	GI tract (10%-20%)
Distribution	Crosses placenta
Metabolism	Urine, unchanged
Excretion	Breast milk
Half-life	8 hr (extended); 14 hr (prompt)

Pharmacodynamics	
Onset	1 hr
Peak	2 hr
Duration	12-24 hr

Interactions

Individual drugs

Alcohol: increased hypotension (large amounts)

Amphotericin B, digoxin, mezlocillin, piperacillin: increased hypokalemia

Lithium: increased toxicity

M

Drug classifications

Antihypertensives: increased antihypertensive effect
Barbiturates, nitrates, opioids: increased hypotension
Glucocorticoids, laxatives (stimulant): increased hypokalemia
NSAIDs, salicylates: decreased action of metolazone

Drug/herb

Aconite: increased toxicity, death
Aloe, buckthorn, cascara sagrada, rhubarb, senna: increased hypokalemia
Astragalus, cola tree: increased or decreased antihypertensive effect
Barberry, betony, black catechu, black cohosh, bloodroot, broom, burdock, cat's claw, dandelion, goldenseal, Irish moss, Jamaican dogwood, kelp, khella, mistletoe, parsley: increased antihypertensive effect
Coltsfoot, guarana, khat, licorice: decreased antihypertensive effect

Drug/lab test

Increased: BSP retention, calcium, amylase, parathyroid test
Decreased: PBI, PSP

NURSING CONSIDERATIONS

Assessment

- Monitor blood glucose if patient is diabetic
- Check for rashes, temp elevation daily
- Monitor patients receiving cardiac glycosides for increased hypokalemia
- Monitor manifestations of hypokalemia; acidic urine, reduced urine, osmolality, nocturia; hypotension, broad T wave, U wave, ectopy, tachycardia, weak pulse; muscle weakness, altered LOC, drowsiness, apathy, lethargy, confusion, depression; anorexia, nausea, cramps, constipation, distention, paralytic ileus; hypoventilation, respiratory muscle weakness
- Monitor for manifestations of hypomagnesemia: agitation, muscle twitching, paresthesias, hyperactive reflexes, positive Babinski reflex, dysphagia, nystagmus seizures, tetany; nausea, vomiting, diarrhea, anorexia, abdominal distention; ectopy, tachycardia, broad, flat, or inverted T-waves, depressed ST segment, prolonged QT interval, decreased cardiac output, hypotension
- Monitor for manifestations of hyponatremia; increased B/P, cold, clammy skin, hypovolemia or hypervolemia; anorexia, nausea, vomiting, diarrhea, abdominal cramps; lethargy, increased ICP, confusion, headache, seizures, coma, fatigue, tremors, hyperreflexia
- Monitor for manifestations of hyperchloremia: weakness, lethargy, coma, deep rapid breathing
- Assess and record fluid volume status: I&O ratios; monitor weight, distended red veins, crackles in lung, color, quality and sp gr of urine, skin turgor, adequacy of pulses, moist mucous membranes, bilateral lung sounds, peripheral pitting edema; dehydration symptoms of decreasing output, thirst, hypotension, dry mouth and mucous membranes should be reported
- Monitor electrolytes: potassium, sodium, calcium, magnesium; also include BUN, blood pH, ABGs, uric acid, CBC, blood glucose
- Assess B/P before and during therapy with patient lying, standing, and sitting as appropriate; orthostatic hypotension can occur rapidly

Nursing diagnoses

- Urinary elimination, impaired (adverse reactions)
- Fluid volume, deficient (adverse reactions)
- Fluid volume, excess (uses)
- Knowledge, deficient (teaching)

Implementation

- Give in AM to avoid interference with sleep
- Provide potassium replacement if potassium level is 3.0; drug may be crushed if patient is unable to swallow
- Give with food; if nausea occurs, absorption may be increased; extended release product is Zaroxolyn; prompt action product is Mykrox; the two formulations are not equivalent

Patient/family education

- Teach patient to take the medication early in the day to prevent nocturia
- Instruct patient to take with food or milk if GI symptoms of nausea and anorexia occur
- Teach patient to maintain a weekly record of weight and notify prescriber of weight loss >5 lb
- Caution patient that this drug causes a loss of potassium, so foods rich in potassium should be added to the diet; refer to a dietitian for assistance in planning
- Caution the patient to rise slowly from sitting or reclining positions, not to exercise in hot weather or stand for prolonged periods, since orthostatic hypotension will be enhanced; lie down if dizziness occurs
- Teach patient not to use alcohol or any OTC medications without prescriber's approval; serious drug reactions may occur
- Emphasize the need to contact prescriber immediately if muscle cramps, weakness, nausea, dizziness, or numbness occurs
- Teach patient to take own B/P and pulse and record
- Advise patient to use sunscreen to prevent burns

- Teach patient to continue taking medication even if feeling better; this drug controls symptoms but does not cure the condition
- Advise patient with hypertension to continue other medical regimen (exercise, weight loss, relaxation techniques, cessation of smoking)

Evaluation

Positive therapeutic outcome

- Decreased edema
- Decreased B/P

Treatment of overdose:

Lavage if taken orally, monitor electrolytes; administer dextrose in saline; monitor hydration, CV, renal status

metoprolol (Rx)

(met-oh-proe'lole)

Betaloc ✤, Betaloc Durules ✤, Lopresor ✤, Lopressor, Lopressor SR ✤, Novometoprol ✤, Nu-Metop ✤, Toprol XL

Func. class.: Antihypertensive, antianginal
Chem. class.: β_1-Adrenergic blocker

Pregnancy category C

Do Not Confuse:

metoprolol/misoprostol

Action: Competitively blocks stimulation of β_1-adrenergic receptor within vascular smooth muscle; produces chronotropic, inotropic activity (decreases rate of SA node discharge, increases recovery time), slows conduction of AV node, decreases heart rate, which decreases O_2 consumption in myocardium; also decreases renin-aldosterone-angiotensin system at high doses

Therapeutic Outcome: Decreased B/P, heart rate, AV conduction

Uses: Mild to moderate hypertension, acute MI to reduce cardiovascular mortality, angina pectoris, New York Heart Association class II, III heart failure

Investigational uses: Atrial ectopy, antipsychotic-induced akathisia, rapid heart rate control, unstable angina, variceal bleeding in portal hypertension, migraine prevention

Dosage and routes

Hypertension

Adult: PO 50 mg bid, or 100 mg daily; may give 200-450 mg in divided doses; ext rel tabs give daily

Elderly: PO 25 mg/day initially, increase weekly as needed

MI

Adult: Early treatment, **IV** bol 5 mg q2 min × 3 doses, then 50 mg PO 15 min after last dose and q6h × 48 hr; late treatment, PO maintenance 100 mg bid for 3 mo

Angina

Adult: PO 100 mg daily as a single dose or in 2 divided doses, increase qwk as needed or 100 mg ext rel tab daily

Migraine prevention (off-label)

Adult: PO 50-100 mg bid-qid

Available forms: Tabs 50, 100 mg; inj 1 mg/ml; ext rel tabs (tartrate) 100 mg; ext rel tabs (succinate) (XL) 25, 50, 100, 200 mg

Adverse effects

CNS: *Insomnia, dizziness,* mental changes, hallucinations, **depression,** anxiety, headaches, nightmares, confusion, fatigue

CV: **CHF,** *palpitations,* dysrhythmias, **cardiac arrest, AV block,** hypotension, **bradycardia, pulmonary edema, chest pain**

EENT: Sore throat, dry burning eyes

GI: *Nausea, vomiting,* colitis, cramps, *diarrhea,* constipation, flatulence, dry mouth, *hiccups*

GU: Impotence

HEMA: **Agranulocytosis, eosinophilia, thrombocytopenic purpura**

INTEG: Rash, purpura, alopecia, dry skin, urticaria, pruritus

RESP: **Bronchospasm,** dyspnea, wheezing

Contraindications: Hypersensitivity to β-blockers, cardiogenic shock, heart block (2nd- and 3rd-degree), sinus bradycardia, bronchial asthma

Precautions: Pregnancy **C,** major surgery, lactation, diabetes mellitus, renal disease, thyroid disease, COPD, CAD, nonallergic bronchospasm, hepatic disease, CHF, elderly

Pharmacokinetics	
Absorption	Well absorbed (PO); completely absorbed (**IV**)
Distribution	Crosses blood-brain barrier, placenta
Metabolism	Liver, extensively
Excretion	Kidneys, breast milk
Half-life	3-4 hr

Pharmacodynamics	PO	IV
Onset	15 min	Immediate
Peak	2-4 hr	20 min
Duration	6-19 hr	5-8 hr

Interactions
Individual drugs
Cimetidine: increased metoprolol level
DOBUTamine: decreased effect of DOBUTamine
DOPamine: decreased DOPamine
EpINEPHrine, hydrALAZINE, methyldopa prazosin, reserpine: increased hypotension, bradycardia
Indomethacin: decreased antihypertensive effect
Insulin: increased hypoglycemia
Drug classifications
Antidiabetics (oral): increased hypoglycemia
Amphetamines, calcium channel blockers, histamine H_2 antagonists: increased hypotension, bradycardia
Barbiturates: decreased metoprolol level
Benzodiazepines: increased effect of benzodiazepines
MAOIs: do not use together
NSAIDs, salicylates: decreased antihypertensive effect
Sulfonylureas: increased hypoglycemic effect
Xanthines: decreased effects of xanthines
Drug/herb
Aconite: increased toxicity, death
Astragalus, cola tree: increased or decreased antihypertensive effect
Barberry, betony, black catechu, black cohosh, bloodroot, broom, burdock, cat's claw, dandelion, goldenseal, Irish moss, Jamaican dogwood, kelp, khella, mistletoe, parsley: increased antihypertensive effect
Coltsfoot, guarana, khat, licorice: increased antihypertensive effect
Drug/food
Increased: absorption with food
Drug/lab test
Increased: BUN, potassium, ANA titer, serum lipoprotein, triglycerides, uric acid, alkaline phosphatase, LDH, AST, ALT

NURSING CONSIDERATIONS
Assessment
- Monitor B/P during beginning treatment, periodically thereafter; pulse q4h; note rate, rhythm, quality; check apical/radial pulse before administration; notify prescriber of any significant changes (pulse <50 bpm)
- Check for baselines in renal, liver function tests before therapy begins and periodically thereafter
- Assess for edema in feet, legs daily; monitor I&O, daily weight; check for jugular vein distention, crackles bilaterally, dyspnea (CHF)
- Monitor skin turgor, dryness of mucous membranes for hydration status, especially elderly

Nursing diagnoses
- Cardiac output, decreased (uses)
- Injury, risk for (adverse reactions)
- Knowledge, deficient (teaching)
- Noncompliance (teaching)

Implementation
PO route
- Do not break, crush, or chew ext rel tabs
- Given ac, at bedtime; tab may be crushed or swallowed whole; give with food to prevent GI upset; reduced dosage in renal dysfunction; take at same time each day
- Store protected from light, moisture; place in cool environment

IV route
- Give by direct **IV** 5 mg/2 min or more × 3 doses at 2 min intervals, start PO 15 min after last **IV** dose

Y-site compatibilities:
Alteplase, meperidine, morphine

Patient/family education
- Teach patient not to discontinue drug abruptly; taper over 2 wk; may cause precipitate angina if stopped abruptly
- Teach patient not to use OTC products containing α-adrenergic stimulants (such as nasal decongestants, cold preparations); to avoid alcohol, smoking and to limit sodium intake as prescribed
- Teach patient how to take pulse and B/P at home; advise when to notify prescriber
- Instruct patient to comply with weight control, dietary adjustments, modified exercise program
- Tell patient to carry/wear emergency ID to identify drug being taken, allergies; tell patient drug controls symptoms but does not cure
- Caution patient to avoid hazardous activities if dizziness, drowsiness is present, to avoid driving until drug response is known
- Teach patient to report symptoms of CHF; difficult breathing, especially with exertion or when lying down, night cough, swelling of extremities or bradycardia, dizziness, confusion, depression, fever
- Teach patient to take drug as prescribed, not to double doses or skip doses; take any missed doses as soon as remembered if at least 4 hr until next dose

Evaluation
Positive therapeutic outcome
- Decreased B/P in hypertension (after 1-2 wk)
- Absence of dysrhythmias

Treatment of overdose: Lavage, **IV** atropine for bradycardia, **IV** theophylline for bronchospasm, digitalis, O_2, diuretic for cardiac failure, hemodialysis, **IV** glucose for hyperglycemia, **IV** diazepam (or phenytoin) for seizures

metronidazole (Rx)

(me-troe-ni'da-zole)

Apo-Metronidazole ✤, Flagyl, Flagyl ER, Flagyl IV, Flagyl IV RTU, Metronidazole, Novonidazole ✤, Protostat, Trikacide ✤

Func. class.: Trichomonacide, amebicide, antiinfective

Chem. class.: Nitroimidazole derivative

Pregnancy category B (2nd, 3rd trimesters)

Action: Direct-acting amebicide/trichomonacide; binds, degrades DNA in organism

Therapeutic Outcome: Trichomonacidal, amebicidal, bactericidal for the following susceptible organisms: *Bacteroides, Clostridium, Trichomonas vaginalis, Giardia lamblia, Entamoeba histolytica*

Uses: Intestinal amebiasis, amebic abscess, trichomoniasis, refractory trichomoniasis, bacterial anaerobic infections, giardiasis; septicemia, endocarditis, bone, joint, and lower respiratory tract infections

Dosage and routes

Trichomoniasis

Adult: PO 250 mg tid × 7 days or 2 g in single dose; do not repeat treatment for 4-6 wk

Child: PO 5 mg/kg/day in tid × 7-10 days

Refractory trichomoniasis

Adult: PO 250 mg bid × 10 days

Amebic hepatic abscess

Adult: PO 500-750 mg tid × 5-10 days

Child: PO 35-50 mg/kg/day in 3 divided doses × 10 days

Intestinal amebiasis

Adult: PO 750 mg tid × 5-10 days

Child: PO 35-50 mg/kg/day in 3 divided doses × 10 days; then oral iodoquinol

Anaerobic bacterial infections

Adult: **IV** inf 15 mg/kg/over 1 hr, then 7.5 mg/kg **IV** or PO q6h, max 4 g/day; first maintenance dose should be administered 6 hr after loading dose

Giardiasis

Adult: PO 250 mg tid × 5 days

Child: PO 5 mg/kg tid × 5 days

Antibiotic-associated pseudomembranous colitis

Adult: PO 250-500 mg 3-4 ×/day × 10-14 days

Child: PO 20 mg/kg/day (max 2 g) divided q6h

Available forms: Tabs 250, 375, 500 mg; ext rel tabs 750 mg; inj 500 mg/100 ml; powder for inj 500 mg single dose

Adverse effects

CNS: *Headache, dizziness,* confusion, irritability, restlessness, ataxia, depression, fatigue, drowsiness, insomnia, paresthesia, peripheral neuropathy, **seizures,** incoordination, depression

CV: Flat T-waves

EENT: Blurred vision, sore throat, retinal edema, dry mouth, metallic taste, furry tongue, glossitis, stomatitis

GI: *Nausea, vomiting, diarrhea,* epigastric distress, *anorexia,* constipation, *abdominal cramps,* metallic taste, **pseudomembranous colitis**

GU: Darkened urine, vaginal dryness, polyuria, **albuminuria,** dysuria, cystitis, decreased libido, **nephrotoxicity,** incontinence, dyspareunia

HEMA: **Leukopenia, bone marrow depression, aplasia**

INTEG: Rash, pruritus, urticaria, flushing

Contraindications: Pregnancy (1st trimester), hypersensitivity to this drug, renal disease, hepatic disease, contracted visual or color fields, blood dyscrasias, lactation, CNS disorders

Precautions: Pregnancy **B** (2nd/3rd trimesters), candidal infections

Pharmacokinetics

Absorption	80% (PO)
Distribution	Widely distributed, crosses placenta
Metabolism	Liver
Excretion	Urine, unchanged; feces
Half-life	6-11 hr

Pharmacodynamics

	PO	IV
Onset	Rapid	Immediate
Peak	1-2 hr	Infusion's end

M

Interactions

Individual drugs

Alcohol: increased disulfiram-like reaction
Azathioprine, fluorouracil: increased leukopenia
Cimetidine, phenobarbital, phenytoin: decreased effect of metronidazole
Warfarin: increased action of warfarin

Drug/lab test

Altered: AST, ALT, LDH

NURSING CONSIDERATIONS

Assessment

- Assess patient for signs and symptoms of infection including characteristics of wounds, WBC >10,000/mm^3, vaginal secretions, fever; obtain baseline information and during treatment
- Obtain C&S before beginning drug therapy to identify if correct treatment has been initiated
- Assess for allergic reactions: rash, urticaria, pruritus
- Identify urine output; if decreasing, notify prescriber (may indicate nephrotoxicity); also check for increased BUN, creatinine
- Assess bowel pattern daily; if severe diarrhea occurs, drug should be discontinued
- Assess for overgrowth of infection: perineal itching, fever, malaise, redness, pain, swelling, drainage, rash, diarrhea, change in cough, sputum

Nursing diagnoses

- Infection, risk for (uses)
- Diarrhea (adverse reactions)
- Injury, risk for (adverse reactions)
- Knowledge, deficient (teaching)
- Noncompliance (teaching)

Implementation

PO route

- Give with or after a meal to avoid GI symptoms, metallic taste; crush tab if needed
- Store in light-resistant container; do not refrigerate

Topical route

- A thin coating should be applied to affected area after cleaning with soap and water and patting dry

IV route

- Give intermittent **IV** prediluted; for Flagyl **IV** dilute with 4.4 ml of sterile water or 0.9% NaCl; must be diluted further with 8 mg/ml or more 0.9% NaCl, D_5W, or LR; must neutralize with 5 mEq of $NaCO_3$/500 mg; CO_2 gas will be generated and may require venting; run over 1 hr or more; primary **IV** must be discontinued; may be given as cont inf; do not use aluminum products; **IV** may require venting

Y-site compatibilities: Acyclovir, allopurinol, amifostine, amiodarone, cefepime, cyclophosphamide, diltiazem, DOPamine, enalaprilat, esmolol, fluconazole, foscarnet, granisetron, heparin, hydromorphone, labetalol, lorazepam, magnesium sulfate, melphalan, meperidine, methylPREDNISolone, midazolam, morphine, perphenazine, piperacillin/tazobactam, sargramostim, tacrolimus, teniposide, theophylline, thiotepa, vinorelbine

Additive compatibilities: Amikacin, aminophylline, cefazolin, cefotaxime, ceftazidime, ceftizoxime, ceftriaxone, cefuroxime, chloramphenicol, ciprofloxacin, clindamycin, disopyramide, floxacillin, fluconazole, gentamicin, heparin, moxalactam, multielectrolyte concentrate, multivitamins, netilmicin, penicillin G potassium, tobramycin

Patient/family education

- Teach patient to report sore throat, bruising, bleeding, joint pain; may indicate blood dyscrasias (rare)
- Advise patient to contact prescriber if vaginal itching, loose foul-smelling stools, furry tongue occur; may indicate superinfection
- Advise patient to notify physician of numbness or tingling of extremities
- Teach trichomoniasis patient that both partners need to be treated; condoms should be used during intercourse to prevent reinfection
- Advise patient of disulfiram-like reaction to alcohol ingestion; alcohol should not be used within 48 hr of this drug
- Inform patient drug has a metallic taste and urine may turn dark
- Advise patient to contact prescriber if pregnancy is suspected
- Advise patient to use sips of water, sugarless gum, candy for dry mouth

Evaluation

Positive therapeutic outcome

- Decreased symptoms of infection

mexiletine (Rx)

(mex-il'e-teen)

Mexitil

Func. class.: Antidysrhythmic (class IB)
Chem. class.: Lidocaine analog

Pregnancy category C

Action: Increases electrical stimulation threshold of ventricle and His-Purkinje system, which stabilizes cardiac membrane and decreases automaticity

Therapeutic Outcome: Decreased ventricular dysrhythmia

Uses: Life-threatening ventricular tachycardia; because of proarrhythmic effects, use with lesser dysrhythmias is not recommended

Investigational uses: Diabetic neuropathy

Dosage and routes

Adult: PO 200-400 mg (loading dose), then 200 mg q8h, then 200-400 mg q8h

Diabetic neuropathy (off-label)

Adult: PO 150 mg/day for 3 days, then 300 mg/day for 3 days followed by 10 mg/kg/day

Available forms: Caps 150, 200, 250 mg

Adverse effects

CNS: Headache, dizziness, confusion, **seizures,** tremors, psychosis, nervousness, paresthesias, weakness, fatigue, coordination difficulties, change in sleep habits

CV: Hypotension, bradycardia, angina, PVCs, **heart block, cardiovascular collapse, arrest,** sinus node slowing, **left ventricular failure,** syncope, **cardiogenic shock, AV conduction disturbances, CHF, atrial dysrhythmias, palpitations, ventricular dysrhythmias, ventricular tachycardia, other ventricular arrhythmias in acute phase of MI**

EENT: Blurred vision, tinnitus

GI: Nausea, vomiting, anorexia, diarrhea, abdominal pain, **hepatitis,** dry mouth, peptic ulcer, altered taste, **GI bleeding,** constipation

GU: Urinary hesitancy, decreased libido

HEMA: **Thrombocytopenia, leukopenia, agranulocytosis**

INTEG: Rash, alopecia, dry skin

MISC: Edema, arthralgia, fever, systemic lupus erythematosus syndrome

RESP: Dyspnea

Contraindications: Hypersensitivity, cardiogenic shock, severe heart block (if no pacemaker)

Precautions: Pregnancy **C,** lactation, children, liver disease, CHF, seizure disorders, hypotension

Pharmacokinetics	
Absorption	Well absorbed
Distribution	Body tissues
Metabolism	Liver, extensively
Excretion	Kidneys, unchanged (10%)
Half-life	12 hr

Pharmacodynamics	
Onset	½-2 hr
Peak	2-3 hr
Duration	8-12 hr

Interactions

Individual drugs

Atropine, aluminum/magnesium hydroxide, phenobarbitol, phenytoin, rifampin: decreased mexiletine levels

Caffeine, theophylline: increased levels of each

Cimetidine: increased or decreased mexiletine effects

Metoclopramide: increased effects of mexiletine

Drug classifications

Acidifers (urinary), opiates: decreased mexiletine levels

Alkalinizers (urinary): increased mexiletine levels

Smoking: decreased mexiletine effect

Drug/herb

Aconite: increased toxicity, death

Aloe, broom, buckthorn (chronic use), cascara sagrada (chronic use), Chinese rhubarb, figwort, fumitory, goldenseal, kudzu, licorice: increased effect

Aloe, buckthorn, cascara sagrada, rhubarb, senna: increased hypokalemia, increased antidysrhythmic action

Coltsfoot: decreased effect

Horehound: increased serotonin effect

Drug/lab test

Increased: CPK

NURSING CONSIDERATIONS

Assessment

- Assess for oxygenation or perfusion deficit: decreased B/P, chest pain, dizziness, loss of consciousness
- Assess respiratory status: auscultate lung fields for bibasilar crackles in patients with advanced CHF
- Assess for urinary retention: check for pain, abdominal absorption, palpate bladder; check males with benign prostatic hypertrophy; anticholinergic reaction may cause retention
- Monitor I&O ratio; electrolytes potassium, sodium, chloride; watch for decreasing urinary output, possible retention
- Monitor liver function studies: AST, ALT, bilirubin, alkaline phosphatase
- Monitor ECG periodically to determine drug effectiveness; measure PR, QRS, QT intervals; check for PVCs, other dysrhythmias; assess B/P for hypotension, hypertension, for rebound hypertension after 1-2 hr; for prolonged

M

PR/QT intervals, QRS complex, if QT or QRS increase by 50% or more, withhold next dose, notify prescriber
- Monitor for dehydration and hypovolemia
- Monitor blood levels (therapeutic level 0.5-2 mcg/ml), notify prescriber of abnormal results
- Assess pulmonary toxicity: dyspnea, fatigue, cough, fever, chest pain; drug should be discontinued
- Assess cardiac rate, respiration: rate, rhythm, character, chest pain, ventricular tachycardia, supraventricular tachycardia, fibrillation

Nursing diagnoses
- Cardiac output, decreased (uses)
- Gas exchange, impaired (adverse reactions)
- Knowledge, deficient (teaching)

Implementation
- Give with meals for GI upset

Patient/family education
- Teach patient to report side effects immediately to prescriber; to take exactly as prescribed; if dose is missed, take when remembered if within 3-4 hr of next dose; do not double doses
- Caution patient to avoid temp extremes; impairment of heat-regulating mechanism can occur
- Encourage patient to complete follow-up appointment with health care provider, including pulmonary function studies, chest x-ray
- Instruct patient that dry mouth may be relieved by frequent sips of water, hard candy, sugarless gum
- Caution patient to make position changes from lying to standing slowly to prevent orthostatic hypotension

Evaluation
Positive therapeutic outcome
- Decreased B/P, dysrhythmias
- Decreased heart rate
- Normal sinus rhythm

Treatment of overdose: O_2, artificial ventilation, ECG monitoring, administer DOPamine for circulatory depression, administer diazepam or thiopental for convulsions, isoproterenol

mezlocillin (Rx)
(mez-loe-sill'in)
Mezlin
Func. class.: Antiinfective—broad-spectrum
Chem. class.: Extended-spectrum penicillin
Pregnancy category B

Do Not Confuse:
mezlocillin/methicillin

Action: Interferes with cell wall replication of susceptible organisms; osmotically unstable cell wall swells, bursts from osmotic pressure

Uses: Infection due to penicillinase-producing staphylococci, streptococci; respiratory tract, skin, skin structure, urinary tract, bone, joint infections; sinusitis, endocarditis, septicemia, meningitis; may be combined with an aminoglycoside for *Pseudomonas* infection

Therapeutic Outcome: Bactericidal effects on the following: gram-positive cocci *Staphylococcus aureus, Streptococcus viridans, Streptococcus faecalis, Streptococcus pneumoniae;* gram-negative coccus *Neisseria gonorrhoeae;* gram-positive bacilli *Clostridium perfringens, Clostridium tetani;* gram-negative bacilli *Bacteroides, Escherichia coli, Haemophilus influenzae, Klebsiella, Morganella morganii, Enterobacter, Serratia, Pseudomonas, Proteus mirabilis, Proteus vulgaris, Proteus rettgeri, Shigella, Citrobacter, Veillonella;* and *Peptococcus, Peptostreptococcus*

Dosage and routes
Adult: IM/**IV** 200-300 mg/kg/day (serious infections) q4-6h or **IV** 500 mg q8h; may give up to 24 g/day for severe infections
Child: IM/**IV** 50 mg/kg q4-6h
Infants >8 days: (>2000 g) 75 mg/kg q6h; <2000 g, 75 mg/kg q8h
Infants <8 days: 75 mg/kg q12h

Renal dose
Adult: IM/**IV** dose reduction indicated if CCr <30 ml/min

Hepatic dose
Adult: Give 50% of dose

Available forms: Powder for inj 1, 2, 3, 4 g; **IV** inf 2, 3, 4 g

Adverse effects
CNS: Lethargy, hallucinations, anxiety, depression, twitching, **coma, seizures**
GI: *Nausea, vomiting, diarrhea,* increased AST, ALT, abdominal pain, glossitis, colitis, abnormal taste
GU: Oliguria, proteinuria, hematuria vaginitis,

moniliasis, **glomerulonephritis,** increased BUN, creatinine
HEMA: Anemia, increased bleeding time, **bone marrow depression, granulocytopenia**
META: Hyperkalemia, hypokalemia, alkalosis, hypernatremia

Contraindications: Hypersensitivity to penicillins

Precautions: Pregnancy **B,** hypersensitivity to cephalosporins, neonates, renal disease

Pharmacokinetics

Absorption	Well absorbed
Distribution	Widely distributed; crosses placenta
Metabolism	Liver, small amounts
Excretion	Kidneys, unchanged (40%-70%); breast milk, bile (15%-30%)
Half-life	50-55 min; increased in renal disease

Pharmacodynamics

	IM	IV
Onset	Rapid	Rapid
Peak	5 min	Inf end

Interactions
Individual drugs
Probenecid: increased mezlocillin levels; decreased renal excretion
Vecuronium: increased effect
Drug classifications
Aminoglycosides: decreased effectiveness of aminoglycosides if mixed together
Oral contraceptives: decreased contraceptive effectiveness
Drug/herb
Khat: decreased absorption, separate by ≥2 hr
Drug/food
Food, carbonated drinks, citrus fruit juices: decreased absorption
Drug/lab test
False positive: urine glucose, urine protein

NURSING CONSIDERATIONS
Assessment
- Assess patient for previous sensitivity reaction to penicillins or other cephalosporins; cross-sensitivity between penicillins and cephalosporins is common
- Assess patient for signs and symptoms of infection including characteristics of wounds, sputum, urine, stool, WBC >10,000/mm^3, fever; obtain baseline information and during treatment
- Obtain C&S before beginning drug therapy to identify if correct treatment has been initiated
- Assess for allergic reactions: rash, urticaria, pruritus, chills, fever, joint pain; angioedema may occur a few days after therapy begins; epINEPHrine, resuscitation equipment should be available for anaphylactic reaction
- Identify urine output; if decreasing, notify prescriber (may indicate nephrotoxicity); also check for increased BUN, creatinine
- Monitor blood studies: AST, ALT, CBC, Hct, bilirubin, LDH, alkaline phosphatase, Coombs' test monthly if patient is on long-term therapy
- Monitor electrolytes: potassium, sodium, chloride monthly if patient is on long-term therapy
- Assess bowel pattern daily; if severe diarrhea occurs, drug should be discontinued; may indicate pseudomembranous colitis
- Assess for symptoms of vaginitis during therapy
- Monitor for bleeding: ecchymosis, bleeding gums, hematuria, stool guaiac daily if on long-term therapy
- Assess for overgrowth of infection: perineal itching, fever, malaise, redness, pain, swelling, drainage, rash, diarrhea, change in cough, sputum
- Assess for possible seizures; use seizure precautions in those receiving high doses

Nursing diagnoses
- Infection, risk for (uses)
- Diarrhea (adverse reactions)
- Injury, risk for (adverse reactions)
- Knowledge, deficient (teaching)
- Noncompliance (teaching)

Implementation
IV route
- Dilute 1 g or less/10 ml of sterile water, for inj; D_5, 0.9% NaCl, for inj; shake, dilute further with D_5W or 0.45 NaCl, give over 3-5 min, change site q48h

Syringe compatibilities: Heparin
Y-site compatibilities: Amifostine, aztreonam, cyclophosphamide, famotidine, fludarabine, granisetron, hydromorphone, morphine, perphenazine, sargramostim, tacrolimus, teniposide, thiotepa

Patient/family education
- Teach patient to report sore throat, bruising, bleeding, joint pain; may indicate blood dyscrasias (rare)
- Advise patient to contact prescriber if vaginal itching, loose foul-smelling stools, furry tongue occur; may indicate superinfection

M

- Advise patient to notify prescriber of diarrhea with blood or pus, which may indicate pseudomembranous colitis

Evaluation

Positive therapeutic outcome

- Absence of signs/symptoms of infection (WBC <10,000/mm^3, temp WNL, absence of red, draining wounds)
- Reported improvement in symptoms of infection

Treatment of anaphylaxis: Withdraw drug, maintain airway, administer epINEPHrine, aminophylline, O_2, **IV** corticosteroids

mibefradil (Rx)

(mi-be-fray'dill)

Posicor

Func. class.: Calcium channel blocker; antihypertensive; antianginal

Chem. class.: Benzimidazole-substituted tetraline derivative

Pregnancy category C

Action: Inhibits calcium ion influx across cell membrane during cardiac depolarization; produces relaxation of coronary vascular smooth muscle; peripheral vascular smooth muscle; dilates coronary vascular arteries; increases myocardial oxygen delivery in patients with vasospastic angina; only calcium channel blocker that blocks both T-type and L-type channels

Therapeutic Outcome: Decreased angina pectoris

Uses: Chronic stable angina pectoris

Dosage and routes

Adult: PO 50-100 mg daily

Available forms: Tabs 50, 100 mg

Adverse effects

CNS: *Headache,* dizziness

CV: Bradycardia, hypotension, palpitation, AV block, Wenckebach episodes

GI: Gastric upset, heartburn

HEMA: **Intravascular hemolysis**

Contraindications: Sick sinus syndrome, 2nd- or 3rd-degree heart block, hypotension less than 90 mm Hg systolic, cardiogenic shock, severe CHF

Precautions: Pregnancy **C**, CHF, hypotension, hepatic injury, lactation, children, renal disease, concomitant β-blocker therapy, elderly

Pharmacokinetics

Absorption	Unknown
Distribution	Unknown
Metabolism	Liver
Excretion	Kidneys
Half-life	27 hr

Pharmacodynamics

Onset	Unknown
Peak	2 hr
Duration	24 hr

Interactions

Drug classifications

β-Adrenergic blockers: increased depressant effects on myocardial contractility

NURSING CONSIDERATIONS

Assessment

- Assess fluid volume status: I&O ratio and record; weight; distended red veins; crackles in lung; color, quality, and sp gr of urine; skin turgor; adequacy of pulses; moist mucous membranes; bilateral lung sounds; peripheral pitting edema; dehydration symptoms of decreasing output, thirst, hypotension, dry mouth, and mucous membranes should be reported
- Monitor if platelets are <150,000/mm^3; if so, drug is usually discontinued and another drug started
- Assess for extravasation: change site q48h
- Monitor cardiac status: B/P, pulse, respiration, ECG

Nursing diagnoses

- Cardiac output, decreased (uses)
- Knowledge, deficient (teaching)

Implementation

- Give once a day, with food for GI symptoms

Patient/family education

- Caution patient to avoid hazardous activities until stabilized on drug, dizziness is no longer a problem
- Instruct patient to limit caffeine consumption; to avoid alcohol and OTC drugs unless directed by prescriber
- Advise patient to comply with medical regimen: diet, exercise, stress reduction, drug therapy; to notify prescriber of irregular heartbeat, shortness of breath, swelling of feet and hands, pronounced dizziness, constipation, nausea, hypotension
- Teach patient to use as directed even if feeling better; may be taken with other cardiovascular drugs (nitrates, β-blockers)

Evaluation

Positive therapeutic outcome

- Decreased anginal pain

Treatment of overdose: Defibrillation, atropine for AV block, vasopressor for hypotension

miconazole 🗝 (OTC)

(mi-kon'a-zole)

Monistat, Monistat I.V.; topical: Micatin, Micatin Liquid, miconazole nitrate, Monistat-Derm, Monistat 3, Monistat 7, Monistat Dual-Pak

Func. class.: Antifungal

Chem. class.: Imidazole

Pregnancy category C

Action: Alters cell membranes, inhibits fungal enzymes, inhibits sterols so intracellular contents are lost, prevents biosynthesis of phospholipids/triglycerides

Therapeutic Outcome: Fungistatic/fungicidal against *Aspergillus, Coccidioides, Cryptococcus, Candida, Dermatophytes, Histoplasma*

Uses: Coccidioidomycosis, candidiasis, cryptococcosis, paracoccidioidomycosis, chronic mucocutaneous candidiasis, fungal meningitis; **IV** used for severe infections only; (top) tinea pedis, tinea cruris, tinea corporis, tinea versicolor, vaginal or vulva candidal infections

Dosage and routes

Adult: **IV** inf 200-3600 mg/day; may be divided in 3 inf at 200-1200 mg/inf; may have to repeat course; IT 20 mg given simultaneously with **IV** for fungal meningitis q1-2 days

Child: **IV** 20-40 mg/kg/day, max 15 mg/kg/day

Adult and child: Top apply to affected area bid × 2-4 wk

Adult: Intravaginal 200 mg supp at bedtime × 3 days or 100 mg supp × 1 wk

Available forms: Inj 10 mg/ml; aerosol 2%; cream 2%; lotion 2%; powder 2%; spray 2%; vag cream 2%; vag supp 100, 200 mg

Adverse effects

CNS: Drowsiness, headache, lethargy

CV: Tachycardia, **dysrhythmias** (rapid **IV**)

GI: Nausea, vomiting, anorexia, diarrhea, cramps

GU: Vulvovaginal burning, itching, hyponatremia, pelvic cramps (topical forms)

HEMA: **Decreased Hct, thrombocytopenia, hyperlipidemia**

INTEG: Pruritus, rash, fever, flushing, hives

SYST: **Anaphylaxis**

Contraindications: Hypersensitivity

Precautions: Pregnancy **C**, renal disease, hepatic disease

Pharmacokinetics

Absorption	Poorly absorbed (PO)
Distribution	Widely distributed (**IV**); bound to serum proteins (90%)
Metabolism	Liver, extensively
Excretion	Unknown
Half-life	Triphasic: 0.4, 2.1, 24 hr

Pharmacodynamics

	IV	TOP	VAG
Onset	Rapid	Unknown	Unknown
Peak	Infusion's end	Unknown	Unknown

Interactions

Individual drugs

Amphotericin B, isoniazid, rifampin: decreased effect of miconazole

Amphotericin B: decreased effect of amphotericin B

Phenytoin: increased effect

Warfarin: increased anticoagulant effect

Drug classifications

Sulfonylureas: increased effect

Drug/lab test

False positive: urine glucose, urine protein

NURSING CONSIDERATIONS

Assessment

- Assess for signs and symptoms of infection: drainage, sore throat, urinary pain, hematuria, fever
- Obtain C&S before beginning treatment; therapy may be started after culture is taken; monitor signs of infection before and throughout treatment
- Monitor bowel pattern before and during treatment; diarrhea may occur
- Monitor cardiac system: B/P, pulse; watch for increasing pulse, cardiac dysrhythmias; drug should be discontinued
- Monitor blood studies: WBC, RBC, Hgb, Hct, bleeding time; patients taking anticoagulants may need a decreased dosage; monitor liver and renal studies periodically for patients on long-term therapy
- Monitor I&O ratio; watch for decreasing urinary output, change in sp gr; discontinue

M

drug to prevent renal damage; patients with renal disease may require lowered dose
- Monitor **IV** site for thrombophlebitis; site should be changed q48-72h
- Monitor for allergies before initiation of treatment and reaction to each medication; highlight allergies on chart; check for allergic reaction: burning, stinging, swelling, redness (top); observe for skin eruptions after administration of drug to 1 wk after discontinuing drug

Nursing diagnoses
- Skin integrity, impaired (uses)
- Infection, risk for (uses)
- Injury, risk for (adverse reactions)
- Knowledge, deficient (teaching)

Implementation
- Have adrenalin, suction, tracheostomy set, endotracheal intubation equipment available

Topical route
- Apply after cleansing area with soap and water before each application; use enough medication to cover lesions completely; dry well
- Store at room temp in dry place

Vaginal route
- Administer 1 applicator full every night high into the vagina
- Store at room temp in dry place

IV route
- Give 200 mg initially to prevent severe hypersensitive reaction
- Give **IV** after diluting ≤1 g/10 ml of sterile water, D_5W, or 0.45% NaCl over 3-5 min
- Give by intermittent **IV** after diluting in 200 ml or more, D_5W or 0.9% NaCl; give over 30-60 min
- Store at room temp; reconstituted sol is stable for 24 hr refrigerated

Y-site compatibilities: Allopurinol, filgrastim, foscarnet, granisetron, melphalan, ondansetron, propofol, sargramostim, teniposide, thiotepa, vinorelbine

Y-site incompatibilities: Fludarabine

Patient/family education
- Inform patient that culture may be performed after completed course of medication
- Advise patient to notify nurse of diarrhea, symptoms of candidal vaginitis

Topical route
- Teach patient to use medical asepsis (hand washing) before, after each application; to apply with glove to prevent further infection; to avoid contact with eyes; not to use occlusive dressings
- Caution patient to avoid use of OTC creams, ointments, lotions unless directed by prescriber
- Instruct patient to notify prescriber if no improvement in condition in 4 wk or if symptoms return in 2 mo; pregnancy or a serious medical condition may be the cause
- Teach patient to use for full prescribed treatment time, or reinfection may occur

Vaginal route
- Instruct patient in asepsis (hand washing) before, after each application
- Teach patient to apply with applicator only; to avoid use of any other vaginal product unless directed by prescriber; sanitary napkin may prevent soiling of undergarments; to abstain from sexual intercourse until treatment is completed; reinfection and irritation may occur
- Instruct patient to notify prescriber if symptoms persist

Evaluation
Positive therapeutic outcome
- Decreasing oral candidiasis, fever, malaise, rash
- Negative C&S for infectious organism
- Decrease in size, number of lesions
- Decrease in itching or white discharge (vaginal)

Treatment of overdose: Withdraw drug; maintain airway; administer epINEPHrine, aminophylline, O_2, **IV** corticosteroids for anaphylaxis

midazolam (Rx)
(mid'ay-zoe-lam)

Versed

Func. class.: Sedative/hypnotic, antianxiety

Chem. class.: Benzodiazepine, short-acting

Pregnancy category D

Controlled substance schedule IV

Do Not Confuse:
Versed/Vepesid, Versed/Vistaril

Action: Depresses subcortical levels in CNS; may act on limbic system, reticular formation; may potentiate GABA by binding to specific benzodiazepine receptors

Therapeutic Outcome: Sedation for anesthesia induction and procedures

Uses: Preoperative sedation, general anesthesia induction, sedation for diagnostic endoscopic procedures, intubation

Investigational uses: Epileptic seizures, refractory status epilepticus

Dosage and routes

Preoperative sedation

Adult and child ≥12 yr: IM 0.07-0.08 mg/kg 30-60 min before general anesthesia

Child 1-6 mo: IM 0.1-0.15 mg/kg, may give up to 0.5 mg/kg if needed

Child 6 mo-5 yr: PO 0.25-1 mg/kg, max 20 mg as a single dose

Child 6 yr-16 yr: PO 0.25-0.5 mg/kg, max 20 mg as a single dose

Induction of general anesthesia

Adult and child 12-16 yr: Unpremedicated patients, **IV** 0.3-0.35 mg/kg over 30 sec, wait 2 min, follow with 25% of initial dose if needed; premedicated patients, 0.15-0.35 mg/kg over 20-30 sec, allow 2 min for effect

Child 6-12 yr: **IV** 0.025-0.05 mg/kg, total dose up to 0.4 mg/kg if needed

Child 6 mo-5 yr: **IV** 0.05-0.1 mg/kg, total dose up to 0.6 mg/kg may be needed

Child <6 mo: Titrate with small increments

Continuous infusion for intubation (critical care)

Adult: **IV** 0.01-0.05 mg/kg over several min; repeat at 10-15 min intervals, until adequate sedation; then 0.02-0.10 mg/kg/hr maintenance, adjust as needed

Child: **IV** 0.05-0.2 mg/kg over 2-3 min then 0.06-0.12 mg/kg/hr by cont inf; adjust as needed

Neonates: **IV** 0.03-0.06 mg/kg/hr titrate using lowest dose

Available forms: Inj 1, 5 mg/ml; syr 2 mg/ml

Adverse effects

CNS: Retrograde amnesia, euphoria, confusion, headache, anxiety, insomnia, slurred speech, paresthesia, tremors, weakness, chills

CV: Hypotension, PVCs, tachycardia, bigeminy, nodal rhythm, **cardiac arrest**

EENT: Blurred vision, nystagmus, diplopia, blocked ears, loss of balance

GI: *Nausea, vomiting,* increased salivation, hiccups

INTEG: Urticaria, pain, swelling at inj site, rash, pruritus

RESP: Coughing, **apnea, bronchospasm, laryngospasm**, dyspnea, **respiratory depression**

Contraindications: Pregnancy **D**, hypersensitivity to benzodiazepines, shock, coma, alcohol intoxication, acute narrow-angle glaucoma

Precautions: COPD, CHF, chronic renal failure, chills, debilitated, elderly, children, lactation, neonates (contains benzyl alcohol)

Pharmacokinetics	
Absorption	Well absorbed
Distribution	Crosses placenta, blood-brain barrier, protein binding 97%
Metabolism	Liver
Excretion	Kidneys, breast milk
Half-life	1-12 hr

Pharmacodynamics	IM	IV
Onset	15 min	3-5 min
Peak	½-1 hr	Unknown
Duration	2-3 hr	<2 hr

Interactions

Individual drugs

Alcohol: increased respiratory depression

Cimetidine, erythromycin, ranitidine, theophylline: decreased midazolam metabolism

Fluvoxamine, indinavir, ritonavir, verapamil: increased respiratory depression

Drug classifications

Antifungals, azole: increased levels of midalozam

Barbiturates, opiate analgesics, other CNS depressants: increased respiratory depression

Oral contraceptives: increased half-life of midazolam

Theophyllines: decreased effect of midazolam

Drug/herb

Black cohosh: increased hypotension

Catnip, chamomile, clary, cowslip, hops, kava, lavender, mistletoe, nettle, pokeweed, poppy, Queen Anne's lace, senega, skullcap, valerian: increased CNS depression

Drug/food

Grapefruit juice: increased midazolam effect

NURSING CONSIDERATIONS

Assessment

- Monitor B/P, pulse, respiration during **IV**; O_2 and emergency equipment should be nearby
- Monitor inj site for redness, pain, swelling
- Assess degree of amnesia in elderly; may be increased
- Assess anterograde amnesia
- Assess vital signs for recovery period in obese patient, since half-life may be extended
- Assess for apnea, respiratory depression, which may be increased in the elderly

M

Nursing diagnoses
- Knowledge, deficient (teaching)

Implementation
PO route
- Remove cap of press-in bottle adaptor and push adaptor into neck of bottle, close with cap, remove cap and insert tip of dispenser and insert into adaptor, turn upside-down and withdraw correct dose, place in mouth

IM route
- Give inj deep into large muscle mass
- Store at room temp; protect from light

IV route
- Give **IV** undiluted or after diluting with D_5W or 0.9% NaCl to a conc of 0.25 mg/ml; give over 2 min (conscious sedation) or over 30 sec (anesthesia induction)
- Ensure immediate availability of resuscitation equipment, O_2 to support airway; do not give by rapid bol

Syringe compatibilities: Alfentanil, atracurium, atropine, benzquinamide, buprenorphine, butorphanol, chlorproMAZINE, cimetadine, cisatracurium, diphenhyDRAMINE, droperidol, fentanyl, glycopyrrolate, hydromorphine, hydrOXYzine, ketamine, meperidine, metoclopramide, morphine, nalbuphine, promazine, promethazine, remifentanil, scopolamine, sufentanil, thiethylperazine, trimethobenzamide

Syringe incompatibilities: Dimenhydrinate, pentobarbital, perphenazine, prochlorperazine, ranitidine

Y-site compatibilities: Abcixmab, alfentamil, amikacin, amiodarone, argatroban, atracurium, atropine, aztreonam, benzotropine, calcium gluconate, cefazolin, cefotaxime, cefoxitine, ceftriaxone, cimetidine, ciprofloxacin, cisplatin, clindamycin, clonidine, cyanocobalamin, cycloSPORINE, dactinomycin, digoxin, diltiazem, diphenhydramine, docetaxal, DOPamine, doxycycline, enalaprilat, epINEPHrine, erythromycin, esmolol, etomidate, etoposide, famotidine, fentanyl, fluconazole, folic acid, gatifloxacin, gemcitabine, gentamicin, glycopyrrolate, granisetron, heparin, hetastarch, hydromorphine, hydromorphone, hydrOXYzine, inamrinone, isoproterenol, labetalol, lactated ringers, levofloxacin, lidocaine, linezolid, lorazepam, magnesium, mannitol, meperidine, methadone, methyldopa, methylPREDNISolone, metoclopromide, metomolol, metronidazole, milrinone, morphine, nalbuphine, naloxone, niCARdipine, nitroglycerin, nitroprusside, norepinephrine, ondansetron, oxacillin, oxytocin, paclitaxel, palonosetron, pancuronium, papaverin, phentolamine, phytonadione, piperacillin, potassium chloride, propanolol, protamine, pyridoxine, ranitidine, remifentanil, sodium nitroprusside, streptokinase, succinylcholine, sufentanil, teniposide, theophylline, thiotepa, ticarcillin, tobramycin, vancomycin, vasopressin, vecuronium, verapamil, voriconazole

Y-site incompatibilities: Foscarnet

Patient/family education
- Inform patient that amnesia occurs; events may not be remembered
- Caution patient to avoid CNS depressants including alcohol for 24 hr after taking this drug

Evaluation
Positive therapeutic outcome
- Induction of sedation, amnesia

Treatment of overdose: O_2, flumazenil

midodrine (Rx)
(mye'doh-dreen)
ProAmatine
Func. class.: Prodrug
Pregnancy category C

Do Not Confuse:
ProAmatine/Protamine

Action: Activates α-adrenergic receptors of arteriolar, venous vasculature; increases vascular tone

Therapeutic Outcome: Decreased feeling of faintness upon rising, absence of significant change in B/P

Uses: Orthostatic hypotension

Dosage and routes
Adult: PO 10 mg tid

Renal dose
Adult: PO 2.5 mg tid

Available forms: Tabs 2.5, 5 mg

Adverse effects
CNS: Drowsiness, restlessness, headache, paresthesia, pain, chills, confusion
CV: **Supine hypertension,** vasodilatation, flushing face
EENT: Dry mouth, blurred vision
GI: Nausea, anorexia
GU: Dysuria
INTEG: Pruritus, piloerection, rash

Contraindications: Hypersensitivity, severe organic heart disease, acute renal disease, urinary retention, pheochromocytoma, thyrotoxicosis, persistent/excessive supine hypertension, thyroid disease, visual disturbance, dialysis, urinary retention

Precautions: Pregnancy **C,** children, lactation, prostatic hypertrophy, hepatic function impairment, orthostatic diabetic patients

Pharmacokinetics

Absorption	Bioavailibility 90%
Distribution	Unknown
Metabolism	Unknown
Excretion	Unknown
Half-life	3-4 hr

Pharmacodynamics

Onset	Unknown
Peak	1-2 hr
Duration	Unknown

Interactions

Individual drugs:

Fludrocortisone: increased supine hypertension

Metformin: increased lactic acidosis

Drug classifications

α-Adrenergic agonists: increased pressor effects

β-Adrenergic blockers, cardiac glycosides, psychotropics, tricyclics: increased bradycardia

NURSING CONSIDERATIONS

Assessment

- Monitor VS, B/P (standing, supine); notify prescriber if B/P supine is increased
- Observe for drowsiness, dizziness, LOC

Nursing diagnoses

- Knowledge, deficient (teaching)

Implementation

- Tablets may be swallowed whole, chewed, or allowed to dissolve
- Administer upon arising, at midday, and in late afternoon (no later than 6 PM)
- Avoid administering if patient is to be supine during day

Patient/family education

- Advise to avoid hazardous activities; activities requiring alertness; dizziness may occur; instruct patient to request assistance with ambulation
- Advise to avoid alcohol, other depressants

Evaluation

Positive therapeutic outcome

- Decreased orthostatic hypotension

mifepristone (Rx)

(mif-ee-press'tone)

Mifeprex

Func. class.: Abortifacient

Chem. class.: Antiprogestational

Pregnancy category C

Action: Stimulates uterine contractions, causing complete abortion

Therapeutic Outcome: Termination of pregnancy

Uses: Abortion through 49 days gestation

Investigational uses: Postcoital contraception/contragestation, intrauterine fetal death, endometriosis, Cushing's syndrome, unresectable meningioma

Dosage and routes

Coadministration of mifepristone/misoprostol

- Day 1: PO single dose 600 mg mifepristone
- Day 3: 400 mcg misoprostol

Available forms: Tabs 200 mg

Adverse effects

CNS: Dizziness, insomnia, anxiety, syncope, fainting, headache

GI: *Nausea, vomiting, diarrhea,* dyspepsia

GU: Uterine cramping, uterine hemorrhage, vaginitis, pelvic pain

MISC: Fatigue, back pain, fever, viral infections, chills, sinusitis

Contraindications: Hypersensitivity, severe hepatic disease, severe renal disease, PID, respiratory disease, cardiac disease, IUD, ectopic pregnancy, chronic adrenal failure, bleeding disorder, inherited porphyrias

Precautions: Pregnancy **C,** asthma, anemia, jaundice, diabetes mellitus, seizure disorders, women >35 yr/smoking ≥10 cigarettes/day, past uterine surgery

Pharmacokinetics

Absorption	Rapidly
Distribution	98% protein binding, albumin, glycoprotein
Metabolism	Unknown
Excretion	Feces, urine
Half-life	Unknown

Pharmacodynamics

Onset	Unknown
Peak	90 min
Duration	Unknown

M

Interactions
Individual drugs
Erythromycin, itraconazole, ketoconazole: decreased metabolism of each specific drug
Drug/herb
St. John's wort: decreased mifepristone action
Drug/food
Grapefruit juice: decreased metabolism of mifepristone

NURSING CONSIDERATIONS
Assessment
- Monitor B/P, pulse; watch for change that may indicate hemorrhage
- Monitor respiratory rate, rhythm, depth; notify prescriber of abnormalities
- Assess for length, duration of contraction; notify prescriber of contractions lasting over 1 min or absence of contractions
- Assess for incomplete abortion, pregnancy must be terminated by another method; drug is teratogenic

Nursing diagnoses
- Pain, acute (adverse reactions)
- Knowledge, deficient (teaching)

Implementation
- Provide emotional support before and after abortion

Patient/family education
- Advise patient to report increased blood loss, abdominal cramps, increased temperature, foul-smelling lochia
- Teach patient some methods of comfort control and pain control
- Advise patient to continue with follow-up
- Advise patient that cramping and vaginal bleeding will occur

Evaluation
Positive therapeutic outcome
- Expulsion of fetus

miglitol (Rx)
(mig'le-tol)
Glyset
Func. class.: Oral hypoglycemic
Chem. class.: α-Glucosidase inhibitor
Pregnancy category B

Action: Delays the digestion of ingested carbohydrates, results in a smaller rise in blood glucose after meals; does not increase insulin production

Therapeutic Outcome: Decreased blood glucose levels in diabetes mellitus

Uses: Type 2 diabetes mellitus

Dosage and routes
Initial dose
Adult: PO 25 mg tid with first bite of meal
Maintenance dose
Adult: PO may be increased to 50 mg tid; may increase to 100 mg tid if needed only in patients >60 kg; dosage adjustment at 4-8 wk intervals

Available forms: Tabs 25, 50, 100 mg

Adverse effects
GI: *Abdominal pain, diarrhea, flatulence,* **hepatotoxicity**
HEMA: Low iron
INTEG: Rash

Contraindications: Hypersensitivity, diabetic ketoacidosis, cirrhosis, inflammatory bowel disease, colonic ulceration, partial intestinal obstruction, chronic intestinal disease

Precautions: Pregnancy **B**, renal disease, lactation, children, hepatic disease

Pharmacokinetics	
Absorption	Unknown
Distribution	Unknown
Metabolism	Not metabolized
Excretion	Kidneys, unchanged drug
Half-life	2 hr

Pharmacodynamics	
Onset	Unknown
Peak	2-3 hr
Duration	Unknown

Interactions
Individual drugs
Digoxin: decreased levels of digoxin
Propranolol: decreased levels of propranolol
Ranitidine: decreased levels of ranitidine
Drug classifications
Adsorbents (intestinal), enzymes (digestive): decreased miglitol levels; do not use together
Drug/herb
Broom, buchu, dandelion, juniper: decreased hypoglycemia
Chromium, fenugreek, ginseng: increased or decreased hypoglycemic effect
Karela: Improved glucose tolerance
Drug/food
Carbohydrates: increased diarrhea

NURSING CONSIDERATIONS
Assessment
- Assess for hypoglycemia, hyperglycemia; even though this drug does not cause hypoglycemia, if taking a sulfonylurea or insulin, hypoglycemia may be additive
- Monitor blood glucose levels, A1C, liver function tests; if hypoglycemia occurs with monotherapy, treat with glucose

Nursing diagnoses
- Nutrition: more than body requirements, imbalanced (uses)
- Nutrition: less than body requirements, imbalanced (adverse reactions)
- Knowledge, deficient (teaching)
- Noncompliance (teaching)

Implementation
- Give tid with first bite of each meal
- Provide storage in airtight container in cool environment

Patient/family education
- Teach patient the symptoms of hypoglycemia, hyperglycemia and what to do about each
- Instruct that medication must be taken as prescribed; explain consequences of discontinuing the medication abruptly; that during periods of stress, infection, surgery, insulin may be required
- Tell patient to avoid OTC medications unless approved by prescriber
- Teach patient that diabetes is a lifelong illness; drug will not cure condition
- Instruct patient to carry/wear emergency ID as diabetic
- Teach patient that diet and exercise regimen must be followed

Evaluation
Positive therapeutic outcome
- Decreased signs, symptoms of diabetes mellitus (polyuria, polydipsia, polyphagia, clear sensorium, absence of dizziness, stable gait)

! HIGH ALERT

milrinone (Rx)
(mill-re′none)

Primacor

Func. class.: Inotropic/vasodilator agent with phosphodiesterase activity

Chem. class.: Bipyridine derivative

Pregnancy category C

Action: Positive inotropic agent with vasodilator properties; increases contractility of cardiac muscle; reduces preload and afterload by direct relaxation of vascular smooth muscle; increases myocardial contractility

Therapeutic Outcome: Increased inotropic effect resulting in increased cardiac output

Uses: Short-term management of advanced CHF that has not responded to other medication; can be used with digitalis products

Dosage and routes
Adult: **IV** bol 50 mcg/kg given over 10 min; start inf of 0.375-0.75 mcg/kg/min; reduce dosage in renal impairment

Available forms: Inj 1 mg/ml; premixed inj 200 mcg/ml in D_5W

Adverse effects
CV: Dysrhythmias, hypotension, chest pain
GI: Nausea, vomiting, anorexia, abdominal pain, **hepatotoxicity,** jaundice
HEMA: **Thrombocytopenia**
MISC: Headache, hypokalemia, tremor

Contraindications: Hypersensitivity to this drug, severe aortic disease, severe pulmonic valvular disease, acute MI

Precautions: Pregnancy **C,** lactation, children, renal disease, hepatic disease, atrial flutter/fibrillation, elderly

M

Pharmacokinetics	
Absorption	Completely absorbed
Distribution	Unknown
Metabolism	Liver (50%)
Excretion	Kidney, unchanged (83%), metabolites (12%)
Half-life	2.4 hr; increased in CHF

Pharmacodynamics	
Onset	2-5 min
Peak	10 min
Duration	Variable

Interactions: None known

NURSING CONSIDERATIONS
Assessment
- Monitor manifestations of hypokalemia: acidic urine, reduced urine, osmolality, nocturia; hypotension, broad T-wave, U-wave, ectopy, tachycardia, weak pulse; muscle weakness, altered LOC, drowsiness, apathy, lethargy, confusion, depression; anorexia, nausea, cramps, constipation, distention, paralytic ileus; hypoventilation, respiratory muscle weakness
- Assess fluid volume status: complete I&O ratio and record; note weight, distended red

veins, crackles in lung, color, quality, and sp gr of urine, skin turgor, adequacy of pulses, moist mucous membranes, bilateral lung sounds, peripheral pitting edema; dehydration symptoms of decreasing output, thirst, hypotension, dry mouth and mucous membranes should be reported

- Monitor electrolytes: potassium, sodium, calcium, magnesium; also include BUN, blood pH, ABGs
- Monitor B/P and pulse, ECG continuously during **IV**, ventricular dysrhythmia can occur, PCWP, CVP, index often during inf; if B/P drops 30 mm Hg, stop inf and call prescriber
- Monitor ALT, AST, bilirubin daily; if these are elevated, hepatoxicity is suspected
- Monitor platelets; if <150,000/mm^3, drug is usually discontinued and another drug started
- Assess for extravasation: change site q48h

Nursing diagnoses

- Cardiac output, decreased (uses)
- Fluid volume, excess (uses)
- Knowledge, deficient (teaching)

Implementation

IV route

- Give **IV** loading dose undiluted over 10 min
- Do not mix directly with glucose sol; chemical reaction occurs over 24 hr; precipitate forms if milrinone and furosemide come in contact
- Administer by direct **IV** into inf through Y-connector or directly into tubing; may give undiluted over 2-3 min
- Give by cont inf diluted with 0.9% NaCl to conc of 1-3 mg/ml, run at prescribed rate; give by infusion pump for doses other than bol
- Administer potassium supplements if ordered for potassium levels <3.0 mg/dl

Syringe compatibilities: Atropine, calcium chloride, digoxin, epINEPHrine, lidocaine, morphine, propranolol, sodium bicarbonate, verapamil

Y-site compatibilities: Digoxin, diltiazem, DOBUTamine, DOPamine, epINEPHrine, fentanyl, heparin, hydromorphone, labetalol, lorazepam, midazolam, morphine, niCARdipine, nitroglycerin, norepinephrine, propranolol, quinidine, ranitidine, thiopental, vecuronium

Additive compatibilities: Quinidine

Patient/family education

- Teach patient reason for medication and expected results
- Instruct patient to make position changes slowly; orthostatic hypotension may occur
- Teach patient signs and symptoms of hypersensitivity reactions and hypokalemia

Evaluation

Positive therapeutic outcome

- Increased cardiac output
- Decreased PCWP, adequate CVP
- Decreased dyspnea, fatigue, edema, ECG

Treatment of overdose: Discontinue drug, support circulation

minocycline (Rx)

(min-oh-sye'kleen)

Arestin, Dynacin, Minocin, Vectrin

Func. class.: Antiinfective

Chem. class.: Tetracycline

Pregnancy category D

Action: Inhibits protein synthesis and phosphorylation in microorganisms by binding to 30S ribosomal subunits and reversibly binding to 50S ribosomal subunits; bacteriostatic

Therapeutic Outcome: Bactericidal action against susceptible organisms, including *Neisseria meningitidis, Neisseria gonorrhoeae, Treponema pallidum, Chlamydia trachomatis, Ureaplasma urealyticum, Mycoplasma pneumoniae, Nocardia, Rickettsia*

Uses: Syphilis, chlamydial infection, gonorrhea, lymphogranuloma venereum, rickettsial infections, inflammatory acne, meningitis carriers, periodontitis

Investigational uses: Rheumatoid arthritis

Dosage and routes

Adult: PO/**IV** 200 mg, then 100 mg q12h or 50 mg q6h, max 400 mg/24 hr **IV**; subgingival insert into periodontal pocket

Child >8 yr: PO/**IV** 4 mg/kg then 4 mg/kg/day PO in divided doses q12h

Gonorrhea

Adult: PO 200 mg, then 100 mg q12h × 4 days

C. trachomatis infection

Adult: PO 100 mg bid × 7 days

Syphilis

Adult: PO 200 mg, then 100 mg q12h × 10-15 days

Uncomplicated gonococcal urethritis in men

Adult: PO 100 mg q12h × 5 days

Rheumatoid arthritis (off-label)

Adult: PO 100 mg bid for ≤48 wk

Available forms: Caps 50, 75, 100 mg; oral susp 50 mg/5 ml; powder for inj 100 mg; caps, pellet filled 50, 100 mg; tabs 50, 75, 100 mg

Adverse effects

CNS: *Dizziness,* fever, lightheadedness, vertigo
CV: Pericarditis
EENT: Dysphagia, glossitis, decreased calcification, permanent discoloration of teeth, oral candidiasis
GI: *Nausea,* abdominal pain, *vomiting, diarrhea,* anorexia, enterocolitis, **hepatotoxicity,** flatulence, abdominal cramps, epigastric burning, stomatitis
GU: Increased BUN, polyuria, polydipsia, **renal failure, nephrotoxicity**
HEMA: **Eosinophilia, neutropenia, thrombocytopenia, hemolytic anemia**
INTEG: *Rash, urticaria, photosensitivity, increased pigmentation,* **exfoliative dermatitis,** pruritus, **angioedema,** blue-gray color of skin and mucous membranes

Contraindications: Pregnancy **D,** hypersensitivity to tetracyclines, children <8 yr

Precautions: Hepatic disease, lactation

Pharmacokinetics

Absorption	Well absorbed (PO)
Distribution	Widely distributed (70%-75% protein bound); some distribution in CSF, crosses placenta
Metabolism	Liver, some
Excretion	Kidneys, unchanged (20%), bile, feces
Half-life	11-17 hr

Pharmacodynamics

	PO	IV
Onset	Rapid	Rapid
Peak	2-3 hr	Infusion's end

Interactions

Individual drugs

Calcium, iron, magnesium: forms chelates, decreased absorption
Carbamazepine, phenytoin: decreased effect
Digoxin: increased effect
Insulin: increased effect
Kaolin/pectin, sodium bicarbonate, cimetidine, iron: decreased minocycline effect
Theophylline: increased effect
Warfarin: increased effect

Drug classifications

Antacids, alkali products: decreased minocycline effect
Anticoagulants (oral): increased effect
Antidiarrheals (adsorbent): decreased absorption
Barbiturates, penicillins: decreased effect
Oral contraceptives: decreased effect of oral contraception

Drug/lab test

False negative: urine glucose with Clinistix, Tes-Tape

NURSING CONSIDERATIONS

Assessment

- Assess patient for previous sensitivity reaction
- Assess patient for signs and symptoms of infection including characteristics of wounds, sputum, urine, stool, WBC >10,000/mm^3, fever; obtain baseline information, before and during treatment
- Obtain C&S before beginning drug therapy to identify if correct treatment has been initiated
- Assess for allergic reactions: rash, urticaria, pruritus
- Monitor blood studies: AST, ALT, CBC, Hct, bilirubin, alkaline phosphatase, amylase monthly if patient is on long-term therapy
- Assess bowel pattern daily; if severe diarrhea occurs, drug should be discontinued
- Monitor for bleeding: ecchymosis, bleeding gums, hematuria, stool guaiac daily if on long-term therapy; blood dyscrasias may occur
- Assess for overgrowth of infection: perineal itching, fever, malaise, redness, pain, swelling, drainage, rash, diarrhea, change in cough, sputum; black, furry tongue

Nursing diagnoses

- Infection, risk for (uses)
- Diarrhea (adverse reactions)
- Knowledge, deficient (teaching)
- Noncompliance (teaching)

Implementation

PO route

- Give around the clock to maintain proper blood levels; give with food to increase absorption of drug; do not give within 3 hr of other agents; drug interactions may occur
- Give with 8 oz of water 1 hr before bedtime to prevent ulceration
- Shake liq preparation well before giving; use calibrated device for proper dosing
- Do not give with iron, calcium, magnesium products, or antacids, which decrease absorption and form insoluble chelate

IV route

- Check for irritation, extravasation, phlebitis daily; change site q72h
- For intermittent inf, dilute each 100 mg/10

ml of 0.9% NaCl, sterile water for inj; further dilute in 500-1000 ml of 0.9% NaCl, D_5W, Ringer's, LR, D_5/LR; give over 6 hr

Y-site compatibilities: Cyclophosphamide, fludarabine, granisetron, heparin, hydrocortisone, magnesium sulfate, melphalan, perphenazine, potassium chloride, sargramostim, sodium succinate, vinorelbine, vit B/C

Y-site incompatibilities: Aztreonam, filgrastim, hydromorphone, meperidine, morphine, teniposide

Patient/family education

- Teach patient to use sunscreen when outdoors to decrease photosensitivity reaction
- Teach patient to report sore throat, bruising, bleeding, joint pain; may indicate blood dyscrasias (rare)
- Advise patient to contact prescriber if vaginal itching, loose foul-smelling stools, furry tongue occur; may indicate superinfection; report itching, rash, pruritus, urticaria
- Instruct patient to take all medication prescribed for the length of time ordered; drug must be taken around the clock to maintain blood levels; do not give medication to others; take with a full glass of water; may take with food; not to use outdated product, Fanconi's syndrome may occur
- Advise patient to use a form of contraception other than hormonal

Evaluation

Positive therapeutic outcome

- Absence of signs/symptoms of infection (WBC <10,000/mm^3, temp WNL, absence of red, draining wounds)
- Reported improvement in symptoms of infection

minoxidil (Rx, OTC)

(mi-nox'i-dill)

Loniten, minoxidil, Rogaine (top)

Func. class.: Antihypertensive, hair growth stimulant

Chem. class.: Vasodilator, peripheral

Pregnancy category C

Do Not Confuse:

Loniten/Lotensin, minoxidil/Monopril

Action: Directly relaxes arteriolar smooth muscle, causing vasodilatation; increased cutaneous blood flow; stimulation of hair follicles

Therapeutic Outcome: Decreased B/P in hypertension; hair growth

Uses: Severe hypertension unresponsive to other therapy (use with diuretic); topically to treat alopecia

Dosage and routes

Severe hypertension

Adult: PO 2.5-5 mg/day max 100 mg daily; usual range 10-40 mg/day in single doses

Elderly: PO 2.5 mg daily, may be increased gradually

Child <12 yr: Initial, 0.2 mg/kg/day; effective range, 0.25-1 mg/kg/day; max, 50 mg/day

Alopecia

Adult: Top 1 ml bid rub into scalp daily, max 2 ml/day

Available forms: Tabs 2.5, 10 mg; top 2% sol

Adverse effects

CNS: Headache, fatigue

CV: ***Severe rebound hypertension (on withdrawal in children),*** tachycardia, angina, increased T-wave, **CHF, pulmonary edema, pericardial effusion,** edema, sodium retention, water retention

GI: Nausea, vomiting

GU: Breast tenderness

HEMA: Hct, Hgb, erythrocyte count may decrease initially

INTEG: Pruritus, **Stevens-Johnson syndrome,** rash, hirsutism

Contraindications: Acute MI, dissecting aortic aneurysm, hypersensitivity, pheochromocytoma

Precautions: Pregnancy **C,** lactation, children, renal disease, CAD, CHF, elderly

Pharmacokinetics

Absorption	Well absorbed (PO); minimally absorbed (top)
Distribution	Widely distributed
Metabolism	Liver
Excretion	Kidneys, breast milk
Half-life	4.2 hr

Pharmacodynamics

	PO	TOP
Onset	½ hr	4 mo
Peak	2-3 hr	Unknown
Duration	75 hr	4 mo

Interactions

Drug classifications

Antihypertensives: increased orthostatic hypotension

Drug/lab test
Increased: renal function studies
Decreased: Hgb, Hct, RBC

NURSING CONSIDERATIONS
Assessment
- ❗ Monitor closely, usually given with β-blocker to prevent tachycardia and increased myocardial workload, usually given with diuretic to prevent serious fluid accumulation, patient should be hospitalized during beginning treatment
- Monitor B/P, pulse, jugular venous distention periodically throughout treatment
- Monitor electrolytes, blood studies: potassium, sodium, chloride, carbon dioxide, CBC, serum glucose
- ❗ Monitor weight daily, I&O; assess edema in feet, legs daily; check skin turgor, dryness of mucous membranes for hydration status
- Assess for crackles, dyspnea, orthopnea, peripheral edema, fatigue, weight gain, jugular vein distention (CHF)
- Assess for signs of hyperglycemia: acetone breath, increased urinary output, severe thirst, lethargy, dizziness

Nursing diagnoses
- Cardiac output, decreased (adverse reactions)
- Injury, risk for (side effects)
- Knowledge, deficient (teaching)

Implementation
PO route
- Give with meals to decrease GI symptoms
- Give with β-blockers and/or diuretic for hypertension
- Store protected from light and heat

Topical route
- Administer 1 ml dose no matter how much balding has occurred; increasing dose does not speed hair growth
- Treatment must continue long term or new hair will be lost again

Patient/family education
Topical route
- Teach patient that new hair will be soft and hardly visible
- Caution patient not to use on other parts of the body; drug is to be used on the scalp only
- Instruct patient that hair should be clean before applying medication; do not get on clothing
- Caution patient not to get medication near mucous membranes (mouth, nose, eyes) and to contact prescriber if burning, stinging, or rash occurs

Evaluation
Positive therapeutic outcome
- Decreased B/P in hypertension
- Hair growth (Top)

mirtazapine (Rx)
(mer-ta'za-peen)
Remeron, Remeron Soltab
Func. class.: Antidepressant
Chem. class.: Tetracyclic

Pregnancy category C

Action: Blocks reuptake of norepinephrine, serotonin into nerve endings, increasing action of norepinephrine, serotonin in nerve cells; has anticholinergic action

Therapeutic Outcome: Decreased symptoms of depression after 2-3 wk

Uses: Depression, dysthymic disorder, bipolar disorder: depression, agitated depression

Dosage and routes
Adult: PO 15 mg/day at bedtime, maintenance to continue for 6 mo, titrate up to 45 mg/day; orally disintegrating tabs, open blister pack, place tab on tongue, allow to disintegrate, swallow

Elderly: PO 7.5 mg nightly, increase by 7.5 mg q1-2 wk to desired dose, max 45 mg/day

Available forms: Tabs 15, 30 mg; orally disintegrating tabs 15, 30, 45 mg

Adverse effects
CNS: *Dizziness, drowsiness,* confusion, headache, anxiety, tremors, stimulation, weakness, insomnia, nightmares, extrapyramidal symptoms (EPS) (elderly), increased psychiatric symptoms, **seizures**

CV: *Orthostatic hypotension, ECG changes, tachycardia, hypertension,* palpitations

EENT: *Blurred vision,* tinnitus, mydriasis

GI: *Diarrhea, dry mouth,* nausea, vomiting, **paralytic ileus,** increased appetite; cramps, epigastric distress, **jaundice, hepatitis,** stomatitis, constipation

GU: *Retention,* **acute renal failure**

HEMA: **Agranulocytosis, thrombocytopenia, eosinophilia, leukopenia**

INTEG: Rash, urticaria, sweating, pruritus, photosensitivity

SYST: Flulike symptoms

Contraindications: Hypersensitivity to tricyclic antidepressants, recovery phase of MI, seizure disorders, prostatic hypertrophy

Precautions: Pregnancy **C**, suicidal patients, severe depression, increased intraocular pressure, narrow-angle glaucoma, urinary retention, cardiac disease, hepatic disease, renal disease, hypothyroidism, hyperthyroidism, electroshock therapy, elective surgery, elderly

Pharmacokinetics	
Absorption	Slow, complete
Distribution	Widely distributed; crosses placenta
Metabolism	Liver, extensively
Excretion	Feces; breast milk
Half-life	20-40 hr

Pharmacodynamics	
Onset	Unknown
Peak	2 hr
Duration	Unknown

Interactions
Individual drugs
Alcohol: increased CNS depression
Drug classifications
Analgesics, antihistamines, sedative/hypnotics: increased CNS depression
Barbiturates, benzodiazepines, CNS depressants (other), contraceptives (oral): increased effects
MAOIs: hypertensive episode, seizures, hyperpyretic crisis
Drug/herb
Belladonna, henbane: increased anticholinergic effect
Chamomile, hops, kava, skullcap, valerian: increased CNS depression
St. John's wort, SAM-e: serotonin syndrome
Scopolia: increased antidepressant effect
Sympathomimetics, indirect acting (epHEDrine): decreased effects
Drug/lab test
Increased: serum bilirubin, blood glucose, alkaline phosphatase
Decreased: VMA, 5-HIAA
False increase: urinary catecholamines

NURSING CONSIDERATIONS
Assessment
- Monitor B/P (with patient lying, standing), pulse q4h during beginning treatment; if systolic B/P drops 20 mm Hg, hold drug, notify prescriber; take VS q4h in patients with CV disease
- Monitor blood studies: CBC, leukocytes, differential, cardiac enzymes if patient is receiving long-term therapy
- Monitor hepatic studies: AST, ALT, bilirubin
- Check weight weekly, drug may increase appetite
- Assess ECG for flattening of T-wave, bundle branch block, AV block, dysrhythmias in cardiac patients
- Assess for EPS primarily in elderly: rigidity, dystonia, akathisia
- Assess mental status: mood, sensorium, affect, suicidal tendencies; assess increase in psychiatric symptoms: depression, panic
- Identify alcohol consumption; if alcohol is consumed, hold dose until AM

Nursing diagnoses
- Coping, ineffective (uses)
- Injury, risk for (side effects)
- Knowledge, deficient (teaching)
- Noncompliance (teaching)

Implementation
- Give with food or milk for GI symptoms; crush if patient is unable to swallow medication whole
- Give dose at bedtime if oversedation occurs during day; may take entire dose at bedtime; elderly may not tolerate once/day dosing
- Store at room temp; do not freeze
- Allow orally disintegrating tablets to dissolve on tongue; no water needed

Patient/family education
- Inform patient that therapeutic effects may take 2-3 wk
- Advise patient to use caution in driving and other activities requiring alertness because of drowsiness, dizziness, blurred vision; to avoid rising quickly from sitting to standing, especially elderly
- Caution patient to avoid alcohol ingestion, other CNS depressants
- Teach patient to increase fluids, bulk in diet if constipation, urinary retention occur, especially elderly
- Teach patient to use gum, hard sugarless candy, or frequent sips of water for dry mouth
- To report immediately urinary retention

Evaluation
Positive therapeutic outcome
- Decrease in depression
- Absence of suicidal thoughts

Treatment of overdose: ECG monitoring, induce emesis, lavage, activated charcoal, administer anticonvulsant

misoprostol (Rx)

(mye-soe-prost'ole)

Cytotec

Func. class.: Gastric mucosa protectant; antiulcer

Chem. class.: Prostaglandin E_1 analog

Pregnancy category X

Do Not Confuse:
Cytotec/Cytoxan, misoprostol/metoprolol

Action: Inhibits gastric acid secretion; may protect gastric mucosa; can increase bicarbonate, mucus production

Therapeutic Outcome: Prevention of gastric ulcers

Uses: Prevention of NSAID-induced gastric ulcers

Dosage and routes

Adult: PO 200 mcg qid with food for duration of NSAID therapy with last dose at bedtime; if 200 mcg is not tolerated, 100 mcg may be given

Available forms: Tabs 100, 200 mcg

Adverse effects

GI: *Diarrhea,* nausea, vomiting, flatulence, constipation, dyspepsia, abdominal pain
GU: Spotting, cramps, hypermenorrhea, menstrual disorders

Contraindications: Pregnancy **X,** hypersensitivity to this drug or prostaglandins

Precautions: Lactation, children, elderly, renal disease

Pharmacokinetics	
Absorption	Well absorbed
Distribution	Unknown
Metabolism	Liver
Excretion	Kidneys
Half-life	½-1 hr

Pharmacodynamics	
Onset	½ hr
Peak	Unknown
Duration	3 hr

Interactions

Drug/food

Decreased absorption with food

NURSING CONSIDERATIONS

Assessment

- Assess patient for GI symptoms: hematemesis, occult or frank blood in stools, also severe abdominal pain, cramping, severe diarrhea
- Obtain a negative pregnancy test in women of childbearing age before starting medication; miscarriages are common

Nursing diagnoses

- Pain, chronic (uses)
- Knowledge, deficient (teaching)

Implementation

- Give with meals for prolonged drug effect; avoid use of magnesium antacids

Patient/family education

- Advise patient to avoid black pepper, caffeine, alcohol, harsh spices, extremes in temp of food, which may aggravate condition
- Caution patient to avoid OTC preparations: aspirin, cough, cold preparations; condition may worsen
- Teach patient that drug must be continued for prescribed time to be effective and taken exactly as prescribed; doses are not to be doubled
- Instruct patient to report to prescriber diarrhea, black tarry stools, abdominal pain, cramping, menstrual disorders
- Caution patient to prevent pregnancy while taking this drug; spontaneous abortion may occur

Evaluation

Positive therapeutic outcome

- Prevention of ulcers

M

! HIGH ALERT

mitomycin (Rx)

(mye-toe-mye'sin)

mitomycin, Mutamycin

Func. class.: Antineoplastic, antibiotic

Pregnancy category D

Action: Inhibits DNA synthesis, primarily; derived from *Streptomyces caespitosus;* appears to cause cross-linking of DNA, a vesicant

Therapeutic Outcome: Prevention of rapidly growing malignant cells

Uses: Pancreas, stomach, head and neck, breast cancer

Investigational uses: Palliative treatment of head, neck, colon, breast, biliary, cervical, lung malignancies

Dosage and routes

Adult: **IV** 10-20 mg/m² q6-8 wk

Available forms: Inj 5, 20, 40 mg/vial

Adverse effects

CNS: Fever, headache, confusion, drowsiness, syncope, fatigue
EENT: Blurred vision
GI: Nausea, vomiting, anorexia, stomatitis, **hepatotoxicity,** diarrhea
GU: Urinary retention, **renal failure,** edema
HEMA: **Thrombocytopenia, leukopenia, anemia**
INTEG: Rash, alopecia, **extravasation**
MISC: **Hemolytic uremic syndrome**
RESP: **Fibrosis, pulmonary infiltrate,** dyspnea

Contraindications: Pregnancy **D** (1st trimester), hypersensitivity, as a single agent, thrombocytopenia, coagulation disorders, lactation

Precautions: Renal disease, bone marrow depression

Pharmacokinetics

Absorption	Complete bioavailability
Distribution	Widely distributed; concentrates in tumor
Metabolism	Liver, extensively
Excretion	Kidneys, unchanged
Half-life	1 hr

Pharmacodynamics

Unknown

Interactions

Individual drugs

Radiation: increased toxicity, bone marrow suppression

Drug classifications

Antineoplastics: increased toxicity, bone marrow suppression

NURSING CONSIDERATIONS

Assessment

- ! Assess for fatal hemolytic uremic syndrome: hypertension, thrombocytopenia, microangiopathic hemolytic anemia, occurs during long-term therapy
- Assess buccal cavity q8h for dryness, sores or ulceration, white patches, oral pain, bleeding, dysphagia; obtain prescription for viscous lidocaine (Xylocaine)
- Assess symptoms indicating severe allergic reaction: rash, pruritus, urticaria, purpuric skin lesions, itching, flushing
- Monitor CBC, differential, platelet count weekly; withhold drug if WBC is <2000/mm^3 or platelet count is <100,000/mm^3 or granulocyte count is <1000/mm^3, notify prescriber of results if WBC <20,000/mm^3, platelets <150,000/mm^3
- Monitor renal function studies: BUN, creatinine, serum uric acid, urine CCr before and during therapy; check I&O ratio; report fall in urine output to <30 ml/hr
- ! Assess for pulmonary fibrosis, bronchospasm, dyspnea, crackles, unproductive cough, chest pain, tachypnea, fatigue, increased pulse, pallor, lethargy
- Monitor temp q4h (may indicate beginning of infection)
- Monitor liver function tests before and during therapy (bilirubin, AST, ALT, LDH) as needed or monthly; check for jaundiced skin and sclera, dark urine, clay-colored stools, itchy skin, abdominal pain, fever, diarrhea
- Assess for bleeding: hematuria, stool guaiac, bruising or petechiae, mucosa or orifices q8h; inflammation of mucosa, breaks in skin
- Identify effects of alopecia on body image; discuss feelings about body changes
- Identify edema in feet, joint pain, stomach pain, shaking; check for inflammation of mucosa, breaks in skin

Nursing diagnoses

- Injury, risk for (adverse reactions)
- Body image, disturbed (adverse reactions)
- Infection, risk for (adverse reactions)
- Knowledge, deficient (teaching)

Implementation

IV route

- Avoid contact with skin, since medication is very irritating; wash completely to remove
- Give fluids **IV** or PO before chemotherapy to hydrate patient
- Provide antacid before oral agent; give drug after evening meal, before bedtime; administer antiemetic 30-60 min before giving drug and prn to prevent vomiting; use antibiotics for prophylaxis of infection
- Give top or syst analgesics for pain
- Give in AM so drug can be eliminated before bedtime
- Provide a liq diet: carbonated beverages; gelatin may be added if patient is not nauseated or vomiting
- Drug should be prepared by experienced personnel using proper precautions in a biologic cabinet using gown, gloves, mask
- Give by direct **IV** after diluting 5 mg/10, or 10 mg/40 ml sterile water for inj; shake, allow to stand, give through Y-tube or 3 way stopcock; give over 5-10 min through running D_5W, 0.9% NaCl **IV**, color of reconstituted sol is gray
- Apply ice compress for extravasation

Syringe compatibilities: Bleomycin, cisplatin, cyclophosphamide, DOXOrubicin, droperidol, fluorouracil, furosemide, heparin, leucovorin, methotrexate, metoclopramide, vinBLAStine, vinCRIStine

Y-site compatibilities: Allopurinol, amifostine, bleomycin, cisplatin, cyclophosphamide, DOXOrubicin, droperidol, fluorouracil, furosemide, granisetron, heparin, leucovorin, melphalan, methotrexate, metoclopramide, ondansetron, teniposide, thiotepa, vinBLAStine, vinCRIStine

Y-site incompatibilities: Sargramostim, vinorelbine

Additive compatibilities: Dexamethasone, hydrocortisone

Additive incompatibilities: Bleomycin

Solution compatibilities: LR, 0.3% NaCl, 0.5% NaCl

Patient/family education

- Encourage patient to rinse mouth tid-qid with water, club soda, brush teeth bid-qid with soft brush or cotton-tipped applicators for stomatitis, use unwaxed dental floss
- Teach patient to avoid use of products containing aspirin or ibuprofen, razors, commercial mouthwash, since bleeding may occur; to report symptoms of bleeding (hematuria, tarry stools)
- Caution patient to report signs of anemia (fatigue, headache, irritability, faintness, shortness of breath)
- Advise patient to report any changes in breathing or coughing even several mo after treatment; to avoid crowds and persons with respiratory tract or other infections
- Inform patient that hair may be lost during treatment; a wig or hairpiece may make patient feel better; new hair may be different in color, texture
- Advise patient not to have any vaccinations without the advice of the prescriber, serious reactions can occur
- Teach patient that contraception is needed during treatment and for several mo after completion of therapy

Evaluation

Positive therapeutic outcome

- Prevention of rapid division of malignant cells

! HIGH ALERT

mitoxantrone (Rx)

(mye-toe-zan'trone)

Novantrone

Func. class.: Antineoplastic-antibiotic, immunomodulator

Chem. class.: Synthetic anthraquinone

Pregnancy category D

Action: DNA reactive agent; cytocidal effect on both proliferating and nonproliferating cells, suggesting lack of cell cycle phase specificity; a vesicant

Therapeutic Outcome: Prevention of rapidly growing malignant cells

Uses: Acute nonlymphocytic leukemia (adult), relapsed leukemia, breast cancer, multiple sclerosis

Investigational uses: Liver malignancies, non-Hodgkin's lymphoma

Dosage and routes

Induction

Adult: **IV** inf 12 mg/m^2/day on days 1-3, and 100 mg/m^2 cytosine arabinoside × 7 days as a cont 24-hr inf

Consolidation

Adult: **IV** inf 12 mg/m^2 given as a short 5-15 min inf

Multiple sclerosis

Adult: **IV** inf 12 mg/m^2 as a 5-15 min infusion q3 mo

Available forms: Inj 2 mg/ml

Adverse effects

CNS: Headache, **seizures**

CV: **CHF, cardiomyopathy, dysrhythmias**

EENT: Conjunctivitis, blue-green sclera

GI: *Nausea, vomiting, diarrhea, anorexia, mucositis,* **hepatoxicity**

HEMA: **Thrombocytopenia, leukopenia, myelosuppression, anemia**

INTEG: *Rash, necrosis at inj site,* alopecia, dermatitis, thrombophlebitis at inj site

MISC: Fever

RESP: Cough, dyspnea

Contraindications: Pregnancy **D,** hypersensitivity

Precautions: Myelosuppression, lactation, cardiac disease, children, renal, hepatic disease, gout

M

Pharmacokinetics

Absorption	Completely absorbed
Distribution	Widely distributed
Metabolism	Liver
Excretion	Bile; kidneys, unchanged (<10%)
Half-life	24-72 hr

Pharmacodynamics

Unknown

Interactions

Individual drugs

Radiation: increased toxicity, bone marrow suppression

Drug classifications

Antineoplastics: increased toxicity, bone marrow suppression

Live virus vaccines: increased adverse reactions

NURSING CONSIDERATIONS

Assessment

- Multiple sclerosis: obtain baseline multigated angiogram, left ventricular ejection fraction (LVEF) if symptoms of CHF occur, repeat LVEF or if cumulative dose is >100 mg/m^2; do not administer to patients who have received a lifetime dose of ≥140 mg/m^2 or if LVEF <50% or significant decrease in LVEF
- Do not administer in multiple sclerosis if neutrophils <1500/mm^3
- Obtain pregnancy test in all women of childbearing age
- ◆ Monitor ECG; watch for ST-T wave changes, low QRS and T, possible dysrhythmias (sinus tachycardia, heart block, PVCs); also monitor ECHO, chest x-ray, RAI angiography to assess ejection fraction before and during treatment, drug is cardiotoxic, may develop during treatment or months to years after treatment
- Assess buccal cavity q8h for dryness, sores or ulceration, white patches, oral pain, bleeding, dysphagia; obtain prescription for viscous lidocaine (Xylocaine)
- Assess symptoms indicating severe allergic reaction: rash, pruritus, urticaria, purpuric skin lesions, itching, flushing
- Assess tachypnea, ECG changes, dyspnea, edema, fatigue
- Monitor CBC, differential, platelet count weekly; withhold drug if WBC is <4000/mm^3 or platelet count is <100,000/mm^3, notify prescriber of results if WBC <20,000/mm^3, platelets <150,000/mm^3
- Assess for increased uric acid levels, swelling, joint pain primarily in extremities; patient should be well hydrated to prevent urate deposits
- Monitor renal function studies: BUN, creatinine, urine CCr before and during therapy; determine I&O ratio
- Monitor temp q4h (may indicate beginning of infection)
- Monitor liver function tests before and during therapy (bilirubin, AST, ALT, LDH) as needed or monthly; check for jaundiced skin and sclera, dark urine, clay-colored stools, itchy skin, abdominal pain, fever, diarrhea
- Assess for bleeding: hematuria, stool guaiac, bruising or petechiae, mucosa or orifices q8h; check for inflammation of mucosa, breaks in skin
- Identify effects of alopecia on body image; discuss feelings about body changes
- ◆ Assess for MS: obtain MUGA, LVEF baselines; repeat LVEF if symptoms of CHF occur or if cumulative dose is >100 mg/m^2; do not give to patients who have received a lifetime dose of ≥140 mg/m^2 or if LVEF <50% or significant LVEF
- ◆ Assess for secondary acute myelogenous leukemia (AML) that can develop after taking this drug

Nursing diagnoses

- Injury, risk for (adverse reactions)
- Body image, disturbed (adverse reactions)
- Infection, risk for (adverse reactions)
- Knowledge, deficient (teaching)

Implementation

- ◆ Do not mix with heparin; precipitate will form
- Avoid contact with skin, since medication is very irritating; wash completely to remove
- Give fluids **IV** or PO before chemotherapy to hydrate patient
- Give antacid before oral agent; give drug after evening meal, before bedtime; provide antiemetic 30-60 min before giving drug and prn to prevent vomiting; administer antibiotics for prophylaxis of infection
- Give top or systemic analgesics for pain
- Liq diet: carbonated beverages; gelatin may be added if patient is not nauseated or vomiting
- Sol should be prepared by qualified personnel only under controlled conditions in a biologic cabinet using mask, gloves, gown
- Use Luer-Lok tubing to prevent leakage; do not let sol come in contact with skin; if contact occurs wash well with soap and water
- Give by direct **IV** after diluting with 50 ml or more of 0.9% NaCl or D_5W; give over 3-5 min, running **IV** of D_5W or 0.9% NaCl

- Intermittent inf may be diluted further in D_5W, 0.9% NaCl and run over 15-30 min; check for extravasation

Y-site compatibilities: Allopurinol, amifostine, cladribine, filgrastim, fludarabine, granisetron, melphalan, ondansetron, sargramostim, teniposide, thiotepa, vinorelbine
Y-site incompatibilities: Paclitaxel
Additive compatibilities: Cyclophosphamide, cytarabine, fluorouracil, hydrocortisone, potassium chloride
Additive incompatibilities: Heparin
Solution compatibilities: D_5/0.9 NaCl, D_5W, 0.9% NaCl

Patient/family education

- Encourage patient to rinse mouth tid-qid with water, club soda, brush teeth bid-qid with soft brush or cotton-tipped applicators for stomatitis, use unwaxed dental floss
- Teach patient to avoid use of products containing aspirin or NSAIDs, razors, commercial mouthwash, since bleeding may occur; to report symptoms of bleeding (hematuria, tarry stools)
- Caution patient to report signs of anemia (fatigue, headache, irritability, faintness, shortness of breath)
- Inform patient that hair may be lost during treatment; a wig or hairpiece may make patient feel better; new hair may be different in color, texture
- Caution patient not to have any vaccinations without the advice of the prescriber; serious reactions can occur
- Advise patient that contraception is needed during treatment and for several mo after completion of therapy
- Advise patient that sclera, urine may turn blue or green
- Advise patient to increase fluids to 2-3 L/day unless contraindicated
- Teach patient to avoid crowds, persons with infections

Evaluation

Positive therapeutic outcome

- Prevention of rapid division of malignant cells

! HIGH ALERT

mivacurium (Rx)

(mi-va-kure'ee-um)

Mivacron

Func. class.: Neuromuscular blocker, nondepolarizing

Pregnancy category C

Do Not Confuse:
Mivacron/Mazicon

Action: Inhibits transmission of nerve impulses by binding with cholinergic receptor sites, antagonizing action of acetylcholine; no analgesic response

Therapeutic Outcome: Paralysis of all skeletal muscles

Uses: Facilitation of endotracheal intubation; skeletal muscle relaxation during mechanical ventilation, surgery, or general anesthesia; reduction of fractures/dislocations

Dosage and routes

Adult: **IV** 0.15 mg/kg; maintenance 0.10 mg/kg q15 min
Child 2-12: **IV** 0.2 mg/kg for a 10-min block

Available forms: 5, 10 ml single-use vial (2 mg/ml); premixed inf in D_5W 50 ml flexible container

Adverse effects

CV: Decreased B/P, bradycardia, tachycardia
EENT: Diplopia
INTEG: Rash, urticaria
MS: Weakness, prolonged skeletal muscle relaxation, **paralysis**
RESP: **Prolonged apnea, bronchospasm, wheezing, respiratory depression**

Contraindications: Hypersensitivity

Precautions: Pregnancy **C**, renal or hepatic disease, lactation, children <3 mo, fluid and electrolyte imbalances, neuromuscular disease, respiratory disease, obesity, elderly

Pharmacokinetics

Absorption	Completely absorbed
Distribution	Extracellular spaces; crosses placenta
Metabolism	Plasma
Excretion	Kidneys
Half-life	2 hr

M

Pharmacodynamics	
Onset	2-2½ min
Peak	2-3 min
Duration	20-30 min

Interactions
Individual drugs
Amphotericin B, bacitracin, carbamazepine, clindamycin, colistin, enflurane, halothane, isoflurane, lidocaine, lincomycin, lithium, magnesium, phenytoin, polymyxin B, procainamide, quinidine: increased paralysis length and intensity
Drug classifications
Anesthetics (local), antibiotics (polymixin), aminoglycosides, diuretics, tetracyclines: increased paralysis length and intensity

NURSING CONSIDERATIONS
Assessment
- Monitor VS (B/P, pulse, respirations, airway) until fully recovered; rate, depth, pattern of respirations, strength of hand grip; patient should be intubated before use
- Monitor for electrolyte imbalances (potassium, magnesium) before drug is used; electrolyte imbalances may lead to increased action of this drug
- Monitor for recovery: decreased paralysis of face, diaphragm, leg, arm, rest of body; residual weakness and respiratory problems may occur during recovery period
- Assess for hypersensitive reactions: rash, fever, respiratory distress, pruritus; drug should be discontinued

Nursing diagnoses
- Breathing pattern, ineffective (uses)
- Communication, verbal, impaired (adverse reactions)
- Fear (adverse reactions)
- Knowledge, deficient (teaching)

Implementation
- Use peripheral nerve stimulator (anesthesiologist) to determine neuromuscular blockade; deep tendon reflexes should be monitored during extended periods
- Give direct **IV** undiluted over 5-15 min
- Give cont **IV** diluted to 0.5 mg ml in D_5W, 0.9% NaCl, D_5/0.9% NaCl, LR, D_5/LR and give as an inf at prescribed rate (only by qualified person, usually an anesthesiologist); do not administer IM
- Store in light-resistant container
- Give anticholinesterase to reverse neuromuscular blockade

Y-site compatibilities: Etomidate, thiopental

Y-site incompatibilities: Barbiturates

Patient/family education
- Provide reassurance if communication is difficult during recovery from neuromuscular blockade
- Provide explanation to patients regarding all procedures or treatments; patient will remain conscious if anesthesia is not given also

Evaluation
Positive therapeutic outcome
- Paralysis of jaw, eyelid, head, neck, rest of body as evaluated by peripheral nerve stimulator

Treatment of overdose: Edrophonium or neostigmine, atropine; monitor VS; may require mechanical ventilation

moexipril (Rx)
(moe-ex′i-pril)

Univasc

Func. class.: Antihypertensive

Chem. class.: Angiotensin-converting enzyme (ACE) inhibitor

Pregnancy category
C (1st trimester),
D (2nd/3rd trimesters)

Action: Selectively suppresses renin-angiotensin-aldosterone system; inhibits ACE; prevents conversion of angiotensin I to angiotensin II; results in dilatation of arterial, venous vessels

Therapeutic Outcome: Decreased B/P in hypertension

Uses: Hypertension, alone or in combination with thiazide diuretics

Dosage and routes
Initial treatment
Adult: PO 7.5 mg 1 hr ac initially, may be increased or divided depending on B/P response

Maintenance
Adult: PO 7.5-30 mg daily in 1-2 divided doses 1 hr ac

Renal dose
Adult: PO CCr <40 ml/min 3.75 mg/day titrate to desired dose

Available forms: Tabs 7.5, 15 mg

Adverse effects
CNS: Fever, chills
CV: Hypotension, postural hypotension
GI: Loss of taste
GU: Impotence, dysuria, nocturia, proteinuria,

nephrotic syndrome, acute reversible renal failure, polyuria, oliguria, frequency
HEMA: **Neutropenia**
INTEG: Rash
META: Hypokalemia
RESP: **Bronchospasm,** dyspnea, dry cough
SYST: **Angioedema, anaphylaxis**

Contraindications: Pregnancy **D** (2nd/3rd trimesters), hypersensitivity, children, lactation, heart block, bilateral renal stenosis

Precautions: Pregnancy **C** (1st trimester), dialysis patients, hypovolemia, leukemia, scleroderma, lupus erythematosus, blood dyscrasias, CHF, diabetes mellitus, renal disease, thyroid disease, COPD, asthma, potassium-sparing diuretics

Pharmacokinetics

Absorption	Unknown
Distribution	Unknown
Metabolism	Liver to metabolites
Excretion	Via kidneys, crosses placenta, excreted in breast milk
Half-life	Unknown

Pharmacodynamics

Unknown

Interactions

Individual drugs

CycloSPORINE: increased hyperkalemia
Digoxin, lithium: increased toxicity

Drug classification

Adrenergic blockers, antihypertensives, diuretics, ganglionic blockers, phenothiazines: increased hypotension
Diuretics (potassium-sparing), potassium supplements, sympathomimetics: do not use together
NSAIDs: decreased antihypertensive effect

Drug/lab test

False positive: urine acetone

NURSING CONSIDERATIONS

Assessment

- Monitor blood studies: neutrophils, decreased platelets
- Monitor B/P
- Monitor renal studies: protein, BUN, creatinine; watch for increased levels that may indicate nephrotic syndrome
- Monitor baselines in renal, liver function tests before therapy begins
- Monitor potassium levels, although hyperkalemia rarely occurs
- Assess edema in feet, legs daily
- Assess allergic reaction: rash, fever, pruritus, urticaria; drug should be discontinued if antihistamines fail to help
- Assess for symptoms of CHF: edema, dyspnea, wet crackles, B/P
- Monitor for renal symptoms: polyuria, oliguria, frequency

Nursing diagnoses

- Knowledge, deficient (teaching)

Implementation

- Give PO 1 hr ac
- Store in airtight container at 86° F or less

Patient/family education

- Instruct patient not to discontinue drug abruptly
- Tell patient not to use OTC (cough, cold, allergy) products unless directed by prescriber
- Teach patient to comply with dosage schedule, even if feeling better
- Encourage patient to rise slowly to sitting or standing position to minimize orthostatic hypotension
- Teach patient to notify prescriber of mouth sores, sore throat, fever, swelling of hands or feet, irregular heartbeat, chest pain, signs of angioedema
- Tell patient that excessive perspiration, dehydration, vomiting, diarrhea may lead to fall in B/P; consult prescriber if this occurs
- Teach patient that dizziness, fainting, lightheadedness may occur during first few days of therapy
- Tell patient that skin rash or impaired perspiration may occur
- Teach patient how to take B/P

Evaluation

Positive therapeutic outcome

- Decreased B/P in hypertension

Treatment of overdose: 0.9% NaCl **IV** inf, hemodialysis

montelukast (Rx)

(mon-teh-loo'kast)
Singulair
Func. class.: Bronchodilator
Chem. class.: Leukotriene antagonist, cysteinyl

Pregnancy category B

Action: Inhibits leukotriene (LTD_4) formation; leukotrienes exert their effects by increasing neutrophil, eosinophil migration; aggregation of neutrophils, monocytes; smooth muscle contraction, capillary permeability;

M

these actions further lead to bronchoconstriction, inflammation, edema

Therapeutic Outcome: Ability to breathe with ease

Uses: Chronic asthma

Investigational uses: Chronic urticaria

Dosage and routes

Asthma

Adult and child ≥15 yr: PO 10 mg daily PM

Child 6-14 yr: PO 5 mg chew tabs daily PM

Child 2-5 yr: PO chew tabs 4 mg daily

Child 12-23 mo: PO 1 packet of granules taken PM

Available forms: Tabs 10 mg; chewable tabs 4, 5 mg; oral granules 4 mg/packet

Adverse effects

CNS: Dizziness, fatigue, headache

GI: Abdominal pain, dyspepsia

INTEG: Rash

MS: Asthenia

RESP: Influenza, cough, nasal congestion

Contraindications: Hypersensitivity

Precautions: Pregnancy **B**, acute attacks of asthma, alcohol consumption, lactation, child <6 yr, aspirin sensitivity

Pharmacokinetics	
Absorption	Rapidly
Distribution	Protein binding 99%
Metabolism	Liver
Excretion	Bile
Half-life	2.7-5.5 hr

Pharmacodynamics	
Onset	Unknown
Peak	3-4 hr
Duration	Unknown

Interactions

Individual drugs

Phenobarbitol, rifampin: decreased montelukast levels

Drug/herb

Tea (green, black), guarana: increased stimulation

Drug/lab test

Increased: ALT, AST

NURSING CONSIDERATIONS

Assessment

- Assess adult patients carefully for symptoms of Churg-Strauss syndrome (rare), including eosinophilia, vasculitic rash, worsening pulmonary symptoms, cardiac complications and/or neuropathy
- Monitor CBC, blood chemistry during treatment
- Assess respiratory rate, rhythm, depth; auscultate lung fields bilaterally; notify prescriber of abnormalities
- Assess allergic reactions: rash, urticaria; drug should be discontinued

Nursing diagnoses

- Airway clearance, ineffective (uses)
- Activity intolerance (uses)
- Knowledge, deficient (teaching)

Implementation

PO route

- Give PO in PM daily
- Do not open packet until ready to use, mix whole dose, give within 15 min
- Granules may be given directly in mouth or mixed with a spoonful of soft food (carrots, applesauce, ice cream, rice)

Patient/family education

- Instruct patient to check OTC and current prescription medications for epHEDrine, which will increase stimulation; to avoid alcohol
- Advise patient to avoid hazardous activities; dizziness may occur
- Teach patient that drug is not to be used for acute asthma attacks
- Advise patient to avoid NSAIDs if sensitive to aspirin
- Advise patient to continue to use inhaled β-agonists if exercise-induced asthma occurs

Evaluation

Positive therapeutic outcome

- Increased ease of breathing
- Decreased bronchospasm

moricizine (Rx)

(more-i'siz-een)

Ethmozine

Func. class.: Antidysrhythmic, group 1A

Chem. class.: Phenothiazine

Pregnancy category B

Action: Decreased rate of rise of action potential, prolonging refractory period and shortening the action potential duration; depression of inward influx if sodium mediates the effects; may slow atrial and AV nodal conduction

Therapeutic Outcome: Resolution of life-threatening dysrhythmias

Uses: Life-threatening ventricular dysrhythmias

Dosage and routes

Hospitalization is required when initiating therapy

Adult: PO 10-15 mg/kg/day or 600-900 mg/day given in 2-3 divided doses

Hepatic dose

Adult: PO 600 mg or less daily

Available forms: Film-coated tabs 200, 250, 300 mg

Adverse effects

CNS: *Dizziness, headache, fatigue, perioral numbness, euphoria,* nervousness, sleep disorders, depression, tinnitus, fatigue, anxiety

CV: Palpitations, chest pain, **CHF,** hypertension, syncope, **dysrythmias,** bradycardia, **MI, thrombophlebitis,** ECG abnormalities, **cardiac arrest**

GI: Nausea, abdominal pain, vomiting, diarrhea

GU: Sexual dysfunction, difficult urination, dysuria, incontinence, urinary retention

MISC: Sweating, musculoskeletal pain, drug fever, blurred vision, dry mouth

RESP: Dyspnea, hyperventilation, **apnea,** asthma, pharyngitis, cough

Contraindications: 2nd- to 3rd-degree AV block, right bundle branch block, cardiogenic shock, hypersensitivity

Precautions: Pregnancy **B,** CHF, hypokalemia, hyperkalemia, sick sinus syndrome, lactation, children, impaired hepatic and renal function, cardiac dysfunction

Pharmacokinetics

Absorption	Well absorbed
Distribution	Plasma protein binding (95%)
Metabolism	Liver, extensively
Excretion	Kidneys, breast milk
Half-life	1½-3½ hr

Pharmacodynamics

Onset	Unknown
Peak	½-2 hr
Duration	8-12 hr

Interactions

Individual drugs

Cimetidine: increased effect of moricizine
Digoxin, propranolol: may increase some cardiac effects of moricizine
Theophylline: decreased effect of theophylline

Drug/herb

Aconite: increased toxicity, death
Aloe, broom, buckthorn (chronic use), cascara sagrada (chronic use), Chinese rhubarb, figwort, fumitory, goldenseal, kudzu, licorice: increased effect
Aloe, buckthorn, cascara sagrada, rhubarb, senna: increased hypokalemia, antidysrhythmic effect
Coltsfoot: decreased effect
Henbane: increased anticholinergic effect
Horehound: increased serotonin effect

Drug/lab test

Increased: CPK

NURSING CONSIDERATIONS

Assessment

- Monitor ECG at baseline and periodically to determine drug effectiveness; measure PR, QRS, QT intervals, check for PVCs, other dysrhythmias; check B/P for hypotension, hypertension and for rebound hypertension after 1-2 hr; check for dehydration or hypovolemia
- ❗ Monitor I&O ratio and electrolytes: potassium, sodium, chloride; check weight daily and for signs of CHF or pulmonary toxicity: dyspnea, fatigue, cough, fever, chest pain; drug should be discontinued
- Monitor liver function studies: AST, ALT, bilirubin, alkaline phosphatase
- Monitor cardiac rate; monitor respiration rate, rhythm, character, and chest pain; watch for ventricular tachycardia, supraventricular tachycardia, or fibrillation
- ❗ Monitor for toxicity: fine tremors, dizziness, emesis, lethargy, coma, syncope, hypotension conduction disturbances

Nursing diagnoses

- Cardiac output, decreased (uses)
- Gas exchange, impaired (adverse reactions)
- Knowledge, deficient (teaching)

Implementation

- Give with meals for GI upset; may be given in 2 divided doses if adverse reactions are minimal
- Make dosage adjustment q3 days or more
- Initiate therapy in hospital

Patient/family education

- Instruct patient to report side effects to prescriber immediately
- Instruct patient to complete follow-up appointment with health care provider including pulmonary function studies, chest x-ray, ophth and otoscopic examinations
- Advise patient to carry/wear emergency ID indicating condition and treatment

M

- Caution patient to avoid driving and other hazardous activities until drug response is determined
- Instruct patient to take medication as prescribed, not to double doses; missed doses may be taken up to 6 hr after previous dose

Evaluation

Positive therapeutic outcome

- Absence of life-threatening ventricular dysrhythmias

Treatment of overdose: O_2, artificial ventilation, ECG, administer DOPamine for circulatory depression, administer diazepam or thiopental for seizures, isoproterenol

! HIGH ALERT

morphine (Rx)

(mor'feen)

Astramorph, Astramorph PF, Avinza, Duramorph, Epimorph ♣, Infumorph, Kadian, Morphine H.P. ♣, morphine sulfate, Morphitec ♣, M.O.S. ♣, M.O.S.-S.R. ♣, MS Contin, MSIR, OMS Concentrate, Oramorph SR, RMS, Roxanol, Roxanol Rescudose, Roxanol-T, Statex ♣

Func. class.: Opioid analgesic

Pregnancy category C

Controlled substance schedule II

Do Not Confuse:
morphine/hydromorphone, Roxanol/Roxicet

Action: Depresses pain impulse transmission at the spinal cord level by interacting with opioid receptors, produces CNS depression

Therapeutic Outcome: Decreased pain

Uses: Severe pain; often given after or during an MI

Dosage and routes

Adult: SUBCUT/IM 5-20 mg q4h prn; PO 10-30 mg q4h prn; ext rel 70 kg patient q8-12h; rec 10-30 mg q4h prn; **IV** 4-10 mg diluted in 4-5 ml of water for inj, over 5 min; PO sus rel cap (Kadian); Kadian is not bioequivalent to other controlled release forms. Avinza, for those with no tolerance to opioids, 30 mg daily; may adjust by no more than 30 mg q4d. May give either total daily oral dose q24h (Kadian, Avinza), 50% of total dose (Oramorph SR, Kadian, MS Contin)

Child: SUBCUT/**IV** 0.1-0.2 mg/kg, max 15 mg; PO 0.2-0.5 mg/kg q4-6h (regular rel), q12h (sus rel)

Available forms: Inj 0.5, 1, 2, 3, 4, 5, 8, 10, 15, 25, 50 mg/ml; sol tabs 10, 15, 30 mg; oral sol 10, 20 mg/5 ml, 20 mg/10 ml, 20 mg/ml; oral tabs 15, 30 mg; rec supp 5, 10, 20, 30 mg; ext rel tabs 15, 30, 60, 100, 200 mg; caps 15, 30 mg; syr 1, 5 mg/ml; cont rel cap pellets (Kadian) 20, 30, 50, 60, 100 mg; ext rel caps (Avinza) 30, 60, 90, 120 mg

Adverse effects

CNS: Drowsiness, dizziness, *confusion*, headache, *sedation*, euphoria
CV: Palpitations, **bradycardia**, change in B/P, **shock, cardiac arrest**
EENT: Tinnitus, blurred vision, miosis, diplopia
GI: Nausea, vomiting, anorexia, *constipation*, cramps, biliary tract pressure
GU: Urinary retention
HEMA: **Thrombocytopenia**
INTEG: Rash, urticaria, bruising, flushing, diaphoresis, pruritus
RESP: **Respiratory depression, respiratory arrest, apnea**

Contraindications: Hypersensitivity, addiction (opioid), hemorrhage, bronchial asthma, increased intracranial pressure

Precautions: Pregnancy **C**, addictive personality, lactation, acute MI, severe heart disease, elderly, respiratory depression, hepatic disease, renal disease, child <18 yr

Pharmacokinetics	
Absorption	Variably absorbed (PO); well absorbed (IM, SUBCUT, rec); completely absorbed (**IV**)
Distribution	Widely distributed; crosses placenta
Metabolism	Liver, extensively
Excretion	Kidneys
Half-life	1½-2 hr

Pharmacodynamics

	PO	PO–EXT REL	IM	SUBCUT	REC	IV	IT
Onset	Variable	Unknown	10-30 min	20 min	Unknown	Rapid	Rapid
Peak	1 hr	Unknown	½-1 hr	1-1½ hr	½-1 hr	20 min	Unknown
Duration	4-5 hr	8-12 hr	3-7 hr	4-5 hr	4-5 hr	4-5 hr	Ext

Interactions
Individual drugs
Alcohol: increased respiratory depression, hypotension, sedation
Rifampin: decreased analgesic action
Drug classifications
Antipsychotics, opiates, sedative/hypnotics, skeletal muscle relaxants: increased effects with other CNS depressants
MAOIs: unpredictable reaction may occur, avoid use
Drug/herb
Chamomile, hops, Jamaican dogwood, kava, lavender, mistletoe, nettle, pokeweed, poppy, senega, skullcap, valerian: increased CNS depression
Corkwood: increased anticholinergic effect
Drug/food
Cranberry juice (excessive amounts), oats: decreased morphine effect
Drug/lab test
Increased: amylase

NURSING CONSIDERATIONS
Assessment
- Assess pain: location, type, character, intensity; give dose before pain becomes extreme
- Monitor I&O ratio; check for decreasing output; may indicate urinary retention; check for constipation; increase fluids, bulk in diet if needed or stool softeners may be prescribed
- Monitor CNS changes: dizziness, drowsiness, hallucinations, euphoria, LOC, pupil reactions
- Monitor allergic reactions: rash, urticaria
- Assess respiratory dysfunction: depression, character, rate, rhythm; notify prescriber if respirations are <10/min

Nursing diagnoses
- Pain, acute (uses)
- Sensory perception, disturbed: visual, auditory (adverse reactions)
- Breathing pattern, ineffective (adverse reactions)
- Knowledge, deficient (teaching)

Implementation
- Give with antiemetic if nausea, vomiting occur
- Administer when pain is beginning to return; determine dosage interval by patient response; continuous dosing of medication is more effective than giving prn
- Withdraw medication slowly after long-term use to prevent withdrawal symptoms
- Store in light-resistant container at room temp

PO route
- Swallow ext rel tabs whole; do not break, crush, or chew
- Kadian tabs may be opened and sprinkled on applesauce immediately before use. Do not break, crush, chew, or dissolve pellets in Kadian cap, which may lead to an overdose. Adjustments may need to be made when converting from another form of morphine.
- May be given with food or milk to lessen GI upset; other forms may be crushed and mixed with food or fluids

IM/SUBCUT route
- Do not give if cloudy or a precipitate has formed

IV route
- Give direct **IV** by diluting with ≥5 ml of sterile water or 0.9% NaCl for inj; give 2.5-15 mg/4-5 min; rapid administration may lead to increased respiratory depression, death
- Give cont inf by adding to D_5W, $D_{10}W$, 0.9% NaCl, 0.45% NaCl, Ringer's, LR, any dextrose/saline sol, or any dextrose/Ringer's, 0.1-1 mg/ml
- Give by infusion pump to deliver correct dosage; titrate to provide adequate pain relief without serious sedation, respiratory depression, hypotension
- May be given by patient-controlled analgesia (PCA) pump in terminal illnesses; patient is able to control amount of morphine
- Administer epidurally with caution in the elderly

Syringe compatibilities: Atropine, benzquinamide, bupivacaine, butorphanol, cimetidine, dimenhyDRINATE, diphenhydrAMINE, droperidol, fentanyl, glycopyrrolate, hydrOXYzine, ketamine, metoclopramide, midazolam, milrinone, pentazocine, perphenazine, promazine, ranitidine, scopolamine

Syringe incompatibilities: Meperidine, thiopental

Y-site compatibilities: Allopurinol, amifostine, amikacin, aminophylline, amiodarone, ampicillin, ampicillin/sulbactam, amsacrine, atenolol, atracurium, aztreonam, bumetanide, calcium chloride, cefamandole, cefazolin, cefmetazole, cefoperazone, cefotaxime, cefotetan, cefoxitin, ceftazidime, ceftizoxime, ceftriaxone, cefuroxime, cephalothin, cephapirin, chloramphenicol, cisplatin, cladribine, clindamycin, cyclophosphamide, cytarabine, dexamethasone, digoxin, diltiazem, dobutamine, DOPamine, doxycycline, enalaprilat, epINEPHrine, erythromycin, esmolol, etomidate, famotidine, fentanyl, filgrastim, fluconazole, fludarabine, foscarnet, gentamicin, granisetron, heparin, hydrocortisone, hydromorphone, IL-2, insulin (regular), kanamycin, labetalol, lidocaine, lorazepam, magnesium sulfate, melphalan, meropenem, methotrexate, methyldopate, methylPREDNISolone, metoclopramide, metoprolol, metronidazole, mezlocillin, midazolam, milrinone, moxalactam, nafcillin, niCARdipine, nitroglycerin, norepinephrine, ondansetron, oxacillin, oxytocin, paclitaxel, pancuronium, penicillin G potassium, piperacillin, piperacillin/tazobactam, potassium chloride, propofol, propranolol, ranitidine, sodium bicarbonate, sodium nitroprusside, teniposide, thiotepa, ticarcillin, ticarcillin/clavulanate, tobramycin, trimethoprim/sulfamethoxazole, vancomycin, vecuronium, vinorelbine, vit B/C, warfarin, zidovudine

Y-site incompatibilities: Furosemide, minocycline, tetracycline

Additive compatibilities: Alteplase, atracurium, baclofen, bupivacaine, DOBUTamine, fluconazole, furosemide, meropenem, metoclopramide, ondansetron, succinylcholine, verapamil

Additive incompatibilities: Aminophylline

Patient/family education

- Advise patient to report any symptoms of CNS changes, allergic reactions
- Caution patients to avoid CNS depressants (alcohol, sedative/hypnotics) for at least 24 hr after taking this drug
- Discuss with patient that dizziness, drowsiness, and confusion are common; to avoid getting up without assistance
- Discuss in detail all aspects of the drug and expected response

Evaluation

Positive therapeutic outcome

- Decreased pain

Treatment of overdose: Naloxone (Narcan) 0.2-0.8 **IV**, O_2, **IV** fluids, vasopressors

moxifloxacin (Rx)

(mox-i-floks'a-sin)

Avelox, Avelox IV

Func. class.: Antiinfective

Chem. class.: Fluoroquinolone

Pregnancy category C

Action: Interferes with conversion of intermediate DNA fragments into high molecular weight DNA in bacteria; DNA gyrase inhibitor

Therapeutic Outcome: Bactericidal action against the following: *Staphylococcus aureus, Streptococcus pneumoniae, Haemophilus influenzae, Haemophilus parainfluenzae, Moraxella catarrhalis, Klebsiella pneumoniae, Mycoplasma pneumoniae, Chlamydia pneumoniae;* uncomplicated skin/skin structure infections: *Staphylococcus aureus, Streptococcus pyogenes*

Uses: Acute bacterial sinusitis, acute bacterial exacerbation of chronic bronchitis, community-acquired pneumonia (mild to moderate)

Dosage and routes

Acute bacterial sinusitis

Adult: PO/**IV** 400 mg q24h × 10 days

Acute bacterial exacerbation of chronic bronchitis

Adult: PO/**IV** 400 mg q24h × 5 days

Community-acquired pneumonia

Adult: PO/**IV** 400 mg q24h × 7-14 days

Uncomplicated skin/skin structure infections

Adult: PO/**IV** 400 mg q24h × 7 days

Available forms: Tabs 400 mg; inj premix 400 mg

Adverse effects

CNS: Headache, dizziness, fatigue, insomnia, depression, restlessness, **seizures,** confusion

CV: Prolonged QT interval, **dysrhythmias**

EENT: Blurred vision, tinnitus

GI: Nausea, constipation, increased ALT, AST, flatulence, heartburn, vomiting, diarrhea, oral candidiasis, dysphagia, **pseudomembranous colitis**

INTEG: Rash, pruritus, urticaria, photosensitivity, flushing, fever, chills

MS: Tremor, arthralgia, tendon rupture

***SYST:* Anaphylaxis, Stevens-Johnson syndrome**

Contraindications: Hypersensitivity to quinolones

Precautions: Pregnancy **C,** lactation, children, renal disease, epilepsy, uncorrected hypokalemia, prolonged QT interval, patients receiving class IA, III antidysrhythmics

Pharmacokinetics

Absorption	Well absorbed (75%) (PO)
Distribution	Widely distributed
Metabolism	Liver
Excretion	Kidneys
Half-life	Increased in renal disease

Pharmacodynamics

	PO
Onset	Rapid
Peak	1 hr

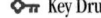

Interactions

Individual drugs

Aluminum hydroxide, calcium, didanosine, iron, sucralfate, zinc sulfate: decreased absorption of moxifloxacin
Caffeine: decreased effect of moxifloxacin
CycloSPORINE: increased cycloSPORINE effect
Probenecid: increased blood levels
Theophylline: increased toxicity
Warfarin: increased warfarin effect

Drug classifications

Antacids (magnesium), iron salts: decreased absorption of moxifloxacin
Antidysrhythmics IA, III: prolonged QT interval

Drug/herb

Cola tree: increased antiinfective effect

Drug/food

Enteral feeding: decreased absorption of moxifloxacin

NURSING CONSIDERATIONS

Assessment

- Assess patient for previous sensitivity reaction
- Assess patient for signs and symptoms of infection including characteristics of wounds, sputum, urine, stool, WBC >10,000/mm^3, fever; baseline and during treatment
- Obtain C&S before beginning drug therapy to identify if correct treatment has been initiated
- Assess for allergic reactions and anaphylaxis: rash, urticaria, pruritus, chills, fever, joint pain; may occur a few days after therapy begins; epINEPHrine and resuscitation equipment should be available for anaphylactic reaction
- Assess for CNS symptoms: headache, dizziness, fatigue, insomnia, depression, **seizures**
- Identify urine output; if decreasing, notify prescriber (may indicate nephrotoxicity); also check for increased BUN, creatinine
- Monitor blood studies: AST, ALT, CBC, Hct, bilirubin, LDH, alkaline phosphatase, Coombs' test monthly if patient is on long-term therapy
- Monitor electrolytes: potassium, sodium chloride monthly if patient is on long-term therapy
- Assess bowel pattern daily; if severe diarrhea occurs, drug should be discontinued
- Monitor for bleeding: ecchymosis, bleeding gums, hematuria, stool guaiac daily if on long-term therapy
- Assess for overgrowth of infection: perineal itching, fever, malaise, redness, pain, swelling, drainage, rash, diarrhea, change in cough, sputum

Nursing diagnoses

- Infection, risk for (uses)
- Diarrhea (side effects)
- Injury, risk for (side effects)
- Knowledge, deficient (teaching)
- Noncompliance (teaching)

Implementation

- Do not use theophylline with this product; may cause toxicity

PO route

- Give once a day for 5-10 days depending on condition

IV route

- Discontinue primary **IV** while administering moxifloxacin
- Do not give SUBCUT, IM

Solution compatibilities: 0.9% NaCl, D_5, D_{10}, LR, sterile water for inj

Patient/family education

- Teach patient to report sore throat, bruising, bleeding, joint pain; may indicate blood dyscrasias (rare)
- Advise patient to contact prescriber if vaginal itching, loose foul-smelling stools, furry tongue occur; may indicate superinfection; report itching, rash, pruritus, urticaria
- Instruct patient to take all medication prescribed for the length of time ordered; do not give medication to others
- Advise patient to notify prescriber of diarrhea with blood or pus
- Advise patient to rinse mouth frequently, use sugarless candy or gum for dry mouth
- Advise patient to take as prescribed, not to double or miss doses

Evaluation

Positive therapeutic outcome

- Absence of signs/symptoms of infection (WBC <10,000/mm^3, temp WNL)
- Reported improvement in symptoms of infection

multivitamins (PO, OTC, IV, Rx)

Adavite, Dayalets, LKV Drops, Multi-75, Multi-Day, One-A-Day, Optilets, Poly-Vi-Sol, Quintabs, Rulets, Sesame Street Vitamins, Tab-A-Vite, Therabid, Theragram, Unicaps, Vita-Bob, Vita-Kid, many other brands

Func. class.: Vitamins, multiple

Pregnancy category A

Do Not Confuse:
Theragran/Phenergan

Action: Needed for adequate metabolism

Therapeutic Outcome: Prevention and treatment of vitamin deficiencies

Uses: Prevention and treatment of vitamin deficiencies

Dosage and routes

Adult and child: PO/**IV**—depends on brand

Available forms: Many forms available

Adverse effects

Rare at recommended dosage

Precautions: Pregnancy **A**

Pharmacokinetics

Absorption	Well absorbed (PO)
Distribution	Widely distributed; crosses placenta
Metabolism	Widely metabolized
Excretion	Kidney, unchanged (water soluble)
Half-life	Unknown

Pharmacodynamics

Unknown

NURSING CONSIDERATIONS

Assessment

- Assess patient for vitamin deficiency; usually more than one vitamin deficiency is present

Nursing diagnoses

- Nutrition: less than body requirements, imbalanced (uses)
- Knowledge, deficient (teaching)

Implementation

PO route

- Liq multivitamins can be diluted or dropped into patients' mouth using dropper provided with some brands
- Chew tabs should be chewed and not swallowed whole

IV route

- Give by cont inf only after diluting 5-10 ml (multivitamins)/500-1000 ml of D_5W, $D_{10}W$, $D_{20}W$, LR, D_5/LR, D_5/0.9% NaCl, 0.9% NaCl, 3% NaCl
- Do not use sol with crystals, precipitate, or color other than bright yellow

Y-site compatibilities: Acyclovir, ampicillin, cefazolin, cephalothin, cephapirin, diltiazem, erythromycin, fludarabine, gentamicin, tacrolimus, tetracycline

Additive compatibilities: Cefoxitin, isoproterenol, methyldopate, metoclopramide, metronidazole, netilmicin, norepinephrine, sodium bicarbonate, verapamil

Additive incompatibilities: Penicillin G, erythromycin, tetracycline, kanamycin, streptomycin, doxycycline, lincomycin should not be admixed

Patient/family education

- Advise patient that adequate nutrition must be maintained to prevent further deficiencies; to comply with treatment regimen
- Advise patient to avoid treating flavored multivitamins as candy; child may overdose
- Caution patient to store vitamins out of children's reach

Evaluation

Positive therapeutic outcome

- Check each individual vitamin for guidelines
- Absence of vitamin deficiencies

muromonab-CD3 (Rx)

(mur-oe-mone'ab)

Orthoclone OKT3

Func. class.: Immunosuppressive

Chem. class.: Murine monoclonal antibody

Pregnancy category C

Action: Reverses graft rejection by blocking T-cell function

Therapeutic Outcome: Prevention of graft rejection

Uses: Acute allograft rejection in renal, cardiac, hepatic transplant patients

Dosage and routes

Adult: **IV** bol 5 mg/day × 10-14 days

Child: **IV** 100 mcg/kg/day × 10-14 day

Cardiac/hepatic allograft rejection, steroid resistant

Adult: **IV** bol 5 mg/day × 10-14 days; begin when it is known that rejection has not been reversed by steroids

Available forms: Inj 5 mg/5 ml

Adverse effects

CNS: *Pyrexia, chills, tremors,* **aseptic meningitis**

CV: *Chest pain*

GI: *Vomiting, nausea, diarrhea*

MISC: **Infection, cytokine release syndrome, anaphylaxis**

RESP: *Dyspnea, wheezing,* **pulmonary edema**

Contraindications: Hypersensitivity to murine origin, fluid overload

Precautions: Pregnancy **C**, child <2 yr, fever

Pharmacokinetics

Absorption	Completely absorbed
Distribution	Unknown
Metabolism	Unknown
Excretion	Unknown
Half-life	Unknown

Pharmacodynamics

Unknown

Interactions

Individual drugs

Azathioprine, cycloSPORINE: increased risk of infection

Indomethacin: increased CNS symptoms

Drug classifications

Corticosteroids: increased risk of infection

Immunosuppressants: increased immunosuppression

Live virus vaccines: decreased antibody response

Drug/herb

Astragalus, echinacea, melatonin: interference with immunosuppression

Ginseng, maitake, mistletoe, schisandra, St. John's wort, turmeric: decreased effect

NURSING CONSIDERATIONS

Assessment

- Assess for cytosine release syndrome (CRS): nausea, vomiting, chills, fever, joint pain, weakness, dizziness, diarrhea, tremors, abdominal pain; occurs 30-60 min after first dose; methylPREDNISolone sodium succinate may be prescribed to lessen this reaction
- Assess for hypersensitivity reaction, anaphylaxis: dyspnea, bronchospasm, urticaria, tachycardia, hypotension, angioedema; discontinue drug; emergency equipment must be nearby
- Assess for headache, photophobia, fever, rigidity; indicate aseptic meningitis has developed
- Assess for sore throat, fever, chills, rash, dysuria, which may indicate infection; therapy may be discontinued
- Assess for fluid overload: edema, pulmonary edema, increasing weight
- Monitor blood studies: CBC with differential, platelets, BUN, creatinine, alkaline phosphatase, bilirubin during treatment monthly
- Monitor AST, ALT, BUN, creatinine, alkaline phosphatase, bilirubin
- Obtain human-mouse antibody; if titer is >1:1000, this drug should not be used
- Monitor T-cells with CD3, CD4, CD8 antigen daily; report should be CD3 positive and T-cells <25/mm^3

Nursing diagnoses

- Infection, risk for (uses)
- Knowledge, deficient (teaching)

Implementation

- Give by direct **IV** undiluted; withdraw with a 0.2-0.22 low–protein binding µm filter; discard and use new needle for administration; give over 1 min
- Give for several days before transplant surgery

Patient/family education

- Instruct patient to report fever, chills, sore throat, fatigue, since serious infections may occur; rash, rapid heartbeat
- Advise patient to use contraceptive measures during treatment and for 12 wk after ending therapy; drug is mutagenic
- Advise patient to avoid crowds and persons with known infections to reduce risk of infection
- Advise patient to report symptoms of cytokine release syndrome, aseptic meningitis, give list of symptoms
- Instruct patient to avoid vaccinations during treatment

Evaluation

Positive therapeutic outcome

- Absence of graft rejection

M

mycophenolate (Rx)

(mie-koe-feen'oh-late)

CellCept, Myfortic

Func. class.: Immunosuppressant

Pregnancy category C

Action: Inhibits inflammatory responses that are mediated by the immune system; prolongs survival of allogenic transplants

Therapeutic Outcome: Absence of graft rejection

Uses: Organ transplants to prevent rejection (renal); prophylaxis of rejection in allogenic cardiac, hepatic, renal transplants

Investigational uses: Refractory uveitis, 2nd-line therapy for Churg-Strauss syndrome, diffuse proliferative lupus nephritis (in combination)

Dosage and routes

Renal transplant

Adult: PO/**IV** give initial dose 72 hr before transplantation; 1 g bid given to renal trans-

plant patients in combination with corticosteroids and cycloSPORINE; ER tab 720 mg bid on empty stomach
Child: PO-ER 400 mg/m^2 bid, max 720 mg bid

Renal dose
Adult: PO/**IV** GFR <25 ml/min, max 2 g/day

Cardiac transplant
Adult: PO/**IV** 1.5 g bid, **IV** can be started ≤24 hr after transplant, switch to PO when able

Hepatic transplant
Adult: PO/**IV** 1.5 g bid, give **IV** over ≥2 hr

Available forms: Caps 250 mg; tabs 500 mg; inj (powder) 500 mg/20 ml vial; powder for oral susp 200 mg/ml; ext rel tab (Myfortic) 180, 360 mg

Adverse effects
CNS: *Tremor, dizziness, insomnia, headache, fever*
CV: *Hypertension, chest pain*
GI: *Nausea, vomiting,* stomatitis, *diarrhea, constipation,* **GI bleeding**
GU: *UTI, hematuria,* **renal tubular necrosis**
HEMA: **Leukopenia, thrombocytopenia, anemia, pancytopenia**
INTEG: *Rash*
META: *Peripheral edema, hypercholesterolemia, hypophosphatemia, edema, hyperkalemia, hypokalemia, hyperglycemia*
MS: Arthralgia, muscle wasting
RESP: *Dyspnea, respiratory infection, increased cough, pharyngitis, bronchitis, pneumonia*
SYST: **Lymphoma, nonmelanoma skin carcinoma, sepsis**

Contraindications: Hypersensitivity to this drug or mycophenolic acid

Precautions: Pregnancy **C,** lymphomas, malignancies, neutropenia, renal disease, lactation

Pharmacokinetics

Absorption	Rapidly and completely absorbed
Distribution	Unknown
Metabolism	To active metabolite (MPA)
Excretion	Urine, feces
Half-life	Unknown

Pharmacodynamics

Unknown

Interactions

Individual drugs
Acyclovir, ganciclovir: increased concentration of both drugs
Azathioprine: avoid use
Cholestyramine: decreased levels of mycophenolate
Phenytoin: increased effects; decreased protein binding of phenytoin
Probenecid: increased levels of mycophenolate
Theophylline: increased effects; decreased protein binding of theophylline

Drug classifications
Antacids: decreased levels of mycophenolate
Contraceptives (oral), live attenuated vaccines: decreased effects
Salicylates: increased levels of mycophenolate

Drug/herb
Astragalus, echinacea, melatonin: interferes with immunosuppression

Drug/food
Decreased absorption if taken with food

NURSING CONSIDERATIONS

Assessment
- Monitor blood studies: CBC monthly during treatment
- Monitor liver function studies: alkaline phosphatase, AST, ALT, bilirubin

Nursing diagnoses
- Infection, risk for (uses)
- Knowledge, deficient (teaching)

Implementation
- Give 72 hr before transplantation; may be given in combination with corticosteroids and cycloSPORINE

PO route
- Do not crush, chew tabs; do not open caps; avoid inhalation or direct contact with skin, mucous membranes; tetratogenic in animals
- Give alone for better absorption

IV route
- Do not give by rapid or bolus inj: reconstitute and dilute to 6 mg/ml with D_5, give over ≥2 hr
- Do not admix with mycophenolate **IV** in infusion catheter or with other **IV** drug or infusion admixtures

Patient/family education
- Teach patient to report fever, rash, severe diarrhea, chills, sore throat, fatigue, since serious infections may occur
- Instruct patient to avoid crowds to reduce risk of infection
- Advise patient that repeated lab tests are necessary

- Advise patient to limit exposure to sunlight/UV light
- Instruct patient to use contraception before, during, and 6 wk after therapy

Evaluation

Positive therapeutic outcome

- Absence of graft rejection

nabumetone (Rx)

(na-byoo'me-tone)

Relafen

Func. class.: Nonsteroidal antiinflammatory

Chem. class.: Acetic acid derivative

Pregnancy category

C (1st trimester)

Action: Inhibits prostaglandin synthesis by decreasing an enzyme needed for biosynthesis; analgesic, antiinflammatory

Therapeutic Outcome: Decreased pain, swelling of joints

Uses: Osteoarthritis, rheumatoid arthritis, acute or chronic treatment

Dosage and routes

Adult: PO 1 g as a single dose; may increase to 1.5-2 g/day if needed; may give daily or bid (as a divided dose)

Available forms: Tabs 500, 750 mg

Adverse effects

CNS: Dizziness, headache, drowsiness, fatigue, tremors, confusion, insomnia, anxiety, depression, nervousness

CV: Tachycardia, peripheral edema, palpitations, **dysrhythmias, CHF**

EENT: Tinnitus, hearing loss, blurred vision

GI: Nausea, anorexia, vomiting, diarrhea, jaundice, cholestatic hepatitis, constipation, flatulence, cramps, dry mouth, peptic ulcer, gastritis, **ulceration, perforation**

GU: **Nephrotoxicity, dysuria, hematuria, oliguria, azotemia,** cystitis

HEMA: **Blood dyscrasias**

INTEG: Purpura, rash, pruritus, sweating, photosensitivity

RESP: Dyspnea, pharyngitis, **bronchospasm**

SYST: **Anaphylaxis, angioneurotic edema**

Contraindications: Avoid in late pregnancy, hypersensitivity to this drug or aspirin, iodides, NSAIDs, asthma, severe renal disease, severe hepatic disease

Precautions: Pregnancy **C** (1st trimester), lactation, children, bleeding disorders, GI disorders, cardiac disorders, renal disorders, hepatic dysfunction, elderly

Pharmacokinetics

Absorption	Well absorbed
Distribution	Unknown
Metabolism	Liver, extensively, to inactive metabolite
Excretion	Unknown
Half-life	22-30 hr

Pharmacodynamics

Onset	Unknown
Peak	2½-4 hr
Duration	Unknown

Interactions

Individual drugs

Alcohol, potassium: increased GI reactions

Cefamandole, cefoperazone, cefotetan, clopidogrel, eptifibatide, plicamycin, ticlopidine, valproic acid: increased risk of bleeding

Radiation: increased risk of hematologic reactions

Drug classifications

Anticoagulants, thrombolytics: increased risk of bleeding

Antihypertensives: decreased effect of antihypertensives

Antineoplastics: increased risk of hematologic reactions

Corticosteroids, NSAIDs, potassium supplements, salicylates: increased GI reactions

Diuretics: decreased effectiveness of diuretics

Drug/herb

Arginine, gossypol: increased gastric irritation

Bearberry, bilberry: increased NSAIDs effect

Bogbean, chondroitin: increased bleeding risk

NURSING CONSIDERATIONS

Assessment

- Assess for pain: frequency, characteristics, location, duration, intensity, relief of pain after medication; and for inflammation of joints, ROM
- Monitor blood counts during therapy; watch for decreasing platelets; if low, therapy may need to be discontinued, restarted after hematologic recovery; check for blood dyscrasias (thrombocytopenia): bruising, fatigue, bleeding, poor healing; monitor liver function tests: AST, ALT, alkaline phosphatase; LDH, blood glucose, WBC, CCr
- Assess for asthma, aspirin sensitivity, nasal polyps; increased hypersensitivity reactions

M

Nursing diagnoses
- Pain, acute (uses)
- Pain, chronic
- Mobility, physical, impaired (uses)
- Injury, risk for (adverse reactions)
- Knowledge, deficient (teaching)

Implementation
- Administer tab to patient crushed or whole
- Give with food or milk to decrease gastric symptoms
- Patient should take with a full glass of water and sit upright

Patient/family education
- Tell patient that drug must be continued for prescribed time to be effective; to avoid aspirin, alcoholic beverages, NSAIDs, and OTC medications unless approved by prescriber
- Caution patient to report bleeding, bruising, fatigue, malaise, since blood dyscrasias do occur
- Instruct patient to use caution when driving; drowsiness, dizziness may occur
- Advise patient to use sunscreen, hat, and other protective clothing to prevent burns
- Advise patient to report dark stools, a change in urine pattern, increased weight, edema, increased pain in joints, fever, blood in urine, blurred vision, ringing or roaring in ears

Evaluation
Positive therapeutic outcome
- Decreased pain
- Decreased inflammation
- Increased mobility

nadolol (Rx)
(nay-doe'lole)

Corgard, Syn-Nadolol

Func. class.: Antihypertensive, antianginal

Chem. class.: β-Adrenergic receptor blocker

Pregnancy category C

Do Not Confuse:
Corgard/Cognex

Action: Competitively blocks stimulation of β-adrenergic receptor within vascular smooth muscle; produces chronotropic, inotropic activity (decreases rate of SA node discharge, increases recovery time), slows conduction of AV node, decreases heart rate, which decreases O_2 consumption in myocardium; also decreases renin-aldosterone-angiotensin system at high doses, inhibits β_2-receptors in bronchial system

Therapeutic Outcome: Decreased B/P, heart rate

Uses: Chronic stable angina pectoris, mild to moderate hypertension

Investigational uses: Tachydysrhythmias, aggression, anxiety, tremors, esophageal varices (rebleeding only), prophylaxis of migraine headaches, hyperthyroidism adjunctive therapy

Dosage and routes
Adult: PO 40 mg daily; increase by 40-80 mg q3-7 days; maintenance 40-240 mg/day for angina, 40-320 mg/day for hypertension

Elderly: PO 20 mg/day, may increase by 20 mg until desired dose

Renal dose

Adult: PO CCr 31-50 ml/min give q24-36h; CCr 10-30 ml/min give q24-48h; CCr <10 ml/min give q40-60h

Available forms: Tabs 20, 40, 80, 120, 160 mg

Adverse effects
CNS: Depression, dizziness, fatigue, lethargy, paresthesia, headache, *weakness,* insomnia, memory loss, nightmares

CV: **Bradycardia,** *hypotension,* **CHF,** palpitations, AV block, chest pain, peripheral ischemia, flushing, edema, vasodilatation, conduction disturbances

EENT: Blurred vision, dry eyes, nasal congestion

ENDO: Hyperglycemia, hypoglycemia

GI: Nausea, vomiting, diarrhea, colitis, constipation, cramps, dry mouth, flatulence, hepatomegaly, **pancreatitis,** taste distortion

GU: *Impotence,* decreased libido

HEMA: **Agranulocytosis, thrombocytopenia**

INTEG: Rash, pruritus, fever, alopecia

RESP: Dyspnea, respiratory dysfunction, **bronchospasm,** cough, wheezing, pharyngitis, **laryngospasm, pulmonary edema**

Contraindications: Hypersensitivity to this drug, cardiac failure, cardiogenic shock, 2nd- or 3rd-degree heart block, bronchospastic disease, sinus bradycardia, CHF, COPD

Precautions: Pregnancy **C,** diabetes mellitus, renal disease, lactation, hyperthyroidism, peripheral vascular disease, myasthenia gravis, major surgery, nonallergic bronchospasm

Pharmacokinetics	
Absorption	Variably absorbed
Distribution	Crosses placenta; minimal concentration in CNS, protein binding 30%
Excretion	Kidneys, unchanged
Half-life	10-24 hr; increased in renal disease

Pharmacodynamics	
Onset	Variable
Peak	3-4 hr
Duration	20-24 hr

Interactions

Individual drugs

Clonidine, epinephrine: increased hypotension, bradycardia
Digoxin: increased bradycardia
Thyroid: decreased β-blocking effect

Drug classifications

Antihypertensives: increased hypotension
Ergots: peripheral ischemia
MAOIs: increased bradycardia; do not use together
NSAIDs: decreased antihypertensive effect
Phenothiazines: increased hypotensive effects

Drug/herb

Aconite: increased toxicity, death
Astragalus, cola tree: increased or decreased antihypertensive effect
Barberry, betony, black catechu, black cohosh, bloodroot, broom, burdock, cat's claw, dandelion, goldenseal, Irish moss, Jamaican dogwood, kelp, khella, mistletoe, parsley: increased antihypertensive effect
Coltsfoot, guarana, khat, licorice: decreased antihypertensive effect

Drug/lab test

Increased: serum potassium, serum uric acid, ALT, AST, alkaline phosphatase, LDH, blood glucose, cholesterol

NURSING CONSIDERATIONS

Assessment

- Monitor B/P at beginning of treatment, periodically thereafter; note rate, rhythm, quality of apical/radial pulse before administration; notify prescriber of any significant changes (pulse <55 bpm), orthostatic hypotension
- Check for baselines in renal, liver function tests before therapy begins
- Assess for edema in feet, legs daily; monitor I&O, daily weight; check for jugular vein distention and crackles bilaterally, dyspnea (CHF)
- Monitor skin turgor, dryness of mucous membranes for hydration status, especially elderly

Nursing diagnoses

- Cardiac output, decreased (uses)
- Injury, risk for (adverse reactions)
- Knowledge, deficient (teaching)
- Noncompliance (teaching)

Implementation

- Given ac, at bedtime, tab may be crushed or swallowed whole; give with food to prevent GI upset; give reduced dosage in renal dysfunction
- Store protected from light, moisture; place in cool environment

Patient/family education

- Teach patient not to discontinue drug abruptly; taper over 2 wk; may cause precipitate angina, serious dysrhythmias if stopped abruptly
- Teach patient not to use OTC products containing α-adrenergic stimulants (such as nasal decongestants, cold preparations); to avoid alcohol, smoking and to limit sodium intake as prescribed
- Teach patient how to take pulse and B/P at home; advise when to notify prescriber
- Instruct patient to comply with weight control, dietary adjustments, modified exercise program
- Advise patient to carry/wear emergency ID to identify drug being taken, allergies; teach patient drug controls symptoms but does not cure condition
- Caution patient to avoid hazardous activities if dizziness, drowsiness present; to rise slowly to prevent orthostatic hypotension
- Teach patient to report symptoms of CHF: difficult breathing, especially on exertion or when lying down, night cough, swelling of extremities or bradycardia, dizziness, confusion, depression, fever
- Teach patient to take drug as prescribed, not to double doses, skip doses; take any missed doses as soon as remembered if at least 4 hr until next dose

Evaluation

Positive therapeutic outcome

- Decreased B/P in hypertension

nafarelin (Rx)

(naf-ah-rell'in)

Synarel

Func. class.: Gonadotropin

Chem. class.: Analog of gonadotropin-releasing hormone

Pregnancy category X

Action: Stimulates the release of LH and FSH, which increases ovarian steroid production; repeated dosing prevents stimulation of the pituitary gland

Therapeutic Outcome: Decreased symptoms of endometriosis; resolution of central precocious puberty

Uses: Endometriosis, gonadotropin-dependent precocious puberty

Dosage and routes

Endometriosis

Adult: Nasal 400 mcg/day as one spray (200 mcg) into one nostril in morning and 1 spray into other nostril in evening; start treatment between days 2 and 4 of menstrual cycle; may increase to 800 mcg/day (1 spray into each nostril twice a day); recommended duration of treatment is 6 mo

Central precocious puberty

Child: Nasal 2 sprays in each nostril AM and PM, may increase to 3 sprays after alternating nostril tid

Available forms: Nasal spray 2 mg/ml (200 mcg/spray)

Adverse effects

CNS: Headache, flushing, depression, insomnia, emotional lability, hot flashes

GU: Decreased libido, vaginal dryness, breast tenderness, increased pubic hair

INTEG: Nasal irritation, acne

MISC: Body odor, seborrhea, rhinitis

SENSITIVITY: Shortness of breath, chest pain, urticaria, pruritus

Contraindications: Pregnancy **X,** hypersensitivity, lactation, undiagnosed abnormal vaginal bleeding

Precautions: Children

Pharmacokinetics

Absorption	Well
Distribution	Unknown
Metabolism	Unknown
Excretion	20%-40% feces, 3% urine, unchanged
Half-life	3 hr

Pharmacodynamics

Onset	Up to 4 wk
Peak	3-4 wk
Duration	Several months

Interactions

Drug classifications

Nasal decongestants (nasal sprays): decreased nafarelin absorbtion

NURSING CONSIDERATIONS

Assessment

- Assess pain in endometriosis during treatment
- Assess endocrine studies, bone age, sex steroids, RHCG, GnRH, baseline q8wk
- Assess for precocious puberty including secondary sex characteristics
- Assess test results: pituitary/hypothalamus dysfunction (decreased LH); postmenopausal (increased LH)

Nursing diagnoses

- Pain, acute (uses)
- Sexual dysfunction (uses, adverse reactions)
- Knowledge, deficient (teaching)

Implementation

- Repeated doses may be necessary to elevate pituitary gonadotropin reserve
- Store at room temperature; protect from light

Patient/family education

- Teach patient to use nonhormonal contraception
- Teach patient about correct nasal use, 1 spray in right nostril AM, 1 in left nostril PM
- Teach patient that medication may cause hot flashes, decreased libido, vaginal dryness

Evaluation

Positive therapeutic outcome

- Decreased symptoms of endometriosis; adequate resolution of central precocious puberty

nafcillin (Rx)

(naf-sill'in)

Nafcillin sodium, Nallpen, Unipen

Func. class.: Antiinfective—broad-spectrum

Chem. class.: Penicillinase-resistant penicillin

Pregnancy category B

Action: Interferes with cell wall replication of susceptible organisms; osmotically unstable cell wall swells, bursts from osmotic pressure

Therapeutic Outcome: Bactericidal effects for gram-positive cocci *Staphylococcus aureus, Streptococcus viridans, Streptococcus pneumoniae* and infections caused by penicillinase-producing *Staphylococcus*

Uses: Infections caused by penicillinase-producing staphylococci, streptococci; respiratory tract, skin, skin structure, urinary tract, bone, joint infections, sinusitis, endocarditis, septicemia, meningitis

Dosage and routes

Adult: **IV** 500-1000 mg q4h

Infant and child >1 mo: **IV** 50-200 mg/kg/day in divided doses q4-6h

Neonates >7 days (weight >2 kg): **IV** 25 mg/kg q8h

Neonates ≤7 days (weight <2 kg): **IV** 25 mg/kg q12h

Meningitis

Adult: **IV** 100-200 mg/kg/day divided q4-6h

Neonates >7 days (weight >2 kg): **IV** 50 mg/kg q6h

Neonates ≤7 days (weight <2 kg): **IV** 50 mg/kg q12h

Available forms: Powder for inj 1, 2, 10 g

Adverse effects

CNS: Lethargy, hallucinations, anxiety, depression, muscle twitching, **coma, seizures**

GI: *Nausea, vomiting, diarrhea,* increased AST, ALT, abdominal pain, glossitis, **pseudomembranous colitis**

GU: Oliguria, **proteinuria, hematuria,** vaginitis, moniliasis, **glomerulonephritis,** interstitial nephritis

HEMA: Anemia, increased bleeding time, **bone marrow depression, granulocytopenia**

SYST: **Anaphylaxis, serum sickness**

Contraindications: Hypersensitivity to penicillins

Precautions: Pregnancy **B**, hypersensitivity to cephalosporins, neonates

Pharmacokinetics

Absorption	Well absorbed (IM); erratic (PO)
Distribution	Widely distributed; crosses placenta
Metabolism	Not metabolized
Excretion	Kidneys, unchanged; breast milk
Half-life	1 hr; increased in renal disease

Pharmacodynamics

	PO	IM	IV
Onset	½ hr	½ hr	Immediate
Peak	1-2 hr	1-2 hr	Inf end

Interactions

Individual drugs

Probenecid: increased nafcillin levels
Disulfiram: increased nafcillin concentrations
Heparin: decreased effect of heparin

Drug classifications

Anticoagulants (oral): decreased anticoagulant effects
Contraceptives (oral): decreased contraceptive effectiveness

Drug/lab test

False positive: urine glucose, urine protein

NURSING CONSIDERATIONS

Assessment

- Assess patient for previous sensitivity reaction to penicillins or other cephalosporins; cross-sensitivity between penicillins and cephalosporins is common
- Assess patient for signs and symptoms of infection including characteristics of wounds, sputum, urine, stool, WBC >10,000/mm^3, earache, fever; obtain baseline information and during treatment
- Obtain C&S before beginning drug therapy to identify if correct treatment has been initiated
- Assess for allergic reactions, anaphylaxis: rash, urticaria, pruritus, chills, fever, dyspnea, laryngeal edema, joint pain; angioedema may occur a few days after therapy begins; epINEPHrine, resuscitation equipment should be available for anaphylactic reaction
- Assess renal studies: urinalysis, protein, blood, BUN, creatinine
- ❗ Identify urine output; if decreasing, notify prescriber (may indicate nephrotoxicity)
- Monitor blood studies: AST, ALT, CBC, Hct, bilirubin, LDH, alkaline phosphatase, Coombs' test monthly if patient is on long-term therapy
- Monitor electrolytes: potassium, sodium, chloride monthly if patient is on long-term therapy
- Assess bowel pattern daily; if severe diarrhea occurs, drug should be discontinued; may indicate pseudomembranous colitis
- Monitor for bleeding: ecchymosis, bleeding gums, hematuria, stool guaiac daily if on long-term therapy

N

• Assess for overgrowth of infection: perineal itching, fever, malaise, redness, pain, swelling, drainage, rash, diarrhea, change in cough, sputum

Nursing diagnoses

• Infection, risk for (uses)
• Diarrhea (adverse reactions)
• Injury, risk for (adverse reactions)
• Knowledge, deficient (teaching)
• Noncompliance (teaching)

Implementation

PO route

• Give in even doses around the clock; if GI upset occurs, give with food; drug must be given for 10-14 days to ensure organism death and prevent superinfection; store in tight container.
• Shake susp; store in refrigerator for 2 wk, 1 wk at room temp

IM route

• Reconstitute 500 mg/1.7-1.8 ml; 1 g/3.4 ml; 2 g/6.6-6.8 ml with sterile water or bacteriostatic water for a conc of 250 mg/ml; store unused portion in refrigerator for up to 7 days
• Give deep in large muscle mass

IV route

• Reconstitute 1 g/3.4 ml, 2 g/6.6-6.8 ml with sterile water or bacteriostatic water for a conc of 250 mg/ml; store unused portion in refrigerator for up to 7 days
• Give by direct **IV** by diluting reconstituted sol with 15-30 ml of sterile water or 0.9% NaCl; give over 5-10 min
• Give by intermittent inf by diluting to a conc of 2-40 mg/ml with 0.9% NaCl, D_5W, $D_{10}W$, D_5/0.9% NaCl, D_5/LR, LR, Ringer's; store in refrigerator for up to 96 hr or 24 hr room temp; run over 30-60 min

Syringe compatibilities: Cimetidine, heparin

Y-site compatibilities: Acyclovir, atropine, cyclophosphamide, diazepam, enalaprilat, esmolol, famotidine, fentanyl, fluconazole, foscarnet, hydromorphone, magnesium sulfate, morphine, perphenazine, propofol, theophylline, zidovudine

Y-site incompatibilities: Droperidol, fentanyl/droperidol, labetalol, nalbuphine, pentazocine, regular insulin, verapamil

Additive compatibilities: Chloramphenicol, chlorothiazide, dexamethasone, diphenhydrAMINE, epHEDrine, heparin, hydrOXYzine, lidocaine, potassium chloride, prochlorperazine, sodium bicarbonate, sodium lactate

Additive incompatibilities: Ascorbic acid, aztreonam, bleomycin, cytarabine, gentamicin, hydrocortisone sodium succinate, methylPREDNISolone sodium succinate, promazine

Patient/family education

• Teach patient to report sore throat, bruising, bleeding, joint pain; may indicate blood dyscrasias (rare)
• Advise patient to contact prescriber if vaginal itching, loose foul-smelling stools, furry tongue occur; may indicate superinfection
• Instruct patient to take all medication prescribed for the length of time ordered
• Advise patient to notify prescriber of diarrhea with blood or pus, which may indicate pseudomembranous colitis
• Advise patient to carry/wear emergency ID if allergic to penicillins

Evaluation

Positive therapeutic outcome

• Absence of signs/symptoms of infection (WBC <10,000/mm^3, temp WNL, absence of red, draining wounds, earache)
• Reported improvement in symptoms of infection

Treatment of anaphylaxis: Withdraw drug, maintain airway, administer epINEPHrine, aminophylline, O_2, **IV** corticosteroids

! HIGH ALERT

nalbuphine (Rx)

(nal'byoo-feen)

Nubain, nalbuphine HCl

Func. class.: Opioid analgesic

Chem. class.: Synthetic opioid agonist/antagonist

Pregnancy category C

Action: Inhibits ascending pain pathways in limbic system, thalamus, midbrain, hypothalamus by binding to opiate receptor sites, thus altering pain perception and response

Therapeutic Outcome: Relief of pain

Uses: Moderate to severe pain, labor analgesia, balanced anesthesia (adjunct)

Dosage and routes

Analgesic

Adult: SUBCUT/IM/**IV** 10-20 mg q3-6h prn, not to exceed 160 mg/day

Balanced anesthesia supplement
Adult: **IV** 0.3-3 mg/kg given over 10-15 min; may give 0.25-0.5 mg/kg as needed (maintenance)

Available forms: Inj 10, 20 mg/ml

Adverse effects
CNS: *Drowsiness, dizziness, confusion, headache, sedation, euphoria,* dysphoria (high doses), hallucinations, increased dreaming, tolerance, physical and psychologic dependency
CV: Palpitations, bradycardia, change in B/P, orthostatic hypotension
EENT: Tinnitus, blurred vision, miosis (high doses), diplopia
GI: *Nausea, vomiting, anorexia, constipation, cramps*
GU: Increased urinary output, dysuria, urinary retention, urgency
INTEG: *Rash,* urticaria, bruising, flushing, *diaphoresis,* pruritus
RESP: **Respiratory depression,** pulmonary edema

Contraindications: Hypersensitivity, addiction (opioid)

Precautions: Pregnancy **C**, addictive personality, lactation, increased intracranial pressure, MI (acute), severe heart disease, respiratory depression, hepatic disease, renal disease

Pharmacokinetics

Absorption	Well absorbed (SUBCUT, IM); completely absorbed (**IV**)
Distribution	Crosses placenta
Metabolism	Liver, extensively
Excretion	Feces, kidneys, unchanged (small amounts); breast milk
Half-life	5 hr

Pharmacodynamics

	IM	SUBCUT	IV
Onset	Up to 15 min	Up to 15 min	Rapid
Peak	1 hr	Unknown	½ hr
Duration	3-6 hr	3-6 hr	3-6 hr

Interactions
Individual drugs
Alcohol: increased respiratory depression, hypotension, sedation
Drug classifications
Antihistamines, CNS depressants, sedative/hypnotics, skeletal muscle relaxants: increased respiratory depression, hypotension
MAOIs: avoid use, results are unpredictable
Opiates: increased effects with other CNS depressants
Drug/herb
Chamomile, hops, Jamaican dogwood, kava, lavender, mistletoe, nettle, pokeweed, poppy, senega, skullcap, valerian: increased CNS depression
Corkwood: increased anticholinergic effect
Drug/lab test
Increased: amylase

NURSING CONSIDERATIONS

Assessment
- Assess pain characteristics (location, intensity, type) before medication administration and after treatment
- Monitor VS after parenteral route; note muscle rigidity, drug history, liver, kidney function tests; respiratory dysfunction: respiratory depression, character, rate, rhythm; notify prescriber if respirations are <10/min
- Monitor CNS changes: dizziness, drowsiness, hallucinations, euphoria, LOC, pupil reaction
- Monitor allergic reactions: rash, urticaria

Nursing diagnoses
- Pain, acute (uses)
- Sensory perception, disturbed: visual, auditory (adverse reactions)
- Breathing pattern, ineffective (adverse reactions)
- Knowledge, deficient (teaching)

Implementation
- Give by inj (IM, **IV**), only with resuscitative equipment available; give slowly to prevent rigidity
- Store in light-resistant area at room temp

IM route
- Give inj deeply in large muscle mass; rotate inj sites

IV route
- Give direct **IV** undiluted 10 mg or less over 3-5 min or more

Syringe compatibilities: Atropine, cimetidine, diphenhydrAMINE, droperidol, glycopyrrolate, hydrOXYzine, lidocaine, midazolam, prochlorperazine, promethazine, ranitidine, scopolamine, trimethobenzamide
Syringe incompatibilities: Diazepam, pentobarbital
Y-site compatibilities: Amifostine, aztreonam, cefmetazole, cladribine, filgrastim, fludarabine, granisetron, melphalan, paclitaxel, propofol, teniposide, thiotepa, vinorelbine
Y-site incompatibilities: Nafcillin, sargramostim

N

Patient/family education

- Instruct patient to report any symptoms of CNS changes, allergic reactions
- Caution patients to avoid CNS depressants: alcohol, sedative/hypnotics for at least 24 hr after taking this drug
- Discuss with patient that dizziness, drowsiness, confusion are common; to avoid getting up without assistance
- Discuss in detail all aspects of the drug: reason for taking drug and expected results
- Instruct patient to change position slowly to prevent orthostatic hypotension
- Teach patient to turn, cough, deep breathe after surgery to prevent atelectasis

Evaluation

Positive therapeutic outcome

- Relief of pain

Treatment of overdose: Naloxone (Narcan) 0.2-0.8 **IV**, O_2, **IV** fluids, vasopressors

naloxone (Rx)

(nal-oks'one)

naloxone HCl, Narcan

Func. class.: Opioid antagonist, antidote

Chem. class.: Thebaine derivative

Pregnancy category B

Do Not Confuse:
Narcan/Norcuron

Action: Competes with opioids at opioid receptor sites

Therapeutic Outcome: Absence of opioid overdose

Uses: Respiratory depression induced by opioids, pentazocine, propoxyphene; refractory circulatory shock

Dosage and routes

Opioid-induced respiratory depression

Adult: **IV**/SUBCUT/IM 0.4-2 mg; repeat q2-3 min if needed

Child: **IV**/SUBCUT/IM 0.01 mg/kg slowly or as an inf titrated to response

Postoperative opioid-induced respiratory depression

Adult: **IV** 0.1-0.2 mg q2-3 min prn

Child: **IV**/IM/SUBCUT 0.01 mg/kg q2-3 min prn

Opioid overdose

Adult: **IV**/SUBCUT/IM 0.4 mg (10 mcg/kg) (not opioid dependent) may repeat q2-3 min; 0.1-0.2 mg q2-3 min (opioid dependent)

Child: **IV**/SUBCUT/IM 10 mcg (0.01 mg/kg) q2-3 min

Available forms: Inj 0.02, 0.4 mg/ml

Adverse effects

CNS: Drowsiness, nervousness

CV: Rapid pulse, **ventricular tachycardia, fibrillation,** increased systolic B/P (high doses)

GI: Nausea, vomiting

RESP: Hyperpnea

Contraindications: Hypersensitivity

Precautions: Pregnancy **B,** children, CV disease, opioid dependency, lactation, seizure disorder

Pharmacokinetics

Absorption	Well absorbed (SUBCUT, IM); completely absorbed (**IV**)
Distribution	Rapidly distributed; crosses placenta
Metabolism	Liver
Excretion	Kidneys
Half-life	1 hr; up to 3 hr (neonates)

Pharmacodynamics

	IV	IM/SUBCUT
Onset	1 min	2-5 min
Peak	Unknown	Unknown
Duration	45 min	45-60 min

Interactions

Drug classifications

Analgesics (opioids): decreased effects of opioid analgesics

Drug/lab test

Interference: urine VMA, 5-HIAA, urine glucose

NURSING CONSIDERATIONS

Assessment

- Assess for signs of opioid withdrawal in drug-dependent individuals: cramping, hypertension, anxiety, vomiting; may occur up to 2 hr after administration
- Monitor VS q3-5 min; ABGs including Po_2, Pco_2
- Assess cardiac status: tachycardia, hypertension; monitor ECG
- Assess for pain: duration, intensity, location before and after administration; may be used for respiratory depression
- Assess for respiratory dysfunction: respiratory depression, character, rate, rhythm; if

respirations are <10/min, probably due to opioid overdose, administer naloxone; monitor LOC

Nursing diagnoses

- Breathing pattern, ineffective (uses)
- Coping, ineffective (uses)
- Pain, acute (adverse reactions)
- Knowledge, deficient (teaching)

Implementation

IV route

- Give by direct **IV** undiluted; give 0.4 mg or less over 15 sec or titrate inf to response
- Give cont inf **IV** further diluted with 0.9% NaCl and D_5 and give as an inf
- Give only with resuscitative equipment, O_2 nearby
- Use only sol prepared within 24 hr
- Store at room temp in darkness

Syringe compatibilities: Benzquinamide, heparin

Y-site compatibilities: Propofol

Additive compatibilities: Verapamil

Patient/family education

- Explain reason for and expected results of medication when patient alert

Evaluation

Positive therapeutic outcome

- Reversal of respiratory depression
- LOC: alert

nandrolone (Rx)

(nan′droe-lone)

Deca-Durabolin, Hybolin Decanoate, Kabolin

Func. class.: Androgenic anabolic steroid, antianemic

Chem. class.: Halogenated testosterone derivative

Pregnancy category X

Controlled substance schedule III

Action: May stimulate bone marrow development, stimulates erythropoietin production

Therapeutic Outcome: Increased Hgb, RBCs

Uses: Anemia associated with renal disease

Dosage and routes

Adult and child ≥14 yr: IM women 50-100 mg qwk; men 100-200 mg qwk

Child 2-13 yr: IM 25-50 mg q 3-4 wk

Available forms: Inj 100, 200 mg/ml

Adverse effects

CNS: Dizziness, headache, fatigue, tremors, paresthesias, flushing, sweating, anxiety, lability, insomnia, carpal tunnel syndrome, chills

CV: Increased B/P

EENT: Conjunctival edema, nasal congestion

ENDO: Abnormal GTT

GI: Nausea, vomiting, constipation, weight gain, **cholestatic jaundice**

GU: **Hematuria**, amenorrhea, vaginitis, decreased libido, decreased breast size, clitoral hypertrophy, testicular atrophy, priapism

INTEG: Rash, acneiform lesions, oily hair/skin, flushing, sweating, acne vulgaris, alopecia, hirsutism

MS: Cramps, spasms

Contraindications: Pregnancy **X**, severe renal, severe cardiac, severe hepatic disease, hypersensitivity, lactation, abnormal genital bleeding, males with cancer of breast, prostate

Precautions: Diabetes mellitus, CV disease, MI

Pharmacokinetics	
Absorption	Well
Distribution	Unknown
Metabolism	Unknown
Excretion	Unknown
Half-life	Unknown

Pharmacodynamics	
Onset	Unknown
Peak	Up to 6 days
Duration	Unknown

Interactions

Drug classifications

Anticoagulants, NSAIDs, salicylates: increased bleeding risk

Hepatotoxics: increased hepatotoxicity

Drug/lab test

Increased: serum cholesterol, blood glucose, urine glucose

Decreased: serum calcium, serum potassium, T_4, T_3, thyroid ^{131}I uptake test, urine 17-OHCS, 17-KS, PBI, BSP

NURSING CONSIDERATIONS

Assessment

- Assess for anemia symptoms: dyspnea, fatigue, weakness, pallor
- Monitor weight daily; notify prescriber if weekly weight gain is >5 lb
- Monitor B/P q4h

N

- Monitor I/O ratio; be alert for decreasing urinary output, increasing edema
- Assess growth rate in children, since growth rate may be uneven (linear/bone growth) with extended use
- Monitor electrolytes: K, Na, Cl, Ca; cholesterol
- Monitor hepatic studies: ALT, AST, bilirubin
- Assess edema, hypertension, cardiac symptoms, jaundice
- Assess mental status: affect, mood, behavioral changes, aggression
- Assess signs of masculinization in female: increased libido, deepening of voice, decreased breast tissue, enlarged clitoris, menstrual irregularities; male: gynecomastia, impotence, testicular atrophy
- Assess hypercalcemia: lethargy, polyuria, polydipsia, nausea, vomiting, constipation, drug may have to be decreased
- Assess for hypoglycemia in diabetics, since oral antidiabetic is increased

Nursing diagnoses
- Knowledge, deficient (teaching)

Implementation
- Give titrated dose; use lowest effective dose
- Inject deeply, use large muscle mass

Patient/family education
- Teach patient that drug must be combined with complete health plan: diet, rest, exercise
- Teach patient to notify prescriber if therapeutic response decreases
- Teach patient not to discontinue abruptly
- Teach patient about changes in sex characteristics
- Teach patient that females should report menstrual irregularities
- Teach patient to increase calories, protein; decrease sodium if edema occurs

Evaluation
Positive therapeutic outcome
- Increased appetite, increased stamina

naproxen (OTC, Rx)
(na-prox'en)

Apo-Naproxen ♣, EC-Naprosyn, Naprelan, Napron X, Naprosyn, Naprosyn-E ♣, Naprosyn-SR ♣, Naxen ♣, Novo-Naprox ♣, Nu-Naprox ♣

naproxen sodium
Aleve, Anaprox, Anaprox DS, Apo-Napro-Na ♣, Apo-Napro-Na DS, Naprelan, Novo-Naprox Sodium ♣, Novo-Naprox Sodium DS ♣, Synflex ♣, Synflex DS ♣

Func. class.: Nonsteroidal antiinflammatory, nonopioid analgesic
Chem. class.: Propionic acid derivative

Pregnancy category
B (1st trimester),
D (2nd/3rd trimesters)

Action: Inhibits prostaglandin synthesis by decreasing enzyme needed for biosynthesis; analgesic, antiinflammatory

Therapeutic Outcome: Decreased pain, inflammation

Uses: Mild to moderate pain, osteoarthritis, rheumatoid arthritis, gouty arthritis, juvenile arthritis, primary dysmenorrhea

Dosage and routes
Antiinflammatory/analgesic/antidysmenorrheal
Adult: PO 250-500 mg bid, max 1.5 g/day; del rel 375-500 mg bid
Child >2 yr: PO 5 mg/kg/day bid

Antigout
Adult: PO 750 mg, then 250 mg q8h

OTC use
Adult: PO 200 mg q8-12h or 400 mg, then 200 mg q12h, max 600 mg/24 hr

Geriatric >65 yr: PO max 200 mg q12h

Available forms: Naproxen tabs: 250, 375, 500 mg; cont rel tabs (Naprelan) 375, 500 mg; del rel tabs (EC-Naprosyn, Naprosyn-E) 250♣, 375, 500 mg; tabs, oral susp 125 mg/5 ml; ext rel tabs (SR) 750 mg♣ naproxen sodium; cont rel tabs, 421.5, 550 mg; tabs 275, 550 mg; supp (Naprosyn, Naxen) 500 mg♣

Adverse effects
CNS: Dizziness, drowsiness, fatigue, tremors, confusion, insomnia, anxiety, depression
CV: Tachycardia, peripheral edema, palpitations, **dysrhythmias**
EENT: Tinnitus, hearing loss, blurred vision
GI: Nausea, anorexia, vomiting, diarrhea, jaundice, **cholestatic hepatitis,** constipation,

flatulence, cramps, dry mouth, peptic ulcer, **GI ulceration, bleeding, perforation**
GU: **Nephrotoxicity: dysuria, hematuria, oliguria, azotemia**
HEMA: **Blood dyscrasias**
INTEG: Purpura, rash, pruritus, sweating
SYST: **Anaphylaxis**

Contraindications: Pregnancy **D** (2nd/3rd trimesters), hypersensitivity, asthma, severe renal disease, severe hepatic disease, ulcer disease

Precautions: Pregnancy **B** (1st trimester), lactation, children <2 yr, bleeding disorders, GI disorders, cardiac disorders, hypersensitivity to other antiinflammatory agents, elderly, CCr <25 ml/min

Pharmacokinetics	
Absorption	Completely absorbed
Distribution	Crosses placenta, 99% protein binding
Metabolism	Liver, extensively
Excretion	Breast milk
Half-life	10-20 hr

Pharmacodynamics	
Onset	1 hr
Peak	2-4 hr
Duration	<7 hr

Interactions
Individual drugs
Alcohol, aspirin: increased risk of GI side effects
Cefamandole, cefoperazone, cefotetan, clopidogrel, eptifibatide, plicamycin, ticlopidine, tirofiban, valproic acid: increased bleeding risk
Lithium: increased toxicity
Methotrexate: increased toxicity
Radiation: increased risk of hematologic toxicity
Drug classifications
ACE inhibitors: possible renal impairment
Anticoagulants, thrombolytics: increased risk of bleeding
Antihypertensives: decreased effect of antihypertensives
Antineoplastics: increased risk of hematologic toxicity
Corticosteroids, NSAIDs: increased risk of GI adverse reactions
Diuretics: decreased effectiveness of diuretics
Drug/herb
Anise, arnica, bogbean, chamomile, chondroitin, clove, dong quai, fenugreek, feverfew, garlic, ginger, ginkgo, ginseng *(Panax)*, licorice: increased bleeding risk
Arginine, gossypol: increased gastric irritation
Bearberry, bilberry: increased NSAIDs effect
Drug/lab test
Increased: BUN, alkaline phosphatase
False: increased 5-HIAA, 17KS

NURSING CONSIDERATIONS
Assessment
- Monitor liver function, renal function, other blood studies: AST, ALT, bilirubin, creatinine, BUN, CBC, Hct, Hgb, protime, LDH, blood glucose, WBC, platelets; if patient is on long-term therapy
- Check I&O ratio; decreasing output may indicate renal failure (long-term therapy)
- Assess hepatotoxicity: dark urine, clay-colored stools, yellowing of the skin and sclera, itching, abdominal pain, fever, diarrhea if patient is on long-term therapy
- Assess for allergic reactions: rash, urticaria; if these occur, drug may have to be discontinued
- Assess for ototoxicity: tinnitus, ringing, roaring in ears; audiometric testing needed before, after long-term therapy
- Assess for visual changes: blurring, halos; may indicate corneal, retinal damage
- Check for edema in feet, ankles, legs
- Identify prior drug history; there are many drug interactions
- Monitor pain: location, frequency, duration, characteristics, type, intensity before dose and 1 hour after; assess ROM before dose and after
- Assess for asthma, aspirin hypersensitivity, or nasal polyps, increased risk of hypersensitivity

Nursing diagnoses
- Pain, acute (uses)
- Pain, chronic
- Mobility, physical, impaired (uses)
- Injury, risk for (adverse reactions)
- Knowledge, deficient (teaching)

Implementation
- Administer to patient crushed or whole
- Give with food or milk to decrease gastric symptoms; give ½ hr ac or 2 hr pc for better absorption
- Patient should take with 8 oz of water and sit upright for 30 min after dose to prevent ulceration

Patient/family education
- Teach patient to report any symptoms of hepatotoxicity, renal toxicity, visual changes, ototoxicity, allergic reactions, bleeding (long-term therapy)
- Caution patient not to exceed recommended dosage; acute poisoning may result; to take as prescribed, do not double dose
- Advise patient to use sunscreen to prevent photosensitivity reactions

• Teach patient to read label on other OTC drugs; many contain other antiinflammatories; caution patient to avoid alcohol ingestion; GI bleeding may occur
• Inform patient that the therapeutic response takes 2 wk (arthritis)
• Teach patient to report tinnitus, confusion, diarrhea, sweating, hyperventilation, blurred vision, fever, joint aches, black stools, flulike symptoms

Evaluation

Positive therapeutic outcome
• Decreased pain
• Decreased inflammation
• Increased mobility

naratriptan (Rx)

(nair'ah-trip-tan)

Amerge

Func. class.: Migraine agent

Chem. class.: 5-HT_1-like receptor agonist

Pregnancy category C

Action: Binds selectively to the vascular 5-HT_1 receptor subtype, exerts antimigraine effect; causes vasoconstriction in cranial arteries

Therapeutic Outcome: Decreased intensity and incidence of migraines

Uses: Acute treatment of migraine with or without aura

Dosage and routes

Adult: PO 1 or 2.5 mg with fluids, if headache returns, repeat once after 4 hr, max 5 mg/24 hr

Hepatic/renal dose

Max 2.5 mg/24 hr

Available forms: Tabs 1, 2.5 mg

Adverse effects

CNS: Dizziness, sedation, fatigue

CV: Increased B/P, palpitations, **tachydysrhythmias, PR, QT_C prolongation, ST/T wave changes, PVCs, atrial flutter, fibrillation, coronary vasospasm**

EENT: EENT infections, photophobia

GI: *Nausea, vomiting*

MISC: Temp change sensations, tightness, pressure sensations

MS: *Weakness, neck stiffness,* myalgia

Contraindications: Angina pectoris, history of MI, documented silent ischemia, ischemic heart disease, concurrent ergotamine-containing preparations, uncontrolled hypertension, hypersensitivity, severe renal disease (CCr <15 ml/min); severe hepatic disease (Child-Pugh grade C), CV syndromes, hemiplegic or basilar migraines

Precautions: Pregnancy **C,** postmenopausal women, men >40 yr, risk factors for CAD, hypercholesterolemia, obesity, diabetes, impaired hepatic or renal function, lactation, children, elderly, peripheral vascular disease

Pharmacokinetics	
Absorption	Unknown
Distribution	28%-31% protein binding
Metabolism	Liver (metabolite)
Excretion	Urine/feces
Half-life	6 hr

Pharmacodynamics	
Onset	Unknown
Peak	2-3 hr
Duration	Unknown

Interactions

Drug classifications

5-HT agonists, ergot derivatives: increased vasospastic effect
MAOIs: increased risk of adverse reactions, do not use together
Selective serotonin release inhibitors: increased weakness, hyperreflexia, incoordination

Drug/herb

Butterbur: increased effect
SAM-e, St. John's wort: increased serotonin syndrome

NURSING CONSIDERATIONS

Assessment

• Assess for stress level, activity, recreation, coping mechanisms
• Assess neurologic status: LOC, blurred vision, nausea, tics preceding headache

Nursing diagnoses

• Pain, acute (uses)
• Knowledge, deficient (teaching)
• Noncompliance (teaching)

Implementation

• Do not use product if another 5-HT agonist or an ergot preparation has been used in past 24 hr
• Give with fluids as soon as symptoms appear, may take another dose after 4 hr; do not take >5 mg in any 24 hr period
• Provide a quiet, calm environment with decreased stimulation for noise, bright light, excessive talking

Patient/family education

• Teach patient to report pain, tightness in chest, neck, throat, or jaw; notify prescriber immediately if sudden, severe abdominal pain occurs

- Teach patient to use contraception while taking drug, to notify prescriber if pregnancy is planned or suspected

Evaluation

Positive therapeutic outcome

- Absence of migraine headaches

nedocromil (Rx)

(ned-o-kroe'mil)

Tilade

Func. class.: Antiasthmatic

Chem. class.: Mast cell stabilizer

Pregnancy category B

Action: Stabilizes the membrane of the sensitized mast cell, preventing release of chemical mediators after an antigen-IgE interaction

Therapeutic Outcome: Reduced symptoms of asthma

Uses: Allergic rhinitis, severe perennial bronchial asthma, exercise-induced bronchospasm (prevention), prevention of acute bronchospasm induced by environmental pollutants, mastocytosis, not for treatment of acute asthma attacks

Dosage and routes

Adult and child >12 yr: 2 inh 2-4 ×/day at regular intervals to provide 14 g/day

Available forms: 1.75 mg of nedocromil per activation in 16.2-g canisters providing at least 112 metered inhalations

Adverse effects

CNS: Headache, dizziness, neuritis, dysphonia

EENT: Throat irritation, cough, nasal congestion, burning eyes, rhinitis

GI: Nausea, vomiting, anorexia, dry mouth, bitter taste

MISC: **Anaphylaxis**

Contraindications: Hypersensitivity to this drug or lactose, status asthmaticus

Precautions: Pregnancy **B**, lactation, children

Pharmacokinetics	
Absorption	Poorly, 3%
Distribution	Unknown
Metabolism	Not usually metabolized
Excretion	Small amounts in bile, urine unchanged
Half-life	80 min

Pharmacodynamics	
Onset	Unknown
Peak	15 min
Duration	4-6 hr

Interactions: None known

NURSING CONSIDERATIONS

Assessment

- Assess pulmonary function testing baseline (asthma)
- Assess respiratory status: respiratory rate, rhythm, characteristics, cough, wheezing, dyspnea

Nursing diagnoses

- Airway clearance, ineffective (uses)
- Knowledge, deficient (teaching)

Implementation

- Give by inh only with spacer device if needed
- Encourage patient to gargle, sip water to decrease irritation in throat

Patient/family education

- Instruct patient to clear mucus before using
- Teach patient proper inhalation technique: exhale; using inhaler, inhale deeply with head tipped back to open airway; remove, hold breath, exhale; use Halermatic or Spinhaler with Intal caps
- Inform patient that therapeutic effect may take up to 4 wk
- Teach patient that drug is preventive only, not restorative

Evaluation

Positive therapeutic outcome

- Decrease in asthmatic symptoms

nelarbine

Arranon

See Appendix A, Selected New Drugs

nelfinavir (Rx)

(nell-fin'a-ver)

Viracept

Func. class.: Antiretroviral

Chem. class.: HIV protease inhibitor

Pregnancy category B

Action: Inhibits HIV-1 protease

Therapeutic Outcome: Prevents maturation of the infectious virus

Uses: HIV-1 in combination with other antiretrovirals

Dosage and routes

HIV Infection

Adult/child >13 yr: PO 750 mg tid or 1250 mg bid

Child 2-13 yr: PO 20-30 mg/kg tid, max 750 mg tid

Prevention of HIV infection after exposure

Adult: PO 750 mg tid with two other antiretroviral agents × 4 wk

Available forms: Tabs 250, 625 mg; oral powder 50 mg/g

Adverse effects

CNS: Headache, asthenia, poor concentration, **seizures, suicidal ideation**
CV: Bleeding
ENDO: Hypoglycemia, hyperlipidemia
GI: Diarrhea, nausea, anorexia, dyspepsia, *flatulence,* **hepatitis, pancreatitis**
HEMA: **Anemia, leukopenia, thrombocytopenia, Hgb abnormalities**
INTEG: Rash, dermatitis
MISC: Asthenia
MS: Pain, arthralgia, myalgia, myopathy
OTHER: **Hypoglycemia,** redistribution of body fat

Contraindications: Hypersensitivity to protease inhibitors

Precautions: Pregnancy **B,** liver disease, lactation, hemophilia, PKU, renal disease, pancreatitis

Pharmacokinetics	
Absorption	Unknown
Distribution	98% protein binding
Metabolism	Liver (minimal)
Excretion	Feces/urine
Half-life	3½-5 hr

Pharmacodynamics	
Onset	Unknown
Peak	2-4 hr
Duration	Unknown

Interactions

Individual drugs

Amiodarone, lovastatin, midazolam, pimozide, quinidine, simvastatin, triazolam: increased serious dysrhythmias
Carbamazepine, nevirapine, phenobarbital, phenytoin, rifamycin: decreased nelfinavir levels
Delavirdine: increased protease inhibitor levels
Indinavir, ketoconazole, ritonavir: increased nelfinavir levels
Rifabutin, azithromycin, atorvaston: increased effect

Drug classifications

Contraceptives (oral), didanosine, methadone, phenytoin: decreased effect
Ergots: increased serious dysrhythmias
HIV protease inhibitors: increased protease inhibitor levels

Drug/herb

St. John's wort: decreased antiretroviral effect

Drug/food

Increased: absorption with food

NURSING CONSIDERATIONS

Assessment

- Assess signs of infection, anemia
- Monitor liver studies: ALT, AST
- Monitor C&S before drug therapy; drug may be taken as soon as culture is performed; repeat C&S after treatment; determine the presence of other sexually transmitted diseases
- Assess bowel pattern before, during treatment; if severe abdominal pain with bleeding occurs, drug should be discontinued; monitor hydration
- Assess skin eruptions, rash, urticaria, itching
- Assess allergies before treatment, reaction of each medication; place allergies on chart
- Monitor viral load, CD_4 cell counts baseline and throughout treatment

Nursing diagnoses

- Infection, risk for (uses)
- Knowledge, deficient (teaching)

Implementation

- Administer with food
- Oral powder can be mixed with fluids, do not mix with juice or acidic fluids, stable mixed for 6 hr

Patient/family education

- Advise patient to take with meal or snack; if dose is missed, take as soon as remembered up to 1 hr before next dose; do not double dose
- Advise patient to avoid taking with other medications, unless directed by prescriber
- Teach patient that drug does not cure, but manages symptoms, does not prevent transmission of HIV to others
- Teach patient to use nonhormonal form of contraception while taking this drug

Evaluation

Positive therapeutic outcome

- Decreasing symptoms of HIV
- Improving viral load and CD4 cell counts

neostigmine (Rx)

(nee-oh-stig'meen)

neostigmine, Prostigmin

Func. class.: Cholinergic stimulant; anticholinesterase

Chem. class.: Quaternary compound

Pregnancy category C

Action: Inhibits destruction of acetylcholine, which increases concentration at sites where acetylcholine is released; this facilitates transmission of impulses across the myoneural junction

Therapeutic Outcome: Increased strength in myasthenia gravis, reversal of nondepolarizing muscular blockers

Uses: Myasthenia gravis, nondepolarizing neuromuscular blocker, antagonist, bladder distention, postoperative ileus

Dosage and routes

Myasthenia gravis

Adult: PO 15 mg q3-4h, may increase to 375 mg/day; IM/**IV** 0.5-2 mg q1-3h

Child: PO 2 mg/kg/day q3-4h

Nondepolarizing neuromuscular blocker antagonist

Adult: **IV** 0.5-2 mg slowly; may repeat if needed (give 0.6-1.2 mg atropine before this drug)

Infant/child: **IV** 0.025-0.1 mg/kg/dose

Abdominal distention/ postoperative ileus

Adult: IM/SUBCUT 0.25-1 mg (1:4000) q4-6h depending on condition × 2-3 days

Renal dose

Adult: PO/IM/**IV** CCr 10-50 ml/min 50% of dose; CCr <10 ml/min 25% of dose

Available forms: Tabs 15 mg; inj 1:1000, 1:2000, 1:4000

Adverse effects

CNS: Dizziness, headache, sweating, weakness, **seizures**, incoordination, **paralysis**, drowsiness, LOC

CV: Tachycardia, **dysrhythmias**, bradycardia, hypotension, AV block, ECG changes, **cardiac arrest**, syncope

EENT: Miosis, blurred vision, lacrimation, visual changes

GI: *Nausea, diarrhea, vomiting, cramps,* increased peristalsis, salivary and gastric secretions

GU: Frequency, incontinence, urgency

INTEG: Rash, urticaria, flushing

RESP: **Respiratory depression, bronchospasm, constriction, laryngospasm, respiratory arrest, dyspnea**

Contraindications: Obstruction of intestine, renal system, bromide sensitivity, peritonitis, urinary tract obstruction, ileus

Precautions: Pregnancy **C**, bradycardia, hypotension, seizure disorders, bronchial asthma, coronary occlusion, hyperthyroidism, dysrhythmias, peptic ulcer, megacolon, poor GI motility, lactation, children

Pharmacokinetics

Absorption	Poorly absorbed (PO), completely absorbed (**IV**)
Distribution	Unknown
Metabolism	Liver
Excretion	Kidneys
Half-life	40-90 min

Pharmacodynamics

	PO	IM	IV
Onset	45-75 min	10-30 min	4-8 min
Peak	Unknown	30 min	30 min
Duration	2½-4 hr	2½-4 hr	2-4 hr

Interactions

Individual drugs

Atropine, disopyramide, haloperidol, quinidine: decreased neostigmine action

Decamethonium, succinylcholine: increased action of each specific drug

Drug classifications

Aminoglycosides, anticholinergics, antidepressants, antihistamines, corticosteroids, local general anesthetics, phenothiazines: decreased neostigmine action

Drug/herb

Pill bearing spurge: increased effect

NURSING CONSIDERATIONS

Assessment

- Monitor VS, respiration during rest
- Monitor for bradycardia, hypotension, bronchospasm, headache, dizziness, seizures, respiratory depression; drug should be discontinued if toxicity occurs

Nursing diagnoses

- Breathing pattern, ineffective (uses)
- Knowledge, deficient (teaching)

Implementation

PO route

- Give only after all other cholinergics have been discontinued
- Increased dosage as ordered may be needed if tolerance develops

N

- Give larger doses as ordered after exercise or fatigue
- Administer on empty stomach for better absorption
- Store at room temp

IV route

- Give direct **IV** undiluted, through Y-tube or 3-way stopcock; give 0.5 mg or less over 1 min
- Give only with atropine sulfate available for cholinergic crisis

Syringe compatibilities: Glycopyrrolate, heparin, pentobarbital, thiopental

Y-site compatibilities: Heparin, hydrocortisone sodium succinate, potassium chloride, vit B/C

Additive compatibilities: Netilmicin

Patient/family education

- Teach patient to carry/wear emergency ID specifying myasthenia gravis, drugs taken, prescriber's phone number

Evaluation

Positive therapeutic outcome

- Increased muscle strength, hand grasp
- Improved gait
- Absence of labored breathing (if severe)

Treatment of overdose: Respiratory support, **IV** atropine 1-4 mg

! HIGH ALERT

nesiritide (Rx)

(nes-eer'ih-tide)

Natrecor

Func. class.: Vasodilator

Chem. class.: Human B-type natriuretic peptide

Pregnancy category C

Action: Uses DNA technology; human B-type natriuretic peptide binds to the receptor in vascular smooth muscle and endothelial cells, leading to smooth muscle relaxation

Therapeutic Outcome: Improvement in symptoms of congestive heart failure (CHF)

Uses: Acutely decompensated CHF

Dosage and routes

Adult: Bol **IV** 2 mcg/kg, then **IV** inf 0.01 mcg/kg/min

Available forms: Powder for inj, 1.5 mg single-use vial

Adverse effects

CNS: Headache, insomnia, dizziness, anxiety, confusion, paresthesia, tremor

CV: *Hypotension,* **tachycardia,** dysrhythmias, bradycardia, ventricular tachycardia, ventricular extrasystoles, **atrial fibrillation**

GI: Vomiting, nausea

INTEG: Rash, sweating, pruritus, inj site reaction

MISC: Back pain, abdominal pain

RESP: Increased cough, hemoptysis, **apnea**

Contraindications: Hypersensitivity, cardiogenic shock or B/P <90 mm Hg as primary therapy

Precautions: Pregnancy **C;** mitral stenosis; significant valvular stenosis, restriction, or obstructive cardiomyopathy, or any condition that depends on venous return; renal disease; lactation; children

Pharmacokinetics	
Absorption	Vascular smooth muscle and endothelial cells
Distribution	Unknown
Metabolism	Unknown
Excretion	Bound to cell surfaces, internalized, and proteolyzed; cleaved by endopeptidases on vascular lumenal surface; renal filtration
Half-life	18 min

Pharmacodynamics	
Onset	15 min
Peak	1 hr
Duration	Unknown

Interactions

Drug classifications

ACE inhibitors: increased symptomatic hypotension

NURSING CONSIDERATIONS

Assessment

- Assess PCWP, RAP, cardiac index, MPAP
- Assess B/P, pulse during treatment until stable

Nursing diagnoses

- Tissue perfusion, ineffective (uses)
- Knowledge, deficient (teaching)

Implementation

IV route

- Do not administer nesiritide through a central heparin-coated catheter; heparin should be administered through a separate catheter
- Prime **IV** fluid with inf of 25 ml before connecting to patient's vascular access port and before bolus dose or **IV** inf
- Reconstitute one 1.5 mg vial/5 ml of diluent from prefilled 250 ml plastic **IV** bag with diluent of choice (D_5, 0.9% NaCl, D_5/0.9%

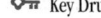

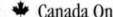

NaCl, D_5/0.2% NaCl); do not shake vial, roll gently; use only clear sol

- Withdraw all contents of reconstituted vial and add to the 250 ml plastic **IV** bag (6 mcg/ml), invert bag several times
- Use within 24 hr of reconstituting

Patient/family education
- Explain purpose of medication and expected results

Evaluation
Positive therapeutic outcome
- Improvement in CHF with improved PCWP, RAP, MPAP

nevirapine (Rx)
(ne-veer'a-peen)
Viramune
Func. class.: Antiretroviral
Chem. class.: Non-nucleoside reverse transcriptase inhibitor (NNRTI)

Pregnancy category C

Do Not Confuse:
nevirapine/nelfinavir
viramune/viracept

Action: Binds directly to reverse transcriptase and blocks RNA, DNA causing a disruption of the enzyme's site

Therapeutic Outcome: Improvement of HIV-1 infection

Uses: HIV-1 in combination with other highly active antiretroviral treatments (HAART)

Dosage and routes
Adult: PO 200 mg daily × 2 wk, then 200 mg bid in combination
Child ≥8 yr: PO 4 mg/kg daily × 2 wk, then 4 mg/kg bid, max 200 mg bid
Child 2 mo-8 yr: PO 4 mg/kg daily × 2 wk, then 7 mg/kg bid

Available forms: Tabs 200 mg; oral susp 50 mg/5 ml

Adverse effects
CNS: *Paresthesia, headache, fever, peripheral neuropathy*
GI: *Diarrhea,* abdominal pain, *nausea, stomatitis,* hepatitis, **hepatotoxicity**
HEMA: **Neutropenia, anemia, thrombocytopenia**
INTEG: *Rash,* **toxic epidermal necrolysis**
MISC: **Stevens-Johnson syndrome**
MS: Pain, myalgia

Contraindications: Hypersensitivity

Precautions: Pregnancy **C**, liver disease, lactation, children, renal disease

Pharmacokinetics
Absorption	Rapid
Distribution	60% bound to plasma proteins
Metabolism	Liver, by hepatic P450 enzyme system
Excretion	91% urine
Half-life	2.5-3 hr

Pharmacodynamics
Peak	4 hr

Interactions
Individual drugs
Cimetidine: increased nevirapine levels
Clonazepam, diazepam, warfarin: decreased nevirapine level
Ketoconazole: decreased effect of ketoconazole
Methadone: decreased effect of methadone
Drug classifications
Anticonvulsants, rifamycins: decreased nevirapine levels
Antiinfectives, macrolides: increased nevirapine levels
Oral contraceptives, protease inhibitors: decreased action
Drug/herb
St. John's wort: decreased nevirapine levels, do not use together
Drug/lab test
Increased: ALT, AST, GGT, bilirubin, Hgb
Decreased: neutrophil count

NURSING CONSIDERATIONS
Assessment
- Assess signs of infection, anemia
- Assess liver, renal, blood studies: ALT, AST; viral load, CD_4, if liver function tests are elevated significantly, drug should be withheld
- Assess C&S before drug therapy; drug may be taken as soon as culture is performed; repeat C&S after treatment; determine the presence of other sexually transmitted disease
- Assess bowel pattern before, during treatment; if severe abdominal pain with bleeding occurs, drug should be discontinued; monitor hydration
- Assess skin eruptions; rash, urticaria, itching; if rash is severe or systemic symptoms occur, discontinue immediately
- Assess allergies before treatment, reaction to each medication

N

Nursing diagnoses
- Infection, risk for (uses)
- Diarrhea (side effects)
- Knowledge, deficient (teaching)

Implementation
- Give without regard to meals
- Give at equal intervals around the clock to maintain blood levels

Patient/family education
- Instruct patient to report any right quadrant pain, jaundice, rash immediately
- Inform patient that drug may be taken with food, antacids, didanosine
- Advise patient to take as prescribed; if dose is missed, take as soon as remembered up to 1 hr before next dose; do not double dose
- Advise patient that drug must be taken in equal intervals around the clock to maintain blood levels for duration of therapy
- Advise patient that drug is not a cure, controls symptoms of HIV
- Instruct patient to avoid OTC agents unless approved by prescriber
- Advise patient to use a nonhormonal form of contraception during treatment

Evaluation
Positive therapeutic outcome
- Decreasing symptoms of HIV
- Improving viral load and CD4 cell counts

niacin
(nye'a-sin)

Edur-Acin, Nia-Bid, Niac, Niacels, Niacor, Niaspan, Nico-400, Nicobid, Nicolar, Nicotinex

nicotinic acid
(nick-oh-tin'ick)

Novo-Niacin ✤, Slo-Niacin, vitamin B

niacinamide
(nye-a-sin'a-mide)

nicotinamide
(nick-oh-tin'ah-mide)

Func. class.: Vitamin B_3
Chem. class.: Water-soluble vitamin, lipid-lowering drug

Pregnancy category C

Do Not Confuse:
Nicobid/Nitro-Bid

Action: Needed for conversion of fats, protein, carbohydrates by oxidation-reduction; acts directly on vascular smooth muscle, causing vasodilatation; reduces LDL, HDL, triglycerides, and lipoprotein A

Therapeutic Outcome: Decreasing cholesterol and LDL levels, B_3 supplementation

Uses: Pellagra, hyperlipidemias (types IV, V), peripheral vascular disease, patients who present a risk for pancreatitis

Dosage and routes
Niacin deficiency
Adult: PO 100-500 mg/day in divided doses; IM/SUBCUT 5-100 mg 5 or more times a day; **IV** 25-100 mg bid or tid
Child: PO up to 300 mg/day in divided doses

Adjunct in hyperlipidemia
Adult: 250 mg after evening meal, may increase dose at 1-4 wk intervals to 1-2 g tid, max 6 g/day; ext rel 500 mg at bedtime, ×4 wk, then 1000 mg at bedtime for wk 5-8, do not increase by more than 500 mg q4wk, max 2000 mg/day

Pellagra
Adult: PO 300-500 mg daily in divided doses
Child: PO 100-300 mg daily in divided doses

Peripheral vascular disease
Adult: PO 250-800 mg daily in divided doses

Available forms: Niacin: tabs 25, 50, 100, 250, 500, 1000 mg; time rel caps 250, 500 mg; time rel tabs 250, 500 mg; elixir 50 mg/5 ml; ext rel caps 250, 400 mg; sus rel tabs 500 mg; cont rel tabs 250, 500, 750 mg; sus rel cap 125, 500 mg; nicotinamide: tabs 100, 250, 500 mg

Adverse effects
CNS: Paresthesias, headache, dizziness, anxiety
CV: Postural hypotension, vasovagal attacks, dysrhythmias, vasodilatation
EENT: Blurred vision, ptosis
GI: Nausea, vomiting, anorexia, flatulence, *jaundice,* diarrhea, peptic ulcer, **hepatotoxicity,** dyspepsia
GU: Hyperuricemia, **glycosuria, hypoalbuminemia**
INTEG: Flushing, dry skin, rash, pruritus, itching, tingling

Contraindications: Hypersensitivity, peptic ulcer, hepatic disease, lactation, hemorrhage, severe hypotension

Precautions: Pregnancy **C**, glaucoma, CV disease, CAD, diabetes mellitus, gout, schizophrenia, lactation

Pharmacokinetics

Absorption	Well absorbed (PO)
Distribution	Widely distributed
Metabolism	Converted to niacinamide
Excretion	Urine, unchanged (30%); breast milk
Half-life	45 min

Pharmacodynamics

	PO	IV
Onset	Unknown	Unknown
Peak	30-70 min	Unknown
Duration	Unknown	Unknown

Interactions

Individual drugs

Alcohol: increased flushing, pruritus, avoid use

Drug classifications

Ganglionic blockers: increased postural hypotension

HMG-CoA reductase inhibitors: increased myopathy, rhabdomyolysis

Drug/lab test

Increased: bilirubin, alkaline phosphatase, liver enzymes, LDH, uric acid, glucose

Decreased: cholesterol

False increase: urinary catecholamines

False positive: urine glucose

NURSING CONSIDERATIONS

Assessment

- Assess for niacin deficiency (pellagra): nausea, vomiting, stomatitis, confusion, hallucinations before and throughout treatment
- Assess for symptoms of niacin deficiency: nausea, vomiting, anemia, poor memory, confusion, dermatitis
- Assess for lipid, triglyceride, cholesterol level, if using for hyperlipidemia
- Assess nutrition: fat, protein, carbohydrates, nutritional analysis should be completed by dietitian
- Monitor liver function studies: AST, ALT, bilirubin, uric acid, alkaline phosphatase; blood glucose before and during treatment; liver dysfunction: clay-colored stools, itching, dark urine, jaundice
- Monitor niacin levels during administration of this drug
- Monitor cardiac status: rate, rhythm, quality; postural hypotension, dysrhythmias
- Monitor nutritional status: liver, yeast, legumes, organ meat, lean poultry; high-level niacin products should be included in the diet
- Assess for CNS symptoms: headache, paresthesias, blurred vision

Nursing diagnoses

- Nutrition: less than body requirements, imbalanced (uses)
- Knowledge, deficient (teaching)
- Noncompliance (teaching)

Implementation

PO route

- Do not break, crush, or chew ext rel products
- Give with meals or milk for GI symptoms, and 81-325 mg of aspirin or NSAIDs ½ hr before dose to decrease flushing

IV route

- Give by direct **IV** after diluting to 2 mg/ml at a rate of ≤2 mg/min
- Give by inf by adding 500 ml of 0.9% NaCl at a rate of ≤2 mg/min

Additive incompatibilities: Acids (strong), alkalis, erythromycin, kanamycin, streptomycin

Additive compatibilities: TPN sol

Patient/family education

- Advise patient that flushing and increase in feelings of warmth will occur several hr after taking drug (PO); after 2 wk of therapy these side effects diminish
- Instruct patient to remain recumbent if postural hypotension occurs; to rise slowly from sitting or recumbent
- Caution patient to abstain from alcohol if drug is prescribed for hyperlipidemia
- Caution patient to avoid sunlight if skin lesions are present
- Advise patient to report clay-colored stools, anorexia, jaundiced sclera, skin, dark urine; hepatotoxicity may occur

Evaluation

Positive therapeutic outcome

- Decreased lipid levels
- Warm extremities
- Absence of numbness in extremities

N

niCARdipine (Rx)

(nye-card'i-peen)

Cardene, Cardene IV, Cardene SR

Func. class.: Calcium channel blocker, antianginal, antihypertensive

Chem. class.: Dihydropyridine

Pregnancy category C

Action: Inhibits calcium ion influx across cell membrane during cardiac depolarization, produces relaxation of coronary vascular smooth muscle and peripheral vascular smooth muscle, dilates coronary arteries, increases myocardial oxygen delivery in patients with vasospastic angina

Therapeutic Outcome: Decreased angina pectoris, decreased B/P in hypertension

Uses: Chronic stable angina pectoris, hypertension

Dosage and routes

Hypertension

Adult: PO 20 mg tid initially; may increase after 3 days (range 20-40 mg tid) or 30 mg bid sus rel, may increase to 60 mg bid **IV** 5 mg/hr, may increase by 2.5 mg/hr q15min, max 15 mg/hr

Angina

Adult: PO 20 mg tid, may be adjusted q3d, may use 20-40 mg tid

Renal dose

Adult: PO 20 mg tid; or 30 mg bid (sus rel)

Hepatic dose

Adult: PO 20 mg bid

Available forms: Caps 20, 30 mg; sus rel caps 30, 45, 60 mg; inj 2.5 mg/ml

Adverse effects

CNS: Headache, dizziness, anxiety, depression, confusion, paresthesia, somnolence
CV: Edema, bradycardia, hypotension, palpitations, **pulmonary edema,** chest pain, tachycardia, increased angina, **arrhythmias, CHF**
GI: Nausea, vomiting, gastric upset, constipation, **hepatitis,** abdominal cramps, dry mouth, sore throat
GU: Nocturia, polyuria, impotence
INTEG: Rash, infusion site discomfort, **acute renal failure, Stevens-Johnson syndrome**
MISC: Blurred vision, flushing, sweating, shortness of breath

Contraindications: Sick sinus syndrome, 2nd- or 3rd-degree heart block, hypersensitivity

Precautions: Pregnancy **C,** CHF, hypotension, hepatic injury, lactation, children, renal disease, elderly

Pharmacokinetics

Absorption	Well absorbed (PO); bioavailability poor
Distribution	Unknown
Metabolism	Liver, extensively
Excretion	Kidneys 60%, feces 35%
Half-life	2-5 hr

Pharmacodynamics

	PO	PO–SUS REL
Onset	½ hr	Unknown
Peak	1-2 hr	2-6 hr
Duration	8 hr	10-12 hr

Interactions

Individual drugs

Alcohol: increased hypotension
Carbamazepine, cycloSPORINE, prazosin, propranolol, quinidine: increased risk of toxicity
Cimetidine: increased nicardipine effects
Digitalis, quinidine, theophylline: increased effects
Rifampin: decreased niCARdipine effect

Drug classifications

Antihypertensives, neuromuscular blocking agents, nitrates: increased hypotension
NSAIDs: decreased antihypertensive effect

Drug/herb

Barberry, betel palm, burdock, goldenseal, khat, khella, lily of the valley, plantain: increased effect
Yohimbe: decreased effect

Drug/food

Grapefruit juice: increased hypotensive effect

NURSING CONSIDERATIONS

Assessment

- Assess fluid volume status (I&O ratio) and record weight, color, quality and sp gr of urine, skin turgor, adequacy of pulses, moist mucous membranes, bilateral lung sounds, peripheral pitting edema; dehydration symptoms of decreasing output, thirst, hypotension, dry mouth, and mucous membranes should be reported
- Monitor for CHF: weight gain, crackles, jugular venous distention, dyspnea
- Monitor B/P and pulse
- Assess anginal pain: intensity, location, duration, alleviating factors
- Monitor potassium, liver function tests, renal studies periodically

Nursing diagnoses

- Cardiac output, decreased (uses)
- Knowledge, deficient (teaching)

Implementation

PO route

- Do not break, crush, chew, or open sus rel caps
- Give with or without regard to meals
- Store in airtight container at room temp

IV route

- Dilute each 25 mg/240 ml of compatible sol (0.1 mg/ml), give slowly, stable for 24 hr at room temp

Solution compatibilities: D_5W, D_5/0.45% NaCl, D_5/0.9% NaCl
Y-site compatibilities: Diltiazem, DOBUTamine, DOPamine, epINEPHrine, fentanyl, hydromorphone, labetalol, loraze-

pam, midazolam, milrinone, morphine, nitroglycerin, norepinephrine, ranitidine, vecuronium

Patient/family education

- Advise patient to avoid hazardous activities until stabilized on drug and dizziness is no longer a problem
- Instruct patient to limit caffeine consumption; to avoid alcohol and OTC drugs unless directed by a prescriber
- Instruct patient to comply in all areas of medical regimen: diet, exercise, stress reduction, drug therapy; to notify prescriber of irregular heart beat, shortness of breath, swelling of feet and hands, pronounced dizziness, constipation, nausea, hypotension
- Teach patient to use medication as directed even if feeling better; may be taken with other cardiovascular drugs (nitrates, β-blockers)
- Teach patient to take medication exactly as prescribed
- Advise patient to contact prescriber if anginal attacks continue or become worse

Evaluation

Positive therapeutic outcome

- Decreased angina attacks
- Decreased B/P

Treatment of overdose: Defibrillation, atropine for AV block, vasopressor for hypotension

nicotinamide

See niacin

nicotine (OTC)

(nik'o-teen)

nicotine chewing gum (OTC)

Nicorette

nicotine inhaler (Rx)

Nicotrol Inhaler

nicotine nasal spray (Rx)

Nicotrol NS

nicotine transdermal (OTC)

Clear Nicoderm CQ, Habitrol, NicoDerm CQ, Nicotrol

Func. class.: Smoking deterrent

Chem. class.: Ganglionic cholinergic agonist

Pregnancy category D (transdermal), X (gum)

Action: Agonist at nicotinic receptors in the peripheral and central nervous systems; acts at sympathetic ganglia, on chemoreceptors of the aorta and carotid bodies; also affects adrenalin-releasing catecholamines

Therapeutic Outcome: Decreased withdrawal effects when smoking cessation is attempted

Uses: Deter cigarette smoking

Investigational uses: Gilles de la Tourette's syndrome

Dosage and routes

Habitrol, NicoDerm

Adult: 21 mg/day × 4-8 wk; 14 mg/day × 2-4 wk; 7 mg/day × 2-4 wk

Nicotine chewing gum

Adult: Gum 1 piece chewed × 30 min as needed to abstain from smoking; not to exceed 30/day

Nicotine inhaler

Adult: Inhale 6 cartridges/day for first 3-6 wk, max 16/day × 12 wk

Nicotine nasal spray

Adult: 1 spray in each nostril 1-2 ×/hr, max 5 ×/hr or 40 ×/day, max 3 mo

Nicotrol

Adult: 15 mg/day × 12 wk; 10 mg/day × 2 wk; 5 mg/day × 2 wk

Nicotrol Inhaler

Adult: Delivers 30% of what a smoker receives from an actual cigarette

Gilles de la Tourette's Syndrome (off-label)

Adult/child: Chewing gum 2 mg chewed × ½ hr bid × 1-6 mo; TD 7 or 10 mg patch daily × 2 days

Available forms: Gum: 2 mg/piece; nicotine transdermal system: (Habitrol, NicoDerm, Nicotine Transdermal System) 7, 14, 21 mg/day delivered; (NicoDerm) 5, 10, 15 mg/day; nicotine inhaler: 4 mg delivered; nasal spray: 0.5 mg of nicotine/actuation

Adverse effects

CNS: Dizziness, vertigo, insomnia, headache, confusion, convulsions, depression, euphoria, numbness, tinnitus, strange dreams

CV: **Dysrhythmias,** tachycardia, palpitations, edema, flushing, hypertension

EENT: Jaw ache, irritation in buccal cavity

GI: *Nausea, vomiting, anorexia, indigestion,* diarrhea, abdominal pain, constipation, eructation

RESP: Breathing difficulty, cough, hoarseness, sneezing, wheezing

N

Contraindications: Pregnancy **X** (gum), **D** (transdermal), hypersensitivity, immediate post-MI recovery period, severe angina pectoris

Precautions: Vasospastic disease, dysrhythmias, diabetes mellitus, hyperthyroidism, pheochromocytoma, coronary disease, esophagitis, peptic ulcer, lactation, hepatic/renal disease

Pharmacokinetics	
Absorption	Slowly absorbed, buccal cavity
Distribution	Unknown
Metabolism	Liver; some by lungs, kidneys
Excretion	Kidneys, unchanged (20%); breast milk
Half-life	1-2 hr

Pharmacodynamics	
Onset	Rapid
Peak	½ hr
Duration	Unknown

Interactions
Individual drugs
Acetaminophen, caffeine, furosemide, imipramine, oxazepam, pentazocine, propranolol: increased effects of each specific drug with cessation of smoking
Glutethimide: decreased absorption
Insulin (SUBCUT): increased absorption
Propoxyphene: decreased propoxyphene metabolism
Theophylline: increased blood levels with cessation of smoking

Drug/herb
Blue cohosh, lobelia: increased effect
Oats: decreased effect

NURSING CONSIDERATIONS
Assessment
- Assess for adverse reaction to gum: irritation of buccal cavity, dislike of taste, jaw ache
- Assess for withdrawal symptoms: headache, fatigue, drowsiness, restlessness, irritability, severe cravings for nicotine products before, during, and after treatment
- Obtain a nicotine assessment: brand of cigarettes, chewing tobacco, cigars, number of each used per day; what increases need or activities performed when each is used
- Gum should not be used if temporomandibular condition exists
- Assess for nicotine toxicity: GI symptoms (nausea, vomiting, diarrhea), cardiopulmonary symptoms (decreased B/P, dyspnea, change in pulse), weakness, abdominal cramping, headache, blurred vision, tinnitus; drug should be discontinued

Nursing diagnoses
- Coping, ineffective (uses)
- Knowledge, deficient (teaching)
- Noncompliance (teaching)

Implementation
- Give only prescribed amount, or toxicity may occur
- Protect gum from light and heat

Patient/family education
- Advise patient to begin drug withdrawal after 3 mo use; do not exceed 6 mo
- Teach patient all aspects of drug; give package insert to patient and explain; caution patient not to exceed prescribed dose
- Caution patient not to use during pregnancy; birth defects may occur

Gum
- Advise patient to chew gum slowly for 30 min to promote buccal absorption of the drug; do not chew over 45 min
- Inform patient that gum will not stick to dentures, dental appliances
- Caution patient that gum is as toxic as cigarettes; it is to be used only to deter smoking

Transdermal patch
- Caution patient that patch is as toxic as cigarettes; to be used only to deter smoking
- Caution patient not to use during pregnancy; birth defects may occur
- Instruct patient to keep used and unused system out of reach of children and pets
- Instruct patient to apply once a day to a nonhairy, clean, dry area of skin on upper body or upper outer arm; to rotate sites to prevent skin irritation
- Instruct patient to stop smoking immediately when beginning patch treatment
- Teach patient to apply promptly after removing from protective pouch; system may lose strength

Inhaler
- Advise patient that puffing on mouthpiece delivers nicotine through the mouth lining

Evaluation
Positive therapeutic outcome
- Decrease in urge to smoke
- Decreased need for gum after 3-6 mo

NIFEdipine (Rx)

(nye-fed'i-peen)

Adalat, Adalat CC, Apo-Nifed ✤, Novo-Nifedin ✤, Nu-Nifedin ✤, NIFEdipine, Procardia, Procardia XL

Func. class.: Calcium channel blocker, antianginal, antihypertensive

Chem. class.: Dihydropyridine

Pregnancy category C

Do Not Confuse:

NIFEdipine/niCARdipine

Action: Inhibits calcium ion influx across cell membrane during cardiac depolarization, produces relaxation of coronary vascular smooth muscle and peripheral vascular smooth muscle, dilates coronary vascular arteries, increases myocardial oxygen delivery in patients with vasospastic angina

Therapeutic Outcome: Decreased angina pectoris, decreased B/P in hypertension

Uses: Chronic stable angina pectoris, vasospastic angina, hypertension

Investigational uses: Migraines, CHF, Raynaud's disease, anal fissures

Dosage and routes

Adult: PO immediate release, 10 mg tid; increase in 10 mg increments q7-14 days, max 180 mg/24 hr or single dose of 30 mg; sus rel, 30-60 mg/day; may increase q7-14 days; doses >120 mg not recommended

Child: PO 0.25-0.5 mg/kg/dose q4-6h, max 1-2 mg/kg/day

Anal fissures (off-label)

Adult: TOP 0.2% gel q12h × 21 days

Available forms: Caps 5, 10, 20 mg; ext rel tabs (CC, XL) 10 ✤, 20 ✤, 30, 60, 90 mg; tabs 10 mg; gel 0.2%

Adverse effects

CNS: *Headache,* fatigue, drowsiness, *dizziness,* anxiety, depression, weakness, insomnia, *lightheadedness,* paresthesia, tinnitus, blurred vision, nervousness, tremor

CV: **Dysrhythmias,** edema, hypotension, palpitations, tachycardia

GI: *Nausea,* vomiting, diarrhea, gastric upset, constipation, increased liver function studies, dry mouth, flatulence, gingival hyperplasia, **hepatotoxicity**

GU: Nocturia, polyuria

INTEG: Rash, pruritus, *flushing,* hair loss

MISC: Sexual difficulties, cough, fever, chills

SYST: **Stevens-Johnson syndrome**

Contraindications: Hypersensitivity

Precautions: Pregnancy **C,** CHF, hypotension, sick sinus syndrome, 2nd- or 3rd-degree heart block, hypotension less than 90 mm Hg systolic, hepatic injury, lactation, children, renal disease

Pharmacokinetics

Absorption	Well absorbed (PO)
Distribution	Unknown
Metabolism	Liver, extensively
Excretion	Unknown
Half-life	2-5 hr

Pharmacodynamics

	PO	PO–EXT REL
Onset	½ hr	Unknown
Peak	Unknown	Unknown
Duration	6-8 hr	24 hr

Interactions

Individual drugs

Carbamazepine, cimetidine, cycloSPORINE, phenytoin, prazosin, ranitidine: increased risk of toxicity

Digoxin: increased digoxin levels, bradycardia, CHF

Quinidine: decreased effects

Smoking: decreased NIFEdipine level

Drug classifications

Antihypertensives, β-adrenergic blockers: increased effects

NSAIDs: decreased antihypertensive effect

Drug/herb

Barberry, betel palm, burdock, goldenseal, khat, khella, lily of the valley, plaintain: increased effect

Yohimbe: decreased effect

Drug/food

Grapefruit juice: increased NIFEdipine level

Drug/lab test

Positive: ANA titer, direct Coombs' test

Increased: CPK, LDH, AST

NURSING CONSIDERATIONS

Assessment

- Assess anginal pain: location, intensity, duration, character, alleviating, aggravating factors
- Monitor potassium, liver function tests, renal studies periodically during treatment
- Assess fluid volume status (I&O ratio) and record weight, distended red veins, crackles in lung, color, quality and sp gr of urine, skin turgor, adequacy of pulses, moist mucous membranes, bilateral lung sounds, peripheral pitting edema; dehydration symptoms of decreasing output, thirst, hypotension, dry

N

mouth, and mucous membranes should be reported
- Monitor ALT, AST, bilirubin daily; if these are elevated, hepatotoxicity is suspected
- Monitor cardiac status: B/P, pulse, respirations, ECG

Nursing diagnoses
- Cardiac output, decreased (uses)
- Pain, acute (uses)
- Knowledge, deficient (teaching)

Implementation
PO route
- Give without regard to meals
- Store in airtight container at room temp

Sublingual route
- Using a sterile needle puncture the cap and squeeze medication in buccal area (not an FDA-approved use)

Patient/family education
- Advise patient to avoid hazardous activities until stabilized on drug and dizziness is no longer a problem
- Instruct patient to limit caffeine consumption; to avoid alcohol and OTC drugs unless directed by prescriber
- Tell patient that ext rel tab has nonabsorbable shell, may appear in stools
- Instruct patient to comply in all areas of medical regimen: diet, exercise, stress reduction, drug therapy; to notify prescriber of irregular heart beat, shortness of breath, swelling of feet and hands, pronounced dizziness, constipation, nausea, hypotension, severe rash
- Teach patient to use as directed even if feeling better; may be taken with other cardiovascular drugs (nitrates, β-blockers)
- Advise patient to increase fluid intake to prevent constipation
- Teach patient to check for gingival hyperplasia and report promptly

Evaluation
Positive therapeutic outcome
- Decreased angina attacks
- Decreased B/P

Treatment of overdose: Defibrillation, atropine for AV block, vasopressor for hypotension

nilutamide (Rx)
(nil-u'ta-mide)

Anandron ♣, Nilandron

Func. class.: Antineoplastic, hormone

Chem. class.: Antiandrogen

Pregnancy category C

Action: Interferes with testosterone uptake in the nucleus or testosterone activity in target tissues; arrests tumor growth in androgen-sensitive tissue, i.e., prostate gland, prostatic carcinoma is androgen-sensitive, so tumor growth is arrested

Therapeutic Outcome: Decreased tumor size

Uses: Metastatic prostatic carcinoma, stage D2 in combination with surgical castration

Dosage and routes
Adult: PO 300 mg daily × 30 days, then 150 mg daily

Available forms: Tabs 100 ♣, 150 mg

Adverse effects
CNS: Hot flashes, drowsiness, insomnia, dizziness, hyperthesia, depression

EENT: Delay in adaptation to dark

GI: Diarrhea, nausea, vomiting, elevated liver function studies, constipation, dyspepsia, **hepatotoxicity**

GU: Decreased libido, impotence, testicular atrophy, UTI, hematuria, nocturia, gynecomastia

HEMA: Anemia

INTEG: Rash, sweating, alopecia, dry skin

MISC: Edema

RESP: Dyspnea, URI, pneumonia, **interstitial pneumonitis**

Contraindications: Hypersensitivity, severe hepatic impairment, severe respiratory disease, women

Precautions: Pregnancy **C**

Pharmacokinetics

Absorption	Rapidly, completely
Distribution	Unknown
Metabolism	Unknown
Excretion	Urine, feces
Half-life	Unknown

Pharmacodynamics
Unknown

Interactions
Individual drugs

Phenytoin, theophylline, vitamin K: increased toxicity

NURSING CONSIDERATIONS
Assessment
- Monitor liver function studies: AST, ALT, alkaline phosphatase, which may be elevated; if elevated 3 × normal, discontinue drug
- Monitor for CNS symptoms: drowsiness, insomnia, dizziness
- Monitor chest x-rays routinely, baseline pulmonary function studies, dyspnea, cough, may indicate interstitial pneumonitis, discontinue treatment if this condition is suspected
- Monitor for hyperglycemia, increased BUN, creatinine, alkaline phosphatase leukopenia

Nursing diagnoses
- Infection, risk for (side effects)
- Knowledge, deficient (teaching)

Implementation
- Administer without regard to meals
- Store at room temp

Patient/family education
- Advise patient to report side effects: decreased libido, impotence, breast enlargement, hot flashes, diarrhea, dyspnea, cough; symptoms of hepatotoxicity (dark urine, abdominal pain, clay-colored stools, jaundiced eyes, skin); notify prescriber immediately if shortness of breath occurs
- Advise patient to wear tinted lens to alleviate delay in adapting to the dark
- Advise patient that drug is started on day of or day after surgical castration
- Advise patient to avoid alcohol consumption

Evaluation
Positive therapeutic outcome
- Decrease in prostatic tumor size, decrease in spread of cancer

Treatment of overdose: Induce vomiting, provide supportive care

nimodipine (Rx)
(ni-moe′dip-een)
Nimotop
Func. class.: Calcium channel blocker
Chem. class.: Dihydropyridine
Pregnancy category C

Action: Unknown, may have greater effect on cerebral arteries

Therapeutic Outcome: Prevention of vascular spasm (subarachnoid hemorrhage)

Uses: Prevention of cerebral vascular spasm in subarachnoid hemorrhage

Dosage and routes
Adult: PO Begin therapy within 96 hr, 60 mg q4h × 21 days

Available forms: Caps 30 mg

Adverse effects
CNS: Headache, fatigue, drowsiness, dizziness, anxiety, depression, weakness, insomnia, confusion, paresthesia, somnolence
CV: Dysrhythmia, edema, CHF, bradycardia, hypotension, palpitations, **MI, pulmonary edema**
GI: Nausea, vomiting, diarrhea, gastric upset, constipation, **hepatitis,** abdominal cramps
GU: Nocturia, polyuria, **acute renal failure**
INTEG: Rash, pruritus, urticaria, photosensitivity, hair loss
MISC: Blurred vision, flushing, nasal congestion, sweating, shortness of breath, gynecomastia, hyperglycemia, sexual difficulties

Contraindications: Sick sinus syndrome, 2nd- or 3rd-degree heart block, hypotension less than 90 mm Hg systolic, hypersensitivity

Precautions: Pregnancy **C,** CHF, hypotension, hepatic injury, lactation, children, renal disease, elderly

Pharmacokinetics	
Absorption	Well absorbed, bioavailability poor
Distribution	Crosses blood-brain barrier
Metabolism	Liver, extensively
Excretion	Kidneys
Half-life	1-2 hr

Pharmacodynamics	
Onset	Unknown
Peak	1 hr
Duration	Unknown

Interactions
Individual drugs
Alcohol: increased hypotension
Digoxin: increased digoxin levels, bradycardia
Phenobarbital, phenytoin: decreased effectiveness
Propranolol: increased toxicity
Drug classifications
Antihypertensives: increased hypotension
β-Adrenergic blockers: increased bradycardia
Nitrates: increased nitrates
Drug/herb
Barberry, betel palm, burdock, goldenseal, khat, khella, lily of the valley, plaintain: increased effect
Yohimbe: decreased effect

N

NURSING CONSIDERATIONS

Assessment

- Assess fluid volume status (I&O ratio) and record weight, distended red veins, crackles in lung, color, quality and sp gr of urine, skin turgor, adequacy of pulses, moist mucous membranes, bilateral lung sounds, peripheral pitting edema; dehydration symptoms of decreasing output, thirst, hypotension, dry mouth and mucous membranes should be reported
- Monitor B/P and pulse; if B/P drops 30 mm Hg, call prescriber
- Monitor ALT, AST, bilirubin daily; if these are elevated, hepatotoxicity is suspected

Nursing diagnoses

- Injury, risk for (uses)
- Knowledge, deficient (teaching)

Implementation

- May puncture cap and dilute in water and give through nasogastric tube; flush tube with 0.9% NaCl
- Store in airtight container at room temp

Evaluation

Positive therapeutic outcome

- Prevention of neurologic damage from subarachnoid hemorrhage

nisoldipine (Rx)

(nye'sol-dye-peen)

Sular

Func. class.: Antihypertensive, calcium channel blocker

Chem. class.: Dihydropyridine

Pregnancy category C

Action: Inhibits calcium ion influx across cell membrane, resulting in dilation of peripheral arteries

Therapeutic Outcome: Decreased B/P in hypertension

Uses: Essential hypertension, alone or with other antihypertensives

Dosage and routes

Adult: PO 20 mg daily initially, may increase by 10 mg/wk, usual dose 20-40 mg daily, max 60 mg/day

Elderly/hepatic dose: PO 10 mg/day, increase by 10 mg/wk

Available forms: Ext rel tabs 10, 20, 30, 40 mg

Adverse effects

CNS: Headache, fatigue, drowsiness, dizziness, anxiety, depression, nervousness, insomnia, light-headedness, paresthesia, tinnitus, psychosis, somnolence, ataxia, confusion, malaise, migraine

CV: **Dysrhythmias**, edema, **CHF**, hypotension, palpitations, **MI, pulmonary edema,** tachycardia, syncope, AV block, angina, chest pain, ECG abnormalities

GI: Nausea, vomiting, diarrhea, gastric upset, constipation, elevated liver function studies, dry mouth, dyspepsia, dysphagia, flatulence

GU: Nocturia, hematuria, dysuria

HEMA: Anemia, leukopenia, petechiae

INTEG: Rash, pruritus

MISC: Sexual difficulties, gingival hyperplasia, chills, fever, gout, sweating, cough, nasal congestion, shortness of breath, wheezing, epistaxis, dyspnea

Contraindications: Hypersensitivity, sick sinus syndrome, 2nd- or 3rd-degree heart block

Precautions: Pregnancy **C**, CHF, hypotension <90 mm Hg systolic, hepatic injury, lactation, children, renal disease, elderly, acute MI, unstable angina

Pharmacokinetics	
Absorption	Well absorbed
Distribution	Highly protein bound
Metabolism	Liver
Excretion	Kidneys
Half-life	Unknown

Pharmacodynamics	
Peak	6-12 hr

Interactions

Individual drugs

Cimetidine, ranitidine: increased nisoldipine level

Digitalis: increased effects

Drug classifications

Antifungals (azole): increased nisoldipine level

Antihypertensives: increased hypotension

β-Adrenergic blockers: increased bradycardia, CHF

Hydantoins: decreased nisoldipine effect

Drug/herb

Barberry, betel palm, burdock, goldenseal, khat, khella, lily of the valley, plaintain: increased effect

Yohimbe: decreased effect

Drug/food

Grapefruit juice: increased hypotension

High-fat: increased nisoldipine level

NURSING CONSIDERATIONS
Assessment
- Assess fluid volume status: I&O ratio and record; weight; skin turgor; adequacy of pulses; moist mucous membranes; bilateral lung sounds; peripheral pitting edema; dehydration symptoms of decreasing output, thirst, hypotension, dry mouth, and mucous membranes should be reported
- Monitor ALT, AST, bilirubin daily, if these are elevated and hepatotoxicity is suspected
- Monitor cardiac status: B/P, pulse, respiration, ECG

Nursing diagnoses
- Cardiac output, decreased (uses)
- Knowledge, deficient (teaching)

Implementation
- Give once a day, with food to decrease GI symptoms, avoid high-fat foods, grapefruit

Patient/family education
- Caution patient to avoid hazardous activities until stabilized on drug and dizziness is no longer a problem
- Instruct patient to limit caffeine consumption; to avoid alcohol and OTC drugs unless directed by prescriber
- Urge patient to comply in all areas of medical regimen: diet, exercise, stress reduction, drug therapy; to notify prescriber of irregular heart beat, shortness of breath, swelling of feet and hands, pronounced dizziness, constipation, nausea, hypotension
- Teach patient to use as directed even if feeling better; may be taken with other cardiovascular drugs (nitrates, β-blockers)
- Advise patient to rise slowly to prevent orthostatic hypotension
- Teach patient to report nausea, dizziness, edema, shortness of breath, palpitations

Evaluation
Positive therapeutic outcome
- Decreased B/P

nitazoxanide (Rx)
(nye-taz-ox'a-nide)
Alinia
Func. class.: Antiprotozoal
Pregnancy category B

Action: Interferes with DNA/RNA synthesis in protozoa

Therapeutic Outcome: C&S negative for organism

Uses: Diarrhea caused by *Cryptosporidium parvum* or *Giardia lamblia*

Dosage and routes
Child 4-11 yr: **PO** 10 ml (200 mg) q12h × 3 days
Child 12-47 mo: **PO** 5 ml (100 mg) q12h × 3 days

Available forms: Powder for oral susp 100 mg/5 ml

Adverse effects
CNS: *Dizziness, fever, headache*
CV: Hypotension
GI: *Nausea,* anorexia, flatulence, increased appetite, enlarged salivary glands, abdominal pain, diarrhea, vomiting
HEMA: Anemia, **leukopenia,** neutropenia
INTEG: Pruritus, sweating
MISC: Increased creatinine, pale yellow eye discoloration, rhinitis, discolored urine, infection, malaise

Contraindications: Hypersensitivity

Precautions: Pregnancy **B,** renal, hepatic disease, lactation, children <1 yr or >11 yr, diabetes mellitus (contains sucrose)

Pharmacokinetics	
Absorption	Unknown
Distribution	Metabolite protein binding >99%
Metabolism	Hydrolyzed to active metabolite, undergoes conjugation
Excretion	Urine, bile, feces
Half-life	Unknown

Pharmacodynamics
Unknown

Interactions
Drug classifications
Other highly protein bound drugs: competes for binding sites

NURSING CONSIDERATIONS
Assessment
- Assess for signs of infection
- Assess bowel pattern before, during treatment

Nursing diagnoses
- Infection, risk for (uses)
- Knowledge, deficient (teaching)

Implementation
PO route
- Give with food

Patient/family education
- Advise to take with food; shake susp well before each dose

N

Evaluation
Positive therapeutic outcome
- C&S negative for organism

nitrofurantoin (Rx)
(nye-troe-fyoor'an-toyn)
Apo-Nitrofurantoin ✤, Furadantin, Macrobid, Macrodantin, nitrofurantoin
Func. class.: Urinary tract antiinfective
Chem. class.: Synthetic nitrofuran derivative
Pregnancy category B

Action: Appears to inhibit bacterial enzymes

Therapeutic Outcome: Resolution of infection

Uses: Urinary tract infections caused by *Escherichia coli, Klebsiella, Pseudomonas, Proteus vulgaris, Proteus morganii, Serratia, Citrobacter, Staphylococcus aureus, Staphylococcus epidermidis, Enterococcus, Salmonella, Shigella*

Dosage and routes
Active infections
Adult and child >12 yr: PO 50-100 mg qid pc or 50-100 mg at bedtime for long-term treatment
Child 1 mo-3 yr: PO 5-7 mg/kg/day in 4 divided doses; 1-3 mg/kg/day for long-term treatment

Chronic suppression
Adult: PO 50-100 mg q PM
Child: PO 1 mg/kg/day q PM

Available forms: Caps 25, 50, 100 mg; tabs 50, 100 mg; susp 25 mg/ml; macrocrystal caps (Macrodantin) 25, 50, 100 mg; cap (Macrobid) 100 mg (25 macrocrystals, 75 monohydrate)

Adverse effects
CNS: *Dizziness, headache,* drowsiness, peripheral neuropathy, chills
GI: *Nausea, vomiting, abdominal pain, diarrhea,* **cholestatic jaundice**, loss of appetite, **pseudomembranous colitis**
INTEG: Pruritus, rash, urticaria, angioedema, alopecia, tooth staining

Contraindications: Hypersensitivity, anuria, severe renal disease, infants <1 mo

Precautions: Pregnancy **B,** lactation, G6PD deficiency, elderly, CCr <60

Pharmacokinetics
Absorption	Readily
Distribution	Crosses placenta, excreted in breast milk
Metabolism	Liver, partially
Excretion	Kidneys, 30%-50% unchanged
Half-life	20-60 min

Pharmacodynamics
Onset	Unknown
Peak	30 min
Duration	6-12 hr

Interactions
Individual drugs
Magnesium trisilicate: decreased absorption
Norfloxacin: antagonist effect
Probenecid: increased nitrofurantoin levels

NURSING CONSIDERATIONS
Assessment
- Monitor blood count during chronic therapy
- Monitor I/O ratio: C&S before treatment, after completion; symptoms of UTI
- Assess CNS symptoms: insomnia, vertigo, headache, drowsiness, convulsions
- Assess allergy: fever, flushing, rash, urticaria, pruritus

Nursing diagnoses
- Infection, risk for (uses)
- Knowledge, deficient (teaching)

Implementation
- Do not break, crush, chew, or open tabs, caps
- Give after clean-catch urine for C&S
- Give two daily doses if urine output is high or if patient has diabetes

Patient/family education
- Teach patient to take with food or milk; avoid alcohol
- Teach patient to protect susp from freezing and shake well before taking
- Teach patient that drug may cause drowsiness; instruct client to seek aid in walking and other activities; advise client not to drive or operate machinery while on medication
- Teach patient that diabetics should monitor blood glucose level
- Teach patient that drug may turn urine rust-yellow to brown
- ⚠ Teach patient to notify prescriber of symptoms of pseudomembranous colitis: fever, diarrhea with mucous, pus, or blood

Evaluation

Positive therapeutic outcome

- Decreased dysuria, fever; negative C&S

nitroglycerin (Rx)

(nye-troe-gli'ser-in)

transmucosal tablets (Rx)

Nitrogard, Nitrogard SR ♣

extended release (Rx)

Nitrocot, Nitroglyn E-R, Nitro-par, Nitro-Time, Nitrong

extended release buccal tabs (Rx)

Nitrogard, Nitrogard SR ♣

intravenous (Rx)

Nitro-Bid IV, Tridil

spray (Rx)

Nitrolingual Translingual Spray

sublingual (Rx)

Nitrostat, NitroQuick

topical ointment (Rx)

Nitro-Bid, Nitrol

transdermal (Rx)

Deponit, Minitran, Nitrek, Nitrocine, Nitrodisc, Nitro-Dur, Transderm-Nitro

Func. class.: Coronary vasodilator, antianginal

Chem. class.: Nitrate

Pregnancy category C

Do Not Confuse:
Nitro-Bid/Nicobid

Action: Decreases preload and afterload, which thus decreases left ventricular end-diastolic pressure and systemic vascular resistance; dilates coronary arteries and improves blood flow through coronary vasculature, dilates arterial, venous beds systemically

Therapeutic Outcome: Prevention of anginal attack

Uses: Chronic stable angina pectoris, prophylaxis of angina pain, CHF associated with acute MI, controlled hypotension in surgical procedures

Dosage and routes

Adult: SL dissolve tab under tongue when pain begins; may repeat q5 min until relief occurs; take no more than 3 tab/15 min; use 1 tab prophylactically 5-10 min before activities; sus rel cap q6-12h on empty stomach; top 1-2 in q8h; increase to 4 in q4h as needed; **IV** 5 mcg/min, then increase by 5 mcg/min q3-5 min; if no response after 20 mcg/min, increase by 10-20 mcg/min until desired response; TD apply a pad daily to a site free from hair; remove patch at bedtime to provide 10-12 hr nitrate-free interval to avoid tolerance

Child: **IV** initial 0.25-0.5 mg/kg/min, titrate to patient response, usual dose 1-3 mg/kg/min

Available forms: Buccal tabs 1, 2, 3 mg; translingual aerosol 0.4 mg/m spray; sus rel caps 2.5, 6.5, 9, 13 mg; sus rel tabs 2.6, 6.5, 9 mg; SL tabs 0.3, 0.4, 0.6 mg; oint 2%; trans syst 0.1, 0.2, 0.3, 0.4, 0.6, 0.8 mg/hr; inj 25 mg/250 ml, 50 mg/250 ml, 100 mg/250 ml, 50 mg/500 ml, 100 mg/500 ml, 200 mg/500 ml

Adverse effects

CNS: *Headache, flushing, dizziness*

CV: *Postural hypotension,* tachycardia, **collapse,** syncope, palpitations

GI: Nausea, vomiting

INTEG: Pallor, sweating, rash

Contraindications: Hypersensitivity to this drug or nitrites, severe anemia, increased ICP, cerebral hemorrhage, closed-angle glaucoma

Precautions: Pregnancy **C,** postural hypotension, lactation, children, severe renal/hepatic disease

Pharmacokinetics

Absorption	Well absorbed (PO, buccal, SL)
Distribution	Unknown
Metabolism	Liver, extensively
Excretion	Kidney
Half-life	1-4 min

Interactions

Individual drugs

Alcohol: increased hypotension, CV collapse
Aspirin: increased nitrate level

Pharmacodynamics

	SUS REL	SL	TD	IV	TRANSMUCOSAL	AEROSOL	TOP OINT
Onset	20-45 min	1-3 min	½-1 hr	1-2 min	1-2 min	2 min	½-1 hr
Peak	Unknown	Unknown	Unknown	Unknown	Unknown	Unknown	Unknown
Duration	3-8 hr	½ hr	12-24 hr	3-5 min	3-5 hr	½-1 hr	2-12 hr

Heparin: decreased effects (with IV nitroglycerin)
Sildenafil, tadalafil, vardenafil: increased hypotension

Drug classifications
Antihypertensives, β-adrenergic blockers, calcium channel blockers, diuretics: increased hypotension

NURSING CONSIDERATIONS

Assessment
- Monitor orthostatic B/P, pulse
- Assess pain: duration, time started, activity being performed, character; check for tolerance if taken over long period
- Monitor for headache, lightheadedness, decreased B/P; may indicate a need for decreased dosage

Nursing diagnoses
- Cardiac output, decreased (uses)
- Poisoning, risk for (uses)
- Tissue perfusion, ineffective (uses)
- Knowledge, deficient (teaching)
- Noncompliance (teaching)

Implementation
PO route
- Swallow sus rel tabs whole; do not break, crush, or chew sus rel tabs
- Give 1 hr ac or 2 hr pc with 8 oz of water

Transmucosal route
- Tab should be placed between cheek and gum line
- Do not take anything PO when tab is in place

Topical route
- Apply ointment using dose-measuring papers supplied; apply to an area without hair; ointment should cover 2-3 in area; may apply an occlusive dressing as directed

Transdermal route
- Apply TD patches to area without hair; press hard to adhere; if patch becomes dislodged, apply a new one

SL route
- Keep tab in original container
- If 3 SL tab in 15 min do not relieve pain, consider diagnosis of MI
- SL tab should be held under tongue until dissolved (a few min); do not take anything by mouth when SL tab is in place

IV route
- Give **IV** diluted in amount specified D_5W, or 0.9% NaCl for inf; use glass inf bottles, non–polyvinyl chloride inf tubing; titrate to patient response; do not use filters

Y-site compatibilities: Amiodarone, amphotericin B cholesteryl, inamrinone, atracurium, cefmetazole, cisatracurium, diltiazem, DOBUTamine, DOPamine, epINEPHrine, esmolol, famotidine, fentanyl, fluconazole, furosemide, haloperidol, heparin, hydromorphone, regular insulin, labetalol, lidocaine, lorazepam, midazolam, milrinone, morphine, niCARdipine, nitroprusside, norepinephrine, pancuronium, ranitidine, remifentanil, streptokinase, tacrolimus, theophylline, vecuronium

Y-site incompatibilities: Alteplase

Additive compatibilities: Alteplase, aminophylline, DOBUTamine, DOPamine, enalaprilat, furosemide, lidocaine, verapamil

Additive incompatibilities: Manufacturer recommends that nitroglycerin not be admixed with other medications

Patient/family education
- Instruct patient to avoid alcohol
- Advise patient that drug may cause headache; tolerance usually develops; use nonopioid analgesic
- Teach patient that drug may be taken before stressful activity, exercise, sexual activity
- Inform patient that SL tab may sting when drug comes in contact with mucous membranes
- Caution patient to avoid hazardous activities if dizziness occurs
- Instruct patient to comply with complete medical regimen
- Advise patient to make position changes slowly to prevent fainting

Evaluation
Positive therapeutic outcome
- Decreased, prevention of anginal pain

! HIGH ALERT

nitroprusside (Rx)
(nye-troe-pruss'ide)

Nitropress, Sodium nitroprusside

Func. class.: Antihypertensive, vasodilator

Pregnancy category C

Action: Directly relaxes arteriolar, venous smooth muscle, resulting in reduction in cardiac preload, afterload

Therapeutic Outcome: Decreased B/P in hypertensive crisis, decreased preload, afterload

Uses: Hypertensive crisis, to decrease bleeding by creating hypotension during surgery, acute CHF

Dosage and routes

Adult: **IV** inf dissolve 50 mg in 2-3 ml of D_5W, then dilute in 250-1000 ml of D_5W; run at 0.5-8 mcg/kg/min

Child: **IV** 0.3-0.5 mg/kg/min, titrate to response

Available forms: Inj 50 mg

Adverse effects

CNS: *Dizziness, headache,* agitation, twitching, decreased reflexes, restlessness

CV: Bradycardia, ECG changes, tachycardia

GI: Nausea, vomiting, abdominal pain

INTEG: Pain, irritation at inj site, sweating

MISC: **Cyanide, thiocyanate toxicity,** flushing, hypothyroidism

Contraindications: Hypersensitivity, hypertension (compensatory) due to aortic coarctation or AV shunting, acute CHF associated with reduced peripheral vascular resistance

Precautions: Pregnancy **C,** lactation, children, fluid, electrolyte imbalances, hepatic disease, renal disease, hypothyroidism, elderly

Pharmacokinetics	
Absorption	Complete bioavailability
Distribution	Not known
Metabolism	RBCs, tissues
Excretion	Kidneys
Half-life	3 days; circulating half-life 2 min

Pharmacodynamics	
Onset	1-2 min
Peak	Rapid
Duration	1-10 min

Interactions

Drug classifications

Circulatory depressants, enflurane, ganglionic blockers, halothane, volatile liquid anesthetics: severe hypotension

Drug/herb

Aconite: increased toxicity, death

Astragalus, cola tree: increased or decreased antihypertensive effect

Barberry, betony, black catechu, black cohosh, bloodroot, broom, burdock, cat's claw, dandelion, goldenseal, Irish moss, Jamaican dogwood, kelp, khella, mistletoe, parsley: increased antihypertensive effect

Coltsfoot, guarana, khat, licorice: decreased antihypertensive effect

NURSING CONSIDERATIONS

Assessment

- Monitor B/P q5 min × 2 hr, then q1h × 2 hr; monitor pulse q4h; monitor jugular venous distention q4h; ECG should be monitored continuously; monitor PCWP; rebound hypertension may occur after nitroprusside is discontinued
- Monitor electrolytes, blood studies: potassium, sodium, chloride, CO_2, CBC, serum glucose, serum methemoglobin if pulmonary oxygen levels are decreased
- Check weight, I&O, edema in feet and legs daily; assess skin turgor, dryness of mucous membranes for hydration status
- Assess for signs of CHF: dyspnea, edema, wet crackles
- Monitor for increased lactate, cyanide, thiocyanate levels if on long-term treatment, thiocyanate level should be ≤1 millimole/L
- Monitor for decrease in bicarbonate, Pco_2 and blood pH; acidosis may occur with this drug

Nursing diagnoses

- Tissue perfusion, ineffective (uses)
- Injury, risk for (adverse reactions)
- Knowledge, deficient (teaching)

Implementation

- Give by cont inf after diluting 50 mg/2-3 ml of D_5W; further dilute in 250 ml of D_5W; use an infusion pump only; wrap bottle with aluminum foil to protect from light; observe for color change in inf; discard if highly discolored (blue, green, red); titrate to patient response; avoid extravasation

Syringe compatibilities: Heparin

Y-site compatibilities: Atracurium, diltiazem, DOBUTamine, DOPamine, enalaprilat, famotidine, inamrinone, lidocaine, nitroglycerin, pancuronium, tacrolimus, theophylline, vecuronium

Additive incompatibilities: Do not give with any other drugs

Patient/family education

- Teach patient to report headache, dizziness, loss of hearing, blurred vision, dyspnea, faintness; may indicate adverse reactions

Evaluation

Positive therapeutic outcome

- Decreased B/P in hypertension
- Absence of bleeding in surgery

Treatment of overdose: Administer amyl nitrate inh until 3% sodium nitrate sol can be prepared for **IV** administration, then inject sodium thiosulfate **IV**; correct drop in B/P with vasopressor

N

nizatidine (Rx, OTC)

(ni-za'ti-deen)

Axid, Axid AR

Func. class.: H_2-Receptor antagonist

Chem. class.: Substituted thiazole

Pregnancy category B

Action: Blocks H_2 receptors thereby reducing gastric acid output

Therapeutic Outcome: Healing of duodenal ulcers or gastric ulcers; prevention of duodenal ulcers; decreases symptoms of gastroesophageal reflex disease (GERD)

Uses: Benign gastric and duodenal ulceration, prevention of duodenal ulcer recurrence, symptomatic relief of gastroesophageal reflux, heartburn prevention

Dosage and routes

Prophylaxis of duodenal ulcer

Adult: PO 150 mg daily at bedtime

Gastric and duodenal ulcer disease

Adult: PO 300 mg at night or 150 mg bid for 4-8 wk; maintenance 150 mg at night

Gastroesophageal reflux

Adult: PO 150 mg bid

Heartburn prevention

Adult: PO 75 mg ac

Renal dose

Adult: PO CCr 20-50 ml/min give 150 mg/day; CCr <20 ml/min give 150 mg every other day

Available forms: Caps 150, 300 mg; tabs 75 mg

Adverse effects

CNS: Headache, somnolence, confusion, abnormal dreams, dizziness

CV: **Dysrhythmias, cardiac arrest**

ENDO: Gynecomastia

GI: Elevated liver enzymes, hepatitis, jaundice, nausea

HEMA: **Thrombocytopenia, agranulocytosis, aplastic anemia**

INTEG: Pruritus, sweating, urticaria, exfoliative dermatitis

META: Hyperuricemia

MS: Myalgia

RESP: **Bronchospasm, laryngeal edema**

Contraindications: Hypersensitivity

Precautions: Pregnancy **B**, renal or hepatic impairment (reduce dose in renal impairment), lactation

Pharmacokinetics

Absorption	PO 70%
Distribution	Breast milk, crosses placenta
Metabolism	Liver, partially
Excretion	Kidney
Half-life	1½ hr

Pharmacodynamics

Onset	Variable
Peak	½-3 hr
Duration	Unknown

NURSING CONSIDERATIONS

Assessment

- Assess patient with ulcers or suspected ulcers: epigastric or abdominal pain, hematemesis, occult blood in stools, blood or gastric aspirate before and throughout treatment, monitor gastric pH (5 should be maintained)
- ◆ Monitor I&O ratio, BUN, creatinine, CBC with differential monthly; agranulocytosis may occur

Nursing diagnoses

- Pain, chronic (uses)
- Knowledge, deficient (teaching)

Implementation

- May be given with or without meals
- Give antacids 1 hr before or 1 hr after this drug

Patient/family education

- Caution patient that gynecomastia, impotence may occur and are reversible after treatment is discontinued
- Advise patient to avoid driving, other hazardous activities until stabilized on this medication; drowsiness or dizziness may occur
- Caution patient to avoid black pepper, caffeine, alcohol, harsh spices, extremes in temp of food; tell patient to avoid OTC preparations: aspirin, cough, cold preparations because condition may worsen
- Caution patient not to take OTC and ℞ forms concurrently
- Inform patient that smoking decreases the effectiveness of the drug; that smoking cessation should be considered
- Instruct patient that drug must be continued for prescribed time to be effective and taken exactly as prescribed; doses should not be doubled; a missed dose should be taken as soon as remembered up to 1 hr before next dose
- Advise patient to report bruising, fatigue, malaise; blood dyscrasias may occur
- Advise patient to report diarrhea, black tarry

stools, sore throat, rash, dizziness, confusion, or delirium to prescriber immediately

Evaluation

Positive therapeutic outcome

- Decreased pain in abdomen
- Healing of ulcers
- Absence of gastroesophageal reflux

norfloxacin (Rx)

(nor-flox'a-sin)

Noroxin

Func. class.: Antiinfective—urinary

Chem. class.: Fluoroquinolone antibacterial

Pregnancy category C

Action: Interferes with conversion intermediate DNA fragments into high-molecular weight DNA in bacteria

Therapeutic Outcome: Bactericidal action against gram-positive *Staphylococcus epidermidis,* methicillin-resistant strains of *Staphylococcus aureus,* group D streptococci; gram-negative *Escherichia coli, Klebsiella pneumoniae, Enterobacter cloacae, Proteus mirabilis, Proteus vulgaris, Providencia rettgeri, Morganella morganii, Pseudomonas aeruginosa, Citrobacter freundii*

Uses: Adult UTIs (including complicated), uncomplicated gonorrhea

Dosage and routes

Uncomplicated infections

Adult: PO 400 mg bid × 3-10 days 1 hr ac or 2 hr pc

Complicated infections

Adult: PO 400 mg bid × 10-21 days; 400 mg daily × 7-10 days in impaired renal function

Uncomplicated gonorrhea

Adult: PO 800 mg as a single dose

Prostatitis

Adult: PO 400 mg bid × 4 wk

Ocular infection

Adult and child: Ophth 1 gtt qid; may increase to 1 gtt q2h for severe infections

Renal dose

Adult: PO CCr ≤30 ml/min 400 mg PO daily

Available forms: Tabs 400 mg

Adverse effects

CNS: *Headache, dizziness,* fatigue, somnolence, depression, insomnia

EENT: Visual disturbances

GI: *Nausea,* constipation, increased ALT, AST, flatulence, heartburn, vomiting, diarrhea, dry mouth

INTEG: Rash

Contraindications: Hypersensitivity to quinolones

Precautions: Pregnancy **C**, lactation, children, renal disease, seizure disorders

Pharmacokinetics

Absorption	30% (PO)
Distribution	Concentration in urinary system
Metabolism	Liver (minimal)
Excretion	Kidneys, unchanged (30%)
Half-life	3-4 hr; increased in renal disease

Pharmacodynamics

	PO
Onset	Unknown
Peak	1 hr

Interactions

Individual drugs

CycloSPORINE: increased serum concentrations

Nitrofurantoin: decreased effectiveness; monitor closely

Probenecid: increased norfloxacin level

Sucralfate: decreased absorption of norfloxacin, give 2 hr apart

Theophylline, caffeine: possible increased levels, toxicity; do not use together

Warfarin: increased anticoagulation

Drug classifications

Antacids, iron salts: decreased absorption of norfloxacin; give 2 hr apart

Anticoagulants (oral): increased effect of anticoagulants

Drug/lab test

Increased: AST, ALT, BUN, creatinine, alkaline phosphatase

NURSING CONSIDERATIONS

Assessment

- Assess patient for previous sensitivity reaction
- Assess patient for signs and symptoms of infection including characteristics of urine, WBC >10,000/mm^3, temp; obtain baseline information before and during treatment
- Obtain C&S before beginning drug therapy to identify if correct treatment has been initiated
- Assess for allergic reactions: rash, urticaria, pruritus
- Monitor blood studies: AST, ALT, BUN, creatinine, alkaline phosphatase monthly if patient is on long-term therapy

N

- Assess bowel pattern daily; if severe diarrhea occurs, drug should be discontinued
- Assess for overgrowth of infection: perineal itching, fever, malaise, redness, pain, swelling, drainage, rash, diarrhea, change in cough, sputum

Nursing diagnoses

- Infection, risk for (uses)
- Diarrhea (adverse reactions)
- Injury, risk for (adverse reactions)
- Knowledge, deficient (teaching)
- Noncompliance (teaching)

Implementation

- Give in equal intervals q12h around the clock to maintain proper blood levels; give with food to increase absorption of drug; do not give within 3 hr of other agents; drug interactions may occur; give with 8 oz of water
- Do not give with iron, zinc products, or antacids, which decrease absorption

Patient/family education

- Instruct patient to take all medication prescribed for the length of time ordered; drug must be taken at same time of day to maintain blood levels; do not give medication to others; do not double doses; take any missed dose when remembered
- Advise patient to increase fluids to 2 L/day to prevent crystalluria
- Caution patient to avoid driving and other hazardous activities until response is known; dizziness may occur
- Instruct patient to use sunglasses to prevent photophobia
- Have patient use hard candy, frequent sips of water for dry mouth
- Teach patient correct instillation procedure (ophth)

Evaluation

Positive therapeutic outcome

- Reported improvement in symptoms of infection
- Absence of red or itching eyes (ophth)

nortriptyline (Rx)

(nor-trip'ti-leen)

Aventyl, Pamelor

Func. class.: Antidepressant, tricyclic

Chem. class.: Dibenzocycloheptene, secondary amine

Pregnancy category C

Do Not Confuse:

nortriptyline/amitriptyline

Action: Blocks reuptake of norepINEPHrine, serotonin into nerve endings, increasing action of norepINEPHrine, serotonin in nerve cells; has anticholinergic effects

Therapeutic Outcome: Decreased symptoms of depression after 2-3 wk

Uses: Major depression

Investigational uses: Chronic pain management

Dosage and routes

Adult: PO 25 mg tid or qid; may increase to 150 mg/day; may give daily dose at bedtime

Elderly: PO 10-25 mg nightly, increase by 10-25 mg at weekly intervals to desired dose; usual maintenance 75 mg daily

Available forms: Caps 10, 25, 50, 75 mg; sol 10 mg/5 ml

Adverse effects

CNS: Dizziness, drowsiness, confusion, headache, anxiety, tremors, stimulation, weakness, insomnia, nightmares, EPS (elderly), increased psychiatric symptoms

CV: Orthostatic hypotension, ECG changes, tachycardia, **hypertension,** palpitations

EENT: Blurred vision, tinnitus, mydriasis

GI: Constipation, dry mouth, nausea, vomiting, **paralytic ileus,** increased appetite, cramps, epigastric distress, jaundice, **hepatitis,** stomatitis

GU: Retention, **acute renal failure**

HEMA: **Agranulocytosis, thrombocytopenia, eosinophilia, leukopenia**

INTEG: Rash, urticaria, sweating, pruritus, photosensitivity

Contraindications: Hypersensitivity to tricyclic antidepressants, recovery phase of MI, seizure disorders, prostatic hypertrophy

Precautions: Pregnancy **C**, suicidal patients, severe depression, increased intraocular pressure, narrow-angle glaucoma, urinary retention, cardiac disease, hepatic disease, hyperthyroidism, electroshock therapy, elective surgery, lactation, children

Pharmacokinetics	
Absorption	Well absorbed
Distribution	Widely distributed; crosses placenta
Metabolism	Liver, extensively
Excretion	Kidneys, breast milk
Half-life	18-28 hr; steady state 4-19 days

Pharmacodynamics
Unknown

Interactions

Individual drugs
Alcohol: increased CNS depression
Clonidine, guanethidine: decreased effects
Smoking (heavy): decreased drug effect

Drug classifications
Barbiturates, benzodiazepines, CNS depressants: increased effects
MAOIs: hypertensive episode, hyperpyretic crisis, convulsions
Sympathomimetics (direct-acting): increased effects
Sympathomimetics, indirect-acting: decreased effects

Drug/herb
Belladonna, corkwood, henbane, jimsonweed: increased anticholinergic effect
Hops, lavender: increased CNS effect
SAM-e, St. John's wort: serotonin syndrome
Scopolia: increased antidepressant action

Drug/lab test
Increased: serum bilirubin, blood glucose, alkaline phosphatase
Decreased: VMA, 5-HIAA
False increase: urinary catecholamines

NURSING CONSIDERATIONS

Assessment
- Monitor B/P (with patient lying, standing), pulse q4h; if systolic B/P drops 20 mm Hg, hold drug, notify prescriber; take VS q4h of patients with CV disease
- Monitor blood studies: CBC, leukocytes, differential, cardiac enzymes if patient is receiving long-term therapy
- Monitor hepatic studies: AST, ALT, bilirubin
- Check weight weekly; appetite may increase with drug
- Assess ECG for flattening of T wave, bundle branch block, AV block, dysrhythmias in cardiac patients
- Assess for extrapyramidal symptoms primarily in elderly: rigidity, dystonia, akathisia
- Assess mental status: mood, sensorium, affect, suicidal tendencies; increase in psychiatric symptoms: depression, panic
- Monitor urinary retention, constipation; constipation is more likely to occur in children or elderly
- ❗ Assess for withdrawal symptoms: headache, nausea, vomiting, muscle pain, weakness; do not usually occur unless drug was discontinued abruptly
- Identify alcohol consumption; if alcohol is consumed, hold dose until AM

Nursing diagnoses
- Coping, ineffective (uses)
- Injury, risk for (adverse reactions)
- Knowledge, deficient (teaching)
- Noncompliance (teaching)

Implementation
- Give with food or milk to decrease GI symptoms; mix conc with water, milk, fruit juice to disguise taste
- Give dose at bedtime if oversedation occurs during day; may take entire dose at bedtime; elderly may not tolerate once/day dosing
- Store at room temp; do not freeze

Patient/family education
- Teach patient that therapeutic effects may take 2-3 wk
- Teach patient to use caution in driving and other activities requiring alertness because of drowsiness, dizziness, blurred vision; to avoid rising quickly from sitting to standing, especially elderly
- Teach patient to avoid alcohol ingestion, other CNS depressants; teach patient not to discontinue medication quickly after long-term use; may cause nausea, headache, malaise
- Teach patient to wear sunscreen or large hat to avoid burns, because photosensitivity occurs
- Teach patient to increase fluids, bulk in diet if constipation, urinary retention occur, especially elderly
- Teach patient to take gum, hard sugarless candy, or frequent sips of water for dry mouth

Evaluation
Positive therapeutic outcome
- Decrease in depression
- Absence of suicidal thoughts

Treatment of overdose: ECG monitoring, induce emesis, lavage, activated charcoal, administer anticonvulsant

nystatin (Rx, OTC)
(nis'ta-tin)

Mycostatin, Pastilles, Nadostine ✤, PMS-Nystatin ✤, nystatin; topical: Mycostatin, Nilstat, Nodostine ✤, Nyoderm ✤, Nystatin, Nystex vaginal
Func. class.: Antiinfective
Chem. class.: Antifungal

Pregnancy category B

Action: Interferes with fungal DNA replication; binds sterols in fungal cell membrane, which increases permeability, resulting in leaking of cell nutrients

Therapeutic Outcome: Fungistatic/fungicidal against *Candida* organisms

N

Uses: *Candida* species causing oral, vaginal, intestinal infections; vag: cutaneous vulvovaginal candidiasis; top: mucocutaneous fungal infections, infant eczema, pruritus ani and vulvae

Dosage and routes

Oral infection

Adult: Susp 400,000-600,000 units qid, use ½ dose in each side of mouth, swish and swallow

Infants: 200,000 units qid (100,000 units in each side of mouth)

Newborn and premature infants: Susp 100,000 units qid

Adult and child: Troches 200,000-400,000 units qid × up to 2 wk

GI infection

Adult: PO 500,000-1,000,000 units tid

Topical

Adult and child: Apply to affected area bid-tid × 14 days, not to exceed 4 wk

Vaginal: 1-2 tabs (100,000 units each) inserted into vagina MUH × 2 wk

Available forms: Tabs 500,000 units; powder 50, 150, 500 million, 1, 2, 5 billion units; troches 200,000 units; susp 100,000 units/ml

Adverse effects

GI: Nausea, vomiting, anorexia, diarrhea, cramps

INTEG: Rash, urticaria (rare)

Contraindication: Hypersensitivity

Precautions: Pregnancy **B**

Pharmacokinetics	
Absorption	Poorly absorbed
Distribution	Unknown
Metabolism	Not metabolized
Excretion	Feces, unchanged
Half-life	Unknown

Pharmacodynamics	
Onset	Rapid
Peak	Unknown
Duration	6-12 hr

Interactions: None known

NURSING CONSIDERATIONS

Assessment

- Assess for allergic reaction: rash, urticaria; drug may have to be discontinued
- Assess for predisposing factors for candidal infection: antibiotic therapy, pregnancy, diabetes mellitus, sexual partner infection (vag infections), AIDS

Nursing diagnoses

- Skin integrity, impaired (uses)
- Infection, risk for (uses)
- Knowledge, deficient (teaching)

Implementation

PO route

- Give oral susp dose by placing ½ in each cheek, swish for several min, then swallow; shake susp before use
- Store oral susp in refrigerator, tab in air-tight, light-resistant containers at room temp

Topical route

- Administer by moistening lesions with a swab coated with cream or ointment; use enough medication to cover lesions completely; give after cleansing with soap, water before each application; dry well

Vaginal route

- Insert vag tab high into vagina with applicator provided; administer in gravid client 3-6 wk before term to decrease candidiasis in the newborn
- Store at room temp in dry place; protect from light, air, heat

Patient/family education

- Instruct patient that long-term therapy may be needed to clear infection; to complete entire course of medication
- Teach patient proper hygiene: use no commercial mouthwashes for mouth infection
- Advise patient to avoid getting preparation on hands
- Instruct patient to wear light-day pad for vag preparations to avoid soiling clothing; to avoid sexual contact during treatment to minimize reinfection
- Instruct patient to notify prescriber if irritation occurs; drug may have to be discontinued
- Inform patient that relief from itching may occur after 24-72 hr

Topical

- Advise patient to discontinue use and notify prescriber if irritation occurs
- Teach patient to apply with glove to prevent further infection; drug may stain
- Caution patient not to use occlusive dressings; to avoid use of OTC creams, ointments, lotions unless directed by prescriber

Evaluation

Positive therapeutic outcome

- Culture negative for *Candida*
- Decrease in size, number of lesions
- Decreased itching, white patches on vulva (vag)

octreotide (Rx)
(ok-tree'-o-tide)
Sandostatin, Sandostatin LAR Depot
Func. class.: Hormone, antidiarrheal
Chem. class.: Octapeptide
Pregnancy category B

Action: Action similar to somatostatin

Therapeutic Outcome: Decreased diarrhea; decreased symptoms of acromegaly, carcinoid tumors, vasoactive intestinal peptide tumors (VIPomas)

Uses: Sandostatin: acromegaly, carcinoid tumors, VIPomas; LAR Depot: long-term maintenance of acromegaly, carcinoid tumors, VIPomas

Investigational uses: GI fistula, variceal bleeding, diarrheal conditions, pancreatic fistula, irritable bowel syndrome, dumping syndrome, acromegaly

Dosage and routes
Acromegaly
Adult: SUBCUT/**IV** 50-100 mcg tid, adjust q2 wk based on growth hormone levels (Sandostatin) or IM 20 mg q4 wk × 3 mo, adjust by growth hormone levels (Sandostatin LAR)

VIPomas
Adult: SUBCUT/**IV** 0.2-0.3 mg daily in 2-4 doses for 2 wk, not to exceed 0.45 mg daily (Sandostatin) or IM 20 mg q2 wk × 2 mo, adjust dose (Sandostatin LAR)

Carcinoid tumors
Adult: SUBCUT/**IV** 0.1-0.6 mg daily in 2-4 doses for 2 wk, titrated to patient response (Sandostatin) or IM 20 mg q4 wk × 2 mo, adjust dose (Sandostatin LAR)

GI fistula
Adult: SUBCUT 50-200 mcg q8h

Irritable bowel syndrome
Adult: SUBCUT 100 mcg single dose to 125 mcg bid

Antidiarrheal in AIDS patients
Adult: SUBCUT/**IV** 100-1800 mcg/day

Dumping syndrome
Adult: SUBCUT 50-150 mcg/day

Variceal bleeding
Adult: **IV** 25-50 mcg/hr cont **IV** inf for 18 hr-5 days

Available forms: Sandostatin: inj 0.05, 0.1, 0.2, 0.5, 1 mg/ml; LAR Depot: inj 10 mg, 20, 30 mg/5 ml

Adverse effects
CNS: *Headache, dizziness, fatigue, weakness,* depression, anxiety, tremors, **seizures,** paranoia
CV: *Sinus bradycardia, conduction abnormalities,* **dysrhythmias,** chest pain, shortness of breath, thrombophlebitis, ischemia, **CHF,** hypertension, palpitations
ENDO: *Hyperglycemia, ketosis, hypothyroidism, hypoglycemia,* galactorrhea, diabetes insipidus
GI: *Diarrhea, nausea, abdominal pain, vomiting, flatulence, distension, constipation,* **hepatitis,** elevated liver function tests, **GI bleeding, pancreatitis**
GU: UTI, pollakiuria
HEMA: Hematoma of inj site, bruise
INTEG: Rash, urticaria, pain, inflammation at inj site
MS: Joint and muscle pain

Contraindications: Hypersensitivity

Precautions: Pregnancy **B,** diabetes mellitus, hypothyroidism, elderly, lactation, children, renal disease

Pharmacokinetics	
Absorption	Rapidly, completely
Distribution	Unknown
Metabolism	Little
Excretion	Urine, unchanged
Half-life	1.7 hr

Pharmacodynamics	
Onset	Unknown
Peak	½ hr
Duration	12 hr

Interactions
Individual drugs
CycloSPORINE: possible increased rejection
Drug/food
Decreased: absorption of dietary fat, vit B_{12} levels

NURSING CONSIDERATIONS
Assessment
- Identify growth hormone antibodies, IGF-1, 1-4 hr intervals for 8-12 hr after dose in acromegaly; 5-HIAA, plasma serotonin, plasma substance P in carcinoid; VIP in VIPomas
- Fecal fat, serum carotene
- Monitor thyroid function tests: T_3, T_4, T_7, TSH to identify hypothyroidism
- Assess for allergic reaction: rash, itching, fever, nausea, wheezing
- Assess for cardiac status: bradycardia, conduction abnormalities, dysrhythmias;

O

monitor ECG for QT prolongation, low voltage, axis shifts, early repolarization, R/S transition, early wave progression

Nursing diagnoses

- Body image, disturbed (uses)
- Knowledge, deficient (teaching)

Implementation

- Store unopened amps, vials in refrigerator; or room temp for 2 wk, protect from light; do not use discolored or cloudy sol

SUBCUT route

- Rotate inj sites, use hip, thigh, abdomen
- Avoid using medication that is cold; allow to reach room temperature

IM route

- Reconstitute with diluent provided; give into gluteal muscle

IV route

- May use **IV** bolus if required; give over 3 min
- To use by intermittent infusion, dilute in 50-200 ml D_5W, 0.9% NaCl, give over 15-30 min

Patient/family education

- Explain reason for medication and expected results
- Advise patient that routine follow-up is needed
- Instruct parents on procedure for medication preparation and inj use; request demonstration, return demonstration; provide written instructions
- Advise patient to change position slowly to prevent orthostatic hypotension

Evaluation

Positive therapeutic outcome

- Decreased symptoms of acromegaly, carcinoid, VIPoma
- Decreased diarrhea in AIDS

ofloxacin (Rx)

(o-flox'a-sin)

Floxin, Ocuflox

Func. class.: Antiinfective

Chem. class.: Fluoroquinolone

Pregnancy category C

Do Not Confuse:

Ocuflex/Ocufen

Action: Interferes with conversion of intermediate DNA fragments into high molecular weight DNA in bacteria

Therapeutic Outcome: Bactericidal action against gram-positive pathogens *Staphylococcus epidermidis,* methicillin-resistant strains of *Staphylococcus aureus, Streptococcus pyogenes, Streptococcus pneumoniae;* gram-negative pathogens *Escherichia coli, Klebsiella* species, *Enterobacter, Salmonella, Shigella, Proteus vulgaris, Proteus rettgeri, Providencia stuartii, Morganella morganii, Pseudomonas aeruginosa, Serratia, Haemophilus* species, *Acinetobacter, Neisseria gonorrhoeae, Neisseria meningitidis, Yersinia, Vibrio, Brucella, Campylobacter,* and *Aeromonas* species; anaerobic pathogens *Bacteroides fragilis intermedius, Clostridium perfringens, Gardnerella vaginalis, Peptococcus niger, Peptostreptococcus* species; *Chlamydia pneumoniae, Chlamydia trachomatis, Legionella pneumoniae, Mycobacterium tuberculosis, Mycoplasma pneumoniae*

Uses: Treatment of lower respiratory tract infections (pneumonia, bronchitis), genitourinary infections (prostatitis, UTIs), skin and skin structure infections, conjunctivitis (ophth)

Dosage and routes

Lower respiratory tract infection/ skin and skin structure infections

Adult: PO/**IV** 400 mg q12h × 10 days

Cervicitis, urethritis

Adult: PO/**IV** 300 mg q12h × 7 days

Prostatitis

Adult: PO 300 mg q12h × 6 wk

Acute, uncomplicated gonorrhea

Adult: PO/**IV** 400 mg as a single dose

Urinary tract infection

Adult: PO/**IV** 200-400 mg q12h × 3-10 days

Conjunctivitis

Adult and child: Ophth 1-2 gtt q2-4h × 2 days, then qid × 5 days

Renal dose

Adult: PO CCr 20-50 ml/min give q24h; CCr <20 ml/min give ½ of dose q24h

Available forms: Tabs 200, 300, 400 mg; inj 20, 40 mg/ml; 200 mg/50 ml, 400 mg/100 ml

Adverse effects

CNS: Dizziness, headache, fatigue, somnolence, depression, insomnia, lethargy, malaise, **seizures**

EENT: Visual disturbances

GI: Diarrhea, nausea, vomiting, anorexia, flatulence, heartburn, dry mouth, increased AST, ALT, abdominal pain, constipation, **pseudomembranous colitis**

INTEG: Rash, pruritus
SYST: **Anaphylaxis, Stevens-Johnson syndrome**

Contraindication: Hypersensitivity to quinolones

Precautions: Pregnancy **C**, lactation, children, elderly, renal disease, seizure disorders, excessive sunlight

Pharmacokinetics

Absorption	Well absorbed (PO)
Distribution	Widely distributed
Excretion	Kidneys, unchanged; breast milk
Half-life	5-9 hr; increased in renal disease

Pharmacodynamics

	PO	IV	OPHTH
Onset	Rapid	Rapid	Unknown
Peak	1-2 hr	Inf end	Unknown

Interactions
Individual drugs
Sucralfate, zinc sulfate: decreased absorption of ofloxacin, separate by 2 hr
Theophylline: increased toxicity, do not use together
Warfarin: increased anticoagulation
Drug classifications
Antacids with aluminum, iron salts, magnesium: decreased absorption of ofloxacin, separate by 2 hr
Antidiabetics: altered blood glucose levels
NSAIDs: increased CNS stimulation, seizures
Drug/herb
Cola nut: increased effect

NURSING CONSIDERATIONS
Assessment
- Assess patient for previous sensitivity reaction
- Assess patient for signs and symptoms of infection including characteristics of wounds, sputum, urine, stool, WBC >10,000/mm^3, fever; obtain baselines and monitor during treatment
- Obtain C&S before beginning drug therapy to identify if correct treatment has been initiated
- Assess for allergic reactions: rash, urticaria, pruritus
- Monitor blood studies: AST, ALT, CBC, serum glucose monthly if patient is on long-term therapy
- Assess bowel pattern daily; if severe diarrhea occurs, drug should be discontinued
- Assess for overgrowth of infection: perineal itching, fever, malaise, redness, pain, swelling, drainage, rash, diarrhea, change in cough, sputum
- Assess for CNS symptoms: seizures, vertigo, drowsiness, agitation, confusion, tremors

Nursing diagnoses
- Infection, risk for (uses)
- Diarrhea (adverse reactions)
- Injury, risk for (adverse reactions)
- Knowledge, deficient (teaching)
- Noncompliance (teaching)

Implementation
PO route
- Give in equal intervals q12h around the clock to maintain proper blood levels; do not give within 2 hr of other agents, since drug interactions are possible: give with 8 oz of water
- Do not give with iron, aluminum, zinc products or antacids, which decrease absorption and form insoluble chelate

IV route
- For intermittent inf, dilute to 4 mg/ml with D_5W, D_5/0.9% NaCl, 0.9% NaCl, D_5/LR, sodium bicarbonate, sodium lactate, D_5/Plasmalyte 56; give over 1 hr or more
- Store for 2 wk refrigerated or 6 mo frozen, after reconstitution

Syringe compatibilities: Cefotaxime
Y-site compatibilities: Ampicillin, cisatracurium, docetaxel, etoposide, gemcitabine, granisetron, linezolid, propofol, remifentanil, thiotepa
Additive compatibilities: Amoxicillin, ceftazidime, clindamycin, gentamicin, piperacillin, tobramycin, vancomycin

Patient/family education
- Instruct patient to take all medication prescribed for the length of time ordered; drug must be taken around the clock to maintain blood levels; do not give medication to others
- Teach patient to use sunscreen when outdoors to decrease phototoxicity
- Advise patient to increase fluids to 2 L/day to prevent crystalluria
- Caution patient to avoid driving and other hazardous activities until response is known; dizziness, confusion, drowsiness may occur

Evaluation
Positive therapeutic outcome
- Absence of signs/symptoms of infection
- Reported improvement in symptoms of infection
- Absence of red or itching eyes (ophth)

olanzapine (Rx)

(oh-lanz'a-peen)

Zyprexa, Zyprexa Zydis

Func. class.: Antipsychotic/neuroleptic

Chem. class.: Thienbenzodiazepine

Pregnancy category C

Action: Unknown; may mediate antipsychotic activity by both dopamine and serotonin type 2 ($5\text{-}HT_2$) antagonism; also, may antagonize muscarinic receptors, histaminic (H_1)- and α-adrenergic receptors

Therapeutic Outcome: Decreased psychotic symptoms

Uses: Schizophrenia, acute manic episodes in bipolar disorder

Investigational uses: Dementia related to Alzheimer's disease

Dosage and routes

Schizophrenia

Adult: PO 5-10 mg initially daily, may increase dosage by 5 mg at 1 wk or more intervals; orally disintegrating tabs: open blister pack, place tab on tongue, let disintegrate, swallow

Elderly: PO 5 mg, may increase cautiously at 1 wk intervals

Bipolar mania

Adult: PO 10-15 mg daily, may increase dose after 24 hr, by 5 mg

Agitation associated with schizophrenia, bipolar I mania

Adult: IM 10 mg

Available forms: Tabs 2.5, 5, 7.5, 10, 15 mg; orally disintegrating tabs 5, 10, 15, 20 mg; powder for injection 10 mg

Adverse effects

CNS: Extrapyramidal symptoms (EPS) (pseudoparkinsonism, akathisia, dystonia, tardive dyskinesia), **seizures,** headache, **neuroleptic malignant syndrome (rare),** somnolence, agitation, nervousness, hostility, dizziness, hypertonia, tremor, euphoria, confusion, *drowsiness,* fatigue, *abnormal gait, insomnia, fever*

CV: Hypotension, tachycardia, chest pain

ENDO: Increased prolactin levels

GI: Dry mouth, nausea, vomiting, anorexia, constipation, abdominal pain, weight gain, appetite, dyspepsia

GU: Urinary retention, urinary frequency, enuresis, impotence, amenorrhea, gynecomastia, breast engorgement, premenstrual syndrome

INTEG: Rash

MISC: Peripheral edema, accidental injury, hypertonia

MS: Joint pain, twitching

RESP: *Cough, pharyngitis*

Contraindications: Hypersensitivity

Precautions: Pregnancy **C,** lactation, hypertension, hepatic disease, cardiac disease, elderly

Pharmacokinetics	
Absorption	Well
Distribution	93% plasma protein binding
Metabolism	Liver
Excretion	Kidneys
Half-life	Unknown

Pharmacodynamics	
Onset	Unknown
Peak	6 hr
Duration	Unknown

Interactions

Individual drugs

Alcohol: increased sedation, hypotension

Bromocriptine, levodopa: decreased antiparkinson activity

Carbamazepine, omeprazole, rifampin: decreased levels of olanzapine

Diazepam: increased hypotension

Fluvoxamine: increased olanzapine levels

Drug classifications

Anesthetics (barbiturates), antidepressants, antihistamines, sedative/hypnotics, CNS depressants: increased sedation

Anticholinergics: increased anticholinergic effects

Antihypertensives: increased hypotension

Dopamine agonists: decreased antiparkinson activity

Drug/herb

Betel palm, kava: increased EPS

Cola tree, hops, nettle, nutmeg: increased action

Drug/lab test

Increased: liver function tests, prolactin, CPK

NURSING CONSIDERATIONS

Assessment

- Assess mental status, orientation, mood, behavior, presence of hallucinations and type before initial administration and monthly
- Monitor swallowing of PO medication: check for hoarding or giving of medication to other patients
- Monitor I&O ratio; palpate bladder if low urinary output occurs, especially in elderly

• Monitor bilirubin, CBC
• Monitor urinalysis; recommended before, during prolonged therapy
• Assess affect, orientation, LOC, reflexes, gait, coordination, sleep pattern disturbances
• Monitor B/P sitting, standing, lying; take pulse and respirations q4h during initial treatment; establish baseline before starting treatment; report drops of 30 mm Hg; obtain baseline ECG
• Assess dizziness, faintness, palpitations, tachycardia on rising
• Assess for neuroleptic malignant syndrome: hyperpyrexia, muscle rigidity, increased CPK, altered mental status, for acute dystonia (check chewing, swallowing, eyes, pin rolling)
• EPS including akathisia (inability to sit still, no pattern to movements), tardive dyskinesia (bizarre movements of the jaw, mouth, tongue, extremities), pseudoparkinsonism (rigidity, tremors, pill rolling, shuffling gait)
• Monitor skin turgor daily
• Monitor constipation, urinary retention daily; increase bulk, H_2O in diet

Nursing diagnoses
• Thought processes, disturbed (uses)
• Knowledge, deficient (teaching)
• Noncompliance (teaching)

Implementation
• Give antiparkinsonian agent for EPS
• Give decreased dose in elderly
• Give PO with full glass of water, milk; or with food to decrease GI upset
• Provide decreased stimuli by dimming light, avoiding loud noises
• Provide supervised ambulation until stabilized on medication; do not involve in strenuous exercise program because fainting is possible; patients should not stand still for long periods
• Give increased fluids to prevent constipation
• Give sips of water, candy, gum for dry mouth
• Store in airtight, light-resistant container
• Give orally disintegrating tabs: open blister pack, place tab on tongue until dissolved, swallow; no water needed

Patient/family education
• Teach patient to use good oral hygiene; frequent rinsing of mouth, candy, ice chips, sugarless gum for dry mouth
• Advise patient to avoid hazardous activities until drug response is determined
• Advise patient that orthostatic hypotension occurs often and to rise from sitting or lying position gradually
• Advise patient to avoid hot tubs, hot showers, tub baths, since hypotension may occur
• Advise patient to avoid abrupt withdrawal of this drug, or EPS may result; drug should be withdrawn slowly
• Advise patient to avoid OTC preparations (cough, hay fever, cold) unless approved by prescriber, since serious drug interactions may occur; avoid use with alcohol, CNS depresssants, increased drowsiness may occur
• Advise patient that in hot weather, heat stroke may occur; take extra precautions to stay cool

Evaluation
Positive therapeutic outcome
• Decrease in emotional excitement, hallucinations, delusions, paranoia, reorganization of patterns of thought, speech

Treatment of overdose: Lavage if orally ingested; provide airway; do not induce vomiting or use epINEPHrine

olmesartan medoxomil (Rx)
(ol-meh-sar'tan)
Benicar
Func. class.: Antihypertensive

Pregnancy category
C (1st trimester),
D (2nd/3rd trimesters)

Action: Blocks the vasoconstrictor and aldosterone-secreting effects of angiotensin II; selectively blocks the binding of angiotensin II to the AT_1 receptor found in tissues

Therapeutic Outcome: Decreased B/P

Uses: Hypertension, alone or in combination with other antihypertensives

Dosage and routes
Adult: **PO** single agent 20 mg daily initially in patients who are not volume depleted, may be increased to 40 mg daily if needed after 2 wk

Available forms: Tabs 5, 20, 40 mg

Adverse effects
CNS: *Dizziness,* fatigue, headache, insomnia
CV: Chest pain, peripheral edema, tachycardia
EENT: Sinusitis, rhinitis, pharyngitis
GI: *Diarrhea,* abdominal pain
MS: Arthralgia, pain
RESP: *Upper respiratory infection,* bronchitis
SYST: **Angioedema**

Contraindications: Pregnancy **D** (2nd/3rd trimesters), hypersensitivity

Precautions: Pregnancy **C** (1st trimester), hypersensitivity to ACE inhibitors; lactation; children; elderly; hepatic disease

O

Pharmacokinetics

Absorption	Unknown
Distribution	Unknown
Metabolism	Unknown
Excretion	Urine, feces
Half-life	Unknown

Pharmacodynamics

Unknown

Interactions
Drug/herb
Aconite: increased toxicity, death
Astragalus, cola tree: increased or decreased antihypertensive effect
Barberry, betony, black catechu, black cohosh, bloodroot, broom, burdock, cat's claw, dandelion, goldenseal, Irish moss, Jamaican dogwood, kelp, khella, mistletoe, parsley: increased antihypertensive effect
Coltsfoot, guarana, khat, licorice: decreased antihypertensive effect

NURSING CONSIDERATIONS
Assessment
- Assess for pregnancy; this drug can cause fetal death when given in pregnancy
- Assess response and adverse reactions, especially in renal disease
- Monitor B/P, pulse q4h; note rate, rhythm, quality; electrolytes: K, Na, Cl; baselines in renal tests, liver function tests before therapy begins
- Assess skin turgor, dryness of mucous membranes for hydration status; for angioedema: facial swelling, dyspnea

Nursing diagnoses
- Tissue perfusion, ineffective (uses)
- Cardiac output, decreased (uses)
- Knowledge, deficient (teaching)
- Noncompliance (teaching)

Implementation
- Give without regard to meals

Patient/family education
- Advise to comply with dosage schedule, even if feeling better
- Advise patient to notify prescriber of mouth sores, fever, swelling of hands or feet, irregular heartbeat, chest pain
- Teach that excessive perspiration, dehydration, vomiting, diarrhea may lead to fall in B/P; to consult prescriber if these occur
- Teach that drug may cause dizziness, fainting; light-headedness may occur
- Advise to rise slowly to sitting or standing position to minimize orthostatic hypotension
- Teach to notify prescriber immediately if pregnant; not to use during lactation
- Advise to avoid all OTC medications, unless approved by prescriber
- Advise to inform all health care providers of medication use
- Advise to use proper technique for obtaining B/P and acceptable parameters

Evaluation
Positive therapeutic outcome
- Decreased B/P

olsalazine (Rx)
(ohl-sal′ah-zeen)
Dipetum ✤
Func. class.: Antiinflammatory
Chem. class.: Salicylate derivative
Pregnancy category C

Action: Bioconverted to 5-aminosalicylic acid, which decreases inflammation

Therapeutic Outcome: Lessening of loose, diarrhea stools and cramping

Uses: Maintenance of remission of ulcerative colitis in patients intolerant to sulfasalazine

Dosage and routes
Adult: PO 500 mg bid

Available forms: Caps 250 mg

Adverse effects
CNS: Headache, hallucinations, depression, vertigo, fatigue, dizziness
GI: Nausea, vomiting, abdominal pain, **hepatitis**, diarrhea, bloating
HEMA: **Leukopenia, neutropenia, thrombocytopenia, agranulocytosis, anemia**
INTEG: Rash, dermatitis, urticaria

Contraindications: Hypersensitivity to salicylates

Precautions: Pregnancy **C,** child <14 yr, lactation; impaired hepatic, renal function; severe allergy; bronchial asthma

Pharmacokinetics

Absorption	Colon 99% converted to mesalamine
Distribution	Colon
Metabolism	Liver
Excretion	Feces
Half-life	0.9 hr

Pharmacodynamics

Onset	Unknown
Peak	1 hr
Duration	12 hr

Interactions

Drug/lab test

False positive: urinary glucose test

NURSING CONSIDERATIONS

Assessment

- Assess for blood dyscrasias: skin rash, fever, sore throat, bruising, bleeding, fatigue, joint pain (rare)
- Assess for allergic reaction: rash, dermatitis, urticaria, pruritus, dyspnea, bronchospasm

Nursing diagnoses

- Pain, acute (uses)
- Diarrhea (uses)
- Knowledge, deficient (teaching)

Implementation

- Give total daily dose evenly spaced to minimize GI intolerance, with food
- Store in tight, light-resistant container at room temperature

Patient/family education

- Advise patient to take as prescribed, take missed dose as soon as remembered
- Inform patient not to operate machinery or drive until effects are known, may cause dizziness
- Advise patient to notify prescriber if symptoms do not improve or if allergic reaction or sore throat occurs

Evaluation

Positive therapeutic outcome

- Absence of fever, mucus in stools

omalizumab (Rx)

(oh-mah-lye-zoo′mab)

Xolair

Func. class.: Monoclonal antibody

Pregnancy category B

Action: Recombinant DNA-derived humanized IgG murine monoclonal antibody that selectively binds to IgE to limit the release of mediators in the allergic response

Therapeutic Outcome: Ability to breathe more easily

Uses: Moderate to severe persistent asthma

Investigational uses: Seasonal allergic rhinitis

Dosage and routes

Adult: **SUBCUT** 150-375 mg × 2-4 wk, divide inj into 2 sites, if dose is >150 mg; dose is adjusted based on IgE levels and significant changes in body weight

Available forms: Powder for inj, lyophilized 202.5 mg (150 mg/1.2 ml after reconstitution)

Adverse effects

INTEG: Pruritus, dermatitis, inj site reactions, rash

MISC: Earache, dizziness, fatigue, pain, **malignancies**, viral infections, **anaphylaxis**

MS: Arthralgia, fracture, leg, arm pain

RESP: Sinusitis, upper respiratory tract infections, pharyngitis

Contraindications: Hypersensitivity to this drug or hamster protein

Precautions: Pregnancy **B,** acute attacks of asthma, lactation, children <12 yr, lymphoma, nephrotic disease

Pharmacokinetics	
Absorption	Slow
Distribution	Unknown
Metabolism	Degradation by liver
Excretion	In bile
Half-life	26 days

Pharmacodynamics	
Onset	Unknown
Peak	7-8 days
Duration	Unknown

Interactions: None known

NURSING CONSIDERATIONS

Assess:

- Monitor respiratory rate, rhythm, depth; auscultate lung fields bilaterally; notify prescriber of abnormalities
- Assess for allergic reactions: rash, urticaria; drug should be discontinued

Nursing diagnoses

- Gas exchange, impaired (uses)
- Knowledge, deficient (teaching)

Implementation

SUBCUT route

- Given q2-4 wk; product is viscous; if >150 mg is given, divide into two sites; the inj may take 5-10 sec to administer
- Do not give more than 150 mg/inj site

Patient/family education

- Advise that improvement will not be immediate
- Teach not to stop taking or decrease current asthma medications unless instructed by prescriber

Evaluation

Positive therapeutic outcome

- Ability to breathe more easily

omeprazole (Rx)

(oh-mep'ra-zole)

Losec ✤, Prilosec

Func. class.: Antiulcer, proton pump inhibitor

Chem. class.: Benzimidazole

Pregnancy category C

Do Not Confuse:

Prilosec/Prinivil, Prilosec/predniSONE, Prilosec/Prozac

Action: Suppresses gastric secretion by inhibiting hydrogen/potassium ATPase enzyme system in the gastric parietal cell; characterized as a gastric acid pump inhibitor, since it blocks the final step of acid production

Therapeutic Outcome: Absence of duodenal ulcers; decreased gastroesophageal reflux

Uses: Gastroesophageal reflux disease (GERD), severe erosive esophagitis, poorly responsive systemic GERD, pathologic hypersecretory conditions (Zollinger-Ellison syndrome, systemic mastocytosis, multiple endocrine adenomas); possibly effective for treatment of duodenal ulcers with or without antiinfectives for *Helicobacter pylori*

Investigational uses: Posterior laryngitis, enhancing pancreatin

Dosage and routes

Active duodenal ulcers

Adult: PO 20 mg daily × 4-8 wk; associated with *H. pylori* 40 mg QAM and clarithromycin 500 mg tid on days 1-14, then 20 mg daily days 15-28

Severe erosive esophagitis/poorly responsive GERD

Adult: PO 20 mg daily × 4-8 wk

Pathologic hypersecretory conditions

Adult: PO 60 mg/day; may increase to 120 mg tid; daily doses >80 mg should be divided

Gastric ulcer

Adult: PO 40 mg daily × 4-8 wk

Elderly: PO max 20 mg/day

Laryngitis (unlabeled)

Adult: PO 20-40 mg nightly × 6-24 wk or 20 mg bid × 4-12 wk

Available forms: Sus rel caps 10, 20, 40 mg

Adverse effects

CNS: *Headache, dizziness, asthenia*

CV: Chest pain, angina, tachycardia, bradycardia, palpitations, peripheral edema

EENT: Tinnitus, taste perversion

GI: *Diarrhea, abdominal pain, vomiting, nausea, constipation, flatulence, acid regurgitation,* abdominal swelling, anorexia, irritable colon, esophageal candidiasis, dry mouth

GU: UTI, frequency, increased creatinine, **proteinuria, hematuria,** testicular pain, glycosuria

HEMA: **Pancytopenia, thrombocytopenia, neutropenia, leukocytosis,** anemia

INTEG: Rash, dry skin, urticaria, pruritus, alopecia

META: Hypoglycemia, increased hepatic enzymes, weight gain

MISC: *Back pain,* fever, fatigue, malaise

RESP: *Upper respiratory tract infections, cough,* epistaxis

Contraindications: Hypersensitivity

Precautions: Pregnancy **C,** lactation, children

Pharmacokinetics	
Absorption	Rapidly absorbed
Distribution	Protein binding (95%); gastric parietal cells
Metabolism	Liver, extensively; by CYP450 enzyme system
Excretion	Kidneys, feces
Half-life	½-1 hr; increased in the elderly, hepatic disease

Pharmacodynamics	
Onset	1 hr
Peak	½-3½ hr
Duration	3-4 days

Interactions

Individual drugs

Ampicillin: decreased ampicillin absorption
Cyanocobalamin: decreased absorption of cyanocobalamin
CycloSPORINE: increased cycloSPORINE levels
Diazepam: increased serum levels of diazepam
Digoxin: increased serum levels, delayed absorption of digoxin
Disulfiram: increased disulfiram levels
Flurazepam: increased flurazepam level
Iron salts: decreased absorption

Ketoconazole: decreased absorption of ketoconazole
Phenytoin: increased serum levels of phenytoin
Triazolam: increased triazolam level
Warfarin: increased bleeding tendencies

Drug classifications
Iron products: decreased absorption of iron

NURSING CONSIDERATIONS
Assessment
- Assess GI system: bowel sounds q8h, abdomen for pain and swelling, anorexia
- Monitor hepatic enzymes: AST, ALT, increased alkaline phosphatase during treatment

Nursing diagnoses
- Pain, chronic (uses)
- Knowledge, deficient (teaching)

Implementation
- Swallow sus rel caps whole; do not break, crush, chew, or open
- Give before patient eats; may give with antacids

Patient/family education
- Advise patient to report severe diarrhea; drug may have to be discontinued
- Caution patient to avoid driving and other hazardous activities until response to drug is known
- Caution patient to avoid alcohol, salicylates, ibuprofen; may cause GI irritation

Evaluation
Positive therapeutic outcome
- Absence of epigastric pain, swelling, fullness

ondansetron (Rx)
(on-dan'sa-tron)
Zofran
Func. class.: Antiemetic
Chem. class.: 5-HT receptor antagonist
Pregnancy category B

Do Not Confuse:
Zofran/Zantac

Action: Prevents nausea, vomiting by blocking serotonin (5-HT) peripherally, centrally, and in the small intestine

Therapeutic Outcome: Control of nausea, vomiting

Uses: Prevention of nausea, vomiting associated with cancer chemotherapy and prevention of postopertive nausea, vomiting

Investigational uses: Bulimia, pruritus (rectal use), alcoholism, hyperemesis gravidarum

Dosage and routes
Prevention of nausea/vomiting associated with cancer chemotherapy
Adult and child 4-18 yr: **IV** 0.15 mg/kg infused over 15 min, 30 min before start of cancer chemotherapy; 0.15 mg/kg is given 4 and 8 hr after first dose or 32 mg as a single dose; dilute in 50 ml of D_5 or 0.9% NaCl before giving; rectal (off-label) 16 mg daily 2 hr before chemotherapy
Adult: **IV** 0.15 mg/kg 15-30 min prior to chemotherapy, repeat 4, 8 hr later or 32 mg single dose ½ hr prior to chemotherapy; PO 8 mg ½ hr prior to chemotherapy, repeat 8 hr later
Child 4-18 yr: **IV** 0.15 mg/kg ½ hr prior to chemotherapy, repeat 4, 8 hr later

Prevention of nausea/vomiting of radiotherapy
Adult: PO 8 mg tid, may repeat q8hr

Prevention of postoperative nausea/vomiting
Adult: **IV** 4 mg undiluted over >30 sec prior to induction of anesthesia
Child 2-12 yr: **IV** 0.1 mg/kg (≤40 kg); 4 mg (≥40 kg) give ≥30 sec

Hepatic dose
Adult: PO/IM/**IV** max dose 8 mg daily

Bulimia (unlabeled)
Adult: PO 4 mg tid (base dose) prn during bingeing/purging

Pruritus (unlabeled)
Adult: PO 4 mg bid

Alcoholism (off-label)
Adult: PO 4 mcg/kg bid

Available forms: Inj 2 mg/ml, 32 mg/50 ml (premixed); tabs 4, 8 mg; oral sol 4 mg/5 ml; oral disintegrating tabs 4, 8 mg

Adverse effects
CNS: *Headache,* dizziness, drowsiness, fatigue, extrapyramidal symptoms (EPS)
GI: *Diarrhea, constipation, abdominal pain*
MISC: Rash, **bronchospasm** (rare), *musculoskeletal pain, wound problems, shivering, fever, hypoxia, urinary retention*

Contraindications: Hypersensitivity

Precautions: Pregnancy **B,** lactation, children, elderly, granisetron hypersensitivity

Pharmacokinetics

Absorption	Completely absorbed (**IV**)
Distribution	Unknown
Metabolism	Liver, extensively
Excretion	Kidneys
Half-life	3.5-4.7 hr

Pharmacodynamics

Unknown

Interactions: Unknown

NURSING CONSIDERATIONS

Assessment

- Assess for absence of nausea, vomiting during chemotherapy
- Assess for hypersensitivity reaction: rash, bronchospasm
- Assess for EPS shuffling gait, tremors, grimacing, rigidity

Nursing diagnoses

- Knowledge, deficient (teaching)
- Noncompliance (teaching)

Implementation

IV route

- Give **IV** after diluting a single dose in 50 ml of 0.9% NaCl or D_5W, 0.45% NaCl; give over 15 min
- Store at room temp for 48 hr after dilution

Y-site compatibilities: Aldesleukin, amifostine, amikacin, aztreonam, bleomycin, carboplatin, carmustine, cefazolin, ceforanide, cefotazime, cefoxitin, ceftazidime, ceftizoxime, cefuroxime, chlorproMAZINE, cimetidine, cisatracurium, cisplatin, cladribine, clindamycin, cyclophosphamide, cytarabine, dacarbazine, dactinomycin, DAUNOrubicin, dexamethasone, diphenhydrAMINE, DOXOrubicin, DOXOrubicin liposome, doxycycline, droperidol, etoposide, famotidine, filgrastim, floxuridine, fluconazole, fludarabine, gentamicin, haloperidol, heparin, hydrocortisone, hydromorphone, hydrOXYzine, ifosfamide, imipenem/cilastatin, magnesium sulfate, mannitol, mechlorethamine, melphalan, meperidine, mesna, methotrexate, metoclopramide, miconazole, mitomycin, mitoxantrone, morphine, paclitaxel, pentostatin, potassium chloride, prochlorperazine, ranitidine, remifentanil, streptozocin, teniposide, thiotepa, ticarcillin, ticarcillin/clavulanate, vancomycin, vinBLAStine, vinCRIStine, vinorelbine, zidovudine

Y-site incompatibilities: Acyclovir, aminophylline, amphotericin B, ampicillin, ampicillin/sulbactam, cefoperazone, furosemide, ganciclovir, lorazepam, methylPREDNISolone, mezlocillin, piperacillin, sargramostim, sodium bicarbonate

Additive compatibilities: Cisplatin, cyclophosphamide, cytarabine, dacarbazine, dexamethasone, DOXOrubicin, etoposide, meperidine, methotrexate

Solution compatibilities: May also be diluted with D_5W, LR, D_5/0.9% NaCl, D_5/0.45% NaCl

Patient/family education

- Instruct patient to report diarrhea, constipation, rash, changes in respirations, or discomfort at insertion site
- Teach patient reason for medication and expected results

Evaluation

Positive therapeutic outcome

- Absence of nausea, vomiting during cancer chemotherapy

orlistat (Rx)

(or-li'-stat)

Xenical

Chem. class.: Weight control agent, lipase inhibitor

Pregnancy category B

Action: Inhibits the absorption of dietary fat

Therapeutic Outcome: Decrease in weight

Uses: Obesity management

Dosage and routes

Adult: PO 120 mg tid with each main meal containing fat

Available forms: Caps 120 mg

Adverse effects

CNS: *Insomnia,* dizziness, headache, depression, anxiety, fatigue

GI: *Oily spotting, flatus with discharge, fecal urgency, fatty/oily stool, oily evacuation, fecal incontinence,* nausea, vomiting, abdominal pain, infectious diarrhea, rectal pain, tooth disorder, hypovitaminosis

GU: UTI, vaginitis, menstrual irregularity

INTEG: Dry skin, rash

MS: Back pain, arthritis, myalgia, tendinitis

RESP: Influenza, upper, lower respiratory tract infection, EENT symptoms

Contraindications: Hypersensitivity, malabsorption syndrome, cholestasis, lactation

Precautions: Pregnancy **B,** hypothyroidism, other organic causes of obesity, children, anorexia nervosa, bulimia, nephrolithiasis

Pharmacokinetics

Absorption	Minimal
Distribution	99% protein binding
Metabolism	Unknown
Excretion	Feces
Half-life	1-2 hr

Pharmacodynamics

Onset	Unknown
Peak	8 hr
Duration	Unknown

Interactions
Individual drugs
Cyclosporine: decreased absorption
Pravastatin: increased lipid-lowering effect
Drug classifications
Fat-soluble vitamins: decreased absorption

NURSING CONSIDERATIONS
Assessment
- Monitor weight weekly, diabetic patients may need reduction in oral hypoglycemics
- Assess for misuse in certain populations (anorexia nervosa, bulimia)

Nursing diagnoses
- Knowledge, deficient (teaching)
- Noncompliance (teaching)

Implementation
- Patient should be on a diet with 30% of calories from fat, omit dose of orlistat if a meal contains no fat

Patient/family education
- Warn patient that safety and effectiveness beyond 2 yr have not been determined
- Instruct patient to read patient's information sheet, discuss unpleasant GI side effects
- Advise patient to avoid hazardous activities until stabilized on medication
- Instruct patient to take a multivitamin containing fat-soluble vitamins, take 2 hr before or after orlistat; psyllium taken with each dose or at bedtime may decrease GI symptoms
- Instruct patient/family to notify prescriber if significant side effects occur
- Advise prescriber if pregnancy is planned or suspected

Evaluation
Positive therapeutic outcome
- Decreased weight

oseltamivir (Rx)
(oh-sell-tam'ih-ver)
Tamiflu
Func. class.: Antiviral
Chem. class.: Neuramidase inhibitor
Pregnancy category C

Action: Inhibits influenza virus neuraminidase with possible alteration of virus particle aggregation and release

Therapeutic Outcome: Decreased symptoms of influenza type A

Uses: Prevention/treatment of influenza type A or B

Investigational uses: Possibly effective for avian flu (H5N1)

Dosage and routes
Treatment
Adult/child >40 kg: PO 75 bid mg × 5 days, begin treatment within 2 days of onset of symptoms
Child 23-40 kg and ≥1 yr: PO 60 mg bid
Child 15-23 kg and ≥1 yr: PO 45 mg bid
Child ≤15 kg and ≥1 yr: PO 30 mg bid
Renal dose
Adult: PO CCr 10-30 ml/min 75 mg daily × 5 days
Prevention
Adult/child ≥13 yr: PO 75 mg daily × ≥7 days; begin treatment within 2 days of contact, max use 6 wk
Renal dose
Adult/child ≥13 yr: PO CCr 10-30 ml/min 75 mg every other day

Available forms: Caps 75 mg; powder for oral susp 12 mg/ml after reconstitution

Adverse effects
CNS: Headache, fatigue, insomnia, dizziness
GI: *Nausea, vomiting,* diarrhea, abdominal pain
RESP: Cough

Contraindications: Hypersensitivity

Precautions: Pregnancy **C**, hepatic disease, renal disease, elderly

Pharmacokinetics

Absorption	Rapidly absorbed
Distribution	Protein binding is low
Metabolism	Converted to oseltamivir carboxylate
Excretion	Eliminated by conversion
Half-life	1-3 hr

O

Pharmacodynamics

Unknown

NURSING CONSIDERATIONS
Assessment
- Assess for symptoms of influenza A: increased temperature, malaise, aches and pains

Nursing diagnoses
- Infection, risk for (uses)
- Knowledge, deficient (teaching)

Implementation
- Give within 2 days of symptoms of influenza; continue for 5 days
- Give at least 4 hr before at bedtime to prevent insomnia
- Administer after meals for better absorption, to decrease GI symptoms: caps may be opened and mixed with food for easy swallowing
- Store in airtight, dry container

Patient/family education
- Teach patient about aspects of drug therapy: the need to report dyspnea, weight gain, dizziness, poor concentration, dysuria, behavioral changes
- Teach patient to avoid hazardous activities if dizziness occurs
- Advise patient to take missed dose as soon as remembered if within 2 hr of next dose

Evaluation
Positive therapeutic outcome
- Absence of fever, malaise, cough, dyspnea in influenza A

oxacillin (Rx)
(ox-a-sill'in)

Bactocill, oxacillin sodium

Func. class.: Broad-spectrum antiinfective

Chem. class.: Penicillinase-resistant penicillin

Pregnancy category B

Action: Interferes with cell wall replication of susceptible organisms; osmotically unstable cell wall swells, bursts from osmotic pressure

Therapeutic Outcome: Bactericidal effects for gram-positive cocci *Staphylococcus aureus, Streptococcus pneumoniae,* infections caused by penicillinase-producing staphylococci

Uses: Infections caused by penicillinase-producing staphylococci, streptococci; respiratory tract, skin, skin structure, urinary tract, bone, joint infections, sinusitis, endocarditis, septicemia, meningitis

Dosage and routes
Adult: PO 2-6 g/day in divided doses q4-6h; IM/**IV** 2-12 g/day in divided doses q4-6h

Child: PO 50-100 mg/kg/day in divided doses q6h; IM/**IV** 50-100 mg/kg/day in divided doses q4-6h

Available forms: Caps 250, 500 mg; powder for oral susp 250 mg/5 ml; powder for inj 250, 500 mg, 1, 2, 4, 10 g

Adverse effects
CNS: Lethargy, hallucinations, anxiety, depression, twitching, **coma, seizures**

GI: *Nausea, vomiting, diarrhea,* increased AST, ALT, abdominal pain, glossitis, colitis, **pseudomembranous colitis**

GU: **Oliguria, proteinuria, hematuria,** vaginitis, moniliasis, **glomerulonephritis**

HEMA: Anemia, increased bleeding time, **bone marrow depression, granulocytopenia**

SYST: **Anaphylaxis, serum sickness**

Contraindications: Hypersensitivity to penicillins

Precautions: Pregnancy **B,** hypersensitivity to cephalosporins, neonates

Pharmacokinetics

Absorption	Rapid, incomplete (PO); well absorbed (IM); completely (**IV**)
Distribution	Widely distributed; crosses placenta
Metabolism	Liver
Excretion	Kidneys, unchanged (51%); breast milk
Half-life	20-50 min; increased in severe hepatic disease

Pharmacodynamics

	PO	IM	IV
Onset	Rapid	Rapid	Rapid
Peak	½-1 hr	½ hr	Inf end

Interactions
Individual drugs

Chloramphenicol, colestipol, cholestyramine: decreased effectiveness of oxacillin

Probenecid: increased oxacillin levels

Rifampin: decreased oxacillin effect

Drug classifications

Contraceptives (oral): decreased contraceptive effectiveness

Erythromycins, tetracyclines: decreased antimicrobial effectiveness

Drug/herb

Acidophilus: do not use with antiinfectives

Khat: decreased absorption, separate by ≥2 hr

Drug/lab test

False positive: urine glucose, urine protein

NURSING CONSIDERATIONS

Assessment

- Assess patient for previous sensitivity reaction to penicillins or other cephalosporins; cross-sensitivity between penicillins and cephalosporins is common
- Assess patient for signs and symptoms of infection including characteristics of wounds, sputum, urine, stool, WBC >10,000/mm^3, fever; obtain baseline information and during treatment
- Obtain C&S before beginning drug therapy to identify if correct treatment has been initiated
- Assess for allergic reactions: rash, urticaria, pruritus, chills, fever, joint pain; angioedema may occur a few days after therapy begins; epINEPHrine, resuscitation equipment should be available for anaphylactic reaction
- Assess urine output; if decreasing, notify prescriber (may indicate nephrotoxicity); also check for increased BUN, creatinine
- Monitor blood studies: AST, ALT, CBC, Hct, bilirubin, LDH, alkaline phosphatase, Coombs' test monthly if patient is on long-term therapy
- Monitor electrolytes: potassium, sodium, chloride monthly if patient is on long-term therapy
- Assess bowel pattern daily; if severe diarrhea occurs, drug should be discontinued; may indicate pseudomembranous colitis
- Monitor for bleeding: ecchymosis, bleeding gums, hematuria, stool guaiac daily if on long-term therapy
- Assess for overgrowth of infection: perineal itching, fever, malaise, redness, pain, swelling, drainage, rash, diarrhea, change in cough, sputum

Nursing diagnoses

- Infection, risk for (uses)
- Diarrhea (adverse reactions)
- Injury, risk for (adverse reactions)
- Knowledge, deficient (teaching)
- Noncompliance (teaching)

Implementation

PO route

- Give in even doses around the clock; if GI upset occurs, give with food; drug must be given for 10-14 days to ensure organism death and prevent superinfection; store in airtight container
- Shake susp; store in refrigerator for 2 wk, 1 wk at room temp

IM route

- Reconstitute 250 mg/1.4 ml, 500 mg/2.7-2.8 ml, 1 g/5.7 ml, 2 g/11.4-11.5 ml, 4 g/21.8-23 ml of sterile water for a conc of 250 mg/1.5 ml; store unused portion in refrigerator for 1 wk or 3 days at room temp
- Inject deeply in large muscle mass

IV route

- Reconstitute 250 mg/1.4 ml, 500 mg/2.7-2.8 ml, 1 g/5.7 ml, 2 g/11.4-11.5 ml, 4 g/21.8-23 ml of sterile water for a conc of 250 mg/1.5 ml; store unused portion in refrigerator for 1 week or 3 days at room temp
- Give direct **IV** by diluting reconstituted sol with 250-500 mg/5 ml, 1 g/10 ml, 2 g/20 ml, 4 g/40 ml of sterile water or 0.9% NaCl, give over 10 min
- Give intermittent inf by diluting to a conc of 0.5-40 mg/ml with D_5W, 0.9% NaCl, D_5/0.9% NaCl, LR; give over 6 hr or less

Y-site compatibilities: Acyclovir, cyclophosphamide, diltiazem, famotidine, fluconazole, foscarnet, heparin, hydrocortisone, hydromorphone, labetalol, magnesium sulfate, meperidine, methotrexate, morphine, perphenazine, potassium chloride, tacrolimus, vit B with C, zidovudine

Y-site incompatibilities: Verapamil

Additive compatibilities: Cephapirin, chloramphenicol, DOPamine, potassium chloride, sodium bicarbonate

Additive incompatibilities: Cytarabine, tetracycline

Patient/family education

- Teach patient to report sore throat, bruising, bleeding, joint pain; may indicate blood dyscrasias (rare)
- Advise patient to contact prescriber if vaginal itching, loose foul-smelling stools, furry tongue occur; may indicate superinfection
- Instruct patient to take all medication prescribed for the length of time ordered
- Advise patient to notify prescriber of diarrhea with blood or pus, which may indicate pseudomembranous colitis

Evaluation

Positive therapeutic outcome

- Absence of signs/symptoms of infection (WBC <10,000/mm^3, temp WNL, absence of red, draining wounds)
- Reported improvement in symptoms of infection

Treatment of anaphylaxis: Withdraw drug, maintain airway, administer epINEPHrine, aminophylline, O_2, **IV** corticosteroids

oxaliplatin (Rx)
(ox-al-i'plat-in)
Eloxitan
Func. class.: Antineoplastic
Pregnancy category D

Action: Forms cross links, inhibiting DNA replication and transcription, cell-cycle nonspecific

Therapeutic Outcome: Decreased size of tumor, spread of malignancy

Uses: Metastatic carcinoma of the colon or rectum in combination with 5-FU/leucovorin

Dosage and routes
Dosage protocols may vary
Adult: **IV** inf *Day 1:* oxaliplatin 85 mg/m^2 in 250-500 ml D_5W and leucovorin 200 mg/m^2 in D_5W, give both over 2 hr at the same time in separate bags using a Y-line, followed by 5-FU 400 mg/m^2 **IV** bol over 2-4 min, then 5-FU 600 mg/m^2 **IV** inf in 500 ml D_5W as a 22-hr cont inf; *Day 2:* leucovorin 200 mg/m^2 **IV** inf over 2 hr, then 5-FU 400 mg/m^2 **IV** bol over 2-4 min, then 5-FU 600 mg/m^2 **IV** inf in 500 D_5W as a 22-hr cont inf; repeat cycle q2wk

Available forms: Powder for inj 50, 100 mg single-use vials

Adverse effects
CNS: Peripheral neuropathy, fatigue, headache, dizziness, insomnia
CV: Cardiac abnormalities
EENT: *Decreased visual acuity, tinnitus, hearing loss*
GI: *Severe nausea, vomiting, diarrhea, weight loss,* stomatitis, anorexia, gastroesophageal reflux, constipation, dyspepsia, mucositis, flatulence
GU: Hematuria, dysuria, creatinine
HEMA: **Thrombocytopenia, leukopenia, pancytopenia, neutropenia, anemia, hemolytic uremic syndrome**
INTEG: *Alopecia,* rash, flushing, extravasation, redness, swelling, pain at inj site
META: Hypokalemia
RESP: **Fibrosis,** dyspnea, cough, rhinitis, URI, pharyngitis
SYST: **Anaphylaxis, angioedema**

Contraindications: Pregnancy **D**, hypersensitivity to this drug or other platinum products, radiation therapy or chemotherapy within 1 mo, thrombocytopenia, smallpox vaccination

Precautions: Pneumococcus vaccination, lactation, children, elderly

Pharmacokinetics

Absorption	Unknown
Distribution	15% of platinum in systemic circulation; 85% is either in tissues or being eliminated in urine
Metabolism	Liver
Excretion	Urine
Half-life	40 days

Pharmacodynamics
Unknown

Interactions
Individual drugs
Alcohol, aspirin: increased risk of bleeding
Radiation: increased myelosuppression
Drug classifications
Aminoglycosides, diuretics (loop): increased nephrotoxicity
Live virus vaccines: decreased antibody response
Myelosuppressives: increased myelosuppression
NSAIDs: increased risk of bleeding

NURSING CONSIDERATIONS
Assessment
For bone marrow depression
- Monitor CBC, differential, platelet count weekly; withhold drug if WBC is <4000 or platelet count is <100,000; notify prescriber of results
- Monitor renal function studies: BUN, creatinine, serum uric acid, urine CCr before, electrolytes during therapy; dose should not be given if BUN <25 mg/dl; creatinine <1.5 mg/dl; I&O ratio; report fall in urine output of <30 ml/hr
- (Alert) Assess for anaphylaxis: wheezing, tachycardia, facial swelling, fainting; discontinue drug and report to prescriber; resuscitation equipment should be nearby
- Monitor temp q4h (may indicate beginning infection)
- Monitor liver function tests before, during therapy (bilirubin, AST, ALT, LDH) as needed or monthly
- Assess for bleeding: hematuria, guaiac, bruising or petechiae, mucosa or orifices q8h; obtain prescription for viscous lidocaine (Xylocaine)
- Assess effects of alopecia on body image; discuss feelings about body changes
- Assess for jaundice of skin, sclera; dark urine; clay-colored stools; itchy skin; abdominal pain; fever; diarrhea
- Assess for edema in feet, joint pain, stomach pain, shaking

Nursing diagnoses
- Infection, risk for (adverse reactions)
- Nutrition: less than body requirements, imbalanced (adverse reactions)
- Knowledge, deficient (teaching)

Implementation
- Provide comprehensive oral hygiene
- Provide all medications PO, if possible, avoid IM inj when platelets <100,000/mm^3
- Increase fluid intake to 2-3 L/day to prevent urate deposits, calculi formation; elimination of drug

IV route
- Do not reconstitute or dilute with sodium chloride or any chloride-containing solutions
- Do not use aluminum equipment during any preparation or administration, will degrade platinum; do not refrigerate unopened powder or solution
- Prepare in biologic cabinet using gown, gloves, mask; do not allow drug to come in contact with skin, use soap and water if contact occurs
- Hydrate patient with 0.9% NaCl over 8-12 hr before treatment
- Have epINEPHrine, antihistamines, corticosteroids for hypersensitivity reaction
- Give antiemetic 30-60 min before giving drug and prn
- Give allopurinol to maintain uric acid levels, alkalinization of urine
- Give diuretic (furosemide 40 mg **IV**) or mannitol after infusion

Patient/family education
- Advise to report signs of infection: increased temp, sore throat, flulike symptoms
- Advise to report signs of anemia: fatigue, headache, faintness, shortness of breath, irritability
- Advise to report bleeding; avoid use of razors, commercial mouthwash
- Advise to avoid aspirin, ibuprofen, NSAIDs, alcohol; may cause GI bleeding
- Advise to report any complaints or side effects to nurse or prescriber
- Advise to report any changes in breathing, coughing
- Advise that hair may be lost during treatment; a wig or hairpiece may make patient feel better; new hair may be different in color, texture
- Advise to report numbness, tingling in face or extremities, poor hearing or joint pain, swelling
- Advise not to receive vaccines during treatment
- Advise to use contraception during treatment and 4 mo after; this drug may cause infertility

Evaluation
Positive therapeutic outcome
- Decreased tumor size, spread of malignancy

oxaprozin (Rx)
(ox-a-proe′zin)

Daypro

Func. class.: Nonsteroidal antiinflammatory, antirheumatic

Chem. class.: Propionic acid derivative

Pregnancy category C

Do Not Confuse:
Daypro/Diupres

Action: Inhibits prostaglandin synthesis by decreasing an enzyme needed for biosynthesis; analgesic, antiinflammatory

Therapeutic Outcome: Decreased pain, inflammation

Uses: Acute and long-term management of osteoarthritis, rheumatoid arthritis, juvenile rheumatoid arthritis

Dosage and routes
Adult: PO 600-1200 mg daily; maximum dose 1800 mg/day or 26 mg/kg, whichever is lower in divided doses

Adult <50 kg: PO 600 mg daily

Available forms: Tabs 600 mg

O

Adverse effects
CNS: Dizziness, headache, drowsiness, fatigue, tremors, confusion, insomnia, anxiety, malaise, depression

CV: Tachycardia, peripheral edema, palpitations, dysrhythmias, CV disease

EENT: Tinnitus, hearing loss, blurred vision

GI: Nausea, *anorexia,* vomiting, *diarrhea,* jaundice, **cholestatic hepatitis,** constipation, flatulence, *cramps,* dry mouth, peptic ulcer, **GI bleeding**

GU: **Nephrotoxicity: dysuria, hematuria, oliguria, azotemia**

HEMA: Increased bleeding time

INTEG: Purpura, rash, pruritus, sweating

SYST: **Anaphylaxis, angioneurotic edema**

Contraindications: Hypersensitivity, asthma, patients in whom aspirin and iodides have induced symptoms of allergic reactions or asthma

Precautions: Pregnancy **C**, avoid in late pregnancy, lactation, children, bleeding disorders, GI disorders, cardiac disorders,

CHF, hypersensitivity to other antiinflammatory agents, severe renal and hepatic disease, elderly

Pharmacokinetics

Absorption	Well absorbed
Distribution	Unknown
Metabolism	Liver, extensively
Excretion	Breast milk
Half-life	40-50 hr

Pharmacodynamics

Onset	Unknown
Peak	2 hr
Duration	Unknown

Interactions

Individual drugs

Alcohol: increased adverse reactions
Aspirin: increased GI adverse reactions, toxicity
Cefamandole, cefoperazone, cefotetan, clopidine, clopidogrel, eptifibatide, plicamycin, ticlodipine, tirofiban: increased bleeding risk
Cyclosporine, methotrexate: increased toxicity
Lithium: increased lithium levels, avoid concomitant use
Phenytoin: increased phenytoin level, avoid concomitant use
Radiation: increased risk of hematologic toxicity

Drug classifications

Anticoagulants, thrombolytics: increased risk of bleeding
Antihypertensives: decreased effect of antihypertensives
Antineoplastics: increased risk of hematologic toxicity
Corticosteroids, NSAIDs: increased adverse reactions
Diuretics: decreased effectiveness of diuretics
Potassium supplements: increased adverse reactions

Drug/herb

Anise, arnica, bogbean, chamomile, chondroitin, clove, dong quai, fenugreek, feverfew, garlic, ginger, ginkgo, ginseng *(Panax)*, licorice: increased bleeding risk
Arginine, gossypol: increased gastric irritation
Bearberry, bilberry: increased NSAIDs effect

Drug/lab test

Increased: BUN, alkaline phosphatase
False positive: increased 5-HIAA
False increase: 17-KS

NURSING CONSIDERATIONS

Assessment

- Assess for pain and ROM: intensity, location, duration
- Monitor blood studies: alkaline phosphatase, LDH, AST, ALT, and bleeding time (may be increased)
- Assess for asthma, aspirin hypersensitivity, nasal polyps; increased hypersensitivity reactions

Nursing diagnoses

- Pain, chronic (uses)
- Mobility, physical, impaired (uses)
- Injury, risk for (adverse reactions)
- Knowledge, deficient (teaching)

Implementation

- Do not break, crush, or chew tabs
- Give with full glass of water to enhance absorption
- Give with food, antacids, milk to decrease gastric symptoms
- Sit upright for 30 min to prevent stomach irritation and ulceration

Patient/family education

- Teach patient that drug must be continued for prescribed time to be effective; to avoid aspirin, alcoholic beverages
- Instruct patient to use caution when driving; drowsiness, dizziness may occur
- Teach patient to take with a full glass of water to enhance absorption; patient should sit upright for 30 min to prevent stomach irritation and ulceration
- Instruct patient to use sunscreen and protective clothing to prevent burns
- Advise patient to report to prescriber severe abdominal pain, rash, itching, yellowing of skin or eyes, depression

Evaluation

Positive therapeutic outcome

- Decreased pain
- Decreased inflammation
- Increased mobility

oxazepam (Rx)

(ox-az'e-pam)

Apo-Oxazepam ✤, Novoxapam ✤, oxazepam

Func. class.: Sedative/hypnotic; antianxiety
Chem. class.: Benzodiazepine

Pregnancy category D

Controlled substance schedule IV

Action: Depresses subcortical levels of CNS, including limbic system, reticular formation; potentiates GABA

Therapeutic Outcome: Decreased anxiety, successful alcohol withdrawal, relaxation

Uses: Anxiety, alcohol withdrawal

Dosage and routes

Anxiety

Adult: PO 10-30 mg tid-qid

Elderly: PO 5 mg daily-bid initially, may increase

Alcohol withdrawal

Adult: PO 15-30 mg tid-qid

Available forms: Caps 10, 15, 30 mg

Adverse effects

CNS: *Dizziness, drowsiness,* confusion, headache, anxiety, tremors, fatigue, depression, insomnia, hallucinations, paradoxic excitement, transient amnesia

CV: *Orthostatic hypotension,* **ECG changes, tachycardia,** hypotension

EENT: *Blurred vision,* tinnitus, mydriasis

GI: Nausea, vomiting, anorexia

HEMA: Leukopenia

INTEG: Rash, dermatitis, itching

Contraindications: Pregnancy **D,** hypersensitivity to benzodiazepines, narrow-angle glaucoma, psychosis, child <12 yr, lactation

Precautions: Elderly, debilitated, hepatic disease, renal disease

Pharmacokinetics	
Absorption	Well absorbed
Distribution	Widely distributed; crosses placenta, blood-brain barrier
Metabolism	Liver
Excretion	Kidneys, breast milk
Half-life	5-15 hr

Pharmacodynamics	
Onset	½-1½ hr
Peak	Unknown
Duration	6-12 hr

Interactions

Individual drugs

Alcohol: increased CNS depression
Disulfiram: increased oxazepam effects
Valproic acid: decreased oxazepam effects

Drug classifications

CNS depressants: increased oxazepam effects
Oral contraceptives: decreased oxazepam effect

Drug/herb

Black cohosh: increased hypotension
Catnip, chamomile, clary, cowslip, hops, kava, lavender, mistletoe, nettle, pokeweed, poppy, Queen Anne's lace, senega, skullcap, valerian: increased CNS depression

Drug/lab test

Increased: AST, ALT, serum bilirubin
Decreased: radioactive iodine uptake
False increase: 17-OHCS

NURSING CONSIDERATIONS

Assessment

- Assess mental status: mood, sensorium, anxiety, affect, sleeping pattern, drowsiness, dizziness, especially elderly; physical dependency, withdrawal symptoms: anxiety, panic attacks, agitation, convulsions, headache, nausea, vomiting, muscle pain, weakness; suicidal tendencies; indications of increasing tolerance and abuse
- Monitor B/P with patient lying, standing, pulse; if systolic B/P drops 20 mm Hg, hold drug, notify prescriber
- Monitor blood studies: CBC during long-term therapy; blood dyscrasias have occurred rarely; decreased hematocrit, neutropenia may occur
- Monitor hepatic studies: AST, ALT, bilirubin, creatinine LDH, alkaline phosphatase if taking long term
- Monitor I&O; indicate renal dysfunction

Nursing diagnoses

- Anxiety (uses)
- Injury, risk for (adverse reactions)
- Knowledge, deficient (teaching)

Implementation

- Give with food or milk for GI symptoms; tab may be crushed if patient is unable to swallow medication whole

Patient/family education

- Teach patient that drug may be taken with food or fluids; tab may be crushed or swallowed whole
- Caution patient not to use for everyday stress or longer than 3 mo unless directed by prescriber; not to take more than prescribed amount; not to double doses or skip doses
- Advise patient to avoid OTC preparations unless approved by prescriber; alcohol and CNS depressants will increase CNS depression
- Caution patient to avoid driving and activities that require alertness, since drowsiness may occur; to avoid alcohol and other psychotropic medications; to rise slowly or fainting may occur, especially elderly; that drowsiness may worsen at beginning of treatment
- Caution patient not to discontinue medication abruptly after long-term use; withdrawal symptoms include vomiting, cramping, tremors, seizures
- Advise patient to use sugarless gum, hard candy, frequent sips of water for dry mouth

O

Evaluation

Positive therapeutic outcome

- Decreased anxiety, restlessness, sleeplessness (short-term treatment only)

Treatment of overdose: Lavage, VS, supportive care

oxcarbazepine (Rx)

(ox'kar-baz'uh-peen)

Trileptal

Func. class.: Anticonvulsant

Pregnancy category C

Action: May inhibit nerve impulses by limiting influx of sodium ions across cell membrane in motor cortex

Therapeutic Outcome: Absence of seizures

Uses: Partial seizures

Investigational uses: Trigeminal neuralgia, atypical panic disorder

Dosage and routes

Seizures adjunctive therapy

Adult: PO 300 mg bid, may be increased to 600 mg/day in divided doses bid; maintenance 1200 mg/day

Child 4-16 yr: PO 8-10 mg/kg/day divided bid, max 600 mg/day; dose is determined by weight

Conversion to monotherapy in partial seizures

Adult: PO 300 mg bid with reduction in other anticonvulsants, increase oxcarbazepine to max 600 mg/day q1wk over 2-4 wk; withdraw other anticonvulsants over 3-6 wk

Initiation of monotherapy in partial seizures

Adult: PO 300 mg bid, increase by 300 mg/day q3 days to 1200 mg divided bid

Renal dose

Adult: PO CCr <30 ml/min 150 mg bid and increase slowly

Available forms: Film-coated tabs, 150, 300, 600 mg; oral susp 300 mg/5 ml

Adverse effects

CNS: *Headache, dizziness, confusion, fatigue,* feeling abnormal, ataxia, abnormal gait, tremors, anxiety, agitation, **worsening of seizures**

CV: *Hypotension,* chest pain, edema

EENT: *Blurred vision, diplopia, nystagmus,* rhinitis, sinusitis

GI: *Nausea, constipation, diarrhea,* anorexia, vomiting, abdominal pain, gastritis, dry mouth, thirst, **rectal hemorrhage**

GU: *Frequency,* UTI, vaginitis

INTEG: Purpura, rash, acne

Contraindications: Hypersensitivity

Precautions: Pregnancy **C**, hypersensitivity to carbamazepine, lactation, child <4 yr, renal disease, fluid restriction

Pharmacokinetics	
Absorption	Unknown
Distribution	Unknown
Metabolism	Liver
Excretion	Unknown
Half-life	Unknown

Pharmacodynamics	
Onset	Unknown
Peak	Unknown
Duration	Unknown

Interactions

Individual drugs

Alcohol: increased CNS depression

Carbamazepine: decreased carbamazepine level

Felodipine: decreased effects of felodipine

Phenobarbital, valproic acid, verapamil: decreased oxcarbazepine level

Phenytoin: decreased oxcarbazepine level

Drug classifications

Contraceptives (oral): decreased oral contraceptive level

Drug/herb

Ginkgo: increased anticonvulsant effect

Ginseng, santonica: decreased anticonvulsant effect

NURSING CONSIDERATIONS

Assessment

- Assess seizure activity including frequency, duration, and aura; provide seizure precautions
- Assess mental status including mood, sensorium, affect, behavioral changes; if mental status changes, notify prescriber
- Assess eye problems: ophthalmic examinations (slit lamp, funduscopy, tonometry) are needed before, during, after treatment
- Assess patient for hypersensitivity to carbamazepine

Nursing diagnoses

- Injury, risk for (side effects)
- Knowledge, deficient (teaching)

Implementation

- Store drug at room temp
- Provide assistance with ambulation during early part of treatment; dizziness may occur

- Give drug with food, milk to decrease GI symptoms

Patient/family education

- Caution patient to avoid driving, other activities that require alertness
- Advise patient not to discontinue medication quickly after long-term use
- Instruct patient to avoid use of alcohol while taking this medication
- Instruct patient to use alternate contraception if using hormonal method
- Advise patient to use hard candy or gum for dry mouth, rinse mouth frequently
- Advise patient to carry/wear emergency ID stating name, drugs taken, condition, prescriber's name and phone number

Evaluation

Positive therapeutic outcome

- Decreased seizure activity

oxtriphylline (Rx)

(ox-trye'fi-lin)

Choledyl SA

Func. class.: Bronchodilator, spasmolytic

Chem. class.: Choline salt of theophylline

Pregnancy category C

Action: Relaxes smooth muscle of respiratory system by blocking phosphodiesterase, which increases cAMP; 64% theophylline

Therapeutic Outcome: Bronchodilatation with ease of breathing

Uses: Acute bronchial asthma, reversible bronchospasm in chronic bronchitis and COPD

Dosage and routes

Adult and child >16 yr: PO 4.7 mg/kg q8h or sus rel q12h

Child 9-16 yr and smokers (adult): 4.7 mg/kg q6h

Child 1-9 yr: 6.2 mg/kg q6h

Available forms: Elixir 100 mg/5 ml ✦; syr 50 mg/5 ml; tabs 100, 200 mg; ext rel tabs 400, 600 mg

Adverse effects

CNS: *Anxiety, restlessness, insomnia, dizziness,* **seizures,** headache, lightheadedness

CV: **Palpitations, sinus tachycardia,** hypotension

GI: Nausea, vomiting, anorexia, diarrhea, bitter taste, dyspepsia

INTEG: Flushing, urticaria, alopecia

RESP: Increased rate, **respiratory arrest**

Contraindications: Hypersensitivity to xanthines, tachydysrhythmias, active peptic ulcer

Precautions: Pregnancy **C,** elderly, CHF, cor pulmonale, hepatic disease, diabetes mellitus, hyperthyroidism, hypertension, children

Pharmacokinetics

Absorption	Well absorbed (PO); slow (PO-SUS REL)
Distribution	Widely distributed; crosses placenta
Metabolism	Liver to caffeine
Excretion	Kidneys, breast milk
Half-life	3-13 hr; increased in renal disease, CHF

Pharmacodynamics

	PO	PO-SUS REL
Onset	15-60 min	Unknown
Peak	1-5 hr	4-8 hr
Duration	6-8 hr	8-12 hr

Interactions

Individual drugs

Allopurinol, cimetidine, disulfiram, mexiletine: decreased metabolism

Cimetidine, disulfiram, fluvoxamine, mexiletine: increased toxicity

Ketoconazole, phenytoin, rifampin: increased metabolism, decreased effect

Lithium: decreased effect of lithium

Nicotine: decreased oxtriphylline level

Drug classifications

Barbiturates: decreased effect of oxtriphylline

β-Adrenergic blockers, fluoroquinolones, glucocorticoids: decreased metabolism, increased toxicity

Calcium channel blockers: increased oxtriphylline level

Contraceptives (oral): increased toxicity

Smoking: increased metabolism; decreased effect

Drug/herb

Cayenne: increased oxtriphylline toxicity

Cola tree: increased action of both

St. John's wort: decreased oxtriphylline level

Drug/food

Caffeinated foods (cola, coffee, tea, chocolate): increased CNS, CV adverse reactions

Charbroiled foods: decreased effect

Drug/lab test

Increased: plasma free fatty acids

O

NURSING CONSIDERATIONS

Assessment

- Monitor blood levels (therapeutic level is 10-20 mcg/ml); toxicity may occur with small increase above 20 mcg/ml, especially elderly; check whether theophylline was given recently (24 hr); watch for toxicity: nausea, vomiting, diarrhea, restlessness, tachycardia
- Monitor I&O; diuresis can occur; dehydration may result in elderly or children
- Monitor respiratory rate, rhythm, depth; auscultate lung fields bilaterally; notify prescriber of abnormalities
- Monitor allergic reactions: rash, urticaria; if these occur, drug should be discontinued
- Monitor pulmonary function studies baseline and during treatment

Nursing diagnoses

- Airway clearance, ineffective (uses)
- Activity intolerance (uses)
- Injury, risk for (uses, adverse reactions)
- Knowledge, deficient (teaching)

Implementation

- Do not break, crush, or chew enteric coated or ext rel tab
- Give PO pc to decrease GI symptoms; absorption may be affected with a full glass of water

Patient/family education

- Teach patient to take doses as prescribed, not to skip dose; to check OTC medications, current prescription medications for epHEDrine, which will increase CNS stimulation; not to drink alcohol or caffeine products (tea, coffee, chocolate, colas)
- Caution patient to avoid hazardous activities; dizziness may occur
- Instruct patient if GI upset occurs, to take drug with food
- Teach patient to notify prescriber of change in smoking habit; a change in dosage may be required
- Teach patient to increase fluids to 2 L/day to decrease viscosity of secretions

Evaluation

Positive therapeutic outcome

- Decreased dyspnea
- Clear lung fields bilaterally

oxybutynin (Rx)

(ox-i-byoo'ti-nin)

Ditropan, Ditropan XL, oxybutynin, Oxytrol

Func. class.: Anticholinergic

Chem. class.: Synthetic tertiary amine

Pregnancy category B

Do Not Confuse:
Ditropan/diazepam

Action: Relaxes smooth muscles in urinary tract by inhibiting acetylcholine at postganglionic sites

Therapeutic Outcome: Decreased symptoms of urgency, nocturia, incontinence

Uses: Antispasmodic for neurogenic bladder

Dosage and routes

Adult: PO 5 mg bid-tid, not to exceed 5 mg qid; ext rel tabs 5 mg daily, may increase by 5 mg, max 30 mg/day; TD apply one patch to abdomen, hip, buttock 2 ×/wk (q3-4 days)

Elderly: PO 2.5-5 mg tid, increase by 2.5 mg q several days

Child >5 yr: PO 5 mg bid, not to exceed 5 mg tid

Child 1-5 yrs: PO 0.2 mg/kg/dose 2-4 ×/day

Available forms: Syr 5 mg/5 ml; tabs 5 mg; ext rel tabs 5, 10, 15 mg; TD 3.9 mg/day

Adverse effects

CNS: *Anxiety, restlessness, dizziness,* **seizures,** headache, drowsiness, confusion

CV: *Palpitations, sinus tachycardia,* hypotension

EENT: Blurred vision, increased intraocular tension, dry mouth, throat

GI: *Nausea, vomiting, anorexia,* abdominal pain, constipation

GU: Dysuria, retention, hesitancy

Contraindications: Hypersensitivity, GI obstruction, GI hemorrhage, GU obstruction, glaucoma, severe colitis, myasthenia gravis, unstable CV status in acute hemorrhage

Precautions: Pregnancy **B,** lactation, suspected glaucoma, children <12 yr, elderly

Pharmacokinetics

Absorption	Rapidly absorbed
Distribution	Unknown
Metabolism	Liver
Excretion	Unknown
Half-life	Unknown

Pharmacodynamics

Onset	½-1 hr
Peak	3-4 hr
Duration	6-10 hr

Interactions

Individual drugs

Acetaminophen: decreased levels of acetaminophen
Atenolol: increased levels of atenolol
Digoxin: increased levels of digoxin
Haloperidol: decreased levels of haloperidol
Levodopa: decreased levels of levodopa
Nitrofurantoin: increased levels of nitrofurantoin

Drug classifications

Phenothiazines: increased or decreased levels of phenothiazines

Drug/herb

Black catechu: increased constipation
Butterbur, jimsonweed, scopolia: increased anticholinergic action
Jamborandi tree, pill-bearing spurge: decreased anticholinergic effect

NURSING CONSIDERATIONS

Assessment

- Assess for allergic reactions: rash, urticaria; if these occur, drug should be discontinued
- Assess urinary patterns: distention, nocturia, frequency, urgency, incontinence; catheterization may be required to remove residual urine

Nursing diagnoses

- Urinary elimination, impaired (uses)
- Pain, acute (uses)
- Knowledge, deficient (teaching)

Implementation

- Do not break, crush, or chew ext rel tabs
- May be given with meals or fluids or given on an empty stomach

Patient/family education

- Advise patient to avoid hazardous activities until response to drug is known; dizziness, blurred vision may occur
- Caution patient to avoid OTC medication with alcohol or other CNS depressants
- Advise patient to prevent photophobia by wearing sunglasses
- Teach patient to use frequent rinsing of mouth, sips of water for dry mouth
- Teach patient to stay cool; avoid hot weather, strenuous activity since overheating may occur; drug decreases perspiration
- Advise patient to report CNS effects: confusion, anxiety, anticholinergic effect in the elderly

Evaluation

Positive therapeutic outcome

- Absence of dysuria, frequency, nocturia, incontinence

! HIGH ALERT

oxycodone (Rx)

(ox-i-koe'done)

Endocodone, M-oxy, OxyContin, OxyFast, Oxyl R, Roxicodone, Roxicodone Supeudol ✤

oxycodone/acetaminophen

Endocet ✤, Oxycocet ✤, Percocet, Roxicet, Roxilox, Tylox

oxycodone/aspirin

Endodan ✤, Oxycodan ✤, Percodan, Percodan-Demi, Roxiprin

Func. class.: Opiate analgesic
Chem. class.: Semisynthetic derivative

Pregnancy category B

Controlled substance schedule II

Do Not Confuse:
Percodan/Decadron, Roxicet/Roxanol, Tylox/Trimox, Tylox/Wymox, Tylox/Xanax

Action: Inhibits ascending pain pathways in CNS, increases pain threshold, alters pain perception

Therapeutic Outcome: Decreased pain

Uses: Moderate to severe pain

O

Investigational uses: Postherpetic neuralgia (cont rel)

Dosage and routes

Adult: PO 10-30 mg q4h (5 mg q6h for Oxyl R, OxyFast) OxyFast conc sol is extremely concentrated, do not use interchangeably
Child: PO 0.05-0.15 mg/kg/dose up to 5 mg/dose q4-6h; not recommended in children

Available forms: Oxycodone: cont rel tabs (OxyContin) 10, 20, 40, 80, 160 mg; immediate rel tabs 15, 30 mg; tabs 5 mg; immediate rel caps 5 mg; oral sol 5 mg/5 ml, 20 mg/ml; oxycodone with acetaminophen: tabs 5 mg/325 mg; caps 5 mg/500 mg; oral sol 5 mg/325 mg/5 ml; oxycodone with aspirin: 2.44, 4.88 mg/325 mg

Adverse effects

CNS: *Drowsiness, dizziness, confusion, headache, sedation, euphoria*
CV: Palpitations, bradycardia, change in B/P
EENT: Tinnitus, blurred vision, miosis, diplopia
GI: *Nausea, vomiting, anorexia, constipation, cramps*

GU: Increased urinary output, dysuria, urinary retention
INTEG: ***Rash,*** urticaria, bruising, flushing, diaphoresis, pruritus
RESP: **Respiratory depression**

Contraindications: Hypersensitivity, addiction (opiate)

Precautions: Pregnancy **B,** addictive personality, lactation, increased ICP, MI (acute), severe heart disease, respiratory depression, hepatic disease, renal disease, child <18 yr

Pharmacokinetics

Absorption	Well absorbed
Distribution	Widely distributed; crosses placenta
Metabolism	Liver, extensively
Excretion	Kidneys, breast milk
Half-life	2-3 hr

Pharmacodynamics

	PO	REC
Onset	15-30 min	Unknown
Peak	½-1 hr	Unknown
Duration	4-6 hr	4-6 hr

Interactions

Individual drugs
Alcohol: increased respiratory depression, hypotension, sedation

Drug classifications
Antipsychotics, CNS depressants, opioids, sedative/hypnotics, skeletal muscle relaxants: increased respiratory depression, hypotension

Drug/herb
Corkwood: increased anticholinergic effect
Jamaican dogwood, lavender, mistletoe, nettle, pokeweed, poppy, senega, valerian: increased sedative effect

Drug/lab test
Increased: amylase

NURSING CONSIDERATIONS

Assessment
- Monitor VS after parenteral route; note muscle rigidity, drug history, liver, kidney function tests, respiratory dysfunction: respiratory depression, character, rate, rhythm; notify prescriber if respirations are <10/min
- Monitor CNS changes: dizziness, drowsiness, hallucinations, euphoria, LOC, pupil reaction
- Monitor allergic reactions: rash, urticaria

Nursing diagnoses
- Pain, acute (uses)
- Pain, chronic
- Sensory perception, disturbed: visual, auditory (adverse reactions)
- Breathing pattern, ineffective (adverse reactions)
- Injury, risk for (adverse reactions)
- Knowledge, deficient (teaching)

Implementation
- Give with antiemetic if nausea, vomiting occur
- Give when pain is beginning to return; determine dosage interval by patient response; continuous dosing of medication is more effective than when given prn
- Medication should be slowly withdrawn after long-term use to prevent withdrawal symptoms
- Store in light-resistant container at room temp

PO route
- Do not break, crush, or chew cont rel tabs
- May be given with food or milk to lessen GI upset
- Use 80, 160 mg cont rel tabs only in opioid-tolerant patients

Rectal route
- Store supp in the refrigerator; run under warm water before insertion

Patient/family education
- Advise patients to avoid CNS depressants: alcohol, sedative/hypnotics
- Discuss with patient that dizziness, drowsiness, and confusion are common; to avoid getting up without assistance
- Discuss in detail all aspects of the drug, including purpose and what to expect
- Advise patient to make position changes slowly to lessen orthostatic hypotension

Evaluation
Positive therapeutic outcome
- Decreased pain

Treatment of overdose: Naloxone 0.2-0.8 **IV**, O_2, **IV** fluids, vasopressors

! HIGH ALERT

oxymorphone (Rx)
(ox-i-mor′fone)
Numorphan
Func. class.: Opiate analgesic
Chem. class.: Semisynthetic phenanthrene derivative

Pregnancy category B

Controlled substance schedule II

Action: Depresses pain impulse transmission at the spinal cord level by interacting with opioid receptors

Therapeutic Outcome: Decreased pain

Uses: Moderate to severe pain

Dosage and routes

Adult: IM/SUBCUT 1-1.5 mg q4-6h prn; **IV** 0.5 mg q4-6h prn; rec 5 mg q4-6h prn

Labor analgesia

Adult: IM 0.5-1 mg

Available forms: Inj 1, 1.5 mg/ml; supp 5 mg

Adverse effects

CNS: *Drowsiness, dizziness, confusion, headache, sedation, euphoria (elderly),* **seizures**

CV: Palpitations, **bradycardia,** change in B/P

EENT: Tinnitus, blurred vision, miosis, diplopia

GI: *Nausea, vomiting, anorexia, constipation, cramps*

GU: Increased urinary output, dysuria, urinary retention

INTEG: *Rash,* urticaria, bruising, flushing, diaphoresis, pruritus

RESP: **Respiratory depression**

Contraindications: Hypersensitivity, addiction (opioid)

Precautions: Pregnancy **B** (short-term), addictive personality, lactation, increased ICP, MI (acute), severe heart disease, respiratory depression, hepatic disease, renal disease, child <18 yr

Pharmacokinetics

Absorption	Well absorbed (rec, IM, SUBCUT); completely absorbed (**IV**)
Distribution	Widely distributed; crosses placenta
Metabolism	Liver, extensively
Excretion	Kidneys
Half-life	2½-4 hr

Pharmacodynamics

	IM/SUBCUT	IV	REC
Onset	15 min	10 min	30 min
Peak	1-1½ hr	15-30 min	Unknown
Duration	3-6 hr	3-4 hr	3-6 hr

Interactions

Individual drugs

Alcohol: increased respiratory depression, hypotension, sedation

Drug classifications

CNS depressants, opiates, antipsychotics, skeletal muscle relaxants, sedative/hypnotics: increased respiratory depression, hypotension

MAOIs: do not use 2 wk before oxymorphone

Drug/herb

Corkwood: increased anticholinergic effect

Jamaican dogwood, lavender, mistletoe, nettle, pokeweed, poppy, senega, valerian: increased sedative effect

Drug/lab test

Increased: amylase

NURSING CONSIDERATIONS

Assessment

- Monitor VS after parenteral route; note muscle rigidity, drug history, liver, kidney function tests, respiratory dysfunction: respiratory depression, character, rate, rhythm; notify prescriber if respirations are <10/min
- Monitor CNS changes: dizziness, drowsiness, hallucinations, euphoria, LOC, pupil reaction
- Monitor allergic reactions: rash, urticaria

Nursing diagnoses

- Pain, acute (uses)
- Sensory perception, disturbed: visual, auditory (adverse reactions)
- Breathing pattern, ineffective (adverse reactions)
- Injury, risk for (adverse reactions)
- Knowledge, deficient (teaching)

Implementation

- Give with antiemetic if nausea, vomiting occur
- Give when pain is beginning to return; determine dosage interval by patient response; continuous dosing of medication is more effective than when given prn
- Medication should be slowly withdrawn after long-term use to prevent withdrawal symptoms
- Store in light-resistant container at room temp

Rectal route

- Store in refrigerator

IV route

- Give by direct **IV** undiluted over 2-3 min

Y-site compatibilities: Glycopyrrolate, hydrOXYzine, ranitidine

Patient/family education

- Advise patients to avoid CNS depressants: alcohol, sedative/hypnotics
- Discuss with patient that dizziness, drowsiness, and confusion are common; to avoid getting up without assistance
- Discuss in detail all aspects of the drug, including purpose and what to expect
- Advise patient to make position changes slowly to lessen orthostatic hypotension

Evaluation

Positive therapeutic outcome

- Decreased pain

O

Treatment of overdose: Naloxone (Narcan) 0.2-0.8 mg **IV**, O_2, **IV** fluids, vasopressors

! HIGH ALERT

oxytocin (Rx)

(ox-i-toe'sin)

Pitocin

Func. class.: Oxytocic hormone

Pregnancy category N/A

Action: Acts directly on myofibrils, producing uterine contraction; stimulates breast milk letdown

Therapeutic Outcome: Stimulation of labor, control of bleeding; stimulation of milk letdown

Uses: Stimulation, induction of labor; missed or incomplete abortion, postpartum bleeding, postpartum breast engorgement

Dosage and routes

Labor induction

Adult: **IV** 1-2 mU/min, increase by 1-2 mU q15-60 min until regular contractions occur, then decrease dosage

Postpartum hemorrhage

Adult: **IV** 10-40 units in 1000 ml nonhydrating diluent infused at 20-40 mU/min

Adult: IM 10 units after placenta delivery

Incomplete abortion

Adult: **IV** inf 10 units/500 ml D_5W or 0.9% NaCl run at 20-40 mU/min; max 30 units/12 hr

Fetal stress test

Adult: **IV** 0.5 mU/min; increase q20 min until 3 contractions occur at 10 min

Available forms: Inj 10 units/ml

Adverse effects

CNS: **Seizures, tetanic contractions**

CV: Hypotension, hypertension, dysrhythmias, increased pulse, bradycardia, tachycardia, premature ventricular contractions

FETUS: Dysrhythmias, jaundice, hypoxia, **intracranial hemorrhage**

GI: Anorexia, nausea, vomiting, constipation

GU: **Abruptio placentae, decreased uterine blood flow**

HEMA: Increased hyperbilirubinemia

INTEG: Rash

RESP: **Asphyxia**

Contraindications: Hypersensitivity, serum toxemia, cephalopelvic disproportion, fetal distress, hypertonic uterus

Precautions: Cervical/uterine surgery, uterine sepsis, primipara >35 yr, 1st, 2nd stage of labor

Pharmacokinetics

Absorption	Well absorbed (nasal); completely absorbed (**IV**)
Distribution	Widely distributed (extracellular fluid)
Metabolism	Liver, rapidly
Excretion	Kidneys
Half-life	3-12 min

Pharmacodynamics

	NASAL	IV	IM
Onset	5 min	Rapid	3-7 min
Peak	Unknown	Unknown	Unknown
Duration	20 min	1 hr	1 hr

Interactions

Drug classifications

Vasopressors: increased hypertension

Drug/herb

Ephedra: hypertension

NURSING CONSIDERATIONS

Assessment

- Assess labor contractions: fetal heart tones, frequency, duration, intensity of contractions; if fetal heart tones increase or decrease significantly or if contractions are longer than 1 min, notify prescriber; turn patient on left side to increase oxygen to fetus
- Assess for water intoxication: confusion, anuria, drowsiness, headache; notify prescriber
- Watch for fetal distress, acceleration, deceleration, fetal presentation, pelvic dimensions
- Monitor B/P, pulse, respiratory rate, rhythm, depth
- Monitor I&O ratio
- Provide an environment conducive to letdown reflex

Nursing diagnoses

- Breastfeeding, ineffective (uses)
- Injury, risk for (uses)
- Knowledge, deficient (teaching)

Implementation

IV route

- Use an infusion pump; rotate sol for mixing; have magnesium sulfate available
- For labor induction administer after diluting 10 units/L of D_5W, 0.9% NaCl, 0.45% NaCl, LR, Ringer's for a conc of 10 units/ml; start at 1-2 units/min (0.1-0.2 ml); may increase by 1-2 units/min q15-30 min until labor begins

- For threatened abortion administer after diluting 10 units/500 ml of D_5W, $D_{10}W$, 0.9% NaCl, 0.45% NaCl, LR, Ringer's for a conc of 20 units/ml; give at 10-40 units/min
- For postpartum bleeding administer after diluting 10-40 units/L of D_5W, $D_{10}W$, 0.9% NaCl, 0.45% NaCl, LR, Ringer's for a conc of 10-40 units/ml; may titrate to response

Y-site compatibilities: Heparin, regular insulin, hydrocortisone, meperidine, morphine, potassium chloride, vit B/C, warfarin

Additive compatibilities: Chloramphenicol, metaraminol, netilmicin, sodium bicarbonate, thiopental, verapamil

Additive incompatibilities: Fibrinolysin, warfarin

Patient/family education

- Teach patient to report increased blood loss, abdominal cramps, increased temp or foul-smelling lochia
- Advise patient that contractions will be similar to menstrual cramps, gradually increasing in intensity

Evaluation

Positive therapeutic outcome

- Stimulation of milk letdown (nasal)
- Induction of labor
- Decreased postpartum bleeding

paclitaxel (Rx)

(pa-kli-tax'el)

Abraxane, Onxol, Taxol

Func. class.: Antineoplastic—miscellaneous

Chem. class.: Natural diterpene, antimicrotubule

Pregnancy category D

Do Not Confuse:

paclitaxel/paroxetine, paclitaxel/Paxil, Taxol/Paxil, Taxol/Taxotera

Action: Inhibits the reorganization of the microtubule network needed for interphase and mitotic cellular functions; also causes abnormal bundles of microtubules during cell cycle and multiple esters of microtubules during mitosis

Therapeutic Outcome: Prevention of rapidly growing malignant cells

Uses: Taxol: metastatic carcinoma of the ovary unresponsive to other treatment, breast carcinoma; AIDS-related Kaposi's sarcoma (2nd-line), non–small cell lung cancer, adjuvant treatment for node-positive breast cancer; Onxol: failure of other treatment in breast cancer, advanced ovarian cancer

Investigational uses: Advanced head, neck, small cell lung cancer; non-Hodgkin's lymphoma, adenocarcinoma of the upper GI tract, hormone-refractory prostate cancer

Dosage and routes

Ovarian carcinoma

Adults: **IV** inf 135 mg/m^2 given over 24 hr q3 wk, then cisplatin 75 mg/m^2 or 175 mg/m^2 over 3 hr q3 wk or 175 mg/m^2 over 3 hr

Advanced ovarian carcinoma

Adult: **IV** inf 175 mg/m^2 with cisplatin 75 mg/m^2 over 3 hr q3 wk

Breast carcinoma

Adult: **IV** inf 175 mg/m^2 over 3 hr q3 wk × 4 courses

AIDS-related Kaposi's sarcoma

Adult: **IV** inf 135 mg/m^2 over 3 hr q3 wk or 100 mg/m^2 over 3 hr q2 wk

1st line non–small cell lung cancer

Adult: Inf 135 mg/m^2/24 hr with cisplatin 75 mg/m^2 × 3 wk

Available forms: Inj 30 mg/5 ml vial (6 mg/ml); powder for inj, lyophilized 100 mg in single-use vials

Adverse effects

CV: *Bradycardia, hypotension, abnormal ECG*

GI: *Nausea, vomiting, diarrhea, mucositis; increased bilirubin, alkaline phosphatase, AST*

HEMA: **Neutropenia, leukopenia, thrombocytopenia, anemia,** bleeding, infections

INTEG: Alopecia

MS: *Arthralgia, myalgia*

NEURO: *Peripheral neuropathy*

SYST: *Hypersensitivity reactions,* **anaphylaxis**

Contraindications: Pregnancy **D**, hypersensitivity to paclitaxel or other drugs with polyoxyethylated castor oil, neutropenia (neutrophils <1500/mm^3)

Precautions: Children, lactation, hepatic disease, CV disease, CNS disorder

Pharmacokinetics

Absorption	Completely absorbed
Distribution	89%-98% protein binding
Metabolism	Liver, extensively
Excretion	Unknown
Half-life	5-17 hr

P

Pharmacodynamics	
Onset	Unknown
Peak	1-2 wk
Duration	3 wk

Interactions

Individual drugs

CycloSPORINE, dexamethasone, diazepam, etoposide, ketoconazole, quinidine, teniposide, testosterone, verapamil, vinCRIStine: decreased metabolism of paclitaxel
DOXOrubicin: increased levels of DOXOrubicin
Radiation: increased myelosuppression

Drug classifications

Antineoplastics: increased myelosuppression
Live virus vaccines: decreased immune response

NURSING CONSIDERATIONS

Assessment

- Assess CNS changes: confusion, paresthesias, psychosis, tremors, seizures, neuropathies; drug should be discontinued
- Check buccal cavity q8h for dryness, sores or ulceration, white patches, oral pain, bleeding, dysphagia; obtain prescription for viscous lidocaine (Xylocaine) to use in mouth
- Assess symptoms indicating severe allergic reaction, anaphylaxis: rash, pruritus, urticaria, purpuric skin lesions, itching, flushing
- Monitor CBC, differential, platelet count weekly; withhold drug if WBC is $<1500/mm^3$ or platelet count is $<100,000/mm^3$, notify prescriber of results
- Monitor renal function studies: BUN, creatinine, serum uric acid, urine CCr before and during therapy; check I&O ratio; report fall in urine output to <30 ml/hr
- Monitor temp q4h (may indicate beginning of infection)
- Monitor liver function tests before and during therapy (bilirubin, AST, ALT, LDH) as needed or monthly; check for jaundice of skin and sclera, dark urine, clay-colored stools, itchy skin, abdominal pain, fever, diarrhea
- Assess for bleeding: hematuria, stool guaiac, bruising or petechiae, mucosa or orifices q8h; check for inflammation of mucosa, breaks in skin
- Assess effects of alopecia on body image; discuss feelings about body changes

Nursing diagnoses

- Injury, risk for (adverse reactions)
- Body image, disturbed (adverse reactions)
- Infection, risk for (adverse reactions)
- Knowledge, deficient (teaching)

Implementation

- Give fluids PO before chemotherapy to hydrate patient
- Give antacid before oral agent; give drug after evening meal, before bedtime; provide antiemetic 30-60 min before giving drug and prn to prevent vomiting; administer antibiotics for prophylaxis of infection
- Give TOP or systemic analgesics for pain to lessen effects of stomatitis
- Give liq diet: carbonated beverages; gelatin may be added if patient is not nauseated or vomiting

IV route

- Give after diluting in 0.9% NaCl, D_5, D_5 and 0.9% NaCl, D_5LR to a concentration of 0.3-1.2 mg/ml
- Use an in-line filter ≤0.22 µm
- Give after premedicating with dexamethasone 20 mg PO 12 and 6 hr before paclitaxel, diphenhydrAMINE 50 mg **IV** ½-1 hr before paclitaxel and cimetidine 300 mg or ranitidine 50 mg **IV** ½-1 hr before paclitaxel
- Use only glass bottles, polypropylene, polyolefin bags and administration sets; do not use PVC infusion bags or sets
- Use gloves and cytotoxic handling precautions

Abraxane

- Reconstitute vial by injecting 20 ml of 0.9% NaCl
- Slowly inject the 20 ml of 0.9% NaCl over at least 1 min to direct the sol flow on wall of vial
- Do not inject 0.9% NaCl directly onto lyophilized cake (foaming will occur)
- Allow vial to sit for at least 5 min to ensure proper wetting of lyophilized cake
- Gently swirl or invert vial slowly for at least 2 min until completely dissolved
- Calculate dosing by: Dosing volume (ml) = total dose (mg) ÷ 5 (mg/ml)

Y-site compatiblilities: Acyclovir, amikacin, aminophylline, bleomycin, butorphanol, calcium chloride, carboplatin, cefepime, cefotetan, ceftazidime, ceftriaxone, cimetidine, cisplatin, cyclophosphamide, cytarabine, dacarbazine, dexamethasone, diphenhydrAMINE, DOXOrubicin, droperidol, etoposide, famotidine, floxuridine, fluconazole, fluorouracil, furosemide, ganciclovir, gentamicin, haloperidol, heparin, mannitol, meperidine, mesna, methotrexate, metoclopramide, morphine, nalbuphine, ondansetron, pentostatin, potassium chloride, prochlorperazine, propofol, ranitidine, sodium bicarbonate, vancomycin, vinBLAStine, vinCRIStine, zidovudine

Patient/family education
- Inform patient that nonhormonal contraceptive measures are recommended during therapy and >4 mo after; teratogenic effects are possible
- Teach patient to avoid use of products containing aspirin or ibuprofen, razors, commercial mouthwash, since bleeding may occur; to report symptoms of bleeding (hematuria, tarry stools)
- Instruct patient to report signs of anemia (fatigue, headache, irritability, faintness, shortness of breath) and CNS reactions (confusion, psychosis, nightmares, seizures, severe headaches)
- Teach patient to rinse mouth tid-qid with water, club soda; brush teeth bid-qid with soft brush or cotton-tipped applicators for stomatitis; use unwaxed dental floss
- Inform patient that hair may be lost during treatment; a wig or hairpiece may make patient feel better; new hair may be different in color, texture
- Inform patient that receiving vaccinations during therapy may cause serious reactions

Evaluation
Positive therapeutic outcome
- Prevention of rapid division of malignant cells

palivizumab (Rx)
(pal-ih-viz'uh-mab)
Synagis
Func. class.: Monoclonal antibody
Pregnancy category C

Action: A humanized monoclonal antibody that exhibits neutralizing and fusion-inhibitory activity against respiratory syncytial virus (RSV)

Therapeutic Outcome: Absence of RSV

Uses: Prevention of serious lower respiratory tract disease caused by RSV in pediatric patients

Dosage and routes
Child: IM 15 mg/kg, those patients who develop RSV should receive monthly doses during RSV season (Nov.-April)

Available forms: Powder for reconstitution 50, 100 mg; solution 50 mg/0.5 ml, 100 mg/1 mg

Adverse effects
CNS: Fever
EENT: Otitis media, rhinitis, pharyngitis
GI: Nausea, vomiting, diarrhea, increased AST
INTEG: Rash, inj site reaction
RESP: Upper respiratory tract infection, **apnea**, cough
SYST: **Anaphylaxis**

Contraindications: Hypersensitivity, adults, cyanotic congenital heart disease

Precautions: Pregnancy **C**, thrombocytopenia, coagulation disorders, established RSV, congenital heart disease, chronic lung disease, systemic allergic reactions

Pharmacokinetics	
Absorption	Unknown
Distribution	Unknown
Metabolism	Unknown
Excretion	Unknown
Half-life	20 days

Pharmacodynamics	
Onset	Unknown
Peak	Unknown
Duration	Unknown

Interactions: Unknown

NURSING CONSIDERATIONS
Assessment
- Assess for presence of RSV infection, drug is given to prevent infection
- Assess for side effects and report if allergic reaction is evident
- Assess for anaphylaxis: difficulty breathing, drug should be discontinued, have emergency equipment nearby

Nursing diagnoses
- Infection, risk for (uses)
- Knowledge, deficient (teaching)

Implementation
- Give IM only
- Give after adding 1 ml of sterile water for inj per 100 mg vial (add 0.6 ml sterile water for inj for 50 mg vial); gently swirl for 30 sec to avoid foaming, do not shake; let stand at room temperature for 20 min until sol clarifies; given within 6 hr of reconstitution

Patient/family education
- Teach patient to report upper respiratory infections, earaches, rash, sore throat

Evaluation
Positive therapeutic outcome
- Absence of RSV

P

palonosetron (Rx)
(pa-lone-o'se-tron)
Aloxi
Func. class.: Antiemetic
Chem. class.: $5\text{-}HT_3$ receptor antagonist
Pregnancy category B

Action: Prevents nausea, vomiting by blocking serotonin peripherally, centrally, and in the small intestine at the $5\text{-}HT_3$ receptor

Therapeutic Outcome: Decreased nausea, vomiting during chemotherapy

Uses: Prevention of nausea, vomiting associated with cancer chemotherapy

Dosage and routes
***Adult:* IV** 0.25 mg as a single dose over 30 sec, 30 min prior to chemotherapy, max 25 mg **IV** over q7d

Available forms: Inj 0.25 mg/5 ml

Adverse effects
CNS: *Headache, dizziness, drowsiness, fatigue, insomnia*
GI: *Diarrhea, constipation,* abdominal pain
MISC: Weakness, hyperkalemia, anxiety, rash, **bronchospasm** (rare), arthralgia, *fever, urinary retention*

Contraindications: Hypersensitivity

Precautions: Pregnancy **B**, lactation, children, elderly, prolongation of QT interval or other cardiac conduction intervals (patients with hypokalemia, hypomagnesemia, taking diuretics, with congenital QT syndrome, and taking antidysrhythmics or other drugs that may prolong QT interval and cumulative high-dose antithramycline therapy)

Pharmacokinetics

Absorption	Unknown
Distribution	62% protein bound
Metabolism	Liver
Excretion	Unchanged drug and metabolites excreted by kidney
Half-life	40 hr

Pharmacodynamics

Onset	Unknown
Peak	Unknown
Duration	Unknown

Interactions: None known

NURSING CONSIDERATIONS
Assessment
- Monitor for absence of nausea, vomiting during chemotherapy
- Assess hypersensitivity reaction: rash, bronchospasm

Nursing diagnoses
Knowledge, deficient (teaching)

Implementation
IV route
- Give as a single dose over 30 sec
- Do not mix with other drugs, flush **IV** line before and after administration
- Store at room temp

Patient/family education
- Teach to report diarrhea, constipation, rash, or changes in respirations or discomfort at insertion site

Evaluation
Positive therapeutic outcome
- Absence of nausea, vomiting during cancer chemotherapy

pamidronate (Rx)
(pam-i-drone'ate)
Aredia
Func. class.: Bone resorption inhibitor, electrolyte modifier
Chem. class.: Bisphosphonate
Pregnancy category D

Do Not Confuse:
Aredia/Adriamycin

Action: Inhibits bone resorption, apparently without inhibiting bone formation and mineralization; absorbs calcium phosphate crystals in bone and may directly block dissolution of hydroxyapatite crystals of bone

Therapeutic Outcome: Serum calcium at normal level

Uses: Moderate to severe Paget's disease associated with malignancy with or without bone metastases; osteolytic bone metastases in breast cancer patients, multiple myeloma

Dosage and routes
Hypercalcemia of malignancy
***Adult:* IV** inf 60-90 mg as a single dose in moderate hypercalcemia, 90 mg in severe hypercalcemia given over 24 hr; dose should be diluted in 1000 ml 0.45% NaCl, 0.9% NaCl, or D_5W; wait 7 days before 2nd course

Osteolytic lesions from multiple myeloma
Adult: **IV** 90 mg/500 ml of D_5W, 0.45% NaCl, or 0.9% NaCl given over 4 hr on a monthly basis

Paget's disease
Adult: **IV** 90-180 mg/treatment, may use 30 mg daily × 3 days

Available forms: Powder for inj 30, 90 mg/vial; inj 3, 6, 9 mg/ml

Adverse effects

CNS: Fatigue, fever, psychosis
CV: *Hypertension*
GI: *Abdominal pain, anorexia, constipation, nausea, vomiting,* diarrhea, dyspepsia
GU: UTI, fluid overload
INTEG: Redness, swelling, induration, pain on palpation at site of catheter insertion
META: Anemia, hypokalemia, hypomagnesemia, hypophosphatemia, hypocalcemia, hyperthyroidism
MS: *Bone pain,* myalgia
RESP: Coughing, dyspnea, URI

Contraindications: Pregnancy **D**, hypersensitivity to bisphosphonates

Precautions: Children, nursing mothers, renal dysfunction

Pharmacokinetics

Absorption	Rapidly cleared from circulation
Distribution	Mainly to bones, primarily in areas of high bone turnover
Metabolism	Unknown
Excretion	Kidneys, unchanged (50%)
Half-life	Biphasic 1½ hr; 27 hr; from bone to 300 days

Pharmacodynamics

Onset	1 day
Peak	1 wk
Duration	Unknown

Interactions:
Individual drugs
Calcium, vitamin D: decreased pamidronate effect
Digoxin: increased hypomagnesemia, hypokalemia

NURSING CONSIDERATIONS
Assessment

- Assess for hypocalcemia: Chvostek's, Trousseau's sign, paresthesia, twitching, laryngospasm
- Monitor manifestations of hypocalcemia: personality changes, anxiety, disturbances, depression, psychosis; nausea, vomiting, constipation, abdominal pain from muscle spasm; decreased contractility, decreased cardiac output, hypotension, lengthened ST segment, prolonged QT interval; scaling eczema, alopecia, hyperpigmentation; tetany, muscle twitching, cramping, grimacing, seizure, altered deep tendon reflexes, spasm
- Monitor manifestations of hypomagnesemia: agitation; muscle twitching, paresthesia, hyperactive reflexes, positive Babinski reflex, dysphagia, nystagmus, seizures, tetany; nausea, vomiting, diarrhea, anorexia, abdominal distention; ectopy, tachycardia, broad, flat, or inverted T waves, depressed ST segment, prolonged QT interval, decreased cardiac output, hypotension
- Monitor manifestations of hypokalemia: acidic urine, reduced urine osmolality, nocturia, polyuria, polydipsia; hypotension, broad T wave, U wave, ectopy, tachycardia, weak pulse; muscle weakness, altered LOC, drowsiness, apathy, lethargy, confusion, depression; anorexia, nausea, cramps, constipation, distention, paralytic ileus; hypoventilation, respiratory muscle weakness
- Assess fluid volume status: check I&O ratio and record, assess for distended red veins, crackles in lung, color, quality, and sp gr of urine, skin turgor, adequacy of pulses, moist mucous membranes, bilateral lung sounds, peripheral pitting edema
- Monitor electrolytes: phosphorus, potassium, sodium, calcium, magnesium; also include BUN, creatinine, CBC, platelets, hemoglobin
- Assess B/P before and during therapy
- Assess for pain: in joints or on exertion, duration and characteristics; analgesics may be ordered
- Assess for phlebitis at **IV** site: swelling, redness, pain, warmth

Nursing diagnoses

- Injury, risk for (uses, adverse reactions)
- Fluid volume, excess (side effects)
- Knowledge, deficient (teaching)

Implementation

- Give by **IV** inf after reconstituting by adding 10 ml of sterile water for inj to each vial, then adding to 1000 ml of sterile 0.45%, 0.9% NaCl, D_5W, run over 24 hr for hypercalcemia or 60 mg ≥4 hr, 90 mg/24 hr; dilute reconstituted sol in 500 ml of 0.9% NaCl, 0.45% NaCl, or D_5W, give over 4 hr (multiple myeloma, Paget's disease)
- Do not mix with calcium-containing infusion sol such as Ringer's sol

P

- Store inf sol for up to 24 hr at room temp
- Reconstituted sol with sterile water may be stored under refrigeration for up to 24 hr

Additive incompatibilities:
Calcium products, sol

Patient/family education

- Advise patient to report hypercalcemic relapse: nausea, vomiting, bone pain, thirst; unusual muscle twitching, muscle spasms, severe diarrhea, constipation
- Advise patient to continue with dietary recommendations, including calcium and vit D
- To obtain an analgesic from provider for bone pain
- That, if nausea/vomiting occur, small, frequent meals may help

Evaluation

Positive therapeutic outcome

- Decreased calcium levels to normal

pancrelipase (Rx)

(pan-kre-li'pase)

Cotazym, Cotazym-65B ✦, Cotazym E.C.S. 8, Cotazym E.C.S. 20, Cotazym Capsules, Cotazym-S, Creon, Ilozyme, Ku-Zyme HP, Lipram-PN16, Lipram-CR20, Lipram-UL12, Lipram-PN10, Pancrease Capsules, Pancrease MT 4, Pancrease MT 10, Pancrease MT 16, Protilase, Ultrase MT 12, Ultrase MT 20, Viokase, Zymase

Func. class.: Digestant
Chem. class.: Pancreatic enzyme (bovine/porcine)

Pregnancy category C

Action: Pancreatic enzyme needed for breakdown of substances released from the pancreas

Therapeutic Outcome: Increases protein, fat, carbohydrate digestion

Uses: Exocrine pancreatic secretion insufficiency, cystic fibrosis (digestive aid), steatorrhea, pancreatic enzyme deficiency

Dosage and routes

Many products listed above are not interchangeable

Adult and child: PO 1-3 cap/tab ac or with meals, or 1 cap/tab with snack or 1-2 powder packets ac

Available forms: Powder 16,800 units lipase/70,000 units protease and amylase; caps 8000 units lipase/30,000 units protease and amylase; delayed rel caps, 4000 units lipase/12,000 units protease and amylase, 4000 units lipase/25,000 units protease/20,000 units amylase, 5000 units lipase/20,000 units protease and amylase, 10,000 units lipase/30,000 units protease and amylase, 12,000 units lipase/24,000 units protease and amylase, 12,000 units lipase/39,000 units protease and amylase, 16,000 units lipase/48,000 units protease and amylase 20,000 units lipase/65,000 units protease and amylase, 24,000 units lipase/78,000 units protease and amylase

Adverse effects

GI: Anorexia, nausea, vomiting, diarrhea
GU: Hyperuricuria, hyperuricemia

Contraindications: Allergy to pork

Precautions: Pregnancy **C**, ileus, pancreatitis, Crohn's disease

Pharmacokinetics

Absorption	Unknown
Distribution	Unknown
Metabolism	Unknown
Excretion	Unknown
Half-life	Unknown

Pharmacodynamics

Unknown

Interactions

Individual drugs
Cimetidine, iron (oral): decreased absorption of pancrelipase

Drug classifications
Antacids: decreased absorption of pancrelipase

NURSING CONSIDERATIONS

Assessment

- Monitor I&O ratio; watch for increasing urinary output
- Monitor fecal fat, nitrogen, protime, during treatment
- Monitor for polyuria, polydipsia, polyphagia (may indicate diabetes mellitus)
- Assess for allergy to pork; patient may also be sensitive to this drug
- Assess for appropriate weight, height, development; there may be a developmental lag
- Check stools for steatorrhea, which signifies undigested fat content

Nursing diagnoses

- Nutrition: less than body requirements, imbalanced (uses)
- Knowledge, deficient (teaching)

Implementation

- Give tab with 8 oz of water and sitting up only; do not let tab sit in mouth
- Give after antacid or cimetidine; decreased pH inactivates drug
- Give powder mixed in prepared fruit for infants, children
- Administer low-fat diet to decrease GI symptoms
- Store in airtight container at room temp

Patient/family education

- Teach patient to take tab with 8 oz or more water, not to let tab sit in mouth; have patient take tab sitting up only
- Advise patient to notify prescriber of allergic reactions, abdominal pain, cramping, or hematuria
- Teach patient not to inhale powder, very irritating to mucous membranes, some powder may irritate skin

Evaluation

Positive therapeutic outcome

- Absence of steatorrhea
- Improved digestion of carbohydrates, proteins, fat

! HIGH ALERT

pancuronium (Rx)

(pan-cure-oh'nee-yum)

pancuronium bromide, Pavulon

Func. class.: Neuromuscular blocker (nondepolarizing)

Chem. class.: Synthetic curariform

Pregnancy category C

Action: Inhibits transmission of nerve impulses by binding with cholinergic receptor sites, antagonizing action of acetylcholine; no analgesic response

Therapeutic Outcome: Paralysis of all skeletal muscles

Uses: Facilitation of endotracheal intubation, skeletal muscle relaxation during mechanical ventilation, surgery, or general anesthesia

Dosage and routes

Adult and child >1 mo: **IV** 0.04-0.1 mg/kg, then 0.01 mg/kg q30-60 min

Child >10 yr: **IV** 0.04-0.1 mg/kg, then 1/5 initial dose q30-60 min

Available forms: Inj 1, 2 mg/ml

Adverse effects

CV: Bradycardia, tachycardia, increased, decreased B/P, ventricular extrasystoles, edema

EENT: Increased secretions

INTEG: Rash, flushing, pruritus, urticaria, sweating, salivation

MS: Weakness to prolonged skeletal muscle relaxation

RESP: **Prolonged apnea, bronchospasm, cyanosis, respiratory depression,** wheezing

SYST: **Anaphylaxis**

Contraindications: Hypersensitivity to bromide ion

Precautions: Pregnancy **C**, renal disease, cardiac disease, lactation, children <2 yr, electrolyte imbalances, dehydration, neuromuscular disease, respiratory disease, hepatic disease

Pharmacokinetics	
Absorption	Complete bioavailability
Distribution	Extracellular space; crosses placenta
Metabolism	Plasma
Excretion	Kidneys, unchanged
Half-life	2 hr

Pharmacodynamics	
Onset	3-5 min, dose dependent
Peak	3-5 min
Duration	35-40 min

Interactions

Individual drugs

Clindamycin, enflurane, isoflurane, lincomycin, lithium, polymyxin B, quinidine: increased neuromuscular blockade

Theophylline: dysrhythmias

Drug classifications

Aminoglycosides, anesthetics (local), analgesics (opioid), thiazides: increased neuromuscular blockade

Drug/lab test

Decreased: cholinesterase

NURSING CONSIDERATIONS

Assessment

- Monitor vital signs (B/P, pulse, respirations, airway) until fully recovered; note rate, depth, pattern of respirations, strength of hand grip; patient should be intubated before use
- Monitor for electrolyte imbalances (potassium, magnesium) before drug is used; electrolyte imbalances may lead to increased action of this drug
- Monitor for recovery: decreased paralysis of face, diaphragm, leg, arm, rest of body;

P

residual weakness and respiratory problems may occur during recovery period

- Assess for hypersensitive reactions, anaphylaxis: rash, fever, respiratory distress, pruritus; drug should be discontinued

Nursing diagnoses

- Breathing pattern, ineffective (uses)
- Communication, verbal, impaired (adverse reactions)
- Fear (adverse reactions)
- Knowledge, deficient (teaching)

Implementation

- Use peripheral nerve stimulator (anesthesiologist) to determine neuromuscular blockade; deep tendon reflexes should be monitored during extended periods
- Give direct **IV** undiluted over 1-2 min, or diluted in D_5W or 0.9% NaCl and give as an inf at prescribed rate; titrate to patient response; should be administered only by qualified person, usually an anesthesiologist; do not administer IM
- Store in light-resistant area
- Give anticholinesterase to reverse neuromuscular blockade

Syringe compatibilities: Heparin
Y-site compatibilities: Aminophylline, cefazolin, cefuroxime, cimetidine, DOBUTamine, DOPamine, epINEPHrine, esmolol, fentanyl, fluconazole, gentamicin, heparin, hydrocortisone, isoproterenol, lorazepam, midazolam, morphine, nitroglycerin, nitroprusside, ranitidine, sulfamethoxazole/trimethoprim, vancomycin
Y-site incompatibilities: Diazepam
Additive compatibilities: Verapamil
Additive incompatibilities: Barbiturates

Patient/family education

- Provide reassurance if communication is difficult during recovery from neuromuscular blockade
- Provide explanation to patients regarding all procedures or treatments; patient will remain conscious if anesthesia is not given also

Evaluation

Positive therapeutic outcome

- Paralysis of jaw, eyelid, head, neck, rest of body as evaluated by peripheral nerve stimulator

Treatment of overdose: Edrophonium or neostigmine, atropine; monitor VS; may require mechanical ventilation

pantoprazole (Rx)

(pan-toe-pray'zole)
Protonix, Protonix IV
Func. class.: Proton pump inhibitor
Chem. class.: Benzimidazole

Pregnancy category C

Action: Suppresses gastric secretion by inhibiting hydrogen/potassium ATPase enzyme system in gastric parietal cell; characterized as gastric acid pump inhibitor, since it blocks final step of acid production

Therapeutic Outcome: Absence of epigastric fullness, pain, swelling

Uses: Gastroesophageal reflux disease (GERD), severe erosive esophagitis, maintenance, long-term pathological hypersecretory conditions including Zollinger-Ellison syndrome

Dosage and routes

GERD

Adult: PO 40 mg daily × 8 wk, may repeat course

Erosive esophagitis

Adult: **IV** 40 mg daily × 7-10 days; PO 40 mg daily × 8 wk; may repeat PO course

Pathological hypersecretory conditions

Adult: **IV** 80 mg q12h; max 240 mg/day

Available forms: Delayed rel tabs, 20, 40 mg; powder for inj, freeze dried 40 mg/vial

Adverse effects

CNS: *Headache,* insomnia
GI: *Diarrhea, abdominal pain,* flatulence
INTEG: *Rash*
META: Hyperglycemia

Contraindications: Hypersensitivity

Precautions: Pregnancy **C**, lactation, children

Pharmacokinetics

Absorption	Unknown
Distribution	Protein binding 97%
Metabolism	Unknown
Excretion	Urine-metabolites, feces, decreased rate in elderly
Half-life	1½ hr

Pharmacodynamics

Onset	Unknown
Peak	2.4 hr
Duration	>24 hr

Interactions
Individual drugs
Clarithromycin, diazepam, flurazepam, phenytoin, triazolam: increased levels of pantoprazole
Sucralfate: decreased absorption of pantoprazole
Warfarin: increased risk of bleeding

NURSING CONSIDERATIONS
Assessment
- Assess GI system: bowel sounds q8h, abdomen for pain, swelling, anorexia
- Monitor hepatic enzymes: AST, ALT, alkaline phosphatase during treatment

Nursing diagnoses
- Knowledge, deficient (teaching)

Implementation
- Swallow del rel tabs whole; do not break, crush, or chew
- May take with or without food

IV route
- Reconstitute with 10 ml of 0.9% NaCl, give required amount slowly over 2 min; or for infusion further dilute reconstituted sol with 100 ml (1 vial) or 80 ml (2 vials) of D_5W, NS or LR for a concentration of 0.4 mg/ml or 0.8 mg/ml respectively; infuse required amount over at least 15 min

Patient/family education
- Advise patient to report severe diarrhea; drug may have to be discontinued
- Advise patient with diabetes that hyperglycemia may occur
- Advise patient to avoid hazardous activities; dizziness may occur
- Advise patient to avoid alcohol, salicylates, ibuprofen; may cause GI irritation

Evaluation
Positive therapeutic outcome
- Absence of epigastric pain, swelling, fullness

paricalcitol (Rx)
(par-ih-cal'sih-tol)
Zemplar
Func. class.: Vitamin D analog
Chem. class.: Fat-soluble vitamin
Pregnancy category C

Action: Reduces parathyroid hormone (PTH) levels; suppresses PTH levels in patients with chronic renal failure with absence of hypercalcemia/hyperphosphatemia; serum PO_4, Ca, calcium-phosphate product (Ca × P) may increase

Therapeutic Outcome: Decreased symptoms of hyperparathyroidism

Uses: Hyperparathyroidism in chronic renal failure

Dosage and routes
Adult: **IV** bol 0.04-0.1 mcg/kg (2.8-7 mcg) no more than every other day during dialysis; may increase by 2-4 mcg q2-4 wk until target serum intact PTH (1.5-3 × nonuremic upper limit of normal) is achieved

Available forms: Inj 5 mcg/ml

Adverse effects
CNS: Light-headedness
CV: Palpitations
GI: Nausea, vomiting, anorexia, dry mouth
MISC: Pneumonia, edema, chills, fever, flu, **sepsis**

Contraindications: Hypersensitivity, hypercalcemia

Precautions: Pregnancy **C**, CV disease, renal calculi, elderly, lactation, children

Pharmacokinetics	
Absorption	Unknown
Distribution	Unknown
Metabolism	Unknown
Excretion	Unknown
Half-life	Unknown

Pharmacodynamics	
Onset	Unknown
Peak	Unknown
Duration	Unknown

Interactions
Individual drugs
Digitalis: increased toxicity

NURSING CONSIDERATIONS
Assessment
- Monitor Ca, PO_4, 2 ×/wk qwk during initial therapy; after dose is established measure calcium and phosphorus q mo

Nursing diagnoses
- Knowledge, deficient (teaching)

Implementation
- Give by **IV** bol only

Patient/family education
- Advise patient to report weakness, lethargy, headache, anorexia, loss of weight
- Teach patient to report nausea, vomiting, palpitations

Evaluation

Positive therapeutic outcome

- Decreased hypoparathyroidism in chronic renal disease

paroxetine (Rx)

(par-ox'e-teen)

Paxil, Paxil CR

Func. class.: Antidepressant, selective serotonin reuptake inhibitor (SSRI)

Chem. class.: Phenylpiperidine derivative

Pregnancy category D

Do Not Confuse:

paroxetine/paclitaxel, Paxil/paclitaxel, Paxil/Taxol

Action: Inhibits CNS neuron reuptake of serotonin but not of norepinephrine or DOPamine

Therapeutic Outcome: Relief of depression

Uses: Major depressive disorder, obsessive-compulsive disorder, panic disorder, generalized anxiety disorder

Investigational uses: Diabetic neuropathy, headache, premature ejaculation, bipolar depression with lithium, fibromyalgia

Dosage and routes

Depression

Adult: PO 20 mg daily in AM; after 4 wk if no clinical improvement is noted, dosage may be increased by 10 mg/day weekly to desired response; not to exceed 60 mg/day; or controlled rel 25 mg/day, may increase by 12.5 mg/day weekly up to 62.5 mg/day

Elderly: PO 10 mg daily, increase by 10 mg to desired dose, max 40 mg/day

Obsessive-compulsive disorder

Adults: PO 20 mg/day in AM; start with 20 mg/day, increase 10 mg/day increments, max 60 mg/day

Panic disorder

Adults: PO 40 mg/day; start with 10 mg/day and increase in 10 mg/day increments, max 60 mg/day or controlled rel 12.5 mg/day max 75 mg/day

Generalized anxiety disorder

Adult: PO 20 mg/day in AM, range 20-50 mg/day

Posttraumatic stress disorder

Adult: PO 20 mg/day, range 20-50 mg/day

Renal dose

Adult: PO 10 mg daily in AM, may increase by 10 mg/day q wk, max 50 mg daily or controlled rel 12.5 mg/day max 50 mg/day

Premenstrual disorders

Adult: Controlled rel 12.5 mg/day in AM

Available forms: Tabs 10, 20, 30, 40 mg; oral susp 10 mg/5 ml; controlled rel 12.5, 25, 37.5 mg

Adverse effects

CNS: *Headache, nervousness, insomnia, drowsiness, anxiety, tremor, dizziness, fatigue, sedation,* abnormal dreams, agitation, apathy, euphoria, hallucinations, delusions, psychosis

CV: Vasodilatation, postural hypotension, palpitations

EENT: Visual changes

GI: *Nausea, diarrhea, constipation, dry mouth, anorexia,* dyspepsia, vomiting, taste changes, flatulence, decreased appetite, cramps

GU: Dysmenorrhea, decreased libido, urinary frequency, UTI, amenorrhea, cystitis, impotence, *abnormal ejaculation* (male)

INTEG: *Sweating,* rash

MS: Pain, arthritis, myalgia, myopathy, myasthenia

RESP: Infection, pharyngitis, nasal congestion, sinus headache, sinusitis, cough, dyspnea

SYST: Asthenia, fever

Contraindications: Hypersensitivity, patients taking MAOIs, alcohol use

Precautions: Pregnancy **D,** lactation, children, elderly, seizure history, patients with history of mania, renal and hepatic disease

Pharmacokinetics	
Absorption	Well absorbed
Distribution	Widely distributed; crosses blood-brain barrier, protein-binding 95%
Metabolism	Liver, mostly by CPY450 enzyme system
Excretion	Kidneys, unchanged (2%); breast milk
Half-life	21 hrs

Pharmacodynamics	
Onset	Unknown
Peak	5.2 hr
Duration	Unknown

Interactions

Individual drugs

Cimetidine: increased paroxetine levels
Digoxin: decreased effect of digoxin
L-tryptophan: increased agitation
Phenobarbital: decreased paroxetine levels
Phenytoin: decreased effect of paroxetine
Theophylline: increased theophylline levels

Thioridazine: do not use with paroxetine, hypertensive crisis, seizures, potentially fatal reactions can occur
Warfarin: increased warfarin levels

Drug classifications

Highly protein-bound drugs: increased side effects
MAOIs: hypertensive crisis, seizures; do not use together, potentially fatal reactions can occur

Drug/herb

Corkwood, jimsonweed: increased anticholinergic effect
Ephedra: hypertensive crisis
Hops, lavender: increased sedation
SAM-e, St. John's wort: possible serotonin syndrome
Yohimbe: increased CNS stimulation

Drug/lab test

Increased: serum bilirubin, blood glucose, alkaline phosphatase
Decreased: VMA, 5-HIAA, blood glucose
False increase: urinary catecholamines

NURSING CONSIDERATIONS

Assessment

- Assess mental status: mood, sensorium, affect, suicidal tendencies; increase in psychiatric symptoms: depression, panic
- Assess for withdrawal symptoms: headache, nausea, vomiting, muscle pain, weakness; do not usually occur unless drug was discontinued abruptly
- Monitor B/P (with patient lying, standing), pulse q4h; if systolic B/P drops 20 mm Hg, hold drug, notify prescriber; take VS q4h in patients with CV disease
- Monitor blood studies: CBC, leukocytes, differential, cardiac enzymes if patient is receiving long-term therapy
- Monitor hepatic studies: AST, ALT, bilirubin
- Check weight weekly; appetite may increase with drug
- Assess ECG for flattening of T wave, bundle branch block, AV block, dysrhythmias in cardiac patients
- Assess for EPS primarily in elderly: rigidity, dystonia, akathisia
- Monitor urinary retention, constipation; constipation is more likely to occur in children or elderly
- Identify alcohol consumption; if alcohol is consumed, hold dose until AM

Nursing diagnoses

- Coping, ineffective (uses)
- Injury, risk for (adverse reactions)
- Knowledge, deficient (teaching)
- Noncompliance (teaching)

Implementation

- Give with food or milk for GI symptoms; store at room temp; do not freeze
- Give crushed if patient is unable to swallow whole

Patient/family education

- Advise patient that therapeutic effects may take 1-4 wk
- Teach patient to use caution in driving and other activities requiring alertness because of drowsiness, dizziness, blurred vision; to avoid rising quickly from sitting to standing, especially elderly
- Caution patient to avoid alcohol ingestion, other CNS depressants, and OTC medication unless prescribed
- Caution patient not to discontinue medication quickly after long-term use; may cause nausea, anxiety, headache, malaise; do not double doses if one is missed
- Advise patient to use gum, hard sugarless candy, or frequent sips of water for dry mouth; if dry mouth continues an artificial saliva product may be used

Evaluation

Positive therapeutic outcome

- Decrease in depression
- Absence of suicidal thoughts

Treatment of overdose: Maintain airway, for seizures give diazepam, symptomatic treatment

pegaptanib (Rx)

(peg-ap'ta-nib)
Macugen
Func. class: Ophthalmic agent—miscellaneous

Pregnancy category B

Action: Binds to vascular endothelial growth factor (VEGF), thereby inhibiting angiogenesis

Therapeutic Outcome: Stabilization of vision in macular degeneration

Uses: Treatment of neovascular (wet) age-related macular degeneration. May be used alone or with photodynamic therapy (PDT).

Dosage and routes

Adult: Intravitreal inj 0.3 mg injected q6 wk

Available forms: Inj 0.3 mg, single glass syringes

Adverse effects

EENT: *Anterior chamber inflammation, blurred vision, conjunctival hemorrhage,* *corneal edema, cataract, eye discharge, eye pain, increased intraocular pressure, punctuate keratitis, reduced visual acuity, vitreous floaters, vitreous opacities, blepharitis, conjunctivitis, photophobia,* retinal detachment, iatrogenic traumatic cataract

Contraindications: Hypersensitivity, ocular or periocular infections

Precautions: Pregnancy **B**, inflammatory eye disease, ocular hypertension

Pharmacokinetics	
Absorption	Unknown
Distribution	Unknown
Metabolism	Unknown
Excretion	Unknown
Half-life	87-100 hr in vitreous humor of the monkey

Pharmacodynamics	
Onset	Unknown
Peak	Unknown
Duration	May remain fully active in the eye for 7-28 days

Interactions: None known

NURSING CONSIDERATIONS

Assessment

- Test visual acuity periodically
- Assess treated eye for increased intraocular pressure, infection, endophthalmitis
- Monitor perfusion of the optic nerve head immediately after injection, tonometry ½ hr after inj, biomicroscopy 2-7 days after inj

Nursing diagnoses

Sensory perception, disturbed: visual (uses)
Knowledge, deficient (teaching)

Implementation

- Administer anesthesia and a broad spectrum anti-infective prior to injection
- The injection should be done under aseptic conditions
- Store at 36°-46° F, do not freeze or shake vigorously

Patient/family education

- Instruct patient to report any inflammation, bleeding, eye discharge, opacities to prescriber.
- Instruct patient to continue with follow up care during treatment

Evaluation

Positive therapeutic outcome

- Macular degeneration stabilized

! HIGH ALERT

pegaspargase (Rx)

(peg-as'per-gase)

Oncaspar, PEG-L-asparaginase

Func. class.: Antineoplastic

Chem. class.: Escherichia coli enzyme

Pregnancy category C

Action: Indirectly inhibits protein synthesis in tumor cells; without amino acid, DNA, RNA synthesis is halted; asparagine, protein synthesis is halted; G_1 phase of cell cycle specific; a nonvesicant

Therapeutic Outcome: Prevention of rapidly growing malignant cells

Uses: Acute lymphocytic leukemia unresponsive to other agents in combination with other antineoplastics

Dosage and routes

In combination

Adult and child with BSA ≥0.6 m²: **IV**/IM 2500 international units/m² q14d, run **IV** over 1-2 hr in 100 ml of NaCl or D_5 through a running **IV**; IM should be no more than 2 ml in one inj site

Child with BSA <0.6 m²: **IV**/IM 82.5 international units/kg q14 days

Sole induction

Adult: **IV** 2500 international units/m² q14d

Available forms: Inj 750 international units/ml in a phosphate-buffered saline sol

Adverse effects

CNS: Neuritis, dizziness, headache, **coma,** depression, fatigue, confusion, hallucinations, **seizures**

CV: Chest pain, **hypertension**

ENDO: Hyperglycemia

GI: *Nausea, vomiting, anorexia, cramps, stomatitis,* **hepatotoxicity, pancreatitis,** *diarrhea*

GU: Urinary retention, **renal failure,** glycosuria, polyuria, azotemia, uric acid neuropathy

HEMA: **Thrombocytopenia, leukopenia, myelosuppression, anemia, decreased clotting factors, pancytopenia**

INTEG: *Rash,* urticaria, chills, fever

RESP: **Fibrosis, pulmonary infiltrate, severe bronchospasm**

SYST: **Anaphylaxis, hypersensitivity**

Contraindications: Hypersensitivity, infants, lactation, pancreatitis

Precautions: Pregnancy **C,** renal disease, hepatic disease, CNS disease

Pharmacokinetics

Absorption	Complete bioavailability
Distribution	Intravascular spaces
Metabolism	Unknown
Excretion	Reticuloendothelial system
Half-life	5½ days

Pharmacodynamics

Onset	Rapid
Peak	Unknown
Duration	2 wk

Interactions
Individual drugs
Aspirin, heparin, warfarin: coagulation factor imbalances
Methotrexate: decreased action of methotrexate
Radiation: do not use together
Drug classifications
NSAIDs: coagulation factor imbalances

NURSING CONSIDERATIONS
Assessment
- Assess for signs and symptoms of pancreatitis (nausea, vomiting, severe abdominal pain), anaphylaxis (bronchospasm, dyspnea), cyanosis; monitor amylase, glucose
- Assess symptoms indicating severe allergic reaction: rash, pruritus, urticaria, purpuric skin lesions, itching, flushing; monitor for joint pain, bronchospasm, hypotension; epINEPHrine and crash carts should be nearby
- Monitor for frequency of stools, characteristics: cramping, acidosis; signs of dehydration: rapid respirations, poor skin turgor, decreased urine output, dry skin, restlessness, weakness
- Monitor CBC, differential, platelet count weekly; withhold drug if WBC is $<4000/mm^3$ or platelet count is $<100{,}000/mm^3$; notify physician of results; also assess protime, PTT, and thrombin time, which may be increased
- Monitor renal function studies: BUN, creatinine, serum uric acid, urine CCr before and during therapy; check I&O ratio; report fall in urine output to <30 ml/hr; patient should be well hydrated with 2-3 L/day to prevent urate deposits
- Monitor temp q4h (may indicate beginning of infection)
- Monitor liver function tests before and during therapy (bilirubin, AST, ALT, LDH) as needed or monthly; check for jaundice of skin and sclera, dark urine, clay-colored stools, itchy skin, abdominal pain, fever, diarrhea; also monitor cholesterol, alkaline phosphatase
- Assess for bleeding: hematuria, stool guaiac, bruising or petechiae, mucosa or orifices q8h; check for inflammation of mucosa, breaks in skin
- Identify edema in feet, joint pain, stomach pain, shaking

Nursing diagnoses
- Injury, risk for (adverse reactions)
- Infection, risk for (adverse reactions)
- Knowledge, deficient (teaching)

Implementation
- Preparation by trained personnel is required in controlled environment
- Give fluids **IV** or PO before chemotherapy to hydrate patient
- Provide antiemetic 30-60 min before giving drug and prn to prevent vomiting; administer antibiotics for prophylaxis of infection
- Provide a liq diet: carbonated beverages; gelatin may be added if patient is not nauseated or vomiting

IM route
- Dilute 10,000 international units/2 ml of 0.9% NaCl with preservatives; give 2 ml or less per site

Intradermal route
- After intradermal skin testing and desensitization, give 0.1 ml (2 international units) intradermally after reconstituting with 5 ml of sterile water or 0.9% NaCl for inj; then add 0.1 ml of reconstituted drug to 9.9 ml of diluent (20 international units/ml); observe for 1 hr, check for wheal; desensitization may be required
- For direct **IV** dilute 10,000 international units/5 ml of sterile water for inj or 0.9% NaCl without preservatives; give through 5-µm filter if fibers are present; do not use if sol cloudy or discolored, give over 30 min through Y-site of full-flowing **IV** of 0.9% NaCl or D_5W; run **IV** sol for at least 2 hr after direct administration
- Give **IV** inf using 21, 23, 25G needle; administer by slow **IV** inf via Y-tube or 3-way stopcock of flowing D_5W or 0.9% NaCl inf over 30 min after diluting 10,000 international units/5 ml of sterile water or 0.9% NaCl (no preservatives) to 2000 international units/ml; filter may be necessary if fibers are present
- Provide allopurinol or sodium bicarbonate to reduce uric acid levels, alkalinization of urine

Patient/family education
- Advise patient that contraceptive measures are recommended during therapy; drug is teratogenic
- Teach patient to avoid use of products containing aspirin or NSAIDs, razors, commer-

P

cial mouthwash, since bleeding may occur; to report symptoms of bleeding (hematuria, tarry stools)
- Teach patient to report signs of anemia (fatigue, headache, irritability, faintness, shortness of breath)
- Tell patient to avoid crowds and persons with respiratory tract infections to prevent patient infection
- Advise patient to avoid vaccinations, since serious reactions can occur
- Teach patient to report nausea, vomiting, bruising, bleeding, stomatitis, severe diarrhea, jaundice, chest pain, abdominal pain, trouble breathing, rash

Evaluation
Positive therapeutic outcome
- Prevention of rapid division of malignant cells

pegfilgrastim (Rx)
(peg-fill-grass'stim)
Neulasta
Func. class.: Hematopoietic agent
Pregnancy category C

Action: Stimulates proliferation and differentiation of neutrophils

Therapeutic Outcome: Absence of infection

Uses: To decrease infection in patients receiving antineoplastics that are myelosuppressive; to increase WBC in patients with drug-induced neutropenia

Dosage and routes
Adult: SUBCUT 6 mg give once per chemotherapy cycle

Available forms: Sol for inj 10 mg/ml

Adverse effects
CNS: Fever, fatigue, headache, dizziness, insomnia, peripheral edema
GI: *Nausea,* vomiting, diarrhea, mucositis, anorexia, constipation, dyspepsia, abdominal pain, stomatitis, **splenic rupture**
HEMA: **Leukocytosis, granulocytopenia, sickle cell crisis**
INTEG: Alopecia
MISC: Chest pain, hyperuricemia, **anaphylaxis**
MS: Skeletal pain
RESP: **Respiratory distress syndrome**

Contraindications: Hypersensitivity to proteins of *E. coli,* filgrastim; ARDS

Precautions: Pregnancy **C,** lactation, myeloid malignancies, sickle cell disease, adolescents, child <45 kg

Pharmacokinetics
Absorption	Unknown
Distribution	Unknown
Metabolism	Unknown
Excretion	Unknown
Half-life	15-80 hr

Pharmacodynamics
Unknown

Interactions
Individual drug
Lithium: increased release of neutrophils
Drug classification
Cytotoxic chemotherapy agents: do not use this drug concomitantly or 2 wk before or 24 hr after administration of cytotoxics
Drug/lab test
Increased: uric acid, LDH, alkaline phosphatase

NURSING CONSIDERATIONS
Assessment
- Assess for allergic reactions, anaphylaxis: rash, urticaria; discontinue this drug, have emergency equipment nearby
- Monitor blood studies: CBC, platelet count before treatment and twice weekly; neutrophil counts may be increased for 2 days after therapy
- Monitor B/P, respirations, pulse before and during therapy
- Assess for bone pain, give mild analgesics

Nursing diagnoses
- Infection, risk for (uses)
- Knowledge, deficient (teaching)

Implementation
- Give using single-use vials; after dose is withdrawn, do not reenter vial
- Do not use 6-mg fixed dose in infants, children, or others <45 kg
- Inspect sol for discoloration, particulates; if present, do not use
- Do not administer in the period 14 days before and 24 hr after cytotoxic chemotherapy
- Store in refrigerator; do not freeze; may store at room temperature up to 6 hr, avoid shaking, protect from light

Patient/family education
- Teach the technique for self-administration: dose, side effects, disposal of containers and needles; provide instruction sheet

Evaluation

Positive therapeutic outcome

- Absence of infection

peginterferon alfa-2a (Rx)

(peg-in-ter-feer'on)

Pegasys

Func. class.: Immunomodulator

Pregnancy category C

Action: Stimulates genes to modulate many biologic effects, including inhibition of viral replication; inhibits ion cell proliferation, immunomodulation, stimulates effector proteins, decreases leukocyte, platelet counts

Therapeutic Outcome: Undetectable viral load; decreasing signs, symptoms of chronic hepatitis C

Uses: Chronic hepatitis C infections in adults with compensated liver disease

Dosage and routes

Adult: SUBCUT 180 mcg qwk × 48 wk; if poorly tolerated, reduce dose to 135 mcg qwk; in some cases reduction to 90 mcg may be needed

Available forms: Inj 180 mcg/ml

Adverse effects

CNS: *Headache, insomnia, dizziness,* anxiety, hostility, lability, nervousness, depression, fatigue, poor concentration, pyrexia

GI: *Abdominal pain, nausea, diarrhea, anorexia, vomiting,* dry mouth

HEMA: **Thrombocytopenia,** neutropenia

INTEG: *Alopecia, pruritus, rash,* dermatitis

MS: *Back pain,* myalgia, arthralgia

Contraindications: Hypersensitivity to interferons, neonates, infants, autoimmune hepatitis, decompensated hepatic disease before use of this drug

Precautions: Pregnancy **C,** thyroid disorders, myelosuppression, hepatic, cardiac disease, lactation, children <18 yr, depression/suicide, preexisting ophthalmologic disorders, pancreatitis, renal disease, elderly

Pharmacokinetics

Absorption	Large variability
Distribution	Large variability
Metabolism	Large variability
Excretion	Large variability
Half-life	15-80 hr

Pharmacodynamics

Unknown

Interactions

Individual drugs

Theophylline: use caution if giving together

Drug classifications

Myelosuppressives: use caution if giving together

NURSING CONSIDERATIONS

Assessment

- Monitor ALT, HCV viral load; patients who show no reduction in ALT, HCV are unlikely to show benefit of treatment after 6 mo
- Monitor platelet counts, heme concentration, ANC, serum creatinine concentration, albumin, bilirubin, TSH, T_4, AFP
- Assess for myelosuppression, hold dose if neutrophil count is $<500 \times 10^6$/L or if platelets are $<50 \times 10^9$/L
- Assess for hypersensitivity: discontinue immediately if hypersensitivity occurs

Nursing diagnoses

- Infection, risk for (uses)
- Knowledge, deficient (teaching)

Implementation

- Give in PM to reduce discomfort, sleep through side effects

Patient/family education

- Provide patient or family member with written, detailed information about drug
- Give instructions for home use if appropriate
- Advise to take in evening to reduce discomfort, sleep through some side effects

Evaluation

Positive therapeutic outcome

- Decreased chronic hepatitis C signs/symptoms, undetectable viral load

P

! HIGH ALERT

pemetrexed (Rx)

(pem-ah-trex'ed)

Alimta

Func. class.: Antineoplastic-antimetabolite

Chem. class.: Folic acid antagonist

Pregnancy category D

Action: Inhibits an enzyme that reduces folic acid, which is needed for cell replication

Therapeutic Outcome: Decreased spread of mesothelioma, decreased tumor size

Uses: Malignant pleural mesothelioma in

combination with cisplatin; non–small cell lung cancer as a single agent

Dosage and routes

Adult: **IV** inf 500 mg/m² given over 10 min on day 1 of a 21-day cycle with cisplatin 75 mg/m² infused over 2 hr beginning ½ hr after end of pemetrexed infusion

Nadir ANC < 500/mm³ and platelets = 50,000/mm³ 75% of previous dose

Available forms: Inj, single use vials, 500 mg

Adverse effects

CNS: *Fatigue, fever, mood alteration, neuropathy*

CV: **Thrombosis/embolism,** *chest pain*

GI: *Nausea, vomiting, anorexia, diarrhea, ulcerative stomatitis, constipation, dysphagia, dehydration*

GU: **Renal failure,** *creatinine elevation*

HEMA: **Neutropenia, leukopenia, thrombocytopenia, myelosuppression, anemia**

INTEG: *Rash, desquamation*

RESP: *Dyspnea*

SYST: **Infection with/without neutropenia**

Contraindications: Pregnancy **D**, hypersensitivity, ANC <1500 cells/mm³, CCr < 45 ml/min, thrombocytopenia (<100,000/mm³), anemia

Precautions: Renal disease, lactation, children, hepatic disease

Pharmacokinetics

Absorption	Unknown
Distribution	81% protein binding
Metabolism	Not metabolized
Excretion	Excreted in urine (unchanged 70-90%) Not known if it is excreted in breast milk
Half-life	3.5 hr

Pharmacodynamics

Unknown

Interactions

Drug classifications

Nephrotoxic drugs (NSAIDs): decreased pemetrexed clearance

NURSING CONSIDERATIONS

Assessment

- ⚠ Monitor CBC, differential, platelet count, monitor for nadir and recovery; a new cycle should not begin if ANC < 1500 cells/mm³, platelets are < 100,000 cells/mm³, creatinine clearance < 45 ml/min
- Monitor renal studies: BUN, serum uric acid, urine CCr, electrolytes before, during therapy
- Monitor I&O ratio; report fall in urine output to <30 ml/hr
- Monitor temp q4h; fever may indicate beginning infection; no rectal temps
- Assess bleeding time, coagulation time during treatment; bleeding: hematuria, guaiac, bruising or petechiae, mucosa or orifices q8h
- Assess buccal cavity q8h for dryness, sores, ulceration, white patches, oral pain, bleeding, dysphagia
- ⚠ Assess for symptoms indicating severe allergic reaction: rash, urticaria, itching, flushing

Nursing diagnoses

- Injury, risk for (adverse reactions)
- Body image, disturbed (adverse reactions)
- Infection, risk for (adverse reactions)
- Knowledge, deficient (teaching)

Implementation

- Administer vit B_{12} and low dose folic acid as a prophylactic measure to treat related hematologic, GI toxicity. At least 5 daily doses of folic acid must be taken in the 7 days preceding first dose
- Premedicate with a corticosteroid (dexamethasone) given PO bid the day before, day of, and day after administration of pemetrexed

IV route

- Use aseptic technique during reconstitution, dilution
- Reconstitute 500 mg vial/20 ml 0.9% NaCl injection (preservative free) = 25 mg/ml, swirl until dissolved, further dilute with 100 ml 0.9% NaCl injection (preservative free) give as **IV** infusion over 10 mg
- Use only 0.9% NaCl injection (preservative free) for reconstitution, dilution
- Follow strict medical asepsis and protective isolation if WBC levels are low
- Use a liquid diet: carbonated beverage, Jell-O; dry toast, crackers may be added when patient is not nauseated or vomiting
- Assist patient with rinsing of mouth tid-qid with water, club soda; brushing of teeth bid-tid with soft brush or cotton-tipped applicators for stomatitis; use unwaxed dental floss
- Store at 77° F, excursions permitted 59°-86° F, not light sensitive, discard unused portions

Patient/family education

- Instruct patient to report any complaints, side effects to nurse or prescriber: black tarry stools, chills, fever, sore throat, bleeding, bruising, cough, shortness of breath, dark or bloody urine

- Instruct patient to avoid foods with citric acid, hot or rough texture if stomatitis is present
- Instruct patient to report stomatitis: any bleeding, white spots, ulcerations in mouth to prescriber; tell patient to examine mouth daily, report symptoms to nurse, use good oral hygiene
- Advise patient that contraceptive measures are recommended during therapy and for at least 8 wk following cessation of therapy, to discontinue breastfeeding; toxicity to infant may occur
- Advise patient to avoid alcohol, salicylates, live vaccines
- Advise patient to avoid use of razors, commercial mouthwash

Evaluation

Positive therapeutic outcome

- Decreased spread of malignancy

PENICILLINS

penicillin G benzathine (Rx)
(pen-i-sill'in)
Bicillin L-A, Megacillin ✤, Permapen
penicillin G (Rx)
Pfizerpen
penicillin G procaine (Rx)
Ayercillin ✤, Duracillin A.S., Wycillin
penicillin V (Rx)
Apo-Pen-VK ✤, Beepen-VK, Nadopen-V ✤, Novopen-VK ✤, Pen-Vee K ✤, PVFK ✤, Veetids
Func. class.: Broad-spectrum antiinfective
Chem. class.: Natural penicillin

Pregnancy category B

Action: Interferes with cell wall replication of susceptible organisms; osmotically unstable cell wall swells and bursts from osmotic pressure, resulting in cell death

Therapeutic Outcome: Bactericidal effects on the gram-positive cocci *Staphylococcus, Streptococcus pyogenes, Streptococcus viridans, Streptococcus faecalis, Streptococcus bovis, Streptococcus pneumoniae;* gram-negative cocci *Neisseria gonorrhoeae;* gram-positive bacilli *Bacillus anthracis, Clostridium perfringens, Clostridium tetani, Corynebacterium diphtheriae, Listeria monocytogenes;* gram-negative bacilli *Escherichia coli, Proteus mirabilis, Salmonella, Shigella, Enterobacter, Streptobacillus moniliformis,* spirochete *Treponema pallidum; Actinomyces*

Uses: Respiratory tract infections, scarlet fever, erysipelas, otitis media, pneumonia, skin and soft tissue infections, gonorrhea; prevention of rheumatic fever, glomerulonephritis

Dosage and routes

Penicillin G benzathine

Early syphilis

Adult: IM 2.4 million units in single dose

Congenital syphilis

Child <2 yr: IM 50,000 units/kg in single dose

Prophylaxis of rheumatic fever, glomerulonephritis

Adult and child: IM 1.2 million units in single dose qmo or 600,000 units q2 wk

Upper respiratory tract infections (group A streptococcal)

Adult: IM 1.2 million units in single dose
Child >27 kg: IM 900,000 units in single dose
Child <27 kg: IM 300,000-600,000 units in single dose

Available forms: Inj 300,000 units/ml; 600,000 units/ml

Penicillin G

Pneumococcal/streptococcal infections (serious)

Adult: IM/**IV** 5-24 million units in divided doses q4-6h
Child <12 yr: **IV** 150,000 units/kg/day in 4-6 divided doses

Renal dose

CCr <10 ml/min, give full loading dose, then ½ of loading dose q8-10h

Available forms: Inj 1, 2, 3 million units/50 ml; powder for inj 1, 5, 20 million units/vial

Penicillin G procaine

Moderate to severe infections

Adult and child: IM 600,000-1.2 million units in 1 or 2 doses/day for 10 days to 2 wk
Newborn: avoid use in newborns

Pneumococcal pneumonia

Adult/child >12 yr: IM 600,000-1.2 million units/day × 7-10 days

Available forms: Inj 600,000, 1,200,000 units/dose

Penicillin V

Pneumococcal/staphylococcal infections

Adult: PO 250-500 mg q6h

P

Child <12 yr: PO 25-50 mg/kg/day in divided doses q6-8h

Streptococcal infections
Adult: PO 125 mg q6-8h × 10 days

Prevention of recurrence of rheumatic fever/chorea
Adult: PO 125-250 mg bid continuously

Vincent's gingivitis/pharyngitis
Adult: PO 250 mg q6-8h

Renal dose
CCr <50 ml/min dosage reduction indicated

Available forms: Tabs 250, 500 mg; powder for oral sol 125, 250 mg/5 ml

Adverse effects

CNS: Lethargy, hallucinations, anxiety, depression, twitching, **coma, seizures**
GI: *Nausea, vomiting, diarrhea,* increased AST, ALT, abdominal pain, glossitis, colitis
GU: **Oliguria, proteinuria, hematuria,** *vaginitis, moniliasis,* **glomerulonephritis**
HEMA: Anemia, increased bleeding time, **bone marrow depression, granulocytopenia**
META: Hyperkalemia, hypokalemia, alkalosis, hypernatremia
MISC: Local pain, tenderness and fever with IM inj, **anaphylaxis serum sickness**

Contraindications: Hypersensitivity to penicillins; neonates

Precautions: Pregnancy **B,** hypersensitivity to cephalosporins, severe renal disease, lactation

Penicillin G benzathine

Pharmacokinetics

Absorption	Delayed; prolonged drug levels
Distribution	Widely distributed; crosses placenta
Metabolism	Liver, minimally
Excretion	Kidneys, unchanged; breast milk
Half-life	½-1 hr

Pharmacodynamics

Onset	Slow
Peak	12-24 hr
Duration	1-4 wk

Penicillin G

Pharmacokinetics

Absorption	Variably absorbed (PO); well absorbed (IM)
Distribution	Widely distributed; crosses placenta
Metabolism	Liver, minimally
Excretion	Kidneys, unchanged; breast milk
Half-life	½-1 hr

Pharmacodynamics

	PO	IM	IV
Onset	Rapid	Rapid	Rapid
Peak	1 hr	¼-½ hr	Immediate

Penicillin G procaine

Pharmacokinetics

Absorption	Delayed; prolonged drug levels
Distribution	Widely distributed; crosses placenta
Metabolism	Liver, minimally
Excretion	Kidneys, unchanged; breast milk
Half-life	½-1 hr

Pharmacodynamics

Onset	Slow
Peak	1-4 hr
Duration	15 hr

Penicillin V

Pharmacokinetics

Absorption	Widely absorbed
Distribution	Widely distributed; crosses placenta
Metabolism	Liver, minimally
Excretion	Kidneys, unchanged; breast milk
Half-life	½-1 hr

Pharmacodynamics

Onset	Rapid
Peak	½ hr

Interactions

Individual drugs
Aspirin, probenecid: increased penicillin levels
Aspirin: decreased renal excretion
Heparin: increased effect of heparin

Drug classifications
Anticoagulants (oral): increased anticoagulant effects
Contraceptives (oral): decreased contraceptive effectiveness
Tetracyclines: decreased antimicrobial effectiveness

Drug/herb
Acidophilus: do not use with antiinfectives
Khat: decreased absorption of penicillin; separate doses by 2 hr or more

Drug/lab test
False positive: urine glucose, urine protein

NURSING CONSIDERATIONS

Assessment

- Assess patient for previous sensitivity reaction to penicillins or cephalosporins; cross-sensitivity between penicillins and cephalosporins is common

- Assess patient for signs and symptoms of infection including characteristics of wounds, sputum, urine, stool, WBC >10,000/mm^3, earache, fever; obtain baseline information and during treatment
- Obtain C&S before beginning drug therapy to identify if correct treatment has been initiated
- Assess for allergic reactions: rash, urticaria, pruritus, chills, fever, joint pain; angioedema may occur a few days after therapy begins; epINEPHrine, resuscitation equipment should be available for anaphylactic reaction
- Identify urine output; if decreasing, notify prescriber (may indicate nephrotoxicity); also check for increased BUN, creatinine
- Monitor blood studies: AST, ALT, CBC, Hct, bilirubin, LDH, alkaline phosphatase, Coombs' test monthly if patient is on long-term therapy
- Monitor electrolytes: potassium, sodium, chloride monthly if patient is on long-term therapy
- Assess bowel pattern daily; if severe diarrhea occurs, drug should be discontinued; may indicate pseudomembranous colitis
- Monitor for bleeding: ecchymosis, bleeding gums, hematuria, stool guaiac daily if on long-term therapy
- Assess for overgrowth of infection: perineal itching, fever, malaise, redness, pain, swelling, drainage, rash, diarrhea, change in cough, sputum

Nursing diagnoses

- Infection, risk for (uses)
- Diarrhea (adverse reactions)
- Injury, risk for (adverse reactions)
- Knowledge, deficient (teaching)
- Noncompliance (teaching)

Implementation

Penicillin G benzathine

PO route

- Give in even doses around the clock; if GI upset occurs, give with food, avoid acidic juices; carbonated beverages may decrease PO absorption; drug must be given for 10-14 days to ensure organism death and prevent superinfection
- Shake susp

IM route

- Do not give **IV**
- Give inj deep in large muscle mass
- Reconstitute with 0.9% NaCl, sterile water for inj, D_5W; refrigerate unused portion

Penicillin G

IM route

- Reconstitute with D_5W, 0.9% NaCl, sterile water for inj; shake well
- Give deep in large muscle mass; massage
- Do not give SUBCUT; may cause severe pain
- If injected near a nerve, loss of function and severe pain may occur

IV route

- Change **IV** sites q48h to prevent pain and phlebitis
- Give by intermittent inf by diluting 3 million units or less/50 ml or more; dilute 3 million units or more/100 ml of D_5W, $D_{10}W$, 0.45% NaCl, 0.9% NaCl, LR, Ringer's, or any combination run over 1-2 hr (adult), 15-30 min (child)
- Give by cont inf by diluting and infusing over 24 hr

Syringe compatibilities: Heparin

Syringe incompatibilities: Metoclopramide

Y-site compatibilities: Acyclovir, amiodarone, cyclophosphamide, diltiazem, enalaprilat, esmolol, fluconazole, foscarnet, heparin, hydromorphone, labetalol, magnesium sulfate, meperidine, morphine, perphenazine, potassium chloride, tacrolimus, theophylline, verapamil, vit B/C

Additive compatibilities: Ascorbic acid, calcium chloride, calcium gluconate, cephapirin, chloramphenicol, cimetidine, clindamycin, colistimethate, corticotropin, dimenhyDRINATE, diphenhydrAMINE, epHEDrine, erythromycin, furosemide, hydrocortisone, kanamycin, lidocaine, magnesium sulfate, methicillin, methylPREDNISolone, metronidazole, polymyxin B, prednisoLONE, potassium chloride, procaine, prochlorperazine, verapamil

Additive incompatibilities: Aminoglycosides, aminophylline, amphotericin B, chlorproMAZINE, DOPamine, floxacillin, hydrOXYzine, metaraminol, oxytetracycline, pentobarbital, prochlorperazine mesylate, promazine, tetracycline, thiopental

Penicillin G procaine

- Do not give **IV**
- Give deeply in large muscle mass
- Reconstitute with 0.9% NaCl, sterile water for inj, D_5W; refrigerate unused portion
- Shake medication before administering
- IM route may include procaine reactions: fear of death, depression, seizures, anxiety, confusion, hallucinations

Penicillin V

- Give in even doses around the clock; if GI upset occurs, give with food; drug must be given for 10-14 days to ensure organism death and prevent superinfection; store in tight container

P

• Shake susp; store in refrigerator for 2 wk or for 1 wk at room temp

Patient/family education

• Teach patient to report sore throat, bruising, bleeding, joint pain; may indicate blood dyscrasias (rare)
• Advise patient to contact prescriber if vaginal itching, loose foul-smelling stools, furry tongue occur; may indicate superinfection
• Instruct patient to take all medication prescribed for the length of time ordered
• Advise patient to notify prescriber of diarrhea with blood or pus, which may indicate pseudomembranous colitis

Evaluation

Positive therapeutic outcome

• Absence of signs/symptoms of infection (WBC <10,000/mm^3, temp WNL, absence of red, draining wounds, earache)
• Reported improvement in symptoms of infection

Treatment of anaphylaxis: Withdraw drug, maintain airway, administer epINEPHrine, aminophylline, O_2, **IV** corticosteroids

pentamidine (Rx)

(pen-tam'i-deen)

Nebupent, Pentam 300, Pentacarinat ✤, Pneumopent ✤

Func. class.: Antiprotozoal

Chem. class.: Aromatic diamide derivative

Pregnancy category C

Action: Interferes with DNA/RNA synthesis in protozoa; has direct effect on islet cells in the pancreas

Therapeutic Outcome: Protozoa death

Uses: Treatment/prevention of *Pneumocystis jiroveci* infections

Investigational uses: Babesiosis, leishmaniasis, African trypanosomiasis

Dosage and routes

Adult and child: **IV**/IM 4 mg/kg/day × 2-3 wk; neb 300 mg via specific nebulizer given q4 wk for prevention

Available forms: Inj; aerosol 300 mg/vial; sol for aerosol 60 mg/vial ✤

Adverse effects

CNS: Disorientation, hallucinations, dizziness, confusion

CV: Hypotension, ventricular tachycardia, ECG abnormalities; **dysrhythmias**

GI: *Nausea, vomiting, anorexia,* increased AST, ALT, **acute pancreatitis,** metallic taste

GU: **Acute renal failure, increased serum creatinine, renal toxicity**

HEMA: Anemia, **leukopenia, thrombocytopenia**

INTEG: Sterile abscess, pain at inj site, pruritus, urticaria, rash

META: Hyperkalemia, hypocalcemia, *hypoglycemia*

MISC: Fatigue, chills, night sweats, **anaphylaxis, Stevens-Johnson syndrome**

RESP: Cough, shortness of breath, **bronchospasm** (with aerosol)

Precautions: Pregnancy **C,** blood dyscrasias, hepatic disease, renal disease, diabetes mellitus, cardiac disease, hypocalcemia, hypertension, hypotension, lactation, children

Pharmacokinetics

Absorption	Well absorbed (IM); minimally absorbed (inh); completely absorbed (**IV**)
Distribution	Widely distributed; does not appear in CSF
Metabolism	Not known
Excretion	Kidneys, unchanged (up to 30%)
Half-life	6½-9½ hr; increased in renal disease

Pharmacodynamics

	IM	IV	INH
Onset	Unknown	Unknown	Unknown
Peak	½-1 hr	Inf end	Unknown

Interactions

Individual drugs

Amphotericin B, cisplatin, vancomycin: increased nephrotoxicity
Erythromycin **IV**: fatal dysrhythmias
Radiation: bone marrow suppression

Drug classifications

Aminoglycosides NSAIDs: increased nephrotoxicity
Antineoplastics: increased bone marrow depression
Class IA, class III antidysrhythmics, phenothiazines: increased QT prolongation

NURSING CONSIDERATIONS

Assessment

◆• Assess any patient with compromised renal system: drug is excreted slowly in poor renal system function; toxicity may occur rapidly
• Assess patient for infection including increased temp, thick sputum, WBC >10,000/mm^3; monitor these signs of infection throughout treatment; obtain C&S before beginning

therapy; treatment may begin after culture is obtained
- Assess respiratory system including rate, rhythm, bilateral lung sounds, shortness of breath, wheezing, dyspnea
- Monitor ECG for cardiac dysrhythmias; ECG and pulse should be checked frequently during treatment, since cardiotoxicity can occur
- Assess for hypoglycemia including nausea, tremors, anxiety, chills, diaphoresis, headache, hunger, cold, pale skin; this side effect can last for several mo after treatment is completed
- Monitor for hyperglycemia including flushed, dry skin, acetone breath, thirst, anorexia, drowsiness, polyuria; this side effect can last for several mo after treatment is completed
- Monitor renal function studies including BUN, urinalysis, creatinine; obtain at baseline and frequently during treatment; nephrotoxicity may occur; check I&O, report hematuria, oliguria
- Monitor blood studies including blood glucose, CBC, platelets; blood glucose fluctuations are common; anemia, leukopenia, thrombocytopenia can occur
- Monitor liver function studies including AST, ALT, alkaline phosphatase, bilirubin before beginning treatment and every 3 days during therapy
- Monitor calcium and magnesium before beginning treatment and every 3 days during therapy; hypocalcemia may occur

Nursing diagnoses
- Infection, risk for (uses)
- Knowledge, deficient (teaching)

Implementation
IM route
- Reconstitute 300 mg/3 ml of sterile water for inj; give deep in large muscle mass by Z-track; IM is a painful route
- Do not mix in normal saline

Inhalation route
- Dilute 300 mg/600 ml sterile water for inj; put reconstituted sol into nebulizer; do not use with other drugs or sol precipitate may occur; sol stable for 48 hr at room temp; protect from light; administer over 30-45 min

IV route
- For intermittent inf reconstitute 300 mg/3-5 ml of sterile water for inj, D_5W; withdraw dose and further dilute in 50-250 ml of D_5W; diluted sol is stable for 48 hr; discard unused sol; give over 1 hr or more

Y-site compatibilities: Zidovudine
Y-site incompatibilities: Foscarnet, fluconazole

Patient/family education
- Teach patient to report sore throat, fever, fatigue; could indicate superinfection
- Advise patient not to drink alcohol or take aspirin, since gastric bleeding may occur
- Teach patient to make position changes slowly to prevent orthostatic hypotension
- Advise patient to maintain adequate fluid intake

Evaluation
Positive therapeutic outcome
- Decreased signs and symptoms of protozoan infections
- Decreased signs and symptoms of *Pneumocystis jiroveci* pneumonia in HIV infections

! HIGH ALERT

pentazocine (Rx)
(pen-taz'oh-seen)
Talwin, Talwin NX
Func. class.: Opiate analgesic
Chem. class.: Synthetic benzomorphan (agonist/antagonist)

Pregnancy category C
Controlled substance schedule IV

Action: Inhibits ascending pain pathways in limbic system, thalamus, midbrain, hypothalamus by binding to opiate receptor sites, altering pain perception and response

Therapeutic Outcome: Relief of pain

Uses: Moderate to severe pain

Dosage and routes
Adult: PO 50-100 mg q3-4h prn, not to exceed 600 mg/day; **IV**/IM/SUBCUT 30 mg q3-4h prn, not to exceed 360 mg/day

Labor
Adult: IM 60 mg; **IV** 30 mg q2-3h when contractions are regular

Renal dose
Adult: CCr 10-50 ml/min reduce dose by 25%; CCr <10 ml/min reduce dose by 50%

Available forms: SUBCUT, IM, **IV** 30 mg/ml; tabs 50 mg

Adverse effects
CNS: *Drowsiness, dizziness, confusion, headache, sedation, euphoria, hallucinations,* dreaming
CV: Palpitations, bradycardia, change in B/P, tachycardia, increased B/P (high doses)
EENT: Tinnitus, blurred vision, miosis, diplopia

P

GI: Nausea, vomiting, anorexia, constipation, cramps, dry mouth
GU: Urinary retention, increased urinary output, dysuria
INTEG: Rash, urticaria, bruising, flushing, diaphoresis, pruritus, severe irritation at inj sites
RESP: **Respiratory depression**

Contraindications: Hypersensitivity, addiction (opioid)

Precautions: Pregnancy **C**, addictive personality, lactation, increased ICP, MI (acute), severe heart disease, respiratory depression, hepatic disease, renal disease, seizure disorder, child <18 yr, head trauma

Pharmacokinetics

Absorption	Well absorbed (PO, SUBCUT, IM); completely absorbed (**IV**)
Distribution	Widely distributed; crosses placenta
Metabolism	Liver, extensively
Excretion	Kidneys, small amounts (unchanged)
Half-life	2-3 hr

Pharmacodynamics

	PO	SUBCUT/IM	IV
Onset	15-30 min	15-30 min	Rapid
Peak	1-3 hr	1-2 hr	15 min
Duration	3 hr	2-4 hr	1 hr

Interactions
Individual drugs
Alcohol: increased side effects
Drug classifications
Antipsychotics, CNS depressants, sedative/hypnotics, skeletal muscle relaxants: increased side effects
MAOIs: use cautiously; results are unpredictable
Opiates: decreased effects
Drug/lab test
Increased: amylase

NURSING CONSIDERATIONS
Assessment
- Assess pain characteristics: location, intensity, type of pain before medication administration and after treatment
- Monitor VS after parenteral route; note muscle rigidity, drug history, liver, kidney function tests, respiratory dysfunction: respiratory depression, character, rate, rhythm; notify prescriber if respirations are <10/min
- Monitor CNS changes: dizziness, drowsiness, hallucinations, euphoria, LOC, pupil reaction
- Monitor allergic reactions: rash, urticaria
- Assess for withdrawal symptoms in opiate-dependent patients

Nursing diagnoses
- Pain, acute (uses)
- Sensory-perceptual, disturbed: visual, auditory (adverse reactions)
- Breathing pattern, ineffective (adverse reactions)
- Knowledge, deficient (teaching)

Implementation
- Give by inj (IM, **IV**), only when resuscitative equipment available; give slowly to prevent rigidity
- Store in light-resistant area at room temp

PO route
- Tabs made in the United States contain naloxone 0.5 mg to prevent abuse if the PO preparation is used **IV**

IM/SUBCUT route
- Give IM inj deeply in large muscle mass; rotate inj sites; repeated SUBCUT inj may cause necrosis

IV route
- Give by direct **IV** after diluting 5 mg/ml of sterile water for inj; give 5 mg or less over 1 min

Syringe compatibilities: Atropine, benzquinamide, butorphanol, chlorproMAZINE, cimetidine, dimenhyDRINATE, diphenhydrAMINE, droperidol, fentanyl, hydromorphone, hydrOXYzine, meperidine, metoclopramide, morphine, perphenazine, prochlorperazine, promazine, promethazine, propiomazine, ranitidine, scopolamine
Syringe incompatibilities: Glycopyrrolate, heparin, pentobarbital, other barbiturates
Y-site compatibilities: Heparin, hydrocortisone, potassium chloride, vit B/C
Y-site incompatibilities: Nafcillin
Additive incompatibilities: Aminophylline, amobarbital, pentobarbital, phenobarbital, secobarbital, sodium bicarbonate

Patient/family education
- Teach patient to report any symptoms of CNS changes, allergic reactions
- Advise patients to avoid CNS depressants: alcohol, sedative/hypnotics for at least 24 hr after taking this drug
- Discuss with patient that dizziness, drowsiness, and confusion are common; to avoid getting up without assistance
- Discuss in detail all aspects of the drug
- Instruct patient to change position slowly to prevent orthostatic hypotension
- Teach patient to turn, cough, deep breathe after surgery to prevent atelectasis

Evaluation
Positive therapeutic outcome
- Relief of pain

Treatment of overdose: Naloxone (Narcan) 0.2-0.8 mg **IV**, O_2, **IV** fluids, vasopressors

! HIGH ALERT

pentobarbital (Rx)
(pen-toe-bar'bi-tal)

Nembutal, Novopentobarb ✦, Nova-Rectal ✦, pentobarbital sodium

Func. class.: Sedative/hypnotic barbiturate; anticonvulsant

Chem. class.: Barbitone, short acting

Pregnancy category D

Controlled substance schedule II (USA), schedule G (Canada)

Do Not Confuse:
pentobarbital/phenobarbital

Action: Depresses activity in brain cells, primarily in reticular activating system in brainstem; also selectively depresses neurons in posterior hypothalamus, limbic structures; may decrease cerebral blood flow, intracranial pressure (**IV**) and cerebral edema; may potentiate GABA, an inhibitory neurotransmitter

Therapeutic Outcome: Sedation, sleep

Uses: Insomnia, sedation, preoperative medication, increased intracranial pressure, dental anesthetic

Dosage and routes
Insomnia

Adult: PO 100-200 mg at bedtime; IM 150-200 mg at bedtime; **IV** 100 mg initially, then up to 500 mg; rec 120-200 mg at bedtime

Child: IM 2-6 mg/kg, not to exceed 100 mg; PO 2-6 mg/kg/day in divided doses; PO preoperatively 2-6 mg/kg, max 100 mg/dose; **IV** 100 mg (hypnotic/anticonvulsant)

Available forms: Caps 50, 100 mg; elixir 20 mg/5 ml; rec supp 25, 30, 50, 60, 120, 200 mg; inj 50 mg/ml

Adverse effects
CNS: *Lethargy, drowsiness, hangover,* dizziness, paradoxic stimulation in elderly and children, light-headedness, dependence, **CNS depression,** mental depression, slurred speech

CV: Hypotension, bradycardia

GI: Nausea, vomiting, diarrhea, constipation

HEMA: **Agranulocytosis, thrombocytopenia, megaloblastic anemia** (long-term treatment)

INTEG: *Rash,* urticaria, pain, abscesses at inj site, **angioedema, thrombophlebitis**

RESP: **Respiratory depression, apnea, laryngospasm, bronchospasm**

SYST: **Stevens-Johnson syndrome**

Contraindications: Pregnancy **D**, hypersensitivity to barbiturates, respiratory depression, addiction to barbiturates, severe liver, renal impairment, porphyria, uncontrolled pain

Precautions: Anemia, lactation, hepatic disease, renal disease, hypertension, elderly, acute/chronic pain

Pharmacokinetics

Absorption	Well absorbed
Distribution	Widely distributed; crosses placenta, enters breast milk
Metabolism	Liver
Excretion	Kidneys, unchanged (minimally)
Half-life	15-48 hr

Pharmacodynamics

	PO	IM	IV	REC
Onset	15-30 min	10-25 min	Immediate	Slow
Peak	3-4 hr	Unknown	1 min	Unknown
Duration	4-6 hr	1-4 hr	15 min	4-6 hr

Interactions:
Individual drugs

Alcohol: increased CNS depression
Doxycycline: increased half-life
Griseofulvin, quinidine: decreased effectiveness

Drug classifications

Anticoagulants: decreased effectiveness
Antihistamines, CNS depressants, MAOIs, opiates, sedative/hypnotics: increased CNS depression
Corticosteroids: decreased effectiveness

Drug/herb

Eucalyptus, Jamaican dogwood, kava, lemon balm, nettle, pill-bearing spurge, poppy, quinine, senega, valerian: increased pentobarbital level

Drug/lab test

False increase: sulfobromophthalein

NURSING CONSIDERATIONS
Assessment
- Assess mental status: mood, sensorium, affect, memory (long, short), especially

P

elderly; if using as a hypnotic, assess sleep patterns during therapy; drug suppresses REM sleep with dreaming; withdrawal insomnia may occur after short-term use; do not start using drug again; insomnia will improve in 1-3 nights; may experience increased dreaming

- Monitor for respiratory dysfunction: respiratory depression, character, rate, rhythm (when using **IV**); hold drug if respirations are <10/min or if pupils are dilated; also check VS q30 min after parenteral route for 2 hr
- Assess for blood dyscrasias: fever, sore throat, bruising, rash, jaundice, epistaxis (long-term treatment only)
- Assess seizure activity including type, location, duration, and character; provide seizure precaution
- Assess for pain in postoperative patients; pain threshold is lowered when patients are taking this medication

Nursing diagnoses

- Injury, risk for (side effects)
- Knowledge, deficient (teaching)

Implementation

- Administer only after removal of cigarettes, to prevent fires
- Reserve use until after trying conservative measures for insomnia

PO route

- Give 30 min before bedtime for expected sleeplessness
- May dilute elixir in juice, milk, or water if needed
- Give on empty stomach for best absorption

IM route

- Give deeply in muscle mass (gluteal) to minimize irritation to tissues; split inj >5 ml into 2 inj since irritation to tissues may occur; do not administer SUBCUT

IV route

- Use large vein to prevent extravasation; if extravasation occurs, use moist heat to the area and 5% procaine sol injected into area; give at 50 mg/1 min or more
- Give **IV** only with resuscitative equipment available (and only by qualified personnel)

Syringe compatibilities: Aminophylline, epHEDrine, hydromorphone, neostigmine, scopolamine, sodium bicarbonate, thiopental

Syringe incompatibilities: Benzquinamide, butorphanol, chlorproMAZINE, cimetidine, dimenhyDRINATE, diphenhydrAMINE, droperidol, fentanyl, glycopyrrolate, hydrOXYzine, meperidine, midazolam, nalbuphine, pentazocine, perphenazine, prochlorperazine, promazine, promethazine, ranitidine

Y-site compatibilities: Acyclovir, propofol, regular insulin

Additive compatibilities: Amikacin, aminophylline, calcium chloride, cephapirin, chloramphenicol, dimenhyDRINATE, erythromycin, lidocaine, thiopental, verapamil

Additive incompatibilities: Chlorpheniramine, codeine, epHEDrine, erythromycin gluceptate, hydrocortisone, hydrOXYzine, levorphanol, methadone, norepinephrine, pentazocine, penicillin G potassium, phenytoin, promazine, promethazine, regular insulin, sodium succinate, streptomycin, triflupromazine, vancomycin

Patient/family education

- Teach patient to carry/wear emergency ID stating name, drugs taken, condition, prescriber's name, phone number
- Caution patient to avoid driving and other activities that require alertness
- Caution patient to avoid alcohol ingestion and CNS depressants; increased sedation may occur
- Teach patient not to discontinue medication quickly after long-term use; taper off over several wk

Evaluation

Positive therapeutic outcome

- Improved sleeping patterns
- Decreased seizure activity
- Improved energy

Treatment of overdose: Lavage, activated charcoal, warming blanket, vital signs, hemodialysis

! HIGH ALERT

pentostatin (Rx)

(pen′toe-sta-tin)

Nipent

Func. class.: Antineoplastic, enzyme inhibitor

Chem. class.: Streptomyces antibioticus derivative

Pregnancy category D

Action: Inhibits the enzyme adenosine deaminase (ADA), which is able to block DNA synthesis and some RNA synthesis

Therapeutic Outcome: Prevention of rapidly growing malignant cells

Uses: α-Interferon–refractory hairy cell leukemia, chronic lymphocytic leukemia

Dosage and routes

Adult: **IV** 4 mg/m^2 every other wk; may be

given **IV** bol or diluted in a larger volume and given over 20-30 min

Available forms: Powder for inj 10 mg/vial

Adverse effects

CNS: Headache, anxiety, confusion, depression, dizziness, insomnia, nervousness, paresthesia

GI: Nausea, vomiting, anorexia, diarrhea, constipation, flatulence, stomatitis, elevated liver function tests

GU: **Hematuria,** dysuria, increased BUN/creatinine

HEMA: **Leukopenia, anemia, thrombocytopenia, ecchymosis, lymphadenopathy,** petechiae

INTEG: Rash, eczema, dry skin, pruritus, sweating, herpes simplex/zoster

RESP: Cough, upper respiratory tract infection, bronchitis, dyspnea, epistaxis, pneumonia, pharyngitis, rhinitis, sinusitis

SYST: Fever, infection, fatigue, pain, allergic reaction, chills, **death, sepsis,** chest pain, flu-like symptoms

Contraindications: Pregnancy **D**, hypersensitivity to this drug or mannitol

Precautions: Renal disease, lactation, children, bone marrow depression

Pharmacokinetics	
Absorption	Completely absorbed
Distribution	Unknown; low protein binding
Metabolism	Unknown
Excretion	Kidneys
Half-life	5-7 hr; increased in renal disease

Pharmacodynamics	
Onset	4-5 mo
Peak	Unknown
Duration	1½-34 mo

Interactions

Individual drugs

Fludarabine: fatal pulmonary reaction
Vidarabine: increased adverse reactions

Drug/lab test

Increased: uric acid

NURSING CONSIDERATIONS

Assessment

- Assess CNS changes: confusion, paresthesias, psychosis, tremors, seizures, neuropathies; drug should be discontinued
- Assess for toxicity: facial flushing, epistaxis, increased protime, thrombocytopenia; drug should be discontinued
- Assess acidosis, signs of dehydration: rapid respirations, poor skin turgor, decreased urine output, dry skin, restlessness, weakness
- Check buccal cavity q8h for dryness, sores or ulceration, white patches, oral pain, bleeding, dysphagia; obtain prescription for viscous lidocaine (Xylocaine) to use in mouth
- Assess symptoms indicating severe allergic reaction: rash, pruritus, urticaria, purpuric skin lesions, itching, flushing
- Assess tachypnea, ECG changes, dyspnea, edema, fatigue; respiratory and cardiovascular reaction can be severe
- Monitor CBC, differential, platelet count weekly; withhold drug if WBC is <2000/mm^3 or platelet count is <100,000/mm^3, notify prescriber of results
- Monitor renal function studies: BUN, creatinine, serum uric acid, urine CCr before and during therapy; I&O ratio; report fall in urine output to <30 ml/hr
- Monitor temp q4h (may indicate beginning of infection)
- Monitor liver function tests before and during therapy (bilirubin, AST, ALT, LDH) as needed or monthly; check for jaundice of skin and sclera, dark urine, clay-colored stools, itchy skin, abdominal pain, fever, diarrhea
- Assess for bleeding: hematuria, stool guaiac, bruising or petechiae, mucosa or orifices q8h; check for inflammation of mucosa, breaks in skin
- Assess effects of alopecia on body image; discuss feelings about body changes

Nursing diagnoses

- Injury, risk for (adverse reactions)
- Body image, disturbed (adverse reactions)
- Infection, risk for (adverse reactions)
- Knowledge, deficient (teaching)

Implementation

- Give fluids **IV** or PO before chemotherapy to hydrate patient
- Give antacid before oral agent, antiemetic 30-60 min before giving drug and prn to prevent vomiting; administer antibiotics for prophylaxis of infection
- Give TOP or systemic analgesics for pain to lessen effects from stomatitis
- Give liq diet: carbonated beverages; gelatin may be added if patient is not nauseated or vomiting
- Preparation should be done by personnel knowledgeable in preparing antineoplastics wearing gloves, gown, mask in biologic cabinet
- Give by direct **IV** by reconstituting 10 mg/5 ml of sterile water for inj (2 mg/ml); shake well

P

- Give over 5 min
- Give by intermittent inf after diluting 10 mg/25-50 ml of 0.9% NaCl, D_5W; give over 30 min
- Diluted sol should be used within 8 hr at room temp

Y-site compatibilities: Fludarabine, melphalan, ondansetron, paclitaxel, sargramostim

Solution compatibilities: D_5W, 0.9% NaCl, LR

Patient/family education

- Teach patient to avoid use of products containing aspirin or NSAIDs, razors, commercial mouthwash, since bleeding may occur; to report symptoms of bleeding (hematuria, tarry stools)
- Encourage patient to rinse mouth tid-qid with water, club soda; brush teeth bid-qid with soft brush or cotton-tipped applicators for stomatitis; use unwaxed dental floss
- Advise patient to report signs of anemia (fatigue, headache, irritability, faintness, shortness of breath); CNS reactions including confusion, psychosis, nightmares, seizures, severe headaches
- Inform patient that hair may be lost during treatment; a wig or hairpiece may make patient feel better; new hair may be different in color, texture
- Advise patient to use sunscreen and protective clothing to prevent photosensitive reactions

Evaluation

Positive therapeutic outcome

- Prevention of rapid division of malignant cells
- Decreased bone marrow hairy cells

pentoxifylline (Rx)

(pen-tox-if′i-lin)

Trental

Func. class.: Hemorheologic agent

Chem. class.: Dimethylxanthine derivative

Pregnancy category C

Action: Decreases blood viscosity, stimulates prostacyclin formation, increases blood flow by increasing flexibility of RBCs; decreases RBC hyperaggregation; reduces platelet aggregation, decreases fibrinogen concentration

Therapeutic Outcome: Decreased claudication and improved blood flow

Uses: Intermittent claudication related to chronic occlusive vascular disease, sickle cell anemia

Investigational uses: Cerebrovascular insufficiency, diabetic neuropathies, TIAs, leg ulcers, CVA, aphthous stomatitis

Dosage and routes

Adult: PO 400 mg tid with meals, may decrease to bid if side effects occur, must be taken for ≥8 wk for maximal effect

Stomatitis (off-label)

Adult: PO 400 mg tid × 1-6 mo

Available forms: Cont rel tabs 400 mg; ext rel tabs 400 mg

Adverse effects

CNS: ***Headache,*** anxiety, ***tremors,*** confusion, ***dizziness***

CV: Angina, dysrhythmias, palpitations, hypotension, chest pain, dyspnea, edema

EENT: Blurred vision, earache, increased salivation, sore throat, conjunctivitis

GI: ***Dyspepsia, nausea, vomiting,*** anorexia, bloating, belching, constipation, cholecystitis, dry mouth, thirst, bad taste

INTEG: Rash, pruritus, urticaria, brittle fingernails

MISC: Epistaxis, flulike symptoms, laryngitis, nasal congestion, **leukopenia,** malaise, weight changes

Contraindications: Hypersensitivity to this drug or xanthines, retinal/cerebral hemorrhage

Precautions: Pregnancy **C,** angina pectoris, cardiac disease, lactation, children, impaired renal function, recent surgery, peptic ulcer, hepatic disease

Pharmacokinetics

Absorption	Well absorbed
Distribution	Unknown
Metabolism	Liver, degradation
Excretion	Kidneys
Half-life	½-1 hr

Pharmacodynamics

Onset	Unknown
Peak	8 wk
Duration	Unknown

Interactions

Individual drugs

Abciximab, eptifibatide, plicamycin, ticlopidine, tirofiban, valproic acid, warfarin: increased bleeding risk

Cimetidine: increased pentoxifylline level

Theophylline: increased theophylline level

Drug classifications

Antihypertensives, nitrates: increased hypotension

NSAIDs, salicylates, thrombolytics: increased bleeding risk

Drug/herb

Anise, arnica, chamomile, clove, dong quai, fenugreek, feverfew, garlic, ginger, ginkgo, ginseng *(Panax)*, licorice: increased bleeding risk

NURSING CONSIDERATIONS

Assessment

- Monitor B/P, respirations in patient taking antihypertensives
- Assess for intermittent claudication baseline and during treatment

Nursing diagnoses

- Pain, chronic (uses)
- Activity intolerance (uses)
- Knowledge, deficient (teaching)
- Noncompliance (teaching)

Implementation

- Do not break, crush, or chew tab
- Give with meals to prevent GI upset

Patient/family education

- Teach patient that therapeutic response may take 2-4 wk
- Instruct patient to observe feet for arterial insufficiency
- Instruct patient to use cotton socks, well-fitted shoes; not to go barefoot
- Advise patient to watch for bleeding, bruises, petechiae, epistaxis

Evaluation

Positive therapeutic outcome

- Decreased pain, cramping
- Increased ambulation

pergolide (Rx)

(per'goe-lide)

Permax

Func. Class.: Antiparkinson agent

Chem. Class.: Dopamine agonist

Pregnancy category B

WITHDRAWN from the market

Do not confuse:

Permax/Pernail

Action: Stimulates postsynaptic dopamine receptors directly. Acts as a dopamine agonist

Therapeutic Outcome: Improved Parkinson's symptoms

Uses: Parkinson's disease with carbidopa/levodopa

Dosage and routes

Adult: **PO** 50 mcg/day × 2 days, then increase by 100-150 mcg/day q3d × 12 days, then increase by 250 mcg/day q3d until desired response, max 5 mg/day

Available forms: Tab 50, 250 mcg, 1 mg

Adverse effects

CNS: *Drowsiness, hallucinations, dyskinesia*

CV: *Orthostatic hypotension,* atrial premature contractions, hypertension, palpitations, **sinus tachycardia, MI**

GI: *Nausea, constipation,* diarrhea, dry mouth, abdominal pain, dyspepsia

META: Weight gain

MS: Arthralgia, chest, back pain

RESP: Dyspnea

Contraindications: Hypersensitivity to this drug or ergots, lactation

Precautions: Pregnancy **B**, psychiatric disorders, children, dysrhythmias

Pharmacokinetics	
Absorption	Well
Distribution	Unknown, protein binding >90%
Metabolism	Liver
Excretion	Urine
Half-life	Unknown

Pharmacodynamics	
Onset	Unknown
Peak	Unknown
Duration	Unknown

Interactions

Individual drugs

Haloperidol, metoclopramide, reserpine: decreased pergolide effect

Drug classifications

Antihypertensives: increased hypotension

Phenothiazines: decreased effects of pergolide

NURSING CONSIDERATIONS

Assessment

- Assess for Parkinson's symptoms: tremor, ataxia, muscle weakness and rigidity; baseline and periodically
- Assess mental status, hallucinations, confusion; notify prescriber
- Monitor cardiac status: B/P, ECG, periodically during beginning treatment

Nursing diagnoses

- Mobility, physical, impaired (uses)
- Injury, risk for (uses, adverse reactions)
- Knowledge, deficient (teaching)

P

Implementation
- Give with meals to prevent nausea; continuing therapy usually reduces or eliminates nausea
- Give a reduced dose of carbidopa/levodopa, cautiously

Patient/family education
- Teach patient to change positions slowly to prevent orthostatic hypotension
- Teach patient to avoid hazardous activities until stabilized; dizziness can occur
- Teach patient to rinse mouth frequently, use sugarless gum to alleviate dry mouth
- Teach patient to take as prescribed, not to miss doses or double doses; take missed dose as soon as remembered, if several hours before next dose

Evaluation
Positive therapeutic outcome
- Improved symptoms in those with Parkinson's disease

perindopril (Rx)
(per-in-doe-pril)
Aceon
Func. class.: Antihypertensive
Chem. class.: Angiotensin-converting enzyme (ACE) inhibitor

Pregnancy category
C (1st trimester),
D (2nd/3rd trimesters)

Action: Selectively suppresses renin-angiotensin-aldosterone system; inhibits ACE; prevents conversion of angiotensin I to angiotensin II, resulting in dilatation of arterial and venous vessels

Therapeutic Outcome: Decreased B/P in hypertension

Uses: Hypertension alone or in combination

Dosage and routes
Hypertension
Adult: PO 4 mg/day, may increase or decrease to desired response; range 4-8 mg/day may give in 2 divided doses or as a single dose, max 16 mg/day

Patients taking diuretics
Discontinue diuretic 2-3 days before perindopril, then resume diuretic if needed

Renal dose
Adult: PO CCr <30 ml/min 2 mg/day, max 8 mg/day

Available forms: Tabs 2, 4, 8 mg

Adverse effects
CNS: *Insomnia, dizziness,* paresthesias, headache, fatigue, anxiety, depression
CV: *Hypotension,* chest pain, tachycardia, dysrhythmias, syncope
EENT: *Tinnitus,* visual changes, sore throat, double vision, dry burning eyes
GI: Nausea, vomiting, colitis, cramps, diarrhea, constipation, flatulence, dry mouth, loss of taste
GU: **Proteinuria, renal failure,** increased frequency of polyuria or oliguria
HEMA: **Agranulocytosis, neutropenia**
INTEG: Rash, purpura, alopecia, hyperhidrosis
META: Hyperkalemia
RESP: Dyspnea, dry cough, crackles
SYST: **Angioedema**

Contraindications: Pregnancy **D** (2nd/3rd trimesters), hypersensitivity, history of angioedema

Precautions: Pregnancy **C** (1st trimester), renal disease, hyperkalemia, lactation, hepatic failure, dehydration, bilateral renal artery stenosis

Pharmacokinetics

Absorption	Well absorbed
Distribution	Unknown
Metabolism	Liver
Excretion	Kidneys
Half-life	Unknown

Pharmacodynamics
Unknown

Interactions
Individual drugs
Allopurinol: increased hypersensitivity
Lithium: increased serum levels
Drug classifications
Antihypertensives, diuretics: increased hypotension
Antihypertensives, neuromuscular blocking agents: increased effects
Diuretics (potassium-sparing), potassium supplements, salt substitutes: hyperkalemia
NSAIDs: decreased effects
Drug/herb
Aconite: increased toxicity, death
Astragalus, cola tree: increased or decreased antihypertensive effect
Barberry, betony, black catechu, black cohosh, bloodroot, broom, burdock, cat's claw, dandelion, goldenseal, Irish moss, Jamaican dog-

wood, kelp, khella, mistletoe, parsley: increased antihypertensive effect
Coltsfoot, guarana, khat, licorice: decreased antihypertensive effect

Drug/lab test
Interference: glucose/insulin tolerance tests

NURSING CONSIDERATIONS

Assessment

- Monitor blood studies: neutrophils, decreased platelets
- Monitor B/P, orthostatic hypotension, syncope; if changes occur dosage change may be required
- Monitor renal studies: protein, BUN, creatinine; increased levels may indicate nephrotic syndrome and renal failure
- Monitor renal symptoms: polyuria, oliguria, frequency, dysuria
- Establish baselines in renal, liver function tests before therapy begins
- Check potassium levels throughout treatment, although hyperkalemia rarely occurs
- Check for edema in feet, legs daily
- Assess for allergic reactions: rash, fever, pruritus, urticaria; drug should be discontinued if antihistamines fail to help

Nursing diagnoses

- Cardiac output, decreased (uses)
- Injury, risk for (adverse reactions)
- Knowledge, deficient (teaching)
- Noncompliance (teaching)

Implementation

- Store in airtight container at 86° F (30° C) or less
- Severe hypotension may occur after 1st dose of this medication; decreased hypotension may be prevented by reducing or discontinuing diuretic therapy 3 days before beginning perindopril therapy
- Give by **IV** inf of 0.9% NaCl (as ordered) to expand fluid volume if severe hypotension occurs

Patient/family education

- Advise patient not to discontinue drug abruptly; advise patient to tell all persons associated with health care
- Teach patient not to use OTC products (cough, cold, allergy medications) unless directed by physician; serious side effects can occur; xanthines, such as coffee, tea, chocolate, cola can prevent action of drug
- Instruct patient on the importance of complying with dosage schedule, even if feeling better; to continue with medical regimen to decrease B/P: exercise, cessation of smoking, decreasing stress, diet modifications
- Emphasize the need to rise slowly to sitting or standing position to minimize orthostatic hypotension; not to exercise in hot weather, which can cause increased hypotension
- Advise patient to notify prescriber of mouth sores, sore throat, fever, swelling of hands or feet, irregular heartbeat, chest pain, coughing, shortness of breath
- Caution patient to report excessive perspiration, dehydration, vomiting, diarrhea; may lead to fall in B/P
- Caution patient that drug may cause dizziness, fainting, light-headedness; may occur during 1st few days of therapy; to avoid activities that may be hazardous
- Teach patient how to take B/P, and normal readings for age-group

Evaluation

Positive therapeutic outcome

- Decreased B/P in hypertension

Treatment of overdose: Lavage, **IV** atropine for bradycardia, **IV** theophylline for bronchospasm, digitalis, O_2; diuretic for cardiac failure, hemodialysis

perphenazine (Rx)

(per-fen'a-zeen)

Apo-Perphenazine ✦, perphenazine, Phenazine ✦, PMS Perphenazine ✦

Func. class.: Antipsychotic/neuroleptic
Chem. class.: Phenothiazine piperidine

Pregnancy category C

P

Action: Depresses cerebral cortex, hypothalamus, limbic system, which control activity, aggression; blocks neurotransmission produced by dopamine at synapse; exhibits strong α-adrenergic, anticholinergic blocking action; as antiemetic inhibits medullary chemoreceptor trigger zone; mechanism for antipsychotic effects is unclear

Therapeutic Outcome: Decreased signs and symptoms of psychosis; decreased nausea and vomiting

Uses: Psychotic disorders, schizophrenia, nausea, vomiting

Dosage and routes

Elderly: PO 2-4 mg daily-bid, increase by 2-4 mg/wk to desired dose

Nausea/vomiting/alcoholism

Adult and child >12 yr: IM 5-10 mg prn, max 15 mg in ambulatory patients, 30 mg in hospitalized patients; PO 8-16 mg/day in divided doses, up to 24 mg; **IV** max 5 mg; give diluted or slow **IV** drip

Psychiatric use in hospitalized patients

Adults: PO 8-16 mg bid-qid, gradually increased to desired dose, max 64 mg/day; IM 5 mg q6h, max 30 mg/day

Child >12 yr: PO 6-12 mg in divided doses

Nonhospitalized patients

Adult: PO 4-8 mg tid

Available forms: Tabs 2, 4, 8, 16 mg; oral conc 16 mg/5 ml; syr 2 mg/5 ml ♣

Adverse effects

CNS: *EPS (pseudoparkinsonism, akathisia, dystonia, tardive dyskinesia),* **neuroleptic malignant syndrome, seizures,** *headache,* dizziness

CV: *Orthostatic hypotension (elderly),* **cardiac arrest,** ECG changes, **tachycardia**

EENT: Blurred vision, glaucoma

GI: *Dry mouth, nausea, vomiting, anorexia, constipation,* diarrhea, jaundice, weight gain

GU: Urinary retention, urinary frequency, enuresis, impotence, amenorrhea, gynecomastia

HEMA: Anemia, **leukopenia, leukocytosis, agranulocytosis**

INTEG: *Rash,* photosensitivity, dermatitis

RESP: **Laryngospasm,** dyspnea, **respiratory depression**

Contraindications: Hypersensitivity, blood dyscrasias, coma, child <12 yr, brain damage, bone marrow depression

Precautions: Pregnancy **C**, lactation, seizure disorders, hypertension, hepatic disease, cardiac disease, elderly, narrow-angle glaucoma

Pharmacokinetics

Absorption	Variably absorbed (PO); well absorbed (IM)
Distribution	Widely distributed; high concentrations in CNS; crosses placenta
Metabolism	Liver, extensively; GI mucosa
Excretion	Kidneys

Pharmacodynamics

	PO	IM	IV
Onset	Erratic	10 min	Rapid
Peak	2-4 hr	1-2 hr	Unknown
Duration	6-12 hr	6-12 hr	Unknown

Interactions

Individual drugs

Alcohol: increased effects of both drugs, oversedation

Aluminum hydroxide, magnesium hydroxide: decreased absorption

Epinephrine: increased toxicity

Levodopa: decreased antiparkinson activity

Lithium: increased risk of EPS

Ritonavir: increased perphenazine effect

Meperidine: increased hypotension

Drug classifications

Anesthetics (barbiturates), CNS depressants, barbiturate anesthetics: increased sedation

Antacids, antidiarrheals (adsorbent): decreased absorption

Anticholinergics: increased anticholinergic effects

Anticoagulants (oral): decreased anticoagulant effect

β-Adrenergic blockers: increased effects of both drugs

Diuretics (thiazide): increased hypotension

Drug/herb

Betel palm, kava: increased extrapyramidal symptoms (EPS)

Cola tree, hops, nettle, nutmeg: increased action

Henbane: increased anticholinergic effect

Drug/lab test

Increased: liver function tests, cardiac enzymes, cholesterol, blood glucose, prolactin, bilirubin, PBI, cholinesterase, iodine

Decreased: hormones (blood and urine)

False positive: pregnancy tests, PKU

False negative: urinary steroids, 17-OHCS

NURSING CONSIDERATIONS

Assessment

- Assess mental status: orientation, mood, behavior, presence and type of hallucinations before initial administration and monthly; this drug should significantly reduce psychotic behavior
- Check for swallowing of PO medication; check for hoarding or giving medication to other patients
- Monitor I&O ratio; palpate bladder if low urinary output occurs, especially in elderly; urinalysis recommended before, during prolonged therapy
- Monitor bilirubin, CBC, liver function studies monthly
- Assess affect, orientation, LOC, reflexes, gait, coordination, sleep pattern disturbances
- Monitor B/P with patient sitting, standing, and lying; take pulse and respirations q4h

during initial treatment; establish baseline before starting treatment; report drops of 30 mm Hg; obtain baseline ECG, with Q- and T-wave changes

- Check for dizziness, faintness, palpitations, tachycardia on rising; severe orthostatic hypotension is common
- Identify for neuroleptic malignant syndrome: hyperpyrexia, muscle rigidity, increased CPK, altered mental status; drug should be discontinued
- Assess for EPS including akathisia (inability to sit still, no pattern to movements), tardive dyskinesia (bizarre movements of the jaw, mouth, tongue, extremities), pseudoparkinsonism (ragged tremors, pill rolling, shuffling gait); an antiparkinsonian drug should be prescribed
- Assess for constipation, urinary retention daily; if these occur, increase bulk, water in diet

Nursing diagnoses

- Thought processes, disturbed (uses)
- Coping, ineffective (uses)
- Knowledge, deficient (teaching)
- Noncompliance (teaching)

Implementation

PO route

- Administer drug in liq form mixed in glass of juice or cola if hoarding is suspected; do not mix in caffeine drinks, tannics, pectins
- Administer decreased dose in elderly, in whom metabolism is slowed
- Administer PO with full glass of water, milk; or give with food to decrease GI upset
- Give antacids 2 hr before or after taking this drug
- Store in airtight, light-resistant container; oral sol in amber bottle

IM route

- Inject in deep muscle mass; do not give SUBCUT; do not administer sol with a precipitate
- Remain lying down after IM inj for at least 30 min

IV route

- Give by direct **IV** after diluting with 0.9% NaCl to a conc of 0.5 mg/1 ml; administer at 1 mg/min; may be further diluted and given as an inf

Syringe compatibilities: Atropine, benztropine, butorphanol, chlorproMAZINE, cimetidine, dimenhyDRINATE, diphenhydrAMINE, droperidol, fentanyl, hydrOXYzine, meperidine, methotrimeprazine, metoclopramide, morphine, pentazocine, prochlorperazine, promethazine, ranitidine, scopolamine

Syringe incompatibilities: Midazolam, opium alkaloids, pentobarbital, thiethylperazine

Y-site compatibilities: Acyclovir, amikacin, ampicillin, azlocillin, cefamandole, cefazolin, cefotaxime, cefoxitin, cefuroxime, cephalothin, cephapirin, chloramphenicol, clindamycin, cotrimoxazole, doxycycline, erythromycin, famotidine, gentamicin, kanamycin, metronidazole, mezlocillin, minocycline, moxalactam, nafcillin, oxacillin, penicillin G potassium, piperacillin, sulfamethoxazole, tacrolimus, ticarcillin, ticarcillin/clavulanate, tobramycin, trimethoprim, vancomycin

Additive compatibilities: Ascorbic acid, ethacrynate, netilmicin

Additive incompatibilities: Cefoperazone

Patient/family education

- Teach patient to use good oral hygiene; frequent rinsing of mouth, sugarless gum for dry mouth
- Advise patient to avoid hazardous activities until drug response is determined, dizziness, blurred vision may occur
- Inform patient that orthostatic hypotension occurs often and to rise from sitting or lying position gradually; to remain lying down after IM inj for at least 30 min; tell patient to avoid hot tubs, hot showers, tub baths, since hypotension may occur; teach patient that in hot weather heat stroke may occur; take extra precautions to stay cool
- Teach patient to avoid abrupt withdrawal of this drug, or EPS may result; drug should be withdrawn slowly
- Teach patient to avoid OTC preparations (cough, hay fever, cold) unless approved by prescriber, since serious drug interactions may occur; avoid use with alcohol, CNS depressants; increased drowsiness may result
- Caution patient to use a sunscreen and sunglasses to prevent burns
- Teach patient about EPS and necessity of meticulous oral hygiene, since oral candidiasis may occur
- Instruct patient to take antacids 2 hr before or after taking this drug
- Teach patient to report sore throat, malaise, fever, bleeding, mouth sores; if these occur, CBC should be performed and drug discontinued
- Teach patient that urine may turn reddish brown

Evaluation

Positive therapeutic outcome

- Decrease in emotional excitement, hallucinations, delusions, paranoia
- Reorganization of patterns of thought, speech

Treatment of overdose: Lavage if orally ingested; provide airway; *do not induce vomiting or use epINEPHrine*

phenazopyridine (Rx, OTC)

(fen-az-o-peer′i-deen)

AZO-Standard, Baridium, Eridium, Geridium, Phenazo ✤, Phenazodine, phenazopyridine, Prodium, Pyridiate, Pyridium, Urodine, Urogesic, Viridium

Func. class.: Nonopioid analgesic, urinary

Chem. class.: Azodye

Pregnancy category B

Action: Exerts analgesic, anesthetic action on the urinary tract mucosa

Uses: Urinary tract irritation, infection (for symptoms only of pain, burning, itching) used with urinary antiinfectives

Dosage and routes

Adult: PO 200 mg tid × 2 days or less when used with antibacterial for UTI

Child 6-12 yr: PO 4 mg/kg tid × 2 days

Renal dose

Adult: PO CCr <50 ml/min do not use

Available forms: Tabs 100, 200 mg

Adverse effects

CNS: Headache

GI: *Nausea, vomiting, diarrhea, heartburn,* anorexia, **hepatic toxicity**

GU: **Renal toxicity,** *orange-red urine*

HEMA: **Thrombocytopenia, agranulocytosis, leukopenia, neutropenia, hemolytic anemia, methemoglobinemia**

INTEG: Rash, pruritus, skin pigmentation

Contraindications: Hypersensitivity, renal insufficiency

Precautions: Pregnancy **B,** lactation, children <12 yr

Pharmacokinetics

Absorption	Well absorbed
Distribution	Unknown; crosses placenta
Metabolism	Unknown
Excretion	Kidneys, unchanged
Half-life	Unknown

Pharmacodynamics

Onset	Unknown
Peak	5-6 hr
Duration	8 hr

Interactions: None known

Drug/lab test

Interference: urinalysis

NURSING CONSIDERATIONS

Assessment

- Assess urinary status: burning, pain, itching, urgency, frequency, hematuria before, during, and after completion of drug therapy
- Monitor liver function studies: AST, ALT, bilirubin if patient is on long-term therapy
- ❗ Assess for hepatotoxicity: dark urine, clay-colored stools, yellowing of skin and sclera, itching, abdominal pain, fever, diarrhea if patient is on long-term therapy
- Assess for allergic reactions: rash, urticaria; if these occur, drug may have to be discontinued

Nursing diagnoses

- Pain, acute (uses)
- Urinary elimination, impaired (uses)
- Knowledge, deficient (teaching)

Implementation

- Give to patient crushed or whole; chew tab should be chewed
- Give with food or milk to decrease gastric symptoms

Patient/family education

- Advise patient to report any symptoms of hepatotoxicity
- Caution patient not to exceed recommended dosage and to take with meals; to read label on other OTC drugs
- Teach patient not to discontinue after pain is relieved but continue to take concurrent prescribed antiinfective until finished
- Inform patient urine may turn red-orange, may stain clothing or contact lens

Evaluation

Positive therapeutic outcome

- Decrease in pain, burning, itching when urinating

Treatment of overdose: Methylene blue 1-2 mg/kg **IV** or vit C 100-200 mg PO

phenelzine (Rx)
(fen′el-zeen)

Nardil

Func. class.: Antidepressant, MAOI

Chem. class.: Hydrazine

Pregnancy category C

Action: Increases concentrations of endogenous epinephrine, norepinephrine, serotonin, dopamine in storage sites in CNS by inhibition of MAO; increased concentration reduces depression

Therapeutic Outcome: Decreased symptoms of depression after 2-3 wk

Uses: Depression, when uncontrolled by other means

Dosage and routes
Adult: PO 45 mg/day in divided doses; may increase to 60 mg/day; dose should be reduced to 15 mg/day, not to exceed 90 mg/day

Elderly: PO 7.5 mg daily, increase by 7.5-15 mg q3-4 days; usual dose 15-60 mg/day in divided doses

Available forms: Tabs 15 mg

Adverse effects
CNS: *Dizziness, drowsiness,* confusion, headache, anxiety, tremors, stimulation, weakness, hyperreflexia, mania, insomnia, fatigue, weight gain

CV: *Orthostatic hypotension, hypertension,* **dysrhythmias, hypertensive crisis,** tachycardia, peripheral edema

EENT: Blurred vision

ENDO: **Syndrome of inappropriate antidiuretic hormone–like syndrome**

GI: Constipation, dry mouth, nausea, vomiting, *anorexia,* diarrhea, weight gain

GU: Change in libido, frequency of urination

HEMA: Anemia

INTEG: Rash, flushing, increased perspiration

Contraindications: Hypersensitivity to MAOIs, hypertension, CHF, severe hepatic disease, pheochromocytoma, severe renal disease, severe cardiac disease, active alcoholism

Precautions: Pregnancy **C,** suicidal patients, seizure disorders, severe depression, schizophrenia, hyperactivity, diabetes mellitus, child <16 yr

Pharmacokinetics

Absorption	Well absorbed
Distribution	Crosses placenta
Metabolism	Liver, extensively
Excretion	Kidneys, breast milk
Half-life	Unknown

Pharmacodynamics
Unknown

Interactions
Individual drugs
Alcohol: increased CNS depression

Clonidine: severe hypotension; avoid use

Guanethidine: decreased effects

Levodopa: increased effect of levodopa

L-Tryptophan: increased confusion, shivering, hyperreflexia

Meperidine: hypertensive crisis, seizures, hypertensive episode

Methylphenidate: seizures, do not use together

Sumatriptan: increased toxicity

Drug classifications
Amphetamines, appetite suppressants, asthma inhalants, nasal decongestants, selective serotonin reuptake inhibitors: increased hyperpyretic crisis, seizures, hypertensive episode

Anticholinergics: increased side effects

Antidepressants (tricyclics), meperidine, methylphenidate, nasal decongestants, sinus medications: hypertensive crisis

Antidepressants (tricyclics), meperidine, nasal decongestants, sinus medications: convulsions

Antidepressants (tricyclics), meperidine, nasal decongestants, sinus medications: selective serotonin reuptake inhibitors: hypertensive episode

Antidiabetics: increased hypoglycemia

Barbiturates: increased effects of barbiturates

Benzodiazepines: increased effects of benzodiazepines

CNS depressants: increased effects of CNS depressants

Diuretics (thiazide): increased hypotension

Rauwolfia alkaloids: decreased serotonin, norepinephrine

Sulfonamides: increased toxicity

Sympathomimetics (direct-acting): increased effects

Sympathomimetics (indirect-acting, mixed): increased pressor effect

Drug/herb
Betel palm, butcher's broom, capsicum peppers, galanthamine, green tea (large amounts), guarana (large amounts), night-

P

blooming cereus: increased sympathomimetic effect
Brewer's yeast, cola tree, khat: increased hypertension
Ginkgo, nutmeg, yohimbe: increased effect
Ginseng: increased tension headache, irritability, visual hallucinations, mania
Jimsonweed: increased anticholinergic effect
Parsley, St. John's wort: serotonin syndrome
Valerian: decreased effect

Drug/food

Caffeine: increased hypertension
Tyramine-containing foods: hypertensive crisis

NURSING CONSIDERATIONS

Assessment

- Monitor B/P (with patient lying, standing), pulse q4h; if systolic B/P drops 20 mm Hg, hold drug, notify prescriber; take VS q4h in patients with CV disease
- Monitor hepatic studies: AST, ALT, bilirubin if patient is on long-term therapy
- Check weight weekly; appetite may increase with drug
- Assess ECG for flattening of T wave, bundle branch block, AV block, dysrhythmias in cardiac patients
- Assess mental status: mood, sensorium, affect, suicidal tendencies; increase in psychiatric symptoms: depression, panic
- Monitor urinary retention, constipation; constipation is more likely to occur in elderly
- Assess for withdrawal symptoms: headache, nausea, vomiting, muscle pain, weakness; do not usually occur unless drug was discontinued abruptly
- Identify alcohol consumption; if alcohol is consumed, hold dose until AM

Nursing diagnoses

- Coping, ineffective (uses)
- Injury, risk for (adverse reactions)
- Knowledge, deficient (teaching)
- Noncompliance (teaching)

Implementation

- Give with food or milk for GI symptoms; crush if patient is unable to swallow medication whole and mix with food or fluids
- Store at room temp; do not freeze

Patient/family education

- Advise patient to use caution in driving and other activities requiring alertness because of drowsiness, dizziness, blurred vision; to avoid rising quickly from sitting to standing, especially elderly
- Caution patient to avoid alcohol ingestion, other CNS depressants; serious reaction can occur
- Advise patient not to discontinue medication quickly after long-term use: may cause nausea, headache, malaise, sweating, hallucinations
- Instruct patient to increase fluids, bulk in diet if constipation, urinary retention occur, especially elderly; a stool softener may be ordered
- Teach patient to take gum, hard sugarless candy, or frequent sips of water for dry mouth
- Teach patient that therapeutic effects may take 1-4 wk
- Teach patient to avoid OTC medications: cold, weight loss, hay fever, cough syrup
- Teach patient to avoid high-tyramine foods: cheese (aged), sour cream, beer, wine, pickled products, liver, raisins, bananas, figs, avocados, meat tenderizers, chocolate, yogurt; increased caffeine, may cause hypertensive reactions
- Teach patient to report headache, palpitations, neck stiffness, dizziness, constriction in chest, throat; rash, insomnia, change in strength, changes in urinary patterns, color of urine

Evaluation

Positive therapeutic outcome

- Decrease in depression
- Absence of suicidal thoughts

Treatment of overdose: Lavage, activated charcoal, monitor electrolytes, VS, diazepam **IV**, sodium bicarbonate

! HIGH ALERT

phenobarbital 🗝 (Rx)

(fee-noe-bar'bit-tal)

Ancalixir ✤, Barbita, Luminal, phenobarbital sodium, Solfoton

Func. class.: Anticonvulsant, sedative/hypnotic

Chem. class.: Barbiturate

Pregnancy category D

Controlled substance schedule IV

Do Not Confuse:
phenobarbital/pentobarbital

Action: Depresses activity in brain cells primarily in reticular activating system in brainstem; also selectively depresses neurons in posterior hypothalamus, limbic structures; able to decrease seizure activity by inhibition of impulses in CNS; decreases motor activity

Therapeutic Outcome: Sedation, anticonvulsant, improved energy

Uses: All forms of epilepsy, status epilepticus, febrile seizures in children, sedation, insomnia

Investigational uses: Hyperbilirubinemia, chronic cholestasis

Dosage and routes

Seizures

Adult: PO 60-200 mg/day in divided doses tid or total dose at bedtime

Child: PO 4-6 mg/kg/day in divided doses q12h; may be given as single dose

Status epilepticus

Adult: **IV** inf 10 mg/kg; run no faster than 50 mg/min; may give up to 20 mg/kg

Child: **IV** inf 5-10 mg/kg; may repeat q10-15 min up to 20 mg/kg; run no faster than 50 mg/min

Insomnia

Adult: PO/IM 100-320 mg

Child: PO/IM 3-5 mg/kg

Sedation

Adult: PO 30-120 mg/day in 2-3 divided doses

Child: PO 3-5 mg/kg/day in 3 divided doses

Preoperative sedation

Adult: IM 100-200 mg 1-1½ hr before surgery

Child: IM 16-100 mg or PO/IM/**IV** 1-3 mg/kg 1-1½ hr before surgery

Available forms: Caps 15 mg; elixir 20 mg/5 ml; tabs 8, 15, 30, 60, 100 mg; inj 30, 60, 65, 130 mg/ml

Adverse effects

CNS: Paradoxic excitement (elderly), drowsiness, lethargy, *hangover headache,* flushing, hallucinations, **coma**

GI: Nausea, vomiting, diarrhea, constipation

INTEG: Rash, urticaria, **Stevens-Johnson syndrome, angioedema,** local pain, swelling, necrosis, **thrombophlebitis**

Contraindications: Pregnancy **D**, hypersensitivity to barbiturates, porphyria, hepatic disease, respiratory disease, nephritis, hyperthyroidism, diabetes mellitus, elderly, lactation

Precautions: Anemia

Pharmacokinetics

Absorption	Slow (70%-90%) (PO/IM/**IV**)
Distribution	Not known; crosses placenta
Metabolism	Liver (75%)
Excretion	Kidneys (25% unchanged)
Half-life	2-6 days

Pharmacodynamics

	PO	IM	IV
Onset	30-60 min	10-30 min	5 min
Peak	Unknown	Unknown	30 min
Duration	6-8 hr	4-6 hr	4-6 hr

Interactions

Individual drugs

Alcohol: increased CNS depression

Chloramphenicol, disulfiram: increased effects

Doxycycline, quinidine, theophylline: decreased effectiveness

Furosemide: increased orthostatic hypotension

Valproic acid: increased sedation

Drug classifications

Anticoagulants, glucocorticoids: decreased effectiveness

Skeletal muscle relaxants (nondepolarizing): increased effects

Sulfonamides: increased effects

Drug/herb

Chamomile, eucalyptus, hops, Jamaican dogwood, kava, lemon balm, nettle, pill-bearing spurge, poppy, senega, skullcap, valerian: increased CNS depression

Quinine: increased phenobarbitol levels

St. John's wort: decreased barbiturate effect

NURSING CONSIDERATIONS

Assessment

- Assess mental status: mood, sensorium, affect, memory (long, short), especially elderly; if using as a hypnotic, assess sleep patterns during therapy; drug suppresses REM sleep with dreaming
- Withdrawal insomnia may occur after short-term use; do not start using drug again; insomnia improves in 1-3 nights; may experience increased dreaming
- Assess respiratory dysfunction: respiratory depression, character, rate, rhythm when using **IV**; hold drug if respirations are <10/min or if pupils are dilated; also check VS q30 min after parenteral route for 2 hr
- Assess for barbiturate toxicity: hypotension, pulmonary constriction, cold, clammy skin, cyanosis of lips, CNS depression, nausea, vomiting, hallucinations, delirium, weakness, coma, pupillary constriction; mild symptoms occur in 8-12 hr without drug
- Assess for pain in postoperative patients; pain threshold is lowered when patients are taking this medication
- Assess for blood dyscrasias: fever, sore throat, bruising, rash, jaundice, epistaxis (long-term treatment only)
- Assess seizure activity including type,

P

location, duration, and character; provide seizure precaution

Nursing diagnoses
- Sleep pattern, disturbed (uses)
- Injury, risk for (adverse reactions)
- Knowledge, deficient (teaching)

Implementation
- Give medication after removal of cigarettes to prevent fires
- Give medication after trying conservative measures for insomnia

PO route
- Tab may be crushed and mixed with food if swallowing is difficult; also may be mixed with other fluids 30-60 min before bedtime for expected sleeplessness; on empty stomach for best absorption

IM route
- Give inj in deep muscle mass (gluteal) to minimize irritation to tissues
- Split inj of >5 ml into two, since irritation to tissues may occur

IV, direct route
- Use large vein to prevent extravasation; if extravasation occurs, use moist heat to the area and 5% procaine sol injected into area; give at 65 mg or less/min; titrate to patient response

Syringe compatibilities: Heparin

Syringe incompatibilities: Benzquinamide, ranitidine

Y-site compatibilities: Enalaprilat, meropenem, propofol, sufentanil

Y-site incompatibilities: Hydromorphone

Additive compatibilities: Amikacin, aminophylline, calcium chloride, calcium gluceptate, cephapirin, colistimethate, dimenhyDRINATE, meropenem, polymyxin B, sodium bicarbonate, thiopental, verapamil

Additive incompatibilities: Cephalothin, chlorproMAZINE, codeine, epHEDrine, hydrALAZINE, hydrocortisone sodium succinate, hydrOXYzine, insulin, levorphanol, meperidine, methadone, morphine, norepinephrine, pentazocine, procaine, prochlorazine mesylate, promazine, promethazine, streptomycin, vancomycin

Solution compatibilities: D_5W, $D_{10}W$, 0.45% NaCl, 0.9% NaCl, Ringer's, dextrose/saline combinations, dextrose/Ringer's, dextrose/LR combinations, sodium lactate

Patient/family education
- Teach patient that hangover is common
- Instruct patient that drug is indicated only for short-term treatment of insomnia and is probably ineffective after 2 wk
- Inform patient that physical dependency may result when used for extended time (45-90 days depending on dosage)
- Teach patient to avoid driving and other activities requiring alertness
- Caution patient to avoid alcohol ingestion and CNS depressants; serious CNS depression may result
- Instruct patient not to discontinue medication quickly after long-term use; may cause seizures; drug should be tapered over 1 wk; take exactly as prescribed
- Emphasize the need to tell all prescribers that a barbiturate is being taken
- Teach the patient to make position changes slowly; orthostatic hypotension may occur
- Teach patient that response may take 4 days to 2 wk
- Instruct patient to notify prescriber immediately if bruising, bleeding occur, which may indicate blood dyscrasias

Evaluation
Positive therapeutic outcome
- Improved sleeping patterns
- Decreased seizure activity
- Sedative preoperatively

Treatment of overdose: Lavage, activated charcoal, warming blanket, VS, hemodialysis, alkalinize urine, give **IV** volume expanders, **IV** fluids

phenolphthalein (OTC)
(fee-nol-thay'leen)

Alophen, Correctol, Espotabs, Evac-U-Gen, Evac-U-Lax, Ex-Lax, Feen-A-Mint, Lax-Pills, Modane, Medilax, Phenolax, Prulet

Func. class.: Laxative, stimulant/irritant

Chem. class.: Diphenylmethane

Pregnancy category C

Action: Directly acts on intestinal smooth muscle by increasing motor activity; thought to irritate colonic intramural plexus; increases fluid in small intestine; alters fluid and electrolytes; action requires presence of bile

Therapeutic Outcome: Decreased constipation

Uses: Constipation, preparation for bowel surgery or examination

Dosage and routes
Adult: PO 30-270 mg at bedtime

Child >6 yr: 30-60 mg/day

Child 2-5 yr: 15-20 mg/day

Available forms: Tabs 60, 90, 97.2, 130

mg; chew tabs 65, 90, 97.2 mg; chew gum 97.2 mg; wafers 64.8 mg; chew wafers 80 mg

Adverse effects

GI: *Nausea, vomiting, anorexia, diarrhea,* abdominal cramps, rectal burning

INTEG: Rash, urticaria, **Stevens-Johnson syndrome**

META: Hypokalemia, electrolyte and fluid imbalances

Contraindications: Hypersensitivity, GI obstructions, abdominal pain, nausea/vomiting, fecal impaction, rectal fissures, hemorrhoids (ulcerated)

Precautions: Pregnancy **C,** lactation

Pharmacokinetics	
Absorption	Minimally absorbed (15%)
Distribution	Unknown
Metabolism	Not metabolized
Excretion	Kidneys, feces
Half-life	Unknown

Pharmacodynamics	
Onset	6-8 hr
Peak	Unknown
Duration	3-4 days

Interactions

Drug classifications

Oral drugs (any): decreased absorption

Drug/lab test

Interference: BSP test

NURSING CONSIDERATIONS

Assessment

- Monitor blood, urine electrolytes if drug used often by patient; check I&O ratio to identify fluid loss
- Assess for cramping, rectal bleeding, nausea, vomiting; if these symptoms occur, drug should be discontinued; identify cause of constipation; identify whether fluids, bulk, or exercise is missing from lifestyle
- Assess stool for color, consistency, amount, presence of flatulence

Nursing diagnoses

- Constipation (uses)
- Diarrhea (adverse reaction)
- Knowledge, deficient (teaching)
- Noncompliance (teaching)

Implementation

- Chew well before swallowing; follow with 4 oz of water to prevent undissolved tab entering small intestine
- Give with 8 oz of water (tab); administer on empty stomach for more rapid results; do not give at bedtime

Patient/family education

- Discuss with patient that adequate fluid consumption is necessary
- Teach patient that normal bowel movements do not always occur daily
- Caution patient not to use in presence of abdominal pain, nausea, vomiting; tell patient to notify prescriber if constipation is unrelieved or if symptoms of electrolyte imbalance occur (muscle cramps, pain, weakness, dizziness, excessive thirst)
- Teach patient not to use laxatives for long-term therapy; bowel tone will be lost
- Teach patient not to take at bedtime as a laxative; may interfere with sleep; also can cause problems with lipid pneumonia
- Teach patient not to use with food or vitamin preparations; delays digestion and absorption of fat-soluble vitamins

Evaluation

Positive therapeutic outcome

- Decreased constipation in 8-10 hr

phentolamine (Rx)

(fen-tole'a-meen)

Regitine, Rogitine ♣

Func. class.: Antihypertensive

Chem. class.: α-Adrenergic blocker

Pregnancy category C

Action: α-Adrenergic blocker, binds to α-adrenergic receptors, dilating peripheral blood vessels, lowering peripheral resistances, lowering blood pressure

Therapeutic Outcome: Decreased B/P, reversal of vasoconstriction (dermal necrosis)

Uses: Hypertension, pheochromocytoma, prevention, treatment of dermal necrosis after extravasation of norepinephrine or DOPamine, impotence

Investigational uses: Impotence, hypertensive crisis due to MAOIs

Dosage and routes

Treatment of hypertensive episodes in pheochromocytoma

Adult: **IV**/IM 5 mg; repeat if necessary

Child: **IV**/IM 1 mg; repeat if necessary

Diagnosis of pheochromocytoma

Adult: **IV** 2.5 mg; if negative, repeat with 5 mg **IV**

P

Child: **IV** 0.05 mg/kg; if negative, repeat with 0.1 mg/kg **IV**

Treatment of necrosis

Adult: 5-10 mg/10 ml NS injected into area of extravasation within 12 hr

Child: 0.1-0.2 mg/kg; max 10 mg

Prevention of dermal necrosis

Adult: **IV** 10 mg/L of norepinephrine-containing sol

Child: **IV** 0.1-0.2 mg/kg, max 10 mg

Available forms: Inj 5 mg/ml

Adverse effects

CNS: *Dizziness,* flushing, weakness, **cerebrovascular spasm**

CV: *Hypotension,* **tachycardia,** *angina,* **dysrhythmias, MI**

EENT: Nasal congestion

GI: *Dry mouth, nausea, vomiting, diarrhea, abdominal pain*

Contraindications: Hypersensitivity, MI, coronary insufficiency, angina

Precautions: Pregnancy **C,** lactation

Pharmacokinetics

Absorption	Well absorbed (IM); completely absorbed (**IV**)
Distribution	Unknown
Metabolism	Unknown
Excretion	Kidneys, unchanged (10%)
Half-life	Unknown

Pharmacodynamics

	IM	IV
Onset	Unknown	Rapid
Peak	20 min	2 min
Duration	½-1 hr	½ hr

Interactions

Individual drugs

EpINEPHrine: increased effects of epINEPHrine

Drug classifications

Antihypertensives: increased effects of antihypertensives

Drug/herb

Aconite: increased toxicity, death

Astragalus, cola tree: increased or decreased antihypertensive effect

Barberry, betony, black catechu, black cohosh, bloodroot, broom, burdock, cat's claw, dandelion, goldenseal, Irish moss, Jamaican dogwood, kelp, khella, mistletoe, parsley: increased antihypertensive effect

Coltsfoot, guarana, khat, licorice: decreased antihypertensive effect

NURSING CONSIDERATIONS

Assessment

- Monitor B/P, orthostatic hypotension, syncope, pulse and ECG until stable

Nursing diagnoses

- Cardiac output, decreased (uses)
- Injury, risk for (adverse reactions)
- Knowledge, deficient (teaching)
- Noncompliance (teaching)

Implementation

- Give with vasopressor nearby

IV route

- Give by direct **IV** after diluting 5 mg/1 ml of sterile water for inj or 0.9% NaCl; give 5 mg or less/min
- Give by cont inf by further diluting 5-10 mg/500 ml of D_5W, titrate to patient response
- Add 10 mg/L to norepINEPHrine in **IV** sol for prevention of dermal necrosis

Syringe compatibilities: Papaverine

Y-site compatibilities: Amiodarone

Additive compatibilities: DOBUTamine, verapamil

Patient/family education

- Caution patient not to discontinue drug abruptly
- Teach patient not to use OTC products (cough, cold, allergy) unless directed by prescriber
- Teach patient the importance of complying with dosage schedule, even if feeling better
- Emphasize the need to rise slowly to sitting or standing position to minimize orthostatic hypotension
- Teach patient to notify prescriber of mouth sores, sore throat, fever, swelling of hands or feet, irregular heartbeat, chest pain
- Caution patient to report excessive perspiration, dehydration, vomiting, diarrhea; may lead to fall in B/P
- Caution patient that drug may cause dizziness, fainting, light-headedness; may occur during 1st few days of therapy
- Teach patient how to take B/P, and normal readings for age-group

Evaluation

Positive therapeutic outcome

- Decreased B/P in hypertension
- Resolution of impotence
- Prevention of dermal necrosis

Treatment of overdose: Administer norepinephrine; discontinue drug

phenylephrine (Rx)
(fen-ill-ef′rin)

Neo-Synephrine

Func. class.: Adrenergic, direct acting
Chem. class.: Direct sympathomimetic amine (α-agonist)

Pregnancy category C

Action: Powerful and selective receptor agonist causing contraction of blood vessels, vasoconstriction of eye arterioles; decreases eye engorgement by stimulation of α-adrenergic receptors

Therapeutic Outcome: Increased B/P, decreased nasal congestion, decreased eye irritation

Uses: Hypotension, paroxysmal supraventricular tachycardia, shock, B/P maintenance during spinal anesthesia, topical ocular vasoconstrictor in uveitis, open-angle glaucoma, preoperatively, diagnostic procedures, refraction without cycloplegia, nasal congestion

Dosage and routes
Hypotension

Adult: SUBCUT/IM 2-5 mg; may repeat q10-15 min if needed, do not exceed initial dose; **IV** 50-100 mcg; may repeat q10-15 min if needed, do not exceed initial dose

Child: IM/SUBCUT 0.1 mg/kg/dose q1-2h prn

Supraventricular tachycardia

Adult: **IV** bol 0.5-1 mg given rapidly, not to exceed prior dose by >0.1 mg; total dose ≤1 mg

Shock

Adult: **IV** inf 10 mg/500 ml of D_5W given 100-180 mcg/min (if 20 gtt/ml device is used), then maintenance of 40-60 mcg/min (if 20 gtt/ml device is used); use infusion pump

Child: **IV** bol 5-20 mcg/kg/dose q10-15 min; **IV** inf 0.1-0.5 mg/kg/min

Available forms: Inj 1% (10 mg/ml)

Adverse effects
CNS: *Headache, dizziness, anxiety, tremor, insomnia*

CV: Reflex bradycardia, **dysrhythmias,** *hypertension,* **tachycardia,** palpitations, ectopic beats, angina

GI: *Nausea, vomiting*

INTEG: Necrosis, tissue sloughing with extravasation, **gangrene**

MISC: **Anaphylaxis**

Contraindications: Hypersensitivity, narrow-angle glaucoma, ventricular fibrillation, tachydysrhythmias, pheochromocytoma, severe hypertension

Precautions: Pregnancy **C,** hyperthyroidism, elderly, severe arteriosclerosis, lactation, arterial embolism, peripheral vascular disease, bradycardia, myocardial disease, partial heart block

Pharmacokinetics

Absorption	Well absorbed (IM); completely absorbed (**IV**); minimally absorbed (nasal, ophth)
Distribution	Unknown
Metabolism	Liver
Excretion	Unknown
Half-life	Unknown

Pharmacodynamics

	IV	SUBCUT/IM
Onset	Rapid	15 min
Peak	Unknown	Unknown
Duration	20-30 min	45-60 min

Interactions
Individual drugs

Bretylium, digoxin: increased dysrhythmias

Drug classifications

α-Blockers: decreased phenylephrine action
Antidepressants (tricyclic), β-adrenergic blockers, H_1 antihistamines: increased pressor effect
General anesthetics: increased dysrhythmias
MAOIs: do not use within 2 wk, hypertensive crisis may result
Oxytocics: increased B/P

P

NURSING CONSIDERATIONS
Assessment
- Monitor I&O ratio; notify prescriber if output <30 ml/hr
- Monitor ECG during administration continuously; if B/P increases, drug is decreased
- Monitor B/P and pulse q5 min after parenteral route; CVP or PWP during inf if possible
- Assess for paresthesias and coldness of extremities; peripheral blood flow may decrease

Nursing diagnoses
- Tissue perfusion, ineffective (uses)
- Cardiac output, decreased (uses)
- Knowledge, deficient (teaching)

Implementation
IV route
- Give plasma expanders for hypovolemia
- Give **IV** after diluting 1 mg/9 ml of sterile water for inj; give dose over 30-60 sec; may be

diluted 10 mg/500 ml of D_5W or 0.9% NaCl; titrate to patient response; low normal B/P; check for extravasation; check site for infiltration; use infusion pump

- Store reconstituted sol in refrigerator for no longer than 24 hr
- Do not use discolored sol

Y-site compatibilities: Amrinone, famotidine, haloperidol, zidovudine

Additive compatibilities: Chloramphenicol, DOBUTamine, lidocaine, potassium chloride, sodium bicarbonate

Patient/family education

- Inform patient of reason for drug administration and expected result
- Advise patient to report pain at inf site immediately
- Instruct patient to report change in vision, blurring, loss of sight; breathing trouble, sweating, flushing

Evaluation

Positive therapeutic outcome

- Increased B/P with stabilization

phenytoin (Rx)

(fen'i-toyn)

Diphenylhydantoin, Dilantin, Dilantin-125, Dilantin Kapseals, Dilantin Infatab, Diphenylan, DPH, Phenytex

Func. class.: Anticonvulsant/antidysrhythmic (class IB)

Chem. class.: Hydantoin

Pregnancy category C

Action: Inhibits spread of seizure activity in motor cortex by altering ion transport; increases AV conduction to decrease dysrhythmias

Therapeutic Outcome: Decreased seizures, absence of dysrhythmias

Uses: Generalized tonic-clonic seizures, status epilepticus, nonepileptic seizures associated with Reye's syndrome or after head trauma, migraines, trigeminal neuralgia, Bell's palsy, ventricular dysrhythmias uncontrolled by antidysrhythmics

Dosage and routes

Seizures

Adult: PO 1 g or 20 mg/kg (ext rel) in 3-4 divided doses given q2h or 400 mg, then 300 mg q2h × 2 doses, maintenance 300-400 mg/day; max 600 mg/day; **IV** 15-20 mg/kg, max 25-50 mg/min then 100 mg q6-8h

Child: PO 5 mg/kg/day in 2-3 divided doses, maintenance 4-8 mg/kg/day in 2-3 divided doses, max 300 mg/day; **IV** 15-20 mg/kg at 1-3 mg/kg/min

Status epilepticus

Adult: **IV** 15-20 mg/kg, max 25-50 mg/min; may give 100 mg q6-8h thereafter

Child: **IV** 15-20 mg/kg, max in divided doses 1-3 mg/kg/min

Neuritic pain

Adult: PO 200-600 mg/day in divided doses

Ventricular dysrhythmias

Adult: PO loading dose 1 g divided over 24 hr, then 500 mg/day × 2 days; **IV** 250 mg given over 5 min until dysrhythmias subside or 1 g is given, or 100 mg q15 min until dysrhythmias subside or 1 g is given

Child: PO 3-8 mg/kg or 250 mg/m^2/day as single dose or divided in 2 doses; **IV** 3-8 mg/kg given over several min, or 250 mg/m^2/day as single dose or divided in 2 doses

Renal dose

Adult: Do not use loading dose CCr <10 ml/min or hepatic failure

Available forms: Susp 30, 125 mg/5 ml; chew tabs 50 mg; inj 50 mg/ml; ext rel caps 30, 100 mg; prompt rel caps 30, 100 mg

Adverse effects

CNS: Drowsiness, dizziness, insomnia, paresthesias, depression, suicidal tendencies, aggression, headache, confusion, slurred speech

CV: Hypotension, **ventricular fibrillation**

EENT: Nystagmus, diplopia, blurred vision

ENDO: Diabetes insipidus

GI: Nausea, vomiting, constipation, anorexia, weight loss, **hepatitis**, jaundice, gingival hyperplasia

GU: **Nephritis**, urine discoloration

HEMA: **Agranulocytosis, leukopenia, aplastic anemia, thrombocytopenia, megaloblastic anemia**

INTEG: Rash, **lupus erythematosus, Stevens-Johnson syndrome**, hirsutism

SYST: Hypocalcemia

Contraindications: Hypersensitivity, psychiatric condition, bradycardia, SA and AV block, Stokes-Adams syndrome, hepatic failure, acute intermittent porphyria

Precautions: Pregnancy **C**, allergies, hepatic disease, renal disease, elderly, petit mal seizures, hypotension, myocardial insufficiency

Pharmacokinetics

Absorption	Slowly absorbed from GI tract; erratic (IM)
Distribution	Crosses placenta, highly protein bound
Metabolism	Liver, extensively
Excretion	Kidneys, minimally; enters breast milk
Half-life	22 hr, dose dependent

Pharmacodynamics

	PO	PO–EXT REL	IM	IV
Onset	2-24 hr	2-24 hr	Erratic	1-2 hr
Peak	1.5-3 hr	4-12 hr	Erratic	Unknown
Duration	6-12 hr	12-36 hr	12-24 hr	12-24 hr

Interactions

Individual drugs

Alcohol (chronic use), carbamazepine, diazoxide, folic acid, rifampin: decreased effects of phenytoin

Chloramphenicol, cimetidine, cycloSERINE, diazepam, valproate: increased phenytoin effect

Drug classifications

Antacids, barbiturates: decreased effect of phenytoin

Antidepressants (tricyclics), benzodiazepines, salicylates: increased phenytoin level

Drug/herb

Aloe, buckthorn, cascara sagrada, senna: increased hypokalemia, antidysrhythmic action

Ginkgo: increased effect

Ginseng, santonica, valerian: decreased anticonvulsant effect

Drug/lab test

Increased: glucose, alkaline phosphatase, BSP

Decreased: dexamethasone, metyrapone test serum, PBI, urinary steroids

NURSING CONSIDERATIONS

Assessment

- Assess drug level: toxic level 30-50 mcg/ml; therapeutic level 7.5-20 mcg/ml, wait ≥1 wk to determine level
- Assess mental status: mood, sensorium, affect, memory (long, short), especially elderly
- Assess for beginning rash that may lead to Stevens-Johnson syndrome or toxic epidermal necrolysis; phenytoin should not be used again
- Assess for blood dyscrasias: fever, sore throat, bruising, rash, jaundice, epistaxis (long-term treatment only)
- Assess seizure activity including type, location, duration, and character; provide seizure precaution
- Assess renal studies: urinalysis, BUN, urine creatinine
- Monitor blood studies: RBC, Hct, Hgb, reticulocyte counts weekly for 4 wk then monthly; also check thyroid function tests, serum calcium
- Monitor hepatic studies: ALT, AST, bilirubin, creatinine; for renal failure
- Assess for signs of physical withdrawal if medication suddenly discontinued
- Assess eye problems: need for ophth exam before, during, after treatment (slit lamp, funduscopy, tonometry)
- Assess allergic reaction: red raised rash, increased temp, lymphadenopathy; if this occurs, drug should be discontinued, usually occurs 3-12 wk after start of treatment; may also cause hepatotoxicity, rhabdomyolysis
- Monitor for toxicity: bone marrow depression, nausea, vomiting, ataxia, diplopia, CV collapse, slurred speech, confusion

Nursing diagnoses

- Injury, risk for (uses, adverse reactions)
- Knowledge, deficient (teaching)
- Noncompliance (teaching)

Implementation

PO route

- Give with meals to decrease GI upset
- Chew tab can be crushed or chewed; cap can be opened and mixed with foods or fluids; cap and tab are not interchangeable, only ext rel cap are to be used for once a day dosing
- Do not take antacids or antidiarrheals within 2-3 hr of taking phenytoin
- Give by gastric/NG tube: dilute susp before administration, flush tube with 20 ml of H_2O after dose
- Shake oral susp well; use measuring device for correct dose
- Allow 7-10 days between dosage changes

IV route

- Administer by direct **IV** after diluting with special diluent provided (1 ml/50 mg, 2.2 ml/100 mg, 5.2 ml/250 mg); shake; give through Y-tube or 3-way stopcock; inject slowly <50 mg/min
- Give intermittent **IV** after diluting to a conc of 1-10 mg/ml
- Clear **IV** tubing first with 0.9% NaCl sol; use in-line filter; discard sol 4 hr after preparation; inject into large veins to prevent purple glove syndrome

Additive compatibilities: Bleomycin, verapamil

Y-site compatibilities: Esmolol, famotidine, fluconazole, foscarnet, tacrolimus

Y-site incompatibilities: Enalaprilat, potassium chloride, vit B/C

P

Patient/family education

- Teach patient to carry/wear emergency ID stating name, drugs taken, condition, prescriber's name and phone number
- Advise patient to avoid driving and other activities that require alertness until drug response is known; dizziness, drowsiness can occur
- Advise patient to avoid alcohol ingestion and CNS depressants unless approved by prescriber; increased sedation may occur
- Teach patient not to discontinue medication quickly after long-term use; taper off over several wk
- Advise patient that urine may turn pink, red, or brown
- Caution patient to avoid antacids or antidiarrheals within 2-3 hr of taking phenytoin
- Instruct patient in proper oral hygiene to prevent gingival hyperplasia; to visit dentist routinely

Evaluation

Positive therapeutic outcome

- Decreased seizure activity
- Decreased dysrhythmias
- Relief of pain

phytonadione (vit K_1) (Rx)

(fye-toe-na-dye'one)

AquaMEPHYTON, Mephyton

Func. class.: Vitamin K_1, fat-soluble vitamin

Pregnancy category C

Action: Needed for adequate blood clotting (factors II, VII, IX, X)

Therapeutic Outcome: Prevention of bleeding

Uses: Vitamin K malabsorption, hypoprothrombinemia, prevention of hypoprothrombinemia caused by oral anticoagulants, prevention of hemorrhagic disease of the newborn

Dosage and routes

Hypoprothrombinemia caused by vitamin K malabsorption

Adult: PO/IM 2.5-25 mg; may repeat or increase to 50 mg

Child: PO/IM 5-10 mg

Infants: PO/IM 2 mg

Prevention of hemorrhagic disease of the newborn

Neonate: IM 0.5-1 mg within 1 hr after birth; repeat in 2-3 wk if required

Hypoprothrombinemia caused by oral anticoagulants

Adult and child: PO/SUBCUT/IM 1-10 mg, may repeat 12-48 hr after PO dose or 6-8 hr after SUBCUT/IM dose, based on protime

Available forms: Tabs 5 mg; inj 2 mg/ml; aqueous colloidal (IM, **IV**); inj aqueous dispersion 10 mg/ml (IM)

Adverse effects

CNS: Headache, **brain damage** (large doses)

GI: Nausea, decreased liver function tests

HEMA: **Hemolytic anemia, hemoglobinuria, hyperbilirubinemia**

INTEG: Rash, urticaria

Contraindications: Hypersensitivity, severe hepatic disease, last few wk of pregnancy

Precautions: Pregnancy **C,** neonates

Pharmacokinetics

Absorption	Well absorbed (PO, IM, SUBCUT)
Distribution	Crosses placenta
Metabolism	Liver, rapidly
Excretion	Breast milk
Half-life	Unknown

Pharmacodynamics

	PO	SUBCUT/IM
Onset	6-12 hr	1-2 hr
Peak	Unknown	6 hr
Duration	Unknown	14 hr

Interactions

Individual drugs

Cholestyramine, mineral oil: decreased action of phytonadione

Drug classifications

Oral anticoagulants: decreased anticoagulant effect

Drug/food

Olestra: decreased vit K levels

NURSING CONSIDERATIONS

Assessment

- Monitor protime during treatment (2-sec deviation from control time, bleeding time, and clotting time); monitor for bleeding, pulse, and B/P
- Assess nutritional status: liver (beef), spinach, tomatoes, coffee, asparagus, broccoli, cabbage, lettuce, greens
- Assess for bleeding or bruising: hematuria, black tarry stools, hematemesis

Nursing diagnoses

- Nutrition: less than body requirements, imbalanced (uses)
- Tissue perfusion, ineffective (uses)
- Knowledge, deficient (teaching)

Implementation

IV route

- Give **IV** after diluting with D_5 NS 10 ml or more; give 1 mg/min or more
- Give **IV** only when other routes not possible (deaths have occurred)
- Store in airtight, light-resistant container

Syringe compatibilities: Doxapram

Y-site compatibilities: Ampicillin, epINEPHrine, famotidine, heparin, hydrocortisone, potassium chloride, tolazoline, vit B/C

Additive compatibilities: Amikacin, calcium gluceptate, cephapirin, chloramphenicol, cimetidine, netilmicin, sodium bicarbonate

Patient/family education

- Teach patient not to take other supplements, unless directed by prescriber; to take this medication as directed
- Teach patient necessary foods high in vit K to be included in diet
- Advise patient to avoid IM inj, hard toothbrush, flossing; use electric razor until treatment is terminated
- Instruct patient to report symptoms of bleeding: bruising, nosebleeds, blood in urine, heavy menstruation, black tarry stools
- Caution patient not to use OTC medications unless approved by prescriber
- Stress the need for periodic lab tests to monitor coagulation levels
- Stress the need for patient to carry/wear emergency ID with condition, treatment, and medications taken

Evaluation

Positive therapeutic outcome

- Decreased bleeding tendencies
- Decreased protime
- Decreased clotting time

pindolol (Rx)

(pin′doe-lole)

Novo-Pindol ♣, Syn-Pindol ♣, Visken

Func. class.: Antihypertensive

Chem. class.: Nonselective β-blocker

Pregnancy category B

Do Not Confuse:
pindolol/Parlodel, pindolol/Plendil

Action: Competitively blocks stimulation of β-adrenergic receptor within vascular smooth muscle; produces chronotropic, inotropic activity (decreases rate of SA node discharge, increases recovery time), slows conduction of AV node, decreases heart rate, which decreases O_2 consumption in myocardium; also decreases renin-aldosterone-angiotensin system and at high doses inhibits β_2 receptors in bronchial system

Therapeutic Outcome: Decreased B/P in hypertension, heart rate

Uses: Mild to moderate hypertension

Dosage and routes

Adult: PO 5 mg bid; usual dose 15 mg/day (5 mg tid); may increase by 10 mg/day q3-4 wk to a max of 60 mg/day

Elderly: PO 5 mg daily increase by 5 mg q3-4 wk

Available forms: Tabs 5, 10 mg

Adverse effects

CNS: *Insomnia, dizziness,* hallucinations, anxiety, fatigue, headache, depression

CV: Hypotension, bradycardia, **CHF**, edema, chest pain, palpitations, claudication, tachycardia, **AV block, pulmonary edema, bradycardia, dysrhythmias**

EENT: *Visual changes,* sore throat, *double vision,* dry burning eyes, nasal stuffiness

GI: *Nausea,* vomiting, **ischemic colitis,** diarrhea, *abdominal pain,* **mesenteric arterial thrombosis,** flatulence, constipation

GU: Impotence, frequency

HEMA: **Agranulocytosis, thrombocytopenia, purpura**

INTEG: Rash, alopecia, pruritus, fever

MISC: *Joint pain, muscle pain*

RESP: **Bronchospasm,** *dyspnea,* cough, crackles

Contraindications: Hypersensitivity to β-blockers, cardiogenic shock, 2nd- or 3rd-degree heart block, sinus bradycardia, CHF, cardiac failure, bronchial asthma, severe COPD

Precautions: Pregnancy **B,** major surgery, lactation, diabetes mellitus, renal disease, thyroid disease, COPD, well-compensated heart failure, CAD, nonallergic bronchospasm, peripheral vascular disease, hepatic disease

Pharmacokinetics	
Absorption	Well absorbed
Distribution	Crosses placenta; some penetration in CNS, protein binding 40%
Metabolism	Liver, moderately (60%-65%)
Excretion	Kidneys, unchanged (30%-45%)
Half-life	3-4 hr

Pharmacodynamics	
Onset	Unknown
Peak	2-4 hr
Duration	8-24 hr

P

Interactions

Individual drugs

Hydralazine, methyldopa, prazosin, reserpine: increased hypotension, bradycardia
Insulin: may alter hypoglycemic effect
Thyroid: decreased effect of β-blockers

Drug classifications

Anticholinergics: increased hypotension, bradycardia
β_2-Adrenergic agonists: increased effect of β-blockers
Calcium channel blockers: increased effects of calcium channel blockers
NSAIDs, sympathomimetics: decreased antihypertensive effect
Oral hypoglycemics: may alter hypoglycemic effect
Theophyllines, β_2-agonists: decreased bronchodilatation

Drug/herb

Aconite: increased toxicity, death
Astragalus, cola tree: increased or decreased antihypertensive effect
Barberry, betony, black catechu, black cohosh, bloodroot, broom, burdock, cat's claw, dandelion, goldenseal, Irish moss, Jamaican dogwood, kelp, khella, mistletoe, parsley: increased antihypertensive effect
Coltsfoot, guarana, khat, licorice: decreased antihypertensive effect

Drug/lab test

Increased: liver function tests, renal function tests
Interference: glucose, insulin tolerance test

NURSING CONSIDERATIONS

Assessment

- Monitor B/P during beginning treatment, periodically thereafter; pulse q4h; note rate, rhythm, quality: apical/radial pulse before administration; notify prescriber of any significant changes (pulse <50 bpm)
- Obtain baselines in renal, liver function tests before therapy begins
- Assess for edema in feet, legs daily; monitor I&O, daily weight; check for jugular vein distention, crackles bilaterally, dyspnea (CHF)
- Monitor skin turgor, dryness of mucous membranes for hydration status, especially elderly

Nursing diagnoses

- Cardiac output, decreased (uses)
- Injury, risk for (adverse reactions)
- Knowledge, deficient (teaching)
- Noncompliance (teaching)

Implementation

- Given ac, at bedtime; tab may be crushed or swallowed whole; give with food to prevent GI upset
- Store protected from light, moisture; place in cool environment

Patient/family education

- ❗ Teach patient not to discontinue drug abruptly; taper over 2 wk; may cause precipitate angina if stopped abruptly
- Teach patient not to use OTC products containing α-adrenergic stimulants (such as nasal decongestants, cold preparations); to avoid alcohol, smoking, and to limit sodium intake as prescribed
- Teach patient how to take pulse and B/P at home; advise when to notify prescriber
- Instruct patient to comply with weight control, dietary adjustments, modified exercise program
- Tell patient to carry/wear emergency ID to identify drug being taken, allergies; tell patient drug controls symptoms but does not cure
- Caution patient to avoid hazardous activities if dizziness, drowsiness present
- Teach patient to report symptoms of CHF: difficult breathing, especially on exertion or when lying down, night cough, swelling of extremities or bradycardia, dizziness, confusion, depression, fever
- Teach patient to take drug as prescribed, not to double doses, skip doses; take any missed doses as soon as remembered if at least 4 hr until next dose; to take with or immediately after meals if GI symptoms occur

Evaluation

Positive therapeutic outcome

- Decreased B/P in hypertension (after 1-2 wk)

Treatment of overdose: Lavage, **IV** atropine for bradycardia, **IV** theophylline for bronchospasm, digitalis, O_2, diuretic for cardiac failure, hemodialysis, **IV** glucose for hyperglycemia, **IV** diazepam (or phenytoin) for seizures

pioglitazone (Rx)

(pie-oh-glye'ta-zone)

Actos

Func. class.: Antidiabetic, oral
Chem. class.: Thiazolidinedione

Pregnancy category C

Action: Specifically targets insulin resistance, an insulin sensitizer; regulates the transcription of a number of insulin responsive genes

Therapeutic Outcome: Decreased symptoms of diabetes mellitus

Uses: Type 2 diabetes mellitus

Dosage and routes

Monotherapy

Adult: PO 15-30 mg daily, may increase to 45 mg/day

Combination therapy

Adult: PO 15-30 mg daily with a sulfonylurea, metformin, or insulin; decrease sulfonylurea dose if hypoglycemia occurs; decrease insulin dose by 10%-25% if hypoglycemia occurs or if plasma glucose is <100 mg/dl, max 45 mg/day

Hepatic dose

Do not use in active liver disease or if ALT >2.5 × ULN

Available forms: Tabs 15, 30, 45 mg

Adverse effects

CNS: *Headache*
ENDO: *Aggravated diabetes mellitus*
MISC: *Myalgia, sinusitis, upper respiratory tract infection, pharyngitis*
MS: Fractures (females)

Contraindications: Hypersensitivity to thiazolidinediones, diabetic ketoacidosis, lactation, children

Precautions: Pregnancy **C**, elderly, thyroid disease, hepatic, renal disease, edema, CHF

Pharmacokinetics	
Absorption	Unknown
Distribution	Unknown
Metabolism	Unknown
Excretion	Kidneys
Half-life	3-7 hr, terminal 16-24 hr

Pharmacodynamics	
Onset	Unknown
Peak	6-12 wk
Duration	Unknown

Interactions

Individual drugs

Ketoconazole: decreased pioglitazone effect

Drug classifications

Oral contraceptives: decreased effect, use an alternative contraceptive method

Drug/herb

Alfalfa, aloe, basil, bay, bilberry, bitter melon, black catechu, buchu, burdock, coriander, dandelion, eyebright (po), fenugreek, garlic, ginseng, glucomannan, glucosamine, goat's rue, gymnema, horehound, horse chestnut, jambul, myrrh, myrtle: increased antidiabetic effect

Bee pollen, blue cohosh, broom, chromium, elecampane, eucalyptus, gotu kola: decreased antidiabetic effect

Chromium, coenzyme Q10, fenugreek: increased hypoglycemia

Glucosamine: decreased blood glucose control

NURSING CONSIDERATIONS

Assessment

- Assess for hypoglycemic reactions (sweating, weakness, dizziness, anxiety, tremors, hunger), hyperglycemic reactions soon after meals
- Check liver function tests periodically; AST, LDH, FBS, glycosylated Hgb, fasting plasma insulin, plasma lipids, lipoproteins, B/P, body weight during treatment

Nursing diagnoses

- Nutrition: more than body requirements, imbalanced (uses)
- Knowledge, deficient (teaching)

Implementation

- Convert from other oral hypoglycemic agents; change may be made with gradual dosage change; monitor serum glucose during conversion
- Give once a day; give with meals to decrease GI upset and provide best absorption
- Give tabs crushed and mixed with meal or fluids for patients with difficulty swallowing
- Store in airtight container in cool environment

Patient/family education

- Teach patient to self-monitor using a blood glucose meter
- Teach patient symptoms of hypo/hyperglycemia, what to do about each
- Advise patient that drug must be continued on daily basis; explain consequence of discontinuing drug abruptly
- Advise patient to avoid OTC medications or herbal preparations unless approved by prescriber
- Advise patient that diabetes is life-long illness; that this drug is not a cure, only controls symptoms
- Advise patient that all food included in diet plan must be eaten to prevent hypoglycemia
- Advise patient to carry/wear emergency ID and glucagon emergency kit for emergencies
- Instruct patient to notify prescriber if oral contraceptives are used
- Teach patient not to use if breastfeeding

P

Evaluation

Positive therapeutic outcome

- Decrease in polyuria, polydipsia, polyphagia; clear sensorium; absence of dizziness; stable gait; blood glucose at normal level

piperacillin (Rx)

(pi-per'a-sill-in)

Pipracil

Func. class.: Broad-spectrum antiinfective

Chem. class.: Extended-spectrum penicillin

Pregnancy category B

Action: Interferes with cell wall replication of susceptible organisms; osmotically unstable cell wall swells and bursts from osmotic pressure

Therapeutic Outcome: Bactericidal effects for gram-positive cocci *Staphylococcus aureus, Streptococcus pyogenes, Streptococcus viridans, Streptococcus faecalis, Streptococcus bovis, Streptococcus pneumoniae;* gram-negative cocci *Neisseria gonorrhoeae, Neisseria meningitidis;* gram-positive bacilli *Clostridium perfringens, Clostridium tetani;* gram-negative bacilli *Bacteroides, Fusobacterium nucleatum, Escherichia coli, Klebsiella, Proteus mirabilis, Proteus vulgaris, Proteus rettgeri, Morganella morganii, Enterobacter, Citrobacter, Pseudomonas aeruginosa, Serratia, Acinetobacter, Peptococcus, Peptostreptococcus, Eubacterium*

Uses: Respiratory tract, skin, skin structure, urinary tract, bone, and joint infections; gonorrhea, pneumonia, endocarditis, septicemia, meningitis, sinusitis; infections caused by penicillinase-producing staphylococci, streptococci; may be combined with an aminoglycoside for *Pseudomonas* infection

Dosage and routes

Urinary tract infections

Adult: **IV** 8-16 g/day (125-200 mg/kg/day) in divided doses q6-8h

Serious systemic infections

Adult and child >12 yr: IM/**IV** 2-4 g q4-6h (2 g/site IM)

Child <12 yr: IM/**IV** 200-300 mg/kg/day in divided doses q4-6h

Neonates <36 wk: **IV** 75 mg/kg q12h in the 1st wk of life, then q8h in 2nd wk

Full term infants: **IV** 75 mg/kg q8h in 1st wk of life, then q6h thereafter

Prophylaxis of surgical infections

Adult: **IV** 2 g 30-60 min before procedure; may be repeated during or after surgery

Renal dose

Adult: **IV** CCr 20-40 ml/min give q8h, CCr <20 ml/min give q12h

Available forms: Powder for inj 2, 3, 4, 40 g

Adverse effects

CNS: Lethargy, hallucinations, anxiety, depression, twitching, **coma, seizures**

GI: *Nausea, vomiting, diarrhea,* increased AST, ALT, abdominal pain, glossitis, colitis, **pseudomembranous colitis**

GU: **Oliguria, proteinuria, hematuria, vaginitis, moniliasis, glomerulonephritis**

HEMA: Anemia, increased bleeding time, **bone marrow depression, thrombocytopenia**

META: Hypokalemia, hypernatremia

SYST: **Serum sickness, anaphylaxis**

Contraindications: Hypersensitivity to penicillins; neonates

Precautions: Pregnancy **B,** hypersensitivity to cephalosporins, CHF, renal disease, seizures, lactation

Pharmacokinetics

Absorption	Well absorbed (80%)
Distribution	Widely distributed; crosses placenta
Metabolism	Not metabolized
Excretion	Kidneys, unchanged (90%); bile (10%); breast milk
Half-life	0.7-1.3 hr

Pharmacodynamics

	IM	IV
Onset	Rapid	Rapid
Peak	30-50 min	Inf end

Interactions

Individual drugs

Aspirin, probenecid: increased piperacillin levels

Drug classifications

Aminoglycosides: decreased antimicrobial effect of piperacillin

Contraceptives (oral): decreased contraceptive effectiveness

Tetracyclines: decreased antimicrobial effectiveness (with high concentrations of piperacillin)

Drug/lab test

False positive: urine glucose, urine protein, Coombs' test

NURSING CONSIDERATIONS

Assessment

- Assess patient for previous sensitivity reaction to penicillins or other cephalosporins; cross-sensitivity between penicillins and cephalosporins is common
- Assess patient for signs and symptoms of infection including characteristics of wounds, sputum, urine, stool, WBC >10,000/mm^3, fever; obtain baseline information and during treatment
- Obtain C&S before beginning drug therapy to identify if correct treatment has been initiated
- Assess for allergic reactions: rash, urticaria, pruritus, chills, fever, joint pain; angioedema may occur a few days after therapy begins; epINEPHrine, resuscitation equipment should be available for anaphylactic reaction
- Identify urine output; if decreasing, notify prescriber (may indicate nephrotoxicity); also check for increased BUN, creatinine
- Monitor blood studies: AST, ALT, CBC, Hct, bilirubin, LDH, alkaline phosphatase, Coombs' test monthly if patient is on long-term therapy
- Monitor electrolytes: potassium, sodium, chloride monthly if patient is on long-term therapy
- Assess bowel pattern daily; if severe diarrhea occurs, drug should be discontinued; may indicate pseudomembranous colitis
- Monitor for bleeding: ecchymosis, bleeding gums, hematuria, stool guaiac daily if on long-term therapy
- Assess for overgrowth of infection: perineal itching, fever, malaise, redness, pain, swelling, drainage, rash, diarrhea, change in cough, sputum

Nursing diagnoses

- Infection, risk for (uses)
- Diarrhea (adverse reactions)
- Injury, risk for (adverse reactions)
- Knowledge, deficient (teaching)
- Noncompliance (teaching)

Implementation

IM route

- Reconstitute 2 g/4 ml, 3 g/6 ml, 4 g/7.8 ml with sterile water, 0.9% NaCl, bacteriostatic water, 0.5% or 1% lidocaine without epINEPHrine
- Inject deep in large muscle mass, massage; split inj >2 g into 2 inj

IV route

- Reconstitute with 5 ml or more 0.9% NaCl, bacteriostatic water; shake sol to dissolve
- Change **IV** sites q48h to prevent phlebitis and pain
- Give direct **IV** over 3-5 min
- Give by intermittent inf by diluting in 50 ml or more D_5W, 0.9% NaCl, D_5/0.9% NaCl, LR, give over 20-30 min by Y-site; discontinue primary inf during intermittent inf

Syringe compatibilities: Heparin

Y-site compatibilities: Acyclovir, aldesleukin, allopurinol, amifostine, aztreonam, ciprofloxacin, cyclophosphamide, diltiazem, enalaprilat, esmolol, famotidine, fludarabine, foscarnet, heparin, hydromorphone, IL-2, labetalol, lorazepam, magnesium sulfate, melphalan, meperidine, midazolam, morphine, perphenazine, propofol, ranitidine, tacrolimus, teniposide, theophylline, thiotepa, verapamil, zidovudine

Y-site incompatibilities: Ondansetron, fluconazole, sargramostim, vinorelbine

Additive compatibilities: Ciprofloxacin, clindamycin, fluconazole, hydrocortisone sodium succinate, ofloxacin, potassium chloride, verapamil

Additive incompatibilities: Aminoglycosides

Patient/family education

- Teach patient to report sore throat, bruising, bleeding, joint pain; may indicate blood dyscrasias (rare)
- Advise patient to contact prescriber if vaginal itching, loose foul-smelling stools, furry tongue occur; may indicate superinfection
- Advise patient to notify prescriber of diarrhea with blood or pus, which may indicate pseudomembranous colitis

Evaluation

Positive therapeutic outcome

- Absence of signs/symptoms of infection (WBC <10,000/mm^3, temp WNL, absence of red, draining wounds)
- Reported improvement in symptoms of infection

Treatment of anaphylaxis: Withdraw drug, maintain airway, administer epINEPHrine, aminophylline, O_2, **IV** corticosteroids

piperacillin/tazobactam (Rx)

Zosyn

Func. class.: Broad-spectrum antiinfective
Chem. class.: Extended-spectrum penicillin

Pregnancy category B

Action: Interferes with cell wall replication of susceptible organisms; osmotically unstable

P

cell wall swells and bursts from osmotic pressure

Therapeutic Outcome: Bactericidal effects for piperacillin-resistant β-lactamase, *Escherichia coli, Staphylococcus aureus, Bacteroides fragilis, Haemophilus influenzae*

Uses: Respiratory tract, skin, skin structure, urinary tract, bone, and joint infections; gonorrhea, pneumonia, infections from penicillinase-producing staphylococci, streptococci

Dosage and routes

Nosocomial pneumonia

Adult: **IV** 3.375 g q6-8h with an aminoglycoside × 1-2 wk; continue aminoglycoside only if *Pseudomonas aeruginosa* is isolated

Other infections

Adult: **IV** inf 6-12 g/day, given 2.25 g q8h to 3.375 g q6h over 30 min × 7-10 days

Renal dose

Adult: **IV** CCr 20-40 ml/min 2.25 g q6h; CCr <20 ml/min 2.25 g q8h

Available forms: Powder for inj 2 g piperacillin/0.25 g tazobactam; 3 g piperacillin/0.375 g tazobactam, 4 g piperacillin/0.5 g tazobactam, 36 g piperacillin/4.5 g tazobactam

Adverse effects

CNS: Headache, insomnia, dizziness, fever, lethargy, hallucinations, anxiety, depression, twitching

GI: *Nausea, vomiting, diarrhea,* increased AST, ALT, abdominal pain, glossitis, constipation, **pseudomembranous colitis**

GU: **Oliguria, proteinuria, hematuria,** *vaginitis, moniliasis,* **glomerulonephritis**

HEMA: Anemia, increased bleeding time, **bone marrow depression**

INTEG: Rash, pruritus

META: Hypokalemia, hypernatremia

SYST: **Serum sickness, anaphylaxis**

Contraindications: Hypersensitivity to penicillins; neonates

Precautions: Pregnancy **B,** CHF, lactation, seizures, hypersensitivity to cephalosporins, renal insufficiency in children

Pharmacokinetics	
Absorption	Well absorbed (80%)
Distribution	Widely distributed; crosses placenta
Metabolism	Not metabolized
Excretion	Kidneys, unchanged (90%); bile (10%); breast milk
Half-life	0.7-1.3 hr

Pharmacodynamics	
Onset	Rapid
Peak	Inf end

Interactions

Individual drugs

Aspirin, probenecid: increased piperacillin levels

Drug classifications

Aminoglycosides(**IV**): decreased piperacillin effect

Anticoagulants (oral): increased anticoagulant effects

Contraceptives (oral): decreased contraceptive effectiveness

Neuromuscular blockers: increased effects

Tetracyclines: decreased antimicrobial effectiveness

Drug/lab test

Increased: platelet count, eosinophilia, neutropenia, leucopenia, serum creatinine, PTT, AST, ALT, alkaline phosphatase, bilirubin, BUN, electrolytes

Decreased: Hct, Hgb, electrolytes

False positive: urine glucose, urine protein, Coombs' test

NURSING CONSIDERATIONS

Assessment

- Assess patient for previous sensitivity reaction to penicillins or other cephalosporins, cross-sensitivity between penicillins and cephalosporins is common
- Assess patient for signs and symptoms of infection including characteristics of wounds, sptum, urine, stool, WBC >10,000/mm^3, fever; obtain baseline information and during treatment
- Obtain C&S before beginning drug therapy to identify if correct treatment has been initiated
- Assess for allergic reactions: rash, urticaria, pruritus, chills, fever, joint pain; angioedema may occur a few days after therapy begins; epINEPHrine, resuscitation equipment should be available for anaphylactic reaction
- (Alert) Identify urine output; if decreasing, notify prescriber (may indicate nephrotoxicity); also check for increased BUN, creatinine
- Monitor blood studies: AST, ALT, CBC, Hct, bilirubin, LDH, alkaline phosphatase, Coombs' test monthly if patient is on long-term therapy
- Monitor electrolytes: potassium, sodium, chloride monthly if patient is on long-term therapy

- Assess bowel pattern daily; if severe diarrhea occurs, drug should be discontinued; may indicate pseudomembranous colitis
- Monitor for bleeding: ecchymosis, bleeding gums, hematuria, stool guaiac daily if on long-term therapy
- Assess for overgrowth of infection: perineal itching, fever, malaise, redness, pain, swelling, drainage, rash, diarrhea, change in cough, sputum

Nursing diagnoses
- Infection, risk for (uses)
- Diarrhea (adverse reactions)
- Injury, risk for (adverse reactions)
- Knowledge, deficient (teaching)
- Noncompliance (teaching)

Implementation
- Reconstitute with 5 ml or more 0.9% NaCl, bacteriostatic water; shake sol to dissolve
- Give by intermittent inf by diluting in 50 ml or more D_5W, 0.9% NaCl, D_5/0.9% NaCl, LR; give over 20-30 min by Y-site; discontinue primary inf during intermittent inf
- Change **IV** sites q48h to prevent phlebitis and pain
- Give direct **IV** over 3-5 min

Y-site compatibilities: Aminophylline, aztreonam, bleomycin, bumetanide, buprenorphine, butorphanol, calcium gluconate, carboplatin, carmustine, cefepime, cimetidine, clindamycin, cyclophosphamide, cytarabine, dexamethasone, diphenhydrAMINE, DOPamine, enalaprilat, etoposide, floxuridine, fluconazole, fludarabine, fluorouracil, furosemide, gallium, granisetron, heparin, hydrocortisone, hydromorphone, ifosfamide, leucovorin, lorazepam, magnesium sulfate, mannitol, meperidine, mesna, methotrexate, methylPREDNISolone, metoclopramide, metronidazole, morphine, ondansetron, plicomycin, potassium chloride, ranitidine, sargramostim, sodium bicarbonate, thiotepa, trimethoprim/sulfamethoxazole, vinBLAStine, vinCRIStine, zidovudine

Y-site incompatibilities: Fluconazole, ondansetron, sargramostim, vinorelbine

Patient/family education
- Teach patient to report sore throat, bruising, bleeding, joint pain; may indicate blood dyscrasias (rare)
- Advise patient to contact prescriber if vaginal itching, loose foul-smelling stools, furry tongue occur; may indicate superinfection
- Advise patient to notify prescriber of diarrhea with blood or pus, which may indicate pseudomembranous colitis

Evaluation
Positive therapeutic outcome
- Absence of signs/symptoms of infection (WBC <10,000/mm^3, temp WNL, absence of red, draining wounds)
- Reported improvement in symptoms of infection

Treatment of anaphylaxis: Withdraw drug, maintain airway, administer epINEPHrine, aminophylline, O_2, **IV** corticosteroids

pirbuterol (Rx)
(peer-byoo'ter-ole)
Maxair
Func. class.: Bronchodilator
Chem. class.: β-Adrenergic agonist
Pregnancy category C

Action: Relaxes bronchial smooth muscle by direct action on β_2-adrenergic receptors, with increased levels of cAMP and increased bronchodilatation, diuresis, and cardiac and CNS stimulation

Therapeutic Outcome: Bronchodilatation with ease of breathing

Uses: Reversible bronchospasm (prevention, treatment), including asthma, may be given with theophylline or steroids

Dosage and routes
Adult and child >12 yr: INH 1-2 (0.4 mg) q4-6h; max 12 inh/day

Available forms: Aerosol delivers 0.2 mg pirbuterol/actuation

Adverse effects
CNS: Tremors, anxiety, insomnia, headache, dizziness, stimulation, restlessness, hallucinations, drowsiness, irritability
CV: Palpitations, tachycardia, hypertension, angina, hypotension, **dysrhythmias**
EENT: Dry nose and mouth, irritation of nose, throat
GI: Gastritis, nausea, vomiting, anorexia
MS: Muscle cramps
RESP: **Paradoxical bronchospasm,** dyspnea, coughing

Contraindications: Hypersensitivity to sympathomimetics, tachycardia

Precautions: Pregnancy **C,** lactation, cardiac disorders, hyperthyroidism, diabetes mellitus, prostatic hypertrophy

P

Pharmacokinetics

Absorption	Minimally absorbed
Distribution	Unknown
Metabolism	Liver
Excretion	Unknown
Half-life	2 hr

Pharmacodynamics

Onset	5-15 min
Peak	1-1½ hr
Duration	5 hr

Interactions
Individual drugs
Levothyroxine: increased pirbuterol action
Drug classifications
Antidepressants (tricyclics), antihistamines: increased pirbuterol action
β-Adrenergic blockers: block therapeutic effect
Bronchodilators, aerosol: increased action of bronchodilator
MAOIs: increased chance of hypertensive crisis
Drug/herb
Cola nut, guarana, yerba maté: increased action of both
Green tea (large amounts), guarana: increased effect

NURSING CONSIDERATIONS
Assessment
- Monitor respiratory function: vital capacity, FEV, ABGs, lung sounds, heart rate, rhythm (baseline)
- Monitor for evidence of allergic reactions, paradoxic bronchospasm (can occur rapidly); withhold dose and notify prescriber

Nursing diagnoses
- Airway clearance, ineffective (uses)
- Gas exchange, impaired (uses)
- Knowledge, deficient (teaching)

Implementation
- Give after shaking; have patient exhale, place mouthpiece in mouth, inhale slowly, hold breath, remove, exhale slowly; allow at least 1 min between inhalations
- Give this medication before other medications and allow at least 1 min between each to prevent overstimulation
- Store in light-resistant container; do not expose to temp over 86° F (30° C)

Patient/family education
- Advise patient not to use OTC medications; extra stimulation may occur; to use this medication before other medications and allow at least 1 min between each to prevent overstimulation
- Teach patient use of inhaler; to avoid getting aerosol in eyes; blurring may result; to wash inhaler in warm water and dry daily; to avoid smoking, smoke-filled rooms, persons with respiratory tract infections; review package insert with patient
- Teach patient that paradoxic bronchospasm may occur and to stop drug immediately and notify prescriber; to limit caffeine products such as chocolate, coffee, tea, and colas
- Instruct patient on administration of dose; not to use more than prescribed; serious side effects may occur

Evaluation
Positive therapeutic outcome
- Absence of dyspnea, wheezing after 1 hr
- Improved airway exchange
- Improved ABGs

Treatment of overdose: Administer a β_2-adrenergic blocker

piroxicam (Rx)
(peer-ox'i-kam)
Apo-Piroxicam ✤, Feldene, Novopirocam ✤, Nu-Pirox, PMS-Piroxicam ✤
Func. class.: Nonsteroidal antiinflammatory
Chem. class.: Oxicam derivative

Pregnancy category B

Action: Inhibits prostaglandin synthesis by decreasing an enzyme needed for biosynthesis; analgesic, antiinflammatory

Therapeutic Outcome: Decreased pain, inflammation

Uses: Mild to moderate pain, osteoarthritis, rheumatoid arthritis

Dosage and routes
Adult: PO 20 mg daily or 10 mg bid

Available forms: Caps 10, 20 mg

Adverse effects
CNS: Dizziness, *drowsiness,* fatigue, tremors, confusion, insomnia, anxiety, depression, *headache*
CV: Tachycardia, peripheral edema, palpitations, **dysrhythmias,** hypertension, **heart failure**
EENT: Tinnitus, hearing loss, blurred vision
GI: *Nausea, anorexia, vomiting, diarrhea,* jaundice, **cholestatic hepatitis,** constipation, flatulence, cramps, dry mouth, peptic ulcer, **bleeding, ulceration, perforation**

GU: **Nephrotoxicity: dysuria, hematuria, oliguria, azotemia**
HEMA: **Blood dyscrasias**
INTEG: Purpura, rash, pruritus, sweating, photosensitivity
SYST: **Anaphylaxis**

Contraindications: Hypersensitivity, asthma, severe renal disease, severe hepatic disease, ulcer disease, cardiac disease

Precautions: Pregnancy **B,** lactation, children, bleeding disorders, GI disorders, cardiac disorders, hypersensitivity to other antiinflammatory agents, CHF, avoid in late pregnancy

Pharmacokinetics

Absorption	Well absorbed
Distribution	Unknown
Metabolism	Liver, extensively
Excretion	Kidneys, minimal; breast milk
Half-life	30-80 hr

Pharmacodynamics

Onset	1 hr
Peak	Unknown
Duration	48-72 hr

Interactions
Individual drugs
Alcohol, aspirin, cycloSPORINE, lithium, methotrexate: increased toxicity
Drug classifications
Anticoagulants (oral), corticosteroids: increased toxicity
Antidiabetics (oral): hypoglycemia
Antihypertensives: decreased effect of antihypertensives
Diuretics: decreased effectiveness of diuretics
Drug/herb
Arginine, gossypol: increased gastric irritation
Bearberry, bilberry: increased NSAIDs effect
Bogbean, chondroitin: increased bleeding risk

NURSING CONSIDERATIONS
Assessment
- Monitor blood counts during therapy; watch for decreasing platelets; if low, therapy may need to be discontinued, restarted after hematologic recovery; check for blood dyscrasia (thrombocytopenia): bruising, fatigue, bleeding, poor healing
- Assess for pain: location, duration, ROM, before and 1-2 hr after administration
- Assess for aspirin sensitivity, asthma, nasal polyps; these may develop into allergic reactions

Nursing diagnoses
- Pain, chronic (uses)
- Mobility, physical, impaired (uses)
- Knowledge, deficient (teaching)
- Injury, risk for (adverse reactions)

Implementation
- Swallow caps whole; do not break, crush, or chew
- Give with food or milk to decrease gastric symptoms, water to enhance absorption

Patient/family education
- Teach patient that drug must be continued for prescribed time to be effective; to avoid aspirin, alcoholic beverages, and other OTC medications unless approved by prescriber
- Caution patient to report bleeding, bruising, fatigue, malaise, since blood dyscrasias do occur
- Instruct patient to use caution when driving; drowsiness, dizziness may occur
- Teach patient to take with a full glass of water to enhance absorption

Evaluation
Positive therapeutic outcome
- Decreased pain
- Decreased inflammation
- Increased mobility

plasma protein fraction (Rx)
Plasmanate, Plasma Plex, Plasmatein, Protenate
Func. class.: Blood derivative
Chem. class.: Human plasma in sodium chloride

Pregnancy category C

Action: Exerts similar oncotic pressure as human plasma, expands blood volume, shifts water from extravascular space to intravascular space

Therapeutic Outcome: Shift of fluid from extravascular into intravascular space

Uses: Hypovolemic shock, hypoproteinemia, ARDS, preoperative cardiopulmonary bypass, acute liver failure, nephrotic syndrome

Dosage and routes
Hypovolemia
Adult: **IV** inf 250-500 ml (12.5-25 g of protein), max 10 ml/min
Child: **IV** inf 22-33 ml/kg at 5-10 ml/min
Hypoproteinemia
Adult: **IV** inf 1000-1500 ml daily, max 8 ml/min

Available forms: Inj 5%

P

Adverse effects

CNS: Fever, chills, headache, paresthesias, flushing
CV: **Fluid overload,** hypotension, erratic pulse
GI: Nausea, vomiting, increased salivation
INTEG: Rash, urticaria, cyanosis
RESP: Altered respirations, dyspnea, **pulmonary edema**

Contraindications: Hypersensitivity, CHF, severe anemia, renal insufficiency

Precautions: Pregnancy **C,** decreased salt intake, decreased cardiac reserve, lack of albumin deficiency, hepatic disease

Pharmacokinetics

Absorption	Completely absorbed
Distribution	Intravascular space
Metabolism	Unknown
Excretion	Unknown
Half-life	Unknown

Pharmacodynamics

Onset	15-30 min
Peak	Unknown
Duration	Unknown

Interactions: None known

Drug/lab test

False increase: alkaline phosphatase

NURSING CONSIDERATIONS

Assessment

- Monitor blood studies: Hct, Hgb; electrolytes, serum protein, if serum protein declines, dyspnea, hypoxemia can result
- Monitor B/P (decreased), pulse (erratic), respiration during inf; CVP, jugular vein distention, PWP (increases if overload occurs); shortness of breath, anxiety, insomnia, expiratory crackles, frothy blood-tinged cough, cyanosis indicate pulmonary overload
- Monitor I&O ratio; urinary output may decrease
- Assess for allergy: fever, rash, itching, chills, flushing, urticaria, nausea, vomiting, or hypotension requires discontinuation of inf; use new lot if therapy reinstituted, premedicate with diphenhydrAMINE

Nursing diagnoses

- Fluid volume, deficient (uses)
- Cardiac output, decreased (uses)
- Fluid volume, excess (adverse reactions)

Implementation

- Give by **IV**; no dilution required; use infusion pump, large-gauge needle (≥20G); discard unused portion; infuse slowly within 4 hr of opening
- Provide adequate hydration before administration
- When storing, check type of albumin, date; may have to refrigerate

Additive compatibilities:

Carbohydrate and electrolyte sol, whole blood, packed RBCs, chloramphenicol, tetracycline

Additive incompatibilities:

Protein hydrolysate sol, amino acids sol, alcohol, norepinephrine

Patient/family education

- Explain reason for and expected result of medication

Evaluation

Positive therapeutic outcome

- Increased B/P
- Decreased edema
- Increased serum albumin

! HIGH ALERT

plicamycin (Rx)

(plik-a-mi'cin)

Mithramycin, Mithracin

Func. class.: Antineoplastic, antibiotic; hypocalcemic

Chem. class.: Crystalline aglycone

Pregnancy category X

Action: Inhibits DNA, RNA, protein synthesis; derived from *Streptomyces plicatus;* replication is decreased by binding to DNA; demonstrates calcium-lowering effect not related to its tumoricidal activity; also acts on osteoclasts and blocks action of parathyroid hormone; a vesicant

Therapeutic Outcome: Prevention of rapidly growing malignant cells, decreased calcium levels

Uses: Testicular cancer, hypercalcemia, hypercalciuria, symptomatic treatment of advanced neoplasms

Dosage and routes

Testicular tumors

Adult: **IV** 25-30 mcg/kg/day × 8-10 days, max 30 mcg/kg/day

Hypercalcemia/hypercalciuria

Adult: **IV** 25 mcg/kg/day × 3-4 days; repeat at intervals of 1 wk

Available forms: Inj 2500 mcg/vial powder

Adverse effects

CNS: *Drowsiness, weakness, lethargy, headache, flushing,* fever, depression
GI: *Nausea, vomiting, anorexia, diarrhea, stomatitis,* increased liver enzymes
GU: Increased BUN, creatinine, **proteinuria**
HEMA: **Hemorrhage, thrombocytopenia,** decreased protime, WBC count
INTEG: *Rash,* cellulitis, **extravasation,** facial flushing
META: Decreased serum calcium, potassium, phosphorus

Contraindications: Pregnancy **X,** hypersensitivity, thrombocytopenia, bone marrow depression, bleeding disorders, child <15 yr

Precautions: Renal disease, hepatic disease, electrolyte imbalances, lactation

Pharmacokinetics

Absorption	Completely absorbed
Distribution	Crosses blood-brain barrier; concentration in bone, liver, renal system
Metabolism	Unknown
Excretion	Kidneys
Half-life	Unknown

Pharmacodynamics

Unknown

Interactions

Individual drugs

Radiation: increased toxicity, bone marrow suppression

Drug classifications

Antineoplastics: increased toxicity, bone marrow suppression

Drug/herb

Anise, arnica, chamomile, clove, dong quai, fenugreek, garlic, ginger, ginkgo, ginseng *(Panax),* licorice: increased bleeding risk

NURSING CONSIDERATIONS

Assessment

- Assess buccal cavity q8h for dryness, sores or ulceration, white patches, oral pain, bleeding, dysphagia; obtain prescription for viscous lidocaine (Xylocaine)
- Assess symptoms indicating severe allergic reaction: rash, pruritus, urticaria, purpuric skin lesions, itching, flushing
- Monitor CBC, differential, platelet count weekly; withhold drug if WBC is $<4000/mm^3$ or platelet count is $<100{,}000/mm^3$; notify prescriber of results if WBC $<20{,}000/mm^3$, platelets $<150{,}000/mm^3$
- Monitor renal function studies: BUN, creatinine, serum uric acid, urine CCr before and during therapy; I&O ratio; report fall in urine output to <30 ml/hr
- Monitor temp q4h (may indicate beginning of infection)
- Monitor liver function tests before and during therapy (bilirubin, AST, ALT, LDH) as needed or monthly; check for jaundice of skin and sclera, dark urine, clay-colored stools, itchy skin, abdominal pain, fever, diarrhea
- Assess for bleeding: hematuria, stool guaiac, bruising or petechiae, mucosa or orifices q8h, may progress to severe bleeding; check for inflammation of mucosa, breaks in skin

Nursing diagnoses

- Injury, risk for (adverse reactions)
- Body image, disturbed (adverse reactions)
- Infection, risk for (adverse reactions)
- Knowledge, deficient (teaching)

Implementation

- Avoid contact with skin; very irritating; wash completely to remove
- Give fluids **IV** or PO before chemotherapy to hydrate patient
- Give antacid before oral agent; give drug after evening meal, before bedtime; provide antiemetic 30-60 min before giving drug and prn to prevent vomiting; administer antibiotics for prophylaxis of infection
- Give TOP or systemic analgesics for pain
- Give in AM so drug can be eliminated before bedtime
- Provide liq diet: carbonated beverages; gelatin may be added if patient is not nauseated or vomiting
- Make sure drug is prepared by experienced personnel using proper precautions
- Give **IV** intermittent inf by diluting 2.5 mg/4.9 ml of sterile water (1 ml = 500 mcg); dilute single dose in 1000 ml of D_5W run over 4-6 hr; give slow **IV** inf using 20G or 21G needle
- Administer EDTA for extravasation; apply ice compress

Y-site compatibilities: Allopurinol, amifostine, aztreonam, filgrastim, melphalan, piperacillin/tazobactam, teniposide, thiotepa, vinorelbine

Patient/family education

- Teach patient to avoid use of products containing aspirin or NSAIDs, razors, commercial mouthwash, since bleeding may occur; to report symptoms of bleeding (hematuria, tarry stools)
- Encourage patient to rinse mouth tid-qid with water, club soda; brush teeth bid-qid with soft brush or cotton-tipped applicators for stomatitis; use unwaxed dental floss

P

- Caution patient to report signs of anemia (fatigue, headache, irritability, faintness, shortness of breath)
- Advise patient to report any changes in breathing or coughing even several mo after treatment; to avoid crowds or persons with respiratory tract and other infections
- Advise patient that hair may be lost during treatment; a wig or hairpiece may make patient feel better; new hair may be different in color, texture
- Caution patient not to have any vaccinations without the advice of the prescriber; serious reactions can occur
- Advise patient that effective contraception is needed during treatment and for several mo after completion of therapy; avoid breastfeeding

Evaluation

Positive therapeutic outcome

- Prevention of rapid division of malignant cells

porfirmer (Rx)

(pour'fur-meer)

Photofrin

Func. class.: Antineoplastic—miscellaneous

Chem. class.: Photosensitizing agent

Pregnancy category C

Action: Used in photodynamic treatment (PDT) of tumors; antitumor and cytotoxic actions are light and O_2 dependent; used with 630 nm laser light

Therapeutic Outcome: Prevention of growth of tumor

Uses: Esophageal cancer (completely obstructing), endobronchial non–small-cell lung cancer

Dosage and routes

Refer to Optiguide for complete instructions

Adult: **IV** 2 mg/kg, then illumination with laser light 40-50 hr after inj; a second laser light application may be given 96-120 hr after inj; may repeat q30 days × 3

Endobronchial cancer

Adult: 200 joules/cm of tumor length

Available forms: Cake/powder for inj 75 mg

Adverse effects

CNS: *Anxiety, confusion, insomnia*

CV: *Hypotension, hypertension,* **atrial fibrillation, cardiac failure,** *tachycardia*

GI: *Abdominal pain, constipation, diarrhea, dyspepsia, dysphagia, eructation, esophageal edema/bleeding, hematemesis, melena, nausea, vomiting, anorexia*

MISC: Dehydration, weight decrease, anemia, photosensitivity reaction, UTI, moniliasis

RESP: **Pleural effusion,** pneumonia, dyspnea, respiratory insufficiency, **tracheoesophageal fistula**

Contraindications: Porphyria, porphyrin allergy (porfirmer); tracheoesophageal, bronchoesophageal fistula; major blood vessels with eroding tumors (PDT)

Precautions: Pregnancy **C,** elderly, lactation, children

Pharmacokinetics

Absorption	Unknown
Distribution	Unknown
Metabolism	Unknown
Excretion	Unknown
Half-life	250 hr

Pharmacodynamics

Unknown

Interactions

Drug classifications

Phenothiazines, sulfonamides, sulfonylureas, tetracyclines, thiazides: increased photosensitivity

NURSING CONSIDERATIONS

Assessment

- Assess for ocular sensitivity; sensitivity to sun, bright lights, car headlights; patients should wear dark sunglasses with an average white light transmittance of <4%
- Assess for chest pain: may be so severe as to necessitate opiate analgesics
- Assess for extravasation at inj site: take care to protect from light

Nursing diagnoses

- Infection, risk for (adverse reactions)
- Knowledge, deficient (teaching)

Implementation

- Give as a single slow **IV** inj over 3-5 min at 2 mg/kg; reconstitute each vial with 31.8 ml of D_5 or 0.9% NaCl (2.5 mg/ml), shake well, do not mix with other drugs or sol, protect from light, and use immediately
- Laser light is initiated 630 nm wavelength laser light
- Wipe spills with damp cloth, avoid skin/eye contact, use rubber gloves, eye protection; dispose of material in polyethylene bag according to policy

Patient/family education
- Advise patient to report chest pain, eye sensitivity
- Advise patient to wear sunglasses; avoid exposure to sunlight or bright light for 30 days

Evaluation
Positive therapeutic outcome
- Reducing number and spread of malignant cells

potassium acetate/ potassium bicarbonate (Rx)
K+Care ET, K-Electrolyte, K-Ide, Klor-Con EF, K-Lyte, K-Vescent

potassium bicarbonate/ potassium chloride (Rx)
Klorvess, Klorvess Effervescent Granules, K-Lyte/Cl, Neo-K ✤

potassium bicarbonate/ potassium citrate (Rx)
Effer-K, K-Lyte DS

potassium chloride (℞)
Apo-K ✤, Cena-K, Gen-K, K+care, K+10, Kalium Durules ✤, Kaochlor, Kaochlor S-F, Kaon-Cl, Kay Ciel, KCl, K-Dur, K-Lease, K-Long ✤, K-Lor, Klor-Con, Klorvess, Klotrix, K-Lyte/Cl powder, K-med, K-Norm, K-Sol, K-Tab, Micro-K, Micro-LS, Potasalan, Roychlor, Rum-K, Slow-K, Ten-K

potassium chloride/ potassium bicarbonate/ potassium citrate
Kaochlor Eff

potassium gluconate
Kaon, Kaylixir, K-G Elixir, Potassium-Rougier ✤

potassium gluconate/ potassium chloride
Kolyum

potassium gluconate/ potassium citrate
Twin-K

Func. class.: Electrolyte, mineral replacement
Chem. class.: Potassium

Pregnancy category C

Action: Needed for adequate transmission of nerve impulses and cardiac contraction, renal function, intracellular ion maintenance

Therapeutic Outcome: Potassium level 3.0-5.0 mg/dl

Uses: Prevention and treatment of hypokalemia

Dosage and routes
Potassium bicarbonate
Adult: PO dissolve 25-50 mEq in water daily-qid

Hypokalemia (prevention)
Adult and child: PO 20 mEq/day in 2-4 divided doses

Potassium acetate—hypokalemia
Adult and child: PO 40-100 mEq/day in divided doses × 2-4 days

Potassium chloride
Adult: PO 40-100 mEq in divided doses tid-qid; **IV** 20 mEq/hr when diluted as 40 mEq/1000 ml, max 150 mEq/day
Child: PO 2-4 mEq/kg/day

Potassium gluconate
Adult: PO 40-100 mEq in divided doses tid-qid

Potassium phosphate
Adult: **IV** 1 mEq/hr in sol of 60 mEq/L, max 150 mEq/day; PO 40-100 mEq/day in divided doses
Child: **IV** max rate of infusion 1 mEq/kg/min

Available forms: Tabs for sol 6.5, 25 mEq; ext rel caps 8, 10 mEq; powder for sol 3.3, 5, 6.7, 10, 13.3 mEq/5 ml; tabs 2, 4, 5, 13.4 mEq; ext rel tabs 6.7, 8, 10 mEq; elixir 6.7 mEq/5 ml; oral sol 2.375 mEq/5 ml; inj for prep of **IV** 1.5, 2, 2.4, 3, 3.2, 4.4, 4.7 mEq

Adverse effects
CNS: Confusion
CV: Bradycardia, *cardiac depression,* **dysrhythmias, arrest, peaking T waves, lowered R and depressed RST, prolonged PR interval, widened QRS complex**
GI: *Nausea, vomiting, cramps,* pain, *diarrhea,* ulceration of small bowel
GU: Oliguria
INTEG: Cold extremities, rash

Contraindications: Renal disease (severe), severe hemolytic disease, Addison's disease, hyperkalemia, acute dehydration, extensive tissue breakdown

Precautions: Pregnancy **C**, cardiac disease, potassium-sparing diuretic therapy, systemic acidosis

Pharmacokinetics	
Absorption	Unknown
Distribution	Unknown
Metabolism	Unknown
Excretion	Kidneys, feces
Half-life	Unknown

P

Pharmacodynamics

	PO	IV
Onset	30 min	Immediate

Interactions

Drug classifications

Angiotensin converting enzyme inhibitors, calcium, diuretics (potassium-sparing), magnesium, potassium phosphate, **IV**, other potassium products: increased hyperkalemia

NURSING CONSIDERATIONS

Assessment

- Assess ECG for peaking T waves, lowered R, depressed RST, prolonged PR interval, widening QRS complex, hyperkalemia; drug should be reduced or discontinued
- Monitor potassium level during treatment (3.5-5.0 mg/dl is normal level)
- Monitor I&O ratio; watch for decreased urinary output; notify prescriber immediately; check urinary pH in patients receiving the drug as a urinary acidifier
- Assess cardiac status: rate, rhythm, CVP, PWP, PAWP if being monitored directly

Nursing diagnoses

- Nutrition: less than body requirements, imbalanced (uses)
- Knowledge, deficient (teaching)

Implementation

PO route

- Do not break, crush, or chew ext rel tabs/caps or enteric-coated products
- Give with meal or pc; take cap with full glass of liq; dissolve effervescent tab, powder in 8 oz of cold water or juice; do not give IM, SUBCUT
- Store at room temp

IV route

- Give through large-bore needle to decrease vein inflammation; check for extravasation; administer in large vein, avoiding scalp vein in child
- After diluting in large volume of **IV** sol give as an **IV** inf slowly to prevent toxicity; never give **IV** bol or IM

Potassium acetate

Additive compatibilities: Metoclopramide

Potassium chloride

Y-site compatibilities: Acyclovir, aldesleukin, allopurinol, amifostine, aminophylline, amiodarone, ampicillin, ininamrinone, atropine, aztreonam, betamethasone, calcium gluconate, cefmetazole, cephalothin, cephapirin, chlordiazepoxide, chlorproMAZINE, ciprofloxacin, cladribine, cyanocobalamin, dexamethasone, digoxin, diltiazem, diphenhydrAMINE, DOBUTamine, DOPamine, droperidol, edrophonium, enalaprilat, epINEPHrine, esmolol, estrogens, ethacrynate, famotidine, fentanyl, filgrastim, fludarabine, fluorouracil, furosemide, gallium, granisetron, heparin, hydrALAZINE, idarubicin, indomethacin, insulin, regular, isoproterenol, kanamycin, labetalol, lidocaine, lorazepam, magnesium sulfate, melphalan, meperidine, methicillin, methoxamine, methylergonovine, midazolam, minocycline, morphine, neostigmine, norepinephrine, ondansetron, oxacillin, oxytocin, paclitaxel, penicillin G potassium, pentazocine, phytonadione, piperacillin/tazobactam, prednisoLONE, procainamide, prochlorperazine, propofol, propranolol, pyridostigmine, sargramostim, scopolamine, sodium bicarbonate, succinylcholine, tacrolimus, teniposide, theophylline, thiotepa, trimethaphan, trimethobenzamide, vinorelbine, zidovudine

Additive compatibilities: Aminophylline, amiodarone, atracurium, bretylium, calcium chloride, cefepime, cephalothin, cephapirin, chloramphenicol, cimetidine, ciprofloxacin, clindamycin, cloxacillin, corticotropin, cytarabine, dimenhyDRINATE, DOPamine, enalaprilat, erythromycin, floxacillin, fluconazole, furosemide, heparin, hydrocortisone, isoproterenol, lidocaine, metaraminol, methicillin, methyldopate, metoclopramide, mitoxantrone, nafcillin, netilmicin, norepinephrine, oxacillin, penicillin G potassium or sodium, phenylephrine, piperacillin, ranitidine, sodium bicarbonate, thiopental, vancomycin, verapamil, vit B/C

Potassium chloride

Y-site compatibilities: Aldesleukin, amifostine, granisetron, lorazepam, midazolam, thiotepa

Patient/family education

- Teach patient to eat foods rich in potassium after medication is discontinued
- Advise patient to avoid OTC products: antacids, salt substitutes, analgesics, vit preparations, unless specifically directed by prescriber
- Advise patient to report hyperkalemia symptoms or continued hypokalemia symptoms
- Tell patient to take cap with full glass of liq; to dissolve powder or tab completely in at least 120 ml of water or juice
- Emphasize importance of regular follow-up

Evaluation

Positive therapeutic outcome

- Absence of fatigue, muscle weakness, and

decreased thirst and urinary output, cardiac changes
- Potassium level normal

pramipexole (Rx)
(pra-mi-pex'ol)
Mirapex
Func. class.: Antiparkinsonian agent
Chem. class.: Dopamine receptor agonist, nonergot

Pregnancy category C

Action: Selective agonist for D_2 receptors (presynaptic/postsynaptic sites); binding at D_3 receptor contributes to antiparkinson effects

Therapeutic Outcome: Decreased symptoms of Parkinson's disease (involuntary movements)

Uses: Parkinsonism

Investigational uses: Restless legs syndrome

Dosage and routes
Initial treatment
Adult: PO from a starting dose of 0.375 mg/day given in 3 divided doses; increase gradually by 0.125 mg/dose at 5-7–day intervals until total daily dose of 4.5 mg is reached

Maintenance treatment
Adult: PO 1.5-4.5 mg daily in 3 divided doses

Renal dose
Adult: PO CCr 35-59 ml/min 0.125 mg bid, may increase q5-7 days to 1.5 mg bid; CCr 15-34 ml/min 0.125 mg daily, may increase q5-7 days to 1.5 mg daily

Restless legs syndrome (off-label)
Adult: PO 0.125-0.375 mg 1-2 hr before bedtime, increase gradually

Available forms: Tabs 0.125, 0.25, 1, 1.5 mg

Adverse effects
CNS: *Agitation, insomnia,* psychosis, hallucinations, depression, dizziness, headache, confusion, **sleep attacks**
CV: *Orthostatic hypotension*, edema, syncope, tachycardia
EENT: Blurred vision
GI: *Nausea, anorexia,* constipation, dysphagia, dry mouth
GU: Impotence, urinary frequency
HEMA: **Hemolytic anemia, leukopenia, agranulocytosis**

Contraindications: Hypersensitivity

Precautions: Pregnancy **C**, renal disease, cardiac disease, MI with dysrhythmias, affective disorders, psychosis, preexisting dyskinesias

Pharmacokinetics

Absorption	Well absorbed
Distribution	Widely distributed
Metabolism	Liver, minimally
Excretion	Kidneys, unchanged
Half-life	8 hr, 12 hr in elderly

Pharmacodynamics

Onset	Unknown
Peak	2 hr
Duration	Unknown

Interactions
Individual drugs
Cimetidine, diltiazem, levodopa, quinidine, ranitidine, triamterine, verapamil: increased pramipexole levels
Metoclopramide: decreased pramipexole levels

Drug classifications
Butyrophenones, DOPamine agonists, phenothiazines: decreased pramipexole effect

Drug/herb
Chaste tree fruit, kava: decreased pramipexole effect

NURSING CONSIDERATIONS
Assessment
- Monitor B/P, ECG, respiration during initial treatment; hypotension or hypertension should be reported
- Assess mental status: affect, mood, behavioral changes, depression; complete suicide assessment
- Monitor renal function studies
- Assess for involuntary movements in parkinsonism: akinesia, tremors, staggering gait, muscle rigidity, drooling; these symptoms should improve with therapy
- Assess for sleep attacks: may fall asleep during activities, without warning; may need to discontinue medication

Nursing diagnoses
- Mobility, physical, impaired (uses)
- Injury, risk for (uses)
- Knowledge, deficient (teaching)
- Noncompliance (teaching)

Implementation
- Adjust dosage to patient response
- Give with meals to decrease GI upset

P

Patient/family education

- Advise patient that therapeutic effects may take several wk to a few mo
- Caution patient to change positions slowly to prevent orthostatic hypotension
- Instruct patient to use drug exactly as prescribed; if drug is discontinued abruptly, parkinsonian crisis may occur; if treatment is to be discontinued, taper over 1 wk; avoid alcohol, OTC sleeping products
- Advise patient to notify prescriber if pregnancy is planned or suspected

Evaluation

Positive therapeutic outcome

- Decreased akathisia, other involuntary movements
- Improved mood

pramlintide

Symlin

See Appendix A, Selected New Drugs

pravastatin (Rx)

(pra'va-sta-tin)

Pravachol

Func. class.: Antilipidemic

Pregnancy category X

Do Not Confuse: Pravachol/Prevacid

Action: Inhibits biosynthesis of VLDL, LDL, which are responsible for cholesterol development, by inhibiting the enzyme HMG-CoA reductase

Therapeutic Outcome: Decreasing cholesterol levels and LDL, increased HDL

Uses: As an adjunct in primary hypercholesterolemia types IIa, IIb, III, IV, artherosclerosis, to reduce the risk of recurrent MI

Dosage and routes

Adult: PO 40-80 mg daily at bedtime (range 20-80 mg daily)
Adolescent 14-18 yr: PO 40 mg daily
Child 8-13 yr: PO 20 mg daily
Elderly/renal/hepatic dose: PO 10 mg/day, initially

Available forms: Tabs 10, 20, 40, 80 mg

Adverse effects

CNS: Headache, dizziness, fatigue
CV: chest pain
EENT: Lens opacities
GI: Nausea, constipation, diarrhea, flatus, abdominal pain, heartburn, **liver dysfunction, pancreatitis, hepatitis**
INTEG: Rash, pruritus, photosensitivity
MS: Muscle cramps, myalgia, **myositis, rhabdomyolysis**
RESP: Common cold, rhinitis, cough

Contraindications: Pregnancy **X,** hypersensitivity, lactation, active liver disease

Precautions: Past liver disease, alcoholism, severe acute infections, trauma, severe metabolic disorders, electrolyte imbalances

Pharmacokinetics

Absorption	Poorly absorbed, erratic
Distribution	Protein binding 80%
Metabolism	Liver, extensively
Excretion	Feces (70%-75%); kidneys, unchanged (20%), breast milk (minimal)
Half-life	2 hr

Pharmacodynamics

Onset	Unknown
Peak	1-1½ hr
Duration	Unknown

Interactions

Individual drugs
Clarithromycin, clofibrate, cycloSPORINE, erythromycin, gemfibrozil, itraconazole, niacin: increased risk for myopathy
Digoxin: increased effects of digoxin
Warfarin: increased bleeding

Drug classifications
Bile acid sequestrants: decreased pravastat in bioavailability
Protease inhibitors: increased risk of myopathy

Drug/herb
Glucomannan: increased effect
Gotu kola: decreased effect

Drug/lab test
Increased: CPK, LFTs
Altered: thyroid function tests

NURSING CONSIDERATIONS

Assessment

- Assess nutrition: fat, protein, carbohydrates; nutritional analysis should be completed by dietitian before treatment
- Monitor triglycerides, esterol, cholesterol at baseline and throughout treatment; LDL and HDL should be watched closely; if increased, drug should be discontinued
- ◆ Assess for muscle tenderness, pain, obtain CPK; rhabdomyolysis may occur, therapy should be discontinued
- Monitor ophthal status qyr

Nursing diagnoses
- Knowledge, deficient (teaching)
- Noncompliance (teaching)

Implementation
- Give at bedtime only; give 1 hr before or 2 hr after bile acid sequestrants
- Store in cool environment in airtight, light-resistant container

Patient/family education
- Inform patient that compliance is needed for positive results to occur; not to double doses or skip doses
- Teach patient that risk factors should be decreased: high-fat diet, smoking, alcohol consumption, absence of exercise
- Advise patient to notify prescriber of weakness, tenderness, or limited mobility
- Explain to patient that contraception is necessary, since drug produces teratogenic effects
- Advise patient to use sunscreen, protective clothing to prevent burns

Evaluation
Positive therapeutic outcome
- Decreased cholesterol, serum triglyceride levels and improved ratio with HDL

prazosin (Rx)
(pra'zoe-sin)

Minipress, prazosin

Func. class.: Antihypertensive

Chem. class.: α_1-Adrenergic blocker

Pregnancy category C

Action: Blocks α-mediated vasoconstriction of adrenergic receptors, inducing peripheral vasodilatation

Therapeutic Outcome: Decreased B/P in hypertension; decreased cardiac preload, afterload

Uses: Hypertension

Investigational uses: Benign prostatic hypertrophy to decreased urine outflow obstruction

Dosage and routes
Hypertension

Adult: PO 1 mg bid or tid, increasing to 20 mg daily in divided doses if required, usual range 6-15 mg/day, not to exceed 1 mg initially; max 20-40 mg/day

Child: PO 0.5-7 mg bid

Benign prostatic hypertrophy

Adult: PO 1-5 mg bid

Available forms: Caps 1, 2, 5 mg

Adverse effects
CNS: *Dizziness, headache, drowsiness,* anxiety, depression, vertigo, weakness, fatigue

CV: *Palpitations, orthostatic hypotension,* tachycardia, edema, rebound hypertension

EENT: Blurred vision, epistaxis, tinnitus, dry mouth, red sclera

GI: *Nausea,* vomiting, diarrhea, constipation, abdominal pain

GU: Urinary frequency, incontinence, impotence, priapism, water and sodium retention

Contraindications: Hypersensitivity

Precautions: Pregnancy **C**, children, lactation

Pharmacokinetics	
Absorption	60%
Distribution	Widely distributed
Metabolism	Liver, extensively; protein binding 97%
Excretion	Kidneys, unchanged (10%), bile (90%)
Half-life	2-3 hr

Pharmacodynamics	
Onset	2 hr
Peak	1-3 hr
Duration	6-12 hr

Interactions
Individual drugs

Alcohol, nitroglycerin, verapamil: increased hypotension

Clonidine: decreased antihypertensive effect

Drug classifications

Antihypertensives, β-adrenergic blockers: increased hypotension

NSAIDs: decreased antihypertensive effect

Drug/herb

Aconite: increased toxicity, death

Astragalus, cola tree: increased or decreased antihypertensive effect

Barberry, betony, black catechu, black cohosh, bloodroot, broom, burdock, cat's claw, dandelion, goldenseal, Irish moss, Jamaican dogwood, kelp, khella, mistletoe, parsley: increased antihypertensive effect

Coltsoot, guarana, khat, licorice: decreased antihypertensive effect

Drug/lab test

Increased: urinary norepinephrine, VMA

NURSING CONSIDERATIONS
Assessment
- Monitor B/P, orthostatic hypotension, syncope; check for edema in feet, legs daily;

P

monitor I&O, weight daily; notify prescriber of changes

- Assess for allergic reactions: rash, fever, pruritus, urticaria; drug should be discontinued if antihistamines fail to help
- Assess for orthostatic hypotension; tell patient to rise slowly from sitting or lying position

Nursing diagnoses

- Cardiac output, decreased (uses)
- Injury, risk for (adverse reactions)
- Knowledge, deficient (teaching)
- Noncompliance (teaching)

Implementation

- Severe hypotension may occur after 1st dose of this medication; hypotension may be prevented by reducing or discontinuing diuretic therapy 3 days before beginning prazosin therapy
- Give same time each day
- Store in airtight container at 86° F (30° C) or less

Patient/family education

- Instruct patient not to discontinue drug abruptly; stress the importance of complying with dosage schedule, even if feeling better; if dose is missed, take as soon as remembered; take at same time each day
- Advise patient not to use OTC products (cough, cold, allergy) unless directed by prescriber; also to avoid large amounts of caffeine
- Emphasize the need to rise slowly to sitting or standing position to minimize orthostatic hypotension
- Teach patient to notify prescriber of mouth sores, sore throat, fever, swelling of hands or feet, irregular heartbeat, chest pain
- Caution patient to report excessive perspiration, dehydration, vomiting, diarrhea; may lead to fall in B/P
- Caution patient that drug may cause dizziness, fainting, light-headedness; may occur during 1st few days of therapy; to avoid hazardous activities
- Teach patient how to take B/P and normal readings for age-group; instruct to take B/P q7 days

Evaluation

Positive therapeutic outcome

- Decreased B/P in hypertension

Treatment of overdose: Administer volume expanders or vasopressors, discontinue drug, place in supine position

prednisoLONE (Rx)

(pred-niss'oh-lone)

Articulose-50, Delta-Cortef, prednisoLONE, Prelone, Key-Pred 25, Key-Pred 50, Predaject-50, Predalone 50, Predcor-25, Predcor-50, Prednisolone Acetate, Orapred, Hydeltrasol, Key-Pred-SP, Pediapred, Hydeltra-T.B.A., Predalone-T.B.A., Prednisol TBA

Func. class.: Corticosteroid, synthetic

Chem. class.: Intermediate-acting glucocorticoid

Pregnancy category C

Do Not Confuse:
prednisoLONE/predniSONE

Action: Decreases inflammation by suppressing migration of polymorphonuclear leukocytes, fibroblasts; reversal to increase capillary permeability and lysosomal stabilization, minimal mineralocorticoid

Therapeutic Outcome: Decreased inflammation, decreased adrenal insufficiency

Uses: Severe inflammation, immunosuppression, neoplasms

Dosage and routes

Adult: PO 2.5-15 mg bid-qid; IM 2-30 mg (acetate, phosphate) q12h; **IV** 2-30 mg (phosphate) q12h, 2-30 mg in joint or soft tissue (phosphate), 4-40 mg in joint of lesion (tebutate)

Asthma/antiinflammatory

Child: PO/**IV** 1 mg/kg q6h × 2 days, then 1-2 mg/kg, max 60 mg/day

Available forms: PrednisoLONE: tabs 5 mg, syr 5 mg/5 ml, 15 mg/5 ml; prednisoLONE acetate: inj 25, 50 mg/ml; prednisoLONE tebutate: inj 20 mg/ml; prednisoLONE phosphate: inj 20 mg/ml, oral liq 5 mg/5 ml; tabs 1, 2.5, 5, 10, 20, 50 mg, oral sol 5 mg/ml, 5 mg/5 ml, syr 5 mg/5 ml

Adverse effects

CNS: *Depression,* flushing, sweating, headache, mood changes

CV: *Hypertension,* **circulatory collapse, thrombophlebitis, embolism,** tachycardia

EENT: Fungal infections, increased intraocular pressure, blurred vision

GI: *Diarrhea, nausea, abdominal distention,* **GI hemorrhage,** increased appetite, **pancreatitis**

HEMA: **Thrombocytopenia**

INTEG: Acne, poor wound healing, ecchymosis, petechiae

MS: Fractures, osteoporosis, weakness

Contraindications: Psychosis, hypersensitivity, idiopathic thrombocytopenia, acute glomerulonephritis, amebiasis, fungal infections, nonasthmatic bronchial disease, child <2 yr

Precautions: Pregnancy **C**, diabetes mellitus, glaucoma, osteoporosis, seizure disorders, ulcerative colitis, CHF, myasthenia gravis

Pharmacokinetics

Absorption	Well absorbed (PO, IM), completely absorbed (**IV**)
Distribution	Widely distributed; crosses placenta
Metabolism	Liver, extensively
Excretion	Kidney, breast milk
Half-life	2-4 hr

Pharmacodynamics

	PO	IM (phosphate)	IV	IA/IL
Onset	1 hr	Rapid	Rapid	Slow
Peak	2 hr	1 hr	Unknown	Unknown
Duration	1½ days	Unknown	Unknown	Up to 1 mo

Interactions

Individual drugs

Alcohol, amphotericin B, cycloSPORINE, digitalis, indomethacin: increased side effects

Ambenonium, isoniazid, neostigmine, somatrem: decreased effects of each specific drug

Cholestyramine, colestipol, epHEDrine, phenytoin, rifampin, theophylline: decreased action of prednisoLONE

Indomethacin, ketoconazole: increased action of prednisoLONE

Piperacillin: increased hypokalemia

Drug classifications

Antibiotics (macrolide), contraceptives (oral), estrogens, salicylates: increased action of prednisoLONE

Anticholinesterases, anticoagulants, anticonvulsants, antidiabetics, salicylates, toxoids, vaccines: decreased effects of each specific drug

Barbiturates: decreased action of prednisoLONE

Diuretics, salicylates: increased side effects

Drug/herb

Aloe, buckthorn, cascara sagrada, Chinese rhubarb, senna: increased hypokalemia

Aloe, licorice, perilla: increased effect

Drug/lab test

Increased: cholesterol, sodium, blood glucose, uric acid, calcium, urine glucose

Decreased: calcium, potassium, T_4, T_3, thyroid ^{131}I uptake test, urine 17-OHCS, 17-KS, PBI

False negative: skin allergy tests

NURSING CONSIDERATIONS

Assessment

- Monitor potassium, blood glucose, urine glucose while patient is on long-term therapy; hypokalemia and hyperglycemia may occur
- Monitor weight daily; notify prescriber of weekly gain >5 lb; monitor I&O ratio; be alert for decreasing urinary output and increasing edema
- Monitor B/P q4h, pulse; notify prescriber if chest pain occurs
- Monitor plasma cortisol levels during long-term therapy (normal level; 138-635 nmol/L [SI units] when measured at 8 AM)
- Assess adrenal function periodically for hypothalamic-pituitary-adrenal axis suppression
- Assess infection: increased temp, WBC even after withdrawal of medication; drug masks infection symptoms
- Assess for potassium depletion: paresthesias, fatigue, nausea, vomiting, depression, polyuria, dysrhythmias, weakness, edema, hypertension, cardiac symptoms
- Assess mental status: affect, mood, behavioral changes, aggression
- Monitor temp; if fever develops, drug should be discontinued
- Assess for systemic absorption: increased temp, inflammation, irritation (top)

Nursing diagnoses

- Infection, risk for (adverse reactions)
- Knowledge, deficient (teaching)
- Noncompliance (teaching)

Implementation

PO route

- Give with food or milk to decrease GI symptoms

IM route

- Give IM inj deep in large muscle mass; rotate sites; avoid deltoid; use 21G needle
- Give in one dose in AM to prevent adrenal suppression; avoid SUBCUT administration; may damage tissue

IV route

- Give by direct **IV** only sodium phosphate product; give over >1 min; may be given by **IV** inf in D_5W, 0.9% NaCl
- Give after shaking susp (parenteral)
- Give titrated dose; use lowest effective dosage

Y-site compatibilities: Ciprofloxacin, potassium chloride, vit B/C

Additive compatibilities: Ascorbic acid, cephalothin, cytarabine, erythromycin, fluorouracil, heparin, methicillin, penicillin G potassium, penicillin G sodium, vit B/C

P

Additive incompatibilities: Calcium gluceptate, methotrexate, polymyxin B sulfate

Patient/family education

- Advise patient to carry/wear emergency ID as steroid user
- Advise patient to notify prescriber if therapeutic response decreases; dosage adjustment may be needed
- Caution patient not to discontinue abruptly; adrenal crisis can result; take exactly as prescribed
- Caution patient to avoid OTC products: salicylates, cough products with alcohol, cold preparations unless directed by prescriber
- Teach patient all aspects of drug usage including cushingoid symptoms
- Teach patient symptoms of adrenal insufficiency: nausea, anorexia, fatigue, dizziness, dyspnea, weakness, joint pain
- Advise patient that long-term therapy may be needed to clear infection (1-2 mo depending on type of infection)

Evaluation

Positive therapeutic outcome

- Decreased inflammation

predniSONE (Rx)

(pred'ni-sone)

Apo-Prednisone ♣, Deltasone, Liquid Pred, Meticorten, Orasone, Panasol-S, Prednicen-M, predniSONE, Sterapred, Winpred

Func. class.: Corticosteroid

Chem. class.: Intermediate-acting glucocorticoid

Pregnancy category C

Do Not Confuse:
predniSONE/methylPREDNISolone, predniSONE/prednisoLONE, predniSONE/Prilosec

Action: Decreases inflammation by suppressing migration of polymorphonuclear leukocytes, fibroblasts; reversal to increase capillary permeability and lysosomal stabilization

Therapeutic Outcome: Decreased inflammation, decreased adrenal insufficiency

Uses: Severe inflammation, immunosuppression, neoplasms, multiple sclerosis, collagen disorders, dermatologic disorders

Dosage and routes

Adult: PO 5-60 mg daily or divided bid-qid

Child: PO 0.05-2 mg/kg/day divided 1-4 ×/day

Nephrosis

Child 18 mo-4 yr: PO 2 mg/kg/day in divided doses, max 28 days, then 1-1.5 mg/kg/day every other day × 4 wk

Multiple sclerosis

Adult: PO 200 mg/day × 1 wk, then 80 mg every other day × 1 mo

Available forms: Tabs 1, 2.5, 5, 10, 20, 50 mg; oral sol 5 mg/5 ml; syr 5 mg/5 ml

Adverse effects

CNS: Depression, flushing, sweating, headache, mood changes

CV: Hypertension, **circulatory collapse, thrombophlebitis, embolism,** tachycardia

EENT: Fungal infections, increased intraocular pressure, blurred vision

GI: Diarrhea, nausea, abdominal distention, **GI hemorrhage,** increased appetite, **pancreatitis**

HEMA: **Thrombocytopenia**

INTEG: Acne, poor wound healing, ecchymosis, petechiae

META: Hyperglycemia

MS: Fractures, osteoporosis, weakness

Contraindications: Psychosis, hypersensitivity, idiopathic thrombocytopenia, acute glomerulonephritis, amebiasis, fungal infections, nonasthmatic bronchial disease, child <2 yr, AIDS, TB

Precautions: Pregnancy **C,** diabetes mellitus, glaucoma, osteoporosis, seizure disorders, ulcerative colitis, CHF, myasthenia gravis, renal disease, esophagitis, peptic ulcer, cataracts, coagulopathy

Pharmacokinetics	
Absorption	Well absorbed
Distribution	Widely distributed; crosses placenta
Metabolism	Liver, extensively
Excretion	Kidney, breast milk
Half-life	3-4 hr

Pharmacodynamics	
Onset	Unknown
Peak	1-2 hr
Duration	1½ days

Interactions

Individual drugs

Alcohol, amphotericin B, cycloSPORINE, digitalis: increased side effects

Ambenonium, isoniazid, neostigmine, somatrem: decreased effects of each specific drug

Cholestyramine, colestipol, epHEDrine, phenytoin, rifampin, theophylline: decreased action of predniSONE
Indomethacin: increased side effects, increased action of predniSONE
Ketoconazole: increased action of predniSONE

Drug classifications

Anticholinesterases, anticoagulants, anticonvulsants, antidiabetics, toxoids, vaccines: decreased effects of each specific drug
Antiinfectives (macrolide), contraceptives (oral), estrogens: increased action of predniSONE
Barbiturates: decreased action of predniSONE
Diuretics: increased side effects
Salicylates: decreased effects of salicylates; increased side effects, action of predniSONE

Drug/herb

Aloe, buckthorn, Chinese rhubarb, senna: increased hypokalemia

Drug/lab test

Increased: cholesterol, sodium, blood glucose, uric acid, calcium, urine glucose
Decreased: calcium, potassium, T_4, T_3, thyroid ^{131}I uptake test, urine 17-OHCS, 17-KS, PBI
False negative: skin allergy tests

NURSING CONSIDERATIONS

Assessment

- Monitor potassium, blood glucose, urine glucose while on long-term therapy; hypokalemia and hyperglycemia may occur
- Monitor weight daily; notify prescriber of weekly gain >5 lb; monitor I&O ratio; be alert for decreasing urinary output and increasing edema
- Monitor B/P q4h, pulse; notify prescriber if chest pain occurs
- Monitor plasma cortisol levels during long-term therapy (normal level 138-635 nmol/L when measured at 8 AM)
- Assess adrenal function periodically for hypothalamic-pituitary-adrenal axis suppression
- Assess infection: increased temp, WBC even after withdrawal of medication; drug masks infection symptoms
- Assess for potassium depletion: paresthesias, fatigue, nausea, vomiting, depression, polyuria, dysrhythmias, weakness, edema, hypertension, cardiac symptoms
- Assess mental status: affect, mood, behavioral changes, aggression
- Monitor temp; if fever develops, drug should be discontinued
- Assess for systemic absorption: increased temp, inflammation, irritation (top)

Nursing diagnoses

- Infection, risk for (adverse reactions)
- Knowledge, deficient (teaching)
- Noncompliance (teaching)

Implementation

- Give with food or milk to decrease GI symptoms; use measuring device for liq route
- For long-term use, alternative drug therapy is recommended, to decrease adverse reactions

Patient/family education

- Advise patient that emergency ID as steroid user should be carried or worn
- Advise patient to notify prescriber if therapeutic response decreases; dosage adjustment may be needed
- Caution patient not to discontinue abruptly; adrenal crisis can result
- Caution patient to avoid OTC products: salicylates, cough products with alcohol, cold preparations unless directed by prescriber
- Teach patient all aspects of drug usage including cushingoid symptoms
- Teach patient symptoms of adrenal insufficiency: nausea, anorexia, fatigue, dizziness, dyspnea, weakness, joint pain
- Advise patient that long-term therapy may be needed to clear infection (1-2 mo depending on type of infection)

Evaluation

Positive therapeutic outcome

- Decreased inflammation

pregabalin

Lyrica

See Appendix A, Selected New Drugs

primidone (Rx)

(pri′mi-done)

Apo-Primidone ♣, Mysoline, PMS-Primidone ♣, primidone, Sertan ♣

Func. class.: Anticonvulsant

Chem. class.: Barbiturate derivative

Pregnancy category D

Action: Raises seizure threshold by conversion of drug to phenobarbital; decreases neuron firing

Therapeutic Outcome: Reduction in seizure activity

Uses: Generalized tonic-clonic (grand mal), complex-partial, psychomotor seizures, essential tremors

Dosage and routes

Adult and child >8 yr: PO 100-125 mg at bedtime on days 1, 2, 3; then 100-125 mg bid on days 4, 5, 6; then 100-125 mg tid on days 7, 8, 9; then maintenance 250 mg tid-qid, max 2 g/day in divided doses

Child <8 yr: PO 50 mg at bedtime on days 1, 2, 3; then 50 mg bid on days 4, 5, 6; then 100 mg bid on days 7, 8, 9; maintenance 125-250 mg tid or 10-25 mg/kg/day in divided doses

Available forms: Tabs 50, 250 mg; susp 250 mg/5 ml; chew tabs 125 mg ♣

Adverse effects

CNS: *Stimulation, drowsiness,* irritability, fatigue, emotional disturbances, mood changes, paranoia, psychosis, ataxia, *vertigo*
EENT: Diplopia, nystagmus, edema of eyelids
GI: *Nausea, vomiting, anorexia,* **hepatitis**
GU: Impotence
HEMA: **Thrombocytopenia, leukopenia, neutropenia, eosinophilia, megaloblastic anemia,** decreased serum folate level, lymphadenopathy
INTEG: Rash, edema, alopecia, lupus-like syndrome

Contraindications: Pregnancy **D,** hypersensitivity, porphyria

Precautions: COPD, hepatic disease, renal disease, hyperactive children

Pharmacokinetics	
Absorption	60%-80%
Distribution	Widely distributed; crosses placenta
Metabolism	Liver, converted to phenobarbital + PEMA
Excretion	Kidneys, breast milk
Half-life	3-12 hr

Pharmacodynamics	
Onset	Unknown
Peak	4 hr
Duration	Unknown

Interactions

Individual drugs

Acebutolol, metoprolol, propranolol: decreased effectiveness
Acetazolamide, carbamazepine: decreased primidone levels
Alcohol, heparin, isoniazid, nicotinamide, phenobarbital, phenytoin: increased primidone levels

Drug classifications

Antidepressants (tricyclic), oral contraceptives, phenothiazines: decreased effectiveness
Hydantoins: increased primidone levels
Succinimides: decreased primidone levels

Drug/herb

Ginkgo: increased effect
Ginseng, santonica: decreased effect

NURSING CONSIDERATIONS

Assessment

- Assess mental status: mood, sensorium, affect, memory (long, short), especially elderly
- Assess for blood dyscrasias: fever, sore throat, bruising, rash, jaundice, epistaxis (long-term treatment only)
- Assess seizure activity including type, location, duration, and character; provide seizure precaution
- Assess renal studies: urinalysis, BUN, urine creatinine
- Monitor blood studies: RBC, Hct, Hgb, reticulocyte counts weekly for 4 wk then monthly
- Monitor hepatic studies: ALT, AST, bilirubin, creatinine
- Monitor drug levels during initial treatment: therapeutic level 5-15 mcg/ml
- Assess for signs of physical withdrawal if medication is suddenly discontinued
- Assess eye problems: need for ophthal exam before, during, after treatment (slit lamp, funduscopy, tonometry)
- Assess allergic reaction: red raised rash; if this occurs, drug should be discontinued
- Monitor for toxicity: bone marrow depression, nausea, vomiting, ataxia, diplopia, CV collapse

Nursing diagnoses

- Injury, risk for (side effects)
- Knowledge, deficient (teaching)

Implementation

- May give with food to decrease gastric irritation
- May crush tab and mix with food or fluid

Patient/family education

- Teach patient to carry/wear emergency ID stating name, drugs taken, condition, prescriber's name, phone number
- Advise patient to avoid driving and other activities that require alertness
- Caution patient to avoid alcohol and CNS depressants; increased sedation may occur
- Teach patient not to discontinue medication quickly after long-term use; taper off over several wk

Evaluation

Positive therapeutic outcome

- Decreased seizure activity

probenecid (Rx)

(proe-ben'e-sid)

Benemid, Benuryl ♣, probenecid

Func. class.: Uricosuric; antigout

Chem. class.: Sulfonamide derivative

Pregnancy category B

Action: Inhibits tubular reabsorption of urates, with increased excretion of uric acids

Therapeutic Outcome: Decreased uric acid levels

Uses: Hyperuricemia in gout, gouty arthritis; adjunct to cephalosporin, cidofovir, or penicillin treatment (gonorrhea)

Dosage and routes

Gonorrhea

Adult: PO 1 g with 3.5 g of ampicillin or 1 g 30 min before 4.8 million units of aqueous penicillin G procaine injected into 2 sites IM

Gout/gouty arthritis

Adult: PO 250 mg bid for 1 wk, then 500 mg bid, not to exceed 2 g/day; maintenance 500 mg/day × 6 mo

Adjunct in penicillin/cephalosporin treatment

Adult and child >50 kg: PO 500 mg qid

Child <50 kg: PO 25 mg/kg, then 40 mg/kg in divided doses qid

Minimize toxicity in cidofovir therapy

Adult: PO 2 g 3 hr prior to cidofovir dose, followed by 1 g at 2 and 8 hr after end of cidofovir infusion

Renal dose

Adult: PO CCr <50 ml/min avoid use

Available forms: Tabs 0.5 g

Adverse effects

CNS: Drowsiness, headache

CV: Bradycardia

GI: *Gastric irritation, nausea, vomiting, anorexia,* **hepatic necrosis**

GU: Glycosuria, thirst, frequency, **nephrotic syndrome**

INTEG: Rash, dermatitis, pruritus, fever

META: *Acidosis, hypokalemia, hyperchloremia,* hyperglycemia

RESP: **Apnea,** irregular respirations

Contraindications: Hypersensitivity, severe hepatic disease, severe renal disease, CCr <50 mg/min, history of uric acid calculus

Precautions: Pregnancy **B,** child <2 yr

Pharmacokinetics

Absorption	Well absorbed
Distribution	Crosses placenta
Metabolism	Liver
Excretion	Kidneys
Half-life	5-8 hr

Pharmacodynamics

Onset	½ hr
Peak	2-4 hr
Duration	8 hr

Interactions

Individual drugs

Acyclovir, allopurinol, dyphylline, zidovudine: increased effect

Clofibrate, dapsone, indomethacin, methotrexate, naproxen, rifampin: increased toxicity

Drug classifications

Barbiturates, benzodiazepines: increased effect

Salicylates: decreased action of probenecid

Sulfa drugs: increased toxicity

Drug/lab test

Increased: BSP/urinary PSP, theophylline levels

False positive: urine glucose with copper sulfate test (Clinitest)

NURSING CONSIDERATIONS

Assessment

- Monitor I&O ratio; observe for decrease in urinary output; increase fluids to 2-3 L/day; urine may be alkalized with sodium bicarbonate acetaZOLAMIDE
- Assess mobility, joint pain, and swelling in the joints
- Monitor CBC, urine pH, uric acid and BUN, creatinine before and periodically during treatment

Nursing diagnoses

- Pain, chronic (uses)
- Mobility, physical, impaired (uses)
- Knowledge, deficient (teaching)

Implementation

- Give with food or antacid to decrease GI upset
- Reduce dosage gradually if uric acid levels are normal after 6 mo

Patient/family education

- Advise patient to increase fluids to 2-3 L/day, avoid caffeine, alcohol
- Caution patient to avoid salicylates; probenecid levels will be decreased
- Advise patient to report any pain, redness, or hard area, usually in legs
- Instruct patient in importance of complying with medical regimen including weight loss program, diet restrictions, and alcohol intake

P

Evaluation

Positive therapeutic outcome

- Decreased pain in joints
- Normal serum uric acid levels
- Increased duration of antiinfectives

procainamide (Rx)

(proe'kane-ah-mide)

Promine, procainamide, Procanbid, Pronestyl, Pronestyl-SR

Func. class.: Antidysrhythmic (class IA)

Chem. class.: procaine HCl amide analog

Pregnancy category C

Action: Depresses excitability of cardiac muscle to electrical stimulation and slows conduction in atrium, bundle of His, and ventricle increases refractory period

Therapeutic Outcome: Prevention of dysrhythmias

Uses: Life-threatening ventricular dysrhythmias

Dosage and routes

Atrial fibrillation/PAT

Adult: PO 1-1.25 g; may give another 750 mg if needed; if no response, 500 mg-1g q2h until desired response; maintenance 50 mg/kg in divided doses q6h

Ventricular tachycardia

Adult: PO 1 g; maintenance 50 mg/kg/day given in 3-hr intervals; sus rel tab 500 mg-1.25 g q6h

Other dysrhythmias

Adult: **IV** bol 100 mg q5 min, given 25-50 mg/min, max 500 mg; or 17 mg/kg total, then **IV** inf 2-6 mg/min

Renal dose

Adult: **IV** CCr 10-50 ml/min give q6-12h; CCr <10 ml/min give q8-24h

Available forms: Caps 250, 375, 500 mg; tabs 250, 375, 500 mg; sus rel tabs 500, 750, 1000 mg; inj **IV** 100, 500 mg/ml

Adverse effects

CNS: Headache, dizziness, confusion, psychosis, restlessness, irritability, weakness

CV: Hypotension, **heart block, cardiovascular collapse, arrest**

GI: Nausea, vomiting, anorexia, diarrhea, hepatomegaly, pain, bitter taste

HEMA: Systemic lupus erythematosus syndrome, **agranulocytosis, thrombocytopenia, neutropenia, hemolytic anemia**

INTEG: Rash, urticaria, edema, swelling (rare), pruritus, flushing

Contraindications: Hypersensitivity, severe heart block, lupus erythromatosis, torsades de pointes

Precautions: Pregnancy **C**, lactation, children, renal disease, liver disease, CHF, respiratory depression, cytopenia, bone marrow failure, dysrhythmia associated with digitalis toxicity, myasthenia gravis, digoxin toxicity

Pharmacokinetics

Absorption	Well absorbed
Distribution	Rapidly distributed
Metabolism	Liver
Excretion	Kidneys, unchanged (50%-70%)
Half-life	2½-4½ hr; increased in renal disease

Pharmacodynamics

	PO	PO–EXT REL	IV
Onset	½ hr	Unknown	Rapid
Peak	1-1½ hr	Unknown	½-1 hr
Duration	3 hr	Up to 8 hr	3-4 hr

Interactions

Individual drugs

Cimetidine, quinidine, ranitidine, trimethoprim: increased procainamide effect

Haloperidol: increased anticholinergic effect

Thioridazine: increased toxicity

Drug classifications

Antidysrhythmics, quinolones: increased toxicity

β-Adrenergic blockers: increased procainamide effects

Neuromuscular blockers: increased neuromuscular blocking effect

Drug/herb

Aconite: increased toxicity, death

Aloe, broom, buckthorn (chronic use), cascara sagrada (chronic use), Chinese rhubarb, figwort, fumitory, goldenseal, kudzu, licorice: increased effect

Coltsfoot: decreased effect

Henbane: increased anticholinergic effect

Horehound: increased serotonin effect

Drug/lab test

Increased: ALT, AST, alkaline phosphatase, LDH, bilirubin

NURSING CONSIDERATIONS

Assessment

- Assess for oxygenation or perfusion deficit: decreased B/P, chest pain, dizziness, loss of consciousness
- Assess respiratory status: auscultate lung

fields for bibasilar crackles in patients with advanced CHF

- Monitor I&O ratio; electrolytes: potassium, sodium, chloride; watch for decreasing urinary output, possible retention
- Monitor liver function studies: AST, ALT, bilirubin, alkaline phosphatase
- Monitor ECG continuously to determine drug effectiveness; measure PR, QRS, QT intervals; check for PVCs, other dysrhythmias; check B/P continuously for hypotension, hypertension; for rebound hypertension after 1-2 hr; prolonged PR/QT intervals, QRS complex; if QT or QRS increases by 50% or more, withhold next dose, notify prescriber
- Monitor ANA titer; during long-term treatment, watch for lupuslike symptoms
- Monitor for dehydration or hypovolemia
- Monitor for CNS symptoms: confusion, seizures, psychosis, numbness, depression, involuntary movements; if these occur, drug should be discontinued
- Monitor blood levels (therapeutic level 3-10 mcg/ml), ANA titer or *N*-acetylprocainamide levels 10-20 mcg/ml; notify prescriber of abnormal results; assess for toxicity: confusion, drowsiness, nausea, vomiting, tachydysrhythmias, oliguria
- Assess cardiac rate, respiration: rate, rhythm, character, chest pain, ventricular tachycardia, supraventricular tachycardia or fibrillation

Nursing diagnoses

- Cardiac output, decreased (uses)
- Gas exchange, impaired (adverse reactions)
- Knowledge, deficient (teaching)

Implementation

PO route

- Do not break, crush, or chew sus rel tab
- Give on an empty stomach with a full glass of water
- May be given with meals if GI irritation occurs; absorption will be decreased
- Tab may be crushed and mixed with fluid or foods for patients with swallowing difficulties

IV route

- Give by direct **IV** after diluting 100 mg/10 ml of D_5W or sterile water for inj; give 50 mg/min or less
- Give by intermittent inf after diluting to a conc of 2-4 mg/ml, 200 mg up to 1 g/50-500 ml of D_5W; give over 30 min (2-6 mg/min maintenance); use infusion pump for correct dosage
- Do not use if sol is dark or if precipitate is present

Y-site compatibilities: Amiodarone, famotidine, heparin, hydrocortisone, potassium chloride, ranitidine, vit B/C

Y-site incompatibilities: Milrinone

Additive compatibilities: Amiodarone, DOBUTamine, flumazenil, lidocaine, netilmicin, verapamil

Additive incompatibilities: Esmolol, ethacrynate, milrinone

Solution compatibilities: D_5W, D_5/0.9% NaCl, 0.45% NaCl, 0.9% NaCl, water for inj

Patient/family education

- Advise patient to report side effects immediately to prescriber; to take exactly as prescribed; if dose is missed take when remembered if within 3-4 hr of next dose, do not double doses
- Caution patient that dark glasses may be needed for photophobia; to use sunscreen or stay out of sun to prevent burns; avoid temp extremes; impairment of heat-regulating mechanism can occur
- Advise patient to complete follow-up appointment with prescriber including pulmonary function studies, chest x-ray
- Instruct patient that dry mouth may be relieved by frequent sips of water, hard candy, sugarless gum
- Caution patient to make position changes from lying to standing slowly to prevent orthostatic hypotension
- Advise prescriber immediately if lupuslike symptoms appear (joint pain, butterfly rash, fever, chills, dyspnea), or leukopenia (sore mouth, gums, throat) or thrombocytopenia (bleeding, bruising)
- Teach patient how to take pulse and when to report to prescriber

Evaluation

Positive therapeutic outcome

- Decreased PVCs, ventricular tachycardia

Treatment of overdose: O_2, artificial ventilation, ECG, administer DOPamine for circulatory depression, diazepam or thiopental for convulsions, isoproterenol

procarbazine (Rx)

(proe-kar'ba-zeen)

Matulane, Natulan ♣

Func. class.: Antineoplastic, alkylating agent

Chem. class.: Hydrazine derivative

Pregnancy category D

Action: Inhibits DNA, RNA, protein synthesis, cell cycle S phase specific; has multiple sites of action; a nonvesicant

Therapeutic Outcome: Prevention of rapidly growing malignant cells

Uses: Lymphoma, Hodgkin's disease, cancers resistant to other therapy

Investigational uses: Brain, lung malignancies, other lymphomas, multiple myeloma, malignant melanoma, polycythemia vera

Dosage and routes

Adult: PO 2-4 mg/kg/day for first wk; maintain dosage of 4-6 mg/kg/day until platelets and WBC fall; after recovery, 1-2 mg/kg/day

Child: PO 50 mg/m^2/day for 7 days, then 100 mg/m^2 until desired response, leukopenia, or thrombocytopenia occurs; 50 mg/day is maintenance after bone marrow recovery

Available forms: Caps 50 mg

Adverse effects

CNS: Headache, dizziness, **seizures,** insomnia, hallucinations, confusion, **coma,** pain, chills, fever, sweating, paresthesias

EENT: Retinal hemorrhage, nystagmus, photophobia, diplopia

GI: *Nausea, vomiting,* anorexia, diarrhea, constipation, dry mouth, stomatitis

GU: Azoospermia, cessation of menses

HEMA: **Thrombocytopenia, anemia, leukopenia, myelosuppression, bleeding tendencies,** purpura, petechiae, epistaxis

INTEG: *Rash,* pruritus, dermatitis, alopecia, herpes, hyperpigmentation

MS: Arthralgias, myalgias

RESP: Cough, pneumonitis

Contraindications: Hypersensitivity, thrombocytopenia, bone marrow depression, pregnancy **D,** lactation

Precautions: Renal disease, hepatic disease, radiation therapy

Pharmacokinetics

Absorption	Well absorbed
Distribution	Widely distributed; crosses blood-brain barrier
Metabolism	Liver
Excretion	Kidneys
Half-life	1 hr

Pharmacodynamics

Unknown

Interactions

Individual drugs

Alcohol: increased CNS depression, disulfiram reaction
Caffeine, guanethidine, levodopa, methyldopa, reserpine: increased hypertension
Insulin: increased hypoglycemia
Meperidine: hypotension; do not use together

Drug classifications

Antidepressants, local anesthetics: increased hypertensive crisis
Antidepressants (tricyclic), MAOIs: disulfiram-like reaction
Antihistamines, barbiturates, CNS depressants, hypotensive agents, opiates, phenothiazines, sedative/hypnotics: increased CNS depression
Hypoglycemics (oral): increased hypoglycemia
Sympathomimetics: disulfiram-like reaction, life-threatening hypertensive crisis

Drug/food

Tyramine-foods: increased disulfiram-like reaction, hypertensive crisis

NURSING CONSIDERATIONS

Assessment

- Monitor CBC, differential, platelet count weekly; withhold drug if WBC is <4000/mm^3 or platelet count is <75,000/mm^3; notify prescriber of results if WBC <20,000/mm^3, platelets <150,000/mm^3
- Monitor pulmonary function tests, chest x-ray films before, during therapy; chest film should be obtained q2 wk during treatment; check for dyspnea, crackles, unproductive cough, chest pain, tachypnea
- Monitor renal function studies: BUN, serum uric acid, urine CCr before, during therapy; I&O ratio; report fall in urine output of 30 ml/hr; check for decreased hyperuricemia
- Monitor for cold, fever, sore throat (may indicate beginning of infection); identify edema in feet, joint and stomach pain, shaking; prescriber should be notified
- Assess for bleeding: hematuria, guaiac, bruising or petechiae, mucosa or orifices q8h, no rectal temp
- Assess for tyramine-containing foods in the diet; hypertensive crisis can occur

Nursing diagnoses

- Injury, risk for (adverse reactions)
- Body image, disturbed (adverse reactions)
- Infection, risk for (adverse reactions)
- Knowledge, deficient (teaching)

Implementation

- Give with foods, fluids for GI upset; open cap and give with food/fluids for swallowing difficulty; administer as directed

Patient/family education

- Teach patient to avoid use of products containing aspirin or NSAIDs, razors, commercial mouthwash, since bleeding may occur; to report symptoms of bleeding (hematuria, tarry stools)

- Caution patient to report signs of anemia (fatigue, headache, irritability, faintness, shortness of breath)
- Advise patient to report any changes in breathing or coughing even several mo after treatment; to avoid crowds and persons with respiratory tract or other infections
- Inform patient hair loss is common; discuss the use of wigs or hairpieces
- Caution patient not to have any vaccinations without the advice of the prescriber; serious reactions can occur
- Advise patient that contraception is needed during treatment and for several mo after the completion of therapy, avoid breast feeding
- To avoid sunlight, or UV exposure, wear sunscreen or protective clothing

Evaluation

Positive therapeutic outcome

- Absence of swelling at night
- Increased appetite, increased weight

prochlorperazine (Rx)

(proe-klor-pair'a-zeen)

Chlorpazine, Compa-Z, Compazine, Contranzine, Provazin ♣, Stemetil ♣, Ultrazine

Func. class.: Antiemetic/antipsychotic

Chem. class.: Phenothiazine, piperazine derivative

Pregnancy category C

Do Not Confuse:
Compazine/Coumadin, prochlorperazine/chlorproMAZINE

Action: Depresses cerebral cortex, hypothalamus, limbic system, which control activity aggression; blocks neurotransmission produced by DOPamine at synapse; exhibits a strong α-adrenergic, anticholinergic blocking action; mechanism for antipsychotic effects is unclear; acts centrally by blocking chemoreceptor trigger zone, which in turn acts on vomiting center

Therapeutic Outcome: Decreased nausea, vomiting, decreased signs and symptoms of psychosis

Uses: Nausea, vomiting, psychosis

Dosage and routes

Postoperative nausea/vomiting

Adult: IM 5-10 mg 1-2 hr before anesthesia; may repeat in 30 min; **IV** 5-10 mg 15-30 min before anesthesia; **IV** inf 20 mg/L D_5W or 0.9% NaCl 15-30 min before anesthesia, max 40 mg/day

Severe nausea/vomiting

Adult: PO 5-10 mg tid-qid; sus rel 15 mg daily in AM or 10 mg q12h; rec 25 mg/bid; IM 5-10 mg; may repeat q4h, max 40 mg/day

Child 18-39 kg: PO 2.5 mg tid or 5 mg bid; max 15 mg/day; IM 0.132 mg/kg

Child 14-17 kg: PO/rec 2.5 mg bid-tid, max 10 mg/day; IM 0.132 mg/kg

Child 9-13 kg: PO/rec 2.5 mg daily-bid, max 7.5 mg/day; IM 0.132 mg/kg

Antipsychotic

Adult and child ≥12 yr: PO 5-10 mg tid-qid; may increase q2-3 day, max 150 mg/day; IM 10-20 mg q2-4h up to 4 doses, then 10-20 mg q4-6h, max 200 mg/day; rec 10 mg tid-qid may increase by 5-10 mg q2-3 days as needed

Child 2-12 yr: PO 2.5 mg bid-tid; IM 0.132 mg/kg, max 10 mg/dose

Antianxiety

Adult and child ≥12 yr: 5 mg tid-qid, max 20 mg/day or >12 wk; IM 5-10 mg q3-4h, max 40 mg/day; **IV** 2.5-10 mg; max 40 mg/day

Child 2-12 yr: IM 132 mcg/kg

Available forms: Syr 5 mg/ml; inj 5 mg/ml; tabs 5, 10, 25 mg; sus rel caps 10, 15, 30 mg; supp 2.5, 5, 25 mg

Adverse effects

CNS: Tardive dyskinesia, *euphoria,* **depression, extrapyramidal symptoms (EPS),** restlessness, tremor, dizziness, **neuroleptic malignant syndrome,** drowsiness

CV: **Circulatory failure, tachycardia**

EENT: Blurred vision

GI: Nausea, vomiting, anorexia, dry mouth, diarrhea, constipation, weight loss, metallic taste, cramps

HEMA: **Agranulocytosis**

RESP: **Respiratory depression**

Contraindications: Hypersensitivity to phenothiazines, coma, seizure, encephalopathy, bone marrow depression, narrow-angle glaucoma

Precautions: Pregnancy **C,** children <2 yr, elderly, lactation

Pharmacokinetics

Absorption	Variably absorbed (PO); well absorbed (IM)
Distribution	Widely distributed; high concentration in CNS; crosses placenta
Metabolism	Liver, extensively; GI mucosa
Excretion	Kidneys, breast milk
Half-life	Unknown

Pharmacodynamics

	PO	PO–SUS REL	REC	IM	IV
Onset	½ hr	½ hr	1 hr	10-20 min	4-5 min
Peak	Unkn	Unkn	Unkn	Unkn	Unkn
Duration	3-4 hr	10-12 hr	3-4 hr	3-4 hr	3-4 hr

Interactions

Drug classifications

Antacids, barbiturates: decreased prochlorperazine effect
Anticholinergics, antidepressants, antiparkinson drugs: increased anticholinergic effects

Drug/herb

Betel palm, kava: increased EPS
Chamomile, cola nut, hops, kava, nettle, nutmeg, skullcap, valerian: increased CNS depression
Henbane, jimsonweed, scopolia: increased anticholinergic effect

Drug/lab test

Increased: liver function tests, cardiac enzymes, cholesterol, blood glucose, prolactin, bilirubin, PBI, ^{131}I, alkaline phosphatase, leukocytes, granulocytes, platelets
Decreased: hormones (blood and urine)
False positive: pregnancy tests, urine bilirubin
False negative: urinary steroids, 17-OHCS, pregnancy tests

NURSING CONSIDERATIONS

Assessment

- Assess mental status: orientation, mood, behavior, presence and type of hallucinations before initial administration and monthly; this drug should significantly reduce psychotic behavior
- Check for swallowing of PO medication; check for hoarding or giving of medication to other patients
- Monitor I&O ratio; palpate bladder if low urinary output occurs, especially in elderly; urinalysis recommended before, during prolonged therapy
- (Alert) Monitor bilirubin, CBC, liver function studies monthly; blood dyscrasias, hepatotoxicity may occur
- Assess affect, orientation, LOC, reflexes, gait, coordination, sleep pattern disturbances
- Monitor B/P with patient sitting, standing, and lying; take pulse and respirations q4h during initial treatment; establish baseline before starting treatment; report drops of 30 mm Hg; obtain baseline ECG, Q-wave and T-wave changes
- Check for dizziness, faintness, palpitations, tachycardia on rising; severe orthostatic hypotension is common
- (Alert) Identify neuroleptic malignant syndrome: hyperpyrexia, muscle rigidity, increased CPK, altered mental status, seizures, fever, tachycardia, dyspnea, fatigue, loss of bladder control; notify prescriber immediately; drug should be discontinued
- Assess for EPS including akathisia (inability to sit still, no pattern to movements), tardive dyskinesia (bizarre movements of the jaw, mouth, tongue, extremities), pseudoparkinsonism (ragged tremors, pill rolling, shuffling gait); an antiparkinsonism drug should be prescribed
- Assess for constipation, urinary retention daily; if these occur, increase bulk, water in diet

Nursing diagnoses

- Thought processes, disturbed (uses)
- Coping, ineffective (uses)
- Knowledge, deficient (teaching)
- Noncompliance (teaching)

Implementation

PO route

- Do not break, crush, or chew sus rel caps
- Give drug in liq form mixed in glass of juice or cola if hoarding is suspected; do not mix in caffeine drinks, tannics, pectins
- Give decreased dosage in elderly since metabolism is slowed
- Give PO with full glass of water, milk; or give with food to decrease GI upset
- Give antacids 2 hr before or after taking this drug
- Store in airtight, light-resistant container; oral sol in amber bottle

IM route

- Inject slowly in deep muscle mass; do not give SUBCUT; aspirate to avoid **IV** administration; do not administer sol with a precipitate; have patient lie down afterward for at least 30 min

IV route

- Give by direct **IV** after diluting **IV** using 0.9% NaCl to 1 mg/1 ml; administer at 1 mg/min or less
- Administer by intermittent inf after diluting

20 mg/L or less LR, Ringer's, dextrose, saline, or any combination

Syringe compatibilities: Atropine, butorphanol, chlorproMAZINE, cimetidine, diamorphine, diphenhydrAMINE, droperidol, fentanyl, glycopyrrolate, hydrOXYzine, meperidine, metoclopramide, nalbuphine, pentazocine, perphenazine, promazine, promethazine, ranitidine, scopolamine, sufentanil

Syringe incompatibilities: DimenhyDRINATE, midazolam, pentobarbital, thiopental

Y-site compatibilities: Amsacrine, calcium gluconate, cisplatin, cladribine, cyclophosphamide, cytarabine, DOXOrubicin, fluconazole, granisetron, heparin, hydrocortisone, melphalan, methotrexate, ondansetron, paclitaxel, potassium chloride, propofol, sargramostim, sufentanil, teniposide, thiotepa, vinorelbine, vit B/C

Y-site incompatibilities: Foscarnet

Additive compatibilities: Amikacin, ascorbic acid, dexamethasone, dimenhydrinate, erythromycin, ethacrynate, lidocaine, nafcillin, netilmicin, sodium bicarbonate, vit B/C

Additive incompatibilities: Aminophylline, amphotericin B, ampicillin, calcium gluceptate, cefoperazone, cephalothin, chloramphenicol, chlorothiazide, floxacillin, furosemide, hydrocortisone sodium succinate, methohexital sodium, penicillin G sodium, phenobarbital, thiopental

Patient/family education

- Teach patient to use good oral hygiene; frequent rinsing of mouth, sugarless gum for dry mouth since oral candidiasis may occur
- Caution patient to avoid hazardous activities until drug response is determined; dizziness, blurred vision may occur
- Inform patient that orthostatic hypotension occurs often and to rise from sitting or lying position gradually; to remain lying down after IM inj for at least 30 min; tell patient to avoid hot tubs, hot showers, tub baths, since hypotension may occur; tell patient that in hot weather heat stroke may occur; take extra precautions to stay cool
- Advise patient to avoid abrupt withdrawal of this drug, or EPS may result; drug should be withdrawn slowly
- Teach patient to avoid OTC preparations (cough, hay fever, cold) unless approved by prescriber, since serious drug interactions may occur; avoid use with alcohol, CNS depressants; increased drowsiness may occur; avoid activities requiring mental alertness
- Instruct patient to avoid sun or use sunscreen, sunglasses and protective clothing to prevent burns
- Advise patient to take antacids 2 hr before or after taking this drug
- Advise patient to report sore throat, malaise, fever, bleeding, mouth sores; if these occur, CBC should be done and drug discontinued
- Teach patient not to double or skip doses
- Teach patient urine may turn pink to reddish brown
- Instruct patient to report dark urine, clay-colored stools, bleeding, bruising, rash, blurred vision

Evaluation

Positive therapeutic outcome

- Relief of nausea and vomiting
- Decrease in emotional excitement, hallucinations, delusions, paranoia
- Reorganization of patterns of thought, speech

Treatment of overdose: Lavage if orally ingested; provide airway; *do not induce vomiting or use epINEPHrine*

progesterone (Rx)

(proe-jess'ter-one)

Crinone, progesterone, Prometrium

Func. class.: Progestogen

Chem. class.: Progesterone derivative

Pregnancy category D

Action: Inhibits secretion of pituitary gonadotropins, which prevents follicular maturation, ovulation; stimulates growth of mammary tissue; antineoplastic action against endometrial cancer

Therapeutic Outcome: Decreased abnormal uterine bleeding, absence of amenorrhea

Uses: Contraception, amenorrhea, premenstrual syndrome, abnormal uterine bleeding, endometrial hyperplasia prevention, assisted reproductive technology (ART) gel

Investigational uses: Corpus luteum dysfunction

Dosage and routes

Infertility

Adult: VAG 90 mg daily

Amenorrhea/uterine bleeding

Adult: IM 5-10 mg daily × 6-8 doses

Endometrial hyperplasia prevention
Adult: PO 200 mg/day

ART
Adult: Gel 90 mg (8%) vaginally daily, for supplementation; 90 mg (8%) vaginally bid for replacement, if pregnancy occurs, continue × 10-12 wk

Available forms: Caps 100, 200 mg; inj 50 mg/ml; powder micronized, vag gel 4%, 8%

Adverse effects
CNS: Dizziness, headache, migraines, depression, fatigue
CV: Hypotension, **thrombophlebitis,** edema, **thromboembolism, stroke, pulmonary embolism, MI**
EENT: Diplopia, retinal thrombosis
GI: *Nausea,* vomiting, anorexia, cramps, increased weight, **cholestatic jaundice**
GU: Amenorrhea, cervical erosion, breakthrough bleeding, dysmenorrhea, vaginal candidiasis, breast changes, *gynecomastia, testicular atrophy, impotence,* endometriosis, **spontaneous abortion**
INTEG: Rash, urticaria, acne, hirsutism, alopecia, oily skin, seborrhea, purpura, melasma
META: Hyperglycemia
SYST: **Angioedema, anaphylaxis**

Contraindications: Pregnancy **D,** breast cancer, hypersensitivity, thromboembolic disorders, reproductive cancer, genital bleeding (abnormal, undiagnosed), cerebral hemorrhage

Precautions: Lactation, hypertension, asthma, blood dyscrasias, gallbladder disease, CHF, diabetes mellitus, bone disease, depression, migraine headache, seizure disorders, hepatic disease, renal disease, family history of breast or reproductive tract cancer

Pharmacokinetics

Absorption	Unknown
Distribution	Unknown
Metabolism	Unknown
Excretion	Breast milk
Half-life	Unknown

Pharmacodynamics

	IM	REC	VAG
Onset	Unknown	Unknown	Unknown
Peak	Unknown	Unknown	Unknown
Duration	24 hr	24 hr	24 hr

Interactions
Drug classifications
Barbiturates, phenytoins: decreased progesterone effect
Drug/herb
Alfalfa: increased hormonal effect
Drug/lab test
Increased: alkaline phosphatase, nitrogen (urine), pregnanediol, amino acids, factors VII, VIII, IX, X
Decreased: GTT, HDL

NURSING CONSIDERATIONS

Assessment
- Monitor B/P at beginning of treatment and periodically; check weight daily; notify prescriber of weekly weight gain >5 lb
- Monitor I&O ratio: be alert for decreasing urinary output, increasing edema, hypertension
- Assess liver function studies: ALT, AST, bilirubin periodically during long-term therapy
- Assess edema, hypertension, cardiac symptoms, jaundice
- Assess mental status: affect, mood, behavioral changes, depression
- Assess for hypercalcemia

Nursing diagnoses
- Sexual dysfunction (uses)
- Tissue perfusion, ineffective (adverse reactions)
- Injury, risk for (adverse reactions)
- Knowledge, deficient (teaching)

Implementation
IM route
- Store in dark area
- Give titrated dose; use lowest effective dosage; give oil sol deep in large muscle mass; rotate sites; use after warming to dissolve crystals

Patient/family education
- Teach patient to report breast lumps, vaginal bleeding, edema, jaundice, dark urine, clay-colored stools, dyspnea, headache, blurred vision, abdominal pain, numbness or stiffness in legs, chest pain
- Teach patient to report suspected pregnancy

Evaluation
Positive therapeutic outcome
- Decreased abnormal uterine bleeding
- Absence of amenorrhea
- Prevented pregnancy

promethazine (Rx)
(proe-meth'a-zeen)

Histanil ✤, Pentazine, Phenadoz, Phenergan, promethazine HCl

Func. class.: Antihistamine, H_1-receptor antagonist; antiemetic; sedative/hypnotic

Chem. class.: Phenothiazine derivative

Pregnancy category C

Do Not Confuse:
Phenergan/Theragran

Action: Acts on blood vessels, GI, respiratory system by competing with histamine for H_1-receptor site; decreases allergic response by blocking histamine; also acts on chemoreceptor trigger zone to decrease vomiting; increases CNS stimulation, has anticholinergic response

Therapeutic Outcome: Absence of allergy symptoms and rhinitis, absence of nausea/vomiting, sedation

Uses: Motion sickness, rhinitis, allergy symptoms, sedation, nausea, preoperative and postoperative sedation

Dosage and routes
Nausea

Adult: PO/IM/**IV**/REC 12.5-25 mg; may repeat 12.5-25 mg q4-6h prn

Child >2 yr: PO/IM/**IV**/REC 0.25-0.5 mg/kg q4-6h

Motion sickness

Adult: PO 25 mg bid; give 30-60 min before departure and q8-12h prn

Child >2 yr: PO/IM/REC 12.5-25 mg bid; give 30-60 min before departure and q8-12h prn

Allergy/rhinitis

Adult: PO 12.5 mg qid, or 25 mg at bedtime

Child >2 yr: PO 6.25-12.5 mg tid or 25 mg at bedtime

Sedation

Adult: PO/IM/**IV**/REC 25-50 mg at bedtime

Child >2 yr: PO/IM/REC 12.5-25 mg at bedtime

Sedation (preoperative/postoperative)

Adult: PO/IM/**IV** 25-50 mg

Child >2 yr: PO/IM/**IV** 0.5-1.1 mg/kg

Available forms: Tabs 12.5, 25, 50 mg; supp 12.5, 25 mg; inj 25, 50 mg/ml; syr 6.25 mg/5 ml

Adverse effects
CNS: *Dizziness, drowsiness,* poor coordination, fatigue, anxiety, euphoria, confusion, paresthesia, neuritis, extrapyramidal symptoms (EPS), **neuroleptic malignant syndrome**

CV: Hypotension, palpitations, tachycardia

EENT: Blurred vision, dilated pupils, tinnitus, nasal stuffiness, dry nose, throat, mouth, photosensitivity

GI: *Constipation,* dry mouth, nausea, vomiting, anorexia, diarrhea

GU: *Retention,* dysuria, frequency

HEMA: **Thrombocytopenia, agranulocytosis, hemolytic anemia**

INTEG: Rash, urticaria, photosensitivity

RESP: Increased thick secretions, wheezing, chest tightness, **apnea in pediatric patients**

Contraindications: Hypersensitivity to H_1-receptor antagonist, sulfite allergy, child <2 yr, acute asthma attack, lower respiratory tract disease

Precautions: Pregnancy **C,** increased intraocular pressure, renal disease, cardiac disease, hypertension, bronchial asthma, seizure disorder, stenosed peptic ulcers, hyperthyroidism, prostatic hypertrophy, bladder neck obstruction

Pharmacokinetics	
Absorption	Well absorbed (PO, IM); erratically absorbed (rec)
Distribution	Widely distributed; crosses the blood-brain barrier, placenta
Metabolism	Liver
Excretion	Kidneys, breast milk
Half-life	Unknown

Pharmacodynamics	PO/IM/REC	IV
Onset	20 min	3-5 min
Peak	Unknown	Unknown
Duration	4-12 hr	4-6 hr

Interactions
Individual drugs

Alcohol: increased CNS depression

Drug classifications

Anticoagulants, oral: decreased anticoagulant effect

Antidepressants (tricyclic), barbiturates, CNS depressants, opiates, sedative/hypnotics: increased CNS depression

Heparin: decreased oral anticoagulant effect

MAOIs: increased promethazine effect

Drug/herb

Henbane, jimsonweed, scopolia: increased anticholinergic effect

Drug/lab test

False negative: skin allergy tests (discontinue antihistamines 3 days before testing)

False-positive: urine pregnancy test

NURSING CONSIDERATIONS

Assessment

- Assess respiratory status: rate, rhythm, increase in bronchial secretions, wheezing, chest tightness; provide fluids to 2 L/day to decrease secretion thickness
- Monitor I&O ratio: be alert for urinary retention, frequency, dysuria, especially elderly; drug should be discontinued if these occur
- Monitor CBC during long-term therapy; blood dyscrasias may occur but are rare

Nursing diagnoses

- Airway clearance, ineffective (uses)
- Injury, risk for (adverse reactions)
- Knowledge, deficient (teaching)
- Noncompliance (teaching, overuse)

Implementation

PO route

- Give 1 hr ac or 2 hr pc to facilitate absorption
- Give with meals to decrease GI upset
- Store in airtight, light-resistant container

IM route

- Give IM inj in large muscle mass; aspirate to avoid **IV** administration; do not give SUBCUT; necrosis may occur

IV route

- Give **IV** directly; give 25 mg or less over 1 min; rapid drop in B/P may occur with rapid administration

Syringe compatibilities: Atropine, butorphanol, chlorproMAZINE, cimetidine, diphenhydramine, droperidol, fentanyl, glycopyrrolate, hydromorphone, hydrOXYzine, meperidine, metoclopramide, midazolam, pentazocine, perphenazine, prochlorperazine, promazine, ranitidine, scopolamine

Syringe incompatibilities: DimenhyDRINATE, heparin, pentobarbital, thiopental

Y-site compatibilities: Amifostine, amsacrine, aztreonam, ciprofloxacin, cisplatin, cladribine, cyclophosphamide, cytarabine, DOXOrubicin, filgrastim, fluconazole, fludarabine, granisetron, melphalan, ondansetron, sargramostim, teniposide, thiotepa, vinorelbine

Y-site incompatibilities: Cefoperazone, foscarnet, heparin

Additive compatibilities: Amikacin, ascorbic acid, chloroquine, hydromorphone, netilmicin, vit B/C

Additive incompatibilities: Aminophylline, carbenicillin, chloramphenicol, chlorothiazide, floxacillin, furosemide, heparin, hydrocortisone sodium succinate, methicillin, methohexital, penicillin G, pentobarbital, phenobarbital, thiopental

Patient/family education

- Inform patient that a false negative result may occur with skin testing; these procedures should not be scheduled until 3 days after discontinuing use
- Advise patient to take 30 min before departure to prevent motion sickness
- Caution patient to avoid hazardous activities, activities requiring alertness, since dizziness may occur; instruct patient to request assistance with ambulation
- Advise patient to avoid alcohol, other depressants; serious CNS depression may occur
- Teach patient all aspects of drug use; to notify prescriber if confusion, sedation, hypotension occur; to avoid driving and other hazardous activity if drowsiness occurs
- Advise patient to take 1 hr ac or 2 hr pc to facilitate absorption
- Caution patient not to exceed recommended dosage; dysrhythmias may occur
- Inform patient hard candy, gum, frequent rinsing of mouth may be used for dryness

Evaluation

Positive therapeutic outcome

- Absence of motion sickness
- Absence of nausea, vomiting

propafenone (Rx)

(pro-faff'e-nown)

Rythmol

Func. class.: Antidysrhythmic (Class IC)

Pregnancy category C

Action: Slows conduction velocity; reduces membrane responsiveness; inhibits automaticity; increases ratio of effective refractory period to action potential duration; β-blocking activity

Uses: Life-threatening dysrhythmias, sustained ventricular tachycardia

Dosage and routes

Adult: PO 150 mg q8h; allow a 3-4 day interval before increasing dose, max 900 mg/day

Available forms: Tabs 150, 225, 300 mg

Adverse effects

CNS: Headache, dizziness, abnormal dreams, syncope, confusion, **seizures**

CV: **Supraventricular dysrhythmia, ventricular dysrhythmia, bradycardia**, prodys-

rhythmia, palpitations, AV block, intraventricular conduction delay, AV dissociation, hypotension, chest pain
EENT: Blurred vision, altered taste, tinnitus
GI: *Nausea, vomiting*, constipation, dyspepsia, cholestasis, **hepatitis**, abnormal hepatic studies, dry mouth
HEMA: **Leukopenia, agranulocytosis, granulocytopenia, thrombocytopenia**, anemia, bruising
INTEG: Rash
RESP: Dyspnea

Contraindications: 2nd-, 3rd-degree AV block, right bundle branch block, cardiogenic shock, hypersensitivity, bradycardia, uncontrolled CHF, sick sinus syndrome, marked hypotension, bronchospastic disorders

Precautions: Pregnancy **C**, CHF, hypokalemia, hyperkalemia, recent MI, nonallergic bronchospasm, lactation, children, hepatic or renal disease, elderly

Pharmacokinetics

Absorption	Well
Distribution	Widely, crosses placenta
Metabolism	Rapid, liver, CYP1A2, CYP2D6, CYP3A4
Excretion	Kidneys
Half-life	2-32 hr

Pharmacodynamics (Antiarrhythmic)

Onset	Hours-several days
Peak	4-5 days
Duration	Several hr

Interactions
Individual drugs
CycloSPORINE, digoxin, metoprolol, propranolol, warfarin: increased serum levels
Drug/herb
Aconite: increased toxicity, death
Aloe, broom, buckthorn (chronic use), cascara sagrada (chronic use), Chinese rhubarb, figwort, fumitory, goldenseal, kudzu, licorice: increased effect
Aloe, buckthorn, cascara sagrada, senna pod/leaf: hypokalemia, increased antidysrhythmic action
Coltsfoot: decreased effect
Horehound: increased serotonin effect
Drug/lab test
Increased: CPK

NURSING CONSIDERATIONS
Assessment
- Monitor GI status: bowel pattern, number of stools
- Assess cardiac status: rate, rhythm, quality; ECG or Holter monitor prior to and during therapy; watch for PR, QT prolongation
- Monitor chest x-ray film, pulmonary function test during treatment
- Monitor I/O ratio; check for decreasing output; daily weight
- Monitor B/P for fluctuations
- Assess lung fields; bilateral crackles, dyspnea, peripheral edema, weight gain, jugular venous distention may occur in CHF patient
- Assess toxicity: fine tremors, dizziness, hypotension, drowsiness, abnormal heart rate

Nursing diagnoses
- Cardiac output, decreased (uses)
- Knowledge, deficient (teaching)

Implementation
- Begin treatment in hospital
- Remove other antiarrhythmics before starting propafenone
- Adjust dosage q3-4days, no sooner

Patient/family education
- Advise patient to avoid hazardous activities until response is known
- Advise patient to report fever, chills, sore throat, bleeding, shortness of breath, chest pain, palpitations, blurred vision
- Advise patient to take medication with food
- Advise patient to carry emergency ID identifying medication and prescriber

Evaluation
Positive therapeutic outcome
- Absence of dysrhythmias

Treatment of overdose: O_2, artificial ventilation, defibrillation ECG; administer DOPamine for circulatory depression, diazepam or thiopental for convulsions, isoproterenol

P

propantheline (Rx)
(proe-pan'the-leen)

Pro-Banthine, Propanthel ✦

Func. class.: GI anticholinergic; antiulcer agent
Chem. class.: Synthetic quaternary ammonium compound

Pregnancy category C

Action: Inhibits muscarinic actions of acetylcholine at postganglionic parasympathetic neuroeffector sites

Therapeutic Outcome: Absence of peptic ulcer disease symptoms

Uses: Treatment of peptic ulcer disease, irritable bowel syndrome, duodenography, urinary incontinence

Investigational uses: Antispasmodic uses

Dosage and routes

Adult: PO 15 mg tid ac, 30 mg at bedtime
Elderly/small patients: PO 7.5 mg tid ac
Child: 0.375 mg/kg (10 mg/m^2) qid

Available forms: Tabs 7.5, 15 mg

Adverse effects

CNS: ***Confusion, stimulation in elderly,*** headache, insomnia, dizziness, drowsiness, anxiety, weakness, hallucinations
CV: Palpitations, tachycardia, orthostatic hypotension (elderly)
EENT: ***Blurred vision,*** photophobia, mydriasis, cycloplegia, increased ocular tension
GI: ***Dry mouth, constipation,*** **paralytic ileus,** heartburn, nausea, vomiting, dysphagia, absence of taste
GU: Hesitancy, retention, impotence
INTEG: Urticaria, rash, pruritus, anhidrosis, fever, allergic reactions

Contraindications: Hypersensitivity to anticholinergics, narrow-angle glaucoma, GI obstruction, myasthenia gravis, paralytic ileus, GI atony, toxic megacolon

Precautions: Pregnancy **C**, hyperthyroidism, CAD, dysrhythmias, CHF, ulcerative colitis, hypertension, hiatal hernia, hepatic disease, renal disease, urinary retention, prostatic hypertrophy, elderly

Pharmacokinetics	
Absorption	Moderately absorbed
Distribution	Unknown
Metabolism	Unknown
Excretion	Unknown
Half-life	Unknown

Pharmacodynamics	
Onset	½ hr
Peak	2-6 hr
Duration	4-6 hr

Interactions

Individual drugs

Amantadine: increased anticholinergic effect
Ketoconazole, levodopa: decreased effects of each drug

Drug classifications

Antidepressants (tricyclic), H_1-antihistamines, MAOIs: increased anticholinergic effect
Phenothiazines: decreased effects

Drug/herb

Henbane, jimsonweed, scopolia: increased anticholinergic effect

NURSING CONSIDERATIONS

Assessment

- Assess for the pain of peptic ulcer disease before, during, and after treatment

Nursing diagnoses

- Pain, chronic (uses)
- Constipation (adverse reactions)
- Thought processes, disturbed (adverse reactions)
- Knowledge, deficient (teaching)

Implementation

- Give 30 min ac and at bedtime; do not give with antacids; separate by at least 1 hr

Patient/family education

- Teach patient to report blurred vision, chest pain, allergic reactions
- Advise patient not to perform strenuous activity in high temp; heat stroke may result due to decreased perspiration
- Instruct patient to take as prescribed; not to skip doses
- Instruct patient to report change in vision; blurring or loss of sight; drug should be discontinued
- Advise patient not to operate machinery or drive if dizziness occurs
- Caution patient not to take OTC products without approval of prescriber

Evaluation

Positive therapeutic outcome

- Decreased pain in peptic ulcer disease

! HIGH ALERT

propofol (Rx)

(pro′poh-fole)

Diprivan, Disoprofol

Func. class.: General anesthetic

Pregnancy category B

Action: Produces dose-dependent CNS depression; action is unknown

Therapeutic Outcome: Induction of anesthesia

Uses: Induction or maintenance of anesthesia as part of balanced anesthetic technique; sedation in mechanically ventilated patients

Dosage and routes

Induction

Adult: **IV** 2-2.5 mg/kg, approximately 40 mg q10 sec until induction onset

Child 3-16 yr: **IV** 2.5-3.5 mg/kg over 20-30 sec

Elderly: **IV** 1-1.5 mg/kg, approximately 20 mg q10 sec until induction onset

Maintenance

Adult: **IV** 0.1-0.2 mg/kg/min (6-12 mg/kg/hr)

Child ≥3 yr: **IV** 0.125-0.3 mg/kg/min (7.5-18 mg/kg/hr)

Elderly: **IV** 0.05-0.1 mg/kg/min (3-6 mg/kg/hr)

ICU sedation

Adult: **IV** 5 mcg/kg/min over 5 min; may give 5-10 mcg/kg/min over 5-10 min until desired response

Available forms: Inj 10 mg/ml in 20 ml ampule, 50 ml and 100 ml vials

Adverse effects

CNS: Involuntary movement, headache, jerking, fever, dizziness, shivering, tremor, confusion, somnolence, paresthesia, agitation, abnormal dreams, euphoria, fatigue, **increased ICP, impaired cerebral flow, seizures**

CV: *Bradycardia, hypotension*, hypertension, PVC, PAC, tachycardia, abnormal ECG, ST segment depression, **asystole**

EENT: Blurred vision, tinnitus, eye pain, strange taste, diplopia

GI: *Nausea, vomiting, abdominal cramping*, dry mouth, swallowing, hypersalivation, **pancreatitis**

GU: Urine retention, green urine, cloudy urine, oliguria

INTEG: *Flushing, phlebitis, hives, burning/stinging at inj site*, rash, pain of extremities

MS: Myalgia

RESP: **Apnea**, *cough, hiccups*, dyspnea, hypoventilation, sneezing, wheezing, tachypnea, hypoxia

Contraindications: Hypersensitivity to drug or soybean oil, egg; hyperlipidemia

Precautions: Pregnancy **B**, elderly, respiratory depression, severe respiratory disorders, cardiac dysrhythmias, labor and delivery, lactation, children

Pharmacokinetics

Absorption	Completely
Distribution	Rapid
Metabolism	Liver, conjugation to active metabolites
Excretion	Urine
Half-life	1-8 min, terminal 5-10 hr

Pharmacodynamics

Onset	15-30 sec
Peak	Unknown
Duration	Unknown

Interactions

Drug classifications

CNS depressants (sedative/hypnotics, opioid analgesics): increased CNS depression

IV fat emulsions: increased hypertriglyceridemia risk

NURSING CONSIDERATIONS

Assessment

- Assess inj site: phlebitis, burning, stinging
- Monitor ECG for changes: PVC, PAC, ST segment changes; monitor VS
- Assess CNS changes: movement, jerking, tremors, dizziness, LOC, pupil reaction
- Assess allergic reactions: hives
- Assess respiratory dysfunction: respiratory depression, character, rate, rhythm; notify prescriber if respirations are <10/min

Nursing diagnoses

- Injury, risk for (adverse reactions)
- Breathing pattern, ineffective (adverse reactions)
- Knowledge, deficient (teaching)

Implementation

- Shake well before use; if diluted, use only D_5W to not less than 2 mg/ml; give over 3-5 min, titrate to needed level of sedation; use only glass containers when mixing, not stable in plastic
- May be given by cont inf; give by inf pump
- Give only with resuscitative equipment available
- Give only by qualified persons trained in anesthesia
- Store in light-resistant area at room temperature; use within 6 hr of opening
- If transferred from original container to another container, complete infusion within 12 hr

Y-site compatibilities: Acyclovir, alfentanil, aminophylline, ampicillin, aztreonam, bumetanide, buprenorphine, butorphanol, calcium gluconate, carboplatin, cefazolin, cefoperazone, cefotaxime, cefotetan, cefoxitin, ceftizoxime, ceftriaxone, cefuroxime, chlorproMAZINE, cimetidine, cisplatin, clindamycin, cyclophosphamide, cycloSPORINE, cytarabine, dexamethasone, diphenhydrAMINE, DOBUTamine, DOPamine, doxycycline, droperidol, enalaprilat, epHEDrine, epINEPHrine, esmolol, famotidine, fentanyl, fluconazole, fluorouracil, furosemide, ganciclovir, glycopyrrolate, granisetron, haloperidol, heparin, hydrocortisone, hydromorphone, hydrOXYzine, ifosfamide, imipenem/cilastatin, inamrinone, insulin (regular), isoproterenol, ketamine, labetalol, levorphanol, lidocaine, lorazepam, magnesium sulfate, mannitol, meperidine, mezlocillin, miconazole, morphine, nafcillin, nalbuphine, naloxone, nitroglycerin, norepinephrine, ofloxacin, paclitaxel, pentobarbital, phenobarbital, piperacillin, potassium chloride, prochlorperazine, propranolol, ranitidine, scopolamine, sodium bicarbonate, sodium nitroprusside, succinylcholine, sufentanil, thiopental, ticarcillin, ticarcillin/clavulanate, vecuronium, verapamil

Solution compatibilities: D_5W, D_5LR, LR, D_5/0.45% NaCl, D_5/0.2% NaCl

Patient/family education

- Teach patient that this medication will cause dizziness, drowsiness, sedation

Evaluation

Positive therapeutic outcome

- Induction of anesthesia

Treatment of overdose: Discontinue drug; administer vasopressor agents or anticholinergics, artificial ventilation

! HIGH ALERT

propoxyphene (Rx)

(proe-pox'i-feen)

Darvon, Darvon-N, Dolene, Novapropoxyn ✦

Func. class.: Opiate analgesics
Chem. class.: Synthetic opiate

Pregnancy category C

Controlled substance schedule IV

Action: Depresses pain impulse transmission at the spinal cord level by interacting with opioid receptors

Therapeutic Outcome: Decreased pain

Uses: Mild to moderate pain

Dosage and routes

Adult: PO 65 mg q4h prn (HCl)

Adult: PO 100 mg q4h prn (napsylate)

Available forms: Propoxyphene HCl: caps 32, 65 mg; propoxyphene napsylate: tabs 100 mg; oral susp 50 mg/5 ml

Adverse effects

CNS: *Drowsiness, dizziness, confusion, headache, sedation,* euphoria, **seizures, hyperthermia** (elderly)
CV: Palpitations, bradycardia, change in B/P, **dysrhythmias**
EENT: Tinnitus, blurred vision, miosis, diplopia
GI: *Nausea, vomiting, anorexia, constipation, cramps*
GU: Urinary retention, dysuria
INTEG: *Rash,* urticaria, bruising, flushing, diaphoresis, pruritus
RESP: **Respiratory depression**

Contraindications: Hypersensitivity to acetylsalicylic acid products (some preparations), addiction (opioid)

Precautions: Pregnancy **C**, addictive personality, lactation, increased ICP, MI (acute), severe heart disease, respiratory depression, hepatic disease, renal disease, child <18 yr, elderly

Pharmacokinetics	
Absorption	Well absorbed
Distribution	Widely distributed; crosses placenta
Metabolism	Liver, extensively
Excretion	Kidneys, breast milk
Half-life	6-12 hr

Pharmacodynamics	
Onset	½-1 hr
Peak	2-2½ hr
Duration	4-6 hr

Interactions

Individual drugs

Alcohol: possible fatal reactions
Nalbuphine, pentazocine: decreased analgesia

Drug classifications

Antipsychotics, CNS depressants, opioids, sedative/hypnotics, skeletal muscle relaxants: increased effects
MAOIs: possible fatal reactions

Drug/herb

Chamomile, hops, kava, Jamaican dogwood, lavender, mistletoe, nettle, pokeweed, poppy, senega, skullcap, valerian: increased CNS depression
Corkwood: increased anticholinergic effects

Drug/lab test

Increased: amylase

NURSING CONSIDERATIONS
Assessment
- Assess pain: location, duration, intensity before and 1 hr after administration
- Monitor CNS changes: dizziness, drowsiness, euphoria, LOC, pupil reaction
- Monitor allergic reactions: rash, urticaria

Nursing diagnoses
- Pain, acute (uses)
- Sensory perception, disturbed: visual, auditory (adverse reactions)
- Breathing pattern, ineffective (adverse reactions)
- Injury, risk for (adverse reactions)
- Knowledge, deficient (teaching)

Implementation
- Give with antiemetic if nausea, vomiting occur
- Give when pain is beginning to return; determine dosage interval by patient response; continuous dosing of medication is more effective than when given prn
- Withdraw medication slowly after long-term use to prevent withdrawal symptoms
- Store in light-resistant container at room temp
- May be given with food or milk to lessen GI upset

Patient/family education
- Teach patient to avoid CNS depressants: alcohol, sedative/hypnotics for at least 24 hr after taking this drug
- Discuss with patient that dizziness, drowsiness, and confusion are common; to avoid getting up without assistance
- Discuss in detail all aspects of the drug, including purpose and what to expect after anesthesia
- Advise patient to make position changes slowly to lessen orthostatic hypotension

Evaluation
Positive therapeutic outcome
- Decreased pain

Treatment of overdose: Naloxone 0.2-0.8 mg **IV**, O_2, **IV** fluids, vasopressors

propranolol (Rx)
(proe-pran'oh-lole)

Apo-Propranolol ✦, Betaclinron E-R ✦, Detensol ✦, Inderal, Inderal LA, NovoPranol ✦, PMS-Propranol, propranolol HCl

Func. class.: Antihypertensive, antianginal, antidysrhythmic (class III)

Chem. class.: β-Adrenergic blocker

Pregnancy category C

Do Not Confuse:
Inderal/Toradol, Inderal LA/IMDUR

Action: Competitively blocks stimulation of β-adrenergic receptor within vascular smooth muscle; produces chronotropic, inotropic activity (decreases rate of SA node discharge, increases recovery time), slows conduction of AV node, decreased heart rate, which decreases O_2 consumption in myocardium; also suppresses renin-aldosterone-angiotensin system at high doses, inhibits β_2-receptors in bronchial system (high doses)

Therapeutic Outcome: Decreased B/P, heart rate

Uses: Chronic stable angina pectoris, hypertension, supraventricular dysrhythmias, migraine prophylaxis, MI, pheochromocytoma, essential tremor, cyanotic spells related to hypertrophic subaortic stenosis

Investigational uses: Parkinson's tremor, prevention of variceal bleeding caused by portal hypertension, akathisia induced by antipsychotics, anxiety

Dosage and routes
Dysrhythmias

Adult: PO 10-30 mg tid-qid; **IV** bol 0.5-3 mg given 1 mg/min; may repeat in 2 min; may repeat q4h thereafter

Child: PO 0.5-1 mg/kg/day divided in 2 doses, **IV** 0.01-0.1 mg/kg over 5 min

Hypertension

Adult: PO 40 mg bid or 80 mg daily (sus rel) initially; usual dosage 120-240 mg/day bid-tid or 120-160 mg daily (sus rel)

Child: PO 0.5-1 mg/kg/day divided q6-12h

Angina

Adult: PO 80-320 mg in divided doses bid-qid or 80 mg daily (sus rel); usual dosage 160 mg daily (sus rel)

MI prophylaxis

Adult: PO 180-240 mg/day tid-qid starting 5 days to 3 wk after MI

P

Pheochromocytoma

Adult: PO 60 mg/day × 3 days preoperatively in divided doses or 30 mg/day in divided doses (inoperable tumor)

Migraine

Adult: PO 80 mg/day (sus rel) or in divided doses; may increase to 160-240 mg/day in divided doses

Child: PO 0.6-1.5 mg/kg/day divided q8h

Essential tremor

Adult: PO 40 mg bid; usual dosage 120 mg/day

Available forms: Sus rel caps 60, 80, 120, 160 mg; tabs 10, 20, 40, 60, 80, 90 mg; inj 1 mg/ml; oral sol 4 mg, 8 mg/ml; conc oral sol 80 mg/ml

Adverse effects

CNS: Depression, hallucinations, dizziness, fatigue, lethargy, paresthesia, bizarre dreams, disorientation

CV: **Bradycardia,** *hypotension,* **CHF,** palpitations, AV block, peripheral vascular insufficiency, vasodilatation, **pulmonary edema, dysrhythmias,** cold extremities

EENT: Sore throat, **laryngospasm,** blurred vision, dry eyes

GI: Nausea, vomiting, diarrhea, colitis, constipation, cramps, dry mouth, hepatomegaly, gastric pain, acute pancreatitis

GU: Impotence, decreased libido, UTIs

HEMA: **Agranulocytosis, thrombocytopenia**

INTEG: Rash, pruritus, fever

META: Hyperglycemia, hypoglycemia

MISC: Facial swelling, weight change, Raynaud's phenomenon

MS: Joint pain, arthralgia, muscle cramps, pain

RESP: Dyspnea, respiratory dysfunction, **bronchospasm,** cough

Contraindications: Hypersensitivity to this drug, cardiac failure, cardiogenic shock, 2nd- or 3rd-degree heart block, bronchospastic disease, sinus bradycardia, CHF, bronchospasm

Precautions: Pregnancy **C,** diabetes mellitus, renal disease, lactation, hyperthyroidism, COPD, hepatic disease, children, myasthenia gravis, peripheral vascular disease, hypotension, CHF

Pharmacokinetics

Absorption	Well absorbed (PO); slowly absorbed (ext rel); completely absorbed **(IV)**
Distribution	Widely distributed; crosses blood-brain barrier, protein binding 90%
Metabolism	Liver, extensively
Excretion	Kidneys
Half-life	3-5 hr; EXT REL 8-11 hr

Pharmacodynamics

	PO	PO–EXT REL	IV
Onset	½ hr	Unknown	Rapid
Peak	1-1½ hr	6 hr	1 min
Duration	6-12 hr	24 hr	4-6 hr

Interactions

Individual drugs

Cimetidine: increased β-blocking effect

Disopyramide: increased negative inotropic effects

Haloperidol, prazosin, quinidine: increased hypotension

Smoking: decreased propranolol levels

Drug classifications

Barbiturates: decreased β-blocking effect

Calcium channel blockers: increased or decreased effect

Neuromuscular blockers: increased effects

Drug/herb

Aconite: increased toxicity, death

Astragalus, cola tree: increased or decreased antihypertensive effect

Barberry, betony, black catechu, black cohosh, bloodroot, broom, burdock, cat's claw, dandelion, goldenseal, Irish moss, Jamaican dogwood, kelp, khella, mistletoe, parsley: increased antihypertensive effect

Coltsfoot, guarana, khat, licorice: decreased antihypertensive effect

Drug/lab test

Increased: serum potassium, serum uric acid, AST, ALT, alkaline phosphatase, LDH

Decreased: blood glucose

Interference: glaucoma testing

NURSING CONSIDERATIONS

Assessment

- Monitor B/P during beginning treatment, periodically thereafter; pulse q4h; note rate, rhythm, quality; check apical/radial pulse before administration; notify prescriber of any significant changes (pulse <50 bpm)
- Check for baselines in renal, liver function tests before therapy begins and periodically thereafter
- Assess for edema in feet, legs daily; monitor

I&O, weight daily; check for jugular vein distention, crackles bilaterally; dyspnea (CHF)
- Monitor skin turgor, dryness of mucous membranes for hydration status, especially elderly

Nursing diagnoses
- Cardiac output, decreased (uses)
- Injury, risk for (adverse reactions)
- Knowledge, deficient (teaching)
- Noncompliance (teaching)

Implementation
PO route
- Do not break, crush, or chew sus rel cap
- Given ac, at bedtime, tab may be crushed or swallowed whole; give with food to prevent GI upset; reduce dosage in renal dysfunction
- May mix oral sol with liquid or semisolid food, rinse container to get entire dose
- Store protected from light, moisture; placed in cool environment

IV route
- Give by direct **IV** undiluted or diluted 1 mg/10 ml of D_5W for inj; administer over 1 min or more
- Give by intermittent inf after diluting in 50 ml of D_5W, 0.9% NaCl, D_5/0.45% NaCl, D_5/0.9% NaCl, LR; administer over 15 min

Y-site compatibilities: Amrinone, heparin, hydrocortisone, meperidine, milrinone, morphine, potassium chloride, tacrolimus, vit B/C
Y-site incompatibilities: Diazoxide
Additive compatibilities: DOBUTamine, verapamil
Solution compatibilities: 0.9% NaCl, 0.45% NaCl, Ringer's, D_5W, D_5/0.9% NaCl, D_5/0.45% NaCl

Patient/family education
- Teach patient not to discontinue drug abruptly, taper over 2 wk; may cause precipitate angina if stopped abruptly
- Teach patient not to use OTC products containing α-adrenergic stimulants (such as nasal decongestants, cold preparations); to avoid alcohol, smoking and to limit sodium intake as prescribed
- Teach patient how to take pulse and B/P at home; advise when to notify prescriber
- Instruct patient to comply with weight control, dietary adjustments, modified exercise program
- Instruct patient to carry/wear emergency ID to identify drug being taken, allergies; tell patient drug controls symptoms but does not cure
- Caution patient to avoid hazardous activities if dizziness, drowsiness is present
- Teach patient to report symptoms of CHF: difficult breathing, especially on exertion or when lying down, night cough, swelling of extremities or bradycardia, dizziness, confusion, depression, fever
- Teach patient to take drug as prescribed, not to double doses, skip doses; take any missed doses as soon as remembered if at least 8 hr until next dose
- Advise patient that sensitivity to cold may occur
- Teach patient to monitor blood glucose, may mask symptoms of hypoglycemia

Evaluation
Positive therapeutic outcome
- Decreased B/P in hypertension (after 1-2 wk)
- Decreased tremors
- Absence of dysrhythmias
- Decreased migraine headaches

Treatment of overdose: Lavage, **IV** atropine for bradycardia, **IV** theophylline for bronchospasm, digitalis, O_2, diuretic for cardiac failure, hemodialysis, **IV** glucose for hyperglycemia, **IV** diazepam (or phenytoin) for seizures

propylthiouracil (Rx)
(proe-pill-thye-oh-yoor'a-sill)
propylthiouracil, Propyl-Thyracil ♣, PTU
Func. class.: Thyroid hormone antagonist (antithyroid)
Chem. class.: Thioamide
Pregnancy category D

Action: Blocks synthesis peripherally of T_3, T_4, inhibits organification of iodine

Therapeutic Outcome: Decreased T_3, T_4 levels, hyperthyroid symptoms

Uses: Preparation for thyroidectomy, thyrotoxic crisis, hyperthyroidism, thyroid storm

Dosage and routes
Thyrotoxic crisis
Adult and child: PO same as hyperthyroidism with iodine and propranolol

Preparation for thyroidectomy
Adult: PO 600-1200 mg/day
Child: PO 10 mg/kg/day in divided doses

Hyperthyroidism
Adult: PO 100 mg tid increasing to 300 mg q8h if condition is severe; continue to euthyroid state, then 100 mg daily-tid
Child >10 yr: PO 100 mg tid; continue to euthyroid state, then 25 mg tid to 100 mg bid

Child 6-10 yr: PO 50-150 mg in divided doses q8h
Neonates: PO 10 mg/kg/day in divided doses

Available forms: Tabs 50, 100 mg

Adverse effects

CNS: *Drowsiness, headache, vertigo, fever,* paresthesias, neuritis
GI: *Nausea, diarrhea, vomiting, jaundice, hepatitis,* loss of taste
GU: **Nephritis**
HEMA: **Agranulocytosis, leukopenia, thrombocytopenia, hypothrombinemia, lymphadenopathy,** bleeding, vasculitis, periarteritis
INTEG: *Rash, urticaria, pruritus, alopecia, hyperpigmentation,* lupus-like syndrome
MS: Myalgia, arthralgia, nocturnal muscle cramps, osteoporosis

Contraindications: Pregnancy **D,** hypersensitivity, lactation

Precautions: Infection, bone marrow depression, hepatic disease

Pharmacokinetics

Absorption	Rapidly absorbed
Distribution	Crosses placenta; concentration in thyroid gland
Metabolism	Liver
Excretion	Urine, bile, breast milk
Half-life	1-2 hr

Pharmacodynamics

Onset	30-40 min
Peak	Unknown
Duration	2-4 hr

Interactions

Individual drugs

Heparin: increased anticoagulant effect
Lithium: increased antithyroid effect
Potassium/sodium iodide: increased effects
Radiation: increased bone marrow depression

Drug classifications

Anticoagulants (oral): increased anticoagulant effect
Antineoplastics: increased bone marrow depression
Phenothiazines: increased agranulocytosis

Drug/lab test

Increased: protime, AST, ALT, alkaline phosphatase

NURSING CONSIDERATIONS

Assessment

- Monitor pulse, B/P, temp; I&O ratio; check for edema (puffy hands, feet, periorbits); indicates hypothyroidism
- Check weight daily with same clothing, scale, time of day
- Monitor T_3, T_4, which are increased; check serum TSH, which is decreased; assess free thyroxine index, which is increased if dosage is too low; discontinue drug 3-4 wk before radioactive iodine uptake test
- Monitor blood work: CBC for blood dyscrasias (leukopenia, thrombocytopenia, agranulocytosis); liver function tests
- (Alert) Assess overdose (peripheral edema, heat intolerance, diaphoresis, palpitations, dysrhythmias, severe tachycardia, increased temp, delirium, CNS irritability); drug should be discontinued
- Assess for hypersensitivity (rash, enlarged cervical lymph nodes); drug may have to be discontinued
- Assess for hypoprothrombinemia (bleeding, petechiae, ecchymosis)
- Monitor clinical response: after 3 wk should include increased weight, decreased pulse, decreased T_4
- Assess for bone marrow depression: sore throat, fever, fatigue

Nursing diagnoses

- Knowledge, deficient (teaching)
- Noncompliance (teaching)

Implementation

- Give with meals to decrease GI upset
- Give at same time each day to maintain drug level
- Give lowest dosage that relieves symptoms
- Store in light-resistant container
- Increase fluids to 3-4 L/day, unless contraindicated

Patient/family education

- Advise patient to abstain from breastfeeding after delivery; drug appears in breast milk
- Teach patient to take pulse daily and to keep graph of weight, pulse, mood
- Advise patient to report redness, swelling, sore throat, mouth lesions, which indicate blood dyscrasias
- Caution patient to avoid OTC products that contain iodine; that seafood, other iodine-containing foods may be restricted by prescriber
- Caution patient not to discontinue this medication abruptly; thyroid crisis may occur; stress patient compliance

- Teach patient that response may take several mo if thyroid is large
- Teach patient symptoms/signs of overdose: periorbital edema, cold intolerance, mental depression; notify prescriber at once
- Teach patient symptoms of inadequate dose: tachycardia, diarrhea, fever, irritability; prescriber should be notified to adjust dosage
- Teach patient to take medication exactly as prescribed, not to skip or double doses; missed doses should be taken when remembered up to 1 hr before next dose
- Instruct patient to carry/wear emergency identification indicating medication taken and condition being treated

Evaluation

Positive therapeutic outcome

- Weight gain
- Decreased pulse
- Decreased T_4
- Decreased B/P

protamine (Rx)

(proe'ta-meen)

Func. class.: Heparin antagonist

Chem. class.: Low-molecular-weight protein

Pregnancy category C

Action: Binds heparin, making it ineffective

Therapeutic Outcome: Prevention of heparin overdose

Uses: Heparin overdose; neutralizes heparin in procedures

Dosage and routes

Adult and child: **IV** 1 mg of protamine/100 units of heparin given or 100 anti-XA units of LMWH; administer slowly over 1-3 min; not to exceed 50 mg/10 min

Available forms: Inj 10 mg/ml

Adverse effects

CNS: Lassitude

CV: Hypotension, bradycardia, **circulatory collapse**

GI: Nausea, vomiting, anorexia

HEMA: Bleeding

INTEG: ***Rash,*** dermatitis, urticaria

RESP: Dyspnea, **pulmonary edema, severe respiratory distress**

SYST: **Anaphylaxis, angioedema**

Contraindication: Hypersensitivity

Precautions: Pregnancy **C**, lactation, children, allergy to salmon, diabetes mellitus

Pharmacokinetics

Absorption	Completely absorbed
Distribution	Unknown
Metabolism	Unknown
Excretion	Unknown
Half-life	Unknown

Pharmacodynamics

Onset	5 min
Peak	Unknown
Duration	2 hr

Interactions: None known

NURSING CONSIDERATIONS

Assessment

- Monitor blood studies (Hct, platelets, occult blood stools) q3 mo
- Monitor coagulation tests (APTT, ACT) 15 min after dose, then in several hr
- Monitor VS, B/P, pulse q30 min, plus 3 hr after dose
- ❗ Assess for hypersensitivity: skin rash, urticaria, dermatitis, cough, wheezing, have emergency equipment nearby; men that have had a vasectomy may be more prone to hypersensitivity
- ❗ Assess for allergy to salmon; use with caution in these patients

Nursing diagnoses

- Injury, risk for (uses)
- Tissue perfusion, ineffective (uses)
- Knowledge, deficient (teaching)

Implementation

- Give by direct **IV** after diluting 50 mg/5 ml of sterile bacteriostatic water for inj; shake; give 20 mg or less over 1-3 min
- Give by intermittent inf after further diluting with equal volume of NaCl or D_5W and run over 2-3 hr; titrate to APTT, ACT; use infusion pump
- Store at 36-46° F (2-8° C)

Additive compatibilities: Cimetidine, ranitidine, verapamil

Additive incompatibilities: Penicillins, cephalosporins

Patient/family education

- Explain reason for medication and expected results
- Caution patient to avoid contact activities that may result in bleeding

Evaluation

Positive therapeutic outcome

- Reversal of heparin overdose

pseudoephedrine (OTC)

(soo-doe-e-fed'rin)

Afrin, Allermed, Canafed, Cenafed, Children's Congestion Relief, Children's Silfedrine, Congestion Relief, Decofed Syrup, DeFed-60, Dorcol Children's Decongestant, Drixoral Non-Drowsy Formula, Dynafed, Efidac/24, Eltor ✤, Genaphed, Halofed, Mini Thin Pseudo, Pedia Care Infant's Decongestant, pseudoepHEDrine HCl, Pseudo, Pseudogest, Seudotabs, Sinustop Pro, Sudafed, Sudafed 12 hour, Sudex, Triaminic AM Decongestant Formula

Func. class.: Adrenergic

Chem. class.: Substituted phenylethylamine

Pregnancy category C

Action: Primary activity through α-adrenergic effects on respiratory mucosal membranes reducing congestion, hyperemia, edema; minimal bronchodilatation secondary to β-adrenergic effects

Therapeutic Outcome: Decreased nasal congestion, swelling

Uses: Nasal decongestant, otitis media adjustment, adjunct with antihistamines

Dosage and routes

Adult and child >12 yr: PO 60 mg q6h; ext rel 120 mg q12h or 240 mg q24h

Elderly: PO 30-60 mg q6h prn

Child 6-12 yr: PO 30 mg q6h, max 120 mg/day

Child 2-6 yr: PO 15 mg q6h, max 60 mg/day

Available forms: Ext rel caps 120, 240 mg; oral sol 15 mg, 30 mg/5 ml; drops 7.5 mg/0.8 ml; tabs 30, 60 mg; caps 60 mg; ext rel tabs 120, 240 mg

Adverse effects

CNS: *Tremors, anxiety,* insomnia, headache, dizziness, hallucinations, **seizures** (elderly)

CV: Palpitations, tachycardia, hypertension, chest pain, **dysrhythmias, CV collapse**

EENT: Dry nose, irritation of nose and throat

GI: *Anorexia, nausea, vomiting,* dry mouth

GU: Dysuria

Contraindications: Hypersensitivity to sympathomimetics, narrow-angle glaucoma

Precautions: Pregnancy **C**, cardiac disorders, hyperthyroidism, diabetes mellitus, prostatic hypertrophy, lactation, hypertension

Pharmacokinetics

Absorption	Well absorbed
Distribution	Enters CSF, crosses placenta
Metabolism	Liver, partially
Excretion	Kidneys, unchanged (75%); breast milk
Half-life	7 hr

Pharmacodynamics

	PO	PO–EXT REL
Onset	15-30 min	1 hr
Peak	Unknown	Unknown
Duration	4-6 hr	12 hr

Interactions

Individual drugs

Methyldopa: decreased effect of pseudoephedrine

Drug classifications

Antidepressants (tricyclics), MAOIs: hypertensive crisis, do not use together

Rauwolfia alkaloids, urinary acidifiers: decreased effect of pseudoephedrine

Urinary alkalizers: increased effect of pseudoephedrine

NURSING CONSIDERATIONS

Assessment

- Assess for CNS side effects in the elderly: excitation, seizures, hallucinations
- Monitor for nasal congestion; auscultate lung sounds; check for tenacious bronchial secretions; children with otitis media should be assessed for eustachian tube congestion
- Monitor B/P and pulse throughout treatment

Nursing diagnoses

- Airway clearance, ineffective (uses)
- Knowledge, deficient (teaching)

Implementation

- Swallow tab and ext rel cap whole; do not break, crush, or chew
- Give several hr before bedtime if insomnia occurs
- Store at room temp

Patient/family education

- Teach patient reason for drug administration and expected results
- Instruct patient not to use continuously, or more than recommended dose; rebound congestion may occur
- Advise patient to check with prescriber before using other drugs, as drug interactions may occur
- Advise patient to avoid taking near bedtime; stimulation can occur
- Caution patient not to use if stimulation, restlessness, tremors occur

- Notify parents of possible excessive agitation in children
- Advise patient to notify prescriber of anxiety, slow or fast heart rate, dyspnea, seizures

Evaluation

Positive therapeutic outcome

- Decreased nasal congestion

psyllium (OTC)

(sill'i-um)

Alramucil, Fiberall, Fiberall Natural Flavor and Orange Flavor, Genifiber, Hydrocil Instant, Karacil ♣, Konsyl, Konsyl Orange, Maalox Daily Fiber Therapy, Metamucil, Metamucil Lemon Lime, Metamucil Orange Flavor, Metamucil Sugar Free, Metamucil Sugar Free Orange Flavor, Modane Bulk, Mylanta Natural Fiber Supplement, Natural Fiber Laxative, Natural Fiber Laxative Sugar Free, Natural Vegetable Reguloid, Perdiem, Prodiem Plain ♣, Reguloid Natural, Reguloid Orange, Reguloid Sugar Free Orange, Reguloid Sugar Free Regular, Restore, Restore Sugar Free, Serutan, Syllact, V-Lax

Func. class.: Laxative, bulk-forming
Chem. class.: Psyllium colloid

Pregnancy category C

Action: Promotes peristalsis by combining with water in the intestine to form a gel-like substance that is easily evacuated

Therapeutic Outcome: Decreased constipation, decreased diarrhea in colitis

Uses: Chronic constipation, ulcerative colitis, irritable bowel syndrome

Dosage and routes

Adult: PO 1-2 tsp in 8 oz of water bid or tid, then 8 oz of water or 1 premeasured packet in 8 oz of water bid or tid, then 8 oz of water

Child >6 yr: 1 tsp in 4 oz of water at bedtime

Available forms: Chew pieces 1.7, 3.4 g/piece; powder effervescent 3.4, 3.7 g/packet; granules 2.5, 4.03 g/tsp; powder 3.3, 3.4, 3.5, 4.94 g/tsp; wafers 3.4 g/wafer

Adverse effects

GI: *Nausea, vomiting, anorexia, diarrhea,* cramps, intestinal/esophageal blockage

Contraindications: Hypersensitivity, intestinal obstruction, abdominal pain, nausea/vomiting, fecal impaction

Precautions: Pregnancy **C**

Pharmacokinetics

Absorption	None
Distribution	None
Excretion	Feces
Half-life	Unknown

Pharmacodynamics

Onset	12-24 hr
Peak	2-4 days
Duration	Unknown

Interactions

Drug classifications

Cardiac glycosides, oral anticoagulants, salicylates: decreased absorption of each specific drug

Drug/herb

Flax, senna: increased laxative

NURSING CONSIDERATIONS

Assessment

- Monitor blood, urine electrolytes if used often by patient; check I&O ratio to identify fluid loss
- Assess for cramping, rectal bleeding, nausea, vomiting; if these symptoms occur, drug should be discontinued; identify cause of constipation; identify whether fluids, bulk, or exercise is missing from lifestyle
- Assess stool for color, consistency, amount, presence of flatulence

Nursing diagnoses

- Constipation (uses)
- Knowledge, deficient (teaching)
- Noncompliance (teaching)

Implementation

- Give alone for better absorption; give after mixing with water immediately before use; administer with 8 oz of water or juice followed by another 8 oz of fluid
- Administer in AM or PM (oral dose)
- Shake susp well

Patient/family education

- Discuss with patient that adequate fluid consumption is necessary
- Teach patient that normal bowel movements do not always occur daily
- Caution patient not to use in presence of abdominal pain, nausea, vomiting; tell patient to notify prescriber if constipation is unrelieved or if symptoms of electrolyte imbalance occur (muscle cramps, pain, weakness, dizziness, excessive thirst)
- Teach patient not to use laxatives for long-term therapy; bowel tone will be lost and will decrease

P

- Teach patient not to take at bedtime as a laxative; may interfere with sleep; also problems with lipid pneumonia
- Teach patient not to use with food or vitamin preparations; delays digestion and absorption of fat-soluble vitamins

Evaluation

Positive therapeutic outcome

- Decreased constipation in 12-24 hr

pyrazinamide (Rx)

(peer-a-zin'a-mide)

PMS Pyrazinamide ✤, pyrazinamide, Tebrazid ✤

Func. class.: Antitubercular agent

Chem. class.: Pyrazinoic acid amine/nicoturimide analog

Pregnancy category C

Action: Bactericidal interference with lipid; nucleic acid biosynthesis is possible

Therapeutic Outcome: Bactericidal for *Mycobacterium* species

Uses: Tuberculosis, as an adjunct when other drugs are not feasible

Dosage and routes

Adult and child: PO 15-30 mg/kg daily, max 2 g/day

Available forms: Tabs 500 mg

Adverse effects

CNS: Headache

GI: **Hepatotoxicity,** abnormal liver function tests, peptic ulcer, nausea, vomiting, anorexia, cramps, diarrhea

GU: Urinary difficulty, increased uric acid

HEMA: **Hemolytic anemia**

INTEG: Photosensitivity, urticaria

Contraindications: Hypersensitivity, severe hepatic damage, acute gout

Precautions: Pregnancy **C,** child <13 yr, renal failure, diabetes, porphyria, chronic gout

Pharmacokinetics	
Absorption	Well absorbed
Distribution	Widely distributed
Metabolism	Liver, extensively
Excretion	Kidneys, breast milk
Half-life	9-10 hr

Pharmacodynamics	
Onset	Unknown
Peak	2 hr
Duration	9½ hr; metabolites 12 hr

Interactions: None known

Drug/lab test

Increased: PBI

Decreased: 17-KS

NURSING CONSIDERATIONS

Assessment

- C&S studies should be done before treatment begins, and periodically during treatment
- Monitor serum uric acid, which may be elevated and cause gout symptoms
- Monitor liver studies weekly: ALT, AST, bilirubin; hepatic status: decreased appetite, jaundice, dark urine, fatigue
- Monitor renal status before treatment and monthly thereafter: BUN, creatinine, output, sp gr, urinalysis, uric acid
- Monitor mental status often: affect, mood, behavioral changes; psychosis may occur

Nursing diagnoses

- Infection, risk for (uses)
- Diarrhea (adverse reactions)
- Injury, risk for (adverse reactions)
- Knowledge, deficient (teaching)
- Noncompliance (teaching)

Implementation

- Give with meals to decrease GI symptoms
- Give antiemetic if vomiting occurs
- May be given with other antitubercular drugs

Patient/family education

- Instruct patient that compliance with dosage schedule, duration is necessary; that scheduled appointments must be kept or relapse may occur
- Advise diabetic patient to use blood glucose monitor to obtain correct result
- Advise patient to report weakness, fatigue, loss of appetite, nausea, vomiting, yellowing of skin or eyes, tingling/numbness of hands/feet

Evaluation

Positive therapeutic outcome

- Decreased symptoms of TB
- Sputum culture negative × 3

pyridostigmine (Rx)

(peer-id-oh-stig'meen)

Mestinon, Mestinon SR, Mestinon Timespan, Regonol

Func. class.: Cholinergic, anticholinesterase

Chem. class.: Tertiary amine carbamate

Pregnancy category C

Action: Inhibits destruction of acetylcholine, which increases concentration at sites where acetylcholine is released; this facilitates transmission of impulses across myoneural junction

Therapeutic Outcome: Decreased action of nondepolarizing muscle relaxant; increased muscle strength in myasthenia gravis

Uses: Nondepolarizing muscle relaxant antagonist, myasthenia gravis

Dosage and routes

Myasthenia gravis

Adult: PO 60-180 mg bid-qid, not to exceed 1.5 g/day; IM/**IV** 2 mg or 1/30 of PO dose; sus rel 180-540 mg daily or bid at intervals of at least 6 hr

Child: 7 mg/kg/day in 5-6 divided doses

Nondepolarizing neuromuscular blocker antagonist

Adult: 0.6-1.2 mg **IV** atropine, then 10-30 mg

Child: 0.1-0.25 mg/kg/dose

Available forms: Tabs 60 mg; ext rel tabs 180 mg; syr 60 mg/5 ml; inj 5 mg/ml

Adverse effects

CNS: Dizziness, headache, sweating, weakness, **seizures,** uncoordination, paralysis, drowsiness, LOC

CV: Tachycardia, dysrhythmias, bradycardia, AV block, hypotension, ECG changes, **cardiac arrest,** syncope

EENT: Miosis, blurred vision, lacrimation, visual changes

GI: *Nausea, diarrhea, vomiting, cramps, increased salivary and gastric secretions, peristalsis*

GU: Frequency, incontinence, urgency

INTEG: Rash, urticaria, flushing

RESP: **Respiratory depression, bronchospasm, constriction, laryngospasm, respiratory arrest**

Contraindications: Bradycardia, hypotension, obstruction of intestine, renal system, bromide sensitivity

Precautions: Pregnancy **C,** seizure disorders, bronchial asthma, coronary occlusion, hyperthyroidism, dysrhythmias, peptic ulcer, megacolon, poor GI motility

Pharmacokinetics

Absorption	Poorly absorbed (PO)
Distribution	Widely distributed; crosses placenta
Metabolism	Liver, plasma cholinesterase
Excretion	Kidneys
Half-life	2 hr (**IV**); 4 hr (PO)

Pharmacodynamics

	PO	IM/IV	PO–EXT REL
Onset	20-30 min	2-15 min	½-1 hr
Peak	Unknown	Unknown	Unknown
Duration	3-6 hr	2-4 hr	3-6 hr

Interactions

Individual drugs

Atropine, gallamine, metocurine, pancuronium, tubocurarine: decreased action

Decamethonium, succinylcholine: increased action of pyridostigmine

Magnesium, mecamylamine, polymyxin, procainamide, quinidine: decreased action of pyridostigmine

Drug classifications

Aminoglycosides, anesthetics, antidysrhythmics, corticosteroids: decreased action of pyridostigmine

Drug/herb

Jaborandi tree, pill-bearing spurge: increased effect

NURSING CONSIDERATIONS

Assessment

- Monitor VS, respiration; increased B/P during test and at baseline
- Monitor diabetic patient carefully, since this drug lowers blood glucose

Nursing diagnoses

- Breathing pattern, ineffective (uses)
- Knowledge, deficient (teaching)

Implementation

PO route

- Give only after all other cholinergics have been discontinued
- Give increased doses as ordered if tolerance occurs
- Give larger doses as ordered after exercise or fatigue
- Give on empty stomach for better absorption
- Store at room temp

IV route

- Give **IV** undiluted, give through Y-tube or 3-way stopcock; give 0.5 mg or less/min
- Give only when atropine sulfate available for cholinergic crisis

Syringe compatibilities: Glycopyrrolate

Y-site compatibilities: Heparin, hydrocortisone, potassium chloride, vit B/C

Patient/family education

- Advise patient to carry/wear emergency ID specifying myasthenia gravis, drugs taken

P

Evaluation

Positive therapeutic outcome
- Increased muscle strength, hand grasp
- Improved gait
- Absence of labored breathing (if severe)

Treatment of overdose: Discontinue drug, atropine 1-4 mg **IV**

pyridoxine (vitamin B_6) (OTC, Rx)

(peer-i-dox'een)

Beesix, Doxine, Nestrex, pyridoxine HCl, Pyri, Rodex, Vitabee 6, Vitamin B_6

Func. class.: Vitamin B_6, water soluble

Pregnancy category A

Action: Needed for fat, protein, carbohydrate metabolism; enhances glycogen release from liver and muscle tissue; needed as coenzyme for metabolic transformations of a variety of amino acids

Therapeutic Outcome: Absence of vit B_6 deficiency

Uses: Vitamin B_6 deficiency associated with the following: inborn errors of metabolism, seizures, cycloSERINE, hydrALAZINE penicillamine, isoniazid therapy, oral contraceptives, alcoholism, polyneuritis

Investigational uses: Palmar-plantar erythrodysesthesia syndrome

Dosage and routes

RDA

Adult: PO male 1.7-2 mg; female 1.4-1.6 mg

Vitamin B_6 deficiency

Adult: PO/IM/**IV** 5-25 mg daily × 3 wk

Child: PO/IM/**IV** 100 mg until desired response

Deficiency caused by isoniazid, cycloSERINE, hydrALAZINE, penicillamine

Adult: PO 6-100 mg daily

Child: PO 5-25 mg/day

Prevention of deficiency caused by isoniazid, cycloSERINE, hydrALAZINE, penicillamine

Adult: PO 6-50 mg daily

Child: PO 0.5-1.5 mg daly

Infant: PO 0.1-0.5 mg daily

Palmar-plantar erythrodysesthesia syndrome (off-label)

Adult: PO 50-150 mg daily

Available forms: Tabs 10, 25, 50, 100 mg; ext rel tabs 100 mg; inj 100 mg/ml; ext rel caps 150 mg

Adverse effects

CNS: Paresthesia, flushing, warmth, lethargy (rare with normal renal function)

INTEG: Pain at inj site

Contraindication: Hypersensitivity

Precautions: Pregnancy **A**, lactation, children, Parkinson's disease, patients taking levodopa should avoid supplemental vitamins with >5 mg pyridoxine

Pharmacokinetics

Absorption	Well absorbed (PO)
Distribution	Stored in liver, muscle, brain; crosses placenta
Metabolism	Unknown
Excretion	Kidneys, unchanged (not used)
Half-life	Unknown

Pharmacodynamics

Unknown

Interactions

Individual drugs

Chloramphenicol, cycloSERINE, hydrALAZINE, isoniazid, penicillamine: decreased effects of pyridoxine

Levodopa: decreased effects of levodopa

Drug classifications

Contraceptives (oral), immunosuppressants: decreased effects of pyridoxine

NURSING CONSIDERATIONS

Assessment
- Monitor pyridoxine levels throughout treatment
- Assess nutritional status: yeast, liver, legumes, bananas, green vegetables, whole grains
- Assess for pyridoxine (B_6) deficiency: nausea, vomiting, dermatitis, cheilosis, seizures, irritability, dermatitis before and during treatment

Nursing diagnoses
- Nutrition: less than body requirements, imbalanced (uses)
- Knowledge, deficient (teaching)
- Noncompliance (teaching, overuse)

Implementation

PO route
- Swallow ext rel cap and ext rel tabs whole; do not break, crush, or chew

IM route
- Rotate sites to avoid pain; burning or

stinging at site may occur; give by Z-track to minimize pain

- Store in airtight, light-resistant container

IV route

- Give **IV** undiluted or added to most **IV** sol; give 50 mg or less/1 min if undiluted

Syringe compatibilities:
Doxapram

Additive incompatibilities:
Erythromycin, iron salts, kanamycin, riboflavin, streptomycin

Patient/family education

- Teach patient to avoid other vitamin supplements unless directed by prescriber
- Advise patient to increase meat, bananas, potatoes, lima beans, whole grain cereals in diet which are high in vit B_6
- Caution patient not to increase dosage, since serious reactions may occur

Evaluation

Positive therapeutic outcome

- Absence of nausea, vomiting, anorexia, skin lesions, glossitis, stomatitis, edema, seizures, restlessness, paresthesia

pyrimethamine (Rx)

(peer-i-meth'a-meen)

Daraprim, Fansidar (with sulfadoxine)

Func. class.: Antimalarial, antiprotozoal

Chem. class.: Folic acid antagonist

Pregnancy category C

Action: Inhibits folic acid metabolism in parasite; prevents transmission by stopping growth of fertilized gametes

Therapeutic Outcome: Prevention of malaria

Uses: Malaria prophylaxis, antiprotozoal action against *Plasmodium vivax*

Investigational uses: *Pneumocystis jiroveci* pneumonia as an adjunct

Dosage and routes

Prophylaxis of malaria

Adult and child >10 yr: PO 25 mg qwk

Child 4-10 yr: PO 12.5 mg qwk

Child <4 yr: PO 6.25 mg qwk

Toxoplasmosis

Adult: PO 100 mg, then 25 mg daily × 4-5 wk, with 1 g sulfADIAZINE q6h

Child: PO 1 mg/kg/day in 2 divided doses or 2 mg/kg/day × 3 days, then 1 mg/kg/day or divided twice daily × 4 wk, max 25 mg/day

Toxoplasmosis in AIDS patients

Adult: PO 100-200 mg/day × 1-2 days, then 50-100 mg/day × 3-6 wk, then 25-50 mg/day for life (given with clindamycin or sulfADIAZINE)

Available forms: Tabs 25 mg; combo tabs 500 mg sulfadoxine/25 mg pyrimethamine

Adverse effects

CNS: Stimulation, irritability, **seizures,** tremors, ataxia, fatigue

CV: **Dysrhythmias**

GI: *Nausea, vomiting, cramps, anorexia,* diarrhea, atrophic glossitis, gastritis

HEMA: **Thrombocytopenia, leukopenia, pancytopenia, megaloblastic anemia,** decreased folic acid, **agranulocytosis**

INTEG: Skin eruptions, photosensitivity

RESP: **Respiratory failure**

Contraindications: Hypersensitivity, chloroquine-resistant malaria, megaloblastic anemia caused by folate deficiency

Precautions: Pregnancy **C**, blood dyscrasias, seizure disorder, lactation, glucose-6-phosphate dehydrogenase disease, renal/hepatic disease

Pharmacokinetics	
Absorption	Well absorbed
Distribution	Widely; crosses placenta
Metabolism	Liver, extensively
Excretion	Kidneys, unchanged (30%); breast milk
Half-life	4 days

Pharmacodynamics	
Onset	Unknown
Peak	2 hr
Duration	Unknown

Interactions

Individual drugs

Folic acid: increased synergistic action

Radiation: increased bone marrow suppression

Drug classifications

Bone marrow depressants: increased bone marrow suppression

NURSING CONSIDERATIONS

Assessment

- C&S studies should be done before treatment begins and periodically during treatment
- Monitor serum uric acid, which may be elevated and cause gout symptoms
- Monitor liver studies weekly: ALT, AST, bilirubin; hepatic status: decreased appetite, jaundice, dark urine, fatigue

P

• Monitor renal status before therapy and monthly thereafter: BUN, creatinine, output, sp gr, urinalysis
• Monitor mental status often: affect, mood, behavioral changes; psychosis may occur

Nursing diagnoses
• Infection, risk for (uses)
• Diarrhea (adverse reactions)
• Injury, risk for (adverse reactions)
• Knowledge, deficient (teaching)
• Noncompliance (teaching)

Implementation
• Give with meals to decrease GI symptoms
• Give antiemetic if vomiting occurs

Patient/family education
• Instruct patient that compliance with dosage schedule, duration is necessary; that scheduled appointments must be kept or relapse may occur
• Advise diabetic patient to use blood glucose monitor to obtain correct result
• Advise patient to report weakness, fatigue, loss of appetite, nausea, vomiting, yellowing of skin or eyes, sore throat, glossitis

Evaluation
Positive therapeutic outcome
• Decreased symptoms of toxoplasmosis
• Decreased symptoms of *Pneumocystis jiroveci* pneumonia

quetiapine (Rx)
(kwe-tie′a-peen)
Seroquel
Func. class.: Antipsychotic
Pregnancy category C

Action: Functions as an antagonist at multiple neurotransmitter receptors in the brain including 5-HT_{1A}, 5-HT_2, dopamine D_1, D_2, H_1, adrenergic α_1, α_2 receptors

Therapeutic Outcome: Decreased hallucination and disorganized thought

Uses: Psychotic disorders

Dosage and routes
Adult: PO 25 mg bid, with incremental increases of 25-50 mg bid-tid on days 2 and 3 to a dose of 300-400 mg daily given bid-tid; max 800 mg/day

Available forms: Tabs 25, 100, 200, 300 mg

Adverse effects
CNS: Extrapyramidal symptoms (EPS), pseudoparkinsonism, akathisia, dystonia, tardive dyskinesia, drowsiness, insomnia, agitation, anxiety, ***headache,*** seizures, **neuroleptic malignant syndrome,** dizziness
CV: Orthostatic hypotension, **tachycardia**
GI: Nausea, anorexia, constipation, abdominal pain, dry mouth
INTEG: Rash
MISC: Asthenia, back pain, fever, ear pain
RESP: Rhinitis

Contraindications: Hypersensitivity

Precautions: Pregnancy **C,** children, lactation, long-term use, seizures, dementia, hepatic disease, elderly, breast cancer

Pharmacokinetics	
Absorption	Rapidly
Distribution	Widely
Metabolism	Liver, extensively; inhibits P450 CYP3A4 enzyme system
Excretion	Urine, feces
Half-life	≥6 hr

Pharmacodynamics	
Onset	Unknown
Peak	1.5 hr
Duration	Up to 12 hr

Interactions
Individual drugs
Alcohol: increased CNS depression
Carbamazepine, phenytoin, rifampin, thioridazine: increased quetiapine clearance
Cimetidine: decreased quetiapine clearance
Levodopa: decreased effect of levodopa
Lorazepam: decreased effect of lorazepam

Drug classifications
Analgesics (opioid), antihistamines, sedative/hypnotics: increased CNS depression
Barbiturates, glucocorticoids: increased clearance of quetiapine
DOPamine agonists: decreased effects of DOPamine agonists

Drug/herb
Cola tree, hops, nettle, nutmeg: increased action
Betel palm, kava: increased EPS

NURSING CONSIDERATIONS
Assessment
• Assess mental status: orientation, mood, behavior, presence and type of hallucinations before initial administration and monthly; this drug should significantly reduce psychotic behavior
• Check that patient swallows all PO medication; check for hoarding or giving of medication to other patients

- Monitor I&O ratio, palpate bladder if low urinary output occurs, especially in elderly; urinalysis recommended before, during prolonged therapy
- Monitor bilirubin, CBC, liver function studies monthly
- Assess affect, orientation, LOC, reflexes, gait, coordination, sleep pattern disturbances
- Monitor B/P with patient in sitting, standing, and lying positions; take pulse and respirations q4h during initial treatment; establish baseline before starting treatment; report drops of 30 mm Hg; obtain baseline ECG and monitor Q- and T-wave changes
- Check for dizziness, faintness, palpitations, tachycardia on rising; severe orthostatic hypotension is common
- Identify for neuroleptic malignant syndrome: hyperpyrexia, muscle rigidity, increased CPK, altered mental status, seizures, tachycardia, diaphoresis, hyper/hypotension, fatigue; drug should be discontinued and prescriber notified immediately
- Assess for EPS including akathisia (inability to sit still, no pattern to movements), tardive dyskinesia (bizarre movements of the jaw, mouth, tongue, extremities), pseudoparkinsonism (rigidity, tremors, pill rolling, shuffling gait); an antiparkinson drug should be prescribed
- Assess for constipation, urinary retention daily; if these occur, increase bulk, water in diet

Nursing diagnoses

- Thought processes, disturbed (uses)
- Coping, ineffective (uses)
- Knowledge, deficient (teaching)
- Noncompliance (teaching)

Implementation

- PO with full glass of water, milk; or give with food to decrease GI upset
- Store in airtight, light-resistant container

Patient/family education

- Teach patient to use good oral hygiene; frequent rinsing of mouth, sugarless gum for dry mouth
- Caution patient to avoid hazardous activities until drug response is determined; dizziness, blurred vision may occur
- Inform patient that orthostatic hypotension occurs often; patient should rise from sitting or lying position gradually; avoid hot tubs, hot showers, and tub baths because hypotension may occur
- Inform patient that heat stroke may occur in hot weather, and to take extra precautions to stay cool
- Advise patient to avoid abrupt withdrawal of this drug or EPS may result; drug should be withdrawn slowly
- Teach patient to avoid OTC preparations (cough, hayfever, cold) unless approved by prescriber; serious drug interactions may occur; avoid use with alcohol, CNS depressants because increased drowsiness may occur

Evaluation

Positive therapeutic outcome

- Decrease in emotional excitement, hallucinations, delusions, paranoia
- Reorganization of patterns of thought, speech

Treatment of overdose: Lavage, provide airway

quinapril (Rx)

(kwin'a-pril)

Accupril

Func. class.: Antihypertensive

Chem. class.: Angiotensin-converting enzyme (ACE) inhibitor

Pregnancy category
C (1st trimester),
D (2nd/3rd trimesters)

Action: Selectively suppresses renin-angiotensin-aldosterone system; inhibits ACE, prevents conversion of angiotensin I to angiotensin II; results in dilation of arterial, venous vessels

Therapeutic Outcome: Decreased B/P in hypertension

Uses: Hypertension, alone or in combination with thiazide diuretics, systolic CHF

Dosage and routes

Hypertension (monotherapy)

Adult: PO 10-20 mg daily initially, then 20-80 mg/day divided bid or daily

Elderly: PO 10 mg daily, titrate to desired response

Congestive heart failure

Adult: PO 5 mg bid, may increase qwk unitl 20-40 mg/day in 2 divided doses

Renal dose

Adult: PO CCr 30-60 ml/min 5 mg/day initially; CCr <30 ml/min 2.5 mg/day initially

Available forms: Tabs 5, 10, 20, 40 mg

Adverse effects

CNS: Headache, dizziness, fatigue, somnolence, depression, malaise, nervousness, vertigo

CV: Hypotension, postural hypotension, syncope, palpitations, angina pectoris, **MI, tachycardia,** vasodilation, chest pain
GI: Nausea, diarrhea, constipation, vomiting, gastritis, GI hemorrhage, dry mouth
GU: Increased BUN, creatinine, decreased libido, impotence
HEMA: **Thrombocytopenia, agranulocytosis**
INTEG: **Angioedema,** rash, sweating, photosensitivity, pruritus
META: Hyperkalemia
MISC: Back pain, amblyopia
MS: Myalgia
RESP: Cough, pharyngitis, dyspnea

Contraindications: Pregnancy **D** (2nd/3rd trimesters), hypersensitivity to ACE inhibitors, children

Precautions: Pregnancy **C** (1st trimester), impaired renal and liver function, dialysis patients, hypovolemia, blood dyscrasias, COPD, asthma, elderly, lactation, bilateral renal stenosis

Pharmacokinetics	
Absorption	Well absorbed
Distribution	Unknown, crosses placenta
Metabolism	Unknown
Excretion	Urine (60%), feces (37%)
Half-life	2 hr

Pharmacodynamics	
Onset	½-1 hr
Peak	2-6 hr
Duration	12-24 hr

Interactions
Individual drugs
Alcohol: increased hypotension (large amounts)
Digoxin, lithium: increased toxicity
Hydralazine, prazosin: use caution
Indomethacin: decreased antihypertensive effect of quinapril
Tetracycline: decreased absorption of tetracycline

Drug classifications
Adrenergic blockers, antihypertensives, diuretics, diuretics (potassium sparing), ganglionic blockers, nitrates, phenothiazines: increased hypotension
Diuretics (potassium sparing), potassium supplements, sympathomimetics, combine vasodilators: use caution

Drug/herb
Aconite: increased toxicity, death
Astragalus, cola tree: increased or decreased antihypertensive effect
Barberry, betony, black catechu, black cohosh, bloodroot, broom, burdock, cat's claw, dandelion, goldenseal, Irish moss, Jamaican dogwood, kelp, khella, mistletoe, parsley: increased antihypertensive effect
Coltsfoot, guarana, khat, licorice: decreased antihypertensive effect

Drug/lab test
False positive: urine acetone, ANA titer

NURSING CONSIDERATIONS
Assessment
- Monitor blood studies: neutrophils, decreased platelets; WBC with differential baseline and periodically q3 mo; if neutrophils $<1000/mm^3$ discontinue treatment
- Monitor B/P, check for orthostatic hypotension, syncope; if changes occur dosage change may be required
- Monitor renal studies (protein, BUN, creatinine); and periodically liver function tests, uric acid, also glucose may be elevated; watch for increased levels that may indicate nephrotic syndrome and renal failure; monitor renal symptoms: polyuria, oliguria, frequency, dysuria
- Check potassium levels throughout treatment, although hyperkalemia rarely occurs
- Check for edema in feet, legs daily, weight daily in CHF
- Assess for allergic reactions: rash, fever, pruritus, urticaria; drug should be discontinued if antihistamines fail to help

Nursing diagnoses
- Cardiac output, decreased (uses)
- Injury, risk for (adverse reactions)
- Knowledge, deficient (teaching)
- Noncompliance (teaching)

Implementation
- Tabs may be crushed if necessary
- Store in airtight container at 86° F (30° C) or less
- Severe hypotension may occur after 1st dose of this medication; may be prevented by reducing or discontinuing diuretic therapy 3 days before beginning quinapril therapy

Patient/family education
- Advise patient not to discontinue drug abruptly; advise patient to tell all persons associated with care
- Teach patient not to use OTC products (cough, cold, allergy) unless directed by physician; serious side effects can occur
- Inform patient that xanthines such as coffee, tea, chocolate, cola can prevent action of drug

- Caution patient on the importance of complying with dosage schedule, even if feeling better; to continue with medical regimen to decrease B/P: exercise, cessation of smoking, decreasing stress, diet modifications
- Emphasize the need to rise slowly to sitting or standing position to minimize orthostatic hypotension; not to exercise in hot weather or increased hypotension can occur
- Teach patient to notify prescriber of mouth sores, sore throat, fever, swelling of hands or feet, irregular heartbeat, chest pain, coughing, shortness of breath
- Caution patient to report excessive perspiration, dehydration, vomiting, diarrhea; may lead to fall in B/P
- Caution patient that drug may cause dizziness, fainting, light-headedness; may occur during 1st few days of therapy; to avoid activities that may be hazardous
- Teach patient how to take B/P, and normal readings for age-group

Evaluation

Positive therapeutic outcome

- Decreased B/P in hypertension

Treatment of overdose: 0.9% NaCl **IV** inf, hemodialysis

quinidine (Rx)
(kwin'i-deen)

quinidine gluconate
Quinaglute Dura-Tabs, Quinalan, Quinate ✦

quinidine polygalacturonate
Cardioquin

quinidine sulfate
Apo-Quinidine ✦, Cin-Quin, Novoquinidine ✦, Quinidex Extentabs, Quinora

Func. class.: Antidysrhythmic (class IA)
Chem. class.: Quinine dextro isomer

Pregnancy category C

Action: Prolongs action potential duration and effective refractory period, thus decreasing myocardial excitability; anticholinergic properties

Therapeutic Outcome: Treatment of dysrhythmias

Uses: Premature ventricular contractions (PVCs), atrial fibrillation, flutter; paroxysmal atrial tachycardia, ventricular tachycardia, malaria/**IV** quinidine gluconate

Dosage and routes

Quinidine sulfate

Atrial fibrillation/flutter

Adult: PO 200 mg q2-3h × 5-8 doses; may increase daily until sinus rhythm is restored; max 4 g/day given only after digitalization, maintenance 200-300 mg tid-qid or 300-600 mg q8-12 hr (sus rel)

Paroxysmal supraventricular tachycardia

Adult: PO 400-600 mg q2-3h, then 200-300 mg q6-8h or 300-600 mg q8-12h (sus rel)

Premature atrial/ventricular contraction

Adult: PO 200-300 mg q6-8h or 300-600 mg (sus rel) q8-12h, not to exceed 4 g/day

Child: PO 30 mg/kg/day or 900 mg/m^2/day in 5 divided doses

Quinidine gluconate

Adult: PO 324-660 mg q6-12h (sus rel); IM 600 mg, then 400 mg q2h; **IV** give 16 mg/min

Available forms: Gluconate: sus rel tabs 324, 330 mg; inj gluconate 80 mg/ml; sulfate: tabs 200, 300 mg; sus rel tabs 300 mg; polygalacturonase: tabs 275 mg

Adverse effects

CNS: *Headache, dizziness,* involuntary movement, confusion, psychosis, restlessness, irritability, syncope, excitement, depression, ataxia

CV: **Hypotension,** *bradycardia, PVCs,* **heart block, cardiovascular collapse, arrest, torsade de pointes,** widening QRS complex, **ventricular tachycardia**

EENT: Cinchonism: tinnitus, blurred vision, hearing loss, mydriasis, disturbed color vision

GI: Nausea, vomiting, anorexia, *diarrhea,* **hepatotoxicity**, abdominal pain

HEMA: **Thrombocytopenia, hemolytic anemia, agranulocytosis,** hypoprothrombinemia

INTEG: Rash, urticaria, **angioedema,** swelling, photosensitivity, flushing with severe pruritus

RESP: Dyspnea, **respiratory depression**

Contraindications: Hypersensitivity or idiosyncratic response, digitalis toxicity, history of long QT syndrome, drug induced torsades de pointes, blood dyscrasias, severe heart block, myasthenia gravis

Precautions: Pregnancy **C,** lactation, children, renal disease, potassium imbalance, liver disease, CHF, respiratory depression, elderly

Q

Pharmacokinetics

Absorption	Well absorbed (PO, IM), slowly absorbed (sus rel)
Distribution	Widely distributed, crosses placenta, protein binding (80%-90%)
Metabolism	Liver
Excretion	Kidney unchanged, 10%-50% breast milk
Half-life	6-8 hr

Interactions

Individual drugs

Amiodarone, cimetidine, nifedipine: increased quinidine level
Digoxin: increased digoxin level
Nifedipine, phenytoin, rifampin, sucralfate: decreased effects of quinidine
Propranolol: increased effect of propranolol
Reserpine: increased cardiac depression
Sodium bicarbonate, verapamil: increased quinidine effect
Warfarin: increased levels of warfarin

Drug classifications

Antacids, carbonic anhydrase inhibitors, diuretics (thiazide), hydroxide suspensions: increased effects of quinidine
Anticholinergic blockers: increased vagolytic effects
Anticoagulants (oral): increased levels of anticoagulant
Antidepressants (tricyclics): increased effect of antidepressant
Antidysrhythmics: increased cardiac depression
Barbiturates, cholinergics: decreased effects of quinidine
Neuromuscular blockers: increased neuromuscular blocking
Phenothiazines: increased cardiac depression

Drug/herb

Aconite: increased toxicity, death
Aloe, broom, buckthorn (chronic use), cascara sagrada (chronic use), Chinese rhubarb, figwort, fumitory, goldenseal, kudzu, licorice: increased effect
Aloe, buckthorn, cascara sagrada, senna: increased hypokalemia, increased antidysrhythmic action
Coltsfoot: decreased effect
Horehound: increased serotonin effect

Drug/food

Grapefruit juice: decreased absorption, decreased metabolism

Drug/lab test

Increased: CPK
Interference: triamterene therapy interferes with quinidine test levels

NURSING CONSIDERATIONS

Assessment

- Monitor ECG continuously to determine drug effectiveness, measure PR, QRS, QT intervals, check for PVCs, other dysrhythmias; monitor B/P continuously for hypotension, hypertension; for rebound hypertension after 1-2 hr; check for dehydration or hypovolemia
- Monitor blood levels (therapeutic level 2-7 mcg/ml)
- Monitor I&O ratio, electrolytes (potassium, sodium, chloride); check weight daily; check for signs of CHF or pulmonary toxicity: dyspnea, fatigue, cough, fever, chest pain; if these occur, drug should be discontinued
- Monitor liver function studies: AST, ALT, bilirubin, alkaline phosphatase
- Assess for CNS symptoms: confusion, psychosis, numbness, depression, involuntary movements; if these occur, drug should be discontinued
- Monitor cardiac rate, respiration: rate, rhythm, character, chest pain; watch for ventricular tachycardia, supraventricular tachycardia, or fibrillation that indicates toxicity

Nursing diagnoses

- Cardiac output, decreased (uses)
- Gas exchange, impaired (adverse reactions)
- Knowledge, deficient (teaching)

Implementation

PO route

- Do not break, crush, or chew sus rel tab
- Give on an empty stomach with a full glass of water
- May be given with meals if GI irritation occurs, absorption will be decreased
- Sus rel forms not interchangeable
- Tab may be crushed and mixed with fluid or foods for patients with swallowing difficulties

IV route

- Give by intermittent inf after diluting 800 mg/50 ml of D_5W; gluconate: (16 mg/ml) give

Pharmacodynamics

	PO (SULFATE)	PO-SUS REL	PO (GLUCONATE)	IM	IV
Onset	½ hr	Unknown	Unknown	½ hr	5 min
Peak	1-1½ hr	4 hr	4 hr	½-1½ hr	Unknown
Duration	6-8 hr	8-12 hr	6-8 hr	6-8 hr	6-8 hr

at 1 ml/min or less using an infusion pump for correct dose

- Do not use colored sol or sol with precipitate
- Diluted quinidine is stable for 24 hr at room temp

Y-site compatibilities: Diazepam, milrinone

Y-site incompatibilities: Furosemide

Additive compatibilities: Bretylium, cimetidine, milrinone, ranitidine, verapamil

Additive incompatibilities: Amiodarone

Patient/family education

- Instruct patient to report adverse effects immediately to prescriber
- Caution patient that sunglasses may be needed for photophobia; to use sunscreen, protective clothing, or stay out of sun to prevent burns
- Instruct patient to complete follow-up appointments with health care provider including pulmonary function studies, chest x-ray, ophth and otoscopic exams

Evaluation

Positive therapeutic outcome

- Resolution of dysrhythmias

quinine (OTC, Rx)

(kwye'nine)

Func. class.: Antimalarial

Chem. class.: Cinchona tree alkaloid

Pregnancy category X

Action: Inhibits parasite replications, transcription of DNA to RNA by forming complexes with DNA of parasite

Therapeutic Outcome: Reduction/death of *Plasmodium falciparum*; decreased leg cramps

Uses: *P. falciparum*, malaria, nocturnal leg cramps

Dosage and routes

Malaria

Adult: PO 650 mg q8h × 3 days, given with tetracycline, doxycycline, sulfadoxine/pyrimethamine, or clindamycin

Child: PO 8.3 mg/kg q8h × 3 days with tetracycline (if over 8 yr old) or sulfadoxine/pyrimethamine or clindamycin

Leg Cramps

Adult: PO 200-300 mg at bedtime; may give an additional 200-300 mg at evening meal

Available forms: Caps 200, 300, 325 mg; tabs 260, 325 mg

Adverse effects

CNS: Headache, stimulation, fatigue, irritability, **seizures**, bad dreams, dizziness, fever, confusion, anxiety

CV: Angina, dysrhythmias, tachycardia, hypotension, **acute circulatory failure**

EENT: *Blurred vision, corneal changes, retinal changes, difficulty focusing*, tinnitus, vertigo, deafness, photophobia, diplopia, night blindness

ENDO: Hypoglycemia

GI: *Nausea, vomiting, anorexia*, diarrhea, epigastric pain

GU: Renal tubular damage, **anuria**

HEMA: **Thrombocytopenia, purpura, hypothrombinemia, hemolysis**

INTEG: Pruritus, pigmentary changes, skin eruptions, lichen planus–like eruptions, flushing, facial edema, sweating

MISC: **Hemolytic uremic syndrome**

RESP: Dyspnea

Contraindications: Pregnancy **X,** hypersensitivity, G6PD deficiency, retinal field changes, lactation

Precautions: Blood dyscrasias, severe GI disease, neurologic disease, severe hepatic disease, psoriasis, cardiac dysrhythmias, tinnitus

Pharmacokinetics	
Absorption	Rapidly, 80%
Distribution	Crosses placenta, excreted breast milk protein binding >90% in malaria
Metabolism	Liver, extensively 80%
Excretion	Urine, 20% unchanged
Half-life	11 hr, increases in malaria

Pharmacodynamics	
Onset	Unknown
Peak	3½-6 hr
Duration	8 hr

Interactions

Individual drugs

Quinidine: increased CV reactions

Mefloxacin: increased seizure risk

Warfarin: increased bleeding risk

Drug classifications

Antacids: decreased absorption of quinine

Neuromuscular blockers: increased effect of neuromuscular blockers

Drug/lab test

Increased: 17-KS

Q

NURSING CONSIDERATIONS

Assessment

- Monitor B/P, pulse; watch for hypotension, tachycardia
- Assess liver studies qwk: ALT, AST, bilirubin
- Assess blood studies, CBC, since blood dyscrasias occur
- Assess for cinchonism: nausea, blurred vision, tinnitus, headache, difficulty focusing; quinidine levels >10 mcg/ml
- Assess for symptoms of malaria and improvement
- Assess frequency/duration of nocturnal leg cramps

Nursing diagnoses

- Infection, risk for (uses)
- Noncompliance (teaching)
- Knowledge, deficient (teaching)

Implementation

- Give before or after meals at same time each day to maintain level
- Store in tight, light-resistant container

Patient/family education

- Advise patient to avoid OTC preparations: cold preparations, tonic water
- Advise patient to take only as prescribed
- Teach patient visual changes may occur, to avoid driving or hazardous activities until response is known
- Teach patient to stop drug and call prescriber if allergic reaction occurs or ringing in the ears, trouble breathing occurs
- Teach patient to use insect repellant, protective clothing if in area with mosquitoes

Evaluation

Positive therapeutic outcome

- Decreased symptoms of malaria

rabeprazole (Rx)

(rab-ee-pray'zole)

Aciphex

Func. class.: Proton pump inhibitor

Chem. class.: Benzimidazole

Pregnancy category C

Action: Suppresses gastric secretion by inhibiting hydrogen/potassium ATPase enzyme system in the gastric parietal cell; characterized as a gastric acid pump inhibitor, since it blocks the final step of acid production

Therapeutic Outcome: Absence of duodenal ulcers; decreased gastroesophageal reflux

Uses: Gastroesophageal reflux disease (GERD), severe erosive esophagitis, poorly responsive systemic GERD, pathologic hypersecretory conditions (Zollinger-Ellison syndrome, systemic mastocytosis, multiple endocrine adenomas); possibly effective for treatment of duodenal ulcers with or without antiinfectives for *Helicobacter pylori;* daytime, nighttime heartburn

Dosage and routes

Healing of duodenal ulcers

Adult: PO 20 mg daily × ≤4 wk, to be taken after breakfast

Erosive esophagitis/GERD

Adult: PO 20 mg daily × 4-8 wk

Pathologic hypersecretory conditions

Adult: PO 60 mg/day; may increase to 120 mg in 2 divided doses

Available forms: Delayed rel tabs, 20 mg

Adverse effects

CNS: *Headache, dizziness, asthenia*

CV: Chest pain, angina, tachycardia, bradycardia, palpitations, peripheral edema

EENT: Tinnitus, taste perversion

GI: *Diarrhea, abdominal pain, vomiting, nausea, constipation, flatulence, acid regurgitation,* abdominal swelling, anorexia, irritable colon, esophageal candidiasis, dry mouth

GU: UTI, frequency, increased creatinine, **proteinuria, hematuria,** testicular pain, glycosuria

HEMA: **Pancytopenia, thrombocytopenia, neutropenia, leukocytosis,** anemia

INTEG: Rash, dry skin, urticaria, pruritus, alopecia

META: Hypoglycemia, increased hepatic enzymes, weight gain

MISC: *Back pain,* fever, fatigue, malaise

RESP: *Upper respiratory tract infections, cough,* epistaxis

Contraindications: Hypersensitivity

Precautions: Pregnancy **C,** lactation, children

Pharmacokinetics

Absorption	Unknown
Distribution	Unknown
Metabolism	Liver, extensively
Excretion	Kidneys, feces
Half-life	Unknown

Pharmacodynamics

Unknown

Interactions
Individual drugs
Clarithromycin, phenytoin: increased levels of rapeprazole
Sucralfate: decreased rapeprazole levels
Drug classifications
Benzodiazepines: increased levels of rapeprazole

NURSING CONSIDERATIONS
Assessment
- Assess GI system: bowel sounds q8h, abdomen for pain and swelling, anorexia
- Monitor hepatic enzymes: AST, ALT, increased alkaline phosphatase during treatment

Nursing diagnoses
- Pain, chronic (uses)
- Knowledge, deficient (teaching)

Implementation
- Do not break, crush, or chew delayed rel tab
- Give after breakfast daily

Patient/family education
- Advise patient to report severe diarrhea; drug may have to be discontinued
- Caution patient to avoid driving and other hazardous activities until response to drug is known
- Caution patient to avoid alcohol, salicylates, NSAIDs; may cause GI irritation
- Advise patient to wear sunscreen, protective clothing to prevent burns

Evaluation
Positive therapeutic outcome
- Absence of epigastric pain, swelling, fullness

raloxifene (Rx)
(ral-ox'ih-feen)
Evista
Func. class.: Bone resorption inhibitor, selective estrogen receptor modulator (SERM)
Chem. class.: Benzothiophene
Pregnancy category X

Action: Reduces resorption of bone and decreases bone turnover; mediated through estrogen receptor binding

Therapeutic Outcome: Absence, or decrease of osteoporosis in postmenopausal women

Uses: Prevention, treatment of osteoporosis in postmenopausal women

Dosage and routes
Hormone replacement
Adult: PO 60 mg daily

Available forms: Tabs 60 mg

Adverse effects
CNS: Insomnia, migraines, depression, fever
CV: Hot flashes, chest pain
GI: **Nausea,** vomiting, diarrhea, anorexia, cramps, dyspepsia
GU: Vaginitis, UTI, leukorrhea, *hot flashes,* cystitis
INTEG: Rash, sweating
META: Weight gain, peripheral edema
MS: Arthralgia, myalgia, *leg cramps,* arthritis
RESP: Sinusitis, pharyngitis, increased cough, pneumonia, laryngitis, rhinitis, bronchitis, **retinal vein occlusion (rare)**

Contraindications: Pregnancy **X,** hypersensitivity, lactation, women with active or history of venous thromboembolic events

Precautions: Venous thromboembolic events, hepatic disease, CV disease, cervical/uterine cancer, elevated triglycerides, pulmonary embolism

Pharmacokinetics	
Absorption	Unknown
Distribution	Highly protein bound
Metabolism	Unknown
Excretion	Feces, breast milk
Half-life	28-32 hr (elimination)

Pharmacodynamics	
Onset	Unknown
Peak	Unknown
Duration	Unknown

Interactions
Individual drugs
Ampicillin, cholestyramine: decreased action of raloxifene
Drug classifications
Anticoagulants: decreased action of anticoagulants
Highly protein-bound drugs: administer cautiously
Drug/lab test
Increased: apolipoprotein, corticosteroid-binding globulin, thyroxine-binding globulin (TBG)
Decreased: lipoprotein, fibrinogen, LDL cholesterol, total cholesterol, calcium, total protein, albumin, platelets

NURSING CONSIDERATIONS

Assessment

- Obtain bone density test baseline and periodically throughout treatment; bone-specific alkaline phosphatase; osteocalcin, collagen breakdown
- Monitor weight daily, notify prescriber of weekly weight gain >5 lb
- Monitor B/P q4h, watch for increase caused by H_2O and sodium retention
- Monitor liver function studies: AST, ALT, bilirubin, alkaline phosphatase
- Monitor I&O ratio; decreasing urinary output, increasing edema

Nursing diagnoses

- Mobility, physical, impaired (uses)
- Knowledge, deficient (teaching)

Implementation

- Administer without regard to meals
- Add calcium supplement, vit D if lacking

Patient/family education

- Teach patient to weigh weekly, report gain >5 lb
- Teach patients to discontinue drug 72 hr before prolonged bedrest
- Advise patient to avoid maintaining one position for long periods
- Advise patient to take calcium supplements, vit D if intake is inadequate
- Advise patient to increase exercise using weights
- Advise patient to stop smoking and to decrease alcohol consumption
- Inform patient that this drug does not help control hot flashes
- Teach patient to report fever, acute migraine, insomnia, emotional distress; UTI or vaginal burning/itching; swelling, warmth, or pain in calves

Evaluation

Positive therapeutic outcome

- Prevention, treatment of osteoporosis

ramipril (Rx)

(ra-mi′pril)

Altace

Func. class.: Antihypertensive

Chem. class.: Angiotensin-converting enzyme (ACE) inhibitor

Pregnancy category
C (1st trimester),
D (2nd/3rd trimesters)

Do Not Confuse:
Altace/alteplase, Altace/Artane, ramipril/enalapril

Action: Selectively suppresses renin-angiotensin-aldosterone system; inhibits ACE; prevents conversion of angiotensin I to angiotensin II; results in dilation of arterial, venous vessels

Therapeutic Outcome: Decreased B/P in hypertension

Uses: Hypertension, alone or in combination with thiazide diuretics; CHF (after MI), reduction in risk of MI, stroke, death from CV disorders

Dosage and routes

Hypertension

Adult: PO 2.5 mg daily initially, then 2.5-20 mg/day divided bid or daily; renal impairment: 1.25 mg daily with CCr <40 ml/min/1.73 m^2, increase as needed to max 5 mg/day

CHF/Post MI

Adult: PO 1.25-2.5 mg bid, may increase to 5 mg bid

Reduction in risk of MI, stroke, death

Adult: PO 2.5 mg daily × 7 days, then 5 mg daily × 21 days, then may increase to 10 mg/day

Renal dose

Adult: PO CCr <40 ml/min 1.73 m^2 50% of dose

Available forms: Caps 1.25, 2.5, 5, 10 mg

Adverse effects

CNS: ***Headache, dizziness,*** anxiety, insomnia, paresthesia, fatigue, depression, malaise, vertigo, **seizures**

CV: ***Hypotension,*** chest pain, palpitations, angina, syncope, **dysrhythmia**

EENT: Hearing loss

GI: Nausea, constipation, vomiting, dyspepsia, dysphagia, anorexia, diarrhea, abdominal pain

GU: **Proteinuria,** increased BUN, creatinine, impotence

HEMA: Decreased Hct, Hgb, **eosinophilia, leukopenia**

INTEG: Rash, sweating, photosensitivity, pruritus

META: Hyperkalemia

MISC: **Angioedema**

MS: Arthralgia, arthritis, myalgia

RESP: Cough, dyspnea

Contraindications: Pregnancy **D** (2nd/3rd trimesters), hypersensitivity to ACE inhibitors, lactation, children, history of angioedema

Precautions: Pregnancy **C** (1st trimester), impaired renal and liver function, dialysis patients, hypovolemia, blood dyscrasias, COPD, CHF, asthma, elderly, renal artery stenosis

Pharmacokinetics

Absorption	Well absorbed
Distribution	Not known, crosses placenta
Metabolism	Liver, extensively, protein binding 73%
Excretion	Urine
Half-life	Ramipril (5 hr), ramiprilat (24 hr)

Pharmacodynamics

Onset	½-1 hr
Peak	6-8 hr
Duration	24-72 hr

Interactions

Individual drugs

Alcohol: increased hypotension (large amounts)
Digoxin, lithium: increased serum levels
Hydralazine, prazocin: increased toxicity
Indomethacin: decreased antihypertensive effect

Drug classifications

Adrenergic blockers, antihypertensives, diuretics, ganglionic blockers, nitrates: increased hypotension
Antacids: decreased absorption
Diuretics (potassium sparing), potassium supplements, sympathomimetics, vasodilators: increased toxicity

Drug/herb

Aconite: increased toxicity, death
Astragalus, cola tree: increased or decreased antihypertensive effect
Barberry, betony, black catechu, black cohosh, bloodroot, broom, burdock, cat's claw, dandelion, goldenseal, Irish moss, Jamaican dogwood, kelp, khella, mistletoe, parsley: increased antihypertensive effect
Coltsfoot, guarana, khat, licorice: decreased antihypertensive effect

Drug/lab test

False positive: urine acetone, ANA titer

NURSING CONSIDERATIONS

Assessment

- Monitor blood studies: neutrophils, decreased platelets; WBC with differential baseline and periodically q3mo, if neutrophils <1000/mm^3, discontinue treatment
- Monitor B/P, check for orthostatic hypotension, syncope; if changes occur, dosage may need to be changed
- Monitor renal studies: protein, BUN, creatinine; watch for increased levels that may indicate nephrotic syndrome and renal failure; monitor renal symptoms: polyuria, oliguria, frequency, dysuria
- Establish baselines in renal, liver function tests before therapy begins and monitor periodically; liver function tests, uric acid, and glucose may be increased
- Check potassium levels throughout treatment, although hyperkalemia rarely occurs
- Check for edema in feet, legs daily, weight daily in CHF
- Assess for allergic reactions: rash, fever, pruritus, urticaria; drug should be discontinued if antihistamines fail to help

Nursing diagnoses

- Cardiac output, decreased (uses)
- Injury, risk for (side effects)
- Knowledge, deficient (teaching)
- Noncompliance (teaching)

Implementation

- Caps can be opened and added to food
- Store in airtight container at 86° F (30° C) or less
- Severe hypotension may occur after 1st dose of this medication; decreased hypotension may be prevented by reducing or discontinuing diuretic therapy 3 days before beginning benazepril therapy
- Give **IV** inf of 0.9% NaCl (as ordered) to expand fluid volume if severe hypotension occurs

Patient/family education

- Caution patient not to discontinue drug abruptly; advise patient to tell all persons associated with care
- Teach patient not to use OTC products (cough, cold, allergy) unless directed by physician; serious side effects can occur; xanthines such as coffee, tea, chocolate, cola can prevent action of drug
- Instruct patient on the importance of complying with dosage schedule, even if feeling better; to continue with medical regimen to decrease B/P: exercise, cessation of smoking, decreasing stress, diet modifications
- Emphasize the need to rise slowly to sitting or standing position to minimize orthostatic hypotension; not to exercise in hot weather because increased hypotension can occur
- Teach patient to notify prescriber of mouth sores, sore throat, fever, swelling of hands or feet, irregular heartbeat, chest pain, coughing, shortness of breath
- Caution patient to report excessive perspira-

tion, dehydration, vomiting, diarrhea; may lead to fall in B/P

- Caution patient that drug may cause dizziness, fainting, lightheadedness; may occur during 1st few days of therapy; to avoid activities that may be hazardous
- Teach patient how to take B/P, and normal readings for age group

Evaluation

Positive therapeutic outcome

- Decreased B/P in hypertension

Treatment of overdose: 0.9% NaCl **IV** inf, hemodialysis

ramelteon

Rozerem

See Appendix A, Selected New Drugs

ranitidine (Rx)

(ra-nit'i-deen)

Apo-Ranitidine ♣, Zantac, Zantac-C ♣, Zantac EFFER-dose, Zantac GELdose

ranitidine bismuth citrate

Tritec

Func. class.: H_2 histamine receptor antagonist

Pregnancy category B

Do Not Confuse:
ranitidine/amantadine, Zantac/Xanax, Zantac/Zofran

Action: Inhibits histamine at H_2 receptor site in the gastric parietal cells, which inhibits gastric acid secretion

Therapeutic Outcome: Healing of duodenal ulcers or gastric ulcers; prevention of duodenal ulcers; decreases symptoms of gastroesophageal reflux disease (GERD) or Zollinger-Ellison syndrome

Uses: Short-term treatment of duodenal and gastric ulcers and maintenance; management of GERD, Zollinger-Ellison syndrome, active duodenal ulcers with *Helicobacter pylori* in combination with clarithromycin

Investigational uses: Prevention of aspiration pneumonitis, stress ulcers, upper GI bleeding

Dosage and routes

Ranitidine

Renal dose

Adult: CCr <50 ml/min PO q24h, IM/**IV** q8-24h

Erosive esophagitis

Adult: PO 150 mg bid, 300 mg at bedtime; IM 50 mg q6-8h; **IV** bol 50 mg diluted to 20 ml over 5 min q6-8h; **IV** intermittent inf 50 mg/100 ml of D_5 over 15-20 min q6-8h

Child: PO 4-5 mg/kg/day divided q8-12h, max 6 mg/kg/day or 300 mg; **IV** 2-4 mg/kg/day divided q6-8h

Duodenal ulcer

Adult: PO 150 mg bid, maintenance 150 mg at bedtime

Zollinger-Ellison syndrome

Adult: PO 150 mg bid, may increase if needed

Gastric ulcer

Adult: PO 150 mg bid × 6 wk, then 150 mg at bedtime

GERD

Adult: PO 150 mg bid

Ranitidine bismuth citrate

Adult: PO 400 mg bid × 4 wk with clarithromycin 500 mg tid × 1st 2 wk

Available forms: Ranitidine: tabs 75, 150, 300 mg; inj 25 mg/ml; caps 150, 300 mg; syr 15 mg/ml; sol for inj 25 mg/ml; effervescent tabs 75, 100 mg; syr 15 mg/ml; effervescent granules 150 mg/packet; ranitidine bismuth citrate: tabs 400 mg

Adverse effects

CNS: Headache, sleeplessness, dizziness, confusion, agitation, depression; hallucination (elderly)

CV: Tachycardia, bradycardia, premature ventricular contractions

EENT: Blurred vision, increased ocular pressure

GI: Constipation, abdominal pain, diarrhea, nausea, vomiting, **hepatotoxicity**

GU: Impotence, gynecomastia

INTEG: Urticaria, rash, fever

Contraindications: Hypersensitivity

Precautions: Pregnancy **B,** lactation, child <12 yr, hepatic disease, renal disease

Pharmacokinetics	
Absorption	Well absorbed (PO, IM), completely absorbed (**IV**)
Distribution	Widely distributed, crosses placenta
Metabolism	Liver (30%)
Excretion	Kidneys unchanged (70%)
Half-life	2-3 hr, increased renal disease

Pharmacodynamics

	PO	IV/IM
Onset	Unknown	Unknown
Peak	2-3 hr	15 min
Duration	8-12 hr	8-12 hr

Interactions

Individual drugs

Diazepam, metoclopramide: decreased absorption of ranitidine

Procainamide: increased absorption, toxicity

Drug classifications

Anticoagulants, sulfonylureas: increased absorption, toxicity

Anticholinergics, antacids: decreased rantidine absorption

Drug/lab test

Increased: alkaline phosphatase, AST, creatinine, ALT, bilirubin

False positive: gastric bleeding test

NURSING CONSIDERATIONS

Assessment

- Assess patient with ulcers or suspected ulcers: epigastric or abdominal pain, hematemesis, occult blood in stools, blood in gastric aspirate before and throughout treatment, monitor gastric pH (5 should be maintained)
- Monitor I&O ratio, BUN, creatinine, CBC with differential monthly

Nursing diagnoses

- Pain, chronic (uses)
- Knowledge, deficient (teaching)

Implementation

PO route

- May be given with or without meals
- Give antacids 1 hr before or 1 hr after this drug

IV, direct route

- Give by direct **IV** after diluting 50 mg/20 ml of 0.9% D_5W, NaCl over 5 min or more

Intermittent IV infusion route

- Give by intermittent inf over 15 min after diluting 50 mg/100 ml of D_5W, 0.9% NaCl

Continuous infusion route

- Give by continuous inf for a concentration 150 mg/250 ml, give 6.25 mg/hr
- Give Zollinger-Ellison patients up to a conc of 2.5 mg/ml at 1 mg/kg/hr initially

Syringe compatibilities: Atropine, cyclizine, dexamethasone, dimenhyDRINATE, diphenhydrAMINE, DOBUTamine, DOPamine, fentanyl, glycopyrrolate, hydromorphone, meperidine, metoclopramide, morphine, nalbuphine, oxymorphone, pentazocine, perphenazine, prochlorperazine, promethazine, scopolamine

Syringe incompatibilities: Hydroxyzine, methotrimeprazine, midazolam, pentobarbital, phenobarbital

Y-site compatibilities: Acyclovir, aldesleukin, allopurinol, amifostine, aminophylline, atracurium, aztreonam, bretylium, DOBUTamine, DOPamine, DOXOrubicin, enalaprilat, epINEPHrine, esmolol, fentanyl, filgrastim, fluconazole, fludarabine, foscarnet, furosemide, gallium, granisetron, heparin, hydromorphone, idarubicin, labetalol, lorazepam, melphalan, meperidine, methotrexate, midazolam, milrinone, morphine, niCARdipine, nitroglycerin, norepinephrine, ondansetron, paclitaxel, pancuronium, piperacillin, piperacillin/tazobactam, procainamide, propofol, sargramostim, vecuronium, zidovudine

Additive compatibilities: Acetazolamide, amikacin, aminophylline, chloramphenicol, chlorothiazide, ciprofloxacin, colistimethate, dexamethasone, digoxin, DOBUTamine, DOPamine, doxycycline, furosemide, gentamicin, heparin, lidocaine, penicillin G sodium, potassium chloride, ticarcillin, tobramycin, vancomycin

Additive incompatibilities: Amphotericin B, clindamycin

Patient/family education

- Caution patient that gynecomastia, impotence may occur and are reversible after treatment is discontinued
- Advise patient to avoid driving, other hazardous activities until stabilized on this medication; drowsiness or dizziness may occur
- Caution patient to avoid black pepper, caffeine, alcohol, harsh spices, extremes in temp of food; tell patient to avoid OTC preparations (aspirin, cough, cold preparations) because condition may worsen
- Inform patient that smoking decreases the effectiveness of the drug; that smoking cessation should be considered
- Instruct patient that drug must be continued for prescribed time to be effective and taken exactly as prescribed; doses should not be doubled; a missed dose should be taken when remembered up to 1 hr before next dose
- Advise patient to report bruising, fatigue, malaise; blood dyscrasias may occur
- Inform patient to report diarrhea, black tarry stools, sore throat, rash, dizziness, confusion, rash, or delirium to prescriber immediately

Evaluation

Positive therapeutic outcome
- Decreased pain in abdomen
- Healing of ulcers
- Absence of gastroesophageal reflux

rasburicase (Rx)

(rass-burr'i-case)

Elitek

Func. class.: Antineoplastic, antimetabolite

Pregnancy category C

Action: Catalyzes enzymatic oxidation of uric acid into an inactive and a soluble metabolite

Therapeutic Outcome: Uric acid levels are decreased

Uses: To reduce uric acid levels in children with leukemia, lymphoma, solid tumor malignancies who are receiving chemotherapy

Dosage and routes

Adult: **IV** inf 0.15 or 0.2 mg/kg as a single daily dose given as **IV** inf over ½ hr

Available forms: Powder for inj 1.5 mg/vial

Adverse effects

CNS: Headache

GI: *Nausea, vomiting, anorexia, diarrhea, abdominal pain, constipation, dyspepsia,* mucositis

HEMA: **Neutropenia with fever**

SYST: Anaphylaxis, hemolysis, **methemoglobinemia, sepsis**

Contraindications: Hypersensitivity, G6PD deficiency, hemolytic reactions, or methemoglobinemia reactions to this drug

Precautions: Pregnancy **C,** lactation, children <2 yr

Pharmacokinetics

Absorption	Unknown
Distribution	Unknown
Metabolism	Unknown
Excretion	Unknown
Half-life	Elimination 18 hr

Pharmacodynamics

Unknown

NURSING CONSIDERATIONS

Assessment

- Monitor renal function studies: BUN, serum uric acid, urine CCr, electrolytes before and during therapy
- Monitor temp q4h; fever may indicate beginning infection; no rectal temps
- Assess for anaphylaxis, have emergency equipment nearby
- Assess for G6PD deficiency, hemolytic reactions, methemoglobinemia; these patients should not be given this agent
- Assess for toxicity: severe diarrhea, nausea, vomiting
- Assess GI symptoms: frequency of stools, cramping; if severe diarrhea occurs, fluid and electrolytes may need to be given

Nursing diagnoses

- Injury, risk for (adverse reactions, uses)
- Knowledge, deficient (teaching)

Implementation

- Give antiemetic 30-60 min before giving drug and prn

Patient/family education

- Advise of reason for therapy, expected results

Evaluation

Positive therapeutic outcome
- Decreased uric acid levels

! HIGH ALERT

remifentanil (Rx)

(re-me-fin'ta-nill)

Ultiva

Func. class.: Opiate agonist analgesic

Chem. class.: µ-Opioid agonist

Pregnancy category C

Controlled substance schedule II

Action: Inhibits ascending pain pathways in limbic system, thalamus, midbrain, hypothalamus

Therapeutic Outcome: Maintenance of anesthesia

Uses: In combination with other drugs in general anesthesia to provide analgesia

Dosage and routes

Adult: Induction **IV** 0.5-1 mcg/kg/min with a hypnotic or volatile agent; maintenance with isoflurane (0.4-1.5 MAC) or propofol (100-200 mcg/kg/min); cont inf 0.25-0.4 mcg/kg/min

Available forms: Powder for inj, lyophilized 1 mg/ml after reconstitution

Adverse effects

CNS: Drowsiness, *dizziness,* confusion,

headache, sedation, euphoria, delirium, agitation, anxiety
CV: Palpitations, **bradycardia,** change in B/P; facial flushing, syncope, **asystole**
EENT: Tinnitus, blurred vision, miosis, diplopia
GI: *Nausea, vomiting,* anorexia, constipation, cramps, dry mouth
GU: Urinary retention, dysuria
INTEG: Rash, urticaria, bruising, flushing, diaphoresis, pruritus
MS: Rigidity
RESP: **Respiratory depression, apnea**

Contraindications: Child <12 yr, hypersensitivity

Precautions: Pregnancy **C,** lactation, increased ICP, acute MI, severe heart disease; renal disease, hepatic disease, asthma, respiratory conditions, seizure disorders, elderly

Pharmacokinetics	
Absorption	Complete
Distribution	Unknown
Metabolism	Unknown
Excretion	Unknown
Half-life	Unknown

Pharmacodynamics	
Onset	Immediate
Peak	Unknown
Duration	Unknown

Interactions
Individual drugs
Alcohol: increased respiratory depression, hypotension, profound sedation
Drug classifications
Antihistamines, CNS depressants, phenothiazines, sedative/hypnotics: increased respiratory depression, hypotension, profound sedation
Drug/herb
Kava: increased CNS depression

NURSING CONSIDERATIONS
Assessment
- Monitor I&O ratio, check for decreasing output; may indicate urinary retention, especially in elderly
- Assess CNS changes: dizziness, drowsiness, hallucinations, euphoria, LOC pupil reaction
- Assess allergic reactions: rash, urticaria
- Assess respiratory dysfunction: respiratory depression, character, rate, rhythm; notify prescriber if respirations are <12/min; CV status, bradycardia, syncope
- Use pain scoring to determine pain perception

Nursing diagnoses
- Knowledge, deficient (teaching)

Implementation
- Add 1 ml diluent per mg remifentanil
- Interruption of infusion results in rapid reversal (no residual opioid effect within 5-10 min)
- Store in light-resistant area at room temperature

Y-site compatibilities: Acyclovir, alfentanil, amikacin, aminophylline, ampicillin, ampicillin/sulbactam, aztreonam, bretylium, bumetanide, buprenorphine, butorphanol, calcium gluconate, cefazolin, cefepime, cefotaxime, cefotetan, cefoxitin, ceftazidime, ceftizoxime, ceftriaxone, cefuroxime, cimetidine, ciprofloxacin, cisatracurium, cisplatin, clindamycin, dactinomycin, dexamethasone, digoxin, diltiazem, diphenhydrAMINE, DOBUTamine, docetaxel, DOPamine, doxacurium, doxycycline, droperidol, enalaprilat, epINEPHrine, esmolol, etoposide, famotidine, fentanyl, fluconazole, furosemide, ganciclovir, gatifloxicin, gemcitabine, gentamicin, granisetron, haloperidol, heparin, hetastarch, hydrocortisone sodium succinate, hydromorphone, hydrOXYzine, imipenem/cilastatin, inamrinone, isoproterenol, ketorolac, levofloxacin, lidocaine, lorazepam, magnesium sulfate, mannitol, meperidine, methlyprednisoLONE sodium succinate, metoclopramide, metronidazole, mezlocillin, midazolam, minocycline, morphine, nalbuphine, netilmicin, nitroglycerin, norepinephrine, ofloxacin, ondansetron, paclitaxel, palonsetron, phenylephrine, pipericillin, potassium chloride, procainamide, prochloroperzine, promethazine, ranitidine, sulfamethoxazole/trimethroprim, sulfentanil, teniposide, theophylline, thiopental, thiotepa, ticarcillin, ticarcillin/clavulate, tobramycin, vancomycin, voriconazole, zidovudine

Solution compatibilities: D_5, 0.45% NaCl, LR

Patient/family education
- Advise patient to call for assistance when ambulating or smoking; drowsiness, dizziness may occur
- Advise patient to make position changes slowly to prevent orthostatic hypotension

Evaluation
Positive therapeutic outcome
- Maintenance of anesthesia

R

repaglinide (Rx)

(re-pag′lih-nide)

Prandin

Func. class.: Antidiabetic

Chem. class.: Meglitinides

Pregnancy category C

Action: Causes functioning β-cells in pancreas to release insulin, leading to drop in blood glucose levels; closes ATP-dependent potassium channels in the β-cell membrane; this leads to opening of calcium channels; increased calcium influx induces insulin secretion

Therapeutic Outcome: Blood glucose controlled

Uses: Type 2 diabetes mellitus

Dosage and routes

Adult: PO 1-2 mg with each meal, max 16 mg/day, adjust at weekly intervals

Available forms: Tabs 0.5, 1, 2 mg

Adverse effects

CNS: *Headache, weakness,* paresthesia

ENDO: **Hypoglycemia**

GI: Nausea, vomiting, diarrhea, constipation, dyspepsia

INTEG: Rash, allergic reactions

MISC: Chest pain, UTI, allergy

MS: Back pains, arthralgia

RESP: URI, sinusitis, rhinitis, bronchitis

Contraindications: Hypersensitivity to meglitinides, diabetic ketoacidosis, type 1 diabetes

Precautions: Pregnancy **C**, elderly, cardiac disease, severe renal disease, severe hepatic disease, thyroid disease, severe hypoglycemic reactions, lactation, children

Pharmacokinetics	
Absorption	Complete
Distribution	98% protein binding, crosses placenta
Metabolism	Liver
Excretion	Urine/feces
Half-life	1 hr

Pharmacodynamics	
Onset	30 min
Peak	1-1½ hr
Duration	<4 hr

Interactions

Individual drugs

Alcohol: disulfiram reaction

Carbamazepine, rifampin: increased repaglinide metabolism

Chloramphenicol, gemfibrozil, probenecid, simvastatin: increased effect of repaglinide

Erythromycin: decreased repaglinide metabolism

Isoniazid, phenobarbital, phenytoin, rifampin: decreased action of repaglinide

Levonorgestrel/ethinyl estradol: increase in both

Drug classifications

Antifungals, macrolides, CYP450 inhibitors: decreased repaglinide metabolism

CYP450 inducers, barbiturates: increased repaglinide metabolism

β-Adrenergic blockers, coumarins, MAOIs, NSAIDs, salicylates, sulfonamides: increased repaglinide effect

Calcium channel blockers, contraceptives (oral), corticosteroids, diuretics (thiazide), estrogens, phenothiazines, sympathomimetics, thyroid preparations: decreased repaglinide effect

Drug/herb

Alfalfa, aloe, basil, bay, bilberry, bitter melon, black catechu, buchu, burdock, coriander, dandelion, eyebright (po), fenugreek, garlic, ginseng, glucomannan, glucosamine, goat's rue, gymnema, horehound, horse chestnut, jambul, myrrh, myrtle: increased antidiabetic effect

Bee pollen, blue cohosh, broom, chromium, elecampane, eucalyptus, gotu kola: decreased antidiabetic effect

Broom, buchu, dandelion, juniper: decreased hypoglycemia

Chromium, fenugreek, ginseng: increased or decreased hypoglycemia

Karela: decreased glucose tolerance

Drug/food

Decreased: repaglinide level, give before meals

NURSING CONSIDERATIONS

Assessment

- ◆ Assess for hypoglycemic or hyperglycemic reaction, which can occur soon after meals; dizziness, weakness, headache, tremor, anxiety, tachycardia, hunger, sweating, abdominal pain
- Monitor A1c, fasting, postprandial glucose during treatment

Nursing diagnoses

- Nutrition: more than body requirements, imbalanced (uses)
- Knowledge, deficient (teaching)
- Noncompliance (teaching)

Implementation

- 15 min before meals: 2, 3, or 4 ×/day preprandially
- Skip dose if meal is skipped; add dose if meal is added
- Store in airtight container in cool environment

Patient/family education

- Advise patient to avoid alcohol; explain disulfiram reaction
- Teach patient technique of blood glucose monitoring using blood glucose meter
- Teach patient the symptoms of hypoglycemia and hyperglycemia; what to do about each
- Teach patient that drug must be continued on daily basis; explain consequence of discontinuing drug abruptly
- Advise patient to avoid OTC medications unless ordered by prescriber
- Advise patient that diabetes is a lifelong illness; drug will not cure disease
- Advise patient to eat all food included in diet plan to prevent hypoglycemia; to have glucagon emergency kit available
- Instruct patient to carry/wear emergency ID for emergency purposes

Evaluation

Positive therapeutic outcome

- Decrease in polyuria, polydipsia, polyphagia, clear sensorium, absence of dizziness, stable gait

Treatment of overdose: Glucose 25 g **IV** via D_{50} sol, 50 ml or 1 mg glucagon

retinoic acid

See tretinoin

Rh_o (D) immune globulin, standard dose IM (Rx)

Gamulin Rh, HypoRho-D, RhoGAM

Rh_o (D) globulin microdose IM

HypoRho-D Mini-Dose, MICRh$_o$GAM, Mini-Gamulin R

Rh_o (D) immune globulin IV (Rx)

WinRho SD, WinRho SDF

Func. class.: Immune globulins

Pregnancy category C

Do Not Confuse:
Gamulin Rh/MICRh$_o$GAM

Action: Suppresses immune response of nonsensitized Rh_o (D or D^u)-negative patients who are exposed to Rh_o (D or D^u)-positive blood

Therapeutic Outcome: Absence of Rh factor and transfusion error

Uses: Prevention of isoimmunization in Rh-negative women exposed to Rh-positive blood given after abortions, miscarriages, amniocentesis

Dosage and routes

After delivery

Adult: IM 1 vial (standard dose) if fetal packed RBCs <15 ml, or 2 vials if fetal packed RBCs >15 ml; given within 72 hr of delivery or miscarriage

Prior to delivery

Adult: IM 1 vial (standard dose) at 26-28 wk, 1 vial (standard dose) 72 hr after delivery

Pregnancy termination <13 wk

Adult: IM 1 vial (micro dose) within 72 hr

Pregnancy termination >13 wk

Adult: IM 1 vial (standard dose) within 72 hr

Fetal-maternal hemorrhage

Adult: IM packed RBCs volume of hemorrhage/15 = needed vials (standard dose)

Transfusion error

Adult: IM (standard dose—1 vial) give within 72 hr

After 34 wk gestation

Adult: IM/**IV** 120 mcg, give within 72 hr (**IV** dose)

Available forms: Inj single-dose vial (50 mcg/vial—microdose, 300 mcg/vial—standard); inj 120, 300 mcg Rh_o(D) immune globulin IV, human

Adverse effects

CNS: Lethargy
INTEG: Irritation at inj site, fever
MS: Myalgia

Contraindications: Previous immunization with this drug, Rh_o (O)-positive/D^u-positive patient

Precautions: Pregnancy **C**

Pharmacokinetics	
Absorption	Well absorbed
Distribution	Unknown
Metabolism	Unknown
Excretion	Unknown
Half-life	Unknown

R

Pharmacodynamics

Onset	Rapid
Peak	Unknown
Duration	Unknown

Interactions

Drug classifications

Live virus vaccines: decreased antibody response to vaccine

NURSING CONSIDERATIONS

Assessment

- ⚠ Assess for allergies, reactions to immunizations; previous immunization with this drug
- Obtain type and cross-match of mother's blood and of neonate's cord blood; neonate must be Rh_o(D)-positive, mother must be Rh_o(D)-negative and (D^u)-negative, medication should be given if there is a doubt
- ⚠ Assess for intravascular hemolysis: back pain, chills, hemoglobinuria, renal insufficiency, idiopathic thrombocytopenic purpura

Nursing diagnoses

- Knowledge, deficient (teaching)

Implementation

IM route

- Reconstitute Rh_o (D) immune globulin IV using 1.25 ml of 0.9% NaCl swirl
- Do not use Rh_o (D) immune globulin or Rh_o (D) immune globulin microdose by **IV**
- Give IM inj in deltoid muscle within 3 hr if possible; aspirate to prevent **IV** administration
- Give only equal lot numbers of drug, crossmatch
- Give only MICRh_oGAM for abortions or miscarriages <13 wk unless fetus or father is Rh-negative
- Store in refrigerator

IV, direct route

- Roconstitute Rh_o (D) immune globulin IV using 2.5 ml of 0.9% NaCl, swirl, give over 3-5 min
- Do not use Rh_o (D) immune globulin or Rh_o (D) immune globulin microdose by **IV**

Patient/family education

- Teach patient how drug works; that drug must be given after subsequent deliveries if subsequent babies are Rh-positive

Evaluation

Positive therapeutic outcome

- Prevention of Rh_o(D) sensitization in transfusion error
- Prevention of erythroblastosis fetalis in subsequent Rh_o(D)-positive neonates

ribavarin (Rx)

(rye-ba-vye'rin)

Virazole

Func. class.: Synthetic antiviral

Chem. class.: Tricyclic amine

Pregnancy category X

Action: Prevents replication of DNA and RNA synthesis

Therapeutic Outcome: Resolution of severe lower respiratory tract infections

Uses: Severe lower respiratory tract infections in infants and children

Investigational uses: Influenza A or B (early)

Dosage and routes

Infants and young children: INH 20 mg/ml × 12-18 hr/day × 3-7 days

Available forms: Powder for reconstitution for aerosol 6 g/vial

Adverse effects

CNS: Dizziness, faintness

CV: Hypotension, cardiac arrest

EENT: Eye irritation, conjunctivitis, blurred vision, photosensitivity

INTEG: Rash

Contraindications: Pregnancy **X**, hypersensitivity, lactation, child <1 yr

Precautions: Epilepsy, hepatic disease, renal disease

Pharmacokinetics

Absorption	Inh (systemic)
Distribution	To respiratory tract
Metabolism	Liver
Excretion	Respiratory tract
Half-life	9½ hr

Pharmacodynamics

Onset	Unknown
Peak	Inh end
Duration	Unknown

Interactions

Individual drugs

Zidovudine: decreased antiviral action, increased toxicity

Drug classification

Cardiac glycosides: increased toxicity

NURSING CONSIDERATIONS

Assessment

- Assess allergies before initiation of treat-

ment, reaction of each medication; list allergies on chart in bright red letters
- Monitor respiratory status: rate, character, wheezing, tightness in chest
- Obtain C&S test results before starting treatment

Nursing diagnoses
- Infection, risk for (uses)
- Gas exchange, impaired (uses)
- Knowledge, deficient (teaching)

Implementation
- Give by the Viratek small particle aerosol generator (SPAG-2), do not use other inhalation equipment
- May be given by an oxygen hood for infants, or a face mask may be attached to the SPAG-2
- Reconstitute 6 g of sterile water for inj or inh, place sol in the Erlenmeyer flask and dilute further to 20 mg/ml

Patient/family education
- Teach patient and parents aspects of drug therapy

Evaluation
Positive therapeutic outcome
- Absence of respiratory syncytial virus (RSV)

riboflavin (vitamin B_2) (OTC)
(rye'boo-flay-vin)

Func. class.: Vitamin B_2, water soluble

Pregnancy category A

Action: Needed for respiratory reactions (catalyzes proteins) and for normal vision

Therapeutic Outcome: Prevention or treatment of riboflavin deficiency

Uses: Vitamin B_2 deficiency or polyneuritis; cheilosis adjunct with thiamine

Dosage and routes
Deficiency

Adult and child >12 yr: PO 5-25 mg daily

Child <12 yr: PO 2-10 mg daily, then 0.6 mg/1000 cal ingested

RDA

Adult: Males 1.4-1.8 mg; females 1.2-1.3 mg

Available forms: Tabs 5, 10, 25, 50, 100, 250 mg

Adverse effects
GU: Yellow discoloration of urine (large doses)

Precautions: Pregnancy **A**

Pharmacokinetics

Absorption	Well absorbed (by active transport)
Distribution	60% protein bound, widely distributed, crosses placenta
Metabolism	Unknown
Excretion	Kidneys (unchanged), excess amounts
Half-life	1-1½ hr

Pharmacodynamics
Unknown

Interactions
Individual drugs

Alcohol, probenecid: increased riboflavin need

Tetracycline: decreased action of tetracycline

Drug classifications

Antidepressants (tricyclic), phenothiazines: increased riboflavin need

Drug/lab test

False increase: urinary catecholamines

NURSING CONSIDERATIONS
Assessment
- Assess patient's nutritional status: liver, eggs, dairy products, yeast, whole grain, green vegetables
- Assess for vit B_2 deficiency: photophobia, cheilosis, stomatitis, ocular swelling

Nursing diagnoses
- Nutrition: less than body requirements, imbalanced (uses)
- Knowledge, deficient (teaching)

Implementation
- Give with food for better absorption
- Store in airtight, light-resistant container

Patient/family education
- Inform patient that urine may turn bright yellow
- Instruct patient about addition of needed foods that are rich in riboflavin

Evaluation
Positive therapeutic outcome
- Absence of headache, GI problems, cheilosis, skin lesions, depression, burning, itchy eyes, anemia

R

rifabutin (Rx)

(riff'a-byoo-tin)

Mycobutin

Func. class.: Antimycobacterial

Chem. class.: Rifamycin S derivative

Pregnancy category B

Do Not Confuse:
rifabutin/rifampin

Action: Inhibits DNA-dependent RNA polymerase in susceptible strains

Therapeutic Outcome: Antimycobacterial death of *Escherichia coli, Bacillus subtilis,* and *Mycobacterium avium*

Uses: Prevention of *M. avium* complex (MAC) in patients with advanced HIV infection

Investigational uses: *Helicobacter pylori* that has not responded to other treatment

Dosage and routes

Adult: PO 300 mg daily (may take as 150 mg bid)

Available forms: Caps 150 mg

Adverse effects

CNS: *Headache,* fatigue, anxiety, confusion, insomnia

GI: *Nausea, vomiting, anorexia, diarrhea,* heartburn, **hepatitis,** discolored saliva

GU: Hematuria, discolored urine

HEMA: **Hemolytic anemia, eosinophilia, thrombocytopenia, leukopenia**

INTEG: *Rash*

MISC: Flulike syndrome, shortness of breath, chest pressure

MS: Asthenia, arthralgia, myalgia

Contraindications: Hypersensitivity, active TB, WBC $<1000/mm^3$, platelets $<50,000/mm^3$

Precautions: Pregnancy **B,** lactation, hepatic disease, blood dyscrasias, children

Pharmacokinetics

Absorption	Well absorbed
Distribution	Widely distributed
Metabolism	Liver
Excretion	Kidney
Half-life	45 hr

Pharmacodynamics

Onset	Unknown
Peak	2-3 hr

Interactions

Individual drugs

Amprenavir, clofibrate, cycloSPORINE, dapsone, delavirdine, digoxin, disopyramide, efavirenz, fluconazole, indinavir, ketoconazole, nelfinavir, nevirapine, phenytoin, quinidine, saquinavir, theophylline, tocainide, verapamil, zidovudine: decreased action of each specific drug

Ritonavir: increased rifabutin level

Drug classifications

Analgesics (opioid), anticoagulants, barbiturates, β-blockers, contraceptives (oral), corticosteroids, estrogens, sulfonylureas: decreased action of each specific drug

Drug/food

High-fat foods: decreased absorption

Drug/lab test

Interference: folate level, vit B_{12}, BSP, gallbladder studies

NURSING CONSIDERATIONS

Assessment

- Assess for active TB: chest x-ray, sputum culture, blood culture, biopsy of lymph nodes, obtain PPD test; drug should be given only for MAC and never for TB
- Monitor CBC for neutropenia, thrombocytopenia, eosinophilia

Nursing diagnoses

- Infection, risk for (uses)
- Diarrhea (adverse reaction)
- Injury, risk for (adverse reaction)
- Knowledge, deficient (teaching)
- Noncompliance (teaching)

Implementation

- Give with meals to decrease GI symptoms; better to take on empty stomach 1 hr ac or 2 hr pc; high-fat food slows absorption
- Give antiemetic if vomiting occurs

Patient/family education

- Caution patient that compliance with dosage schedule and duration is necessary
- Instruct patient that scheduled appointments must be kept or relapse may occur
- Instruct patient to notify prescriber if hepatitis, neutropenia, or thrombocytopenia occurs: sore throat, fever, bleeding, bruising, yellow sclera, anorexia, nausea, vomiting, fatigue, weakness; myositis: muscle or bone pain
- Advise patient that urine, feces, saliva, sputum, sweat, tears may be colored red-orange; soft contact lens may become permanently stained
- Caution patients using oral contraceptives to use a nonhormonal method of birth control

because rifabutin may decrease efficiency of oral contraceptives

Evaluation

Positive therapeutic outcome

- Decreased symptoms of *M. avium* in patients with HIV

rifampin (Rx)

(rif'am-pin)

Rifadin, Rimactane, Rofact ♣

Func. class.: Antitubercular

Chem. class.: Rifamycin B derivative

Pregnancy category C

Do Not Confuse: rifampin/rifabutin

Action: Inhibits DNA-dependent polymerase, decreases replication

Therapeutic Outcome: Bactericidal against the following organisms: mycobacteria, *Staphylococcus aureus, Haemophilus influenzae, Neisseria meningitidis, Legionella pneumophila*

Uses: Pulmonary TB, meningococcal carriers (prevention)

Dosage and routes

Tuberculosis

Adult: PO/**IV** max 600 mg/day as single dose 1 hr ac or 2 hr pc or 10 mg/kg/day 2-3 ×/wk

Child >5 yr: PO/**IV** 10-20 mg/kg/day as single dose 1 hr ac or 2 hr pc, max 600 mg/day, with other antitubercular drugs

6-mo regimen: 2-mo treatment of isoniazid, rifampin, pyrazinamide, and possibly streptomycin or ethambutol; then rifampin and isoniazid × 4 mo

9-mo regimen: Rifampin and isoniazid supplemented with pyrazinamide, or streptomycin or ethambutol

Meningococcal carriers

Adult: PO/**IV** 600 mg bid × 2 days

Child >5 yr: PO/**IV** 10-20 mg/kg bid × 2 days, max 600 mg/dose

Infant 3 mo-1 yr: PO 5 mg/kg bid for 2 days

Prevention of* H. influenzae *type B infection

Adult: PO 600 mg/day × 4 days

Child: PO 20 mg/kg/day × 4 days

Available forms: Caps 150, 300 mg; powder for inj 600 mg/vial

Adverse effects

CNS: Headache, fatigue, anxiety, drowsiness, confusion

EENT: Visual disturbances

GI: *Nausea, vomiting, anorexia, diarrhea,* **pseudomembranous colitis,** *heartburn,* sore mouth and tongue, **pancreatitis,** elevated liver function tests

GU: **Hematuria, acute renal failure, hemoglobinuria**

HEMA: **Hemolytic anemia, eosinophilia, thrombocytopenia, leukopenia**

INTEG: Rash, pruritus, urticaria

MISC: Flulike syndrome, menstrual disturbances, edema, shortness of breath

MS: Ataxia, weakness

Contraindications: Hypersensitivity

Precautions: Pregnancy **C,** lactation, hepatic disease, blood dyscrasias, child <5 yr

Pharmacokinetics

Absorption	Well absorbed (PO), completely absorbed (**IV**)
Distribution	Widely distributed, crosses placenta
Metabolism	Liver—extensively
Excretion	Feces
Half-life	3 hr

Pharmacodynamics

	PO	IV
Onset	Rapid	Rapid
Peak	2-3 hr	Inf end

Interactions

Individual drugs

Acetaminophen: decreased action of acetaminophen
Alcohol: decreased action of alcohol
Chloramphenicol: decreased effect of chloramphenicol
Clofibrate: decreased action of clofibrate
CycloSPORINE: decreased action of cycloSPORINE
Dapsone: decreased action of dapsone
Digoxin: decreased action of digoxin
Diltiazem: decreased action of diltiazem
Doxycycline: decreased action of doxycycline
Haloperidol: decreased action of haloperidol
Imidazole: decreased antifungal action
Isoniazid: increased hepatotoxicity
Lithium: increased lithium toxicity
Nifedipine: decreased action of nifedipine
Phenytoin: decreased effect of phenytoin
Sodium lactate: drugs are incompatible
Theophylline: decreased effect of theophylline
Verapamil: decreased effect of verapamil
Zidovudine: decreased action of zidovudine

R

Drug classifications
Anticoagulants: decreased action of anticoagulants
Antidiabetics: decreased action of antidiabetics
Barbiturates: decreased action of barbiturates
Benzodiazepines: decreased action of benzodiazepines
β-blockers: decreased action of β-blockers
Contraceptives (oral), glucocorticoids: decreased effect
Fluroquinolones: decreased action of fluoroquinolones
Hormones: decreased action of hormones
Imidazole antifungals: decreased antifungal action
Sulfonamides: decreased action of sulfonamides
Protease inhibitors: decreased action of protease inhibitors

Drug/lab test
Interference: folate level, vit B_{12} gallbladder studies, dexamethasone suppression test
False positive: direct Coombs' test

NURSING CONSIDERATIONS
Assessment
- Monitor liver studies qmo: ALT, AST, bilirubin
- Monitor renal status: before, qmo: BUN, creatinine, output, sp gr, urinalysis
- Monitor mental status often: affect, mood, behavioral changes; psychosis may occur
- Monitor hepatic status: decreased appetite, jaundice, dark urine, fatigue
- Assess for infection: sputum culture, lung sounds
- C&S should be performed before beginning treatment, during, and after therapy is completed

Nursing diagnoses
- Infection, risk for (uses)
- Diarrhea (adverse reactions)
- Injury, risk for (adverse reactions)
- Knowledge, deficient (teaching)
- Noncompliance (teaching)

Implementation
- Administer with meals to decrease GI symptoms; better to take on empty stomach 1 hr ac or 2 hr pc, with full glass of water

Intermittent IV route
- Give by intermittent inf after reconstituting 600 mg/10 ml of sterile water for inj, agitate gently; dilute further in 100 or 500 ml of 0.9% NaCl or D_5W; give 100 ml/30 min or 500 ml/3 hr
- Do not mix with other drugs or sols

Patient/family education
- Instruct patient that compliance with dosage schedule, duration is necessary
- Instruct patient that scheduled appointments must be kept or relapse may occur
- Instruct patient to notify prescriber if hepatitis, neutropenia, or thrombocytopenia occurs: sore throat, fever, bleeding, bruising, yellow sclera, anorexia, nausea, vomiting, fatigue, weakness
- Advise patient that urine, feces, saliva, sputum, sweat, tears may be colored red-orange; soft contact lens may be permanently stained
- Caution patients using oral contraceptives to use a nonhormonal method of birth control because rifabutin may decrease the efficiency of oral contraceptives
- Advise patient to avoid alcohol, hepatotoxicity may occur

Evaluation
Positive therapeutic outcome
- Decreased symptoms of TB

rifapentine (Rx)
(riff'ah-pen-teen)
Priftin
Func. class.: Antitubercular
Chem. class.: Rifamycin derivative
Pregnancy category C

Action: Inhibits DNA-dependent polymerase, decreases tubercule bacilli replication

Therapeutic Outcome: Resolution of pulmonary TB

Uses: Pulmonary TB; must be used with at least one other antitubercular drug

Dosage and routes
Intensive phase
Adult: PO 600 mg (4 150 mg tabs 2 ×/wk), with an interval of 72 hr between doses × 2 mo; must be given with at least one other antitubercular drug

Continuation phase
Adult: 600 mg qwk × 4 mo in combination with isoniazid or other appropriate antitubercular drug

Available forms: Tabs 150 mg

Adverse effects
CNS: Headache, fatigue, anxiety, dizziness
EENT: Visual disturbances
GI: *Nausea, vomiting, anorexia, diarrhea,* bilirubinemia, hepatitis, increased ALT, AST, *heartburn,* **pancreatitis**

GU: **Hematuria,** pyuria, proteinuria, urinary casts, urine discoloration
HEMA: **Thrombocytopenia, leukopenia, neutropenia, lymphopenia,** anemia, **leukocytosis,** purpura, hematoma
INTEG: Rash, pruritus, urticaria, acne
MISC: Edema, aggressive reaction, increased B/P
MS: Gout, arthrosis

Contraindications: Hypersensitivity to rifamycins, porphyria

Precautions: Pregnancy **C,** lactation, hepatic disease, blood dyscrasias, children <12 yr, HIV, elderly

Pharmacokinetics	
Absorption	Unknown
Distribution	Unknown
Metabolism	Unknown
Excretion	Unknown
Half-life	Unknown

Pharmacodynamics	
Onset	Unknown
Peak	Unknown
Duration	Unknown

Interactions

Individual drugs

Amitriptyline, chloramphenicol, clarithromycin, clofibrate, cycloSPORINE, dapsone, delaviridine, diazepam, digoxin, diltiazam, disopyramide, doxycycline, fentanyl, fluconazole, haloperidol, indinavir, itraconazole, ketoconazole, methadone, mexiletine, nelfinavir, NIFEdipine, nortriptyline, phenytoin, quinidine, quinine, ritonavir, saquinavir, sildenafil, tacrolimus, theophylline, tocainide, verapamil, warfarin, zidovudine: decreased action of each specific drug

Drug classifications

Anticoagulants, antidiabetics, barbiturates, β-adrenergic blockers, corticosteroids, fluoroquinolones, oral contraceptives, phenothiazines, progestins, thyroid preparations: decreased action of each drug class
Protease inhibitors: use extreme caution

Drug/food

Food: increased absorption with food

Drug/lab test

Interference: folate level, vit B_{12}

NURSING CONSIDERATIONS

Assessment

- Obtain baselines in CBC, AST, ALT, bilirubin, platelets
- Assess for infection: sputum culture, lung sounds
- Assess signs of anemia: Hct, Hgb, fatigue
- Monitor liver studies qmo: ALT, AST, bilirubin
- Monitor renal status qmo: BUN, creatinine, output, sp gr, urinalysis
- Assess hepatic status: decreased appetite, jaundice, dark urine, fatigue

Nursing diagnoses

- Infection, risk for (uses)
- Diarrhea (side effects)
- Knowledge, deficient (teaching)
- Noncompliance (teaching)

Implementation

- May be given with food for GI upset
- Give antiemetic if vomiting occurs
- Administer after C&S is completed; qmo to detect resistance

Patient/family education

- Advise patient that compliance with dosage schedule, duration is necessary
- Instruct patient that scheduled appointments must be kept; relapse may occur
- Teach patient that urine, feces, saliva, sputum, sweat, tears may be colored red-orange; soft contact lenses, dentures may be permanently stained
- Teach patient to use alternative method of contraception, oral contraceptive action may be decreased
- Teach patient to report flulike symptoms: excessive fatigue, anorexia, vomiting, sore throat; unusual bleeding, jaundice of skin, eyes

Evaluation

Positive therapeutic outcome

- Decreased symptoms of TB
- Negative culture

R

rifaximin (Rx)

(rif-ax'i-min)
Xifaxan
Func. class: Misc. antiinfective
Chem. class: Analog of rifampin
Pregnancy category C

Action: Binds to bacterial DNA dependent RNA polymerase, thereby inhibiting bacterial R synthesis.

Therapeutic Outcome: Bacterial action against *E. coli*

Uses: Traveler's diarrhea in those ≥12 yrs old, caused by *E. coli*

Dosage and routes

Adult and child ≥12 yr: PO 200 mg tid × 3 days without regard to meals

Available forms: Tabs 200 mg

Adverse effects

CNS: Abnormal dreams, dizziness, insomnia
GI: *Abdominal pain, constipation, defecation urgency, flatulence, nausea, rectal tenesmus,* vomiting
MISC: *Headache, pyrexia*

Contraindications: Hypersensitivity

Precautions: Pregnancy **C**, lactation, children

Pharmacokinetics

Absorption	Unknown
Distribution	Unknown
Metabolism	Induces P450 3A4 (CYP3A4)
Excretion	Feces
Half-life	6 hr

Pharmacodynamics

Unknown

Interactions: None known

NURSING CONSIDERATIONS

Assessment

- Assess for GI symptoms: amount character of diarrhea, abdominal pain, nausea, vomiting
- ◆ Assess for overgrowth of infection and pseudomembranous colitis

Nursing diagnoses

- Infection, risk for (uses)
- Noncompliance (teaching)
- Knowledge, deficient (teaching)

Implementation

- May be administered without regard to food

Patient/family education

- Instruct patient to discontinue rifaximin and notify prescriber if diarrhea persists for more than 24-48 hrs, if diarrhea worsens, or if blood is in stools and fever is present

Evaluation

Positive therapeutic outcome

- Absence of infection

riluzole (Rx)

(ri-loo′zole)

Rilutek

Func. class.: Amyotropic lateral sclerosis (ALS) agent

Chem. class.: Benzathiazole

Pregnancy category C

Action: Unknown; may act by inhibiting glutamate, interfering with binding of amino acid receptors, inactivation of voltage-dependent sodium channels

Therapeutic Outcome: Decreased symptoms of ALS

Uses: ALS

Dosage and routes

Adult: PO 50 mg q12h, take 1 hr ac or 2 hr pc

Available forms: Tabs 50 mg

Adverse effects

CNS: Hypertonia, depression, dizziness, insomnia, somnolence, vertigo
CV: Hypertension, tachycardia, phlebitis, palpitation, postural hypertension
GI: Nausea, vomiting, dyspepsia, anorexia, diarrhea, flatulence, stomatitis, dry mouth, increased LFTs, jaundice
GU: UTI, dysuria
HEMA: **Neutropenia**
INTEG: Pruritus, eczema, alopecia, **exfoliative dermatitis**
RESP: Decreased lung function; rhinitis, increased cough

Contraindications: Hypersensitivity

Precautions: Pregnancy **C**, neutropenia, renal disease, hepatic disease, elderly, lactation, children, cigarette smoking

Pharmacokinetics

Absorption	Well
Distribution	Unknown
Metabolism	Extensively—live
Excretion	Urine, feces
Half-life	Unknown

Pharmacodynamics

Unknown

Interactions

Individual drugs

Allopurinol, leflunomide, methotrexate, methyldopa, sulfasalazine, tacrine: increased hepatic injury

Amitriptyline, caffeine, theophylline: decreased elimination of riluzole
Carbamazepine: increased LFTs
Cigarette smoke, omeprazole, rifampin: increased elimination of riluzole
Drug classifications
Barbiturates: increased LFTs
Quinolones: decreased elimination of riluzole
Drug/food
Charcoal-broiled foods: increased elimination of riluzole
High-fat meal: decreased absorption

NURSING CONSIDERATIONS
Assessment
- Monitor liver function tests: AST, ALT, bilirubin, GGT, baseline and qmo × 3 mo, then q3 mo
- Assess for neutropenia (neutrophils <500/mm^3)

Nursing diagnoses
- Mobility, physical, impaired (uses)
- Knowledge, deficient (teaching)

Implementation
- Give 1 hr ac or 2 hr pc; a high-fat meal decreases absorption

Patient/family education
- Advise to report febrile illness, may indicate neutropenia
- Teach reason for drug and expected results

Evaluation
Positive therapeutic outcome
- Decreasing symptoms of ALS

rimantadine (Rx)
(ri-man′ti-deen)
Flumadine
Func. class.: Synthetic antiviral
Chem. class.: Tricyclic amine
Pregnancy category C

Do Not Confuse:
rimantadine/amantadine/ranitidine

Action: Prevents uncoating of nucleic acid in viral cell, preventing penetration of virus to host; causes release of dopamine from neurons

Therapeutic Outcome: Prevention of influenza type A

Uses: Prophylaxis or treatment of influenza type A

Dosage and routes
Renal/hepatic dose
Reduce as needed

Influenza type A prophylaxis
Adult and child 1-10 yr: PO 100 mg bid; in renal or hepatic disease, lower dose to 100 mg/day × 5-7 days
Child 1-10 yr: PO 5 mg/kg/day, max 150 mg

Treatment
Adult: PO 100 mg bid; in renal or hepatic disease, lower dose to 100 mg/day; start treatment at onset of symptoms, continue for at least 1 wk
Elderly: PO 100 mg/day × 5-7 days

Available forms: Tabs 100 mg; syr 50 mg/5 ml

Adverse effects
CNS: *Headache, dizziness,* fatigue, depression, hallucinations, tremors, **seizures,** insomnia, poor concentration, asthenia, gait abnormalities, anxiety, confusion
CV: Pallor, palpitations, edema
EENT: Tinnitus, taste abnormality, eye pain
GI: *Nausea, vomiting,* constipation, *dry mouth, anorexia, abdominal pain, diarrhea,* dyspepsia
INTEG: Rash

Contraindications: Hypersensitivity to drugs of adamantine class (this drug, amantadine)

Precautions: Pregnancy **C,** epilepsy, hepatic disease, renal disease, lactation, child <1 yr

Pharmacokinetics

Absorption	Minimally absorbed (PO)
Distribution	Widely distributed, crosses placenta, CSF concentration 50% plasma
Metabolism	Liver
Excretion	95% unchanged—kidneys
Half-life	2-3.5 hr, increased in renal disease

Pharmacodynamics

	PO
Onset	Unknown
Peak	1½-2½

Interactions
Individual drugs
Acetaminophen, aspirin: decreased peak concentration of rimantadine
Cimetidine: increased rimantidine concentration

R

NURSING CONSIDERATIONS

Assessment

- Assess for seizures; if seizures occur, drug should be discontinued
- Assess allergies before initiation of treatment, patient's reaction to each medication; list allergies on chart
- Monitor respiratory status: rate, character, wheezing, tightness in chest

Nursing diagnoses

- Infection, risk for (uses)
- Knowledge, deficient (teaching)

Implementation

- Give before exposure to influenza; continue for 10 days after contact
- Give at least 4 hr before bedtime to prevent insomnia
- Administer pc for better absorption, to decrease GI symptoms; cap may be opened and mixed with food for easy swallowing
- Give in divided doses to prevent CNS disturbances: headache, dizziness, fatigue, drowsiness
- Store in airtight, dry container

Patient/family education

- Instruct patient about aspects of drug therapy: need to report dyspnea, dizziness, poor concentration, behavioral changes
- Advise patient to avoid hazardous activities if dizziness occurs
- Caution patient to consult prescriber before taking OTC medications, alcohol; serious drug interactions may result

Evaluation

Positive therapeutic outcome

- Absence of fever, malaise, cough, dyspnea

risedronate (Rx)

(rih-sed'roh-nate)

Actonel

Func. class: Bone resorption inhibitor

Chem. class.: Bisphosphonate

Pregnancy category C

Action: Inhibits bone resorption; absorbs calcium phosphate crystal in bone and may directly block dissolution of hydroxyapatite crystals of bone

Therapeutic Outcome: Increased bone mass, activity without fractures

Uses: Paget's disease, prevention, treatment of osteoporosis in postmenopausal women, glucocorticoid-induced osteoporosis

Dosage and routes

Paget's disease

Adult: PO 30 mg daily × 2 mo; give calcium and vit D if dietary intake is lacking; if relapse occurs, retreatment is advised

Postmenopausal osteoporosis/ glucocorticoid-induced osteoporosis

Adult: PO 35 mg qwk (postmenopausal osteoporosis) or 5 mg daily

Available forms: Tabs 5, 30, 35 mg

Adverse effects

CNS: Dizziness, headache, depression

CV: Chest pain, hypertension

GI: *Abdominal pain, anorexia,* diarrhea, *nausea,* constipation

MS: *Bone pain,* arthralgia

MISC: Rash, UTI, pharyngitis

Contraindications: Hypersensitivity to bisphosphonates, inability to stand or sit upright for ≥30 min

Precautions: Pregnancy **C,** children, lactation, renal disease, active upper GI disorders

Pharmacokinetics	
Absorption	Unknown
Distribution	To bones
Metabolism	Unknown
Excretion	Kidneys
Half-life	Unknown

Pharmacodynamics	
Onset	Unknown
Peak	Unknown
Duration	Unknown

Interactions

Drug classifications

Antacids, calcium supplements: decreased absorption of risedronate

NSAIDs, salicylates: increased GI irritation

Drug/food

Food: decreased bioavailability; take ½ hr before food or drinks other than water

Drug/lab test

Increased: bone imaging agents

NURSING CONSIDERATIONS

Assessment

- Assess for symptoms of Paget's disease: headache, bone pain, increased head circumference
- Monitor electrolytes; renal function studies (calcium, phosphorus, magnesium, potassium)

- Assess for hypercalcemia: paresthesia, twitching, laryngospasm, Chvostek's/ Trousseau's signs

Nursing diagnoses
- Mobility, physical, impaired (uses)
- Nutrition: less than body requirements, imbalanced (uses)
- Knowledge, deficient (teaching)

Implementation
- Give PO for 2 mo to be effective in Paget's disease
- Give with a full glass of water; patient should be in upright position
- Administer supplemental calcium and vit D in Paget's disease
- Give daily ≥30 min ac
- Store in cool environment, out of direct sunlight

Patient/family education
- Advise patient to sit upright for ½ hr after dose to prevent irritation
- Instruct patient to comply with dietary restrictions
- Advise patient to notify prescriber if pregnancy is planned or suspected

Evaluation
Positive therapeutic outcome
- Increased bone mass, absence of fractures

risperidone (Rx)
(res-pare'a-done)
Risperdal, Risperdal M-TAB
Func. class: Antipsychotic
Chem. class.: Benzisoxazole derivative
Pregnancy category C

Do Not Confuse:
Risperdal/reserpine

Action: Unknown; may be mediated through both dopamine type 2 (D_2) and serotonin type 2 (5-HT_2) antagonism

Therapeutic Outcome: Decreased hallucinations and disorganized thought

Uses: Psychotic disorders

Dosage and routes
Adult: PO 1 mg bid, with incremental increases of 1 mg bid on days 2 and 3 to a dose of 3 mg bid by day 3; then do not increase dose for at least 1 wk
Elderly: PO 0.5 mg daily-bid increase by 1 mg qwk
Hepatic dose/renal dose
Adult: PO 0.5 mg, increase by 0.5 mg bid, then increase to 1.5 mg bid

Available forms: Tabs 1, 2, 3, 4 mg; oral sol 1 mg/ml; orally disintegrating tabs 0.5, 1, 2 mg

Adverse effects
CNS: *EPS (pseudoparkinsonism, akathisia, dystonia, tardive dyskinesia), drowsiness, insomnia, agitation, anxiety, headache,* **neuroleptic malignant syndrome,** dizziness, **seizures**
CV: Orthostatic hypotension, **tachycardia**
EENT: Blurred vision
GI: *Nausea,* vomiting, *anorexia, constipation,* jaundice, weight gain
RESP: Rhinitis

Contraindications: Hypersensitivity, lactation, seizure disorders

Precautions: Pregnancy **C,** children, renal disease, hepatic disease, elderly, breast cancer

Pharmacokinetics	
Absorption	Unknown
Distribution	Unknown
Metabolism	Liver, extensively
Excretion	Unknown
Half-life	Unknown

Pharmacodynamics	
Onset	Unknown
Peak	Unknown
Duration	Up to 12 hr

Interactions
Individual drugs
Alcohol: increased effects of both drugs, oversedation
Carbamazepine: increased risperidone excretion
Levodopa: decreased levodopa effect
Drug classifications
Antipsychotics: increased EPS
CNS depressants: increased sedation
Drug/herb
Betel palm, kava: increased extrapyramidal symptoms (EPS)
Cola tree, hops, nettle, nutmeg: increased action
Kava: increased CNS depression
Drug/lab test
Increased: prolactin levels

NURSING CONSIDERATIONS
Assessment
- Assess mental status: orientation, mood,

behavior, presence and type of hallucinations before initial administration and monthly; this drug should significantly reduce psychotic behavior
- Check that patient swallows all PO medication; check for hoarding or giving of medication to other patients
- Monitor I&O ratio, palpate bladder if low urinary output occurs, especially in elderly; urinalysis recommended before, during prolonged therapy
- Monitor bilirubin, CBC, liver function studies monthly
- Assess affect, orientation, LOC, reflexes, gait, coordination, sleep pattern disturbances
- Monitor B/P with patient in sitting, standing, and lying positions; take pulse and respirations q4h during initial treatment; establish baseline before starting treatment; report drops of 30 mm Hg; obtain baseline ECG and monitor Q- and T-wave changes
- Check for dizziness, faintness, palpitations, tachycardia on rising; severe orthostatic hypotension is common
- ◆ Identify for neuroleptic malignant syndrome: hyperpyrexia, muscle rigidity, increased CPK, altered mental status; drug should be discontinued
- Assess for EPS including akathisia (inability to sit still, no pattern to movements), tardive dyskinesia (bizarre movements of the jaw, mouth, tongue, extremities), pseudoparkinsonism (rigidity, tremors, pill rolling, shuffling gait); an antiparkinsonian drug should be prescribed
- Assess for constipation, urinary retention daily; if these occur, increase bulk, water in diet

Nursing diagnoses
- Thought processes, disturbed (uses)
- Coping, ineffective (uses)
- Knowledge, deficient (teaching)
- Noncompliance (teaching)

Implementation
- PO with full glass of water, milk; or give with food to decrease GI upset
- Do not open blister pack or orally disintegrating tabs until ready to use. Tear one of the four units apart at perforation; bend corner where indicated; peel back foil; do not push tab through foil; remove from pack and place on tongue; tab disintegrates in seconds and can be swallowed with or without liquids
- Store in airtight, light-resistant container
- Patient should lie down 30 min after IM inj

Patient/family education
- Teach patient to use good oral hygiene; frequent rinsing of mouth, sugarless gum for dry mouth
- Caution patient to avoid hazardous activities until drug response is determined; dizziness, blurred vision may occur
- Inform patient that orthostatic hypotension occurs often; patient should rise from sitting or lying position gradually and remain lying down for at least 30 min after IM inj
- Instruct patient to avoid hot tubs, hot showers, tub baths; hypotension may occur
- Inform patient that heat stroke may occur in hot weather, and to take extra precautions to stay cool
- Advise patient to avoid abrupt withdrawal of this drug, or EPS may result; drug should be withdrawn slowly
- Teach patient to avoid OTC preparations (cough, hay fever, cold) unless approved by prescriber; serious drug interactions may occur; avoid use with alcohol, CNS depressants because increased drowsiness may occur
- Advise patient to use contraception, to inform prescriber if pregnancy is planned or suspected

Evaluation
Positive therapeutic outcome
- Decrease in emotional excitement, hallucinations, delusions, paranoia
- Reorganization of patterns of thought, speech

Treatment of overdose: Lavage, provide airway

ritonavir (Rx)
(ri-toe'na-veer)
Norvir
Func. class.: Antiretroviral
Chem. class.: Protease inhibitor
Pregnancy category B

Do Not Confuse:
ritonavir/retrovir

Action: Inhibits HIV-1 protease and prevents maturation of the infectious virus

Therapeutic Outcome: Improvement of HIV-1 infection

Uses: HIV-1 in combination with other antiretrovirals

Dosage and routes
Adult: PO 600 mg bid; if nausea occurs, begin dose at ½ and gradually increase
Child 2-16 yr: PO 400 mg/m^2 bid up to 1200 mg/day

Available forms: Caps 100 mg; oral sol 80 mg/ml

Adverse effects

CNS: Paresthesia, headache, **seizures**, dizziness, insomnia, headache, fever
GI: *Diarrhea,* buccal mucosa ulceration, abdominal pain, *nausea,* taste perversion, dry mouth, anorexia
INTEG: Rash
MISC: Asthenia, **angioedema, anaphylaxis, Stevens-Johnson syndrome,** increased lipids, lipodystrophy
MS: Pain

Contraindications: Hypersensitivity

Precautions: Pregnancy **B,** liver disease, lactation, children, pancreatitis, diabetes

Pharmacokinetics	
Absorption	Well
Distribution	Unknown
Metabolism	98% protein binding, liver
Excretion	Unknown
Half-life	3-5 hr

Pharmacodynamics	
Peak	2-4 hr

Interactions

Individual drugs

Amiodarone, bepridil, bupropion, clozapine, desipramine, dihydroergotamine, encainide, ergotamine, flecainide, meperedine, midazolam, pimozide, piroxicam, propafenone, propoxyphene, quinidine, saquinavir, terfenadine, trazolam, zolpidem: toxicity, do not use together
Atovaquone: decreased levels of atovaquone
Clarithromycin: increased level of both drugs
ddI: increased levels of both drugs
Fluconazole: increased ritonavir level
Divalproex: decreased levels of divalproex
Ethinyl estradiol: decreased levels of ethinyl estradiol
Lamotrigine: decreased levels of lamotrigine
Nevirapine, phenytoin: decreased ritonavir levels
Phenytoin: decreased levels of phenytoin
Sulfamethoxazole: decreased levels of sulfamethoxazole
Theophylline: decreased levels of theophylline
Zidovudine: decreased levels of zidovudine

Drug classifications

Anticoagulants: decreased levels of anticoagulants
Azole antifungals, benzodiazepines, HMG-CoA reductase inhibitors, interleukins: toxicity, do not use together
Barbiturates, rifamycins: decreased ritonavir level

Drug/herb

St. John's wort: decreased ritonavir levels, avoid concurrent use

Drug/lab test

Increased: ALT, GGT, AST, CPK, cholesterol, triglycerides, uric acid
Decreased: Hct, RBC, Hgb, neutrophils, WBC

NURSING CONSIDERATIONS

Assessment

- Assess signs of infection, anemia
- Monitor viral load and CD4 baseline and throughout therapy
- Assess liver function studies: ALT, AST
- Monitor C&S before drug therapy; drug may be taken as soon as culture is done; repeat C&S after treatment; determine the presence of other sexually transmitted diseases
- Assess bowel pattern before, during treatment; if severe abdominal pain with bleeding occurs, drug should be discontinued; monitor hydration
- Assess skin eruptions, rash
- Assess allergies before treatment, reaction to each medication; place allergies on chart

Nursing diagnoses

- Infection, risk for (uses)
- Knowledge, deficient (teaching)

Implementation

- Administer with food at equal intervals around the clock
- Mix oral powder with high-calorie drink
- Store caps in refrigerator

Patient/family education

- Teach patient to take as prescribed; if dose is missed, take as soon as remembered up to 1 hr before next dose; do not double dose
- Teach patient that drug must be taken in equal intervals around the clock to maintain blood levels for duration of therapy
- Teach patient that drug is not a cure for HIV; opportunistic infections may continue to be acquired, and others may continue to contract HIV from the patient
- Advise patient not to use St. John's wort, that it decreases this drug's effect
- Inform that redistribution of body fat or accumulation of body fat may occur

Evaluation

Positive therapeutic outcome

- Decreasing symptoms of HIV
- Improving viral load and CD4 cell counts

R

rituximab (Rx)

(rih-tuks'ih-mab)

Rituxan

Func. class.: Antineoplastic—miscellaneous

Chem. class.: Murine/human monoclonal antibody

Pregnancy category C

Action: Directed against the CD20 antigen that is found on malignant B lymphocytes; CD20 regulates a portion of cell cycle initiation/differentiation

Therapeutic Outcome: Decreased tumor size, prevention of spread of cancer

Uses: Non-Hodgkin's lymphoma (CD20 positive, B-cell), bulky disease (tumors >10 cm)

Dosage and routes

Adult: **IV** inf 375 mg/m^2 qwk × 4 doses; give at 50 mg/hr for 1st inf; if hypersensitivity does not occur, increase rate by 50 mg/hr q½h, max 400 mg/hr; slow/interrupt inf if hypersensitivity occurs; other inf can be given at 100 mg/hr and increased by 100 mg/hr, max 400 mg/hr

Available forms: Inj 10 mg/ml

Adverse effects

CNS: **Life-threatening brain infection**

CV: **Cardiac dysrhythmias**

GI: *Nausea, vomiting, anorexia*

GU: **Renal failure**

HEMA: **Leukopenia, neutropenia, thrombocytopenia**

INTEG: *Irritation at inj site, rash,* **fatal mucocutaneous infections (rare)**

MISC: Fever, chills, asthenia, headache, **angioedema,** hypotension, myalgia, bronchospasm

SYST: **Stevens-Johnson syndrome**

Contraindications: Hypersensitivity, murine proteins

Precautions: Pregnancy **C,** lactation, children, elderly, cardiac conditions

Pharmacokinetics

Absorption	Unknown
Distribution	Unknown
Metabolism	Unknown
Excretion	Unknown
Half-life	42-79 min

Pharmacodynamics

Onset	Unknown
Peak	Unknown
Duration	Unknown

Interactions: None known

NURSING CONSIDERATIONS

Assessment

- ⚠ Assess for signs of fatal infusion reaction: hypoxia, pulmonary infiltrates, acute respiratory distress syndrome, MI, ventricular fibrillation, cardiogenic shock; most fatal infusion reactions occur with 1st inf, discontinue drug
- ⚠ Assess for signs of severe mucocutaneous reactions: Stevens-Johnson syndrome, lichenoid dermatitis, toxic epidermal lysis; signs occur 1-13 wk after drug was given
- ⚠ Assess for tumor lysis syndrome: acute renal failure requiring hemodialysis, hyperkalemia, hypocalcemia, hyperuricemia, hyperphosphatasemia
- Monitor CBC, differential, platelet count weekly; withhold drug if WBC is <3500/mm^3, or platelet count <100,000/mm^3; notify prescriber of these results; drug should be discontinued
- Assess food preferences: list likes, dislikes
- Assess GI symptoms: frequency of stools
- Assess signs of dehydration: rapid respirations, poor skin turgor, decreased urine output, dry skin, restlessness, weakness

Nursing diagnoses

- Injury, risk for (side effects)
- Knowledge, deficient (teaching)

Implementation

IV route

- Administer after diluting to a final conc of 1-4 mg/ml; use 0.9% NaCl, D_5W, gently invert bag to mix; do not mix with other drugs
- Increase fluid intake to 2-3 L/day to prevent dehydration, unless contraindicated
- Change **IV** site q48h
- Provide nutritious diet with iron, vitamin supplement, low fiber, few dairy products
- Store vials at 36°-40° F, protect vials from direct sunlight, inf sol is stable at 36°-46° F × 24 hr and room temp for another 12 hr

Patient/family education

- Teach patient to report adverse reactions

Evaluation

Positive therapeutic outcome

- Decrease in tumor size, decrease in spread of cancer

rivastigmine (Rx)

(riv-as-tig'mine)

Exelon

Func. class.: Anti-Alzheimer agent

Chem. class.: Cholinesterase inhibitor

Pregnancy category B

Action: May enhance cholinergic functioning by increasing acetylcholine

Therapeutic Outcome: Decreased signs and symptoms of Alzheimer's dementia

Uses: Mild-moderate Alzheimer's dementia

Dosage and routes

Adult: PO 1.5 mg bid for 2 wk or more, may increase to 3 mg bid after 2 wk or more; may increase to 4.5 mg bid and thereafter 6 mg bid, max 12 mg/day

Available forms: Caps 1.5, 3, 4.5, 6 mg; sol 2 mg/ml

Adverse effects

CNS: *Tremors, confusion, insomnia,* psychosis, hallucination, depression, dizziness, headache, anxiety, somnolence, fatigue, syncope

GI: *Nausea, vomiting, anorexia, abdominal distress, flatulence,* diarrhea, constipation, dyspepsia

MISC: UTI, asthenia, increased sweating, hypertension, influenza-like syncope, weight change

Contraindications: Hypersensitivity to this drug, other carbamates; narrow-angle glaucoma, undiagnosed skin lesions

Precautions: Pregnancy **B,** renal disease, hepatic disease, respiratory disease, seizure disorder, asthma, lactation, children, cardiac disease, urinary obstruction, asthma

Pharmacokinetics

Absorption	Rapidly, completely
Distribution	Not known
Metabolism	To decarbamylated metabolite
Excretion	Kidney—metabolites, clearance lowered in elderly, hepatic disease, increased nicotine use
Half-life	1½ hr

Pharmacodynamics

Unknown

Interactions

Drug classifications

Cholinesterase inhibitors: increased synergistic effect

Drug/herb

Pill-bearing spurge: increased effect

NURSING CONSIDERATIONS

Assessment

- Monitor liver function studies: AST, ALT, alkaline phosphatase, LDH, bilirubin, CBC
- Assess for severe GI effects: nausea, vomiting, anorexia, weight loss
- Monitor B/P, respiration during initial treatment; hypo/hypertension should be reported
- Assess mental status: affect, mood, behavioral changes, depression; complete suicide assessment

Nursing diagnoses

- Knowledge, deficient (teaching)

Implementation

- Give with meals; take with AM and PM meal even though absorption may be decreased
- Provide assistance with ambulation during beginning therapy
- Discontinue treatment for several doses and restart at same or next lower dosage level if adverse reactions cause intolerance
- If treatment is interrupted for longer than several days treatment should be initiated with the lowest daily dose and titrate as indicated above

Patient/family education

- Teach patient procedure for giving oral sol; use instruction sheet provided
- Teach patient to notify prescriber of severe GI effects

Evaluation

Positive therapeutic outcome

- Increased coherence, decreased symptoms of Alzheimer's disease

R

rizatriptan (Rx)

(rye-zah-trip'tan)

Maxalt, Maxalt-MLT

Func. class.: Migraine agent

Chem. class.: 5-HT_1-like receptor agonist

Pregnancy category C

Action: Binds selectively to the vascular serotonin type 1 (5-HT_1) receptor, exerts antimigraine effect; causes vasoconstriction in cranial arteries

Therapeutic Outcome: After treatment, relief of migraine

Uses: Acute treatment of migraine

Dosage and routes

Adult: **PO** 5-10 mg single dose, redosing separate by 2 hr or more; max 30 mg/24 hr, use 5 mg in patient on propanolol; max 15 mg/24 hr

Available forms: Tabs (Maxalt) 5, 10 mg; orally disintegrating tabs (Maxalt-MLT) 5, 10 mg

Adverse effects

CNS: *Dizziness,* drowsiness, ***headache,*** *fatigue,* warm/cold sensation, flushing, hot flashes

CV: **MI, ventricular fibrillation, ventricular tachycardia, coronary artery vasospasm**

ENDO: Hot flashes, mild increase in growth hormone

GI: *Nausea,* dry mouth, diarrhea, abdominal pain

RESP: Chest tightness, pressure, dyspnea

Contraindications: Angina pectoris, history of MI, documented silent ischemia, Prinzmetal's angina, ischemic heart disease, concurrent ergotamine-containing preparations, uncontrolled hypertension, hypersensitivity, basilar or hemiplegic migraine

Precautions: Pregnancy **C**, postmenopausal women, men >40 yr, risk factors for CAD, hypercholesterolemia, obesity, diabetes, impaired hepatic or renal function, lactation, children, elderly

Pharmacokinetics

Absorption	Unknown
Distribution	Unknown
Metabolism	Liver (metabolite)
Excretion	Urine/feces
Half-life	2-3 hr

Pharmacodynamics

Onset	10 min-2 hr
Peak	Unknown
Duration	Unknown

Interactions

Individual drugs

Cimetidine, isocarboxazide, pargyline, phenelzine, propranolol, trancyclomine: increased rizatriptan action

Ergot: increased vasospastic effects

Drug classifications

Contraceptives (oral), MAOIs, MAOIs (nonselective types A and B): increased rizatriptan action

Ergot derivatives, 5-HT_1 receptor agonists: increased vasospastic effects

Selective serotonin reuptake inhibitors: increased weakness, hyperreflexia, incoordination

Drug/herb

SAM-e, St. John's wort: serotonin syndrome

Butterbur: increased effect

NURSING CONSIDERATIONS

Assessment

- Assess for stress level, activity, recreation, coping mechanisms
- Assess neurologic status: LOC, blurring vision, nausea, vomiting, tingling in extremities preceding headache
- Monitor for ingestion of tyramine-containing foods (pickled products, beer, wine, aged cheese), food additives, preservatives, colorings, artificial sweeteners, chocolate, caffeine, which may precipitate these types of headaches

Nursing diagnoses

- Pain, acute (uses)
- Knowledge, deficient (teaching)

Implementation

- Provide quiet, calm environment with decreased stimulation for noise, bright light, excessive talking
- Do not open blister pack until ready to use
- Put orally disintegrating tab on tongue to dissolve; swallow with saliva

Patient/family education

- Teach patient use of orally disintegrating tab: instruct patient not to open blister until use, to peel blister open with dry hands, to place tab on tongue, where it will dissolve, and to swallow with saliva (contains phenylalanine)
- Advise patient to report any side effects to prescriber
- Advise patient to use alternate contraception while taking drug if oral contraceptives are being used

Evaluation

Positive therapeutic outcome

- Decrease in frequency, severity of headache

ropinirole (Rx)

(roe-pin′e-role)

Requip

Func. class.: Antiparkinsonian agent

Chem. class.: Dopamine-receptor agonist, nonergot

Pregnancy category C

Action: Selective agonist for dopamine D_2 receptors (presynaptic/postsynaptic sites); binding at D_3 receptor contributes to antiparkinson effects

Therapeutic Outcome: Decreased symptoms of Parkinson's disease (involuntary movements)

Uses: Parkinsonism, restless legs syndrome

Dosage and routes

Adult: PO 0.25 mg tid, titrate weekly to max of 24 mg/day

Restless legs syndrome

Adult: PO 0.25 mg at bedtime, may increase until symptoms resolve

Available forms: Tabs 0.25, 0.5, 1, 2, 4, 5 mg

Adverse effects

CNS: Dystonia, *agitation, insomnia,* dizziness, psychosis, hallucinations, depression, somnolence, **sleep attacks**

CV: *Orthostatic hypotension,* hypotension, syncope, palpitations, **tachycardia,** hypertension

EENT: Blurred vision

GI: *Nausea, vomiting, anorexia, dry mouth,* constipation, dyspepsia, flatulence

GU: Impotence, urinary frequency

HEMA: **Hemolytic anemia, leukopenia, agranulocytosis**

INTEG: Rash, sweating

RESP: Pharyngitis, rhinitis, sinusitis, bronchitis, dyspnea

Contraindications: Hypersensitivity

Precautions: Pregnancy **C,** renal disease, cardiac disease, dysrhythmias, affective disorders, psychosis, hepatic disease

Pharmacokinetics

Absorption	Well absorbed
Distribution	Widely distributed
Metabolism	Liver, extensively by the liver by CYP450 CYP1A2 enzyme system
Excretion	Kidneys
Half-life	6 hr

Pharmacodynamics

Unknown

Interactions

Individual drugs

Cimetidine, ciprofloxacin, digoxin, diltiazem, enoxacin, erythromycin, fluvoxamine, levodopa, mexiletine, norfloxacin, tacrine, theophylline: increased effect of ropinirole

Metoclopramide: decreased ropinirole effect

Drug classifications

Butyrophenones, phenothiazines, thioxanthenes: decreased ropinirole effect

Drug/herb

Chaste tree fruit, kava: decreased ropinirole action

NURSING CONSIDERATIONS

Assessment

- Monitor B/P, respiration during initial treatment; hypotension or hypertension should be reported
- Assess mental status: affect, mood, behavioral changes, depression; complete suicide assessment
- Assess for involuntary movements in parkinsonism: akinesia, tremors, staggering gait, muscle rigidity, drooling; these symptoms should improve with therapy
- Assess for sleep attacks, drowsiness, falling asleep without warning even during hazardous activities

Nursing diagnoses

- Mobility, physical, impaired (uses)
- Injury, risk for (uses)
- Knowledge, deficient (teaching)
- Noncompliance (teaching)

Implementation

- Give drug until NPO before surgery
- Adjust dosage to patient response
- Give with meals to decrease GI upset

Patient/family education

- Advise patient that therapeutic effects may take several wk to a few mo
- Caution patient to change positions slowly to prevent orthostatic hypotension
- Instruct patient to use drug exactly as prescribed; if drug is discontinued abruptly, parkinsonian crisis may occur

Evaluation

Positive therapeutic outcome

- Decreased akathisia, other involuntary movements
- Increased mood

R

ropivacaine (Rx)

(roe-pi'va-kane)

Naropin

Func. class.: Local anesthetic

Chem. class.: Amide

Pregnancy category B

Action: Competes with calcium for sites in nerve membrane that control sodium transport across cell membrane; decreases rise of depolarization phase of action potential

Therapeutic Outcome: Maintenance of local anesthesia

Uses: Peripheral nerve block, caudal anesthesia, central neural block, vaginal, epidural, spinal block

Dosage and routes

Lumbar epidural block for C-section

Adult: 20-30 ml of 0.5% sol, or 15-20 ml of 0.75% sol

Thoracic epidural

Adult: 5-15 ml of 0.5%-0.75%

Major nerve block

Adult: 35-50 ml of 0.5% sol or 10-40 ml of 0.75% sol

Labor pain epidural

Adult: 10-20 ml of 0.2% sol, then 6-14 ml/hr

Postoperative (lumbar/thoracic epidural)

Adult: 6-14 ml/hr of 0.2%

Infiltration/minor nerve block

Adult: 1-100 ml of 0.2% sol or 1-40 ml of 0.5% sol

Available forms: Inj 2, 5, 7.5 mg/ml

Adverse effects

CNS: Anxiety, restlessness, **seizures, loss of consciousness,** drowsiness, disorientation, tremors, shivering, paresthesia

CV: **Myocardial depression, cardiac arrest, dysrhythmias,** bradycardia, hypotension, hypertension, **fetal bradycardia**

EENT: Blurred vision, tinnitus, pupil constriction

ENDO: Hypokalemia

GI: Nausea, vomiting

GU: Urinary retention

INTEG: Rash, urticaria, allergic reactions, edema, burning, skin discoloration at injection site, tissue necrosis

RESP: **Status asthmaticus, respiratory arrest, anaphylaxis**

Contraindications: Hypersensitivity to amide local anesthetics, child <12 yr, elderly, severe liver disease, severe hypotension, complete heart block

Precautions: Pregnancy **B,** severe drug allergies, hyperthyroidism, cardiovascular disease, hepatic disease, neurological disease

Pharmacokinetics

Absorption	Complete
Distribution	Unknown
Metabolism	Liver
Excretion	Kidneys
Half-life	Unknown

Pharmacodynamics

Onset	2-8 min
Peak	Unknown
Duration	3 hr, varies with inj site

Interactions

Individual drugs

Amiodarone, ciprofloxacin, fluvoxamine: increased effect

Chloroprocaine: decreased action of ropivacaine

Enflurane, epINEPHrine, halothane: increased dysrhythmias

Drug classifications

Antidepressants (tricyclic), MAOIs, phenothiazines: increased hypertension

Azole antifungals: increased effect

NURSING CONSIDERATIONS

Assessment

- Assess B/P, pulse, respiration during treatment
- Assess fetal heart tones during labor
- Assess allergic reactions: rash, urticaria, itching
- Assess cardiac status: ECG for dysrhythmias, pulse, B/P during anesthesia

Nursing diagnoses

- Knowledge, deficient (teaching)

Implementation

- Give only with resuscitative equipment nearby
- Give only drugs without preservatives for epidural or caudal anesthesia
- Use new sol; discard unused portions

Evaluation

Positive therapeutic outcome

- Anesthesia necessary for procedure

Treatment of overdose: Airway, O_2, vasopressor, **IV** fluids, anticonvulsants for seizures

rosiglitazone (Rx)

(roes-i-glye'ta-zone)

Avandia

Func. class.: Antidiabetic, oral

Chem. class.: Thiazolidinedione

Pregnancy category C

Action: Improves insulin resistance by hepatic glucose metabolism, insulin receptor kinase activity, insulin receptor phosphorylation

Therapeutic Outcome: Decreased symptoms of diabetes mellitus

Uses: Stable type 2 diabetes mellitus alone or in combination with sulfonylureas, metformin, or insulin

Dosage and routes

Monotherapy

Adult: PO 4 mg daily or in 2 divided doses, may increase to 8 mg daily or in 2 divided doses after 12 wk

Combination therapy

Adult: PO this drug should be added to metformin, sulfonylureas at the adult dose

Available forms: Tabs 2, 4, 8 mg

Adverse effects

CNS: Fatigue, headache

ENDO: Hyper/hypoglycemia

MISC: Accidental injury, upper respiratory tract infection, sinusitis, anemia, back pain, diarrhea, edema

Contraindications: Hypersensitivity to thiazolidinediones, children, lactation, diabetic ketoacidosis

Precautions: Pregnancy **C**, elderly, thyroid disease, hepatic, renal disease

Pharmacokinetics	
Absorption	Unknown
Distribution	Protein binding 99.8%
Metabolism	Unknown
Excretion	Urine, feces, breast milk
Half-life	Elimination 3-4 hr

Pharmacodynamics	
Onset	Unknown
Peak	6-12 wk
Duration	Unknown

Interactions

Drug classification

Contraceptives (oral): may decrease effect of oral contraceptive, alternative method advised

Drug/herb

Alfalfa, aloe, basil, bay, bilberry, bitter melon, black catechu, buchu, burdock, coriander, dandelion, eyebright (po), fenugreek, garlic, ginseng, glucomannan, goat's rue, gymnema, horehound, horse chestnut, jambul, myrrh, myrtle: increased antidiabetic effect

Bee pollen, blue cohosh, broom, chromium, elecampane, eucalyptus, gotu kola: decreased antidiabetic effect

Chromium, coenzyme Q10, fenugreek: hypoglycemia

Glucosamine: decreased glucose control

NURSING CONSIDERATIONS

Assessment

- Assess for hypoglycemic reactions (sweating, weakness, dizziness, anxiety, tremors, hunger), hyperglycemic reactions soon after meals
- Check liver function tests periodically; AST, FBS, ALT (if ALT >2.5 × ULN, do not use), HbA_{2c}, fasting plasma insulin, plasma lipids, lipoproteins, B/P, body weight during treatment

Nursing diagnoses

- Nutrition: more than body requirements, imbalanced (uses)
- Knowledge, deficient (teaching)

Implementation

- Convert from other oral hypoglycemic agents if needed; change may be made without gradual dosage change; monitor serum or urine glucose and ketones tid during conversion
- Give tabs crushed and mixed with meal or fluids for patients with difficulty swallowing
- Store in airtight container in cool environment

Patient/family education

- Teach patient to monitor capillary blood glucose test
- Teach patient symptoms of hypo/hyperglycemia, what to do about each
- Advise patient that drug must be continued on daily basis; explain consequence of discontinuing drug abruptly
- Advise patient to avoid OTC medications or herbal preparations unless approved by prescriber
- Advise patient that diabetes is lifelong illness; that this drug is not a cure, only controls symptoms
- Advise patient that all food included in diet plan must be eaten to prevent hypoglycemia
- Advise patient to carry/wear emergency ID and glucagon emergency kit for emergencies
- Instruct patient to notify prescriber if oral contraceptives are used
- Teach patient not to use if breastfeeding, may be secreted in breast milk

Evaluation

Positive therapeutic outcome

- Decrease in polyuria, polydipsia, polyphagia; clear sensorium; absence of dizziness; stable gait; blood glucose at normal level

R

rosuvastatin (Rx)
(roe-soo'va-sta-tin)
Crestor
Func. class.: Antilipemic
Chem. class.: HMG-CoA reductase inhibitor
Pregnancy category X

Action: Inhibits HMG-CoA reductase enzyme, which reduces cholesterol synthesis

Therapeutic Outcome: Decreasing cholesterol levels

Uses: As an adjunct in primary hypercholesterolemia (types IIa, IIb), mixed dyslipidemia elevated serum triglycerides, homozygous familial hypercholesterolemia (FH)

Dosage and routes
Patient should first be placed on a cholesterol-lowering diet

Hypercholesterolemia
Adult: PO 5-40 mg daily; initial dose 10 mg daily, reanalyze lipid levels at 2-4 wk and adjust dosage accordingly

Homozygous FH
Adult: PO 20 mg daily, max 40 mg

Dose in patients taking cycloSPORINE
Adult: 5 mg daily

Dose when taken with gemfibrozil
Adult: 10 mg daily

Available forms: Tabs 5, 10, 20, 40 mg

Adverse effects
CNS: *Headache, dizziness,* insomnia, paresthesia
GI: *Nausea, constipation, abdominal pain, flatus, diarrhea, dyspepsia, heartburn,* **kidney failure, liver dysfunction**, vomiting
HEMA: **Thrombocytopenia, hemolytic anemia, leukopenia**
INTEG: *Rash, pruritus,* photosensitivity
MS: *Asthenia, muscle cramps, arthritis, arthralgia, myalgia,* **myositis, rhabdomyolysis,** leg, shoulder or localized pain
RESP: Rhinitis, sinusitis, *pharyngitis,* bronchitis, increased cough

Contraindications: Pregnancy **X**, hypersensitivity, lactation, active liver disease

Precautions: Past liver disease, alcoholism, severe acute infections, trauma, hypotension, uncontrolled seizure disorders, severe metabolic disorders, electrolyte imbalances, children, severe renal impairment, elderly, hypothyroidism

Pharmacokinetics

Absorption	Unknown
Distribution	88% protein bound, crosses placenta
Metabolism	Minimal liver metabolism (about 10%)
Excretion	Primarily in feces (90%)
Half-life	19 hr

Pharmacodynamics

Onset	Unknown
Peak	3-5 hr
Duration	Unknown

Interactions
Individual drugs
Clofibrate, cycloSPORINE, gemfibrozil, niacin: increased myalgia, myositis
Warfarin: increased bleeding

Drug classifications
Antifungals (azole): increased myalgia, myositis
Bile acid sequestrants: increased effects

Drug/food
Grapefruit juice: possible toxicity

Drug/lab test
Increased: CPK, LFTs

NURSING CONSIDERATIONS
Assessment
- Assess diet: obtain diet history including fat, cholesterol in diet
- Monitor fasting cholesterol, LDL, HDL, triglycerides periodically during treatment
- Monitor liver function tests q1-2 mo during the first 1½ yr of treatment; AST, ALT, liver function tests may increase
- Monitor renal function in patients with compromised renal system: BUN, creatinine, I&O ratio
- Obtain ophthalmic exam before, 1 mo after treatment begins, annually; lens opacities may occur
- (Alert) Assess for muscle pain, tenderness, obtain CPK; if these occur, drug may need to be discontinued

Nursing diagnoses
- Knowledge, deficient (teaching)
- Noncompliance (teaching)

Implementation
- May be taken at any time of day, with or without food
- Store in cool environment in airtight, light-resistant container

Patient/family education
- Advise to report suspected pregnancy

- Advise that blood work and ophthalmic exam will be necessary during treatment
- Teach to report blurred vision, severe GI symptoms, dizziness, headache, muscle pain, weakness
- Teach to use sunscreen or stay out of the sun to prevent photosensitivity
- Teach that previously prescribed regimen will continue: low-cholesterol diet, exercise program, smoking cessation

Evaluation

Positive therapeutic outcome

- Cholesterol at desired level after 8 wk

rotavirus vaccine

RotaTeq

See Appendix A, Selected New Drugs

salmeterol (Rx)

(sal-met'er-ole)

Serevent

Func. class.: Adrenergic β_2 agonist, bronchodilator

Pregnancy category C

Action: Causes bronchodilatation by action on β_2 (pulmonary) receptors by increasing levels of cAMP, which relaxes smooth muscle; with very little effect on heart rate, maintains improvement in FEV from 3 to 12 hr; prevents nocturnal asthma symptoms

Therapeutic Outcome: Ease of breathing

Uses: Prevention of exercise-induced asthma, bronchospasm, COPD

Dosage and routes

Adult: INH 50 mcg (one inhalation as dry powder); exercise-induced bronchospasm: 50 mcg (2 inh) ½-1 hr prior to exercise

Child 4-12 yr: INH 50 mcg as dry powder bid; exercise-induced bronchospasm 50 mcg as dry powder ½-1 hr prior to exercise

Available forms: Inhalation powder 50 mcg/blister

Adverse effects

CNS: Tremors, anxiety, insomnia, headache, dizziness, stimulation, restlessness, hallucinations, flushing, irritability

CV: Palpitations, **tachycardia,** hypertension, angina, hypotension, **dysrhythmias**

EENT: Dry nose, irritation of nose and throat

GI: Heartburn, nausea, vomiting

MS: Muscle cramps

RESP: **Bronchospasm**

Contraindications: Hypersensitivity to sympathomimetics, tachydysrhythmias, severe cardiac disease

Precautions: Pregnancy **C**, lactation, cardiac disorders, hyperthyroidism, diabetes mellitus, hypertension, prostatic hypertrophy, narrow-angle glaucoma, seizures, acute asthma, as a substitute for corticosteroids

Pharmacokinetics	
Absorption	Unknown
Distribution	Unknown
Metabolism	Unknown
Excretion	Unknown
Half-life	Unknown

Pharmacodynamics	
Onset	5-15 min
Peak	4 hr
Duration	12 hr

Interactions

Drug classifications

Antidepressants (tricyclics): increased salmeterol action

β-Adrenergic blockers: block therapeutic effect

Bronchodilators, aerosol: increased action of bronchodilator

MAOIs: increased action of salmeterol

Drug/herb

Betel palm, butterbur, coffee, cola nut, figwort, fumitory, guarana, hawthorn, lily of the valley, motherwort, plantain, tea (black, green), yerba maté: increased stimulation

NURSING CONSIDERATIONS

Assessment

- Monitor respiratory function: vital capacity, FEV, ABGs, lung sounds, heart rate, rhythm (baseline)

Nursing diagnoses

- Airway clearance, ineffective (uses)
- Gas exchange, impaired (uses)
- Knowledge, deficient (teaching)

Implementation

- Shake aerosol container, ask patient to exhale, then place mouthpiece in mouth, inhale slowly, hold breath, remove, exhale slowly; allow at least 1 min between inhalations
- Use this medication before other medications and allow at least 1 min between each
- Use spacing device for pediatric/elderly patients
- Store in light-resistant container, do not expose to temp over 86° F (30° C)

S

Patient/family education

- Caution patient not to use OTC medications because extra stimulation may occur
- Instruct patient to use this medication before other medications and to allow at least 1 min between each, to prevent overstimulation
- Teach patient how to use inhaler; to avoid getting aerosol in eyes; blurring may result; to wash inhaler in warm water daily and dry; to avoid smoking, smoke-filled rooms, and persons with respiratory infections; review package insert with patient
- Instruct patient on administration of dose, not to use more than prescribed; serious side effects may occur

Evaluation

Positive therapeutic outcome

- Absence of dyspnea, wheezing
- Improved airway exchange
- Improved ABGs

Treatment of overdose: Administer a β_2-adrenergic blocker

salsalate (Rx)

(sal-sa'late)

Amigesic, Anaflex, Disalcid, Marthritic, Mono-Gesic, Salflex, Salgesic, Salsalate, Salsitab

Func. class.: Nonopioid analgesic; nonsteroidal antiinflammatory agent

Chem. class.: Salicylate

Pregnancy category C

Action: Blocks formation of peripheral prostaglandins, which cause pain and inflammation; antipyretic action results from inhibition of hypothalamic heat-regulating center; does not inhibit platelet aggregation

Therapeutic Outcome: Decreased pain, inflammation

Uses: Mild to moderate pain or fever, including arthritis, juvenile rheumatoid arthritis

Dosage and routes

Adult: PO 3 g/day in divided doses

Available forms: Caps 500 mg; tabs 500, 750 mg

Adverse effects

CNS: Stimulation, drowsiness, dizziness, confusion, **seizures,** headache, flushing, hallucinations, coma

CV: Rapid pulse, **pulmonary edema**

EENT: Tinnitus, hearing loss

ENDO: Hypoglycemia, hyponatremia, hypokalemia, alteration in acid-base balance

GI: *Nausea, vomiting, GI bleeding, diarrhea, heartburn,* anorexia, **hepatotoxicity**

HEMA: **Thrombocytopenia, agranulocytosis, leukopenia, neutropenia, hemolytic anemia,** increased protime

INTEG: *Rash,* urticaria, bruising

RESP: Wheezing, hyperpnea

Contraindications: Hypersensitivity to salicylates, NSAIDs, GI bleeding, bleeding disorders, children <3 yr, vit K deficiency

Precautions: Pregnancy **C** (1st trimester), anemia, hepatic disease, renal disease, Hodgkin's disease, lactation, elderly

Pharmacokinetics	
Absorption	Absorbed in small intestine
Distribution	Rapidly and widely distributed, crosses placenta
Metabolism	Not metabolized
Excretion	Unchanged—kidneys
Half-life	2-3 hr (low doses), 15-30 hr (high doses)

Pharmacodynamics	
Onset	30 min
Peak	1-3 hr
Duration	3-6 hr

Interactions

Individual drugs

Alcohol, heparin, ibuprofen, warfarin: increased bleeding

Insulin, methotrexate, phenytoin, probenecid: increased effects

p-Aminobenzoic acid: increased toxic effects

Spironolactone, sulfinpyrazone: decreased effects

Drug classifications

Antacids, steroids, urinary alkalizers: decreased effects of salsalate

Anticoagulants, penicillins: increased effects

Salicylates: decreased blood glucose levels

Diuretics (loop), sulfonylamides: decreased effects

NSAIDs: increased bleeding risk

Drug/food

Foods causing acidic urine may increase level

Drug/lab test

Increased: coagulation studies, liver function studies, serum uric acid, amylase, CO_2, urinary protein

Decreased: serum potassium, PBI, cholesterol, blood glucose

Interference: urine catecholamines, pregnancy test

NURSING CONSIDERATIONS

Assessment

- Monitor liver function studies: AST, ALT, bilirubin, creatinine if patient is on long-term therapy
- Monitor renal function studies: BUN, urine creatinine if patient is on long-term therapy
- Monitor blood studies: CBC, Hct, Hgb, Pro-time if patient is on long-term therapy
- Check I&O ratio; decreasing output may indicate renal failure if patient is on long-term therapy
- Assess hepatotoxicity: dark urine, clay-colored stools, yellowing of the skin and sclera, itching, abdominal pain, fever, diarrhea if patient is on long-term therapy
- Assess for allergic reactions: rash, urticaria; if these occur, drug may have to be discontinued; assess for asthma, aspirin sensitivity, nasal polyps, may develop hypersensitivity
- Assess for ototoxicity: tinnitus, ringing, roaring in ears; audiometric testing needed before, after long-term therapy
- Assess for visual changes: blurring, halos; corneal, retinal damage
- Check edema in feet, ankles, legs
- Identify prior drug history; many drug interactions are possible
- Monitor pain: location, duration, type, intensity, prior to dose and 1 hr after
- Monitor musculoskeletal status: ROM before dose
- Identify fever, length of time, and related symptoms

Nursing diagnoses

- Pain, chronic (uses)
- Mobility, physical, impaired (uses)
- Knowledge, deficient (teaching)
- Injury, risk for (side effects)

Implementation

- Administer to patient crushed or whole; chewable tab may be chewed
- Give with 8 oz of water and sit upright ½ hr after dose; with food or milk to decrease gastric symptoms
- Give antacids 1-2 hr after enteric products

Patient/family education

- Advise patient to report any symptoms of hepatotoxicity, renal toxicity, visual changes, ototoxicity, allergic reactions, bleeding (long-term therapy)
- Instruct patient to take with 8 oz of water and sit upright for ½ hr after dose
- Caution patient not to exceed recommended dosage; acute poisoning may result
- Advise patient to read label on other OTC drugs; many contain aspirin
- Inform patient that the therapeutic response takes 2 wk (arthritis)
- Teach patient to report tinnitus, confusion, diarrhea, sweating, hyperventilation
- Caution patient to avoid alcohol ingestion; GI bleeding may occur
- Inform patient that patients who have allergies may develop allergic reactions

Evaluation

Positive therapeutic outcome

- Decreased pain
- Decreased inflammation

Treatment of overdose: Lavage, activated charcoal, monitor electrolytes, VS

saquinavir (Rx)

(sa-quen'a-ver)

Fortovase, Invirase

Func. class.: Antiretroviral

Chem. class.: Protease inhibitor

Pregnancy category B

Action: Inhibits HIV-1 protease

Therapeutic Outcome: Prevents maturation of the infectious virus

Uses: HIV-1 in combination with other antiretrovirals

Dosage and routes

Adult: PO 600 mg (hard cap, Invirase) or 1200 mg (soft cap, Fortovase) tid within 2 hr after a full meal

Available forms: Caps 200 mg (soft); 200, 500 mg (hard)

Adverse effects

CNS: *Paresthesia*, headache

GI: *Diarrhea*, buccal mucosa ulceration, *abdominal pain, nausea,* vomiting

INTEG: *Rash*

MISC: Asthenia, *hyperglycemia*

MS: Pain

Contraindications: Hypersensitivity

Precautions: Pregnancy **B,** liver disease, lactation, children, diabetes, pancreatitis

Pharmacokinetics	
Absorption	Increased with food
Distribution	Protein-binding 98%
Metabolism	Extensively
Excretion	Unknown
Half-life	Terminal 12 hr

S

Pharmacodynamics

Unknown

Interactions

Individual drugs

Clarithromycin, delavirdine, indinavir, ketoconazole, nelfinavir, ritonavir: increased saquinavir level
Carbamazepine, dexamethasone, nevirapine, phenobarbital, phenytoin, rifamycins: decreased saquinavir levels
Clindamycin, dapsone, quinidine: increased toxicity
Midazolam, triazolam: increased toxicity, increased CNS depression; do not use concurrently

Drug classifications

Calcium channel blockers, ergot derivatives: increased toxicity
Ergot derivatives: increased vasoconstriction, do not use together
HMG-CoA reductase inhibitors: avoid use with saquinavir

Drug/herb

St. John's wort: decreased saquinavir level, avoid concurrent use

Drug/food

Increased: bioavailability after high-fat meal
Grapefruit juice: increased saquinivir level

Drug/lab test

Interference: CPK, glucose (low)

NURSING CONSIDERATIONS

Assessment

- Assess signs of infection, anemia
- Monitor liver function studies: ALT, AST
- Monitor C&S before drug therapy; drug may be taken as soon as culture is done; repeat C&S after treatment; determine the presence of other sexually transmitted diseases
- Assess bowel pattern before, during treatment; if severe abdominal pain with bleeding occurs, drug should be discontinued; monitor hydration
- Assess skin eruptions, rash, urticaria, itching
- Assess allergies before treatment, reaction of each medication; place allergies on chart

Nursing diagnoses

- Infection, risk for (uses)
- Knowledge, deficient (teaching)

Implementation

- Give in equal intervals around the clock for duration of therapy

Patient/family education

- Advise patient to take as prescribed within 2 hr of a full meal; if dose is missed, take as soon as remembered up to 1 hr before next dose; do not double dose
- Advise patient that drug must be taken in equal intervals around the clock to maintain blood levels for duration of therapy, that Invirase and Fortovase are not interchangeable

Evaluation

Positive therapeutic outcome

- Decreasing symptoms of HIV
- Improving viral load and CD4 cell counts

sargramostim (Rx)

(sar-gram'oh-stim)

Leukine, rhu GM-CSF

Func. class.: Biologic modifier: cytokine

Chem. class.: Granulocyte/macrophage colony stimulating factor (GM-CSF)

Pregnancy category C

Do Not Confuse:

Leukine/leucovorin, Leukine/Leukeran

Action: Stimulates proliferation and differentiation of hematopoietic progenitor cells (granulocyte, macrophage)

Uses: Acceleration of myeloid recovery in patients with non-Hodgkin's lymphoma, acute lymphoblastic leukemia, autologous bone marrow transplantation in Hodgkin's disease; bone marrow transplantation failure or engraftment delay; mobilization and transplant of peripheral blood progenitor cells (PBPCs)

Dosage and routes

Myeloid reconstitution after autologous bone marrow transplantation

Adult: **IV** 250 mcg/m^2/day × 3 wk; give over 2 hr, 2-4 hr after autologous bone marrow inf, and not less than 24 hr after last dose of antineoplastics and 12 hr after last dose of radiotherapy, bone marrow transplantation failure, or engraftment delay

Acceleration of myeloid recovery

Adult: **IV** 250 mcg/m^2/day × 14 days; give over 2 hr; may repeat in 7 days, may repeat 500 mcg/m^2/day × 14 days after another 7 days if no improvement

Mobilization of PBPCs

Adult: **IV**/SUBCUT 250 mcg/m^2/day during collection of PBPCs

After PBPC transplantation

Adult: **IV**/SUBCUT 250 mcg/m^2/day until ANC >1500/mm^3 × 3 days

Available forms: Powder for inj lyophilized 250, 500 mcg; liq 500 mcg/ml

Adverse effects

CNS: Fever, malaise, CNS disorder, weakness, chills, dizziness, syncope
CV: **Transient supraventricular tachycardia,** peripheral edema, **pericardial effusion**
GI: Nausea, vomiting, diarrhea, anorexia, **GI hemorrhage,** stomatitis, **liver damage**
GU: Urinary tract disorder, abnormal kidney function
HEMA: **Blood dyscrasias, hemorrhage**
INTEG: Alopecia, rash, peripheral edema
RESP: Dyspnea

Contraindications: Hypersensitivity to GM-CSF, benzyl alcohol, yeast products; excessive leukemic myeloid blast in the bone marrow or peripheral blood, neonates

Precautions: Pregnancy **C,** lactation, children; renal, hepatic, lung disease; cardiac disease; pleural, pericardial effusions, peripheral edema

Pharmacokinetics	
Absorption	Completely absorbed
Distribution	Unknown
Metabolism	Unknown
Excretion	Unknown
Half-life	2 hr

Pharmacodynamics	
Onset	Rapid
Peak	2 hr
Duration	Unknown

Interactions

Individual drugs

Lithium: increased myeloproliferation

Drug classifications

Antineoplastics: do not use together
Corticosteroids: increased myeloproliferation

NURSING CONSIDERATIONS

Assessment

- Monitor blood studies: CBC, differential count before treatment and twice weekly; leukocytosis may occur (WBC >50,000 cells/mm^3, ANC >20,000 cells/mm^3), platelets; if ANC >20,000/mm^3 or 10,000/mm^3 after nadir has occurred, or platelets >500,000/mm^3 reduce dose by ½ or discontinue; if blast cells occur, discontinue
- Monitor renal and hepatic studies before treatment: BUN, creatinine, urinalysis; AST, ALT, alkaline phosphatase; monitoring is needed twice a week in renal, hepatic disease
- Assess for hypersensitivity reactions/rashes, and local inj site reactions; usually transient
- Assess for increased fluid retention in cardiac disease
- Assess for myalgia, arthralgia in legs, feet; use analgesics

Nursing diagnoses

- Infection, risk for (uses)
- Knowledge, deficient (teaching)

Implementation

- Reconstitute with 1 ml of sterile water for inj without preservative; do not reenter vial; discard unused portion; direct reconstitution sol at side of vial; rotate contents; do not shake

SUBCUT route

- Use reconstituted sol

IV route

- Give by intermittent inf after diluting in 0.9% NaCl inj to prepare **IV** inf; if final conc is <10 mcg/ml, add human albumin to make a final conc of 0.1% to the NaCl before adding sargramostim to prevent absorption; for a final conc of 0.1% albumin, add 1 mg of human albumin/1 ml of 0.9% NaCl inj; run over 2 hr (bone marrow transplant or failure of graft); over 4 hr (chemotherapy for acute myeloid leukemia); over 24 hr as cont inf (PBPCs); give within 6 hr after reconstitution
- Store in refrigerator; do not freeze

Y-site compatibilities: Amikacin, aminophylline, aztreonam, bleomycin, butorphanol, calcium gluconate, carboplatin, carmustine, cefazolin, cefepime, cefotaxime, cefotetan, ceftizoxime, ceftriaxone, cefuroxime, cimetidine, cisplatin, clindamycin, cyclophosphamide, cycloSPORINE, cytarabine, dacarbazine, dactinomycin, dexamethasone, diphenhydrAMINE, DOPamine, DOXOrubicin, doxycycline, droperidol, etoposide, famotidine, fentanyl, floxuridine, fluconazole, fluorouracil, furosemide, gentamicin, granisetron, heparin, idarubicin, ifosfamide, immune globulin, magnesium sulfate, mannitol, mechlorethamine, meperidine, mesna, methotrexate, metoclopramide, metronidazole, mezlocillin, miconazole, minocycline, mitoxantrone, netilmicin, pentostatin, piperacillin/tazobactam, potassium chloride, prochlorperazine, promethazine, ranitidine, teniposide, ticarcillin, ticarcillin/clavulanate, trimethoprim/sulfamethoxazole, vinBLAStine, vinCRIStine, zidovudine

Y-site incompatibilities: Acyclovir, ampicillin, ampicillin/sulbactam, cefonicid, cefoperazine, ceftazidime, chlorproMAZINE, ganciclovir, haloperidol, hydrocortisone, hydromorphone, hydrOXYzine, idarubicin,

S

imipenem/cilastatin, lorazepam, methylPREDNISolone sodium succinate, mitomycin, morphine, nalbuphine, ondansetron, piperacillin, sodium bicarbonate, tobramycin

Patient/family education

- Teach patient reason for medication and expected results
- Advise patient to notify nurse or prescriber of side effects

Evaluation

Positive therapeutic outcome

- WBC and differential recovery
- Absence of infection

scopolamine (Rx)

(skoe-pol'a-meen)

Transderm-Scop, Transderm-V

Func. class.: Antiemetic, anticholinergic, mydriatic

Chem. class.: Belladonna alkaloid

Pregnancy category C

Action: Inhibits acetylcholine at receptor sites in autonomic nervous system, which controls secretions, free acids in stomach; blocks central muscarinic receptors, which decreases involuntary movements; blocks response of iris sphincter muscle, muscle of accommodation of ciliary body to cholinergic stimulation, resulting in dilatation, paralysis of accommodation

Therapeutic Outcome: Absence of vomiting, secretions (preoperatively), involuntary movements

Uses: Reduction of secretions before surgery, calm delirium, uveitis, iritis, cycloplegia, mydriasis; prevention of motion sickness, parkinson symptoms

Investigational uses: Drooling (TD)

Dosage and routes

Ophthalmic route

Adult: Instill 1-2 gtt before refraction or 1-2 gtt daily-tid for iritis or uveitis

Child: Instill 1 gtt bid × 2 days before refraction

Prevention of motion sickness

Adult: TD 1 patch placed behind ear 4-5 hr before travel, reapply q3d, alternate ears

Not recommended for children

Parkinson symptoms

Adult: IM/SUBCUT/**IV** 0.3-0.6 mg tid-qid diluted using dilution provided

Preoperatively

Adult: SUBCUT 0.4-0.6 mg

Nausea and vomiting

Child: SUBCUT 0.006 mg/kg or 0.2 mg/m^2

Drooling (off-label)

Adult: TD 1.5 mg patch q3 days

Available forms: Patch 0.5, 1 mg delivered in 72 hr; inj 0.3, 0.4, 0.86, 1 mg/ml

Adverse effects

CNS: Confusion, drowsiness, disorientation, hallucinations, sedation, depression, incoherence, dizziness, excitement, delirium, flushing, weakness, **TD,** memory disturbances

CV: Palpitations, **tachycardia,** postural hypotension, paradoxical bradycardia

EENT TD: Blurred vision, photophobia, dilated pupils, difficulty swallowing, mydriasis, cycloplegia, altered depth perception, *dry mouth,* dry, itchy red eyes, narrow-angle glaucoma

GI: *Dryness of mouth, constipation,* nausea, vomiting, abdominal distress, **paralytic ileus**

GU: Hesitancy, retention

INTEG: Rash, erythema (patch)

MISC: Suppression of lactation, nasal congestion, decreased sweating

Contraindications: Hypersensitivity, narrow-angle glaucoma, myasthenia gravis, GI/GU obstruction, hypersensitivity to belladonna, barbiturates

Precautions: Pregnancy **C,** elderly, lactation, prostatic hypertrophy, CHF, hypertension, dysrhythmias, children, gastric ulcer; TD: pyloric urinary, bladder neck, intestinal obstruction; liver, kidney disease

Pharmacokinetics

Absorption	Well absorbed (IM, SUBCUT, TD)
Distribution	Crosses placenta, blood-brain barrier
Metabolism	Liver
Excretion	Unknown
Half-life	8 hr

Pharmacodynamics

	SUBCUT/IM	IV	TD	OPHTH
Onset	30-45 min	10-15 min	4-5 hr	Unknown
Peak	1 hr	1 hr	Unknown	20-30 min
Duration	6 hr	4 hr	72 hr	3-7 days

Interactions

Individual drugs

Alcohol: increased anticholinergic effect

Drug classifications
Antidepressants, antidepressants (tricyclic), antihistamines: increased anticholinergic effect

NURSING CONSIDERATIONS
Assessment
- Assess for eye pain; discontinue use (opticue)
- Monitor I&O ratio; retention commonly causes decreased urinary output
- Assess for parkinsonism, extrapyramidal symptoms (EPS): shuffling gait, muscle rigidity, involuntary movements
- Assess for urinary hesitancy, retention; palpate bladder if retention occurs
- Assess for constipation; increase fluids, bulk, exercise if this occurs
- Assess for tolerance over long-term therapy; dose may have to be increased or changed
- Assess mental status: affect, mood, CNS depression, worsening of mental symptoms during early therapy

Nursing diagnoses
- Fluid volume, deficient (uses)
- Knowledge, deficient (teaching)

Implementation
IM/SUBCUT/IV route
- Administer parenteral dose with patient recumbent to prevent postural hypotension

TD route
- Instruct patient to wash, dry hands before and after applying to surface behind ear; to change patch q72h; to apply at least 4 hr before traveling

Ophthalmic route
- Apply pressure on lacrimal sac for 1 min; do not touch dropper to eye
- Wait 5 min to use other drops; blink more than usual

IV route
- Give by direct **IV** after diluting with sterile water; give slowly

Syringe compatibilities: Atropine, benzquinamide, butorphanol, chlorproMAZINE, cimetidine, dimenhyDRINATE, diphenhydrAMINE, droperidol, fentanyl, glycopyrrolate, hydromorphone, hydrOXYzine, meperidine, metoclopramide, midazolam, morphine, nalbuphine, pentazocine, pentobarbital, perphenazine, prochlorperazine, promazine, promethazine, ranitidine, sufentanil, thiopental

Y-site compatibilities: Heparin, hydrocortisone, potassium chloride, propofol, sufentanil, vit B/C

Additive compatibilities: Floxacillin, furosemide, meperidine, succinylcholine

Patient/family education
- Tell patient to avoid hazardous activities, activities requiring alertness; dizziness may occur
- Advise patient to discontinue use if blurred vision, severe dizziness, drowsiness occurs; another type of antiemetic may be used or the patch rotated to the other ear
- Instruct patient to read labels of all OTC medications; if any scopolamine is found in product, avoid use
- Advise patient to keep medication out of children's reach
- Caution patient to report change in vision, blurring or loss of sight, trouble breathing, inhibition of sweating, flushing
- Teach patient method of ophthalmic instillation
- Inform patient that blurred vision will decrease with repeated use of ophthalmic drug
- Caution patient not to discontinue this drug abruptly; to taper off over 1 wk

Evaluation
Positive therapeutic outcome
- Decrease in inflammation, cycloplegic refraction
- Decreased secretions
- Absence of motion sickness

selegiline (Rx)
(se-le'ji-leen)
Apo-Selegiline, Carbex, Eldepryl, Gen-Selegiline, Novo-Selegiline ♣, Nu-Selegiline, SD-Deprenyl
Func. class.: Antiparkinson agent
Chem. class.: MAOI, type B
Pregnancy category C

Do Not Confuse:
Eldepryl/enalapril

Action: Increased dopaminergic activity by inhibition of MAO type B activity; not fully understood

Therapeutic Outcome: Decreased symptoms of Parkinson's disease

Uses: Adjunct management of Parkinson's disease in patients being treated with levodopa/carbidopa who have responded poorly to therapy

Investigational use: Alzheimer's disease

Dosage and routes
Adult: PO 10 mg/day in divided doses, 5 mg at breakfast and lunch with levodopa/

S

carbidopa; after 2-3 days begin to reduce the dose of levodopa/carbidopa 10%-30%

Alzheimer's disease (off-label)
Adult: PO 5 mg bid AM, PM

Available forms: Tabs 5 mg, caps 5 mg

Adverse effects

CNS: Increased tremors, chorea, restlessness, blepharospasm, increased bradykinesia, grimacing, tardive dyskinesia, dystonic symptoms, involuntary movements, increased apraxia, hallucinations, dizziness, mood changes, nightmares, delusions, lethargy, apathy, overstimulation, sleep disturbances, headache, migraine, numbness, muscle cramps, confusion, anxiety, tiredness, vertigo, personality change, back/leg pain
CV: Orthostatic hypotension, hypertension, **dysrhythmia,** palpitations; angina pectoris, hypotension, tachycardia, edema, sinus bradycardia, syncope, **hypertensive crisis**
EENT: Diplopia, dry mouth, blurred vision, tinnitus
GI: *Nausea,* vomiting, constipation, weight loss, anorexia, diarrhea, heartburn, rectal bleeding, poor appetite, dysphagia, xerostomia
GU: Slow urination, nocturia, prostatic hypertrophy, hesitation, retention, frequency, sexual dysfunction
INTEG: Increased sweating, alopecia, hematoma, rash, photosensitivity, facial hair
RESP: Asthma, shortness of breath

Contraindications: Hypersensitivity

Precautions: Pregnancy **C,** lactation, children

Pharmacokinetics	
Absorption	Well absorbed
Distribution	Widely distributed
Metabolism	Rapidly, liver
Excretion	Metabolites-N-desmethyldeprenyl, amphetamine, methamphetamine
Half-life	9 min

Pharmacodynamics	
Onset	Unknown
Peak	½-2 hr
Duration	Unknown

Interactions

Individual drugs
Fluoxetine, fluvoxamine, paroxetine, sertraline: increased serotonin syndrome (confusion, seizures, fever, hypertension, agitation) discontinue 5 wk before selegiline
Levodopa/carbidopa: increased side effects
Meperidine: do not use, fatal reaction

Drug classifications
Antidepressants (tricyclics), opioids: do not use, fatal reaction

Drug/herb
Chaste tree fruit, kava: decreased selegiline action

Drug/food
Avoid foods high in tyramine

Drug/lab test
Decreased: VMA
False positive: urine ketones, urine glucose
False negative: urine glucose (glucose oxidase)
False: increased uric acid, increased urine protein

NURSING CONSIDERATIONS

Assessment
- Monitor B/P, respiration throughout treatment
- Assess mental status: affect, mood, behavioral changes, depression; perform suicide assessment
- Assess for decreased Parkinson's symptoms: rigidity, unsteady gait, weakness, tremors; these should decrease in severity

Nursing diagnoses
- Mobility, physical, impaired (uses)
- Knowledge, deficient (teaching)

Implementation
- Adjust dosage to patient response
- Give with meals; limit protein taken with drug
- Give at doses <10 mg/day because of risks associated with nonselective inhibition of MAO

Patient/family education
- Caution patient to change positions slowly to prevent orthostatic hypotension
- Advise patient to report side effects: twitching, eye spasms; may indicate overdose
- Caution patient to use drug exactly as prescribed; if drug is discontinued abruptly, parkinsonian crisis may occur
- Instruct patient to avoid foods high in tyramine: cheese, pickled products, wine, beer, large amounts of caffeine
- Instruct patient not to exceed recommended dose of 10 mg; might precipitate a hypertensive crisis; report severe headache or other unusual symptoms

Evaluation
Positive therapeutic outcome
- Decreased symptoms of Parkinson's disease

Treatment of overdose: **IV** fluids for hypertension, **IV** dilute pressure agent for B/P titration

senna, sennosides (OTC)
(sin'na)

Black Draught, Dr. Caldwell Dosalax, Ex-Lax Gentle, Fletcher's Castoria, Gentlax, Senexon, Senna-Gen, Senokot, Senokotxtra, Senolax

Func. class.: Laxative-stimulant

Chem. class.: Anthraquinone

Pregnancy category C

Action: Stimulates peristalsis by action on Auerbach's plexus; softens feces by increasing water and electrolytes in large intestine

Therapeutic Outcome: Decreased constipation

Uses: Acute constipation; bowel preparation for surgery or exam

Dosage and routes

Adult: PO (Senokot) 1-8 tabs/day or ½ to 4 tsp of granules added to water or juice; rec supp 1-2 at bedtime; syr 1-4 tsp at bedtime (1 tsp = 4 ml), 7.5-15 ml; (Black Draught) ¾ oz dissolved in 2.5 oz of liq given between 2-4 PM the day before procedure (X-Prep)

Child >27 kg: PO ½ adult dose; do not use Black Draught for children

Child 1 mo-1 yr: Syr 1.25-2.5 ml (Senokot) at bedtime

Available forms: Supp 625 mg, 30 mg sennosides; powder 662 mg/g, 6, 15 mg sennosides/3 g; tabs 8.6 sennosides, 180 mg; oral sol 3 mg sennosides/ml

Adverse effects

GI: *Nausea, vomiting, anorexia, abdominal cramps,* diarrhea, flatulence

GU: Pink-red or brown-black discoloration of urine

META: Hypocalcemia, enteropathy, alkalosis, hypokalemia, **tetany**

Contraindications: Hypersensitivity, GI bleeding, intestinal obstruction, CHF, lactation, abdominal pain, nausea/vomiting, appendicitis, acute surgical abdomen

Precautions: Pregnancy **C**

Pharmacokinetics

Absorption	Minimally absorbed (PO)
Distribution	Unknown
Metabolism	Not metabolized
Excretion	Kidneys, feces
Half-life	Unknown

Pharmacodynamics

	PO	REC
Onset	6-24 hr	Unknown
Peak	Unknown	Unknown
Duration	3-4 days	Unknown

Interactions

Individual drugs

Disulfiram: do not use together

Drug/herb

Flax, senna: increased laxative effect

NURSING CONSIDERATIONS

Assessment

- Monitor blood, urine electrolytes if used often by patient; check I&O ratio to identify fluid loss
- Assess cramping, rectal bleeding, nausea, vomiting; if these symptoms occur, drug should be discontinued; identify cause of constipation; identify whether fluids, bulk, or exercise is missing from lifestyle
- Assess for magnesium toxicity: thirst, confusion, decrease in reflexes
- Monitor blood ammonia level (30-70 mg/100 ml); monitor for clearing of confusion, lethargy, restlessness, irritability (hepatic encephalopathy)

Nursing diagnoses

- Constipation (uses)
- Diarrhea (side effects)
- Knowledge, deficient (teaching)
- Noncompliance (teaching)

Implementation

PO route

- Administer on empty stomach for more rapid results
- Give with a full glass of water in AM or PM (oral dose); evacuation occurs 6-12 hr later
- Dissolve granules in water or juice before administration
- Shake oral sol before giving

Patient/family education

- Discuss with patient that adequate fluid consumption is necessary
- Inform patient that normal bowel movements do not always occur daily
- Teach patient not to use in presence of abdominal pain, nausea, vomiting; tell patient to notify prescriber if constipation is unrelieved or if symptoms of electrolyte imbalance occur: muscle cramps, pain, weakness, dizziness, excessive thirst

Evaluation

Positive therapeutic outcome

- Decreased constipation in 8-10 hr

S

sertraline (Rx)
(ser'tra-leen)
Zoloft
Func. class.: Antidepressant
Chem. class.: Selective serotonin reuptake inhibitor (SSRI)
Pregnancy category B

Do Not Confuse:
Zoloft/Zocor

Action: Inhibits serotonin reuptake in CNS, thus increasing action of serotonin; does not affect dopamine, norepinephrine

Therapeutic Outcome: Relief of depression, obsessive-compulsive disorder (OCD), posttraumatic stress disorder (PTSD), panic disorder

Uses: Major depression, OCD, PTSD, social anxiety disorder, panic disorder, premenstrual dysphoric disorder (PMDD)

Investigational uses: Extended interval dosing

Dosage and routes
Adult: PO 50 mg daily; may increase to a maximum of 200 mg/day, do not change dose at intervals of <1 wk; administer daily in AM or PM; or 100 mg 3 ×/wk
Elderly: PO 25 mg daily, increase by 25 mg q3 days to desired dose
Child 6-12 yr: PO 25 mg daily
Child 13-17 yr: PO 50 mg daily

Premenstrual disorders
Adult: PO 50-150 mg nightly

Available forms: Tabs 25, 50, 100 mg; oral conc 20 mg/ml

Adverse effects
CNS: *Insomnia, agitation, somnolence, dizziness, headache, tremor, fatigue,* paresthesia, twitching, confusion, ataxia, fever, gait abnormality (elderly)
CV: Palpitations, chest pain
EENT: Vision abnormalities
ENDO: Syndrome of inappropriate antidiuretic hormone (elderly)
GI: *Diarrhea, nausea, constipation, anorexia, dry mouth,* dyspepsia, *vomiting, flatulence*
GU: *Male sexual dysfunction,* micturition disorder
INTEG: Increased sweating, rash, hot flashes

Contraindications: Hypersensitivity to this drug or SSRIs

Precautions: Pregnancy **B,** lactation, elderly, hepatic, renal disease, epilepsy, recent MI; latex sensitivity (dropper of oral conc)

Pharmacokinetics	
Absorption	Well absorbed
Distribution	Unknown, steady state 1 wk
Metabolism	Liver, extensively
Excretion	Feces (14%)
Half-life	1-4 days

Pharmacodynamics	
Onset	Unknown
Peak	4.5-8.4 hr
Duration	Unknown

Interactions
Individual drugs
Cimetidine, warfarin: increased sertraline effect
Diazepam: increased diazepam effect
Disulfiram: disulfiram reaction with oral conc due to alcohol content
Lithium: altered lithium levels
Pimozide: sertraline is contraindicated with pimozide
Sumatriptan: increased sumatriptan effects
TOLBUTamide: increased effect of TOLBUTamide
Warfarin: increased warfarin effect

Drug classifications
Antidepressants (tricyclic), benzodiazepines: increased effect
Highly protein-bound drugs: increased sertraline levels
MAOIs: fatal reactions

Drug/herb
Corkwood, jimsonweed: increased anticholinergic effect
Ephedra: hypertensive crisis
Hops, lavender: increased CNS effect
SAM-e, St. John's wort: increased effect of SSRIs, serotonin syndrome; do not use together

Drug/lab test
Increased: AST, ALT

NURSING CONSIDERATIONS
Assessment
- Assess mental status: mood, sensorium, affect, suicidal tendencies; increase in psychiatric symptoms: depression, panic
- Identify alcohol consumption; if alcohol is consumed, hold dose until AM

Nursing diagnoses
- Coping, ineffective (uses)
- Injury, risk for (adverse reactions)

- Knowledge, deficient (teaching)
- Noncompliance (teaching)

Implementation

- Administer dosage at bedtime if oversedation occurs during day; may take entire dose at bedtime; may crush
- Store at room temp; do not freeze

Patient/family education

- Teach patient that therapeutic effects may take 1 wk or longer
- Instruct patient to use caution in driving or other activities requiring alertness because of drowsiness, dizziness, blurred vision; to avoid rising quickly from sitting to standing, especially elderly
- Advise patient to avoid alcohol ingestion, other CNS depressants
- Teach patient not to discontinue medication quickly after long-term use: may cause nausea, headache, malaise
- Caution patient to wear sunscreen or large hat because photosensitivity can occur
- Teach patient to increase fluids, bulk in diet if constipation, urinary retention occur, especially elderly
- Instruct patient to take gum, hard sugarless candy, or frequent sips of water for dry mouth

Evaluation

Positive therapeutic outcome

- Decrease in depression, OCD
- Absence of suicidal thoughts

Treatment of overdose: ECG monitoring, induce emesis, lavage, activated charcoal, administer anticonvulsant

sildenafil (Rx)

(sil-den'a-fill)

Viagra

Func. class.: Erectile agent

Chem. class.: Selective inhibitor of cGMP-PDE5

Pregnancy category B

Action: Enhances the effect of nitric oxide (NO) by inhibiting phosphodiesterase type 5 (PDE5), which is necessary for degrading cGMP in the carpus cavernosum

Therapeutic Outcome: Ability to achieve and maintain erection

Uses: Treatment of erectile dysfunction

Dosage and routes

Adult: PO 50 mg 1 hr before sexual activity or may be taken ½-4 hr before sexual activity; may be increased to 100 mg or decreased to 25 mg; max once/day

Renal/hepatic dose

Adult: PO 25 mg, take 1 hr before sexual activity, do not use more than 1 ×/day

Available forms: Tabs 25, 50, 100 mg

Adverse effects

CNS: *Headache, flushing, dizziness*

CV: **MI, sudden death, CV collapse**

MISC: *Dyspepsia, nasal congestion, UTI, abnormal vision, diarrhea, rash,* **NAION (non-arteritic ischemic optic neuropathy)**

Contraindications: Hypersensitivity to nitrates

Precautions: Pregnancy **B**, anatomical penile deformities, sickle cell anemia, leukemia, multiple myeloma, retinitis pigmentosa

Pharmacokinetics	
Absorption	Rapidly, bioavailability (40%)
Distribution	Unknown
Metabolism	Liver (active metabolites)
Excretion	Feces, urine
Half-life	4 hr

Pharmacodynamics	
Onset	Unknown
Peak	½-1½ hr
Duration	Unknown

Interactions

Individual drugs

Amlodipine: decreased B/P

Cimetidine, erythromycin, itraconazole, ketoconazole: increased sildenafil levels

Drug classifications

Antiretroviral protease inhibitors: increased sildenafil levels

Barbiturates: decreased sildenafil levels

α-Blockers: decreased B/P

Nitrates: fatal reaction, do not use together

Rifampin: decreased sildenafil levels

NURSING CONSIDERATIONS

Assessment

- Identify organic nitrates that should not be used with this drug
- Assess for any severe loss of vision while taking this or any similar products; these products should not be used if vision loss has occurred

Nursing diagnoses

- Noncompliance (teaching)
- Knowledge, deficient (teaching)

Implementation
- Give approximately 1 hr before sexual activity, do not use more than once a day
- Tab may be split

Patient/family education
- Teach patient that drug does not protect against sexually transmitted diseases, including HIV
- Teach patient that drug absorption is reduced with a high-fat meal
- Teach patient that drug should not be used with nitrates in any form
- Teach patient that tab may be split
- Teach patient to notify prescriber immediately and stop taking product if vision loss occurs

Evaluation
Positive therapeutic outcome
- Ability to achieve and maintain an erection

simethicone (OTC)
(si-meth'i-kone)

Extra Strength Gas-X, Extra Strength Maalox Anti-Gas, Extra Strength Maalox GRF Gas Relief Formula ✤, Flatulex, Gas Relief, Gas-X, Genasyme, Maalox Anti-Gas, Maalox GRF Gas Relief Formula ✤, Maximum Strength Gas Relief, Maximum Strength Mylanta Gas Relief, Maximum Strength Phazyme, Mylanta Gas, Mylicon, Ovol ✤, Phazyme, Phazyme-95, Phazyme-125

Func. class.: Antiflatulent

Pregnancy category C

Do Not Confuse:
Mylicon/Mylanta Gas

Action: Disperses, prevents gas pockets in GI system; does not decrease gas production

Therapeutic Outcome: Belching or flatus

Uses: Flatulence

Dosage and routes
Adult and child >12 yr: PO 40-100 mg pc, at bedtime

Child <2 yr: PO 20 mg qid

Available forms: Chew tabs 40, 80, 125 mg; tabs 60, 80, 95 mg; drops 40 mg/0.6 ml, 40 mg/ml, 95 mg/1.425 ml; caps 95, 125 mg; caps, soft gel 125 mg

Adverse effects
GI: Belching, rectal flatus

Contraindications: Hypersensitivity, GI obstruction/perforation

Precautions: Pregnancy **C**, abdominal pain, fistula, hiatal hernia

Pharmacokinetics	
Absorption	None
Distribution	None
Metabolism	None
Excretion	None
Half-life	Unknown

Pharmacodynamics	
Onset	Rapid
Peak	Unknown
Duration	3 hr

Interactions: None known

NURSING CONSIDERATIONS
Assessment
- Identify the reason for excess gas production: decreased bowel sounds, recent surgery, other GI conditions

Nursing diagnoses
- Pain, acute (uses)
- Knowledge, deficient (teaching)

Implementation
- Give pc and at bedtime
- Shake susp well before administration
- Chew tab should be chewed and not swallowed whole

Patient/family education
- Caution patient that tab must be chewed; to shake susp well before pouring

Evaluation
Positive therapeutic outcome
- Absence of flatulence

simvastatin (Rx)
(sim-va-stat'in)

Zocor

Func. class.: Antilipidemic

Chem. class.: HMG-CoA reductase inhibitor

Pregnancy category X

Do Not Confuse:
Zocor/Cozaar, Zocor/Zoloft

Action: Inhibits HMG-CoA reductase enzyme, which reduces cholesterol synthesis; this enzyme is needed for cholesterol production

Therapeutic Outcome: Decreasing cholesterol levels and LDLs, increased HDLs

Uses: As an adjunct in primary hypercholesterolemia (types IIa, IIb), mixed hyperlipidemia, CAD, isolated hypertriglyceridemia (Frederickson type IV) and type III hyperlipoproteinemia

Dosage and routes

Adult: PO 5-20 mg daily in PM initially, usual range 5-40 mg/day daily in PM, not to exceed 80 mg/day; dosage adjustments may be made at 4-wk intervals or more; those taking verapamil, max 20 mg/day

Elderly/renal dose/those taking cycloSPORINE: PO 5 mg/day, initially

Available forms: Tabs 5, 10, 20, 40, 80 mg

Adverse effects

CNS: Headache

EENT: Lens opacities

GI: Nausea, constipation, diarrhea, dyspepsia, flatus, abdominal pain, **liver dysfunction, pancreatitis**

INTEG: Rash, pruritus, photosensitivity

MS: Muscle cramps, myalgia, **myositis, rhabdomyolysis**

RESP: Upper respiratory tract infection

Contraindications: Pregnancy **X,** hypersensitivity, lactation, active liver disease

Precautions: Past liver disease, alcoholism, severe acute infections, trauma, severe metabolic disorders, electrolyte imbalances, elderly, renal disease

Pharmacokinetics	
Absorption	85%
Distribution	Unknown
Metabolism	Liver—extensively
Excretion	70% feces, 20% kidneys
Half-life	3 hr

Pharmacodynamics	
Onset	Unknown
Peak	Unknown
Duration	Unknown

Interactions

Individual drugs

Clarithromycin, clofibrate, cycloSPORINE, erythromycin, gemfibrozil, itraconazole, ketoconazole, niacin: increased myalgia, myositis

Digoxin: increased digoxin levels

Warfarin: increased risk of bleeding

Drug classifications

Protease inhibitors: increased myalgia, myositis

Drug/herb

Glucomannan: increased effect

Gotu kola: decreased effect

Drug/lab test

Increased: CPK, liver function tests

NURSING CONSIDERATIONS

Assessment

- Assess nutrition: fat, protein, carbohydrates; nutritional analysis should be completed by dietitian before treatment is initiated
- Assess for rhabdomyolysis: muscle tenderness, increased CPK levels; therapy should be discontinued
- Monitor bowel pattern daily; diarrhea may be a problem
- Monitor triglycerides, cholesterol baseline and throughout treatment; LDL, HDL, triglycerides and cholesterol at 6-8 wk and q6 mo should be watched closely; if increased, drug should be discontinued

Nursing diagnoses

- Diarrhea (adverse reactions)
- Knowledge, deficient (teaching)
- Noncompliance (teaching)

Implementation

- Give 30 min before AM and PM meals

Patient/family education

- Inform patient that compliance is needed for positive results to occur; not to double doses
- Advise patient to lower risk factors: high-fat diet, smoking, alcohol consumption, absence of exercise
- Advise patient to notify health care prescriber if the GI symptoms of diarrhea, abdominal or epigastric pain, nausea, vomiting occur; or if chills, fever, sore throat occur

Evaluation

Positive therapeutic outcome

- Decreased cholesterol levels, serum triglycerides and improved ratio with HDLs

S

sirolimus (Rx)

(seer-roe'-li-mus)

Rapamune

Func. class.: Immunosuppressant

Chem. class.: Macrolide

Pregnancy category C

Action: Produces immunosuppression by inhibiting T-lymphocyte activation and proliferation

Therapeutic Outcome: Prevention of rejection in organ transplant

Uses: Organ transplants: to prevent rejection, recommended use is with cycloSPORINE and corticosteroids

Investigational uses: Psoriasis

Dosage and routes

Adult: PO 2 mg daily with 6 mg loading dose, may use 5 mg daily with a 15 mg loading dose

Child >13 yr <40 kg (88 lb): PO 1 mg/m^2/day, 3 mg/m^2/loading dose

Hepatic dose

Adult/child ≥13 yr <40 kg: PO reduce by 33% in maintenance dose

Available forms: Oral sol 1 mg/ml

Adverse effects

CNS: *Tremors, headache, insomnia,* paresthesia, chills, fever

CV: Hypertension, **atrial fibrillation, CHF,** hypotension, palpitations, **tachycardia**

EENT: Blurred vision, photophobia

GI: Nausea, vomiting, diarrhea, constipation

GU: UTI, **albuminuria, hematuria, proteinuria, renal failure**

HEMA: Anemia, **thrombocytopenia purpura, leukopenia**

INTEG: *Rash, acne,* photosensitivity

META: Increased creatinine, edema, hypercholesterolemia, *hyperlipemia,* hypophosphatemia, weight gain, hyperglycemia, hyperkalemia, hyperuricemia, hypokalemia, hypomagnesemia

RESP: **Pleural effusion, atelectasis,** *dyspnea*

SYST: **Lymphoma**

Contraindications: Hypersensitivity to this drug or to components of the drug, lactation

Precautions: Pregnancy **C**, severe renal disease, severe hepatic disease, diabetes mellitus, hyperkalemia, hyperuricemia, lymphomas, child <13 yr, hypertension, infection, other malignancies

Pharmacokinetics

Absorption	Rapidly absorbed
Distribution	92% protein binding
Metabolism	Liver; extensively by CYP3A4 enzyme system
Excretion	Unknown
Half-life	Unknown

Pharmacodynamics

	PO
Onset	Unknown
Peak	1 hr single dose, 2 hr multiple dosing
Duration	Unknown

Interactions

Individual drugs

Bromocriptine, cimetidine, cycloSPORINE, danazol, erythromycin, metoclopramide: increased blood level

Carbamazepine, phenobarbital, phenytoin, rifamycin, rifapentine: decreased blood levels

Drug classifications

Antifungal agents, calcium channel blockers, HIV protease inhibitors: increased blood levels

Live virus vaccines: decreased effect of vaccines

Drug/herb

Astragalus, echinacea, melatonin: decreased immunosuppression

Ginseng, maitake, mistletoe: increased effect

St. John's wort: decreased sirolimus effect

Drug/food

Food: alters bioavailability, use consistently with or without food

Grapefruit juice: do not use with grapefruit juice

NURSING CONSIDERATIONS

Assessment

- Monitor blood studies: Hgb, WBC, platelets monthly during treatment; if leukocytes are <3000/mm^3, or platelets <100,000/mm^3, drug should be discontinued or reduced; decreased Hgb level may indicate bone marrow suppression
- Monitor blood levels in those who may have altered metabolism, trough levels ≥15 ng/ml are associated with increased adverse reactions
- Monitor lipid profile: cholesterol, triglycerides; a lipid-lowering agent may be needed
- Assess for infection and development of lymphoma
- Monitor liver function studies: alkaline phosphatase, AST, ALT, amylase, bilirubin, and for hepatotoxicity: dark urine, jaundice, itching, light-colored stools; drug should be discontinued

Nursing diagnoses

- Infection, risk for (uses)
- Knowledge, deficient (teaching)

Implementation

- Administer prophylaxis for *Pneumocystis jiroveci* pneumonia for 1 yr after transplantation; prophylaxis for cytomegalovirus (CMV) is recommended for 90 days after transplantation in those at increased risk for CMV
- Use amber oral dose syringe and withdraw amount of oral sol needed from the bottle,

empty correct dose into plastic/glass container holding 60 ml of water/orange juice, stir vigorously and have patient drink at once, refill container with additional 120 ml of water/orange juice, stir vigorously, and have patient drink at once; if using a pouch squeeze entire contents into container and follow above directions

- Give all medications PO if possible; avoid IM inj because bleeding may occur
- Give for 3 days before transplant surgery; patients should be placed in protective isolation
- Store protected from light, refrigerate, stable for 24 months

Patient/family education

- Instruct patient to report fever, rash, severe diarrhea, chills, sore throat, fatigue because serious infections may occur; clay-colored stools, cramping may indicate hepatotoxicity
- Caution patient to avoid crowds or persons with known infections to reduce risk of infection
- Teach patient to use contraception before, during, and 12 wk after drug has been discontinued, avoid breastfeeding
- Teach patient to use sunscreen, protective clothing to prevent burns

Evaluation

Positive therapeutic outcome

- Absence of graft rejection

sodium bicarbonate (OTC)

baking soda, Bell/ans, Citrocarbonate, Neut, Soda Mint

Func. class.: Alkalinizer; antacid

Pregnancy category C

Action: Orally neutralizes gastric acid, which forms water, NaCl, CO_2; increases plasma bicarbonate, which buffers H^+ ion concentration; reverses acidosis **IV**

Therapeutic Outcome: Correction of acidosis, gastric acid neutralization

Uses: Acidosis (metabolic), cardiac arrest, alkalinization (systemic/urinary); antacid (PO)

Dosage and routes

Acidosis, metabolic

Adult and child: **IV** inf 2-5 mEq/kg over 4-8 hr depending on CO_2, pH

Cardiac arrest

Adult and child: **IV** bol 1 mEq/kg of 7.5% or 8.4% sol, then 0.5 mEq/kg q10 min, then doses based on ABGs

Infant: **IV** inf not to exceed 8 mEq/kg/day based on ABGs (4.2% sol)

Alkalinization of urine

Adult: PO 325 mg-2 g qid or 48 mEq/kg (4 g), then 12-24 mEq q4h

Child: PO 12-120 mg/kg/day (1-10 mEq/kg)

Antacid

Adult: PO 300 mg-2 g chewed, taken with water daily-qid

Available forms: Tabs 300, 325, 600, 650 mg; inj 4.2%, 5%, 7.5%, 8.4%

Adverse effects

CNS: Irritability, headache, confusion, stimulation, tremors, *twitching, hyperreflexia,* **tetany**, weakness, **seizures** caused by alkalosis

CV: Irregular pulse, **cardiac arrest,** water retention, edema, weight gain

GI: Flatulence, *belching, distention,* **paralytic ileus,** acid rebound

GU: Calculi

META: *Alkalosis*

RESP: Shallow, slow respirations, cyanosis, **apnea**

Contraindications: Hypertension, peptic ulcer, renal disease, hypocalcemia

Precautions: Pregnancy **C**, CHF, cirrhosis, toxemia, renal disease

Pharmacokinetics	
Absorption	Unknown
Distribution	Widely distributed—extracellular fluids
Metabolism	Unknown
Excretion	Kidneys
Half-life	Unknown

Pharmacodynamics	PO	IV
Onset	2 min	Rapid
Peak	½ hr	Rapid
Duration	1-3 hr	Unknown

Interactions

Individual drugs

Chlorpropamide, lithium: decreased effect of each specific drug

Flecainide, mecamylamine, pseudoephedrine, quinidine, quinine: increased effects of each specific drug

Drug classifications

Amphetamines, anorexiants: increased effects

Barbiturates: decreased effects of barbiturates

Benzodiazepines: decreased effects

S

Corticosteroids: increased sodium; decreased potassium
Salicylates: decreased effect of salicylates

Drug/herb

Oak bark: decreased action of sodium bicarbonate

Drug/lab test

Increased: urinary urobilinogen
False positive: urinary protein, blood lactate

NURSING CONSIDERATIONS

Assessment

- Assess respiratory and pulse rate, rhythm, depth, lung sounds; notify prescriber of abnormalities
- Assess for CO_2 in GI tract; may lead to perforation if ulcer is severe
- Monitor fluid balance (I&O ratio, weight daily, edema); notify prescriber of fluid overload
- Monitor electrolytes, blood pH, PO_2, HCO_3, during beginning treatment; ABGs frequently during emergencies
- Monitor urine pH, urinary output, during beginning treatment
- Monitor extravasation with **IV** administration (tissue sloughing, ulceration, and necrosis)
- Assess for alkalosis: irritability, confusion, twitching, hyperreflexia, stimulation, slow respirations, cyanosis, irregular pulse
- Monitor manifestations of hypokalemia: *RENAL:* acidic urine, reduced urine osmolality, nocturia, polyuria, polydipsia; *CV:* hypotension, broad T wave, U wave, ectopy, tachycardia, weak pulse; *NEURO:* muscle weakness, altered LOC, drowsiness, apathy, lethargy, confusion, depression; *GI:* anorexia, nausea, cramps, constipation, distention, paralytic ileus; *RESP:* hypoventilation, respiratory muscle weakness
- Monitor for manifestations of hyponatremia: *CV:* increased B/P, cold, clammy skin, hypo- or hypervolemia; *GI:* anorexia, nausea, vomiting, diarrhea, abdominal cramps; *NEURO:* lethargy, increased ICP, confusion, headache, seizures, coma, fatigue, tremors, hyperreflexia
- ◆ Assess for milk-alkali syndrome: confusion, headache, nausea, vomiting, anorexia, urinary stones, hypercalcemia

Nursing diagnoses

- Gas exchange, impaired (uses)
- Fluid volume, excess (adverse reactions)
- Knowledge, deficient (teaching)

Implementation

PO route

- Antacid tab must be chewed and taken with 8 oz of water
- Dissolve effervescent tab in water
- May be used to neutralize gastric acid in peptic ulcer disease, given 1 and 3 hr pc and at bedtime

IV route

- Give **IV** bol in cardiac arrest, may be repeated q10 min
- Give by intermittent or continuous inf in prepared sol or diluted in an equal amount of any dextrose/saline combination; administer 2-5 mEq/kg over 4-8 hr, not to exceed 50 mEq/hr; slower rate in children

Syringe compatibilities: Milrinone, pentobarbital

Syringe incompatibilities: Glycopyrrolate, metoclopramide, thiopental

Y-site compatibilities: Acyclovir, amifostine, asparaginase, aztreonam, cefepime, cefmetazole, ceftriaxone, cladribine, cyclophosphamide, cytarabine, DAUNOrubicin, dexamethasone, dexchlorpheniramine, DOXOrubicin, etoposide, famotidine, filgrastim, fludarabine, gallium, granisetron, heparin, ifosfamide, indomethacin, insulin, melphalan, mesna, methylPREDNISolone, morphine, paclitaxel, piperacillin/tazobactam, potassium chloride, propofol, tacrolimus, teniposide, thiotepa, tolazoline, vancomycin, vit B/C

Y-site incompatibilities: Calcium chloride, idarubicin, imanrinone, sargramostim, verapamil, vinorelbine

Additive compatibilities: Amikacin, aminophylline, amobarbital, amphotericin B, atropine, bretylium, calcium gluceptate, cefoxitin, ceftazidime, cephalothin, cephapirin, chloramphenicol, chlorothiazide, cimetidine, clindamycin, cytarabine, droperidol/fentanyl, ergonovine, erythromycin, esmolol, floxacillin, furosemide, heparin, hyaluronidase, hydrocortisone, kanamycin, lidocaine, mannitol, metaraminol, methotrexate, methyldopate, multivitamins, nafcillin, nalmefene, netilmicin, nizatidine, ofloxacin, oxacillin, oxytocin, phenobarbital, phenylephrine, phenytoin, phytonadione, potassium chloride, prochlorperazine, thiopental, verapamil

Additive incompatibilities: Amoxicillin, ascorbic acid, carboplatin, carmustine, cefotaxime, cisplatin, codeine, DOBUTamine, epINEPHrine, hydromorphone, imipenem/cilastatin, insulin, isoproterenol, labetalol, levorphanol, magnesium sulfate, methadone, morphine, norepinephrine, pentazocine, pentobarbital, procaine, secobarbital, streptomycin, succinylcholine, tetracycline, vit B/C

Patient/family education

- Instruct patient to chew antacid tab and drink 8 oz of water; not to take antacid with milk because milk-alkali syndrome may result; not to use antacid for more than 2 wk
- Advise patient to notify prescriber if indigestion is accompanied by chest pain; dyspnea; diarrhea; dark, tarry stools
- Teach patient about sodium-restricted diet; to avoid use of baking soda for indigestion

Evaluation

Positive therapeutic outcome

- ABGs, electrolytes, blood pH, HCO_3 normal levels
- Decreased gastric pain

sodium biphosphate/ sodium phosphate (OTC)

Fleet Enema, Phospho-soda

Func. class.: Laxative, saline

Pregnancy category C

Action: Increases water absorption in the small intestine by osmotic action; laxative effect occurs by increased peristalsis and water retention

Therapeutic Outcome: Absence of constipation

Uses: Constipation, bowel or rectal preparation for surgery, examination

Dosage and routes

Adult: PO 20-30 ml (Phospho-soda)

Child: PO 5-15 ml (Phospho-soda)

Adult and child >12 yr: REC enema (118 ml)

Child 2-12 yr: REC ½ enema (59 ml)

Available forms: Enema 7 g/phosphate and 19 g/biphosphate/118 ml; oral sol 18 g phosphate/48 g biphosphate/100 ml

Adverse effects

CV: **Dysrhythmias, cardiac arrest,** hypotension, widening QRS complex

GI: *Nausea, cramps,* diarrhea

META: Electrolyte, fluid imbalances

Contraindications: Hypersensitivity, rectal fissures, abdominal pain, nausea/vomiting, appendicitis, acute surgical abdomen, ulcerated hemorrhoids, Na-restricted diets, renal failure, hyperphosphatemia, hypocalcemia, hypokalemia, hypernatremia, Addison's disease, CHF, ascites, bowel perforation

Precautions: Pregnancy **C**

Pharmacokinetics

Absorption	Up to 20% (rec)
Distribution	Unknown
Metabolism	Unknown
Excretion	Kidneys
Half-life	Unknown

Pharmacodynamics

	PO	REC
Onset	½-3 hr	5 min
Peak	Unknown	Unknown
Duration	Unknown	Unknown

Interactions: None known

NURSING CONSIDERATIONS

Assessment

- Assess stools: color, amount, consistency
- Assess for bowel pattern, bowel sounds (frequency, intensity), flatulence, distention, increased temp, dietary patterns (fluid, bulk), exercise
- Assess for cramping, rectal bleeding, nausea, vomiting; if these symptoms occur, drug should be discontinued

Nursing diagnoses

- Constipation (uses)
- Knowledge, deficient (teaching)

Implementation

PO route

- Give on empty stomach
- Mix oral sol in cold water
- Take alone for better absorption; do not take within 1 hr of other drugs

Patient/family education

- Advise patient not to use laxatives or enema for long-term therapy; bowel tone will be lost
- Teach patient that normal bowel movements do not always occur daily
- Caution patient not to use in presence of abdominal pain, nausea, vomiting
- Caution patient to notify prescriber if constipation is unrelieved or if symptoms of electrolyte imbalance occur: muscle cramps, pain, weakness, dizziness, excessive thirst
- Instruct patient to maintain adequate fluid consumption to help prevent constipation

Evaluation

Positive therapeutic outcome

- Decrease in constipation

S

sodium polystyrene sulfonate (Rx)

(po-lee-stye'reen)

Kayexalate, K-Exit ✤, Kionex, PMS Sodium Polystyrene Sulfonate ✤, SPS

Func. class.: Potassium-removing resin

Chem. class.: Cation exchange resin

Pregnancy category C

Action: Removes potassium by exchanging sodium for potassium in body; occurs primarily in large intestine

Therapeutic Outcome: Potassium levels within accepted range

Uses: Hyperkalemia in conjunction with other measures

Dosage and routes

Adult: PO 15 g daily-qid; rec enema 30-50 g/100 ml of sorbitol warmed to body temp q6h

Child: PO/rec 1 mEq of K exchanged/g of resin, approximate dose 1 g/kg q6h

Available forms: Susp, 15 g polystyrene sulfonate, 21.5 ml sorbitol, 15 g (65 mEq) sodium/60 ml; powder 15 g/4 level tsp

Adverse effects

GI: ***Constipation,*** anorexia, nausea, vomiting, diarrhea (sorbitol), ***fecal impaction,*** gastric irritation

META: Hypocalcemia, hypokalemia, hypomagnesemia, sodium retention

Contraindications: Hypersensitivity to saccharin or parabens that may be in some products; ileus

Precautions: Pregnancy **C**, renal failure, CHF, severe edema, severe hypertension, elderly, sodium restriction, constipation

Pharmacokinetics

Absorption	None
Distribution	None
Metabolism	None
Excretion	Feces
Half-life	Unknown

Pharmacodynamics

	PO	REC
Onset	2-12 hr	2-12 hr
Peak	Unknown	Unknown
Duration	6-24 hr	4-6 hr

Interactions

Drug classifications

Antacids (calcium or magnesium), laxatives: decreased effect of sodium polystyrene

Diuretics (loop): increased hypokalemia

NURSING CONSIDERATIONS

Assessment

- Assess bowel function daily: amount of stool, color, characteristics
- Assess for hypotension: confusion, irritability, muscular pain, weakness
- Monitor for manifestations of hypokalemia: *RENAL:* acidic urine, reduced urine osmolality, nocturia, polyuria, polydipsia; *CV:* hypotension, broad T wave, U wave, ectopy, tachycardia, weak pulse; *NEURO:* muscle weakness, altered LOC, drowsiness, apathy, lethargy, confusion, depression; *GI:* anorexia, nausea, cramps, constipation, distention, paralytic ileus; *RESP:* hypoventilation, respiratory muscle weakness
- Monitor for manifestations of hyperkalemia: confusion, dyspnea, weakness, dysrhythmias
- Monitor for manifestations of hypocalcemia: *CNS:* personality changes, anxiety, disturbances, depression, psychosis, nausea, vomiting, *GI:* constipation, abdominal pain from muscle spasm; *CV:* decreased contractility, decreased cardiac output, hypotension, lengthened ST segment, prolonged QT interval; *INTEG:* scaling eczema, alopecia, hyperpigmentation; *NEURO:* tetany, muscle twitching, cramping grimacing, seizure, altered deep tendon reflexes, spasm
- Monitor for manifestations of hypomagnesemia; *CNS:* agitation; *NEURO:* muscle twitching, paresthesias, hyperactive reflexes, positive Babinski reflex, dysphagia, nystagmus, seizures, tetany; *GI:* nausea, vomiting, diarrhea, anorexia, abdominal distention; *CV:* ectopy; tachycardia, broad, flat, or inverted T waves; depressed ST segment; prolonged QT interval; decreased cardiac output; hypotension
- Monitor electrolytes: potassium, sodium, calcium, magnesium; I&O ratio, weight daily
- Monitor ECG for spiked T waves, depressed ST segments, prolonged QT interval and widening QRS complex

Nursing diagnoses

- Constipation (adverse reactions)
- Diarrhea (adverse reactions)
- Knowledge, deficient (teaching)

Implementation

PO route

- Give oral dose as susp mixed with H_2O or syr (20-100 ml)
- Give mild laxative as ordered to prevent constipation and fecal impaction; sorbitol as ordered to prevent constipation

Rectal route

- Give by retention enema after mixing with

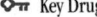

warm water; introduce by gravity, continue stirring, flush with 100 ml of fluid, clamp, and leave in place for at least ½-1 hr

- Complete irrigation of colon after enema with 1-2 qt of nonsodium sol, drain
- Store freshly prepared sol for 24 hr at room temp

Patient/family education

- Explain reason for medication and expected results

Evaluation

Positive therapeutic outcome

- Potassium level 3.5-5 mg/dl

solifenacin (Rx)

(sol-i-fen'a-sin)

VESIcare

Func. class.: Overactive bladder product, anticholinergic

Chem. class.: Muscarinic receptor antagonist

Pregnancy category C

Action: Relaxes smooth muscles in urinary tract by inhibiting acetylcholine at postganglionic sites

Therapeutic Outcome: Decreased dysuria, frequency, nocturia, incontinence

Uses: Overactive bladder (urinary frequency, urgency, incontinence)

Dosage and routes

Adult: PO 5 mg daily, max 10 mg daily

Renal/hepatic dose

Adult: PO CCr <30 ml/min 5 mg daily

Available forms: Tabs 5, 10 mg

Adverse effects

CNS: Anxiety, paresthesia, fatigue, *dizziness,* headache

CV: Chest pain, hypertension

EENT: *Vision abnormalities, xerophthalmia*

GI: *Nausea, vomiting, anorexia,* abdominal pain, *constipation*, dry mouth, dyspepsia

GU: Dysuria, urinary retention, frequency, UTI

INTEG: Rash, pruritus

RESP: Bronchitis, cough, pharyngitis, URI

Contraindications: Hypersensitivity, uncontrolled narrow-angle glaucoma, urinary retention, gastric retention

Precautions: Pregnancy **C**, lactation, children, renal/hepatic disease, controlled narrow-angle glaucoma

Pharmacokinetics

Absorption	Rapid
Distribution	98% highly protein bound
Metabolism	Extensively metabolized by CYP3A4
Excretion	Excreted in urine/feces
Half-life	Terminal half-life 45-68 hr

Pharmacodynamics

Unknown

Interactions

Drug classifications

CYP3A4 inducers (ketoconazole): increased action of solifenacin (dose >5 mg is not recommended)

NURSING CONSIDERATIONS

Assessment

- Assess urinary patterns: distention, nocturia, frequency, urgency, incontinence
- Assess for allergic reactions: rash; if this occurs, drug should be discontinued

Nursing diagnoses

- Urinary incontinence (uses)
- Knowledge, deficient (teaching)

Patient/family education

- Caution patient to avoid hazardous activities; dizziness may occur
- Advise patient that constipation, blurred vision may occur
- Instruct patient to call prescriber if severe abdominal pain or constipation lasts for 3 or more days
- Advise patient that heat prostration may occur if used in a hot environment

Evaluation

Positive therapeutic outcome

- Urinary status: dysuria, frequency, nocturia, incontinence

S

somatropin (Rx)

(soe-ma-troe'pin)

Genotropin, Humatrope, Norditropin, Nutropin, Nutropin AQ, Nutropin Depot, Saizen, Serostim

Func. class.: Pituitary hormone

Chem. class.: Growth hormone

Pregnancy category C

Action: Stimulates growth; similar to natural growth hormone—both preparations are developed by recombinant DNA technique

Therapeutic Outcome: Increase in height as a result of skeletal growth in pituitary growth hormone deficiency

Uses: Pituitary growth hormone deficiency (hypopituitary dwarfism), children with human growth hormone deficiency, AIDS wasting syndrome, cachexia, adults with somatropin deficiency syndrome (SDS)

Dosage and routes

Genotropin: SUBCUT 0.16-0.24 mg/kg/wk, divided into 6 or 7 inj, give in abdomen, thigh, buttocks

Humatrope: SUBCUT/IM 0.18 mg/kg divided into equal doses either on 3 alternate days or 6 ×/wk, max wk dose is 0.3 mg/kg

Growth hormone deficiency

Nutropin/Nutropin AQ: SUBCUT 0.3 mg/kg/wk

Serostim: SUBCUT at bedtime >55 kg 6 mg, 45-55 kg 5 mg, 35-45 kg 4 mg

Norditropin: SUBCUT 0.024-0.034 mg/kg 6-7 ×/wk

Available forms: Powder for inj (lyophilized) 1.5 mg (4 international units/ml), 4 mg (12 international units/vial), 5 mg (13 international units/vial), 5 mg (15 international units/vial), 5 mg (15 international units/vial) rDNA origin, 5.8 mg (15 international units/ml), 6 mg (18 international units/ml), 8 mg (24 international units/vial), 10 mg (26 international units/vial), inj 10 mg (30 international units/vial); 5, 10, 15 mg/1.5 ml

Adverse effects

CNS: Headache, **growth of intracranial tumor**

ENDO: *Hyperglycemia, ketosis, hypothyroidism*

GU: *Hypercalciuria*

INTEG: Rash, urticaria, pain, inflammation at inj site

MS: Tissue swelling, joint and muscle pain

SYST: *Antibodies to growth hormone*

Contraindications: Hypersensitivity to benzyl alcohol, closed epiphyses, intracranial lesions

Precautions: Pregnancy **C**, diabetes mellitus, hypothyroidism, lactation

Pharmacokinetics

Absorption	Well absorbed (SUBCUT/IM)
Distribution	Unknown
Metabolism	Unknown
Half-life	15-60 min

Pharmacodynamics

	IM/SUBCUT (GROWTH)
Onset	Unknown
Peak	Unknown
Duration	7 days

Interactions

Drug classifications

Androgens, thyroid hormones: increased epiphyseal closure

Glucocorticosteroids: decreased growth

NURSING CONSIDERATIONS

Assessment

- Identify growth hormone antibodies if patient fails to respond to therapy
- Monitor thyroid function tests: T_3, T_4, T_7, TSH to identify hypothyroidism
- Assess for allergic reaction: rash, itching, fever, nausea, wheezing
- Assess for hypercalciuria: urinary stones; groin, flank pain; nausea, vomiting, frequency, hematuria, chills
- Monitor growth rate of child at intervals during treatment

Nursing diagnoses

- Body image, disturbed (uses)
- Knowledge, deficient (teaching)

Implementation

- Store in refrigerator for <1 mo; if reconstituted, <1 wk; do not use discolored or cloudy sol

IM route

- Norditropin: After reconstituting 4-8 mg/2 ml diluent
- Humetrope: 5 mg/1.5-5 ml dilute, do not shake
- Nutropin/Nutropin AQ: Reconstitute 5 mg/1-5 ml or 10 mg/1-10 ml of bacteriostatic water for inj (benzyl alcohol preserved)

Patient/family education

- Explain reason for medication and expected results; that treatment may continue for yr
- Advise patient that routine follow-up is needed to monitor growth rate
- Instruct parents on procedure for medication preparation and inj use; request demonstration, return demonstration; provide written instructions
- Teach patient to maintain growth record, report knee, hip pain or limping
- Advise patient treatment is very expensive

Evaluation

Positive therapeutic outcome

- Growth in children until epiphyseal plates close

sorafenib

Nexavar

See Appendix A, Selected New Drugs

sotalol (Rx)

(soe-ta'lole)

Betapace, Betapace AF, Sotacar ♣

Func. class.: Antidysrhythmic, group III

Chem. class.: Nonselective β-blocker

Pregnancy category B

Action: Competitively blocks stimulation of β-adrenergic receptor within vascular smooth muscle; produces chronotropic, inotropic activity (decreases rate of SA node discharge, increases recovery time), slows conduction of AV node, decreases heart rate, which decreases O_2 consumption in myocardium; also decreases renin-aldosterone-angiotensin system at high doses, inhibits β_2 receptors in bronchial system (high doses)

Therapeutic Outcome: Decreased B/P, heart rate, AV conduction

Uses: Life-threatening ventricular dysrhythmias; Betapace AF: to maintain sinus rhythm in symptomatic atrial fibrillation/flutter

Dosage and routes

Adult: PO initial 80 mg bid, may increase to total of 240-320 mg/day

Renal dose

Adult: PO CCr 30-60 ml/min q24h; CCr 10-29 ml/min q36-48h; CCr <10 ml/min individualize dose

Betapace AF

Adult: PO initial 80 mg bid, titrate upward to 120 mg bid during initial hospitalization

Renal dose (Betapace AF)

CCr >60 ml/min q12h; CCr 40-60 ml/min q24h; CCr <40 ml/min do not use

Available forms: Tabs 80, 120, 160, 240 mg; (Betapace AF) 80, 120, 160 mg

Adverse effects

CNS: Dizziness, mental changes, drowsiness, fatigue, headache, catatonia, depression, anxiety, nightmares, paresthesia, lethargy, insomnia, decreased concentration

CV: Orthostatic hypotension, bradycardia, **CHF**, chest pain, **ventricular dysrhythmias**, AV block, peripheral vascular insufficiency, palpitations, **prodysrhythmia, torsades de pointes; Betapace AF: life-threatening ventricular dysrhythmias**

EENT: Tinnitus, visual changes, sore throat, double vision, dry, burning eyes

GI: Nausea, vomiting, diarrhea, dry mouth, flatulence, constipation, anorexia

GU: Impotence, dysuria, ejaculatory failure, urinary retention

HEMA: **Agranulocytosis, thrombocytopenic purpura (rare), thrombocytopenia, leukopenia**

INTEG: Rash, alopecia, urticaria, pruritus, fever

MISC: Facial swelling, decreased exercise tolerance, weight change, Raynaud's disease

MS: Joint pain, arthralgia, muscle cramps, pain

RESP: **Bronchospasm**, dyspnea, wheezing, nasal stuffiness, pharyngitis

Contraindications: Hypersensitivity to β-blockers, cardiogenic shock, heart block (2nd or 3rd degree), sinus bradycardia, CHF, bronchial asthma, congenital or acquired long QT syndrome, CCr >40 ml/min

Precautions: Pregnancy **B**, major surgery, lactation, diabetes mellitus, renal disease, thyroid disease, COPD, well-compensated heart failure, CAD, nonallergic bronchospasm, electrolyte disturbances, bradycardia, cardiac dysrhythmias, peripheral vascular disease

Pharmacokinetics	
Absorption	Variable (30%)
Distribution	Crosses placenta, minimal penetration in CNS
Metabolism	Liver, protein binding 0%
Excretion	70% unchanged—kidneys
Half-life	10-24 hr, increased in renal disease

Pharmacodynamics	
Onset	Several hr
Peak	Unknown
Duration	Unknown

Interactions

Individual drugs

Insulin: increased hypoglycemia

Lidocaine: increased effects of lidocaine

Nitroglycerin: increased hypotension

Theophylline: decreased bronchodilating effects of theophylline

Drug classifications

Antihypertensives, diuretics: increased hypotension

β_2-Agonists: decreased bronchodilating effects

Sulfonylureas: decreased hypoglycemic effects

Sympathomimetics: decreased β-blocker effects

Drug/herb
Aconite: increased toxicity, death
Aloe, buckthorn, cascara sagrada, senna hypokalemia: increased antidysrhythmic effect
Broom, Chinese rhubarb, figwort, fumitory, goldenseal, kudzu, licorice: increased effect
Coltsfoot: decreased effect
Horehound: increased serotonin effect

Drug/lab test
False: increased urinary catecholamines
Interference: glucose, insulin tolerance tests

NURSING CONSIDERATIONS

Assessment

- Monitor B/P during beginning treatment, periodically thereafter; pulse q4h; note rate, rhythm, quality: apical/radial pulse before administration; notify prescriber of any significant changes (pulse <50 bpm); monitor ECG continuously (Betapace AF); use QT interval to determine patient eligibility; baseline QT must be ≤450 msec
- Check for baselines in renal studies, before therapy begins
- Assess for edema in feet, legs daily, monitor I&O ratio, daily weight; check for jugular vein distention, crackles, bilaterally, dyspnea (CHF)
- Monitor skin turgor, dryness of mucous membranes for hydration status, especially in elderly

Nursing diagnoses

- Cardiac output, decreased (uses)
- Injury, risk for (adverse reactions)
- Knowledge, deficient (teaching)
- Noncompliance (teaching)

Implementation

- Given ac, at bedtime, tab may be crushed or swallowed whole; give with food to prevent GI upset; reduce dosage in renal dysfunction
- Betapace and Betapace AF are not interchangeable
- Store protected from light, moisture; place in cool environment

Patient/family education

- Teach patient not to discontinue drug abruptly, taper over 2 wk; may cause precipitate angina if stopped abruptly
- Teach patient not to use OTC products containing α-adrenergic stimulants (such as nasal decongestants, cold preparations); to avoid alcohol and smoking and to limit sodium intake as prescribed
- Teach patient how to take pulse and B/P at home, advise when to notify prescriber
- Instruct patient to comply with weight control, dietary adjustments, modified exercise program
- Caution patient to carry/wear emergency ID to identify drug being taken, allergies
- Inform patient that drug controls symptoms but does not cure
- Caution patient to avoid hazardous activities if dizziness, drowsiness is present
- Teach patient to report symptoms of CHF: difficulty breathing, especially on exertion or when lying down; night cough; swelling of extremities; bradycardia; dizziness; confusion; depression; fever
- Teach patient to take drug as prescribed, not to double or skip doses; take any missed doses as soon as remembered if at least 4 hr until next dose

Evaluation

Positive therapeutic outcome

- Absence of dysrhythmias

Treatment of overdose: Lavage; **IV** atropine for bradycardia; **IV** theophylline for bronchospasm; digitalis, O_2, diuretic for cardiac failure; hemodialysis; **IV** glucose for hyperglycemia; **IV** diazepam (or phenytoin) for seizures

sparfloxacin (Rx)

(spar-floks'a-sin)
Zagam
Func. class.: Antiinfective
Chem. class.: Fluoroquinolone antibacterial

Pregnancy category C

Action: Interferes with conversion of intermediate DNA fragments into high molecular weight DNA in bacteria; DNA gyrase inhibitor

Therapeutic Outcome: Bactericidal action against the following organisms: *Chlamydia pneumoniae, Haemophilus influenzae, Haemophilus parainfluenzae, Moraxella catarrhalis*

Uses: Adult infections (including complicated): lower respiratory, community-acquired pneumonia, chronic bronchitis

Dosage and routes

Adult: PO 400 mg loading dose, then 200 mg q24h × 10 days

Renal dose

Adult: PO 400 mg on day 1 if CCr <50 ml/min; then 200 mg every other day on days 2-10

Available forms: Tabs 200 mg

Adverse effects

CNS: *Headache, dizziness, insomnia*
CV: QT interval prolongation, vasodilation
GI: *Nausea,* flatulence, abdominal pain, **pseudomembranous colitis,** *vomiting,* diarrhea
HEMA: **Leukopenia,** eosinophilia, anemia
INTEG: Rash, pruritus, photosensitivity
SYST: **Anaphylaxis, Stevens-Johnson syndrome**

Contraindications: Hypersensitivity to quinolones, photosensitivity

Precautions: Pregnancy **C,** lactation, children, renal disease, seizure disorder

Pharmacokinetics

Absorption	Slow-erratic
Distribution	Widely distributed
Metabolism	Liver
Excretion	Kidneys, feces
Half-life	20 hr

Pharmacodynamics

Unknown

Interactions

Individual drugs

Amiodarone, bepridil, disopyramide, erythromycin, pentamine: increased torsades de pointes
CycloSPORINE: increased nephrotoxicity
Sucralfate, zinc sulfate: decreased absorption of sparfloxacin, give 4 hr apart
Warfarin: increased warfarin level

Drug classifications

Antacids with aluminum, magnesium; iron products: decreased absorption of sparfloxacin, give 4 hr apart
Antidepressants (tricyclic), antidysrhythmics (class IA/III), phenothiazines: increased torsades de pointes

Drug/herb

Cola tree: increased effect

Drug/lab test

Increased: AST, ALT

NURSING CONSIDERATIONS

Assessment

- Assess patient for previous sensitivity reaction
- Assess patient for signs and symptoms of infection including characteristics of wounds, sputum, urine, stool, WBC >10,000/mm^3, fever; obtain baseline information before and monitor during treatment
- Obtain C&S before beginning drug therapy to identify if correct treatment has been initiated
- Assess for allergic reactions, anaphylaxis: rash, urticaria, pruritus, chills, fever, joint pain; may occur a few days after therapy begins; epINEPHrine and resuscitation equipment should be available for anaphylactic reaction
- Identify urine output; if decreasing, notify prescriber (may indicate nephrotoxicity); also check for increased BUN, creatinine
- Monitor blood studies: AST, ALT, CBC, Hct, bilirubin, LDH, alkaline phosphatase, Coombs' test monthly if patient is on long-term therapy
- Assess bowel pattern daily; if severe diarrhea occurs, drug should be discontinued
- Monitor for bleeding: ecchymosis, bleeding gums, hematuria, stool guaiac daily if on long-term therapy
- Assess for overgrowth of infection: perineal itching, fever, malaise, redness, pain, swelling, drainage, rash, diarrhea, change in cough, sputum

Nursing diagnoses

- Infection, risk for (uses)
- Diarrhea (side effects)
- Injury, risk for (side effects)
- Knowledge, deficient (teaching)
- Noncompliance (teaching)

Implementation

PO route

- Give around the clock to maintain proper blood levels
- Give 4 hr before or after antacids/calcium
- Do not use theophylline with this product

IV route

- Check for irritation, extravasation, phlebitis daily
- For intermittent inf, dilute to 1-2 mg/ml of D_5W, 0.9% NaCl; give over 60 min; sol will remain stable under refrigeration for 2 wk

Patient/family education

- Advise patient to contact prescriber if vaginal itching, loose foul-smelling stools, furry tongue occur; may indicate superinfection; report itching, rash, pruritus, urticaria
- Instruct patient to take all medication prescribed for the length of time ordered; drug must be taken around the clock to maintain blood levels; do not give medication to others
- Teach patient to avoid direct sunlight or use sunscreen to prevent phototoxicity
- Advise patient to drink plenty of fluids, take 4 hr before or after antacids/calcium

- Advise patient to notify prescriber of diarrhea with blood or pus
- Advise patient to increase fluid intake to 2 L/day to prevent crystalluria
- Advise patient to avoid hazardous activities until response is known
- Instruct patient to rinse mouth frequently, use sugarless candy or gum for dry mouth

Evaluation

Positive therapeutic outcome

- Absence of signs/symptoms of infection (WBC <10,000/mm^3, temp WNL)
- Reported improvement in symptoms of infection
- C&S negative for organism

spironolactone (Rx)

(speer'on-oh-lak'tone)

Aldactone, Novospiroton ♣

Func. class: Potassium-sparing diuretic

Chem. class.: Aldosterone antagonist

Pregnancy category D

Action: Competes with aldosterone at receptor sites in the distal tubule in the renal system, resulting in excretion of sodium, chloride, water, bicarbonate, and calcium; potassium, phosphate, and hydrogen are retained

Therapeutic Outcome: Diuretic and antihypertensive effect while retaining potassium; lowered aldosterone levels

Uses: Edema of CHF, hypertension, diuretic-induced hypokalemia, primary hyperaldosteronism (diagnosis, short-term treatment, long-term treatment), edema of nephrotic syndrome, cirrhosis of the liver with ascites

Investigational uses: CHF

Dosage and routes

Edema/hypertension

Adult: PO 25-400 mg/daily in single or divided doses

CHF

Adult: PO 12.5-25 mg/day

Edema

Child: PO 3.3 mg/kg/day in single or divided doses

Hypertension

Child: PO 1-2 mg/kg bid

Hypokalemia

Adult: PO 25-100 mg/day; if PO, potassium supplements must not be used

Primary hyperaldosteronism diagnosis

Adult: PO 400 mg/day × 4 days or 4 wk depending on the test, then 100-400 mg/day maintenance

Available forms: Tabs 25, 50, 100 mg

Adverse effects

CNS: Headache, confusion, drowsiness, lethargy, ataxia

ELECT: Hyperchloremic metabolic acidosis, **hyperkalemia,** hyponatremia

ENDO: Impotence, gynecomastia, irregular menses, amenorrhea, postmenopausal bleeding, hirsutism, deepening voice

GI: Diarrhea, cramps, bleeding, gastritis, vomiting, anorexia, nausea

HEMA: **Agranulocytosis**

INTEG: *Rash, pruritus,* urticaria

Contraindications: Pregnancy **D,** hypersensitivity, anuria, severe renal disease, hyperkalemia

Precautions: Dehydration, hepatic disease, lactation, renal disease, electrolyte imbalances

Pharmacokinetics	
Absorption	GI tract; well absorbed
Distribution	Crosses placenta
Metabolism	Liver to canrenone (active metabolite)
Excretion	Renal; breast milk
Half-life	12-24 hr (canrenone)

Pharmacodynamics	
Onset	24-48 hr
Peak	48-72 hr
Duration	Unknown

Interactions

Individual drugs

Aspirin: decreased action of spironolactone

Digoxin: increased digoxin action

Lithium: increased action, toxicity

Drug classifications

ACE inhibitors, diuretics (potassium-sparing), potassium products, salt substitute: increased hyperkalemia

Anticoagulants: decreased effects of anticoagulants

Antihypertensives: increased action

Drug/herb

Bearberry, gossypol: hypokalemia

Cucumber, dandelion, horsetail, licorice nettle, pumpkin, Queen Anne's lace: increased effect

Khella: increased hypotension

St. John's wort: severe photosensitivity

Arginine: fatal hypokalemia

Drug/lab test
Interference: 17-OHCS, 17-KS, radioimmunoassay, digoxin assay

NURSING CONSIDERATIONS
Assessment
- Monitor for manifestations of hyperkalemia: *MS:* fatigue, muscle weakness; *CV:* arrhythmias, hypotension, *NEURO:* paresthesias, confusion, *RESP:* dyspnea
- Monitor for manifestations of hyponatremia: *CV:* increased B/P, cold, clammy skin, hypo- or hypervolemia; *GI:* anorexia, nausea, vomiting, diarrhea, abdominal cramps; *NEURO:* lethargy, increased ICP, confusion, headache, seizures, coma, fatigue, tremors, hyperreflexia
- Monitor for manifestations of hyperchloremia: *NEURO:* weakness, lethargy, coma; *RESP:* deep rapid breathing
- Assess fluid volume status: I&O ratios and record, count or weigh diapers as appropriate, weight, distended red veins, crackles in lung, color, quality, and sp gr of urine, skin turgor, adequacy of pulses, moist mucous membranes, bilateral lung sounds, peripheral pitting edema; dehydration symptoms of decreasing output, thirst, hypotension, dry mouth and mucous membranes should be reported
- Monitor electrolytes: potassium, sodium, calcium, magnesium; also include BUN, ABGs, uric acid, CBC, blood glucose

Nursing diagnoses
- Urinary elimination, impaired (adverse reactions)
- Fluid volume, deficient (adverse reactions)
- Fluid volume, excess (uses)
- Knowledge, deficient (teaching)

Implementation
- Give in AM to avoid interference with sleep
- With food, if nausea occurs, absorption may be increased; take at same time each day

Patient/family education
- Teach patient to take medication early in day to prevent nocturia
- Instruct patient to take with food or milk if GI symptoms of nausea and anorexia occur
- Teach patient to maintain a record of weight on a weekly basis and notify prescriber of weight loss of >5 lb
- Caution patient that this drug causes an increase in potassium levels, that foods high in potassium should be avoided; refer to dietitian for assistance planning
- Teach patient not to use alcohol, or any OTC medications without prescriber's approval; serious drug reactions may occur
- Emphasize the need to contact prescriber immediately if muscle cramps, weakness, nausea, dizziness, or numbness occurs
- Teach patient to take own B/P and pulse and record
- Advise patient that dizziness and confusion may occur; avoid driving or other hazardous activities if alertness is decreased
- Teach patient to continue taking medication even if feeling better; this drug controls symptoms but does not cure the condition
- Advise patient with hypertension to continue other treatment (exercise, weight loss, relaxation techniques, cessation of smoking)

Evaluation
Positive therapeutic outcome
- Prevention of hypokalemia (diuretic use)
- Decreased edema
- Decreased B/P
- Decreased aldosterone levels
- Increased diuresis

Treatment of overdose:
- Lavage if taken orally, monitor electrolytes
- Administer sodium bicarbonate
- Monitor hydration, CV, renal status

stavudine (Rx)
(sta'vu-deen)
d4T, Zerit
Func. class.: Antiretroviral
Chem. class.: Nucleoside reverse transcriptase inhibitor
Pregnancy category C

Action: Prevents replication of HIV-1 by the inhibition of the enzyme reverse transcriptase

Therapeutic Outcome: Decreasing diarrhea, fatigue, night sweats; increased body weight

Uses: Treatment of HIV-1; used in combination with other antiretrovirals

Dosage and routes
Adult >60 kg: PO 40 mg q12h
Adult <60 kg: 30 mg q12h
Child <30 kg: PO 1 mg/kg q12h
Child ≥30 kg ≤60 kg: PO 30 mg q12h
Child >60 kg: PO 40 mg q12h

Renal dose
Adult >60 kg: CCr 26-50 ml/min 20 mg q12h; CCr 10-25 ml/min 20 mg q24h
Adult <60 kg: CCr 26-50 ml/min 15 mg q12h; CCr 10-25 ml/min 15 mg q24h

Available forms: Caps 15, 20, 30, 40 mg; oral powder for sol 1 mg/ml

S

Adverse effects

CNS: *Peripheral neuropathy,* insomnia, anxiety, neuropathy, depression, dizziness, confusion, headache, chills/fever, malaise
CV: Chest pain, vasodilatation, hypertension
EENT: Conjunctivitis, abnormal vision
GI: **Hepatotoxicity,** diarrhea, nausea, vomiting, anorexia, dyspepsia, constipation, stomatitis, **pancreatitis**
HEMA: **Bone marrow suppression**
INTEG: Rash, sweating, pruritus, benign neoplasms
MISC: **Lactic acidosis,** asthenia, lipodystrophy
MS: Myalgia, arthralgia
RESP: Dyspnea, pneumonia, asthma

Contraindications: Hypersensitivity to this drug or zidovudine, didanosine, zalcitabine; severe peripheral neuropathy

Precautions: Pregnancy **C,** advanced HIV infections, lactation, bone marrow suppression, renal disease, liver disease, peripheral neuropathy, osteoporosis

Pharmacokinetics

Absorption	Rapidly absorbed, 82% bioavailability
Distribution	Cerebrospinal fluid
Metabolism	Unknown
Excretion	Kidneys, breast milk
Half-life	Elimination: 1-1.6 hr, intracellular: 3-3.5 hr

Pharmacodynamics

Onset	Unknown
Peak	1 hr
Duration	Unknown

Interactions

Individual drugs

Antineoplastics, antifungal, chloramphenicol, cisplatin, dapsone, didanosine, ethambutol, hydrALAZINE, lithium, phenytoin, vinCRIStine, zalcitabine: increased peripheral neuropathy
Methadose: decreased stavudine effect

Drug classifications

Myelosuppressants: increased myelosuppression

NURSING CONSIDERATIONS

Assessment

- ◆ Assess for lactic acidosis and severe hepatomegaly with steatosis; death may result
- Monitor viral load and CD4 counts baseline and throughout treatment
- Monitor for peripheral neuropathy: tingling, pain in extremities; if these occur discontinue drug
- Monitor for pancreatitis: severe upper abdominal pain, nausea, vomiting throughout treatment; if these occur discontinue drug
- Monitor blood studies: WBC, differential, RBC, Hct, Hgb, platelets
- Monitor renal studies: urinalysis, protein, blood
- Obtain C&S before drug therapy; drug may be taken as soon as culture is performed; repeat C&S after therapy
- Monitor bowel pattern before, during treatment
- Monitor fluid overload; drug requires large volume to stay in sol
- Assess for weakness, tremors, confusion, dizziness, psychosis; if these occur, drug may have to be decreased or discontinued

Nursing diagnoses

- Infection, risk for (uses)
- Knowledge, deficient (teaching)

Implementation

- Give with or without meals; absorption does not appear to be lowered when taken with food
- Give drug q4h around the clock, even during night

Patient/family education

- Teach patient signs of peripheral neuropathy: burning, weakness, pain, pricking feeling in the extremities
- Caution patient that this drug should not be given with antineoplastics
- Inform patient that GI complaints and insomnia resolve after 3-4 wk of treatment
- Inform patient that drug is not a cure for AIDS, but will control symptoms
- Advise patient to call prescriber if sore throat, swollen lymph nodes, malaise, fever occur; may indicate presence of other infections
- Caution patient that even with drug administration, virus is still infective and may be passed on to others
- Caution patient that follow-up visits must be continued because serious toxicity may occur; blood counts must be done q2 wk
- Teach patient that drug must be taken q4h around the clock even during night
- Caution patient that serious drug interactions with other medications may occur, check with prescriber first if taking chloramphenicol, dapsone, cisplatin, didanosine, ethambutol, lithium, antifungals
- Inform patient that other drugs may be necessary to prevent other infections
- Inform patient that drug may cause fainting or dizziness

Evaluation

Positive therapeutic outcome

- Decreased symptoms of HIV infection

! HIGH ALERT

streptokinase (Rx)

(strep-toe-kye'nase)

Kabikinase, Streptase

Func. class.: Thrombolytic enzyme

Chem. class.: β-Hemolytic *Streptococcus* filtrate (purified)

Pregnancy category C

Action: Activates conversion of plasminogen to plasmin (fibrinolysin): plasmin breaks down clots (fibrin), fibrinogen, factors V, VII; occlusion of venous access lines

Therapeutic Outcome: Lysis of emboli, or thrombosis in various parts of the body

Uses: Deep vein thrombosis (DVT), pulmonary embolism, arterial thrombosis, arterial embolism, arteriovenous cannula occlusion, lysis of coronary artery thrombi after MI, acute evolving transmural MI

Dosage and routes

Lysis of coronary artery thrombi

Adult: IC 20,000 international units, then 2000 international units/min over 1 hr as **IV** inf

Arteriovenous cannula occlusion

Adult: **IV** inf 250,000 international units/2 ml sol into occluded limb of cannula run over ½ hr; clamp for 2 hr; aspirate contents; flush with NaCl sol and reconnect

Thrombosis/embolism/DVT/pulmonary embolism

Adult: **IV** inf 250,000 international units over ½ hr, then 100,000 international units/hr for 72 hr for deep thrombosis; 100,000 international units/hr over 24-72 hr for pulmonary embolism; 100,000 international units/hr × 24-72 hr for arterial thrombosis or embolism

Acute evolving transmural MI

Adult: **IV** inf 1,500,000 international units diluted to a volume of 45 ml; give within 1 hr; intracoronary inf 20,000 international units by bol, then 2000 international units/min × 1 hr, total dose 140,000 international units

Available forms: Powder for inj, lyophilized 250,000, 600,000, 750,000, 1,500,000 international units/vial

Adverse effects

CNS: Headache, fever

CV: **Dysrhythmias,** hypotension, noncardiogenic pulmonary edema, **pulmonary embolism**

EENT: Periorbital edema

GI: Nausea

HEMA: Decreased Hct, **bleeding**

INTEG: Rash, urticaria, phlebitis at infusion site, itching, flushing

MS: Low back pain

RESP: Altered respirations, shortness of breath, **bronchospasm**

SYST: **GI, GU, intracranial retroperitoneal bleeding, surface bleeding, anaphylaxis**

Contraindications: Hypersensitivity, active internal bleeding, intraspinal surgery, CNS neoplasms, uncontrolled severe hypertension, recent CVA, intracranial, intrapleural surgery, lactation, children

Precautions: Pregnancy **C,** arterial emboli from left side of heart, ulcerative colitis, enteritis, severe renal disease, hepatic disease, hypocoagulation, COPD, subacute bacterial endocarditis, rheumatic valvular disease, cerebral embolism/thrombosis/hemorrhage, intraarterial diagnostic procedure or surgery (10 days), recent major surgery

Pharmacokinetics	
Absorption	Completely absorbed
Distribution	Unknown
Metabolism	>80%—liver, rapidly cleared by reticuloendothelial system
Excretion	Kidneys
Half-life	35 min

Pharmacodynamics	
Onset	Immediate
Peak	Rapid
Duration	<12 hr

S

Interaction

Individual drugs

Abciximab, aspirin, clopidogrel, dipyridamole, eptifibatide, indomethacin, phenylbutazone, plicamycin, ticlopidine, tirofiban, valproic acid: increased bleeding risk

Drug classifications

Anticoagulants (oral), cephalosporins (some), glycoprotein IIb/IIIa inhibitors, NSAIDs: increased bleeding risk

Drug/lab test

Increased: protime, APTT, TT

Decreased: plasminogen, fibrinogen

NURSING CONSIDERATIONS

Assessment

- Monitor VS, B/P, pulse, respirations (including peripheral), neurologic signs, temp at least q4h; temp >104° F (40° C) indicates internal bleeding; monitor rhythm closely; ventricular dysrhythmias may occur with hyperfusion; monitor heart, breath sounds, neurologic status, peripheral pulses
- ❗ Assess for bleeding during first hr of treatment: hematuria, hematemesis, bleeding from mucous membranes, epistaxis, ecchymosis; guaiac, all body fluids, stools; may require transfusion (rare); blood studies (Hct, platelets, PTT, protime, TT, APTT) before starting therapy; protime or APTT must be less than 2 × control before starting therapy; TT or protime q3-4h during treatment
- Assess allergy: fever, rash, itching, chills; mild reaction may be treated with antihistamines; report to prescriber
- Monitor ECG on monitor, watch for segment changes, changes in rhythm; sinus bradycardia, ventricular tachycardia, accelerated idioventricular rhythm may occur as a result of reperfusion (coronary thrombosis); cardiac enzymes, radionuclide myocardial scanning/coronary angiography
- Monitor ABGs, respiratory rate (depth, characteristics), pulse, B/P, hemodynamics (pulmonary embolism)
- Monitor peripheral pulses, assess Homan's sign, check for redness, swelling qh; notify prescriber of changes; B/P should not be taken in extremities (deep vein thrombosis)
- Check catheter for ability to aspirate blood from port; patient must exhale and hold breath when inserting and removing syringe to prevent air embolism (catheter/cannula occlusion)
- Assess for Guillain-Barré syndrome that may occur after treatment with this drug
- Assess for respiratory depression

Nursing diagnoses

- Tissue perfusion, ineffective (uses)
- Injury, risk for (adverse reactions)
- Gas exchange, impaired (uses)
- Knowledge, deficient (teaching)

Implementation

- Give after reconstituting with provided diluent; add appropriate amount of sterile water for inj (no preservatives) 20-mg vial/20 ml or 50 mg-vial/50 ml to make 1 mg/ml, mix by slow inversion or dilute with NaCl, D_5W to a concentration of 0.5 mg/ml; further dilution, 1.5-<0.5 mg/ml may result in precipitation of drug; use 18G needle; flush line with NaCl after administration; reconstituted **IV** sol within 8 hr; within 6 hr of coronary occlusion for best results
- Give **IV** loading dose over 30 min to avoid hypotension
- Give **IV** over 1 hr after dilution with 4-5 g/250 ml of 0.9% NaCl, D_5W, LR; may give by continuous inf after loading dose(s) of 1 g/hr diluted in 50-100 ml of compatible sol; use infusion pump; do not give by direct **IV**
- Give heparin therapy after thrombolytic therapy is discontinued, TT, ACT, or APTT less than 2 × control (about 3-4 hr); **IV** heparin with loading dose is recommended after discontinuing streptokinase to prevent redevelopment of thrombis
- Avoid invasive procedures, injection, taking temp via rectal route
- Apply pressure for 30 sec to minor bleeding sites; 30 min to sites of atrial puncture, followed by pressure dressing; inform prescriber if this does not attain hemostasis; apply pressure dressing
- Store powder at room temp or refrigerate; protect from excessive light

Y-site compatibilities: Dobutamine, DOPamine, heparin, lidocaine, nitroglycerin

Additive incompatibilities: Do not mix with other medications

Patient/family education

- Teach patient reason for medication, signs and symptoms of bleeding, allergic reactions, when to notify prescriber
- Explain that patient is to continue bed rest to avoid injury

Evaluation

Positive therapeutic outcome

- Lysis of thrombi or emboli

streptomycin (Rx)

(strep-toe-mye'sin)

Func. class.: Antiinfective, antituberculosis

Chem. class.: Aminoglycoside

Pregnancy category D

Action: Interferes with protein synthesis in bacterial cell by binding to ribosomal subunit, causing inaccurate peptide sequence to form in protein chain, resulting in bacterial death

Therapeutic Outcome: Bactericidal effects for the following organisms: sensitive strains of *Mycobacterium tuberculosis,* nontuberculous infections caused by sensitive strains of *Yersinia pestis, Brucella, Hae-*

mophilus influenzae, Klebsiella pneumoniae, Escherichia coli, Enterobacter aerogenes, Streptococcus viridans, Francisella tularensis, Proteus

Uses: Active TB; used in combination for streptococcal and enterococcal infections; endocarditis, tularemia, plague

Dosage and routes

Tuberculosis

Adult: IM 15 mg/kg (max 1 g) daily × 2-3 mo, then 1 g 2-3 ×/wk given with other antitubercular drugs

Child: IM 20-40 mg/kg/day in divided doses given with other antituberculosis drugs; max 15 mg/kg/day

Streptococcal endocarditis

Adult: IM 1 g q12h × 1 wk with penicillin, then 500 mg bid × 1 wk

Enterococcal endocarditis

Adult: IM 1 g q12h × 2 wk, then 500 mg q12h × 4 wk with penicillin, max 15 mg/kg/day

Available forms: Inj 500 mg ✤, 1 g/ml

Adverse effects

CNS: Confusion, dizziness, depression, numbness, tremors, **seizures**, muscle twitching, **neurotoxicity**

CV: Hypotension, myocarditis, palpitations

EENT: *Ototoxicity,* tinnitus, deafness, visual disturbances

GI: *Nausea, vomiting, anorexia,* increased ALT, AST, bilirubin, hepatomegaly, **hepatic necrosis,** splenomegaly

GU: **Oliguria, hematuria, renal damage, azotemia, renal failure, nephrotoxicity**

HEMA: **Agranulocytosis, thrombocytopenia, leukopenia, eosinophilia, anemia**

INTEG: *Rash,* burning, urticaria, dermatitis, alopecia

Contraindications: Pregnancy **D**, severe renal disease, hypersensitivity

Precautions: Neonates, mild renal disease, myasthenia gravis, lactation, hearing deficits, elderly, Parkinson's disease

Pharmacokinetics

Absorption	Well absorbed
Distribution	Widely distributed in extracellular fluids, poorly distributed in CSF; crosses placenta
Metabolism	Minimal—liver
Excretion	Mostly unchanged (>90%) kidneys
Half-life	2-2½ hr, increase in renal disease

Pharmacodynamics

Onset	Rapid
Peak	1-2 hr

Interactions

Individual drugs

Amphotericin B, bacitracin, cisplatin, ethacrynic acid, furosemide, mannitol, methoxyflurane, polymyxin, vancomycin: increased ototoxicity, neurotoxicity, nephrotoxicity

Lysine (large amounts): increased toxicity

Succinylcholine, warfarin: increased effects of streptomycin

Drug classifications

Aminoglycosides, cephalosporins: increased ototoxicity, neurotoxicity, nephrotoxicity

Nondepolarizing neuromuscular blockers: increased effects of streptomycin

NURSING CONSIDERATIONS

Assessment

- Assess patient for previous sensitivity reaction
- Assess patient for signs and symptoms of infection including characteristics of sputum, urine, stool WBC >10,000/mm^3, temp
- Obtain baseline information before and during treatment
- Complete C&S testing before and after drug therapy to identify if correct treatment has been initiated
- Assess for allergic reactions: rash, urticaria, pruritus, chills, fever, joint pain; angioedema may occur a few days after therapy begins; epINEPHrine, resuscitation equipment should be available for anaphylactic reaction
- Identify urine output; if decreasing, notify prescriber (may indicate nephrotoxicity); also increased BUN, creatinine, urine CCr <80 ml/min
- Monitor blood studies: AST, ALT, CBC, Hct, bilirubin, LDH, alkaline phosphatase, Coombs' test monthly if patient is on long-term therapy
- Monitor electrolytes: potassium, sodium, chloride, magnesium monthly if patient is on long-term therapy
- Monitor for bleeding: ecchymosis, bleeding gums, hematuria, stool guaiac daily if on long-term therapy
- Assess for overgrowth of infection: perineal itching, fever, malaise, redness, pain, swelling, drainage, rash, diarrhea, change in cough, sputum
- Obtain weight before treatment; calculation of dosage is usually based on ideal body weight, but may be calculated on actual body weight
- Monitor I&O ratio; urinalysis daily for

proteinuria, cells, casts; report sudden change in urine output
- Obtain serum peak 60 min after IM inj, trough level obtained just before next dose; blood level should be 2-4 × bacteriostatic level
- Monitor for deafness by audiometric testing, ringing, roaring in ears, vertigo; assess hearing before, during, after treatment
- Monitor for dehydration: high sp gr, decrease in skin turgor, dry mucous membranes, dark urine

Nursing diagnoses
- Infection, risk for (uses)
- Diarrhea (adverse reactions)
- Injury, risk for (adverse reactions)
- Knowledge, deficient (teaching)
- Noncompliance (teaching)

Implementation
- Give deeply in large muscle mass
- Reconstitute with 4.2-4.5 ml of sterile water for inj or 0.9% NaCl/1 g (200 mg/ml), 3.2-3.5 ml/1 g (250 mg/ml), 17 ml/5 g (250 mg/ml); give at 500 mg/ml or less

Syringe compatibilities: Penicillin G sodium
Syringe incompatibilities: Heparin
Y-site compatibilities: Esmolol
Additive compatibilities: Bleomycin

Patient/family education
- Teach patient to report sore throat, bruising, bleeding, joint pain, may indicate blood dyscrasias (rare); ringing, roaring in the ears
- Advise patient to contact prescriber if vaginal itching, loose foul-smelling stools, furry tongue occur; may indicate superinfection

Evaluation
Positive therapeutic outcome
- Absence of signs/symptoms of infection
- Reported improvement in symptoms of infection

Treatment of overdose: Withdraw drug, hemodialysis, monitor serum levels of drug, may give ticarcillin or carbenicillin

succimer (Rx)
(sux'i-mer)
Chemet
Func. class: Heavy metal antagonist
Chem. class.: Chelating agent
Pregnancy category C

Action: Binds with ions of lead to form a water-soluble complex that is excreted by kidneys

Therapeutic Outcome: Removal of lead from the body

Uses: Lead poisoning in children with lead levels above 45 mcg/dl; may be beneficial in mercury, arsenic poisoning

Dosage and routes
Child: PO 10 mg/kg or 350 mg/m^2 q8h × 5 days, then 10 mg/kg or 350 mg/m^2 q12h × 2 wk; another course may be required depending on lead levels; allow 2 wk between courses

Available forms: Caps 100 mg

Adverse effects
CNS: Drowsiness, dizziness, paresthesia, sensorimotor neuropathy
EENT: Otitis media, watery eyes, film in eyes, plugged ears
GI: *Nausea, vomiting, diarrhea, metallic taste, anorexia*
GU: **Proteinuria,** decreased urination, voiding difficulties
HEMA: **Increased platelets, intermittent eosinophilia**
INTEG: Rash, urticaria, pruritus
META: Increased AST, ALT, alkaline phosphatase, cholesterol
RESP: Sore throat, rhinorrhea, nasal congestion, cough
SYST: Back, stomach, head, rib, flank pain; abdominal cramps; chills; fever; flulike symptoms, head cold; headache

Contraindications: Hypersensitivity

Precautions: Pregnancy **C**, lactation, children <1 yr

Pharmacokinetics	
Absorption	Rapidly absorbed
Distribution	Unknown
Metabolism	Liver—extensively
Excretion	Kidneys—unchanged
Half-life	2 days

Pharmacodynamics	
Onset	Up to 2 hr
Peak	2-4 hr
Duration	8-12 hr

Interactions
Drug classifications
Heavy metal antagonist, others: do not use together

NURSING CONSIDERATIONS
Assessment
- Assess VS, B/P, pulse, respirations, weigh daily

- Monitor I&O ratio, kidney function studies, BUN, creatinine, CCr; watch for decreasing urine output
- Assess neurologic status: watch for paresthesias, beginning of seizures
- Monitor urine: pH, albumin, casts, blood, coproporphyrins, calcium
- Assess for febrile reactions that may occur 4-8 hr after drug therapy
- Monitor for cardiac abnormalities: dysrhythmias, hypotension, tachycardia
- Assess for allergic reactions (rash, urticaria); if these occur, drug should be discontinued

Nursing diagnoses

- Poisoning, risk for (uses)
- Injury, risk for (uses, adverse reactions)
- Knowledge, deficient (teaching)

Implementation

- Give whole or cap contents mixed with food or fluid

Patient/family education

- Explain reason for medication and expected results
- Provide a referral to health department to assess lead levels in home or workplace
- Teach patient to increase fluid intake

Evaluation

Positive therapeutic outcome

- Decreased symptoms of lead intoxication
- Decreased lead level <50 mcg/dl

! HIGH ALERT

succinylcholine (Rx)

(suk-sin-ill-koe'leen)

Anectine, Anectine Flo-Pack, Quelicin, succinylcholine chloride, Sucostrin, Suxamethonium

Func. class.: Neuromuscular blocker (depolarizing—ultra short)

Pregnancy category C

Action: Inhibits transmission of nerve impulses by binding with cholinergic receptor sites, antagonizing action of acetylcholine; causes release of histamine

Therapeutic Outcome: Paralysis of skeletal muscles

Uses: Facilitation of endotracheal intubation, skeletal muscle relaxation during orthopedic manipulations

Dosage and routes

Adult: **IV** 0.3-1.1 mg/kg, then 0.5-10 kg/min; IM 3-4 mg/kg, max 150 mg

Child: **IV**/IM 1-4 mg/kg

Available forms: Inj 20, 50, 100 mg/ml; powder for inj 100, 500 mg/vial, 1 g/vial

Adverse effects

CV: Bradycardia, tachycardia; increased, decreased B/P, **sinus arrest, dysrhythmias**

EENT: Increased secretions, increased intraocular pressure

HEMA: **Myoglobulinemia**

INTEG: Rash, flushing, pruritus, urticaria

MS: Weakness, muscle pain, fasciculation, prolonged relaxation

RESP: **Prolonged apnea, bronchospasm, cyanosis, respiratory depression,** wheezing

Contraindications: Hypersensitivity, malignant hyperthermia, decreased plasma pseudocholinesterase, penetrating eye injuries, acute narrow-angle glaucoma

Precautions: Pregnancy **C**, cardiac disease, severe burns, fractures (fasciculation may increase damage), lactation, children <2 yr, electrolyte imbalances, dehydration, neuromuscular disease, respiratory disease, collagen diseases, glaucoma, eye surgery, penetrating eye wounds, elderly or debilitated patients, renal/hepatic disease

Pharmacokinetics

Absorption	Well absorbed (IM)
Distribution	Widely distributed, crosses placenta
Metabolism	Plasma (90%)
Excretion	Hydrolyzed in blood, excreted in urine (active/inactive metabolites)
Half-life	Unknown

Pharmacodynamics

	IV	IM
Onset	1 min	2-3 min
Peak	2-3 min	Unknown
Duration	6-10 min	10-30 min

Interactions

Individual drugs

Clindamycin, enflurane, isoflurane, lincomycin, lithium, oxytocin, procainamide, quinidine: increased neuromuscular blockade

Theophylline: dysrhythmias

Drug classifications

Aminoglycosides, anesthetics (local), antibiotics (polymyxin), β-adrenergic blockers, cardiac glycosides, magnesium salts, opioids, thiazides: increased neuromuscular blockade

Drug/herb

Melatonin: blocks succinylcholine

S

NURSING CONSIDERATIONS

Assessment

- Assess for electrolyte imbalances (potassium, magnesium); may lead to increased action of this drug
- Monitor VS (B/P, pulse, respirations, airway) until fully recovered; rate, depth, pattern of respirations, strength of hand grip
- Monitor I&O ratio; check for urinary retention, frequency, hesitancy
- Assess for recovery: decreased paralysis of face, diaphragm, leg, arm, rest of body
- Assess for allergic reactions: rash, fever, respiratory distress, pruritus; drug should be discontinued if these occur

Nursing diagnoses

- Communication, verbal, impaired (adverse reactions)
- Breathing pattern, ineffective (uses)

Implementation

IM route

- Give inj deep IM, preferably high in deltoid muscle
- Store in refrigerator; store powder at room temp; close container tightly

IV route

- Use nerve stimulator by anesthesiologist to determine neuromuscular blockade
- Give anticholinesterase to reverse neuromuscular blockade
- Give by **IV** inf; dilute 1-2 mg/ml in D_5, isotonic saline sol, give 0.5-10 mg/min, titrate to patient response; may be given directly over 1 min

Syringe compatibilities: Heparin

Y-site compatibilities: Etomidate, heparin, potassium chloride, propofol, vit B/C

Additive compatibilities: Amikacin, cephapirin, isoproterenol, meperidine, methyldopate, morphine, norepinephrine, scopolamine

Additive incompatibilities: Barbiturates, nafcillin, sodium bicarbonate

Patient/family education

- Explain reason for medication and expected results
- Provide reassurance if communication is difficult during recovery from neuromuscular blockade; postoperative stiffness is normal, soon subsides

Evaluation

Positive therapeutic outcome

- Paralysis of jaw, eyelid, head, neck, rest of body

Treatment of overdose: Edrophonium or neostigmine, atropine, monitor VS; may require mechanical ventilation

sucralfate (Rx)

(soo-kral'fate)

Carafate, Sulcrate ✤

Func. class.: Protectant; antiulcer

Chem. class.: Aluminum hydroxide/sulfated sucrose

Pregnancy category B

Do Not Confuse: Carafate/Cafergot

Action: Forms a complex that adheres to ulcer site, adsorbs pepsin

Therapeutic Outcome: Healing of ulcers

Uses: Duodenal ulcer, oral mucositis, stomatitis after radiation of head and neck

Investigational uses: Gastric ulcers, gastroesophageal reflux

Dosage and routes

Ulcers

Adult: PO 1 g qid 1 hr ac, at bedtime

Child: PO 40-80 mg/kg/day

Gastroesophageal reflux disease (GERD)

Adult: PO 1 g qid 1 hr ac and at bedtime

Child: PO 500 mg-1g qid, 1 hr ac and at bedtime

Available forms: Tabs 1 g; oral susp 1 g/10 ml

Adverse effects

CNS: Drowsiness, dizziness

GI: *Dry mouth, constipation,* nausea, gastric pain, vomiting

INTEG: Urticaria, rash, pruritus

Contraindications: Hypersensitivity

Precautions: Pregnancy **B,** lactation, children, renal failure

Pharmacokinetics	
Absorption	Minimally absorbed
Distribution	Unknown
Metabolism	Not metabolized
Excretion	Feces (90%)
Half-life	6-20 hr

Pharmacodynamics	
Onset	½ hr
Peak	Unknown
Duration	6 hr

Interactions

Individual drugs

Cimetidine, digoxin, ketoconazole, phenytoin, ranitidine, tetracycline, theophylline: decreased action of each specific drug

Drug classifications
Antacids: decreased absorption of sucralfate
Fat-soluble vitamins: decreased action of fat-soluble vitamins
Fluoroquinolones: decreased absorption

NURSING CONSIDERATIONS
Assessment
- Monitor gastric pH (>5 should be maintained); blood in stools

Nursing diagnoses
- Pain, chronic (uses)
- Pain, acute (uses)
- Constipation (adverse reactions)
- Knowledge, deficient (teaching)

Implementation
- Do not break, crush, or chew tabs
- Give on empty stomach 1 hr ac and at bedtime
- Avoid antacids ½ hr before or 1 hr after taking this drug
- Store at room temp

Patient/family education
- Instruct patient to take medication on empty stomach
- Caution patient to take full course of therapy, not to use over 8 wk, to avoid smoking
- Caution patient to avoid antacids within ½ hr of drug or 1 hr after this drug

Evaluation
Positive therapeutic outcome
- Absence of pain or GI complaints

sulfamethoxazole
See also trimethoprim/sulfamethoxazole

sulfamethoxazole (Rx)
(sul-fa-meth-ox'a-zole)
Apo-Sulfamethoxazole ✤, Gantanol, Urobak
Func. class.: Antiinfective
Chem. class.: Sulfonamide, intermediate-acting
Pregnancy category C

Action: Interferes with bacterial biosynthesis of proteins by competitive antagonism of *p*-aminobenzoic acid (PABA)

Therapeutic Outcome: Bactericidal action against susceptible organisms: streptococci and staphylococci, *Clostridium perfringens, Clostridium tetani, Nocardia asteroides;* gram-negative pathogens, including *Enterobacter, Escherichia coli, Klebsiella, Proteus mirabilis, Proteus vulgaris, Salmonella, Shigella*

Uses: UTIs, chancroid, inclusion conjunctivitis, malaria, meningococcal meningitis, nocardiosis, acute otitis media, toxoplasmosis, trachoma

Dosage and routes
Adult: PO 2 g, then 1 g bid or tid for 7-10 days
Child >2 mo: PO 50-60 mg/kg × 1 dose, then 25-30 mg/kg bid, max 75 mg/kg/day

Renal dose
Adult: PO CCr <50 ml/min 50% of dose

Available forms: Tabs 500 mg; oral susp 500 mg/5 ml

Adverse effects
CNS: Headache, insomnia, hallucinations, depression, vertigo, fatigue, anxiety, seizures, drug fever, chills, drowsiness
CV: **Allergic myocarditis**
GI: *Nausea, vomiting, abdominal pain,* stomatitis, **hepatitis,** glossitis, **pancreatitis,** diarrhea, **enterocolitis,** anorexia
GU: **Renal failure, toxic nephrosis,** increased BUN, creatinine, crystalluria, hematuria, proteinuria
HEMA: **Leukopenia, thrombocytopenia, agranulocytosis, hemolytic anemia, aplastic anemia**
INTEG: Rash, dermatitis, urticaria, erythema, photosensitivity, alopecia
SYST: **Anaphylaxis, Stevens-Johnson syndrome**

Contraindications: Hypersensitivity to sulfonamides, sulfonylureas, thiazide and loop diuretics, salicylates, sunscreen with PABA, lactation, infants <2 mo (except congenital toxoplasmosis), pregnancy at term, porphyria, G6PD deficiency

Precautions: Pregnancy **C,** impaired hepatic/renal function, severe allergy, bronchial asthma

Pharmacokinetics

Absorption	Well absorbed
Distribution	Widely distributed, crosses placenta
Metabolism	Liver, large amounts
Excretion	Unchanged kidneys (20%), enters breast milk
Half-life	7-12 hr

S

Pharmacodynamics

Onset	1 hr
Peak	3-4 hr

Interactions

Individual drugs

Cyclosporine: increased nephrotoxicity
Indomethacin, probenecid: increased drug-free concentrations
Methotrexate: decreased renal excretion of methotrexate
Phenytoin: decreased hepatic clearance of phenytoin
Warfarin: increased anticoagulant effect

Drug classifications

Barbiturates, uricosuric agents: increased effects
Diuretics (thiazide): increased thrombocytopenia
Salicylates: increased drug-free concentrations
Sulfonylurea agents: increased hypoglycemic response

NURSING CONSIDERATIONS

Assessment

- Assess patient for previous sensitivity reaction
- Assess patient for signs and symptoms of infection including characteristics of wounds, sputum, urine, stool, WBC >10,000/mm^3, elevated temp; obtain baseline information before and during treatment
- Complete C&S studies before beginning drug therapy to identify if correct treatment has been initiated
- Assess for allergic reactions: rash, urticaria, pruritus, chills, fever, joint pain; angioedema may occur a few days after therapy begins; epINEPHrine, resuscitation equipment should be on unit for anaphylactic reaction; AIDS patients are more susceptible
- Monitor blood studies: CBC, Hct, bilirubin, alkaline phosphatase monthly if patient is on long-term therapy
- Monitor for bleeding: ecchymosis, bleeding gums, hematuria, stool guaiac daily if patient is on long-term therapy
- Assess for overgrowth of infection: perineal itching, fever, malaise, redness, pain, swelling, drainage, rash, diarrhea, change in cough, sputum

Nursing diagnoses

- Infection, risk for (uses)
- Diarrhea (adverse reactions)
- Injury, risk for (adverse reactions)
- Knowledge, deficient (teaching)
- Noncompliance (teaching)

Implementation

- Give around the clock to maintain proper blood levels; give on empty stomach to increase absorption of drug; do not give within 3 hr of other agents, drug actions may occur

Patient/family education

- Teach patient to report sore throat, bruising, bleeding, joint pain; may indicate blood dyscrasias (rare)
- Instruct patient to take with 8 oz of water to prevent crystalluria
- Advise patient to contact prescriber if vaginal itching, loose foul-smelling stools, furry tongue occur; may indicate superinfection; report itching, rash, pruritus, urticaria
- Instruct patient to take all medication prescribed for the length of time ordered; drug must be taken around the clock to maintain blood levels; do not give medication to others

Evaluation

Positive therapeutic outcome

- Absence of signs/symptoms of infection (WBC <10,000/mm^3, temp WNL, absence of urinary pain, hematuria)
- Reported improvement in symptoms of infection
- Negative C&S

sulfasalazine (Rx)

(sul-fa-sal′a-zeen)

Azulfidine, Azulfidine EN-tabs, PMS-Sulfusalazine ✦, S.A.S. ✦, Salazopyrin ✦, sulfasalazine

Func. class.: GI Antiinflammatory, antirheumatic (DMARD)

Chem. class.: GI Sulfonamide

Pregnancy category C

Do Not Confuse:

sulfasalazine/sulfiSOXAZOLE

Action: Prodrug to deliver sulfapyridine and 5-aminosalicylic acid to colon; antinflammatory in connective tissue

Therapeutic Outcome: Treatment of ulcerative colitis, rheumatoid arthritis

Uses: Ulcerative colitis, rheumatoid arthritis (delayed rel tab) in patients who inadequately respond to or are intolerant of analgesics/NSAIDs, juvenile rheumatoid arthritis (Azulfidine EN-tabs)

Investigational uses: Ankylosing spondylitis, Crohn's disease, psoriasis, granulomatous colitis, regional enteritis

Dosage and routes

Bowel disease

Adult: PO 3-4 g/day in divided doses; maintenance 2 g/day in divided doses q6h

Child ≥6 yr: PO 40-60 mg/kg/day in 4-6 divided doses, then 30 mg/kg/day in 4 doses, max 2 g/day

Rheumatoid arthritis

Adult: PO 2 g/day in evenly divided doses, initiate treatment with a lower dose of enteric-coated tab

Juvenile rheumatoid arthritis

Child ≥6 yr: PO 30-50 mg/kg/24 hr, divided into 2 doses

Renal dose

Adult: PO CCr 10-30 ml/min bid; CCr <10 ml/min daily

Available forms: Tabs 500 mg; oral susp 250 mg/5 ml; delayed rel tabs 500 mg

Adverse effects

CNS: Headache, confusion, insomnia, hallucinations, depression, vertigo, fatigue, anxiety, **seizures,** drug fever, chills

CV: **Allergic myocarditis**

GI: *Nausea, vomiting, abdominal pain,* stomatitis, **hepatitis,** glossitis, **pancreatitis,** diarrhea

GU: **Renal failure, toxic nephrosis,** increased BUN, creatinine, crystalluria

HEMA: **Leukopenia, neutropenia, thrombocytopenia, agranulocytosis, hemolytic anemia**

INTEG: Rash, dermatitis, **Stevens-Johnson syndrome,** erythema, photosensitivity

SYST: **Anaphylaxis**

Contraindications: Hypersensitivity to sulfonamides or salicylates, pregnancy at term, child <2 yr, intestinal, urinary obstruction, porphyria

Precautions: Pregnancy **C,** lactation, impaired hepatic function, severe allergy, bronchial asthma, impaired renal function, megaloblastic anemia

Pharmacokinetics	
Absorption	Partially absorbed
Distribution	Crosses placenta
Metabolism	Liver
Excretion	Kidneys, breast milk
Half-life	6 hr

Pharmacodynamics	
Onset	1 hr
Peak	1½-6 hr
Duration	6-12 hr

Interactions

Individual drugs

Azathioprine, mercaptopurine: increased leucopenia risk

Digoxin: decreased digoxin effect

Folic acid: decreased folic acid effect

Methotrexate: decreased renal excretion

Drug classifications

Anticoagulants (oral): increased anticoagulant effect

Hypoglycemics (oral): increased hypoglycemic response

Drug/food

Iron, folic acid will be poorly absorbed

Drug/lab test

False positive: urinary glucose test

NURSING CONSIDERATIONS

Assessment

- Monitor I&O ratio; note color, amount, character, pH of urine if drug administered for UTIs; output should be 800 ml less than intake; if urine is highly acidic, alkalization may be needed
- Monitor kidney function studies: BUN, creatinine, urinalysis if on long-term therapy
- Monitor blood dyscrasias: skin rash, fever, sore throat, bruising, bleeding, fatigue, joint pain; monitor CBC before, during therapy (q3 mo)
- Assess for allergic reaction: rash, dermatitis, urticaria, pruritus, dyspnea, bronchospasm

Nursing diagnoses

- Injury, risk for (uses)
- Knowledge, deficient (teaching)

Implementation

- Give with full glass of water to maintain adequate hydration; increase fluids to 2 L/day to decrease crystallization in kidneys; contact lens, urine, skin may be yellow-orange
- Give total daily dose in evenly spaced doses and after meals to help minimize GI intolerance
- Give rectal susp at bedtime
- Store in airtight, light-resistant container at room temp

Patient/family education

- Advise patient to take each oral dose with full glass of water to prevent crystalluria
- Teach patient to avoid sunlight or to use sunscreen to prevent burns

- Teach patient to avoid OTC medication (aspirin, vit C) unless directed by prescriber
- Advise patient to notify prescriber if skin rash, sore throat, fever, mouth sores, unusual bruising, bleeding occur
- Advise patient to use rectal susp at bedtime and retain all night

Evaluation

Positive therapeutic outcome

- Absence of fever, mucus in stools or pain in joints

sulfinpyrazone (Rx)

(sul-fin-peer'a-zone)

Anturan ✤, Anturane, sulfinpyrazone

Func. class.: Uricosuric

Chem. class.: Pyrazolone

Pregnancy category C

Action: Inhibits tubular reabsorption of urates, with increased excretion of uric acid; inhibits prostaglandin synthesis, which decreases platelet aggregation

Therapeutic Outcome: Decreased uric acid levels, absence of platelet aggregation

Uses: Gout, gouty arthritis

Dosage and routes

Gout/gouty arthritis

Adult: PO 100-200 mg bid × 1 wk, then 200-400 mg bid, not to exceed 800 mg/day

Child: PO 10 mg/kg/day in 3-4 divided doses

Renal dose

CCr <50 ml/min; avoid use

Available forms: Tabs 100 mg; caps 200 mg

Adverse effects

CNS: Dizziness, **seizures, coma**

EENT: Tinnitus

GI: *Gastric irritation, nausea, vomiting, anorexia,* **hepatic necrosis, GI bleeding**

GU: Renal calculi, hypoglycemia

HEMA: **Agranulocytosis** (rare)

INTEG: Rash, dermatitis, pruritus, fever, photosensitivity

RESP: **Apnea,** irregular respirations

Contraindications: Hypersensitivity to pyrazolone derivatives, salicylates, blood dyscrasias, CCr <50 ml/min, active peptic ulcer, GI inflammation, nephrolithiasis

Precautions: Pregnancy **C,** renal disease, NSAIDs hypersensitivity

Pharmacokinetics	
Absorption	Well absorbed
Distribution	Unknown
Metabolism	Liver
Excretion	Feces (metabolites/active drug)
Half-life	4 hr

Pharmacodynamics	
Onset	Unknown
Peak	1-2 hr
Duration	4-6 hr

Interactions

Individual drugs

Acetaminophen: increased toxicity

Niacin: decreased effects of sulfinpyrazone

Theophylline, verapamil: decreased effect of each specific drug

TOLBUTamide, warfarin: increased effect of each specific drug

Drug classifications

NSAIDs: increased bleeding risk

Salicylates: decreased effect of sulfinpyrazone

Drug/lab test

Increased: PSP, aminohippuric acid

False positive: Clinitest

NURSING CONSIDERATIONS

Assessment

- Monitor I&O ratio; observe for decrease in urinary output; increase fluids to 2-3 L/day
- Monitor CBC, platelets, reticulocytes before, during therapy (q3 mo)
- Assess mobility, joint pain, and swelling in the joints

Nursing diagnoses

- Pain, chronic (uses)
- Mobility, physical, impaired (uses)
- Knowledge, deficient (teaching)

Implementation

- Give with food or antacid to decrease GI upset
- Reduce dose gradually if uric acid levels are normal after 6 mo

Patient/family education

- Advise patient to increase fluids to 3-4 L/day
- Caution patient to avoid alcohol, OTC preparations that contain alcohol; skin rashes may occur
- Advise patient to report any pain, redness, or hard area, usually in legs
- Instruct patient on importance of complying with medical regimen; bone marrow depression may occur

Evaluation

Positive therapeutic outcome

- Decreased pain in joints
- Normal serum uric acid levels
- Increased duration of antiinfectives

sulfiSOXAZOLE (Rx)

(sul-fi-sox'a-zole)

Gantrisin, Gantrisin Pediatric, Novo-Soxazole ✤, sulfiSOXAZOLE

Func. class.: Antiinfective

Chem. class.: Sulfonamide, short-acting

Pregnancy category C

Do Not Confuse:
sulfiSOXAZOLE/sulfasalazine
sulfiSOXAZOLE/sulfADIAZINE

Action: Interferes with bacterial biosynthesis of proteins by competitive antagonism of *p*-aminobenzoic acid (PABA)

Therapeutic Outcome: Bactericidal action against susceptible organisms: gram-positive pathogens, including streptococci and staphylococci, *Clostridium perfringens, Clostridium tetani, Nocardia asteroides;* gram-negative pathogens, including *Enterobacter, Escherichia coli, Klebsiella, Proteus mirabilis, Proteus vulgaris, Salmonella, Shigella*

Uses: UTIs; chancroid, trachoma, toxoplasmosis, acute otitis media, malaria, *Haemophilus influenzae* meningitis, meningococcal meningitis, nocardiosis

Dosage and routes

UTIs, other systemic infections

Adult: PO 2-4 g loading dose, then 1-2 g qid × 7-10 days

Child >2 mo: PO 75 mg/kg or 2 g/m^2 loading dose, then 120-150 mg/kg/day or 4 g/m^2/day in divided doses q6h, max 6 g/day

Chlamydia trachomatis

Adult: PO 500 mg-1 g qid × 3 wk

Renal dose

Adult: PO CCr 10-50 ml/min q8-12h; CCr <10 ml/min q12-24h

Available forms: Tabs 500 mg; sulfiSOXAZOLE acetyl: liq 500 mg/5 ml

Adverse effects

CNS: Headache, insomnia, hallucinations, depression, vertigo, fatigue, anxiety, **seizures,** drug fever, chills, drowsiness

CV: **Allergic myocarditis**

GI: *Nausea, vomiting, abdominal pain,* stomatitis, **hepatitis,** glossitis, pancreatitis, diarrhea, **enterocolitis,** anorexia

GU: **Renal failure, toxic nephrosis,** increased BUN, creatinine, crystalluria, hematuria, proteinuria

HEMA: **Leukopenia, thrombocytopenia, agranulocytosis, hemolytic anemia, aplastic anemia**

INTEG: Rash, dermatitis, urticaria, erythema, photosensitivity, alopecia

SYST: **Anaphylaxis, Stevens-Johnson syndrome**

Contraindications: Hypersensitivity to sulfonamides and sulfonylureas, thiazide and loop diuretics, salicylates; sunscreen with PABA, lactation, infants <2 mo (except congenital toxoplasmosis); pregnancy at term, porphyria

Precautions: Pregnancy **C**, lactation, impaired hepatic/renal function, severe allergy, bronchial asthma

Pharmacokinetics

Absorption	Well absorbed
Distribution	Widely distributed, crosses placenta
Metabolism	Liver, mostly
Excretion	Breast milk
Half-life	4-7 hr

Pharmacodynamics

Onset	Unknown
Peak	2-4 hr

Interactions

Individual drugs

CycloSPORINE: increased nephrotoxicity

Indomethacin, probenecid: increased drug-free concentrations

Methotrexate: decreased renal excretion of methotrexate

Phenytoin: decreased hepatic clearance of phenytoin

TOLBUTamide: increased effects of TOLBUTamide

Warfarin: increased anticoagulant effect

Drug classifications

Barbiturates, uricosuric agents: increased effects of each specific drug

Diuretics (thiazide): increased thrombocytopenia

Salicylates: increased drug-free concentrations

Sulfonylurea agents: increased hypoglycemic response

Drug/lab test

False positive: urinary glucose test

NURSING CONSIDERATIONS
Assessment
- Assess patient for previous sensitivity reaction
- Assess patient for signs and symptoms of infection including characteristics of wounds, sputum, urine, stool, WBC >10,000/mm^3, temp; obtain baseline information before and during treatment
- Complete C&S testing before beginning drug therapy to identify if correct treatment has been initiated
- Assess for allergic reactions: rash, urticaria, pruritus, chills, fever, joint pain; angioedema may occur a few days after therapy begins; epINEPHrine, resuscitation equipment should be available for anaphylactic reaction
- Monitor blood studies: CBC, Hct, bilirubin, alkaline phosphatase monthly if patient is on long-term therapy
- Monitor for bleeding: ecchymosis, bleeding gums, hematuria, stool guaiac daily if on long-term therapy
- Assess for overgrowth of infection: perineal itching, fever, malaise, redness, pain, swelling, drainage, rash, diarrhea, change in cough, sputum

Nursing diagnoses
- Infection, risk for (uses)
- Diarrhea (adverse reactions)
- Injury, risk for (adverse reactions)
- Knowledge, deficient (teaching)
- Noncompliance (teaching)

Implementation
- Give around the clock to maintain proper blood levels; give on an empty stomach to increase absorption of drug; do not give within 3 hr of other agents; drug interactions may occur
- Give with 8 oz of water

Patient/family education
- Teach patient to report sore throat, bruising, bleeding, joint pain; may indicate blood dyscrasias (rare)
- Advise patient to contact prescriber if vaginal itching; loose foul-smelling stools; or furry tongue occur; may indicate superinfection; report itching, rash, pruritus, urticaria
- Instruct patient to take all medication prescribed for the length of time ordered; drug must be taken around the clock to maintain blood levels; medication should not be shared with others

Evaluation
Positive therapeutic outcome
- Absence of signs/symptoms of infection (WBC <10,000/mm^3, temp WNL, absence of urinary pain, hematuria)
- Reported improvement in symptoms of infection
- Negative C&S

sulindac (Rx)
(sul-in'dak)

Apo-Sulin ✤, Clinoril, Novosundac ✤, sulindac

Func. class.: Nonsteroidal antiinflammatory, antirheumatic

Chem. class.: Indeneacetic acid derivative

Pregnancy category C

Do Not Confuse:
Clinoril/Clozaril, Clinoril/Oruvail

Action: Inhibits prostaglandin synthesis by decreasing an enzyme needed for biosynthesis; analgesic, antiinflammatory, antipyretic

Therapeutic Outcome: Decreased pain, inflammation

Uses: Mild to moderate pain, osteoarthritis, rheumatoid, gouty arthritis, ankylosing spondylitis, bursitis, arthritis

Dosage and routes
Arthritis

Adult: PO 150 mg bid, may increase to 200 mg bid

Bursitis/acute arthritis

Adult: PO 200 mg bid × 1-2 wk, then reduce dose

Child: PO 2-4 mg/kg/day in divided doses, max 6 mg/kg/day or 200 mg bid, whichever is less (safe/effective dose not established)

Available forms: Tabs 150, 200 mg

Adverse effects
CNS: Dizziness, drowsiness, fatigue, tremors, confusion, insomnia, anxiety, depression, *headache*

CV: Tachycardia, peripheral edema, palpitations, dysrhythmias

EENT: Tinnitus, hearing loss, blurred vision

GI: *Nausea, anorexia, vomiting, diarrhea,* jaundice, **cholestatic hepatitis,** constipation, flatulence, cramps, dry mouth, peptic ulcer, **bleeding, ulceration, perforation**

GU: **Nephrotoxicity: dysuria, hematuria, oliguria, azotemia**

HEMA: **Blood dyscrasias with prolonged use**

INTEG: Purpura, *rash, pruritus,* sweating, photosensitivity

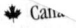

Contraindications: Hypersensitivity, asthma, severe renal disease, severe hepatic disease, active ulcers

Precautions: Pregnancy **C** (1st trimester), lactation, children, bleeding disorders, GI disorders, cardiac, renal disorders, hypersensitivity to other antiinflammatory agents

Pharmacokinetics	
Absorption	Well absorbed
Distribution	Not known
Metabolism	Converted to active drug—liver
Excretion	Minimal unchanged kidneys, breast milk
Half-life	7.8 hr; 16.4 hr active metabolite

Pharmacodynamics	
Onset	Unknown
Peak	2 hr
Duration	Unknown

Interactions

Individual drugs

Aspirin: increased GI reactions
Clopidogrel, eptifibatide, plicamycin, ticlopidine, tirofiban, valproic acid: increased bleeding risk
CycloSPORINE: increased nephrotoxicity
Diflunisal: decreased sulindac effect; do not use together
Methotrexate, probenecid: increased toxicity

Drug classifications

Anticoagulants, cephalosporins, thrombolytics: increased bleeding risk
Glucocorticoids, NSAIDs: increased GI reactions
Sulfonamides, sulfonylurea: increased toxicity

Drug/herb

Arginine, gossypol: increased gastric irritation
Bearberry, bilberry: increased NSAIDs effect
Bogbean, chondroitin: increased bleeding risk

NURSING CONSIDERATIONS

Assessment

- Monitor blood counts during therapy; watch for decreasing platelets; if low, therapy may need to be discontinued, restarted after hematologic recovery; and for blood dyscrasia (thrombocytopenia): bruising, fatigue, bleeding, poor healing
- Assess pain: frequency, intensity, characteristics, relief 1-2 hr after medication
- Assess for asthma, aspirin hypersensitivity, nasal polyps; hypersensitivity may develop

Nursing diagnoses

- Pain, chronic (uses)
- Mobility, physical, impaired (uses)
- Knowledge, deficient (teaching)
- Injury, risk for (adverse reactions)

Implementation

- Do not break, crush, or chew tabs
- Give with full glass of water to enhance absorption
- Administer with food or milk to decrease gastric symptoms; food slows absorption slightly, does not decrease absorption

Patient/family education

- Advise patient that drug must be continued for prescribed time to be effective; to avoid aspirin, alcoholic beverages
- Caution patient to report bleeding, bruising, fatigue, malaise because blood dyscrasias do occur
- Instruct patient to use caution when driving; drowsiness, dizziness may occur
- Teach patient to take with a full glass of water to enhance absorption

Evaluation

Positive therapeutic outcome

- Decreased pain
- Decreased inflammation
- Increased mobility

sumatriptan (Rx)

(soo-ma-trip'tan)
Imitrex
Func. class.: Antimigraine agent
Chem. class.: 5-HT_1 receptor agonist

Pregnancy category C

Action: Binds selectively to the vascular 5-HT_1 receptor subtype and exerts antimigraine effect; causes vasoconstriction in cranial arteries

Therapeutic Outcome: Absence of migraines

Uses: Acute treatment of migraine with or without aura and cluster headache

Dosage and routes

Adult: SUBCUT 6 mg or less; may repeat in 1 hr; not to exceed 12 mg/24 hr; PO 25 mg with fluids if no relief in 2 hr, give another dose, max 200 mg/day; nasal: 1 dose of 5, 10, or 20 mg in one nostril, may repeat in 2 hr, max 40 mg/24 hr

Hepatic dose

Adult: PO 25 mg, if no response after 2 hr, give up to 50 mg

Available forms: Inj 6 mg (12 mg/ml); tabs 25, 50, 100 mg; nasal spray 5 mg/100

mcl-units dose spray device 20 mg/100 mcl-units

Adverse effects

CNS: *Tingling, hot sensation, burning, feeling of pressure, tightness, numbness, dizziness, sedation,* headache, anxiety, fatigue, cold sensation
CV: *Flushing,* **MI**
EENT: Throat, mouth, nasal discomfort, vision changes
GI: Abdominal discomfort
INTEG: *Inj site reaction,* sweating
MS: *Weakness, neck stiffness,* myalgia
RESP: Chest tightness, pressure

Contraindications: Angina pectoris, history of MI, documented silent ischemia, Prinzmetal's angina, ischemic heart disease, **IV** use, concurrent ergotamine-containing preparations, uncontrolled hypertension, hypersensitivity, basilar or hemiplegic migraine

Precautions: Pregnancy **C**, postmenopausal women, men >40 yr, risk factors for CAD, hypercholesterolemia, obesity, diabetes, impaired hepatic or renal function, lactation, children <18 yr, elderly

Pharmacokinetics

Absorption	Well absorbed (SUBCUT)
Distribution	10%-20% plasma protein binding
Metabolism	Liver (metabolite)
Excretion	Urine, feces
Half-life	2 hr

Pharmacodynamics

	SUBCUT
Onset	10-20 min
Peak	10 min-2 hr
Duration	Up to 24 hr (pain relief)

Interactions

Individual drugs

Ergotamine: increased risk of vasospastic reaction

Drug classifications

Ergot derivatives: extended vasospastic effects
MAOIs, SSRIs: increased sumatriptan levels

Drug/herb

Butterbur: increased effect
SAM-e, St. John's wort: serotonin syndrome

NURSING CONSIDERATIONS

Assessment

- Assess for tingling, hot sensation, burning, feeling of pressure, numbness, flushing, inj site reaction
- Assess B/P; signs/symptoms of coronary vasospasm
- Monitor stress level, activity, reaction, coping mechanisms of patient
- Assess neurologic status: LOC, blurring vision, nausea, vomiting, tingling in extremities preceding headache
- Assess for ingestion of tyramine-containing foods (pickled products, beer, wine, aged cheese), food additives, preservatives, colorings, artificial sweeteners, chocolate, caffeine, which may precipitate these types of headaches

Nursing diagnoses

- Pain, chronic (uses)
- Knowledge, deficient (teaching)

Implementation

PO route

- Swallow tab whole; do not break, crush, or chew
- Take with fluids as soon as symptoms appear; may take a second dose >4 hr, max 200 mg/24 hr

SUBCUT route

- Give by SUBCUT route only, avoid IM or **IV** administration, use only for actual migraine attack

Nasal route

- Spray once in 1 nostril, may repeat if headache returns, do not repeat if pain continues after 1st dose

Patient/family education

- Caution patient not to take more than 2 doses/day or 12 mg/day; allow at least 1 hr between doses
- Caution patient to avoid driving or hazardous activities if dizziness or drowsiness occurs
- Teach patient to report chest tightness, heat, flushing, drowsiness, dizziness, fatigue, sudden severe abdominal pain or any allergic reactions that occur to prescriber immediately
- Inform patient to report any side effects to prescriber
- Caution patient to use contraception when taking drug, to notify prescriber if pregnancy is suspected or planned

Evaluation

Positive therapeutic outcome

- Decrease in frequency, severity of headache

tacrine (Rx)
(tack'rin)
Cognex
Func. class.: Anti-Alzheimer agent
Chem. class.: Reversible cholinesterase inhibitor

Pregnancy category C

Do Not Confuse:
Cognex/Corgard

Action: Elevates acetylcholine concentrations (cerebral cortex) by slowing degrading of acetylcholine released in cholinergic neurons; does not alter underlying dementia

Therapeutic Outcome: Improvement in symptoms of dementia in Alzheimer's disease

Uses: Treatment of mild to moderate dementia in Alzheimer's disease

Dosage and routes
Adult: PO 10 mg qid × 4 wk, then 20 mg qid × 4 wk, increase at 4-wk intervals if patient tolerates drug well and if transaminase is within normal limits, then titrate to higher doses (30-40 mg qid) at 4 wk intervals

Available forms: Caps 10, 20, 30, 40 mg

Adverse effects
CNS: *Dizziness, confusion, insomnia,* tremor, *ataxia, somnolence, anxiety, agitation, depression, hallucinations, hostility, abnormal thinking,* chills, fever, headache, **seizures**
CV: Hypotension or hypertension, **bradycardia, heart block**
GI: *Nausea, vomiting, anorexia, abdominal pain, constipation,* dyspepsia, flatulence, **hepatotoxicity, GI bleeding,** diarrhea
GU: *Frequency, UTI, incontinence*
INTEG: *Rash,* flushing
OTHER: Myalgia
RESP: *Rhinitis, upper respiratory tract infection, cough,* pharyngitis

Contraindications: Hypersensitivity to this drug or acridine derivatives, patients treated with this drug who developed jaundice with a total bilirubin of >3 mg/dl

Precautions: Pregnancy **C,** sick sinus syndrome, history of ulcers, GI bleeding, hepatic disease, bladder obstruction, asthma, lactation, children, seizure disorder, history of bradyarrhythmias

Pharmacokinetics

Absorption	Rapidly absorbed, low
Distribution	55% plasma protein bound
Metabolism	Liver, extensively by CYP450 enzyme system
Excretion	Unknown
Half-life	2-4 hr

Pharmacodynamics
Unknown

Interactions
Individual drugs
Cimetidine, ciprofloxacin, fluvoxamine, ritonavir: increased tacrine level
Succinylcholine: synergistic effect
Theophylline: increased elimination half-life of theophylline
Smoking: may decrease drug level

Drug classifications
Anticholinergics: decreased activity of anticholinergics
Cholinergic agonists, cholinesterase inhibitors: synergistic effect
NSAIDs: increased bleeding risk

Drug/food
May delay absorption, give 1 hr ac

NURSING CONSIDERATIONS
Assessment
- Monitor ALT qowk × 4-16 wk, then q3 mo; weekly ALT × 6 wk if dose is increased
- Monitor B/P for hypotension or hypertension
- Assess mental status: affect, mood, behavioral changes, depression, hallucinations, confusion; conduct suicide assessment
- Assess GI status: nausea, vomiting, anorexia, constipation, abdominal pain; add bulk and increase fluids for constipation
- Assess GU status: urinary frequency, incontinence
- Jaundice confirmed by significant increase in bilirubin (>3 mg/dl) and/or those with hypersensitivity (rash/fever) with increased ALT; should be immediately, permanently discontinued

Nursing diagnoses
- Injury, risk for (uses)
- Thought processes, disturbed (uses)
- Knowledge, deficient (teaching)

Implementation
- Give dosage adjusted to patient's response no more than q4 wk
- Provide assistance with ambulation if needed during beginning therapy; dizziness, ataxia may occur

T

• Give between meals; if GI symptoms occur, may be given with meals

Patient/family education

• Advise patient to report side effects: severe nausea, vomiting, sweating, salivation, bradycardia, hypotension, collapse, seizures; may indicate overdose
• Instruct patient to use drug exactly as prescribed at regular intervals, preferably between meals; may be taken with meals for GI upset; drug is not a cure
• Advise patient to notify prescriber of nausea, vomiting, diarrhea (dose increased or beginning treatment) or rash, very dark or very light stools, jaundice (delayed onset)
• Caution patient not to increase or abruptly decrease dose; serious consequences may result

Evaluation

Positive therapeutic outcome

• Decrease in confusion, improved mood

Treatment of overdose: Withdraw drug, administer tertiary anticholinergics, provide supportive care

tacrolimus (Rx)

(tak-roe'li-mus)

Prograf

tacrolimus topical

Protopic

Func. class.: Immunosuppressant
Chem. clas.: Macrolide

Pregnancy category C

Action: Produces immunosuppression by inhibiting lymphocytes (T)

Therapeutic Outcome: Prevention of rejection in organ transplant

Uses: Organ transplants, to prevent rejection; topical: atopic dermatitis

Investigational uses: Autoimmune diseases, severe recalcitrant psoriasis

Dosage and routes

Adult and child: **IV** 0.03-0.05 mg/kg/day × 3 days then PO 0.15 mg/kg bid; adjust dose in renal impairment

Adult/child ≥2 yr: Apply ointment bid × 7 days

Available forms: Inj **IV** 5 mg/ml; caps 0.5, 1, 5 mg; ointment 0.03%, 0.1%

Adverse effects

CNS: *Tremors, headache,* insomnia, paresthesia, chills, fever, **seizures**
CV: Hypertension
EENT: Blurred vision, photophobia
GI: Nausea, vomiting, diarrhea, constipation, GI bleeding
GU: Urinary tract infections, **albuminuria, hematuria, proteinuria, renal failure**
HEMA: Anemia, **leukocytosis, thrombocytopenia purpura**
INTEG: Rash, flushing, itching, alopecia
META: Hirsutism, hyperglycemia, hyperkalemia, hyperuricemia, hypokalemia, hypomagnesemia
RESP: **Pleural effusion, atelectasis,** dyspnea
SYST: **Anaphylaxis**

Contraindications: Hypersensitivity to this drug or to some kinds of castor oil

Precautions: Pregnancy **C,** severe renal disease, severe hepatic disease, diabetes mellitus, hyperkalemia, hyperuricemia, lymphomas, lactation, children <12 yr; hypertension

Pharmacokinetics

Absorption	Erractically absorbed (PO), completely absorbed (**IV**)
Distribution	Crosses placenta, 75% protein binding
Metabolism	Liver to metabolite
Excretion	Kidney—minimal, breast milk, bile
Half-life	10 hr

Pharmacodynamics

	PO	IV
Onset	Unknown	Unknown
Peak	1-4 hr	Unknown
Duration	12 hr	12 hr

Interactions

Individual drugs

Carbamazepine, phenobarbital, phenytoin, rifamycin: decreased blood levels
Cimetidine, danazol, erythromycin, mycophenolate, mofetil: increased blood levels
Cisplatin, cycloSPORINE: increased toxicity
Ibuprofen: increased oliguria

Drug classifications

Aminoglycosides: increased toxicity
Antifungals, calcium channel blockers: increased blood levels
Vaccines: decreased effect

Drug/herb

Astragalus, echinacea, melatonin: decreased immunosuppression
Ginseng, maitake, mistletoe: decreased effect

NURSING CONSIDERATIONS
Assessment

- Monitor blood studies: Hgb, WBC, platelets during treatment monthly; if WBC is <3000/mm^3, or platelet count <100,000/mm^3, drug should be discontinued or reduced; decreased Hgb level may indicate bone marrow suppression
- Monitor liver function studies: alkaline phosphatase, AST, ALT, amylase, bilirubin, and for hepatotoxicity: dark urine, jaundice, itching, light-colored stools; drug should be discontinued
- Assess for anaphylaxis: rash, pruritus, wheezing, laryngeal edema; stop infusion, initiate emergency procedures

Nursing diagnoses

- Infection, risk for (uses)
- Knowledge, deficient (teaching)

Implementation

PO route

- Give all medications PO if possible; avoid IM inj because bleeding may occur
- Give with meals to reduce GI upset; nausea is common
- Give for several days before transplant surgery; patients should be placed in protective isolation

IV route

- Give after diluting in 0.9% NaCl or D_5W to a concentration of 0.004-0.02 mg/ml as a cont inf

Y-site compatibilities: Acyclovir, aminophylline, amphotericin B, ampicillin, ampicillin/sulbactam, benztropine, calcium gluconate, cefazolin, cefotetan, ceftazidime, ceftriaxone, cefuroxime, chloramphenicol, cimetidine, ciprofloxacin, clindamycin, dexamethasone, digoxin, diphenhydrAMINE, DOBUTamine, DOPamine, doxycycline, erythromycin, esmolol, fluconazole, furosemide, ganciclovir, gentamicin, haloperidol, heparin, hydrocortisone, imipenem/cilastatin, insulin (regular), isoproterenol, leucovorin, lorazepam, methylPREDNISolone, metoclopramide, metronidazole, mezlocillin, multivitamins, nitroglycerin, nitroprusside, oxacillin, penicillin G potassium, perphenazine, phenytoin, piperacillin, potassium chloride, propranolol, ranitidine, sodium bicarbonate, trimethoprim/sulfamethoxazole, vancomycin

Patient/family education

- Instruct patient to report fever, rash, severe diarrhea, chills, sore throat, fatigue because serious infections may occur; clay-colored stools, cramping may indicate hepatotoxicity
- Caution patient to avoid crowds or persons with known infections to reduce risk of infection

Evaluation

Positive therapeutic outcome

- Absence of graft rejection
- Immunosuppression in autoimmune disorders

tadalafil (Rx)

(tah-dal'a-fil)

Cialis

Func. class.: Impotence agent

Chem. class.: Phosphodiesterase type 5 inhibitor

Action: Inhibits phosphodiesterase type 5 (PDE5); enhances erectile function by increasing the amount of cGMP, which causes smooth muscle relaxation and increased blood flow into the corpus cavernosum; improves erectile function for up to 36 hr

Therapeutic Outcome: Erection

Uses: Treatment of erectile dysfunction

Dosage and routes

Adult: PO 10 mg, taken prior to sexual activity, dose may be reduced to 5 mg or increased to a max of 20 mg; usual max dosing frequency is once per day

Renal dose

Adult (CCr 31-50 ml/min): PO 5 mg/daily, max 10 mg q48hr; CCr <30 ml/min, max 5 mg

Hepatic dose

Adult (Child-Pugh class A, B): PO max 10 mg daily; Child-Pugh class C, not recommended

Concomitant medications

Ketoconazole, ritonavir, max 10 mg q72hr

Available forms: Tabs 5, 10, 20 mg

Adverse effects

CNS: *Headache, flushing, dizziness*

CV: **MI, sudden death, CV collapse**

MISC: Back pain/myalgia, *dyspepsia, nasal congestion, UTI,* blurred vision, changes in color vision, *diarrhea,* pruritus

Contraindications: Hypersensitivity, patients taking organic nitrates regularly or intermittently, patients taking any α-adrenergic antagonist other than 0.4 mg once daily tamsulosin

Precautions: Anatomic penile deformities, sickle cell anemia, leukemia, multiple

T

myeloma; tadalafil is not indicated for use in newborns, children, or women

Pharmacokinetics

Absorption	Rapid; rate and extent of absorption of tadalafil are not influenced by food
Distribution	94% protein bound
Metabolism	Liver
Excretion	Excreted primarily as metabolites, feces, urine; plasma concentration 61% in feces, 36% in urine
Half-life	17.5 hr

Pharmacodynamics

Onset	Rapid
Peak	6 hr
Duration	Unknown

Interactions

Individual drugs

Ketoconazole, ritonavir: increased levels (although not studied, may also include other HIV protease inhibitors)

Drug classifications

Do not use with nitrates because of unsafe drop in B/P that could result in heart attack or stroke

Antihypertensive medications: decreased B/P

NURSING CONSIDERATIONS

Assessment

- Assess for organic nitrates that should not be used with this drug

Nursing diagnoses

- Sexual dysfunction (uses)
- Knowledge, deficient (teaching)

Implementation

- Before sexual activity; do not use more than once a day

Patient/family education

- Advise that drug does not protect against STDs, including HIV
- Instruct to tell physician if patient has a bleeding problem
- Advise that drug should not be used with nitrates in any form
- Advise that drug has no effect in the absence of sexual stimulation
- Instruct to seek medical help if an erection lasts more than 4 hr
- Advise to tell physician of all medicines, vitamins, and herbs patient is taking, especially α-blockers, erythromycin, indinavir, itraconazole, ketoconozole, nitrates, ritonavir
- Advise that tadalafil is contraindicated for use with α-blockers except 0.4 mg/daily tamsulosin

Evaluation

Positive therapeutic outcome

- Sustainable erection

tamoxifen (Rx)

(ta-mox'i-fen)

Alpha-Tamoxifen ✤, Med Tamoxifen ✤, Nolvadex, Nolvadex-D ✤, Novo-Tamoxifen ✤, Tamofen ✤, Tamone ✤, Tamoplex ✤

Func. class.: Antineoplastic

Chem. class.: Antiestrogen hormone

Pregnancy category D

Action: Inhibits cell division by binding to cytoplasmic estrogen receptors; resembles normal cell complex but inhibits DNA synthesis and estrogen response of target tissue

Therapeutic Outcome: Prevention of rapidly growing malignant cells

Uses: Advanced breast carcinoma that has not responded to other therapy in estrogen receptor-positive patients (usually postmenopausal), prevention of breast cancer, after breast surgery/radiation in ductal carcinoma in situ

Investigational uses: Mastalgia, pain/size of gynecomastia, ovulation stimulation, malignant carcinoid tumor, carcinoid syndrome

Dosage and routes

Breast cancer

Adult: PO 20-40 mg daily, doses >20 mg/day divide AM/PM

High risk for breast cancer

Adult: PO 20 mg daily × 5 yr

Ductal carcinoma in situ

Adult: PO 20 mg daily × 5 yr

Available forms: Tabs 10, 20 mg

Adverse effects

CNS: *Hot flashes, headache, lightheadedness,* depression
CV: Chest pain
EENT: Ocular lesions, retinopathy, corneal opacity, blurred vision (high doses)
GI: *Nausea, vomiting,* altered taste (anorexia)
GU: Vaginal bleeding, pruritus vulvae
HEMA: **Thrombocytopenia, leukopenia,** deep vein thrombosis, **pulmonary embolism**
INTEG: *Rash,* alopecia
META: Hypercalcemia

Contraindications: Pregnancy **D**, hypersensitivity, lactation

Precautions: Leukopenia, thrombocytopenia, cataracts

Pharmacokinetics	
Absorption	Adequately absorbed
Distribution	Unknown
Metabolism	Liver—extensively
Excretion	Feces—slowly, small amounts (kidneys)
Half-life	1 wk

Pharmacodynamics	
Onset	Unknown
Peak	4-7 hr
Duration	Unknown

Interactions

Individual drugs

Aminoglutethimide, medroxyprogesterone, rifamycin: decreased tamoxifen levels
Bromocriptine: increased tamoxifen level
Letrozole: decreased levels of letrozole
Radiation: increased myelosuppression

Drug classifications

Anticoagulants: increased risk of bleeding
Antineoplastics: increased thromboembolic action

Drug/lab test

Increased: serum calcium

NURSING CONSIDERATIONS

Assessment

- Monitor CBC, differential, platelet count weekly; withhold drug if WBC is <4000/mm^3 or platelet count is <75,000/mm^3; notify prescriber of results; monitor calcium levels (hypercalcemia is common)
- Assess for tumor flare: increase in bone, tumor pain during beginning treatment; give analgesics as ordered to decrease pain
- Assess for bleeding: hematuria, guaiac, bruising or petechiae, mucosa or orifices q8h, no rectal temp
- Assess for uterine malignancies: Symptoms of stroke, pulmonary embolism that may occur in women with ductal carcinoma in situ (DCIS) and women at high risk for breast cancer

Nursing diagnoses

- Injury, risk for (adverse reactions)
- Knowledge, deficient (teaching)

Implementation

- Do not break, crush, or chew tabs
- Give with food or fluids for GI upset; repeat dose may be needed if vomiting occurs
- Store in light-resistant container at room temp

Patient/family education

- Instruct patient to report any complaints, side effects to prescriber; if dose is missed, do not double next dose
- Advise patient that vaginal bleeding, pruritus, hot flashes can occur and are reversible after discontinuing treatment
- Instruct patient to report immediately decreased visual acuity, which may be irreversible; stress need for routine eye exams
- Inform patient about who should be told about tamoxifen therapy
- Advise patient to report vaginal bleeding immediately; that tumor flare (increase in size or tumor, increased bone pain) may occur and will subside rapidly; may take analgesics for pain; that premenopausal women must use mechanical birth control method because ovulation may be induced (teratogenic drug)
- Caution patient to use sunscreen and protective clothing to prevent burns because photosensitivity is common
- Teach patient that hair loss may occur during treatment; a wig or hairpiece may make patient feel better; new hair may be different in color, texture
- Inform patient rash or lesions are temporary and may become large during beginning therapy
- Advise patient to increase fluids to 2 L/day unless contraindicated

Evaluation

Positive therapeutic outcome

- Decreased spread of malignant cells in breast cancer

tamsulosin (Rx)

(tam-sue-lo'sen)

Flomax

Func. class.: Selective α-adrenergic blocker
Chem. class.: Sulfamoyl phenethylamine derivative

Pregnancy category B

Do Not Confuse:
Flomax/Fosamax/Volmax

Therapeutic Outcome: Decreased symptoms of benign prostatic hyperplasia (BPH)

Uses: Symptoms of BPH

Dosage and routes

Adult: PO 0.4 mg daily, increasing to 0.8 mg daily if required

Available forms: Caps 0.4 mg

Adverse effects

CNS: *Dizziness, headache,* asthenia, insomnia
CV: Chest pain
EENT: Amblyopia
GI: Nausea, diarrhea
GU: Decreased libido, abnormal ejaculation
MS: Back pain
RESP: Rhinitis, pharyngitis, cough

Contraindications: Hypersensitivity

Precautions: Pregnancy **B,** children, lactation, hepatic disease, coronary artery disease, severe renal disease

Pharmacokinetics

Absorption	Well absorbed
Distribution	Not known; 98% plasma protein bound
Metabolism	Liver, extensively
Excretion	Kidneys
Half-life	9-15 hr

Pharmacodynamics

Unknown

Interactions

Individual drugs

Cimetidine: increased toxicity
Doxazosin, prazosin, terazosin, vardenafil: do not use together

Drug classifications

β-Adrenergic blockers: do not use together

Drug/food

Decreased: absorption with food

NURSING CONSIDERATIONS

Assessment

- Monitor CBC with differential and liver function studies; B/P and heart rate
- Monitor urodynamic studies/urinary flow rates, residual volume
- Assess for BPH: change in urinary patterns, baseline and throughout treatment
- Monitor I&O ratios, weight daily, edema, report weight gain or edema

Nursing diagnoses

- Cardiac output, decreased (uses)
- Injury, risk for (side effects)
- Knowledge, deficient (teaching)
- Noncompliance (teaching)

Implementation

- Swallow caps whole; do not break, crush, or chew
- Store in airtight container at 86° F (30° C) or less
- May be given with food to prevent GI symptoms; ½ hr after same meal each day

Patient/family education

- Teach patient not to discontinue drug abruptly; emphasize the importance of complying with dosage schedule, even if feeling better; if dose is missed take as soon as remembered; take at same time each day
- Teach patient not to use OTC products (cough, cold, allergy) unless directed by prescriber; also to avoid large amounts of caffeine
- Caution patient that drug may cause dizziness, may occur during 1st few days of therapy; to avoid hazardous activities

Evaluation

Positive therapeutic outcome

- Decreased symptoms of BPH

tazobactam

See piperacillin/tazobactam

tegaserod (Rx)

(teg-as′er-odd)

Zelnorm

Func. class.: 5-HT$_4$ receptor partial agonist, GI agent—miscellaneous

Pregnancy category B

WITHDRAWN from the market

Action: A 5-HT$_4$ receptor partial agonist that binds 5-HT$_4$ receptors, stimulating peristalsis and intestinal secretion

Therapeutic Outcome: Decreased constipation in irritable bowel syndrome (IBS)

Uses: IBS where primary bowel symptom is constipation

Dosage and routes

Adult: **PO** 6 mg bid before meals × 4-6 wk, another 4-6 wk course may be used

WITHDRAWN from the market

Available forms: Tabs 2, 6 mg

Adverse effects

CNS: *Headache, dizziness, depression, vertigo, fatigue,* suicide attempt, poor concentration
CV: Hypotension, angina, **dysrhythmias, bundle branch block, supraventricular tachycardia**
GI: *Nausea, abdominal pain, increased appetite, eructation, increased AST, in-*

creased ALT, diarrhea, irritable colon, tenesmus, flatulence
GU: Polyuria, renal pain, ovarian cyst, miscarriage, albuminuria
MISC: Pain, facial edema, increased CPK, asthma, breast carcinoma
MS: Back pain, arthralgia
***SYST:* Anaphylaxis**

Contraindications: Hypersensitivity, severe renal disease, moderate to severe hepatic disease, history of bowel obstruction, gallbladder disease, abdominal adhesions, sphincter of Oddi dysfunction, hypotension

Precautions: Pregnancy **B,** lactation, children, diarrhea

Pharmacokinetics

Absorption	Unknown
Distribution	98% protein binding
Metabolism	Unknown
Excretion	2/3 unchanged in feces, remainder in urine as metabolites
Half-life	11 hr

Pharmacodynamics

Onset	Unknown
Peak	1 hr
Duration	Unknown

Interactions
Individual drug
Digoxin: decreased effect of digoxin
Drug classification
Antimuscarinics: decreased tegaserod effect
Oral contraceptives: decreased effect of oral contraceptives
Drug/food
Food: decreased absorption, but is minimized when taken ½ hr before a meal

NURSING CONSIDERATIONS
Assessment
- Assess GI symptoms: nausea, abdominal pain
- Assess CV status: B/P, pulse, chest pain

Nursing diagnoses
- Constipation, (uses)
- Knowledge, deficient (teaching)

Implementation
- Give before meals, bid
- Store at room temp

Patient/family education
- Advise to notify prescriber of GI symptoms, hypersensitivity reactions

Evaluation
Positive therapeutic outcome
- Decreased constipation in IBS

telithromycin (Rx)
(teh-lih-throw-my'sin)
Ketek
Func. class.: Antiinfective
Chem. class.: Ketolides

Pregnancy category C

Action: Binds to 50S ribosomal subunits of susceptible bacteria and suppresses protein synthesis

Therapeutic Outcome: Bacterial action against *Streptococcus pneumoniae, Haemophilus influenzae, Moraxella catarrhalis, Staphylococcus aureus*

Uses: Acute bacterial exacerbation of chronic bronchitis caused by *Streptococcus pneumoniae, Haemophilus influenzae, Moraxella catarrhalis*; acute bacterial sinusitis caused by *S. pnuemoniae, H. influenzae, M. catarrhalis, Staphylococcus aureus*, community acquired pneumonia

Dosage and routes
Acute bacterial exacerbation of bronchitis
Adult: PO 800 mg daily × 5 days

Acute bacterial sinusitis
Adult: PO 800 mg daily × 5 days

Community-acquired pneumonia
Adult: PO 800 mg daily × 7-10 days

Available forms: Tabs 400 mg

Adverse effects
CNS: Dizziness, headache, insomnia, increased sweating
EENT: Blurred vision, diplopia, difficulty focusing
GI: *Nausea, vomiting, diarrhea*, hepatitis, abdominal pain/distension, stomatitis, anorexia
GU: *Vaginitis, moniliasis*
INTEG: Rash, urticaria
MISC: Atrial dysrythymias
MS: Muscle cramps
***SYST:* Anaphylaxis**

Contraindications: Hypersensitivity

Precautions: Pregnancy **C,** lactation, children, elderly, myasthenia gravis, ongoing prodysrrhymias, hepatic disease

Pharmacokinetics

Absorption	Unknown
Distribution	Protein binding 60%-70%
Metabolism	Liver
Excretion	Bile, feces
Half-life	Unknown

T

Pharmacodynamics

Onset	Unknown
Peak	1 hr
Duration	Unknown

Interactions
Individual drugs
Atorvastatin, digoxin, ergots, lovastatin, metoprolol, midazolam, simvastatin, theophylline: increased action, toxicity
Pimozide: serious dysrhythmias; do not use together
Carbamazepine, phenobarbital, phenytoin, rifampin: decreased action of telithromycin
Sotalol: decreased action
Itraconazole, ketoconazole: increased telithromycin
Drug/herb
Do not use acidophilus with antiinfectives
Drug/lab test
Increased: AST/ALT

NURSING CONSIDERATIONS
Assessment
- Assess for infection: temp, sputum, WBCs, baseline and periodically
- Assess for oliguria in renal disease
- Monitor hepatic studies: AST, ALT, if patient is on long-term therapy
- Monitor C&S before drug therapy; drug may be given as soon as culture is taken; C&S may be repeated after treatment
- Monitor bowel pattern before, during treatment
- Assess for skin eruptions, itching

Nursing diagnoses
- Infection, risk for (uses)

Implementation
- May take without regard to food
- Store at room temperature
- Provide adequate intake of fluids (2 L) during diarrhea episodes

Patient/family education
- Teach patient to report sore throat, fever, fatigue (could indicate superinfection)
- Teach patient to notify nurse of diarrhea stools, dark urine, pale stools, jaundice of eyes or skin, and severe abdominal pain
- Teach patient to report blurred vision, if interfering with daily activities
- Advise patient to avoid driving, hazardous activities if blurred vision occurs
- Instruct patient to take as prescribed, do not double or skip doses
- Instruct patient not to use this drug if using Class 1A or III antidysrhythmics
- Advise patient to avoid simvastatin, lovastatin or atorvastatin
- Inform patient that medication may be taken without regard to meals

Evaluation
Positive therapeutic outcome
- Decreased symptoms of infection

Treatment of hypersensitivity:
Withdraw drug; maintain airway; administer epINEPHrine, aminophylline, O_2, **IV** corticosteroids

telmisartan (Rx)
(tel-mih-sar'tan)
Micardis
Func. class.: Antihypertensive
Chem. class.: Angiotensin II receptor (type AT_1)

Pregnancy category
C (1st trimester),
D (2nd/3rd trimesters)

Action: Blocks the vasoconstrictor and aldosterone-secreting effects of angiotensin II; selectively blocks the binding of angiotensin II to the AT_1 receptor found in tissues

Therapeutic Outcome: Decreased B/P

Uses: Hypertension, alone or in combination

Investigational uses: Heart failure

Dosage and routes
Adult: PO 40 mg daily; range 20-80 mg

Available forms: Tabs 20, 40, 80 mg

Adverse effects
CNS: Dizziness, insomnia, *anxiety,* headache, fatigue
GI: *Diarrhea,* dyspepsia, *anorexia, vomiting*
MS: *Myalgia, pain*
RESP: Cough, *upper respiratory tract infection,* sinusitis, pharyngitis

Contraindications: Pregnancy **D** (2nd/3rd trimesters), hypersensitivity

Precautions: Pregnancy **C** (1st trimester); hypersensitivity to angiotensin-converting enzyme (ACE) inhibitors; lactation, children, elderly

Pharmacokinetics

Absorption	Unknown
Distribution	Highly protein bound
Metabolism	Liver (extensively)
Excretion	Urine/feces
Half-life	Terminal 24 hr

Pharmacodynamics

Onset	Unknown
Peak	Unknown
Duration	Unknown

Interactions
Digoxin: increased digoxin peak, trough concentrations

Drug classifications

Antihypertensives, diuretics: increased antihypertensive action
Potassium-sparing diuretics, potassium salt substitutes: increased hyperkalemia

Drug/herb

Aconite: increased toxicity, death
Astragalus, cola tree: increased or decreased antihypertensive effect
Barberry, betony, black catechu, black cohosh, bloodroot, broom, burdock, cat's claw, dandelion, goldenseal, Irish moss, Jamaican dogwood, kelp, khella, mistletoe, parsley: increased antihypertensive effect
Coltsfoot, guarana, khat, licorice: decreased antihypertensive effect

NURSING CONSIDERATIONS
Assessment
- Monitor B/P, pulse q4h; note rate, rhythm, quality
- Monitor electrolytes: potassium, sodium, chloride
- Monitor baselines in renal, liver function tests before therapy begins
- Assess edema in feet, legs daily
- Assess skin turgor, dryness of mucous membranes for hydration status

Nursing diagnoses
- Tissue perfusion, ineffective (uses)
- Knowledge, deficient (teaching)
- Noncompliance (teaching)

Implementation
- Give without regard to meals
- Give increased dose to African-American patients, B/P response may be reduced

Patient/family education
- Instruct patient to comply with dosage schedule, even if feeling better
- Advise patient to notify prescriber of mouth sores, fever, swelling of hands or feet, irregular heartbeat, chest pain
- Teach patient that excessive perspiration, dehydration, vomiting, diarrhea may lead to fall in blood pressure; consult prescriber if these occur
- Teach patient that drug may cause dizziness, fainting; light-headedness may occur
- Advise patient to use contraception while taking this drug
- Teach patient to notify prescriber of all prescriptions, OTC preparations, and supplements taken

Evaluation
Positive therapeutic outcome
- Decreased B/P

temazepam (Rx)
(tem-az'a-pam)

Razepam, Restoril, Temazepam
Func. class.: Sedative/hypnotic
Chem. class.: Benzodiazepine

Pregnancy category X

Controlled substance schedule IV (USA), schedule F (Canada)

Action: Produces CNS depression at limbic, thalamic, hypothalamic levels of the CNS; may be mediated by neurotransmitter γ-aminobutyric acid (GABA); results are sedation, hypnosis, skeletal muscle relaxation, anticonvulsant activity, anxiolytic action

Therapeutic Outcome: Decreased insomnia

Uses: Insomnia (short-term)

Dosage and routes
Adult: PO 15-30 mg at bedtime
Elderly: PO 7.5 mg at bedtime

Available forms: Caps 7.5, 15, 30 mg

Adverse effects
CNS: *Lethargy, drowsiness, daytime sedation,* dizziness, confusion, lightheadedness, headache, anxiety, irritability
CV: Chest pain, pulse changes
GI: Nausea, vomiting, diarrhea, heartburn, abdominal pain, constipation, anorexia
HEMA: **Leukopenia, granulocytopenia** (rare)

Contraindications: Pregnancy **X,** hypersensitivity to benzodiazepines, lactation, intermittent porphyria

Precautions: Anemia, hepatic disease, renal disease, suicidal individuals, drug abuse, elderly, psychosis, child <15 yr, acute narrow-angle glaucoma, seizure disorders

T

Pharmacokinetics

Absorption	Well absorbed
Distribution	Widely distributed, crosses placenta, crosses blood-brain barrier
Metabolism	Liver
Excretion	Kidneys, breast milk
Half-life	10-20 hr

Pharmacodynamics

Onset	½ hr
Peak	2-3 hr
Duration	6-8 hr

Interactions
Individual drugs
Alcohol: increased actions of both drugs
Cimetidine, disulfiram: increased effect of each specific drug
Rifampin: decreased action of rifampin
Theophylline: decreased effects of theophylline
Drug classifications
Contraceptives (oral): increased effect
CNS depressants: increased action of both drugs
Drug/herb
Black cohosh: increased hypotension
Catnip, chamomile, clary, cowslip, hops, kava, lavender, mistletoe, nettle, pokeweed, poppy, Queen Anne's lace, senega, skullcap, valerian: increased CNS depression
Drug/lab test
Increased: AST/ALT, serum bilirubin
Decreased: radioactive iodine uptake
False increase: 17-OHCS

NURSING CONSIDERATIONS
Assessment
- Assess mental status: mood, sensorium, anxiety, affect, sleeping pattern, drowsiness, dizziness, especially elderly; physical dependency, withdrawal symptoms: anxiety, panic attacks, agitation, seizures, headache, nausea, vomiting, muscle pain, weakness; suicidal tendencies; for indications of increasing tolerance and abuse
- Monitor B/P (lying, standing), pulse; if systolic B/P drops 20 mm Hg, hold drug, notify prescriber
- Monitor blood studies: CBC during long-term therapy; blood dyscrasias have occurred rarely; decreased hematocrit, neutropenia may occur
- Monitor hepatic studies: AST, ALT, bilirubin, creatinine LDH, alkaline phosphatase
- Monitor I&O ratio; indicate renal dysfunction

Nursing diagnoses
- Anxiety (uses)
- Injury, risk for (adverse reactions)
- Knowledge, deficient (teaching)

Implementation
- Give with food or milk to decrease GI symptoms; if patient is unable to swallow medication whole, tab may be crushed and mixed with foods or fluids
- Give sugarless gum, hard candy, frequent sips of water for dry mouth

Patient/family education
- Inform patient that drug may be taken with food, and that fluids and tab may be crushed or swallowed whole
- Advise patient not to use for everyday stress or longer than 3 mo unless directed by prescriber; not to take more than prescribed amount; may be habit forming; not to double or skip doses
- Caution patient to avoid OTC preparations unless approved by prescriber; alcohol and CNS depressants will increase CNS depression
- Advise patient to avoid driving, activities that require alertness, because drowsiness may occur; to avoid alcohol ingestion or other psychotropic medications; to rise slowly or fainting may occur, especially in elderly; that drowsiness may worsen at beginning of treatment
- Caution patient not to discontinue medication abruptly after long-term use; withdrawal symptoms include vomiting, cramping, tremors, seizures
- Advise patient to use contraception while taking this drug

Evaluation
Positive therapeutic outcome
- Decreased anxiety, restlessness, sleeplessness (short-term treatment only)

Treatment of overdose: Lavage, VS, supportive care

temozolomide (Rx)
(tem-oo-zole'oo-mide)
Temodar
Func. class.: Antineoplastic alkylating agents
Chem. class.: Imidazotetrazine derivative
Pregnancy category D

Action: A prodrug that undergoes conversion to 5-(3-methyl-1-triazeno) imidazole-4-carboxamide (MTIC); MTIC action prevents DNA transcription

Therapeutic Outcome: Prevention of rapidly growing malignant cells

Uses: Anaplastic astrocytoma with relapse, glioblastoma multiforme

Investigational uses: Metastatic melanoma

Dosage and routes

Anaplastic astrocytoma

Adult: PO adjust dose based on nadir neutrophil and platelet counts 150 mg/m^2/day × 5 days during 28-day cycle

Glioblastoma multiforme

Adult: PO 75 mg/m^2/day × 42 days with focal radiotherapy, then maintenance of 6 cycles

Available forms: Caps 5, 20, 100, 250 mg

Adverse effects

CNS: **Seizures,** *hemiparesis, dizziness, poor coordination, amnesia, insomnia, paresthesia, somnolence, paresis, ataxia, anxiety, dysphagia, depression, confusion*
GI: *Nausea, anorexia, vomiting*
GU: *Urinary incontinence, UTI, frequency*
HEMA: **Thrombocytopenia, leukopenia,** anemia
INTEG: *Rash, pruritus*
MISC: *Headache, fatigue, asthenia, fever, edema, back pain, weight increase, diplopia*
RESP: *Upper respiratory tract infection, pharyngitis, sinusitis, coughing*

Contraindications: Pregnancy **D,** hypersensitivity to this drug or dacarbazine, lactation

Precautions: Radiation therapy, renal, hepatic disease

Pharmacokinetics	
Absorption	Rapid, complete
Distribution	Crosses blood-brain barrier
Metabolism	To MTIC and metabolite
Excretion	Urine, feces
Half-life	1.8 hr

Pharmacodynamics	
Onset	Unknown
Peak	1 hr
Duration	Unknown

Interactions

Individual drugs

Radiation: increased toxicity, bone marrow suppression

Drug classifications

Antineoplastics, bone marrow–suppressing drugs: increased bone marrow suppression
Live virus vaccines: increased adverse reactions, decreased antibody reaction

NURSING CONSIDERATIONS

Assessment

- Assess symptoms indicating severe allergic reaction: rash, pruritus, urticaria, purpuric skin lesions, itching, flushing; drug should be discontinued
- Obtain CBC on day 22 (21 days after 1st dose), CBC weekly until recovery if ANC is $<1.5 \times 10^9$/L and platelets $<100 \times 10^9$/L, do not administer to patients that do not tolerate 100 mg/m^2; myelosuppression usually occurs late in the treatment cycle
- Assess for seizures throughout treatment
- Monitor renal function studies: BUN, creatinine, urine CCr before and during therapy; I&O ratio; report fall in urine output to <30 ml/hr
- Monitor temp q4h (may indicate beginning of infection)
- Monitor liver function tests before and during therapy (bilirubin, AST, ALT, LDH) as needed or monthly; note jaundice of skin or sclera, dark urine, clay-colored stools, itchy skin, abdominal pain, fever, diarrhea; hepatotoxicity can be serious and fatal
- Assess for bleeding: hematuria, stool guaiac, bruising or petechiae, mucosa or orifices q8h; check for inflammation of mucosa, breaks in skin

Nursing diagnoses

- Injury, risk for (adverse reactions)
- Body image, disturbed (adverse reactions)
- Infection, risk for (adverse reactions)
- Knowledge, deficient (teaching)

Implementation

- Give fluids **IV** or PO before chemotherapy to hydrate patient
- Give antiemetic 30-60 min before giving drug to prevent vomiting, and prn; antibiotics for prophylaxis of infection
- Provide liq diet: carbonated beverages; gelatin may be added if patient is not nauseated or vomiting
- Capsules should not be opened, if accidentally damaged, do not allow contact with skin, or inhale; take caps one at a time with 8 oz of water at the same time of day
- Give on empty stomach to prevent nausea/vomiting

Patient/family education

- Teach patient to avoid use of products containing aspirin or NSAIDs, razors, commercial mouthwash, since bleeding may occur; to

report symptoms of bleeding (hematuria, tarry stools)
- Instruct patient to report signs of anemia (fatigue, headache, irritability, faintness, shortness of breath)
- Caution patient not to have any vaccinations without the advice of prescriber; serious reactions can occur
- Advise patient contraception is needed during treatment and for several months after completion of therapy; drug has teratogenic properties

Evaluation

Positive therapeutic outcome
- Prevention of rapid division of malignant cells

! HIGH ALERT

tenecteplase (Rx)

(ten-ek'ta-place)

TNKase

Func. class.: Thrombolytic enzyme

Chem. class.: Tissue plasminogen activator

Pregnancy category C

Action: Activates conversion of plasminogen to plasmin (fibrinolysin): plasmin breaks down clots (fibrin), fibrinogen, factors V, VII; occlusion of venous access lines

Therapeutic Outcome: Resolution of MI

Uses: Acute MI

Dosage and routes

Adult <60 kg: **IV** bol 30 mg, give over 5 sec

Adult ≥60-<70 kg: **IV** bol 35 mg, give over 5 sec

Adult ≥70-<80 kg: **IV** bol 40 mg, give over 5 sec

Adult ≥80-<90 kg: **IV** bol 45 mg, give over 5 sec

Adult ≥90 kg: **IV** bol 50 mg, give over 5 sec

Available forms: Powder for inj, lyophilized 50 mg

Adverse effects

CV: Dysrhythmias, hypotension, pulmonary edema, **pulmonary embolism, cardiogenic shock, cardiac arrest, heart failure, myocardial reinfarction, myocardial rupture, tamponade, pericarditis, pericardial effusion, thrombosis**

HEMA: Decreased Hct, **bleeding**

INTEG: Rash, urticaria, phlebitis at **IV** inf site, itching, flushing

SYST: **GI, GU, intracranial, retroperitoneal bleeding, surface bleeding, anaphylaxis**

Contraindications: Hypersensitivity, arteriovenous malformation, aneurysm, active bleeding, intracranial, intraspinal surgery, CNS neoplasms, severe hypertension, severe renal disease, hepatic disease, history of CVA

Precautions: Pregnancy **C**, arterial emboli from left side of heart, lactation, children, ulcerative colitis, enteritis, hypocoagulation, COPD, subacute bacterial endocarditis, rheumatic valvular disease, cerebral embolism/thrombosis/hemorrhage, intraarterial diagnostic procedure or surgery (10 days), recent major surgery, elderly

Pharmacokinetics	
Absorption	Unknown
Distribution	Unknown
Metabolism	Liver
Excretion	Unknown
Half-life	20-24 min

Pharmacodynamics	
Onset	Immediate
Peak	Unknown
Duration	Unknown

Interactions

Individual drugs

Aspirin, dipyridamole, glycoprotein IIb, indomethacin, IIIa inhibitors, phenylbutazone: increased bleeding potential

Drug classifications

Anticoagulants, antithrombolytics: increased bleeding potential

Drug/herb

Agrimony, alfalfa, angelica, anise, basil, bay, bilberry, black haw, bogbean, bromelain, buchu, chondroitin, cinchona bark, dong quai, fenugreek, feverfew, garlic, ginger, ginkgo, ginseng, horse chestnut, Irish moss, kelp, kelpware, khella, lovage, lungwort, meadowsweet, motherwort, mugwort, nettle, papaya, parsley (large amounts), pau d'arco, pineapple, poplar, prickly ash, safflower, saw palmetto, tonka bean, turmeric, wintergreen, yarrow: increased risk of bleeding

Chamomile, coenzyme Q10, flax, glucomannan, goldenseal, guar gum: decreased anticoagulant effect

Drug/lab test

Increased: protime, APTT, TT

Decreased: plasminogen, fibrinogen

NURSING CONSIDERATIONS

Assessment

- Assess for allergy: fever, rash, itching, chills; mild reaction may be treated with antihistamines
- ❗Assess for bleeding during 1st hr of treatment; hematuria, hematemesis, bleeding from mucous membranes, epistaxis, ecchymosis; may require transfusion (rare), continue to assess for bleeding for 24 hr
- Monitor blood studies (Hct, platelets, PTT, protime, TT, APTT) before starting therapy; protime or APTT must be less than 2 × control before starting therapy; PTT or protime q3-4h during treatment
- Assess for hypersensitive reactions: fever, rash, dyspnea; drug should be discontinued
- Monitor VS, B/P, pulse, respirations, neurologic signs, temp at least q4h; temp >104° F (40° C) indicates internal bleeding; systolic pressure increase >25 mm Hg should be reported to prescriber
- ❗Assess for neurologic changes that may indicate intracranial bleeding
- ❗Assess for retroperitoneal bleeding: back pain, leg weakness, diminished pulses

Nursing diagnoses

- Knowledge, deficient (teaching)
- Cardiac output, decreased (uses)

Implementation

IV route

- Give as soon as thrombi identified; not useful for thrombi >1 wk old
- Administer cryoprecipitate or fresh frozen plasma if bleeding occurs
- Give heparin after fibrinogen level >100 mg/dl; heparin infusion to increase PTT to 1.5-2 × baseline for 3-7 days; **IV** heparin with loading dose is recommended
- Aseptically withdraw 10 ml of sterile H_2O for inj from diluent vial, use red cannula syringe-filling device, inject all contents of syringe into drug vial, direct into powder, swirl, withdraw correct dose, discard any unused solution; stand the shield with dose vertically on flat surface and passively recap the red cannula, remove entire shield assembly by twisting counterclockwise, give by **IV** bol
- **IV** therapy: use upper extremity vessel that is accessible to manual compression
- Provide bed rest during entire course of treatment
- Avoid venous or arterial puncture, inj, rectal temp; any invasive treatment
- Treat fever with acetaminophen or aspirin
- Apply pressure for 30 sec to minor bleeding sites; inform prescriber if this does not attain hemostasis; apply pressure dressing

Evaluation

Positive therapeutic outcome

- Resolution of myocardial infarction

tenofovir (Rx)

(ten-oh-foh'veer)

Viread

Func. class.: Antiretroviral

Chem. class.: Nucleoside analog reverse transcriptase inhibitor

Pregnancy category B

Action: Inhibits replication of HIV-1 virus by competing with the natural substrate and then incorporating into cellular DNA by viral reverse transcriptase, thereby terminating cellular DNA chain

Therapeutic Outcome: Improved symptoms of HIV-1 infection

Uses: HIV-1 infection with other antiretrovirals

Dosage and routes

Adult: PO 300 mg with meal; if used with didanosine, give tenofovir 2 hr before or 1 hr after didanosine

Renal dose

CCr 30-49 mg/min 300 mg q48h
CCr 10-29 ml/min 300 mg 2 ×/wk
CCr <10 ml/min not recommended

Available forms: Tabs 300 mg (300 mg of fumarate salt equivalent to 245 mg tenofovir disoproxil)

Adverse effects

CNS: *Headache*

GI: *Nausea, vomiting, diarrhea,* anorexia, *flatulence, abdominal pain*

SYST: Change in body fat distribution

Contraindications: Hypersensitivity

Precautions: Pregnancy **B,** lactation, children, elderly, renal disease, hepatic insufficiency, CCr <60 ml/min, osteoporosis

Pharmacokinetics

Absorption	Rapidly absorbed
Distribution	Extravascular space; bound to serum plasma <0.7%; to serum proteins <7.2%
Metabolism	Unknown
Excretion	Urine, unchanged (70%-80%)
Half-life	Terminal 17h

T

Pharmacodynamics

Onset	Unknown
Peak	0.6-1.4 hr
Duration	Unknown

Interactions
Individual drugs
Acyclovir, cidofovir, ganciclovir, valacyclovir, valganciclovir: increased level of tenofovir
Didanosine: increased level of didanosine when coadministered with tenofovir
Drug classifications
Increased: levels of tenofovir with any drug that decreased renal function

NURSING CONSIDERATIONS
Assessment
- Assess liver studies: AST, ALT, bilirubin; amylase, lipase, triglycerides periodically during treatment
- Assess for bone, renal toxicity: if bone abnormalities are suspected, obtain tests: serum phosphorus, creatinine
- Assess for lactic acidosis, severe hepatomegaly with steatosis

Nursing diagnoses
- Infection, risk for (uses)
- Injury, risk for (adverse reactions)
- Knowledge, deficient (teaching)

Implementation
- Administer PO daily with meal
- Store at 25° C (77° F)
- Give drug 2 hr before or 1 hr after taking didanosine (if used)

Patient/family education
- Instruct patient to take this drug 2 hr before or 1 hr after taking didanosine (if used)
- Instruct patient to take drug with meal
- Advise patients that GI complaints resolve after 3-4 wk of treatment
- Caution patient not to breastfeed while taking this drug
- Inform patient that drug must be taken daily even if patient feels better
- Advise patient to continue follow-up visits since serious toxicity may occur; blood counts must be done q2 wk
- Inform patient that drug will control symptoms but is not a cure for HIV; patient is still infectious, may pass HIV virus on to others
- Advise patient that other drugs may be necessary to prevent other infections
- Advise patient that changes in body fat distribution may occur

Evaluation
Positive therapeutic outcome
- Decrease in signs/symptoms of HIV

terazosin (Rx)
(ter-ay′zoe-sin)
Hytrin
Func. class.: Antihypertensive
Chem. class.: α-Adrenergic blocker (peripherally acting)
Pregnancy category C

Action: Peripheral blood vessels are dilated, peripheral resistance lowered; reduction in blood pressure results from α-adrenergic receptors being blocked

Therapeutic Outcome: Decreased B/P in hypertension, decreased symptoms of benign prostatic hyperplasia (BPH)

Uses: Hypertension, as a single agent or in combination with diuretics or β-blockers, BPH

Dosage and routes
Hypertension
Adult: PO 1 mg at bedtime, may increase doses slowly to desired response; max 20 mg/day
Benign prostatic hyperplasia
Adult: PO 1 mg at bedtime, gradually increase up to 5-10 mg

Available forms: Tabs 1, 2, 5, 10 mg

Adverse effects
CNS: *Dizziness, headache, drowsiness,* anxiety, depression, vertigo, weakness, fatigue
CV: Palpitations, orthostatic hypotension, tachycardia, edema, rebound hypertension
EENT: Blurred vision, epistaxis, tinnitus, dry mouth, red sclera, nasal congestion, sinusitis
GI: *Nausea,* vomiting, diarrhea, constipation, abdominal pain
GU: Urinary frequency, incontinence, impotence, priapism
RESP: Dyspnea, cough, pharyngitis

Contraindications: Hypersensitivity

Precautions: Pregnancy **C**, children, lactation

Pharmacokinetics

Absorption	Well absorbed
Distribution	Not known
Metabolism	Liver—50%
Excretion	Kidneys unchanged—10%, feces unchanged—20%
Half-life	9-12 hr

Pharmacodynamics

Onset	15 min
Peak	1 hr
Duration	24 hr

Interactions

Individual drugs

Alcohol, nitroglycerin, verapamil: increased hypotensive effects

Drug classifications

Antihypertensives (other): increased hypotension

β-Blockers: increased hypotensive effects

Estrogens, NSAIDs, sympathomimetics: decreased antihypertensive effect

NURSING CONSIDERATIONS

Assessment

- Monitor B/P, orthostatic hypotension, syncope; check for edema in feet, legs daily; I&O ratio; weight daily; notify prescriber of changes
- Assess for allergic reactions: rash, fever, pruritus, urticaria; drug should be discontinued if antihistamines fail to help

Nursing diagnoses

- Cardiac output, decreased (uses)
- Injury, risk for (adverse reactions)
- Knowledge, deficient (teaching)
- Noncompliance (teaching)

Implementation

- May be used in combination with other antihypertensives
- Give at same time each day
- May be given with food to prevent GI symptoms
- Store in airtight container at 86° F (30° C) or less

Patient/family education

- Caution patient not to discontinue drug abruptly; the importance of complying with dosage schedule, even if feeling better; if dose is missed take as soon as remembered; take medication at same time each day
- Teach patient not to use OTC products (cough, cold, allergy) unless directed by prescriber; also to avoid large amounts of caffeine
- Emphasize the need to rise slowly to sitting or standing position to minimize orthostatic hypotension
- Teach patient to notify prescriber of mouth sores, sore throat, fever, swelling of hands or feet, irregular heartbeat, chest pain
- Caution patient to report excessive perspiration, dehydration, vomiting, diarrhea; may lead to fall in B/P
- Caution patient that drug may cause dizziness, fainting, light-headedness; may occur during 1st few days of therapy; to avoid hazardous activities
- Teach patient how to take B/P, and normal readings for age-group; to take B/P q7 days

Evaluation

Positive therapeutic outcome

- Decreased B/P in hypertension
- Decreased symptoms of BPH

Treatment of overdose: Administer volume expanders or vasopressors; discontinue drug; place patient in supine position

terbinafine (Rx)

(ter-bin′a-feen)

Lamisil

Func. class.: Antifungal, systemic

Chem. class.: Synthetic allylamine derivative

Pregnancy category B

Do Not Confuse:
lamotrigine/Lamisil

Action: Interferes with cell membrane permeability in fungi such as *Trichophyton rubrum, Trichophyton mentagrophytes, Trichophyton tonsurans, Epidermophyton floccosum, Microsporum canis, Microsporum audouinii, Microsporum gypseum, Candida*, broad-spectrum antifungal

Therapeutic Outcome: Resolution of fungal infection

Uses: (Oral) onychomycosis of the toenail or fingernail due to dermatophytes

Investigational uses: Cutaneous candidiasis, tinea versicolor

Dosage and routes

Fingernail: 250 mg/day × 6 wk

Toenail: 250 mg/day × 12 wk

Available forms: Tabs 250 mg

Adverse effects

GI: Diarrhea, dyspepsia, abdominal pain, nausea, hepatitis

HEMA: **Neutropenia**

INTEG: Rash, pruritus, urticaria, **Stevens-Johnson syndrome**

MISC: Headache, hepatic enzyme changes, taste, visual disturbance

Contraindications: Hypersensitivity, chronic/active hepatic disease, renal disease GFR ≤50 mg/min

Precautions: Pregnancy **B,** lactation, children, renal disease

T

Pharmacokinetics

Absorption	80%
Distribution	Extensive, most to hair, scalp, nails, excreted in breast milk, protein binding 99%
Metabolism	Liver, extensively
Excretion	Unknown
Half-life	22 days or longer

Pharmacodynamics (antifungal)

Onset	Up to 1 wk
Peak	Several days-weeks
Duration	Several weeks

Interactions:
Individual drugs
Alcohol: increased hepatotoxicity risk
Cimetidine: increased effect
Drug classifications
Hepatotoxics: increased hepatotoxicity risk
Rifamycins: decreased effect

NURSING CONSIDERATIONS
Assessment
- Assess hepatic studies (ALT, AST) prior to beginning treatment; do not use in presence of liver disease
- Monitor CBC in treatment >6 wk
- Assess for continuing infection

Nursing diagnoses
- Infection, risk for (uses)
- Noncompliance (teaching)
- Knowledge, deficient (teaching)

Patient/family education
- Teach patient to notify prescriber of nausea, vomiting, fatigue, jaundice, dark urine, clay-colored stool, RUQ pain, that may indicate hepatic dysfunction
- Teach patient to avoid using OTC medication unless approved by prescriber

Evaluation
Positive therapeutic outcome
- Decrease in size, number of lesions

terbutaline (Rx)
(ter-byoo′te-leen)
Brethine, Bricanyl
Func. class.: Selective β_2-agonist; bronchodilator
Chem. class.: Catecholamine
Pregnancy category B

Action: Relaxes bronchial smooth muscle by direct action on β_2-adrenergic receptors through accumulation of cAMP at β-adrenergic receptor sites; results are bronchodilation, diuresis, and CNS and cardiac stimulation; relaxes uterine smooth muscle

Therapeutic Outcome: Bronchodilation with ease of breathing

Uses: Bronchospasm

Investigational uses: Premature labor, hyperkalemia

Dosage and routes
Bronchospasm
Adult and child >12 yr: INH 2 puffs q1 min, then q4-6h; PO 2.5-5 mg q8h; SUBCUT 0.25 mg q15-30 min, max 0.5 mg in 4 hr
Bronchodilation
Adult/child >15 yr: PO 2.5-5 mg q6h during day, max 15 mg/24 hr
Child 12-15 yr: PO 2.5 mg tid
Tocolytic (preterm labor) (off-label)
Adult: PO 2.5 mg q4-6h until delivery
Renal dose
Adult: PO GFR 10-50 ml/min 50% of dose
Severe renal failure
Adult: PO avoid if GFR <10 ml/min

Available forms: Tabs 2.5, 5 mg; aerosol 0.2 mg/actuation; inj 1 mg/ml

Adverse effects
CNS: Tremors, anxiety, insomnia, headache, dizziness, stimulation
CV: Palpitations, tachycardia, hypertension, dysrhythmias, **cardiac arrest**
GI: Nausea, vomiting

Contraindications: Hypersensitivity to sympathomimetics; narrow-angle glaucoma, tachydysrhythmias

Precautions: Pregnancy **B,** cardiac disorders, hyperthyroidism, diabetes mellitus, prostatic hypertension, lactation, elderly, hypertension, seizure disorder

Pharmacokinetics

Absorption	Well absorbed (SUBCUT), partially absorbed (PO)
Distribution	Unknown
Metabolism	Liver—partially
Excretion	Unknown
Half-life	Unknown

Pharmacodynamics

	PO	INH	SUBCUT	IV
Onset	½ hr	5-15 min	10-15 min	Rapid
Peak	1-2 hr	1-2 hr	½-1 hr	Unknown
Duration	4-8 hr	4-6 hr	1½-4 hr	Unknown

Interactions

Individual drugs

Bleomycin: drugs are incompatible

Drug classifications

β-Adrenergic blockers: block therapeutic effect

MAOIs: increased chance of hypertensive crisis

Sympathomimetics: increased effects of both drugs

Drug/herb

Green tea (large amounts), guarana: increased effect

NURSING CONSIDERATIONS

Assessment

- Monitor respiratory function: vital capacity, FEV, ABGs, lung sounds, heart rate, rhythm (baseline)
- Determine that patient has not received theophylline therapy before giving dose; assess client's ability to self-medicate
- Monitor for evidence of allergic reactions; withhold dose and notify prescriber
- Assess for paradoxical bronchospasm: dyspnea, wheezing, keep emergency resuscitative equipment nearby
- Assess for labor: maternal heart rate, B/P, contractions, fetal heart rate

Nursing diagnoses

- Airway clearance, ineffective (uses)
- Gas exchange, impaired (uses)
- Knowledge, deficient (teaching)
- Noncompliance (teaching)

Implementation

- Use this medication before other medications and allow 5 min between each to prevent overstimulation

PO route

- Give PO with meals to decrease gastric irritation; tab may be crushed and mixed with foods and fluids

SUBCUT route

- May give by SUBCUT route; do not give by IM route

Aerosol route

- Give after shaking; ask patient to exhale, place mouthpiece in mouth, then inhale slowly; hold breath, remove, exhale slowly; allow at least 1 min between inhalations
- Store in light-resistant container, do not expose to temp over 86° F (30° C)

IV route

- Give at 5 mcg q10 min until contractions are stopped, use infusion pump for correct dose; after ½-1 hr with no contraction decrease dose by 5 mcg; switch to PO dose when possible

Syringe compatibilities: Doxapram

Y-site compatibilities: Regular insulin

Additive compatibilities: Aminophylline

Additive incompatibilities: Bleomycin

Patient/family education

- Advise patient not to use OTC medications; extra stimulation may occur; to use this medication before other medications and allow at least 5 min between each to prevent overstimulation
- Teach patient how to use inhaler; to avoid getting aerosol in eyes because blurring may result; to wash inhaler in warm water daily and dry; to avoid smoking, smoke-filled rooms, persons with respiratory infections; review package insert with patient
- Teach patient that paradoxical bronchospasm may occur; to stop drug immediately and notify prescriber; to limit caffeine products such as chocolate, coffee, tea, and colas
- Instruct patient on administration of dose, not to use more than prescribed; serious side effects may occur; if taking PO regularly and dose is missed, take when remembered; space other doses on new time schedule

Evaluation

Positive therapeutic outcome

- Absence of dyspnea, wheezing after 1 hr
- Improved airway exchange
- Improved ABGs

Treatment of overdose: Administer a β_2-adrenergic blocker

T

teriparatide (Rx)
(tah-ree-par'ah-tide)
Forteo
Func. class.: Parathyroid hormone (rDNA)

Pregnancy category C

Action: Contains human recombinant parathyroid hormone, which stimulates new bone growth

Therapeutic Outcome: Calcium levels at 9-10 mg/dl, decreased symptoms of hypocalcemia, hypoparathyroidism

Uses: Postmenopausal women with osteoporosis, men with primary or hypogonadal osteoporosis who are at high risk for fracture

Dosage and routes
Adult: **SUBCUT** 20 mcg daily

Available forms: Prefilled pen delivery device (delivers 20 mcg/day)

Adverse effects
CNS: Dizziness, headache, insomnia, depression, vertigo
CV: Hypertension, angina, syncope
GI: Nausea, diarrhea, dyspepsia, vomiting, constipation
INTEG: Rash, sweating
MISC: Pain, asthenia
MS: Arthralgia, leg cramps
RESP: Rhinitis, cough, pharyngitis, pneumonia, dyspnea

Contraindications: Hypersensitivity, increased baseline risk of osteosarcoma (Paget's disease, open epiphyses, previous bone radiation), bone metastases, history of skeletal malignancies, other metabolic bone diseases, preexisting hypercalcemia

Precautions: Pregnancy **C**, lactation, urolithiasis, hypotension, use >2 yr

Pharmacokinetics

Absorption	Extensively, rapidly
Distribution	Unknown
Metabolism	Liver
Excretion	Kidneys
Half-life	Unknown

Pharmacodynamics
Unknown

Interactions
Individual drug
Digoxin: increased digoxin toxicity
Drug/lab test
Calcium: increased levels

NURSING CONSIDERATIONS
Assessment
- Uric acid, chloride, magnesium, electrolytes, urine pH, vit D, phosphate for normal serum levels. Serum calcium may be transiently increased after dosing (max at 4-6 hrs post-dose)
- For bone pain, headache, fatigue, changes in LOC, leg cramps
- For signs of persistent hypercalcemia: nausea, vomiting, constipation, lethargy, muscle weakness
- Nutritional status: diet for sources of vit D (milk, some seafood), calcium (dairy products, dark green vegetables), phosphates (dairy products)

Nursing diagnoses
- Injury, risk for (uses)
- Mobility, physical, impaired (uses)
- Knowledge, deficient (teaching)

Implementation
- Store refrigerated, do not freeze

SUBCUT route
- Give by SUBCUT only, rotate inj sites

Patient/family education
- Advise patient of the symptoms of hypercalcemia
- Teach about foods rich in calcium
- Teach how to use delivery device, dispose of needles, not to share pen with others
- To sit or lie down if dizziness or fast heartbeat occurs after the first few doses

Evaluation
Positive therapeutic outcome
- Increased bone mineral density

testosterone ⚷ (Rx)
(tess-toss'te-rone)

testosterone, long acting

testosterone enanthate
Andro LA, Andropository, Andryl, Delatest, Delatestryl, Everone, Malog-x ♣, Testone LA, Testrin-PA

testosterone cypionate
Andro-Cyp, Andronate, depAndro, Depotest, Depo-Testosterone, Dura-test, T-Cypionate, Testa-C, Testred, Testoject-LA, Virilon IM

testosterone pellets
Testopel

testosterone transdermal
Androderm, Testoderm, Testoderm TTS, Testoderm with Adhesive

testosterone gel
AndroGel 1%, Testim

Func. class.: Androgenic anabolic steroid
Chem. class.: Halogenated testosterone derivative

testosterone buccal (Rx)
Striant

Pregnancy category X

Controlled substance schedule III

Action: Increases weight by building body tissue; increases potassium, phosphorus, chloride, nitrogen levels; increases bone development; responsible for maintenance of secondary sex characteristics (male)

Therapeutic Outcome: Increased hormone levels in eunuchoidism, decreased tumor growth in female breast cancer, onset of male puberty

Uses: Female breast cancer, eunuchoidism, male climacteric, oligospermia, impotence, osteoporosis, weight loss in AIDS patients, vulvar dystrophies, low testosterone levels, delayed male puberty (Inj)

Dosage and routes

Replacement

Adult: **IM** 25-50 mg 2-3 ×/wk (base or propionate) or 50-400 mg q2-4 wk (enanthate or cypionate); TD (Testoderm) 4-6 mg applied q24h; (Androderm, AndroGel) 5 mg applied q24h; once daily (gel); buccal: 1 buccal system (30 mg) to the gum region q12h ac/PM

Breast cancer

Adult: IM 50-100 mg 3 ×/wk (propionate) or 200-400 mg q2-4 wk (cypionate or enanthate)

Delayed male puberty

Child >12 yr: IM up to 100 mg/mo for up to 6 mo

Available forms: Enanthate: inj 200 mg/ml; cypionate: inj 100, 200 mg/ml; pellets 75 mg; TD 2.5, 4, 5, 6 mg/24 hr; gel 1% buccal system 30 mg

Adverse effects

CNS: Dizziness, headache, fatigue, tremors, paresthesias, flushing, sweating, anxiety, lability, insomnia, carpal tunnel syndrome
CV: Increased B/P
EENT: Conjunctival edema, nasal congestion
ENDO: Abnormal GTT
GI: Nausea, vomiting, constipation, weight gain, **cholestatic jaundice**
GU: Hematuria, amenorrhea, vaginitis, decreased libido, decreased breast size, clitoral hypertrophy, testicular atrophy
INTEG: Rash, acneiform lesions, oily hair and skin, flushing, sweating, acne vulgaris, alopecia, hirsutism
MS: Cramps, spasms

Contraindications: Pregnancy **X**, severe renal disease, severe cardiac disease, severe hepatic disease, hypersensitivity, lactation, genital bleeding (rare)

Precautions: Diabetes mellitus, CV disease, MI

Pharmacokinetics

Absorption	Well but slowly absorbed
Distribution	Crosses placenta
Metabolism	Liver
Excretion	Kidneys, breast milk
Half-life	8 days (cypionate) 10-100 min (base)

Pharmacodynamics

	IM (base)	IM (cypionate)	IM (enanthate)	IM (propionate)
Onset	Unknown	Unknown	Unknown	Unknown
Peak	Unknown	Unknown	Unknown	Unknown
Duration	1-3 days	2-4 wk	2-4 wk	1-3 days

Interactions

Individual drugs

ACTH: increased edema
Insulin: decreased glucose levels may alter need for insulin
Oxyphenbutazone: increased effects of oxyphenbutazone

Drug classifications

Adrenal steroids: increased edema
Anticoagulants: increased protime

Antidiabetics, oral: decreased need for oral antidiabetics

Drug/lab test

Increased: serum cholesterol, blood glucose, urine glucose

Decreased: serum Ca, serum K, T_4, T_3, thyroid ^{131}I uptake test, urine 17-OHCS, 17-KS, PBI

NURSING CONSIDERATIONS

Assessment

- Monitor patient's weight daily; notify prescriber if weekly weight gain is >5 lb; assess I&O ratio; be alert for decreasing urinary output, increasing edema
- Monitor B/P q4h
- Assess growth rate in adolescent because growth rate may be uneven (linear/bone growth) if used for extended periods
- Monitor electrolytes: potassium, sodium, chloride, calcium; cholesterol
- Monitor liver function studies: ALT, AST, bilirubin
- Assess edema, hypertension, cardiac symptoms, jaundice
- Assess mental status: affect, mood, behavioral changes, aggression
- Assess signs of masculinization in female: increased libido, deepening of voice, decreased breast tissue, enlarged clitoris, menstrual irregularities; male: gynecomastia, impotence, testicular atrophy
- Assess hypercalcemia: lethargy, polyuria, polydipsia, nausea, vomiting, constipation; drug may have to be decreased
- Assess hypoglycemia in diabetics because oral antidiabetic action is increased

Nursing diagnoses

- Infection, risk for (adverse reactions)
- Injury, risk for (adverse reactions)
- Knowledge, deficient (teaching)

Implementation

- Administer diet with increased calories, protein; decreased sodium if edema occurs
- Administer supportive drug if anemia occurs
- Give titrated dose; use lowest effective dose
- Give IM inj deep into upper outer quadrant of gluteal muscle; route can be painful

Transdermal route

- Apply Testoderm to skin of scrotum, Androderm to skin of back, upper arms, thighs, abdomen; area must be clean and dry, free of hair

Patient/family education

- Inform patient that drug needs to be combined with complete health plan: diet, rest, exercise
- Caution patient to notify prescriber if therapeutic response decreases; not to discontinue this medication abruptly
- Inform women patients to report menstrual irregularities; about changes in sex characteristics
- Discuss that 1-3 mo course is necessary for response in breast cancer
- Inform patient about application of TD patches: Testoderm to skin of scrotum, Androderm to skin of back, upper arms, thighs, abdomen; area must be dry and free of hair; may be reapplied after bathing, swimming

Evaluation

Positive therapeutic outcome

- Decrease size of tumor in breast cancer
- Increased androgen levels

tetracycline (Rx)

(tet-ra-sye'kleen)

Achromycin V, Actisite (dental product), Apo-Tetra ✤, Novotetra ✤, Nu-Tetra ✤, Panmycin, Robitet, Sumycin, Teline, Tetracap, tetracycline HCl, Tetracyn, Tetralan, Tetram

Func. class.: Antiinfective—broad-spectrum

Chem. class.: Tetracycline

Pregnancy category D

Action: Inhibits protein synthesis and phosphorylation in microorganisms; bacteriostatic

Therapeutic Outcome: Bactericidal action against susceptible organisms: gram-positive pathogens *Bacillus anthracis, Clostridium perfringens, Clostridium tetani, Listeria monocytogenes, Nocardia, Propionibacterium acnes, Actinomyces israelii;* gram-negative pathogens *Haemophilus influenzae, Legionella pneumophila, Yersinia entercolitica, Yersinia pestis, Neisseria gonorrhoeae, Neisseria meningitidis*

Uses: Syphilis, Chlamydia trachomatis, gonorrhea, lymphogranuloma venereum, uncommon gram-positive, gram-negative organisms, rickettsial infections

Dosage and routes

Susceptible gram-positive/gram-negative infections

Adult: PO 250-500 mg q6h

Child >8 yr: PO 25-50 mg/kg/day in divided doses q6h

Gonorrhea

Adult: PO 1.5 g, then 500 mg qid for a total of 9 g over 7 days

Chlamydia trachomatis
Adult: PO 500 mg qid × 7 days

Syphilis
Adult and adolescent: PO 500 mg qid × 2 wk; if syphilis duration >1 yr, must treat 30 days

Brucellosis
Adult: PO 500 mg qid × 3 wk with 1 g of streptomycin IM 2 ×/day × 1 wk, and 1 ×/day the 2nd wk

Urethral, endocervical rectal infections (C. trachomatis)
Adult: PO 500 mg qid × 7 days

Acne
Adult and adolescent: PO 250 mg q6h, then 125-500 mg daily or every other day

Available forms: Oral susp 125 mg/5 ml, caps 250, 500 mg

Adverse effects

CNS: Fever, headache, paresthesia
CV: **Pericarditis**
EENT: Dysphagia, glossitis, decreased calcification (permanent discoloration) of deciduous teeth, oral candidiasis, oral ulcers
GI: Nausea, abdominal pain, *vomiting, diarrhea,* anorexia, enterocolitis, **hepatotoxicity,** flatulence, abdominal cramps, epigastric burning, stomatitis
GU: Increased BUN
HEMA: **Eosinophilia, neutropenia, thrombocytopenia, leukocytosis, hemolytic anemia**
INTEG: Rash, urticaria, photosensitivity, increased pigmentation, **exfoliative dermatitis,** pruritus, **angioedema**

Contraindications: Pregnancy **D**, hypersensitivity to tetracyclines, children <8 yr, lactation

Precautions: Renal disease, hepatic disease

Pharmacokinetics	
Absorption	60%-80% (PO), lower (IM)
Distribution	Widely distributed, some in CSF; crosses placenta
Metabolism	Not metabolized
Excretion	Unchanged—kidneys
Half-life	6-10 hr

Pharmacodynamics	
Onset	1-2 hr
Peak	2-3 hr

Interactions

Individual drugs
Cimetidine, $NaHCO_3$: decreased tetracycline effect
Digoxin: increased digoxin effect
Iron: forms chelates, decreased absorption
Methoxyflurane: nephrotoxicity
Warfarin: increased warfarin effect

Drug classifications
Alkali products, antacids: decreased tetracycline effect
Contraceptives (oral): decreased oral contraceptive effect
Penicillins: decreased penicillin effect

Drug/herb
Dong quai: increased photosensitivity

Drug/food
Decreased: absorption with dairy products; forms insoluble chelate

Drug/lab test
False increase: urinary catecholamines

NURSING CONSIDERATIONS

Assessment

- Assess patient for previous sensitivity reaction
- Assess patient for signs and symptoms of infection including characteristics of wounds, sputum, urine, stool, WBC >10,000/mm^3, temp; obtain baseline information before and during treatment
- Complete C&S testing before beginning drug therapy to identify if correct treatment has been initiated
- Assess for allergic reactions: rash, urticaria, pruritus, chills, fever, joint pain; angioedema may occur a few days after therapy begins; epINEPHrine, resuscitation equipment should be available for anaphylactic reaction
- Identify urine output; if decreasing, notify prescriber (may indicate nephrotoxicity); also, increased BUN, creatinine
- Monitor blood studies: AST, ALT, CBC, Hct, bilirubin, LDH, alkaline phosphatase, monthly if patient is on long-term therapy
- Assess bowel pattern daily; if severe diarrhea occurs, drug should be discontinued
- Monitor for bleeding: ecchymosis, bleeding gums, hematuria, stool guaiac daily if on long-term therapy; blood dyscrasias may occur
- Assess for overgrowth of infection: perineal itching, fever, malaise, redness, pain, swelling, drainage, rash, diarrhea, change in cough, sputum

Nursing diagnoses

- Infection, risk for (uses)
- Diarrhea (adverse reactions)
- Injury, risk for (adverse reactions)

T

- Knowledge, deficient (teaching)
- Noncompliance (teaching)

Implementation

PO route

- Give around the clock to maintain proper blood levels; give with food to increase absorption of drug; do not give within 3 hr of other agents; drug actions may occur; take on an empty stomach
- Give with 8 oz of water
- Shake liq preparation well before giving; use calibrated device for proper dosing

Patient/family education

- Teach patient to report sore throat, bruising, bleeding, joint pain; may indicate blood dyscrasias (rare)
- Advise patient to use sunscreen when outdoors to decrease photosensitivity reaction
- Advise patient to contact prescriber if vaginal itching; loose foul-smelling stools, furry tongue occur; may indicate superinfection; report itching, rash, pruritus, urticaria
- Instruct patient to take all medication prescribed for the length of time ordered; drug must be taken around the clock to maintain blood levels; do not give medication to others

Evaluation

Positive therapeutic outcome

- Absence of signs/symptoms of infection (WBC <10,000/mm^3, temp WNL, absence of red, draining wounds)
- Reported improvement in symptoms of infection

theophylline 🗝 (Rx)

(thee-off'i-lin)

Accurbron, Aquaphyllin, Asmalix, Bronkodyl, Elixomin, Elixophyllin, Lanophyllin, Quibron-T Dividose, Quibron-T/SR, Respbid, Slo-bid Gyrocaps, Slo-Phyllin, Sustaire, Theo-24, Theobid Duracaps, Theochron, Theoclear-80, Theoclear L.A., Theo-Dur, Theolair-SR,Theo-Sav, Theospan-SR, Theostat 80, Theovent, Theo-X, T-Phy, Uni-Dur, Uniphyl

Func. class.: Spasmolytic, bronchodilator

Chem. class.: Xanthine, ethylenediamine

Pregnancy category C

Action: Relaxes smooth muscle of respiratory system by blocking phosphodiesterase, which increases cAMP, which increases bronchodilatation, diuresis, circulation, CNS stimulation

Therapeutic Outcome: Ability to breathe without difficulty

Uses: Bronchial asthma, bronchospasm of COPD, chronic bronchitis

Dosage and routes

Hepatic dose

Adult: PO 6 mg/kg loading dose, then 2 mg/kg q8h ×2 doses, then 1-2 mg/kg q12h

Adult: **IV** 4.7 mg/kg then 0.39 mg/kg/hr for 12 hr, then 0.08-0.16 mg/kg/hr maintenance

Bronchospasm, bronchial asthma

Adult: PO 100-200 mg q6h; dosage must be individualized

Child: PO 50-100 mg q6h, max 12 mg/kg/24 hr

COPD, chronic bronchitis

Adult: PO 330-660 q6-8h pc

Child 1-9 yr: PO 5 mg/kg loading dose, then 4 mg/kg q6h

Child 9-16 yr: PO 5 mg/kg loading dose, then 3 mg/kg q6h

Apnea of prematurity

Neonate: 2-10 mg/kg/day divided q8-12h (usual loading dose is 4 mg/kg)

Available forms: Caps 50, 100, 200, 250 mg; tabs 100, 125, 200, 225, 250, 300 mg; time rel tabs 100, 200, 250, 300, 400, 500 mg; time rel caps 50, 65, 100, 125, 130, 200, 250, 260, 300, 400, 500 mg; elixir 80, 11.25 mg/15 mg; sol 80 mg/15 ml; liq 80, 150, 160 mg/15 ml; susp 300 mg/15 ml

Adverse effects

CNS: *Anxiety, restlessness, insomnia, dizziness, seizures,* headache, light-headedness, muscle twitching, tremors

CV: *Palpitations, sinus tachycardia,* hypotension, **dysrhythmias,** fluid retention with tachycardia

ENDO: Hyperglycemia

GI: *Nausea, vomiting, anorexia,* diarrhea, bitter taste, dyspepsia, gastric distress

INTEG: Flushing, urticaria

RESP: Increased rate

Contraindications: Hypersensitivity to xanthines, tachydysrhythmias

Precautions: Pregnancy **C**, elderly, CHF, cor pulmonale, hepatic disease, active peptic ulcer disease, diabetes mellitus, hyperthyroidism, hypertension, children

Pharmacokinetics

Absorption	Well absorbed (PO), slowly absorbed (ext rel)
Distribution	Crosses placenta, widely distributed
Metabolism	Liver
Excretion	Kidneys, breast milk
Half-life	3-13, increased in liver disease, CHF, elderly

Pharmacodynamics

	PO	PO–TIME REL	IV
Onset	Rapid	Slow	Immediate
Peak	1 hr	4-8 hr	Inf end
Duration	6 hr	12-24 hr	6-8 hr

Interactions
Individual drugs
Carbamazepine: decreased theophylline level
Cimetidine, ciprofloxacin, disulfiram, erythromycin, fluvoxamine, influenza vaccine, mexiletine, propranolol: increased theophylline action
Lithium: decreased effect of lithium
Phenobarbital, phenytoin, rifampin: decreased theophylline
Drug classifications
Anticoagulants: increased anticoagulant level
β-Adrenergic blockers: cardiotoxicity
Contraceptives (oral), corticosteroids, fluoroquinolones, interferons: increased theophylline action
Smoking: decreased theophylline level
Drug/herb
Coffee, cola nut, guarana, tea (black, green), yerba maté: increased toxicity
St. John's wort: decreased theophylline level
Ma Huang (ephedra): increased toxicity

NURSING CONSIDERATIONS
Assessment
- Monitor theophylline blood levels (therapeutic level is 5-15 mcg/ml); toxicity may occur with small increase above 15 mcg/ml
- Monitor I&O; diuresis occurs; dehydration may result in elderly or children
- Assess for signs of toxicity: irritability, insomnia, restlessness, tremors, nausea, vomiting
- Monitor respiratory rate, rhythm, depth; auscultate lung fields bilaterally; notify prescriber of abnormalities
- Assess for allergic reactions: rash, urticaria; if these occur, drug should be discontinued

Nursing diagnoses
- Airway clearance, ineffective (uses)
- Knowledge, deficient (teaching)

Implementation
PO route
- Do not break, crush, or chew time release products
- Give PO with 8 oz water; to decrease GI symptoms; avoid food, absorption may be affected
- Contents of bead-filled cap may be sprinkled over food for children's use

IV route
- Give loading dose over 20-30 min, max 20-25 mg/min, do not give by rapid **IV**, use only by cont inf

Y-site compatibilities: Acyclovir, ampicillin, aztreonam, cefazolin, cefotetan, ceftazidime, ceftriaxone, cimetidine, clindamycin, dexamethasone, diltiazem, DOBUTamine, DOPamine, doxycycline, erythromycin, famotidine, fluconazole, gentamicin, haloperidol, heparin, hydrocortisone, lidocaine, methyldopate, methylPREDNISolone, metronidazole, midazolam, nafcillin, nitroglycerin, nitroprusside, penicillin G potassium, piperacillin, potassium chloride, ranitidine, ticarcillin, ticarcillin/clavulanate, tobramycin, vancomycin

Additive compatibilities: Cefepime, chlorproMAZINE, fluconazole, methylPREDNISolone, verapamil

Patient/family education
- Advise patient to check OTC medications, current prescription medications for epHEDrine, which will increase stimulation, and to avoid alcohol, caffeine
- Caution patient to avoid hazardous activities; dizziness may occur
- Inform patient that if GI upset occurs, to take drug with 8 oz of water; avoid food; absorption may be decreased
- Advise patient to notify prescriber of toxicity: nausea, vomiting, anxiety, insomnia, seizures
- Advise patient to notify prescriber of change in smoking habit; dosage may have to be changed

Evaluation
Positive therapeutic outcome
- Ability to breathe more easily

thiamine (vitamin B_1) (PO, OTC; **IV**, Rx)

Betaxin ✤, Betalin S, Biamine, Revitonus, Thiamilate, thiamine HCl

Func. class.: Vitamin B_1

Chem. class.: Water soluble

Pregnancy category A

Pharmacokinetics

Absorption	Well absorbed (PO, IM), completely absorbed (**IV**)
Distribution	Widely distributed
Metabolism	Liver
Excretion	Kidneys (unchanged—excess amounts)
Half-life	Unknown

Pharmacodynamics

Unknown

Do Not Confuse:

thiamine/Tenormin

Action: Needed for pyruvate metabolism, carbohydrate metabolism

Therapeutic Outcome: Prevention and treatment of thiamine deficiency

Uses: Vit B_1 deficiency or polyneuritis, cheilosis adjunct with thiamine beriberi, Wernicke-Korsakoff syndrome, pellagra, metabolic disorders

Dosage and routes

RDA

Adult: Male 1.2-1.5 mg; females 1.1 mg; pregnancy 1.5 mg; lactation 1.6 mg

Child 7-10 yr: 1.3 mg

Child 4-6 yr: 0.9 mg

Child 1-3 yr: 0.7 mg

Infants 6 mo-1 yr: 0.4 mg

Neonates and infants to 6 mo: 0.3 mg

Beriberi

Adult: IM 10-20 mg tid × 2 wk, then 5-10 mg daily × 1 mo

Beriberi with cardiac failure

Adult and child: **IV** 10-30 mg tid

Available forms: Tabs 50, 100, 250, 500 mg; inj 100 mg/ml; enteric-coated tabs 20 mg

Adverse effects

CNS: Weakness, restlessness

CV: **Collapse, pulmonary edema,** hypotension

EENT: Tightness of throat

GI: Hemorrhage, *nausea, diarrhea*

INTEG: **Angioneurotic edema,** cyanosis, sweating, warmth

SYST: **Anaphylaxis**

Contraindications: Hypersensitivity

Precautions: Pregnancy **A**

Interactions: None known

NURSING CONSIDERATIONS

Assessment

- Assess nutritional status: yeast, beef, liver, whole or enriched grains, legumes

Nursing diagnoses

- Nutrition: less than body requirements, imbalanced (uses)
- Knowledge, deficient (teaching)

Implementation

IM route

- Give by IM inj; rotate sites if pain and inflammation occur; do not mix with alkaline sol; Z-track to minimize pain
- Application of cold compress may decrease pain
- Store in airtight, light-resistant container

IV route

- **IV** undiluted given over 5 min or diluted with **IV** sol and given as an inf at a rate of 100 mg or less/5 min or more

Syringe compatibilities: Doxapram

Y-site compatibilities: Famotidine

Additive incompatibilities: Barbiturates; sol with neutral or alkaline pH, such as carbonates, bicarbonates, citrates and acetates; erythromycin, kanamycin, or streptomycin

Patient/family education

- Teach patient necessary foods to be included in diet: yeast, beef, liver, legumes, whole grains

Evaluation

Positive therapeutic outcome

- Absence of nausea, vomiting, anorexia, insomnia, tachycardia, paresthesias, depression, muscle weakness

thiethylperazine (Rx)
(thye-eth-il-per'a-zeen)
Norzine, Torecan
Func. class.: Antiemetic
Chem. class.: Phenothiazine, piperazine derivative

Pregnancy category X

Do Not Confuse:
Torecan/Toradol

Action: Acts centrally by blocking chemoreceptor trigger zone, which in turn acts on vomiting center

Therapeutic Outcome: Control of nausea, vomiting

Uses: Nausea, vomiting

Dosage and routes
Adult: PO/IM 10 mg/daily-tid

Available forms: Tabs 10 mg; inj 5 mg/ml

Adverse effects
CNS: *Euphoria, depression,* restlessness, tremor, extrapyramidal symptoms (EPS), **seizures,** drowsiness, confusion, **neuroleptic malignant syndrome**
CV: **Circulatory failure, tachycardia,** postural hypotension, ECG changes
GI: Nausea, vomiting, anorexia, dry mouth, diarrhea, constipation, weight loss, metallic taste, cramps
GU: Urinary retention, dark urine
HEMA: **Agranulocytosis, leukopenia**
RESP: **Respiratory depression**

Contraindications: Pregnancy **X,** hypersensitivity to phenothiazines, coma, seizure, encephalopathy, bone marrow depression

Precautions: Children <2 yr, elderly, lactation, Parkinson's disease

Pharmacokinetics

Absorption	Readily absorbed
Distribution	Crosses placenta
Metabolism	Liver
Excretion	Kidneys, breast milk
Half-life	Unknown

Pharmacodynamics

	PO	IM
Onset	45-60 min	Unknown
Peak	Unknown	Unknown
Duration	4 hr	Unknown

Interactions
Individual drugs
Ethanol: increased sedation
Drug classifications
Anesthetics (general), anxiolytics, sedatives/hypnotics, benzodiazepines, opiate agonists: increased sedation
Antacids: decreased effect of thiethylperzaine
Anticholinergics, antiparkinson drugs, antidepressants (tricylic): increased anticholinergic action
Barbiturates: decreased effect of thiethylperazine, increased sedation
Phenothiazines: avoid use, seizures may occur

NURSING CONSIDERATIONS
Assessment
- Monitor I&O ratio, palpate bladder if low urinary output occurs, especially in elderly; urinalysis recommended before, during prolonged therapy
- Monitor bilirubin, CBC, liver function studies monthly
- Assess affect, orientation, LOC, reflexes, gait, coordination, sleep pattern disturbances
- Monitor B/P with patient in sitting, standing, and lying positions; take pulse and respirations q4h during initial treatment; establish baseline before starting treatment; report drops of 30 mm Hg
- Check for dizziness, faintness, palpitations, tachycardia on rising; severe orthostatic hypotension is common
- ❗ Identify for neuroleptic malignant syndrome: hyperpyrexia, muscle rigidity, increased CPK, altered mental status, seizures, fatigue, loss of urinary control, tachycardia; drug should be discontinued; have emergency equipment nearby
- Assess for EPS including akathisia (inability to sit still, no pattern to movements), tardive dyskinesia (bizarre movements of the jaw, mouth, tongue, extremities), pseudoparkinsonism (tremors, pill rolling, shuffling gait); antiparkinsonian drug should be prescribed
- Assess for constipation, urinary retention daily; if these occur, increase bulk, water in diet

Nursing diagnoses
- Thought processes, disturbed (uses)
- Coping, ineffective (uses)
- Knowledge, deficient (teaching)
- Noncompliance (teaching)

Implementation
IM route
- Give IM inj in large muscle mass; aspirate to avoid **IV** administration; give slowly; have

T

patient remain supine for at least 30 min after administration

Syringe compatibilities: Butorphanol, hydromorphone, midazolam, ranitidine

Y-site compatibilities: Aldesleukin

Patient/family education

- Teach patient to use good oral hygiene; frequent rinsing of mouth, sugarless gum for dry mouth
- Caution patient to avoid hazardous activities until drug response is determined; dizziness, blurred vision may occur
- Inform patient that orthostatic hypotension often occurs and to rise gradually from sitting or lying position; avoid hot tubs, hot showers, and tub baths since hypotension may occur
- Instruct patient to remain lying down after IM inj for at least 30 min
- Inform patient that heat stroke may occur in hot weather, and to take extra precautions to stay cool
- Teach patient to avoid OTC preparations (cough, hay fever, cold) unless approved by prescriber because serious drug interactions may occur; avoid use with alcohol, CNS depressants because increased drowsiness may occur
- Inform patient to use sunglasses and sunscreen to prevent burns
- Teach patient about EPS
- Instruct patient to report sore throat, malaise, fever, bleeding, mouth sores; if these occur, CBC should be performed and drug discontinued

Evaluation

Positive therapeutic outcome

- Absence of nausea, vomiting

thioridazine (Rx)

(thye-or-rid'a-zeen)

Apo-Thioridazine ♣, Mellaril, Mellaril Concentrate, Mellaril-5, Novo-Ridazine ♣, PMS-Thioridazine ♣, thioridazine HCl

Func. class.: Antipsychotic/neuroleptic

Chem. class.: Phenothiazine, piperidine

Pregnancy category C

Do Not Confuse:

Mellaril/Elavil

Action: Depresses cerebral cortex, hypothalamus, limbic system, which control activity, aggression; blocks neurotransmission produced by dopamine at synapse; exhibits strong α-adrenergic, anticholinergic blocking action; mechanism for antipsychotic effects is unclear

Therapeutic Outcome: Decreased signs and symptoms of psychosis

Uses: Psychotic disorders, schizophrenia, behavioral problems in children, alcohol withdrawal as adjunct, anxiety, major depressive disorders, organic brain syndrome, dementia in elderly

Dosage and routes

Psychosis

Adult: PO 25-100 mg tid, max dose 800 mg/day; dose is gradually increased to desired response, then reduced to minimum maintenance

Depression/behavioral problems/organic brain syndrome

Adult: PO 25 tid, range from 10 mg bid-qid to 50 mg tid-qid

Elderly: PO 10-25 mg daily-bid, increase 4-7 days by 10-25 mg to desired dose

Child 2-12 yr: PO 0.5-3 mg/kg/day in divided doses

Available forms: Tabs 10, 15, 25, 50, 100, 150, 200 mg; conc 30, 100 mg/ml; susp 25, 100 mg/5 ml; syr 10 mg/15 ml

Adverse effects

CNS: *Extrapyramidal symptoms (EPS) (rare) (pseudoparkinsonism, akathisia, dystonia, tardive dyskinesia),* **seizures,** *headache,* confusion, **neuroleptic malignant syndrome, dizziness**

CV: Orthostatic hypotension, **cardiac arrest,** ECG changes, **tachycardia**

EENT: Blurred vision, glaucoma, dry eyes

GI: *Dry mouth, nausea, vomiting, anorexia, constipation,* diarrhea, jaundice, weight gain

GU: Urinary retention, urinary frequency, enuresis, impotence, amenorrhea, gynecomastia

HEMA: Anemia, **leukopenia, leukocytosis, agranulocytosis**

INTEG: *Rash,* photosensitivity, dermatitis

RESP: **Laryngospasm,** dyspnea, **respiratory depression**

Contraindications: Hypersensitivity, blood dyscrasias, coma, child <2 yr, brain damage, bone marrow depression

Precautions: Pregnancy **C,** lactation, seizure disorders, hypertension, hepatic disease, cardiac disease

Pharmacokinetics

Absorption	Variably absorbed (tab)
Distribution	Widely distributed, high concentrations in CNS, crosses placenta
Metabolism	Liver, extensively, GI mucosa
Excretion	Kidneys, breast milk
Half-life	26-36 hr

Pharmacodynamics

Onset	Erratic
Peak	2-4 hr
Duration	8-12 hr

Interactions

Individual drugs

Alcohol: oversedation
Aluminum hydroxide, magnesium hydroxide: decreased absorption
Lithium: decreased thioridazine levels

Drug classifications

Anesthetics (barbiturate), CNS depressants: oversedation
Antacids: decreased absorption
Anticholinergics: increased anticholinergic effects
Barbiturates: decreased thioridazine effect
Centrally acting antihypertensives: decreased antihypertensive effect

Drug/herb

Betel palm, kava: increased EPS
Cola tree, hops, nettle, nutmeg: increased effect
Kava: increased CNS depression

Drug/lab test

Increased: liver function tests, cardiac enzymes, cholesterol, blood glucose, prolactin, bilirubin, PBI, cholinesterase, ^{131}I
Decreased: hormones (blood and urine)
False positive: pregnancy tests, PKU
False negative: urinary steroids, pregnancy test

NURSING CONSIDERATIONS

Assessment

- Assess mental status: orientation, mood, behavior, presence of hallucinations, and type before initial administration and monthly; this drug should significantly reduce psychotic behavior
- Check for swallowing of PO medication; check for hoarding or giving of medication to other patients
- Monitor I&O ratio, palpate bladder if low urinary output occurs, especially in elderly; urinalysis recommended before, during prolonged therapy
- Monitor bilirubin, CBC, liver function studies monthly
- Assess affect, orientation, LOC, reflexes, gait, coordination, sleep pattern disturbances
- Monitor B/P sitting, standing, and lying, take pulse and respirations q4h during initial treatment; establish baseline before starting treatment; report drops of 30 mm Hg; obtain baseline ECG, monitor Q- and T-wave changes
- Check for dizziness, faintness, palpitations, tachycardia on rising; severe orthostatic hypotension is common
- (!) Identify for neuroleptic malignant syndrome: hyperpyrexia, muscle rigidity, increased CPK, altered mental status, dyspnea, fatigue; drug should be discontinued
- Assess for EPS including akathisia (inability to sit still, no pattern to movements), tardive dyskinesia (bizarre movements of the jaw, mouth, tongue, extremities), pseudoparkinsonism (ragged tremors, pill rolling, shuffling gate); an antiparkinsonian drug should be prescribed
- Assess for constipation, urinary retention daily; if these occur, increase bulk, water in diet

Nursing diagnoses

- Thought processes, disturbed (uses)
- Coping, ineffective (uses)
- Knowledge, deficient (teaching)
- Noncompliance (teaching)

Implementation

- Administer drug in liq form mixed in glass of juice if hoarding is suspected; do not mix in caffeine drinks, tannics, pectins
- Decrease dose in elderly because metabolism is slowed
- Administer PO with full glass of water, milk; or give with food to decrease GI upset
- Give antacids 2 hr before or after this drug
- Store in airtight, light-resistant container, oral sol in amber bottle

Patient/family education

- Teach patient to use good oral hygiene; frequent rinsing of mouth, sugarless gum for dry mouth
- Advise patient to avoid hazardous activities until drug response is determined; dizziness, blurred vision are common
- Inform patient that orthostatic hypotension occurs often and to rise from sitting or lying position gradually; to avoid hot tubs, hot showers, tub baths because hypotension may occur
- Instruct patient that in hot weather, heat stroke may occur; take extra precautions to stay cool
- Caution patient to avoid abrupt withdrawal

of this drug, or EPS may result; drug should be withdrawn slowly
- Teach patient to avoid OTC preparations (cough, hay fever, cold) unless approved by prescriber; serious drug interactions may occur; avoid use with alcohol, CNS depressants; increased drowsiness may occur
- Advise patient to use sunglasses and sunscreen to prevent burns
- Teach patient about EPS and necessity for meticulous oral hygiene because oral candidiasis may occur
- Advise patient to take antacids 2 hr before or after this drug
- Instruct patient to report sore throat, malaise, fever, bleeding, mouth sores; if these occur, CBC should be performed and drug discontinued; may cause vision impairment, report to prescriber
- Advise patient that urine may be discolored

Evaluation

Positive therapeutic outcome
- Decrease in emotional excitement, hallucinations, delusions, paranoia
- Reorganization of patterns of thought, speech

Treatment of overdose: Lavage if orally ingested; provide airway; *do not induce vomiting or use epINEPHrine,* CV monitoring, continuous ECG

thyroid USP (desiccated) (Rx)

(thye'roid)

Armour Thyroid, Thyrar, Thyroid Strong, Westhroid

Func. class.: Thyroid hormone

Chem. class.: Active thyroid hormone in natural state and ratio

Pregnancy category A

Do Not Confuse:
Thyrar/Thyrolar

Action: Increases metabolic rates; controls protein synthesis; increases cardiac output, renal blood flow, O_2 consumption, body temp, blood volume, growth, development at cellular level

Therapeutic Outcome: Correction of lack of thyroid hormone

Uses: Hypothyroidism, cretinism (juvenile hypothyroidism), myxedema

Dosage and routes

Hypothyroidism

Adult: PO 65 mg daily, increased by 65 mg q30 days until desired response; maintenance dose 65-195 mg daily

Elderly: PO 7.5-15 mg daily, double dose q6-8 wk until desired response

Cretinism/juvenile hypothyroidism

Child over 1 yr: PO up to 180 mg daily titrated to response

Child 4-12 mo: PO 30-60 mg daily

Child 1-4 mo: PO 15-30 mg daily; may increase q2 wk; titrated to response; maintenance dose 30-45 mg daily

Myxedema

Adult: PO 16 mg daily, double dose q2 wk, maintenance 65-195 mg/day

Available forms: Tabs 16, 32, 65, 98, 130, 195, 260, 325 mg; enteric-coated tabs 32, 65, 130 mg; sugar-coated tabs 32, 65, 130, 195 mg; caps 65, 130, 195, 325 mg

Adverse effects

CNS: *Insomnia, tremors,* headache, thyroid storm

CV: *Tachycardia, palpitations, angina,* **dysrhythmias,** hypertension, **cardiac arrest**

GI: Nausea, diarrhea, increased or decreased appetite, cramps

MISC: Menstrual irregularities, weight loss, sweating, heat intolerance, fever

Contraindications: Adrenal insufficiency, MI, thyrotoxicosis

Precautions: Pregnancy **A,** elderly, angina pectoris, hypertension, ischemia, cardiac disease, lactation

Pharmacokinetics	
Absorption	Well absorbed
Distribution	Widely distributed, does not cross placenta
Metabolism	Liver, tissues
Excretion	Feces via bile, breast milk
Half-life	T_3—2 days; T_4—1 wk

Pharmacodynamics	
Onset	1 hr
Peak	12-48 hr
Duration	Unknown

Interactions

Individual drugs

Digoxin: decreased effect of digoxin

Insulin: increased requirement for insulin

Drug classifications

Anticoagulants, oral: increased effects of anticoagulants
Antidepressants (tricyclic): increased antidepressants (tricylic) effect
Bile acid sequestrants: decreased thyroid absorption
Catecholamines: increased effects of catecholamines
Estrogens: decreased thyroid hormone effect
Hypoglycemics: decreased effect of hypoglycemics
Sympathomimetics: increased effects of sympathomimetics

Drug/herb

Agar, bugleweed, carnitine, kelpware, soy, spirulina: decreased thyroid effect

Drug/food

Avoid iodine-containing food

Drug/lab test

Increased: CPK, LDH, AST, PBI, blood glucose
Decreased: thyroid function tests

NURSING CONSIDERATIONS

Assessment

- Identify if the patient is taking anticoagulants, antidiabetic agents; document on chart
- Take B/P, pulse before each dose; monitor I&O ratio and weight every day in same clothing, using same scale, at same time of day
- Monitor height, weight, psychomotor development, and growth rate if given to a child
- Monitor T_3, T_4, FTIs, which are decreased; radioimmunoassay of TSH, which is increased; radioactive iodine uptake (RAIU), which is increased if patient's dose of medication is too low
- Monitor protime; patient may require decreased dosage of anticoagulant; check for bleeding, bruising
- Assess for increased nervousness, excitability, irritability, which may indicate that dose of medication is too high, usually after 1-3 wk of treatment
- Assess cardiac status: angina, palpitation, chest pain, change in VS; the elderly patient may have undetected cardiac problems and baseline ECG should be completed before treatment

Nursing diagnoses

- Knowledge, deficient (teaching)
- Noncompliance (teaching)

Implementation

- Give in AM if possible as a single dose to decrease sleeplessness; at same time each day to maintain drug level
- Do not give with food as absorption will be decreased
- Give only for hormone imbalances; not to be used for obesity, male infertility, menstrual conditions, lethargy; give lowest dose that relieves symptoms; lower dose to the elderly and in cardiac diseases
- Store in airtight, light-resistant container
- Wean patient off medication 4 wk before RAIU test

Patient/family education

- Teach patient that drug is not a cure but controls symptoms and that treatment is long-term
- Instruct patient to report excitability, irritability, anxiety, sweating, heat intolerance, chest pain, palpitations, which indicate overdose
- Advise patient not to switch brands unless approved by prescriber; bioavailability may differ; do not take with food; absorption will be decreased
- Teach patient that drug may be discontinued after giving birth; thyroid panel will be evaluated after 1-2 mo
- Teach patient that hyperthyroid child will show almost immediate behavior/personality change; that hair loss will occur in child and is temporary
- Caution patient that drug is not to be taken to reduce weight
- Caution patient to avoid OTC preparations containing iodine; read labels; other medications should not be used unless approved by prescriber
- Teach patient to avoid iodine-containing food: iodized salt, soybeans, tofu, turnips, certain kinds of seafood and bread

Evaluation

Positive therapeutic outcome

- Absence of depression
- Weight loss, increased diuresis, pulse, appetite
- Absence of constipation, peripheral edema, cold intolerance, pale, cool dry skin, brittle nails, alopecia, coarse hair, menorrhagia, night blindness, paresthesias, syncope, stupor, coma, rosy cheeks
- Improved levels of T_3, T_4 by laboratory tests
- Child: Age-appropriate weight, height, and psychomotor development

Treatment of overdose: Withhold dose for up to 1 wk, acute overdose—gastric lavage or induce emesis, then activated charcoal; provide supportive treatment to control symptoms

tiagabine (Rx)

(tie-ah-ga′been)

Gabitril

Func. class.: Anticonvulsant

Pregnancy category C

Action: Mechanism unknown; may increase seizure threshold

Uses: Adjunct treatment of partial seizures

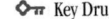

Dosage and routes

Adult: PO 4 mg daily, may increase by 4-8 mg qwk until desired response, max 56 mg/day

Child 12-18 yr: PO 4 mg daily, may increase by 4 mg at beginning of wk 2, may increase by 4-8 mg qwk until desired response, max 32 mg/day

Available forms: Tabs 2, 4, 12, 16 mg

Adverse effects

CNS: *Dizziness, anxiety,* somnolence, ataxia, confusion, *asthenia,* unsteady gait, depression

CV: Vasodilatation

GI: Nausea, diarrhea, vomiting

INTEG: Pruritus, rash

RESP: Pharyngitis, coughing

Contraindications: Hypersensitivity to this drug

Precautions: Pregnancy **C,** hepatic disease, renal disease, lactation, child <12 yr, elderly

Pharmacokinetics

Absorption	>95%
Distribution	Unknown
Metabolism	Liver
Excretion	Kidneys
Half-life	7-9 hr

Pharmacodynamics

Unknown

Interactions

Individual drugs

Carbamazepine, phenobarbital, phenytoin, primidone: decreased effect of these drugs

Drug classifications

CNS depressants: increased CNS depression

Drug/food

High fat meal: decreased rate of absorption

Valproate: lower dose of tiagabine may be required

NURSING CONSIDERATIONS

Assessment

- Monitor renal studies: urinalysis, BUN, urine creatinine q3 mo
- Monitor hepatic studies: ALT, AST, bilirubin
- Assess description of seizures: location, duration, presence of aura
- Assess mental status: mood, sensorium, affect, behavioral changes; if mental status changes, notify prescriber

Nursing diagnoses

- Injury, risk for (uses, adverse reactions)
- Knowledge, deficient (teaching)
- Noncompliance (teaching)

Implementation

- Store at room temp away from heat and light
- Provide assistance with ambulation during early part of treatment; dizziness occurs
- Provide seizure precautions: padded side rails; move objects that may harm patient

Patient/family education

- Advise patient to carry/wear emergency ID stating patient's name, drugs taken, condition, prescriber's name and phone number
- Advise patient to avoid driving, other activities that require alertness
- Teach patient not to discontinue medication quickly after long-term use

Evaluation

Positive therapeutic outcome

- Decreased seizure activity; document on patient's chart

Treatment of overdose: Lavage, VS

ticarcillin (Rx)

(tye-kar-sill′in)

Ticar

Func. class.: Broad-spectrum antiinfective

Chem. class.: Extended-spectrum penicillin

Pregnancy category B

Action: Interferes with cell wall replication of susceptible organisms; osmotically unstable cell wall swells, bursts from osmotic pressure

Therapeutic Outcome: Decreased symptoms of infection

Uses: Respiratory, soft tissue, urinary tract infections, bacterial septicemia; effective for gram-positive cocci *(Staphylococcus aureus, Streptococcus faecalis, Streptococcus pneumoniae)*, gram-negative cocci *(Neisseria gonorrhoeae)*, gram-positive bacilli *(Clostridium perfringens, Clostridium tetani)*, gram-negative bacilli *(Bacteroides, Fusobacterium nucleatum, Escherichia coli, Proteus mirabilis, Salmonella, Morganella morganii, Proteus rettgeri, Enterobacter, Pseudomonas aeruginosa, Serratia; and Peptococcus, Peptostreptococcus, Eubacterium)*

Dosage and routes

Bacterial septicemia, respiratory, skin, soft tissue, intraabdominal, reproductive infections

Adult: **IV** inf 200-300 mg/kg/day in divided doses q4-6h

Child <40 kg: **IV** inf 200-300 mg/kg/day in divided doses q4-6h

Urinary tract complicated infections

Adult/child: **IV** inf 150-200 mg/kg/day in divided doses q4-6h

Uncomplicated urinary infections

Adult: **IV** direct/IM 1 g q6h

Child <40 kg: **IV** direct/IM 50-100 mg/kg/day q6-8h

Severe infections **(Pseudomonas, Proteus, E. coli)**

Neonates: IM/**IV** <2 kg: 75 mg/kg q8-12h; IM/**IV** >2 kg 75-100 mg/kg q8h

Renal dose/hepatic dose

Adult: CCr >60 ml/min 3 g q4h; CCr 30-60 ml/min 2 g q4h; CCr 10-30 ml/min 2 g q8h; CCr <10 ml/min 2 g q12h or 1 g q6h; CCr <10 ml/min and hepatic dysfunction 2 g q24h or 1 g q12h

Available forms: Inj 1, 3, 6, 20, 30 g

Adverse effects

CNS: Lethargy, hallucinations, anxiety, depression, twitching, **coma, seizures**

GI: *Nausea, vomiting, diarrhea;* increased AST, ALT, abdominal pain, glossitis, colitis

GU: Oliguria, proteinuria, hematuria, *vaginitis, moniliasis,* **glomerulonephritis**

HEMA: Anemia, increased bleeding time, **bone marrow depression, granulocytopenia**

INTEG: Rash

META: Hypokalemia

SYST: **Anaphylaxis**

Contraindications: Hypersensitivity to penicillins

Precautions: Pregnancy **B,** hypersensitivity to cephalosporins, lactation, renal disease

Pharmacokinetics

Absorption	Unknown
Distribution	Widely, breast milk
Metabolism	Liver, small amount
Excretion	Kidneys
Half-life	70 min

Pharmacodynamics

	IM	IV
Onset	Unknown	Unknown
Peak	1 hr	30-45 min
Duration	4-6 hr	4 hr

Interactions

Individual drugs

Aspirin, probenecid: increased ticarcillin concentration

Erythromycin: decreased effect of erthromycin

Heparin: increased effect of heparin

Drug classifications

Aminoglycosides (**IV**), tetracyclines: decreased effect of ticarcillin

Contraceptives (oral): decreased effect of oral contraceptives

Neuromuscular blockers: increased effect of neuromuscular blockers

Drug/lab test

False positive: urine glucose, urine protein

NURSING CONSIDERATIONS

Assessment

- Monitor I&O ratio; report hematuria, oliguria, since penicillin in high doses is nephrotoxic
- Monitor any patient with compromised renal system, since drug is excreted slowly in poor renal system function; toxicity may occur rapidly
- Monitor liver function tests: AST, ALT
- Monitor blood studies: WBC, RBC, Hgb, Hct, bleeding time
- Monitor renal function studies: urinalysis, protein, blood, BUN, creatinine
- Monitor C&S before drug therapy; drug may be given as soon as culture is performed
- Assess bowel pattern before, during treatment
- Check for skin eruptions after administration of penicillin to 1 wk after discontinuing drug
- Assess for anaphylaxis: wheezing, rash, pruritus, laryngeal edema, keep emergency equipment nearby
- Assess allergies before initiation of treatment, reaction of each medication

Nursing diagnoses

- Infection, risk for (uses)
- Knowledge, deficient (teaching)

Implementation

- Give drug after C&S has been completed
- Have adrenalin, suction, tracheostomy set, endotracheal intubation equipment
- Provide adequate fluid intake (2 L) during diarrhea episodes

- Provide scratch test to assess allergy on order from prescriber; usually done when penicillin is only drug of choice
- Store at room temp, reconstituted sol 72 hr at room temp

IM route
- Inject into well-developed muscle
- Reconstitute ticarcillin 1 g/2 ml sterile water for inj, NaCl inj, 1% lidocaine HCl without epINEPHrine (385 mg/ml)

IV route
- Give **IV** after diluting 1 g or less/4 ml of sterile H_2O for inj; dilute further with 10-20 ml or more D_5W, 0.9% NaCl, or sterile H_2O for inj sol; give 1 g or less/5 min or more or by intermittent inf over ½-2 hr or by continuous inf at prescribed rate

Y-site compatibilities: Acyclovir, allopurinol, amifostine, aztreonam, cyclophosphamide, diltiazem, famotidine, filgrastim, fludarabine, granisetron, hydromorphone, heparin, IL-2, insulin (regular), magnesium sulfate, melphalan, meperidine, morphine, ondansetron, perphenazine, propofol, sargramostim, teniposide, theophylline, thiotepa, verapamil, vinorelbine

Additive compatibilities: Ranitidine, verapamil

Patient/family education
- Advise patient that culture may be done after completed course of medication
- Teach patient to report sore throat, fever, fatigue (may indicate superinfection)
- Teach patient to carry/wear emergency ID if allergic to penicillins
- Advise patient to notify nurse of diarrhea

Evaluation
Positive therapeutic outcome
- Absence of fever, purulent drainage, redness, inflammation

Treatment of overdose: Withdraw drug, maintain airway, administer epINEPHrine, aminophylline, O_2, **IV** corticosteroids for anaphylaxis

ticarcillin/clavulanate (Rx)
(tye-kar-sill'in)

Timentin

Func. class.: Extended-spectrum penicillin

Chem. class: Antiinfective—broad-spectrum

Pregnancy category B

Action: Interferes with cell wall replication of susceptible organisms; osmotically unstable cell wall swells, bursts from osmotic pressure

Therapeutic Outcome: Resolution of infection

Uses: Respiratory, soft tissue, urinary tract infections; bacterial septicemia; effective for gram-positive cocci *(Staphylococcus aureus, Streptococcus faecalis, Streptococcus pneumoniae)*, gram-negative cocci *(Neisseria gonorrhoeae)*, gram-positive bacilli *(Clostridium perfringens, Clostridium tetani)*, gram-negative bacilli *(Bacteroides, Fusobacterium nucleatum, Escherichia coli, Proteus mirabilis, Salmonella, Morganella morganii, Proteus rettgeri, Enterobacter, Pseudomonas aeruginosa, Serratia, Peptococcus, Peptostreptococcus, Eubacterium)*

Dosage and routes
Renal dose

Adult: CCr 60 ml/min 3.1 g q4h; CCr 30-60 ml/min 2 g q4h; CCr 10-30 ml/min 2g q8h; CCr <10 ml/min 2 g q12h; CCr <10 ml/min with hepatic dysfunction 2 g q24h

Systemic/urinary tract infections, serious infections

Adult ≥60 kg: **IV** inf 3.1 g q4-6h

Adult <60 kg: **IV** inf 200-300 mg/kg/day q4-6h

Child >60 kg: **IV** inf 3.1 g q4h

Child <60 kg: **IV** inf 300 mg/kg/day q4h

Mild/moderate infections

Child ≥60 kg: **IV** inf 3.1 g q6h

Child <60 kg: **IV** inf 200 mg/kg/day q6h

Available forms: Inj IM, **IV** 3 g ticarcillin and 0.1 g clavulanate; **IV** inf 3 g ticarcillin and 0.1 g clavulanate; powder for inj 3 g ticarcillin, 0.1 g clavulanate

Adverse effects
CNS: Lethargy, hallucinations, anxiety, depression, twitching, **coma, seizures**

GI: *Nausea, vomiting, diarrhea,* increased AST, ALT, abdominal pain, glossitis, colitis

GU: Oliguria, proteinuria, hematuria, *vaginitis, moniliasis,* **glomerulonephritis**

HEMA: Anemia, increased bleeding time, **bone marrow depression, granulocytopenia**

META: Hypokalemia, hyperkalemia, alkalosis, hypernatremia

SYST: **Anaphylaxis**

Contraindications: Hypersensitivity to penicillins; neonates

Precautions: Pregnancy **B,** hypersensitivity to cephalosporins, renal disease

Pharmacokinetics

Absorption	Completely absorbed (**IV**)
Distribution	Widely distributed, crosses blood-brain barrier
Metabolism	Liver
Excretion	Kidneys
Half-life	64-68 min

Pharmacodynamics

	IV
Onset	Unknown
Peak	30-45 min
Duration	4 hr

Interactions

Individual drugs

Aspirin, probenecid: increased ticarcillin concentration

Heparin: increased effect of heparin

Drug classifications

Aminoglycosides (**IV**): decreased antimicrobial effect of ticarcillin

Contraceptives (oral): decreased effect of oral contraceptives

Erythromycins: decreased absorption

Neuromuscular blockers: increased neuromuscular blocking

Tetracyclines: decreased ticarcillin effect

Drug/lab test

False positive: urine glucose, urine protein, Coombs' test

NURSING CONSIDERATIONS

Assessment

- Monitor I&O ratio; report hematuria, oliguria because penicillin in high doses is nephrotoxic
- Monitor any patient with compromised renal system because drug is excreted slowly in poor renal system function; toxicity may occur rapidly
- Monitor liver function tests: AST, ALT
- Monitor blood studies: WBC, RBC, Hgb, Hct, bleeding time
- Monitor renal function studies: urinalysis, protein, blood
- Obtain C&S test results before initiating drug therapy; drug may be given as soon as culture is performed
- Assess bowel pattern before, during treatment
- Assess skin eruptions after administration of penicillin to 1 wk after discontinuing drug
- Assess for anaphylaxis: wheezing, rash, laryngeal edema; have emergency equipment nearby
- Assess allergies before initiation of treatment, reaction of each medication

Nursing diagnoses

- Infection, risk for (uses)
- Knowledge, deficient (teaching)

Implementation

- Give drug after C&S has been completed
- Have adrenalin, suction, tracheostomy set, endotracheal intubation equipment available
- Give adequate fluid intake (2 L) during diarrhea episodes
- Obtain scratch test results to assess allergy after securing order from prescriber; usually done when penicillin is only drug of choice
- Store at room temp, reconstituted sol for 12-24 hr or 3-7 days refrigerated

IV route

- Give **IV** after diluting 3.1 g or less/13 ml of sterile H_2O or NaCl (200 mg/ml), shake; may further dilute in 50-100 ml or more 0.9% NaCl, D_5W, or LR sol and run over ½ hr

Y-site compatibilities: Allopurinol, aztreonam, cefepime, cyclophosphamide, diltiazem, famotidine, filgrastim, fluconazole, fludarabine, foscarnet, heparin, insulin (regular), melphalan, meperidine, morphine, ondansetron, perphenazine, sargramostim, teniposide, theophylline, vinorelbine

Patient/family education

- Advise patient that C&S may be performed after completed course of medication
- Instruct patient to report sore throat, fever, fatigue (may indicate superinfection)
- Advise patient to carry/wear emergency ID if allergic to penicillins

Evaluation

Positive therapeutic outcome

- Absence of fever, purulent drainage, redness, inflammation

Treatment of overdose: Withdraw drug, maintain airway, administer epINEPHrine, aminophylline, O_2, **IV** corticosteroids for anaphylaxis

T

ticlopidine (Rx)

(tye-cloe'pi-deen)

Ticlid

Func. class.: Platelet aggregation inhibitor

Chem. class.: Thienopyridine compound

Pregnancy category B

Action: Irreversible inhibition of platelet aggregation through antagonism of ADP

Therapeutic Outcome: Decreased stroke by decreasing platelet aggregation

Uses: Reducing the risk of stroke in high-risk patients

Investigational uses: Intermittent claudication, chronic arterial occlusion, subarachnoid hemorrhage, uremic patients with AV shunts/fistulas, open heart surgery, coronary artery bypass grafts, primary glomerulonephritis, diabetic neuropathy

Dosage and routes

Adult: PO 250 mg bid with food

Available forms: Tabs 250 mg

Adverse effects

CNS: Dizziness

GI: Nausea, vomiting, diarrhea, GI discomfort, **cholestatic jaundice, hepatitis,** increased cholesterol LDL, VLDL, TG

HEMA: **Bleeding (epistaxis, hematuria, conjunctival hemorrhage, GI bleeding), agranulocytosis, neutropenia, thrombocytopenia, thrombotic thrombocytopenic purpura**

INTEG: Rash, pruritus

Contraindications: Hypersensitivity, severe liver disease, blood dyscrasias, active bleeding, coagulopathy

Precautions: Pregnancy **B,** past liver disease, renal disease, elderly, lactation, children, increased bleeding risk, anemia, peptic ulcer disease, surgery

Pharmacokinetics	
Absorption	Well absorbed
Distribution	Unknown
Metabolism	Liver—extensively, 98% protein binding
Excretion	Kidneys—unchanged drug
Half-life	Increased with repeat dosing; 4-5 days (multiple doses)

Pharmacodynamics	
Onset	Unknown
Peak	1-3 hr
Duration	Unknown

Interactions

Individual drugs

Cimetidine: increased effects of ticlopidine
Digoxin: decreased plasma levels of digoxin
Phenytoin: increased levels of phenytoin
Theophylline: increased effects of theophylline

Drug classifications

Antacids: decreased plasma levels of ticlopidine
Anticoagulants, NSAIDs, salicylates, thrombolytics: increased bleeding risk

NURSING CONSIDERATIONS

Assessment

- Monitor liver function studies: AST, ALT, bilirubin, creatinine if patient is on long-term therapy (4 mo or more)
- Monitor blood studies: CBC, Hct, Hgb, protime if patient is on long-term therapy; CBC q2 wk × 3 mo therapy; thrombocytopenia, neutropenia may occur
- Monitor bleeding time baseline and throughout therapy, levels may be 2-5 × normal limit

Nursing diagnoses

- Injury, risk for (uses)
- Knowledge, deficient (teaching)

Implementation

- Give with food or after eating to decrease GI effects

Patient/family education

- Advise patient that blood studies will be necessary during treatment
- Advise patient to report any unusual bleeding to prescriber
- Instruct patient to take with food or just after eating to minimize GI discomfort
- Caution patient to report side effects such as diarrhea, skin rashes, subcutaneous bleeding, signs of cholestasis (yellow skin and sclera, dark urine, light-colored stools)

Evaluation

Positive therapeutic outcome

- Absence of stroke

tigecycline

Tygacil

See Appendix A, Selected New Drugs

tiludronate (Rx)

(till-oo'droe-nate)

Skelid

Func. class.: Bone resorption inhibitor

Chem. class.: Bisphosphonate

Pregnancy category C

Action: Decreases bone reabsorption and new bone development

Therapeutic Outcome: Decreased bone reabsorption and reduced calcium levels WNL

Uses: Paget's disease in those with alkaline phosphatase at 2 × upper limit, patients at risk of future complications of Paget's disease

Dosage and routes

Adult: PO 400 mg daily, with 8 oz of water × 3 mo

Available forms: Tabs 240 mg (equivalent to 200 mg tiludronic acid)

Adverse effects

CNS: Headache, somnolence, dizziness, anxiety, vertigo, nervousness, involuntary movements
CV: Chest pain, edema, hypertension, peripheral edema
ENDO: Hyperparathyroidism
GI: *Nausea, diarrhea,* dry mouth, gastritis, vomiting, flatulence, gastric ulcers, dyspepsia
GU: **Nephrotoxicity,** UTI
INTEG: Rash, epidermal necrosis, pruritus, sweating
MS: *Bone pain,* decreased mineralization of nonaffected bones, pathologic fractures
RESP: Bronchitis, rhinitis, crackles, sinusitis, upper respiratory tract infection

Contraindications: Hypersensitivity to bisphosphonates, severe renal disease with creatinine >5 mg/dl

Precautions: Pregnancy **C,** renal disease, lactation, restricted vit D/Ca, GI disease

Pharmacokinetics	
Absorption	Rapid
Distribution	Unknown, steady state 10 days
Metabolism	Protein binding 90%
Excretion	Feces (unabsorbed), kidney (unchanged)
Half-life	150 hr

Pharmacodynamics	
Onset	Up to 4 wk
Peak	Unknown
Duration	Unknown

Interactions

Individual drugs

Aspirin: decreased tiludronate absorption
Indomethacin: increased effect of tiludronate

Drug classifications

Antacids, mineral supplements with magnesium, calcium, or aluminum: decreased absorption of tiludronate, separate by ≥2 hr

NURSING CONSIDERATIONS

Assessment

- Assess for GI symptoms, polyuria, flushing, head swelling, tingling, headache; may indicate hypercalcemia; nervousness, irritability, twitching, seizures, spasm, paresthesia indicates hypocalcemia at start of treatment
- Identify nutritional status; evaluate diet for sources of vit D (milk, some seafood), calcium (dairy products, dark green vegetables), phosphates
- Monitor BUN, creatinine, uric acid, chloride, electrolytes, urine pH, urinary calcium, magnesium, phosphate, urinalysis (calcium should be kept at 9-10 mg/dl), albumin, alkaline phosphatase baseline and q3-6 mo; check urine sediment for casts throughout treatment
- Assess for increased drug level; toxic reactions occur rapidly; have calcium chloride or gluconate on hand if calcium level drops too low; check for tetany

Nursing diagnoses

- Injury, risk for (adverse reactions)
- Pain, chronic (uses)
- Knowledge, deficient (teaching)

Implementation

- Administer on empty stomach to improve absorption (2 hr ac), with 6-8 oz of water; take calcium or mineral supplements 2 hr before or 2 hr after tiludronate; take aluminum or magnesium antacids ≥2 hr after tiludronate; do not take indomethacin within 2 hr
- Remove tabs from foil strip immediately before use

Patient/family education

- Caution patient to notify prescriber of hypercalcemic relapse: renal calculi, nausea, vomiting, thirst, lethargy, deep bone or flank pain
- Teach patient to follow a low-calcium diet as prescribed (Paget's disease, hypercalcemia)
- Advise patient to notify prescriber of diarrhea, nausea; dose may be divided to lessen these symptoms

Evaluation

Positive therapeutic outcome

- Calcium levels 9-10 mg/dl
- Decreasing symptoms of Paget's disease including pain

timolol (Rx)
(tye'moe-lole)

Apo-Timol ✤, Blocadren, Novo-Timol ✤, timolol maleate, Timoptic

Func. class.: Antihypertensive; antiglaucoma

Chem. class.: Nonselective β-blocker

Pregnancy category C

Do Not Confuse:
Timoptic/Viroptic

Action: Competitively blocks stimulation of β-adrenergic receptor within vascular smooth muscle (decreases rate of SA node discharge, increases recovery time), slows conduction of AV node, decreases heart rate, which decreases O_2 consumption in myocardium; also decreases renin-aldosterone-angiotensin system; at high doses inhibits β_2 receptors in bronchial system

Therapeutic Outcome: Decreased B/P, decreased arrhythmias, absence of death from MI, decreased aqueous humor in the eye, absence of migraine headaches

Uses: Mild to moderate hypertension

Investigational uses: Mitral valve prolapse, hypertrophic cardiomyopathy, thyrotoxicosis, tremors, anxiety, pheochromocytoma, tachyarrhythmias, angina pectoris

Dosage and routes
Hypertension
Adult: PO 10 mg bid, or 20 mg daily, may increase by 10 mg q7 days, not to exceed 60 mg/day

Myocardial infarction
Adult: 10 mg bid beginning 1-4 wk after MI

Glaucoma
Adult: Ophth 1 gtt daily or bid

Child: Ophth 1 gtt daily or bid (0.25% sol only)

Migraine headache prevention
Adult: PO 10 mg bid, or 20 mg daily, may increase to 30 mg/day, 20 mg in AM, 10 mg in PM, discontinue if not effective after 8 wk

Available forms: Tabs 5, 10, 20 mg; ophth sol 0.25%, 0.5%

Adverse effects
CNS: *Insomnia, dizziness,* hallucinations, anxiety, fatigue, depression

CV: Hypotension, bradycardia, **CHF**, edema, chest pain, bradycardia, claudication, angina, AV block, ventricular dysrhythmias

EENT: *Visual changes,* sore throat, *double vision,* dry burning eyes

GI: *Nausea,* vomiting, **ischemic colitis,** diarrhea, *abdominal pain,* **mesenteric arterial thrombosis,** flatulence, constipation

GU: Impotence, urinary frequency

HEMA: **Agranulocytosis, thrombocytopenia, purpura**

INTEG: Rash, alopecia, pruritus, fever

META: Hypoglycemia

MUSC: *Joint pain, muscle pain*

RESP: **Bronchospasm,** dyspnea, cough, crackles, nasal stuffiness

Contraindications: Hypersensitivity to β-blockers, cardiogenic shock, heart block (2nd or 3rd degree), sinus bradycardia, CHF, cardiac failure, severe COPD

Precautions: Pregnancy **C,** major surgery, lactation, diabetes mellitus, renal disease, thyroid disease, COPD, well-compensated heart failure, CAD, nonallergic bronchospasm, peripheral vascular disease, hepatic disease

Pharmacokinetics	
Absorption	Well absorbed (PO), ophth (minimal)
Distribution	Protein binding <10%
Metabolism	Liver—extensively
Excretion	Breast milk
Half-life	3 hr

Pharmacodynamics	PO
Onset	Unknown
Peak	2-4 hr
Duration	12-24 hr

Interactions
Individual drugs
Alcohol: increased hypotension, bradycardia (large amounts)

HydrALAZINE, methyldopa, prazosin, reserpine: increased hypotension, bradycardia

Insulin: decreased hypoglycemia

Thyroid hormones: decreased effect of timolol

Drug classifications
Anticholinergics, antihypertensives, nitrates: increased hypotension, increased bradycardia

β_2-Adrenergic agonists: increased β-blocking effect

Calcium channel blockers: increased effects of calcium channel blockers

NSAIDs, sympathomimetics: decreased antihypertensive effect

Sulfonylureas: decreased hypoglycemic effect

Theophyllines: decreased bronchodilatation

Drug/herb
Aconite: increased toxicity, death

Astragalus, cola tree: increased or decreased antihypertensive effect

Barberry, betony, black catechu, black cohosh,

bloodroot, broom, burdock, cat's claw, dandelion, goldenseal, Irish moss, Jamaican dogwood, kelp, khella, mistletoe, parsley: increased antihypertensive effect
Coltsfoot, guarana, khat, licorice: decreased antihypertensive effect

Drug/lab test
Increased: liver function tests, renal function tests, potassium, uric acid
Decreased: Hct, Hgb, HDL
Interference: glucose, insulin tolerance test

NURSING CONSIDERATIONS

Assessment

- Assess for headaches: location, severity, duration, frequency baseline and throughout treatment
- Monitor B/P during beginning treatment, periodically thereafter; pulse q4h; note rate, rhythm, quality: apical/radial pulse before administration; notify prescriber of any significant changes (pulse <50 bpm)
- Check for baselines in renal, liver function tests before therapy begins
- Assess for edema in feet, legs daily, monitor I&O ratio, daily weight; check for jugular vein distention, crackles, bilaterally, dyspnea (CHF)
- Monitor skin turgor, dryness of mucous membranes for hydration status, especially elderly

Nursing diagnoses

- Cardiac output, decreased (uses)
- Injury, risk for (side effects)
- Knowledge, deficient (teaching)
- Noncompliance (teaching)

Implementation

- Given ac, at bedtime; tab may be crushed or swallowed whole; give with food to prevent GI upset; reduced dosage in renal dysfunction
- Store protected from light, moisture; place in cool environment

Patient/family education

- Teach patient not to discontinue drug abruptly; taper over 2 wk; may cause precipitate angina if stopped abruptly
- Advise patient not to use OTC products containing α-adrenergic stimulants (such as nasal decongestants, cold preparations); to avoid alcohol, smoking and to limit sodium intake as prescribed
- Teach patient how to take pulse and B/P at home; advise patient when to notify prescriber
- Instruct patient to comply with weight control, dietary adjustments, modified exercise program
- Advise patient to carry/wear emergency ID to identify drug being taken, any allergies; tell patient drug controls symptoms but does not cure
- Caution patient to avoid hazardous activities if dizziness, drowsiness is present
- Teach patient to report symptoms of CHF; difficult breathing, especially on exertion or when lying down; night cough; swelling of extremities or bradycardia; dizziness; confusion; depression; fever
- Teach patient to take drug as prescribed, not to double dose, skip doses; take any missed doses as soon as remembered if at least 4 hr until next dose

Evaluation

Positive therapeutic outcome

- Decreased B/P in hypertension (after 1-2 wk)
- Absence of dysrhythmias

Treatment of overdose: Lavage, **IV** atropine for bradycardia, **IV** theophylline for bronchospasm, digitalis, O_2, diuretic for cardiac failure, hemodialysis, **IV** glucose for hyperglycemia, **IV** diazepam (or phenytoin) for seizures

tinidazole (Rx)

(tye-ni'da-zole)
Tindamax
Func. class.: Antiprotozoal
Chem. class.: Nitroimidazole derivative
Pregnancy category C

Action: Interferes with DNA/RNA synthesis in protozoa

Therapeutic Outcome: Decrease in infection

Uses: Amebiasis, giardiasis, trichomoniasis

Dosage and routes

Amebiasis
Adult: PO 2 g /day × 3-5 days
Child >3 yrs: PO 50 mg/kg/day × 3-5 days, max 2 g

Giardiasis
Adult: PO 2 g as a single dose
Child >3 yrs: PO 50 mg/kg as a single dose, max 2 g

Trichomoniasis
Adult: PO 2 g as a single dose

Available forms: Tabs 250, 500 mg

Adverse effects

CNS: *Dizziness, headache,* **seizures,** *peripheral neuropathy*
GI: *Nausea, vomiting,* anorexia, increased AST and ALT, constipation, abdominal pain

T

HEMA: **Leukopenia,** neutropenia
INTEG: Pruritus, urticaria, *rash*, oral monilia
SYST: **Angioedema**

Contraindications: Hypersensitivity to this product or nitroimidazole derivative, pregnancy 1st trimester

Precautions: Pregnancy **C,** hepatic disease, lactation, children, elderly, CNS depression

Pharmacokinetics

Absorption	Unknown
Distribution	Crosses blood/brain barrier
Metabolism	Extensively in the liver
Excretion	Unchanged (20-25%) in urine, (12%) feces
Half-life	12-14 hr

Pharmacodynamics

Unknown

Interactions

Individual drugs

Do not use within 2 wk of taking disulfiram
CycloSPORINE, tacrolimus, fluorouracil, lithium: increased action

Drug classifications

Anticoagulants, hydantoins: increased action
CYP 3A4 inducers (phenobarbital, rifampin, phenytoin); cholestyramine, oxytetracycline: decreased action of tinidazole
CYP 3A4 inhibitors (cimetidine, ketoconazole): increased action of tinidazole

NURSING CONSIDERATIONS

Assessment

- Assess for signs of infection, anemia
- Assess bowel pattern before, during treatment

Nursing diagnoses

- Infection, risk for (uses)
- Knowledge, deficient (teaching)

Implementation

- Administer to those over 3 yr old
- Give with food

Patient/family education

- Instruct patient to take with food to increase plasma concentrations, minimize epigastric distress and other GI effects; not to use alcoholic beverages during or for 3 days afterward
- Advise patient that in cases of trichomoniasis, both partners should be treated

Evaluation

Positive therapeutic outcome

- Decreased in infection as evidenced by negative culture

! HIGH ALERT

tinzaparin (Rx)

(tin-zay-par′in)

Innohep

Func. class.: Anticoagulant

Chem. class.: Unfractionated porcine heparin

Pregnancy category C

Action: Prevents conversion of fibrinogen to fibrin and prothrombin to thrombin by enhancing inhibitory effects of antithrombin III; produces higher ratio of antifactor Xa to antifactor IIa

Therapeutic Outcome: Resolution of deep vein thrombosis

Uses: Treatment of deep vein thrombosis, pulmonary emboli when given with warfarin

Dosage and routes

Adult: SUBCUT 175 anti-Xa international units/kg daily ≥6 days and until adequate anticoagulation with warfarin (INR ≥2 for 2 consecutive days)

Available forms: Inj 40,000 international units/2 ml

Adverse effects

CNS: Fever, confusion, dizziness, insomnia
CV: Angina, dysrhythmias, peripheral edema
GI: Nausea, constipation, flatulence, dyspepsia, **hepatitis**
GU: UTI, hematuria, urinary retention, dysuria
HEMA: Hemorrhage, **hypochromic anemia, thrombocytopenia,** bleeding
INTEG: Ecchymosis
MISC: Headache, chest pain

Contraindications: Hypersensitivity to this drug, heparin, pork or benzyl alcohol, sulfites; hemophilia, leukemia with bleeding, peptic ulcer disease, thrombocytopenic purpura, heparin-induced thrombocytopenia

Precautions: Pregnancy **C,** alcoholism, elderly, hepatic disease (severe), renal disease (severe), blood dyscrasias, severe uncontrolled hypertension, subacute bacterial endocarditis, acute nephritis, lactation, children

Pharmacokinetics

Absorption	Unknown
Distribution	Unknown
Metabolism	Unknown
Excretion	Unknown
Half-life	4.5 hr

Pharmacodynamics	
Onset	Unknown
Peak	3-5 hr (max antithrombin activity)
Duration	Unknown

Interactions
Individual drug
Ticlopidine: increased tinzaparin action
Drug classifications
Anticoagulants (oral), NSAIDs, platelet inhibitors, salicylates, thrombolytics: increased tinzaparin action
Drug/herb
Agrimony, alfalfa, angelica, anise, basil, bay, bilberry, black haw, bogbean, bromelain, buchu, chondroitin, cinchona bark, dong quai, fenugreek, feverfew, garlic, ginger, ginkgo, ginseng, horse chestnut, Irish moss, kelp, kelpware, khella, lovage, lungwort, meadowsweet, motherwort, mugwort, nettle, papaya, parsley (large amounts), pau d'arco, pineapple, poplar, prickly ash, safflower, saw palmetto, tonka bean, turmeric, wintergreen, yarrow: increased risk of bleeding
Chamomile, coenzyme Q10, flax, glucomannan, goldenseal, guar gum: decreased anticoagulant effect

NURSING CONSIDERATIONS
Assessment
- Monitor blood studies (Hct, platelets, occult blood in stools), anti-Xa; thrombocytopenia may occur
- Assess for bleeding gums, petechiae, ecchymosis, black tarry stools, hematuria

Nursing diagnoses
- Cardiac output, decreased (uses)
- Knowledge, deficient (teaching)

Implementation
- Give only after screening patient for bleeding disorders
- Give SUBCUT only; do not give IM
- Give SUBCUT to recumbent patient; rotate inj sites (left/right anterolateral, left/right posterolateral abdominal wall)
- Insert whole length of needle into skin fold held with thumb and forefinger
- Use only this drug when ordered; not interchangeable with heparin or LMWHs
- Give at same time each day to maintain steady blood levels
- Do not massage area or aspirate when giving SUBCUT inj
- Avoid all IM inj that may cause bleeding
- Do not mix with other drugs or infusion fluids
- Store at 77° F (25° C); do not freeze

Patient/family education
- Advise patient to use soft-bristle toothbrush to avoid bleeding gums, to use electric razor
- Instruct patient to report any signs of bleeding: gums, under skin, urine, stools

Evaluation
Positive therapeutic outcome
- Resolution of deep vein thrombosis

Treatment of overdose: Protamine 1 mg/100 anti-Xa international units of tinzaparin

tiotropium (Rx)
(ty-oh'tro-pee-um)
Spiriva
Func. class.: Anticholinergic, bronchodilator
Chem. class.: Synthetic quaternary ammonium compound

Pregnancy category C

Action: Inhibits interaction of acetylcholine at receptor sites on the bronchial smooth muscle, resulting in decreased cGMP and bronchodilation

Therapeutic Outcome: Improved breathing

Uses: COPD, for long-term treatment, once daily maintenance of bronchospasm, associated with COPD including chronic bronchitis and emphysema

Dosage and routes
Adult: Inh content of 1 cap daily using HandiHaler inhalation device

Available forms: Powder for inhalation 18 mcg in blister packs containing 6 caps with inhaler

Adverse effects
CNS: Depression
CV: Chest pain, increased heart rate
EENT: Dry mouth, blurred vision, glaucoma
GI: *Vomiting,* abdominal pain, constipation, dyspepsia
INTEG: Rash
MISC: Urinary difficulty, urinary retention
RESP: *Cough, worsening of symptoms,* sinusitis, URI, epistaxis, pharyngitis

Contraindications: Hypersensitivity to this drug, atropine or its derivatives

Precautions: Pregnancy **C**, lactation, children, narrow-angle glaucoma, prostatic hypertrophy, bladder neck obstruction, elderly

T

Pharmacokinetics

Absorption	Unknown
Distribution	Does not cross blood-brain barrier
Metabolism	Very little metabolized in the liver
Excretion	Excreted in urine
Half-life	5-6 days in animals

Pharmacodynamics

Unknown

Interactions

Drug classifications

Anticholinergics: avoid use with other anticholinergics

Drug/herb

Black catechu: increased constipation
Butterbur, jimsonweed: increased anticholinergic effect
Green tea (large amts), guarana: increased bronchodilator effect
Jaborandi tree, pill-bearing spurge: decreased anticholinergic effect

NURSING CONSIDERATIONS

Assessment

- For tolerance over long-term therapy; dose may have to be increased or changed

Nursing diagnoses

- Breathing pattern, ineffective (uses)
- Knowledge, deficient (teaching)

Implementation

- Caps are for INH only; do not swallow
- Immediately prior to administration, peel back foil until cap is visable; until "stop" line, open dust cap of HandiHaler by pulling upwards, then open mouthpiece
- Place cap in center chamber; firmly close mouthpiece until it clicks, leaving dust cap open
- Hold HandiHaler with mouthpiece upward; press button in once, completely, and release; this allows for medication to be released
- Breathe out completely; do not breathe into mouthpiece at any time
- Raise device to mouth and close lips tightly around mouthpiece
- With head upright, breathe in slowly/deeply, but allowing the cap to vibrate; breathe until lungs fill; hold breath and remove mouthpiece; resume normal breathing
- Repeat
- Remove used capsule and dispose; close the mouthpiece and dust cap; store

Patient/family education

- Teach patient how to use Handihaler
- Teach patient signs of narrow angle glaucoma
- Advise patient that drug is used for long term maintenance, not for immediate relief of breathing problems
- Caution patient to avoid getting the powder in the eyes; may cause blurred vision and pupil dilation

Evaluation

Positive therapeutic outcome

- Ability to breathe easier

tipranavir

Aptivus

See Appendix A, Selected New Drugs

! HIGH ALERT

tirofiban (Rx)

(tie-roh-fee'ban)

Aggrastat

Func. class.: Antiplatelet

Chem. class.: Glycoprotein IIb/IIIa inhibitor

Pregnancy category B

Action: Antagonist of platelet glycoprotein (GP) IIb/IIIa receptor that leads to binding of fibrinogen and von Willebrand's factor, which inhibits platelet aggregation

Therapeutic Outcome: Decreased platelet count

Uses: Acute coronary syndrome in combination with heparin

Dosage and routes

Adult: **IV** 0.4 mcg/kg/min × 30 min, then 0.1 mcg/kg/min for 12-24 hr after angioplasty or atherectomy

Renal dose

Adult: **IV** CCr <30 ml/min 0.2 mcg/kg/min × 30 min, then 0.05 mcg/kg/min, during angiography and for up to 24 hr after angioplasty

Available forms: Inj for sol 250 mcg/ml, inj 50 mcg/ml

Adverse effects

CNS: Dizziness, headache
CV: Bradycardia
GI: Nausea, vomiting
HEMA: Bleeding, **thrombocytopenia**
INTEG: *Rash*
MISC: Dissection, coronary artery edema, pain in legs/pelvis, sweating

Contraindications: Hypersensitivity, active internal bleeding, stroke, major surgery, severe trauma, intracranial neoplasm, aneurysm, hemorrhage, acute pericarditis, platelets <100,000/mm^3, history of thrombocytopenia, coagulopathy

Precautions: Pregnancy **B,** lactation, elderly, renal disease, bleeding tendencies, children, hypertension

Pharmacokinetics	
Absorption	Unknown
Distribution	Plasma clearance 20%-25%
Metabolism	Liver
Excretion	Urine/feces
Half-life	2 hr

Pharmacodynamics	
Onset	Unknown
Peak	Unknown
Duration	Unknown

Interactions

Individual drugs

Abciximab, aspirin, cefamandole, cefoperazone, cefotetan, clopidogrel, dipyridamole, eptifibatide, heparin, ticlopidine, valproic acid: increased bleeding risk

Drug classifications

NSAIDs: increased bleeding risk

Drug/herb

Agrimony, alfalfa, angelica, anise, basil, bay, bilberry, black haw, bogbean, bromelain, buchu, chondroitin, cinchona bark, dong quai, fenugreek, feverfew, garlic, ginger, ginkgo, ginseng, green tea, horse chestnut, Irish moss, kelp, kelpware, khella, lovage, lungwort, meadowsweet, motherwort, mugwort, nettle, papaya, parsley (large amounts), pau d'arco, pineapple, poplar, prickly ash, safflower, saw palmetto, tonka bean, turmeric, wintergreen, yarrow: increased risk of bleeding

Chamomile, coenzyme Q10, flax, glucomannan, goldenseal, guar gum: decreased anticoagulant effect

NURSING CONSIDERATIONS

Assessment

- Monitor platelet counts, Hct, Hgb, before treatment, within 6 hr of loading dose and at least daily thereafter; watch for bleeding from puncture sites, catheters or in stools, urine

Nursing diagnoses

- Tissue perfusion, ineffective (uses)

Implementation

- Dilute inj: withdraw and discard 100 ml from a 500 ml bag of sterile 0.9% NaCl or D_5 and replace this vol with 100 ml of tirofiban inj from two vials
- Tirofiban inj for sol is premixed in containers of 500 ml 0.9% NaCl (50 mg/ml)
- Minimize other arterial/venous punctures IM inj, catheter use, intubation, to reduce bleeding risks

Y-site compatibility: Heparin

Patient/family education

- Advise patient that it is necessary to quit smoking to prevent excessive vasoconstriction

Evaluation

Positive therapeutic outcome

- Treatment of acute coronary syndrome

tizanidine (Rx)

(tye-za′na-deen)

Zanaflex

Func. class.: Skeletal muscle relaxant, central acting

Chem. class.: Imidazole

Pregnancy category C

Action: Unknown; possesses central α_2-adrenergic agonist properties; reduces excitation of spinal cord interneurons; also acts on the basal ganglia, producing muscle relaxation

Therapeutic Outcome: Decreased spasticity of muscles

Uses: Spinal cord injury, spasticity in multiple sclerosis, tension headache

Dosage and routes

Adult: PO 4-8 mg q6-8h increase gradually by 2-4 mg increments, may repeat q6-8h up to 3 doses/24 hr, max 36 mg/day

Available forms: Tabs 2, 4 mg; caps 2, 4, 6 mg

Adverse effects

CNS: *Dizziness,* somnolence, speech disorder, dyskinesia, nervousness, hallucination, psychosis

CV: Hypotension, bradycardia

GI: *Constipation, vomiting, dry mouth,* increased ALT, abnormal liver function tests

GU: Urinary frequency

OTHER: Blurred vision, flulike symptoms, pharyngitis, rhinitis, tremor, rash, muscle weakness

Contraindications: Hypersensitivity

Precautions: Pregnancy **C,** renal disease, hepatic disease, elderly, hypotension, lactation, children

T

Pharmacokinetics

Absorption	Complete
Distribution	Widely
Metabolism	Liver, extensively
Excretion	Kidneys, feces
Half-life	2½ hr

Pharmacodynamics

Onset	Unknown
Peak	1-2 hr
Duration	3-6 hr

Interactions
Individual drugs
Alcohol: CNS depression
Drug classifications
Contraceptives (oral): decreased clearance of tizanidine
Drug/lab test
Increased: AST, alkaline phosphatase, ALT, serum glucose

NURSING CONSIDERATIONS
Assessment
- Assess for muscle spasticity baseline and throughout treatment
- Monitor B/P, heart rate
- Perform neurologic exam in spasticity: deep tendon reflexes, muscle tone, clonus, sensory function
- Monitor liver, renal function tests, electrolytes, CBC with differential during long-term treatment
- Assess for allergic reactions: rash, fever, respiratory distress; severe weakness, numbness in extremities
- Assess CNS depression: dizziness, drowsiness, psychiatric symptoms
- Check dosage, as individual titration is required

Nursing diagnoses
- Mobility, physical, impaired
- Injury, risk for (adverse reactions)
- Knowledge, deficient (teaching)

Implementation
- Give with meals for GI symptoms
- Store in airtight container at room temp
- Give consistently either with or without food; food may affect absorption
- Titrate dose carefully

Patient/family education
- Advise patient not to discontinue medication quickly; spasticity, will occur; drug should be tapered off over 1-2 wk
- Advise patient not to take with alcohol, other CNS depressants, take as directed, if dose is missed, take as soon as remembered, unless it is almost time for next dose
- Caution patient to avoid altering activities while taking this drug; to avoid hazardous activities if drowsiness or dizziness occurs; to rise from sitting or lying slowly to prevent fainting
- Teach patient to use gum, frequent sips of water for dry mouth
- Advise patient to avoid using OTC medications (cough preparations, antihistamines) unless directed by prescriber
- Notify prescriber if fainting, hallucinations, dark urine, stomach pain, yellowing of skin/eyes occurs

Evaluation
Positive therapeutic outcome
- Decreased pain, spasticity

tobramycin (Rx)
(toe-bra-mye'sin)

Nebcin, tobramycin sulfate, TOBI

Func. class.: Antiinfective

Chem. class.: Aminoglycoside

Pregnancy category D

Do Not Confuse:
Tobrex/Tobra Dex

Action: Interferes with protein synthesis in bacterial cell by binding to ribosomal subunit, causing inaccurate peptide sequence to form in protein chain, causing bacterial death

Therapeutic Outcome: Bactericidal effects for the following organisms: *Pseudomonas aeruginosa, Enterobacter, Escherichia coli, Providencia, Citrobacter, Staphylococcus, Proteus, Klebsiella, Serratia*

Uses: Severe systemic infections of CNS, respiratory, GI, urinary tract, bone, skin, soft tissues, eye, cystic fibrosis (nebulizer) for *P. aeruginosa*

Dosage and routes
Adult: IM/**IV** 3 mg/kg/day in divided doses q8h; may give up to 5 mg/kg/day in divided doses q6-8h; once daily dosing is an option

Child: IM/**IV** 6-7.5 mg/kg/day in 3-4 equal divided doses

Child ≥6 yr: NEB 300 mg bid in repeating cycles of 28 days on/28 days off; give inh over 10-15 min using a hand-held PARI LC PLUS reusable nebulizer with a DeVilbiss Pulmo-Aid compressor

Neonates <1 wk: IM up to 4 mg/kg/day in divided doses q12h; **IV** up to 4 mg/kg/day in divided doses q12h diluted in 50-100 mg NS or D_5W; give over 30-60 min

Renal dose

Adult: IM/**IV** 1 mg/kg, then dose determined by blood levels

Available forms: Inj 10, 40 mg/ml; powder for inj 1.2 g; neb sol 300 mg/5 ml

Adverse effects

CNS: Confusion, depression, numbness, tremors, **seizures,** muscle twitching, **neurotoxicity,** dizziness, vertigo

CV: Hypotension, hypertension, palpitations

EENT: *Ototoxicity,* deafness, visual disturbances, tinnitus

GI: *Nausea, vomiting, anorexia,* increased ALT, AST, bilirubin, hepatomegaly, **hepatic necrosis,** splenomegaly

GU: **Oliguria, hematuria, renal damage, azotemia, renal failure, nephrotoxicity**

HEMA: **Agranulocytosis, thrombocytopenia, leukopenia, eosinophilia,** anemia

INTEG: *Rash,* burning, urticaria, dermatitis, alopecia

Contraindications: Pregnancy **D,** severe renal disease, hypersensitivity to aminoglycosides

Precautions: Neonates, mild renal disease, myasthenia gravis, lactation, hearing deficits, Parkinson's disease, elderly

Pharmacokinetics

Absorption	Well absorbed (IM), completely absorbed (**IV**)
Distribution	Widely distributed in extracellular fluids
Metabolism	Minimal—liver
Excretion	Mostly unchanged (>90%) kidneys
Half-life	2-3 hr, increased in renal disease, neonates

Pharmacodynamics

	IM	IV	OPHTH
Onset	Rapid	Rapid	Rapid
Peak	1 hr	Inf end	Unknown

Interactions

Individual drugs

Acyclovir, amphotericin B, bacitracin, cisplatin, ethacrynic acid, furosemide, mannitol, methoxyflurane, polymyxin, vancomycin: increased ototoxicity, neurotoxicity, nephrotoxicity

Drug classifications

Aminoglycosides, cephalosporins, penicillins: increased otoxicity, neurotoxicity, nephrotoxicity

Drug/herb

Lysine (large amounts): increased toxicity

NURSING CONSIDERATIONS

Assessment

- Assess patient for previous sensitivity reaction

Systemic route

- Assess patient for signs and symptoms of infection including characteristics of wounds, sputum, urine, stool WBC >10,000/mm^3, temp; baseline and during treatment
- Complete C&S testing before beginning drug therapy to identify if correct treatment has been initiated
- Assess for allergic reactions: rash, urticaria, pruritus, chills, fever, joint pain
- Identify urine output; if decreasing, notify prescriber (may indicate nephrotoxicity); also, obtain BUN, creatinine, urine CCr (<80 ml/min) values; urinalysis daily for proteinuria, cells, casts; report sudden change in urine output
- Monitor blood studies: AST, ALT, CBC, Hct, bilirubin, LDH, alkaline phosphatase, Coombs' test monthly if patient is on long-term therapy
- Monitor electrolytes: potassium, sodium, chloride, magnesium monthly if patient is on long-term therapy
- Monitor for bleeding: ecchymosis, bleeding gums, hematuria, stool guaiac daily if patient is on long-term therapy
- Assess for overgrowth of infection: perineal itching, fever, malaise, redness, pain, swelling, drainage, rash, diarrhea, change in cough, sputum
- Obtain weight before treatment; calculation of dosage is usually based on ideal body weight, but may be calculated on actual body weight
- Monitor VS during inf, watch for hypotension, change in pulse
- Assess **IV** site for thrombophlebitis including pain, redness, swelling q30 min, change site if needed; apply warm compresses to discontinued site
- Obtain serum peak, drawn at 30-60 min after **IV** inf or 60 min after IM inj, trough level drawn just before next dose; peak 4-12 mcg/ml, trough 1-2 mcg/ml
- Monitor for deafness by audiometric testing, ringing, roaring in ears, vertigo; assess hearing before, during, after treatment
- Monitor for dehydration: high sp gr, decrease in skin turgor, dry mucous membranes, dark urine

T

• Monitor for overgrowth of infection including increased temp, malaise, redness, pain, swelling, perineal itching, diarrhea, stomatitis, change in cough, sputum

Nursing diagnoses

• Infection, risk for (uses)
• Diarrhea (adverse reactions)
• Injury, risk for (adverse reactions)
• Knowledge, deficient (teaching)
• Noncompliance (teaching)

Implementation

IM route

• Give inj deeply in large muscle mass

Nebulizer route

• Give as close to q12h apart as possible; do not use <6 hr apart
• Do not mix with dornase alfa in the nebulizer
• Inhale sitting or standing, breathe normally through the mouthpiece, may use nose clips

IV route

• Give **IV** diluted in 50-100 ml of 0.9% NaCl, $D_{10}W$, D_5/0.9% NaCl, 0.9% NaCl, Ringer's, LR, D_5W (adult), infuse over 20-60 min
• Flush after inf with D_5W, 0.9% NaCl
• Separate aminoglycosides and penicillins by ≥1 hr

Syringe compatibilities: Doxapram

Syringe incompatibilities: Cefamandole, clindamycin, heparin, sargramostim

Y-site compatibilities: Acyclovir, amifostine, amiodarone, amsacrine, aztreonam, ciprofloxacin, cyclophosphamide, diltiazem, enalaprilat, esmolol, filgrastim, fluconazole, fludarabine, foscarnet, furosemide, granisetron, hydromorphone, IL-2, insulin (regular), labetalol, magnesium sulfate, melphalan, meperidine, midazolam, morphine, perphenazine, tacrolimus, teniposide, theophylline, thiotepa, tolazoline, vinorelbine, zidovudine

Additive compatibilities: Aztreonam, bleomycin, calcium gluconate, cefoxitin, ciprofloxacin, clindamycin, furosemide, metronidazole, ofloxacin, ranitidine, verapamil

Additive incompatibilities: Cefamandole, floxacillin

Patient/family education

• Advise patient to use multiple therapies first, then tobramycin
• Teach patient to report sore throat, bruising, bleeding, joint pain; may indicate blood dyscrasias (rare)
• Advise patient to contact prescriber if vaginal itching, loose foul-smelling stools, furry tongue occur; may indicate superinfection
• Advise patient to notify prescriber of diarrhea with blood or pus; may indicate pseudomembranous colitis

Evaluation

Positive therapeutic outcome

• Absence of signs/symptoms of infection (WBC <10,000/mm^3, temp WNL, absence of red, draining wounds)
• Reported improvement in symptoms of infection

Treatment of overdose: Withdraw drug, hemodialysis, exchange transfusion in the newborn, monitor serum levels of drug, may give ticarcillin or carbenicillin

tocainide (Rx)

(toe-kay'nide)

Tonocard

Func. class.: Antidysrhythmic (class IB)

Chem. class.: Lidocaine analog

Pregnancy category C

Action: Produces dose-dependent decreases in sodium and potassium conduction, thereby decreasing the excitability of myocardial cells; does not affect heart rate or B/P

Therapeutic Outcome: Decreased ventricular dysrhythmia

Uses: Life-threatening ventricular dysrhythmias (multifocal/unifocal premature ventricular contractions [PVCs]), ventricular tachycardia

Dosage and routes

Adult: PO 400 mg q8h, may increase to 1.2-1.8 g/day in divided doses q8-12h

Available forms: Tabs 400, 600 mg

Adverse effects

CNS: *Headache, dizziness,* involuntary movement, confusion, psychosis, restlessness, irritability, paresthesias, tremors, **seizures**

CV: *Hypotension, bradycardia,* angina, PVCs, **heart block, CV collapse, sinus arrest, CHF,** chest pain, tachycardia, prodysrhythmias

EENT: Tinnitus, blurred vision, hearing loss

GI: Nausea, vomiting, anorexia, diarrhea, hepatitis

HEMA: **Blood dyscrasias: leukopenia, agranulocytosis, hypoplastic anemia, thrombocytopenia,** bone marrow depression

INTEG: Rash, urticaria, lupus, alopecia, sweating

RESP: Dyspnea, **respiratory depression,**

pulmonary fibrosis, pulmonary edema, interstitial pneumonitis pneumonia

Contraindications: Hypersensitivity to amides, severe heart block

Precautions: Pregnancy **C**, lactation, children, renal disease, liver disease, CHF, myasthenia gravis, blood dyscrasias, pulmonary disease, hypokalemia, atrial flutter/fibrillation, elderly

Pharmacokinetics

Absorption	Well absorbed
Distribution	Widely distributed, crossed blood-brain barrier
Metabolism	Liver
Excretion	Kidney (up to 40% unchanged)
Half-life	10-17 hr

Pharmacodynamics

Onset	1 hr
Peak	½-2 hr
Duration	8-12 hr

Interactions

Individual drugs

Cimetidine, rifampin: decreased effects of tocainide

Metropolol: increased tocainide effects

Drug/herb

Aconite: increased toxicity, death

Aloe, broom, buckthorn (chronic use), cascara sagrada (chronic use), Chinese rhubarb, figwort, fumitory, goldenseal, kudzu, licorice: increased effect

Coltsfoot: decreased effect

Horehound: increased serotonin effect

Drug/lab test

Increased: CPK

False positive: ANA titer

NURSING CONSIDERATIONS

Assessment

- Assess for oxygenation or perfusion deficit: decreased B/P, chest pain, dizziness, loss of consciousness
- Assess respiratory status: auscultate lung fields for bibasilar crackles in patients with advanced CHF
- Assess for urinary retention: check for pain, abdominal absorption, palpate bladder; check males with benign prostatic hypertrophy; anticholinergic reaction may cause retention
- Monitor I&O ratio; electrolytes (potassium, sodium, chloride); watch for decreasing urinary output, possible retention
- Monitor liver function studies: AST, ALT, bilirubin, alkaline phosphatase
- Monitor ECG to determine drug effectiveness; measure PR, QRS, QT intervals; check for PVCs, other dysrhythmias; monitor B/P for hypotension, hypertension; for rebound hypertension after 1-2 hr
- Monitor patient for CNS symptoms: confusion, psychosis, numbness, depression, involuntary movements; if these occur, drug should be discontinued
- Assess pulmonary toxicity: dyspnea, fatigue, cough, fever, chest pain; drug should be discontinued if these occur
- Assess cardiac rate, respiration (rate, rhythm, character), chest pain, ventricular tachycardia, supraventricular tachycardia or fibrillation

Nursing diagnoses

- Cardiac output, decreased (uses)
- Gas exchange, impaired (adverse reactions)
- Knowledge, deficient (teaching)

Implementation

- Give with meals to decrease GI upset

Patient/family education

- Inform patient or family of reason for medication and expected results
- Teach patient method for taking pulse at home and what to report to prescriber
- Advise patient to avoid hazardous activities until drug response is known; dizziness, confusion, sedation may occur
- Advise patient to carry/wear emergency ID indicating medications taken, condition, and prescriber's name and phone number
- Instruct patient to report bleeding, bruising, respiratory symptoms, chills, fever, sore throat to prescriber

Evaluation

Positive therapeutic outcome

- Decreased dysrhythmias

Treatment of overdose: Defibrillation, vasopressor for hypotension

tolcapone (Rx)

(toll'cah-pone)

Tasmar

Func. class.: Antiparkinson agent

Chem. class.: Catecholamine inhibitor (COMT)

Pregnancy category C

Action: Selective, reversible inhibitor of catecholamine; used as adjunct to levodopa/carbidopa therapy

T

Therapeutic Outcome: Increased ability to move and speak

Uses: Parkinsonism

Dosage and routes

Adult: PO 100-200 mg tid, with levodopa/carbidopa therapy; max 600 mg/day; discontinue if no benefit in 3 wk

Renal dose

Adult: PO 100 mg tid or less

Available forms: Tabs 100, 200 mg

Adverse effects

CNS: Dystonia, dyskinesia, dreaming, *fatigue, headache, confusion,* psychosis, hallucination, dizziness

CV: *Orthostatic hypotension,* chest pain, hypotension

EENT: Cataract, eye inflammation

GI: *Nausea, vomiting, abdominal distress,* diarrhea, constipation, **fatal liver failure,** elevated liver function tests

GU: UTI, urine discoloration, uterine tumor, micturition disorder, hematuria

HEMA: **Hemolytic anemia, leukopenia, agranulocytosis**

INTEG: Sweating, alopecia

Contraindications: Hypersensitivity

Precautions: Pregnancy **C,** renal disease, cardiac disease, hepatic disease, hypertension, asthma, lactation

Pharmacokinetics	
Absorption	Rapidly
Distribution	Protein binding 99%
Metabolism	Liver (extensively)
Excretion	Urine (60%), feces (40%)
Half-life	2-3 hr

Pharmacodynamics	
Onset	Unknown
Peak	2 hr
Duration	Unknown

Interactions

Individual drugs

Apomorphine, DOBUTamine, isoproterenol, α-methyldopa: may influence pharmacokinetics

Drug classifications

MAOIs: decreased normal catecholamine metabolism; MAO-B inhibitor may be used

Drug/herb

Kava: decreased effect

NURSING CONSIDERATIONS

Assessment

- Monitor liver function enzymes: AST, ALT, alkaline phosphatase, LDH, bilirubin, CBC
- Assess involuntary movements in parkinsonism: akinesia, tremors, staggering gait, muscle rigidity, drooling
- Monitor B/P, respiration during initial treatment; hypo/hypertension should be reported
- Monitor mental status: affect, mood, behavioral changes

Nursing diagnoses

- Mobility, physical, impaired (uses)
- Injury, risk for (uses)
- Knowledge, deficient (teaching)

Implementation

- Administer tid with levodopa/carbidopa therapy
- Food taken within 1 hr ac or 2 hr pc increases action of drug by 20%
- Provide assistance with ambulation during beginning therapy

Patient/family education

- Advise patient to change positions slowly to prevent orthostatic hypotension
- Advise patient that urine, sweat may change color
- Teach patient to report nausea, vomiting, anorexia

Evaluation

Positive therapeutic outcome

- Decrease in akathisia, increased mood

tolterodine (Rx)

(tol-tehr'oh-deen)

Detrol, Detrol LA

Func. class.: Overactive bladder product

Chem. class.: Muscarinic receptor antagonist

Pregnancy category C

Action: Relaxes smooth muscles in urinary tract by inhibiting acetylcholine at postganglionic sites

Therapeutic Outcome: Decreased symptoms of overactive bladder

Uses: Overactive bladder (frequency, urgency)

Dosage and routes

Adult: **PO** 2 mg bid, hepatic disease 1 mg bid; 4 mg daily, may decrease to 2 mg if needed, max 4 mg/day

Renal dose
Adult: PO CCr ≤30 ml/min reduce by 50%

Available forms: Tabs 1, 2 mg; ext rel caps 2, 4 mg

Adverse effects
CNS: *Anxiety,* paresthesia, fatigue, *dizziness,* headache
CV: Chest pain, hypertension
EENT: Vision abnormalities, xerophthalmia
GI: *Nausea, vomiting, anorexia,* abdominal pain, constipation, dry mouth, dyspepsia
GU: Dysuria, retention, frequency, UTI
INTEG: Rash, pruritus
RESP: Bronchitis, cough, pharyngitis, upper respiratory tract infection

Contraindications: Hypersensitivity, uncontrolled narrow-angle glaucoma, urinary retention, gastric retention

Precautions: Pregnancy **C,** lactation, children, renal/hepatic disease, controlled narrow-angle glaucoma

Pharmacokinetics	
Absorption	Rapidly
Distribution	Highly protein bound
Metabolism	Liver (extensively)
Excretion	Urine/feces
Half-life	Unknown

Pharmacodynamics	
Onset	Unknown
Peak	Unknown
Duration	Unknown

Interactions
Drug classifications
Antibiotics (macrolide), antifungal agents: increased action of tolterodine
Drug/food
Increased: bioavailability of tolterodine

NURSING CONSIDERATIONS
Assessment
- Assess urinary patterns: distension, nocturia, frequency, urgency, incontinence
- Assess allergic reactions: rash; if this occurs, drug should be discontinued

Nursing diagnoses
- Urinary elimination, impaired (uses)
- Incontinence, urinary, functional (uses)
- Knowledge, deficient (teaching)
- Activity intolerance (uses)

Patient/family education
- Advise patient to avoid hazardous activities; dizziness may occur

Evaluation
Positive therapeutic outcome
- Decreased urinary frequency, urgency

topiramate (Rx)
(to-pi-ra'mate)
Topamax
Func. class.: Anticonvulsant—miscellaneous
Chem. class.: Monosaccharide derivative
Pregnancy category C

Action: Mechanism of action unknown; may prevent seizure spread as opposed to an elevation of seizure threshold

Therapeutic Outcome: Absence of seizures

Uses: Partial seizures in adults and children 2-16 yr old; tonic-clonic seizures; seizures in Lennox-Gastaut syndrome

Investigational uses: Cluster headache, infantile spasms

Dosage and routes
Adjunctive therapy
Adult: PO 25-50 mg/day initially, titrate by 25-50 mg/wk, up to 400 mg/day in 2 divided doses

Renal dose
Adult: PO CCr <70 ml/min ½ dose

Available forms: Tabs 25, 100, 200 mg; sprinkle caps 15, 25 mg

Adverse effects
CNS: Dizziness, fatigue, cognitive disorder, *insomnia,* anxiety, depression, paresthesia
EENT: Diplopia, vision abnormality
GI: *Diarrhea, anorexia,* nausea, dyspepsia, abdominal pain, constipation, dry mouth
GU: Breast pain, dysmenorrhea, menstrual disorder
INTEG: Rash
MISC: Weight loss, leukopenia
RESP: Upper respiratory tract infection, pharyngitis

Contraindications: Hypersensitivity

Precautions: Pregnancy **C,** hepatic disease, renal disease, lactation, children, acute myopia, secondary angle closure glaucoma

T

Pharmacokinetics

Absorption	Well absorbed
Distribution	Crosses placenta, plasma protein binding (9%-17%); steady state 4 days
Metabolism	Unknown
Excretion	Kidneys unchanged 55%-97%
Half-life	19-25 hr

Pharmacodynamics

Onset	Unknown
Peak	2-4 hr
Duration	Unknown

Interactions
Individual drugs
Alcohol: increased CNS depression
Carbamazepine, phenytoin: decreased levels of topiramate
Digoxin: decreased levels of digoxin
Metformin: increased topiramate levels
Valproic acid: decreased levels of both drugs
Drug classifications
Carbonic anhydrase inhibitors: increased kidney stone formation
Contraceptives, oral: decreased level of oral contraceptives
CNS depressants: increased CNS depression
Drug/herb
Ginkgo: increased effect
Ginseng, santonica: decreased effect

NURSING CONSIDERATIONS
Assessment
- Assess mental status: mood, sensorium, affect, memory (long, short), especially in elderly
- Assess for blood dyscrasias: fever, sore throat, bruising, rash, jaundice, epistaxis (long-term treatment only)
- Assess seizure activity including type, location, duration, and character; provide seizure precaution
- Monitor CBC during long-term therapy
- Assess body weight and evidence of cognitive disorder

Nursing diagnoses
- Injury, risk for (side effects)
- Knowledge, deficient (teaching)

Implementation
- Do not break, crush, or chew tabs; very bitter
- May take without regard to meals
- Sprinkle cap can be given whole or opened and sprinkled on soft food; do not chew

Patient/family education
- Teach patient to carry/wear emergency ID stating name, drugs taken, condition, prescriber's name and phone number
- Advise patient to avoid driving, other activities that require alertness
- Teach patient not to discontinue medication abruptly after long-term use

Evaluation
Positive therapeutic outcome
- Decreased seizure activity

Treatment of overdose: Lavage, VS

! HIGH ALERT

topotecan (Rx)
(to-poe′ti-kan)
Hycamtin
Func. class: Antineoplastic hormone
Chem. class: Semisynthetic derivative of camptothecin (topoisomerase inhibitor)

Pregnancy category D

Action: Antitumor drug with topoisomerase I–inhibitory activity; topoisomerase I relieves torsional strain in DNA by causing single-strand breaks; causes double-strand DNA damage

Therapeutic Outcome: Decreased tumor size

Uses: Metastatic carcinoma of the ovary after failure of traditional chemotherapy; relapsed small cell lung cancer

Dosage and routes
Adult: **IV** inf 1.5 mg/m^2 over 30 min daily × 5 days starting on day 1 of a 21-day course × 4 courses; may be reduced to 0.25 mg/m^2 for subsequent courses if severe neutropenia occurs

Renal dose
Adult: **IV** CCr 20-39 ml/min 0.75 mg/m^2/day × 5 days on day 1 of a 21-day course

Available forms: Lyophilized powder for inj 4 mg

Adverse effects
CNS: Arthralgia, asthenia, headache, myalgia, pain
GI: Abdominal pain, constipation, diarrhea, obstruction, nausea, stomatitis, vomiting, increased ALT, AST, anorexia
HEMA: **Neutropenia, leukopenia, thrombocytopenia, anemia, sepsis**
INTEG: Total alopecia
RESP: Dyspnea

Contraindications: Pregnancy **D**, hypersensitivity, lactation, severe bone marrow depression

Precautions: Children

Pharmacokinetics

Absorption	Rapidly/completely
Distribution	Unknown
Metabolism	Liver
Excretion	Urine, feces to metabolites
Half-life	8 hr

Pharmacodynamics

Unknown

Interactions

Individual drugs

Cisplatin: increased myelosuppression

Granulocyte colony-stimulating factor: increased duration of neutropenia

NURSING CONSIDERATIONS

Assessment

- Monitor liver function studies: AST, ALT, alkaline phosphatase, which may be elevated
- Monitor for CNS symptoms: drowsiness, confusion, depression, anxiety
- Monitor CBC, differential, platelet count weekly; withhold drug if WBC is <3500/mm^3 or platelet count is <100,000/mm^3; notify prescriber of these results; drug should be discontinued
- Assess buccal cavity q8h for dryness, sores or ulceration, white patches, oral pain, bleeding, dysphagia
- Assess GI symptoms: frequency of stools, cramping
- Assess signs of dehydration: rapid respiration, poor skin turgor, decreased urine output, dry skin, restlessness, weakness

Nursing diagnoses

- Infection, risk for (adverse reactions)
- Knowledge, deficient (teaching)

Implementation

- Provide increased fluid intake to 2-3 L/day to prevent dehydration, unless contraindicated
- Change **IV** site q48h

Patient/family education

- Advise patient to avoid foods with citric acid or hot or rough texture if stomatitis is present; to drink adequate fluids
- Provide patient with nutritious diet of iron, vit K supplements, low fiber, few dairy products
- Advise patient that total alopecia may occur; hair grows back but may be different in color and texture
- Advise patient to report stomatitis; any bleeding, white spots, ulcerations in mouth; tell patient to examine mouth daily; report symptoms
- Assess patient to report signs of anemia; fatigue, headache, faintness, shortness of breath, irritability
- Teach patient to rinse mouth tid-qid with water, club soda; brush teeth bid-tid with soft brush or cotton-tipped applicator for stomatitis; use unwaxed dental floss
- Teach patient to use effective contraception during treatment, avoid breastfeeding

Evaluation

Positive therapeutic outcome

- Decreased tumor size, spread of malignancy

toremifene (Rx)

(tore′me-feen)

Fareston

Func. class.: Antineoplastic

Chem. class.: Antiestrogen hormone

Pregnancy category D

Action: Inhibits cell division by binding to cytoplasmic estrogen receptors; resembles normal cell complex but inhibits DNA synthesis and estrogen response of target tissue

Therapeutic Outcome: Prevention of rapidly growing malignant cells

Uses: Advanced breast carcinoma that has not responded to other therapy in estrogen-receptor-positive patients (usually postmenopausal)

Dosage and routes

Adult: PO 60 mg daily

Available forms: Tabs 60 mg

Adverse effects

CNS: *Hot flashes, headache, lightheadedness,* depression

CV: Chest pain, **CHF, MI, pulmonary embolism**

EENT: Ocular lesions, retinopathy, corneal opacity, blurred vision (high doses)

GI: *Nausea, vomiting,* altered taste (anorexia)

GU: Vaginal bleeding, pruritus vulvae

HEMA: **Thrombocytopenia, leukopenia**

INTEG: *Rash,* alopecia

META: Hypercalcemia

Contraindications: Pregnancy **D**, hypersensitivity, history of thromboembolism

T

Precautions: Leukopenia, thrombocytopenia, lactation, cataracts

Pharmacokinetics

Absorption	Adequately absorbed
Distribution	Unknown
Metabolism	Liver, extensively
Excretion	Feces, slowly, small amounts (kidneys)
Half-life	Unknown

Pharmacodynamics

Onset	Unknown
Peak	3 hr
Duration	Unknown

Interactions
Individual drugs

Warfarin: increased warfarin effect

Drug/lab test

Increased: serum Ca

NURSING CONSIDERATIONS
Assessment
- Monitor CBC, differential, platelet count weekly; withhold drug if WBC is <4000/mm^3 or platelet count is <75,000/mm^3; notify prescriber of results; monitor calcium levels (hypercalcemia is common)
- Assess for tumor flare: increase in bone, tumor pain during beginning treatment; give analgesics as ordered to decrease pain
- Assess for bleeding: hematuria, guaiac, bruising or petechiae, mucosa or orifices q8h, no rectal temp

Nursing diagnoses
- Injury, risk for (adverse reactions)
- Knowledge, deficient (teaching)

Implementation
- Do not break, crush, or chew tabs
- Give with food or fluids to decrease GI upset; repeat dose may be needed if vomiting occurs
- Store in light-resistant container at room temp

Patient/family education
- Instruct patient to report any complaints, side effects to prescriber; if dose is missed, do not double next dose
- Advise patient that vaginal bleeding, pruritus, hot flashes can occur and are reversible after discontinuing treatment
- Instruct patient to report immediately decreased visual acuity, which may be irreversible; stress need for routine eye exams
- Inform patient about who should be told about toremifene therapy
- Advise patient to report vaginal bleeding immediately; that tumor flare (increase in size of tumor, increased bone pain) may occur and will subside rapidly; may take analgesics for pain; that premenopausal women must use mechanical birth control method because ovulation may be induced (teratogenic drug)
- Caution patient to use sunscreen and protective clothing to prevent burns because photosensitivity is common
- Teach patient that hair loss may occur during treatment; a wig or hairpiece may make patient feel better; new hair may be different in color, texture
- Inform patient rash or lesions are temporary and may become large during beginning therapy

Evaluation
Positive therapeutic outcome
- Decreased spread of malignant cells in breast cancer

trace elements (chromium, copper, iodide, manganese, selenium, zinc) (Rx)

Concentrated Multiple Trace Elements, ConTE-PAK-4, M.T.E.-4, M.T.E.-4 Concentrated, M.T.E.-5, M.T.E.-5 Concentrated, M.T.E.-6, M.T.E.-6 Concentrated, M.T.E.-7, MulTE-PAK-4, MulTE-PAK-5, Multiple Trace Element, Multiple Trace Element Neonatal, Multiple Trace Element Pediatric, Neotrace 4, Ped TE-PAK-4, Pedtrice-4, P.T.E.-4, P.T.E.-5

Func. class.: Mineral supplement

Pregnancy category C

Action: Needed for adequate absorption and synthesis of amino acids

Therapeutic Outcome: Replacement for mineral deficiencies

Uses: Prevention of trace element deficiency, a component of TPN

Dosage and routes
Usual dosage may be given in TPN sol

Chromium
- *Adult:* **IV** 10-15 mcg daily
- *Child:* **IV** 0.14-0.20 mcg/ kg/day

Copper
- *Adult:* **IV** 0.5-1.5 mg/day
- *Child:* **IV**.05-0.2 mg/kg/day

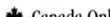

Iodide
- *Adult:* **IV** 1 mcg/kg/day

Manganese
Adult: **IV** 1-3 mg/day
Selenium
Adult: 40-120 mcg/day
Child: 3 mcg/kg/day
Zinc
Adult: **IV** 2-4 mg/day
Child: **IV** 0.05 mg/kg/day

Available forms: Many forms available; see particular elements

Adverse effects
CHROMIUM: **Seizures, coma,** nausea, vomiting, ulcers, **renal/hepatic toxicity**
COPPER: Personality changes, diarrhea, weakness, photophobia, muscle weakness
IODINE: Headache, edema of eyelids, acne, metallic taste, sore mouth, runny nose
MANGANESE: Incoordination, headache, irritability, lability, slurred speech, impotence
SELENIUM: Alopecia, depression, vomiting, GI cramping, nervousness, garlic smell
ZINC: Vomiting, oliguria, **hypothermia,** vision changes, **tachycardia,** jaundice, **coma**

Precautions: Pregnancy **C,** liver, biliary disease, lactation, vomiting or diarrhea

Pharmacokinetics	
Absorption	Completely absorbed
Distribution	Widely distributed
Metabolism	Unknown
Excretion	Depends on element
Half-life	Unknown

Pharmacodynamics
Unknown

Interactions: None known

NURSING CONSIDERATIONS
Assessment
- Assess trace element levels; notify prescriber if low copper 0.07-0.15 mg/ml, zinc 0.05-0.15 mg/100 ml, manganese 4-20 mcg/100 ml, selenium 0.1-0.19 mcg/ml
- Assess trace element deficiency if patient is receiving TPN for extended period
- Obtain calorie count to identify nutritional deficiencies
- Assess for toxicity to individual element (see Adverse effects)

Nursing diagnoses
- Nutrition: less than body requirements, imbalanced (uses)
- Knowledge, deficient (teaching)

Implementation
- Give by **IV** inf, often mixed with TPN sol
- Discard unused portions
- Give by continuous inf diluted in 1 L or more **IV** sol; give at prescribed rate

Patient/family education
- Explain to patient reason for and expected results of medication

Evaluation
Positive therapeutic outcome
- Absence of element deficiency

tramadol (Rx)
(trah'mah-dol)
Ultram
Func. class.: Central analgesic
Pregnancy category C

Do Not Confuse:
tramadol/Toradol

Action: Not completely understood, binds to opioid receptors and inhibits reuptake of norepinephrine, serotonin; does not cause histamine release or affect heart rate

Therapeutic Outcome: Relief of pain

Uses: Management of moderate to severe pain

Dosage and routes
Adult: PO 50-100 mg prn q4-6h, max 400 mg/day
Elderly >75 yr: PO <300 mg/day in divided dose
Hepatic dose
Adult: PO 50 mg q12h
Renal dose
Adult: PO CCr <30 ml/min q12h, max 200 mg/day

Available forms: Tabs 50 mg

Adverse effects
CNS: Dizziness, CNS stimulation, somnolence, headache, anxiety, confusion, euphoria, **seizures,** hallucinations
CV: Vasodilatation, orthostatic hypotension, tachycardia, hypertension, abnormal ECG
GI: Nausea, constipation, vomiting, dry mouth, diarrhea, abdominal pain, anorexia, flatulence, GI bleeding
GU: Urinary retention/frequency, menopausal symptoms, dysuria, menstrual disorder
INTEG: Pruritus, rash, urticaria, vesicles

Contraindications: Hypersensitivity, acute intoxication with any CNS depressant

Precautions: Pregnancy **C,** seizure disorder, lactation, children, elderly, renal, hepatic disease, respiratory depression, head trauma, increased ICP, acute abdominal condition, drug abuse

Pharmacokinetics

Absorption	Rapidly, almost completely absorbed
Distribution	Steady state 2 days
Metabolism	Extensively in liver, may cross blood-brain barrier
Excretion	Unchanged drug 30% in urine
Half-life	Unknown

Pharmacodynamics

Unknown

Interactions

Individual drugs

Alcohol: increased CNS depression
Carbamazepine: decreased tramadol level

Drug classifications

MAOIs: inhibition of norepinephrine and serotonin reuptake; use together with caution
Opiates, sedative/hypnotics: increased CNS depression
SSRIs: increased serotonin syndrome

Drug/herb

Chamomile, hops, kava, skullcap, valerian: increased CNS depression

Drug/lab test

Increased: creatinine, liver enzymes
Decreased: Hgb

NURSING CONSIDERATIONS

Assessment

- Assess pain: location, type, character; give before pain becomes extreme
- Assess for increased side effects in hepatic, renal disease
- Monitor I&O ratio: check for decreasing output; may indicate urinary retention
- Assess need for drug
- Assess for constipation and bowel pattern; increase fluids, bulk in diet
- Monitor CNS changes: dizziness, drowsiness, hallucinations, euphoria, LOC, pupil reaction
- Determine allergic reactions: rash, urticaria

Nursing diagnoses

- Pain, acute (uses)
- Pain, chronic (uses)
- Sensory perception, disturbed: visual, auditory (adverse reactions)
- Injury, risk for (adverse reactions)
- Knowledge, deficient (teaching)

Implementation

- Give with antiemetic for nausea, vomiting
- Administer when pain is beginning to return; determine dosage interval by patient response
- Store in cool environment, protect from sunlight

Patient/family education

- Teach patient to report any symptoms of CNS changes, allergic reactions
- Teach patient that drowsiness, dizziness, and confusion may occur; to call for assistance
- Instruct patient to make position changes slowly; orthostatic hypotension may occur
- Tell patient to avoid OTC medication and alcohol unless approved by prescriber

Evaluation

Positive therapeutic outcome

- Decreased pain

trandolapril (Rx)

(tran-doe'la-prill)

Mavik

Func. class.: Antihypertensive
Chem. class.: Angiotensin-converting enzyme (ACE) inhibitor

Pregnancy category
C (1st trimester),
D (2nd/3rd trimesters)

Action: Selectively suppresses renin-angiotensin-aldosterone system; inhibits ACE; prevents conversion of angiotensin I to angiotensin II, resulting in dilatation of arterial and venous vessels and lowered B/P

Therapeutic Outcome: Decreased B/P in hypertension

Uses: Hypertension alone or in combination, heart failure, after MI/left ventricular dysfunction after MI

Dosage and routes

Hypertension

Adult: PO 1 mg/day, 2 mg/day in African Americans, make dosage adjustment ≥wk; up to 8 mg/day

Heart failure (after MI/left ventricular dysfunction)

Adult: PO 1 mg/day, titrate upward to 4 mg/day if tolerated

Renal dose/hepatic dose

Adult: PO CCr <30 ml/min 0.5 mg/day, may increase gradually up to 4 mg/day

Available forms: Tabs 1, 2, 4 mg

Adverse effects
CNS: *Dizziness,* paresthesias, headache, *syncope,* fatigue, drowsiness, depression, sleep disturbances, anxiety
CV: *Hypotension,* **MI,** palpitations, angina, TIAs, **stroke,** bradycardia, dysrhythmias
GI: Nausea, vomiting, cramps, diarrhea, constipation, pancreatitis, *dyspepsia*
GU: **Proteinuria, renal failure**
HEMA: **Agranulocytosis, neutropenia, leukopenia,** anemia
INTEG: Rash, purpura, pruritus
MISC: Hyperkalemia, hyponatremia, impotence, *myalgia,* **angioedema,** muscle cramps, asthenia, hypocalcemia, gout
RESP: Dyspnea, cough

Contraindications: Pregnancy **D** (2nd/3rd trimesters), hypersensitivity, history of angioedema

Precautions: Pregnancy **C** (1st trimester), hyperkalemia, hepatic disease, bilateral renal stenosis, post kidney transplant, aortal/mitral valve stenosis, cirrhosis, severe renal disease, untreated CHF, autoimmune diseases, severe hypertension

Pharmacokinetics	
Absorption	40-60%
Distribution	Unknown
Metabolism	Liver
Excretion	Kidneys, feces
Half-life	0.6-1.1 hr, 16-24 hr

Pharmacodynamics	
Onset	½ hr
Peak	4-10 hr
Duration	>8 days

Interactions
Individual drugs
Levodopa, reserpine: increased effect of each specific drug
Drug classifications
Antacids: decreased absorption
Antihypertensives, diuretics: increased severe hypotension
Barbiturates, ergots, hypoglycemics, neuromuscular blocking agents: increased effects of each specific drug
Diuretics (potassium-sparing): increased toxicity
Phenothiazines: increased antihypertensive effects
Potassium supplements: increased toxicity of potassium
Salt substitutes: increased potassium levels
Drug/herb
Aconite: increased toxicity, death
Astragalus, cola tree: increased or decreased antihypertensive effect
Barberry, betony, black catechu, black cohosh, bloodroot, broom, burdock, cat's claw, dandelion, goldenseal, Irish moss, Jamaican dogwood, kelp, khella, mistletoe, parsley: increased antihypertensive effect
Coltsfoot, guarana, khat, licorice: decreased antihypertensive effect

NURSING CONSIDERATIONS
Assessment
- Monitor blood studies: neutrophils, decreased platelets
- Monitor B/P, orthostatic hypotension, syncope; if changes occur dosage change may be required
- Monitor renal studies: protein, BUN, creatinine; increased levels may indicate nephrotic syndrome and renal failure
- Monitor renal symptoms: polyuria, oliguria, frequency, dysuria
- Establish baselines in renal, liver function tests before therapy begins
- Check potassium levels throughout treatment, although hyperkalemia rarely occurs
- Check for edema in feet, legs daily
- Assess for allergic reactions: rash, fever, pruritus, urticaria; drug should be discontinued if antihistamines fail to help

Nursing diagnoses
- Cardiac output, decreased (uses)
- Injury, risk for (adverse reactions)
- Knowledge, deficient (teaching)
- Noncompliance (teaching)

Implementation
- Store in airtight container at ≤77° F (≤25° C) or less

Patient/family education
- Advise patient not to discontinue drug abruptly; advise patient to tell all persons associated with health care
- Teach patient not to use OTC products (cough, cold, allergy medications) unless directed by physician; serious side effects can occur; xanthines, such as coffee, tea, chocolate, cola, can prevent action of drug
- Instruct patient on the importance of complying with dosage schedule, even if feeling better; to continue with medical regimen to decrease B/P: exercise, cessation of smoking, decreasing stress, diet modifications
- Emphasize the need to rise slowly to sitting or standing position to minimize orthostatic

hypotension; not to exercise in hot weather, which can cause increased hypotension
- Advise patient to notify prescriber of mouth sores, sore throat, fever, swelling of hands or feet, irregular heartbeat, chest pain, coughing, shortness of breath
- Caution patient to report excessive perspiration, dehydration, vomiting, diarrhea; may lead to fall in B/P
- Caution patient that drug may cause dizziness, fainting, light-headedness; may occur during 1st few days of therapy; to avoid activities that may be hazardous
- Teach patient how to take B/P, and normal readings for age-group

Evaluation
Positive therapeutic outcome
- Decreased B/P in hypertension

Treatment of overdose: Lavage, **IV** atropine for bradycardia, **IV** theophylline for bronchospasm, digitalis, O_2, diuretic for cardiac failure, hemodialysis

tranylcypromine (Rx)
(tran-ill-sip′roe-meen)
Parnate
Func. class: Antidepressant—MAOI
Chem. class: Nonhydrazine

Pregnancy category C

Action: Increases concentrations of endogenous epinephrine, norepinephrine, serotonin, dopamine in storage sites in CNS by inhibition of MAO; increased concentration reduces depression

Therapeutic Outcome: Decreased symptoms of depression after 2-3 wk

Uses: Depression, when uncontrolled by other means

Investigational uses: Bulimia, cocaine addiction, migraines, seasonal affective disorder, panic disorder

Dosages and routes
Adult: PO 10 mg bid; may increase to 30 mg/day after 2 wk; up to 60 mg/day

Available forms: Tabs 10 mg

Adverse effects
CNS: *Dizziness, drowsiness,* confusion, headache, anxiety, tremors, stimulation, weakness, hyperreflexia, mania, insomnia, fatigue
CV: *Orthostatic hypotension, hypertension,* **dysrhythmias, hypertensive crisis**
EENT: Blurred vision
ENDO: **Syndrome of inappropriate antidiuretic hormone-like symptoms**
GI: Constipation, dry mouth, nausea, vomiting, *anorexia,* diarrhea, weight gain
GU: Change in libido, frequency
HEMA: Anemia
INTEG: Rash, flushing, increased perspiration

Contraindications: Hypersensitivity to MAOIs, elderly, uncontrolled hypertension, CHF, severe hepatic disease, pheochromocytoma, severe renal disease, severe cardiac disease

Precautions: Pregnancy **C,** suicidal patients, seizure disorders, severe depression, schizophrenia, hyperactivity, diabetes mellitus, child <16 yr, lactation

Pharmacokinetics

Absorption	Well absorbed
Distribution	Crosses placenta
Metabolism	Liver, extensively
Excretion	Kidneys, breast milk
Half-life	Unknown

Pharmacodynamics
Unknown

Interactions
Individual drugs
Alcohol: increased CNS depression
Buspirone, clonidine, guanethidine: increased pressor effect
Dextromethorphan, meperidine, methylphenidate: increased hypertensive crisis
Fluoxetine, fluvoxamine, paroxetine, sertraline: serotonin syndrome, do not use together
Levodopa, methyldopa, sumatriptan: increased effects of each specific drug

Drug classifications
Antidepressants (tricyclic), appetite suppressants, asthma inhalants, decongestants, sinus medications: increased hypertensive crisis
Antidiabetics, β-adrenergic blockers, rauwolfia alkaloids, sulfonamides: increased effects
Barbiturates, benzodiazepines, diuretics (thiazides), CNS depressants: increased effects of each specific drug
Dibenzazepine agents: hypertensive crisis
Sympathomimetics (direct-acting—epINEPHrine): increased effects of sympathomimetics (direct-acting)
Sympathomimetics (indirect-acting—epHEDrine): increased pressor effects

Drug/herb
Betel palm, butcher's broom, capsicum

peppers, galanthamine, green tea (large amounts), guarana (large amounts), night-blooming cereus: hypertensive crisis
Ginseng: mania
Parsley: serotonin syndrome

Drug/food
Foods containing tyramine: increased hypertensive crisis; avoid all

NURSING CONSIDERATIONS
Assessment
- Monitor B/P (lying, standing), pulse q4h; if systolic B/P drops 20 mm Hg hold drug, notify prescriber; take vital signs q4h in patients with CV disease
- Monitor hepatic studies: AST, ALT, bilirubin
- Check weight qwk; appetite may increase with drug
- Assess mental status: mood, sensorium, affect, suicidal tendencies; increase in psychiatric symptoms: depression, panic
- Monitor urinary retention, constipation; constipation is more likely to occur in children or elderly
- Assess for withdrawal symptoms: headache, nausea, vomiting, muscle pain, weakness; do not usually occur unless drug was discontinued abruptly
- Identify alcohol consumption; if alcohol is consumed, hold dose until AM

Nursing diagnoses
- Coping, ineffective (uses)
- Injury, risk for (side effects)
- Knowledge, deficient (teaching)
- Noncompliance (teaching)

Implementation
- Give with food or milk for GI symptoms; crush if patient is unable to swallow medication whole
- Store at room temp; do not freeze

Patient/family education
- Advise patient that therapeutic effects may take 48 hr-3 wk
- Teach patient to use caution in driving or other activities requiring alertness because of drowsiness, dizziness, blurred vision; to avoid rising quickly from sitting to standing, especially elderly
- Caution patient to avoid alcohol ingestion, other CNS depressants, increased effect may occur
- Advise patient not to discontinue medication quickly after long-term use: may cause nausea, headache, malaise
- Advise patient to increase fluids, bulk in diet if constipation, urinary retention occur, especially elderly
- Teach patient to take gum, hard sugarless candy, or frequent sips of water for dry mouth
- Teach patient to avoid high-tyramine foods; cheese (aged), sour cream, beer, wine, pickled products, liver, raisins, bananas, figs, avocados, meat tenderizers, chocolate, yogurt; increased caffeine, ginseng
- Teach patient to report headache, palpitation, neck stiffness
- Instruct patient to carry/wear emergency ID with medications taken, condition treated, and prescriber's name and phone number
- Advise patient to rise slowly to prevent postural hypotension

Evaluation
Positive therapeutic outcome
- Decrease in depression
- Absence of suicidal thoughts

Treatment of overdose: Lavage, activated charcoal, monitor electrolytes, VS, diazepam **IV**, $NaHCO_3$

! HIGH ALERT

trastuzumab (Rx)
(tras-tuz'uh-mab)
Herceptin
Func. class.: Antineoplastic—miscellaneous
Chem. class.: Humanized monoclonal antibody

Pregnancy category B

Action: DNA-derived monoclonal antibody selectively binds to extracellular portion of human epidermal growth factor receptor 2 (HER2); it inhibits proliferation of cancer cells

Therapeutic Outcome: Decreasing symptoms of breast cancer

Uses: Breast cancer; metastatic with overexpression of HER2

Dosage and routes
Adult: **IV** 4 mg/kg given over 90 min, then maintenance 2 mg/kg given over 30 min; do not give as **IV** push or bol

Available forms: Lyophilized powder 440 mg

Adverse effects
CNS: *Dizziness, numbness, paresthesias,* depression, insomnia, neuropathy, peripheral neuritis
CV: **Tachycardia, CHF**
GI: Nausea, vomiting, anorexia, diarrhea
HEMA: Anemia, **leukopenia**
INTEG: *Rash,* acne, herpes simplex

T

META: Edema, peripheral edema
MISC: *Flulike symptoms; fever, headache, chills*
MS: Arthralgia, bone pain
RESP: Cough, dyspnea, pharyngitis, rhinitis, sinusitis
SYST: **Anaphylaxis, angioedema**

Contraindications: Hypersensitivity to this drug, Chinese hamster ovary cell protein

Precautions: Pregnancy **B,** lactation, children, elderly, cardiac disease, anemia, leukopenia

Pharmacokinetics

Absorption	Unknown
Distribution	Unknown
Metabolism	Unknown
Excretion	Unknown
Half-life	1.7-12 days

Pharmacodynamics

Onset	Unknown
Peak	Unknown
Duration	Unknown

Interactions
Individual drugs
Cyclophosphamide: increased cardiomyopathy risk; avoid use
Drug classifications
Anthracyclines: increased cardiomyopathy risk

NURSING CONSIDERATIONS
Assessment
- Assess for symptoms of infection; may be masked by drug
- Assess CNS reaction: LOC, mental status, dizziness, confusion
- Assess for CHF and other cardiac symptoms: dyspnea, coughing, gallop; obtain a full cardiac workup including ECG, echocardiogram, multigated angiogram
- Assess for hypersensitivity reactions, anaphylaxis
- Monitor for potentially fatal infusion reactions: fever, chills, nausea, vomiting, pain, headache, dizziness, hypotension; discontinue drug

Nursing diagnoses
- Infection, risk for (side effects)
- Nutrition: less than body requirements, imbalanced (side effects)
- Knowledge, deficient (teaching)

Implementation
- Give acetaminophen as ordered to alleviate fever and headache
- Increase fluid intake to 2-3 L/day

IV route
- Administer after reconstituting vial with 20 ml of bacteriostatic water for inj, 1.1% benzyl alcohol preserved (supplied) to yield 21 mg/ml, mark date on vial 28 days from reconstitution date, if patient is allergic to benzyl alcohol, reconstitute with sterile water for inj; use immediately
- Do not mix or dilute with other drugs or dextrose sol

Patient/family education
- Advise patient to take acetaminophen for fever
- Teach patient to avoid hazardous tasks, since confusion, dizziness may occur
- Teach patient to report signs of infection: sore throat, fever, diarrhea, vomiting
- Inform patient that emotional lability is common; instruct patient to notify prescriber if severe or incapacitating

Evaluation
Positive therapeutic outcome
- Decrease in size of tumors

trazodone (Rx)
(tray′zoe-done)
Desyrel, Desyrel Dividose, trazodone HCl, Trazon, Trialodine
Func. class.: Antidepressant—miscellaneous
Chem. class.: Triazolopyridine
Pregnancy category C

Action: Selectively inhibits serotonin, norepinephrine uptake by brain, potentiates behavioral changes

Therapeutic Outcome: Decreased symptoms of depression after 2-3 wk

Uses: Depression

Investigational uses: Chronic pain syndromes

Dosage and routes:
Adult: PO 150 mg/day in divided doses; may increase by 50 mg/day q3-4 days, not to exceed 600 mg/day
Elderly: PO 25-50 at bedtime, increase by 25-50 mg q3-7 days to desired dose, usual 75-150 mg/day
Child 6-18 yr: PO 1.5-2 mg/kg/day in divided doses, may increase q3-4 days up to 6 mg/kg/day

Available forms: Tabs 50, 100, 150, 300 mg

Adverse effects

CNS: *Dizziness, drowsiness,* confusion, headache, anxiety, tremors, stimulation, weakness, insomnia, nightmares, extrapyramidal symptoms (EPS) (elderly), increase in psychiatric symptoms
CV: *Orthostatic hypotension, ECG changes, tachycardia,* **hypertension,** palpitations
EENT: *Blurred vision,* tinnitus, mydriasis
GI: *Diarrhea, dry mouth,* nausea, vomiting, **paralytic ileus,** increased appetite, cramps, epigastric distress, jaundice, **hepatitis,** stomatitis, constipation
GU: *Retention,* **acute renal failure, priapism**
HEMA: **Agranulocytosis, thrombocytopenia, eosinophilia, leukopenia**
INTEG: Rash, urticaria, sweating, pruritus, photosensitivity

Contraindications: Hypersensitivity to tricyclic antidepressants, recovery phase of MI, seizure disorders, prostatic hypertrophy

Precautions: Pregnancy **C,** suicidal patients, severe depression, increased intraocular pressure, narrow-angle glaucoma, urinary retention, cardiac disease, hepatic disease, hyperthyroidism, electroshock therapy, elective surgery

Pharmacokinetics

Absorption	Well absorbed
Distribution	Widely distributed
Metabolism	Liver, extensively
Excretion	Kidneys—unchanged minimally
Half-life	4½-7½ hr

Pharmacodynamics

Unknown

Interactions

Individual drugs

Alcohol, digoxin, phenytoin: increased effect of each drug
Clonidine: decreased effects of clonidine
Fluoxetine: increased levels, increased toxicity
Guanethidine: decreased effects

Drug classifications

Barbiturates, benzodiazepines, CNS depressants: increased effects
MAOIs: increased hyperpyretic crisis, seizures, hypertensive episode
Phenothiazines: increased toxicity
Sympathomimetics (direct-acting): increased sympathomimetic effects
Sympathomimetics (indirect-acting): decreased effects

Drug/herb

Chamomile, hops, kava, lavender, skullcap, valerian: increased CNS depression
Corkwood, jimsonweed: increased anticholinergic effect
SAM-e, St. John's wort: increased serotonin syndrome

Drug/lab test

Increased: serum bilirubin, blood glucose, alkaline phosphatase
Decreased: VMA, 5-HIAA
False increase: urinary catecholamines

NURSING CONSIDERATIONS

Assessment

- Assess for pain: location, duration, intensity before and 1-2 hr after medication
- Monitor B/P (lying, standing), pulse q4h; if systolic B/P drops 20 mm Hg hold drug, notify prescriber; take vital signs q4h in patients with CV disease
- Monitor blood studies: CBC, leukocytes, differential, cardiac enzymes if patient is receiving long-term therapy
- Monitor hepatic function studies: AST, ALT, bilirubin
- Check weight qwk; appetite may increase with drug
- Assess ECG for flattening of T wave, bundle branch block, AV block, dysrhythmias in cardiac patients
- Assess for EPS primarily in elderly: rigidity, dystonia, akathisia
- Assess mental status: mood, sensorium, affect, suicidal tendencies; increase in psychiatric symptoms: depression, panic
- Monitor urinary retention, constipation; constipation is more likely to occur in children or elderly
- Assess for withdrawal symptoms: headache, nausea, vomiting, muscle pain, weakness; do not usually occur unless drug was discontinued abruptly
- Identify alcohol consumption; if alcohol is consumed, hold dose until AM

Nursing diagnoses

- Coping, ineffective (uses)
- Injury, risk for (adverse reactions)
- Knowledge, deficient (teaching)
- Noncompliance (teaching)

Implementation

- Give with food or milk for GI symptoms; crush if patient is unable to swallow medication whole
- Give dosage at bedtime if oversedation occurs during day; may take entire dose at

T

bedtime; elderly may not tolerate once/day dosing
• Store at room temp; do not freeze

Patient/family education
• Teach patient that therapeutic effects may take 2-3 wk
• Teach patient to use caution in driving or other activities requiring alertness because of drowsiness, dizziness, blurred vision; to avoid rising quickly from sitting to standing, especially elderly
• Caution patient to avoid alcohol ingestion, other CNS depressants
• Teach patient not to discontinue medication quickly after long-term use: may cause nausea, headache, malaise
• Advise patient to wear sunscreen or large hat because photosensitivity occurs
• Teach patient to increase fluids, bulk in diet if constipation, urinary retention occur, especially elderly
• Advise patient to take gum, hard sugarless candy, or frequent sips of water for dry mouth
• Teach family to watch for suicidal ideation or tendencies

Evaluation
Positive therapeutic outcome
• Decrease in depression
• Absence of suicidal thoughts

Treatment of overdose: ECG monitoring, induce emesis, lavage, activated charcoal, administer anticonvulsant

treprostinil (Rx)
(treh-prah'stin-ill)
Remodulin
Func. class.: Antiplatelet agent
Chem. class.: Tricyclic benzidine prostacyclin analog
Pregnancy category B

Action: Direct vasodilatation of pulmonary, systemic arterial vascular beds, inhibition of platelet aggregation

Therapeutic Outcome: Decreased pulmonary arterial hypertension (PAH)

Uses: Pulmonary arterial hypertension (PAH) NYHA class II through IV

Dosage and routes
Adult: SUBCUT inf 1.25 ng/kg/min by cont inf, may reduce to 0.625 mg if not tolerated; may increase by 1.25 ng/kg/min qwk for first 4 wk, then 2.5 ng/kg/min/wk for remainder of infusion

Hepatic dose
Adult: SUBCUT INFUSION 0.625 ng/kg ideal body weight/min and increase cautiously

Available forms: Inj 1, 2.5, 5, 10 mg/ml

Adverse effects
CNS: Dizziness, headache
CV: Vasodilatation, hypotension, edema
GI: Nausea, *diarrhea*
INTEG: *Rash,* pruritus
OTHER: Jaw pain
SYST: Infusion site reactions, infusion site pain

Contraindications: Hypersensitivity

Precautions: Pregnancy **B,** past liver disease, renal disease, elderly, lactation, children

Pharmacokinetics	
Absorption	Unknown
Distribution	Unknown
Metabolism	Liver, 90% protein binding
Excretion	Urine, feces
Half-life	2-4 hr, terminal

Pharmacodynamics
Unknown

Interactions
Individual drug
Aspirin: increased risk of bleeding
Drug classifications
Anticoagulants: increased risk of bleeding
Antihypertensives, diuretics, vasodilators: increased hypotension

NURSING CONSIDERATIONS
Assessment
• Monitor liver function tests: AST, ALT, bilirubin, creatinine (long-term therapy)
[Alert] • Monitor blood studies: CBC; CBC q2 wk × 3 mo, Hct, Hgb, protime (long-term therapy)
[Alert] • Monitor bleed time baseline and throughout; levels may be 2-5 × normal limit

Nursing diagnoses
• Tissue perfusion, ineffective (uses)
• Knowledge, deficient (teaching)

Implementation
• Give by continuous SUBCUT infusion or surgically placed indwelling central venous catheter via infusion pump

Patient/family education
• Teach patient that blood work will be necessary during treatment
• Teach patient to report side effects such as diarrhea, skin rashes

- Teach patient that therapy will be needed for prolonged periods of time, sometimes years
- Advise patient that aseptic technique must be used in preparing and administration to prevent infection

Evaluation

Positive therapeutic outcome

- Decreased pulmonary arterial hypertension (PAH)

tretinoin (vitamin A acid, retinoic acid) (Rx)

(tret'i-noyn)

Retin-A, Stievaa ✤, Tretinoin LF IV, Vesanoid

Func. class.: Vitamin A acid/acne product, antineoplastic—miscellaneous

Chem. class.: Tretinoin derivative

Pregnancy category

C (TOP), D (PO)

Action: Decreases cohesiveness of follicular epithelium, decreases microcomedone formation (TOP); induces maturation of acute promyelocytic leukemia, exact action is unknown (PO)

Therapeutic Outcome: Decreased signs/symptoms of leukemia

Uses: Acne vulgaris (grades 1-3) (TOP); acute promylocytic leukemia (PO)

Investigational uses: Skin cancer

Dosage and routes

Adult and child: Top cleanse area, apply at bedtime; cover lightly

Promyelocytic leukemia

Adult: PO 45 mg/m^2/day given as 2 evenly divided doses until remission, discontinue treatment 30 days after remission or after 90 days of treatment, whichever is first

Available forms: TOP cream 0.05%, 0.01%; TOP gel 0.025%, 0.01%; TOP liq 0.05%; caps 10 mg

Adverse effects

PO route

CNS: Headache, fever, sweating

GI: Nausea, vomiting, **hemorrhage,** abdominal pain, diarrhea, constipation, dyspepsia, distention, **hepatitis**

Topical route

INTEG: Rash, stinging, warmth, redness, erythema, blistering, crusting, peeling, contact dermatitis, hypopigmentation, hyperpigmentation

Contraindications: Pregnancy **D** (PO), hypersensitivity to retinoids or sensitive to parabens

Precautions: Pregnancy **C** (TOP), lactation, eczema, sunburn

Pharmacokinetics

Absorption	Small amounts
Distribution	Unknown
Metabolism	Unknown
Excretion	Kidneys
Half-life	Unknown

Pharmacodynamics

Unknown

Interactions

Individual drugs

Benzoyl peroxide, resorcinol, salicylic acid (TOP), sulfur: increased peeling

Ketoconazole: increased plasma concentrations of tretinoin (oral)

Drug classifications

Abrasive soaps, alcohol, astringents, cleansers with drying effect: use with caution (TOP)

Diuretics (thiazide), phenothiazines, quinolones, retinoids, sulfonamides, sulfonylureas: increased photosensitivity

Tetracyclines: increased ICP, risk of pseudotumor cerebri; do not use together

NURSING CONSIDERATIONS

Assessment

Topical route

- Assess part of body involved, including time involved, what helps or aggravates condition, cysts, dryness, itching; lesions may become worse at beginning of treatment

Nursing diagnoses

- Skin integrity, impaired (uses)
- Body image, disturbed (uses)
- Knowledge, deficient (teaching)

Implementation

Topical route

- Apply using gloves or cotton, once daily before bedtime; cover area lightly using gauze
- Store at room temp
- Wash hands after application
- Apply only to affected areas

Patient/family education

Topical route

- Instruct patient to avoid application on normal skin, and to avoid getting cream in eyes, nose, other mucous membranes
- Advise patient to avoid sunlight, sunlamps or

T

to use protective clothing or sunscreen to prevent burns

- Advise patient that treatment may cause warmth, stinging; dryness; peeling will occur
- Inform patient that cosmetics may be used over drug; not to use shaving lotions
- Inform patient that rash may occur during first 1-3 wk of therapy
- Caution patient that drug does not cure condition; only relieves symptoms; that therapeutic results may be seen in 2-3 wk but may not be optimal until after 6 wk

Evaluation

Positive therapeutic outcome

- Decrease in size and number of lesions

triamcinolone (Rx)

(trye-am-sin'oh-lone)

Amcort, Aristocort, Aristocort Forte, Aristocort Intralesional, Aristospan Intra-Articular, Aristospan Intralesional, Articulose L.A., Atolone, Azmacort, Cenocort A-40, Cenocort Forte, Kenacort, Kenaject-40, Kenalog, Kenalog-10, Kenalog-40, Tac-3, Tac-40, Triam-A, triamcinolone, triamcinolone acetonide, Triam Forte, Triamolone 40, Triamonide 40, Tri-Kort, Trilog, Trilone, Trisoject

Func. class.: Corticosteroid, synthetic; antiinflammatory

Chem. class.: Glucocorticoid, intermediate-acting

Pregnancy category C

Action: Decreases inflammation by suppression of migration of polymorphonuclear leukocytes, fibroblasts, reversal of increased capillary permeability and lysosomal stabilization

Therapeutic Outcome: Decreased inflammation, normal immune response

Uses: Severe inflammation, immunosuppression, neoplasms, asthma (steroid dependent), collagen, respiratory, dermatologic disorders

Dosage and routes

Adult: PO 4-12 mg/day in divided doses daily-qid; IM 40 mg qwk (acetonide, or diacetate), 5-48 mg into neoplasms (diacetate, acetonide), 2-40 mg into joint or soft tissue (diacetate, acetonide), 0.5 mg/sq in of affected intralesional skin (hexacetonide), 2-20 mg into joint or soft tissue (hexacetonide)

Child: PO 117 mcg/kg/day in divided doses

Asthma

Adult: INH 2 tid-qid, max 16 inh/day

Child 6-12 yr: INH 1-2 tid-qid, max 12 inh/day

Available forms: Tabs 1, 2, 4, 8 mg; syr 2, 4.85 mg/5 ml; inj 25, 40 mg/ml diacetate; inj 3, 10, 40 mg/ml acetonide; inj 5, 20 mg/ml hexacetonide; inh 100 mcg/spray

Adverse effects

CNS: *Depression, flushing, sweating,* headache, mood changes

CV: *Hypertension,* **circulatory collapse, thrombophlebitis, embolism,** tachycardia, edema

EENT: Fungal infections, increased intraocular pressure, blurred vision

GI: *Diarrhea, nausea, abdominal distention,* **GI hemorrhage,** *increased appetite,* **pancreatitis**

HEMA: **Thrombocytopenia**

INTEG: Acne, poor wound healing, ecchymosis, petechiae

MS: Fractures, osteoporosis, weakness

Contraindications: Psychosis, hypersensitivity, idiopathic thrombocytopenia, acute glomerulonephritis, amebiasis, fungal infections, nonasthmatic bronchial disease, child <2 yr, AIDS, TB, adrenal insufficiency

Precautions: Pregnancy **C**, diabetes mellitus, glaucoma, osteoporosis, seizure disorders, ulcerative colitis, CHF, myasthenia gravis, renal disease, esophagitis, peptic ulcer, lactation, acne, cataracts, coagulopathy

Interactions

Individual drugs

Alcohol, amphotericin B, cycloSPORINE, digitalis, indomethacin: increased side effects

Ambenonium, isoniazid, neostigmine, somatrem: decreased effects of each specific drug

Cholestyramine, colestipol, epHEDrine, phenytoin, rifampin, theophylline: decreased action of triamcinolone

Indomethacin, ketoconazole: increased action of triamcinolone

Drug classifications

Anticholinesterases, anticoagulants, anticonvulsants, antidiabetics, salicylates: decreased effects of each specific drug

Antiinfectives (macrolide), contraceptives (oral), estrogens, salicylates: increased action of triamcinolone

Barbiturates: decreased action of triamcinolone

Diuretics, salicylates: increased side effects

Hypoglycemic agents: increased need for hypoglycemic agents
Toxoids, vaccines: decreased effects of toxoids, vaccines

Drug/herb

Aloe, buckthorn, cascara sagrada, Chinese rhubarb, senna: increased hypokalemia

Drug/lab test

Increased: cholesterol, sodium, blood glucose, uric acid, calcium, urine glucose
Decreased: calcium, potassium, T_4, T_3, thyroid ^{131}I uptake test, urine 17-OHCS, 17-KS, PBI
False negative: skin allergy tests

Pharmacokinetics

Absorption	Well absorbed (PO, IM)
Distribution	Crosses placenta, widely distributed
Metabolism	Liver—extensively
Excretion	Kidney, breast milk
Half-life	2-5 hr, adrenal suppression 3-4 days

NURSING CONSIDERATIONS

Assessment

- Monitor potassium, blood glucose, urine glucose while on long-term therapy; hypokalemia and hyperglycemia
- Monitor weight daily; notify prescriber of weekly gain >5 lb; I&O ratio; be alert for decreasing urinary output and increasing edema
- Monitor B/P q4h, pulse; notify prescriber if chest pain occurs
- Monitor plasma cortisol levels during long-term therapy (normal level; 138-635 nmol/L [SI units] when measured at 8 AM); adrenal function periodically for hypothalamic-pituitary-adrenal axis suppression
- Assess for infection: increased temp, WBC even after withdrawal of medication; drug masks infection symptoms
- Assess for potassium depletion: paresthesias, fatigue, nausea, vomiting, depression, polyuria, dysrhythmias, weakness
- Assess mental status: affect, mood, behavioral changes, aggression
- Assess nasal passages during long-term treatment for changes in mucus (nasal)
- Monitor temp; if fever develops, drug should be discontinued
- Assess for systemic absorption: increased temp, inflammation, irritation (TOP)

Nursing diagnoses

- Infection, risk for (adverse reactions)
- Knowledge, deficient (teaching)
- Noncompliance (teaching)

Implementation

PO route

- Give with food or milk to decrease GI symptoms, tablet may be crushed

IM route

- Give IM inj deeply in large muscle mass, rotate sites, avoid deltoid, use 21G needle
- Give in one dose in AM to prevent adrenal suppression; avoid SUBCUT administration; may damage tissue

Inhalation route

- Use spacer device for elderly
- Give inh with water to decrease possibility of fungal infections; titrated dose, use lowest effective dose
- Give after cleaning aerosol top daily with warm water, dry thoroughly
- Store in cool environment; do not puncture or incinerate container

Topical route

- Apply only to affected areas; do not get in eyes
- Apply medication, then cover with occlusive dressing (only if prescribed), seal to normal skin, change q12h; systemic absorption may occur
- Apply only to dermatoses; do not use on weeping, denuded, or infected areas
- Cleanse skin before applying drug
- Continue treatment for a few days after area has cleared
- Store at room temp

Nasal route

- Have patient clear nasal passages before administration; use decongestant if needed; shake inhaler, invert, tilt head backward, insert nozzle into nostril, away from septum; hold other nostril closed and depress activator, inhale through nose, exhale through mouth

Patient/family education

- Advise patient that emergency ID as steroid user should be carried/worn

Pharmacodynamics

	PO	IM	TOP	INH	INTRANASAL
Onset	Unknown	Unknown	Min to hr	1-2 wk	Unknown
Peak	1-2 hr	1-2 hr	Hr to days	Unknown	2-3 wk
Duration	3 days	Unknown	Hr to days	Unknown	Unknown

- Instruct patient to notify prescriber if therapeutic response decreases; dosage adjustment may be needed; not to discontinue abruptly; adrenal crisis can result
- Caution patient to avoid OTC products: salicylates, alcohol in cough products, cold preparations unless directed by prescriber
- Advise patient on all aspects of drug usage including cushingoid symptoms
- Teach patient symptoms of adrenal insufficiency: nausea, anorexia, fatigue, dizziness, dyspnea, weakness, joint pain
- Teach patient that long-term therapy may be needed to clear infection (1-2 mo depending on type of infection)

Inhalation route
- Teach patient proper administration technique; to wash inhaler with warm water and dry after each use
- Teach patient all aspects of drug usage including cushingoid symptoms

Topical route
- Instruct patient to avoid sunlight on affected area; burns may occur

Nasal route
- Instruct patient to clear nasal passages if sneezing attack occurs, repeat dose
- Advise patient to continue using product even if mild nasal bleeding occurs; is usually transient
- Teach patient method of instillation after providing written instruction from manufacturer

Evaluation
Positive therapeutic outcome
- Decrease in runny nose (nasal)
- Decreased dyspnea, wheezing, dry crackles on auscultation (inh)
- Ease of respirations, decreased inflammation
- Absence of severe itching, patches on skin, flaking (TOP)

triamterene (Rx)
(try-am'ter-een)
Dyrenium
Func. class.: Potassium-sparing diuretic
Chem. class.: Pteridine derivative
Pregnancy category B

Action: Acts primarily on distal tubule to inhibit reabsorption of sodium, chloride; increase potassium retention and conserve hydrogen ions

Therapeutic Outcome: Diuretic and antihypertensive effect while retaining potassium

Uses: Edema, hypertension, diuretic-induced hypokalemia

Dosage and routes
Adult: PO 100 mg bid pc, max 300 mg/day
Elderly: PO 50 mg daily, max 100 mg/day

Available forms: Caps 50, 100 mg

Adverse effects
CNS: Weakness, headache, dizziness, fatigue
ELECT: Hyperkalemia, hyponatremia, hypochloremia
GI: Nausea, diarrhea, vomiting, dry mouth, jaundice, **liver disease**
GU: **Azotemia, interstitial nephritis,** increased BUN, creatinine, renal stones, bluish discoloration of urine
HEMA: **Thrombocytopenia, megaloblastic anemia,** low folic acid levels
INTEG: Photosensitivity, rash

Contraindications: Hypersensitivity, anuria, severe renal, hepatic disease; hyperkalemia, lactation

Precautions: Pregnancy **B**, dehydration, hepatic disease, CHF, renal disease, cirrhosis

Pharmacokinetics	
Absorption	GI tract; well absorbed
Distribution	Crosses placenta
Metabolism	Liver
Excretion	Renal; breast milk
Half-life	3 hr

Pharmacodynamics	
Onset	2 hr
Peak	6-8 hr
Duration	12-16 hr

Interactions
Individual drugs
Amantadine: increased amantadine toxicity
Cimetidine: decreased renal clearance of triamterene
Indomethacin: increased nephrotoxicity

Drug classifications
Angiotensin-converting enzyme inhibitors, diuretics (potassium-sparing), potassium products, salt substitutes: increased hyperkalemia
Antihypertensives: increased action

Drug/herb
Arginine: fatal hypokalemia
Bearberry, gossypol: increased hypokalemia
Cucumber, dandelion, horsetail, licorice,

nettle, pumpkin, Queen Anne's lace: increased diuretic effect
St. John's wort: severe photosensitivity

Drug/lab test
Interference: quinidine serum levels, LDH

NURSING CONSIDERATIONS

Assessment

- Monitor for manifestations of hyperkalemia: *RENAL:* acidic urine, reduced urine osmolality, nocturia, polyuria, polydipsia; *CV:* hypotension, broad T wave, U wave, ectopy, tachycardia, weak pulse; *NEURO:* muscle weakness, altered LOC, drowsiness, apathy, lethargy, confusion, depression, anorexia, nausea, cramps, constipation, distention, paralytic ileus, hypoventilation, respiratory muscle weakness
- Monitor for manifestations of hyponatremia: *CV:* increased B/P, cold, clammy skin, hypo/hypervolemia; *GI:* anorexia, nausea, vomiting, diarrhea, abdominal cramps; *NEURO:* lethargy, increased ICP, confusion, headache, seizures, coma, fatigue, tremors, hyperreflexia
- Monitor for manifestations of hyperchloremia: *NEURO:* weakness, lethargy, coma; *RESP:* deep rapid breathing
- Assess fluid volume status: I&O ratios and record, weight, distended red veins, crackles in lung, color, quality, and sp gr of urine, skin turgor, adequacy of pulses, moist mucous membranes, bilateral lung sounds, peripheral pitting edema; dehydration symptoms of decreasing output, thirst, hypotension, dry mouth and mucous membranes should be reported
- Monitor electrolytes: potassium, sodium, calcium, magnesium; also include BUN, ABGs, uric acid, CBC, blood glucose

Nursing diagnoses

- Urinary elmination, impaired (adverse reactions)
- Fluid volume, deficient (adverse reactions)
- Fluid volume, excess (uses)
- Knowledge, deficient (teaching)

Implementation

- Give in AM to avoid interference with sleep
- With food or milk, if nausea occurs

Patient/family education

- Teach patient to take medication early in the day to prevent nocturia
- Instruct the patient to take with food or milk if GI symptoms of nausea and anorexia occur
- Teach patient to maintain a record of weight on a weekly basis and notify prescriber of weight loss of 5 lb
- Caution the patient that this drug causes an increase in potassium levels, that foods high in potassium should be avoided; refer to dietitian for assistance planning
- Caution the patient not to exercise in hot weather, stand for prolonged periods of time because orthostatic hypotension will be enhanced
- Advise patient to wear protective clothing and sunscreen in the sun to prevent photosensitivity
- Teach patient not to use alcohol or any OTC medications without prescriber's approval because serious drug reactions may occur
- Emphasize the need to contact prescriber immediately if muscle cramps, weakness, nausea, dizziness, or numbness occur
- Teach patient to take own B/P and pulse and record
- Advise patient that dizziness and confusion may occur; avoid driving or other hazardous activities if alertness is decreased
- Teach patient to continue taking medication even if feeling better; this drug controls symptoms but does not cure the condition
- Advise the patient with hypertension to continue other medical treatment (exercise, weight loss, relaxation techniques, cessation of smoking)

Evaluation

Positive therapeutic outcome

- Prevention of hypokalemia (diuretic use)
- Decreased edema
- Decreased B/P
- Increased diuresis

Treatment of overdose: Lavage if taken orally; monitor electrolytes; administer sodium bicarbonate for potassium 6.5 mEq/L; monitor hydration, CV, renal status

triazolam (Rx)

(trye-az'oh-lam)

Apo-Triazo ♣, Gen-Triazolam ♣, Halcion, Novotriolam ♣, Nu-Triazol ♣

Func. class.: Sedative-hypnotic, antianxiety
Chem. class.: Benzodiazepine

Pregnancy category X

Controlled substance schedule IV (USA), schedule F (Canada)

Action: Produces CNS depression at limbic, thalamic, hypothalamic levels of CNS; may be mediated by neurotransmitter; γ-aminobutyric acid (GABA); results are sedation, hypnosis, skeletal muscle relaxation, anticonvulsant activity, anxiolytic action

Therapeutic Outcome: Decreased anxiety, insomnia

Uses: Insomnia (short-term), sedative/hypnotic

Dosage and routes

Adult: PO 0.125-0.5 mg at bedtime

Elderly: PO 0.625-0.125 mg at bedtime

Available forms: Tabs 0.125, 0.25 mg

Adverse effects

CNS: ***Headache, lethargy, drowsiness, daytime sedation,*** dizziness, confusion, lightheadedness, anxiety, irritability, amnesia, poor coordination

CV: Chest pain, pulse changes

GI: Nausea, vomiting, diarrhea, heartburn, abdominal pain, constipation

HEMA: **Leukopenia, granulocytopenia** (rare)

Contraindications: Pregnancy **X,** hypersensitivity to benzodiazepines, lactation, intermittent porphyria

Precautions: Anemia, hepatic disease, renal disease, suicidal individuals, drug abuse, elderly, psychosis, child <15 yr, acute narrow-angle glaucoma, seizure disorders

Pharmacokinetics	
Absorption	Well absorbed
Distribution	Widely distributed, crosses placenta, crosses blood-brain barrier
Metabolism	Liver
Excretion	Kidneys, breast milk
Half-life	2-3 hr

Pharmacodynamics	
Onset	½ hr
Peak	Unknown
Duration	6-8 hr

Interactions

Individual drugs

Alcohol: increased action of both drugs
Cimetidine, disulfiram, isoniazid: increased action, do not use concurrently
Erythromycin, probenecid: increased effects, do not use concurrently
Rifampin: decreased action of rifampin
Theophylline: decreased effects of theophylline

Drug classifications

Antacids: decreased effects of antacids
Antiinfectives (macrolide): increased effects
CNS depressants: increased effects of both drugs
Contraceptives (oral): increased effects; do not use concurrently
Smoking: decreased hypnotic effects

Drug/herb

Black cohosh: increased hypotension
Catnip, clary, chamomile, hops, kava, lavender, mistletoe, nettle, pokeweed, poppy, Queen Anne's lace, senega, skullcap, valerian: increased CNS depression

Drug/lab test

Increased: AST, ALT, serum bilirubin
Decreased: radioactive iodine uptake
False increase: 17-OHCS

NURSING CONSIDERATIONS

Assessment

- Assess patient's mental status: mood, sensorium, anxiety, affect, sleeping pattern, drowsiness, dizziness, especially elderly; physical dependency, withdrawal symptoms: anxiety, panic attacks, agitation, seizures, headache, nausea, vomiting, muscle pain, weakness; suicidal tendencies; for indications of increasing tolerance and abuse
- Monitor patient's B/P (lying, standing), pulse; if systolic B/P drops 20 mm Hg, hold drug, notify prescriber
- Monitor blood studies: CBC during long-term therapy; blood dycrasias have occurred rarely; decreased hematocrit, neutropenia may occur
- Monitor hepatic function studies: AST, ALT, bilirubin, creatinine LDH, alkaline phosphatase
- Monitor I&O ratio; indicate renal dysfunction

Nursing diagnoses

- Anxiety (uses)
- Injury, risk for (adverse reactions)
- Knowledge, deficient (teaching)

Implementation

- Give with food or milk to decrease GI symptoms; if patient is unable to swallow medication whole, tab may be crushed and mixed with foods or fluids
- Give sugarless gum, hard candy, frequent sips of water for dry mouth

Patient/family education

- Advise patient that drug may be taken with food or fluids, and tab may be crushed or swallowed whole
- Caution patient not to use for everyday stress or longer than 3 mo unless directed by prescriber; not to take more than prescribed amount; may be habit forming; not to double doses or skip doses
- Instruct patient to avoid OTC preparations

unless approved by prescriber; alcohol and CNS depressants will increase CNS depression
- Caution patient to avoid driving, activities that require alertness because drowsiness may occur; to avoid alcohol ingestion or other psychotropic medications; to rise slowly or fainting may occur, especially elderly; that drowsiness may worsen at beginning of treatment
- Advise patient not to discontinue medication abruptly after long-term use; withdrawal symptoms include vomiting, cramping, tremors, seizures

Evaluation

Positive therapeutic outcome
- Decreased anxiety, restlessness, sleeplessness (short-term treatment only)

Treatment of overdose: Lavage, VS, supportive care

trifluoperazine (Rx)

(trye-floo-oh-per'a-zeen)

Apo-Trifluoperazine ♣, Novoflurazine ♣, Solazine ♣, Suprazine, Terfluzine, trifluoperazine HCl, Triflurin

Func. class.: Antipsychotic/neuroleptic
Chem. class.: Phenothiazine, piperazine

Pregnancy category C

Do Not Confuse:
trifluoperazine/trihexyphenidyl

Action: Depresses cerebral cortex, hypothalamus, limbic system, which control activity, aggression; blocks neurotransmission produced by DOPamine at synapse; exhibits strong α-adrenergic, anticholinergic blocking action; mechanism for antipsychotic effects is unclear

Therapeutic Outcome: Decreased signs and symptoms of psychosis

Uses: Psychotic disorders, nonpsychotic anxiety, schizophrenia

Dosage and routes

Psychotic disorders

Adult: PO 2-5 mg bid, usual range 15-20 mg/day, may require 40 mg/day or more; IM 1-2 mg q4-6h

Elderly: PO 0.5-1 mg daily-bid, increase q4-7 days by 0.5-1 mg/day to desired dose

Child >6 yr: PO 1 mg daily or bid; IM *not recommended for children,* but 1 mg may be given daily or bid

Nonpsychotic anxiety

Adult: PO 1-2 mg bid, not to exceed 6 mg/day; do not give longer than 12 wk

Available forms: Tabs 1, 2, 5, 10 mg; conc 10 mg/ml; inj 2 mg/ml

Adverse effects

CNS: *EPS (pseudoparkinsonism, akathisia, dystonia, tardive dyskinesia),* **seizures,** *headache,* **neuroleptic malignant syndrome,** dizziness
CV: *Orthostatic hypotension,* hypertension, **cardiac arrest,** ECG changes, **tachycardia**
EENT: Blurred vision, glaucoma, dry eyes
GI: *Dry mouth, nausea, vomiting, anorexia, constipation,* diarrhea, jaundice, weight gain
GU: Urinary retention, urinary frequency, enuresis, impotence, amenorrhea, gynecomastia
HEMA: Anemia, **leukopenia, leukocytosis, agranulocytosis**
INTEG: *Rash,* photosensitivity, dermatitis
RESP: **Laryngospasm,** dyspnea, **respiratory depression**

Contraindications: Hypersensitivity, CV disease, coma, blood dyscrasias, severe hepatic disease, child <6 yr, narrow-angle glaucoma

Precautions: Pregnancy **C,** breast cancer, seizure disorders, lactation, diabetes mellitus, respiratory conditions, prostatic hypertrophy, elderly

Pharmacokinetics

Absorption	Variably absorbed (PO), well absorbed (IM)
Distribution	Widely distributed, high concentrations in CNS, crosses placenta
Metabolism	Liver—extensively
Excretion	Kidneys, breast milk
Half-life	Unknown

Pharmacodynamics

	PO	IM
Onset	Rapid	Immediate
Peak	2-3 hr	1 hr
Duration	12 hr	12 hr

T

Interactions

Individual drugs

Alcohol: increased effects of both drugs, oversedation
Aluminum hydroxide, magnesium hydroxide: decreased absorption
Levodopa: decreased antiparkinson activity
Lithium: decreased effects of lithium

Drug classifications

Anesthetics (barbiturate): oversedation
Anesthetics (general), opiates, sedative/hypnotics: increased CNS depression

Antacids: decreased absorption
Anticholinergics: increased anticholinergic effects
Anticonvulsants: decreased effects of anticonvulsants
β-Adrenergic blockers: increased effects of both drugs

Drug/herb

Chamomile, hops, kava, skullcap, valerian: increased CNS depression
Betel palm, kava: increased extrapyramidal symptoms (EPS)
Cola tree, hops, nettle, nutmeg: increased action

Drug/lab test

Increased: LFTs, cardiac enzymes, cholesterol, blood glucose, prolactin, bilirubin, PBI, cholinesterase, alkaline phosphatase, leukocytes, granulocytes, platelets
Decreased: hormones (blood and urine)
False positive: pregnancy tests, PKU, urine bilirubin
False negative: urinary steroids, 17-OHCS

NURSING CONSIDERATIONS

Assessment

- Assess mental status: orientation, mood, behavior, presence of hallucinations and type before initial administration and monthly; drug should significantly reduce psychotic behavior
- Check for swallowing of PO medication; check for hoarding or giving of medication to other patients
- Monitor I&O ratio, palpate bladder if low urinary output occurs, especially in elderly; urinalysis recommended before, during prolonged therapy
- Monitor bilirubin, CBC, liver function studies monthly
- Assess affect, orientation, LOC, reflexes, gait, coordination, sleep pattern disturbances
- Monitor B/P sitting, standing, and lying, take pulse and respirations q4h during initial treatment; establish baseline before starting treatment; report drops of 30 mm Hg; obtain baseline ECG, monitor Q- and T-wave changes
- Check for dizziness, faintness, palpitations, tachycardia on rising; severe orthostatic hypotension is common
- ◆ Identify for neuroleptic malignant syndrome: hyperpyrexia, muscle rigidity, increased CPK, altered mental status; drug should be discontinued
- Assess for EPS including akathisia (inability to sit still, no pattern to movements), tardive dyskinesia (bizarre movements of the jaw, mouth, tongue, extremities), pseudoparkinsonism (ragged tremors, pill rolling, shuffling gait); an antiparkinson drug should be prescribed
- Assess for constipation, urinary retention daily; if these occur, increase bulk, water in diet
- Assess for hypo/hyperglycemia; appetite patterns

Nursing diagnoses

- Thought processes, disturbed (uses)
- Coping, ineffective (uses)
- Knowledge, deficient (teaching)
- Noncompliance (teaching)

Implementation

PO route

- Give drug in liq form mixed in glass of juice if hoarding is suspected; do not mix in caffeine drinks, tannics, pectins
- Give decreased dose in elderly; metabolism is slowed in the elderly
- Give PO with full glass of water, milk; or give with food to decrease GI upset
- Give antacids 2 hr before or after this drug
- Store in airtight, light-resistant container, oral sol in amber bottle

IM route

- Inj in deep muscle mass, do not give SUBCUT; do not administer sol with a precipitate
- Patient should lie down for 30 min after IM inj

IV route

- Give **IV** after diluting 10 mg/9 ml of 0.9% NaCl; give 1 mg or less/2 min

Syringe compatibilities: Glycopyrrolate
Additive compatibilities: Meperidine, netilmicin

Patient/family education

- Teach patient to use good oral hygiene; frequent rinsing of mouth, sugarless gum for dry mouth; oral candidasis may occur
- Caution patient to avoid hazardous activities until drug response is determined; dizziness, blurred vision is common
- Inform patient that orthostatic hypotension occurs often; to rise from sitting or lying position gradually; avoid tubs, hot showers, and tub baths because hypotension may occur
- Teach patient to remain lying down after IM inj for at least 30 min
- Instruct patient that heat stroke may occur in hot weather, so take extra precautions to stay cool
- Advise patient to avoid abrupt withdrawal of this drug, or EPS may result; drug should be withdrawn slowly
- Teach patient to avoid OTC preparations (cough, hay fever, cold) unless approved by

prescriber because serious drug interactions may occur; avoid use with alcohol, CNS depressants because increased drowsiness may occur
- Advise patient to use sunglasses and sunscreen to prevent burns
- Instruct patient to report sore throat, malaise, fever, bleeding, mouth sores; if these occur, CBC should be performed and drug discontinued

Evaluation
Positive therapeutic outcome
- Decrease in emotional excitement, hallucinations, delusions, paranoia
- Reorganization of patterns of thought, speech

Treatment of overdose: Lavage if orally ingested; provide airway; *do not induce vomiting or use epINEPHrine*

trihexyphenidyl (Rx)
(trye-hex-ee-fen'i-dill)

Apo-Trihex ♣, Artane, Artane Sequels, Novohexidyl ♣, PMS-Trihexyphenidyl ♣, Trihexy-2, Trihexy-5, trihexyphenidyl HCl, Trihexane

Func. class.: Cholinergic blocker; antiparkinson

Chem. class.: Synthetic tertiary amine

Pregnancy category C

Do Not Confuse:
Artane/Altace, trihexyphenidyl/trifluoperazine

Action: Blocks central muscarinic receptors, which decreases involuntary movements, sweating, salivation

Therapeutic Outcome: Decreased involuntary movements

Uses: Parkinsonian symptoms, drug-induced extrapyramidal symptoms (EPS)

Dosage and routes
Parkinsonian symptoms

Adult: PO 1 mg, increased by 2 mg q3-5 days to a total of 6-10 mg/day, given in 3-4 divided doses; give ext rel cap q12h

Drug-induced EPS

Adult: PO 1 mg/day; usual dose 5-15 mg/day, given in 3-4 divided doses, give ext rel q12h

Available forms: Tabs 2, 5 mg; ext rel caps 5 mg; elixir 2 mg/5 ml

Adverse effects
CNS: Confusion, anxiety, restlessness, irritability, delusions, hallucinations, headache, sedation, depression, incoherence, dizziness, flushing, weakness

CV: Palpitations, tachycardia, postural hypotension

EENT: Blurred vision, photophobia, dilated pupils, difficulty swallowing, dry eyes, increased intraocular tension, angle-closure glaucoma

GI: *Dryness of mouth, constipation,* nausea, vomiting, abdominal distress, **paralytic ileus**

GU: Urinary hesitancy, urinary retention, dysuria

INTEG: Urticaria, rash

MISC: Suppression of lactation, nasal congestion, decreased sweating, increased temp, hyperthermia, heat stroke, numbness of fingers

MS: Weakness, cramping

Contraindications: Hypersensitivity, narrow-angle glaucoma, myasthenia gravis, GI/GU obstruction, myocardial ischemia, unstable CV disease, prostatic hypertrophy

Precautions: Pregnancy **C,** elderly, lactation, tachycardia, abdominal obstruction, infection, children, gastric ulcer

Pharmacokinetics

Absorption	Well absorbed
Distribution	Unknown
Metabolism	Unknown
Excretion	Unknown
Half-life	5-10 hr

Pharmacodynamics

	PO	PO-EXT REL
Onset	1 hr	Unknown
Peak	2-3 hr	Unknown
Duration	6-12 hr	Up to 24 hr

Interactions
Individual drugs

Alcohol: increased CNS depression
Amantadine: increased cholinergic effects
Digoxin: increased levels of digoxin
Haloperidol: decreased action of haloperidol

Drug classifications

Analgesics, antihistamines, opioids, sedative/hypnotics: increased CNS depression
Antihistamines, phenothiazines: increased anticholinergic effects

NURSING CONSIDERATIONS
Assessment
- Monitor I&O ratio; retention commonly causes decreased urinary output, distention, frequency, incontinence

T

- Assess for parkinsonism, EPS: shuffling gait, muscle rigidity, involuntary movements, pill rolling, muscle spasms, drooling before and during treatment
- Monitor for urinary hesitancy, retention; palpate bladder if retention occurs
- Monitor for constipation, cramping, pain in abdomen, abdominal distention; increase fluids, bulk, exercise if this occurs
- Assess for tolerance over long-term therapy; dose may have to be increased or changed
- Assess for mental status: affect, mood, CNS depression, worsening of mental symptoms during early therapy

Nursing diagnoses
- Mobility, physical, impaired (uses)
- Knowledge, deficient (teaching)

Implementation
- Give with or after meals to prevent GI upset; may give with fluids other than water
- Give at bedtime to avoid daytime drowsiness in patient with parkinsonism
- Store at room temp

Patient/family education
- Teach patient to use caution in hot weather; drug may increase susceptibility to stroke because perspiration is decreased; patient should remain indoors
- Teach patient not to discontinue this drug abruptly; to taper off over 1 wk to prevent withdrawal symptoms (insomnia, involuntary movements, anxiety, tachycardias)
- Caution patient to avoid driving or other hazardous activities; drowsiness, dizziness may occur
- Advise patient to avoid OTC medications (cough, cold preparations with alcohol, antihistamines) unless directed by prescriber; increased CNS depression may occur
- Instruct patient to rise from sitting or recumbent position slowly to minimize orthostatic hypotension
- Advise patient to use gum, hard candy, frequent sips of water to decrease dry mouth; if dry mouth continues, saliva substitutes may be prescribed
- Instruct patient that doses should not be doubled, but missed dose may be taken up to 2 hr before next dose

Evaluation
Positive therapeutic outcome
- Absence of involuntary movements (pill rolling, tremors, muscle spasms)

trimethobenzamide (Rx)
(trye-meth-oh-ben′za-mide)

Arrestin, Benzacot, Brogan, Stemetic, T-Gen, Tebamide, Ticon, Tigan, Tijet-20, Triban, Trimazide, trimethobenzamide, trimethobenzamide HCl

Func. class.: Antiemetic, anticholinergic
Chem. class.: Ethanolamine derivative

Pregnancy category C

Action: Acts centrally by blocking chemoreceptor trigger zone, which in turn acts on vomiting center

Therapeutic Outcome: Absence of nausea and vomiting

Uses: Nausea, vomiting, prevention of postoperative vomiting

Dosage and routes
Postoperative vomiting
Adult: IM/rec 200 mg before or during surgery; may repeat 3 hr after

Discontinuing anesthesia
Child 13-40 kg: PO/rec 100-200 mg tid-qid
Child <13 kg: PO/rec 100 mg tid-qid

Nausea/vomiting
Adult: PO 250-300 mg tid-qid; IM/rec 200 mg tid-qid

Available forms: Caps 100, 250, 300, mg; supp 100 (pediatric), 200 (adult) mg; inj 100 mg/ml

Adverse effects
CNS: *Drowsiness,* restlessness, headache, dizziness, insomnia, confusion, nervousness, tingling, *vertigo,* extrapyramidal symptoms (EPS)
CV: Hypertension, hypotension, palpitations
EENT: Dry mouth, blurred vision, diplopia, nasal congestion, photosensitivity
GI: Nausea, anorexia, diarrhea, vomiting, constipation
INTEG: Rash, urticaria, fever, chills, flushing

Contraindications: Hypersensitivity to opioids, shock, children (parenterally)

Precautions: Pregnancy **C,** children, cardiac dysrhythmias, elderly, asthma, prostatic hypertrophy, bladder-neck obstruction, narrow-angle glaucoma, stenosing peptic ulcer, pyloroduodenal obstruction

Pharmacokinetics

Absorption	Unknown
Distribution	Unknown
Metabolism	Liver, extensively
Excretion	Kidneys
Half-life	Unknown

Pharmacodynamics

	PO	IM	REC
Onset	20-40 min	15 min	10-40 min
Peak	Unknown	Unknown	Unknown
Duration	3-4 hr	2-3 hr	3-4 hr

Interactions
Individual drugs
Alcohol: increased CNS depression
Drug classifications
Analgesics, antidepressants, antihistamines, CNS depressants, sedative/hypnotics: increased CNS effect
Antibiotics: may mask ototoxic symptoms

NURSING CONSIDERATIONS
Assessment
- Monitor VS, B/P; check patients with cardiac disease more often
- Assess for signs of toxicity of other drugs or masking of symptoms of disease: brain tumor, intestinal obstructions
- Observe for drowsiness, dizziness
- Assess for nausea, vomiting before and after treatment

Nursing diagnoses
- Knowledge, deficient (teaching)

Implementation
PO route
- Cap may be swallowed whole or opened and mixed with food or fluids

IM route
- Administer IM inj in large muscle mass; aspirate to avoid **IV** administration
- Patient should remain lying down for 30 min after IM inj

Syringe compatibilities: Glycopyrrolate, hydromorphone, midazolam, nalbuphine
Y-site compatibilities: Heparin, hydrocortisone, potassium chloride, vit B/C

Patient/family education
- Teach patient to use good oral hygiene; frequent rinsing of mouth, sugarless gum for dry mouth
- Caution patient to avoid hazardous activities until drug response is determined, drowsiness may occur
- Inform patient that orthostatic hypotension occurs often and to rise from sitting or lying position gradually; avoid hot tubs, hot showers, and tub baths because hypotension may occur
- Teach patient to remain lying down after IM inj for at least 30 min
- Inform patient that in hot weather, heat stroke may occur; take extra precautions to stay cool
- Teach patient to avoid OTC preparations (cough, hayfever, cold) unless approved by prescriber because serious drug interactions may occur; avoid use with alcohol, CNS depressants because increased drowsiness may occur
- Teach patient about EPS
- Instruct patient to report sore throat, malaise, fever, bleeding, mouth sores; if these occur, CBC should be performed and drug discontinued

Evaluation
Positive therapeutic outcome
- Decreased nausea, vomiting

trimethoprim/ sulfamethoxazole (cotrimoxazole) (Rx)
(trye-meth'oh-prim/sul-fa-meth-ox'a-zole [ko-trye-mox'a-zole])
Apo-Sulfatrim*, Apo-Sulfatrim DS ✤, Bactrim, Bactrim IV, Bethaprim, Cotrim, Novo-Trimel ✤, Novo-Trimel DS ✤, Nu-Cotrimox ✤, Nu-Cotrimox DS ✤, Roubac ✤, Septra, Septra DS, SMZ/TMP, Sulfatrim
Func. class.: Antiinfective
Chem. class.: Sulfonamide—miscellaneous
Pregnancy category C

Action: Sulfamethoxazole (SMZ) interferes with bacterial biosynthesis of proteins by competitive antagonism of PABA when adequate levels are maintained; trimethoprim (TMP) blocks synthesis of tetrahydrofolic acid; combination blocks two consecutive steps in bacterial synthesis of essential nucleic acids, protein

Therapeutic Outcome: Absence of infection, based on C&S

Uses: UTI, otitis media, acute and chronic prostatitis, shigellosis, *Pneumocystis jiroveci* pneumonitis, chronic bronchitis, chancroid, traveler's diarrhea

Dosage and routes

UTI

Adult: PO 160 mg TMP/q12h × 10-14 days
Child: PO 8 mg/kg TMP/daily in 2 divided doses q12h

Otitis media

Child: PO 8 mg/kg TMP/daily in 2 divided doses q12h × 10 days

Chronic bronchitis

Adult: PO 160 mg TMP/q12h × 14 days

Pneumocystis jiroveci pneumonitis

Adult and child: PO 20 mg/kg TMP daily in 4 divided doses q6h × 14 days; **IV** 15-20 mg/kg/day (based on TMP) in 3-4 divided doses for up to 14 days

Renal dose

Dosage reduction necessary in moderate to severe renal impairment (CCr <30 ml/min)

Available forms: Tabs 80 mg trimethoprim (TMP)/400 mg sulfamethoxazole (SMZ), 160 mg TMP/800 mg SMZ; susp 40 mg/200 mg/5 ml; **IV** 16 mg/80 mg/ml

Adverse effects

CNS: Headache, insomnia, hallucinations, depression, vertigo, fatigue, anxiety, seizures, drug fever, chills, **aseptic meningitis**
CV: **Allergic myocarditis**
GI: *Nausea, vomiting, abdominal pain,* stomatitis, **hepatitis,** glossitis, pancreatitis, diarrhea, **enterocolitis,** anorexia
GU: **Renal failure, toxic nephrosis;** increased BUN, creatinine; crystalluria
HEMA: **Leukopenia, neutropenia, thrombocytopenia, agranulocytosis, hemolytic anemia, hypoprothrombinemia, Henoch-Schönlein purpura, methemoglobinemia, eosinophilia I**
INTEG: Rash, dermatitis, urticaria, erythema, photosensitivity, pain, inflammation at injection site, **toxic epidermal necrolysis, erythema multiforme**
RESP: Cough, shortness of breath
SYST: **Anaphylaxis, systemic lupus erythematosus, Stevens-Johnson syndrome**

Contraindications: Hypersensitivity to trimethoprim or sulfonamides, pregnancy at term, megaloblastic anemia, infants <2 mo, CCr <15 ml/min, lactation, porphyria

Precautions: Pregnancy **C,** renal disease, elderly, glucose-6-phosphate dehydrogenase deficiency, impaired hepatic/renal function, possible folate deficiency, severe allergy, bronchial asthma

Pharmacokinetics	
Absorption	Rapid
Distribution	Breast milk, crosses placenta, 68% protein bound
Metabolism	Liver
Excretion	Kidneys
Half-life	8-13 hr

Pharmacodynamics	
Onset	Unknown
Peak	1-4 hr
Duration	Unknown

Interactions

Individual drugs

CycloSPORINE: decreased response
Methotrexate: increased bone marrow depression
Phenytoin: decreased hepatic clearance of phenytoin

Drug classifications

Anticoagulants (oral): increased anticoagulant effect
Diuretics (thiazide): increased thrombocytopenia
Sulfonylureas: increased hypoglycemic response

Drug/lab test

Increased: alkaline phosphatase, creatinine, bilirubin

NURSING CONSIDERATIONS

Assessment

- Assess allergic reactions: rash, fever (AIDS patients more susceptible)
- Monitor I&O ratio; note color, character, pH of urine if drug administered for UTI; output should be 800 ml less than intake; if urine is highly acidic, alkalization may be needed
- Monitor kidney function studies: BUN, creatinine, urinalysis (long-term therapy)
- Assess type of infection; obtain C&S before starting therapy
- Assess blood dyscrasias, skin rash, fever, sore throat, bruising, bleeding, fatigue, joint pain
- Assess allergic reaction: rash, dermatitis, urticaria, pruritus, dyspnea, bronchospasm

Nursing diagnoses

- Infection, risk for (uses)
- Knowledge, deficient (teaching)
- Noncompliance (teaching)

Implementation

- Give with full glass of water to maintain adequate hydration; increase fluids to 2 L/day to decrease crystallization in kidneys

- Give medication after C&S; repeat C&S after full course of medication
- Store in airtight, light-resistant container at room temp

IV route

- Dilute 5 ml ampule/100-125 ml of D_5W, stable for 6 hr, give over 1½ hr, do not refrigerate

Syringe compatibilities: Heparin

Y-site compatibilities: Acyclovir, aldesleukin, allopurinol, amifostine, atracurium, aztreonam, cefepime, cyclophosphamide, diltiazem, enalaprilat, esmolol, filgrastim, fludarabine, gallium, granisetron, hydromorphone, labetalol, lorazepam, magnesium sulfate, melphalan, meperidine, morphine, pancuronium, perphenazine, piperacillin/tazobactam, sargramostim, tacrolimus, teniposide, thiotepa, vecuronium, zidovudine

Patient family education

- Teach patient to take each oral dose with full glass of water to prevent crystalluria; drink 8-10 glasses of water/day
- Teach patient to complete course of full treatment to prevent superinfection
- Teach patient to avoid sunlight or use sunscreen to prevent burns
- Teach patient to avoid OTC medications (aspirin, vit C) unless directed by prescriber
- If diabetic, teach patient to use Clinistix or Tes-Tape
- Teach patient to use alternative contraceptive measures; decreased effectiveness of oral contraceptives may result
- Teach patient to notify prescriber if skin rash, sore throat, fever, mouth sores, unusual bruising, bleeding occur

Evaluation

Positive therapeutic outcome

Absence of pain, fever, C&S negative

triptorelin (Rx)

(trip-toe'rel-in)

Trelstar Depot

Func. class.: Gonadotropin-releasing hormone antagonist

Chem. class.: Synthetic decapeptide analog of LHRH

Pregnancy category X

Action: Inhibitor of pituitary gonadotropin secretion; initially increases LH and FSH, with increases in testosterone, reduction in sex steroid levels

Therapeutic Outcome: Decreased signs/symptoms of advanced prostate cancer

Uses: Advanced prostate cancer

Dosage and routes

Adult: IM 3.75 mg qmo

Available forms: Microgranules, depot inj 3.75 mg

Adverse effects

CNS: Headache, insomnia, dizziness, lability, fatigue

CV: *Hypertension*

ENDO: Gynecomastia, breast tenderness, hot flashes

GI: Nausea, vomiting, diarrhea

GU: Impotence, urinary retention, UTI

INTEG: Rash, pain on injection, pruritus, hypersensitivity

MISC: **Anaphylaxis, angioedema**

MS: Osteoneuralgia

Contraindications: Pregnancy **X**, hypersensitivity to this product or other LHRH agonists or LHRH, lactation

Pharmacokinetics

Absorption	Unknown
Distribution	Unknown
Metabolism	CYP/450
Excretion	Liver, kidneys
Half-life	3 hr

Pharmacodynamics

Unknown

Interactions None known

Drug/lab test

Increased: alkaline phosphatase, estradiol, FSH, LH, testosterone levels

Decreased: testosterone levels, progesterone

NURSING CONSIDERATIONS

Assessment

- Assess for severe hypersensitivity: discontinue drug and give antihistamines, have emergency equipment nearby
- Monitor I&O ratios; palpate bladder for distention in urinary obstruction
- Monitor for relief of bone pain (back pain)
- Assess levels of testosterone and prostate-specific antigen (PSA)

Nursing diagnoses

- Diarrhea (adverse reactions)
- Knowledge, deficient (teaching)

T

Implementation
- Give IM using implant, inserted by qualified person
- Use syringe with 20-G needle, withdraw 2 ml of sterile water for inj, inject into vial, shake well, withdraw vial contents, inject immediately

Patient/family education
- Teach patient that gynecomastia may occur but will decrease after treatment is discontinued
- Advise patient to report allergic reaction immediately
- Teach patient that disease flare may occur at beginning of therapy

Evaluation
Positive therapeutic outcome
- More normal levels of PSA, acid phosphatase, alk phosphatase; testosterone level of <25 ng/dl

trospium (Rx)
(trose'pee-um)

Sanctura

Func. class.: Anticholinergic, overactive bladder product

Chem. class.: Muscarinic receptor antagonist

Pregnancy category C

Action: Relaxes smooth muscles in bladder by inhibiting acetylcholine effect on muscarinic receptors

Therapeutic Outcome: Absence of urinary distention, nocturia, frequency, urgency, incontinence

Uses: Overactive bladder (urinary frequency, urgency)

Dosage and routes
Adult: PO 20 mg bid, give 5 ml ≥1 hr prior to meals

Renal dose

Adult: PO CCr < 30 ml/min 20 mg daily at bedtime

Elderly ≥75 yr: PO titrate down to 20 mg daily based on response and tolerance

Available forms: Tabs 20 mg

Adverse effects
CNS: Fatigue, dizziness, headache

EENT: Dry eyes, vision abnormalities

GI: Flatulence, abdominal pain, *constipation, dry mouth*, dyspepsia

Contraindications: Hypersensitivity, uncontrolled narrow-angle glaucoma, urinary retention, gastric retention

Precautions: Pregnancy **C**, lactation, children, renal/hepatic disease, controlled narrow-angle glaucoma, ulcerative colitis, intestinal atony, myasthenia gravis

Pharmacokinetics

Absorption	Rapidly absorbed (10%)
Distribution	Protein bound (50–85%)
Metabolism	Not fully understood in humans Extensively metabolized
Excretion	Urine (6%)/feces (85%) Excreted in urine by active tubular secretion
Half-life	Unknown

Pharmacodynamics
Unknown

Interactions
Individual drugs

Alcohol: increased drowsiness

Drug/food

High fat meal: decreased absorption

NURSING CONSIDERATIONS
Assessment
- Assess urinary patterns: distention, nocturia, frequency, urgency, incontinence

Nursing diagnoses
- Urinary incontinence (uses)
- Knowledge, deficient (teaching)

Implementation
- Take 1 hr prior to meals or on empty stomach

Patient/family education
- Advise patient to avoid hazardous activities; dizziness may occur
- Caution patient that alcohol may increase drowsiness
- Inform patient about anticholinergic effects that may occur

Evaluation
Positive therapeutic outcome
- Correction of urinary status: absence of dysuria, frequency, nocturia, incontinence

! HIGH ALERT

tubocurarine (Rx)

(too-boh-cure'a-reen)

Tubarine ♣, Tubocuraine

Func. class.: Neuromuscular blocker non-depolarizing

Chem. class.: Synthetic curariform

Pregnancy category C

Action: Inhibits transmission of nerve impulses by binding with cholinergic receptor sites, antagonizing action of acetylcholine; no analgesic response

Therapeutic Outcome: Skeletal muscle paralysis during anesthesia

Uses: Facilitation of endotracheal intubation, skeletal muscle relaxation during mechanical ventilation, surgery, or general anesthesia

Dosage and routes

Adult: **IV** bol 0.2-0.6 mg/kg, then 0.04-0.1 mg/kg 20-45 min after 1st dose if needed for prolonged procedures

Available forms: Inj 3 mg/ml (20 U/ml)

Adverse effects

CV: Bradycardia, tachycardia, increased, decreased B/P

EENT: Increased secretions

INTEG: Rash, flushing, pruritus, urticaria

RESP: **Prolonged apnea, bronchospasm, cyanosis, respiratory depression,** wheezing

Contraindications: Hypersensitivity

Precautions: Pregnancy **C**, cardiac disease, lactation, children <2 yr, electrolyte imbalances, dehydration, neuromuscular disease, respiratory disease, renal/hepatic disease

Pharmacokinetics

Absorption	Complete bioavailability
Distribution	Extensive, crosses placenta
Metabolism	Liver, small amount
Excretion	Kidneys—unchanged (30%-75%), bile (11%)
Half-life	1-3 hr

Pharmacodynamics

	IV	IM
Onset	3-5 min, dose dependent	15-30 min
Peak	2-3 min	Unknown
Duration	½-1½ hr	Unknown

Interactions

Individual drugs

Amphotericin B, clindamycin, lidocaine, lithium, magnesium, polymyxin B, quindine, verapamil: increased paralysis, length and intensity

Enflurane, isoflurane, lincomycin, trimethaphan: increased neuromuscular blockade

Theophylline: dysrhythmias

Drug classifications

Aminoglycosides, loop diuretics: increased paralysis, length and intensity

Analgesics (opioid), anesthetics (local), antiinfectives (polymyxin), thiazides: increased neuromuscular blockade

NURSING CONSIDERATIONS

Assessment

- Monitor for electrolyte imbalances (potassium, magnesium) before drug is used; electrolyte imbalances may lead to increased action of this drug
- Monitor VS (B/P, pulse, respirations, airway) until fully recovered; rate, depth, pattern of respirations, strength of hand grip; patient should be intubated before use
- Monitor recovery: decreased paralysis of face, diaphragm, leg, arm, rest of body; residual weakness and respiratory problems may occur during recovery period
- Monitor allergic reactions: rash, fever, respiratory distress, pruritus; drug should be discontinued

Nursing diagnoses

- Breathing pattern, ineffective (uses)
- Communication, verbal, impaired (adverse reactions)
- Fear (adverse reactions)
- Knowledge, deficient (teaching)

Implementation

- Use peripheral nerve stimulator by anesthesiologist to determine neuromuscular blockade; deep tendon reflexes should be monitored during extended periods
- Give **IV** undiluted by direct **IV** over 1-1½ min (only by qualified person, usually an anesthesiologist)

Syringe compatibilities: Pentobarbital, thiopental

Additive incompatibilities: Barbiturates, sodium bicarbonate

Solution compatibilities: D_5, $D_{10}W$, 0.9% NaCl, 0.45% NaCl, Ringer's, LR, dextrose/Ringer's or dextrose/LR combinations

Patient/family education
- Provide patient reassurance if communication is difficult during recovery from neuromuscular blockade
- Provide explanation to patient regarding all procedures or treatments; patient will remain conscious if anesthesia is not given also

Evaluation
Positive therapeutic outcome
- Paralysis of jaw, eyelid, head, neck, rest of body as evaluated by peripheral nerve stimulator

Treatment of overdose: Edrophonium or neostigmine, atropine, monitor VS; patient may require mechanical ventilation

! HIGH ALERT

urokinase (Rx)
(yoor-oh-kin'ase)

Abbokinase, Abbokinase Open-Cath

Func. class.: Thrombolytic enzyme

Chem. class.: β-Hemolytic *Streptococcus* filtrate (purified)

Pregnancy category B

Action: Promotes thrombolysis by directly converting plasminogen to plasmin

Therapeutic Outcome: Lysis of emboli, or thrombosis in various parts of the body

Uses: Venous thrombosis, pulmonary embolism, arterial thrombosis, arterial embolism, arteriovenous cannula occlusion, lysis of coronary artery thrombi after MI

Dosage and routes
Lysis of pulmonary emboli

Adult and child: **IV** 4400 international units/kg/hr × 12-24 hr, not to exceed 200 ml; then **IV** heparin, then anticoagulants

Coronary artery thrombosis

Adult: Instill 6000 international units/min into occluded artery for 1-2 hr after giving **IV** bol of heparin 2500-10,000 units; may also give as **IV** inf of 2-3 million units over 45-90 min

Venous catheter occlusion

Adult and child: Instill 5000 international units into line, wait 5 min, then aspirate; repeat aspiration attempts q5 min × ½ hr; if occlusion has not been removed, then cap line and wait ½-1 hr, then aspirate; may need 2nd dose if still occluded

Available forms: Powder for inj, lyophilized: 250,000 international units/vial; powder for catheter clearance

Adverse effects
CNS: *Headache,* fever

CV: Hypotension, dysrhythmias

GI: *Nausea,* vomiting

HEMA: *Decreased Hct,* **bleeding**

INTEG: *Rash, urticaria,* phlebitis at **IV** inf site, itching, flushing

MS: Low back pain

RESP: Altered respirations, cyanosis, shortness of breath, **bronchospasm**

SYST: **GI, GU, intracranial, retroperitoneal bleeding**; surface bleeding; **anaphylaxis** (rare)

Contraindications: Hypersensitivity, internal active bleeding, intraspinal surgery, neoplasms of CNS, ulcerative colitis/enteritis, severe uncontrolled hypertension, renal disease, hepatic disease, hypocoagulation, COPD, subacute bacterial endocarditis, rheumatic valvular disease, cerebral embolism/thrombosis/hemorrhage, intraarterial diagnostic procedure or surgery (10 days), recent major surgery/trauma, aneurysm, AV malformation

Precautions: Pregnancy **B,** arterial emboli from left side of heart, hepatic disease

Pharmacokinetics	
Absorption	Completely
Distribution	Unknown
Metabolism	Liver
Excretion	Kidneys
Half-life	10-20 min

Pharmacodynamics	
Onset	Rapid
Peak	Rapid
Duration	12 hr

Interactions
Individual drugs

Abciximab, aspirin, clopidogrel, dipyridamole, eptifibatide, heparin, indomethacin, phenylbutazone, plicamycin, ticlopidine, tirofiban, valproic acid: increased bleeding potential

Drug classifications

Anticoagulants (oral), cephalosporins (some), NSAIDs: increased bleeding potential

Glycoprotein IIb, IIIa inhibitors: increased bleeding risk

Drug/lab test

Increased: protime, APTT, TT

NURSING CONSIDERATIONS

Assessment

- Monitor VS, B/P, pulse, respirations (including peripheral), neurologic signs, temp at least q4h; temp >104° F (40° C) indicates internal bleeding; monitor rhythm closely; ventricular dysrhythmias may occur with hyperfusion; monitor heart, breath sounds, neurologic status, peripheral pulses
- Assess for bleeding during 1st hr of treatment: hematuria, hematemesis, bleeding from mucous membranes, epistaxis, ecchymosis; guaiac, all body fluids, stools; blood studies (Hct, platelets, PTT, protime, TT, APTT) before starting therapy (protime or APTT must be less than 2 × control); TT or protime q3-4h during treatment
- Assess hypersensitivity: fever, rash, itching, chills, facial swelling, dyspnea; mild reaction may be treated with antihistamines; notify prescriber of severe reactions, stop drug, keep resuscitative equipment nearby
- Monitor ECG on monitor, watch for segment changes, changes in rhythm; sinus bradycardia, ventricular tachycardia, accelerated idioventricular rhythm may occur because of reperfusion

Nursing diagnoses

- Tissue perfusion, ineffective (uses)
- Injury, risk for (adverse reactions)
- Gas exchange, impaired (uses)

Implementation

Intermittent IV route

- Give **IV** loading dose over 30 min to avoid hypotension
- **IV** after dilution with 4-5 g/250 ml of 0.9% NaCl, D_5W, LR, give over 1 hr; may give by continuous inf after loading dose(s) of 1 g/hr diluted in 50-100 ml of compatible sol; use infusion pump; do not give by direct **IV**
- Give heparin therapy after thrombolytic therapy is discontinued, TT, ACT, or APTT less than 2 × control (about 3-4 hr)
- Avoid invasive procedures, inj, rectal temp
- Apply pressure for 30 sec to minor bleeding sites, 30 min to sites of atrial puncture, followed by pressure dressing; inform prescriber if this does not attain hemostasis
- Store powder at room temp or refrigerate; protect from excessive light

Additive incompatibilities: Do not mix with other medications

Patient/family education

- Teach patient reason for medication, signs and symptoms of bleeding, allergic reactions, when to notify health care prescriber

Evaluation

Positive therapeutic outcome

- Lysis of thrombi or emboli

valacyclovir (Rx)

(val-a-sye'kloh-vir)

Valtrex

Func. class.: Antiviral

Chem. class.: Acyclic purine nucleoside analog

Pregnancy category B

Do Not Confuse:
Valtrex/Valcyte, valacyclovir/valganciclovir

Action: Interferes with DNA synthesis by conversion to acyclovir, causing decreased viral replication, time of lesional healing

Therapeutic Outcome: Absence of itching, painful lesions; crusting and healing of lesions

Uses: Treatment or suppression of herpes zoster, recurrent genital herpes, herpes labialis

Investigational uses: Prevention of cytomegalovirus infection, in advanced HIV posttransplant patients

Dosage and routes

Genital herpes (suppressive initial)

Adult: PO 1 g bid × 10 days initially

Genital herpes (recurrent episodes)

Adult: PO 500 mg bid × 3 days

Genital herpes (suppressive therapy)

Adult: PO 1 g daily with normal immune function; 500 mg daily for those with ≤9 recurrences/yr; 500 mg bid in HIV-infected patients with CD4 ≥100

Herpes zoster

Adult: PO 1 g tid × 1 wk

Herpes labialis

Adult: PO 2 g bid × 1 day

Renal dose

Adult: PO CCr 30-49 ml/min 1g q12h (herpes zoster); 1 g q12h × 1 day (herpes labalis); CCr 10-29 ml/min 1 g q24h (genital herpes/herpes zoster); 500 mg q24h (recurrent genital herpes); CCr <10 ml/min 500 mg q24h (genital herpes/herpes zoster), 500 mg q24h (recurrent genital herpes)

Available forms: Tabs 500, 1000 mg

Adverse effects

CNS: Tremors, lethargy, *dizziness, headache, weakness,* depression
ENDO: *Dysmennorhea*
GI: *Nausea, vomiting, diarrhea, abdominal pain, constipation,* increased AST
HEMA: Thrombocytopenic purpura, hemolytic uremic syndrome
INTEG: *Rash*

Contraindications: Hypersensitivity to this drug or acyclovir

Precautions: Pregnancy **B,** lactation, hepatic disease, renal disease, electrolyte imbalance, dehydration, elderly

Pharmacokinetics	
Absorption	Unknown
Distribution	Crosses placenta, enters breast milk
Metabolism	Converts to acyclovir
Excretion	Urine, as acyclovir
Half-life	2½-3½ hr

Pharmacodynamics	
Onset	Unknown
Peak	Unknown
Duration	Unknown

Interactions
Individual drugs
Cimetidine, probenecid: increased blood levels of valacyclovir

NURSING CONSIDERATIONS
Assessment
- Assess for signs of infection; characteristics of lesions; therapy should be started at first sign of herpes and is most effective within 72 h of outbreak
- Assess C&S before drug therapy; drug may be performed as soon as culture is performed; repeat C&S after treatment; determine the presence of other sexually transmitted diseases
- Assess bowel pattern before, during treatment
- Assess for skin eruptions: rash
- Assess allergies before treatment, reaction of each medication
- ❗ Assess for thrombocytopenic purpura, hemolytic uremic syndrome, may be fatal

Nursing diagnoses
- Infection, risk for (uses)

Implementation
- Give within 72 hr of outbreak
- Give orally before infection occurs

Patient/family education
- Advise patient to take as prescribed; if dose is missed, take as soon as remembered up to 2 hr before next dose; do not double dose
- Instruct patient to take drug orally before infection occurs; drug should be taken when itching or pain occurs, usually before eruptions
- Inform patient that partners need to be told that patient has herpes; they can become infected; condoms must be worn to prevent reinfections
- Tell patient that drug does not cure infection, just controls symptoms and does not prevent infection to others

Evaluation
Positive therapeutic outcome
- Absence of itching, painful lesions; crusting and healed lesions

Treatment of overdose:
- Discontinue drug
- Provide hemodialysis, resuscitation if needed

valganciclovir (Rx)
(val-gan-sy'kloh-veer)
Valcyte
Func. class: Antiviral
Chem. class: Synthetic nucleoside analog
Pregnancy category C

Do Not Confuse:
Valcyte/Valtrex, valganciclovir/valacyclovir

Action: Valganciclovir is metabolized to ganciclovir; inhibits replication of human cytomegalovirus in vivo and in vitro by selectively inhibiting viral DNA synthesis

Therapeutic Outcome: Decreased proliferation of virus responsible for CMV retinitis

Uses: Cytomegalovirus (CMV) retinitis in immunocompromised persons, including those with AIDS, after indirect ophthalmoscopy confirms diagnosis; prevention of CMV in transplantation

Dosage and routes
Treatment of CMV
Adult: PO induction 900 mg bid × 21 days with food; maintenance 900 mg daily with food

Transplant
Adult: PO 900 mg daily with food starting within 10 days of transplantation until 100 days post transplantation

Renal dose

CCr ≥60 ml/min same dosage as above; CCr 40-59 ml/min 450 mg bid, then 450 mg daily; CCr 25-39 ml/min 450 mg daily, then 450 mg q2 days; CCr 10-24 ml/min 450 mg q2 days, then 450 mg 2×/ week

Available forms: Tabs 450 mg

Adverse effects

CNS: *Fever*, chills, **coma**, *confusion*, abnormal thoughts, dizziness, bizarre dreams, *headache*, psychosis, tremors, somnolence, *paresthesia, weakness,* **seizures**
EENT: Retinal detachment in CMV retinitis
GI: *Abnormal liver function tests, nausea, vomiting, anorexia, diarrhea, abdominal pain,* **hemorrhage**
GU: **Hematuria**, increased creatinine, BUN
HEMA: **Granulocytopenia, thrombocytopenia, irreversible neutropenia, anemia, eosinophilia**
INTEG: *Rash*, alopecia, *pruritus*, urticaria, pain at inj site, phlebitis, **Stevens-Johnson syndrome**
MISC: Local and systemic infections and sepsis

Contraindications: Hypersensitivity to acyclovir or ganciclovir, absolute neutrophil count <500/mm^3, platelet count <25,000/mm^3, hemodialysis

Precautions: Pregnancy **C**, preexisting cytopenias, renal function impairment, lactation, children <6 mo, elderly

Pharmacokinetics	
Absorption	Well absorbed from GI tract
Distribution	Plasma protein binding unknown; crosses blood-brain barrier, CSF
Metabolism	Rapidly metabolized in intestinal wall and liver to ganciclovir
Excretion	Kidneys (ganciclovir)
Half-life	3-4½ hr

Pharmacodynamics	
Onset	Unknown
Peak	1-3 hr
Duration	Unknown

Interactions

Individual drugs

Adriamycin, amphotericin B, cycloSPORINE, dapsone, DOXOrubicin, flucytosine, pentamidine, trimethoprim/sulfamethoxazole, vinBLAStine, vinCRIStine: increased toxicity
Didanosine: decreased effect
Imipenem/cilastatin: increased seizures
Probenecid: decreased renal clearance of valganciclovir
Radiation, zidovudine: severe granulocytopenia; do not coadminister

Drug classifications

Antineoplastics: severe granulocytopenia; do not coadminister
Nucleoside analogs, other: increased toxicity

NURSING CONSIDERATIONS

Assessment

- Assess for leukopenia/neutropenia/thrombocytopenia: WBCs, platelets q2 days during 2×/day dosing and then qwk
- Assess for leukopenia daily with WBC count in patients with prior leukopenia using other nucleoside analogs or for whom leukopenia counts are <1000 cells/mm^3 at start of treatment
- Assess serum creatinine or CCr ≥q2 wk

Nursing diagnoses

- Infection, risk for (uses)
- Injury, risk for (uses, adverse reactions)
- Knowledge, deficient (teaching)

Implementation

- Give with food

Patient/family education

- Inform patient that drug does not cure condition, that regular ophthalmologic and blood tests are necessary
- Caution patient that major toxicities may necessitate discontinuing drug
- Caution patient to use contraception during treatment and that infertility may occur; men should use barrier contraception for 90 days after treatment
- Instruct patient to take with food
- Instruct patient to report infection: fever, chills, sore throat; blood dyscrasias: bruising, bleeding, petechiae
- Advise patient to avoid crowds, persons with respiratory infections
- Caution patient to use sunscreen to prevent burns

Evaluation

Positive therapeutic outcome

- Decreased symptoms of CMV

Treatment of overdose: Maintain adequate hydration; dialysis may help reduce serum concentrations; consider use of hematopoietic growth factors

V

valproate (Rx)
(val-proh'ate)
Depacon

valproic acid (Rx)
Depakene, Myproic acid

divalproex sodium (Rx)
Depakote, Depakote ER, Epival
Func. class.: Anticonvulsant
Chem. class.: Carboxylic acid derivative

Pregnancy category D

Action: Increases levels of γ-aminobutyric acid (GABA) in brain, which decreases seizure activity

Therapeutic Outcome: Decreased symptoms of epilepsy, bipolar disorder

Uses: Simple (petit mal), complex (petit mal), absence, mixed seizures, manic episode associated with bipolar disorder, prophylaxis of migraine, adjunct in schizophrenia, tardive dyskinesia, aggression in children with ADHD, organic brain syndrome

Investigational uses: Tonic-clonic (grand mal), myoclonic seizures; rectal (valproic acid) for seizures

Dosage and routes
Epilepsy
Adult and child: PO 10-15 mg/kg/day divided in 2-3 doses, may increase by 5-10 mg/kg/day qwk, max 60 mg/kg/day in 2-3 divided doses; **IV** ≤20 mg/min over 1 hr

Mania (divalproex sodium)
Adult: PO 750 mg daily in divided doses, max 60 mg/kg/day

Migraine (divalproex sodium)
Adult: PO 250 mg bid, may increase to 1000 mg/day; or 500 mg (Depakote ER) daily × 7 days, then 1000 mg daily

Available forms: Valproic acid: caps 250 mg; divalproex: delayed rel tabs 125, 250, 500 mg; ext rel tabs 250, 500 mg; sprinkle caps 125 mg; valproate: inj 100 mg/ml; syr 250 mg/5 ml

Adverse effects
CNS: *Sedation, drowsiness,* dizziness, headache, incoordination, depression, hallucinations, behavioral changes, tremors, aggression, weakness
EENT: Visual disturbances, taste perversion
GI: *Nausea, vomiting, constipation, diarrhea, dyspepsia,* anorexia, cramps, **hepatic failure, pancreatitis, toxic hepatitis,** stomatitis
GU: Enuresis, irregular menses
HEMA: **Thrombocytopenia, leukopenia, lymphocytosis,** increased protime, bruising, epistaxis
INTEG: *Rash,* alopecia, photosensitivity, dry skin

Contraindications: Pregnancy **D**, hypersensitivity, hepatic disease

Precautions: Lactation, child <2 yr, elderly

Pharmacokinetics	
Absorption	Unknown
Distribution	Breast milk, crosses placenta, widely distributed
Metabolism	Liver
Excretion	Kidneys
Half-life	9-16 hr

Pharmacodynamics	
Onset	15-30 min
Peak	1-4 hr
Duration	4-6 hr

Interactions
Individual drugs
Abciximab, cefamandole, cefoperazone, cefotetan, eptifibatide, heparin, tirofiban: increased bleeding risk
Alcohol: increased CNS depression
Carbamazipine, ethosuximide, lamotrigine, zidovudine: increased toxicity of these drugs
Cimetidine: decreased metabolism of valproic acid
Chlorpromazine, erythromycin, felbamate: increased valproic acid
Phenytoin: increased action of phenytoin
Rifampin, carbamazepine, lamotrigine: decreased valproic acid level
Warfarin: increased warfarin effect

Drug classifications
Antihistamines, barbiturates, MAOIs, opioids, sedative/hypnotics: increased CNS depression
Antiplatelets, NSAIDs, thrombolytics: increased bleeding risk
Salicylates: increased valproic acid effect

Drug/lab test
False positive: ketones
Interference: thyroid function tests

NURSING CONSIDERATIONS
Assessment
- Monitor blood studies: Hct, Hgb, RBC, serum folate, platelets, protime, vit D if on long-term therapy
- Monitor hepatic studies: AST, ALT, bilirubin, creatinine, failure

- Monitor blood levels: therapeutic level 50-100 mcg/ml
- Assess seizure disorder: location, aura, activity, duration; seizure precautions should be in place
- Assess bipolar disorder: mood, activity, sleeping, eating, behavior
- Assess migraines: frequency, intensity
- Assess respiratory dysfunction: respiratory depression, character, rate, rhythm; hold drug if respirations are <12/min or if pupils are dilated

Nursing diagnoses
- Injury, risk for (uses, adverse reactions)
- Knowledge, deficient

Implementation
- Swallow tabs and caps whole; do not break, crush, or chew
- Give elixir alone; do not dilute with carbonated beverage; do not give syrup to patients on sodium restriction
- Give with food or milk to decrease GI symptoms

Patient/family education
- Teach patient that physical dependency may result from extended use
- Instruct patient to avoid driving, other activities that require alertness
- Advise patient not to discontinue medication quickly after long-term use; seizures may result
- Advise patient to report visual disturbances, rash, diarrhea, light-colored stools, jaundice, protracted vomiting to prescriber

Evaluation
Positive therapeutic outcome
- Decreased seizures

valrubicin (Rx)
(val-roo'bih-sin)
Valstar
Func. class.: Antineoplastic, antibiotic
Chem. class.: Anthracycline glycoside
Pregnancy category C

Action: A semisynthetic analog of DOXOrubicin that inhibits DNA synthesis primarily; replication is decreased by binding to DNA, which causes strand splitting; active throughout entire cell cycle; a vesicant

Therapeutic Outcome: Decreased symptoms of breast cancer

Uses: Bladder cancer

Dosage and routes
Adult: Intravesically 800 mg qwk × 6 wk, delay administration ≥2 wk after transurethral resection or fulguration

Available forms: Sol for intravesical instillation 40 mg/ml

Adverse effects
CV: *Chest pain*
GI: *Nausea, vomiting, anorexia, diarrhea*
GU: *UTI, urinary retention, hematuria*
HEMA: **Thrombocytopenia, leukopenia,** *anemia*
INTEG: *Rash*

Contraindications: Hypersensitivity to anthracyclines or Cremophor EL, urinary tract infection, small bladder

Precautions: Pregnancy **C**, lactation, children

Pharmacokinetics	
Absorption	Unknown
Distribution	Penetrates bladder wall
Metabolism	Unknown
Excretion	Unknown
Half-life	Unknown

Pharmacodynamics	
Onset	Unknown
Peak	Unknown
Duration	Unknown

Interactions: Unknown

NURSING CONSIDERATIONS
Assessment
- Monitor I&O ratio; report fall in urine output of <30 ml/hr
- Monitor temp q4h; fever may indicate beginning of infection
- Monitor local irritation, pain, burning at injection site

Nursing diagnoses
- Infection, risk for (side effects)
- Nutrition: less than body requirements, imbalanced (side effects)
- Knowledge, deficient (teaching)

Implementation
- Administer after urinary catheter is inserted under aseptic conditions, drain bladder and instill the diluted 75 ml of valrubicin by gravity for several min, withdraw catheter; drug should be retained for 2 hr, then void
- Use procedure for handling and disposal of cytotoxic agents

V

- Do not use polyvinyl chloride (PVC) **IV** tubing
- Prepare/store valrubicin sol in glass, polypropylene, or polyolefin tubing/containers
- For instillation, 5-ml vials (200 mg valrubicin/5-ml vial) should be warmed to room temp, withdraw 20 ml from the 4 vials and dilute with 55 ml of 0.9% NaCl inj to 75 ml of diluted valrubicin sol
- Valrubicin sol is clear red, at lower temps a waxy precipitate may form, warm in hand until sol is clear
- Perform strict hand-washing technique; use gloves, protective clothing
- Provide increased fluid intake to 2 L/day to prevent urate, calculi formation
- Store at room temp for 12 hr after reconstituting

Patient/family education
- Advise patient to report any complaints, side effects to nurse or prescriber
- Advise patient to consume fluids to 2 L/day unless contraindicated
- Teach patient that urine and other body fluids may be red-orange for 48 hr
- Teach patient that contraceptive measures are recommended during therapy

Evaluation
Positive therapeutic outcome
- Decreased tumor size, spread of malignancy

valsartan (Rx)
(val-zar'tan)
Diovan
Func. class.: Antihypertensive
Chem. class.: Angiotensin II receptor antagonist (type AT_1)
Pregnancy category D

Action: Blocks the vasoconstrictor and aldosterone-secreting effects of angiotensin II; selectively blocks the binding of angiotensin II to the AT_1 receptor found in tissues

Therapeutic Outcome: Decreased B/P

Uses: Hypertension, alone or in combination, CHF

Dosage and routes
Adult: PO 80-160 mg daily alone or in combination with other antihypertensives, may increase to 320 mg CHF

CHF
Adult: PO 40 mg bid, up to 60 mg bid

Available forms: Tabs 80, 160, 320 mg

Adverse effects
CNS: *Dizziness, insomnia,* drowsiness, vertigo, headache, fatigue
CV: Angina pectoris, 2nd-degree AV block, **cerebrovascular accident,** hypotension, **MI, dysrhythmias**
EENT: Conjunctivitis
GI: Diarrhea, abdominal pain, nausea, **hepatotoxicity**
GU: Impotence, **nephrotoxicity**
HEMA: *Anemia,* neutropenia
META: Hyperkalemia
MS: Cramps, myalgia, pain, stiffness
RESP: *Cough*

Contraindications: Pregnancy **D** (2nd/3rd trimester), hypersensitivity, severe hepatic disease, bilateral renal artery stenosis

Precautions: Hypersensitivity to angiotensin-converting enzyme inhibitors, CHF, hypertrophic cardiomyopathy, aortic/mitral valve stenosis, CAD; lactation, children, elderly

Pharmacokinetics	
Absorption	Well absorbed
Distribution	Bound to plasma proteins
Metabolism	Extensive
Excretion	Feces, urine, breast milk
Half-life	9 hr

Pharmacodynamics	
Onset	Unknown
Peak	2 hr
Duration	24 hr

Interactions: None significant

Drug/herb
Aconite: increased toxicity, death
Astragalus, cola tree: increased or decreased antihypertensive effect
Barberry, betony, black catechu, black cohosh, bloodroot, broom, burdock, cat's claw, dandelion, goldenseal, Irish moss, Jamaican dogwood, kelp, khella, mistletoe, parsley: increased antihypertensive effect
Coltsfoot, guarana, khat, licorice: decreased antihypertensive effect

NURSING CONSIDERATIONS
Assessment
- Assess B/P, pulse q4h; note rate, rhythm, quality
- Monitor electrolytes: potassium, sodium, chloride; total CO_2
- Obtain baselines in renal, liver function tests before therapy begins

- Assess blood studies: BUN, creatinine, before treatment
- Monitor for edema in feet, legs daily
- Assess for skin turgor, dryness of mucous membranes for hydration status

Nursing diagnoses
- Fluid volume, deficient (side effects)
- Noncompliance (teaching)
- Knowledge, deficient (teaching)

Implementation
- Administer without regard to meals

Patient/family education
- Teach patient not to take this drug if breast-feeding or pregnant, or have had an allergic reaction to this drug
- If a dose is missed, instruct patient to take as soon as possible, unless it is within an hour before next dose
- Advise patient to comply with dosage schedule, even if feeling better
- Teach patient to notify prescriber of fever, swelling of hands or feet, irregular heartbeat, chest pain
- Advise patient excessive perspiration, dehydration, diarrhea may lead to fall in blood pressure; consult prescriber if these occur
- Inform patient that drug may cause dizziness, fainting; light-headedness may occur
- Caution patient to rise slowly to sitting or standing position to minimize orthostatic hypotension

Evaluation
Positive therapeutic outcome
- Decreased B/P

vancomycin
(van-koe-mye'sin)

Lyphocin, Vancocin, Vancoled, vancomycin HCl

Func. clas.: Antiinfective—miscellaneous
Chem. class.: Tricyclic glycopeptide

Pregnancy category C

Action: Inhibits bacterial cell wall synthesis

Therapeutic Outcome: Bactericidal for the following organisms: staphylococci, streptococci, *Corynebacterium, Clostridium*

Uses: Resistant staphylococcal infections, pseudomembranous colitis, staphylococcal enterocolitis, group A β-hemolytic streptococci, endocarditis prophylaxis for dental procedures, diphtheroid endocarditis

Dosage and routes
Serious staphylococcal infections
Adult: **IV** 500 mg (7.5 mg/kg) q6-8h or 1 g (15 mg/kg) q12h
Child: **IV** 40 mg/kg/day divided q6-8h
Neonates: **IV** 15 mg/kg initially followed by 10 mg/kg q8-24h

Pseudomembranous/ staphylococcal enterocolitis
Adult: PO 500 mg in 3 divided doses for 7-10 days
Child: PO 40 mg/kg/day divided q6h, max 2 g/day

Endocarditis prophylaxis for dental procedure
Adult: **IV** 1 g over 1 hr, 1 hr before dental procedure
Child: **IV** 20 mg/kg over 1 hr, 1 hr before procedure

Available forms: Pulvules 125, 250 mg; powder for oral sol 1, 10 g; powder for inj **IV** 500 mg; vials 1, 5, 10 g

Adverse effects
CV: **Cardiac arrest, vascular collapse** (rare)
EENT: *Ototoxicity, permanent deafness,* tinnitus
GI: **Nausea, pseudomembranous colitis**
GU: **Nephrotoxicity: increased BUN, creatinine, albumin, fatal uremia**
HEMA: **Leukopenia, eosinophilia, neutropenia**
INTEG: Chills, fever, rash, thrombophlebitis at inj site, urticaria, pruritus, necrosis (Red man's syndrome)
RESP: Wheezing, dyspnea
SYST: **Anaphylaxis**

Contraindications: Hypersensitivity, previous hearing loss

Precautions: Pregnancy **C,** renal disease, lactation, elderly, neonates

Pharmacokinetics	
Absorption	Poorly absorbed (PO), completely absorbed (**IV**)
Distribution	Widely distributed, crosses placenta
Metabolism	Liver
Excretion	PO—feces, **IV**—kidneys
Half-life	4-8 hr

Pharmacodynamics

	IV
Onset	Immediate
Peak	Inf end

Interactions
Individual drugs
Amphotericin B, bacitracin, cisplatin, colistin, polymyxin B: increased ototoxicity or nephrotoxicity
Drug classifications
Aminoglycosides, cephalosporins, nondepolarizing muscle relaxants: increased ototoxicity or nephrotoxicity

NURSING CONSIDERATIONS
Assessment
- Monitor I&O ratio; report hematuria, oliguria because nephrotoxicity may occur
- Monitor any patient with compromised renal system (BUN, creatinine); drug is excreted slowly in poor renal system function; toxicity may occur rapidly
- Monitor blood studies: WBC; serum levels; peak 1 hr after 1-hr inf 25-40 mg/ml; trough before next dose 5-10 mg/ml
- Obtain C&S before drug therapy; drug may be given as soon as culture is performed
- Assess auditory function during, after treatment; hearing loss, ringing, roaring in ears; drug should be discontinued
- Monitor B/P during administration; sudden drop may indicate Red man's syndrome
- Assess for signs of infection
- Assess respiratory status: rate, character, wheezing, tightness in chest
- Identify allergies before treatment, reaction of each medication

Nursing diagnoses
- Infection, risk for (uses)
- Knowledge, deficient (teaching)

Implementation
- Give antihistamine if Red man's syndrome occurs: decreased B/P, flushing of neck, face
- Give dose based on serum concentration
- Give in equal intervals around the clock to maintain blood levels
- Store at room temp for up to 2 wk after reconstitution
- Have adrenalin, suction, tracheostomy set, endotracheal intubation equipment on unit; anaphylaxis may occur
- Provide adequate intake of fluids (2 L) to prevent nephrotoxicity

IV route
- Give after reconstitution with 10 ml of sterile water for inj (500 mg/10 ml); further dilution is needed for **IV**, 500 mg/100 ml of 0.9% NaCl, D_5W given as intermittent inf over 1 hr; decrease rate of infusion if red man's syndrome occurs

Y-site compatibilities: Acyclovir, allopurinol, amiodarone, amsacrine, atracurium, cyclophosphamide, diltiazem, enalaprilat, esmolol, filgrastim, fluconazole, fludarabine, gallium, granisetron, hydromorphone, insulin (regular), labetalol, lorazepam, magnesium sulfate, melphalan, meperidine, meropenem, midazolam, morphine, ondansetron, paclitaxel, pancuronium, perphenazine, propofol, sodium bicarbonate, tacrolimus, teniposide, theophylline, thiotepa, tolazoline, vecuronium, vinorelbine, warfarin, zidovudine

Additive compatibilities: Amikacin, atracurium, calcium gluconate, cefepime, cimetidine, corticotropin, dimenhyDRINATE, hydrocortisone, meropenem, ofloxacin, potassium chloride, ranitidine, verapamil, vit B/C

Patient/family education
- Teach patient aspects of drug therapy: need to complete entire course of medication to ensure organism death (7-10 days); culture may be performed after completed course of medication
- Advise patient to report sore throat, fever, fatigue; could indicate superinfection
- Instruct patient that drug must be taken in equal intervals around clock to maintain blood levels

Evaluation
Positive therapeutic outcome
- Absence of fever, sore throat
- Negative culture after treatment

vardenafil (Rx)
(var-den'a-fil)

Levitra

Func. class.: Impotence agent

Chem. class.: Phosphodiesterase type 5 inhibitor

Pregnancy category B

Action: Inhibits phosphodiesterase type 5 (PDE5); enhances erectile function by increasing the amount of cGMP, which causes smooth muscle relaxation and increased blood flow into the corpus cavernosum

Therapeutic Outcome: Erection

Uses: Treatment of erectile dysfunction

Dosage and routes

Adult: PO 10 mg, taken 1 hr before sexual activity, dose may be reduced to 5 mg or increased to a max of 20 mg; max dosing frequency is once daily

Elderly >65 yr: PO 5 mg initially

Hepatic dose (Child-Pugh B)

Adult: PO 5 mg, max 10 mg

Concomitant medications

Ritonavir, max 2.5 mg q72 hr; for indinavir, ketoconazole 400 mg/day and itraconazole 400 mg/day, max 2.5 mg/day; for ketoconazole 200 mg/day, itraconazole 200 mg/day and erythromycin max 5 mg/day

Available forms: Tabs 2.5, 5, 10, 20 mg

Adverse effects

CNS: *Headache, flushing, dizziness, insomnia*

CV: Hypertension, **MI, CV collapse**

EENT: Conjunctivitis, tinnitus, photophobia, diminished vision, glaucoma

GU: Abnormal ejaculation, priapism

MISC: Rash, GERD, GGTP increased, **NAION (nonarteritic ischemic optic neuropathy)**

MS: Myalgia, arthralgia, neck pain

RESP: Rhinitis, sinusitis, dyspnea, pharyngitis, epistaxis

Contraindications: Hypersensitivity, coadministration of α-blockers or nitrates, renal failure

Precautions: Pregnancy **B**, hepatic impairment, retinitis pigmentosa, cardiovascular disease including congenital or acquired QT prolongation, anatomic penile deformities, sickle cell anemia, leukemia, multiple myeloma, not indicated for women, children, or newborns

Pharmacokinetics	
Absorption	Rapid; reduced absorption with high-fat meal
Distribution	Bioavailability 15%; protein binding 95%
Metabolism	Liver
Excretion	Primarily in feces (91%-95%)
Half-life	4-5 hr

Pharmacodynamics	
Onset	20 min
Peak	½-1½ hr
Duration	<5 hr

Interactions

Individual drugs

Cimetidine, erythromycin, itraconazole, ketoconazole: increased levels

Indinavir, ritonavir: decreased protease inhibitor effect

NIFEdipine: decreased B/P

Drug classifications

α-Blockers, protease inhibitors: do not use concurrently

Do not use with nitrates because of unsafe decrease in B/P that could result in heart attack or stroke

NURSING CONSIDERATIONS

Assessment

- Assess for use of organic nitrates that should not be used with this drug
- Assess for severe loss of vision while taking this or any similar products; these products should not be used if vision loss has occurred

Nursing diagnoses

- Sexual dysfunction (uses)
- Knowledge, deficient (teaching)

Implementation

- Give approximately 1 hr before sexual activity, do not use more than once a day

Patient/family education

- Advise that drug does not protect against sexually transmitted diseases, including HIV
- Teach that drug absorption is reduced with a high-fat meal
- Instruct that drug should not be used with nitrates in any form
- Inform that drug has no effect in the absence of sexual stimulation
- Teach that patient should seek immediate medical attention if erections last for more than 4 hr
- Advise to inform physician of all medications being taken
- Teach patient to notify prescriber immediately and stop taking product if vision loss occurs

Evaluation

Positive therapeutic outcome

- Sustainable erection

vasopressin (Rx)

(vay-soe-press'in)

Pitressin Synthetic

Func. class.: Pituitary hormone

Chem. class.: Lysine vasopressin

Pregnancy category C

Action: Promotes reabsorption of water by action on renal tubular epithelium, causes vasoconstriction on muscles in the GI system

Therapeutic Outcome: Increased

V

osmolality, decreased urine output in diabetes insipidus

Uses: Diabetes insipidus (nonnephrogenic/nonpsychogenic), abdominal distention postoperatively, bleeding esophageal varices

Dosage and routes

Diabetes insipidus

Adult: IM/SUBCUT 5-10 units bid-qid prn; IM/SUBCUT 2.5-5 units q2-3 days (Pitressin Tannate) for chronic therapy

Child: IM/SUBCUT 2.5-10 units bid-qid prn; IM/SUBCUT 1.25-2.5 units q2-3 days (Pitressin Tannate) for chronic therapy

Abdominal distention

Adult: IM 5 units, then q3-4 hr, increasing to 10 units if needed (aqueous)

Available forms: Inj 20, 5 units/ml (tannate), spray, cotton pledgets

Adverse effects

CNS: Drowsiness, headache, lethargy, flushing
CV: Increased B/P
EENT: Nasal irritation, congestion, rhinitis
GI: Nausea, heartburn, cramps
GU: Vulval pain, uterine cramping
MISC: Tremor, sweating, vertigo, urticaria, bronchial constriction

Contraindications: Hypersensitivity, chronic nephritis

Precautions: Pregnancy **C**, CAD, lactation

Pharmacokinetics

Absorption	Erratically absorbed (IM)
Distribution	Widely distributed extracellular fluid
Metabolism	Liver—rapidly
Excretion	Kidneys—unchanged
Half-life	10-20 min

Pharmacodynamics

	IV	IM
Onset	Unknown	1 hr
Peak	Unknown	Unknown
Duration	3-8 hr	3-8 hr

NURSING CONSIDERATIONS

Assessment

- Monitor nasal mucosa for irritation if given by intranasal spray
- Assess intranasal use: nausea, congestion, cramps, headache; usually decreased with decreased dose
- Monitor pulse, B/P when giving drug **IV** or SUBCUT
- Monitor I&O ratio, weight daily; check for edema in extremities; if water retention is severe, diuretic may be prescribed; check for water intoxication: lethargy, behavioral changes, disorientation, neuromuscular excitability

Nursing diagnoses

- Fluid volume, excess (side effects)
- Fluid volume, deficit (uses)
- Knowledge, deficient (teaching)

Implementation

IM/SUBCUT route

- May be given IM/SUBCUT for diagnosis of diabetes insipidus
- Give patient 16 oz water at administration to prevent nausea, vomiting, cramping

Patient/family education

- Teach patient technique for nasal instillation: to insert tube into nasal cavity to instill drug
- Caution patient to avoid OTC products for cough, hay fever because these preparations may contain epINEPHrine, decrease drug response; do not use with alcohol
- Advise patient to carry/wear emergency ID specifying therapy, disease process (diabetes insipidus)
- Teach patient to measure/record I&O
- Teach patient to avoid alcohol, all OTC medications unless approved by prescription

Evaluation

Positive therapeutic outcome

- Absence of severe thirst
- Decreased urine output, osmolality

! HIGH ALERT

vecuronium (Rx)

(ve-kure-oh'nee-yum)

Norcuron

Func. class.: Neuromuscular blocker, non-depolarizing

Chem. class.: Synthetic curariform

Pregnancy category C

Do Not Confuse:

Nocuron/Narcan

Action: Inhibits transmission of nerve impulses by binding with cholinergic receptor sites, antagonizing action of acetylcholine; no analgesic response

Therapeutic Outcome: Skeletal muscle paralysis during anesthesia

Uses: Facilitation of endotracheal intubation; skeletal muscle relaxation during mechanical ventilation, surgery, or general anesthesia

Dosage and routes

Adult and child **>9 yr:** **IV** bol 0.08-0.10 mg/kg, then 0.010-0.015 mg/kg for prolonged procedures

Available forms: 10 mg/5 ml vial

Adverse effects

CNS: Skeletal muscle weakness or paralysis (rarely)

INTEG: Urticaria

RESP: **Prolonged apnea, possible respiratory paralysis,** bronchospasm, tachycardia, flushing, wheezing

SYST: **Anaphylaxis**

Contraindications: Hypersensitivity

Precautions: Pregnancy **C**, cardiac disease, lactation, children <2 yr, electrolyte imbalances, dehydration, neuromuscular disease, respiratory, hepatic disease

Pharmacokinetics	
Absorption	Completely absorbed
Distribution	Rapid—to extracellular fluids
Metabolism	Liver (20%)
Excretion	Kidneys—unchanged (35%)
Half-life	1½ hr, increased in liver disease

Pharmacodynamics	
Onset	1 min
Peak	3-5 min
Duration	15-25 min (recovery index)

Interactions

Individual drugs

Amphotericin B, clindamycin, lithium, phenytoin, piperacillin, polymyxin B, quinidine, succinylcholine, verapamil: increased paralysis, length and intensity

Enflurane, isoflurane, lincomycin: increased neuromuscular blockade

Theophylline: dysrhythmias

Drug classifications

Aminoglycosides: increased paralysis, length and intensity

Analgesics (opioid), local anesthetics, thiazides: increased neuromuscular blockade

NURSING CONSIDERATIONS

Assessment

- Monitor for electrolyte imbalances (potassium, magnesium) before drug is used; electrolyte imbalances may lead to increased action of this drug
- Monitor patient's vital signs (B/P, pulse, respirations, airway) until fully recovered; rate, depth, pattern of respirations, strength of hand grip; patient should be intubated before use
- Monitor patient's recovery: decreased paralysis of face, diaphragm, leg, arm, rest of body; residual weakness and respiratory problems may occur during recovery period
- Monitor allergic reactions: rash, fever, respiratory distress, pruritus; drug should be discontinued

Nursing diagnoses

- Breathing pattern, ineffective (uses)
- Communication, verbal, impaired (adverse reactions)
- Fear (adverse reactions)
- Knowledge, deficient (teaching)

Implementation

- Use peripheral nerve stimulator by anesthesiologist to determine neuromuscular blockade; deep tendon reflexes should be monitored during extended periods
- Give by direct **IV** after reconstituting with bacteriostatic water, over 5 min, D_5W, 0.9% NaCl or LR
- Give by direct **IV** after reconstituting dose in 5-10 ml of provided diluent; give by titrating to patient response
- Give by continuous inf after diluting to 10-20 mg/100 ml and by titrating to patient response (only by qualified person, usually an anesthesiologist); do not administer IM
- Store in light-resistant area

Syringe incompatibilities: Barbiturates

Y-site compatibilities: Aminophylline, cefazolin, cefuroxime, cimetidine, diltiazem, DOBUTamine, DOPamine, epINEPHrine, esmolol, fentanyl, fluconazole, gentamicin, heparin, hydrocortisone, hydromorphone, isoproterenol, labetalol, lorazepam, midazolam, milrinone, morphine, niCARdipine, nitroglycerin, nitroprusside, norepinephrine, propofol, ranitidine, trimethoprim/sulfamethoxazole, vancomycin

Y-site incompatibilities: Barbiturates

Patient/family education

- Provide patient reassurance if communication is difficult during recovery from neuromuscular blockade
- Provide explanation to patients regarding all procedures or treatments; patient will remain conscious if anesthesia is not given also

Evaluation

Positive therapeutic outcome

- Paralysis of jaw, eyelid, head, neck, rest of body as evaluated by peripheral nerve stimulator

V

Treatment of overdose: Edrophonium or neostigmine, atropine, monitor VS; may require mechanical ventilation

venlafaxine (Rx)

(ven-la-fax'een)

Effexor, Effexor XR

Func. class.: Second-generation antidepressant—miscellaneous

Pregnancy category C

Action: Potent inhibitor of neuronal serotonin and norepinephrine uptake, weak inhibitor of dopamine; no muscarinic, histaminergic, or α-adrenergic receptors in vitro

Therapeutic Outcome: Relief of depression

Uses: Prevention/treatment of major depression, to treat depression at end of life, long-term treatment of generalized anxiety disorder, social anxiety disorder

Investigational uses: Hot flashes, obsessive-compulsive disorder (OCD), premenstrual dysphoric disorder (PMDD), posttraumatic stress disorder (PTSD)

Dosage and routes

Depression

Adult: PO 75 mg/day in 2 or 3 divided doses; taken with food, may be increased to 150 mg/day; if needed may be further increased to 225 mg/day; increments of 75 mg/day should be made at intervals of no less than 4 days; some hospitalized patients may require up to 375 mg/day in 3 divided doses; ext rel 37.5-75 mg PO daily, max 225 mg/day; give Effexor XR daily

Hepatic dose

Moderate impairment 50% of dose

Renal dose

Mild to moderate impairment 75% of dose

Hot flashes (investigational)

Adult: PO 12.5 mg bid × 4 wk or ext rel cap 37.5 mg × 4 wk

Available forms: Tabs scored (Effexor) 25, 37.5, 50, 75, 100 mg; ext rel caps (Effexor XR) 37.5, 75, 150 mg

Adverse effects

CNS: *Emotional lability, vertigo,* apathy, ataxia, CNS stimulation, euphoria, hallucinations, hostility, increased libido, hypertonia, hypotonia, psychosis, insomnia, anxiety, **suicidal ideation in children/adolescents, seizures**

CV: *Migraine,* angina pectoris, extrasystoles, postural hypotension, syncope, thrombophlebitis, hypertension

EENT: *Abnormal vision,* taste, *ear pain,* cataract, conjunctivitis, corneal lesions, dry eyes, otitis media, photophobia

GI: *Dysphagia, eructation,* colitis, gastritis, gingivitis, **rectal hemorrhage,** stomatitis, stomach and mouth ulceration, nausea, anorexia, dry mouth

GU: *Anorgasmia,* abnormal ejaculation, *dysuria, hematuria, metrorrhagia, vaginitis, impaired urination,* albuminuria, amenorrhea, kidney calculus, cystitis, nocturia, breast and bladder pain, polyuria, **uterine hemorrhage, vaginal hemorrhage,** moniliasis

INTEG: Ecchymosis, acne, alopecia, brittle nails, dry skin, photosensitivity

META: *Peripheral edema, weight loss or gain,* diabetes mellitus, edema, glycosuria, hyperlipemia, hypokalemia

MS: Arthritis, bone pain, bursitis, myasthenia tenosynovitis, arthralgia

RESP: *Bronchitis, dyspnea,* asthma, chest congestion, epistaxis, hyperventilation, laryngitis

SYST: *Malaise, neck pain,* enlarged abdomen, cyst, facial edema, hangover effect, hernia

Contraindications: Hypersensitivity, bipolar disorder

Precautions: Pregnancy **C,** mania, lactation, children, elderly, recent MI, cardiac disease, seizure disorder, hypertension

Pharmacokinetics

Absorption	Well absorbed
Distribution	Widely distributed, 27% protein binding
Metabolism	Liver—extensively
Excretion	Kidneys, 87%
Half-life	5-7 hr, 11-13 hr (active metabolite)

Pharmacodynamics

Unknown

Interactions

Individual drugs

Alcohol: increased CNS depression

Cimetidine: increased venlafaxine effect

Clozapine, desipramine, haloperidol, warfarin: increased levels of these drugs

Cyproheptadine: decreased venlafaxine effect

Indinavir: decreased effect of indinavir

Sibutramine, sumatriptan, trazadone: increased serotonin syndrome

Drug classifications
Antihistamines, opioids, sedative/hypnotics: increased CNS depression
MAOIs: hyperthermia, rigidity, rapid fluctuations of vital signs, mental status changes, neuroleptic malignant syndrome
Phenothiazines: increased toxicity

Drug/herb
Chamomile, hops, kava, lavender, skullcap, valerian: increased CNS depression
Corkwood, jimsonweed: increased anticholinergic effect
SAM-e, St. John's wort: serotonin syndrome
Yohimbe: increased hypertension

Drug/lab test
Increased: alkaline phosphatase, bilirubin, AST, ALT, BUN, creatinine, serum cholesterol, CPK, LDH

NURSING CONSIDERATIONS
Assessment
- Monitor B/P (lying, standing), pulse q4h; if systolic B/P drops 20 mm Hg hold drug, notify prescriber; take vital signs q4h in patients with CV disease
- Monitor blood studies: CBC, leukocytes, differential, cardiac enzymes if patient is receiving long-term therapy
- Monitor hepatic studies: AST, ALT, bilirubin
- Check weight qwk; weight loss or gain; appetite may increase, peripheral edema may occur
- Assess mental status: mood, sensorium, affect; increase in psychiatric symptoms: depression, panic; for suicidal ideation in children/adolescents
- Monitor urinary retention, constipation; constipation is more likely to occur in children or elderly
- Assess for withdrawal symptoms: headache, nausea, vomiting, muscle pain, weakness; do not usually occur unless drug was discontinued abruptly
- Identify alcohol consumption; if alcohol is consumed, hold dose

Nursing diagnoses
- Coping, ineffective (uses)
- Injury, risk for (side effects)
- Knowledge, deficient (teaching)
- Noncompliance (teaching)

Implementation
- Give with food or milk for GI symptoms
- Crush if patient is unable to swallow medication whole
- Store at room temp; do not freeze

Patient/family education
- Advise patient to notify prescriber of rash, hives, or allergic reactions
- Teach patient that therapeutic effects may take 2-3 wk
- Teach patient to use caution in driving or other activities requiring alertness because of drowsiness, dizziness, blurred vision; to avoid rising quickly from sitting to standing, especially elderly
- Teach patient to avoid alcohol ingestion, other CNS depressants
- Advise patient to avoid pregnancy, breastfeeding while taking this product

Evaluation
Positive therapeutic outcome
- Decreased depression
- Absence of suicidal thoughts

Treatment of overdose: ECG monitoring, induce emesis, lavage, activated charcoal, administer anticonvulsant

verapamil (Rx)
(ver-ap'a-mil)
Apo-Verap, Calan, Calan SR, Covera-HS, Isoptin, Isoptin SR, verapamil HCl, verapamil HCl SR, Verelan PM
Func. class.: Calcium-channel blocker; antihypertensive; antianginal
Chem. class.: Diphenylalkylamine
Pregnancy category C

Action: Inhibits calcium ion influx across cell membrane during cardiac depolarization; produces relaxation of coronary vascular smooth muscle; peripheral vascular smooth muscle; dilates coronary vascular arteries; increases myocardial oxygen delivery in patients with vasospastic angina

Therapeutic Outcome: Decreased angina pectoris, dysrhythmias, B/P

Uses: Chronic stable vasospastic, unstable angina; dysrhythmias, hypertension, supraventricular tachycardia, atrial flutter or fibrillation

Investigational uses: Prevention of migraine headaches, ventricular outflow obstruction in hypertrophic cardiomyopathy, recumbent nocturnal leg cramps

Dosage and routes
Angina
Adult: PO 80-120 mg tid, increase qwk

Dysrhythmias
Adult: PO 240-320 mg/day in 3-4 divided doses in digitalized patients

V

Adult: **IV** bol 5-10 mg (0.075-0.15 mg/kg) over 2 min, may repeat 10 mg (0.15 mg/kg) ½ hr after first dose
Child 1-15 yr: **IV** bol 0.1-0.3 mg/kg over >2 min, repeat in 30 min, not to exceed 5 mg in a single dose
Child 0-1 yr: **IV** bol 0.1-0.2 mg/kg over ≥2 min, may repeat after 30 min

Hypertension
Adult: PO 80 mg tid, may titrate upward; ext rel 120-240 mg/day as a single dose, may increase to 240-480 mg/day

Available forms: Tabs 40, 80, 120 mg; ext rel tabs, 120, 180, 240 mg; inj 2.5 mg/ml; ext rel caps: 100, 120, 180, 200, 240, 300 mg

Adverse effects
CNS: *Headache, drowsiness,* dizziness, anxiety, depression, weakness, asthenia, fatigue, insomnia, confusion, light-headedness
CV: *Edema,* **CHF,** bradycardia, hypotension, palpitations, AV block
GI: *Nausea,* diarrhea, gastric upset, *constipation,* elevated liver function studies
GU: Impotence, nocturia, polyuria, gynecomastia
INTEG: Rash, bruising
MISC: Gingival hyperplasia
SYST: **Stevens-Johnson syndrome**

Contraindications: Sick sinus syndrome, 2nd- or 3rd-degree heart block, hypotension <90 mm Hg systolic, cardiogenic shock, severe CHF

Precautions: Pregnancy **C**, CHF, hypotension, hepatic injury, lactation, children, renal disease, concomitant β-blocker therapy, elderly

Pharmacokinetics

Absorption	Well absorbed (PO)
Distribution	Not known
Metabolism	Liver—extensively
Excretion	Kidneys, (70%)
Half-life	Biphasic 4 min, 3-7 hr

Pharmacodynamics

	PO	PO-EXT REL	IV
Onset	1-2 hr	Unknown	1-5 min
Peak	½-1½ hr	5-7 hr	3-5 min
Duration	3-7 hr	24 hr	2 hr

Interactions
Individual drugs
Carbamazepine, cycloSPORINE, digoxin, theophylline: increased levels of each specific drug
Cimetidine: increased effect of verapamil
Fentanyl, prazosin, quinidine: increased hypotension
Lithium: decreased lithium levels
Drug classifications
Antihypertensive, nitrates, β-adrenergic blockers: increased effects of verapamil
Nondepolarizing muscle relaxants: increased effect
NSAIDs: decreased antihypertensive effect
Drug/herb
Barberry, betel palm, burdock, goldenseal, khat, lily of the valley, plantain: increased effect
Yohimbe: decreased effect
Drug/food
Grapefruit juice: increased hypotension
Drug/lab test
Increased: LFT, alkaline phosphatase, AST, ALT, BUN, creatinine, serum cholesterol

NURSING CONSIDERATIONS
Assessment
- Assess fluid volume status: I&O ratio and record; weight; distended red veins; crackles in lung; color; quality, sp gr of urine; skin turgor; adequacy of pulses; moist mucous membranes; bilateral lung sounds; peripheral pitting edema; dehydration symptoms of decreasing output, thirst, hypotension, dry mouth, and mucous membranes should be reported
- Monitor B/P and pulse, pulmonary capillary wedge pressure (PCWP), central venous pressure, index, often during inf; if B/P drops 30 mm Hg, stop inf and call prescriber
- Monitor ALT, AST, bilirubin daily; if these are elevated, hepatotoxicity is suspected
- Monitor if platelets are <150,000/mm^3, if so, drug is usually discontinued and another drug started
- Assess for extravasation; change site q48h
- Monitor cardiac status: B/P, pulse, respiration, ECG
- Monitor renal/hepatic studies during long-term treatment, serum potassium, periodically

Nursing diagnoses
- Cardiac output, decreased (uses)
- Knowledge, deficient (teaching)

Implementation
PO route
- Do not crush or chew ext rel products
- Cap may be opened and contents sprinkled on food; do not disscolve chew cap
- Give once a day before meals at bedtime; sus rel give with food to decrease GI symptoms

IV route

- Give by direct **IV** undiluted (Y-site, 3-way stopcock) over at least 2 min, or 3 min elderly; discard unused solution; to prevent serious hypotension, patient should be recumbent for 1 hr or more

Syringe compatibilities: Amrinone, heparin, milrinone

Y-site compatibilities: Aprofloxacin, dobutamine, DOPamine, famotidine, hydrALAZINE, inamrinone, meperidine, methicillin, milrinone, penicillin G potassium, piperacillin, propofol, ticarcillin

Y-site incompatibilities: Albumin, ampicillin, mezlocillin, nafcillin, oxacillin, sodium bicarbonate

Additive compatibilities: Amikacin, amiodarone, ascorbic acid, atropine, bretylium, calcium chloride, calcium gluconate, cefamandole, cefazolin, cefotaxime, cefoxitin, cephapirin, chloramphenicol, cimetidine, clindamycin, dexamethasone, diazepam, digoxin, DOPamine, epINEPHrine, erythromycin, gentamicin, heparin, hydrocortisone, hydromorphone, hydrocortisone sodium phosphate, insulin (regular), isoproterenol, lidocaine, magnesium sulfate, mannitol, meperidine, metaraminol, methicillin, methyldopate, methylPREDNISolone, metoclopramide, mezlocillin, morphine, moxalactam, multivitamins, naloxone, nitroglycerin, norepinephrine, oxytocin, pancuronium, penicillin G potassium, penicillin G sodium, pentobarbital, phenobarbital, phentolamine, phenytoin, piperacillin, potassium chloride, potassium phosphates, procainamide, propranolol, protamine, quinidine, sodium bicarbonate, sodium nitroprusside, theophylline, ticarcillin, tobramycin, tolazoline, vancomycin, vasopressin, vit B/C

Patient/family education

- Advise patient to increase fluids/fiber to counteract constipation
- Caution patient to avoid hazardous activities until stabilized on drug and dizziness is no longer a problem
- Instruct patient to limit caffeine consumption; to avoid alcohol and OTC drugs unless directed by prescriber
- Advise patient to comply with medical regimen: diet, exercise, stress reduction, drug therapy; to notify prescriber of irregular heartbeat, shortness of breath, swelling of feet and hands, pronounced dizziness, constipation, nausea, hypotension, **IV** calcium
- Teach patient to use as directed even if feeling better; may be taken with other CV drugs (nitrates, β-blockers)

Evaluation

Positive therapeutic outcome

- Decreased anginal pain
- Decreased dysrhythmias
- Decreased B/P

Treatment of overdose: Defibrillation, atropine for AV block, vasopressor for hypotension, **IV** calcium

! HIGH ALERT

vinBLAStine (VLB) (Rx)

(vin-blast'een)

Velban, Velbe ♣, vinBLAStine sulfate

Func. class.: Antineoplastic

Chem. class.: Vinca rosea alkaloid

Pregnancy category D

Do Not Confuse:
vinBLAStine/vinCRIStine

Action: Inhibits mitotic activity, arrests cell cycle at metaphase; inhibits RNA synthesis, blocks cellular use of glutamic acid needed for purine synthesis; a vesicant

Therapeutic Outcome: Prevention of rapid growth of malignant cells, immunosuppressive

Uses: Breast, testicular cancer; lymphomas; neuroblastoma; Hodgkin's, non-Hodgkin's lymphomas; mycosis fungoides; histiocytosis; Kaposi's sarcoma

Dosage and routes

Adult: **IV** 0.1 mg/kg or 3.7 mg/m^2 qwk or q2 wk, max 0.5 mg/kg or 18.5 mg/m^2 qwk

Child: **IV** 2.5 mg/m^2 then dose of 3.75, 5.0, 6.25, and 7.5 at 7-day intervals

Available forms: Inj powder 10 mg for 10 ml **IV** inj

Adverse effects

CNS: Paresthesias, peripheral neuropathy, depression, headache, **seizures**

CV: Tachycardia, orthostatic hypotension

GI: *Nausea, vomiting,* ileus, *anorexia, stomatitis,* constipation, abdominal pain, GI and rectal bleeding, **hepatotoxicity,** pharyngitis

GU: Urinary retention, **renal failure**

HEMA: **Thrombocytopenia, leukopenia, myelosuppression**

INTEG: *Rash,* alopecia, photosensitivity

META: Syndrome of inappropriate diuretic hormone

V

RESP: **Fibrosis, pulmonary infiltrate, bronchospasm**

Contraindications: Pregnancy **D**, hypersensitivity, infants, leukopenia, granulocytopenia, lactation

Precautions: Renal disease, hepatic disease

Pharmacokinetics

Absorption	Complete bioavailability
Distribution	Crosses blood-brain barrier slightly
Metabolism	Liver—active antineoplastic
Excretion	Biliary, kidneys
Half-life	Triphasic—35 min, 53 min, 19 hr

Pharmacodynamics

Unknown

Interactions

Individual drugs

Bleomycin: increased synergism
Methotrexate: increased methotrexate action
Mitomycin: increased bronchospasm
Phenytoin: decreased phenytoin level
Radiation: increased toxicity, bone marrow suppression, do not use together

Drug classifications

Antineoplastics: increased toxicity, bone marrow suppression
Live virus vaccines: increased adverse reactions

NURSING CONSIDERATIONS

Assessment

- Monitor B/P (baseline and q15 min) during administration
- Monitor CBC, differential, platelet count weekly; withhold drug if WBC is <2000/mm^3 or platelet count is <75,000/mm^3; notify prescriber of results, recovery will take 3 wk
- Assess for dyspnea, crackles, unproductive cough, chest pain, tachypnea
- Monitor renal function studies: BUN, serum uric acid, urine CCr before, during therapy; I&O ratio; report fall in urine output of 30 ml/hr; for decreased hyperuricemia
- Monitor for cold, fever, sore throat (may indicate beginning of infection); notify prescriber if these occur
- Assess for bleeding: hematuria, guaiac, bruising or petechiae, mucosa or orifices q8h, no rectal temp; avoid IM inj; use pressure to venipuncture sites
- Identify nutritional status: an antiemetic may need to be prescribed
- Assess for symptoms indicating severe allergic reactions: rash, pruritus, urticaria, itching, flushing, bronchospasm, hypotension; epINEPHrine and resuscitative equipment should be nearby

Nursing diagnoses

- Injury, risk for (adverse reactions)
- Body image, disturbed (adverse reactions)
- Infection, risk for (adverse reactions)
- Knowledge, deficient (teaching)

Implementation

- Give by intermittent inf
- Sol should be prepared by qualified personnel only under controlled conditions
- Use Luer-Lok tubing to prevent leakage; do not let sol come in contact with skin; if contact occurs, wash well with soap and water
- Administer **IV** after diluting 10 mg/10 ml NaCl; give through Y-tube or 3-way stopcock or directly over 1 min
- Give hyaluronidase 150 units/ml in 1 ml of NaCl, warm compress for extravasation for vesicant activity treatment

Syringe compatibilities: Bleomycin, cisplatin, cyclophosphamide, droperidol, fluorouracil, leucovorin, methotrexate, metoclopramide, mitomycin, vinCRIStine

Y-site compatibilities: Allopurinol, amifostine, aztreonam, bleomycin, cisplatin, cyclophosphamide, DOXOrubicin, droperidol, filgrastim, fludarabine, fluorouracil, granisetron, heparin, leucovorin, melphalan, methotrexate, metoclopramide, mitomycin, ondansetron, paclitaxel, piperacillin/tazobactam, sargramostim, teniposide, thiotepa, vinCRIStine, vinorelbine

Y-site incompatibilities: Furosemide

Additive compatibilities: Bleomycin

Patient/family education

- Teach patient to avoid use of products containing aspirin or NSAIDs, razors, commercial mouthwash because bleeding may occur; to report symptoms of bleeding (hematuria, tarry stools)
- Instruct patient to report signs of anemia, (fatigue, headache, irritability, faintness, shortness of breath)
- Caution patient to report any changes in breathing or coughing even several mo after treatment
- Advise patient that contraception will be necessary during treatment; teratogenesis may occur
- Advise patient to use sunscreen, wear protective clothing, and sunglasses
- Inform patient that hair may be lost during treatment; a wig or hairpiece may make patient feel better; new hair will be different in color, texture

- Advise patient to avoid vaccinations during treatment; serious reactions may occur
- Teach patient to report signs/symptoms of infection: fever, chills, sore throat; patient should avoid crowds and persons with known infections

Evaluation
Positive therapeutic outcome
- Decreased spread of malignant cells

! HIGH ALERT

vinCRIStine (VCR) (Rx)
(vin-kris'teen)

Oncovin, Vincasar PFS, vinCRIStine sulfate
Func. class.: Antineoplastic—miscellaneous
Chem. class.: Vinca alkaloid

Pregnancy category D

Do Not Confuse:
vinCRIStine/vinBLAStine

Action: Inhibits mitotic activity, arrests cell cycle at metaphase; inhibits RNA synthesis, blocks cellular use of glutamic acid needed for purine synthesis; a vesicant

Therapeutic Outcome: Prevention of rapid growth of malignant cells, immunosuppression

Uses: Breast, lung cancer; lymphomas; neuroblastomas; Hodgkin's disease; acute lymphoblastic and other leukemias; rhabdomyosarcoma, Wilms' tumor; osteogenic and other sarcomas

Dosage and routes
Adult: **IV** 1-2 mg/m^2/wk, max 2 mg
Child: **IV** 1.5-2 mg/m^2/wk, max 2 mg

Available forms: Inj 1 mg/ml; powder for inj 5 mg/vial

Adverse effects
CNS: *Decreased reflexes, numbness, weakness, motor difficulties,* CNS depression, cranial nerve paralysis, **seizures**
CV: Orthostatic hypotension
GI: *Nausea, vomiting, anorexia, stomatitis, constipation,* **paralytic ileus, abdominal pain, hepatotoxicity**
HEMA: **Thrombocytopenia, leukopenia, myelosuppression, anemia**
INTEG: *Alopecia*

Contraindications: Pregnancy **D**, hypersensitivity, infants, radiation therapy, lactation

Precautions: Renal disease, hepatic disease, hypertension, neuromuscular disease

Pharmacokinetics
Absorption	Complete bioavailability
Distribution	Rapidly, widely distributed; blood-brain barrier
Metabolism	Liver
Excretion	Biliary, in feces, crosses placenta
Half-life	Triphasic 0.85 min, 7.4 min, 1.64 min

Pharmacodynamics
Onset	Unknown
Peak	Unknown
Duration	1 wk

Interactions
Individual drugs
L-Asparaginase: decreased action of vinCRIStine
Digoxin: decreased digoxin level
Methotrexate: increased action of methotrexate
Mitomycin-C: increased acute pulmonary reactions
Radiation: increased toxicity, bone marrow suppression; do not use together

Drug classifications
Anticoagulants: increased action of anticoagulants
Peripheral nervous system drugs: neurotoxicity

NURSING CONSIDERATIONS
Assessment
- Monitor CBC, differential, platelet count weekly; withhold drug if WBC is <4000/mm^3 or platelet count is <75,000/mm^3; notify prescriber of results; platelets may increase or decrease
- Assess neurologic status: paresthesia, weakness, cranial nerve palsies, orthostatic hypotension, lethargy, agitation, psychosis; notify prescriber
- Monitor renal function studies: BUN, serum uric acid, urine CCr before, during therapy; I&O ratio; report fall in urine output of 30 ml/hr; for decreased hyperuricemia, hyponatremia, and increased fluid retention (syndrome of inappropriate antidiuretic hormone)
- Monitor for cold, fever, sore throat (may indicate beginning of infection)
- Identify for increased uric acid levels, joint pain in extremities; increase fluid intake to 2-3 L/day unless contraindicated

Nursing diagnoses
- Injury, risk for (adverse reactions)
- Body image, disturbed (adverse reactions)
- Infection, risk for (adverse reactions)
- Knowledge, deficient (teaching)

Implementation

• Administer **IV** after diluting with diluent provided or 1 mg/10 ml of sterile water or 0.9% NaCl; give through Y-tube or 3-way stopcock or directly over 1 min
• Hyaluronidase 150 units/ml in 1 ml of NaCl; apply warm compress for extravasation

Syringe compatibilities: Bleomycin, cisplatin, cyclophosphamide, doxapram, DOXOrubicin, droperidol, fluorouracil, heparin, leucovorin, methotrexate, metoclopramide, mitomycin, ondansetron, vinCRIStine

Syringe incompatibilities: Furosemide

Y-site compatibilities: Allopurinol, amifostine, aztreonam, bleomycin, cisplatin, cladribine, cyclophosphamide, DOXOrubicin, droperidol, filgrastim, fludarabine, fluorouracil, granisetron, heparin, leucovorin, methotrexate, metoclopramide, mitomycin, ondansetron, paclitaxel, sargramostim, teniposide, thiotepa, vinCRIStine, vinorelbine

Y-site incompatibilities: Furosemide

Patient/family education

• Teach patient to avoid use of products containing aspirin or NSAIDs, razors, commercial mouthwash because bleeding may occur; to report symptoms of bleeding (hematuria, tarry stools)
• Instruct patient to report signs of anemia (fatigue, headache, irritability, faintness, shortness of breath)
• Caution patient to report any changes in breathing or coughing, even several mo after treatment
• Advise patient that contraception will be necessary during treatment; teratogenesis may occur
• Inform patient that hair may be lost during treatment; a wig or hairpiece may make patient feel better; new hair will be different in color, texture
• Advise patient to avoid vaccinations during treatment; serious reactions may occur
• Teach patient to report signs/symptoms of infection: fever, chills, sore throat; patient should avoid crowds or persons with known infections
• Advise patient to increase fluids, bulk in diet, exercise to prevent constipation

Evaluation

Positive therapeutic outcome
• Decreased spread of malignancies

! HIGH ALERT

vinorelbine (Rx)

(vi-nor'el-bine)
Navelbine
Func. class.: Antineoplastic—miscellaneous
Chem. class.: Semisynthetic vinca alkaloid
Pregnancy category D

Action: Inhibits mitotic activity, arrests cell cycle at metaphase; inhibits RNA synthesis, blocks cellular use of glutamic acid needed for purine synthesis; a vesicant

Therapeutic Outcome: Decreased spread of malignancy

Uses: Breast cancer; unresectable, advanced non–small-cell lung cancer (NSCLC) stage IV; may be used alone or in combination with cisplatin for stage III or IV NSCLC

Dosage and routes

Adult: **IV** 30 mg/m^2 qwk

Hepatic dose

Adult: **IV** total bilirubin 2.1-3 mg/dl 15 mg/m^2 qwk; total bilirubin ≥3 mg/dl 7.5 mg/m^2 daily

Available forms: Inj 10 mg/ml

Adverse effects

CNS: Paresthesias, peripheral neuropathy, depression, headache, **seizures,** weakness, jaw pain
CV: Chest pain
GI: *Nausea, vomiting,* ileus, *anorexia, stomatitis,* constipation, abdominal pain, GI, diarrhea, **hepatotoxicity**
HEMA: **Neutropenia, anemia, thrombocytopenia, granulocytopenia**
INTEG: *Rash,* alopecia, photosensitivity
META: Syndrome of inappropriate diuretic hormone
MS: Myalgia
RESP: Shortness of breath

Contraindications: Pregnancy **D,** hypersensitivity, infants, granulocyte count <1000 cells/mm^3 pretreatment, lactation

Precautions: Renal disease, hepatic disease, elderly, children

Pharmacokinetics	
Absorption	Poor bioavailability (<50%)
Distribution	Unknown
Metabolism	Liver—to metabolite
Excretion	Bile
Half-life	43 hr

Pharmacodynamics	
Onset	Unknown
Peak	1-2 hr
Duration	Unknown

Interactions
Individual drugs
Fluorouracil: increased toxicity a possibility

NURSING CONSIDERATIONS
Assessment
- Monitor B/P (baseline and q15 min) during administration
- Monitor CBC, differential, platelet count weekly; withhold drug if WBC is <4000/mm^3 or platelet count is <75,000/mm^3; notify prescriber of results, recovery will take 3 wk
- Assess for dyspnea, crackles, unproductive cough, chest pain, tachypnea
- Monitor renal function studies: BUN, serum uric acid, urine CCr before, during therapy, I&O ratio; report fall in urine output of 30 ml/hr; for decreased hyperuricemia
- Monitor for cold, fever, sore throat (may indicate beginning infection); notify health care prescriber if these occur; effects of alopecia on body image
- Assess for bleeding: hematuria, guaiac, bruising or petechiae, mucosa or orifices q8h: no rectal temp; avoid IM inj; use pressure on venipuncture sites
- Identify nutritional status: an antiemetic may need to be prescribed
- Assess for symptoms indicating severe allergic reactions: rash, pruritus, urticaria, itching, flushing, bronchospasm, hypotension; epINEPHrine and resuscitative equipment should be nearby

Nursing diagnoses
- Injury, risk for (adverse reactions)
- Body image, disturbed (adverse reactions)
- Infection, risk for (adverse reactions)
- Knowledge, deficient (teaching)

Implementation
- Hyaluronidase 150 units/ml in 1 ml of NaCl, warm compress for extravasation for vesicant activity treatment
- Antacid before oral agent; give drug after evening meal before bedtime
- Antiemetic 30-60 min before giving drug and prn to prevent vomiting

Continuous infusion
- Give 40 mg/m^2 q3 wk after **IV** bol of 8 mg/m^2; may be given in combination with DOXOrubicin, fluorouracil, cisplatin

Y-site compatibilities: Amikacin, aztreonam, bleomycin, buprenorphine, butorphanol, calcium gluconate, carboplatin, cefotaxime, cisplatin, cimetidine, clindamycin, dexamethasone, enalaprilat, etoposide, famotidine, filgrastim, fluconazole, fludarabine, gentamicin, hydrocortisone, lorazepam, meperidine, morphine, netilmicin, ondansetron, plicamycin, streptozocin, teniposide, ticarcillin, tobramycin, vancomycin, vinBLAStine, vinCRIStine, zidovudine

Patient/family education
- Teach patient to use liq diet: cola, Jell-O; dry toast or crackers may be added if patient is not nauseated or vomiting
- Advise patient to rinse mouth 3-4 ×/day with water and brush teeth 2-3 ×/day with soft brush or cotton-tipped applicators for stomatitis; use unwaxed dental floss
- Inform patient that a nutritious diet with iron, vitamin supplements is necessary
- Advise patient to avoid crowds, people with infections, vaccinations
- Advise patient to use effective contraception, avoid breast feeding
- Teach patient hair may be lost but will grow back; new hair may be different texture, color

Evaluation
Positive therapeutic outcome
- Decreased spread of malignant cells

vitamin A (PO, OTC; IM, Rx)
Aquasol A, Del-Vi-A, Vitamin A

Func. class.: Vitamin, fat-soluble

Chem. class.: Retinol

Pregnancy category C

Action: Needed for normal bone and tooth development, visual dark adaptation, skin disease, mucosa tissue repair, assists in production of adrenal steroids, cholesterol, RNA

Therapeutic Outcome: Prevention, absence of vit A deficiency

Uses: Vit A deficiency

Dosage and routes
Adult and child >8 yr: PO 100,000-500,000 international units daily × 3 days, then 50,000 daily × 2 wk; dose based on severity of deficiency; maintenance 10,000-20,000 international units for 2 mo

Child 1-8 yr: IM 5000-15,000 international units daily × 10 days

Infants <1 yr: IM 5000-15,000 international units × 10 days

V

Maintenance
Child 4-8 yr: IM 15,000 international units daily × 2 mo
Child <4 yr: IM 10,000 international units daily × 2 mo

Available forms: Caps 10,000, 25,000, 50,000 international units; drops 5000 international units; inj 50,000 international units/ml; tabs 10,000, 25,000, 50,000 international units

Adverse effects

CNS: Headache, **increased ICP, intracranial hypertension**, lethargy, malaise
EENT: Gingivitis, papilledema, exophthalmos, inflammation of tongue and lips
GI: Nausea, vomiting, anorexia, abdominal pain, *jaundice*
INTEG: Drying of skin, pruritus, increased pigmentation, night sweats, alopecia
META: Hypomenorrhea, hypercalcemia
MS: Arthralgia, retarded growth, hard areas on bone

Contraindications: Hypersensitivity to vit A, malabsorption syndrome (PO)

Precautions: Pregnancy **C,** lactation, impaired renal function

Pharmacokinetics

Absorption	Rapidly absorbed
Distribution	Stored in liver, kidneys, lungs
Metabolism	Liver
Excretion	Breast milk
Half-life	Unknown

Pharmacodynamics

Unknown

Interactions

Individual drugs
Cholestyramine, colestipol, mineral oil: decreased absorption of vit A
Drug classifications
Contraceptives (oral), corticosteroids: increased levels of vit A
Drug/lab test
False increase: bilirubin, serum cholesterol

NURSING CONSIDERATIONS

Assessment

- Assess nutritional status: increase intake of yellow and dark green vegetables, yellow/orange fruits, vit A–fortified foods, liver, egg yolks
- Assess vit A deficiency: decreased growth; night blindness; dry, brittle nails; hair loss; urinary stones; increased infection; hyperkeratosis of skin; drying of cornea
- Identify vit A deficiency by plasma vit A, carotene level
- Assess for chronic vit A toxicity: increased calcium, BUN, glucose, cholesterol, triglyceride level

Nursing diagnoses

- Nutrition: less than body requirements, imbalances (uses)
- Knowledge, deficient (teaching)

Implementation

PO route
- Give with food (PO) for better absorption; do not give **IV** because anaphylaxis may occur, IM only
- Oral preparations are not indicated for vit A deficiency in those with malabsorption syndrome
- Store in airtight, light-resistant container

Patient/family education

- Instruct patient that if dose is missed, it should be omitted
- Inform patient that ophth exams may be required periodically throughout therapy
- Instruct patient not to use mineral oil while taking this drug because absorption will be decreased
- Advise patient to notify prescriber of nausea, vomiting, lip cracking, loss of hair, headache
- Caution patient not to take more than the prescribed amount

Evaluation

Positive therapeutic outcome
- Increase in growth rate, weight
- Absence of dry skin and mucous membranes, night blindness

Treatment of overdose: Discontinue drug

vitamin A acid

See tretinoin

vitamin B_1

See thiamine

(vitamin B_{12}) cyanocobalamin (PO, OTC; IM/SUBCUT, Rx)

(sye-an-oh-koe-bal'a-min)

Alphamin, Anacobin ✦, Bedoz ✦, B_{12}, Resin, Cobex, Cobolin-M Crystamine, Hydro-Crysti-1000, Cyanabin ✦ Cyanoject, Cyomin, Ener-B, Hydrobexan, Hydro Cobex, Hydro-Crysti-12

Func. class.: Vitamin B_{12}, water-soluble vitamin

(vitamin B_{12}a) hydroxocobalamin (vit B_{12}) (Rx)

(hye-drox'-o-ko-bal'-a-min)

Acti-B_{12} ✦, Alphamin, Hydro-Crysti12, Hydroxo-12, Hydroxycobalamin, LA-12

Pregnancy category A

Action: Needed for adequate nerve functioning, protein and carbohydrate metabolism, normal growth, RBC development and cell reproduction

Therapeutic Outcome: Prevention, correction of vit B_{12} deficiency

Uses: Vit B_{12} deficiency; pernicious anemia; vit B_{12} malabsorption syndrome; Schilling test; increased requirements with pregnancy, thyrotoxicosis, hemolytic anemia, hemorrhage, renal and hepatic disease

Dosage and routes

Cyanocobalamin

Adult: PO up to 1000 mcg/day SUBCUT/IM 30-100 mcg/day × 1 wk, then 100-200 mcg/mo

Shilling test

Adult and child: IM 1000 mcg in 1 dose

Child: PO up to 1000 mcg/day SUBCUT/IM 30-50 mcg/day × 2 wk, then 100 mcg/mo; NASAL 500 mcg qwk

Hydroxocobalamin

Adult: SUBCUT/IM 30-50 mcg/day × 5-10 days, then 100-200 mcg/mo

Child: SUBCUT/IM 30-50 mcg/day × 5-10 days, then 100 mcg/mo

Available forms: Cyanocobalamin: tabs 25, 50, 100, 250, 500, 1000, 5000 mcg; ext rel tabs 100, 200, 500, 1000 mcg; lozenges: 100, 250, 500 mcg; nasal gel 500 mcg/spray; inj 100, 1000 mcg/ml; hydroxocobalamin: inj 1000 mcg/ml

Adverse effects

CNS: Flushing, optic nerve atrophy

CV: **CHF**, peripheral vascular thrombosis, **pulmonary edema**

GI: *Diarrhea*

INTEG: Itching, rash, pain at site

META: Hypokalemia

SYST: **Anaphylactic shock**

Contraindications: Hypersensitivity, optic nerve atrophy

Precautions: Pregnancy **A,** lactation, children

Pharmacokinetics

Absorption	Well absorbed (IM, SUBCUT)
Distribution	Crosses placenta
Metabolism	Stored in liver, kidney, stomach
Excretion	50%-90% (urine), breast milk
Half-life	Unknown

Pharmacodynamics

Unknown

Interactions

Individual drugs

Alcohol, aminosalicylic acid, chloramphenicol, cimetidine, colchicine: decreased absorption

Prednisone: increased absorption

Drug classifications

Aminoglycosides, anticonvulsants, potassium products: decreased absorption

Drug/herb

Goldenseal: decreased vit B_{12} absorption

Drug/lab test

False positive: intrinsic factor

NURSING CONSIDERATIONS

Assessment

- Assess for deficiency: anorexia, dyspepsia on exertion, palpitations, paresthesias, psychosis, visual disturbances, pallor, red inflamed tongue, neuropathy, edema of legs
- Monitor potassium levels during beginning treatment in patients with megaloblastic anemia
- Monitor CBC for increase in reticulocyte count during 1st wk of therapy, then increase in RBC and hemoglobin; folic acid levels, vit B_{12} levels
- Assess nutritional status: egg yolks, fish, organ meats, dairy products, clams, oysters, which are good sources for vit B_{12}
- Monitor for pulmonary edema or worsening of CHF in cardiac patients

V

Nursing diagnoses

- Nutrition: less than body requirements, imbalanced (uses)
- Knowledge, deficient (teaching)
- Noncompliance (teaching) (overuse)

Implementation

PO route

- Give with fruit juice to disguise taste; administer immediately after mixing
- Give with meals if possible for better absorption

IM route

- Give by IM inj for pernicious anemia for life unless contraindicated

IV route

- May be mixed with TPN sol, but **IV** route is not recommended

Y-site compatibilities: Heparin, hydrocortisone sodium succinate, potassium chloride

Solution compatibilities: Dextrose/Ringer's or lactated Ringer's combinations, dextrose/saline combinations, D_5W, $D_{10}W$, 0.45% NaCl, Ringer's or lactated Ringer's sol, ascorbic acid

Patient/family education

- Instruct patient that treatment must continue for life if diagnosed as having pernicious anemia
- Advise patient to eat well-balanced diet from the food pyramid and comply with dietary recommendation
- Caution patient not to exceed the RDA of vit B_{12} because adverse reactions may occur

Evaluation

Positive therapeutic outcome

- Decreased anorexia, dyspnea on exertion, palpitations, paresthesias, psychosis, visual disturbances, edema of legs
- Prevention or correction of vit B_{12} deficiency

Treatment of overdose: Discontinue drug

vitamin D (cholecalciferol, vitamin D_3 or ergocalciferol, vitamin D_2) (Rx, OTC)

Calciferol, Delta-D, Drisdol, Radiostol ♣, Radiostol Forte ♣, vitamin D, vitamin D_3

Func. class.: Vitamin D

Chem. class: Fat-soluble vitamin

Pregnancy category C

Do Not Confuse:
Calciferol/calcitriol

Action: Needed for regulation of calcium, phosphate levels; normal bone development; parathyroid activity; neuromuscular functioning

Therapeutic Outcome: Prevention of rickets, osteomalacia, normal calcium/phosphate levels

Uses: Vit D deficiency, rickets, renal osteodystrophy, hypoparathyroidism, hypophosphatemia, psoriasis, rheumatoid arthritis

Dosage and routes

Deficiency

Adult: PO/IM 12,000 international units daily, then increased to 500,000 international units/day

Child: PO/IM 1500-5000 international units daily × 2-4 wk, may repeat after 2 wk or 600,000 international units as single dose

Hypoparathyroidism

Adult and child: PO/IM 200,000 international units given with 4 g calcium tab

Available forms: Tabs 400, 1000, 50,000 international units; caps 25,000, 50,000; oral sol 8000 international units/ml; inj 500,000 international units/ml, 500,000 international units/5 ml

Adverse effects

CNS: Fatigue, weakness, drowsiness, **seizures,** headache, psychosis

CV: Hypertension, dysrhythmias

GI: Nausea, vomiting, anorexia, cramps, diarrhea, constipation, metallic taste, dry mouth

GU: Polyuria, nocturia, **hematuria, albuminuria, renal failure,** decreased libido

INTEG: Pruritus, photophobia

MS: Decreased bone growth, early joint pain, early muscle pain

Contraindications: Hypersensitivity, hypercalcemia, renal dysfunction, hyperphosphatemia

Precautions: Pregnancy **C,** CV disease, renal calculi

Pharmacokinetics

Absorption	Well absorbed
Distribution	Stored in liver
Metabolism	Liver, sun
Excretion	Bile, kidney
Half-life	12-22 hr

Pharmacodynamics

	PO	IM
Onset	Unknown	Unknown
Peak	4 hr	Unknown
Duration	15-20 days	Unknown

Interactions
Individual drugs
Cholestyramine, colestipol, phenobarbital, phenytoin: decreased effects of vit D
Verapamil: increased toxicity
Drug classifications
Antacids, diuretics (thiazide): increased toxicity

NURSING CONSIDERATIONS
Assessment
- Monitor BUN, urinary calcium, AST, ALT, cholesterol, creatinine, uric acid, chloride, magnesium, electrolytes, urine pH, phosphate—may increase; calcium should be kept at 9-10 mg/dl; vit D at 50-135 international units/dl, phosphate at 70 mg/dl; alkaline phosphatase may be decreased
- Monitor for increased blood level; toxic reactions may occur rapidly
- Assess for dry mouth, metallic taste, polyuria, bone pain, muscle weakness, headache, fatigue, tinnitus, change in LOC, irregular pulse, dysrhythmias, increased respirations, anorexia, nausea, vomiting, cramps, diarrhea, constipation; may indicate hypercalcemia
- Assess renal status: decreased urinary output (oliguria, anuria), edema in extremities, weight gain 5 lb, periorbital edema
- Assess nutritional status, diet for sources of vit D (milk, cod, halibut, salmon, sardines, egg yolk) calcium (dairy products, dark green vegetables), phosphates (dairy products)

Nursing diagnoses
- Nutrition, less than body requirements, imbalanced (uses)
- Knowledge, deficient (teaching)

Implementation
PO route
- PO may be increased q4 wk depending on blood level
- Store in airtight, light-resistant container at room temp

IM route
- Give inj deeply in large muscle mass, administer slowly, aspirate to avoid **IV** administration, rotate inj site

Patient/family education
- Advise patient to omit dose if missed; to avoid vitamin supplements unless directed by prescriber
- Inform patient of necessary foods to be included in diet
- Advise patient to keep appointments for evaluation because therapeutic and toxic levels are narrow
- Instruct patient to report weakness, lethargy, headache, anorexia, loss of weight; to report nausea, vomiting, abdominal cramps, diarrhea, constipation, excessive thirst, polyuria, muscle and bone pain
- Caution patient to decrease intake of antacids and laxatives containing magnesium

Evaluation
Positive therapeutic outcome
- Calcium levels 9-10 ml/dl
- Decreasing symptoms of bone disease

vitamin E (OTC)
Amino-Opti-E, Aquasol E, Daltose ♣, E-Complex-600, E-Ferol, E-Vitamin Succinate, E-200 I.U. Softgels, Gordo-Vite E, Tocopherol, vitamin E, Vita-Plus E Softgells, Vitec

Func. class.: Vitamin E
Chem. class.: Fat-soluble vitamin

Pregnancy category A

Action: Needed for digestion and metabolism of polyunsaturated fats, decreases platelet aggregation, decreases blood clot formation, promotes normal growth and development of muscle tissue, prostaglandin synthesis

Therapeutic Outcome: Prevention and treatment of vit E deficiency

Uses: Vit E deficiency, impaired fat absorption, hemolytic anemia in premature neonates, prevention of retrolental fibroplasia, sickle cell anemia, supplement in malabsorption syndrome

Dosage and routes
Deficiency
Adult: PO 60-75 international units daily
Child: PO 1 mg/0.6 g of dietary fat
Prevention of deficiency
Adult: PO 30 units/day
Infant: PO 5 international units/day
Topical route
Adult and child: TOP apply to affected areas as needed

Available forms: Caps 100, 200, 400, 500, 600, 1000 international units; tabs 100, 200, 400 international units; drops 50 mg/ml; chew tabs 400 units; ointment, cream, lotion, oil

Adverse effects
CNS: Headache, fatigue
CV: Increased risk of thrombophlebitis
EENT: Blurred vision
GI: Nausea, cramps, diarrhea

V

GU: Gonadal dysfunction
INTEG: Sterile abscess, contact dermatitis
META: Altered metabolism of hormones, thyroid, pituitary, adrenal, altered immunity
MS: Weakness

Contraindications: IV use in infants

Precautions: Pregnancy **A**

Pharmacokinetics

Absorption	20%-80% (PO)
Distribution	Widely distributed, stored in fat
Metabolism	Liver
Excretion	Bile
Half-life	Unknown

Pharmacodynamics

Unknown

Interactions

Individual drugs

Cholestyramine, colestipol, mineral oil, sucralfate: decreased absorption

Drug classification

Anticoagulants (oral): increased action of anticoagulants

NURSING CONSIDERATIONS

Assessment

- Assess nutritional status: intake of wheat germ, dark green leafy vegetables, nuts, eggs, liver, vegetable oils, dairy products, cereals
- Assess for vit E deficiency (usually in neonates): irritability, restlessness, hemolytic anemia

Nursing diagnoses

- Nutrition: less than body requirements, imbalanced (uses)
- Knowledge, deficient (teaching)

Implementation

PO route

- Chew chewable tabs well
- Sol: may be dropped in mouth or mixed with food
- Store in airtight, light-resistant container

Topical route

- Apply TOP to moisturize dry skin

Patient/family education

- Inform patient necessary foods to be included in diet high in vit E
- Instruct patient to omit if dose missed
- Instruct patient to avoid vit supplements unless directed by prescriber because overdose may occur

Evaluation

Positive therapeutic outcome

- Absence of hemolytic anemia
- Adequate vit E levels
- Improvement in skin lesions
- Decrease in edema

voriconazole (Rx)

(vohr-i-kahn'a-zol)

Vfend

Func. class: Antifungal

Pregnancy category D

Action: Inhibits fungal CYP450-mediation demethylation, needed for biosynthesis

Therapeutic Outcome: Decreasing signs, symptoms of infection

Uses: Invasive aspergillosis, serious fungal infections (*Scedosporium apiospermum, Fusarium* sp.)

Dosage and routes

Adult: PO Give 1 hr ac or pc; ≥40 kg: 200 mg q12h; <40 kg: 100 mg q12h
Adult: **IV** Loading dose 6 mg/kg q12h × 2 dose, then 4 mg/kg q12h; may switch to oral dosing

Available forms: Tabs 50, 200 mg; powder for inj, lyophilized 200 mg voriconazole, 3200 mg sulfobutyl ester β-cyclodextrin sodium (SBECD), powder for oral susp 45 g (40 mg/ml after reconstitution)

Adverse effects

CNS: *Headache,* paresthesias, peripheral neuropathy, hallucinations, psychosis, extrapyramidal symptoms (EPS), depression, Guillain-Barré syndrome, insomnia, suicidal ideation, dizziness
CV: **Tachycardia,** hyper/hypotension, vasodilatation, **atrial dysrhythmias, atrial fibrillation, AV block, bradycardia, CHF, MI**
EENT: Blurred vision, eye hemorrhage
INTEG: *Burning, irritation,* pain, necrosis at inj site with extravasation, dermatitis, rash, photosensitivity
GI: *Nausea, vomiting, anorexia,* diarrhea, cramps, **hemorrhagic gastroenteritis, acute liver failure, hepatitis, intestinal perforation, pancreatitis**
GU: *Hypokalemia,* azotemia, **renal tubular necrosis, permanent renal impairment, anuria, oliguria**
HEMA: Anemia, **eosinophilia,** hypomagnesemia, **thrombocytopenia, leukopenia, pancytopenia**

MISC: Respiratory disorder
SYST: **Stevens-Johnson syndrome, toxic epidermal necrolysis, sepsis**

Contraindications: Pregnancy **D**, hypersensitivity, severe bone marrow depression, lactation, children, severe hepatic disease

Precautions: Renal disease **(IV)**

Pharmacokinetics

Absorption	Unknown
Distribution	Protein binding 58%
Metabolism	By CYP45 enzyme
Excretion	Via hepatic metabolism
Half-life	Unknown

Pharmacodynamics

Onset	Unknown
Peak	1-2 hr
Duration	Unknown

Interactions

Individual drugs

Cisplatin, cycloSPORINE, polymyxin B, vancomycin: increased nephrotoxicity
Digitalis: increased hypokalemia
CycloSPORINE, phenytoin, pimozide, prednisolone, quinidine, rifabutin, sirolimus, tacrolimus, warfarin: increased effects of each specific drug

Drug classifications

Aminoglycosides: increased nephrotoxicity
Benzodiazepines, calcium channel blockers, ergots, HMG-CoA reductase inhibitors, nonnucleoside reverse transcriptase inhibitors, protease inhibitors, proton pump inhibitors, sulfonylureas, vinca alkaloids: increased effects of each specific drug
Corticosteroids, diuretics (thiazide), skeletal muscle relaxants: increased hypokalemia

Drug/herb

Gossypol: increased nephrotoxicity

Drug/food

High-fat foods: avoid use with high-fat meals

NURSING CONSIDERATIONS

Assessment

- Monitor VS q15-30 min during first infusion; note changes in pulse, B/P
- Monitor I&O ratio; watch for decreasing urinary output, change in specific gravity; discontinue drug to prevent permanent damage to renal tubules
- Monitor blood studies: CBC, K, Na, Ca, Mg q2 wk; BUN, creatinine weekly
- Monitor weight weekly; if weight increases over 2 lb/wk, edema is present; renal damage should be considered
- Assess for renal toxicity: increasing BUN, serum creatinine; if BUN is >40 mg/dl or if serum creatinine >3 mg/dl, drug may be discontinued or dosage reduced
- Assess for hepatotoxicity: increasing AST, ALT, alkaline phosphatase, bilirubin
- Assess for allergic reaction: dermatitis, rash; drug should be discontinued, antihistamines (mild reaction) or epINEPHrine (severe reaction) administered
- Assess for hypokalemia: anorexia, drowsiness, weakness, decreased reflexes, dizziness, increased urinary output, increased thirst, paresthesias
- Assess for ototoxicity: tinnitus (ringing, roaring in ears), vertigo, loss of hearing (rare)

Nursing diagnoses

- Infection, risk for (uses)
- Injury, risk for (uses, adverse reactions)
- Knowledge, deficient (teaching)

Implementation

- Give 1 hr before or after meals
- Store at room temp (powder, tabs)

IV route

- Give drug only after C&S confirms organism, drug needed to treat condition; make sure drug is used in life-threatening infections
- Reconstitute powder with 19 ml water for inj to 10 mg/ml, shake until dissolved; infuse over 1-2 hr at a conc of 5 mg/ml or less; do not admix with other drugs, 4.2% sodium bicarbonate inf

Patient/family education

- Teach that long-term therapy may be needed to clear infection (2 wk-3 mo depending on type of infection)
- Advise patient to notify prescriber of bleeding, bruising, or soft tissue swelling
- Teach to take 1 hr before or after meal
- Advise patient not to drive at night because of vision changes
- Advise to avoid strong, direct sunlight
- Advise that women of childbearing age should use effective contraceptive

Evaluation

Positive therapeutic outcome

- Decreased fever, malaise, rash, negative C&S for infecting organism

! HIGH ALERT

warfarin (Rx)

(war'far-in)

Coumadin, warfarin sodium, Warfilone ✦

Func. class.: Anticoagulant

Pregnancy category X

Do Not Confuse:
Coumadin/Cardura, Coumadin/Compazine

Action: Interferes with blood clotting by indirect means; depresses hepatic synthesis of vit K–dependent coagulation factors (II, VII, IX, X)

Therapeutic Outcome: Prevention of clotting

Uses: Pulmonary emboli, deep vein thrombosis, prevention or treatment of venous thrombosis, pulmonary embolism, thromboembolic complications associated with atrial fibrillation or cardiac valve replacement, after MI to reduce risk of death

Dosage and routes

Adult: PO/**IV** 2.5-10 mg/day × 3 days, then titrated to Pro-time or INR daily

Elderly: PO/**IV** 2-10 mg/day

Child: PO 0.1 mg/kg/day titrated to INR

Available forms: Tabs 1, 2, 2.5, 3, 4, 5, 6, 7.5, 10 mg; 5.4 mg powder for inj

Adverse effects

CNS: *Fever*

GI: *Diarrhea,* nausea, vomiting, anorexia, stomatitis, cramps, **hepatitis**

GU: **Hematuria**

HEMA: **Hemorrhage, agranulocytosis, leukopenia, eosinophilia**

INTEG: *Rash,* dermatitis, urticaria, alopecia, pruritus

Contraindications: Pregnancy **X,** hypersensitivity, hemophilia, leukemia with bleeding, peptic ulcer disease, thrombocytopenic purpura, hepatic disease (severe), malignant hypertension, subacute bacterial endocarditis, acute nephritis, blood dyscrasias, eclampsia, preeclampsia, lactation

Precautions: Alcoholism, elderly , CHF

Pharmacokinetics

Absorption	Well absorbed (PO), completely absorbed
Distribution	Crosses placenta, 99% plasma protein binding
Metabolism	Liver
Excretion	Kidney, feces (active, inactive metabolites)
Half-life	Effective ½-2½ days

Pharmacodynamics

	PO
Onset	12-24 hr
Peak	½-4 days
Duration	3-5 days

Interactions

Individual drugs

Allopurinol, amiodarone, cefamandole, chloral hydrate, chloramphenicol, cimetidine, clofibrate, clotrimoxazole, diflunisal, disulfiram, erythromycin, furosemide, glucagon, heparin, indomethacin, isoniazid, mefenamic acid, metronidazole, phenylbutazone, quinidine, sulfinpyrazone, sulindac, thyroid: increased warfarin action

Carbamazepine, dicloxicillin, ethchlorvynol, griseofulvin, nafcillin, phenytoin, rifampin, sucralfate, vitamin K: decreased warfarin action

Phenytoin: increased toxicity

Drug classifications

Antidepressants (tricyclic), ethacrynic acids, HMG-CoA reductase inhibitors, NSAIDs, oxyphenbutazones, COX-2 selective inhibitors, penicillins, quinolones, salicylates, SSRIs, steroids, sulfonamides, thrombolytics: increased warfarin action

Barbiturates, contraceptives (oral), estrogens: decreased warfarin action

Sulfonylureas (oral): increased toxicity

Drug/herb

Agrimony, alfalfa, angelica, anise, basil, bay, bilberry, black haw, bogbean, bromelain, buchu, chondroitin, cinchona bark, dong quai, fenugreek, feverfew, garlic, ginger, ginkgo, ginseng, horse chestnut, Irish moss, kelp, kelpware, khella, lovage, lungwort, meadowsweet, motherwort, mugwort, nettle, papaya, parsley (large amounts), pau d'arco, pineapple, poplar, prickly ash, safflower, saw palmetto, tonka bean, turmeric, wintergreen, yarrow: increased risk of bleeding

Chamomile, coenzyme Q10, flax, glucomannan, goldenseal, guar gum: decreased anticoagulant effect

Drug/food

Vit K foods: decreased warfarin action

Drug/lab test

Increased: T_3 uptake

Decreased: uric acid

NURSING CONSIDERATIONS

Assessment

- Monitor blood studies (Hct, occult blood in stools) q3 mo; partial protime, which should be 1½-2 × control, PTT; often done daily,

APTT, ACT; platelet count q2-3 days; thrombocytopenia may occur
- Monitor B/P, watch for increasing signs of hypertension
- Assess for bleeding: bleeding gums, petechiae, ecchymosis, black tarry stools, hematuria, epistaxis; decreased B/P may indicate bleeding and possible hemorrhage
- Assess for fever, skin rash, urticaria
- Assess for needed dosage change q1-2 wk

Assess patients carefully for symptoms of Churg-Strauss syndrome (rare): eosinophilia, vasculitis, rash, worsening pulmonary symptoms, cardiac complications, neuropathy

Nursing diagnoses
- Injury, risk for (uses, adverse reactions)
- Tissue perfusion, ineffective (uses)
- Knowledge, deficient (teaching)

Implementation
PO route
- Warfarin is usually given with **IV** heparin for 3 or more days, warfarin blood level may take several days

IV route
- Reconstitute with 2.7 ml of sterile water for inj; do not use solution that is discolored or has particulates
- Give over 1-2 min into peripheral vein

Y-site compatibilities: Cefazolin, ceftriaxone, DOPamine, heparin, lidocaine, morphine, nitroglycerin, potassium chloride, ranitidine

Patient/family education
- Caution patient to avoid OTC preparations unless directed by prescriber; may cause serious drug interactions
- Advise patient that drug may be withheld during active bleeding (menstruation), depending on condition
- Advise patient to use soft-bristle toothbrush to avoid bleeding gums, avoid contact sports, use electric razor, avoid IM inj
- Instruct patient to carry/wear emergency ID identifying drug taken
- Advise patient to report any signs of bleeding: gums, under skin, urine, stools
- Teach patient to read food labels; limited intake of vit K foods (green leafy vegetables) is necessary to maintain consistent prothrombin levels

Evaluation
Positive therapeutic outcome
- Decrease of deep vein thrombosis
- Protime (1.3-2.0 × control)

zafirlukast (Rx)
(za-feer'loo-cast)
Accolate
Func. class.: Bronchodilator
Chem. class: Leukotriene receptor antagonist
Pregnancy category B

Action: Antagonizes the contractile action of leukotrienes (LTC_4, LTD_4, LTE_4) in airway smooth muscle; inhibits bronchoconstriction caused by antigens

Therapeutic Outcome: Ability to breathe more easily

Uses: Prophylaxis and chronic treatment of asthma in adults/children >12 yr

Investigational uses: Chronic urticaria

Dosage and routes
Adult/child ≥12 yr: PO 20 mg bid, take 1 hr ac or 2 hr pc
Child 5-11 yr: PO 10 mg bid

Available forms: Tabs 10, 20 mg

Adverse effects
CNS: Headache, dizziness
GI: Nausea, diarrhea, abdominal pain, vomiting, dyspepsia
MISC: Infections, pain, asthenia, myalgia, fever, increased ALT, urticaria, rash, **angioedema**

Contraindications: Hypersensitivity

Precautions: Pregnancy **B**, elderly, lactation, children, hepatic disease

Pharmacokinetics	
Absorption	Rapidly
Distribution	Unknown
Metabolism	Extensively by CYP450 2C9, 3A4 enzyme systems, protein binding (99%)
Excretion	Feces
Half-life	10 hr

Pharmacodynamics	
Onset	Unknown
Peak	3 hr
Duration	Unknown

Interactions
Individual drugs
Aspirin: increased plasma levels of zafirlukast
Erythromycin, theophylline: decreased plasma levels of zafirlukast
Warfarin: increased protime

Drug/herb
Green tea (large amounts), guarana: increased effect
Drug/food
Decreased: bioavailability of zafirlukast

NURSING CONSIDERATIONS
Assessment
- Assess respiratory rate, rhythm, depth; auscultate lung fields bilaterally; notify prescriber of abnormalities

Nursing diagnoses
- Breathing pattern, ineffective (uses)
- Knowledge, deficient (teaching)
- Noncompliance (teaching)

Implementation
- Give PO 1 hr ac or 2 hr pc; absorption may be decreased if given with food
- Give with 8 oz of water if GI upset occurs

Patient/family education
- Advise patient to check OTC medications, current prescription medications, which will increase stimulation
- Advise patient to avoid hazardous activities; dizziness may occur
- Advise patient that if GI upset occurs, to take drug with 8 oz of water; avoid food if possible, absorption may be decreased
- Advise to take even if symptom free
- Advise patient to notify prescriber of nausea, vomiting, diarrhea, abdominal pain, fatigue, jaundice, anorexia, flulike symptoms (hepatic dysfunction)
- Advise patient not to use for acute asthma episodes, or to use while breastfeeding

Evaluation
Positive therapeutic outcome
- Ability to breathe more easily

zalcitabine (Rx)
(zal-sit′a-bin)
ddC, dideoxycitidine, HIVID
Func. class.: Antiretroviral
Chem. class.: (NRTI) Nucleoside reverse transcriptase inhibitor
Pregnancy category C

Action: Inhibits HIV-1 replication by the conversion of this drug by cellular enzymes to an active antiviral metabolite; a chain terminator

Therapeutic Outcome: Improved symptoms of HIV-1 infection

Uses: HIV-1 infections in combination in adults and children >13 yr

Dosage and routes
Adult: PO 0.75 mg q8h in combination with other antiretrovirals; in presence of peripheral neuropathy initiate dose at 0.375 mg q8h of zalcitabine
Renal dose
Adult: PO CCr 10-40 ml/min 0.75 mg q12h; CCr <10 ml/min 0.75 mg q24h

Available forms: Tabs 0.375, 0.75 mg

Adverse effects
CNS: *Headache, peripheral neuropathy,* **seizures,** confusion, anxiety, hypertonia, abnormal thinking, asthenia, insomnia, CNS depression, pain, *dizziness,* chills, *fever*
CV: Hypertension, vasodilatation, dysrhythmia, syncope, palpitation, tachycardia, **cardiomyopathy, CHF**
EENT: Ear pain, otitis, photophobia, visual impairment
ENDO: Hypoglycemia, hyponatremia, hyperbilirubinemia, hyperglycemia
GI: **Pancreatitis,** *diarrhea, nausea, vomiting,* abdominal pain, constipation, stomatitis, dysplasia, liver abnormalities, *oral ulcers,* flatulence, taste perversion, dry mouth, oral thrush, melena, *increased ALT, AST, alkaline phosphatase, amylase*
GU: Uric acid, **toxic nephropathy,** polyuria
HEMA: **Leukopenia, granulocytopenia, thrombocytopenia,** anemia
INTEG: *Rash, pruritus,* alopecia, sweating, acne
MS: *Myalgia,* arthritis, myopathy, muscular atrophy
RESP: *Cough,* pneumonia, dyspnea, asthma, hypoventilation
SYST: **Lactic acidosis**

Contraindications: Hypersensitivity

Precautions: Pregnancy **C,** renal, hepatic, disease, lactation, children <13 yr, patients with peripheral neuropathy, heart failure

Pharmacokinetics	
Absorption	Minimally absorbed
Distribution	Unknown
Metabolism	Liver
Excretion	Kidneys
Half-life	1-3 hr, increased in renal disease

Pharmacodynamics	
Onset	Unknown
Peak	0.5-2 hr
Duration	Unknown

Interactions

Individual drugs

Amphotericin B, chloramphenicol, cimetidine, cisplatin, dapsone, disulfiram, ethionamide, foscarnet, glutethimide, gold, hydrALAZINE, iodoquinol, isoniazid, metronidazole, nitrofurantoin, phenytoin, probenecid, ribavirin, vinCRIStine: increased peripheral neuropathy
ddI, d4T: increased pancreatitis risk
Ketoconazole, dapsone, metoclopramide: decreased absorption

Drug classifications

Aminoglycosides: increased peripheral neuropathy
Antacids: decreased absorption
Nucleoside analogs: increased peripheral neuropathy risk

NURSING CONSIDERATIONS

Assessment

- Assess for peripheral neuropathy: tingling or pain in hands and feet, distal numbness; if these occur during therapy, drug may be decreased or discontinued
- Assess for lactic acidosis; severe hepatomegaly with steatosis, which can be fatal; drug should be discontinued
- Assess for pancreatitis: abdominal pain, nausea, vomiting, elevated liver enzymes; drug should be discontinued because condition can be fatal
- Assess children by dilated retinal examination q6 mo to rule out retinal depigmentation
- Monitor CBC, differential, platelet count qmo; withhold drug if WBC is $<4000/mm^3$ or platelet count is $<75,000/mm^3$; notify prescriber of results
- Monitor renal function studies (BUN, serum uric acid, urine CCr) before, during therapy; these may be elevated throughout treatment
- Monitor temp q4h, may indicate beginning of infection
- Monitor liver function tests (bilirubin, AST, ALT, amylase, alkaline phosphatase, triglycerides) before, during therapy as needed or qmo
- Monitor viral load, CD4 baseline and throughout treatment

Nursing diagnoses

- Infection, risk for (uses)
- Injury, risk for (adverse reactions)
- Knowledge, deficient (teaching)

Implementation

- Give on empty stomach, q8h around the clock
- Give on empty stomach 1 hr prior or 2 hr after a meal
- Do not take dapsone at same time as ddC

Patient/family education

- Advise patient to take on empty stomach 1 hr prior or 2h after a meal; not to take dapsone at same time as ddC; to use exactly as prescribed
- Instruct patient to report signs of infection: increased temp, sore throat, flulike symptoms; to avoid crowds and those with known infections
- Caution patient to report signs of anemia: fatigue, headache, faintness, shortness of breath, irritability
- Advise patient to report bleeding; avoid use of razors or commercial mouthwash
- Inform patient that hair may be lost during therapy (rare); a wig or hairpiece may make patient feel better
- Caution patient to avoid OTC products or other medications without approval of prescriber
- Caution patient not to have any sexual contact without use of a condom; that needles should not be shared; that blood from infected individual should not come in contact with another's mucous membranes

Evaluation

Positive therapeutic outcome

- Absence of infection; symptoms of HIV infection

zaleplon (Rx)

(zale'plon)
Sonata
Func. class.: Sedative-hypnotic, antianxiety
Chem. class.: Pyrazolopyrimidine

Pregnancy category C

Controlled substance schedule IV

Action: Binds selectively to ω-1 receptor of the γ-aminobutyric acid type A ($GABA_A$) receptor complex; results are sedation, hypnosis, skeletal muscle relaxation, anticonvulsant activity, anxiolytic action

Therapeutic Outcome: Ability to sleep

Uses: Insomnia

Dosage and routes

Adult: PO 10 mg at bedtime; may increase dose to 20 mg at bedtime if needed; 5 mg may be used in low weight persons
Elderly: PO 15 mg at bedtime; may increase if needed

Available forms: Caps 5, 10 mg

Adverse effects

CNS: *Drowsiness,* amnesia, depersonalization,

hallucinations, hypesthesia, paresthesia, somnolence, tremor, vertigo, dizziness, anxiety, *lethargy, daytime sedation,* confusion
EENT: Vision changes, ear/eye pain, hyperacusis, parosmia
GI: Nausea, anorexia, colitis, dyspepsia, dry mouth, constipation, abdominal pain
MISC: Asthenia, fever, headache, myalgia, dysmenorrhea

Contraindications: Hypersensitivity

Precautions: Pregnancy **C**, hepatic disease, renal disease, elderly, psychosis, child <15 yr, lactation

Pharmacokinetics	
Absorption	Rapidly absorbed
Distribution	Extravascular tissues, crosses blood-brain barrier; crosses placenta
Metabolism	Extensively, liver to inactive metabolites
Excretion	Kidneys
Half-life	1 hr

Pharmacodynamics	
Onset	Rapid
Peak	1 hr
Duration	Unknown

Interactions
Individual drugs
Cimetidine: increased action of zaleplon
Rifampin: decreased zaleplon levels
Drug/herb
Black cohosh: increased hypotension
Catnip, chamomile, clary, cowslip, hops, kava, lavender, mistletoe, nettle, pokeweed, poppy, Queen Anne's lace, senega, skullcap, valerian: increased CNS depression
Drug/food
High-fat/heavy meal: prolonged absorption, sleep onset reduced

NURSING CONSIDERATIONS
Assessment
- Assess for previous drug dependence or tolerance; if drug dependent or tolerant, amount of medication should be restricted
- Monitor patient's mental status: mood, sensorium, affect, sleeping patterns, drowsiness, dizziness, suicidal tendencies

Nursing diagnoses
- Sleep pattern, disturbed (uses)
- Knowledge, deficient (teaching)
- Noncompliance (teaching)

Implementation
- Give ½-1 hr before bedtime for sleeplessness; give on empty stomach

Patient/family education
- Inform patient that drug is for short-term use only
- Teach patient to take immediately before going to bed
- Advise patient that drug may cause memory problems, dependence (if used for longer periods of time), changes in behavior/thinking
- Advise patient not to ingest a high-fat/heavy meal before taking
- Advise patient to avoid OTC preparations unless approved by a physician, to avoid alcohol ingestion or other psychotropic medications unless prescribed by a health care provider, that 1-2 wk of therapy may be required before therapeutic effects occur
- Caution patient to avoid driving, activities requiring alertness; drowsiness may occur; until medication response is known, tell patient that drowsiness may worsen at beginning of treatment
- Instruct patient not to discontinue medication abruptly after long-term use

Evaluation
Positive therapeutic outcome
- Decreased sleeplessness

zanamivir (Rx)
(zan-a-mee'veer)
Relenza
Func. class.: Antiviral
Chem class.: Nevramidase inhibitor

Pregnancy category C

Action: Inhibits neuramidase enzyme needed for influenza virus replication

Therapeutic Outcome: Decreased symptoms of influenza types A and B for those who have been symptomatic for no more than 2 days

Uses: Treatment of influenza types A and B

Investigational uses: Prophylaxis against influenza A and B infections; avian flu (H5N1)

Dosage and routes
Adult and child >7 yr: INH 2 inhalations (two 5 mg blisters) q12h × 5 days, on the 1st day 2 doses should be taken with at least 2 hr between doses

Available forms: Blisters of powder for inhalation 5 mg

Adverse effects
CNS: *Headache, dizziness,* fatigue
EENT: Ear, nose, throat infections
GI: *Nausea, vomiting, diarrhea*
RESP: Nasal symptoms, cough, sinusitis, bronchitis

Contraindications: Hypersensitivity

Precautions: Pregnancy **C**, elderly, lactation, children <7 yr, respiratory disease,

Pharmacokinetics

Absorption	4%-17% absorbed
Distribution	<10% protein binding
Metabolism	Not metabolized
Excretion	Kidneys unchanged
Half-life	2½-5 hr

Pharmacodynamics
Unknown

Interactions: None known

NURSING CONSIDERATIONS
Assessment
- Assess for symptoms of influenza A: increased temp, malaise, aches and pains
- Assess for skin eruptions, photosensitivity after administration of drug
- Monitor respiratory status: rate, character, wheezing, tightness in chest
- Assess for allergies before initiation of treatment, reaction of each medication

Nursing diagnoses
- Infection, risk for (uses)
- Knowledge, deficient (teaching)

Implementation
- Give before exposure to influenza; continue for 5 days after contact
- Store in airtight, dry container

Patient/family education
- Give patient "Patient's instruction for use" and review all points before using delivery system
- Teach patient to avoid hazardous activities if dizziness occurs
- Teach patient to take drug exactly as prescribed; to use for the entire 5 days
- Inform patient that this drug does not reduce transmission risk of influenza to others
- Advise patients with asthma or COPD to carry a fast-acting inhaled bronchodilator since bronchospasm may occur; to use scheduled inhaled bronchodilators before using this drug

Evaluation
Positive therapeutic outcome
- Absence of fever, malaise, cough, dyspnea in influenza A

zidovudine (Rx)
(zye-doe'vue-deen)
Apo-Zidovudine ♣, Azidothymidine, AZT, Novo-AZT ♣, Retrovir
Func. class.: Antiretroviral
Chem. class.: (NRTI) Nucleoside reverse transcriptase inhibitor

Pregnancy category C

Action: Inhibits replication of HIV-1 by incorporating into cellular DNA by viral reverse transcriptase, thereby terminating the cellular DNA chain

Therapeutic Outcome: Decreased symptoms of HIV-1 infection

Uses: Used in combination with other antiretrovirals for HIV-1 infection

Dosage and routes
Adult: PO 600 mg daily in divided doses, either 200 mg tid or 300 mg bid in combination with other antiretrovirals; **IV** 1-2 mg/kg q4h, initiate PO as soon as possible, up to 1000 mg

Child 6 wk-12 yr: PO 160 mg/m² q8h (480 mg/m²/day, max 200 mg q8h) in combination with other antiretrovirals; **IV** same as adult

Neonates: PO 2-3 mg/kg/dose q6h; **IV** 1.5 mg/kg infused over 30 min q6h

Prevention of maternal-fetal HIV transmission

Neonatal: PO 2 mg/kg/dose q6h × 6 wk beginning 8-12 hr after birth; **IV** 1.5 mg/kg/dose over 30 min q6h until able to take PO

Maternal (>14 wk gestation): PO 100 mg 5 ×/day until start of labor, then during labor/delivery **IV** 2 mg/kg over 1 hr followed by **IV** inf 1 mg/kg/hr until umbilical cord clamped

Symptomatic HIV infection

Child 3 mo-12 yr: PO 90-180 mg/m² q6h, max 200 mg q6h; **IV** 1-2 mg/kg over 1 hr q4h

Adult: PO 100 mg q4h; **IV** 1-2 mg/kg over 1 hr q4h

Prevention of HIV after needlestick

Adult: PO 200 mg tid plus lamivudine 150

mg bid, plus a protease inhibitor for high-risk exposure; begin within 2 hr of exposure

Available forms: Caps 100 mg; tabs 300 mg; inj 200 mg/20 ml; oral syr 50 mg/5 ml

Adverse effects

CNS: *Fever, headache, malaise,* diaphoresis, *dizziness, insomnia,* paresthesia, somnolence, chills, tremor, twitching, anxiety, confusion, depression, lability, vertigo, loss of mental acuity, **seizures**

EENT: Taste change, hearing loss, photophobia

GI: *Nausea, vomiting, diarrhea,* anorexia, cramps, *dyspepsia,* constipation, dysphagia, *flatulence,* rectal bleeding, mouth ulcer, abdominal pain

GU: Dysuria, polyuria, frequency, hesitancy

HEMA: **Granulocytopenia, anemia**

INTEG: *Rash,* acne, pruritus, urticaria

MS: Myalgia, arthralgia, muscle spasm

RESP: Dyspnea

Contraindications: Hypersensitivity

Precautions: Pregnancy **C,** granulocyte count <1000/mm^3 or Hgb <9.5 g/dl, lactation, children, severe renal disease, impaired hepatic function, anemia

Pharmacokinetics

Absorption	Well absorbed (PO), completely absorbed (**IV**)
Distribution	Widely distributed—crosses placenta, CSF, protein binding 38%
Metabolism	Liver—mostly
Excretion	Kidneys
Half-life	Terminal ½-3 hr

Pharmacodynamics

	PO	IV
Onset	Unknown	Rapid
Peak	½-1½ hr	Inf end
Duration	Unknown	Unknown

Interactions

Individual drugs

Fluconazole, probenecid: increased toxicity

Ganciclovir, radiation, valganciclovir, SMX/TMP: increased bone marrow suppression

Methadone: increased zidovudine

Drug classifications

Antineoplastics: increased bone marrow suppression

NURSING CONSIDERATIONS

Assessment

- Assess for peripheral neuropathy: tingling or pain in hands and feet, distal numbness; if these occur, drug may be decreased or discontinued
- Assess for pancreatitis: abdominal pain, nausea, vomiting, elevated liver enzymes; drug should be discontinued because condition can be fatal
- Assess children by dilated retinal examination q6 mo to rule out retinal depigmentation
- Monitor CBC, differential, platelet count qmo; withhold drug if WBC is <4000/mm^3 or platelet count is <75,000/mm^3; notify prescriber of results; monitor viral load, CD4 counts baseline and throughout treatment
- Monitor renal function studies: BUN, serum uric acid, urine CCr before, during therapy; these may be elevated throughout treatment
- Monitor temp q4h, may indicate beginning of infection
- Monitor liver function tests before, during therapy (bilirubin, AST, ALT amylase, alkaline phosphatase) prn or qmo

Nursing diagnoses

- Infection, risk for (uses)
- Injury, risk for (adverse reactions)
- Knowledge, deficient (teaching)

Implementation

PO route

- Give on empty stomach, bid or tid
- Do not take dapsone at same time as didanosine

IV route

- Give by intermittent inf after diluting with D_5W; give over 1 hr (<4 mg/ml), do not give by direct **IV**

Y-site compatibilities: Acyclovir, allopurinol, amikacin, amphotericin B, aztreonam, ceftazidime, ceftriaxone, cimetidine, clindamycin, dexamethasone, DOBUTamine, DOPamine, erythromycin, fluconazole, fludarabine, gentamicin, heparin, imipenem/cilastatin, lorazepam, metoclopramide, morphine, nafcillin, ondansetron, oxacillin, pentamidine, phenylephrine, piperacillin, potassium chloride, ranitidine, sargramostim, tobramycin, trimethoprim/sulfamethoxazole, vancomycin

Additive incompatibilities: Blood products or protein solutions

Patient/family education

- Caution patient to take on empty stomach; to use exactly as prescribed
- Advise patient to report signs of infection: increased temp, sore throat, flulike symptoms; to avoid crowds and those with known infections
- Instruct patient to report signs of anemia:

fatigue, headache, faintness, shortness of breath, irritability
- Advise patient to report bleeding; avoid use of razors or commercial mouthwash
- Inform patient that hair may be lost during therapy (rare); a wig or hairpiece may make patient feel better
- Caution patient to avoid OTC products or other medications without approval of prescriber
- Caution patient not to have any sexual contact without use of a condom; needles should not be shared; blood from infected individual should not come in contact with another's mucous membranes

Evaluation
Positive therapeutic outcome
- Decreased infection; symptoms of HIV infection

zileuton (Rx)
(zye-loo'tahn)
Zyflo
Func. class.: Bronchodilator
Chem. class.: 5-Lipoxygenase inhibitor, leukotriene pathway inhibitor
Pregnancy category C

Action: Inhibits leukotriene (LT) formation; leukotrienes exert their effects by increasing neutrophil, eosinophil migration; aggregation of neutrophils, monocytes; smooth muscle contraction, capillary permeability; these actions further lead to bronchoconstriction, inflammation, edema

Therapeutic Outcome: Ability to breathe more easily

Uses: Asthma

Investigational uses: Ulcerative colitis, rheumatoid arthritis

Dosage and routes
Asthma
Adult and child >12 yr: PO 600 mg qid, may be given with meal and at bedtime
Ulcerative colitis (off-label)
Adult: PO 600 mg bid

Available forms: Tabs 600 mg

Adverse effects
CNS: Dizziness, insomnia, fatigue, paresthesias, headache
GI: Nausea, abdominal pain, dyspepsia, diarrhea, liver function test abnormalities
INTEG: Hives
MS: Myalgia, asthenia

Contraindications: Active hepatic disease, elevations in liver function tests 3 × upper limits, hypersensitivity

Precautions: Pregnancy **C**, acute attacks of asthma, alcohol consumption, lactation, history of hepatic disease

Pharmacokinetics	
Absorption	Rapid
Distribution	Protein binding 93%
Metabolism	Liver
Excretion	Urine
Half-life	2.1-2.5 hr

Pharmacodynamics	
Onset	Unknown
Peak	1-3 hr
Duration	Unknown

Interactions
Individual drugs
Propranolol: increased propranolol effects
Theophylline: increased theophylline effects
Warfarin: increased warfarin effect
Drug/herb
Green tea (large amounts), guarana: increased effect

NURSING CONSIDERATIONS
Assessment
- Assess CBC, blood chemistry, during treatment
- Assess liver function tests before and qmo × 3 mo, then q2-3 mo during first year treatment
- Assess respiratory rate, rhythm, depth; auscultate lung fields bilaterally; notify prescriber of abnormalities
- Assess allergic reactions: rash, urticaria; drug should be discontinued

Nursing diagnoses
- Breathing pattern, ineffective (uses)
- Knowledge, deficient (teaching)
- Noncompliance (teaching)

Implementation
- Give PO with water or food to decrease GI symptoms

Patient/family education
- Advise patient to check OTC medications, current prescription medications for epHEDrine, which will increase stimulation; to avoid alcohol

- Advise patient to avoid hazardous activities; dizziness may occur
- Advise patient that if GI upset occurs, to take drug with 8 oz of water or food
- Advise patient to notify prescriber of nausea, vomiting, anxiety, insomnia
- Advise to take even without symptoms
- Advise not to use for acute asthma attack

Evaluation
Positive therapeutic outcome
- Ability to breathe more easily

zinc sulfate
(PO, OTC; **IV**, Rx)
(zink sul'fate)

Orazinc, PMS Egozine ✱, Verazinc, Zinca-Pak, Zincate, Zinc 15, Zinc-220, zinc sulfate

Func. class.: Trace element; nutritional supplement

Pregnancy category A

Action: Needed for adequate healing, bone and joint development, taste and smell (23% zinc)

Therapeutic Outcome: Replacement of zinc

Uses: Prevention of zinc deficiency, adjunct to vit A therapy

Investigational uses: Wound healing

Dosage and routes
Dietary supplement
Adult: PO 25-50 mg/day

***Nutritional supplement* (IV)**
Adult: 2.5-4 mg/day, may increase by 2 mg/day if needed
Child to 5 yr: **IV** 100 mcg/kg/day
Infants: <1500 g-3 kg: **IV** 300 mcg/kg/day

Wound healing
Adult: PO 50 mg daily × 1-2 mo

Available forms: Tabs 66, 110 mg; caps 220 mg; inj 1, 5 mg/ml

Adverse effects
GI: Nausea, vomiting, cramps, heartburn, ulcer formation
OVERDOSE: Diarrhea, rash, dehydration, restlessness

Precautions: Pregnancy **A**

Pharmacokinetics

Absorption	Poorly absorbed (PO), completely absorbed (**IV**)
Distribution	Widely distributed
Metabolism	Liver
Excretion	90%—feces, 10%—kidneys
Half-life	Unknown

Pharmacodynamics
Unknown

Interactions
Drug classification
Fluoroquinolones, tetracyclines: decreased absorption

NURSING CONSIDERATIONS
Assessment
- Monitor zinc levels during treatment

Nursing diagnoses
- Nutrition: less than body requirements, imbalanced (uses)
- Knowledge, deficient (teaching)

Implementation
PO route
- Give with meals to decrease gastric upset; restrict dairy products, caffeine, which decrease absorption

IV route
- Part of TPN

Patient/family education
- Inform patient that element must be taken for 3 mo to be effective
- Advise patient to report immediately nausea, diarrhea, rash, severe vomiting, restlessness, abdominal pain, tarry stools

Evaluation
Positive therapeutic outcome
- Absence of zinc deficiency
- Improved wound healing

ziprasidone (Rx)
(zi-praz'ih-dohn)

Geodon

Func. class.: Antipsychotic/neuroleptic
Chem. class.: Benzisoxazole derivative

Pregnancy category C

Action: Unknown; may be mediated through both dopamine type 2 (D_2) and serotonin type 2 (5-HT_2) antagonism

Therapeutic Outcome: Decreased signs/symptoms of psychosis

Uses: Schizophrenia, acute agitation

Dosage and routes

Adult: PO 20 mg bid with food, adjust dosage every 2 days upward to max of 80 mg bid; IM 10-20 mg; may give 10 mg q2h, doses of 20 mg may be given q4h, max 40 mg/day

Available forms: Tabs 20, 40, 60, 80 mg; inj 20 mg/ml

Adverse effects

CNS: *EPS (pseudoparkinsonism, akathisia, dystonia, tardive dyskinesia), drowsiness, insomnia, agitation, anxiety, headache,* **seizures, neuroleptic malignant syndrome,** dizziness, tremor

CV: Orthostatic hypotension, **tachycardia, prolonged QT/QTc, sudden death,** hypertension

EENT: Blurred vision

GI: *Nausea,* vomiting, *anorexia, constipation,* jaundice, weight gain, diarrhea, dry mouth, abdominal pain

RESP: Rhinitis, dyspnea

Contraindications: Hypersensitivity, lactation, seizure disorders

Precautions: Pregnancy **C,** children, renal disease, hepatic disease, elderly, breast cancer

Pharmacokinetics

Absorption	Unknown
Distribution	Protein binding 90%
Metabolism	Liver—extensively to metabolite
Excretion	Unknown
Half-life	Unknown

Pharmacodynamics

Unknown

Interactions

Individual drugs

Alcohol: increased sedation

Carbamazepine: increased excretion of ziprasidone

Ketoconazole: increased ziprasidone level

Lithium: increased extrapyramidal symptoms (EPS)

Drug classifications

Antihypertensives: increased hypotension

Antipsychotics: increased EPS

CNS depressants: increased sedation

Drug/herb

Betel palm, kava: increased EPS

Chamomile, hops, kava, skullcap, valerian: increased CNS depression

Cola tree, hops, nettle, nutmeg: increased action

NURSING CONSIDERATIONS

Assessment

- Assess mental status before initial administration
- Check swallowing of PO medication; check for hoarding or giving of medication to other patients
- Monitor I&O ratio; palpate bladder if urinary output is low
- Monitor bilirubin, CBC, liver function studies qmo
- Monitor urinalysis before, during prolonged therapy
- Assess affect, orientation, LOC, reflexes, gait, coordination, sleep pattern disturbances
- Monitor B/P standing and lying; also pulse, respirations; take these q4h during initial treatment; establish baseline before starting treatment; report drops of 30 mm Hg; watch for ECG changes
- Assess dizziness, faintness, palpitations, tachycardia on rising
- Assess EPS, including akathisia (inability to sit still, no pattern to movements), tardive dyskinesia (bizarre movements of the jaw, mouth, tongue, extremities), pseudoparkinsonism (rigidity, tremors, pill rolling, shuffling gait)
- ❗ Assess for neuroleptic malignant syndrome: hyperthermia, increased CPK, altered mental status, muscle rigidity
- Assess skin turgor daily
- Assess constipation, urinary retention daily; if these occur, increase bulk and water in diet

Nursing diagnoses

- Thought processes, disturbed (uses)
- Coping, ineffective (uses)
- Knowledge, deficient (teaching)
- Noncompliance (teaching)

Implementation

- Give reduced dose in elderly
- Give antiparkinsonian agent on order from prescriber, to be used for EPS
- Provide decreased stimulus by dimming lights, avoiding loud noises
- Provide supervised ambulation until patient is stabilized on medication; do not involve in strenuous exercise program because fainting is possible; patient should not stand still for a long time
- Store in airtight, light-resistant container

IM route

- Add 1.2 ml sterile water for inj to vial, shake vigorously until drug is dissolved, do not admix

Patient/family education

- Advise patient that orthostatic hypotension

may occur and to rise from sitting or lying position gradually; avoid hot tubs, hot showers, tub baths because hypotension may occur
- Advise patient to avoid abrupt withdrawal of this drug; EPS may result; drug should be withdrawn slowly
- Advise patient to avoid OTC preparations (cough, hay fever, cold) unless approved by prescriber, since serious drug interactions may occur; avoid use with alcohol, CNS depressants; increased drowsiness may occur
- Teach patient to avoid hazardous activities if drowsy or dizzy
- Advise patient to increase fluids to prevent constipation
- Teach patient to use sips of water, candy, gum for dry mouth
- Teach patient compliance with drug regimen
- Teach patient to report impaired vision, tremors, muscle twitching
- Teach patient that in hot weather, heat stroke may occur; take extra precautions to stay cool

Evaluation

Positive therapeutic outcome

- Decrease in emotional excitement, hallucinations, delusions, paranoia; reorganization of patterns of thought, speech

Treatment of overdose: Lavage if orally ingested; provide airway; *do not induce vomiting*

zoledronic acid (Rx)

(zoh'leh-drah'nick ass'id))

Zometa

Func. class.: Bone-resorption inhibitor

Chem. class.: Bisphosphonate

Pregnancy category D

Action: Inhibits normal and abnormal bone resorption; potent inhibitor of osteoclastic bone resorption; inhibits osteoclastic activity, reduces bone resorption and inhibits skeletal calcium release caused by stimulating factors released by tumors; reduction of abnormal bone resorption is responsible for therapeutic effect in hypercalcemia; may directly block dissolution of hydroxyapatite bone crystals

Therapeutic Outcome: Serum calcium at normal level

Uses: Moderate to severe hypercalcemia associated with malignancy; multiple myeloma; bone metastases from solid tumors (used with antineoplastics)

Dosage and routes

Hypercalemia of malignancy

Adult: **IV** inf 4 mg, given as a single inf over ≥15 min, may re-treat with 4 mg if serum calcium does not return to normal within 1 wk

Multiple myeloma/metastatic bone lesions

Adult: **IV** inf 4 mg, given over 15 min q3-4 wk; may continue treatment for 9-15 mo, depending on condition

Available forms: Powder for inj 4 mg

Adverse effects

CNS: Dizziness, headache, anxiety, confusion, insomnia, agitation

CV: Hypotension, leg edema

GI: Abdominal pain, anorexia, constipation, nausea, diarrhea, vomiting, micositis

GU: UTI, possible reduced renal function

META: Anemia, hypokalemia, hypomagnesemia, hypophosphatemia, hypocalcemia, increased serum creatinine

MISC: *Fever, chills, flulike symptoms*

MS: Bone pain, *arthralgias, myalgias*

Contraindications: Pregnancy **D,** hypersensitivity to this drug or bisphosphonates

Precautions: Children, nursing mothers, renal dysfunction, aspirin-sensitive asthmatic patients

Pharmacokinetics	
Absorption	Rapidly cleared from circulation
Distribution	Taken up mainly by bones; plasma protein binding ~22%
Metabolism	Not metabolized
Excretion	Kidneys (~50% eliminated in urine within 24 hr)
Half-life	146 hr

Pharmacodynamics	
Onset	Unknown
Peak	15 min
Duration	Max effect 7 days

Interactions

Individual drugs

Calcium, vitamin D: decreased zoledronic acid effect

Digoxin: hypomagnesemia, hypokalemia infusion solutions (calcium-containing): do not mix with Ca-containing infusion sol such as Ringer's sol

Drug classifications

Aminoglycosides, loop diuretics: decreased serum calcium

NURSING CONSIDERATIONS

Assessment

- Assess renal studies and Ca, P, Mg, K, creatinine, if creatinine is elevated hold treatment
- Assess for hypercalcemia: paresthesia, twitching, laryngospasm; Chvostek's, Trousseau's signs

Nursing diagnoses

- Injury, risk for (uses, adverse reactions)
- Fluid, volume excess (side effects)
- Knowledge, deficient (teaching)

Implementation

- Saline hydration must be performed before administration; urine output should be 2 L/day during treatment, do not overhydrate
- Sol reconstituted with sterile water may be stored under refrigeration for up to 24 hr **IV**
- Administer in separate **IV** line from all other drugs
- Administer after reconstituting by adding 5 ml of sterile water for inj to each vial, then add up to ≥100 ml of sterile 0.9% NaCl, D_5W, run over ≥15 min

Patient/family education

- Instruct patient to report hypercalcemic relapse: nausea, vomiting, bone pain, thirst
- Advise patient to continue with dietary recommendations including calcium and vit D; take a multiple vitamin daily, 500 mg of calcium 400 international units vit D in multiple myeloma
- Teach patient if nausea/vomiting occur, eat small meals, use lozenges, or chewing gum
- Advise patient if bone pain occurs, notify prescriber to obtain analgesic
- Advise patient to avoid pregnancy

Evaluation

Positive therapeutic outcome

- Calcium levels decreased to normal

Treatment of overdose: Correct clinically relevant reductions in serum calcium by administering **IV** calcium gluconate; in serum phosphorus, with potassium or sodium phosphate; in serum magnesium, with magnesium sulfate

zolmitriptan (Rx)

(zole-mih-trip'tan)

Zomig, Zomig-ZMT

Func. class.: Migraine agent

Chem. class.: 5-HT_1 receptor agonist

Pregnancy category C

Action: Binds selectively to the vascular serotonin type 1 (5-HT_1) receptor subtype, exerts antimigraine effect; causes vasoconstriction in cranial arteries

Therapeutic Outcome: Decreased severity, frequency of headache

Uses: Acute treatment of migraine with or without aura

Dosage and routes:

Adult: PO Start at 2.5 mg or lower (tab may be broken), may repeat after 2 hr, max 10 mg/24 hr; nasal 1 spray in each nostril at onset of migraine, repeat in 2 hr if no relief

Available forms: Tabs 2.5, 5 mg; orally disintegrating tabs 2.5, 5 mg; nasal spray 5 mg

Adverse effects

CNS: *Tingling, hot sensation, burning, feeling of pressure, tightness, numbness, dizziness, sedation*

CV: Palpitations, chest pain

GI: Abdominal discomfort, nausea, dry mouth, dyspepsia, dysphagia

MISC: Odd taste (spray)

MS: *Weakness, neck stiffness,* myalgia

RESP: Chest tightness, pressure

Contraindications: Angina pectoris, history of MI, documented silent ischemia, ischemic heart disease, concurrent ergotamine-containing preparations, uncontrolled hypertension, hypersensitivity, basilar or hemiplegic migraine, risk of CV events

Precautions: Pregnancy **C,** postmenopausal women, men >40 yr, risk factors for CAD, hypercholesterolemia, obesity, diabetes, impaired hepatic or renal function, lactation, children, elderly

Pharmacokinetics	
Absorption	Unknown
Distribution	25% plasma protein binding
Metabolism	Liver
Excretion	Urine, feces
Half-life	3-3½ hr

Pharmacodynamics	
Onset	Unknown
Peak	Unknown
Duration	2-3½ hr

Interactions

Individual drugs

Cimetidine: increased half-life of zolmitriptan
Ergot: increased vasospastic effects
Fluoxetine, fluvoxamine, paroxetine, sertraline: increased weakness, hyperreflexia, incoordination

Drug classifications

Contraceptives (oral): increased half-life of zolmitriptan
Ergot derivatives: increased vasospastic effects
MAOIs: do not use within 2 wk
Selective serotonin reuptake inhibitors (SSRIs): increased weakness, hyperreflexia, incoordination

Drug/herb

Butterbur: increased effect
SAM-e, St. John's wort: serotonin syndrome

NURSING CONSIDERATIONS

Assessment

- Assess tingling, hot sensation, burning, feeling of pressure, numbness, flushing
- Assess for stress level, activity, recreation, coping mechanisms
- Assess neurologic status: LOC, blurring vision, nausea, vomiting, tingling in extremities preceding headache
- Monitor ingestion of tyramine foods (pickled products, beer, wine, aged cheese), food additives, preservatives, colorings, artifical sweeteners, chocolate, caffeine, which may precipitate these types of headaches
- Assess for serotonin syndrome, if also taking an SSRI

Nursing diagnoses

- Pain, acute (uses)
- Noncompliance (teaching)
- Knowledge, deficient (teaching)

Implementation

- Give with fluids as soon as symptoms of migraine occur
- Provide quiet, calm environment with decreased stimulation for noise, bright light, excessive talking

Patient/family education

- Teach patient to report any side effects to prescriber
- Advise patient to use contraception while taking drug

Evaluation

Positive therapeutic outcome

- Decrease in frequency, severity of headache

zolpidem (Rx)

(zole-pi'dem)

Ambien

Func. class.: Sedative-hypnotic
Chem. class.: Nonbenzodiazepine of imidazopyridine class

Pregnancy category B

Controlled substance schedule IV

Action: Produces CNS depression at limbic, thalamic, hypothalamic levels of CNS; may be mediated by neurotransmitter γ-aminobutyric acid (GABA); results are sedation, hypnosis, skeletal muscle relaxation, anticonvulsant activity, anxiolytic action

Therapeutic Outcome: Ability to sleep, sedation

Uses: Insomnia, short-term treatment

Dosage and routes

Adult: PO 10 mg at bedtime × 7-10 days only; total dose should not exceed 10 mg
Elderly: PO 5 mg at bedtime

Available forms: Tabs 5, 10 mg

Adverse effects

CNS: Headache, lethargy, drowsiness, daytime sedation, dizziness, confusion, lightheadedness, anxiety, irritability, amnesia, poor coordination
CV: Chest pain, palpitation
GI: Nausea, vomiting, diarrhea, heartburn, abdominal pain, constipation
HEMA: **Leukopenia, granulocytopenia** (rare)

Contraindications: Hypersensitivity to benzodiazepines

Precautions: Pregnancy **B,** anemia, hepatic disease, renal disease, suicidal individuals, drug abuse, elderly, psychosis, child <18 yr, seizure disorders, lactation

Pharmacokinetics	
Absorption	Rapidly absorbed
Distribution	Unknown
Metabolism	Liver—inactive metabolite
Excretion	Kidneys, breast milk
Half-life	2½ hr, increased in elderly

Pharmacodynamics

Unknown

Interactions

Individual drugs

Alcohol: increased action of both drugs

Drug classifications

CNS depressants: increased action of both drugs

Drug/herb

Chamomile, hops, kava, skullcap, valerian: increased CNS depression

Drug/lab test

Increased: ALT, AST, serum bilirubin
Decreased: radioactive iodine uptake
False increase: urinary 17-OHCS

NURSING CONSIDERATIONS

Assessment

- Assess mental status: mood, sensorium, anxiety, affect, sleeping pattern, drowsiness, dizziness, especially elderly; physical dependency, withdrawal symptoms: anxiety, panic attacks, agitation, seizures, headache, nausea, vomiting, muscle pain, weakness; suicidal tendencies; for indications of increasing tolerance and abuse
- Monitor B/P (lying, standing), pulse; if systolic B/P drops 20 mm Hg, hold drug, notify prescriber
- Monitor blood studies: CBC during long-term therapy; blood dycrasias have occurred rarely; decreased hematocrit, neutropenia may occur
- Monitor hepatic studies: AST, ALT, bilirubin, creatinine LDH, alkaline phosphatase
- Monitor I&O ratio for renal dysfunction

Nursing diagnoses

- Anxiety (uses)
- Injury, risk for (adverse reactions)
- Knowledge, deficient (teaching)

Implementation

- Give ½-1 hr before bedtime for sleeplessness; give several hr before patient is to arise (to avoid hangover)
- Give with food or fluids; tab may be crushed or swallowed whole
- Store in airtight container in cool environment

Patient/family education

- Instruct patient that drug may be taken with food or fluids
- Caution patient not to use for everyday stress or longer than 3 mo unless directed by prescriber; not to take more than prescribed amount; may be habit forming; not to double or skip doses
- Caution patient to avoid OTC preparations unless approved by prescriber; alcohol and CNS depressants will increase CNS depression
- Advise patient to avoid driving, activities that require alertness, because drowsiness may occur; to avoid alcohol ingestion or other psychotropic medications; to rise slowly or fainting may occur, especially elderly; that drowsiness may worsen at beginning of treatment
- Instruct patient not to discontinue medication abruptly after long-term use; withdrawal symptoms include vomiting, cramping, tremors, seizures

Evaluation

Positive therapeutic outcome

- Ability to sleep at night
- Decreased amount of early morning awakening if taking drug for insomnia

Treatment of overdose: Lavage, VS, supportive care

zonisamide (Rx)

(zone-is'a-mide)

Zonegran

Func. class.: Anticonvulsant
Chem. class.: Sulfonamides

Pregnancy category C

Action: May act through sodium and calcium channels, but exact action is unknown

Therapeutic Outcome: Decreased seizures

Uses: Epilepsy, adjunctive therapy of partial seizures

Dosage and routes

Adults and child >16 yr: PO 100 mg daily, may increase after 2 wk to 200 mg/day, may increase q2 wk, max dose 600 mg/day

Available forms: Caps 25, 50, 100 mg

Adverse effects

CNS: Dizziness, insomnia, paresthesias, depression, fatigue, headache, confusion, somnolence, agitation, irritability
EENT: Diplopia, verbal difficulty, speech abnormalities, taste perversion
GI: Nausea, constipation, anorexia, weight loss, diarrhea, dyspepsia
HEMA: **Aplastic anemia, granulocytopenia** (rare)
INTEG: Rash
SYST: **Stevens-Johnson syndrome**

Contraindications: Hypersensitivity to this drug or sulfonamides, psychiatric condition, hepatic failure

Precautions: Pregnancy **C,** allergies, hepatic disease, renal disease, elderly, lactation, child <16 yr

Pharmacokinetics	
Absorption	Unknown
Distribution	Unknown
Metabolism	Liver
Excretion	Kidneys
Half-life	63 hr

Pharmacodynamics	
Onset	Unknown
Peak	2-6 hr
Duration	Unknown

Interactions

Drugs inducing CYP450 enzyme (carbamazepine, phenytoin, phenobarbital): decreased half-life of zonisamide

NURSING CONSIDERATIONS

Assessment

- Assess for seizures: duration, type, intensity, precipitating factors
- Renal function: albumin conc
- Assess mental status: mood, sensorium, affect, memory (long, short)

Nursing diagnoses

- Injury, risk for (uses, adverse reactions)
- Knowledge, deficient (teaching)
- Noncompliance (teaching)

Patient/family education

- Advise patient not to discontinue drug abruptly; seizures may occur
- Advise patient to avoid hazardous activities until stabilized on drug
- Advise patient to carry/wear emergency ID stating drug use

Evaluation

Positive therapeutic outcome

- Decrease in severity of seizures

ALPHA-ADRENERGIC BLOCKERS

Action: Binds to α-adrenergic receptors, causing dilatation of peripheral blood vessels; lowers peripheral resistance, resulting in decreased blood pressure.

Uses: Used for pheochromocytoma, prevention of tissue necrosis, and sloughing associated with extravasation of IV vasopressors.

Adverse effects: The most common side effects are hypotension, tachycardia, nasal stuffiness, nausea, vomiting, and diarrhea.

Contraindications: Hypersensitive reactions may occur, and allergies should be identified before these products are given. Patients with myocardial infarction, coronary insufficiency, angina, or other evidence of coronary artery disease should not use these products.

Pharmacokinetics: Onset, peak, and duration vary among products.

Interactions: Vasoconstrictive and hypertensive effects of epinephrine are antagonized by α-adrenergic blockers.

NURSING CONSIDERATIONS

Assessment

- Monitor electrolytes: potassium, sodium chloride, carbon dioxide
- Monitor weight daily, I&O
- Monitor B/P with patient lying, standing before starting treatment, q4h thereafter
- Assess for nausea, vomiting, diarrhea
- Assess for skin turgor, dryness of mucous membranes for hydration status

Nursing diagnoses

- Tissue perfusion, ineffective (uses)
- Injury, risk for (adverse reactions)
- Sleep pattern, disturbed (adverse reactions)

Implementation

PO route

- Start with low dose, gradually increasing to prevent side effects
- Give with food or milk for GI symptoms

Evaluation

- Therapeutic response: decreased B/P, increased peripheral pulses

Patient/family education

- Caution patient to avoid alcoholic beverages
- Advise patient to report dizziness, palpitations, fainting
- Instruct patient to change position slowly or fainting may occur
- Teach patient to take drug exactly as prescribed; to avoid all OTC products (cough, cold, allergy) unless directed by prescriber

Generic Names

phentolamine

ANESTHETICS—GENERAL/LOCAL

Action: Anesthetics (general) act on the CNS to produce tranquilization and sleep before invasive procedures. Anesthetics (local) inhibit conduction of nerve impulses from sensory nerves.

Uses: General anesthetics are used to premedicate for surgery, and for induction and maintenance in general anesthesia. For local anesthetics, refer to individual product listing for indications.

Adverse effects: The most common side effects are dystonia, akathisia, flexion of arms, fine tremors, drowsiness, restlessness, and hypotension. Also common are chills, respiratory depression, and laryngospasm.

Contraindications: Persons with CVA, increased intracranial pressure, severe hypertension, cardiac decompensation should not use these products, since severe adverse reactions can occur.

Precautions: Anesthetics (general) should be used with caution in the elderly, cardiovascular disease (hypotension, bradydysrhythmias), renal disease, liver disease, Parkinson's disease, children <2 yr. The precaution for anesthetics (local) is pregnancy.

Pharmacokinetics: Onset, peak, and duration vary widely among products. Most products are metabolized in the liver and excreted in urine.

Interactions: MAOIs, tricyclics, phenothiazines may cause severe hypotension or hypertension when used with local anesthetics. CNS depressants will potentiate general and local anesthetics.

NURSING CONSIDERATIONS

Assessment

- Monitor VS q10 min during **IV** administration, q30 min after IM dose

Nursing diagnoses

General

- Injury, risk for (adverse reactions)
- Knowledge, deficient (teaching)

Local

- Pain, acute (uses)
- Knowledge, deficient (teaching)

Implementation

- Give anticholinergic preoperatively to decrease secretions
- Administer only with resuscitative equipment nearby
- Provide quiet environment for recovery to decrease psychotic symptoms

Evaluation

- Therapeutic response: maintenance of anesthesia, decreased pain

---

Generic Names

General anesthetics:
droperidol (high alert)
etomidate
fentanyl (high alert)
fentanyl transdermal
midazolam
propofol (high alert)

Local anesthetics:
🔑 **lidocaine, parenteral** (high alert)
ropivacaine
tetracaine

ANTACIDS

Action: Antacids are basic compounds that neutralize gastric acidity and decrease the rate of gastric emptying. Products are divided into those containing aluminum, magnesium, calcium, or a combination of these.

Uses: Hyperacidity is decreased by antacids in conditions such as peptic ulcer disease, reflux esophagitis, gastritis, or hiatal hernia.

Adverse effects: The most common side effect caused by aluminum-containing antacids is constipation, which may lead to fecal impaction and bowel obstruction. Diarrhea occurs often when magnesium products are given. Alkalosis may occur when systemic products are used. Constipation occurs more frequently than laxation with calcium carbonate. The release of CO_2 from carbonate-containing antacids causes belching, abdominal distention, and flatulence. Sodium bicarbonate may act as a systemic antacid and produce systemic electrolyte disturbances and alkalosis. Calcium carbonate and sodium bicarbonate may cause rebound hyperacidity and milk-alkali syndrome. Alkaluria may occur when products are used on a long-term basis, particularly in persons with abnormal renal function.

Contraindications: Sensitivity to aluminum or magnesium products may cause hypersensitive reactions. Aluminum products should not be used by persons sensitive to aluminum; magnesium products should not be used by persons sensitive to magnesium. Check for sensitivity before administering.

Precautions: Magnesium products should be given cautiously to patients with renal insufficiency, during pregnancy, or lactation. Sodium content of antacids may be significant; use with caution for patients with hypertension, CHF, or those on a low-sodium diet.

Pharmacokinetics: Duration is 20-40 min. If ingested 1 hr pc, acidity is reduced for at least 3 hr.

Interactions: Drugs whose effects may be increased by some antacids: quinidine, amphetamines, pseudoephedrine, levodopa, valproic acid, dicumarol. Drugs whose effects may be decreased by some antacids: cimetidine, corticosteroids, ranitidine, iron salts, phenothiazines, phenytoin, digoxin, tetracyclines, ketoconazole, salicylates, isoniazid.

NURSING CONSIDERATIONS

Assessment

- Assess for aggravating and alleviating factors of epigastric pain or hyperacidity; identify the location, duration, and characteristics of epigastric pain
- Assess GI symptoms, including constipation, diarrhea, abdominal pain; if severe abdominal pain with fever occurs, these drugs should not be given
- Assess renal symptoms, including increasing urinary pH, electrolytes

Nursing diagnoses

- Pain, chronic (uses)
- Constipation (adverse reactions)
- Diarrhea (adverse reactions)

Implementation

- Give all products with an 8-oz glass of water to ensure absorption in the stomach
- Give another antacid if constipation occurs with aluminum products
- Advise patient not to take other drugs within 1-2 hr of antacid administration, since antacids may impair absorption of other drugs

Evaluation

- Therapeutic response: absence of epigastric pain, decreased acidity

Generic Names

aluminum hydroxide
bismuth subsalicylate
calcium carbonate
magaldrate
magnesium oxide
sodium bicarbonate

ANTIANGINALS

Action: The antianginals are divided into the nitrates, calcium channel blockers, and β-adrenergic blockers. The nitrates dilate coronary arteries, causing decreased preload, and dilate systemic arteries, causing decreased afterload. Calcium channel blockers dilate coronary arteries, decrease SA/AV node conduction. β-Adrenergic blockers decrease heart rate so that myocardial O_2 use is decreased. Dipyridamole selectively dilates coronary arteries to increase coronary blood flow.

Uses: Antianginals are used in chronic stable angina pectoris, unstable angina, vasospastic angina. Some (i.e., calcium channel blockers and β-blockers) may be used as dysrhythmias and in hypertension.

Adverse effects: The most common side effects are postural hypotension, headache, flushing, dizziness, nausea, edema, and drowsiness. Also common are rash, dysrhythmias, and fatigue.

Contraindications: Persons with known hypersensitivity, increased intracranial pressure, or cerebral hemorrhage should not use some of these products.

Precautions: Antianginals should be used with caution in postural hypotension, pregnancy, lactation, children, renal disease, and hepatic injury.

Pharmacokinetics: Onset, peak, and duration vary widely among coronary products. Most products are metabolized in the liver and excreted in urine.

Interactions: Please check individual monographs, since interactions vary widely among products.

NURSING CONSIDERATIONS

Assessment

- Orthostatic B/P, pulse
- Assess for pain: duration, time started, activity being performed, character
- Assess for tolerance if taken over long period
- Assess for headache, lightheadedness, decreased B/P; may indicate a need for decreased dosage

Nursing diagnoses

- Tissue perfusion, ineffective (uses)
- Pain, chronic (uses)
- Injury, risk for (uses)
- Knowledge, deficient (teaching)
- Cardiac output, decreased (adverse reactions)

Implementation

- Store protected from light, moisture; place in cool environment

Evaluation

- Therapeutic response: decreased, prevention of anginal pain

Patient/family education

- Instruct patient to keep tabs in original container
- Instruct patient not to use OTC products unless directed by prescriber
- Advise patient to report bradycardia, dizziness, confusion, depression, fever
- Teach patient to take pulse at home; advise when to notify prescriber
- Advise patient to avoid alcohol, smoking, sodium intake
- Advise patient to comply with weight control, dietary adjustments, modified exercise program
- Teach patient to carry/wear emergency ID to identify drug being taken, allergies
- Caution patient to make position changes slowly to prevent fainting

Generic Names

Nitrates:
amyl nitrite
isosorbide
nitroglycerin

β-Adrenergic blockers:
atenolol
dipyridamole
metoprolol
nadolol
propranolol

Calcium channel blockers:
amlodipine
bepridil
diltiazem (high alert)
niCARdipine
NIFEdipine
verapamil

ANTICHOLINERGICS

Action: Anticholinergics inhibit the muscarinic actions of acetylcholine at receptor sites in the autonomic nervous system; anticholinergics are also known as antimuscarinic drugs.

Uses: Anticholinergics are used for a variety of conditions: gastrointestinal anticholinergics are used to decrease motility (smooth muscle tone) in the GI, biliary, and urinary tracts and for their ability to decrease gastric secretions (propantheline, glycopyrrolate); decreasing involuntary movements in parkinsonism (benztropine, trihexyphenidyl); bradydysrhythmias (atropine); nausea and vomiting (scopolamine); and as cycloplegic mydriatics (atropine, hematropine, scopalamine, cyclopentolate, tropicamide).

Adverse effects: The most common side effects are dry mouth, constipation, urinary retention, urinary hesitancy, headache, and dizziness. Also common is paralytic ileus.

Contraindications: Persons with narrow-angle glaucoma, myasthenia gravis, or GI/GU obstruction should not use some of these products.

Precautions: Anticholinergics should be used with caution in patients who are elderly, pregnant, or lactating or in those with prostatic hypertrophy, CHF, or hypertension; use with caution in presence of high environmental temp.

Pharmacokinetics: Onset, peak, and duration vary widely among products. Most products are metabolized in the liver and excreted in urine.

Interactions: Increased anticholinergic effects may occur when used with MAOIs and tricyclic antidepressants and amantadine. Anticholinergics may cause a decreased effect of phenothiazines and levodopa.

NURSING CONSIDERATIONS

Assessment

- Assess I&O ratio; retention commonly causes decreased urinary output
- Assess for urinary hesitancy, retention; palpate bladder if retention occurs
- Assess for constipation; increase fluids, bulk, exercise if this occurs
- Identify tolerance over long-term therapy; dosage may need to be increased or changed
- Assess mental status: affect, mood, CNS depression, worsening of mental symptoms during early therapy

Nursing diagnoses

- Cardiac output, decreased (uses)
- Constipation (adverse reactions)
- Knowledge, deficient (teaching)

Implementation

IM/IV routes

- Give parenteral dose with patient recumbent to prevent postural hypotension
- Give parenteral dose slowly; keep in bed for at least 1 hr after dose; monitor VS
- Give after checking dose carefully; even slight overdose could lead to toxicity

PO route

- Give with or after meals to prevent GI upset; may give with fluids other than water
- Store at room temp
- Give hard candy, frequent drinks, sugarless gum to relieve dry mouth

Evaluation

- Therapeutic response: decreased sécretions, absence of nausea and vomiting

Patient/family education

- Caution patient to avoid driving and other hazardous activities; drowsiness may occur
- Advise patient to avoid OTC medication: cough, cold preparations with alcohol, antihistamines unless directed by prescriber

Generic Names

Key Drug **atropine** (high alert)
Key Drug benztropine
biperiden
glycopyrrolate
hyoscyamine
propantheline
scopolamine (transdermal)
solifenacin
trihexyphenidyl

ANTICOAGULANTS

Action: Anticoagulants interfere with blood clotting by preventing clot formation.

Uses: Anticoagulants are used for deep vein thrombosis, pulmonary emboli, myocardial infarction, open heart surgery, disseminated intravascular clotting syndrome, atrial fibrillation with embolization, and in transfusion and dialysis.

Adverse effects: The most serious adverse reactions are hemorrhage, agranulocytosis, leukopenia, eosinophilia, and thrombocytopenia, depending on the specific product. The most common side effects are diarrhea, rash, and fever.

Contraindications: Persons with hemophilia, leukemia with bleeding, peptic ulcer disease, thrombocytopenic purpura, blood dyscrasias, acute nephritis, and subacute bacterial endocarditis should not use these products.

Precautions: Anticoagulants should be used with caution in alcoholism, elderly, and pregnancy.

Pharmacokinetics: Onset, peak, and duration vary widely among products. Most products are metabolized in the liver and excreted in urine.

Interactions: Salicylates, steroids, and nonsteroidal antiinflammatories will potentiate the action of anticoagulants. Anticoagulants may cause serious effects; please check individual monographs.

NURSING CONSIDERATIONS

Assessment

- Monitor blood studies (Hct, platelets, occult blood in stools) q3 mo
- Monitor partial prothrombin time, which should be 1½-2 × control, PPT; often daily, APTT, ACT, INR
- Monitor B/P; watch for increasing signs of hypertension
- Monitor for bleeding gums, petechiae, ecchymosis, black tarry stools, hematuria
- Monitor for fever, skin rash, urticaria
- Monitor for needed dosage change q1-2 wk

Nursing diagnoses

- Tissue perfusion, ineffective (uses)
- Injury, risk for (side effects)
- Knowledge, deficient (teaching)

Implementation

SUBCUT route

- Give at same time each day to maintain steady blood levels
- Do not massage area or aspirate when giving SUBCUT inj; give in abdomen between pelvic bones; rotate sites; do not pull back on plunger, leave in for 10 sec; apply gentle pressure for 1 min
- Do not change needles
- Avoid all IM inj that may cause bleeding
- Store in tight container (PO dose)

Evaluation

- Therapeutic response: decrease of deep vein thrombosis

Patient/family education

- Advise patient to avoid OTC preparations that may cause serious drug interactions unless directed by prescriber
- Inform patient that drug may be held during active bleeding (menstruation), depending on condition
- Caution patient to use soft-bristle toothbrush to avoid bleeding gums; avoid contact sports; use electric razor
- Instruct patient to carry/wear emergency ID identifying drug taken
- Instruct patient to report any signs of bleeding: gums, under skin, urine, stools

Generic Names

ardeparin (high alert)
argatroban
dalteparin (high alert)
danaparoid (high alert)
desirudin
enoxaparin (high alert)
fondaparinux
🔑 **heparin** (high alert)
lepirudin (high alert)
tinzaparin (high alert)
🔑 **warfarin** (high alert)

ANTICONVULSANTS

Action: Anticonvulsants are divided into the barbiturates (p. 1010), benzodiazepines (p. 1010), hydantoins, succinimides, and miscellaneous products. Barbiturates and benzodiazepines are discussed in separate sections. Hydantoins act by inhibiting the spread of seizure activity in the motor cortex. Succinimides act by inhibiting spike and wave formation; they also decrease amplitude, frequency, duration, and spread of discharge in seizures.

Uses: Hydantoins are used in generalized tonic-clonic seizures, status epilepticus, and psychomotor seizures. Succinimides are used for absence of (petit mal) seizures. Barbiturates are used in generalized tonic-clonic and cortical focal seizures.

Adverse effects: Bone marrow depression is the most life-threatening adverse reaction associated with hydantoins or succinimides. The most common side effects are GI symptoms. Other common side effects for hydantoins are gingival hyperplasia and CNS effects such as nystagmus, ataxia, slurred speech, and confusion.

Contraindications: Hypersensitive reactions may occur, and allergies should be identified before these products are given.

Precautions: Persons with renal or hepatic disease should be watched closely.

Pharmacokinetics: Onset, peak, and duration vary widely among products. Most products are metabolized in the liver and excreted in urine, bile, and feces.

Interactions: Decreased effects of estrogens, oral contraceptives (hydantoins).

NURSING CONSIDERATIONS
Assessment
- Monitor renal function studies, including BUN, creatinine, serum uric acid, urine CCr before and during therapy
- Monitor blood studies: RBC, Hct, Hgb, reticulocyte counts weekly for 4 wk then monthly
- Monitor hepatic studies: AST, ALT, bilirubin, creatinine
- Assess mental status, including mood, sensorium, affect, behavioral changes; if mental status changes, notify prescriber
- Assess for eye problems, including need for ophth examinations before, during, and after treatment (slit lamp, fundoscopy, tonometry)
- Assess for allergic reaction, including red, raised rash; if this occurs, drug should be discontinued
- Assess for blood dyscrasias, including fever, sore throat, bruising, rash, jaundice
- Monitor toxicity, including bone marrow depression, nausea, vomiting, ataxia, diplopia, cardiovascular collapse, Stevens-Johnson syndrome

Nursing diagnoses
- Injury, risk for (uses)
- Noncompliance (teaching)
- Sleep pattern, disturbed (adverse reactions)

Implementation
PO route
- Give with food, milk to decrease GI symptoms
- Good oral hygiene is important for patients taking hydantoins

Evaluation
- Therapeutic response, including decreased seizure activity; document on patient's chart

Patient/family education
- Advise patient to carry/wear emergency ID stating drugs taken, condition, prescriber's name, phone number
- Advise patient to avoid driving, other activities that require alertness

Generic Names
Hydantoins:
fosphenytoin
phenytoin (Key Drug)

Miscellaneous:
acetazolamide
carbamazepine
clonazepam
diazepam (Key Drug)
felbamate
gabapentin
lamotrigine
magnesium sulfate (high alert)
tiagabine
topiramate
valproate/valproic acid/divalproex sodium
zonisamide

Barbiturates:
phenobarbital (high alert) (Key Drug)
primidone
thiopental (high alert)

ANTIDEPRESSANTS

Action: Antidepressants are divided into the tricyclics, MAOIs, and miscellaneous antidepressants. The tricyclics work by blocking reuptake of norepinephrine and serotonin into nerve endings and increasing action of norepinephrine and serotonin in nerve cells. MAOIs act by increasing concentrations of endogenous epinephrine, norepinephrine, serotonin, dopamine in storage sites in CNS by inhibition of MAO; increased concentration reduces depression.

Uses: Antidepressants are used for depression and in some cases enuresis in children.

Adverse effects: The most serious adverse reactions are paralytic ileus, acute renal failure, hypertension, and hypertensive crisis, depending on the specific product. Common side effects are dizziness, drowsiness, diarrhea, dry mouth, urinary retention, and orthostatic hypotension.

Contraindications: The contraindications for antidepressants are convulsive disorders, prostatic hypertrophy, severe renal, hepatic, cardiac disease depending on the type of medication.

Precautions: Antidepressants should be used cautiously in suicidal patients, severe depression, schizophrenia, hyperactivity, diabetes mellitus, pregnancy, and the elderly.

Pharmacokinetics: Onset, peak, and duration vary widely among products. Most products are metabolized in the liver and excreted in urine.

Interactions: Please check individual monographs, since interactions vary widely among products.

NURSING CONSIDERATIONS

Assessment

- Monitor B/P (lying, standing), pulse q4h; if systolic B/P drops 20 mm Hg, hold drug, notify prescriber; take VS q4h in patients with cardiovascular disease
- Monitor blood studies: CBC, leukocytes, differential, cardiac enzymes if patient is receiving long-term therapy
- Monitor hepatic studies: AST, ALT, bilirubin, creatinine
- Monitor weight weekly; appetite may increase with drug
- Monitor for extrapyramidal symptoms (EPS) primarily in elderly: rigidity, dystonia, akathisia
- Assess mental status: mood, sensorium, affect, suicidal tendencies, increase in psychiatric symptoms (depression, panic)
- Check for urinary retention, constipation; constipation is more likely to occur in children, elderly
- Assess for withdrawal symptoms: headache, nausea, vomiting, muscle pain, weakness; do not usually occur unless drug was discontinued abruptly
- Identify alcohol consumption; if alcohol is consumed, hold dose until AM

Nursing diagnoses

- Coping, ineffective (uses)
- Injury, risk for (uses/adverse reactions)
- Knowledge, deficient (teaching)

Implementation

PO Route

- Give increased fluids, bulk in diet if constipation, urinary retention occur
- Give with food or milk for GI symptoms
- Give gum, hard candy, or frequent sips of water for dry mouth
- Store in airtight container at room temp; do not refreeze
- Provide assistance with ambulation during beginning therapy, since drowsiness/dizziness occurs

Evaluation

- Therapeutic response: decreased depression

Patient/family education

- Teach patient that therapeutic effects may take 2-3 wk
- Advise patient to use caution in driving or other activities requiring alertness because of drowsiness, dizziness, blurred vision
- Caution patient to avoid alcohol ingestion, other CNS depressants
- Instruct patient not to discontinue medication quickly after long-term use; may cause nausea, headache, malaise
- Instruct patient to wear sunscreen or large hat, since photosensitivity may occur

---

Generic Names

Tetracyclic:
mirtazapine

Tricyclics:
amitriptyline
amoxapine
clomiPRAMINE
desipramine
doxepin
🔑 imipramine
nortriptyline
trimipramine

Miscellaneous:
buPROPion
trazodone
venlafaxine

MAOIs:
phenelzine
tranylcypromine

SSRIs
citalopram
escitalopram
fluoxetine
paroxetine
sertraline

ANTIDIABETICS

Action: Antidiabetics are divided into the insulins that decrease blood glucose, phosphate, and potassium and increase blood pyruvate and lactate; and oral antidiabetics that cause functioning β-cells in the pancreas to release insulin, improves the effect of endogenous and exogenous insulin.

Uses: Insulins are used for ketoacidosis and diabetes mellitus types 1 and 2; oral antidiabetics are used for diabetes mellitus type 2.

Adverse effects: The most common side effect of insulin and oral antidiabetics is hypoglycemia. Other adverse reactions for oral antidiabetics include blood dyscrasias, hepatotoxicity, and, rarely, cholestatic jaundice. Adverse reactions for insulin products include allergic responses and, more rarely, anaphylaxis.

Contraindications: Hypersensitive reactions may occur, and allergies should be identified before these products are given. Oral antidiabetics should not be used in juvenile or brittle diabetes, diabetic ketoacidosis, severe renal disease, or severe hepatic disease.

Precautions: Oral antidiabetics should be used with caution in the elderly, in cardiac disease, pregnancy, lactation, and in the presence of alcohol.

Pharmacokinetics: Onset, peak, and duration vary widely among products. Oral antidiabetics are metabolized in the liver, with metabolites excreted in urine, bile, and feces.

Interactions: Interactions vary widely among products. Check individual monograph for specific information.

NURSING CONSIDERATIONS

Assessment

- Monitor blood, urine glucose levels during treatment to determine diabetes control (oral products)
- Monitor fasting blood glucose, 2 hr PP (60-100 mg/dl normal fasting level) (70-130 mg/dl—normal 2-hr level)
- Assess for hypoglycemic reaction that can occur during peak time

Nursing diagnoses

- Nutrition, imbalanced: more than body requirements (uses)

Implementation

SUBCUT route

- Give insulin after warming to room temp by rotating in palms to prevent lipodystrophy from injecting cold insulin
- Give human insulin to those allergic to beef or pork
- Rotate inj sites when giving insulin; use abdomen, upper back, thighs, upper arm, buttocks; keep a record of sites

PO route

- Give oral antidiabetic 30 min ac

Evaluation

- Therapeutic response, including decrease in polyuria, polydipsia, polyphagia, clear sensorium, absence of dizziness, stable gait

Patient/family education

- Advise patient to avoid alcohol and salicylates except on advice of prescriber
- Teach patient symptoms of ketoacidosis: nausea, thirst, polyuria, dry mouth, decreased B/P, dry, flushed skin, acetone breath, drowsiness, Kussmaul respirations
- Teach patient symptoms of hypoglycemia: headache, tremors, fatigue, weakness; and that candy or sugar should be carried to treat hypoglycemia
- Advise patient to test urine for glucose/ketones tid if this drug is replacing insulin
- Advise patient to continue weight control, dietary restrictions, exercise, hygiene

Generic Names

chlorproPAMIDE
glipiZIDE
glyBURIDE
insulin, aspart (high alert)
insulin, glargine (high alert)
insulin, glulisine (high alert)
insulin, lispro (high alert)
🔑 **insulin, regular** (high alert)
insulin, regular concentrated (high alert)
insulin, zinc suspension (Lente) (high alert)
insulin, zinc suspension extended, (Ultralente) (high alert)
metformin
miglitol
pioglitazone
repaglinide
rosiglitazone

ANTIDIARRHEALS

Action: Antidiarrheals work by various actions including direct action on intestinal muscles to decrease GI peristalsis; or by inhibiting prostaglandin synthesis responsible for GI hypermotility; acting on mucosal receptors responsible for peristalsis; or decreasing water content of stools.

Uses: Antidiarrheals are used for diarrhea of undetermined causes.

Adverse effects: The most serious adverse reactions of some products are paralytic ileus, toxic megacolon, and angioneurotic edema. The most common side effects are constipation, nausea, dry mouth, and abdominal pain.

Contraindications: Persons with severe ulcerative colitis, pseudomembranous colitis with some products.

Precautions: Antidiarrheal should be used with caution in the elderly, pregnancy, lactation, children, dehydration.

Pharmacokinetics: Onset, peak, and duration vary widely among products. Most products are metabolized in the liver and excreted in urine.

Interactions: Please check individual monographs, since interactions vary widely among products.

NURSING CONSIDERATIONS

Assessment

- Monitor electrolytes (potassium, sodium, chloride) if on long-term therapy
- Monitor bowel pattern before; for rebound constipation after termination of medication
- Assess response after 48 hr; if no response, drug should be discontinued
- Identify dehydration in children

Nursing diagnoses

- Diarrhea (uses)
- Constipation (adverse reactions)
- Fluid volume, deficient (adverse reactions)
- Knowledge, deficient (teaching)

Implementation

PO route

- Give for 48 hr only

Evaluation

- Therapeutic response: decreased diarrhea

Patient/family education

- Advise patient to avoid OTC products
- Caution patient not to exceed recommended dose

Generic Names

bismuth subsalicylate
kaolin/pectin
loperamide

ANTIDYSRHYTHMICS

Action: Antidysrhythmics are divided into four classes and miscellaneous antidysrhythmics:

- Class I increases the action potential duration and the effective refractory period and reduces disparity in the refractory period between a normal and infarcted myocardium; further subclasses include Ia, Ib, Ic
- Class II decreases the rate of SA node discharge, increases recovery time, slows conduction through the AV node, and decreases heart rate, which decreases O_2 consumption in the myocardium
- Class III increases the action potential duration and the effective refractory period
- Class IV inhibits calcium ion influx across the cell membrane during cardiac depolarization; decreases SA node discharge, decreases conduction velocity through the AV node
- Miscellaneous antidysrhythmics include those such as adenosine, which slows conduction through the AV node, and digoxin, which decreases conduction velocity and prolongs the effective refractory period in the AV node

Uses: These products are used for PVCs, tachycardia, hypertension, atrial fibrillation, angina pectoris.

Adverse effects: Side effects and adverse reactions vary widely among products.

Contraindications: Contraindications vary widely among products.

Precautions: Precautions vary widely among products.

Pharmacokinetics: Onset, peak, and duration vary widely among products.

Interactions: Interactions vary widely among products; check individual monograph for specific information.

NURSING CONSIDERATIONS

Assessment

- Monitor ECG continuously to determine drug effectiveness, PVCs, or other dysrhythmias
- Assess for dehydration or hypovolemia
- Monitor B/P continuously for hypotension, hypertension
- Monitor I&O ratio
- Monitor serum potassium
- Assess for edema in feet and legs daily

Nursing diagnoses

- Tissue perfusion, ineffective (uses)
- Cardiac output, decreased (uses)
- Diarrhea (adverse reactions)
- Gas exchange, impaired (adverse reactions)

Evaluation

- Therapeutic response, including decrease in B/P in hypertension, decreased B/P, edema, moist rales in CHF

Patient/family education

- Advise patient to comply with dosage schedule, even if patient is feeling better
- Instruct patient to report bradycardia, dizziness, confusion, depression, fever

Generic Names

Class I:
moricizine

Class Ia:
disopyramide
procainamide (Key Drug)
quinidine (Key Drug)

Class Ib:
lidocaine, parenteral (high alert)
mexiletine
phenytoin (Key Drug)
tocainide

Class Ic:
flecainide
propafenone

Class II:
acebutolol
esmolol
propranolol (Key Drug)
sotalol

Class III:
amiodarone (high alert)
bretylium (high alert) (Key Drug)
ibutilide (high alert)

Class IV:
verapamil (Key Drug)

Miscellaneous:
adenosine (high alert)
atropine (high alert) (Key Drug)
digoxin (high alert) (Key Drug)

ANTIFUNGALS (SYSTEMIC)

Action: Antifungals act by increasing cell membrane permeability in susceptible organisms by binding sterols and decreasing potassium, sodium, and nutrients in the cell.

Uses: Antifungals are used for infections of histoplasmosis, blastomycosis, coccidioidomycosis, cryptococcosis, aspergillosis, phycomycosis, candidiasis, sporotrichosis causing severe meningitis, septicemia, and skin infections.

Adverse effects: The most serious adverse reactions include renal tubular acidosis, permanent renal impairment, anuria, oliguria, hemorrhagic gastroenteritis, acute liver failure, and blood dyscrasias. Some common side effects include hypokalemia, nausea, vomiting, anorexia, headache, fever, and chills.

Contraindications: Persons with severe bone depression or hypersensitivity should not use these products.

Precautions: Antifungals should be used with caution in renal disease, pregnancy, and hepatic disease.

Pharmacokinetics: Onset, peak, and duration vary widely among products. Most products are metabolized in the liver and excreted in urine.

Interactions: Please check individual monographs, since interactions vary widely among products.

NURSING CONSIDERATIONS

Assessment

- Monitor VS q15-30 min during first inf; note changes in pulse, B/P
- Monitor I&O ratio; watch for decreasing urinary output, change in sp gr; discontinue drug to prevent permanent damage to renal tubules
- Monitor blood studies; CBC, potassium, sodium, calcium, magnesium q2 wk
- Monitor weight weekly; if weight increases over 2 lb/wk, edema is present; renal damage should be considered
- Assess for renal toxicity: increasing BUN, is >40 mg/dl or if serum creatinine >3 mg/dl; drug may be discontinued or dosage reduced
- Assess for hepatotoxicity: increasing AST, ALT, alkaline phosphatase, bilirubin
- Assess for allergic reaction: dermatitis, rash; drug should be discontinued; antihistamines (mild reaction) or epinephrine (severe reaction) administered
- Assess for hypokalemia: anorexia, drowsiness, weakness, decreased reflexes, dizziness, increased urinary output, increased thirst, paresthesias
- Assess for ototoxicity: tinnitus (ringing, roaring in ears), vertigo, loss of hearing (rare)

Nursing diagnoses

- Infection, risk for (uses)
- Injury, risk for (adverse reactions)
- Knowledge, deficient (teaching)

Implementation

IV route

- Give by **IV** using in-line filter (mean pore diameter >1 μm) using distal veins; check for extravasation, necrosis q8h
- Give drug only after C&S confirms organism, drug needed to treat condition; make sure drug is used in life-threatening infections
- Provide protection from light during inf; cover with foil
- Give symptomatic treatment as ordered for adverse reactions: aspirin, antihistamines, antiemetics, antispasmodics

- Store protected from moisture and light; diluted sol is stable for 24 hr

Evaluation

- Therapeutic response: decreased fever, malaise, rash, negative C&S for infecting organism

Patient/family education

- Teach patient that long-term therapy may be needed to clear infection (2 wk-3 mo depending on type of infection)

Generic Names

amphotericin B
fluconazole
griseofulvin
itraconazole
ketoconazole
nystatin
voriconazole

ANTIHISTAMINES

Action: Antihistamines compete with histamines for H_1 receptor sites. They antagonize in varying degrees most of the pharmacologic effects of histamines.

Uses: Products are used to control the symptoms of allergies, rhinitis, and pruritus.

Adverse effects: Most products cause drowsiness; however, two of the newer products, loratadine and fexofenadine, produce little, if any, drowsiness. Other common side effects are headache and thickening of bronchial secretions. Serious blood dyscrasias may occur, but are rare. Urinary retention, GI effects occur with many of these products.

Contraindications: Hypersensitivity to H_1-receptor antagonists occurs rarely. Patients with acute asthma and lower respiratory tract disease should not use these products, since thick secretions may result. Other contraindications include narrow-angle glaucoma, bladder neck obstruction, stenosing peptic ulcer, symptomatic prostatic hypertrophy, newborn, lactation.

Precautions: These products must be used cautiously in conjunction with intraocular pressure, since they increase intraocular pressure. Caution should also be used in patients with renal and cardiac disease, hypertension, and seizure disorders, pregnancy, lactation, and in the elderly.

Pharmacokinetics: Onset varies from 20-60 min, with duration lasting 4-12 hr. In general, pharmacokinetics vary widely among products.

Interactions: Barbiturates, opioids, hypnotics, tricyclic antidepressants, and alcohol can increase CNS depression when taken with antihistamines.

NURSING CONSIDERATIONS

Assessment

- Check I&O ratio; be alert for urinary retention, frequency, dysuria; drug should be discontinued if these occur
- Assess for blood dyscrasias: thrombocytopenia, agranulocytosis (rare)
- Assess for respiratory status, including rate rhythm, increase in bronchial secretions, wheezing, chest tightness
- Assess for cardiac status, including palpitations, increased pulse, hypotension
- Assess CBC during long-term therapy, since hemolytic anemia, although rare, may occur
- Administer with food or milk to decrease GI symptoms; absorption may be decreased slightly
- Administer whole (sus rel tab)
- Provide hard candy, gum, frequent rinsing of mouth for dryness

Nursing diagnoses

- Airway clearance, ineffective (uses)

Evaluation

- Therapeutic response: absence of allergy symptoms, itching

Patient/family education

- Advise patient to notify prescriber if confusion, sedation, hypotension occur
- Caution patient to avoid driving and other hazardous activity if drowsiness occurs
- Instruct patient to avoid concurrent use of alcohol and other CNS depressants
- Inform patient to discontinue a few days before skin testing

---

Generic Names

brompheniramine
budesonide
cetirizine
chlorpheniramine
cyproheptadine
desloratadine
diphenhydrAMINE
fexofenadine
loratadine
promethazine

ANTIHYPERTENSIVES

Action: Antihypertensives are divided into angiotensin converting enzyme (ACE) inhibitors, β-adrenergic blockers, calcium channel blockers, centrally acting adrenergics, diuretics, peripherally acting antiadrenergics, and vasodilators. β-Blockers, calcium channel blockers, and diuretics are discussed in separate sections. ACE inhibitors selectively suppress conversion of renin-angiotensin I to angiotensin II; dilatation of arterial and venous vessels occurs. Centrally acting adrenergics act by inhibiting the sympathetic vasomotor center in the CNS, which reduces impulses in the sympathetic nervous system; blood pressure, pulse rate, and cardiac output decrease. Peripherally acting antiadrenergics inhibit sympathetic vasoconstriction by inhibiting release of norepinephrine and/or depleting norepinephrine stores in adrenergic nerve endings. Vasodilators act on arteriolar smooth muscle by producing direct relaxation or vasodilatation; a reduction in blood pressure, with concomitant increases in heart rate and cardiac output, occurs.

Uses: Used for hypertension and for heart failure not responsive to conventional therapy. Some products are used in hypertensive crisis, angina, and for some cardiac dysrhythmias.

Adverse effects: The most common side effects are marked hypotension, bradycardia, tachycardia, headache, nausea, and vomiting. Side effects and adverse reactions may vary widely between classes and specific products.

Contraindications: Hypersensitive reactions may occur, and allergies should be identified before these products are given. Antihypertensives should not be used in patients with heart block or in children.

Precautions: Antihypertensives should be used with caution in the elderly, in dialysis patients, and in the presence of hypovolemia, leukemia, and electrolyte imbalances.

Pharmacokinetics: Onset, peak, and duration vary widely among products. Most products are metabolized in the liver, with metabolites excreted in urine, bile, and feces.

Interactions: Interactions vary widely among products; check individual monograph for specific information.

NURSING CONSIDERATIONS
Assessment

- Monitor blood studies: neutrophil; decreased platelets occur with many of the products
- Monitor renal studies: protein, BUN, creatinine; watch for increased levels, which may indicate nephrotic syndrome; obtain baselines in renal and liver function studies before beginning treatment
- Assess for edema in feet and legs daily
- Identify allergic reaction, including rash, fever, pruritus, urticaria: drug should be discontinued if antihistamines fail to help
- Identify symptoms of CHF: edema, dyspnea, wet crackles, B/P
- Assess for renal symptoms: polyuria, oliguria, frequency

Nursing diagnoses

- Tissue perfusion, ineffective (uses)
- Cardiac output, decreased (uses)
- Diarrhea (adverse reactions)
- Gas exchange, impaired (adverse reactions)

Implementation

- Place patient in supine or Trendelenburg position for severe hypotension

Evaluation

- Therapeutic response: decrease in B/P in hypotension; decreased B/P, edema, moist crackles in CHF

Patient/family education

- Instruct patient to comply with dosage schedule, even if feeling better
- Advise patient to rise slowly to sitting or standing position to minimize orthostatic hypotension

---

Generic Names

Aldosterone receptor antagonist:
eplerone

Angiotensin-converting enzyme inhibitors:
benazepril
enalapril
fosinopril
lisinopril
quinapril
ramipril
trandolapril

Angiotensin II receptor blockers:
candesartan
eprosartan
irbesartan
losartan
olmesartan
telmisartan
valsartan

Centrally acting adrenergics:
(Key Drug) clonidine
guanfacine
methyldopa

Peripherally acting antiadrenergics:
doxazosin
🔑 prazosin
reserpine
terazosin

Vasodilators:
diazoxide
fenoldopam
hydrALAZINE
minoxidil
nitroprusside (high alert)

Antiadrenergic: Combined α/β-blocker:
labetalol

ANTIINFECTIVES

Action: Antiinfectives are divided into several groups, which include but are not limited to penicillins, cephalosporins, aminoglycosides, sulfonamides, tetracyclines, monobactam, erythromycins, and quinolones. These drugs inhibit the growth and replication of susceptible bacterial organisms.

Uses: Used for infections of susceptible organisms. These products are effective against bacterial, rickettsial, and spirochete infections.

Adverse effects: The most common side effects are nausea, vomiting, and diarrhea. Adverse reactions include bone marrow depression and anaphylaxis.

Contraindications: Hypersensitive reactions may occur, and allergies should be identified before these products are given. Cross-sensitivity can occur between products of different classes (penicillins or cephalosporins). Often persons allergic to penicillins are also allergic to cephalosporins.

Precautions: Antiinfectives should be used with caution in persons with renal and liver disease.

Pharmacokinetics: Onset, peak, and duration vary widely among products. Most products are metabolized in the liver, and metabolites are excreted in urine, bile, and feces.

Interactions: Interactions vary widely among products; check individual monograph for specific information.

NURSING CONSIDERATIONS

Assessment

- Assess for nephrotoxicity, including increased BUN, creatinine
- Monitor blood studies: AST, ALT, CBC, Hct, bilirubin; test monthly if patient is on long-term therapy
- Monitor bowel pattern daily; if severe diarrhea occurs, drug should be discontinued
- Monitor urine output; if decreasing, notify prescriber; may indicate nephrotoxicity
- Assess for allergic reaction, including rash, fever, pruritus, urticaria; drug should be discontinued
- Assess for bleeding: ecchymosis, bleeding gums, hematuria, stool guaiac daily
- Assess for overgrowth of infection: perineal itching, fever, malaise, redness, pain, swelling, drainage, rash, diarrhea, change in cough, sputum

Nursing diagnoses

- Infection, risk for (uses)
- Diarrhea (adverse reactions)

Implementation

- Give for 10-14 days to ensure organism death, prevention of superinfection
- Give after C&S completed; drug may be taken as soon as culture is obtained

Evaluation

- Therapeutic response: absence of fever, fatigue, malaise, draining wounds

Patient/family education

- Teach patient to comply with dosage schedule, even if feeling better
- Advise patient to report sore throat, bruising, bleeding, joint pain; may indicate blood dyscrasias (rare)

Generic Names

Aminoglycosides:
amikacin
azithromycin
clarithromycin
gentamicin
kanamycin
neomycin
streptomycin
tobramycin

Cephalosporins:
cefaclor
cefadroxil
cefazolin
cefdinir
cefditoren
cefepime
cefmetazole
cefonicid
cefoperazone

cefotaxime
cefprozil
ceftibuten
cefuroxime
🔑 cephalexin
cephapirin
cephradine

Fluoroquinolones:
alatrofloxacin/trovafloxacin
ciprofloxacin
enoxacin
gemifloxacin
levofloxacin
lomefloxacin
norfloxacin
ofloxacin
sparfloxacin

Ketolides:
telithromycin

Miscellaneous:
adefovir
dipivoxil
daptomycin
ertapenem
meropenem
peginterferon alfa-2a

Penicillins:
amoxicillin/clavulanate
ampicillin/sulbactam
cloxacillin
dicloxacillin
imipenem/cilastatin
mezlocillin
nafcillin
oxacillin
penicillin G benzathine
penicillin G
penicillin G procaine
penicillin V
piperacillin
ticarcillin
ticarcillin/clavulanate

Sulfonamides:
sulfasalazine
sulfiSOXAZOLE

Tetracyclines:
doxycycline
minocycline
tetracycline

ANTINEOPLASTICS

Action: Antineoplastics are divided into alkylating agents, antimetabolites, antibiotic agents, hormonal agents, and miscellaneous agents. Alkylating agents act by cross-linking strands of DNA. Antimetabolites act by inhibiting DNA synthesis. Antibiotic agents act by inhibiting RNA synthesis and by delaying or inhibiting mitosis. Hormones alter the effect of androgens, luteinizing hormone, follicle-stimulating hormone, or estrogen by changing the hormonal environment.

Uses: Uses vary widely among products and classes of drugs. They are used to treat leukemia, Hodgkin's disease, lymphomas, and other tumors throughout the body.

Adverse effects: Most products cause thrombocytopenia, leukopenia, and anemia, and, if these reactions occur, the drug may need to be stopped until the problem is corrected. Other side effects include nausea, vomiting, glossitis, and hair loss. Some products also cause hepatotoxicity, nephrotoxicity, and cardiotoxicity.

Contraindications: Hypersensitive reactions may occur, and allergies should be identified before these products are given. Also, persons with severe liver and kidney disease should not use these products unless the benefits outweigh the risks.

Precautions: Persons with bleeding, severe bone marrow depression, or renal or hepatic disease should be watched closely.

Pharmacokinetics: Onset, peak, and duration vary widely among products. Most products cross the placenta and are excreted in breast milk and in urine.

Interactions: Toxicity may occur when used with other antineoplastics or radiation.

NURSING CONSIDERATIONS
Assessment

- Monitor CBC, differential, platelet count weekly; withhold drug if WBC is <4000 or platelet count is <75,000; notify prescriber of results
- Monitor renal function studies, including BUN, creatinine, serum uric acid, and urine creatinine clearance before and during therapy
- Monitor I&O ratio; report fall in urine output of 30 ml/hr
- Monitor temp q4h (may indicate beginning infection)
- Monitor liver function tests before and during therapy (bilirubin, AST, ALT, LDH) prn or monthly
- Assess for bleeding, including hematuria, guaiac, bruising or petechiae, mucosa, or orifices q8h; obtain prescription for viscous lidocaine (Xylocaine)

- Identify jaundice of skin, sclera, dark urine, clay-colored stools, itchy skin, abdominal pain, fever, diarrhea
- Assess for edema in feet, joint pain, stomach pain, shaking
- Assess for inflammation of mucosa, breaks in skin

Nursing diagnoses
- Infection, risk for (adverse reactions)
- Nutrition: less than body requirements, imbalanced (adverse reactions)
- Oral mucous membrane, impaired (adverse reactions)

Implementation
- Check **IV** site for irritation; phlebitis
- Have epinephrine available for hypersensitivity reaction
- Give antibiotics for prophylaxis of infection
- Provide strict medical asepsis, protective isolation if WBC levels are low
- Provide comprehensive oral hygiene, using careful technique and soft-bristle brush

Evaluation
- Therapeutic response: decreased tumor size

Patient/family education
- Advise patient to report signs of infection, including increased temp, sore throat, malaise
- Instruct patient to report signs of anemia, including fatigue, headache, faintness, shortness of breath, irritability
- Instruct patient to report bleeding and to avoid use of razors and commercial mouthwash

---

Generic Names
Alkylating agents:
busulfan (high alert)
carboplatin (high alert)
carmustine (high alert)
chlorambucil
cisplatin (high alert)
cyclophosphamide (high alert)
dacarbazine (high alert)
lomustine
mechlorethamine
melphalan (high alert)
oxaliplatin
thiotepa

Antimetabolites:
capecitabine
cytarabine (high alert)
etoposide (high alert)
fludarabine
fluorouracil (high alert)
mercaptopurine
pemetrexed
thioguanine (6-TG)

Antibiotic agents:
bleomycin (high alert)
dactinomycin (high alert)
DAUNOrubicin (high alert)
DOXOrubicin (high alert)
epirubicin (high alert)
methotrexate (high alert)
mitomycin (high alert)
mitoxantrone (high alert)
plicamycin (high alert)

Hormonal agents:
flutamide
fulvestrant
goserelin
irinotecan (high alert)
leuprolide (high alert)
megestrol
mitotane
nilutamide
tamoxifen
testolactone
topotecan (high alert)

Miscellaneous agents:
alemtuzumab
altretamine
anastrozole
arsenic trioxide
asparaginase (high alert)
bortezomib
cetuximab
cladribine
gefitinib (Appx A)
gemcitabine
ibritumomab tiuxetan
imatinib
interferon alfa-2a
interferon alfa-2b
irinotecan (high alert)
pentostatin (high alert)
porfimer
procarbazine
rituximab
vinBLAStine (high alert)
vinCRIStine (high alert)
vinorelbine (high alert)

ANTIPARKINSONIAN AGENTS

Action: Antiparkinsonian agents are divided into cholinergics and dopamine agonists. Cholinergics work by the blocking or competing at central acetylcholine receptors; dopamine agonists work by decarboxylation to dopamine or by activation of dopamine receptors; monoamine oxidase type B inhibitors increase dopamine activity by inhibiting MAO type B activity.

Uses: These agents are used alone or in combination for patients with Parkinson's disease.

Adverse effects: Side effects and adverse reactions vary widely among products. The most common side effects include involuntary movements, headache, numbness, insomnia, nightmares, nausea, vomiting, dry mouth, and orthostatic hypotension.

Contraindications: Persons with hypersensitivity, narrow-angle glaucoma, and undiagnosed skin lesions should not use these products.

Precautions: Antiparkinsonian agents should be used with caution in pregnancy, lactation, children, renal, cardiac, hepatic disease, and affective disorder.

Pharmacokinetics: Onset, peak, and duration vary widely among products. Most products are metabolized in the liver and excreted in urine.

Interactions: Please check individual monographs, since interactions vary widely among products.

NURSING CONSIDERATIONS

Assessment

- Monitor B/P, respiration
- Assess mental status: affect, behavioral changes, depression, complete suicide assessment

Nursing diagnoses

- Injury, risk for (uses)
- Mobility, physical, impaired (uses)
- Knowledge, deficient (teaching)

Implementation

- Give drug up until NPO before surgery
- Adjust dosage depending on patient response
- Give with meals; limit protein taken with drug
- Give only after MAOIs have been discontinued for 2 wk
- Assist with ambulation, during beginning therapy if needed
- Test for diabetes mellitus and acromegaly if on long-term therapy

Evaluation

- Therapeutic response: decrease in akathisia, improvement in mood

Patient/family education

- Advise patient to change positions slowly to prevent orthostatic hypotension
- Instruct patient to report side effects: twitching, eye spasm; indicate overdose
- Advise patient to use drug exactly as prescribed; if drug is discontinued abruptly, parkinsonian crisis may occur

Generic Names

amantadine
apomorphine
(Key Drug) benztropine
biperiden
bromocriptine
cabergoline
carbidopa-levodopa
(Key Drug) levodopa
pramipexole
selegiline
tolcapone
trihexyphenidyl

ANTIPSYCHOTICS

Action: Antipsychotics/neuroleptics are divided into several subgroups: phenothiazines, thioxanthenes, butyrophenones, dibenzoxazepines, dibenzodiazepines, and indolones and other heterocyclic compounds. Although chemically different, these subgroups share many pharmacologic and clinical properties. All antipsychotics work to block postsynaptic dopamine receptors in the brain that are responsible for psychotic behavior, including hallucinations, delusions, and paranoia.

Uses: Antipsychotic behavior is decreased in conditions such as schizophrenia, paranoia, and mania. These agents are also effective for severe anxiety, intractable hiccups, nausea, vomiting, behavioral problems in children, and before surgery for relaxation.

Adverse effects: The most common side effects include extrapyramidal symptoms (EPS) such as pseudoparkinsonism, akathisia, dystonia, and tardive dyskinesia, which may be controlled by use of antiparkinsonian agents. Serious adverse reactions such as hypotension, agranulocytosis, cardiac arrest, and laryngospasm have occurred. Other common side effects include dry mouth and photosensitivity.

Contraindications: Persons with liver damage, severe hypertension or coronary disease, cerebral arteriosclerosis, blood dyscrasias, bone marrow depression, parkinsonism, severe depression, or narrow-angle glaucoma, children <12 yr, or persons withdrawing from alcohol or barbiturates should not use antipsychotics until these conditions are corrected.

Precautions: Caution must be used when antipsychotics are given to the elderly, since metabolism is slowed and adverse reactions can occur rapidly. Hepatic and renal disease may cause poor metabolism and excretion of the drug. Seizure threshold is decreased with these products; increases in the dose of anticonvulsants may be required. Persons with diabetes mellitus, prostatic hypertrophy, chronic respiratory disease, and peptic ulcer disease should be monitored closely.

Pharmacokinetics: Onset, peak, and duration vary widely with different products and routes. Products are metabolized by the liver, are excreted in urine as metabolites, are highly bound to plasma proteins, cross the placenta, and enter breast milk. Half-life can be extended over 3 days.

Interactions: Because other CNS depressants can cause oversedation, these combinations should be used carefully. Anticholinergics may decrease the therapeutic actions of phenothiazines and also cause increased anticholinergic effects.

NURSING CONSIDERATIONS

Assessment

- Monitor bilirubin, CBC, liver function studies monthly, since these drugs are metabolized in the liver and excreted in urine
- Monitor I&O ratio: palpate bladder if low urinary output occurs, since urinary retention occurs with many of these products
- Assess affect, orientation, LOC, reflexes, gait, coordination, sleep pattern disturbances
- Assess dizziness, faintness, palpitations, tachycardia on rising
- Check B/P with patient lying and standing; wide fluctuations between lying and standing B/P may require dosage or product change, since orthostatic hypotension is occurring
- Assess for EPS, including akathisia, tardive dyskinesia, pseudoparkinsonism

Nursing diagnoses

- Thought processes, disturbed (uses)
- Sensory perception, disturbed (uses)

Implementation

- Give antiparkinsonian agent if EPS occur
- Administer liq conc mixed in glass of juice or cola, since taste is unpleasant; avoid contact with skin when preparing liq conc or parenteral medications
- Supervise ambulation until stabilized on medication; do not involve in strenuous exercise program, since fainting is possible; patient should not stand still for long periods
- Increase fluids to prevent constipation
- Give sips of water, candy, gum for dry mouth
- Patient should remain lying down for at least 30 min after IM inj

Evaluation

- Therapeutic response: decrease in excitement, hallucinations, delusions, paranoia, reorganization of thought patterns, speech

Patient/family education

- Advise patient to rise from sitting or lying position gradually, since fainting may occur
- Caution patient to avoid hot tubs, hot showers, or tub baths, since hypotension may occur
- Advise patient to wear sunscreen or protective clothing to prevent burns
- Advise patient to take extra precautions during hot weather to stay cool; heat stroke can occur
- Caution patient to avoid driving and other activities requiring alertness until response to medication is known
- Inform patient that drowsiness or impaired mental/motor activity is evident the first 2 wk, but tends to decrease over time

Generic Names

Phenothiazines:
chlorproMAZINE
fluphenazine
perphenazine
prochlorperazine
thioridazine
thiothixene
trifluoperazine

Butyrophenone:
haloperidol

Miscellaneous:
aripiprazole
loxapine
molindone
olanzapine
quetiapine
risperidone
ziprasidone

ANTITUBERCULARS

Action: Antituberculars act by inhibiting RNA or DNA, or interfering with lipid and protein synthesis, thereby decreasing tubercle bacilli replication.

Uses: Antituberculars are used for pulmonary tuberculosis.

Adverse effects: They vary widely among products. Most products can cause nausea, vomiting, anorexia, and rash. Serious adverse reactions include renal failure, nephrotoxicity, ototoxicity, and hepatic necrosis.

Contraindications: Persons with severe renal disease or hypersensitivity should not use these products.

Precautions: Antituberculars should be used with caution in pregnancy, lactation, and hepatic disease.

Pharmacokinetics: Onset, peak, and duration vary widely among products. Most products are metabolized in the liver and excreted in urine.

Interactions: Please check individual monographs, since interactions vary widely among products.

NURSING CONSIDERATIONS

Assessment

- Assess for signs of anemia: Hct, Hgb, fatigue
- Monitor liver studies weekly: ALT, AST, bilirubin
- Monitor renal status before treatment and monthly thereafter: BUN, creatinine, output, sp gr, urinalysis
- Monitor hepatic status: decreased appetite, jaundice, dark urine, fatigue

Nursing diagnoses

- Infection, risk for (uses)
- Injury, risk for (adverse reactions)
- Knowledge, deficient (teaching)
- Noncompliance (teaching)

Implementation

- Give some of these agents on empty stomach, 1 hr ac (only for isoniazid and rifampin) or 2 hr pc
- Give antiemetic if vomiting occurs
- Give after C&S is completed; monthly to detect resistance

Evaluation

- Therapeutic response: decreased symptoms of TB, culture negative

Patient/family education

- Teach patient that compliance with dosage schedule, duration is necessary
- Teach patient that scheduled appointments must be kept; relapse may occur
- Advise patient to avoid alcohol while taking drug
- Advise patient to report flulike symptoms: excessive fatigue, anorexia, vomiting, sore throat; unusual bleeding, yellowish discoloration of skin/eyes

Generic Names

ethambutol
🔑 isoniazid
pyrazinamide
rifabutin
rifampin
streptomycin

ANTITUSSIVES/EXPECTORANTS

Action: Antitussives suppress the cough reflex by direct action on the cough center in the medulla. Expectorants act by liquefying and reducing the viscosity of thick, tenacious secretions.

Uses: Antitussives/expectorants are used to treat cough occurring in pneumonia, bronchitis, TB, cystic fibrosis, and emphysema; as an adjunct in atelectasis (expectorants); and for nonproductive cough (antitussives).

Adverse effects: The most common side effects are drowsiness, dizziness, and nausea.

Contraindications: Some products are contraindicated in hypothyroidism, iodine sensitivity, pregnancy, and lactation.

Precautions: Some products should be used cautiously in asthma, elderly, and debilitated patients.

Pharmacokinetics: Onset, peak, and duration vary widely among products. Some products are metabolized in the liver and excreted in urine.

Interactions: Please check individual monographs, since interactions vary widely among products.

NURSING CONSIDERATIONS

Assessment

- Assess cough: type, frequency, character including sputum

Nursing diagnoses:

- Breathing pattern, ineffective (uses)
- Airway clearance, ineffective (uses)
- Knowledge, deficient (teaching)

Implementation

- Give decreased dosage to elderly patients; their metabolism may be slowed
- Increase fluids to liquefy secretions
- Humidify patient's room

Evaluation

- Therapeutic response: absence of cough

Patient/family education

- Advise patient to avoid driving and other

hazardous activities until stabilized on this medication
- Caution patient to avoid smoking, smoke-filled rooms, perfumes, dust, environmental pollutants, cleaners that increase cough

Generic Names

acetylcysteine
benzonatate
codeine
dextromethorphan
diphenhydrAMINE
guaifenesin
hydrocodone

ANTIVIRALS/ANTIRETROVIRALS

Action: Antivirals/antiretrovirals act by interfering with DNA synthesis that is needed for viral replication.

Uses: Antivirals/antiretrovirals are used for mucocutaneous herpes simplex virus, herpes genitalis (HSV_1, HSV_2), advanced HIV infections, herpes simplex virus encephalitis, varicella-zoster encephalomyelitis.

Adverse effects: Serious adverse reactions are fatal metabolic encephalopathy, blood dyscrasias, and acute renal failure. Common side effects are nausea, vomiting, anorexia, diarrhea, headache, vaginitis, and moniliasis.

Contraindications: Persons with hypersensitivity and immunosuppressed individuals with herpes zoster should not use these products.

Precautions: Antivirals/antiretrovirals should be used with caution in renal disease, liver disease, lactation, pregnancy, and dehydration.

Pharmacokinetics: Onset, peak, and duration vary widely among products. Most products are metabolized in the liver and excreted in urine.

Interactions: Please check individual monographs, since interactions vary widely among products.

NURSING CONSIDERATIONS

Assessment

- Assess for signs of infection, anemia
- Monitor I&O ratio; report hematuria, oliguria, fatigue, weakness; may indicate nephrotoxicity; check for protein in urine during treatment
- Monitor any patient with compromised renal system, since drug is excreted slowly in poor renal system function; toxicity may occur rapidly
- Check liver studies: AST, ALT
- Check blood studies: WBC, RBC, Hct, Hgb, bleeding time; blood dyscrasias may occur; drug should be discontinued
- Check renal studies: urinalysis, protein, BUN, creatinine, CCr
- Obtain C&S before drug therapy; drug may be taken as soon as culture is obtained; repeat C&S after treatment
- Assess bowel pattern before, during treatment; if severe abdominal pain with bleeding occurs, drug should be discontinued
- Identify skin eruptions: rash, urticaria, itching
- Assess for allergies before treatment, reaction of each medication; place allergies on chart

Nursing diagnoses

- Infection, risk for (uses)
- Injury, risk for (adverse reactions)
- Knowledge, deficient (teaching)

Implementation

- Give increased fluids to 3 L/day to decrease crystalluria when given IB
- Store at room temp for up to 12 hr after reconstitution
- Give adequate intake of fluids (2000 ml) to prevent deposit in kidneys

Evaluation

- Therapeutic response: absence of or control of infection

Patient/family education

- Inform patient that drug does not cure infection, just controls symptoms
- Instruct patient to report sore throat, fever, fatigue; could indicate superinfection
- Advise patient that drug must be taken in equal intervals around the clock to maintain blood levels for duration of therapy
- Advise patient to notify prescriber of side effects of bruising, bleeding, fatigue, malaise; may indicate blood dyscrasias

Generic Names

abacavir
acyclovir
amantadine
atazanvir
cidofovir
delavirdine
didanosine
emtricitabine

enfuvirtide
famciclovir
fosamprenavir
foscarnet
ganciclovir
indinavir
nelfinavir
nevirapine
rimantadine
ritonavir
saquinavir
stavudine
tenofovir
valganciclovir
zalcitabine
🔑 zidovudine

BARBITURATES

Action: Barbiturates act by decreasing impulse transmission to the cerebral cortex.

Uses: All forms of epilepsy can be controlled, since the seizure threshold is increased. Uses also include febrile seizures in children, sedation, insomnia, hyperbilirubinemia, chronic cholestasis with some of these products. Ultra–short-acting barbiturates are used as anesthetics.

Adverse effects: The most common side effects are drowsiness and nausea. Serious adverse reactions such as Stevens-Johnson syndrome and blood dyscrasias may occur with high doses and long-term treatment.

Contraindications: Hypersensitivity may occur, and allergies should be identified before administering. Barbiturates are identified as pregnancy category **D** and should not be used in pregnancy. Other contraindications include porphyria and marked impairment of liver function.

Precautions: Caution must be used when these products are given to the elderly or debilitated; usually smaller doses are needed, since metabolism is slowed. Persons with renal and hepatic disease may show delayed excretion. Barbiturates may produce excitability in children.

Pharmacokinetics: Onset of action can be slow, up to 1 hr, with a peak of 8 hr and a duration of 3-10 hr. These drugs are metabolized by the liver, excreted by the kidneys, cross the placenta, and enter breast milk.

Interactions: Increased CNS depressant effect may occur with alcohol, MAOIs, sedatives, or opioids. These products should be used together cautiously. Oral anticoagulants, corticosteroids, griseofulvin, quinidine, oral contraceptives, and theophylline may show a decreased effect when used with barbiturates.

NURSING CONSIDERATIONS

Assessment

- Monitor hepatic and renal studies: AST, ALT, bilirubin, creatinine, LDH, alkaline phosphatase, BUN if patient is on long-term therapy, since these products are metabolized and excreted by the liver and kidney
- Monitor blood studies: CBC, hematocrit, hemoglobin, and prothrombin time if patient is on long-term therapy, since these products increase the possibility of bleeding and blood dyscrasias
- Identify barbiturate toxicity: hypotension, pulmonary constriction, cold, clammy skin, cyanosis of lips, insomnia, nausea, vomiting, hallucinations, delirium, weakness

Nursing diagnoses

- Sleep pattern, disturbed (uses)
- Injury, risk for (adverse reactions)

Evaluation

- Therapeutic response: appropriate sedation or seizure control

Patient/family education

- Inform patient that physical dependency may result when used for extended periods (45-90 days, depending on dosage)
- Advise patient to avoid driving and activities that require alertness, since drowsiness and dizziness may occur
- Caution patient to abstain from alcohol and other psychotropic medications unless prescribed by prescriber
- Instruct patient not to discontinue medication abruptly after long-term use; withdrawal symptoms will occur

Generic Names

pentobarbital (high alert)
🔑 phenobarbital
secobarbital (high alert)
thiopental (high alert)

BENZODIAZEPINES

Action: Benzodiazepines potentiate the effects of GABA, including any other inhibitory transmitters in the CNS, resulting in decreased anxiety.

Uses: Anxiety is relieved in conditions such as phobic disorders. Benzodiazepines are also used for acute alcohol withdrawal to relieve the possibility of delirium tremens, and some products are used before surgery for relaxation.

Adverse effects: The most common side effects are dizziness, drowsiness, blurred vision, and orthostatic hypotension. Most adverse effects are mediated through the CNS. There is a risk for physical dependence and abuse.

Contraindications: Hypersensitivity, acute narrow-angle glaucoma, children <6 months, liver disease (clonazepam), lactation (diazepam).

Precautions: Caution must be used when these products are given to the elderly or debilitated; usually smaller dosages are needed, since metabolism is slowed. Persons with renal and hepatic disease may show delayed excretion. Clonazepam may increase incidence of seizures.

Pharmacokinetics: Onset of action is ½-1 hr, with a peak of 1-2 hr and a duration of 4-6 hr. These drugs are metabolized by the liver, excreted by the kidneys, cross the placenta, and enter breast milk.

Interactions: Increased CNS depressant effect may occur with other CNS depressants. These products should be used together cautiously. Alcohol should not be used; fatal reactions can occur. The serum concentration and toxicity of digoxin may be increased.

NURSING CONSIDERATIONS

Assessment

- Monitor B/P (with patient lying, standing), pulse; if systolic B/P drops 20 mm Hg, hold drug, notify prescriber; orthostatic hypotension is severe
- Monitor hepatic and renal studies: AST, ALT, bilirubin, creatinine, LDH, alkaline phosphatase
- Assess for physical dependency, withdrawal symptoms, including headache, nausea, vomiting, muscle pain, weakness after long-term use

Nursing diagnoses

- Anxiety (uses)
- Injury, risk for (adverse reactions)

Implementation

- Give with food or milk for GI symptoms; may give crushed if patient is unable to swallow medication whole

Evaluation

- Therapeutic response: relaxation or decreased anxiety

Patient/family education

- Teach patient that drug should not be used for everyday stress or long term; not to take more than prescribed amount, since drug is habit forming
- Caution patient to avoid driving and activities that require alertness, since drowsiness and dizziness occur
- Caution patient to abstain from alcohol and other psychotropic medications except on advice of prescriber
- Advise patient not to discontinue medication abruptly after long-term use; withdrawal symptoms will occur

---

Generic Names

alprazolam
chlordiazepoxide
clonazepam
diazepam
flurazepam
lorazepam
midazolam
oxazepam
temazepam
triazolam

β-ADRENERGIC BLOCKERS

Action: β-Blockers are divided into selective and nonselective blockers. Nonselective blockers produce a fall in blood pressure without reflex tachycardia or reduction in heart rate through a mixture of β-blocking effects; elevated plasma renins are reduced. Selective β-blockers competitively block stimulation of β_1-receptors in cardiac smooth muscle; these drugs produce chronotropic and inotropic effects.

Uses: β-Blockers are used for hypertension, ventricular dysrhythmias, and prophylaxis of angina pectoris.

Adverse effects: The most common side effects are orthostatic hypotension, bradycardia, diarrhea, nausea, vomiting. Serious adverse reactions include blood dyscrasias, bronchospasm, and CHF.

Contraindications: Hypersensitive reactions may occur, and allergies should be identified before these products are given. β-Adrenergic blockers should not be used in heart block, CHF, or cardiogenic shock.

Precautions: β-Blockers should be used with caution in the elderly or in renal and thyroid disease, COPD, CAD, diabetes mellitus, pregnancy, or asthma.

Pharmacokinetics: Onset, peak, and duration vary widely among products. Most products are metabolized in the liver, with metabolites excreted in urine, bile, and feces.

Interactions: Interactions vary widely among products; check individual monograph for specific information.

NURSING CONSIDERATIONS

Assessment

- Monitor renal studies, including protein, BUN, creatinine; watch for increased levels that may indicate nephrotic syndrome; obtain baselines in renal and liver function studies before beginning treatment
- Monitor I&O ratio, weight daily
- Monitor B/P during beginning treatment and periodically thereafter, pulse q4h; note rate, rhythm, quality
- Monitor apical/radial pulse before administration; notify prescriber of significant changes
- Check for edema in feet and legs daily

Nursing diagnoses

- Tissue perfusion, ineffective (uses)
- Cardiac output, decreased (uses)
- Diarrhea (adverse reactions)
- Gas exchange, impaired (adverse reactions)

Implementation

- Give PO ac, at bedtime; tab may be crushed or swallowed whole
- Give reduced dosage in renal dysfunction

Evaluation

- Therapeutic response: decrease in B/P in hypertension; decreased B/P, edema, moist crackles in CHF

Patient/family education

- Instruct patient to comply with dosage schedule, even if feeling better
- Caution patient to rise slowly to sitting or standing position to minimize orthostatic hypotension
- Advise patient to report bradycardia, dizziness, confusion, depression, fever
- Teach patient to take pulse at home; advise when to notify prescriber
- Instruct patient to comply with weight control, dietary adjustment, modified exercise program
- Advise patient to wear support hose to minimize effects of orthostatic hypotension
- Advise patient not to discontinue drug abruptly; taper over 2 wk; may precipitate angina

---

Generic Names

Selective β_1-receptor blockers:
acebutolol
atenolol
esmolol
metoprolol

Nonselective β_1 and β_2-blockers:
carteolol
nadolol
pindolol
(Key Drug) propranolol
timolol

Combined α_1, β_1, and β_2-receptor blocker:
labetalol

BRONCHODILATORS

Action: Bronchodilators are divided into anticholinergics, α/β-adrenergic agonists, β-adrenergic agonists, and phosphodiesterase inhibitors. Anticholinergics act by inhibiting interaction of acetylcholine at receptor sites on bronchial smooth muscle; α/β-adrenergic agonists by relaxing bronchial smooth muscle and increasing diameter of nasal passages; β-adrenergic agonists by action on β_2-receptors, which relaxes bronchial smooth muscle; phosphodiesterase inhibitors by blocking phosphodiesterase and increasing cAMP, which mediates smooth muscle relaxation in the respiratory system.

Uses: Bronchodilators are used for bronchial asthma, bronchospasm associated with bronchitis, emphysema, other obstructive pulmonary diseases, and Cheyne-Stokes respirations, as well as prevention of exercise-induced asthma.

Adverse effects: The most common side effects are tremors, anxiety, nausea, vomiting, and irritation in the throat. The most serious adverse reactions include bronchospasm and dyspnea.

Contraindications: Persons with hypersensitivity, narrow-angle glaucoma, tachydysrhythmias, and severe cardiac disease should not use some of these products.

Precautions: Bronchodilators should be used with caution in lactation, pregnancy, hyperthyroidism, hypertension, prostatic hypertrophy, and seizure disorders.

Pharmacokinetics: Onset, peak, and

duration vary widely among products. Most products are metabolized in the liver and excreted in urine.

Interactions: Please check individual monographs, since interactions vary widely among products.

NURSING CONSIDERATIONS

Assessment

- Monitor respiratory function: vital capacity, FEV, ABGs, lung sounds, heart rate and rhythm

Nursing diagnoses

- Airway clearance, ineffective (uses)
- Activity intolerance (uses)
- Injury, risk for (adverse reactions)
- Knowledge, deficient (teaching)

Implementation

- Give after shaking; exhale, place mouthpiece in mouth, inhale slowly, hold breath, remove, exhale slowly
- Give gum, sips of water for dry mouth
- Give PO with meals to decrease gastric irritation
- Store in light-resistant container; do not expose to temp over 86° F

Evaluation

- Therapeutic response: absence of dyspnea, wheezing

Patient/family education

- Advise patient not to use OTC medications; extra stimulation may occur
- Teach patient use of inhaler; review package insert with patient; to wash inhaler in warm water daily and dry
- Advise patient to avoid getting aerosol in eyes
- Caution patient to avoid smoking, smoke-filled rooms, persons with respiratory tract infections

---

Generic Names

albuterol
aminophylline
atropine
dyphylline
epHEDrine (high alert)
epINEPHrine (high alert)
formoterol
ipratropium
isoproterenol
levalbuterol
metaproterenol
mibefradil
oxtriphylline
pirbuterol
terbutaline
theophylline
tiotropium

CALCIUM CHANNEL BLOCKERS

Action: These products inhibit calcium ion influx across the cell membrane in cardiac and vascular smooth muscle. This action produces relaxation of coronary vascular smooth muscle, dilates coronary arteries, slows SA/AV node conduction, and dilates peripheral arteries.

Uses: These products are used for chronic stable angina pectoris, vasospastic angina, dysrhythmias, hypertension, and unstable angina.

Adverse effects: The most common side effects are dysrhythmias and edema. Also common are headache, fatigue, drowsiness, and flushing.

Contraindications: Persons with 2nd- or 3rd-degree heart block, sick sinus syndrome, hypotension of <90 mm Hg systolic, Wolff-Parkinson-White syndrome, or cardiogenic shock should not use these products, since worsening of those conditions may occur.

Precautions: CHF may worsen, since edema may be increased. Hypotension may worsen, since B/P is decreased. Patients with renal and liver disease should use these products cautiously, since they are metabolized in the liver and excreted by the kidneys.

Pharmacokinetics: Onset, peak, and duration vary widely with route of administration. Drugs are metabolized by the liver and excreted in the urine primarily as metabolites.

Interactions: Increased levels of digoxin and theophylline may occur when used with these products. Increased effects of β-blockers and antihypertensives may occur with calcium channel blockers.

NURSING CONSIDERATIONS

Assessment

- Monitor cardiac system, including B/P, pulse, respirations, ECG intervals (PR, QRS, QT)

Nursing diagnoses

- Tissue perfusion, ineffective (uses)
- Cardiac output, decreased (adverse reactions)

Implementation

- Give PO ac and at bedtime

Evaluation
- Therapeutic response: decreased anginal pain, decreased B/P, dysrhythmias

Patient/family education
- Teach patient how to take pulse before taking drug; patient should record or graph pulses to identify changes
- Advise patient to avoid hazardous activities until stabilized on this drug, since dizziness occurs frequently
- Inform patient of need for compliance to all areas of medical regimen, including diet, exercise, stress reduction, drug therapy

Generic Names
amlodipine
diltiazem (high alert)
felodipine
isradipine
niCARdipine
NIFEdipine
verapamil

CARDIAC GLYCOSIDES

Action: Products act by inhibiting sodium and potassium ATPase and then making more calcium available to activate contracted proteins. Cardiac contractility and cardiac output are increased.

Uses: These products are used for CHF, atrial fibrillation, atrial flutter, atrial tachycardia, and rapid digitalization in these disorders.

Adverse effects: The most common side effects are cardiac disturbances, headache, hypotension, GI symptoms. Also common are blurred vision and yellow-green halos.

Contraindications: Hypersensitive reactions may occur, and allergies should be identified before these products are given. Also, persons with ventricular tachycardia, ventricular fibrillation, and carotid sinus syndrome should not use these products.

Precautions: Persons with acute MI and those who have or may develop serum potassium, calcium, or magnesium imbalances should use these products cautiously. Also, persons with AV block, severe respiratory disease, hypothyroidism, renal and liver disease, and the elderly should exercise caution when these drugs are prescribed.

Pharmacokinetics: Onset, peak, and duration vary widely with the route of administration. Digitoxin is inactivated by the liver, and inactive metabolites are excreted in urine. Digoxin is excreted in urine mainly as the parent drug and metabolites.

Interactions: Toxicity may occur when used with diuretics, succinylcholine, quinidine, and thioamines. Increased blood levels may occur with propantheline bromide, spironolactone, quinidine, verapamil, aminoglycosides (PO), amiodarone, anticholinergics, and quinine. Diuretics may increase toxicity.

NURSING CONSIDERATIONS
Assessment
- Montior cardiac system, including B/P, pulse, respirations, and increased urine output
- Monitor apical pulse for 1 min before giving drug; if pulse <60, take again in 1 hr; if <60 notify prescriber
- Monitor electrolytes, including potassium, sodium, chloride, calcium, magnesium; renal function studies, including BUN and creatinine; and blood studies, including AST, ALT, bilirubin
- Monitor I&O ratio, daily weights
- Monitor therapeutic drug levels

Nursing diagnoses
- Tissue perfusion, ineffective (uses)
- Cardiac output, decreased (adverse reactions)

Implementation
- Give potassium supplements if ordered for potassium levels <3

Evaluation
- Therapeutic response: decreased weight, edema, pulse, respiration, and increased urine output

Patient/family education
- Teach patient how to take pulse before taking drug; patient should record or graph pulse to identify changes
- Advise patient to avoid hazardous activities until stabilized on this drug, since dizziness occurs frequently
- Inform patient of need for compliance to all areas of medical regimen, including diet, exercise, stress reduction, drug therapy

Generic Names
digoxin (high alert)

CHOLINERGICS

Action: Cholinergics act by preventing destruction of acetylcholine, which increases concentration at sites where acetylcholine is released; this exaggerates the effects of acetylcholine and facilitates transmission of impulses across myoneural junction. Cholinergics may also act by stimulating receptors for acetylcholine.

Uses: Cholinergics are used for myasthenia gravis, as antagonists of nondepolarizing neuromuscular blockade, postoperative bladder distention and urinary distention, postoperative ileus.

Adverse effects: The most serious adverse reactions are respiratory depression, bronchospasm, constriction, laryngospasm, respiratory arrest, convulsions, and paralysis. The most common side effects are nausea, diarrhea, and vomiting.

Contraindications: Persons with obstruction of the intestine or renal system should not use these products.

Precautions: Caution should be used in patients with bradycardia, hypotension, seizure disorders, bronchial asthma, coronary occlusion, hyperthyroidism, and in lactation and children.

Pharmacokinetics: Onset, peak, and duration vary widely among products. Most products are metabolized in the liver and excreted in urine.

Interactions: Please check individual monographs since interactions vary widely among products.

NURSING CONSIDERATIONS

Assessment

- Monitor VS, respiration q8h
- Monitor I&O ratio; check for urinary retention or incontinence
- Assess for bradycardia, hypotension, bronchospasm, headache, dizziness, convulsions, respiratory depression; drug should be discontinued if toxicity occurs

Nursing diagnoses

- Urinary elimination, impaired (uses)
- Breathing pattern, ineffective (uses)
- Knowledge, deficient (teaching)
- Noncompliance (teaching)

Implementation

- Give only with atropine sulfate available for cholinergic crisis
- Give only after all other cholinergics have been discontinued
- Give increased dosages if tolerance occurs
- Give larger doses after exercise or fatigue
- Give on empty stomach for better absorption
- Store at room temp

Evaluation

- Therapeutic response: increased muscle strength, hand grasp, improved muscle gait, absence of labored breathing (if severe)

Patient/family education

- Inform patient that drug is not a cure; it only relieves symptoms (myasthenia gravis)
- Advise patient to carry/wear emergency ID specifying myasthenia gravis, drugs taken

---

Generic Names

bethanechol
edrophonium
neostigmine
physostigmine
pyridostigmine

CHOLINERGIC BLOCKERS

Action: Cholinergic blockers inhibit or block acetylcholine at receptor sites in the autonomic nervous system.

Uses: Many products are used to decrease secretions before surgery, to reverse neuromuscular blockade, and to decrease motility of GI, biliary, urinary tracts. Other products are used for parkinsonian symptoms, including dystonia associated with neuroleptic drugs.

Adverse effects: The most common side effects are dryness of the mouth and constipation, which can be prevented by frequent rinsing of the mouth and increasing water and bulk in the diet.

Contraindications: Hypersensitivity can occur, and allergies should be identified before administering these products. Persons with GI and GU obstruction should not use these products, since constipation and urinary retention may occur. They are also contraindicated in angle closure glaucoma and myasthenia gravis.

Precautions: Caution must be used when these products are given to the elderly, since metabolism is slowed. Also, persons with tachycardia or prostatic hypertrophy should use these products with caution.

Pharmacokinetics: Onset, peak, and duration vary with route.

Interactions: Increase in anticholinergic effect occurs when used with opioids, barbiturates, antihistamines, MAOIs, phenothiazines, amantadine.

NURSING CONSIDERATIONS

Assessment

- Assess I&O ratio; be alert for urinary retention, frequency, dysuria; drug should be discontinued if these occur
- Assess urinary hesitancy, retention; palpate bladder if retention occurs
- Assess constipation; increase fluids, bulk, exercise
- Assess for tolerance over long-term therapy; dosage may need to be changed
- Assess mental status: affect, mood, CNS depression, worsening of mental symptoms during early therapy

Nursing diagnoses

- Mobility, physical, impaired (uses)
- Pain, acute (uses)
- Pain, chronic (uses)

Implementation

- Give with food or milk to decrease GI symptoms
- Give parenteral dose with patient recumbent to prevent postural hypotension; give dose slowly, monitoring VS
- Give hard candy, gum, frequent rinsing of mouth for dryness

Evaluation

- Therapeutic response: absence of cramps, absence of extrapyramidal symptoms (EPS)

Patient/family education

- Caution patient to avoid driving and other hazardous activity if drowsiness occurs
- Advise patient to avoid concurrent use of cough, cold preparations with alcohol, antihistamines unless directed by prescriber
- Caution patient to use with caution in hot weather, since medication may increase susceptibility to heat stroke

Generic Names

On **atropine** (high alert)
On benztropine
biperiden
glycopyrrolate
scopolamine
trihexyphenidyl

CORTICOSTEROIDS

Action: Corticosteroids are divided into glucocorticoids and mineralocorticoids. Glucocorticoids decrease inflammation by the suppression of migration of polymorphonuclear leukocytes, fibroblasts, increased capillary permeability, and lysosomal stabilization. They also have varied metabolic effects and modify the body's immune responses to many different stimuli. Mineralocorticoids act by increasing resorption of sodium by increasing hydrogen and potassium excretion in the distal tubule.

Uses: Glucocorticoids are used to decrease inflammation and for immunosuppression. In addition, some products may be given for allergy, adrenal insufficiency, or cerebral edema. Mineralocorticoids are given for adrenal insufficiency or adrenogenital syndrome.

Adverse effects: The most common side effects include change in behavior, including insomnia and euphoria; GI irritation, including peptic ulcer; metabolic reactions, including hypokalemia, hyperglycemia, and carbohydrate intolerance; and sodium and fluid retention. Most adverse reactions are dose dependent.

Contraindications: Hypersensitivity may occur and should be identified before administering. Since these products mask infection, they should not be used in systemic fungal infections or amebiasis. Mothers taking pharmacologic doses of corticosteroids should not nurse.

Precautions: Caution must be used when these products are prescribed for diabetic patients, since hyperglycemia may occur. Also, patients with glaucoma, seizure disorders, peptic ulcer, impaired renal function, CHF, hypertension, ulcerative colitis, or myasthenia gravis should be monitored closely if corticosteroids are given. Use with caution in children and the elderly and during pregnancy.

Pharmacokinetics: For oral preparations the onset of action occurs between 1-2 hr, and duration can be up to 2 days, with a half-life of 2-4 days. Pharmacokinetics vary widely among products. These products cross the placenta and appear in breast milk.

Interactions: Decreased corticosteroid effect may occur with barbiturates, rifampin, phenytoin; corticosteroid dosage may need to be increased. There is a possibility of GI bleeding when used with salicylates, indomethacin. Steroids may reduce salicylate levels. When using with digitalis glycosides, potassium-depleting diuretics, and amphotericin, serum potassium levels should be monitored.

NURSING CONSIDERATIONS

Assessment

- Monitor potassium, blood glucose, urine glucose while on long-term therapy; hypokalemia and hyperglycemia are common
- Monitor weight daily; notify prescriber if weekly gain of >5 lb, since these products alter fluid and electrolyte balance
- Assess for potassium depletion, including paresthesias, fatigue, nausea, vomiting, depression, polyuria, dysrhythmias, weakness
- Assess for mental status, including affect, mood, behavioral changes, aggression; if severe personality changes occur, including depression, drug may need to be tapered and then discontinued
- Monitor I&O ratio; be alert for decreasing urinary output and increasing edema
- Monitor plasma cortisol levels during long-term therapy (normal level is 138-635 nmol/L when drawn at 8 AM)
- Assess for infection, including increased temp, WBC, even after withdrawal of medication; drug masks symptoms of infection
- Assess for adrenal insufficiency: nausea, anorexia, fatigue, dizziness, dyspnea, weakness, joint pain

Nursing diagnoses

- Infection, risk for (adverse reactions)
- Body image, disturbed (adverse reactions)
- Suicide, risk for (adverse reactions)

Implementation

- Give with food or milk to decrease GI symptoms
- Give single daily or alternate-day doses in the morning before 9 AM (for replacement therapy)

Evaluation

- Therapeutic response: decreased inflammation

Patient/family education

- Advise patient that emergency ID as steroid user should be carried/worn
- Advise patient not to discontinue this medication abruptly or adrenal crisis can result
- Teach patient all aspects of drug use, including cushingoid symptoms
- Instruct patient to take with meals or a snack

Generic Names

Glucocorticoids:
beclomethasone
betamethasone
cortisone
dexamethasone
hydrocortisone
methylPREDNISolone
predniSOLONE
predniSONE
triamcinolone

Mineralocorticoid:
fludrocortisone

DIURETICS

Action: Diuretics are divided into subgroups: thiazides and thiazide-like diuretics, loop diuretics, carbonic anhydrase inhibitors, osmotic diuretics, and potassium-sparing diuretics. Each one of these subgroups differs in its mechanism of action. Thiazides and thiazide-like diuretics increase excretion of water and sodium by inhibiting resorption in the early distal tubule. Loop diuretics inhibit resorption of sodium and chloride in the thick ascending limb of the loop of Henle. Carbonic anhydrase inhibitors increase sodium excretion by decreasing sodium-hydrogen ion exchange throughout the renal tubule. Carbonic anhydrase inhibitors also decrease secretion of aqueous humor in the eye and thus decrease intraocular pressure. Osmotic diuretics increase the osmotic pressure of glomerular filtrate, thus decreasing net absorption of sodium. The potassium-sparing diuretics interfere with sodium resorption at the distal tubule, thus decreasing potassium excretion.

Uses: Blood pressure is reduced in hypertension; edema is reduced in CHF; intraocular pressure is decreased in glaucoma.

Adverse effects: Hypokalemia, hyperuricemia, and hyperglycemia occur most frequently with thiazide diuretics. Aplastic anemia, blood dyscrasias, volume depletion, and dehydration may occur when thiazide-like diuretics, loop diuretics, or carbonic anhydrase inhibitors are given. Side effects and adverse reactions vary widely for the miscellaneous products.

Contraindications: Persons with electrolyte imbalances (sodium, chloride, potassium), dehydration, or anuria should not be given these products until the problem is corrected.

Precautions: Caution must be used when diuretics are given to the elderly, since electrolyte disturbances and dehydration can occur rapidly. Hepatic and renal disorders may cause poor metabolism and excretion of the drug.

Pharmacokinetics: Onset, peak, and duration vary widely among the different subgroups of these drugs.

Interactions: Cholestyramine and colestipol decrease the absorption of thiazide diuretics. Concurrent use of thiazides with diazoxide may increase hyperuricemia, hyperglycemia, and antihypertensive effects of thiazides. Ototoxicity may occur when loop diuretics are used with aminoglycosides. Thiazide and loop diuretics may increase therapeutic and toxic effects of lithium.

NURSING CONSIDERATIONS

Assessment

- Monitor weight, I&O ratio daily to determine fluid loss; check skin turgor for dehydration
- Monitor electrolytes: potassium, sodium, chloride: include BUN, blood glucose, CBC, serum creatinine, blood pH, ABGs, uric acid, calcium; electrolyte imbalances may occur quickly
- Monitor B/P with patient lying, standing; postural hypotension may occur, since fluid loss occurs from intravascular spaces first
- Assess for signs of metabolic alkalosis, including drowsiness and restlessness
- Assess for signs of hypokalemia with some products, including postural hypotension, malaise, fatigue, tachycardia, leg cramps, weakness

Nursing diagnoses

- Fluid volume, excess (uses)
- Cardiac output, decreased (adverse reactions)

Implementation

- Give in AM to avoid interference with sleep if using drug as a diuretic
- Give potassium replacement if potassium is less than 3 mg/dl

Evaluation

- Therapeutic reponse: improvement in edema of feet, legs, sacral area daily if medication is being used in CHF; improvement in B/P if medication is being used as a diuretic; improvement in intraocular pressure if medication is being used to decrease aqueous humor in the eye

Patient/family education

- Teach patient to take drug early in the day (diuretic) to prevent nocturia

Generic Names

Thiazides:
chlorothiazide
🔑 hydrochlorothiazide

Thiazide-like:
chlorthalidone
indapamide
metolazone

Loop:
bumetanide
🔑 furosemide
torsemide

Carbonic anhydrase inhibitors:
acetaZOLAMIDE

Potassium-sparing:
amiloride
spironolactone
triamterene

Osmotic:
mannitol

HISTAMINE H_2 ANTAGONISTS

Action: Histamine H_2 antagonists act by inhibiting histamine at H_2 receptor site in parietal cells, which inhibits gastric acid secretion.

Uses: Histamine H_2 antagonists are used for short-term treatment of duodenal and gastric ulcers and maintenance therapy for duodenal ulcer; and for gastroesophageal reflux disease.

Adverse effects: The most serious adverse reactions are agranulocytosis, thrombocytopenia, neutropenia, aplastic anemia, and exfoliative dermatitis. The most common side effects are confusion (not with rantidine), headache and diarrhea.

Contraindications: Persons with hypersensitivity should not use these products.

Precautions: Caution should be used in pregnancy, lactation, children <16 yr, organic brain syndrome, hepatic disease, renal disease.

Pharmacokinetics: Onset, peak, and duration vary widely among products. Most products are metabolized in the liver and excreted in urine.

Interactions: Antacids interfere with absorption of histamine H_2 antagonists. Check individual monographs for other interactions.

NURSING CONSIDERATIONS

Assessment

- Monitor gastric pH (>5 should be maintained)
- Monitor I&O ratio, BUN, creatinine

Nursing diagnoses

- Pain, chronic (uses)
- Injury, risk for (bleeding)
- Knowledge, deficient (teaching)

Implementation

- Give with meals for prolonged drug effect
- Give antacids 1 hr before or 1 hr after cimetidine
- Give **IV** slowly; bradycardia may occur; give over 30 min
- Store diluted sol at room temp for up to 48 hr

Evaluation

- Therapeutic response: decreased pain in abdomen

Patient/family education

- Advise patient that gynecomastia, impotence may occur, but is reversible
- Caution patient to avoid driving and other hazardous activities until patient is stabilized on this medication
- Caution patient to avoid black pepper, caffeine, alcohol, harsh spices, extremes in temp of food
- Caution patient to avoid OTC preparations: aspirin, cough, cold preparations
- Inform patient that drug must be continued for prescribed time to be effective
- Advise patient to report bruising, fatigue, malaise; blood dyscrasias may occur

Generic Names

Key: cimetidine
famotidine
ranitidine

IMMUNOSUPPRESSANTS

Action: Immunosuppressants produce immunosuppression by inhibiting T lymphocytes.

Uses: Most products are used for organ transplants to prevent rejection.

Adverse effects: The most serious adverse reactions are albuminuria, hematuria, proteinuria, renal failure, and hepatotoxicity. The most common side effects are oral *Candida* infection, gum hyperplasia, tremors, and headache. The most serious adverse reactions for azathioprine are hematologic (leukopenia and thrombocytopenia) and GI (nausea and vomiting). There is a risk of secondary infection.

Contraindications: Products are contraindicated in hypersensitivity.

Precautions: Caution should be used in severe renal disease, severe hepatic disease, and pregnancy.

Pharmacokinetics: Onset, peak, and duration vary widely among products. Most products are metabolized in the liver and excreted in urine.

Interactions: Please check individual monographs, since interactions vary widely among products.

NURSING CONSIDERATIONS

Assessment

- Monitor renal studies: BUN, creatinine at least monthly during treatment, 3 mo after treatment
- Monitor liver function studies: alkaline phosphatase, AST, ALT, bilirubin
- Monitor drug blood levels during treatment
- Assess for hepatotoxicity: dark urine, jaundice, itching, light-colored stools; drug should be discontinued

Nursing diagnoses

- Infection, risk for (adverse reactions)
- Injury, risk for (uses)
- Knowledge, deficient (teaching)

Implementation

- Give for several days before transplant surgery
- Give with meals for GI upset or place drug in chocolate milk
- Give with oral antifungal for *Candida* infections

Evaluation

- Therapeutic response: absence of rejection

Patient/family education

- Advise patient to report fever, chills, sore throat, fatigue, since serious infections may occur
- Caution patient to use contraceptive measures during treatment and for 12 wk after ending therapy

Generic Names

Key: azathioprine
basiliximab (high alert)
cycloSPORINE
muromonab-CD3
sirolimus
tacrolimus

LAXATIVES

Action: Laxatives are divided into bulk products, lubricants, osmotics, saline laxative stimulants, and stool softeners. Bulks work by absorbing water and expanding to increase moisture content and bulk in the stool. Lubricants increase water retention in the stool, causing reabsorption of water in the bowel. Stimulants act by increasing peristalsis by direct effect on the intestine. Saline draws water into the intestinal lumen. Osmotics increase distention and promote peristalsis. Stool softeners reduce surface tension of liq in the bowel.

Uses: Laxatives are used as a preparation for bowel, rectal examination, constipation, or as stool softeners.

Adverse effects: The most common side effects are nausea, abdominal cramps, and diarrhea.

Contraindications: Persons with GI obstruction, perforation, gastric retention, toxic colitis, megacolon, abdominal pain, nausea, vomiting, and fecal impaction should not use these products.

Precautions: Caution should be used in rectal bleeding, large hemorrhoids, and anal excoriation.

Pharmacokinetics: Onset, peak, and duration vary among products.

Interactions: Please check individual monographs, since interactions vary widely among products.

NURSING CONSIDERATIONS

Assessment

- Monitor blood, urine electrolytes if drug is used often by patient
- Monitor I&O ratio to identify fluid loss
- Determine cause of constipation; identify whether fluids, bulk, or exercise is missing from lifestyle
- Assess for cramping, rectal bleeding, nausea, vomiting; if these symptoms occur, drug should be discontinued

Nursing diagnoses

- Constipation (uses)
- Diarrhea (adverse reactions)
- Knowledge, deficient (teaching)

Implementation

- Give alone only with water for better absorption; do not take within 1 hr of antacids, milk, or cimetidine
- Swallow tab whole; do not break, crush, or chew

Evaluation

- Therapeutic response: decrease in constipation

Patient/family education

- Caution patient not to use laxatives for long-term therapy; bowel tone will be lost; that normal bowel movements do not always occur daily
- Caution patient not to use in presence of abdominal pain, nausea, vomiting
- Advise patient to notify prescriber of abdominal pain, nausea, vomiting
- Advise patient to notify prescriber if constipation is unrelieved or if symptoms of electrolyte imbalance occur: muscle cramps, pain, weakness, dizziness

Generic Names

Bulk laxatives:
calcium polycarbophil
psyllium

Osmotic agents:
glycerin
lactulose

Saline laxatives:
magnesium salts
sodium biphosphate/phosphate

Stimulants:
bisacodyl
cascara sagrada
phenolphthalein
senna

Stool softeners:
docusate

NEUROMUSCULAR BLOCKING AGENTS

Action: Neuromuscular blocking agents are divided into depolarizing and nondepolarizing blockers. They act by inhibiting transmission of nerve impulses by binding with cholinergic receptor sites.

Uses: Neuromuscular blocking agents are used to facilitate endotracheal intubation and skeletal muscle relaxation during mechanical ventilation, surgery, or general anesthesia.

Adverse effects: The most serious adverse reactions are prolonged apnea, bronchospasm, cyanosis, respiratory depression, and malignant hyperthermia. The most common side effects are bradycardia and decreased motility.

Contraindications: Persons that are hypersensitive should not be given this product.

Precautions: Caution should be used in pregnancy, thyroid disease, collagen disease, cardiac disease, lactation, children <2 yr, electrolyte imbalances, dehydration, neuromuscular disease (myasthenia gravis), and respiratory disease.

Pharmacokinetics: Onset, peak, and duration vary widely among products. Most products are metabolized in the liver and excreted in urine.

Interactions: Aminoglycosides potentiate neuromuscular blockade. See individual monographs.

NURSING CONSIDERATIONS
Assessment

- Monitor for electrolyte imbalances (potassium, magnesium); may lead to increased action of this drug
- Monitor VS (B/P, pulse, respirations, airway) q15 min until fully recovered; rate, depth, pattern of respirations, strength of hand grip
- Monitor I&O ratio; check for urinary retention, frequency, hesitancy
- Assess for recovery: decreased paralysis of face, diaphragm, leg, arm, rest of body
- Assess for allergic reactions: rash, fever, respiratory distress, pruritus; drug should be discontinued

Nursing diagnoses

- Breathing pattern, ineffective (uses)
- Injury, risk for (adverse reactions)
- Knowledge, deficient (teaching)

Implementation

- Administer using nerve stimulator by anesthesiologist to determine neuromuscular blockade
- Administer anticholinesterase to reverse neuromuscular blockade
- Administer **IV** undiluted over 1-2 min (only by qualified person, usually an anesthesiologist)
- Store in light-resistant, cool area
- Reassure if communication is difficult during recovery from neuromuscular blockade

Evaluation

- Therapeutic response: paralysis of jaw, eyelid, head, neck, rest of body

Generic Names

atracurium
mivacurium (high alert)
pancuronium (high alert)
pipecuronium (high alert)
succinylcholine (high alert)
tubocurarine (high alert)
vecuronium (high alert)

NONSTEROIDAL ANTIINFLAMMATORIES

Action: Nonsteroidal antiinflammatories decrease prostaglandin synthesis by inhibiting an enzyme needed for biosynthesis.

Uses: Nonsteroidal antiinflammatories are used to treat mild to moderate pain, osteoarthritis, rheumatoid arthritis, and dysmenorrhea.

Adverse effects: The most serious adverse reactions are nephrotoxicity (dysuria, hematuria, oliguria, azotemia), blood dyscrasias, and cholestatic hepatitis. The most common side effects are nausea, abdominal pain, anorexia, dizziness, and drowsiness.

Contraindications: Persons with hypersensitivity, asthma, severe renal disease, and severe hepatic disease should not use these products.

Precautions: Caution should be used in pregnancy, lactation, children, bleeding disorders, GI disorders, cardiac disorders, hypersensitivity to other antiinflammatory agents, and the elderly.

Pharmacokinetics: Onset, peak, and duration vary widely among products. Most products are metabolized in the liver and excreted in urine.

Interactions: Please check individual monographs, since interactions vary widely among products.

NURSING CONSIDERATIONS
Assessment

- Monitor renal, liver, blood studies: BUN, creatinine, AST, ALT, Hgb, before treatment, periodically thereafter
- Monitor audiometric, ophth examination before, during, and after treatment.
- Check for eye, ear problems: blurred vision, tinnitus, may indicate toxicity

Nursing diagnoses

- Pain, chronic (uses)
- Mobility, physical, impaired (uses)
- Knowledge, deficient (teaching)
- Noncompliance (teaching)

Implementation

- Give with food to decrease GI symptoms; however, best to take on empty stomach to facilitate absorption
- Store at room temp

Evaluation

- Therapeutic response: decreased pain, stiffness in joints, decreased swelling in joints, ability to move more easily

Patient/family education

- Advise patient to report blurred vision, ringing, roaring in ears; may indicate toxicity
- Caution patient to avoid driving, other hazardous activities if dizziness, drowsiness occurs, especially elderly
- Advise patient to report change in urine pattern, increased weight, edema, increased pain in joints, fever, blood in urine; indicate nephrotoxicity
- Inform patient that therapeutic effects may take up to 1 mo

---

Generic Names

celecoxib
diclofenac
etodolac
🔑 ibuprofen
indomethacin
ketoprofen
ketorolac
nabumetone
naproxen
piroxicam
sulindac

OPIOID ANALGESICS

Action: These agents depress pain impulse transmission at the spinal cord level by interacting with opioid receptors. Products are divided into opiates and nonopiates.

Uses: Most products are used to control moderate to severe pain and are used before and after surgery.

Adverse effects: GI symptoms, including nausea, vomiting, anorexia, constipation, and cramps are the most common side effects. Other common side effects include lightheadedness, dizziness, sedation. Serious adverse reactions such as respiratory depression, respiratory arrest, circulatory depression, and increased intracranial pressure may result, but are less common and usually dose dependent.

Contraindications: Hypersensitive reactions occur frequently. Check for sensitivity before administering. These drugs should not be used if opioid addiction is suspected, and they are also contraindicated in acute bronchial asthma and upper airway obstruction.

Precautions: Caution must be used when these products are given to persons with an addictive personality, since the possibility of addiction is so great. Also, persons with increased intracranial pressure may experience an even greater increase in intracranial pressure. Persons with severe heart disease, hepatic or renal disease, respiratory conditions, and seizure disorders should be monitored closely for worsening condition.

Pharmacokinetics: Onset of action is immediate by **IV** route and rapid by IM and PO routes. Peak occurs from 1-2 hr, depending on route, with a duration of 2-8 hr. These agents cross the placenta and appear in breast milk.

Interactions: Barbiturates, other opioids, hypnotics, antipsychotics, or alcohol can increase CNS depression when taken with opioids.

NURSING CONSIDERATIONS

Assessment

- Monitor I&O ratio; be alert for urinary retention, frequency, dysuria; drug should be discontinued if these occur
- Assess for respiratory dysfunction, including respiratory depression, rate, rhythm, character; notify prescriber if respirations are <12/min
- Assess for CNS changes: dizziness, drowsiness, hallucinations, euphoria, LOC, pupil reaction
- Assess for allergic reactions: rash, urticaria
- Assess for need for pain medication, use pain scoring

Nursing diagnoses

- Pain, acute (uses)
- Gas exchange, impaired (adverse reactions)

Implementation

- Give with antiemetic if nausea or vomiting occurs
- Give when pain is beginning to return; determine dosage interval by patient response
- Provide assistance with ambulation; patient should not be ambulating during drug peak

Evaluation

- Therapeutic response: decrease in pain

Patient/family education
- Advise patient to report any symptoms of CNS changes, allergic reactions, or shortness of breath
- Caution patient that physical dependency may result when used for extended periods
- Teach patient that withdrawal symptoms may occur, including nausea, vomiting, cramps, fever, faintness, anorexia
- Advise patient to avoid alcohol and other CNS depressants

Generic Names

buprenorphine
butorphanol
🔑 codeine
fentanyl (high alert)
fentanyl transdermal
hydromorphone (high alert)
🔑 **meperidine** (high alert)
methadone (high alert)
🔑 **morphine** (high alert)
nalbuphine
oxycodone (high alert)
oxymorphone (high alert)
pentazocine (high alert)
propoxyphene (high alert)
remifentanil (high alert)

SALICYLATES

Action: Salicylates have analgesic, antipyretic, and antiinflammatory effects. The antiinflammatory and analgesic activities may be mediated through the inhibition of prostaglandin synthesis. Antipyretic action results from inhibition of the hypothalamic heat-regulating center.

Uses: The primary uses of salicylates are relief of mild to moderate pain and fever and in inflammatory conditions such as arthritis, thromboembolic disorders, and rheumatic fever.

Adverse effects: The most common side effects are GI symptoms and rash. Serious blood dyscrasias and hepatotoxicity may result when used for long periods at high doses. Tinnitus or impaired hearing may indicate that blood salicylate levels are reaching or exceeding the upper limit of the therapeutic range.

Contraindications: Hypersensitivity to salicylates is common. Check for sensitivity before administering. Persons with bleeding disorders, GI bleeding, and vit K deficiency should not use these products, since salicylates increase prothrombin time. Children should not use these products, since salicylates have been associated with Reye's syndrome.

Precautions: Caution is needed when salicylates are given to patients with anemia, hepatic or renal disease, or Hodgkin's disease. Caution should also be exercised in pregnancy and lactation.

Pharmacokinetics: Onset of action occurs in 15-30 min, with a peak of 1-2 hr and a duration up to 6 hr. These drugs are metabolized by the liver and excreted by the kidneys.

Interactions: Increased effects of anticoagulants, insulin, methotrexate, heparin, valproic acid, and oral sulfonylureas may occur when used with salicylates. Aspirin may decrease serum concentrations of nonsteroidal antiinflammatory agents.

NURSING CONSIDERATIONS
Assessment
- Monitor hepatic and renal studies: AST, ALT, bilirubin, creatinine, LDH, alkaline phosphatase, BUN if patient is on long-term therapy, since these products are metabolized and excreted by the liver and kidney
- Monitor blood studies: CBC, Hct, Hgb, and prothrombin time if patient is on long-term therapy, since these products increase the possibility of bleeding and blood dyscrasias
- Assess for hepatotoxicity: dark urine, clay-colored stools, jaundiced skin and sclera, itching, abdominal pain, fever, diarrhea, which may occur with long-term use
- Assess for ototoxicity: tinnitus, ringing, roaring in ears; audiometric testing is needed before and after long-term therapy

Nursing diagnoses
- Pain, acute (uses)
- Pain, chronic (uses)
- Mobility, physical, impaired (uses)
- Activity intolerance (uses)
- Sensory perception, disturbed (adverse reactions)
- Thermoregulation, ineffective (uses)

Implementation
- Give with food or milk to decrease gastric irritation; give 30 min ac or 1 hr pc with a full glass of water

Evaluation
- Therapeutic response: decreased pain, fever

Patient/family education
- Advise patient that blood sugar levels should be monitored closely, if patient is diabetic
- Caution patient not to exceed recommended dosage; acute poisoning may result

• Inform patient that therapeutic response takes 2 wk in arthritis
• Caution patient to avoid use of alcohol, since GI bleeding may result
• Advise patient to notify prescriber if ringing in the ears or persistent GI pain occurs
• Advise patient to take with full glass of water to reduce risk of lodging in esophagus

Generic Names

🔑 aspirin
choline salicylate
magnesium salicylate
salsalate

THROMBOLYTICS

Action: Thrombolytics activate conversion of plasminogen to plasmin (fibrinolysin): plasmin is able to break down clots (fibrin).

Uses: Thrombolytics are used to treat deep vein thrombosis, pulmonary embolism, arterial thrombosis, arterial embolism, arteriovenous cannula occlusion, lysis of coronary artery thrombi after MI, acute evolving transmural MI.

Adverse effects: Serious adverse reactions include GI, GU, intracranial, and retroperitoneal bleeding, and anaphylaxis. The most common side effects are decreased Hct, urticaria, headache, and nausea.

Contraindications: Persons with hypersensitivity, active bleeding, intraspinal surgery, neoplasms of the CNS, ulcerative colitis/enteritis, severe hypertension, renal disease, hepatic disease, hypocoagulation, COPD, subacute bacterial endocarditis, rheumatic valvular disease, cerebral embolism/thrombosis/hemorrhage, intraarterial diagnostic procedure or surgery (10 days), and recent major surgery should not use these products.

Precautions: Caution should be used in arterial emboli from left side of heart and pregnancy.

Pharmacokinetics: Onset, peak, and duration vary widely among products. Most products are metabolized in the liver and excreted in urine.

Interactions: Please check individual monographs, since interactions vary widely among products.

NURSING CONSIDERATIONS

Assessment

• Monitor VS, B/P, pulse, respirations, neurologic signs, temp at least q4h, temp is an indicator of internal bleeding, cardiac rhythm following intracoronary administration; systolic pressure increase of >25 mm Hg should be reported to prescriber
• Assess for neurologic changes that may indicate intracranial bleeding
• Assess retroperitoneal bleeding: back pain, leg weakness, diminished pulses
• Assess for allergy: fever, rash, itching, chills; mild reaction may be treated with antihistamines
• Assess for bleeding during 1st hr of treatment: hematuria, hematemesis, bleeding from mucous membranes, epistaxis, ecchymosis
• Monitor blood studies (Hct, platelets, PTT, PT, TT, APTT) before starting therapy; PT or APTT must be less than 2 times control before starting therapy TT or PT q3-4h during treatment

Nursing diagnoses

• Injury, risk for (uses)

Implementation

• Administer as soon as thrombi identified; not useful for thrombi over 1 wk old
• Administer cryoprecipitate or fresh, frozen plasma if bleeding occurs
• Administer loading dose at beginning of therapy; may require increased loading doses
• Give heparin after fibrinogen level is over 100 mg/dl; heparin inf to increase PTT to 1.5-2 times baseline for 3-7 days
• About 10% of patients have high streptococcal antibody titers requiring increased loading doses
• Give **IV** therapy using 0.8-μm filter
• Store reconstituted sol in refrigerator; discard after 24 hr
• Provide bed rest during entire course of treatment
• Avoid venous or arterial puncture, injection, rec temp
• Provide treatment of fever with acetaminophen or aspirin
• Apply pressure for 30 sec to minor bleeding sites; inform prescriber if this does not attain hemostasis; apply pressure dressing

Evaluation

• Therapeutic response: resolution of thrombosis, embolism

Generic Names

alteplase (high alert)
anistreplase (high alert)
drotrecogin alfa
🔑 **streptokinase** (high alert)

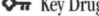

tenecteplase (high alert)
urokinase (high alert)

THYROID HORMONES

Action: Increase metabolic rates, resulting in increased cardiac output, O_2 consumption, body temp, blood volume, growth, development at cellular level, respiratory rate, enzyme system activity

Uses: Products are used for thyroid replacement.

Adverse effects: The most common side effects include insomnia, tremors, tachycardia, palpitations, angina, dysrhythmias, weight loss, and changes in appetite. Serious adverse reactions include thyroid storm.

Contraindications: Persons with adrenal insufficiency, myocardial infarction, or thyrotoxicosis should not use these products.

Precautions: The elderly and patients with angina pectoris, hypertension, ischemia, cardiac disease, or diabetes mellitus or insipidus should be watched closely when using these products. Caution should be used in pregnancy and lactation.

Pharmacokinetics: Pharmacokinetics vary widely among products; check specific monographs.

Interactions

- Impaired absorption of thyroid products may occur when administered with cholestyramine (separate by 4-5 hr)
- Increased effects of anticoagulants, sympathomimetics, tricyclic antidepressants, catecholamines may occur
- Decreased effects of digitalis, glycosides, insulin, hypoglycemics may occur
- Decreased effects of thyroid products may occur with estrogens

NURSING CONSIDERATIONS

Assessment

- Monitor B/P, pulse before each dose
- Monitor I&O ratio
- Monitor weight daily in same clothing, using same scale, at same time of day
- Monitor height, growth rate if given to a child
- Monitor T_3, T_4, which are decreased; radioimmunoassay of TSH, which is increased; ratio uptake, which is decreased if patient is on too low a dosage of medication
- Assess for increased nervousness, excitability, irritability; may indicate too high a dosage of medication usually after 1-3 wk of treatment
- Assess for cardiac status: angina, palpitation, chest pain, change in VS

Nursing diagnoses

- Knowledge, deficient (teaching)
- Noncompliance (teaching)
- Body image, disturbed (adverse reactions)

Implementation

- Give at same time each day to maintain drug level
- Give only for hormone imbalances; not to be used for obesity, male infertility, menstrual conditions, lethargy
- Remove medication 4 wk before RAIU test

Evaluation

- Therapeutic response: absence of depression; increased weight loss, diuresis, pulse, appetite; absence of constipation, peripheral edema, cold intolerance, pale, cool, dry skin, brittle nails, alopecia, coarse hair, menorrhagia, night blindness, paresthesias, syncope, stupor, coma, rosy cheeks

Patient/family education

- Advise patient that hair loss will occur in child and is temporary
- Advise patient to report excitability, irritability, anxiety; indicates overdose
- Caution patient not to switch brands unless directed by prescriber
- Caution patient that hypothyroid child will show almost immediate behavior/personality change
- Advise patient that treatment drug is not to be taken to reduce weight
- Advise patient to avoid OTC preparations with iodine; read labels; to avoid iodine-containing food, iodinized salt, soybeans, tofu, turnips, some seafood, some bread

Generic Names

levothyroxine (T_4)
liothyronine (T_3)
liotrix
thyroid USP

VASODILATORS

Action: Vasodilators act in various ways. Please check individual monograph for specific action.

Uses: Vasodilators are used to treat intermittent claudication, arteriosclerosis obliterans, vasospasm and muscular ischemia, ischemic cerebral vascular disease, hypertension, and angina.

Adverse effects: The most common side effects are headache, nausea, hypotension or hypertension, and ECG changes.

Contraindications: Some drugs are contraindicated in acute MI, paroxysmal tachycardia, and thyrotoxicosis.

Precautions: Caution should be used in uncompensated heart disease or peptic ulcer disease.

Pharmacokinetics: Onset, peak, and duration vary widely among products. Most products are metabolized in the liver and excreted in urine.

Interactions: Please check individual monographs, since interactions vary widely among products.

NURSING CONSIDERATIONS

Assessment

- Assess bleeding time in individuals with bleeding disorders
- Assess cardiac status: B/P, pulse, rate, rhythm, character; watch for increasing pulse

Nursing diagnoses

- Cardiac output, decreased (uses)
- Tissue perfusion, ineffective (uses)
- Knowledge, deficient (teaching)

Implementation

- Give with meals to reduce GI symptoms
- Store in tight container at room temp

Evaluation

- Therapeutic response: ability to walk without pain, increased temp in extremities, increased pulse volume

Patient/family education

- Inform patient that medication is not cure, may need to be taken continuously
- Advise patient that it is necessary to quit smoking to prevent excessive vasoconstriction
- Advise patient that improvement may be sudden, but usually occurs gradually over several wk
- Instruct patient to report headache, weakness, increased pulse, since drug may need to be decreased or discontinued
- Instruct patient to avoid hazardous activities until stabilized on medication; dizziness may occur

---

Generic Names

amyl nitrite
bosentan
dipyridamole
hydrALAZINE
midodrine
minoxidil
nesiritide
papaverine

VITAMINS

Action: Action varies widely among products and classes; check specific monographs.

Uses: Vitamins are used to correct and prevent vitamin deficiencies.

Adverse effects: There is an absence of side effects or adverse reactions with the water-soluble vitamins (C, B). However, fat-soluble vitamins (A, D, E, K) may accumulate in the body and cause adverse reactions (refer to specific monographs).

Contraindications: Hypersensitive reactions may occur, and allergies should be identified before these products are given.

Pharmacokinetics: Onset, peak, and duration vary widely among products; check individual monograph for specific information.

NURSING CONSIDERATIONS

Nursing diagnoses

- Nutrition: less than body requirements, imbalanced (uses)

Implementation

- Give PO with food for better absorption
- Store in tight, light-resistant container

Evaluation

- Therapeutic response: absence of vitamin deficiency

Patient/family education

- Advise patient not to take more than prescribed amount

Generic Names

Fat-soluble:
phytonadione (vitamin K_1)
vitamin A
vitamin D
vitamin E

Water-soluble:
ascorbic acid (C)
pyridoxine (B_6)
riboflavin (B_2)
thiamine (B_1)

Miscellaneous:
multivitamins

Appendix A

Selected New Drugs

abatacept (Rx)
(ab-a-ta'sept)
Orencia
Func. class.: Antirheumatic agent (disease modifying); biologic response modifier
Pregnancy category C

Action: A selective costimulation modulator, inhibits T-lymphocytes, inhibits tumor necrosis factor (TNF-α), interferon-γ, interleukin-2, that is involved in immune and inflammatory reactions

Therapeutic Outcome: Decreased pain, inflammation in joints

Uses: Acute, chronic rheumatoid arthritis that has not responded to other disease-modifying agents, may use in combination with DMARDs; do not use with TNF antagonists (adalimumab, etanercept, infliximab) or anakinra

Dosage and routes
Adult >100 kg: **IV** inf 1 g
Adult 60-100 kg: **IV** inf 750 mg
Adult <60 kg: **IV** inf 500 mg over 30 min; give 2-4 wk after 1st inf, then q4wk

Available forms: Lyophilized powder, single-use vials 250 mg

Adverse effects
CNS: Headache, asthenia, dizziness
CV: *Hypertension, hypotension*
GI: Abdominal pain, dyspepsia, nausea
INTEG: Rash, *inj site reaction*, flushing, urticaria, pruritus
RESP: *Pharyngitis, cough, URI,* non-URI, *rhinitis*, wheezing
SYST: **Anaphylaxis, malignancies, angioedema**

Contraindications: Hypersensitivity, TB

Precautions: Pregnancy **C**, lactation, children, elderly, recurrent infections, COPD

Pharmacokinetics

Absorption	Unknown
Distribution	Unknown
Metabolism	Unknown
Excretion	Unknown
Half-life	Terminal 13-16 days, steady state 60 days

Pharmacodynamics
Unknown

Interactions
Individual drugs
Anakinra: do not use
Drug classifications
Do not give concurrently with vaccines; immunizations should be brought up to date before treatment
Corticosteroids, immunosuppressives: do not use concurrently
TNF antagonists (adalimumab, etanercept, infliximab): do not use

NURSING CONSIDERATIONS
Assessment
- Assess for latent/active TB before beginning treatment
- Assess for pain, stiffness, ROM, swelling of joints during treatment
- Assess for inj site pain, swelling
- Monitor patient's overall health on each visit; product should not be given with active infections

Nursing diagnoses
- Pain, chronic (uses)
- Knowledge, deficient (teaching)

Implementation
- To reconstitute, remove plastic flip top from vial and wipe the top with alcohol wipe; insert syringe needle into vial and direct stream of sterile water for inj on the wall of vial; rotate vial until mixed; vent with needle to rid foam after reconstitution 25 mg/ml; further dilute in 100 ml from a 100 ml infusion bag/bottle; withdraw the needed volume (2 vials remove 20 mg; 3 vials remove 30 ml, 4 vials remove 40 ml); slowly add the reconstituted Orencia sol from each vial into the infusion bag/bottle using the same disposable syringe supplied; mix gently, discard unused portions of vials; do not use if particulate is present or discolored; give over 30 min; use non-protein binding filter (0.2-1.2 mcg)

- Do not admix with other sol or medications
- Store in refrigerator; do not use expired vials

Patient/family education

- Teach patient that drug must be continued for prescribed time to be effective
- Advise patient to use caution when driving; dizziness may occur
- Advise patient not to have vaccinations while taking this product
- Discuss with patient information included in packaging

Evaluation

Positive therapeutic outcome

- Decreased inflammation, pain in joints; decreased erythrocyte sedimentation rate (ESR)

entecavir (Rx)

(en-te'ka-veer)

Baraclude

Func. class.: Antiviral

Chem. class.: Guanosine nucleoside analog

Pregnancy category C

Action: Inhibits hepatitis B virus DNA polymerase by competing with natural substrates and by causing DNA termination after its incorporation into viral DNA; causes viral DNA death

Therapeutic Outcome: Improved liver function tests in chronic hepatitis B (HBV)

Uses: Chronic hepatitis B (HBV)

Dosage and routes

Chronic hepatitis B (nucleoside treatment–naive)

Adult and adolescent ≥16 yr: PO 0.5 mg daily

Chronic hepatitis B while receiving lamivudine or known lamivudine resistance mutations

Adult and adolescent ≥16 yr: PO 1 mg daily

Renal dose

Adult: PO CCr ≥50 ml/min 0.5 mg daily; CCr 30-49 ml/min 0.25 mg daily, 0.5 mg daily for lamivudine refractory patient; CCr 10-29 ml/min 0.15 daily, 0.3 for lamivudine refractory patient; CCr <10 ml/min 0.05 mg PO daily, 0.1 mg for lamivudine refractory patient

Available forms: Tabs, film coated 0.5, 1 mg; oral sol 0.05 mg/ml

Adverse effects

CNS: Headache, fatigue, dizziness, insomnia

GI: Dyspepsia, nausea, vomiting, diarrhea

***SYST:* Lactic acidosis, severe hepatomegaly with stenosis**

Contraindications: Hypersensitivity

Precautions: Pregnancy **C**, lactation, child, severe renal disease, elderly

Pharmacokinetics	
Absorption	100%
Distribution	Extensively to tissues, protein binding 13%
Metabolism	Unknown
Excretion	Unchanged 62%-73% via kidneys
Half-life	Terminal 128-149 hr

Pharmacodynamics	
Onset	Unknown
Peak	0.5-1.5 hr
Duration	Unknown

Interactions: None known

Drug/lab test

Increased: ALT, AST, total bilirubin, amylase, lipase, creatinine, blood glucose, urine glucose

Decreased: platelets, albumin

NURSING CONSIDERATIONS

Assessment

- Assess for nephrotoxicity: increasing CCr, BUN
- Assess for HIV before beginning treatment because HIV resistance may occur in chronic hepatitis B patients
- ⚠ Assess for lactic acidosis, severe hepatomegaly with stenosis
- Monitor elderly patients more carefully; may develop renal, cardiac symptoms more rapidly
- Assess for exacerbations of hepatitis after discontinuing treatment, monitor LFTs

Nursing diagnoses

- Infection, risk for (uses)
- Injury, risk for (uses, adverse reactions)

Implementation

- Give by mouth on empty stomach 2 hr before or after food
- Store in cool environment; protect from light

Patient/family education

- Teach patient not to take with food
- Teach patient to take exactly as prescribed
- Advise patient not to stop medication without approval of prescriber

• Advise that optimal duration of treatment is unknown
• Teach patient to avoid use with other medications unless approved by prescriber
• Teach patient to notify prescriber of decreased urinary output, blood in urine
• Teach patient symptoms of lactic acidosis: muscle pain, severe tiredness, weakness, trouble breathing, stomach pain with nausea/vomiting, coldness in arms/legs, fast/irregular heartbeat, dizziness
• Teach patient symptoms of hepatotoxicity: eyes/skin turns yellow, dark urine, light bowel movements, no appetite for days, nausea, stomach pain
• Advise patient that product does not cure, but lowers the amount of HBV in body
• Teach patient that product does not stop the spreading of HBV to others by sex, sharing needles, or being exposed to blood

Evaluation

Positive therapeutic outcome

• Decreased symptoms of chronic hepatitis B, improving LFTs

exenatide (Rx)

(ex-en′a-tide)

Byetta

Func. class.: Antidiabetic

Chem. class.: Incretin mimetic

Pregnancy category C

Action: Binds and activates known human GLP-1 receptor, mimics natural physiology for self-regulating glycemic control

Therapeutic Outcome: Decreased polyuria, polydipsia, polyphagia; improved A1c

Uses: Type 2 diabetes mellitus given in combination with metformin or a sulfonylurea

Dosage and routes

Adult: SUBCUT 5 mcg bid 1 hr before morning and evening meal; may increase to 10 mcg bid after 1 mo of therapy

Available forms: Inj 250 mcg/ml pen injector

Adverse effects

CNS: *Headache, dizziness,* feeling jittery, restlessness, weakness

ENDO: **Hypoglycemia**

GI: Nausea, vomiting, diarrhea, dyspepsia, anorexia, gastroesophageal reflux, weight loss

Contraindications: Hypersensitivity

Precautions: Pregnancy **C,** elderly, severe renal disease, severe hepatic disease, severe GI disease

Pharmacokinetics

Absorption	Unknown
Distribution	Unknown
Metabolism	Unknown
Excretion	Glomerular filtration
Half-life	Unknown

Pharmacodynamics

Onset	Unknown
Peak	2.1 hr
Duration	Unknown

Interactions

Individual drugs

Acetaminophen: may increase the effect of acetaminophen
Acetaminophen (elixir), digoxin, lovastatin: decreased action of these drugs
Alcohol, disopyramide: increased hypoglycemia
Dextrothyroxine, niacin, triamterene: decreased hypoglycemia
Erythromycin, metoclopramide: do not use with exenatide
Exenatide: increased action

Drug classifications

ACE inhibitors, anabolic steroids, androgens, corticosteroids, fibric acid derivatives: increased hypoglycemia
Estrogens, MAOIs, oral contraceptives, progestins, thiazide diuretics: decreased hypoglycemia
Phenothiazines: increased hyperglycemia

NURSING CONSIDERATIONS

Assessment

• Monitor fasting blood, glucose, A1c levels, postprandial glucose during treatment to determine diabetes control
• Assess for hypo/hyperglycemic reaction that can occur soon after meals; for severe hypoglycemia give **IV** $D_{50}W$, then **IV** dextrose solution

Nursing diagnoses

• Injury, risk for (uses)
• Knowledge, deficient (teaching)
• Noncompliance (teaching)

Implementation

• Give 1 hr before meals; if patient is NPO, may need to hold dose to prevent hypoglycemia
• Store in refrigerator

Patient/family education
- Teach patient symptoms of hypo/hyperglycemia, what to do about each; to have glucagon emergency kit available; to carry a glucose source (candy, sugar cube) to treat hypoglycemia
- Advise patient that drug must be continued on daily basis; explain consequences of discontinuing drug abruptly
- Teach patient that diabetes is a lifelong illness; drug will not cure disease
- Advise that all food in diet plan must be eaten to prevent hypoglycemia
- Advise patient to carry emergency ID with prescriber and medications
- Advise patient to continue weight control, dietary restrictions, exercise, hygiene
- Inform patient that regular blood glucose monitoring and A1c testing is needed
- Advise patient to notify prescriber if pregnant or intend to become pregnant
- Advise patient to read "Information for the Patient" and "Pen User Manual"

Evaluation
Positive therapeutic outcome
- Decrease in polyuria, polydipsia, polyphagia, clear sensorium; improved A1c, weight; absence of dizziness, stable gait

RARELY USED

galsulfase (Rx)
Func. class.: Miscellaneous drug

Dosage and routes
Adult and child ≥5 yr: **IV** 1 mg/kg infused over ≥4h once per week

Uses: Mucopolysaccharidosis VI (MPS VI); Maroteaux-Lamy syndrome

Contraindications: Hypersensitivity

! HIGH ALERT

insulin, inhaled (Rx)
Exubera

Func. class.: Antidiabetic, pancreatic hormone, inhaled

Chem. class.: Exogenous unmodified insulin

Pregnancy category C

Action: Decreases blood glucose; by transport of glucose into cells and the conversion of glucose to glycogen, indirectly increases blood pyruvate and lactate, decreases phosphate and potassium; processed by recombinant DNA technologies

Therapeutic Outcome: Decreased polyuria, polydipsia, polyphagia; improved A1c

Uses: Adult patients with type 1 or type 2 diabetes mellitus

Dosage and routes
Adult: INH Insert dose in hand-held inhalation device and inhale 10 min before meal

Available forms: Inhaled, dry powder 1, 3 mg unit dose blisters (3 of the 1 mg blister packs is not equal to 1, 3 mg blister pack)

Adverse effects
EENT: Blurred vision, dry mouth, cough
GI: Nausea, vomiting, weight gain
META: *Hypoglycemia,* insulin resistance
RESP: **Bronchospasm,** laryngitis, dyspnea, epistaxis, rhinitis, sinusitis
SYST: **Anaphylaxis,** antibody formation

Contraindications: Hypersensitivity; poorly controlled, unstable lung disease; smokers; those who have quit smoking within the last 6 mo, diabetic ketoacidosis, hyperosmolar hyperglycemic state (HHS), hypoglycemia, mannitol hypersensitivity

Precautions: Pregnancy **C;** chronic lung disorders (asthma, bronchitis, emphysema); hepatic, renal disease; cystic fibrosis

Pharmacokinetics	
Absorption	10% of regular insulin (SUBCUT)
Distribution	Unknown
Metabolism	Unknown
Excretion	Unknown
Half-life	Unknown

Pharmacodynamics	
Onset	10-20 min
Peak	Peak 49 min; range 30-90 min
Duration	6 hr

Interactions
Individual drugs
Alcohol, guanethidine, salicylate, sulfinpyrazone: increased hypoglycemia

Drug classifications
ACE inhibitors, anabolic steroids, β-blockers, fibric acid derivatives, MAOIs, oral hypoglycemics: increased hypoglycemia
Atypical psychotics, corticosteroids, estrogens, oral contraceptives, progestins, thiazides, thyroid hormones: decreased hypoglycemia

NURSING CONSIDERATIONS
Assessment
- Monitor fasting blood glucose, 2 hr PP (80-150 mg/dl, normal fasting level; 70-130

mg/dl, normal 2 hr level); also A1c may be drawn to identify treatment effectiveness

- Assess for hypoglycemic reaction that can occur during peak time (sweating, weakness, dizziness, chills, confusion, headache, nausea, rapid weak pulse, fatigue, tachycardia, memory lapses, slurred speech, staggering gait, anxiety, tremors, hunger)
- Assess for hyperglycemia: acetone breath, polyuria, fatigue, polydipsia, flushed, dry skin, lethargy

Nursing diagnoses
- Injury, risk for (uses)
- Knowledge, deficient (teaching)
- Noncompliance (teaching)

Implementation
- Give 10 min before meal
- 1 mg and 3 mg blisters are used in combination, consecutive inhalation of 3 (1 mg blisters) is associated with 30%-40% greater insulin exposure than 1 (3 mg blister); they are not interchangeable
- SUBCUT regular insulin 3 units = 1 mg Exubera (1 blister pack)

Patient/family education
- Advise patient that if blurred vision occurs, not to change corrective lens until vision is stabilized 1-2 mo
- Advise patient to keep insulin, equipment available at all times
- Teach patient that drug does not cure diabetes but controls symptoms
- Advise patient to carry emergency ID as diabetic
- Teach patient to recognize hypoglycemia reaction: headache, tremors, fatigue, weakness
- Teach patient the dosage, route, mixing instructions, if any diet restrictions, disease process
- Advise patient to carry candy or lump sugar to treat hypoglycemia
- Advise patient of symptoms of ketoacidosis: nausea; thirst; polyuria; dry mouth; decreased B/P; dry, flushed skin; acetone breath; drowsiness; Kussmaul respirations
- Teach patient that a plan is necessary for diet, exercise; all food on diet should be eaten; exercise routine should not vary
- Teach patient about blood glucose testing; make sure patient is able to determine glucose level in order to self monitor
- Advise patient to avoid OTC drugs unless directed by prescriber

Evaluation
Positive therapeutic outcome
- Decrease in polyuria, polydipsia, polyphagia, clear sensorium; improved A1c; absence of dizziness, stable gait

Treatment of overdose: Glucose 25 g **IV**, via dextrose 50% sol, 50 ml or glucagon 1 mg

mecasermin (Rx)
(mec-a′sir-men)

Increlex

Func. class.: Biologic response modifier; insulin-like growth factor

Pregnancy category C

Action: Stimulates growth; IGF-1 is the principal hormonal mediator of statural growth. GH binds to its receptor in the liver and other tissues

Therapeutic Outcome: Increased height

Uses: Growth failure in children with severe primary insulin-like growth factor-1 (IGF-1) deficiency (primary IGFD) or with growth hormone (GH) gene deletion who have developed neutralizing antibodies to GH

Investigational uses: ALS

Dosage and routes
Child: SUBCUT 0.04-0.08 mg/kg (40-80 mcg/kg) bid; if well tolerated for 1 wk, may increase by 0.04 mg/kg/dose, max 0.12 mg/kg bid

Available forms: Inj 10 mg/ml

Adverse effects
CNS: Headache, **seizures**, dizziness, cardiac valvulopathy
CV: Cardiac murmur
EENT: Ear pain, otitis media, abnormal tympanometry, papilledema, visual impairment
ENDO: **Hypoglycemia, ketosis, hypothyroidism**
GU: Vomiting
HEMA: Thymus hypertrophy
META: Hypoglycemic
MISC: Bruising, lipohypertrophy, hypersensitivity reactions
MS: Arthralgia, joint pain
RESP: Snoring, tonsillar hypertrophy, **apnea**
SYST: **Antibodies to growth hormone**

Contraindications: Hypersensitivity, benzyl alcohol, closed epiphyses, active/suspected neoplasia, **IV** use

Precautions: Pregnancy **C,** diabetes mellitus, hypothyroidism, lactation, child <2 yr, increased intracranial pressure, malnutrition, scoliosis, sleep apnea

Pharmacokinetics

Absorption	Near 100%
Distribution	Unknown
Metabolism	Liver/kidneys
Excretion	Unknown
Half-life	5.8 hr

Pharmacodynamics

Unknown

Interactions
Drug classifications
Antidiabetics, corticosteroids: increased hypoglycemia

NURSING CONSIDERATIONS
Assessment
- Monitor preprandial glucose at beginning of treatment and until well tolerated
- Monitor by funduscopic exam at beginning and periodically during treatment
- Assess for allergic reactions; if present, interrupt treatment and notify prescriber
- Assess growth rate of child at intervals during treatment

Nursing diagnoses
- Knowledge, deficient (teaching)

Implementation
SUBCUT route
- Rotate inj site; use sterile, disposable syringe/needles; use small-volume syringe for accurate measurement
- Give shortly before or after a meal or snack to lessen hypoglycemia
- Store in refrigerator before opening, avoid freezing; after opening, stable for 30 days after initial vial entry, store in refrigerator, do not use if particulate matter is present, avoid direct light, do not use after expiration date

Patient/family education
- Teach patient that treatment may continue for years; regular assessments are required
- Advise patient to avoid hazardous activities, driving within 2-3 hr of dosing
- Teach patient correct administration and needle disposal

Evaluation
Positive therapeutic outcome
- Growth in children

nelarabine (Rx)
(nella-ra'ben)

Arranon

Func. class.: Antineoplastic

Chem. class.: Purine analog

Pregnancy category D

Action: Leukemic blasts allow for incorporation into DNA, thus interfering with cell replication lending to cell death

Therapeutic Outcome: Decreased growth of malignant cells

Uses: T-cell lymphoblastic leukemia, T-cell lymphoblastic lymphoma post relapse or treatment failure with at least two chemotherapeutic agents

Dosage and routes
Adult: **IV** 1500 mg/m^2 over 2 hr on days 1, 3, 5 repeated q 21 days

Child: **IV** 650 mg/m^2 over 1 hr daily × 5 days, repeated q 21 days

Available forms: Sol for inj 5 mg/ml

Adverse effects
CNS: Dizziness, *fatigue,* insomnia, rigors, **seizures,** peripheral neuropathy, **paralysis,** confusion, headache

CV: Edema

GI: *Nausea, vomiting, anorexia, diarrhea, stomatitis, constipation*

HEMA: **Neutropenia**, leukopenia, **thrombocytopenia**, anemia

META: Decreased potassium, calcium, magnesium, glucose, albumin, bilirubin, AST, ALT, hyperuricemia; increased glucose

MS: Myalgia, arthralgia, back pain, weakness

RESP: **Pleural effusion**, cough, dyspnea, wheezing, epistaxis

Contraindications: Pregnancy **D**, hypersensitivity, severe neurotoxicity

Precautions: Renal disease, hepatic disease, lactation, children, elderly

Pharmacokinetics

Absorption	Unknown
Distribution	Unknown
Metabolism	Liver
Excretion	Kidneys
Half-life	30 min-3hr

Pharmacodynamics

Unknown

Interactions

Drug classifications

Do not use with live virus vaccinations

NURSING CONSIDERATIONS

Assessment

- Monitor CBC (RBC, Hct, Hgb), differential platelet count weekly; withhold drugs if WBC is $<4000/mm^3$, platelet count is $<75{,}000/mm^3$, or RBC, Hct, Hgb low; notify prescriber of these results
- Monitor renal studies: BUN, serum uric acid, urine CCr, electrolytes before and during therapy
- Monitor temp q4h; fever may indicate beginning infection; no rectal temps
- Monitor hepatic studies before and during therapy: bilirubin, ALT, AST, alkaline phosphatase as needed or monthly
- Assess for bleeding: hematuria, heme-positive stools, bruising or petechiae, mucosa or orifices q8h
- Assess for neurotoxicity: somnolence, confusion, seizures, ataxia, paraesthesias, hypoesthesia, coma, status epilepticus, craniospinal demyelination; contact prescriber immediately
- Assess for dyspnea, crackles, unproductive cough, chest pain, tachypnea, fatigue, increased pulse, pallor, lethargy, personality changes
- Assess buccal cavity q8h for dryness, sores or ulceration, white patches, oral pain, bleeding, dysphagia
- Assess for GI symptoms: frequency of stools, cramping, if severe diarrhea occurs, fluid and electrolytes may need to be given

Nursing diagnoses

- Injury, risk for (uses, adverse reactions)

Implementation

- Provide **IV** hydration, and allopurinol in risk of hyperuricemia
- Use procedures for proper handling/disposal of anticancer drugs
- Provide for rinsing of mouth tid-qid with water, club soda; brushing of teeth bid-tid with soft brush or cotton-tipped applicators for stomatitis; use unwaxed dental floss
- Store at room temp

Patient/family education

- Advise patient to avoid foods with citric acid, hot or rough texture if stomatitis is present
- Advise patient to use contraception while taking this product
- Advise patient to avoid using while lactating
- Teach patient to report signs of infection: increased temp, sore throat, flulike symptoms
- Teach patient to report signs of anemia: fatigue, headache, faintness, shortness of breath, irritability
- Teach patient to report bleeding; to avoid use of razors, commercial mouthwash
- Advise patient that seizures may occur, do not operate machinery or drive until effects are known
- Advise patient not to receive vaccinations while taking this product

Evaluation

Positive therapeutic outcome

- Decreased spread of malignancy

pramlintide (Rx)

(pram'lin-tide)

Symlin

Func. class.: Antidiabetic

Chem. class.: Synthetic human amylin analog

Pregnancy category C

Action: Modulates and slows stomach emptying, prevents postprandial rise in plasma glucagon, decreases appetite, leads to decreased caloric intake and weight loss

Therapeutic Outcome: Decreased polyuria, polydipsia, polyphagia; improved A1c

Uses: Type 1 diabetes mellitus, type 2 diabetes mellitus as an adjunct to insulin therapy with uncontrolled type 1 or type 2 diabetes

Dosage and routes

Adult: SUBCUT 15 mcg, may increase by 15 mcg to 30-60 mcg, max 120 mcg/dose

Available forms: Inj 5 ml vials (0.6 mg/ml)

Adverse effects

CNS: Headache, fatigue, dizziness

GI: Nausea, vomiting, anorexia, abdominal pain

INTEG: Inj site reactions

META: Hypoglycemia (while used with insulin)

MS: Arthralgia

RESP: Cough, pharyngitis

SYST: Systemic allergy

Contraindications: Hypersensitivity to this product or metacresol, gastroparesis

Precautions: Pregnancy **C,** lactation

Pharmacokinetics

Absorption	30%-40%
Distribution	Extensively bound to blood cells or albumin
Metabolism	Kidneys
Excretion	Unknown
Half-life	48 min

Pharmacodynamics

Unknown

Interactions
Individual drugs
Acetaminophen: may increase effect of acetaminophen
Alcohol, disopyramide: increased hypoglycemia
Dextrothyroxine, niacin, triamterene: decreased hypoglycemia
Diphenoxylate, loperamide, octreotide: increased pramlintide action
Erythromycin, metoclopramide: do not use
Drug classifications
ACE inhibitors, anabolic steroids, androgens, corticosteroids, fibric acid derivatives: increased hypoglycemia
α-Glucosidase inhibitors, antimuscarinics, opiate agonist, tricyclic antidepressants: increased pramlintide action
Estrogens, MAOIs, oral contraceptives, progestins, thiazide diuretics: decreased hypoglycemia
Phenothiazines: increased hyperglycemia

NURSING CONSIDERATIONS
Assessment
- Monitor fasting blood glucose, 2 hr PP (80-150 mg/dl, normal fasting level; 70-130 mg/dl, normal 2 hr level); A1c may also be drawn to identify treatment effectiveness; also monitor weight, appetite
- Assess for hypoglycemic reaction (sweating, weakness, dizziness, chills, confusion, headache, nausea, rapid weak pulse, fatigue, tachycardia, memory lapses, slurred speech, staggering gait, anxiety, tremors, hunger)
- Assess for hyperglycemia: acetone breath, polyuria, fatigue, polydipsia, flushed, dry skin, lethargy

Nursing diagnoses
- Injury, risk for (uses)
- Knowledge, deficient (teaching)
- Noncompliance (teaching)

Implementation
SUBCUT route
- Give prior to mealtime, or if 30 g of carbohydrates will be consumed
- Do not use if a meal is skipped
- Do not use if discolored
- Store at room temperature, keep away from heat and sunlight; refrigerate all other supply

Syringe compatibilities: Do not mix with insulin, give separately

Patient/family education
- Advise patient that drug does not cure diabetes but controls symptoms
- Advise patient to carry emergency ID as diabetic
- Teach patient to recognize hypoglycemia reaction: headache, fatigue, weakness
- Teach patient the dosage, route, mixing instructions, if any diet restrictions, disease process
- Advise patient to carry a glucose source (candy or lump sugar) to treat hypoglycemia
- Teach patient symptoms of ketoacidosis: nausea, thirst, polyuria, dry mouth, decreased B/P, dry, flushed skin, acetone breath, drowsiness, Kussmaul respirations
- Advise patient that a plan is necessary for diet, exercise; all food on diet should be eaten; exercise routine should not vary
- Teach patient about blood glucose testing; make sure patient is able to determine glucose level
- Advise patient to avoid OTC drugs unless directed by prescriber, alcohol
- Advise patient not to operate machinery or drive until effect is known

Evaluation
Positive therapeutic outcome
- Decrease in polyuria, polydipsia, polyphagia, clear sensorium; improved A1c; absence of dizziness, stable gait

Treatment of overdose: Glucose 25 g **IV**, via dextrose 50% sol, 50 ml or glucagon 1 mg SUBCUT

pregabalin (Rx)
(pre-gab'a-lin)
Lyrica
Func. class.: Anticonvulsant
Controlled substance schedule V
Pregnancy category C

Action: Binds to high-voltage–gated calcium channels in CNS tissues; this may lead to anticonvulsant action, similar to the inhibitory neurotransmitter GABA, anxiolytic, analgesics, and antiepileptic properties

Therapeutic Outcome: Decreased seizure activity, decreased neuropathic pain

Uses: Neuropathic pain associated with diabetic peripheral neuropathy, partial onset seizures, postherpetic neuralgia

Investigational uses: Generalized anxiety disorder (GAD), moderate pain, social anxiety disorder

Dosage and routes

Diabetic peripheral neuropathic pain

Adult: PO 50 mg tid, may increase to 300 mg/day (max) within 1 wk, adjust in renal disease

Partial onset seizures

Adult: PO 75 mg bid or 50 mg tid; may increase to 600 mg/day (max)

Postherpetic neuralgia

Adult: PO 75-150 mg bid or 50-100 mg tid in patient with CCr ≥60 ml/min, initially give 75 mg bid or 50 mg tid and may increase to 600 mg/day (max) within 1 wk

Available forms: Caps 25, 50, 75, 100, 150, 200, 225, 300 mg

Adverse effects

CNS: Dizziness, fatigue, confusion, euphoria, incoordination, nervousness, neuropathy, tremor, vertigo, somnolence, ataxia, amnesia, abnormal thinking

EENT: Dry mouth, blurred vision, nystagmus, amblyopia

GI: Constipation, flatulence, abdominal pain, weight gain

HEMA: Ecchymosis

MS: Back pain

OTHER: Pruritus, impotence

RESP: Dyspnea

Contraindications: Hypersensitivity, abrupt discontinuation

Precautions: Pregnancy **C,** renal disease, lactation, children <12 yr, elderly, PR interval prolongation, creatine kinase elevations, CHF (class III, IV), decreased platelets, drug abuse, dependence, glaucoma, myopathy

Pharmacokinetics	
Absorption	Well, decreased by food
Distribution	Not bound to plasma proteins
Metabolism	Negligible
Excretion	90% unchanged, urine
Half-life	6 hr

Pharmacodynamics
Unknown

Interactions

Drug classifications

Anxiolytics, barbiturates, general anesthetics, hypnotics, opiate agonists, phenothiazines, sedating H_1 blockers, sedatives, thiazolidinediones, tricyclic antidepressants: increased CNS depression

Thiazolidinediones: increased weight gain/fluid retention; avoid use if possible

NURSING CONSIDERATIONS

Assessment

- Assess for seizures: aura, location, duration, activity at onset
- Assess for pain: location, duration, characteristics if using for diabetic neuropathy
- Monitor renal studies: urinalysis, BUN, urine creatinine q3mo, creatine kinase; if markedly increased, discontinue
- Assess mental status: mood, sensorium, affect, behavioral changes; if mental status changes, notify prescriber

Nursing diagnoses

- Pain, chronic (uses)
- Knowledge, deficient (teaching)

Implementation

- Do not crush or chew caps; caps may be opened and contents put in applesauce or dissolved in juice
- Give without regard to meals
- Gradually withdraw over 7 days; abrupt withdrawal may precipitate seizures
- Store at room temperature away from heat and light
- Give hard candy, frequent rinsing of mouth, gum for dry mouth
- Provide assistance with ambulation during early part of treatment; dizziness occurs
- Provide seizure precautions: padded side rails; move objects that may harm patient
- Provide increased fluids, bulk in diet for constipation

Patient/family education

- Advise patient to carry emergency ID stating patient's name, drugs taken, condition, prescriber's name and phone number
- Advise patient to avoid driving, other activities that require alertness: dizziness, drowsiness may occur
- Teach patient not to discontinue medication quickly after long-term use, taper over ≥1 wk; withdrawal-precipitated seizures may occur, not to double doses if dose is missed, take if 2 hr or more before next dose
- Teach patient to notify prescriber if pregnancy planned or suspected; avoid breastfeeding

- Teach patient to report muscle pain, tenderness, weakness, when accompanied by fever, malaise
- Advise patient to avoid alcohol

Evaluation

Positive therapeutic outcome

- Decreased seizure activity; decrease in neuropathic pain

Treatment of overdose: Lavage, VS, hemodialysis

ramelteon (Rx)

(rah-mel′tee-on)

Rozerem

Func. class.: Sedative/hypnotic, antianxiety

Chem. class.: Melatonin receptor agonist

Pregnancy category C

Action: Binds selectively to melatonin receptors (MT_1, MT_2); thought to be involved in circadian rhythm and the normal sleep/wake cycle

Therapeutic Outcome: Ability to fall asleep easily and decrease early morning awakenings

Uses: Insomnia

Dosage and routes

Adult: PO 8 mg at bedtime

Hepatic dose

Do not use in severe hepatic disease; use with caution in mild to moderate hepatic disease

Available forms: Tabs 8 mg

Adverse Effects

CNS: Dizziness, somnolence, fatigue, headache, insomnia, depression

GI: Nausea, diarrhea, dysgeusia, vomiting

MISC: Myalgia, arthralgia, decreased blood cortisol, influenza, upper respiratory tract infection

Contraindications: Hypersensitivity, children, infants, lactation, alcohol intoxication, hepatic encephalopathy

Precautions: Pregnancy **C**, hepatic disease, alcoholism, COPD, seizure disorder, sleep apnea, suicidal ideation

Pharmacokinetics	
Absorption	Rapidly
Distribution	Protein binding 82%
Metabolism	Rapid first pass metabolism, liver
Excretion	84% urine, 4% feces
Half-life	2-5 hr

Pharmacodynamics	
Onset	Unknown
Peak	0.75 hr
Duration	Unknown

Interactions

Individual drugs

Alcohol, fluconazole, fluvoxamine, ketoconazole: increased ramelteon effect

Rifampin: decreased effect of ramelteon

Drug classifications

Antiretroviral protease inhibitors: possible toxicity

Anxiolytics, azole antifungals, barbiturates, hypnotics, sedatives: increased ramelteon effect

Drug/herb

Do not use with melatonin

Catnip, chamomile, clary, cowslip, hops, kava, lavender, mistletoe, nettle, pokeweed, poppy, Queen Anne's lace, senega, skullcap, valerian: increased CNS depression

Drug/food

High-fat/heavy meal: prolonged absorption, sleep onset reduced

NURSING CONSIDERATIONS

Assessment

- Assess mental status: mood, sensorium, affect, memory (long, short)
- Assess type of sleep problem: falling asleep, staying asleep

Nursing diagnoses

- Sleep pattern, disturbed (uses)
- Injury, risk for (adverse reactions)
- Knowledge, deficient (teaching)

Implementation

- Give after removal of cigarettes to prevent fires
- Give after trying conservative measures for insomnia
- Give within 30 min of bedtime for sleeplessness
- Give on empty stomach for fast onset
- Provide assistance with ambulation after receiving dose
- Provide safety measure: nightlight, call bell within easy reach
- Check to see if PO medication has been swallowed
- Store in tight container in cool environment

Patient/family education

- Advise patient to avoid driving or other activities requiring alertness until drug is stabilized

- Advise patient to avoid alcohol ingestion or CNS depressants
- Teach patient alternative measures to improve sleep: reading, exercise several hr before bedtime, warm bath, warm milk, TV, self-hypnosis, deep breathing
- Advise patient to take immediately before going to bed
- Advise patient not to ingest a high-fat/heavy meal before taking
- Teach patient to report cessation of menses, galactorrhea (women), decreased libido, infertility; worsening of insomnia, or behavioral changes

Evaluation

Positive therapeutic outcome

- Ability to sleep at night, decreased amount of early morning awakening

rotavirus vaccine (Rx)

(rota-vi'rus vak'seen)

RotaTeq

Func. class: Vaccine, rotavirus

Action: A live, oral vaccine; protects against serotypes G1, G2, G3, G4, P1

Therapeutic Outcome: Prevention of rotavirus

Uses: Prevents rotavirus gastroenteritis in infants

Dosage and routes

Infants: PO 3 doses given between 6 and 32 wk of age; the first dose should be given between 6-12 wk; subsequent doses every 4-10 wk

Available forms: Single dose (PO)

Adverse Effects

EENT: Runny nose, sore throat, ear infection
GI: Diarrhea, vomiting, **gastroenteritis**
GU: **Urinary tract infection**
RESP: Wheezing, coughing, **pneumonia, pyrexia**

Contraindications: Hypersensitivity, immunocompromised; bone marrow, lymphatic disorders; blood products given within 6 wk

Pharmacokinetics

Unknown

Pharmacodynamics

Unknown

Interactions

Drug classifications

Antineoplastics, corticosteroids, radiation therapy: do not give with rotavirus vaccine

NURSING CONSIDERATIONS

Assessment

- Assess for age of infant; should only be given between 6 and 32 wk of age
- Assess for urinary tract infection, pneumonia, which can be serious
- Assess for intussusception, which was associated with a previously licensed product

Nursing diagnoses

- Injury, risk for (uses)
- Knowledge, deficient (teaching)

Implementation

- Give only during 6-32 wk of age
- May be given during well-baby checks at 2, 4, 6 mo

Patient/family education

- Teach patient to report coughing, wheezing, painful or scant urination

Evaluation

Positive therapeutic outcome

- Absence of rotavirus infection

sorafenib (Rx)

(sore-ah-fen'ib)

Nexavar

Func. class.: Antineoplastic—miscellaneous
Chem. class.: Multikinase inhibitor, signal transduction inhibitor

Pregnancy category D

Action: Multikinase inhibitor that decreases tumor cell proliferation

Therapeutic Outcome: Prevent spread of malignancy

Uses: Advanced/metastatic murine renal cell carcinoma

Dosage and routes

Adult: PO 400 mg bid without food, continue until no longer benefiting or until unacceptable toxicity occurs

Available forms: Tabs 200 mg

Adverse effects

CNS: Fatigue, weight loss, headache
CV: **Hypertension, cardiac ischemia, infarction**
GI: *Nausea, diarrhea, vomiting,* anorexia, **pancreatitis,** mouth ulceration, abdominal pain, constipation

HEMA: **Hemorrhage, leukopenia, lymphopenia, anemia, neutropenia, thrombocytopenia**
INTEG: *Rash,* pruritus, *dry skin,* erythema, hand-foot rash, **exfoliative dermatitis,** acne, flushing, alopecia
META: *Hypophosphatemia*
MS: *Arthralgia, myalgia*
RESP: *Hoarseness*

Contraindications: Pregnancy **D**, hypersensitivity

Precautions: Lactation, children, elderly, hepatic disease

Pharmacokinetics

Absorption	38%-49%, high fat meal decreases bioavailability
Distribution	Protein binding 99.5%
Metabolism	Liver, oxidative metabolism by CYP3A4, glucuronidation by UGT1A9
Excretion	77% feces
Half-life	Elimination 25-48 hr

Pharmacodynamics

Onset	Unknown
Peak	3 hr
Duration	Unknown

Interactions
Individual drugs
Carbamazepine, cimetidine, dexamethasone, phenobarbital, phenytoin, ranitidine, rifampin, sodium bicarbonate: may decrease sorafenib levels
Drug classifications
UGT1A1 drugs (irinotecan, DOXOrubicin, gemcitabine, oxaliplatin): increased effect of sorafenib
Drug/lab test
Increased: lipase, amylase

NURSING CONSIDERATIONS
Assessment
- Assess for skin toxicities: Grade 1, continue therapy, topical treatment for relief; grade 2 (1st episode), continue therapy, if no improvement after 7 days, delay treatment until resolved to grade ≤1, resume dose by one dose level; grade 2 (2nd or 3rd episode), delay treatment until resolved to grade ≤1, resume dose by one dose level; grade 2 (4th episode), discontinue therapy; grade 3 (1st or 2nd episode), delay treatment until resolved to grade ≤1, resume dose by one dose level; grade 3 (3rd episode), discontinue therapy.

Nursing diagnoses
- Injury, risk for (uses, adverse reactions)

Implementation
- Swallow tab whole; do not break, crush, or chew
- Give on empty stomach 1 hr before or 2 hr after meal
- Store in room temp, in dry place

Patient/family education
- ❗ Teach patient to report adverse reactions immediately
- Teach patient the reason for treatment, expected results
- Advise patient to use contraception during treatment, birth defects may occur; avoid breastfeeding
- Advise patient not to double dose if missed

Evaluation
Positive therapeutic outcome
- Decrease in renal cell carcinoma progression

tigecycline (Rx)
(tye-ge-sye'kleen)
Tygacil
Func. class.: Broad-spectrum antiinfective
Chem. class.: Glycylcyclines
Pregnancy category D

Action: Inhibits protein synthesis and phosphorylation in microorganisms; bacteriostatic structurally similar to the tetracyclines

Therapeutic Outcome: Resolution of infection

Uses: Complicated skin/skin structure infections (*Escherichia coli, Enterococcus faecalis* (vancomycin-susceptible only) *Staphylococcus aureus, Streptococcus agalactiae, S. anginosus* group, *S. pyogenes, Bacteroides fragilis*; complicated intraabdominal infections *(Citrobacter freundii), Enterobacter cloacae, E. coli, Klebsiella oxytoca, K. pneumoniae, E. faecalis* (vancomycin-susceptible only), *S. aureus* (methicillin-susceptible only), *S. anginosus* group, *B. fragilis, Bacteroides thetaiotaomicron, B. uniformis, B. vulgatus, Clostridium perfringens, Peptostreptococcus micros*

Dosage and routes
Adult: **IV** 100 mg, then 50 mg q12h, **IV** inf is given over 30 min to 60 min q12 hr; given for 5-14 days depending on infection

Hepatic dose (Child-Pugh C)
Adult: **IV** 100 mg, then 25 mg q12h

Available forms: Powder for inj, lyophilized 50 mg

Adverse effects

CNS: Headache, dizziness, insomnia
CV: Hyper/hypotension, phlebitis
GI: *Nausea, vomiting, diarrhea,* anorexia, constipation, dyspepsia
HEMA: **Anemia, leukocytosis, thrombocytopenia**
INTEG: *Rash*, pruritus, sweating, photosensitivity
META: Increased ALT, AST, BUN, lactic acid, alkaline phosphatase, amylase, hyperglycemia, hypokalemia, hypoproteinemia, bilirubinemia
MISC: Back pain, fever, abnormal healing, abdominal pain, abscess, asthenia, infection, pain, peripheral edema, local reactions
RESP: Cough, dyspnea

Contraindications: Pregnancy **D**, hypersensitivity to tigecycline, children <18 yr, lactation

Precautions: Renal disease, hepatic disease, hypersensitivity to tetracyclines

Pharmacokinetics

Absorption	Unknown
Distribution	Unknown
Metabolism	Not extensively
Excretion	22% unchanged, urine; primarily biliarily excreted
Half-life	Terminal 42 hr

Pharmacodynamics

Unknown

Interactions

Individual drugs

Warfarin: increased effect of tigecycline

Drug classifications

Oral contraceptives: decreased effect of tigecycline

NURSING CONSIDERATIONS

Assessment

- Assess for pseudomembranous colitis
- Assess for signs of anemia: Hct, Hgb, fatigue
- Monitor blood studies: PT, CBC, AST, ALT, BUN creatinine
- Assess for allergic reactions: rash, itching, pruritus, angioedema
- Assess for nausea, vomiting, diarrhea; administer antiemetic, antacids as ordered
- Assess for overgrowth of infection: fever, malaise, redness, pain, swelling, drainage, perineal itching, diarrhea, changes in cough or sputum

Nursing diagnoses

- Infection, risk for (use)
- Knowledge, deficient (teaching)

Implementation

- Give after C&S obtained

IV route

- Reconstitute each vial with 5.3 ml of 0.9% NaCl, or D_5 (10 mg/ml); swirl to dissolve; immediately withdraw 5 ml of the reconstituted sol and add to a 100 ml **IV** bag for inf (1 mg/ml); may be yellow or orange, if not, sol should be discarded; do not give if particulate matter is present
- Store in tight, light-resistant container at room temperature

Patient/family education

- Teach patient to avoid sun exposure; sunscreen does not seem to decrease photosensitivity
- Teach patient to avoid pregnancy while taking this product; fetal harm may occur

Evaluation

Positive therapeutic outcome

- Decreased temp, absence of lesions, negative C&S

tipranavir (Rx)

(ti-pran'a-veer)

Aptivus

Func. class.: Antiretroviral
Chem. class.: Protease inhibitor

Pregnancy category C

Action: Inhibits human immunodeficiency virus (HIV) protease; this prevents the maturation of virus

Therapeutic Outcome: Prevent worsening of HIV

Uses: HIV in combination with other antiretrovirals

Dosage and routes

Reduce dose in mild or moderate hepatic impairment and ketoconazole coadministration

Adult: PO 500 mg coadministered with ritonavir 200 mg bid with food

Available forms: Caps 250 mg

Adverse effects

CNS: *Headache, insomnia,* dizziness, somnolence, fatigue
GI: *Diarrhea, abdominal pain, nausea,*

vomiting, anorexia, dry mouth, **hepatitis B or C, fatalities when given with ritonavir**
GU: Nephrolithiasis
INTEG: Rash
MS: Pain
OTHER: Asthenia, **insulin-resistant hyperglycemia,** hyperlipidemia, **ketoacidosis**

Contraindications: Hypersensitivity, hepatic disease (Child-Pugh B to C)

Precautions: Pregnancy **C,** lactation, children, renal disease, history of renal stones, sulfa allergy, hemophilia, diabetes mellitus

Pharmacokinetics

Absorption	Unknown
Distribution	Protein binding, 99.9%, steady state 7-10 days
Metabolism	CYP3A4
Excretion	80% feces
Half-life	Terminal 6 hr

Pharmacodynamics

Unknown

Interactions

Individual drugs

Clarithromycin, zidovudine: increased levels of both drugs
Delavirdine, itraconazole, ketoconazole: increased tipranavir levels
Efavirenz, fluconazole, nevirapine: decreased tipranavir levels
Lovastatin, simvastatin: increased myopathy
Midazolam, rifampin, triazolam: life-threatening dysrhythmias

Drug classifications

Ergots: life-threatening dysrhythmias
Oral contraceptives: increased levels of tipranavir
Rifamycins: decreased tipranavir levels

Drug/herb

St. John's wort: decreased tipranavir levels; avoid concurrent use

Drug/food

Grapefruit juice, high-fat, high-protein foods: decreased tipranavir absorption

NURSING CONSIDERATIONS

Assessment

- Monitor for complaints of lower back, flank pain; indicates kidney stones
- Assess for signs of infection, anemia, the presence of other sexually transmitted diseases
- Assess for hepatic studies: ALT, AST; total bilirubin, amylase, all may be elevated
- Monitor viral load, CD4 during treatment
- Monitor bowel pattern before, during treatment; if severe abdominal pain with bleeding occurs, drug should be discontinued; monitor hydration
- Monitor skin eruptions; rash, urticaria, itching
- Assess for allergies before treatment, reaction of each medication; place allergies on chart

Nursing Diagnoses

- Infection, risk for (use, adverse reactions)
- Knowledge, deficient (teaching)

Implementation

- Swallow cap whole; do not break, crush, or chew
- Give after meals
- Give in equal intervals around the clock to maintain blood levels

Patient/family education

- Teach patient to take as prescribed; if dose is missed, take as soon as remembered up to 1 hr before next dose; do not double dose
- Teach patient that drug must be taken in equal intervals around the clock to maintain blood levels for duration of therapy
- ◆ That hyperglycemia may occur; watch for increased thirst, weight loss, hunger, dry, itchy skin; notify prescriber
- Teach patient to increase fluids to prevent kidney stones, if stone formation occurs, treatment may need to be interrupted
- Advise patient that drug dose not cure AIDS, only controls symptoms; not to donate blood

Evaluation

Positive therapeutic outcome

- Prevention of viral replication

Appendix B

Recent FDA Drug Approvals

GENERIC NAME	TRADE NAME	USE
conivaptan	Vaprisol	Euvolemic hyponatremia
lenalidomide	Revlimid	Transfusion-dependent anemia
lubiprostone	Amitiza	Chronic idiopathic constipation
nitisinone	Orfadin	Hereditary tyrosinemia type 1
ranolazine	Ranexa	Chronic angina
sunitinib	Sutent	GI treatment of stromal tumor, advanced renal carcinoma

Appendix C

High-Alert Drugs

The Institute for Safe Medication Practices (ISMP) recently compiled a list of the medications with the greatest potential for patient harm if they are used in error. These high-alert medications include drugs in the 19 classes listed below, as well as the specific drugs listed below. To help nurses identify these drugs, each specific drug monograph is clearly identified in this book. Although care should be taken in giving any medication, nurses are advised to exercise extra precautions when administering these high-risk drugs.

Class/Category of Medications

adrenergic agonists, **IV** (e.g., epINEPHrine)
adrenergic antagonists, **IV** (e.g., propranolol)
anesthetic agents, general, inhaled, and **IV** (e.g., propofol)
cardioplegic solutions
chemotherapeutic agents, parenteral and oral
dextrose, hypertonic, 20% or greater
dialysis solutions, peritoneal and hemodialysis
epidural or intrathecal medications
glycoprotein IIb/IIIa inhibitors (e.g., eptifibatide)
hypoglycemics, oral
inotropic medications, **IV** (e.g., digoxin, milrinone)
liposomal forms of drugs (e.g., liposomal amphotericin B)
moderate sedation agents, **IV** (e.g., midazolam)
moderate sedation agents, oral, for children (e.g., chloral hydrate)
narcotics/opiates, **IV**, and oral (including liquid concentrates, immediate- and sustained-release)
neuromuscular blocking agents (e.g., succinylcholine)
opioids, **IV** and oral (including liquid concentrates and immediate- and sustained-release)
radiocontrast agents, **IV**
thrombolytics/fibrinolytics, **IV** (e.g., tenecteplase)
total parenteral nutrition solutions

Individual Medications

abciximab
adenosine
aldesleukin
alteplase
amiodarone
anistreplase
antihemophilic factor VIII (AHF)
ardeparin
argatroban
arsenic trioxide
asparaginase
atropine
azacitidine
basiliximab
bevacizumab
bivalirudin
bleomycin
bretylium
busulfan
carboplatin
carmustine
celecoxib
cisplatin
coagulation factor VIIa, recombinant
cyclophosphamide
cytarabine
dacarbazine
daclizumab
dactinomycin
dalteparin
DAUNOrubicin
digoxin
diltiazem
DOPamine

DOXOrubicin
droperidol
enoxaparin
epHEDrine
epINEPHrine
epirubicin
eptifibatide
etoposide
factor IX complex (human)/factor IV
fentanyl
fluorouracil
gemtuzumab
heparin
hydromorphone
ibutilide
idarubicin
ifosfamide
inamrinone
insulin
irinotecan
ketamine
lepirudin
leuprolide
lidocaine, parenteral
magnesium sulfate
melphalan
meperidine
methadone
methotrexate
milrinone
mitomycin
mitoxantrone
mivacurium
morphine
nalbuphine
nesiritide
nitroprusside
oxycodone
oxymorphone
oxytocin
pancuronium
pegaspargase
pemetrexed
pentazocine
pentobarbital
pentostatin
phenobarbital
pipecuronium
plicamycin
poractant alfa
propofol
propoxyphene
remifentanil
secobarbital
streptokinase
succinylcholine
tenecteplase
thiopental
tinzaparin
tirofiban
topotecan
trastuzumab
tubocurarine
urokinase
vecuronium
vinBLAStine
vinCRIStine
vinorelbine
warfarin

1. Cohen MR, Kilo CM: High-alert medications: safeguarding against errors. In Cohen MR, editor: *Medication Errors,* Washington, D.C., 1999, American Pharmaceutical Association.
2. Joint Commission on Accreditation of Healthcare Organizations: High-alert medications and patient safety, *Sentinel Event Alert,* Nov, 1999, accessed on 2/1/06 at www.jcaho.org/about+us/news+letters/sentinel+event+alert/sea_11.htm [Accessed on 4/30/02].
3. ISMP's List of High-Alert Medications, accessed on 2/1/06 at http: //www.ismp.org/Tools/highalertmedications.pdf.

Appendix D

Ophthalmic, Nasal, Topical, and Otic Products

OPHTHALMIC PRODUCTS

α-ADRENERGIC BLOCKER

dapiprazole (Rx)
(da-pip′ra-zole)
Rev-Eyes

ANESTHETICS

proparacaine (Rx)
(proe-par′a-kane)
Alcaine, Diocaine ✤, Ophthaine, Ophthestic

tetracaine (Rx)
(tet′ra-kane)
Pontocaine, Tetracaine

ANTIHISTAMINES

azelastine (Rx)
(ay-zell′ah-steen)
Optivar

emedastine (Rx)
(ee-med′-a-steen)
Emadine

epinastine (Rx)
(ep-een-as′teen)
Elestat

ketotifen (Rx)
(kee-toh-tif′en)
Zaditor

olopatadine (Rx)
(oh-loh-pat′ah-deen)
Patanol

ANTIINFECTIVES

chloramphenicol (Rx)
(klor-am-fen′i-kole)
AK-Chlor, Chloramphenicol, Chloromycetin Ophthalmic, Chloroptic, Chloroptic S.O.P., Fenicol ✤, Isopto Fenical ✤, Pentamycin ✤

ciprofloxacin (Rx)
(sip-ro-floks′a-sin)
Ciloxan

erythromycin (Rx)
(er-ith-roe-mye′sin)
Erythromycin, Ilotycin

fomivirsen (Rx)
(foh-muh-vir′sun)
Vitravene

ganciclovir (Rx)
(gan-sye′kloe-vir)
Vitrasert

gatifloxacin (Rx)
(gat-ih-floks′ah-sin)
Zymar

gentamicin (Rx)
(jen-ta-mye′sin)
Garamycin Ophthalmic, Genoptic Ophthalmic, Genoptic S.O.P., Gentacidin, Gentamicin Ophthalmic, Gentak

idoxuridine-IDU (Rx)
(eye-dox-yoor′i-deen)
Herplex

levofloxacin (Rx)
(lee-voh-flock′sah-sin)
Quixin

moxifloxacin (Rx)
Vigamox

natamycin (Rx)
(nat-a-mye′sin)
Natacyn

norfloxacin (Rx)
(nor-floks′a-sin)
Chibroxin

ofloxacin (Rx)
(oh-floks′a-sin)
Ocuflox

polymyxin B (Rx)
(pol-ee-mix′in)
Polymyxin B Sulfate Sterile

silver nitrate 1% (Rx)

silver nitrate

sulfacetamide sodium (Rx)
(sul-fa-seet′a-mide)
AK-Sulf, Bleph-10, Bleph-10 S.O.P., Cetamide, Isopto Cetamide, Ocusulf-10, Sodium Sulamyd, Sodium Sulfacetamide, Storz sulf, Sulf-10, Sulster

sulfiSOXAZOLE diolamine (Rx)
(sul-fih-sox′ah-zohl)
Gantrisin

tobramycin (Rx)
(toe-bra-mye′sin)
AKTob, Defy, Tobrex

trifluridine (Rx)
(trye-floor′i-deen)
Viroptic

vidarabine (Rx)
(vye-dare′a-been)
Vira-A

β-ADRENERGIC BLOCKERS

betaxolol (Rx)
(beh-tax′oh-lole)
Betoptic, Betoptic S

carteolol (Rx)
(kar-tee′oh-lole)
Carteolol HCl, Ocupress

levobetaxolol (Rx)
(lee-voh-beh-tax′oh-lohl)
Betaxon

levobunolol (Rx)
(lee-voe-byoo′no-lole)
AK Beta, Betagen

metipranolol (Rx)
(met-ee-pran′oh-lole)
OptiPranolol

timolol (Rx)
(tym′-moe-lole)
Apo-Timop ♣, Betimol, Timoptic, Timoptic-XE

CARBONIC ANHYDRASE INHIBITORS

brinzolamide (Rx)
(brin-zoh′la-mide)
Azopt

dorzolamide (Rx)
(dor-zol′a-mide)
Trusopt

CHOLINERGICS (Direct-acting)

acetylcholine (Rx)
(ah-see-til-koe′leen)
Miochol-E

carbachol (Rx)
(kar′ba-kole)
Carbastat, Carboptic, Isopto Carbachol, Miostat

pilocarpine (Rx)
(pye-loe-kar′peen)
Adsorbocarpine, Akarpine, Isopto Carpine, Ocu-Carpine, Ocusert Pilo-20, Ocusert Pilo-40, Pilagan, Pilocar, pilocarpine, Pilopine HS, Piloptic-½, Piloptic-1, Piloptic-2, Piloptic-3, Piloptic-4, Piloptic-6, Pilostat, Pilopto-Carpine

CHOLINESTERASE INHIBITORS

demecarium (Rx)
(dem-e-kare′ee-um)
Humorsol

ecothiophate (Rx)
(ek-oh-thye′oh-fate)
Phospholine Iodide

CORTICOSTEROIDS

dexamethasone (Rx)
(dex-a-meth′a-sone)
AK-Dex, Decadron Phosphate, Dexamethasone Ophthalmic Suspension, Maxidex

fluorometholone (Rx)
(flure-oh-meth′oh-lone)
Flarex, Fluor-Op, FML, FML Forte, FML S.O.P.

loteprednol (Rx)
(loe-tee-pred-nole)
Alrex, Lotemax

medrysone (Rx)
(me′dri-sone)
HMS

prednisoLONE (Rx)
(pred-niss′oh-lone)
Econopred, Econopred Plus, AK-Pred, Inflamase Forte, Inflamase Mild, PredForte

rimexolone (Rx)
(ri-mex′a-lone)
Vexol

MYDRIATICS

atropine (Rx)
(a′troe-peen)
Atropine-1, Atropine Care, Atropine Sulfate Ophthalmic, Atropisol, Isopto Atropine

cyclopentolate (Rx)
(sye-kloe-pen′toe-late)
AK-Pentolate, Cyclogyl, Cyclopentolate HCl

homatropine (Rx)
(home-a′troe-peen)
Isopto Homatropine, Minims Homatropine ♣, Homatropine HBr

hydroxyamphetamine HBr (Rx)
(hy-drox-ee-am-fet'a-meen)
Paredrine

phenylephrine (OTC)
(fen-ill-ef'rin)
AK-Dilate, AK-Nefrin, Isopto Frin, Neo-Synephrine 2.5%, Neo-Synephrine 10%, phenylephrine HCl, 2.5% Mydfrin, Phenoptic, Relief, Prefrin

scopolamine (Rx)
(skoe-pol'a-meen)
Isopto Hyoscine

tropicamide (Rx)
(troe-pik'a-mide)
Mydriacyl, Opticyl, Tropicacyl, Tropicamide

NONSTEROIDAL ANTIINFLAMMATORIES

diclofenac (Rx)
(dye-kloe'fen-ak)
Voltaran

flurbiprofen (Rx)
(flure-bi'-pro-fen)
Ocufen

ketorolac (Rx)
(kee-toe'role-ak)
Acular

suprofen (Rx)
(soo-proe'fen)
Profenal

SYMPATHOMIMETICS

apraclonidine (Rx)
(a-pra-klon'i-deen)
Iopidine

brimonidine (Rx)
(brem-on'-i-dine)
Alphagan, Alphagan P

dipivefrin (Rx)
(dye-pi'vef-rin)
Propine, AKPro

epINEPHrine/epinephryl borate (Rx)
(ep-i-nef'rin)
Epifrin, Glaucon/Epinal, Eppy ♣

OPHTHALMIC DECONGESTANTS/ VASOCONSTRICTORS

levocabastine (Rx)
(lee-voh-cab'ah-steen)
Livostin

lodoxamide
(loe-dox'ah-mide)
Alomide

naphazoline (OTC, Rx)
(naf-az'oh-leen)
20/20 Eye Drops, AK-Con, Allergy Drops, Albalon, Allerest Eye Drops, Clear Eyes, Clear Eyes ACR, Comfort Eye Drops, Degest 2, Maximum Strength Allergy Drops, Nafazair, naphazoline HCl, Naphcon, Naphcon Forte, Opcon, Vasoclear, Vasocon Regular

oxymetazoline (Rx)
(ox-i-met-ah-zoh'leen)
OcuClear, Visine L.R.

tetrahydrozoline (OTC)
(tet-ra-hye-dro'zoe-leen)
Collyrium Fresh, Eyesine, Geneye, Geneye Extra, Mallazine Eye Drops, Murine Plus, Optigene 3, tetrahydrozoline HCl, Tetrasine, Tetrasine Extra, Visine Moisturizing

MISCELLANEOUS OPHTHALMICS

bimatoprost (Rx)
(by-mat'oh-praat bedtimet)
Lumigan

brinzolamide (Rx)
(brin-zole'aa-mide)
Azopt

dorzolamide (Rx)
(dor-zol'a-mid)
Trusopt

latanoprost (Rx)
(la-tan'oh-proest)
Xalatan

travoprost (Rx)
(trav'oh-prahst)
Travatan

unoprostone (Rx)
(yoo-noh-prahs'tohn)
Rescula

Pregnancy category:
Demecarium, isoflurophate X; apraclonidine, cyclopentolate, ecothipate, glucocorticoids, levobunalol, metipranolol, pilocarpine, proparacaine, suprofen, tetracaine C; dapiprazole, dipivefrin B

β-Adrenergic blockers
Action: Reduces production of aqueous humor by unknown mechanism

Uses: Ocular hypertension, chronic open-angle glaucoma

Anesthetics

Action: Decreases ion permeability by stabilizing neuronal membrane

Uses: Cataract extraction, tonometry, gonioscopy, removal of foreign objects, corneal suture removal, glaucoma surgery (ophthalmic); pruritus, sunburn, toothache, sore throat, cold sores, oral pain, rectal pain and irritation, control of gagging (topical)

Antiinfectives

Action: Inhibits folic acid synthesis by preventing PABA use, which is necessary for bacterial growth

Uses: Conjunctivitis, superficial eye infections, corneal ulcers, prophylaxis against infection after removal of foreign matter from the eye

Antiinflammatories

Action: Decreases inflammation, resulting in decreased pain, photophobia, hyperemia, cellular infiltration

Uses: Inflammation of eye, eyelids, conjunctiva, cornea; uveitis, iridocyclitis, allergic conditions, burns, foreign bodies, postoperatively in cataract

Carbonic anhydrase inhibitor

Action: Converted to epinephrine, which decreases aqueous production and increases outflow

Uses: Open-angle glaucoma, ocular hypertension

Direct-acting miotic

Action: Acts directly on cholinergic receptor sites; induces miosis, spasm of accommodation, fall in intraocular pressure, caused by stimulation of ciliary, pupillary sphincter muscles, which leads to pulling away of iris from filtration angle, resulting in increased outflow of aqueous humor

Uses: Primary glaucoma, early stages of wide-angle glaucoma (less useful in advanced stages), chronic open-angle glaucoma, acute narrow-angle glaucoma before emergency surgery; also neutralizes mydriatics used during eye exam; may be used alternately with mydriatics to break adhesions between iris and lens

Adverse effects

CNS: Headache
CV: Hypertension, tachycardia, dysrhythmias
EENT: Burning, stinging
GI: Bitter taste

Contraindications: Hypersensitivity

Precautions: Pregnancy, lactation, children, aphakia, hypersensitivity to carbonic anhydrase inhibitors, sulfonamides, thiazide diuretics, ocular inhibitors, hepatic and renal insufficiency

NURSING CONSIDERATIONS

Assessment

- Monitor ophthalmic exams and intraocular pressure readings
- Monitor blood counts; liver, renal function tests and serum electrolytes during long-term treatment

Nursing diagnoses

- Sensory perception, disturbed: visual (uses)
- Knowledge, deficient (teaching)

Implementation

- Storage at room temp away from light

Patient/family education

- Teach how to instill drops
- Advise patient that drug may cause burning, itching, blurring, dryness of eye area

Evaluation

Positive therapeutic outcome

- Absence of increased intraocular pressure

NASAL AGENTS

NASAL DECONGESTANTS

azelastine (Rx)
(ay-zell′ah-steen)
Astelin

desoxyephedrine (OTC)
(des-oxy-e-fed′rin)
Vicks Inhaler

epHEDrine (OTC)
(e-fed′rin)
Pretz-D

epINEPHrine (OTC)
(ep-i-neff′rin)
Adrenalin

naphazoline (OTC)
(naff-a-zoe′leen)
Privine

oxymetazoline (OTC)
(ox-i-met-az′oh-leen)
12 Hour Nasal, Afrin 12 Hour Original, Afrin 12-Hour Original Pump Mist, Afrin Severe Congestion With Menthol, Afrin Sinus With Vapornase, Afrin No-Drip 12-Hour, Afrin No-Drip 12-Hour Extra Moisturizing, Dristan, Duramist Plus, Duration, Genasal, Nafrine ✦, Neo-Synephrine 12 Hour, Nostrilla, oxymetazoline HCl, Nasal Relief, Nasal Decongestant, Maximum Strength, Vicks Sinex 12 Hour Long-Acting, Vicks Sinex 12-Hour Ultra Fine Mist for Sinus Relief

phenylephrine (OTC)
(fen-ill-eff′rin)
Alconefrin 12, Children's Nostril, Neo-Synephrine, Sinex

propylhexadrine (OTC)
(proe-pil-hex′a-dreen)
Benzedrex Inhaler

tetrahydrozoline (OTC)
(tet-ra-hye-dro′zoe-leen)
Tyzine, Tyzine Pediatric

xylometazoline (OTC)
(zye-loh-meh-tazz′oh-leen)
Natru-vent, Otrivin, Otrivin Pediatric Nasal

NASAL STEROIDS

beclomethasone (Rx)
(be-kloe-meth′a-sone)
Beconase AQ Nasal, Beconase Inhalation, Vancenase AQ Nasal, Vancenase Pocket Inhaler

budesonide (Rx)
(byoo-des′oh-nide)
Rhiocort, Rhinocort Aqua

flunisolide (Rx)
(floo-niss′oh-lide)
Nasalide, Nasarel

fluticasone (Rx)
(floo-tic′a-son)
Flonase

mometasone (Rx)
(mo-met′a-sone)
Nasonex

triamcinolone (Rx)
(trye-am-sin′oh-lone)
Nasacort AQ

Pregnancy category C

Action: Produces vasoconstriction (rapid, long acting) of arterioles, thereby decreasing fluid exudation, mucosal engorgement by stimulation of α-adrenergic receptors in vascular smooth muscle

Therapeutic Outcome: Absence of nasal congestion

Uses: Nasal congestion

Dosage and routes

Desoxyephedrine

Adult and child >6 yr: 1-2 INH in each nostril q2h or less

EpHEDrine

Adult: Fill dropper to the level marked, then use in each nostril q4h or less

EpINEPHrine

Adult and child >6 yr: Apply with swab, drops, spray prn

Naphazoline

Adult and child >6 yr: 1-2 drops/spray q6h or less

Oxymetazoline

Adult and child >6 yr: INSTILL 2-3 gtt or sprays to each nostril bid

Child 2-6 yr: INSTILL 2-3 gtt or sprays 0.025 sol bid, not to exceed 3 days

Phenylephrine

Adult and child >12 yr: 2-3 drops/spray (0.25-0.5) in each nostril: q3-4h or less; or 2-3 drops/spray (1%) in each nostril q4h or less

Child 6-12 yr: 2-3 drops/spray (0.25%) in each nostril q3-4h

Infant >6 mo: 1-2 drops (0.16%) in each nostril q3h

Propylhexadrine

Adult and child >6 yr: 1-2 INH in each nostril q2h or less

Tetrahydrozoline

Adult and child >6 yr: 2-4 drops (0.1%) q3-4h prn or 3-4 sprays in each nostril q4h prn

Child 2-6 yr: 2-3 drops (0.05%) in each nostril q4-6h prn

Xylometazoline

Adult and child >12 yr: 2-3 drops/spray (0.1%) in each nostril q8-10h

Child 2-12 yr: 2-3 drops (0.05%) in each nostril q8-10h

Available forms: Nasal sol 0.025%, 0.05%

Adverse effects

CNS: Anxiety, restlessness, tremors, weakness, insomnia, dizziness, fever, headache

EENT: Irritation, burning, sneezing, stinging, dryness, rebound congestion

GI: Nausea, vomiting, anorexia

INTEG: Contact dermatitis

Contraindications: Hypersensitivity to sympathomimetic amines

Precautions: Pregnancy **C,** children <6 yr, elderly, diabetes, cardiovascular disease, hypertension, hyperthyroidism, increased intracranial pressure, prostatic hypertrophy, glaucoma

NURSING CONSIDERATIONS

Assessment

- Assess for redness, swelling, pain in nasal passages before and during treatment
- Assess for syst absorption; hypertension, tachycardia; notify prescriber; syst absorption occurs at high doses or after prolonged use

Nursing diagnoses

- Airway clearance, ineffective (uses)
- Knowledge, deficient (teaching)
- Noncompliance (teaching)

Implementation

- Have patient tilt head back, squeeze bulb to create a vacuum, and draw correct amount of sol into dropper; insert 2 gtt of sol into nostril; repeat in other nostril
- Store in light-resistant container; do not expose to high temp or let sol come into contact with aluminum
- Give for <4 consecutive days
- Provide environmental humidification to decrease nasal congestion, dryness

Patient/family education

- Advise patient that stinging may occur for several applications; drying of mucosa may be decreased by environmental humidification
- Caution patient to notify prescriber if irregular pulse, insomnia, dizziness, or tremors occur
- Teach patient proper administration to avoid syst absorption
- Advise patient to rinse dropper with very hot water to prevent contamination

Evaluation

Positive therapeutic outcome

- Decreased nasal congestion

TOPICAL GLUCOCORTICOIDS

alclometasone (Rx)
(al-kloe-met'a-sone)
Adovate

amcinonide (Rx)
(am-sin'oh-nide)
Cyclocort

betamethasone (Rx)
(bay-ta-meth'a-sone)
Alphatrex, Beben ✤, Betacort ✤, Betatrex, Beta-Val, Bethovate ✤, Celestoderm ✤, Diprosone, Ectosonel ✤, Luxiq, Maxivate, Metaderm ✤, Psorion, Valisone

betamethasone (augmented) (Rx)
(bay-ta-meth'a-sone)
Diprolene, Diprolene AF

clobetasol (Rx)
(kloe-bay'ta-sol)
Cormax, Dermovate ✤, Embeline E 0.05%, Temovate

clocortolone (Rx)
(kloe-kore'toe-lone)
Cloderm

desonide (Rx)
(dess'oh-nide)
Desonide, Des Owen, Tridesilon

desoximetasone (Rx)
(dess-ox-i-met'a-sone)
Topicort, Topicort LP

dexamethasone (Rx)
(dex-a-meth'a-sone)
Aeroseb-Dex, Decaspray

diflorasone (Rx)
(dye-flor'a-sone)
Florone, Maxiflor, Psorcon

fluocinolone (Rx)
(floo-oh-sin'oh-lone)
Fluocin, Licon, Lidemol ✤, Lidex, Lyderm ✤, Topsyn ✤, Vasoderm

flurandrenolide (Rx)
(flure-an-dren'oh-lide)
Cordran, Cordran SP, Drenison 1/4 ✤, Drenison Tape ✤

fluticasone (Rx)
(floo-tik'a-sone)
Cutivate

halcinonide (Rx)
(hal-sin'oh-nide)
Halog, Halog-E

halobetasol (Rx)
(hal-oh-bay'ta-sol)
Ultravate

hydrocortisone (Rx)
(hye-droe-kor′ti-sone)
Actiocort, Aeroseb-HC, Ala-Cort, Allercort, Alphaderm, Anusol HC, Bactine, Barriere-HC ✤, CaldeCORT Anti-Itch, Carmol HC, Cetacort, Cortacet ✤, Cortaid, Cortate ✤, Cort-Dome, Cortef ✤, Corticaine, Corticreme ✤, Cortifair, Cortizone, Cortoderm ✤, Cortril, Delcort, Dermacort, DemiCort, Dermtex HC, Emo-Cort, Epifoam, FoilleCort, Gly-Cort, Gynecort, Hi-Cor, Hycort, Hyderm ✤, Hydro-Tex, Hytone, Lacti-Care-HC, Lanacort, Lemoderm, Locoid, My Cort, Novoehydrocort ✤, Nutracort Pharm, Pharmacort, Pentacort, Rederm, Rhulicort S-T Cort, Synacort, Sarna HC ✤, Texa-Cort, Unicort ✤, Westcort

methylPREDNISolone (Rx)
(meth-il-pred-niss′oh-lone)

mometasone (Rx)
(moe-met′a-sone)
Elocon

prednicarbate (Rx)
(pred-ni-kar′bate)
Dermatop

triamcinolone (Rx)
(trye-am-sin′oh-lone)
Aristocort, Delta-Tritex, Flutex, Kenac, Kenalog, Kenonel, Triaderm, Trianide ✤, Triderm, Trymex

Pregnancy category C

Action: Antipruritic, antiinflammatory

Therapeutic Outcome: Decreased itching, inflammation

Uses: Psoriasis, eczema, contact dermatitis, pruritus; usually reserved for severe dermatoses that have not responded to less potent formulation

Dosage and routes

Adult and child: Apply to affected area

Adverse effects

INTEG: *Acne, atrophy, epidermal thinning, purpura, striae*

Contraindications: Hypersensitivity, viral infections, fungal infections

Precautions: Pregnancy **C**

NURSING CONSIDERATIONS
Assessment

- Temp; if fever develops, drug should be discontinued
- For systemic absorption, increased temp, inflammation, irritation

Nursing diagnoses

- Pain, chronic (uses)
- Knowledge, deficient (teaching)
- Skin integrity, impaired (uses)

Implementation

- Apply only to affected areas; do not get in eyes
- Apply and leave site uncovered or lightly covered; occlusive dressing is not recommended—systemic absorption may occur
- Use only on dermatoses; do not use on weeping, denuded, or infected area
- Cleanse area before application of drug
- Continue treatment for a few days after area has cleared
- Store at room temp

Patient/family education

- Teach patient to avoid sunlight on affected area, burns may occur
- Teach patient to limit treatment to 14 days

Evaluation

Positive therapeutic outcome

- Absence of severe itching, patches on skin, flaking

TOPICAL ANTIFUNGALS

amphotericin B (OTC)
(am-foe-ter′i-sin)
Fungizone

butenafine (Rx)
(byoo-tin′a-feen)
Lotrimin Ultra, Mentex

ciclopirox (OTC)
(sye-kloe-peer′ox)
Loprox, Penlac Nail Lacquer

clioquinol (OTC)
(klye-oh-kwin′ole)
Vioforim

clotrimazole (OTC)
(kloe-trye′ma-zole)
Canestew ✤, Clotrimaderm ✤, Clotrimazole, Cruex, Desenex, Lotrimin AF, Myclo ✤, Neozol ✤

econazole (OTC)
(ee-kon′a-zole)
Spectazole

haloprogin (OTC)
(hal-oh-proe′jin)
Halotex

ketoconazole (OTC)
(kee-toe-kon'a-zole)
Nizoral
miconazole (OTC)
(mye-kon'a-zole)
Absorbine Antifungal Foot Powder, Breeze Mist Antifungal, Fungoid Tincture, Lotrimin AF, Maximum Strength Desenex Antifungal, Micatin, Monistat-Derm, Ony-Clear Tetterine, ZeaSob-AF
naftifine (OTC)
(naf f'ti-feen)
Naftin
nystatin (OTC)
(nye-stat'in)
Mycostatin, Nodostine ✦, Nilstat, Nyoderm ✦, Nystex
oxiconazole (OTC)
(ox-i-kon'a-zole)
Oxistat
selenium (OTC)
(see-leen'ee-um)
Exsel, Head and Shoulders Intensive Treatment, Selenium Sulfide, Selsun, Selsun Blue
sertaconazole (Rx)
(ser-tah-koe'na-zole)
Ertaczo
terbinafine (OTC)
(ter-bin'a-feen)
Lamisil
tolnaftate (OTC)
(tole-naf'tate)
Absorbine Athlete's Foot Cream, Aftate for Athlete's Foot, Aftate for Jock Itch, Genaspor, Quinsana Plus, Tinactin, Ting, tolnaftate
undecylenic acid (OTC)
(un-deh-sih-len'ik)
Blis-To-Sol, Breeze Mist, Caldesene, Cruex, Decylenes, Desenex, Desenex Maximum Strength, Pedi-Pro, Phicon F, Protectol

Pregnancy category B

Action: Interferes with fungal cell membrane permeability

Therapeutic Outcome: Absence of itching and white patches of the skin

Uses: Tinea cruris, tinea pedis, diaper rash, minor skin irritations; amphotericin B is used for *Candida* infections

Dosage and routes
Massage into affected area, surrounding area daily or bid, continue for 7-14 days, not to exceed 4 wk

Adverse effects
INTEG: Burning, stinging, dryness, itching, local irritation

Contraindications: Hypersensitivity

Precautions: Pregnancy **B,** lactation, children

Interactions: None known

NURSING CONSIDERATIONS
Assessment
- Assess skin for fungal infections; peeling, dryness, itching before and throughout treatment
- Assess for continuing infection; increased size, number of lesions

Nursing diagnoses
- Skin integrity, impaired (uses)
- Infection, risk for (uses)
- Knowledge, deficient (teaching)

Implementation
- Apply to affected area, surrounding area; do not cover with occlusive dressings
- Store below 30° C (86° F)

Teach patient/family
- Instruct to apply with glove to prevent further infection; not to cover with occlusive dressings
- Teach patient that long-term therapy may be needed to clear infection (2 wk-6 mo depending on organism); compliance is needed even after feeling better
- Teach patient proper hygiene; hand-washing technique, nail care, use of concomitant top agents if prescribed
- Caution patient to avoid use of OTC creams, ointments, lotions unless directed by prescriber
- Instruct patient to use medical asepsis (hand washing) before, after each application; to change socks and shoes once a day during treatment of tinea pedis
- Advise patient to report to health care prescriber if infection persists or recurs; if blisters, burning, oozing, swelling occur
- Caution patient to avoid alcohol because nausea, vomiting, hypertension may occur
- Caution patient to use sunscreen or avoid direct sunlight to prevent photosensitivity
- Advise patient to notify prescriber of sore throat, fever, skin rash, which may indicate overgrowth of organisms

Evaluation
Positive therapeutic outcome
- Decrease in size, number of lesions

TOPICAL ANTIINFECTIVES

azelaic acid (Rx)
(a-zuh-lay'ic)
Azelex, Finacea
bacitracin (OTC)
(bass-i-tray'sin)
Bacitin ✤, Bacitracin
clindamycin (Rx)
(klin-da-my'sin)
Cleocin T, Clindets, Clindagel, ClindaMax
erythromycin (OTC, Rx)
(er-ith-roe-mye'sin)
A/T/S, Akne-Mycin, Eryderm, Erygel, Erythromycin, Staticin, T-Statd
gentamicin (Rx)
(jen-ta-mye'sin)
Gentamicin
mafenide (Rx)
(ma'fe-nide)
Sulfamylon
metronidazole (Rx)
(met-roh-nye'da-zole)
MetroGel, MetroCream, MetroLotion, Noritate
mupirocin (Rx)
(myoo-peer'oh-sin)
Bactroban
neomycin (OTC)
(nee-oh-mye'sin)
Neomycin Sulfate
nitrofurazone (Rx)
(nye-troe-fyoor'a-zone)
Furacin, Nitrofurazone
silver sulfADIAZINE (Rx)
(sul-fa-dye'a-zeen)
Flamazine ✤, Silvadene, SSD, SSD AF, Thermazene
Pregnancy category C

Action: Interferes with bacterial protein synthesis

Therapeutic Outcome: Resolution of infection

Uses: Skin infections, minor burns, wounds, skin grafts, primary pyodermas, otitis externa

Adverse effects
INTEG: Rash, urticaria, scaling, redness

Contraindications: Hypersensitivity, large areas, burns, ulcerations

Precautions: Pregnancy **C,** lactation, impaired renal function, external ear or perforated eardrum

NURSING CONSIDERATIONS
Assessment
- Assess for allergic reaction: burning, stinging, swelling, redness
- Assess for signs of nephrotoxicity or ototoxicity

Nursing diagnoses
- Infection, risk for (uses)
- Skin integrity (uses)
- Knowledge, deficient (teaching)

Implementation
- Apply enough medication to cover lesions completely
- Apply after cleansing with soap, water before each application; dry well
- Apply to less than 20% of body surface area when patient has impaired renal function
- Store at room temp in dry place

Evaluation
Positive therapeutic outcome
- Decrease in size, number of lesions

TOPICAL ANTIVIRALS

acyclovir (Rx)
(ay-sye'kloe-ver)
Zovirax
penciclovir (Rx)
(pen-sye'kloe-ver)
Denavir
Pregnancy category C

Action: Interferes with viral DNA replication

Therapeutic Outcome: Resolution of infection

Uses: Simple mucocutaneous herpes simplex, in immunocompromised clients with initial herpes genitalis

Adverse effects
INTEG: Rash, urticaria, stinging, burning, pruritus, vulvitis

Contraindications: Hypersensitivity

Precautions: Pregnancy **C,** lactation

NURSING CONSIDERATIONS
Assessment
- Assess for allergic reaction: burning, stinging, swelling, redness, rash, vulvitis, pruritus

- Assess for signs of nephrotoxicity or ototoxicity

Nursing diagnoses
- Infection, risk for (uses)
- Skin integrity (uses)
- Knowledge, deficient (teaching)

Implementation
- Apply with finger cot or rubber glove to prevent further infection
- Apply enough medication to cover lesions completely
- Apply after cleansing with soap, water before each application; dry well
- Storage at room temp in dry place

Patient/family education
- Teach patient not to use in eyes or when there is no evidence of infection
- Advise patient to apply with glove to prevent further infection
- Advise patient to avoid use of OTC creams, ointments, lotions unless directed by prescriber
- Advise patient to use medical asepsis (hand washing) before, after each application and avoid contact with eyes
- Advise patient to adhere strictly to prescribed regimen to maximize successful treatment outcome
- Advise patient to begin taking drug when symptoms arise

Evaluation
Positive therapeutic outcome
- Decrease in size, number of lesions

TOPICAL ANESTHETICS

benzocaine (OTC)
(ben′zoe-kane)
Americaine Anesthetic, Anbesol Maximum Strength, Baby Anbesol, Biozene, Boil-Ease, Children's Chloraseptic, Dermoplast, Foille, Foille Plus, Hurricaine, Lanacaine, Medamint, Orabase, Oracin, Ora-Jel

dibucaine (OTC)
(dye′byoo-kane)
Dibucaine, Nupercainal

lidocaine (OTC, Rx)
(lye′doe-kane)
Anestacon, Burn-O-Jel, Dentipatch, Derma Flex, ELA-Max, Lidocaine HCl Topical, Lidocaine Viscous, Numby Staff, Solarcaine Aloe Extra Burn Relief, Xylocaine, Xylocaine 10% Oral, Xylocaine Viscous, Zilactin-L

pramoxine (OTC)
(pra-mox′een)
Itch-X, PrameGel, Prax, Tronothane

tetracaine (OTC, Rx)
(tet′ra-cane)
Pontocaine, Viractin

Pregnancy category C

Action: Inhibits conduction of nerve impulses from sensory nerves

Therapeutic Outcome: Decreasing inflammation, itching, pain

Uses: Oral irritation, sore throat, toothache, cold sore, canker sore, sunburn, minor cuts, insect bites, pain, itching

Dosage and routes
Adult and child: Top apply qid as needed; RECT insert tid and after each BM

Adverse effects
INTEG: Rash, irritation, sensitization

Contraindications: Hypersensitivity, infants <1 yr, application to large areas

Precautions: Pregnancy **C**, child <6 yr, sepsis, denuded skin

NURSING CONSIDERATIONS
Assessment
- Assess pain: location, duration, characteristics before and after administration
- Assess for infection: redness, drainage, inflammation; this drug should not be used until infection is treated

Implementation
- Store in tight, light-resistant container; do not freeze, puncture, or incinerate aerosol container

Patient/family education
- Teach patient to avoid contact with eyes
- Teach patient not to use for prolonged periods: use for <1 wk; if condition remains, prescriber should be contacted

Evaluation
Positive therapeutic outcome
- Decreased redness, swelling, pain

TOPICAL MISCELLANEOUS

docosanol (OTC)
(doh-koh'sah-nohl)
Abreva
pimecrolimus (Rx)
(pim-eh-kroh-ly'mus)
Elidel
Pregnancy category C

Action: Docosanol unknown; pimecrolimus may bind with macrophilin and inhibit calcium-dependent phosphatase

Therapeutic Outcome: Decreased redness, swelling, pain

Uses: Docosanol applied to fever blisters to promote more rapid healing; pimecrolimus used to treat mild to moderate atopic dermatitis in nonimmunocompromised patients ≥2 yr who are unresponsive to other treatment

Dosage and routes
Docosanol
Adult: TOP rub into blisters 5×/day until healing occurs

Pimecrolimus
Adult and child ≥2 yr: TOP apply thin layer 2×/day and rub in, use as long as needed

Adverse effects
Docosanol
None known

Pimecrolimus
INTEG: Burning

Contraindications: Hypersensitivity

Precautions: Pregnancy **C**, lactation, dermal infections

NURSING CONSIDERATIONS
Assessment
- Assess skin condition (color, pain, inflammation) before and after administration
- Assess for signs and symptoms of skin infections (redness, draining lesions); if present, avoid use of product (pimecrolimus)

Nursing diagnoses
- Skin integrity, impaired (uses)
- Infection, risk for (uses)
- Knowledge, deficient (teaching)

Implementation
- Apply to skin, rub in gently

Patient/family education
- Advise patient to avoid contact between medication and eyes
- Instruct patient to discontinue use of product when condition clears

Evaluation
Positive therapeutic outcome
- Decreased inflammation, redness

VAGINAL ANTIFUNGALS

butoconazole (OTC)
(byoo-toh-kone'ah-zole)
Femstat-3, Gynazol-1, Mycelex-3
clotrimazole (OTC)
(kloe-trye'ma-zole)
Canesten ✤, Clotriamazole, Gyne-Lotrimin 3, Gyne-Lotrimin 7, Mycelex 7, Myclo ✤
miconazole (OTC)
(mye-kon'a-zole)
Femizole-M, Monistat, Monistat 3, Monistat 7, Monistat Dual Pak, M-Zole 7 Dual Pack
nystatin (OTC)
(nye-stat'in)
Nystatin
terconazole (OTC)
(ter-kone'ah-zole)
Terazol 7, Tetrazol 3
tioconazole (OTC)
(tye-oh-kone'ah-zole)
Gyne-Trosyd ✤, Monistat 1, Vagistat-1
Pregnancy category:
Nystatin A;
clotrimazole B;
butoconazole, terconazole, tioconazole C

Action: Interferes with fungal DNA replication; binds sterols in fungal cell membranes, which increases permeability, leaking of nutrients

Therapeutic Outcome: Fungistatic/fungicidal against susceptible organisms: *Candida* only

Uses: Vaginal, vulval, vulvovaginal candidiasis (moniliasis)

Dosage and routes
Butoconazole
Adult: VAG 5 g (1 applicator) at bedtime × 3-6 days

Clotrimazole
Adult: 100 mg (1 vag tab, 100 mg) at bedtime × 1 wk, or 200 mg (2 vag tab, 100 mg) at bedtime × 3 nights, or 500 mg (1 vag tab, 500 mg); or 5 g (1 applicator) at bedtime × 1-2 wk

Miconazole
Adult: 200 mg supp at bedtime × 3 days or 100 mg supp × 1 wk

Nystatin
Adult: 100,000 units daily × 2 wk

Terconazole
Adult: VAG 5 g (1 applicator) at bedtime × 7 days

Tioconazole
Adult: 1 applicator at bedtime × 1 wk

Adverse effects
GU: Vulvovaginal burning, itching, pelvic cramps
INTEG: Rash, urticaria, stinging, burning
MISC: *Headache,* body pain

Contraindications: Hypersensitivity

Precautions: Children <2 yr, pregnancy, lactation

Interactions: None known

NURSING CONSIDERATIONS
Assessment
- Assess for allergic reaction: burning, stinging, itching, discharge, soreness

Nursing diagnoses
- Skin integrity, impaired (uses)
- Infection, risk for (uses)
- Knowledge, deficient (teaching)

Implementation
Topical route
- Administer one full applicator every night high into the vagina
- Store at room temp in dry place

Patient/family education
- Instruct patient in asepsis (hand washing) before, after each application
- Teach patient to apply with applicator only; to avoid use of any other vaginal product unless directed by prescriber; sanitary napkin may prevent soiling of undergarments
- Instruct patient to abstain from sexual intercourse until treatment is completed; reinfection and irritation may occur
- Advise patient to notify prescriber if symptoms persist

Evaluation
Positive therapeutic outcome
- Decrease in itching or white discharge (vaginal)

OTIC ANTIINFECTIVES

boric acid (OTC)
Auro-Dri, Dri/Ear, Ear Dry
chloramphenicol (Rx)
(klor-am-fen′i-kole)
Chloromycetin Otic
Pregnancy category C

Action: Inhibits protein synthesis in susceptible microorganisms

Uses: Ear infection (external), short-term use

Adverse effects
EENT: Itching, irritation in ear
INTEG: Rash, urticaria

Contraindications: Hypersensitivity, perforated eardrum

Precautions: Pregnancy **C**

NURSING CONSIDERATIONS
Assess:
- For redness, swelling, fever, pain in ear, which indicates superinfection

Administer:
- After removing impacted cerumen by irrigation
- After cleaning stopper with alcohol
- After restraining child if necessary
- After warming sol to body temp

Evaluation
Positive therapeutic outcome
- Decreased ear pain

Patient/family education
- The correct method of instillation using aseptic technique, including not touching dropper to ear
- That dizziness may occur after instillation

Appendix E

Combination Products

A-200 Shampoo:
0.33% pyrethrins
4% piperonyl butoxide
Uses: Scabicide, pediculicide
Accuretic 10/12.5:
quinapril 10 mg
hydrochlorthiazide 12.5 mg
Uses: Antihypertensive
Accuretic 20/12.5:
quinapril 20 mg
hydrochlorthiazide 12.5 mg
Uses: Antihypertensive
Accuretic 20/25:
quinapril 20 mg
hydrochlorthiazide 25 mg
Uses: Antihypertensive
Aceta w/Codeine:
acetaminophen 300 mg
codeine 30 mg
Uses: Opioid analgesic
Acid-X:
acetaminophen 500 mg
calcium carbonate 250 mg
Uses: Analgesic, antacid
Actagen C Cough Syrup:
Per 5 ml:
triprolidine 1.25 mg
pseudoephedrine 30 mg
codeine 10 mg
Uses: Antihistamine, adrenergic, antitussive
Actifed:
pseudoephedrine 60 mg
triprolidine 2.5 mg
Uses: Decongestant
Actifed Allergy, Daytime:
pseudoephedrine 30 mg
Uses: Adrenergic
Actifed Allergy, Nighttime:
pseudoephedrine 30 mg
diphenhydrAMINE 25 mg
Uses: Decongestant, antihistamine
Actifed with Codeine:
pseudoephedrine 30 mg
triprolidine 1.25 mg
codeine 10 mg
Uses: Adrenergic, antihistamine, antitussive
Actifed with Codeine Cough Syrup:
Per 3 ml:
pseudoephedrine 30 mg
triprolidine 1.25 mg
codeine 10 mg
Uses: Adrenergic, antihistamine, antitussive
Actifed Cold and Allergy:
pseudoephedrine 60 mg
triprolidine 2.5 mg
Uses: Adrenergic, antihistamine
Actifed Cold and Sinus:
chlorpheniramine 2 mg
pseudoephedrine 30 mg
acetaminophen 500 mg
Uses: antihistamine, adrenergic, analgesic
Actifed Plus:
pseudoephedrine 30 mg
triprolidine 1.25 mg
acetaminophen 500 mg
Uses: Decongestant, antihistamine
Actifed Plus ES Caplets:
pseudoephedrine 60 mg
triprolidine 2.5 mg
acetaminophen 500 mg
Uses: Adrenergic, antihistamine, analgesic
Actifed Sinus Daytime:
pseudoephedrine 30 mg
acetaminophen 500 mg
Uses: Decongestant
Actifed Sinus Nighttime:
pseudoephedrine 30 mg
diphenhydrAMINE 25 mg
acetaminophen 500 mg
Uses: Decongestant, antihistamine
Actifed Syrup:
Per 5 ml:
triprolidine 1.25 mg
pseudoephedrine 30 mg
Uses: Antihistamine, adrenergic
Activella Tablets:
estriol 1 mg
norethindrone 0.5 mg
Uses: Menopause
Adderall 5 mg:
dextroamphetamine sulfate 1.25 mg
dextroamphetamine saccharate 1.25 mg
amphetamine sulfate 1.25 mg
amphetamine aspartate 1.25 mg
Uses: CNS stimulant
Adderall 10 mg:
dextroamphetamine sulfate 5 mg
dextroamphetamine saccharate 2.5 mg
amphetamine sulfate 2.5 mg
amphetamine aspartate 2.5 mg
Uses: CNS stimulant
Adderall 20 mg:
dextroamphetamine sulfate 5 mg
dextroamphetamine saccharate 5 mg
amphetamine sulfate 5 mg
amphetamine aspartate 5 mg
Uses: CNS stimulant
Adderall 30 mg:
dextroamphetamine sulfate 7.5 mg
dextroamphetamine saccharate 7.5 mg
amphetamine sulfate 7.5 mg
amphetamine aspartate 7.5 mg

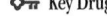

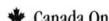

Uses: CNS stimulant
Adderall XR 10 mg:
dextroamphetamine sulfate 2.5 mg
dextroamphetamine saccharate 2.5 mg
amphetamine sulfate 2.5 mg
amphetamine aspartate 2.5 mg
Uses: CNS stimulant
Adderall XR 20 mg:
dextroamphetamine sulfate 5 mg
dextroamphetamine saccharate 5 mg
amphetamine sulfate 5 mg
amphetamine aspartate 5 mg
Uses: CNS stimulant
Adderall XR 30 mg:
dextroamphetamine sulfate 7.5 mg
dextroamphetamine saccharate 7.5 mg
amphetamine sulfate 7.5 mg
amphetamine aspartate 7.5 mg
Uses: CNS stimulant
Advair Diskus 100:
fluticasone 100 mcg
salmetrol 50 mcg
Uses: Corticosteroid, bronchodilator
Advair Diskus 250:
fluticasone 250 mcg
salmeterol 50 mcg
Uses: Corticosteroid, bronchodilator
Advair Diskus 500:
fluticasone 500 mcg
salmeterol 50 mcg
Uses: Corticosteroid, bronchodilator
Advicor 500:
niacin 500 mg
lovastatin 20 mg
Uses: Antilipidemic
Advicor 750:
niacin 750 mg
lovastatin 20 mg
Uses: Antilipidemic
Advicor 1000:
niacin 1000 mg
lovastatin 20 mg
Uses: Antilipidemic
Advil Cold & Sinus Caplets:
pseudoephedrine 30 mg
ibuprofen 200 mg
Uses: Decongestant
Aggrenox:
200 mg ext rel dipyridamole
25 mg aspirin
Uses: Antiplatelet
AK-Cide Ophthalmic Suspension/Ointment:
10% sulfacetamide sodium
0.5% prednisoLONE acetate
Uses: Ophthalmic antiinfective, antiinflammatory
Aldactazide 25/25:
spironolactone 25 mg
hydrochlorothiazide 25 mg
Uses: Diuretic
Aldactazide 50/50:
spironolactone 50 mg
hydrochlorothiazide 50 mg
Uses: Diuretic
Aldoclor-150:
methyldopa 250 mg
chlorothiazide 150 mg
Uses: Antihypertensive
Aldoclor-250:
methyldopa 250 mg
chlorothiazide 250 mg
Uses: Antihypertensive
Aldori 15:
methyldopa 250 mg
hydrochlorothiazide 15 mg
Uses: Antihypertensive
Aldoril 25:
methyldopa 250 mg
hydrochlorothiazide 25 mg
Uses: Antihypertensive
Aldoril D30
hydrochlorothiazide 30 mg
methyldopa 500 mg
Uses: Antihypertensive
Aldoril D50:
hydrochlorothiazide 50 mg
methyldopa 500 mg
Uses: Antihypertensive
Aleve Cold & Sinus:
naproxen 200 mg
ER pseudoephedrine 120 mg
Uses: Analgesic, adrenergic
Alka-Seltzer Cold:
sodium bicarbonate 958 mg
citric acid 832 mg
potassium bicarbonate 312 mg
Uses: Antacid, adsorbent
Alka-Seltzer Effervescent, Original:
sodium bicarbonate 1916 mg
citric acid 1000 mg
aspirin 325 mg
Uses: Antacid, adsorbent, antiflatulent
Alka-Seltzer Plus Cold & Cough Effervescent Tablets:
dextromethorphan 10 mg
chlorpheniramine 2 mg
phenylephrine 5 mg
Uses: Antitussive, antihistamine, decongestant
Alka-Seltzer Plus Cold & Flu Liqui-Gels:
dextromethorphan 10 mg
pseudoephedrine 30 mg
acetaminophen 325 mg
Uses: Antitussive, decongestant, analgesic
Alka-Seltzer Plus Cold Liqui-Gels:
pseudoephedrine 30 mg
chlorpheniramine 2 mg
acetaminophen 250 mg
Uses: Decongestant, antihistamine
Alka-Seltzer Plus Flu Liqui-Gels
dextromethorphan 10 mg
pseudoephedrine 30 mg
acetaminophen 325 mg
Uses: Antitussive, decongestant, analgesic
Alka-Seltzer Plus Night-Time Cold Effervescent Tablets:
dextromethorphan 10 mg
doxylamine 6.25 mg
phenylephrine 5 mg
Uses: Antitussive, antihistamine, decongestant

Alka-Seltzer Plus Night-Time Cold Liqui-Gels:
doxylamine 6.25 mg
dextromethorphan 10 mg
pseudoephedrine 30 mg
acetaminophen 325 mg
Uses: Antitussive, decongestant, antihistamine, analgesic
Allegra-D:
fexofenadine 60 mg
pseudoephedrine 120 mg
Uses: Antihistamine, adrenergic
Allercon Tablets:
triprolidine 2.5 mg
pseudoephedrine 60 mg
Uses: Antihistamine, adrenergic
Allerest Headache Strength Advanced Formula:
pseudoephedrine 30 mg
chlorpheniramine 2 mg
acetaminophen 325 mg
Uses: Decongestant, antihistamine
Allerest Maximum Strength Tablets:
pseudoephedrine 30 mg
chlorpheniramine 2 mg
Uses: Decongestant, antihistamine
Allerest No-Drowsiness:
pseudoephedrine 30 mg
acetaminophen 325 mg
Uses: Decongestant, analgesic
Allerest Sinus Pain Formula:
pseudoephedrine 30 mg
chlorpheniramine 2 mg
acetaminophen 500 mg
Uses: Decongestant, antihistamine, analgesic
Allerfrim Syrup:
Per 5 ml:
triprolidine 1.25 mg
pseudoephedrine 30 mg
Uses: Antihistamine, adrenergic
Allerfrim Tablets:
triprolidine 2.5 mg
pseudoephedrine 60 mg
Uses: Antihistamine, adrenergic
All-Nite Cold Formula Liquid:
Per 5 ml:
pseudoephedrine 10 mg
doxylamine 1.25 mg
dextromethorphan 5 mg
acetaminophen 167 mg
Uses: Decongestant, antihistamine, analgesic
Alor 5/500:
hydrocodone 5 mg
aspirin 500 mg
Uses: Analgesic
Amaphen:
acetaminophen 325 mg
butalbital 50 mg
caffeine 40 mg
Uses: Analgesic, barbiturates
Ambenyl Cough Syrup:
Per 5 ml:
bromodiphenhydramine 12.5 mg
codeine 10 mg
5% alcohol
Uses: Antihistamine, opioid analgesic
Anacin:
aspirin 400 mg
caffeine 32 mg
Uses: Analgesic
Anacin Maximum Strength:
aspirin 500 mg
caffeine 32 mg
Uses: Analgesic
Anacin PM (Aspirin Free):
diphenhydrAMINE 25 mg
acetaminophen 500 mg
Uses: Analgesic
Anacin w/Codeine:
aspirin 325 mg
codeine 8 mg
caffeine 32 mg
Uses: Opioid analgesic
Anaplex HD Syrup:
Per 5 ml:
hydrocodone 1.7 mg
phenylephrine 5 mg
chlorpheniramine 2 mg
Uses: Analgesic, adrenergic, antihistamine
Anaplex Liquid:
Per 5 ml:
chlorpheniramine 2 mg
pseudoephedrine 30 mg
Uses: Antihistamine, decongestant
Anatuss LA:
pseudoephedrine 120 mg
guaifenesin 400 mg
Uses: Adrenergic, expectorant
Anexsia 5/500:
hydrocodone 5 mg
acetaminophen 500 mg
Uses: Analgesic
Anexsia 7.5/650:
hydrocodone 7.5 mg
acetaminophen 650 mg
Uses: Analgesic
Apresazide 25/25:
hydrALAZINE 25 mg
hydrochlorothiazide 25 mg
Uses: Antihypertensive
Apresazide 50/50:
hydrALAZINE 50 mg
hydrochlorothiazide 50 mg
Uses: Antihypertensive
Apri:
desorgestrel 0.15 mg
ethinyl estradiol 30 mcg
Uses: Estrogen, progestin
Arthritis Pain Formula:
aspirin 500 mg
aluminum hydroxide 27 mg
magnesium hydroxide 100 mg
Uses: Analgesic, antacid
Arthrotec:
diclofenac 50 or 75 mg
misoprostol 200 mcg
Uses: NSAID, gastric protectant
Ascriptin:
aspirin 325 mg
magnesium hydroxide 50 mg

aluminum hydroxide 50 mg
calcium carbonate 50 mg
Uses: Nonopioid analgesic, antipyretic
Ascriptin A/D:
aspirin 325 mg
aluminum hydroxide 75 mg
magnesium hydroxide 75 mg
calcium carbonate 75 mg
Uses: Analgesic
Aspirin-Free Bayer Select Allergy Sinus:
pseudoephedrine 30 mg
chlorpheniramine 2 mg
acetaminophen 500 mg
Uses: Adrenergic, antihistamine, analgesic
Aspirin Free Excedrin:
acetaminophen 500 mg
caffeine 65 mg
Uses: Analgesic
Aspirin Free Excedrin Dual:
acetaminophen 500 mg
calcium carbonate 111 mg
magnesium carbonate 64 mg
magnesium oxide 30 mg
Uses: Analgesic, antacid
Atacand HCT 16:
candesartan 16 mg
hydrochlorthiazide 12.5 mg
Uses: Antihypertensive
Atacand HCT 32:
candesartan 32 mg
hydrochlorthiazide 12.5 mg
Uses: Antihypertensive
Augmentin 250:
amoxicillin 250 mg
clavulanic acid 125 mg
Uses: Antiinfective
Augmentin 500:
amoxicillin 500 mg
clavulanic acid 125 mg
Uses: Antiinfective
Augmentin 875:
amoxicillin 875 mg
clavulanic acid 125 mg
Uses: Antiinfective
Augmentin 125 Chewable:
amoxicillin 125 mg
clavulanic acid 31.25 mg
Uses: Antiinfective
Augmentin 200 Chewable:
amoxicillin 200 mg
clavulanic acid 28.5 mg
Uses: Antiinfective
Augmentin 250 Chewable:
amoxicillin 250 mg
clavulanic acid 62.5 mg
Uses: Antiinfective
Augmentin 400 Chewable:
amoxicillin 400 mg
clavulanic acid 57 mg
Uses: Antiinfective
Augmentin 125 mg/5 ml Suspension:
Per 5 ml:
amoxicillin 125 mg
clavulanic acid 31.25 mg
Uses: Antiinfective
Augmentin 200 mg/5 ml Suspension:
Per 5 ml:
amoxicillin 200 mg
clavulanic acid 28.5 mg
Uses: Antiinfective
Augmentin 250 mg/5 ml Suspension:
Per 5 ml:
amoxicillin 250 mg
clavulanic acid 62.5 mg
Uses: Antiinfective
Augmentin 400 mg/5 ml Suspension:
Per 5 ml:
amoxicillin 400 mg
clavulanic acid 57 mg
Uses: Antiinfective
Auralgan Otic Solution:
5.4% antipyrine
1.4% benzocaine
Uses: Otic analgesic
Avalide:
hydrochlorthiazide 12.5 mg
irbesartan 150 mg
Uses: Antihypertensive
Avalide 300:
hydrochlorthiazide 12.5 mg
irbesartan 300 mg
Uses: Antihypertensive
Avandamet:
rosiglitazone/metformin
1 mg/500 mg
2 mg/500 mg
2 mg/1000 mg
4 mg/500 mg
4 mg/1000 mg
Uses: Diabetes mellitus
Azo-Gantanol:
sulfamethoxazole 500 mg
phenazopyridine 100 mg
Uses: Sulfonamide
Azo-Gantrisin:
sulfiSOXAZOLE 500 mg
phenazopyridine 50 mg
Uses: Sulfonamide
Azo-Sulfamethoxazole:
sulfamethoxazole 500 mg
phenazopyridine 100 mg
Uses: Sulfonamide
Azo-SulfiSOXAZOLE:
sulfiSOXAZOLE 500 mg
phenazopyridine 50 mg
Uses: Sulfonamide
B&O Supprettes No. 15A Supps:
belladonna extract 15 mg
opium 30 mg
Uses: Anticholinergic, opioid analgesic
B&O Supprettes No. 16A Supps:
belladonna extract 16.2 mg
opium 60 mg
Uses: Anticholinergic, opioid analgesic
Bactrim:
trimethoprim 80 mg
sulfamethoxazole 400 mg
Uses: Antiinfective
Bactrim DS:
trimethoprim 160 mg

sulfamethoxazole 800 mg
Uses: Antiinfective
Bactrim I.V.:
Per 5 ml:
trimethoprim 80 mg
sulfamethoxazole 400 mg
Uses: Antiinfective
Bancap HC:
acetaminophen 500 mg
hydrocodone 5 mg
Uses: Analgesic
Bayer Plus, Extra Strength:
aspirin 500 mg
calcium carbonate 250 mg
Uses: Analgesic, antacid
Bayer Select Chest Cold:
dextromethorphan 15 mg
acetaminophen 500 mg
Uses: Antitussive, analgesic
Bayer Select Flu Relief:
acetaminophen 500 mg
pseudoephedrine 30 mg
dextromethorphan 15 mg
chlorpheniramine 2 mg
Uses: Analgesic, adrenergic, antitussive, antihistamine
Bayer Select Head Cold:
pseudoephedrine 30 mg
acetaminophen 500 mg
Uses: Adrenergic, analgesic
Bayer Select Maximum Strength Headache:
acetaminophen 500 mg
caffeine 65 mg
Uses: Nonopioid analgesic
Bayer Select Maximum Strength Menstrual:
acetaminophen 500 mg
pamabrom 25 mg
Uses: Nonopioid analgesic
Bayer Select Maximum Strength Night-Time Pain Relief:
acetaminophen 500 mg
diphenhydrAMINE 25 mg
Uses: Analgesic, antihistamine
Bayer Select Maximum Strength Sinus Pain Relief:
acetaminophen 500 mg
pseudoephedrine 30 mg
Uses: Analgesic, adrenergic
Bayer Select Night Time Cold:
acetaminophen 500 mg
pseudoephedrine 30 mg
dextromethorphan 15 mg
triprolidine 1.25 mg
Uses: Analgesic, adrenergic, antitussive, antihistamine
Bellatal:
phenobarbital 16.2 mg
hyoscyamine sulfate 0.1037 mg
atropine sulfate 0.0194 mg
scopolamine hydrobromide 0.0065 mg
Uses: Barbiturate, anticholinergic
Bellergal-S:
ergotamine 0.6 mg
belladonna alkaloids 0.2 mg
phenobarbital 40 mg
Uses: α-Adrenergic blocker, anticholinergic, barbiturate
Bel-Phen-Ergot-SR:
phenobarbital 40 mg
ergotamine tartrate 0.6 mg
belladonna alkaloids 0.2 mg
Uses: α-Adrenergic blocker, anticholinergic, barbiturate
Benadryl Allergy Decongestant Liquid:
Per 5 ml:
diphenhydrAMINE 12.5 mg
pseudoephedrine 30 mg
Uses: Antihistamine, adrenergic
Benadryl Allergy/Sinus Headache Caplets:
diphenhydrAMINE 12.5 mg
pseudoephedrine 30 mg
acetaminophen 500 mg
Uses: Antihistamine, adrenergic, analgesic
Benadryl Decongestant Allergy:
pseudoephedrine 60 mg
diphenhydrAMINE 25 mg
Uses: Adrenergic, antihistamine
Benylin Expectorant Liquid:
Per 5 ml:
dextromethorphan 5 mg
guaifenesin 100 mg
5% alcohol
Uses: Expectorant, antitussive
Benylin Multi-Symptom Liquid:
Per 5 ml:
dextromethorphan 5 mg
pseudoephedrine 15 mg
guaifenesin 100 mg
Uses: Antitussive, adrenergic, expectorant
Benzamycin:
benzoyl peroxide 5%
erythromycin 3%
Uses: Antiinfective
BenzaClin:
clindamycin 10%
benzoyl peroxide 5%
Uses: Antiinfective
BiDil:
isosorbide 20 mg
Hydralazine 37.5 mg
Uses: Vasodilator
Blephamide Ophthalmic Suspension/Ointment:
0.2% prednisoLONE
10% sodium sulfacetamide
Uses: Ophthalmic antiinfective, antiinflammatory
Bromfed Capsules:
pseudoephedrine 120 mg
brompheniramine 12 mg
Uses: Antihistamine, adrenergic
Bromfed-PD Capsules:
pseudoephedrine 60 mg
brompheniramine 6 mg
Uses: Adrenergic, antihistamine
Bromfed Tablets:
pseudoephedrine 60 mg
brompheniramine 4 mg
Uses: Antihistamine, adrenergic

Bromfenex:
brompheniramine 12 mg
pseudoephedrine 120 mg
Uses: Antihistamine, adrenergic
Bromfenex PD:
brompheniramine 6 mg
pseudoephedrine 60 mg
Uses: Antihistamine, adrenergic
Bromo-Seltzer:
sodium bicarbonate 2781 mg
acetaminophen 325 mg
citric acid 2224 mg
Uses: Antacid, analgesic
Bufferin:
aspirin 325 mg
calcium carbonate 158 mg
magnesium oxide 63 mg
magnesium carbonate 34 mg
Uses: Analgesic, antacid
Bufferin AF Nite-Time:
acetaminophen 500 mg
diphenhydrAMINE 38 mg
Uses: Analgesic, antihistamine
Butibel:
belladonna extract 15 mg
butabarbital 15 mg
Uses: Anticholinergic, barbiturate
Caduet:
amlodipine 5 mg
atorvastatin 10, 20, 40, 80 mg
amlodipine 10 mg
atorvastatin 10, 20, 40, 80 mg
Uses: Antihyperlipidemic/antihypertension
Cafatine PB:
ergotamine 1 mg
caffeine 100 mg
belladonna alkaloids 0.125 mg
pentobarbital 30 mg
Uses: Migraine agent
Cafergot:
ergotamine 1 mg
caffeine 100 mg
Uses: Adrenergic blocker
Cafergot Suppositories:
ergotamine 2 mg
caffeine 100 mg
Uses: Adrenergic blocker
Caladryl:
8% calamine, camphor
2.2% alcohol
1% pramoxine
Uses: Top antihistamine
Calcet:
calcium 152.8 mg
vitamin D 100 international units
Uses: Supplement
Caltrate 600+D:
vitamin D 200 international units
calcium 600 mg
Uses: Supplement
Cama Arthritis Pain Reliever:
aspirin 500 mg
magnesium oxide 150 mg
aluminum hydroxide 125 mg
Uses: Nonopioid analgesic, antacid
Capital w/Codeine:
Per 5 ml:
acetaminophen 120 mg
codeine 12 mg
Uses: Opioid analgesic
Capozide 25/15:
captopril 25 mg
hydrochlorothiazide 15 mg
Uses: Antihypertensive
Capozide 25/25:
captopril 25 mg
hydrochorothiazide 25 mg
Uses: Antihypertensive
Capozide 50/15:
captopril 50 mg
hydrochlorothiazide 15 mg
Uses: Antihypertensive
Capozide 50/25:
captopril 50 mg
hydrochlorothiazide 25 mg
Uses: Antihypertensive
Cardec DM Syrup:
Per 5 ml:
pseudoephedrine 60 mg
carbinoxamine 4 mg
dextromethorphan 15 mg
Uses: Adrenergic, antitussive
Cenafed Plus Tablets:
triprolidine 2.5 mg
pseudoephedrine 60 mg
Uses: Antihistamine, adrenergic
Cetapred Ophthalmic Ointment:
0.25% prednisoLONE
10% sodium sulfacetamide
Uses: Ophthalmic antiinfective, antiinflammatory
Cheracol D Cough Formula Syrup:
dextromethorphan 10 mg
guaifenesin 100 mg
Uses: Antitussive, expectorant
Cheracol Syrup:
Per 5 ml:
codeine 10 mg
guaifenesin 100 mg
Uses: Analgesic, expectorant
Children's Cepacol Liquid:
Per 5 ml:
acetaminophen 160 mg
pseudoephedrine 15 mg
Uses: Analgesic, adrenergic
Chlor-Trimeton Allergy 4 Hour Decongestant:
pseudoephedrine 60 mg
chlorpheniramine 4 mg
Uses: Antihistamine, adrenergic
Chlor-Trimeton 12 Hour Relief Tablets:
pseudoephedrine 120 mg
chlorpheniramine 8 mg
Uses: Antihistamine, adrenergic
Chromagen:
ferrous fumarate 66 mg
vitamin B_{12} 10 mcg
vitamin C 250 mg
intrinsic factor 100 mg
Uses: Supplement

Cipro HC Otic:
Per 1 ml:
ciprofloxacin 2 mg
hydrocortisone 10 mg
Uses: Antiinfective/antiinflammatory
Claritin-D 12 Hour:
loratidine 5 mg
pseudoephedrine 120 mg
Uses: Antihistamine, adrenergic
Claritin-D 24-Hour:
loratidine 10 mg
pseudoephedrine 240 mg
Uses: Antihistamine, adrenergic
Clindex:
chlordiazepoxide 5 mg
clidinium 2.5 mg
Uses: Antianxiety, anticholinergic
Clomycin Ointment:
bacitracin 500 units
neomycin sulfate 3.5 g
polymyxin B sulfate 500 units
lidocaine 40 mg
Uses: Antiinfective, local anesthetic
Co-Apap:
pseudoephedrine 30 mg
chlorpheniramine 2 mg
dextromethorphan 15 mg
acetaminophen 325 mg
Uses: Adrenergic, antihistamine, antitussive, analgesic
Co-Gesic:
acetaminophen 500 mg
hydrocodone 5 mg
Uses: Analgesic
Codeprex:
Codeine:
Chlorpheniramine:
Uses: Cough, rhinitis
Codiclear DH Syrup:
Per 5 ml:
hydrocodone 5 mg
guaifenesin 100 mg
Uses: Analgesic, expectorant
Codimal:
pseudoephedrine 30 mg
chlorpheniramine 2 mg
acetaminophen 500 mg
Uses: Adrenergic, antihistamine, analgesic
Codimal DH Syrup:
Per 5 ml:
hydrocodone 1.66 mg
phenylephrine 5 mg
pyrilamine 8.33 mg
Uses: Analgesic, adrenergic
Codimal DM Syrup:
Per 5 ml:
phenylephrine 5 mg
pyrilamine 8.33 mg
dextromethorphan 10 mg
Uses: Adrenergic, antitussive
Codimal-LA:
chlorpheniramine 8 mg
pseudoephedrine 120 mg
Uses: Antihistamine, adrenergic
Codimal PH Syrup:
Per 5 ml:
codeine 10 mg
phenylephrine 5 mg
pyrilamine 8.33 mg
Uses: Analgesic, adrenergic
Col-Probenecid:
probenecid 500 mg
colchicine 0.5 mg
Uses: Antigout agent
ColBenemid:
probenecid 500 mg
colchicine 0.5 mg
Uses: Antigout agent
Coldrine:
pseudoephedrine 30 mg
acetaminophen 500 mg
Uses: Decongestant, nonopioid analgesic
Col-Probenecid:
probenecid 500 mg
colchicine 0.5 mg
Uses: Antigout
Coly-Mycin S Otic Suspension:
1% hydrocortisone
neomycin base 3.3 mg/ml
colistin 3 mg/ml
0.05% thonzonium bromide
Uses: Otic antiinfective
CombiPatch 0.05/0.14:
estradiol 0.05 mg/day
norethindrone 0.14 mg/day
Uses: Estrogen, progestin
CombiPatch 0.05/0.25:
estradiol 0.05 mg/day
norethindrone 0.25 mg/day
Uses: Estrogen, progestin
Combipres 0.1:
chlorthalidone 15 mg
clonidine 0.1 mg
Uses: Antihypertensive
Combipres 0.2:
chlorthalidone 15 mg
clonidine 0.2 mg
Uses: Antihypertensive
Combipres 0.3:
chlorthalidone 15 mg
clonidine 0.3 mg
Uses: Antihypertensive
Combisor:
mometasone 0.1%
salicylic acid 5%
Uses: Corticosteroid
Combivent:
ipratropium bromide 18 mcg
albuterol 103 mcg/actuation
Uses: Bronchodilator
Combivir:
lamivudine 150 mg
zidovudine 300 mg
Uses: Antiviral
Comtrex Allergy-Sinus:
chlorpheniramine 2 mg
acetaminophen 500 mg
pseudoephedrine 30 mg
Uses: Antihistamine, analgesic, decongestant

Comtrex Liquid:
Per 5 ml:
chlorpheniramine 0.67 mg
acetaminophen 108.3 mg
dextromethorphan 3.3 mg
pseudoephedrine 10 mg
Uses: Antihistamine, analgesic, antitussive, decongestant
Comtrex Maximum Strength
Caplets:
acetaminophen 500 mg
pseudoephedrine 30 mg
chlorpheniramine 2 mg
dextromethorphan 15 mg
Uses: Analgesic, decongestant, antihistamine, antitussive
Comtrex Maximum Strength Multi-Symptoms Cold, Flu Relief:
pseudoephedrine 30 mg
dextromethorphan 15 mg
chlorpheniramine 2 mg
acetaminophen 500 mg
Uses: Analgesic, decongestant, antihistamine, antitussive
Comtrex Maximum Strength Non-Drowsy Caplets:
acetaminophen 500 mg
pseudoephedrine 30 mg
dextromethorphan 15 mg
Uses: Analagesic, decongestant, antitussive
Congess SR:
guaifenesin 250 mg
pseudoephedrine 120 mg
Uses: Expectorant, decongestant
Congestac:
guaifenesin 400 mg
pseudoephedrine 60 mg
Uses: Expectorant, decongestant
Contac Cough & Chest Cold Liquid:
Per 5 ml:
pseudoephedrine 15 mg
dextromethorphan 5 mg
guaifenesin 50 mg
acetaminophen 125 mg
Uses: Decongestant, antitussive, expectorant, analgesic
Contac Cough & Sore Throat Liquid:
Per 5 ml:
dextromethorphan 5 mg
acetaminophen 125 mg
Uses: Antitussive, analgesic
Contac Day Allergy/Sinus:
pseudoephedrine 60 mg
acetaminophen 650 mg
Uses: Decongestant, analgesic
Contac Day Cold and Flu:
pseudoephedrine 60 mg
dextromethorphan 30 mg
acetaminophen 650 mg
Uses: Decongestant, antitussive, analgesic
Contac Night Allergy Sinus:
pseudoephedrine 60 mg
diphenhydrAMINE 50 mg
acetaminophen 650 mg
Uses: Decongestant, antihistamine, analgesic
Contac Night Cold and Flu Caplets:
pseudoephedrine 60 mg
diphenhydrAMINE 50 mg
acetaminophen 650 mg
Uses: Decongestant, antihistamine, antitussive, analgesic
Contac Non-Drowsy Maximum Strength 12 Hour:
pseudoephedrine 120 mg
Uses: Adrenergic
Contac Severe Cold & Flu Nighttime Liquid:
Per 5 ml:
pseudoephedrine 10 mg
chlorpheniramine 0.67 mg
dextromethorphan 5 mg
acetaminophen 167 mg
18.5% alcohol
Uses: Decongestant, antihistamine, antitussive, analgesic
Coricidin:
chlorpheniramine 2 mg
acetaminophen 325 mg
Uses: Antihistamine, analgesic
Coricidin D Tablets:
chlorpheniramine 2 mg
acetaminophen 325 mg
Uses: Antihistamine, analgesic
Coricidin D Cold, Flu & Sinus:
chlorpheniramine 2 mg
acetaminophen 325 mg
pseudoephedrine sulfate 30 mg
Uses: Antihistamine, analgesic, decongestant
Coricidin HBP Congestion & Cough Softgels Capsules:
dextromethorphan 10 mg
guaifenesin 200 mg
Uses: Antitussive, expectorant
Corcidin HBP Cough and Cold:
chlorpheniramine 4 mg
dextromethorphan 30 mg
Uses: Antihistamine, expectorant
Corcidin HBP Maximum Strength Flu:
acetaminophen 500 mg
chlorpheniramine 2 mg
dextromethorphan 15 mg
Uses: Analgesic, antihistamine, expectorant
Cortisporin Ophthalmic/Otic Suspension:
0.35% neomycin polymyxin B 10,000 units/ml
1% hydrocortisone
Uses: Ophthalmic antiinfective, antiinflammatory
Cortisporin Ophthalmic Ointment:
0.35% neomycin base
bacitracin 400 units
polymyxin B 10,000 units
1% hydrocortisone
Uses: Ophthalmic antiinfective
Cortisporin Topical Cream:
0.5% neomycin sulfate
polymyxin B 10,000 units
0.5% hydrocortisone
Uses: Topical antiinfective

Cortisporin Topical Ointment:
0.5% neomycin sulfate
bacitracin 400 units
polymyxin B 5000 units
1% hydrocortisone
Uses: Topical antiinfective
Corzide 40/5:
nadolol 40 mg
bendroflumethiazide 5 mg
Uses: Antihypertensive
Corzide 80/5:
nadolol 80 mg
bendroflumethiazide 5 mg
Uses: Antihypertensive
Cosopt:
dorzolamide 2%
timolol 0.5%
Uses: Antihypertensive
Cough-X:
dextromethorphan 5 mg
benzocaine 2 mg
Uses: Antitussive, local anesthetic
Creon:
lipase 8000 units
amylase 30,000 units
protease 13,000 units
pancreatin 300 mg
Uses: Digestive enzyme
Cyclomydril Ophthalmic Solution:
0.2% cyclopentolate
1% phenylephrine
Uses: Mydriatic
Dallergy Caplets:
chlorpheniramine 8 mg
phenylephrine 20 mg
methscopolamine 2.5 mg
Uses: Antihistamine, adrenergic
Dallergy Syrup:
Per 5 ml:
chlorpheniramine 2 mg
phenylephrine 10 mg
methscopolamine 0.625 mg
Uses: Antihistamine, adrenergic
Dallergy Tablets:
chlorpheniramine 4 mg
phenylephrine 10 mg
methscopolamine 1.25 mg
Uses: Antihistamine, adrenergic
Dallergy-D Syrup:
Per 5 ml:
phenylephrine 5 mg
chlorpheniramine 2 mg
Uses: Antihistamine, adrenergic
Damason-P:
hydrocodone 5 mg
aspirin 500 mg
Uses: Analgesic
Darvocet-N 100:
propoxyphene-N 100 mg
acetaminophen 650 mg
Uses: Analgesic
Darvon Compound-65:
propoxyphene 65 mg
aspirin 389 mg
caffeine 32.4 mg
Uses: Analgesic
♣Darvon-N Compound:
aspirin 375 mg
propoxyphene 100 mg
caffeine 30 mg
Uses: Analgesic
♣Darvon-N w/A.S.A.:
aspirin 325 mg
propoxyphene 100 mg
Uses: Analgesic
Deconamine:
pseudoephedrine 60 mg
chlorpheniramine 4 mg
Uses: Antihistamine, decongestant
Deconamine CX:
hydrocodone 5 mg
pseudoephedrine 30 mg
guaifenesin 300 mg
Uses: Analgesic, decongestant, expectorant
Deconamine SR:
pseudoephedrine 120 mg
chlorpheniramine 8 mg
Uses: Antihistamine, decongestant
Deconamine Syrup:
Per 5 ml:
pseudoephedrine 30 mg
chlorpheniramine 2 mg
Uses: Antihistamine, decongestant
Defen-LA:
pseudoephedrine 60 mg
guaifenesin 600 mg
Uses: Decongestant, expectorant
Demi-Regroton:
chlorthalidone 25 mg
reserpine 0.125 mg
Uses: Antihypertensive
Demulen 1/35:
ethinyl estradiol 35 mcg
ethynodiol diacetate 1 mg
Uses: Oral contraceptive
Demulen 1/50:
ethinyl estradiol 50 mcg
ethynodiol diacetate 1 mg
Uses: Oral contraceptive
Depo-Testadiol:
estradiol cypionate 2 mg
testosterone cypionate 50 mg
Uses: Menopause
Desogen:
ethinyl estradiol 30 mcg
desorgestrel 0.15 mg
Uses: Estrogen, progestin
Dexacidin Ophthalmic Ointment/Suspension:
Per ml:
0.1% dexamethasone
0.35% neomycin
polymyxin B 10,000 units/g
Uses: Ophthalmic, antiinfective/antiinflammatory
Dexasporin Ophthalmic Ointment:
Per gram:
0.1% dexamethasone
0.35% neomycin
polymyxin B 10,000 units

Uses: Ophthalmic, antiinfective/antiinflammatory
DHC Plus:
dihydrocodeine 16 mg
acetaminophen 356.4 mg
caffeine 30 mg
Uses: Analgesic
Dialose Plus:
docusate sodium 100 mg
yellow phenolphthalein 65 mg
Uses: Laxative
Di-Gel Advanced Formula:
magnesium hydroxide 128 mg
calcium carbonate 280 mg
simethicone 20 mg
Uses: Antacid, adsorbent, antiflatulent
Di-Gel Liquid:
Per 5 ml:
aluminum hydroxide 200 mg
magnesium hydroxide 200 mg
simethicone 20 mg
Uses: Antacid, adsorbent, antiflatulent
Dihistine DH Liquid:
Per 5 ml:
pseudoephedrine 30 mg
chlorpheniramine 2 mg
codeine 10 mg
Uses: Decongestant, antihistamine, analgesic
Dilaudid Cough Syrup:
Per 5 ml:
guaifenesin 100 mg
hydromorphone 1 mg
5% alcohol
Uses: Expectorant, analgesic
Dilor-G:
dyphylline 200 mg
guaifenesin 200 mg
Uses: Bronchodilator, expectorant
Dimetane Decongestant:
brompheniramine 4 mg
phenylephrine 10 mg
Uses: Antihistamine, adrenergic
Dimetane-DX Cough Syrup:
Per 5 ml:
brompheniramine 2 mg
pseudoephedrine 30 mg
dextromethorphan 10 mg
Uses: Antihistamine, decongestant, antitussive
Dimetapp DM Elixir:
Per 5 ml:
pseudoephedrine 5 mg
brompheniramine 2 mg
dextromethorphan 10 mg
Uses: Antihistamine, adrenergic, expectorant
Dimetapp Long Acting Cough Plus Cold Syrup:
dextromethorphan 7.5 mg
pseudoephedrine 15 mg
Uses: Antitussive, decongestant
Dimetapp Sinus:
pseudoephedrine 30 mg
ibuprofen 200 mg
Uses: Decongestant, analgesic
Diovan 80 HCT:
valsartan 80 mg
hydrochlorthiazide 12.5 mg
Uses: Antihypertensive
Diovan 160 HCT:
valsartan 160 mg
hydrochlorthiazide 12.5 mg
Uses: Antihypertensive
Diurigen w/Reserpine:
chlorothiazide 250 mg
reserpine 0.125 mg
Uses: Antihypertensive
Diutensin-R:
methylclothiazide 2.5 mg
reserpine 0.1 mg
Uses: Antihypertensive
Doan's PM Extra Strength:
magnesium salicylate 500 mg
diphenhydrAMINE 25 mg
Uses: Analgesic, antihistamine
Dolacet:
hydrocodone 5 mg
acetaminophen 500 mg
Uses: Analgesic
Donnatal:
phenobarbital 16.2 mg
hyoscyamine 0.1037 mg
atropine 0.0194 mg
scopolamine 0.0065 mg
Uses: Anticholinergic, barbiturate
Donnatal Elixir:
Per 5 ml:
phenobarbital 16.2 mg
hyoscyamine 0.1037 mg
atropine 0.0194 mg
scopolamine 0.0065 mg
23% alcohol
Uses: Anticholinergic, barbiturate
Donnatal Extentabs:
phenobarbital 48.6 mg
hyoscyamine 0.3111 mg
atropine 0.0582 mg
scopolamine 0.0195 mg
Uses: Anticholinergic, barbiturate
Donnazyme:
pancreatin 500 mg
lipase 1000 units
protease 12,500 units
amylase 12,500 units
Uses: Pancreatic enzymes
Dorcol Children's Cold Formula Liquid:
Per 5 ml:
pseudoephedrine 15 mg
chlorpheniramine 1 mg
Uses: Decongestant, antihistamine
Doxidan:
docusate calcium 60 mg
phenolphthalein 65 mg
Uses: Stool softener
Dristan Cold:
pseudoephedrine 30 mg
acetaminophen 500 mg
Uses: Decongestant, analgesic
Dristan Cold Maximum Strength Caplets:
pseudoephedrine 30 mg
brompheniramine 2 mg
acetaminophen 500 mg

Uses: Decongestant, antihistamine, analgesic
Dristan Cold Multi-Symptom Formula:
acetaminophen 325 mg
phenylephrine 5 mg
chlorpheniramine 2 mg
Uses: Analgesic, adrenergic, antihistamine
Dristan Sinus:
pseudoephedrine 30 mg
ibuprofen 200 mg
Uses: Decongestant, analgesic
Drixoral Allergy Sinus:
pseudoephedrine 60 mg
dexbrompheniramine 3 mg
acetaminophen 500 mg
Uses: Decongestant, antihistamine, analgesic
Drixoral Cold & Allergy:
pseudoephedrine 120 mg
dexbrompheniramine 6 mg
Uses: Decongestant, antihistamine
Drixoral Cold & Flu:
pseudoephedrine 60 mg
dexbrompheniramine 3 mg
acetaminophen 500 mg
Uses: Decongestant, antihistamine, analgesic
Drixoral Nasal Decongestant:
pseudoephedrine 120 mg
Uses: Decongestant
DT:
Per 5 ml dose:
diphtheria toxoid 2LfU
tetanus toxoid 5LfU
Uses: Vaccine
DTP:
Per 0.5 ml dose:
diphtheria toxoid 6.5LfU
tetanus toxoid 5LfU
pertussis 4LfU
Uses: Vaccine
DuoNeb:
Per 3 ml:
albuterol 3 mg
ipratropium 0.5 mg
Uses: Bronchodilator
Dura-Vent/DA:
phenylephrine 20 mg
chlorpheniramine 8 mg
methscopolamine 2.5 mg
Uses: Adrenergic, antihistamine
Dyazide:
hydrochlorothiazide 25 mg
triamterene 37.5 mg
Uses: Diuretic
Dylline-GG Tablets:
dyphylline 200 mg
guaifenesin 200 mg
Uses: Bronchodilator, expectorant
Dynafed Asthma Relief:
epHEDrine 25 mg
guaifenesin 200 mg
Uses: Adrenergic, expectorant
Dynafed Plus Maximum Strength:
pseudoephedrine 30 mg
acetaminophen 500 mg
Uses: Decongestant, analgesic
Dyphylline-GG Elixir:
Per 5 ml:
dyphylline 100 mg
guaifenesin 100 mg
Uses: Bronchodilator, expectorant
E-Lor:
acetaminophen 650 mg
propoxyphene 65 mg
Uses: Analgesic
E-Pilo-1 Ophthalmic Solution:
1% epINEPHrine
1% pilocarpine
Uses: Mydriatic, miotic
E-Pilo-2 Ophthalmic Solution:
1% epINEPHrine
2% pilocarpine
Uses: Mydriatic, miotic
E-Pilo-4 Ophthalmic Solution:
1% epINEPHrine
4% pilocarpine
Uses: Mydriatic, miotic
E-Pilo-6 Ophthalmic Solution:
1% epINEPHrine
6% pilocarpine
Uses: Mydriatic, miotic
Elase Ointment:
Per gram:
fibrinolysin 1 unit
desoxyribonuclease 666.6 units
Uses: Enzyme
Elixophyllin GG Liquid:
Per 5 ml:
theophylline 100 mg
guaifenesin 100 mg
Uses: Expectorant, bronchodilator
EMLA Cream:
lidocaine 2.5 mg
prilocaine 2.5 mg
Uses: Local anesthetic
Empirin w/Codeine #3:
aspirin 325 mg
codeine phosphate 30 mg
Uses: Analgesic
Empirin w/Codeine #4:
aspirin 325 mg
codeine phosphate 60 mg
Uses: Analgesic
✱Empracet-60:
acetaminophen 300 mg
codeine 60 mg
Uses: Analgesic
Endocet:
acetaminophen 325 mg
oxycodone 5 mg
Uses: Analgesic
✱Endodan:
aspirin 325 mg
oxycodone 5 mg
Uses: Analgesic
Enduronyl:
methyclothiazide 5 mg
deserpidine 0.25 mg
Uses: Antihypertensive

Enduronyl Forte:
methyclothiazide 5.0 mg
deserpidine 0.5 mg
Uses: Antihypertensive
Entex PSE:
pseudoephedrine 120 mg
guaifenesin 600 mg
Uses: Adrenergic, expectorant
Epifoam Aerosol Foam:
1% hydrocortisone
1% pramoxine
Uses: Topical corticosteroid
Epzicom:
abacavir 600 mg
lamivudine 300 mg
Uses: HIV infection
Equagesic:
meprobamate 200 mg
aspirin 325 mg
Uses: Antianxiety
Eryzole:
Per 5 ml:
erythromycin 200 mg
sulfisoxazole 600 mg
Uses: Macrolide antiinfective
Esgic-Plus:
butalbital 50 mg
acetaminophen 500 mg
caffeine 40 mg
Uses: Barbiturate, analgesic
Esimil:
guanethidine 10 mg
hydrochlorothiazide 25 mg
Uses: Antihypertensive
Estratest:
esterified estrogens 1.25 mg
methyltestosterone 2.5 mg
Uses: Menopause
Estratest HS:
esterified estrogens 1.25 mg
methyltestosterone 2.5 mg
Uses: Menopause
Etrafon:
perphenazine 2 mg
amitriptyline 25 mg
Uses: Antipsychotic, antidepressant
Etrafon 2-10:
perphenazine 2 mg
amitriptyline 10 mg
Uses: Antidepressant
Etrafon A:
perphenazine 4 mg
amitriptyline 10 mg
Uses: Antidepressant
Etrafon Forte:
perphenazine 4 mg
amitriptyline 25 mg
Uses: Antipsychotic, antidepressant
Excedrin Migraine:
aspirin 250 mg
acetaminophen 250 mg
caffeine 65 mg
Uses: Migraine agent
Excedrin P.M.:
acetaminophen 500 mg
diphenhydrAMINE citrate 38 mg
Uses: Analgesic, antihistamine
Excedrin P.M. Liquigels:
acetaminophen 500 mg
diphenhydrAMINE 25 mg
Uses: Analgesic, antihistamine
Excedrin Sinus Extra Strength:
pseudoephedrine 30 mg
acetaminophen 500 mg
Uses: Decongestant, analgesic
Fansidar:
sulfidoxine 500 mg
pyrimethamine 25 mg
Uses: Antimalarial
Fedahist:
pseudoephedrine 60 mg
chlorpheniramine 4 mg
Uses: Decongestant, antihistamine
Fedahist Expectorant Syrup:
Per 5 ml:
guaifenesin 200 mg
pseudoephedrine 20 mg
Uses: Expectorant, decongestant
Fedahist Gyrocaps:
pseudoephedrine 65 mg
chlorpheniramine 10 mg
Uses: Decongestant, antihistamine
Fedahist Timecaps:
pseudoephedrine 120 mg
chlorpheniramine 8 mg
Uses: Decongestant, antihistamine
Feen-A-Mint Pills:
docusate sodium 100 mg
phenolphthalein 65 mg
Uses: Laxative
Fem-1:
acetaminophen 500 mg
pamabrom 25 mg
Uses: Nonopioid analgesic
Fembrt 1/5:
norethindrone 1 mg
ethinyl estradiol 5 mcg
Uses: Menopause
Ferro-Sequels:
docusate sodium 100 mg
ferrous fumarate 150 mg
Uses: Laxative, hematinic
Fioricet:
acetaminophen 325 mg
caffeine 40 mg
butalbital 50 mg
Uses: Analgesic, barbiturate
Fioricet w/Codeine:
acetaminophen 325 mg
caffeine 40 mg
butalbital 50 mg
codeine 30 mg
Uses: Analgesic, barbiturate
Fiorinal:
aspirin 325 mg
caffeine 40 mg
butalbital 50 mg
Uses: Analgesic, barbiturate
Fiorinal w/Codeine:
aspirin 325 mg

caffeine 40 mg
butalbital 50 mg
codeine 30 mg
Uses: Analgesic, barbiturate
FML-S Ophthalmic Suspension:
0.1% flurometholone
10% sulfacetamide
Uses: Ophthalmic, antiinfective/antiinflammatory
Gas-Ban:
calcium carbonate 500 mg
simethicone 40 mg
Uses: Antiflatulent, antacid
Gas-Ban DS Liquid:
Per 5 ml:
aluminum hydroxide 400 mg
magnesium hydroxide 400 mg
simethicone 40 mg
Uses: Antiflatulent, antacid
Gaviscon:
magnesium trisilicate 20 mg
aluminum hydroxide 80 mg
Uses: Antacid, adsorbent, antiflatulent
Gaviscon Liquid:
Per 5 ml:
aluminum hydroxide 31.7 mg
magnesium carbonate 119.3 mg
Uses: Antacid, adsorbent, antiflatulent
Gelprin:
acetaminophen 125 mg
aspirin 240 mg
caffeine 32 mg
Uses: Analgesic
Gelusil:
aluminum hydroxide 200 mg
magnesium hydroxide 200 mg
simethicone 25 mg
Uses: Antacid, adsorbent, antiflatulent
Genac Tablets:
triprolidine 2.5 mg
pseudoephedrine 60 mg
Uses: Antihistamine
Genatuss DM Syrup:
Per 5 ml:
guaifenesin 100 mg
dextromethorphan 10 mg
Uses: Expectorant, antitussive
Glucovance 1.25:
glyBURIDE: 1.25 mg
metformin: 250 mg
Uses: Antidiabetic
Glucovance 2.50:
glyBURIDE: 2.5 mg
metformin: 500 mg
Uses: Antidiabetic
Glucovance 5:
glyBURIDE: 5 mg
metformin: 500 mg
Uses: Antidiabetic
Granulex Aerosol:
Per 0.82 ml:
trypsin 0.1 mg
balsam peru 72.5 mg
castor oil 650 mg
Uses: Top enzyme
Guaifenex PSE 60:
pseudoephedrine 60 mg
guaifenesin 600 mg
Uses: Decongestant, expectorant
Guaifenex PSE 120:
pseudoephedrine 120 mg
guaifenesin 600 mg
Uses: Decongestant, expectorant
Guaituss AC:
Per 5 ml:
codeine 10 mg
guafenesin 100 mg
Uses: Analgesic, expectorant
Haley's M-O Liquid:
Per 15 ml:
magnesium hydroxide 900 mg
mineral oil 3.75 ml
Uses: Laxative
Halotussin-DM Sugar Free Liquid:
Per 5 ml:
guaifenesin 100 mg
dextromethorphan 10 mg
Uses: Expectorant, antitussive
Helidac:
In a compliance package:
bismuth subsalicylate 262.4 mg tabs
metronidazole 250 mg tabs
tetracycline 500 mg caps
Uses: Antiinfective
Hemate P:
AHF/VWF 250 units/500 units, 500 units/1000 units, 1000 units/2000 units
Uses: Hemophilia, von Willebrand disease
Humalog Mix 50/50:
insulin lispro protamine 50%
insulin lispro (rDNA) 50%
Uses: Antidiabetic
Humalog Mix 75/25:
insulin lispro protamine 75%
insulin lispro (rDNA) 25%
Uses: Antidiabetic
Humibid DM Sprinkle Caps:
dextromethorphan 15 mg
guaifenesin 300 mg
Uses: Expectorant, antitussive
Humibid DM Tablets:
dextromethorphan 30 mg
guaifenesin 600 mg
Uses: Expectorant, antitussive
HycoClear Tuss:
Per 5 ml:
hydrocodone 5 mg
guaifenesin 100 mg
Uses: Analgesic, expectorant
Hycodan:
hydrocodone 5 mg
homatropine 1.5 mg
Uses: Analgesic, mydriatic
Hycodan Syrup:
Per 5 ml:
hydrocodone 5 mg
homatropine 1.5 mg
Uses: Analgesic, mydriatic
Hycomine Compound:
chlorpheniramine 2 mg

acetaminophen 250 mg
phenylephrine 10 mg
hydrocodone 5 mg
caffeine 30 mg
Uses: Antihistamine, analgesic, adrenergic

Hycotuss Expectorant Syrup:
Per 5 ml:
guaifenesin 100 mg
hydrocodone 5 mg
10% alcohol
Uses: Expectorant

Hydergine:
dihydroergocornine 0.167 mg
dihydroergocristine 0.167 mg
dihydroergocryptine 0.167 mg
Uses: Adrenergic blocker

Hydrocet:
hydrocodone 5 mg
acetaminophen 500 mg
Uses: Opioid analgesic

Hydrogesic:
hydrocodone 5 mg
acetaminophen 500 mg
Uses: Opioid analgesic

Hydropres-50:
hydrochlorothiazide 50 mg
reserpine 0.125 mg
Uses: Antihypertensive

Hydroserpine:
hydrochlorothiazide 25 mg
reserpine 0.125 mg
Uses: Antihypertensive

Hydroserpine:
hydrochlorothiazide 50 mg
reserpine 0.125 mg
Uses: Antihypertensive

Hyzaar:
losartan potassium 50 mg
hydrochlorothiazide 12.5 mg
potassium 4.24 mg
Uses: Antihypertensive

Imodium Advanced:
loperamide 2 mg
simethicone 125 mg
Uses: Antidiarrheal, antiflatulent

Inderide 40/25:
propranolol 40 mg
hydrochlorothiazide 25 mg
Uses: Antihypertensive

Inderide 80/25:
propranolol 80 mg
hydrochlorothiazide 25 mg
Uses: Antihypertensive

Inderide LA 80/50:
propranolol 80 mg
hydrochlorothiazide 50 mg
Uses: Antihypertensive

Inderide LA 120/50:
propranolol 120 mg
hydrochlorothiazide 50 mg
Uses: Antihypertensive

Inderide LA 160/50:
propranolol 160 mg
hydrochlorothiazide 50 mg
Uses: Antihypertensive

Innovar:
Per ml:
droperidol 2.5 mg
fentanyl 0.05 mg
Uses: Opioid analgesic, general anesthetic

Iofed:
brompheniramine 12 mg
pseudoephedrine 120 mg
Uses: Antihistamine, adrenergic

Iofed PD:
brompheniramine 6 mg
pseudoephedrine 60 mg
Uses: Antihistamine, adrenergic

Isopap:
isometheptene 65 mg
APAP 325 mg
dicloral-phenazone 100 mg
Uses: Migraine agent

Kaletra Capsules:
lopinavir 133.3 mg
ritonavir 33.3 mg
Uses: HIV

Kaletra Solution:
Per 1 ml:
lopinavir 80 mg
ritonavir 20 mg
Uses: HIV

Lactinex:
Mixed culture of:
Lactobacillus acidophilus and
Lactobacillus bulgaricus
Uses: Supplement

Lenoltec w/Codeine No. 1:
acetaminophen 650 mg
hydrocodone 10 mg
Uses: Analgesic

Levlite:
levonorgestrel 0.100 mg
ethinyl estradiol 20 mcg
Uses: Estrogen, progestin

Levsin PB Drops:
Per ml:
hyoscyamine 0.125 mg
phenobarbital 15 mg
5% alcohol
Uses: Anticholinergic, barbiturate

Levsin w/Phenobarbital:
hyoscyamine 0.125 mg
phenobarbital 15 mg
Uses: Anticholinergic, barbiturate

Lexxel 1:
enalapril 5 mg
felodipine 5 mg
Uses: Antihypertensive

Lexxel 2:
enalapril 5 mg
felodipine 2.5 mg
Uses: Antihypertensive

Librax:
chlordiazepoxide 5 mg
clidinium 2.5 mg
Uses: Antianxiety, anticholinergic

Lida-Mantel-HC-Cream:
0.5% hydrocortisone
3% lidocaine

Uses: Antiinflammatory, analgesic
Limbitrol DS 10-25:
chlordiazepoxide 10 mg
amitriptyline 25 mg
Uses: Antidepressant, antianxiety
Lobac:
salicylamide 200 mg
phenyltoloxamine 20 mg
acetaminophen 300 mg
Uses: Skeletal muscle relaxant, analgesic
Loestrin Fe 1/20:
norethindrone acetate 1 mg/tablet
ethinyl estradiol 20 mcg/tablet
with 7 tablets of ferrous fumarate 75 mg/ container
Uses: Oral contraceptive
Loestrin Fe 1.5/30:
norethindrone acetate 1.5 mg
ethinyl estradiol 30 mcg
Uses: Oral contraceptive
Lomotil:
diphenoxylate 2.5 mg
atropine 0.025 mg
Uses: Antidiarrheal, anticholinergic
Lomotil Liquid:
Per 5 ml:
diphenoxylate 2.5 mg
atropine 0.025 mg
Uses: Antidiarrheal, anticholinergic
Lo Ovral:
ethinyl estradiol 30 mcg
norgestrel 0.3 mg
Uses: Oral contraceptive
Lopressor HCT 50/25:
metoprolol 50 mg
hydrochlorothiazide 25 mg
Uses: Antihypertensive
Lopressor HCT 100/25:
metoprolol 100 mg
hydrochlorothiazide 25 mg
Uses: Antihypertensive
Lopressor HCT 100/50:
metoprolol 100 mg
hydrochlorothiazide 50 mg
Uses: Antihypertensive
Lorcet 10/650:
acetaminophen 650 mg
hydrocodone 10 mg
Uses: Analgesic
Lorcet-HD:
hydrocodone 10 mg
acetaminophen 300 mg
Uses: Analgesic
Lorcet Plus:
acetaminophen 650 mg
hydrocodone 7.5 mg
Uses: Analgesic
Lortab 2.5/500:
hydrocodone 2.5 mg
acetaminophen 500 mg
Uses: Analgesic
Lortab 5/500:
hydrocodone 5 mg
acetaminophen 500 mg
Uses: Analgesic
Lortab 7.5/500:
hydrocodone 7.5 mg
acetaminophen 500 mg
Uses: Analgesic
Lortab 10/500:
hydrocodone 10 mg
acetaminophen 500 mg
Uses: Analgesic
Lortab ASA:
aspirin 500 mg
hydrocodone 5 mg
Uses: Analgesic
Lortab Elixir:
Per 5 ml:
hydrocodone 2.5 mg
acetaminophen 167 mg
Uses: Analgesic
Losec 1-2-3A:
omeprazole 20 mg
clarithromycin 500 mg
amoxicillin 1 g
Uses: Antiinfective
Losec 1-2-3M:
omeprazole 20 mg
clarithromycin 250 mg
medtronidazole 500 mg
Uses: Antiinfective
Lotensin HCT 5/6.25:
benazepril 5 mg
hydrochlorothiazide 6.25 mg
Uses: Antihypertensive
Lotensin HCT 10/12.5:
benazepril 10 mg
hydrochlorothiazide 12.5 mg
Uses: Antihypertensive
Lotensin HCT 20/12.5:
benazepril 20 mg
hydrochlorothiazide 12.5 mg
Uses: Antihypertensive
Lotensin HCT 20/25:
benazepril 20 mg
hydrochlorothiazide 25 mg
Uses: Antihypertensive
Lotrel 2.5/10:
amlopidine 2.5 mg
benazepril 10 mg
Uses: Antihypertensive
Lotrel 5/10:
amlodipine 5 mg
benazepril 10 mg
Uses: Antihypertensive
Lotrel 5/20:
amlodipine 5 mg
benazepril 20 mg
Uses: Antihypertensive
Lotrisone Topical:
0.05% betamethasone
1% clotrimazole
Uses: Local antiinfective, antiinflammatory
Lufyllin-EPG Elixir:
Per 5 ml:
dyphylline 150 mg
epHEDrine 24 mg
guaifenesin 300 mg
phenobarbital 24 mg

Uses: Bronchodilator, expectorant

Lufyllin-GG:
dyphylline 200 mg
guaifenesin 200 mg
Uses: Bronchodilator, expectorant

Lunelle Monthly Contraceptive Injection:
25 mg medroxyprogesterone
5 mg estradiol/0.5 ml
Uses: Contraceptive

M-M-R-II:
measles
mumps
rubella
Uses: Vaccine, toxoid

Maalox:
aluminum hydroxide 200 mg
magnesium hydroxide 200 mg
Uses: Antacid, adsorbent, antiflatulent

Maalox Plus:
aluminum hydroxide 200 mg
magnesium hydroxide 200 mg
simethicone 25 mg
Uses: Antacid, adsorbent, antiflatulent

Maalox Plus Extra Strength Suspension:
Per 5 ml:
aluminum hydroxide 500 mg
magnesium hydroxide 450 mg
simethicone 40 mg
Uses: Antacid, adsorbent, antiflatulent

Maalox Suspension:
Per 5 ml:
aluminum hydroxide 225 mg
magnesium hydroxide 200 mg
Uses: Antacid, adsorbent, antiflatulent

Macrobid:
nitrofurantoin macrocrystals 25 mg
nitrofurantoin monohydrate 75 mg
Uses: Antiinfective

Magnaprin:
aspirin 325 mg
magnesium hydroxide 50 mg
aluminum hydroxide 50 mg
calcium carbonate 50 mg
Uses: Nonopioid analgesic

Magnaprin Arthritis Strength:
aspirin 325 mg
magnesium hydroxide 75 mg
aluminum hydroxide 75 mg
calcium carbonate 75 mg
Uses: Nonopioid analgesic

Malarone:
250 mg atovaquone
100 mg proguanil
Uses: Malaria

Malarone Pediatric:
62.5 mg atovaquone
25 mg proguanil
Uses: Malaria

Mapap Cold Formula:
acetaminophen 325 mg
chlorpheniramine 2 mg
pseudoephedrine 30 mg
dextromethorphan 15 mg
Uses: Bronchodilator, expectorant

Marax:
epHEDrine 25 mg
theophylline 130 mg
hydrOXYzine 10 mg
Uses: Bronchodilator, sedative/hypnotic

Maxitrol Ophthalmic Suspension/Ointment:
Per ml:
0.35% neomycin
0.1% dexamethasone
polymyxin B 10,000 units
Uses: Ophthalmic antiinfective, antiinflammatory

Maxzide:
hydrochlorothiazide 50 mg
triamterene 75 mg
Uses: Antihypertensive, diuretic

Maxzide-25 MG:
hydrochlorothiazide 25 mg
triamterene 37.5 mg
Uses: Diuretic

Medi-Flu Liquid:
Per 5 ml:
pseudoephedrine 10 mg
chlorpheniramine 0.67 mg
dextromethorphan 5 mg
acetaminophen 167 mg
18.5% alcohol
Uses: Decongestant, antihistamine, antitussive, analgesic

Medigesic:
acetaminophen 325 mg
caffeine 40 mg
butalbital 50 mg
Uses: Nonopioid analgesic

Mepergan Fortis:
meperidine 50 mg
promethazine 25 mg
Uses: Analgesic, antihistamine

Mepergan Injection:
meperidine 25 mg
promethazine 25 mg
Uses: Analgesic

Metaglip:
glipiZIDE/metformin 2.5 mg/250 mg, 2.5 mg/500 mg, 5 mg/500 mg
Uses: Diabetes mellitus

Metimyd Ophthalmic Suspension/Ointment:
0.5% prednisoLONE
10% sodium sulfacetamide
Uses: Ophthalmic antiinfective, antiinflammatory

Micardis HCT 40:
telmesartan 40 mg
hydrochlorthiazide 12.5 mg
Uses: Antihypertensive

Micardis HCT 80:
telmesartan 80 mg
hydrochlorthiazide 12.5 mg
Uses: Antihypertensive

Microgestin Fe 1/20:
norethindrone 1 mg
ethinyl estradiol 20 mcg
ferrous fumarate 75 mg in container
Uses: Estrogen, progestin

Microgestin Fe 1.5/30:
norethindrone 1.5 mg
ethinyl estradiol 30 mcg
ferrous fumarate 75 mg in container
Uses: Estrogen, progestin
Midol Maximum Strength Multi-Symptom Menstrual Gelcaps:
acetaminophen 500 mg
pyrilamine 15 mg
caffeine 60 mg
Uses: Analgesic
Midol PM:
acetaminophen 500 mg
diphenhydrAMINE 25 mg
Uses: Analgesic, antihistamine
Midol PMS Maximum Strength Caplets:
acetaminophen 500 mg
pyrilamine 15 mg
pamabrom 25 mg
Uses: Analgesic
Midol, Teen:
acetaminophen 400 mg
pamabrom 25 mg
Uses: Analgesic
Midrin:
isometheptene 65 mg
acetaminophen 325 mg
dichloralphenazone 100 mg
Uses: Analgesic
Minizide 1:
prazosin 1 mg
polythiazide 0.5 mg
Uses: Antihypertensive
Minizide 2:
prazosin 2 mg
polythiazide 0.5 mg
Uses: Antihypertensive
Minizide 5:
prazosin 5 mg
polythiazide 0.5 mg
Uses: Antihypertensive
Moduretic:
hydrochlorothiazide 50 mg
amiloride 5 mg
Uses: Diuretic
Monopril-HCT 10:
fosinopril 10 mg
hydrochlorthiazine 12.5 mg
Uses: Antihypertensive
Monopril-HCT 20:
fosinopril 20 mg
hydrochlorthiazine 12.5 mg
Uses: Antihypertensive
Motrin Children's Cold Suspension:
Per 5 ml:
ibuprofen 100 mg
pseudoephedrine 15 mg
Uses: Nonopioid analgesic, decongestant
Motrin IB Sinus:
pseudoephedrine 30 mg
ibuprofen 200 mg
Uses: Adrenergic, analgesic
Mucinex:
guaifenesin 600 mg or 1200 mg
Uses: Cough suppressant, expectorant
Mucinex D:
guaifenesin/pseudoephedrine 1200 mg/120 mg, 600 mg/60 mg
Uses: Expectorant, decongestant
Mucinex DM:
dextromethorphan 30 mg
guaifenesin 600 mg
Uses: Antitussive, expectorant
Murocoll-2 Ophthalmic Drops:
0.3% scopolamine
10% phenylephrine
Uses: Ophthalmic anticholinergic, mydriatic
Mycolog II Topical:
Per gram:
0.1% triamcinolone acetonide
nystatin 100,000 units
Uses: Local antiinfective, antiinflammatory
Mylanta:
aluminum hydroxide 200 mg
magnesium hydroxide 200 mg
simethicone 20 mg
Uses: Antacid, adsorbent, antiflatulent
Mylanta Double Strength Liquid:
Per 5 ml:
aluminum hydroxide 400 mg
magnesium hydroxide 400 mg
simethicone 40 mg
Uses: Antacid, adsorbent, antiflatulent
Mylanta Gelcaps:
calcium carbonate 311 mg
magnesium carbonate 232 mg
Uses: Antacid, adsorbent, antiflatulent
Naldecon Senior DX Liquid:
Per 5 ml:
dextromethorphan 10 mg
guaifenesin 200 mg
Uses: Expectorant, antitussive
Naphcon-A Ophthalmic Solution:
0.25% naphazoline
0.3% pheniramine
Uses: Ophthalmic vasoconstrictor
Nasatab LA:
guaifenesin 500 mg
pseudoephedrine 120 mg
Uses: Expectorant, decongestant
NeoDecadron Ophthalmic Ointment:
0.35% neomycin
0.05% dexamethasone
Uses: Ophthalmic antiinfective, antiinflammatory
NeoDecadron Ophthalmic Solution:
0.35% neomycin
0.1% dexamethasone
Uses: Ophthalmic antiinfective, antiinflammatory
Neosporin Cream:
Per gram:
polymyxin B 10,000 units
neomycin 3.5 mg
Uses: Top antiinfective
Neosporin G.U. Irrigant:
Per ml:
neomycin 40 mg
polymyxin B 200,000 units

Uses: Antiinfective
Neosporin Ointment:
Per gram:
polymyxin B 5000 units
bacitracin zinc 400 units
neomycin 3.5 mg
Uses: Top antiinfective
Neosporin Ophthalmic Solution:
Per ml:
neomycin 1.75 mg
polymyxin B 10,000 units
gramicidin 0.025 mg
Uses: Ophthalmic antiinfective
Neosporin Ophthalmic Ointment:
Per gram:
neomycin 3.5 mg
polymyxin B 10,000 units
bacitracin zinc 400 units
Uses: Ophthalmic antiinfective
Neosporin Plus Cream:
polymyxin B 10,000 units
neomycin 3.5 mg
lidocaine 40 mg
Uses: Top antiinfective
Niferex-150 Forte:
ferrous sulfate 150 mg
vitamin B_{12} 25 mcg
folic acid 1 mg
Uses: Supplement
Norco 5/325:
hydrocodone 5 mg
acetaminophen 325 mg
Uses: Analgesic, opioid, nonopioid
Norco:
hydrocodone 10 mg
acetaminophen 325 mg
Uses: Analgesic, opioid, nonopioid
Norgesic:
orphenadrine 25 mg
aspirin 385 mg
caffeine 30 mg
Uses: Skeletal muscle relaxant, analgesic
Norgesic Forte:
orphenadrine 50 mg
aspirin 770 mg
caffeine 60 mg
Uses: Skeletal muscle relaxant, analgesic
Novacet Lotion:
sodium sulfacetamine 10%
sulfur 5%
Uses: Acne agent
Novafed A:
pseudoephedrine 120 mg
chlorpheniramine 8 mg
Uses: Adrenergic, antihistamine
Novahistone Elixir:
Per 5 ml:
phenylephrine 5 mg
chlorpheniramine 2 mg
5% alcohol
Uses: Antihistamine
Novo-Gesic 🍁 C8:
acetaminophen 300 mg
codeine 8 mg
caffeine 15 mg
Uses: Analgesic
NuLytely:
PEG 3350/420 g
sodium bicarbonate 5.72 g
sodium chloride 11.2 g
potassium chloride 1.48 g
Uses: Laxative
NyQuil Hot Therapy:
Per packet:
acetaminophen 1000 mg
pseudoephedrine 60 mg
dextromethorphan 30 mg
doxylamine 12.5 mg
Uses: Analgesic, adrenergic, antitussive
NyQuil Nightime Cold/Flu Medicine Liquid:
Per 5 ml:
pseudoephedrine 10 mg
doxylamine 1.25 mg
dextromethorphan 5 mg
acetaminophen 167 mg
25% alcohol
Uses: Adrenergic, antitussive, analgesic
Octicair Otic Suspension:
1% hydrocortisone
neomycin 5 mg/ml
polymyxin B 10,000 units/ml
Uses: Otic antiinflammatory, antiinfective
Opcon-A Ophthalmic Solution:
0.027% naphazoline
0.315% pheniramine
Uses: Ophthalmic vasoconstrictor
Ornade Spansules:
phenylpropanolamine 75 mg
chlorpheniramine 12 mg
Uses: Antihistamine, decongestant
Ornex:
pseudoephedrine 30 mg
acetaminophen 500 mg
Uses: Adrenergic, analgesic
Ornex No Drowsiness Caplets:
acetaminophen 325 mg
pseudoephedrine 30 mg
Uses: Adrenergic, analgesic
Orphengesic:
orphenadrine 25 mg
aspirin 385 mg
caffeine 30 mg
Uses: Analgesic
Orphengesic Forte:
orphenadrine 50 mg
aspirin 770 mg
caffeine 60 mg
Uses: Analgesic
Ortho-cept:
ethinyl estradiol 30 mcg
desogestrel 0.15 mg
Uses: Oral contraceptive
Ortho-cyclen:
ethinyl estradiol 35 mcg
norgestimate 0.25 mg
Uses: Oral contraceptive
Ortho-Novum 7/7/7:
Phase I:
0.5 mg norethindrone
35 mcg ethinyl estradiol

Phase II:
0.75 mg norethindrone
35 mcg ethinyl estradiol
Phase III:
1 mg norethinidrone
35 mcg estradiol
Uses: Oral contraceptive
Ortho-Prefest:
estradiol 1 mg (15)
norgestimate 0.09 mg (15)
Uses: Menopause
Ovcon-50:
ethinyl estradiol 50 mcg
norethindrone 1 mg
Uses: Oral contraceptive
✤Oxycocet:
acetaminophen 325 mg
oxycodone 5 mg
Uses: Analgesic
P-A-C Analgesic:
aspirin 400 mg
caffeine 32 mg
Uses: Nonopioid analgesic
Pain-X Topical:
0.05% capsaicin
5% menthol
4% camphor
Uses: Top analgesic
Pamprin Maximum Pain Relief:
acetaminophen 250 mg
pamabrom 25 mg
magnesium salicylate 250 mg
Uses: Analgesic
Pamprin Multi-Symptom:
acetaminophen 500 mg
pamabrom 25 mg
pyrilamine 15 mg
Uses: Analgesic
Panacet 5/500:
hydrocodone 5 mg
acetaminophen 500 mg
Uses: Analgesic
Panasal 5/500:
hydrocodone 5 mg
aspirin 500 mg
Uses: Analgesic
Pancrease Capsules:
amylase 20,000 units
protease 25,000 units
lipase 4500 units (microspheres)
Uses: Digestive enzyme
Parcopa:
carbidopa/levodopa 10 mg/100 mg, 25 mg/100 mg/25 mg/250 mg
Uses: Parkinson's disease
Pedia Care Cold-Allergy Chewable:
pseudoephedrine 15 mg
chlorpheniramine 1 mg
Uses: Adrenergic, antihistamine
Pedia Care Cough-Cold Liquid:
Per 5 ml:
pseudoephedrine 15 mg
chlorpheniramine 1 mg
dextromethorphan 5 mg
Uses: Adrenergic, antihistamine, antitussive
Pedia Care NightRest Cough-Cold Liquid:
Per 5 ml:
pseudoephedrine 15 mg
chlorpheniramine 1 mg
dextromethorphan 7.5 mg
Uses: Adrenergic, antihistamine, antitussive
Pediacof Syrup:
Per 5 ml:
codeine 5 mg
phenylephrine 2.5 mg
chlorpheniramine 0.75 mg
potassium iodide 75 mg
5% alcohol
Uses: Opioid, narcotic analgesic, antihistamine
Pediazole Suspension:
Per 5 ml:
erythromycin 200 mg
sulfiSOXAZOLE 600 mg
Uses: Antiinfective
Pepcid Complete:
calcium carbonate 800 mg
magnesium hydroxide 165 mg
famotidine 10 mg
Uses: Antiulcer agent
Percocet 2.5/325:
oxycodone 2.5 mg
acetaminophen 325 mg
Uses: Analgesic
Percocet 5/325:
oxycodone 5 mg
acetaminophen 325 mg
Uses: Analgesic
Percocet 7.5/500:
oxycodone 7.5 mg
acetaminophen 500 mg
Uses: Analgesic
Percocet 10/650:
oxycodone 10 mg
acetaminophen 650 mg
Uses: Analgesic
Percodan:
oxycodone 4.88 mg
aspirin 325 mg
Uses: Analgesic
Percodan-Demi:
aspirin 325 mg
oxycodone HCl 2.25 mg
oxycodone terephthalate 0.19 mg
Uses: Analgesic
Percodan-Demi:
aspirin 325 mg
oxycodone 2.5 mg
Uses: Analgesic
Percogesic:
phenyltoloxamine 30 mg
acetaminophen 325 mg
Uses: Analgesic
Perdiem Granules:
Per teaspoon:
senna 0.74 g
psyllium 3.25 g
sodium 1.8 mg
potassium 35.5 mg
Uses: Laxative

Peri-Colace:
docusate sodium 100 mg
casanthranol 30 mg
Uses: Laxative
Peri-Colace Syrup:
Per 15 ml:
docusate sodium 60 mg
casanthranol 30 mg
Uses: Laxative
Phenaphen w/Codeine No. 3:
aspirin 325 mg
codeine 30 mg
Uses: Analgesic
Phenaphen w/Codeine No. 4:
aspirin 325 mg
codeine 60 mg
Uses: Analgesic
Phenerbel-S:
ergotamine tartrate 0.6 mg
belladonna alkaloids 0.2 mg
phenobarbital 40 mg
Uses: α-Adrenergic blocker, anticholinergic
Phenergan VC Syrup:
Per 5 ml:
phenylephrine 5 mg
promethazine 6.25 mg
Uses: Adrenergic, antihistamine
Phenergan VC w/Codeine Syrup:
Per 5 ml:
phenylephrine 5 mg
promethazine 6.25 mg
codeine 10 mg
Uses: Adrenergic, antihistamine, opioid analgesic
Phenergan w/Codeine Syrup:
Per 5 ml:
promethazine 6.25 mg
codeine 10 mg
Uses: Antihistamine, analgesic
Pherazine DM Syrup:
Per 5 ml:
dextromethorphan 15 mg
promethazine 6.25 mg
7% alcohol
Uses: Antitussive, antihistamine
Phillips' Laxative Gelcaps:
docusate sodium 83 mg
phenolphthalein 90 mg
Uses: Laxative
PMB-400:
conjugated estrogens 0.45 mg
meprobamate 400 mg
Uses: Oral contraceptive
Polaramine Expectorant Liquid:
Per 5 ml:
guaifenesin 100 mg
dexchlorpheniramine 2 mg
pseudoephedrine 20 mg
7.5% alcohol
Uses: Expectorant
Polycillin-PRB Oral Suspension:
Per single dose:
ampicillin 3.5 g
probenecid 1 g
Uses: Antiinfective
Polycitra Syrup:
Per 5 ml:
potassium citrate 550 mg
sodium citrate 500 mg
citric acid 334 mg
Uses: Laxative
Poly-Histine Elixir:
Per 5 ml:
pheniramine 4 mg
pyrilamine 4 mg
phenyltoloxamine 4 mg
4% alcohol
Uses: Antihistamine
Polysporin Ophthalmic Ointment:
Per gram:
polymyxin B 10,000 units
bacitracin zinc 500 units
Uses: Ophthalmic antiinfective
Polysporin Topical Ointment:
Per gram:
polymyxin B 10,000 units
bacitracin zinc 500 units
Uses: Top antiinfective
Polytrim Ophthalmic Solution:
Per ml:
trimethoprim 1 mg
polymyxin B 10,000 units
Uses: Ophthalmic antiinfective
Pravigard PAC:
aspirin 81 mg
pravastin 20, 40, 80 mg
aspirin 325 mg
pravastin 20, 40, 80 mg
Uses: Antihyperlipidemic, antithrombotic
Premphase:
In a compliance package:
conjugated estrogens 0.625 mg
medroxyPROGESTERone 5 mg
Uses: Menopause
Prempro:
In a compliance package:
conjugated estrogens 0.625 mg
medroxyPROGESTERone 2.5 mg
Uses: Menopause
Premsyn PMS:
acetaminophen 500 mg
pamabrom 25 mg
pyrilamine 15 mg
Uses: Analgesic
Prevpac:
In a compliance package:
amoxicillin 500 mg caps
clarithromycin 500 mg tabs
lansoprazole 30 mg caps
Uses: Antiinfective
Primatene:
theophylline 130 mg
epHEDrine 24 mg
phenobarbital 7.5 mg
Uses: Bronchodilator, barbiturate
Primaxin 250 mg IV for Injection:
imipenem 250 mg
cilastatin sodium 250 mg
Uses: Antiinfective

Primaxin 500 mg IV for Injection:
imipenem 500 mg
cilastatin sodium 500 mg
Uses: Antiinfective
Prinzide 10-12.5:
lisinopril 10 mg
hydrochlorothiazide 12.5 mg
Uses: Antihypertensive
Prinzide 20-12.5:
lisinopril 20 mg
hydrochlorothiazide 12.5 mg
Uses: Antihypertensive
Prinzide 20-25:
lisinopril 20 mg
hydrochlorothiazide 25 mg
Uses: Antihypertensive
Probampacin Oral Suspension:
Per single dose:
ampicillin 3.5 g
probenecid 1 g
Uses: Antiinfective
Proben-C:
colchicine 0.5 mg
probenecid 500 mg
Uses: Antigout agent
Proctofoam-HC Aerosol Foam:
1% hydrocortisone
1% pramoxine
Uses: Topical corticosteroid
Prometh w/Codeine Syrup:
codeine 10 mg
promethazine 6.25 mg/5 ml
Uses: Antitussive, antihistamine
Prometh VCW/Codeine Syrup:
codeine 10 mg
promethazine 6.25 mg
phenylephrine 5 mg/5 ml
Uses: Antitussive, antihistamine, decongestant
Propacet 100:
propoxyphene-N 100 mg
acetaminophen 650 mg
Uses: Analgesic
Pseudo-Chlor:
pseudoephedrine 120 mg
chlorpheniramine 8 mg
Uses: Antihistamine
Pseudo-Gest Plus:
pseudoephedrine 60 mg
chlorpheniramine 4 mg
Uses: Antihistamine
P-V-Tussin:
phenindamine 25 mg
guaifenesin 200 mg
hydrocodone 5 mg
Uses: Antihistamine, analgesic
P-V-Tussin Syrup:
Per 5 ml:
chlorpheniramine 2 mg
phenindamine 5 mg
phenylephrine 5 mg
pyrilamine 6 mg
Uses: Antihistamine, decongestant
Quadrinal:
epHEDrine 24 mg
theophylline 65 mg
potassium iodide 320 mg
phenobarbital 24 mg
Uses: Adrenergic, bronchodilator, barbiturate
Quelidrine Cough Syrup:
Per 5 ml:
dextromethorphan 10 mg
phenylephrine 5 mg
epHEDrine 5 mg
chlorpheniramine 2 mg
ammonium chloride 40 mg
ipecac 0.005 ml
Uses: Expectorant, adrenergic, antihistamine
Quibron-300:
theophylline 300 mg
guaifenesin 180 mg
Uses: Bronchodilator, expectorant
Quibron:
theophylline 150 mg
guaifenesin 90 mg
Uses: Bronchodilator, expectorant
Quinaretic:
quinapril/hydrochlorothiazide 10 mg/12.5 mg or 20 mg/12.5 mg
Uses: Hypertension
R&C Shampoo:
0.3% pyrethrins
3% piperonyl butoxide
Uses: Scabicide, pediculicide
Rauzide:
bendroflumethiazide 4 mg
powdered *Rauwolfia serpentina* 50 mg
Uses: Diuretic, antihypertensive
Rebetron:
interferon alfa-2b 3 million units/0.5 ml
ribavirin, PO 200 mg
Uses: Biologic response modifier, antiviral
Regroton:
chlorthalidone 50 mg
reserpine 0.25 mg
Uses: Diuretic, antihypertensive
Regulace:
docusate sodium 100 mg
casanthranol 30 mg
Uses: Laxative
Renese-R:
polythiazide 2 mg
reserpine 0.25 mg
Uses: Diuretic, antihypertensive
Repan:
acetaminophen 325 mg
caffeine 40 mg
butalbital 50 mg
Uses: Nonopioid analgesic
Respahist:
pseudoephedrine 60 mg
brompheniramine 6 mg
Uses: Adrenergic, antihistamine
Respaire-60:
guaifenesin 200 mg
pseudoephedrine 60 mg
Uses: Expectorant, adrenergic
RID Mousse:
pyrethrins 0.33%
piperonyl butoxide 4%
Uses: Scabicide, pediculicide

RID Shampoo:
0.3% pyrethrins
3% piperonyl butoxide
Uses: Scabicide, pediculicide
Rifamate:
isoniazid 150 mg
rifampin 300 mg
Uses: Antitubercular, antileprotic
Rifater:
rifampin 120 mg
isoniazid 50 mg
pyrazinamide 300 mg
Uses: Antitubercular
Rimactane/INH Dual Pack:
isoniazid 300 mg (30 tabs)
rifampin 300 mg (60 caps)
Uses: Antitubercular
Riopan Plus Suspension:
Per 5 ml:
magaldrate 540 mg
simethicone 40 mg
Uses: Antacid, adsorbent, antiflatulent
Robaxisal:
methocarbamol 400 mg
aspirin 325 mg
Uses: Skeletal muscle relaxant, analgesic
Robitussin Allergy & Cough Liquid:
dextromethorphan 10 mg
brompheniramine 2 mg
pseudoephedrine 30 mg
Uses: Antitussive, antihistamine, decongestant
Robitussin Cold & Cough Softgels:
pseudoephedrine 30 mg
guaifenesin 200 mg
dextromethorphan 10 mg
Uses: Antitussive, expectorant, decongestant
Robitussin Cold, Multi-Symptom Cold & Flu Tablets:
dextromethorphan 10 mg
guaifenesin 200 mg
pseudoephedrine 30 mg
acetaminophen 325 mg
Uses: Antitussive, expectorant, decongestant, analgesic
Robitussin Cough & Cold Infant Drops:
pseudoephedrine 6 mg/ml
dextromethorphan 2 mg/ml
guaifenesin 40 mg/ml
Uses: Decongestant, antitussive, expectorant
Robitussin Cough & Congestion Formula:
dextromethorphan 10 mg
guaifenesin 200 mg
Uses: Antitussive, expectorant
Robitussin-DM Infant Drops:
dextromethorphan 2 mg/ml
guaifenesin 40 mg/ml
Uses: Antitussive, expectorant
Robitussin-DM Liquid:
Per 5 ml:
guaifenesin 100 mg
dextromethorphan 10 mg
Uses: Expectorant, antitussive
Robitussin Flu Liquid:
dextromethorphan 5 mg
chlorpheniramine 1 mg
pseudoephedrine 15 mg
acetaminophen 160 mg
Uses: Antitussive, antihistamine, decongestant, analgesic
Robitussin Honey Cough & Cold Liquid:
dextromethorphan 10 mg
pseudoephedrine 15 mg
Uses: Antitussive, decongestant
Robitussin Honey Flu Multi-Symptom Liquid:
dextromethorphan 6.6 mg
pseudoephedrine 20 mg
acetaminophen 166.7
Uses: Antitussive, decongestant, analgesic
Robitussin Honey Flu Night-Time Syrup:
dextromethorphan 20 mg
chlorpheniramine 4 mg
pseudoephedrine 60 mg
acetaminophen 500 mg
Uses: Antitussive, antihistamine, decongestant, analgesic
Robitussin Honey Flu Non-Drowsy Syrup:
dextromethorphan 20 mg
pseudoephedrine 60 mg
acetaminophen 500 mg
Uses: Antitussive, decongestant, analgesic
Robitussin Maximum Strength Cough and Cold Syrup:
dextromethorphan 15 mg
pseudoephedrine 30 mg
Uses: Antitussive, adrenergic
Robitussin Night Relief Liquid:
dextromethorphan 5 mg
pyrilamine 8.3 mg
pseudoephedrine 10 mg
acetaminophen 108.3 mg
Uses: Antitussive, adrenergic
Robitussin Pediatric Cough & Cold Liquid:
Per 5 ml:
pseudoephedrine 15 mg
dextromethorphan 7.5 mg
Uses: Antitussive, adrenergic
Robitussin Pediatric Night Relief Cough & Cold Liquid:
pseudoephedrine 15 mg
chlorpheniramine 1 mg
dextromethorphan 7.5 mg
Uses: Decongestant, antihistamine, antitussive
Robitussin PM Cough & Cold Liquid:
dextromethorphan 7.5 mg
chlorpheniramine 1 mg
pseudoephedrine 15 mg
Uses: Antitussive, antihistamine, decongestant
Robitussin Sugar Free Cough Liquid:
dextromethorphan 10 mg
guaifenesin 100 mg
Uses: Antitussive, expectorant
Rolaids Calcium Rich:
magnesium hydroxide 80 mg
calcium carbonate 412 mg
Uses: Antacid, adsorbent, antiflatulent
Rondec:
pseudoephedrine 60 mg
carbinoxamine 4 mg
Uses: Adrenergic

Rondec DM Drops:
Per ml:
pseudoephedrine 25 mg
carbinoxamine 2 mg
dextromethorphan 4 mg
Uses: Adrenergic, antitussive
Rondec DM Syrup:
Per 5 ml:
pseudoephedrine 60 mg
carbinoxamine 4 mg
dextromethorphan 15 mg
Uses: Adrenergic, antitussive
Rondec Oral Drops:
Per 5 ml:
pseudoephedrine 25 mg
carbinoxamine 2 mg
Uses: Adrenergic
Roxicet:
Per 5 ml:
acetaminophen 325 mg
oxycodone 5 mg
Uses: Opioid analgesic
Roxicet 5/500:
oxycodone 5 mg
acetaminophen 500 mg
Uses: Opioid analgesic
Roxicet Oral Solution:
Per 5 ml:
acetaminophen 325 mg
oxycodone 5 mg
Uses: Analgesic
Roxiprin:
aspirin 325 mg
oxycodone HCl 4.5 mg
oxycodone terephthalate 0.38 mg
Uses: Analgesic
Ru-Tuss DE:
pseudoephedrine 120 mg
guaifenesin 600 mg
Uses: Adrenergic, expectorant
Ru-Tuss Expectorant Liquid:
Per 5 ml:
guaifenesin 100 mg
pseudoephedrine 30 mg
dextromethorphan 10 mg
10% alcohol
Uses: Adrenergic, expectorant, antitussive
Ru-Tuss with Hydrocodone Liquid:
Per 5 ml:
hydrocodone: 1.7 mg
phenylephrine 5 mg
pyrilamine 3.3 mg
pheniramine 3.3 mg
phenylpropanolamine 3.3 mg
5% alcohol
Uses: Antihistamine, analgesic, decongestant
Ryna-C Liquid:
Per 5 ml:
pseudoephedrine 30 mg
chlorpheniramine 2 mg
codeine 10 mg
Uses: Adrenergic, antihistamine, analgesic
Ryna Liquid:
Per 5 ml:
pseudoephedrine 30 mg
chlorpheniramine 2 mg
Uses: Adrenergic, antihistamine
Rynatan:
phenylephrine 25 mg
chlorpheniramine 8 mg
pyrilamine 25 mg
Uses: Adrenergic, antihistamine
Rynatan Pediatric Suspension:
Per 5 ml:
phenylephrine 5 mg
chlorpheniramine 2 mg
pyrilamine 12.5 mg
Uses: Adrenergic, antihistamine
Rynatuss:
epHEDrine 10 mg
carbetapentane 60 mg
chlorpheniramine 5 mg
phenylephrine 10 mg
Uses: Adrenergic, antihistamine
Saleto Tablets:
acetaminophen 115 mg
aspirin 210 mg
salicylamide 65 mg
caffeine 16 mg
Uses: Nonopioid analgesic
Salutensin:
hydroflumethiazide 50 mg
reserpine 0.125 mg
Uses: Antihypertensive
Salutensin Demi:
hydroflumethiazide 25 mg
reserpine 0.125 mg
Uses: Antihypertensive
Scot-Tussin DM Liquid:
Per 5 ml:
chlorpheniramine 2 mg
dextromethorphan 15 mg
Uses: Antihistamine, antitussive
Scot-Tussin Original 5-Action Liquid:
phenylephrine 4.2 mg
pheniramine 13.3 mg
sodium citrate 83.3 mg
sodium salicylate 83.3 mg
caffeine citrate 25 mg
Uses: Adrenergic, analgesic
Scot-Tussin Senior Clear Liquid:
Per 5 ml:
guaifenesin 200 mg
dextromethorphan 15 mg
Uses: Antitussive, expectorant
Sedapap-10:
acetaminophen 650 mg
butalbital 50 mg
Uses: Analgesic, barbiturate
Semprex-D:
acrivastine 8 mg
pseudoephedrine 60 mg
Uses: Adrenergic, bronchodilator
Senokot-S:
docusate 50 mg
senna concentrate 187 mg
Uses: Laxative
Septra:
sulfamethoxazole 400 mg

trimethroprim 80 mg
Uses: Antiinfective
Septra DS:
sulfamethoxazole 800 mg
trimethroprim 160 mg
Uses: Antiinfective
Septra I.V. for Injection:
Per 5 ml:
trimethoprim 80 mg
sulfamethoxazole 400 mg
Uses: Antiinfective
Septra Suspension:
Per 5 ml:
trimethoprim 40 mg
sulfamethoxazole 200 mg
Uses: Antiinfective
Ser-A-Gen:
hydrochlorothiazide 15 mg
hydrALAZINE 25 mg
reserpine 0.1 mg
Uses: Antihypertensive
Ser-Ap-Es:
hydrochlorothiazide 15 mg
reserpine 0.1 mg
hydrALAZINE 25 mg
Uses: Diuretic, antihypertensive
Silafed Syrup:
Per 5 ml:
pseudoephedrine 30 mg
triprolidine 1.25 mg
Uses: Adrenergic, antihistamine
Silaminic Cold Syrup:
Per 5 ml:
phenylpropanolamine 12.5 mg
chlorpheniramine 2 mg
Uses: Antihistamine, decongestant
Sinarest Extra Strength:
pseudoephedrine 30 mg
chlorpheniramine 2 mg
acetaminophen 500 mg
Uses: Adrenergic, antihistamine, analgesic
Sinarest No Drowsiness:
pseudoephedrine 30 mg
acetaminophen 500 mg
Uses: Adrenergic, analgesic
Sinarest Sinus:
pseudoephedrine 30 mg
chlorpheniramine 2 mg
acetaminophen 325 mg
Uses: Adrenergic, antihistamine, analgesic
Sine-Aid IB:
pseudoephedrine 30 mg
ibuprofen 200 mg
Uses: Adrenergic, analgesic
Sine-Aid Maximum Strength:
pseudoephedrine 30 mg
acetaminophen 500 mg
Uses: Adrenergic, analgesic
Sinemet 10/100:
carbidopa 10 mg
levodopa 100 mg
Uses: Antiparkinsonian
Sinemet 25/100:
carbidopa 25 mg
levodopa 100 mg
Uses: Antiparkinsonian
Sinemet 25/250:
carbidopa 25 mg
levodopa 250 mg
Uses: Antiparkinsonian
Sinemet CR 25-100:
carbidopa 25 mg
levodopa 100 mg
Uses: Antiparkinsonian
Sinemet CR 50-200:
carbidopa 50 mg
levodopa 200 mg
Uses: Antiparkinsonian
Sine-Off Maximum Strength No Drowsiness Formula Caplets:
pseudoephedrine 30 mg
acetaminophen 500 mg
Uses: Adrenergic, analgesic
Sine-Off Sinus Medicine:
pseudoephedrine 30 mg
chlorpheniramine 2 mg
acetaminophen 500 mg
Uses: Adrenergic, antihistamine, analgesic
Sinus-Relief:
acetaminophen 325 mg
pseudoephedrine 30 mg
Uses: Nonopioid analgesic
Sinutab:
acetaminophen 325 mg
chlorpheniramine 2 mg
pseudoephedrine 30 mg
Uses: Nonopioid analgesic
Sinutab Maximum Strength Sinus Allergy:
acetaminophen 500 mg
pseudoephedrine 30 mg
chlorpheniramine 2 mg
Uses: Analgesic, adrenergic, antihistamine
Sinutab Maximum Strength Without Drowsiness:
acetaminophen 500 mg
pseudoephedrine 30 mg
Uses: Analgesic, adrenergic
Sinutab Non-Drying:
pseudoepedrine 30 mg
guaifenesin 200 mg
Uses: Adrenergic, expectorant
Slo-Phyllin GG Syrup:
theophylline 150 mg
guaifenesin 90 mg
Uses: Bronchodilator, expectorant
Slow-Salt-K:
sodium chloride 410 mg
potassium chloride 15 mg
Uses: Potassium, sodium supplement
Solage:
mequinol 2%
tretinoin 0.01%
Uses: Antineoplastic
Soma Compound w/Codeine:
carisoprodol 200 mg
aspirin 325 mg
codeine 16 mg
Uses: Skeletal muscle relaxant

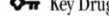

Soma Compound:
carisoprodol 200 mg
aspirin 325 mg
Uses: Skeletal muscle relaxant, analgesic
Spec-T Lozenge:
dextromethorphan 10 mg
benzocaine 10 mg
Uses: Antitussive, topical anesthetic
Stalevo 50:
carbidopa 12.5 mg
levodopa 50 mg
entacapone 200 mg
Uses: Parkinsonism
Stalevo 100:
carbidopa 25 mg
levodopa 100 mg
entacapone 200 mg
Uses: Parkinsonism
Stalevo 150:
carbidopa 37.5 mg
levodopa 150 mg
entacapone 200 mg
Uses: Parkinsonism
Sudafed Cold & Allergy:
pseudoephedrine 60 mg
chlorpheniramine 4 mg
Uses: Adrenergic, antihistamine
Sudafed Cold & Cough Liquicaps:
pseudoephedrine 30 mg
dextromethorphan 10 mg
guaifenesin 100 mg
acetaminophen 250 mg
Uses: Adrenergic, antitussive, expectorant, analgesic
Sudafed Cold & Sinus:
pseudoephedrine 30 mg
acetaminophen 325 mg
Uses: Adrenergic, analgesic
Sudafed Plus:
pseudoephedrine 60 mg
chlorpheniramine 4 mg
Uses: Adrenergic, antihistamine
Sudafed Severe Cold:
pseudoephedrine 30 mg
dextromethorphan 15 mg
Uses: Adrenergic, antitussive
Sudafed Sinus Maximum Strength:
pseudoephedrine 30 mg
acetaminophen 500 mg
Uses: Adrenergic, analgesic
Sudal 60/500:
pseudoephedrine 60 mg
guaifenesin 500 mg
Uses: Adrenergic, expectorant
Sudal 120/600:
pseudoephedrine 120 mg
guaifenesin 600 mg
Uses: Adrenergic, expectorant
Sulfimycin Suspension:
Per 5 ml:
erythromycin 200 mg
sulfiSOXAZOLE 600 mg
Uses: Macrolide antiinfective
Sultrin Triple Sulfa Vaginal Cream:
3.42% sulfathiazole
2.86% sulfacetamine
3.7% sulfabenzamide
Uses: Antiinfective
Sultrin Triple Sulfa Vaginal Tablets:
sulfathiazole 172.5 mg
sulfacetamide 143.75
sulfabenzamide 184 mg
Uses: Antiinfective
Symbyax:
olanzapine 6 mg
fluoxetine 25 mg
olanzapine 6 mg
fluoxetine 50 mg
olanzapine 12 mg
fluoxetine 25 mg
olanzapine 12 mg
fluoxetine 50 mg
Uses: Bipolar disorder
Synalgos-DC:
aspirin 356.4 mg
caffeine 30 mg
dihydrocodeine 16 mg
Uses: Analgesic
Synercid:
quinupristin 150 mg
dalfopristin 350 mg
Uses: Antiinfective
Syntest D.S.:
esterified estrogens 1.25 mg
methylTESTOSTERone 2.5 mg
Uses: Menopause
Synophylate-GG Syrup:
theophylline 150 mg
guaifenesin 100 mg
15% alcohol
Uses: Bronchodilator, expectorant
Syntest H.S.:
esterified estrogens 0.625 mg
methylTESTOSTERone 1.25 mg
Uses: Menopause
Talacen:
acetaminophen 650 mg
pentazocine 25 mg
Uses: Analgesic
Talwin Compound:
aspirin 325 mg
pentazocine 12.5 mg
Uses: Analgesic
Talwin NX:
pentazocine 50 mg
naloxone 0.5 mg
Uses: Analgesic, opioid antagonist
Tarka 182:
trandolapril 2 mg (immed rel)
verapamil 180 mg (sus rel)
Uses: Antihypertensive, calcium channel blocker
Tarka 241:
trandolapril 1 mg (immed rel)
verapamil 240 mg (sus rel)
Uses: Antihypertensive, calcium channel blocker
Tarka 242:
trandolapril 2 mg (immed rel)
verapamil 240 mg (sus rel)

Uses: Antihypertensive, calcium channel blocker
Tarka 244:
trandolapril 4 mg (immed rel)
verapamil 240 mg (sus rel)
Uses: Antihypertensive, calcium channel blocker
Tavist Allergy/Sinus Headache:
clemastine 0.335 mg
pseudoephedrine 30 mg
acetaminophen 500 mg
Uses: Antihistamine, adrenergic, analgesic
Tavist Sinus:
acetaminophen 500 mg
pseudoephedrine 30 mg
Uses: Analgesic, adrenergic
♣ **Tecnal:**
aspirin 330 mg
caffeine 40 mg
butalbital 50 mg
Uses: Nonopioid analgesic
Teczem:
enalapril 5 mg (extended release)
diltiazem 180 mg (extended release)
Uses: Antihypertensive, calcium channel blocker
Tedrigen:
epHEDrine 22.5 mg
theophylline 120 mg
phenobarbital 7.5 mg
Uses: Adrenergic, bronchodilator, barbiturate
Tegrin-LT Shampoo:
0.33% pyrethrins
3.15% piperonyl butoxide
Uses: Scabicide, pediculicide
Tenoretic 50:
atenolol 50 mg
chlorthalidone 25 mg
Uses: Antihypertensive
Tenoretic 100:
atenolol 100 mg
chlorthalidone 25 mg
Uses: Antihypertensive
Terra-Cortril Ophthalmic Suspension:
1.5% hydrocortisone acetate
0.5% oxytetracycline
Uses: Ophthalmic antiinflammatory, antiinfective
Terramycin w/Polymycin B Sulfate Ophthalmic Ointment:
Per gram:
polymyxin B 10,000 units
oxytetracycline 5 mg
Uses: Ophthalmic antiinfective
T-Gesic:
hydrocodone 5 mg
acetaminophen 500 mg
Uses: Analgesic
Theodrine:
epHEDrine 22.5 mg
theophylline 120 mg
Uses: Adrenergic, bronchodilator
Thera-Flu Cold & Cough Powder:
Per packet:
pseudoephedrine 60 mg
chlorpheniramine 4 mg
dextromethorphan 20 mg
acetaminophen 650 mg
Uses: Adrenergic, antihistamine, antitussive, analgesic
Thera-Flu Flu & Chest Congestion Non-Drowsy Powder:
dextromethorphan 30 mg
guaifenesin 400 mg
pseudoephedrine 60 mg
acetaminophen 1000 mg
Uses: Antitussive, expectorant, decongestant, analgesic
Thera-Flu Flu, Cold, Cough & Sore Throat Maximum Strength Powder:
dextromethorphan 30 mg
chlorpheniramine 4 mg
pseudoephedrine 60 mg
acetaminophen 1000 mg
Uses: Antitussive, antihistamine, decongestant, analgesic
Thera-Flu Maximum Strength Flu, Cold & Cough Powder:
dextromethorphan 30 mg
guaifenesin 400 mg
pseudoephedrine 60 mg
acetaminophen 1000 mg
Uses: Antitussive, expectorant, decongestant, analgesic
Thera-Flu Non-Drowsy Flu, Cold & Cough Maximum Strength Powder:
Per packet:
pseudoephedrine 60 mg
dextromethorphan 30 mg
acetaminophen 1000 mg
Uses: Decongestant, antitussive, analgesic
Thera-Flu Severe Cold & Congestion Night-Time Maximum Strength Powder:
Per packet:
pseudoephedrine 60 mg
chlorpheniramine 4 mg
dextromethorphan 30 mg
acetaminophen 1000 mg
Uses: Decongestant, antihistamine, antitussive, analgesic
Thera-Flu Severe Cold & Congestion Non-Drowsy Maximum Strength Powder:
dextromethorphan 30 mg
pseudoephedrine 60 mg
acetaminophen 1000 mg
Uses: Antitussive, decongestant, acetaminophen
Thera-Flu Severe Cold & Cough Powder:
dextromethorphan 30 mg
chlorpheniramine 4 mg
pseudoephedrine 60 mg
acetaminophen 1000 mg
Uses: Antitussive, antihistamine, decongestant, analgesic
Thera-Flu Severe Cold Non-Drowsy Packet:
dextromethorphan 30 mg
pseudoephedrine 60 mg
acetaminophen 1000 mg
Uses: Antitussive, decongestant, acetaminophen
Thera-Flu Severe Cold Non-Drowsy Tablets:
dextromethorphan 15 mg

pseudoephedrine 30 mg
acetaminophen 500 mg
Uses: Antitussive, decongestant, analgesic

Thera-Flu Severe Cold Tablets:
dextromethorphan 15 mg
chlorpheniramine 2 mg
pseudoephedrine 30 mg
acetaminophen 500 mg
Uses: Antitussive, antihistamine, decongestant, analgesic

Timentin for Injection:
Per 3.1-g vial:
ticarcillin 3 g
clavulanic acid 0.1 g
Uses: Antiinfective

Timolide 10/25:
timolol 10 mg
hydrochlorothiazide 25 mg
Uses: Antihypertensive

Titralac Plus:
calcium carbonate 420 mg
simethicone 21 mg
Uses: Antacid, adsorbent, antiflatulent

Tobra Dex Ophthalmic Suspension/Ointment:
tobramycin 0.3%
dexamethasone 0.1%
Uses: Ophthalmic antiinfective, antiinflammatory

Triacin-C Cough Syrup:
Per 5 ml:
codeine 10 mg
pseudoephedrine 30 mg
triprolidine 1.25 mg
Uses: Analgesic, adrenergic, antihistamine

Triad:
acetaminophen 325 mg
caffeine 40 mg
butalbital 50 mg
Uses: Nonopioid analgesic

Tri-Hydroserpine:
hydrALAZINE 25 mg
hydrochlorothiazide 15 mg
reserpine 0.1 mg
Uses: Antihypertensive

Tri-Levlen:
Phase I:
levonorgestrel 0.05 mg
ethinyl estradiol 30 mcg
Phase II:
levonorgestrel 0.075 mg
ethinyl estradiol 40 mcg;
Phase III:
levonorgestrel 0.125 mg
ethinyl estradiol 30 mcg
Uses: Oral contraceptive

Triaminic AM Cough & Decongestant Formula Liquid:
Per 5 ml:
pseudoephedrine 15 mg
dextromethorphan 7.5 mg
Uses: Adrenergic, antitussive

Triaminic Nite Light Liquid:
Per 5 ml:
pseudoephedrine 15 mg
chlorpheniramine 1 mg
dextromethorphan 7.5 mg
Uses: Adrenergic, antihistamine, antitussive

Triaminic Sore Throat Formula Liquid:
Per 5 ml:
pseudoephedrine 15 mg
dextromethorphan 7.5 mg
acetaminophen 160 mg
Uses: Adrenergic, antitussive

Triavil 2-10:
perphenazine 2 mg
amitriptyline 10 mg
Uses: Antipsychotic, antidepressant

Triavil 2-25:
perphenazine 2 mg
amitriptyline 25 mg
Uses: Antipsychotic, antidepressant

Triavil 4-10:
perphenazine 4 mg
amitriptyline 10 mg

Triavil 4-25:
perphenazine 4 mg
amitriptyline 25 mg
Uses: Antipsychotic, antidepressant

Triavil 4-50:
perphenazine 4 mg
amitriptyline 50 mg
Uses: Antipsychotic, antidepressant

Trinalin Repetabs:
azatadine maleate 1 mg
pseudoephedrine 120 mg
Uses: Antihistamine

Triphasil:
Phase I:
levonorgestrel 0.05 mg
ethinyl estradiol 30 mcg
Phase II:
levonorgestrel 0.075 mg
ethinyl estradiol 40 mcg
Phase III:
levonorgestrel 0.125 mg
ethinyl estradiol 30 mcg
Uses: Oral contraceptive

Triple Antibiotic Ophthalmic Ointment:
Per gram:
polymyxin B 10,000 units
neomycin 3.5 mg
bacitracin 400 units
Uses: Antiinfective

Triprolidine/Pseudoephedrine Syrup (generic):
Per 5 ml
triprolidine 1.25 mg
pseudoephedrine 50 mg
Uses: Antihistamine, decongestant

Triprolidine/Pseudoephedrine Tablets (generic):
triprolidine 2.5 mg
pseudoephedrine 60 mg
Uses: Antihistamine, decongestant

Triposed Tablets:
triprolidine 150 mg
pseudoephedrine 60 mg
Uses: Decongestant, antihistamine

Trizivir:
300 mg abacavir
150 mg lamivudine
300 mg zidovudine
Uses: HIV

Truvada:
emtricitabine 200 mg
tenofovir 300 mg
Uses: HIV

Tuinal 100 mg:
amobarbital 50 mg
secobarbital 50 mg
Uses: Sedative-hypnotic

Tuinal 200 mg:
amobarbital 100 mg
secobarbital 100 mg
Uses: Sedative-hypnotic

Tusibron-DM Syrup:
Per 5 ml:
guaifenesin 100 mg
dextromethorphan 15 mg
Uses: Expectorant, antitussive

Tussionex Pennkinetic Suspension:
Per 5 ml:
chlorpheniramine 8 mg
hydrocodone 10 mg
Uses: Antihistamine, analgesic

Tussi-Organidin NR Liquid:
Per 5 ml:
codeine 10 mg
guaifenesin 100 mg
Uses: Analgesic, expectorant

Tussi-Organidin DM NR Liquid:
Per 5 ml:
guaifenesin 100 mg
dextromethorphan 10 mg
Uses: Expectorant, antitussive

Twinrix:
hepatitis A vaccine
hepatitis B vaccine
Uses: Vaccine

Two-Dyne:
acetaminophen 325 mg
caffeine 40 mg
butalbital 50 mg
Uses: Nonopioid analgesic

Tylenol Allergy Sinus, Maximum Strength Gelcaps:
acetaminophen 500 mg
chlorpheniramine 2 mg
pseudoephedrine 30 mg
Uses: Antihistamine, adrenergic, analgesic

Tylenol Children's Cold:
acetaminophen 80 mg
chlorpheniramine 0.5 mg
pseudoephedrine 7.5 mg
Uses: Antihistamine, adrenergic, analgesic

Tylenol Children's Cold Liquid:
Per 5 ml:
acetaminophen 160 mg
chlorpheniramine 1 mg
pseudoephedrine 15 mg
Uses: Antihistamine, adrenergic, analgesic

Tylenol Children's Cold Multi-Symptom Plus Cough Liquid:
Per 5 ml:
acetaminophen 160 mg
dextromethorphan 5 mg
chlorpheniramine 1 mg
pseudoephedrine 15 mg
Uses: Antihistamine, adrenergic, analgesic

Tylenol Children's Cold Plus Cough Chewable:
acetaminophen 80 mg
pseudoephedrine 7.5 mg
dextromethorphan 2.5 mg
chlorpheniramine 0.5 mg
Uses: Antihistamine, adrenergic, analgesic

Tylenol Children's Cold Plus Cough Suspension:
pseudoephedrine 15 mg
chlorpheniramine 1 mg
dextromethorphan 5 mg
acetaminophen 160 mg
Uses: Decongestant, antihistamine, antitussive, analgesic

Tylenol Children's Flu Suspension:
pseudoephedrine 15 mg
chlorpheniramine 1 mg
dextromethorphan 7.5 mg
acetaminophen 160 mg
Uses: Decongestant, antihistamine, antitussive, analgesic

Tylenol Cold Complete Formula Tablets:
acetaminophen 325 mg
chlorpheniramine 2 mg
pseudoephedrine 30 mg
dextromethorphan 15 mg
Uses: Antihistamine, adrenergic, analgesic

Tylenol Cold & Flu Severe DayTime Liquid:
dextromethorphan 5 mg
pseudoephedrine 10 mg
acetaminophen 166.7 mg
Uses: Antitussive, decongestant, analgesic

Tylenol Cold Severe Congestion Tablets:
dextromethorphan 15 mg
guaifenesin 200 mg
pseudoephedrine 32 mg
acetaminophen 325 mg
Uses: Antitussive, expectorant, decongestant, analgesic

Tylenol Cough & Sore Throat DayTime Liquid:
dextromethorphan 5 mg
acetaminophen 166.7 mg
Uses: Antitussive, analgesic

Tylenol Flu Maximum Strength Non-Drowsy Gelcaps:
dextromethorphan 15 mg
pseudoephedrine 30 mg
acetaminophen 500 mg
Uses: Analgesic, adrenergic, antitussive

Tylenol Flu NightTime Maximum Strength Liquid:
dextromethorphan 5 mg
doxylamine 2.1 mg
pseudoephedrine 10 mg
acetaminophen 167 mg

Uses: Antitussive, antihistamine, decongestant, acetaminophen
Tylenol Headache Plus, Extra Strength:
acetaminophen 500 mg
calcium carbonate 250 mg
Uses: Analgesic, antacid
Tylenol PM, Extra Strength:
acetaminophen 500 mg
diphenhydrAMINE 25 mg
Uses: Analgesic, antihistamine
Tylenol Severe Allergy:
diphenhydrAMINE 12.5 mg
acetaminophen 500 mg
Uses: Analgesic, antihistamine
Tylenol Sinus Maximum Strength:
pseudoephedrine 30 mg
acetaminophen 500 mg
Uses: Adrenergic, analgesic
Tylenol w/Codeine Elixir:
Per 5 ml:
acetaminophen 120 mg
codeine 12 mg
Uses: Analgesic
Tylenol w/Codeine No. 1:
acetaminophen 300 mg
codeine 7.5 mg
Uses: Analgesic
Tylenol w/Codeine No. 2:
acetaminophen 300 mg
codeine 15 mg
Uses: Analgesic
Tylenol w/Codeine No. 3:
acetaminophen 300 mg
codeine 30 mg
Uses: Analgesic
Tylenol w/Codeine No. 4:
acetaminophen 300 mg
codeine 60 mg
Uses: Analgesic
Tylox:
oxycodone 5 mg
acetaminophen 500 mg
Uses: Analgesic
Tyrodone Liquid:
Per 5 ml:
hydrocodone 5 mg
pseudoephedrine 60 mg
5% alcohol
Uses: Analgesic, adrenergic
Ultracet:
tramadol 37.5 mg
acetaminophen 325 mg
Uses: Analgesic
Unasyn for Injection 3 g:
ampicillin 2 g
sulbactam 1 g
Uses: Antiinfective
Uniretic:
moexipril 7.5 mg
hydrochlorothiazide 12.5 mg
or moexipril 15 mg
hydrochlorothiazide 25 mg
Uses: Antihypertensive, diuretic
Unituss HC Syrup:
hydrocodone 2.5 mg
phenylephrine 5 mg
chlorpheniramine 2 mg
Uses: Analgesic, adrenergic, antihistamine
Urised:
methenamine 40.8 mg
phenylsalicylate 18.1 mg
atropine 0.03 mg
hyoscyamine 0.03 mg
benzoic acid 4.5 mg
methylene blue 5.4 mg
Uses: Antiinfective
Urobiotic 250:
oxytetracycline 250 mg
sulfamethizole 250 mg
phenazopyridine 50 mg
Uses: Antiinfective
Vanquish:
aspirin 227 mg
acetaminophen 194 mg
caffeine 33 mg
aluminum hydroxide 25 mg
magnesium hydroxide 50 mg
Uses: Nonopioid analgesic
Vaseretic 5-12.5:
enalapril 5 mg
hydrochlorthiazide 12.5 mg
Uses: Antihypertensive diuretic
Vaseretic 10-25:
enalapril 10 mg
hydrochlorothiazide 25 mg
Uses: Antihypertensive, diuretic
Vasocidin Ophthalmic Ointment:
sulfacetamide 10%
prednisoLONE 0.5%
Uses: Ophthalmic antiinfective, antiinflammatory
Vasocidin Ophthalmic Solution:
sulfacetamide 10%
prednisoLONE 0.25%
Uses: Ophthalmic antiinfective, antiinflammatory
Vasocon-A Ophthalmic Solution:
naphazoline 0.05%
antazoline 0.5%
Uses: Ophthalmic vasoconstrictor
Vicks 44D Cough & Head Congestion Liquid:
Per 5 ml:
dextromethorphan 10 mg
pseudoephedrine 20 mg
Uses: Antitussive, adrenergic
Vicks 44E Liquid:
Per 5 ml:
dextromethorphan 6.7 mg
guaifenesin 66.7 mg
Uses: Antitussive, expectorant
Vicks 44M Cold, Flu, & Cough LiquiCaps:
dextromethorphan 10 mg
pseudoephedrine 30 mg
chlorpheniramine 2 mg
acetaminophen 250 mg
Uses: Antitussive, adrenergic, antihistamine, analgesic

Vicks 44 Non-Drowsy Cold & Cough LiquiCaps:
dextromethorphan 30 mg
pseudoephedrine 60 mg
Uses: Antitussive, adrenergic
Vicks Children's NyQuil Nighttime Cough/ Cold Liquid:
Per 5 ml:
pseudoephedrine 10 mg
chlorpheniramine 0.67 mg
dextromethorphan 5 mg
Uses: Adrenergic, antihistamine, antitussive
Vicks Cough Silencers:
dextromethorphan 2.5 mg
benzocaine 1 mg
Uses: Antitussive, top anesthetic
Vicks DayQuil Liquid:
Per 5 ml:
dextromethorphan 3.3 mg
pseudoephedrine 10 mg
acetaminophen 108.3 mg
guaifenesin 33.3 mg
Uses: Antitussive, adrenergic, analgesic, expectorant
Vicks DayQuil Multi-Symptom Cold/Flu Relief Liquid:
dextromethorphan 33 mg
pseudoephedrine 10 mg
acetaminophen 108.3 mg
Uses: Antitussive, decongestant, analgesic
Vicks DayQuil Sinus Pressure & Pain Relief:
pseudoephedrine 30 mg
acetaminophen 500 mg
Uses: Adrenergic, analgesic
Vicks NyQuil Liquicaps:
pseudoephedrine 30 mg
doxylamine 6.25 mg
dextromethorphan 10 mg
acetaminophen 250 mg
Uses: Adrenergic, antihistamine, antitussive, analgesic
Vicks NyQuil Multi-Symptom Cold Flu Relief Liquid:
pseudoephedrine 10 mg
doxylamine 2.1 mg
dextromethorphan 5 mg
acetaminophen 167 mg
Uses: Adrenergic, antihistamine, antitussive, analgesic
Vicks Pediatric Formula 44e Cough & Chest Congestion Relief Liquid:
Per 5 ml:
dextromethorphan 3.3 mg
guaifenesin 33.3 mg
Uses: Expectorant, antitussive
Vicks Pediatric Formula 44m Multi-Symptom Cough & Cold Liquid:
pseudoephedrine 10 mg
chlorpheniramine 0.67 mg
dextromethorphan 5 mg
Uses: Adrenergic, antihistamine, antitussive
Vicodin:
acetaminophen 500 mg
hydrocodone 5 mg
Uses: Analgesic
Vicodin ES:
acetaminophen 750 mg
hydrocodone 7.5 mg
Uses: Analgesic
Vicodin HP:
hydrocodone 10 mg
acetaminophen 660 mg
Uses: Analgesic
VicodinTuss:
Per 5 ml:
hydrocodone 5 mg
guaifenesin 100 mg
Uses: Analgesic, expectorant
Vicoprofen:
hydrocodone 7.5 mg
ibuprofen 200 mg
Uses: Analgesic
Vytorin:
ezetimibe: 10, 10, 10, 10 mg
simvastatin: 10, 20, 40, 80 mg
Uses: Antihyperlipidemic
Wigraine Suppositories:
ergotamine 2 mg
caffeine 100 mg
Uses: α-Adrenergic blocker
Yasmin 28:
ethinyl estadiol 30 mcg
dropirenone 3 mg
Uses: Oral contraceptive
Zestoretic 10/12.5:
lisinopril 10 mg
hydrochlorothiazide 12.5 mg
Uses: Antihypertensive
Zestoretic 20/12.5:
lisinopril 20 mg
hydrochlorothiazide 12.5 mg
Uses: Antihypertensive
Zestoretic 20/25:
lisinopril 20 mg
hydrochlorothiazide 25 mg
Uses: Antihypertensive
Ziac 2.5:
bisoprolol 2.5 mg
hydrochlorothiazide 6.25 mg
Uses: Antihypertensive
Ziac 5:
bisoprolol 5 mg
hydrochlorothiazide 6.25 mg
Uses: Antihypertensive
Ziac 10:
bisoprolol 10 mg
hydrochlorothiazide 6.25 mg
Uses: Antihypertensive
Ziks Cream:
methyl salicylate 12%
menthol 1%
capsaicin 0.025%
Uses: Analgesic, decongestant
Zydone:
hydrocodone 5 mg
acetaminophen 500 mg
Uses: Analgesic

Appendix F

Rarely Used Drugs

! HIGH ALERT

abciximab (Rx)

Func. class.: Platelet aggregation inhibitor

Dosage and routes

Percutaneous coronary intervention (PCI)

Adult: **IV** bol 250 mcg (0.25 mg)/kg 10-60 min before PCI, followed by 125 mcg/kg/min cont inf for 12 hr

MI

Adult: **IV** bol 0.25 mg over 5 min, then 0.125 mcg/kg/min, max 10 mcg/min; **IV** inf for 12 hr unless complications

Uses: Used with heparin and aspirin to prevent acute cardiac ischemia following PTCA in patients at high risk for reclosure of affected arteries

Contraindications: Hypersensitivity to this drug or murine protein; GI, GU bleeding; CVA within 2 yr, bleeding disorders, intracranial neoplasm, intracranial arteriovenous malformations, intracranial aneurysm, platelet count <100,000 cells/mm^3, recent surgery, aneurysm, uncontrolled severe hypertension, vasculitis coagulopathy

agalsidase beta (Rx)

Func. class.: Drug—miscellaneous

Dosage and routes

Adult: **IV** inffl mg/kg q2 wk, run at ≤0.25 mg/min (15 mg/hr), slow if infusion-associated reaction occurs

Uses: Fabry disease

Contraindications: Hypersensitivity

alefacept (Rx)

Func. class.: Immunosuppressive

Dosage and routes

Adult: **IV** BOL 7.5 mg q wk or IM 15 mg q wk, for 12 wk

Uses: Adults with moderate to severe plaque psoriasis

Contraindications: Hypersensitivity

alfentanil (Rx)

Func. class.: Opioid analgesic

Controlled substance schedule II

Dosage and routes

Anesthesia <30 min

Combination

Adult: **IV** 8-50 mcg/kg, may increase by 3-15 mcg/kg

Anesthetic induction

Adult: **IV** 3-5 mcg/kg, then 0.5-1.5 mcg/kg/min; total dose is 8-40 mcg/kg

Anesthesia 30-60 min

Induction

Adult: **IV** 20-50 mcg/kg

Maintenance

Adult: **IV** 5-15 mcg/kg; may give up to 75 mcg/kg total dose

Continuous anesthesia >45 min

Induction

Adult: **IV** 50-75 mcg/kg

Maintenance

Adult: **IV** 0.5-3.0 mcg/kg/min; rate should be decreased by 30%-50% after 1 hr maintenance inf; may be increased to 4 mcg/kg/min or bol doses of 7 mcg/kg

Induction of anesthesia >45 min

Adult: **IV** 130-245 mcg/kg, then 0.5-1.5 mcg/kg/min

MAC

Induction

Adult: **IV** duration ≤½ hr 3-8 mcg/kg

Maintenance

Adult: 3-5 mcg/kg q5-20min to 1 mcg/kg/min, total dose 3-40 mcg/kg

Uses: In combination with other drugs in general anesthesia, as a primary anesthetic in general surgery, monitored anesthesia care (MAC)

Contraindications: Child <12 yr, hypersensitivity

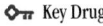

alprostadil (Rx)

Func. class.: Hormone

Dosage and routes

Patent ductus arteriosus

Infants: **IV** inf 0.1 mcg/kg/min, until desired response, then reduce to lowest effective amount, 0.4 mcg/kg/min not likely to produce greater beneficial effects

Erectile dysfunction of vasculogenic or mixed etiology, psychogenic

Men: Intracavernosal 2.5 mcg may increase by 2.5 mcg; may then increase by 5-10 mcg until adequate response occurs; intraurethral administer as needed to achieve erection

Uses: To maintain patent ductus arteriosus (temporary treatment), erectile dysfunction

Contraindications: Hypersensitivity, respiratory distress syndrome (RDS)

altretamine (Rx)

Func. class.: Antineoplastic—miscellaneous

Dosage and routes

Adult: PO 260 mg/m^2 day for 14 or 21 days in a 28-day cycle; give in 4 divided doses pc and at bedtime

Uses: Palliative treatment of recurrent, persistent ovarian cancer following first-line treatment with cisplatin or alkylating agent–based combination

Contraindications: Pregnancy **D**, hypersensitivity, severe bone marrow depression, severe neurologic toxicity

amantadine (Rx)

Func. class.: Antiviral, antiparkinsonian agent

Do Not Confuse:
amantadine/ranitidine, amantadine/rimantidine, Symmetrel/Synthroid

Dosage and routes

Influenza type A

Adult and child >12 yr: PO 200 mg/day in single dose or divided bid, max 400 mg/day

Child 9-12 yr: PO 100 mg bid

Child 1-9 yr: PO 5 mg/kg/day divided bid-tid, not to exceed 150 mg/day

Elderly: PO no more than 100 mg daily

Extrapyramidal reaction/ parkinsonism

Adult: PO 100 mg bid, up to 400 mg/day in extrapyramidal symptoms (EPS); give for 1 wk, then 100 mg as needed up to 400 mg in parkinsonism

MS-associated fatigue (off-label)

Adult: PO 200 mg daily or 100 mg bid

Neuroleptic malignant syndrome (off-label)

Adult: PO 100 mg bid × 3 wk

Renal dose

CCr 40-50 ml/min 100 mg/day; CCr 30 ml/min 200 mg 2×/wk; CCr 20 ml/min 100 mg 3×/wk; CCr <10 ml/min 100 mg alternating with 200 mg q7d

Uses: Prophylaxis or treatment of influenza type A, extrapyramidal symptoms (EPS), parkinsonism, Parkinson's disease

Contraindications: Hypersensitivity, lactation, child <1 yr, eczematic rash

aminocaproic acid (Rx)

Func. class.: Hemostatic

Dosage and routes

Adult: PO/**IV** 5 g loading dose, then 1-1.25 g q1h

Uses: Hemorrhage from hyperfibrinolysis; adjunctive therapy in hemophilia

Contraindications: Hypersensitivity, abnormal bleeding, postpartum bleeding, DIC, upper urinary tract bleeding, new burns

aminoglutethimide (Rx)

Func. class.: Antineoplastic, adrenal steroid inhibitor

Dosage and routes

Adult: PO 250 mg qid at 6 hr intervals, may increase by 250 mg/day q1-2 wk, not to exceed 2 g/day; concurrent hydrocortisone supplementation is recommended

Uses: Suppression of adrenal function in Cushing's syndrome, adrenal cancer

Contraindications: Pregnancy **D**, hypersensitivity, hypothyroidism

aminolevulinic acid (Rx)
Func. class.: Photochemotherapy

Dosage and routes
Adult: TOP 1 application of solution and 1 dose of illumination/treatment site × 8 wk

Uses: Face/scalp nonhyperkeratotic actinic keratoses

Contraindications: Hypersensitivity to porphyrins

ammonium chloride (PO-OTC, IV-Rx)
Func. class.: Acidifier

Dosage and routes
Alkalosis
Adult and child: **IV** Inf 0.9-1.3 ml/min of a 2.14% sol, not to exceed 5 ml/min
Acidifier
Adult: PO 4-12 g/day in divided doses
Child: PO 75 mg/kg/day in divided doses
Expectorant
Adult: PO 250-500 mg q2-4h as needed

Uses: Alkalosis (metabolic), systemic and urinary acidifier, expectorant, diuretic

Contraindications: Hypersensitivity, severe hepatic disease, severe renal disease

amyl nitrite (Rx)
Func. class.: Coronary vasodilator

Dosage and routes
Angina
Adult: INH 0.18-0.3 ml as needed, 1-6 puffs from 1 cap; may repeat in 3-5 min
Cyanide poisoning
Adult: INH 0.3 ml ampule 15 sec until preparation of sodium nitrite inf is ready

Uses: Acute angina pectoris, cyanide poisoning

Investigational uses: Cardiac murmur diagnosis

Contraindications: Pregnancy **X**, hypersensitivity to nitrites, severe anemia, increased intracranial pressure, hypertension

atracurium (Rx)
Func. class.: Neuromuscular blocker (nondepolarizing)

Dosage and routes
Adult and child >2 yr: **IV** bol 0.3-0.5 mg/kg, then 0.08-0.10 mg/kg 20-45 min after first dose if needed for prolonged procedures
Child, 1 mo-2 yr: **IV** bol 0.3-0.4 mg/kg

Uses: Facilitation of endotracheal intubation, skeletal muscle relaxation during mechanical ventilation, surgery, or general anesthesia

Contraindications: Hypersensitivity

auranofin (Rx)
Func. class.: Antiinflammatory

Do Not Confuse:
Ridaura/Cardura

Dosage and routes
Adult: PO 6 mg daily or 3 mg bid; may increase to 9 mg/day after 3 mo

Uses: Rheumatoid arthritis; not for first-line therapy

Investigational uses: SLE, psoriatic arthritis, pemphigus

Contraindications: Hypersensitivity to gold, necrotizing enterocolitis, bone marrow aplasia, child <6 yr, lactation, pulmonary fibrosis, exfoliative dermatitis, blood dyscrasias, recent radiation therapy, renal/hepatic disease, marked hypertension, uncontrolled CHF

aurothioglucose/gold sodium thiomalate (Rx)
Func. class.: Antiinflammatory (gold)

Dosage and routes
Aurothioglucose
Adult: IM 10 mg; then 25 mg weekly × 2-3 wk; then 50 mg/wk until total of 1 g is administered; then 25-50 mg q3-4 wk if there is improvement without toxicity; total of 800 mg-1 g
Child 6-12 yr: IM 0.25 mg/kg/wk 1st wk, increase by 0.25 mg/kg/wk up to 0.75-1 mg/kg/wk, max 25 mg/dose; give for 20 wk
Gold sodium thiomalate
Adult: IM 10 mg, then 25 mg after 1 wk, then 50 mg weekly for total of 14-20 doses; then 50 mg q2 wk × 4; then 50 mg q3 wk × 4; then 50 mg monthly for maintenance

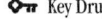

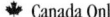

Child* <6 *yr: IM 10 mg 1st wk, then 1 mg/kg, max 50 mg/dose; space doses as per adult dosing schedule if improvement without toxicity

Uses: Rheumatoid arthritis, psoriatic arthritis

Contraindications: Hypersensitivity to gold, SLE, uncontrolled diabetes mellitus, marked hypertension, recent radiation therapy, CHF, lactation, renal disease, hepatic disease

aztreonam (Rx)

Func. class.: Antiinfective—miscellaneous

Dosage and routes

Urinary tract infections

Adult: **IV**/IM 500 mg-1 g q8-12h

Systemic infections

Adult: **IV**/IM 1-2 g q8-12h

Child: **IV**/IM 90-120 mg/kg/day divided q6-8h

Severe systemic infections

Adult: **IV**/IM 2 g q6-8h; do not exceed 8 g/day

Continue treatment for 48 hr after negative culture or until patient is asymptomatic

Uses: Urinary tract infection; septicemia; skin, muscle, bone, lower respiratory tract, intraabdominal infections, and other infections caused by gram-negative organisms

Contraindications: Hypersensitivity to this drug, penicillins, cephalosporins

bacitracin (Rx)

Func. class.: Antiinfective—miscellaneous

Dosage and routes

Infant* >*2.5 kg: IM 1000 units/kg/day in divided doses q8-12h

Infant* ≤*2.5 kg: IM 900 units/kg/day in divided doses q8-12h

Uses: Staphylococcal pneumonia, empyema

Contraindications: Hypersensitivity, severe renal disease (IM use)

benzonatate (Rx)

Func. class.: Antitussive, nonopioid

Dosage and routes

Adult and child: PO 100 mg tid, not to exceed 600 mg/day

Uses: Nonproductive cough

Contraindications: Hypersensitivity

benzoyl peroxide (OTC)

Func. class.: Antiacne medication

Dosage and routes

Adult and child: TOP apply to affected area daily or bid

Uses: Mild to moderate acne

Contraindications: Hypersensitivity to benzoic acid derivatives

beractant (Rx)

Func. class.: Natural lung surfactant

Dosage and routes

Newborn intratracheal instill: 4 doses can be administered in the 1st 48 hr of life; give doses no more frequently than q6h; each dose is 100 mg of phospholipids/kg birth weight (4 ml/kg)

Uses: Prevention and treatment (rescue) of respiratory distress syndrome in premature infants

bitolterol (Rx)

Func. class.: Bronchodilator, adrenergic β_2-agonist

Dosage and routes

Inhaler

Adult and child* >*12 yr: INH 2 puffs, wait 1-3 min before 3rd puff if needed, not to exceed 3 INH q6h or 2 INH q4h

Nebulization

Adult and child* >*12 yr: INH 0.5 ml (1 mg) tid by intermittent flow or 1.25 mg tid by cont flow, max 8 mg (intermittent), 14 mg (cont)

Uses: Asthma, bronchospasm

Contraindications: Hypersensitivity to bitolterol products

cabergoline (Rx)

Func. class.: Dopamine receptor/agonist

Dosage and routes

Hyperprolactinemic indications

Adult: PO 0.25 mg 2×/wk, may increase by 0.25 mg 2×/wk at 4 wk intervals, max 1 mg

2×/wk; maintenance therapy may be needed for 6 mo

Uses: Reduced prolactin/secretion in postpartum lactation

Contraindications: Hypersensitivity, uncontrolled hypertension

chlorproPAMIDE (Rx)

Func. class.: Antidiabetic, oral

Dosage and routes

Adult: PO 100-250 mg daily initially, then 100-500 mg maintenance according to response; not to exceed 750 mg/day

Uses: Type 2 diabetes mellitus

Contraindications: Pregnancy **D**, hypersensitivity to sulfonylureas, juvenile or brittle diabetes, renal failure, lactation

cladribine (CdA) (Rx)

Func. class.: Antineoplastic antiinfective

Dosage and routes

Adult: **IV** 0.09 mg/kg diluted with 0.9% NaCl qs to 100 ml; pass through 0.22 mcg microfilter, given for cont inf × 5-7 days

Uses: Treatment of active hairy cell leukemia; may be useful in chronic lymphocytic leukemia, non-Hodgkin's lymphomas, acute myeloid leukemia, autoimmune hemolytic anemia

Contraindications: Hypersensitivity, lactation

clocortolone (Rx)

Func. class.: Topical corticosteroid

Dosage and routes

Adult and child: Top apply to affected area tid-qid

Uses: Psoriasis, eczema, contact dermatitis, pruritus

Contraindications: Hypersensitivity to corticosteroids, fungal infections

clofazimine (Rx)

Func. class.: Leprostatic

Dosage and routes

Erythema nodosum leprosum

Adult: PO 100-200 mg daily × 3 mo, then taper dosage to 100 mg when disease is controlled; do not exceed 200 mg/day

Dapsone-resistant leprosy

Adult: PO 100 mg/day in combination with at least one other antileprosy drug × 3 yr, then 100 mg daily clofazimine (only)

Uses: Lepromatous leprosy, dapsone-resistant leprosy, lepromatous leprosy complicated by erythema nodosum leprosum

Contraindications: Hypersensitivity to this drug

clotrimazole (Rx) (OTC)

Func. class.: Local antiinfective

Dosage and routes

Adult and child: Massage into affected area, surrounding area daily or bid, continue for 7-14 days, not to exceed 4 wk; loz dissolve in mouth 5 times/day × 2 wk; intravag 1 applicator/1 tab × 1-2 wk at bedtime; oral troches 10 mg 5 times/day × 14 days

Uses: Tinea pedis, tinea cruris, tinea corporis, tinea versicolor, *Candida albicans* infection of the vagina, vulva, throat, mouth

Contraindications: Hypersensitivity

corticotropin (ACTH) (Rx)

Func. class.: Pituitary hormone

Dosage and routes

Acute exacerbations of multiple sclerosis

Adult: IM 80-120 units/day × 14-21 days

Infantile spasms

Infant: IM Gel 20 units/day × 2 wk, increase if needed

Uses: Testing adrenocortical function, treatment of adrenal insufficiency caused by administration of corticosteroids (long term), multiple sclerosis, infantile spasms

Contraindications: Hypersensitivity, scleroderma, osteoporosis, CHF, peptic ulcer disease, hypertension, systemic fungal infections, smallpox vaccination, recent surgery, ocular herpes simplex, primary adrenocortical insufficiency/hyperfunction

cosyntropin (Rx)

Func. class.: Pituitary hormone

Dosage and routes

Adult and child >2 yr: IM/ **IV** 0.25-1 mg between blood sampling

Child <2 yr: IM/**IV** 0.125 mg

Uses: Testing adrenocortical function

Contraindications: Hypersensitivity

crotamiton (Rx)

Func. class.: Scabicide

Dosage and routes

Scabies

Adult and child: Cream wash area with soap, water; remove visible crusts, apply cream, apply another coat in 24 hr, remove with soap, water in 48 hr

Pruritus: Massage into affected area, repeat as necessary

Uses: Scabies, pruritus

Contraindications: Hypersensitivity, skin inflammation, abrasions, breaks in skin, mucous membranes

dapsone (DDS) (Rx)

Func. class.: Leprostatic

Dosage and routes

Hansen's disease

Adult: PO 100 mg daily with rifampin 600 mg daily × 6 mo, then dapsone alone for 3-10 yr

Child: PO 1-2 mg/kg/day

PCP

Adult: PO 50-100 mg/day usually given with trimethoprim 20 mg/kg/day in 4 divided doses for 3 wk

Child: PO 2 mg/kg/day

Uses: Hansen's disease, PCP (*Pneumocystis jiroveci* pneumonia), malaria, dermatitis herpetiformis

Contraindications: Hypersensitivity to sulfones, severe anemia

deferoxamine (Rx)

Func. class.: Heavy metal antagonist

Do Not Confuse:
deferoxamine/cefuroxime

Dosage and routes

Acute iron toxicity

Adult and child: IM/**IV** 1 g; then 500 mg q4h × 2 doses; then 500 mg q4-12h × 2 doses, not to exceed 15 mg/kg/hr or 6 g/24 hr

Chronic iron toxicity

Adult and child: IM 500 mg-1 g/day plus **IV** inf 2 g given by separate line with each blood transfusion, not to exceed 15 mg/kg/hr or 6 g/24 hr; SUBCUT 1-2 g over 8-24 hr by SUBCUT infusion pump

Uses: Acute, chronic iron intoxication, hemochromatosis, hemosiderosis

Contraindications: Hypersensitivity, anuria, severe renal disease, child <3 yr

demeclocycline (Rx)

Func. class.: Antiinfective

Dosage and routes

Adult: PO 150 mg q6h or 300 mg q12h

Child >8 yr: PO 6-12 mg/kg/day in divided doses q6-12h

Gonorrhea

Adult: PO 600 mg, then 300 mg q12h × 4 days, total 3 g

Uses: Uncommon gram-positive/gram-negative bacteria, protozoa, *Rickettsia, Mycoplasma, Haemophilus ducreyi, Yersinia pestis, Campylobacter fetus, Chlamydia trachomatis,* psittacosis, granuloma inguinale

Contraindications: Pregnancy **D,** hypersensitivity to tetracyclines, children <8 yr

desipramine

Func. class.: Antidepressant, tricyclic

Dosage and routes

Adult: PO 75-150 mg/day in divided doses; may increase to 300 mg/day or may give daily dose at bedtime

Adolescent and elderly: PO 25-50 mg/day, may increase to 100 mg/day

Uses: Depression

Contraindications: Hypersensitivity to tricyclics, recovery phase of myocardial infarction, narrow-angle glaucoma, convulsive disorders, prostatic hypertrophy, child <12 yr

dicyclomine (Rx)

Func. class.: Gastrointestinal anticholinergic

Dosage and routes

Adult: PO 10-20 mg tid-qid; IM 20 mg q4-6h
Child >2 yr: PO 10 mg tid-qid
Child 6 mo-2 yr: PO 5 mg tid-qid

Uses: Treatment of peptic ulcer disease in combination with other drugs; infant colic, urinary incontinence, IBS

Contraindications: Hypersensitivity to anticholinergics, narrow-angle glaucoma, GI obstruction, myasthenia gravis, paralytic ileus, GI atony, toxic megacolon

diflunisal (Rx)

Func. class.: Nonsteroidal anti-inflammatory/analgesic (nonopioid)

Dosage and routes

Adult: PO loading dose 1 g; then 500-1000 mg/day in 2 divided doses, q12h, not to exceed 1500 mg/day

Geriatric: PO ½ adult dose

Uses: Mild to moderate pain or fever including arthritis; 3-4 × more potent than aspirin

Contraindications: Hypersensitivity to salicylates, GI bleeding, bleeding disorders, children <12 yr, vit K deficiency

dimercaprol (Rx)

Func. class.: Heavy metal antagonist

Dosage and routes

Severe gold/arsenic poisoning

Adult: IM 3 mg/kg q4h × 2 days, then qid × 1 day, then bid × 10 days

Mild gold/arsenic poisoning

Adult: IM 2.5 mg/kg qid × 2 days, then bid × 1 day, then daily × 10 days

Acute lead poisoning

Adult: IM 4 mg/kg; then q4h with edetate calcium disodium 12.5 mg/kg IM; not to exceed 5 mg/kg/dose

Mercury poisoning

Adult: IM 5 mg/kg; then 2.5 mg/kg/day or bid × 10 days

Uses: Arsenic, gold, mercury, lead poisoning

Contraindications: Pregnancy **D**, hypersensitivity, anuria, hepatic insufficiency, poisoning with other metals, severe renal disease, child <3 yr

disulfiram (Rx)

Func. class.: Alcohol deterrent

Dosage and routes

Adult: PO 250-500 mg daily × 1-2 wk, then 125-500 mg daily until fully socially recovered

Uses: Chronic alcoholism (as adjunct)

Contraindications: Pregnancy **X**, hypersensitivity, alcohol intoxication, psychoses, CV disease, lactation

! HIGH ALERT

doxacurium (Rx)

Func. class.: Neuromuscular blocker (nondepolarizing)

Dosage and routes

Adult: **IV** 0.05 mg/kg; 0.08 mg/kg is used for prolonged neuromuscular blockade; maintenance 0.005-0.01 mg/kg
Child 2-12 yr: **IV** 0.03-0.05 mg/kg; may decrease for maintenance dose

Uses: Facilitation of endotracheal intubation, skeletal muscle relaxation during mechanical ventilation, surgery, or general anesthesia

Contraindications: Hypersensitivity, neonates

edetate calcium disodium (Rx)

Func. class.: Heavy metal antagonist; antidote

Dosage and routes

Acute lead encephalopathy

Adult and child: 1.5 g/m^2/day × 3-5 days in 2-3 divided doses IM or slow **IV** with dimercaprol; may be given again after 4 days off drug

Lead poisoning

Adult: **IV** 1 g/250-500 ml D_5W or 0.9% NaCl over 1-2 hr or q12h × 3-5 days; may repeat after 2 days; not to exceed 50 mg/kg/day; may be given as a cont inf over 8-24 hr
Adult: IM 35 mg/kg bid
Child: IM 35 mg/kg/day in divided doses q8-12h, not to exceed 50 mg/kg/day; may give for 3-5 days, off 4 days before next course

Uses: Lead poisoning, acute lead encephalopathy

Contraindications: Hypersensitivity,

anuria, poisoning of other metals, severe renal disease, child <3 yr

edetate disodium (Rx)

Func. class.: Metal antagonist

Dosage and routes

Adult and child: **IV** inf 15-50 mg/kg/day in 2 divided doses, diluted in 500 ml D_5W or 0.9% NaCl, given over 3-4 hr, not to exceed 3 g/day (adult) or 70 mg/kg/day (child); allow 5 days between courses (child), 2 days (adult)

Uses: Hypercalcemic crisis, control of ventricular dysrhythmias associated with digitalis toxicity

Contraindications: Hypersensitivity, anuria, hepatic insufficiency, poisoning of other metals, severe renal disease, child <3 yr, seizure disorders, active/inactive TB

efalizumab (Rx)

Func. class.: Immunosuppressive

Dosage and routes

Adult: SUBCUT 0.7 mg/kg as a conditioning dose, then SUBCUT 1 mg/kg qwk, max single dose 200 mg

Uses: Adults 18 years of age and older with moderate to severe plaque psoriasis

Contraindications: Hypersensitivity

estramustine

Func. class.: Antineoplastic

Dosage and routes

Adult: PO 10-16 mg/kg in 3-4 divided doses/day; treatment may continue for ≥3 mo or 600 mg/m^2/day in 3 divided doses

Uses: Metastatic prostate cancer

Contraindications: Pregnancy **D**, hypersensitivity to estradiol, thromboembolic disorders

ethosuximide (Rx)

Func. class.: Anticonvulsant

Dosage and routes

Adult and child >6 yr: PO 250 mg bid initially; may increase by 250 mg q4-7d, max 2 g/day

Child 3-6 yr: PO 250 mg/day or 125 mg bid; may increase by 250 mg q4-7d

Uses: Absence seizures, partial seizures, tonic-clonic seizures

Contraindications: Hypersensitivity

etomidate (Rx)

Func. class.: General anesthetic

Dosage and routes

Adult and child >10 yr: **IV** 0.2-0.6 mg/kg over ½-1 min

Uses: Induction of general anesthesia

Contraindications: Hypersensitivity, labor/delivery

felbamate (Rx)

Func. class.: Anticonvulsant

Dosage and routes

Adjunctive therapy

Adult or child >14 yr: PO add 1.2 g/day in 3-4 divided doses; reduce other anticonvulsants (valproic acid, phenytoin, carbamazepine, and derivatives) by 20% to control plasma concentrations; may increase felbamate in 1.2 g/day increments qwk, up to 3.6 g/day

Monotherapy

Adult: PO 1.2 g/day in 3-4 divided doses; titrate with close supervision; increase dose in 600 mg increments q2 wk to 3.6 g/day if needed

Lennox-Gastaut syndrome adjunctive therapy

Child (2-14 yr): PO add 15 mg/kg/day in 3-4 divided doses; reduce other anticonvulsants (valproic acid, phenytoin, carbamazepine, and derivatives) by 20% to control plasma concentrations; may increase felbamate 15 mg/kg/day q wk up to 45 mg/day

Uses: Partial seizures, with or without generalization in adults; partial and generalized seizures in children with Lennox-Gastaut syndrome

Contraindications: Hypersensitivity to this drug, other carbamates, history of blood dyscrasia, aplastic anemia, hepatic disease

fenoprofen (Rx)

Func. class.: Nonsteroidal antiinflammatory/nonopioid analgesic

Dosage and routes

Pain

Adult: PO 200 mg q4-6h prn

Arthritis

Adult: PO 300-600 mg qid, not to exceed 3.2 g/day

Uses: Mild to moderate pain, osteoarthritis, rheumatoid arthritis, acute gout, arthritis, inflammation

Contraindications: Hypersensitivity, asthma, severe renal disease, severe hepatic disease

flavoxate (Rx)

Func. class.: Spasmolytic

Dosage and routes

Adult and child >12 yr: PO 100-200 mg tid-qid

Uses: Relief of nocturia, incontinence, suprapubic pain, dysuria, frequency associated with urologic conditions (symptomatic only)

Contraindications: Hypersensitivity, GI obstruction, GI hemorrhage, GU obstruction

floxuridine (Rx)

Func. class.: Antineoplastic, antimetabolite

Dosage and routes

Adult: Intraarterial by cont inf 0.1-0.6 mg/kg/day × 1-6 wk; hepatic artery inj 0.4-0.6 mg/kg/day × 1-6 wk

Uses: GI adenocarcinoma metastatic to liver; cancer of breast, head, neck, liver, brain, gallbladder, bile duct

Contraindications: Pregnancy **D**, hypersensitivity, myelosuppression, poor nutritional status, serious infections

fludarabine (Rx)

Func. class.: Antineoplastic, antimetabolite

Dosage and routes

Adult: **IV** 25 mg/m^2 over 30 min daily × 5 days, may repeat q28 days; reconstitute with 2 ml of sterile water for inj; dissolution should occur in <15 sec

Uses: Chronic lymphocytic leukemia; non-Hodgkin's lymphoma

Contraindications: Pregnancy **D**, hypersensitivity, lactation

gallamine (Rx)

Func. class.: Neuromuscular blocker (nondepolarizing)

Dosage and routes

Adult and child >1 mo: **IV** 1 mg/kg, not to exceed 100 mg, then 0.5-1 mg/kg q30-40 min

Child <1 mo, >5 kg: **IV** 0.25-0.75 mg/kg, then 0.01-0.05 mg/kg q30-40 min

Uses: Facilitation of endotracheal intubation, skeletal muscle relaxation during mechanical ventilation, surgery, or general anesthesia

Contraindications: Hypersensitivity to iodides

glycerin (OTC)

Func. class.: Laxative, hyperosmotic, antiglaucoma agent

Dosage and routes

Laxative

Adult and child >6 yr: REC SUPP 3 g; enema 5-15 ml

Child <6 yr: REC SUPP 1-1.5 g; enema 2-5 ml

Intraocular pressure reduction

Adult: PO 1-1.5 g/kg once, then may be given 500 mg/kg q6h

Child: PO 1-1.5 g/kg daily once, then 500 mg/kg 4-8 hr after first dose

Uses: Constipation, intraocular pressure in glaucoma; ICP, edema in the superficial layers of the cornea

Contraindications: Hypersensitivity

griseofulvin microsize/ultramicrosize (Rx)

Func. class.: Antifungal

Dosage and routes

Adult: PO 500-1000 mg daily in single or divided doses (microsize), 125-165 mg bid (ultramicrosize), or 250-330 mg daily; may need 500-660 mg in divided doses for severe infections

Child: PO 10 mg/kg/day or 30 mg/m^2/day (microsize) or 5 mg/kg/day (ultramicrosize)

Uses: Mycotic infections: tinea corporis, tinea pedis, tinea cruris, tinea barbae, tinea capitis, tinea unguium if caused by *Epidermophyton, Microsporum, Trichophyton*

Contraindications: Hypersensitivity, porphyria, hepatic disease, lupus erythematosus

guanfacine (Rx)

Func. class.: Antihypertensive

Dosage and routes

Adult: PO 1 mg/day at bedtime; may increase dose in 3-4 wk to 2 mg/day, max 4 mg daily

Uses: Hypertension in individual using a thiazide diuretic or other antihypertensives

Investigational uses: Heroin withdrawal

Contraindications: Hypersensitivity

halcinonide (Rx)

Func. class.: Corticosteroid, synthetic

Dosage and routes

Adult: TOP apply to affected area bid-tid (not around eyes)

Uses: Inflammation of corticosteroid-responsive dermatoses

Contraindications: Hypersensitivity, viral infections, fungal infections

hyaluronidase (Rx)

Func. class.: Enzyme

Dosage and routes

Adjunct

Adult and child: Inj 150 units with other drug

Urography

Adult and child: SUBCUT 75 units over scapula, then contrast medium injected at same site

Hypodermoclysis

Adult and child >3 yr: SUBCUT 150 units/L of lysis sol

Uses: Hypodermoclysis, subcutaneous urography; adjunct to dispersion of other drugs

Contraindications: Hypersensitivity to bovine products, CHF, hypoproteinemia, around infected/inflamed or cancerous area

hydroxychloroquine (Rx)

Func. class.: Antimalarial, antiarthritic

Dosage and routes

Malaria

Adult: PO suppression or prevention 200 mg qwk, begin 1-2 wk before travel, continue 4 wk after returning; treatment 400 mg, then 200 mg at 6, 24, 48 hr after 1st dose

Child: PO suppression or prevention 5 mg/kg qwk, begin 1-2 wk before travel, continue 4 wk after returning; treatment 10 mg/kg, then 5 mg/kg at 6, 24, 48 hr after 1st dose

Lupus erythematosus

Adult: PO 400 mg daily-bid; length depends on patient response; maintenance 200-400 mg daily

Rheumatoid arthritis

Adult: PO 400-600 mg daily for 4-12 wk, then 200-300 mg daily after good response

Child: PO 3-5 mg/kg/day max 400 mg/day

Uses: Malaria caused by *Plasmodium vivax, P. malariae, P. ovale, P. falciparum* (some strains); SLE, rheumatoid arthritis

Contraindications: Hypersensitivity, retinal field changes, children (long term)

isoproterenol (Rx)

Func. class.: β-Adrenergic agonist, antidysrhythmic, inotropic

Dosage and routes

Asthma, bronchospasm

Adult: SL tab 10-20 mg q6-8h, max 60 mg/day; inh 1 puff; may repeat in 2-5 min; maintenance 1-2 puffs 4-6 ×/day; **IV** 1020 mcg during anesthesia

Child: SL tab 5-10 mg q6-8h; inh 1 puff; may repeat in 2-5 min; maintenance 1-2 puffs 4-6 ×/day

Shock

Adult: **IV** inf 0.5-5 mcg/min (1 mg/500 ml of D_5W) titrate to B/P, CVP, hourly urine output

Uses: Bronchospasm, asthma, heart block, ventricular dysrhythmias, shock

Contraindications: Hypersensitivity to sympathomimetics, narrow-angle glaucoma, tachydysrhythmias

isotretinoin (Rx)

Func. class.: Dermatologic antiacne agent

Dosage and routes
Adult: PO 0.5-2 mg/kg/day in 2 divided doses × 15-20 wk; if relapse occurs, repeat after 2 mo off drug

Uses: Severe recalcitrant cystic acne

Contraindications: Pregnancy **X**, hypersensitivity, inflamed skin

kanamycin (Rx)

Func. class.: Antiinfective

Dosage and routes
Severe systemic infections
Adult and child: **IV** inf 15 mg/kg/day in divided doses q8-12h; diluted 500 mg/200 ml of NS or D_5W given over 30-60 min, not to exceed 1.5 g/day; IM 15 mg/kg/day in divided doses q8-12h, not to exceed 1.5 g/day; irrigation not to exceed 1.5 g/day; inh 250 mg qid

Preoperative bowel sterilization
Adult: PO 1 g qh × 4 doses, then q6h × 36-72 hr

Renal dose
Adult: IM/**IV** 7.5 mg/kg, may increase or decrease dose based on renal status

Uses: Severe systemic infections of CNS; respiratory, GI, urinary tract; bone, skin, soft tissues caused by *Escherichia coli, Acinetobacter, Proteus, Klebsiella pneumoniae, Pseudomonas aeruginosa;* also as an adjunct in hepatic coma, peritonitis, preoperatively to sterilize bowel; decreases ammonia-producing bacteria in bowel and IP after fecal spill during surgery

Contraindications: Pregnancy **D**, bowel obstruction, severe renal disease, hypersensitivity

laronidase (Rx)

Func. class.: Drug—miscellaneous

Dosage and routes
Adult: **IV** inf 0.58 mg/kg qwk; pretreat with antipyretic and/or antihistamines 1 hr prior to **IV** inf

Uses: Mucopolysaccharidosis I (MPSI), patients with Hurler and Hurler-Scheie forms of MPSI

Contraindications: Hypersensitivity

levobupivacaine (Rx)

Func. class.: Local anesthetic

Dosage and routes
Varies with route of anesthesia

Uses: Local, regional anesthesia, surgical anesthesia, pain management, continuous epidural analgesia

Contraindications: Hypersensitivity, children <12 yr, elderly, severe hepatic disease

miglustat (Rx)

Func. class.: Agent—miscellaneous

Dosage and routes
Adult: PO 100 mg tid, without regard to food

Uses: Adults with mild to moderate type 1 Gaucher disease

Contraindications: Pregnancy **X**, hypersensitivity

mitotane (Rx)

Func. class.: Antineoplastic

Dosage and routes
Adult: PO 9-10 g/day in divided doses tid or qid; may have to decrease dosage if severe reactions occur

Uses: Adrenocortical carcinoma

Contraindications: Hypersensitivity

modafinil (Rx)

Func. class.: Cerebral stimulant
Controlled substance schedule IV

Dosage and routes
Adult: PO 200 mg daily in the AM, may increase to 400 mg daily if needed

Hepatic dose
Reduce dose by 50%

Uses: Narcolepsy, sleep apnea

Investigational uses: Fatigue

Contraindications: Hypersensitivity, hyperthyroidism, hypertension, glaucoma, severe arteriosclerosis, drug abuse, CV disease, anxiety

neomycin (Rx)
Func. class.: Antiinfective

Dosage and routes
Hepatic encephalopathy
Adult: PO 4-12 g/day in divided doses × 5-6 days
Child: PO 50-100 mg/kg/day in divided doses

Preoperative intestinal antisepsis
Adult: PO on 3rd day of a 3-day regimen; give 1 g early PM; repeat in 1 hr; repeat at bedtime (given with erythromycin); give saline cathartic before giving this drug
Child: PO 14.7 mg/kg or 4.7 mg/m^2 q4h × 3 days

Uses: Severe systemic infections of CNS, respiratory tract, GI tract, urinary tract, eye, bone, skin, soft tissues, also used for hepatic coma, preoperatively to sterilize bowel, infectious diarrhea; minor skin infections (TOP)

Contraindications: Bowel obstruction (PO use), severe renal disease, hypersensitivity, infants, children

papaverine (Rx)
Func. class.: Peripheral vasodilator

Dosage and routes
Adult: Sus rel cap 150-300 mg q8-12h; IM/**IV** 30-120 mg

Uses: Arterial spasm resulting in cerebral and peripheral ischemia, myocardial ischemia associated with vascular spasm or dysrhythmias, angina pectoris, peripheral pulmonary embolism, visceral spasm as in ureteral, biliary, GI colic, peripheral vascular disease

Contraindications: Hypersensitivity, complete AV heart block

paraldehyde (Rx)
Func. class.: Anticonvulsant

Dosage and routes
Seizures
Adult: IM 5-10 ml; divide 10 ml into 2 inj; **IV** 0.2-0.4 ml/kg in NS inj
Child: IM 0.15 ml/kg; rect 0.3 ml/kg q4-6h or 1 ml/yr of age, not to exceed 5 ml; may repeat in 1 hr prn; **IV** 5 ml/90 ml NS inj; begin infusion at 5 ml/hr; titrate to patient response

Alcohol withdrawal
Adult: PO/rect 5-10 ml, not to exceed 60 ml; IM 5 ml q4-6h × 24 hr, then q6h on following days, not to exceed 30 ml

Sedation
Adult: PO/rec 4-10 ml; IM 5 ml; **IV** 3-5 ml in emergency only
Child: PO/rec/IM 0.15 ml/kg

Tetanus
Adult: **IV** 4-5 ml or 12 ml by gastric tube q4h diluted with water; IM 5-10 ml prn

Uses: Refractory seizures, status epilepticus, sedation, insomnia, alcohol withdrawal, tetanus, eclampsia

Contraindications: Hypersensitivity, gastroenteritis with ulceration

paromomycin (Rx)
Func. class.: Amebicide

Dosage and routes
Intestinal amebiasis
Adult and child: PO 25-35 mg/kg/day in 3 divided doses × 5-10 day pc

Hepatic coma
Adult: PO 4 g daily in divided doses × 5-6 day

Uses: Intestinal amebiasis, adjunct in hepatic coma

Contraindications: Hypersensitivity, renal disease, GI obstruction

pegvisomant (Rx)
Func. class.: Agent—miscellaneous

Dosage and routes
Adult: SUBCUT loading dose of 40 mg, under supervision of prescriber, then SUBCUT 10 mg daily; measure IGF-I levels q4-6 wk

Uses: Acromegaly, in those patients who have an inadequate response to other treatment

Contraindications: Hypersensitivity, latex allergy

penicillamine (Rx)
Func. class.: Heavy metal antagonist

Dosage and routes
Cystinuria
Adult: PO 250 mg qid ac, not to exceed 5 g/day
Child: PO 30 mg/kg/day in divided doses qid ac

Wilson's disease
Adult: PO 250 mg qid ac
Child: PO 20 mg/kg/day in divided doses ac

Rheumatoid arthritis
Adult: PO 125-250 mg/day, then increase 250 mg q2-3 mo if needed, not to exceed 1 g/day
Child: PO 3 mg/kg/day × 3 mo, then 6 mg/kg/day in divided doses × 3 mo, then increase to max 10 mg/kg/day

Uses: Wilson's disease, rheumatoid arthritis, cystinuria, heavy metal poisoning (lead, mercury, gold)

Contraindications: Pregnancy **D**, hypersensitivity to penicillins, anuria, agranulocytosis, severe renal disease, lactation

perflutren lipid microsphere (Rx)

Func. class.: Diagnostic drug

Dosage and routes: Use only after activation in the Vialmix apparatus
Adult: **IV** bol 10 μl/kg of the activated product within 30-60 sec, followed by 10 ml saline flush, may repeat
Adult: **IV** inf 1.3 ml/50 ml preservative-free saline, give at 4 ml/min, not to exceed 10 ml/min

Uses: Contrast enhancement during echocardiographic procedures

Contraindications: Hypersensitivity to octafluoropropane, known cardiac shunts, administration by direct intraarterial inj

permethrin (OTC, Rx)

Func. class.: Pediculicide

Dosage and routes
Lice (head)
Adult and child: Wash hair, towel dry; apply liberally to hair, leave on 10 min, rinse with water

Scabies
Adult and child: TOP 5% cream applied and massaged into all skin surfaces; leave cream on 8-14 hr, then wash

Uses: Lice, nits, ticks, flea nits

Contraindications: Hypersensitivity

phendimetrazine (Rx)

Func. class.: Anorexiant

Dosage and routes
Adult: PO 35 mg bid-tid 1 hr ac, not to exceed 70 mg tid; sus rel 105 mg daily ac AM

Uses: Exogenous obesity

Contraindications: Hypersensitivity, hyperthyroidism, hypertension, glaucoma, severe arteriosclerosis, severe cardiovascular disease, children <12 yr, agitated states, drug abuse, MAOI use within 14 days

phenoxybenzamine (Rx)

Func. class.: Antihypertensive

Dosage and routes
Adult: PO 10 mg daily; increase by 10 mg every other day; usual range 20-40 mg bid-tid
Child: PO 0.2 mg/kg or 6 mg/m^2/day, max 10 mg, may increase at 4-day intervals; maintenance dosage 0.4-1.2 mg/kg/day or 12-36 mg/m^2/day given in divided doses tid or qid

Uses: Pheochromocytoma

Contraindications: Hypersensitivity, CHF, angina, cerebral vascular insufficiency, coronary arteriosclerosis

physostigmine (Rx)

Func. class.: Antidote, reversible anticholinesterase

Dosage and routes
Overdose of anticholinergics
Adult: IM/**IV** 2 mg; give no more than 1 mg/min; may repeat
Child: IM/**IV** inj 0.02 mg/kg, not more than 0.5 mg/min; may repeat at 5-10 min intervals until max dose of 2 mg

Postanesthesia
Adult: IM/**IV** 0.5-1 mg; give no more than 1 mg/min (**IV**); can repeat at 10-30 min intervals

Uses: To reverse CNS effects of anticholinergic

Contraindications: Hypotension, obstruction of intestine or renal system, asthma, gangrene, CV disease, choline esters, depolarizing neuromuscular blocking agents, diabetes

! HIGH ALERT

pipecuronium (Rx)

Func. class.: Neuromuscular blocker (nondepolarizing)

Dosage and routes:
Adult: **IV** dosage is individualized; in patients with normal renal function who are not obese, initial dose is 70-85 mcg/kg; maintenance dose ranges from 10-15 mcg/kg
Child 1-14 yr: **IV** 57 mcg/kg
Child 3 mo-1 yr: **IV** 40 mcg/kg

Uses: Facilitation of endotracheal intubation; skeletal muscle relaxation during mechanical ventilation, surgery, or general anesthesia

Contraindications: Hypersensitivity to bromide ion

! HIGH ALERT

poractant alfa (Rx)

Func. class.: Lung surfactant extract

Dosage and routes
Premature infant: Intratracheal instill 2.5 ml/kg birth weight, up to 2 subsequent doses of 1.25 ml/kg birth weight can be administered at 12-hr intervals, max 5 ml/kg

Uses: Treatment (rescue) of respiratory distress syndrome (RDS) in premature infants

pralidoxime (Rx)

Func. class.: Cholinesterase reactivator

Dosage and routes
Anticholinesterase overdose
Adult: **IV** 1-2 g, then 250 mg q5 min until desired response

Organophosphate poisoning
Adult: **IV** inf 1-2 g/100 ml 0.9% NaCl over 15-30 min; may repeat in 1 hr; PO 1-3 g q5h
Child: **IV** inf 20-40 mg/kg/dose diluted in 100 ml 0.9% NaCl over 15-30 min

Uses: Cholinergic crisis in myasthenia gravis, organophosphate poisoning antidote (early), relief of paralysis of respiratory muscles; used as an adjunct to systemic atropine administration

Contraindications: Hypersensitivity, carbamate insecticide poisoning

reserpine (Rx)

Func. class.: Antihypertensive, antiadrenergic agent, peripherally action

Do Not Confuse:
reserpine/Risperdal

Dosage and routes
Adult: PO 0.05-0.1 mg daily × 1-2 wk, then 0.1-0.25 mg daily for maintenance
Elderly: PO 0.05 mg daily, increase by 0.05 weekly to desired dose

Uses: Hypertension

Contraindications: Pregnancy **D**, hypersensitivity, depression, suicidal patients, active peptic ulcer disease, ulcerative colitis, Parkinson's disease

! HIGH ALERT

secobarbital (Rx)

Func. class.: Sedative/hypnotic-barbiturate

Controlled substance schedule II (USA), schedule G (CDSA IV) (Canada)

Dosage and routes
Insomnia
Adult: PO/IM 100-200 mg at bedtime
Child: IM 3-5 mg/kg, max 100 mg, do not inject >5 ml in one site

Sedation/preoperatively
Adult: PO 200-300 mg 1-2 hr preoperatively
Child: PO 50-100 mg 1-2 hr preoperatively

Status epilepticus
Adult and child: IM/**IV** 250-350 mg

Acute psychotic agitation
Adult and child: IM/**IV** 5.5 mg/kg q3-4h

Uses: Insomnia, sedation, preoperative medication, status epilepticus, acute tetanus seizures

Contraindications: Pregnancy **D**, hypersensitivity to barbiturates, respiratory depression, addiction to barbiturates, severe liver impairment, porphyria, uncontrolled severe pain

sevelamer (Rx)

Func. class.: Polymeric phosphate binder

Dosage and routes
Reduction of serum phosphorus in adults not taking phosphate binders
Adult: PO initially 800-1600 mg tid with

meals based on serum phosphorus level (see below); adjust dose gradually at 2-wk intervals until serum phosphorus 6 mg/dl

Adult, serum phosphorus ≥9 mg/dl: 1600 mg tid with meals

Adult, serum phosphorus ≥7.5 and <9 mg/dl: 1200-1600 mg tid with meals

Adult, serum phosphorus >6 and <7.5 mg/dl: 800 mg tid with meals

Uses: End-stage renal disease (ESRD)

Contraindications: Hypophosphatemia, bowel obstruction, hypersensitivity

sibutramine (Rx)

Func. class.: Appetite suppressant

Controlled substance schedule IV

Dosage and routes

Adult: PO 10 mg daily; may be increased to 15 mg daily after 4 wk, or lowered to 5 mg daily depending on response

Uses: Obesity in conjunction with other treatments

Contraindications: Hypersensitivity, hypothyroidism, anorexia nervosa, severe hepatic/renal disease, uncontrolled hypertension, history of CAD, CHF, dysrhythmias, lactation, CVA

teniposide (Rx)

Func. class.: Antineoplastic

Dosage and routes

Child: **IV** inf combo teniposide 165 mg/m^2 and cytarabine 300 mg/m^2 2×/wk × 8-9 doses or combo teniposide 250 mg/m^2 and vinCRIStine 1.5 mg/m^2 qwk × 4-8 wk and predniSONE 40 mg/m^2 PO × 28 days

Uses: Childhood acute lymphoblastic leukemia (ALL), refractory childhood acute lymphocytic leukemia

Contraindications: Pregnancy **D**, hypersensitivity, bone marrow depression, severe hepatic disease, severe renal disease, bacterial infection

thioguanine (6-TG) (Rx)

Func. class.: Antineoplastic-antimetabolite

Dosage and routes

Adult and child: PO 2 mg/kg/day, then increase slowly to 3 mg/kg/day after 4 wk

Uses: Acute leukemias, chronic granulocytic leukemia, lymphomas, multiple myeloma, solid tumors

Contraindications: Pregnancy **D**, prior drug resistance, leukopenia (WBC <2500/mm^3), thrombocytopenia (platelets <100,000/mm^3), anemia

! HIGH ALERT

thiopental (Rx)

Func. class.: General anesthetic

Controlled substance schedule III

Dosage and routes

Narcoanalysis

Adult: **IV** 100 mg/min, not to exceed 50 ml/min

Sedation or narcosis

Adult: Rec 12-20 mg/lb

Increased intracranial pressure

Adult: 1.5-3.5 mg/kg

Uses: Short, general anesthesia; narcoanalysis, induction anesthesia before other anesthetics

Investigational uses: Increased intracranial pressure

Contraindications: Hypersensitivity, status asthmaticus, porphyrias

thiotepa (Rx)

Func. class.: Antineoplastic

Dosage and routes

Adult: **IV** 0.3-0.4 mg/kg at 1-4 wk intervals

Neoplastic effusions

Adult: Intracavity 0.6-0.8 mg/kg

Bladder cancer

Adult: Instill 60 mg/30-60 ml water for inj instilled in bladder for 2 hr once/wk × 4 wk

Uses: Hodgkin's disease, lymphomas; breast, ovarian, lung, bladder cancer; neoplastic effusions

Contraindications: Pregnancy **D**, hypersensitivity

thiothixene (Rx)

Func. class.: Antipsychotic/neuroleptic

Dosage and routes

Adult: PO 2-5 mg bid-qid depending on severity of condition; dose gradually increased to 15-30 mg if needed; IM 4 mg bid-qid; max dose 30 mg daily; administer PO dose as soon as possible

Elderly: PO 1-2 mg daily-bid, increase by 1-2 mg q4-7 days to desired dose

Uses: Psychotic disorders, schizophrenia, acute agitation

Contraindications: Hypersensitivity, blood dyscrasias, child <12 yr, bone marrow depression, circulatory collapse, CNS depression, coma, alcoholism, CV disease, hepatic disease, Reye's syndrome, narrow-angle glaucoma

Appendix G Less Frequently Used Antihistamines

GENERIC NAME	TRADE NAME(S)	USES	DOSAGES AND ROUTES	AVAILABLE FORMS	INTERACTIONS	CONTRAINDICATIONS
acrivastine/ pseudoephedrine (Rx)	Semprex-D	• Rhinitis • Allergy symptoms • Chronic idiopathic urticaria	• Adult, child >12 yr: PO 8 mg q4-6h	• Caps 8 mg/60 mg	• Increased CNS depression: alcohol, opioids, sedatives, hypnotics • Hypertensive crisis: MAOIs • May increase CNS depression: kava • May increase anticholinergic effect: henbane leaf	• Hypersensitivity to this drug or triprolidine • Severe hypertension • Cardiac disease
azatadine (Rx)	Optimine	• Allergy symptoms • Rhinitis • Chronic urticaria	• Adult: PO 1-2 mg bid, not to exceed 4 mg/day • Elderly: PO 1 mg daily-bid	• Tabs 1 mg	• Increased CNS depression: barbiturates, opioids, hypnotics, tricyclic antidepressants, alcohol • Decreased effect of: oral anticoagulants • Increased effect of azatadine: MAOIs • Increased CNS depression: kava • Increased anticholinergic effect: henbane leaf	• Hypersensitivity to H_1-receptor antagonists • Acute asthma attack • Lower respiratory tract disease • Child <12 yr
buclizine (Rx)	Bucladin-S, Softabs	• Motion sickness • Dizziness • Nausea • Vomiting • Antihistamine	• Adult: PO 25-50 mg prn ½ hr before travel; may be repeated q4-6h prn	• Tabs 50 mg	• Increased anticholinergic effect: henbane leaf • Increased CNS depression: kava	• Hypersensitivity to cyclizines • Shock

clemastine (Rx)	Contac Allergy 12 Hour, Tavist, Antihist-1	• Allergy symptoms • Rhinitis • Angioedema • Urticaria • Common cold	• Adult/child >12 yr: PO 1.34-2.68 mg bid-tid, not to exceed 8.04 mg/day	• Tabs 1.34, 2.68 mg • Syr 0.67 mg/ml	• Increased CNS depression: barbiturates, opiates, hypnotics, tricyclics, alcohol • Increased effect of clemastine: MAOIs • Increased CNS depression: kava • Increased anticholinergic effect: henbane leaf	• Hypersensitivity to H_1-receptor antagonists • Acute asthma attack • Lower respiratory tract disease
cyclizine (OTC, Rx)	Marezine	• Motion sickness • Prevention of postoperative vomiting • Antihistamine	*Vomiting* • Adult: IM 25-50 mg ½ hr before termination of surgery, then q4-6h prn (lactate) • Child: IM 3 mg/kg divided in 3 equal doses *Motion sickness* • Adult: PO 50 mg then q4-6h prn, not to exceed 200 mg/day (HCl) • Child: PO 25 mg q4-6h prn	• Tabs (HCl) 50 mg • Inj (lactate) 50 mg/ml	• May increase CNS effect: alcohol, tranquilizers, opioids • Increased CNS depression: kava	• Hypersensitivity to cyclizines • Shock
dexchlorpheniramine (Rx)	Dexchlor, dexclorpheniramine maleate, Poladex, Polaramine	• Allergy symptoms • Rhinitis • Pruritus • Contact dermatitis	• Adult: PO 1-2 mg tid-qid; repeat action 4-6 mg bid-tid • Child 6-11 yr: PO 1 mg q4-6h, or time rel 4 mg at bedtime • Child 2-5 yr: PO 0.5 mg q4-6h; do not use repeat action form	• Tabs 2 mg • Repeat action tabs 4, 6 mg • Syr 2 mg/5 ml	• Increased CNS depression: barbiturates, opioids, hypnotics, tricyclic antidepressants, alcohol • Decreased effect: oral anticoagulants, heparin • Increased effect of dexchlorpheniramine: MAOIs • Increased anticholinergic effect: henbane leaf	• Hypersensitivity to H_1-receptor antagonists • Acute asthma attack • Lower respiratory tract disease

Continued

Appendix G Less Frequently Used Antihistamines—cont'd

GENERIC NAME	TRADE NAME(S)	USES	DOSAGES AND ROUTES	AVAILABLE FORMS	INTERACTIONS	CONTRAINDICATIONS
trimeprazine (Rx)	Panectyl ♣, Temaril	• Pruritus	• Adult: PO 2.5 mg qid; time-rel 5 mg bid • Elderly: PO 2.5 mg bid • Child 3-12 yr: PO 2.5 mg tid or at bedtime • Child 6 mo-1 yr: PO 1.25 mg tid or at bedtime	• Tabs 2.5 mg • Time rel spanules 5 mg • Syr 2.5 mg/5 ml	• Increased CNS depression: barbiturates, opioids, hypnotics, tricyclic antidepressants, alcohol • Decreased effect of oral anticoagulants, heparin • Increased effect of trimeprazine: MAOIs • Increased anticholinergic effect: henbane leaf	• Hypersensitivity to H_1-receptor antagonists • Acute asthma attack • Lower respiratory tract disease
tripelennamine (Rx)	PBZ, PBZ-SR, Pelamine, tripelennamine HCl	• Rhinitis • Allergy symptoms	• Adults: PO 25-50 mg q4-6h, not to exceed 600 mg/day; time-rel 100 mg bid-tid, not to exceed 600 mg/day • Child >5 yr: PO time-rel 50 mg q8-12h, not to exceed 300 mg/day • Child <5 yr: PO 5 mg/kg/day in 4-6 divided doses, not to exceed 300 mg/day	• Tabs 25, 50 mg • Time-rel tabs 100 mg • Elix 37.5 mg/5 ml	• Increased CNS depression: barbiturates, opioids, hypnotics, tricyclic antidepressants, alcohol • Decreased effect of oral anticoagulants, heparin • Increased effect of tripelennamine: MAOIs • Increased anticholinergic effect: henbane leaf	• Hypersensitivity to H_1-receptor antagonists • Acute asthma attack • Lower respiratory tract disease

◆ Alert ♣ Canada Only 🔑 Key Drug

Appendix H Vaccines and Toxoids

GENERIC NAME	TRADE NAME	USES	DOSAGES AND ROUTES	CONTRAINDICATIONS
BCG vaccine	TICE BCG	TB exposure	Adult/child >1 mo: 0.2-0.3 ml Child <1 mo: Reduce dose by 50% using 2 ml of sterile water after reconstituting	Hypersensitivity, hypogammaglobulinemia, positive TB test, burns
cholera vaccine	No trade name	Immunization for cholera in other countries	Adult/child >10 yr: IM/SUBCUT 2× of 0.5 ml, 7-30 days before traveling to areas with cholera Booster is used q6 mo 0.5 ml prn	Hypersensitivity, acute febrile illness
diphtheria and tetanus toxoids, adsorbed	No trade name	Induces antitoxins to provide immunity to diphtheria, tetanus	Adult/child ≥7 yr: IM (adult strength) 0.5 ml q4-8 wk × 2 doses, then 3rd dose 6-12 mo after 2nd dose, booster IM 0.5 ml q10 yr Child 1-6 yr: IM (pediatric strength) 0.5 ml q4 wk × 2 doses, booster 6-12 mo after 2nd dose Infant 6 wk-1 yr: IM (pediatric strength) 0.5 ml q4 wk × 3 doses, booster 6-12 mo after 3rd dose	Hypersensitivity to mercury, thimerosal, immunocompromised patients, radiation, corticosteroids, acute illness
diphtheria and tetanus toxoids and whole-cell pertussis vaccine (DPT, DTP)	DTwP, Tr-Immunol	Prevention of diphtheria, tetanus, pertussis	Adult: booster dose q10 yr Child >6 wk-6 yr: IM 0.5 ml at 2, 4, 6 mo, 1-½ yr; booster needed 0.5 ml at age 6	Hypersensitivity, active infection, poliomyelitis outbreak, immunosuppression, febrile illness
diphtheria and tetanus toxoids and acellular pertussis vaccine	Acel-Imune, DTaP, Tripedia			

TB, Tuberculosis; *DPT*, diphtheria-pertussis-tetanus (vaccine); *DTP*, diphtheria and tetanus toxoids and pertussis vaccine.

Continued

GENERIC NAME	TRADE NAME	USES	DOSAGES AND ROUTES	CONTRAINDICATIONS
haemophilus b conjugate vaccine, diphtheria CRM_{197} protein conjugate (HbOC) haemophilus b conjugate vaccine, meningococcal protein conjugate (PRP-OMP)	HibTITER PedvaxHIB	Polysaccharide immunization of children 2-6 yr against *H. influenzae b*, conjugate immunization of child 2, 4, 6 mo	**HibTITER (IM only)** Child: IM 0.5 ml Child 2-6 mo: 0.5 ml q2 mo × 3 inj Child 7-11 mo: Previously unvaccinated 0.5 ml q2mo inj Child 12-14 mo: previously unvaccinated 0.5 ml × 1 inj **PEDVAXHIB (IM only)** Child 2-14 mo: 0.5 ml × 2 inj at 2, 4 mo of age (6 mo dose not needed), then booster at 12-18 mo against invasive disease Child ≥15 mo: Previously unvaccinated 0.5 ml inj	Hypersensitivity, febrile illness, active infection
hepatitis A vaccine, inactivated	Havrix, Vaqta	Active immunization against hepatitis A virus	Adults: IM 1, 440 EL units (Havrix) or 50 units (Vaqta) as a single dose, booster dose is the same given at 6, 12 mo Child 2-18 yr: IM 720 EL units (Havrix) or 25 units (Vaqta) as a single dose, booster dose is the same given at 6, 12 mo	Hypersensitivity
hepatitis B vaccine, recombinant	Engerix-B, Recombivax HB	Immunization against all subtypes of hepatitis B virus	Varies widely	Hypersensitivity to this vaccine or yeast

influenza virus vaccine, trivalent A and B (whole virus/split virus)	Fluogen, FluShield, Fluviral ✤, Fluvirin, Fluzone, influenza virus vaccine, trivalent	Prevention of Russian, Chilean, Philippine influenza	Adult/child >12 yr: IM 0.5 ml in 1 dose Child 3-12 yr: IM 0.5 ml, repeat in 1 mo (split) unless 1978-1985 vaccine was given Child 6 mo to 3 yr: IM 0.25 ml, repeat in 1 mo (split) unless 1978-1985 vaccine was given	Hypersensitivity, active infection, chicken egg allergy, Guillain-Barré syndrome, active neurologic disorders
Japanese encephalitis virus vaccine, inactivated	JE-VAX	Active immunity against Japanese encephalitis (JE)	Adult/child ≥3 yr: SUBCUT 1 ml, days 0, 7, 30; booster SUBCUT 1 ml 2 yr after last dose Child 1-3 yr: SUBCUT 0.5 ml, days 0, 7, 30; booster SUBCUT 0.5 ml 2 yr after last dose	Hypersensitivity to murine, thimerosal; allergic reactions to previous dose
Lyme disease vaccine (recombinant OspA)	LYMErix	Immunization against Lyme disease	Adult and adolescent 15-70: IM 30 mcg in deltoid, repeat at 1, 12 mo after first dose	Hypersensitivity, antibiotic refractory Lyme arthritis
measles and rubella virus vaccine, live attenuated	M-R-Vax II	Immunity to measles and rubella by antibody production	Adult/child ≥15 mo: SUBCUT 0.5 ml (1000 units)	Hypersensitivity, immunocompromised patients, active untreated TB, cancer, blood dyscrasias, radiation, corticosteroids, pregnancy; allergic reactions to neomycin, eggs
measles, mumps, and rubella vaccine, live	M-M-R-II	Prevention of measles, mumps, rubella	Adult: SUBCUT 1 vial; 2 vials separated by 1 mo, in person born after 1957 Child >15 mo and adult: SUBCUT 0.5 ml	Hypersensitivity, blood dyscrasias, anemia, active infection, immunosuppression; egg, chicken allergy; pregnancy, febrile illness, neomycin allergy, neoplasms

◆ Alert ✤ Canada Only 🗝 Key Drug

Continued

GENERIC NAME	TRADE NAME	USES	DOSAGES AND ROUTES	CONTRAINDICATIONS
measles virus vaccine, live attenuated	Attenuvax	Immunity to measles by antibody production	Adult/child ≥15 mo: SUBCUT 0.5 ml (1000 units), one dose 15 mo, 2nd dose age 4-6 or 11, or 12	Hypersensitivity to eggs, neomycin; cancer, radiation, corticosteroids, pregnancy, immunocompromised patients, blood dyscrasias, active untreated TB
meningococcal polysaccharide vaccine	Menomune-A/C/Y/W-135	Prophylaxis to meningococcal meningitis	Adult/child >2 yr: SUBCUT 0.5 ml	Hypersensitivity to thimerosal, pregnancy, acute illness
mumps virus vaccine, live	Mumpsvax	Active immunity to mumps	Adult/child ≥1 yr: SUBCUT 0.5 ml (20,000 units)	Hypersensitivity to eggs, neomycin; cancer, radiation, corticosteroids, pregnancy, immunocompromised patients, blood dyscrasias, active untreated TB
plague vaccine	No trade name	Active immunity to *Yersinia pestis* plague	Adult: IM 1 ml, then 0.2 ml in 4-12 wk, then 0.2 ml 5-6 mo after 2nd dose; booster 0.1-0.2 ml q6 mo when in area where plague is present	Hypersensitivity to phenol, sulfites, formaldehyde, beef, soy, casein; pregnancy, coagulation disorders
pneumococcal 7-valent conjugate vaccine	Prevnar	Immunity against *Streptococcus pneumoniae*	Child: IM 0.5 ml × 3 doses (7-11 mo); × 2 doses (12-23 mo); × 1 dose >2-9 yr	Hypersensitivity to diphtheria toxoid or this product
pneumococcal vaccine, polyvalent	Pneumovax 23, Pnu-Imune 23	Pneumococcal immunization	Adult/child >2 yr: IM/SUBCUT 0.5 ml	Hypersensitivity, Hodgkin's disease, ARDS
poliovirus vaccine, live, oral, trivalent (TOPV) poliovirus vaccine (IPV)	Orimune, IPOL	Prevention of polio	Adult/child >2 yr: PO 0.5 ml, given q8 wk × 2 doses, then 0.5 ml ½-1 yr after dose 2 Infant: PO 0.5 at 2,4, 18 mo; booster at 4-6 yr; may also be given IPV at 2, 4 mo, then TOPV at 12-18 mo, booster at 4-6 yr	Hypersensitivity, active infection, allergy to neomycin/streptomycin, immunosuppression, vomiting, diarrhea

rabies vaccine, adsorbed	No trade name	Active immunity to rabies	**Preexposure** Adult/child: IM 1 ml day 0, 7, 21, or 28 days (total 3 doses); booster IM 1 ml prn q2-5 yr **Postexposure** Adult/child not vaccinated: IM 20 international units/kg of HRIG and 5 1 ml inj of rabies vaccine on days 0, 7, 14, 28	Severe hypersensitivity to previous inj of vaccine, thimerosal
rabies vaccine, HDCV	IMOVax Rabies, IM-OVax Rabies I.D.	Active immunity to rabies	**Preexposure** Adult/child: IM 1 ml day 0, 7, 21 or 28 **Postexposure** Adult/child: IM 1 ml on day 0, 3, 7, 14, 28	No contraindications
rubella and mumps virus vaccine, live	Biavax II	Immunity to rubella and mumps by antibody production	Adult/child ≥1 yr: SUBCUT 0.5 ml	Hypersensitivity to eggs, neomycin; cancer, radiation, corticosteroids, pregnancy, immunocompromised patients, blood dyscrasias, active untreated TB
rubella virus vaccine, live attenuated (RA 27/3)	Meruvax II	Immunity to rubella by antibody production	Adult/child ≥1 yr: SUBCUT 0.5 ml (1000 units)	Hypersensitivity to eggs, neomycin; cancer, radiation, corticosteroids
tetanus toxoid, adsorbed/tetanus toxoid	No trade name	Tetanus toxoid: used for prophylactic treatment of wounds	Adult/child: IM 0.5 ml q4-6 wk × 2 doses, then 0.5 ml 1 yr after dose 2 (adsorbed); SUBCUT/IM 0.5 ml q4-8 wk × 3 doses, then 0.5 ml 1/2-1 yr after dose 3, booster dose 0.5 ml q10 yr	Hypersensitivity, active infection, poliomyelitis outbreak, immunosuppression

ARDS, Acute respiratory distress syndrome; *HRIG,* human rabies immune globulin; *HDCV,* human diploid cell vaccine.

Continued

GENERIC NAME	TRADE NAME	USES	DOSAGES AND ROUTES	CONTRAINDICATIONS
typhoid vaccine, parenteral typhoid vaccine, oral	No trade name Vivotif Berna Vaccine	Active immunity to typhoid fever	Adult: PO 1 cap 1 hr before meals × 4 doses, booster q5 yr Adult/child >10 yr: SUBCUT 0.5 ml, repeat in 4 wk, booster q3 yr Child 6 mo-10 yr: SUBCUT 0.25 ml, repeat in 4 wk, booster q3 yr	Parenteral: systemic or allergic reaction, acute respiratory or other acute infection, intensive physical exercise in high temp Oral: hypersensitivity, acute febrile illness, suppressive or antibiotic drugs
typhoid Vi polysaccharide vaccine	Typhim Vi	Active immunity to typhoid fever	Adult/child ≥2 yr: IM 0.5 ml as a single dose, reimmunize q2 yr 0.5 ml IM, if needed	Hypersensitivity, chronic typhoid carriers
varicella virus vaccine	Varivax	Prevention of varicella-zoster (chickenpox)	Adult/child ≥13 yr: SUBCUT 0.5 ml, 2nd dose SUBCUT 0.5 ml 4-8 wk later	Hypersensitivity to neomycin; blood dyscrasias, immunosuppression, active untreated TB, acute illness, pregnancy, diseases of lymphatic system
yellow fever vaccine	YF-Vax	Active immunity to yellow fever	Adult/child ≥9 mo: SUBCUT 0.5 ml deeply, booster q10 yr Child 6-9 mo: same as above if exposed	Hypersensitivity to egg or chicken embryo protein, pregnancy, child <6 mo, immunodeficiency

Appendix I

Herbal Products

acidophilus

Uses: Diarrhea, vaginal and other candida infections, urinary tract infections, atopic dermatitis (eczema), atopic disease, IBS, respiratory tract infections

alfalfa

Uses:
- *External:* Boils and insect bites
- *Internal:* Constipation, arthritis, increase blood clotting, diuretic, relieve inflammation of the prostate, treat acute or chronic cystitis, nutrient source

aloe

Uses of aloe vera gel: Minor burns, skin irritations, minor wounds, frostbite, radiation-caused injuries

angelica

Uses: Poor blood flow to the extremities, headaches, backaches, osteoporosis, asthma, allergies, skin disorders, diuretic, antispasmodic, cholagogue, stomach cancer, mild antiseptic, expectorant, bronchitis, ease rheumatic pains, stomach cramps, muscle spasms

anise

Uses:
- *External:* Treat catarrhs of respiratory system (asthma, bronchitis), cancer, cholera, colic, dysmenorrheal, epilepsy, indigestion, insomnia, lice, migraine, nausea, neuralgia, rash, scabies; given to children to reduce gas, colic, and respiratory symptoms
- *Internal:* Expectorant, bronchitis, emphysema, whooping cough, antibacterial, antispasmodic, abortifacient (large quantities), diaphoretic, diuretic, stimulant, tonic, flavoring in food

astragalus

Uses: Bronchitis, COPD, colds, flu, gastrointestinal conditions, weakness, fatigue, chronic hepatitis, ulcers, hypertension and viral myocarditis, immune stimulant, aphrodisiac, and improve sperm motility

bilberry

Uses: Improve night vision, prevent cataracts, macular degeneration, glaucoma, varicose veins, hemorrhoids, diabetic retinopathy, myopia, mild diarrhea, dyspepsia in adults or children, controlling insulin levels, diuretic, urinary antiseptic

black cohosh

Uses: Smooth-muscle relaxant, antispasmodic, antitussive, astringent, diuretic, antidiarrheal, antiarthritic, hormone balancer in perimenopausal women, decrease uterine spasms in first trimester of pregnancy, antiabortion agent, dysmenorrheal

Adapted from Skidmore-Roth L: *Mosby's Handbook of Herbs & Natural Supplements, ed 3,* St. Louis, 2006, Elsevier.

buckthorn

Uses: Powerful laxative

capsicum peppers

Uses:
- *External:* Diabetic neuropathy, psoriasis, postmastectomy pain, Raynaud's disease, herpes zoster, arthritic, muscular pain, poor peripheral circulation
- *Internal:* Cardiovascular health, CAD, reduce cholesterol and blood clotting, peptic ulcer disease, cold, flu

cascara

Uses: Laxative

chamomile

Uses:
- *External:* As an antiseptic and soothing agent for inflamed skin and minor wounds
- *Internal:* As an antispasmodic, antianxiety, gas-relieving, and antiinflammatory agent for the treatment of digestive problems; light sleep aid and sedative

chondroitin

Uses: Alone or in combination with glucosamine for joint conditions, as an antithrombotic, extravasation therapy agent, for ischemic heart disease, hyperlipidemia

chromium

Uses: Essential trace mineral required for proper metabolic functioning, decreases glucose tolerance, arteriosclerosis, elevated cholesterol, glaucoma, hypoglycemia, diabetes, obesity

coenzyme Q10

Uses: Ischemic heart disease, congestive heart failure (CHF), angina pectoris, hypertension, arrhythmias, diabetes mellitus, deafness, Bell's palsy, decreased immunity, mitral valve prolapse, periodontal disease, infertility

dong quai

Uses: Menopausal symptoms, menstrual irregularities, headache neuralgia, herpes infections, malaria, vitiligo, anemia

echinacea

Uses:
- *External:* Wound healing, bruises, burns, scratches, leg ulcers
- *Internal:* Immune stimulant, prophylaxis for colds, influenzae, other infections

eyebright

Uses: Internally and externally to relieve eye fatigue, redness, sty and eye infections, nasal catarrh in sinusitis and hay fever

feverfew

Uses: Menstrual irregularities, threatened spontaneous abortion, arthritis, fever

flax

Uses:
- *External*: Inflammatory
- *Internal*: Laxative anticholesteremic

garlic

Uses: Antilipidemic, antimicrobial, antiasthmatic, antiinflammatory, possible antihypertensive, treatment for some heavy metal poisonings

ginger

Uses: Antioxidant, nausea, motion sickness, vomiting, sore throat, migraine headaches

ginkgo

Uses: Poor circulation, age-related decline in cognition, memory; vascular disease, antioxidant, depressive mood disorders, sexual dysfunction, asthma, glaucoma, menopausal symptoms, multiple sclerosis, headaches, tinnitus, dizziness, arthritis, altitude sickness, intermittent claudication

ginseng

Uses: Physical and mental exhaustion, stress, sluggishness, fatigue, weak immunity, as a tonic

goldenseal

Uses: Gastritis, gastrointestinal ulceration, peptic ulcer disease, mouth ulcer, bladder infection, sore throat, postpartum hemorrhage, skin disorders, cancer, tuberculosis, wound healing, antiinflammatory, in combination with echinacea for cold and flu

green tea

Uses: Antioxidant, anticancer agent, diuretic, stimulant, antibacterial, antilipidemic, antiatherosclerotic

hops

Uses: Analgesic, hyperactivity, anthelmintic, mild sedative, insomnia, menopausal symptoms

kava

Uses: Anxiolytic, antiepileptic, antidepressant, antipsychotic, nervous anxiety, hyperactivity, restlessness, sleep disturbances, headache, muscle relaxant, wound healing

khat

Uses: Fatigue, obesity, gastric ulcers, depression

lemon balm

Uses:
- *External:* Cold sores
- *Internal:* Insomnia, anxiety, gastric conditions, psychiatric conditions, Graves' disease, attention deficit disorder (ADD)

licorice

Uses: Allergies, arthritis, asthma, constipation, esophagitis, gastritis, hepatitis, inflammatory conditions, peptic ulcers, poor adrenal function, poor appetite

lysine

Uses: Cold sores, herpes infections, Bell's palsy, rheumatoid arthritis, detoxify opiates

maitake

Uses: Diabetes, hypertension, high cholesterol, obesity, cancer

melatonin

Uses: Insomnia, inhibit cataract formation, increase longevity, epilepsy, hypertension, various cancers, jet lag, cancer protection, oral contraceptive

panax ginseng

Uses: Physical and mental exhaustion, stress, sluggishness, fatigue, weak immunity, as a tonic

papaya

Uses:

- *External:* Debridement of worms
- *Internal:* Intestinal worms, gastrointestinal disorders, injection in a herniated lumbar intervertebral disk

raspberry

Uses:

- *External:* Leaves promote diuresis, treat inflammation, cough, wounds
- *Internal:* UTIs, renal calculi, antimicrobial action, morning sickness and speed, ease labor in pregnancy

red clover

Uses: Antispasmodic, expectorant, sedative, psoriasis, eczema, amenorrhea

St. John's wort

Uses:

- *External:* Antiinflammatory, relieve hemorrhoids, treat vitiligo, burns
- *Internal:* Depression, anxiety

SAM-e

Uses: Depression, Alzheimer's disease, migraine headache, hypersensitivity, chronic liver disease, fibromyalgia pain, inflammation in osteoarthritis

saw palmetto

Uses: Benign prostatic hypertrophy, mild diuretic, chronic and subacute cystitis, increase breast size, sperm count, sexual potency

senna

Uses: Laxative

siberian ginseng

Uses: Increase immunity, energy and performance, decrease inflammation and insomnia

turmeric

Uses: Menstrual disorders, colic, inflammation, bruising, dyspepsia, hematuria, flatulence

valerian

Uses: Sedative

wintergreen

Uses:

- *External:* Sore, inflamed muscles and joints
- *Internal:* Bladder inflammation, urinary tract diseases, diseases of prostate and kidney

yohimbe

Uses: Aphrodisiac, hallucinogenic

Appendix J

FDA Pregnancy Categories

A No risk demonstrated to the fetus in any trimester
B No adverse effects in animals, no human studies available
C Only given after risks to the fetus are considered; animal studies have shown adverse reactions, no human studies available
D Definite fetal risks, may be given in spite of risks if needed in life-threatening conditions
X Absolute fetal abnormalities; not to be used anytime during pregnancy

Note: **UK** = Unknown fetal risk (used in this text but not an official FDA pregnancy category).

Appendix K

Controlled Substance Chart

DRUGS	UNITED STATES*
Heroin, LSD, peyote, marijuana, mescaline	Schedule I • High abuse potential • No currently accepted medical use
Opium (morphine), meperidine, amphetamines, cocaine, short-acting barbiturates (secobarbital)	Schedule II • High abuse potential; potentially severe psychologic or physical dependence • Currently accepted medical use but may be severely restricted • Telephone orders only in emergencies if written Rx follows promptly • No refills
Glutethimide, paregoric, phendimetrazine	Schedule III • Abuse potential less than the drugs/substances in Schedules I and II; potentially moderate or low physical dependence or high psychologic dependence • Currently accepted medical use • Telephone orders permitted • Prescriber may authorize limited refills
Chloral hydrate, chlordiazepoxide, diazepam, mazindol, meprobamate, phenobarbital	Schedule IV • Low abuse potential relative to drugs/substances in Schedule III; potentially limited physical or psychologic dependence • Currently accepted medical use • Telephone orders permitted • Prescriber may authorize limited refills
Antidiarrheals with opium, antitussives	Schedule V • Lowest abuse potential; potentially very limited physical or psychologic dependence • Currently accepted medical use • Prescriber determines refills • Some products containing limited amounts of Schedule V substances (e.g., cough suppressants) available OTC to patients >18 yr

*See appendix N for Canadian controlled substance chart

Appendix L

Commonly Used Abbreviations

abd abdomen
ABG arterial blood gas
ac before meals
ACE angiotensin-converting enzyme
ACT activated clotting time
ADA American Diabetes Association
ADH antidiuretic hormone
ALT alanine aminotransferase
ANA antinuclear antibody
AP anteroposterior
APTT activated partial thromboplastin time
ASA acetylsalicylic acid, aspirin
ASHD arteriosclerotic heart disease
AST aspartate aminotransferase (SGOT)
AV atrioventricular
bid twice a day
BM bowel movement
BMR basal metabolic rate
B/P blood pressure
BPH benign prostatic hypertrophy
BPM beats per minute
BS blood sugar
BUN blood urea nitrogen
C Celsius (centigrade)
Ca cancer
CAD coronary artery disease
cap capsule
Cath catheterization or catheterize
CBC complete blood cell count
CC chief complaint
CHF congestive heart failure
cm centimeter
CNS central nervous system
CO_2 carbon dioxide
cont continuous
COPD chronic obstructive pulmonary disease
CPAP continuous positive airway pressure
CPK creatinine phosphokinase
CPR cardiopulmonary resuscitation
CCr creatinine clearance
C&S culture and sensitivity
C sect cesarean section
CSF cerebrospinal fluid
CV cardiovascular
CVA cerebrovascular accident
CVP central venous pressure
D&C dilatation and curettage
dir inf direct infusion
dr dram
D_5W 5% glucose in distilled water
ECG electrocardiogram (EKG)
EDTA ethylenediamine tetraacetic acid
EEG electroencephalogram
EENT ear, eye, nose, and throat
EPS extrapyramidal symptoms
ESR erythrocyte sedimentation rate
ext rel extended release
EXTRA STREN extra strength
susp suspension
FBS fasting blood sugar
FHT fetal heart tones
FSH follicle-stimulating hormone
g gram
GABA γ-aminobutyric acid
GI gastrointestinal
gr grain
GTT glucose tolerance test
gtt drops
GU genitourinary
H_2 histamine$_2$
hCG human chorionic gonadotropin
Hct hematocrit
HDCV human diploid cell rabies vaccine

Hgb hemoglobin
H&H hematocrit and hemoglobin
5-HIAA 5-hydroxyindoleacetic acid
HIV human immunodeficiency virus (AIDS)
H_2O water
HOB head of bed
HR heart rate
hr hour
IgG immunoglobulin G
IM intramuscular
inf infusion
INH inhalation
inj injection
I&O intake and output
IPPB intermittent positive-pressure breathing
ITP idiopathic thrombocytopenic purpura
IUD intrauterine device
IV intravenous
IVP intravenous pyelogram
K potassium
kg kilogram
L liter
lb pound
LDH lactic dehydrogenase
LE lupus erythematosus
LH luteinizing hormone
LLQ left lower quadrant
LMP last menstrual period
LOC level of consciousness
LR lactated Ringer's solution
LUQ left upper quadrant
M meter
m minim
m^2 square meter
MAOI monoamine oxidase inhibitor
mcg microgram
mEq milliequivalent
mg milligram
MI myocardial infarction
min minute
ml milliliter
mm millimeter
mo month
Na sodium
neg negative
NPO nothing by mouth (Lat. *nulla per os*)
NS normal saline
O_2 oxygen
OBS organic brain syndrome
OD right eye
OR operating room
OS left eye
OTC over-the-counter
OU each eye
oz ounce
$\bar{p}$ after
P56 Plasma-Lyte 56
$PaCO_2$ arterial carbon dioxide tension (pressure)
PaO_2 arterial oxygen tension (pressure)
PAT paroxysmal atrial tachycardia
PBI protein-bound iodine
pc after meals
PCWP pulmonary capillary wedge pressure
PEEP positive end-expiratory pressure
PERRLA pupils equal, round, react to light and accommodation
pH hydrogen ion concentration
PO by mouth
postop postoperative
PP postprandial
preop preoperative
prn as required
PT prothrombin time
PTT partial thromboplastin time
PVC premature ventricular contraction
q every
qAM every morning
qh every hour
q2h every 2 hours
q3h every 3 hours
q4h every 4 hours
q6h every 6 hours
q12h every 12 hours
qid four times daily
qPM every night
qs sufficient quantity
qt quart
R right
RAIU radioactive iodine uptake
RBC red blood count or cell
RLQ right lower quadrant
ROM range of motion
RUQ right upper quadrant
Rx prescription
SIMV synchronous intermittent mandatory ventilation
SL sublingual

SLE systemic lupus erythematosus
SOB shortness of breath
sol solution
sp gr specific gravity
ss one half
SUBCUT subcutaneous
supp suppository
sus rel sustained release
syr syrup
T&A tonsillectomy and adenoidectomy
tab tablet
tbsp tablespoon
temp temperature
tid three times daily
tinc tincture
TPN total parenteral nutrition
top topical
TRANS transdermal
TSH thyroid-stimulating hormone
tsp teaspoon
TT thrombin time
UA urinalysis
UTI urinary tract infection
UV ultraviolet
vag vaginal
VMA vanillylmandelic acid
vol volume
VS vital sign
WBC white blood cell count
wk week
wt weight
yr year
> greater than
< less than
= equal
° degree
% percent
α alpha
γ gamma
β beta

• For a list of The Institute for Safe Medicine Practices (ISMP) error prone abbreviations, symbols, and dose designations, please see http://www.ismp.org/tools/errorproneabbreviations.pdf.
• For frequently asked questions regarding the 2006 National Patient Safety Goals, please visit the Joint Commission on Accreditation of Healthcare Organizations (JCAHO) website at http://www.jcaho.org/accredited+organizations/patient+safety

Appendix M

High-Alert Canadian Medications

High-alert medications are medications that have a narrow margin of safety and when misused have the greatest potential to cause significant client harm. The Institute for Safe Medication Practices Canada (ISMP Canada) is a national nonprofit organization that independently reviews voluntary reports of medication errors and develops recommendations for safe medication practices throughout Canada to reduce the harm to clients. In 2003, the ISMP compiled a list of high-alert medications that includes medications in the 19 classes listed below, as well as the specific medications listed below. When these drugs appear in this book, each specific drug monograph is highlighted with a light color screen to help nurses identify them. While care should be taken in giving any medication, nurses are advised to exercise extra precautions when administering these high-risk drugs.

Class/Category of Medications
adrenergic agonists, **IV** (e.g., epINEPHrine)
adrenergic antagonists, **IV** (e.g., propranolol)
anesthetic agents, general, inhaled and **IV** (e.g., propofol)
cardioplegic solutions
chemotherapeutic agents, parenteral and oral
dextrose, hypertonic, 20% or greater
dialysis solutions, peritoneal and hemodialysis
epidural or intrathecal medications
glycoprotein IIb/IIIa inhibitors (e.g., eptifibatide)
hypoglycemics, oral
inotropic medications, **IV** (e.g., digoxin, milrinone)
liposomal forms of drugs (e.g., liposomal amphotericin B)
moderate sedation agents, **IV** (e.g., midazolam)
moderate sedation agents, oral, for children (e.g., chloral hydrate)
narcotics/opiates, **IV** and oral (including liquid concentrates, immediate- and sustained-release)
neuromuscular blocking agents (e.g., succinylcholine)
radiocontrast agents, **IV**
thrombolytics/fibrinolytics, **IV** (e.g., tenecteplase)
total parenteral nutrition solutions

Individual Medications
amiodarone, **IV**
colchicine injection
heparin, low molecular weight, injection
heparin, unfractionated, **IV**
insulin, subcutaneous and **IV**
lidocaine, **IV**
magnesium sulfate, injection
methotrexate, oral, nononcologic use
nesiritide
nitroprusside, sodium, for injection
potassium chloride, concentrate, for injection
potassium phosphates, injection
sodium chloride, hypertonic, more than 0.9% concentration, injection
warfarin

1. Cohen MR, Kilo CM: High-alert medications: safeguarding against errors. In Cohen MR, editor: *Medication errors,* Washington, DC, 1999, American Pharmaceutical Association.
2. High-alert medications and patient safety, *Sentinel Event Alert* 11, Nov 1999.
3. ISMP's list of high-alert medications, accessed 12/28/04 at http://www.ismp.org/MSAarticles/highalert.htm
4. ISMP Canada accessed 12/28/04 at http://www.ismp-canada.org/index.htm.

Appendix N

Canadian Controlled Substance Chart

DRUGS	CANADA
LSD, mescaline (peyote), harmaline, psilocin & psilocybin (magic mushrooms)	**Part J of the Food and Drug Regulation (FDR)** • Considered "restricted drugs" • High misuse potential • No recognized medical use • Marihuana exemption from FDR if produced for medical reasons
Sedatives such as barbiturates and derivatives (secobarbital), thiobarbiturates (pentothal sodium); anabolic steroids (androstanolone), weight reduction drugs (anorexiants)	**Part G of the FDR** • Controlled drugs • Misuse potential • Verbal and written prescriptions under certain conditions • Only prescribed if required for medical condition • Specified number of refills (conditions apply) • Records must be kept • May be administered under emergency situations (conditions apply)
Amphetamines; benzaphetamine; methamphetamine; phenmetrazine; phendimetrazine	**Part G of the FDR** • Designated controlled drug • May be used for designated medical conditions outlined in FDR
Benzodiazepine tranquilizers such as diazepam, lorazepam, flunitrazepam, zolpidem	**Benzodiazepines and Other Targeted Substances Regulations** • Misuse potential • Verbal and written prescriptions under certain conditions • Only prescribed if required for medical condition • Specified number of refills (conditions apply) • Records must be kept • May be administered under emergency situations (conditions apply)
Opiates: heroin, morphine, codeine >8 mg, amidones (methadone), coca and derivatives (cocaine), phencyclidine (PCP), benzazocines (analgesics such as pentazocine), fentanyls	**Narcotic Control Regulation** • High misuse potential • Written prescriptions for specific medical conditions* • Records of opiate prescription file must be kept • No refills (limited amounts in a prescription) • Heroin and methadone are subject to specific controls
Chloral hydrate, chlordiazepoxide	**Schedule F of the FDR** • Low misuse potential

*Verbal prescriptions are permitted for certain opioid preparations (such as Tylenol No. 2 and No. 3), but not for opiate alone, or opiates with 1 other active non-opioid ingredient.

Explanation of Controlled Drugs and Substances Chart for Canada

The *Canadian Controlled Drugs and Substances Act (CDSA)* is a "legislative framework for the control of substances that can alter mental processes and that may produce harm to the health of an individual and to society when diverted or misused" (*Canada Gazette*, 2003, paragraph 5) that is under the jurisdiction of Health Canada. A "controlled substance" means a substance included in Schedules I to VI. Schedules VII and VIII specify amounts of substances in Schedule II (e.g., cannabis and cannabis resin) associated of the FDR or the *Benzodiazepines and Other Targeted Substances Regulations* (Targeted Substances Regulations). Different levels of control measures are found within the various regulations that apply to licensed dealers, pharmacists, practitioners, and hospitals. Part J of the FDR regulates the use of controlled substances with no recognized medical use; substances listed in the schedule to Part J of the FDR are defined as "restricted drugs" and include such substances as LSD and mescaline. Controlled substances included in CDSA Schedules III and IV that have some therapeutic use are regulated under either Part G of the FDR or the Targeted Substances Regulations with the former having more stringent controls over distribution.

Canada Gazette. (2003). Order amending schedule III to the controlled drugs and substances act. Retrieved January 3, 2005 from http://canadagazette.gc.ca/partII/2003/20031231/html/sor412-e.html.

Department of Justice Canada. (2004). *Narcotic Control Regulations*. Retrieved January 6, 2005 from http://laws.justice.gc.ca/en/C-38.8/C.R.C.-c.1041/76122.html.

Department of Justice Canada. (2004). Controlled Drugs *and Substances Act*. Retrieved December 31, 2004 from http://laws.justice.gc.ca/en/C-38.8/.

Health Canada. (2004). *Food and Drugs Act*. Part G–Controlled Drugs. Part J–Restricted Drugs. Schedule F. Retrieved January 6, 2005 from http://www.hc-sc.gc.ca/food-aliment/friia-raaii/food_drugs-aliments_drogues/act-loi/e_index.html.

National Association of Pharmacy Regulatory Authorities (NAPRA). *Controlled Drugs and Substances Act and Regulations*. Retrieved January 6, 2005 from http://www.napra.org/docs/0/93/143.asp.

NAPRA. (2003). *Maribuana Exception (Food and Drugs Act) Regulations*. Retrieved January 6, 2005 from http://www.napra.ca/pdfs/fedleg/0307marihuanaexemption.pdf.

NAPRA. *Benzodiazepines and Other Targeted Substances Regulations*. Retrieved January 6, 2005 from http://www.napra.ca/pdfs/fedleg/benzodiaz.pdf.

Appendix O

Canadian Recommended Immunization Schedules for Infants and Children

	MONTHS					YEARS		
VACCINE	2	4	6	12	18	4 TO 6	9 TO 13	14 TO 16
Hepatitis B*	3 doses	3 doses	3 doses	3 doses	3 doses	3 doses	3 doses	
Diphtheria, Pertussis, and Tetanus (DPT)	DPT	DPT	DPT		DPT	DPT		Td **
Haemophilus influenzae type b *** (Hib)	Hib	Hib	Hib		Hib			
Polio (inactivated polio vaccine/oral polio vaccine)	Polio	Polio	Polio ****		Polio	Polio		Polio ****
Measles, Mumps, and Rubella ***** (MMR)				MMR	MMR *****	MMr *****		

* Adolescents who have not received hepatitis B vaccine in infancy should receive it through school programs according to the provincial and territorial policies.

** Td (tetanus and diphtheria toxoids, adult formulation).

*** Recommended schedule for both Hib-TITER® and ActHIB®.

**** If oral polio vaccine is used exclusively, boosters at 6 months and 14 to 16 years of age may be omitted.

***** The second dose of MMR is routinely recommended at either 18 months or at 4 to 6 years of age. It should be given any time before school entry provided that there is at least a 1-month interval between receipt of the first and second doses.

Disorders Index

A

Acne, recalcitrant
isotretinoin for, 1096
Agammaglobulinemia
immune globulin for, 501-502
Alzheimer's
donepezil for, 335-336
galantamine for, 444-445
memantine for, 588-589
selegiline for, 843-844, 1006
Amyotrophic lateral sclerosis
diazepam for, 305-307, 996, 1011, 1117, 1123
pyridostigmine for, 798-800, 1015
quinidine for, 805-807, 1000
Anemia, aplastic
cyclophosphamide for, 270-272, 1005, 1042
Anemia, iron deficiency
ferrous sulfate for, 408-410
iron dextran for, 522-523
Angina pectoris
amlodipine for, 83-84, 993, 1014
amyl nitrite for, 993, 1026, 1088
atenolol for, 114-116, 993, 1012
bepridil for, 993, 1014
isosorbide for, 993
metoprolol for, 617-619, 993, 1012
nadolol for, 654-655, 993, 1012
nicardipine for, 671-673, 993, 1014
nifedipine for, 675-676, 993, 1014
nitroglycerin for, 681-682, 993
propranolol for, 791-793, 993, 1000, 1012
verapamil for, 963-965, 993, 1000, 1014
Arthritis
anakinra for, 97-98
aspirin for, 111-113, 1024
celecoxib for, 190-192, 1022, 1042
diclofenac for, 1022, 1046, 1047
hydroxychloroquine for, 484-485, 1095
ibuprofen for, 491-492, 1022
ketoprofen for, 531-533, 1022
methotrexate for, 603-605, 1005, 1043, 1121
naproxen for, 662-664, 1022
rofecoxib for, 1022
valdecoxib for, 1022
Asthma
albuterol for, 52-54, 1013
dyphylline for, 352-353, 1013
formoterol for, 431-432, 1013
omalizumab for, 695-696
terbutaline for, 893-894, 1013
theophylline for, 898-899, 1013
Atrial fibrillation/flutter
digoxin for, 313-315, 1000, 1014, 1042
diltiazem for, 318-319, 993, 1014, 1042
Atrial tachycardia
digoxin for, 313-315, 1000, 1014, 1042
diltiazem for, 318-319, 993, 1014, 1042
Attention deficit hyperactivity disorder (ADD/ADHD)
atomoxetine for, 116-117
dexmethylphenidate for, 300-301
methylphenidate for, 608-610

B

Bipolar disorder
divalproex for, 329, 954-955
lithium for, 562-564
Bronchitis, chronic
cefditoren for, 1003
cephalosporins—2nd generation for, 196-202
cephalosporins—3rd generation for, 202-210
lomefloxacin for, 564-565, 1004
Bronchospasm
formoterol for, 431-432, 1013
isoproterenol for, 1013, 1095
levalbuterol for, 547-548, 1013

C

Cancer, adrenocortical
aminoglutethimide for, 1087
mitotane for, 1005, 1096
Cancer, breast
doxorubicin for, 343-345, 1005, 1043
fulvestrant for, 439-440
letrozole for, 543-544
megestrol for, 584-585, 1005
toremifene for, 925-926
Cancer, colorectal
fluorouracil for, 419-421, 1005, 1043
oxaliplatin for, 702-703
Cancer, ovarian
altretamine for, 1005, 1087
cisplatin for, 240-242, 1005, 1042
doxorubicin for, 343-345, 1005, 1043
paclitaxel for, 713-715
Cancer, prostate
flutamide for, 427, 1005
Cancer, renal cell
aldesleukin for, 54-56, 1042
Cancer, testicular
cisplatin for, 240-242, 1005, 1042
plicamycin for, 764-766, 1005, 1043
Candidiasis
fluconazole for, 416-417, 1001
nystatin for, 687-688, 1001
Cardiogenic shock
digoxin for, 313-315, 1000, 1014, 1042
CMV retinitis
foscarnet for, 432-434, 1010
ganciclovir for, 446-448, 1010
idoxuridine for, 1010
valganciclovir for, 952-953, 1010
Congestive heart failure (CHF)
digoxin for, 313-315, 1000, 1014, 1042
furosemide for, 440-443, 1018
nesiritide for, 668-669, 1026, 1043, 1121
nitroglycerin for, 681-682, 993
nitroprusside for, 682-683, 1003, 1043

D

Deep vein thrombosis (DVT)
ardeparin for, 995, 1042
danaparoid for, 282-284, 995, 1042
desirudin for, 294, 995
enoxaparin for, 361-363, 995, 1043
heparin for, 470-472, 995, 1043

warfarin for, 976-977, 995, 1043
Depression
bupropion for, 160-161, 997
escitalopram for, 381-382
fluoxetine for, 421-423, 997
imipramine for, 499-501, 997
mirtazapine for, 635-636, 997
paroxetine for, 722-723, 997
sertraline for, 846-847, 997
trazodone for, 932-934, 997
venlafaxine for, 962-963, 997
Diabetes mellitus
acarbose for, 35-36
glipizide for, 459-460, 998
glyburide for, 460-462, 998
insulins for, 510-512
miglitol for, 630-631, 998
rosiglitazone for, 834-835, 998
Dysmenorrhea
diclofenac for, 1022, 1046, 1047
ibuprofen for, 491-492, 1022
ketoprofen for, 531-533, 1022
naproxen for, 662-664, 1022
Dysrhythmias
acebutolol for, 36-38, 1000, 1012
adenosine for, 48-49, 1000, 1042
amiodarone for, 79-81, 1000, 1042, 1121
amlodipine for, 83-84, 993, 1014
atropine for, 119-121, 994, 1000, 1013, 1016, 1042
bepridil for, 993, 1014
bretylium for, 151-152, 1000, 1042
digoxin for, 313-315, 1000, 1014, 1042
diltiazem for, 318-319, 993, 1014, 1042
disopyramide for, 328-329, 1000
esmolol for, 383-384, 1000, 1012
flecainide for, 415-416, 1000
ibutilide for, 492-493, 1000, 1043
isoproterenol for, 1013, 1095
lidocaine for, 1000, 1121
mexiletine for, 620-622, 1000
moricizine for, 644-646, 1000
nifedipine for, 675-676, 993, 1014
nicardipine for, 671-673, 993, 1014
phenytoin for, 752-754, 996, 1000
procainamide for, 778-779, 1000
propranolol for, 791-793, 993, 1000, 1012
quinidine for, 805-807, 1000
sotalol for, 857-858, 1000
tocainide for, 920-921, 1000
verapamil for, 963-965, 993, 1000, 1014

E

Emphysema
azithromycin for, 125-127, 1004
hydrocortisone for, 480-482, 1017
theophylline for, 898-899, 1013
Endometriosis
goserelin for, 464
leuprolide for, 545-547, 1005, 1043
Epilepsy
diazepam for, 305-307, 996, 1011, 1117, 1123
fosphenytoin for, 437-438, 996
phenobarbital for, 746-748, 996, 1010, 1043, 1117
phenytoin for, 752-753, 996, 1000
tiagabine for, 996
topiramate for, 923-924, 996

F

Folic acid deficiency
folic acid for, 429-430
leucovorin for, 544-545

G

Gastroesophageal reflux disease (GERD)
cimetidine for, 234-236, 1019
esomeprazole for, 384-385
famotidine for, 399-401, 1019
ranitidine for, 812-813, 1019
Glaucoma
acetazolamide for, 39-42, 996, 1018
carbachol for, 1045, 1047
glycerin for, 1020, 1094

H

Hemophilia A
antihemophilic factor for, 101-102, 1042
Hemophilia B
factor IX complex (human)/factor IV for, 397-398, 1043
Hepatitis C
interferon alfa-2B for, 1005
peginterferon alfa-2a for, 727
Herpes simplex keratitis
idoxuridine for, 1010
HIV/AIDS infection
abacavir for, 33-34, 1009
acyclovir for, 44-46, 1009
atazanavir for, 113-114, 1009
cidofovir for, 232-233, 1009
delavirdine for, 290-291, 1009
didanosine for, 311-312, 1009
emtricitabine for, 356-357, 1009
enfuvirtide for, 359-360, 1009
fosamprenavir for, 434-435, 1010
foscarnet for, 432-434, 1010
ganciclovir for, 446-448, 1010
indinavir for, 506-507, 1010
nelfinavir for, 665-666, 1010
nevirapine for, 669-670, 1010
ritonavir for, 828-829, 1010
saquinavir for, 839-840, 1010
tenofovir for, 889-890, 1010
zalcitabine for, 978-979, 1010
zidovudine for, 981-983, 1010
Hodgkin's disease
doxorubicin for, 343-345, 1005, 1043
procarbazine for, 779-781, 1005
Hydatid mole
methotrexate for, 603-605, 1005, 1043, 1121
Hyperbilirubinemia
albumin for, 51-52
Hypercalcemia
calcitonin for, 166-168
zoledronic acid for, 986-987
Hyperlipidemia
ezetimibe for, 396
fluvastatin for, 428-429
rosuvastatin for, 836-837
simvastatin for, 848-849
Hyperplasia, benign prostatic (BPH)
doxazosin for, 339-340, 1003
dutasteride for, 351
tamsulosin for, 881-882
terazosin for, 890-891, 1003

Hypertension
acebutolol for, 36-38, 1000, 1012
atenolol for, 114-116, 993, 1012
benazepril for, 131-133, 1002
bisoprolol for, 144-146
candesartan for, 173-174, 1002
captopril for, 175-177, 1002
carteolol for, 186-187, 1012, 1045, 1046-1047
clonidine for, 253-255, 1002
doxazosin for, 339-340, 1003
enalapril/enalaprilat for, 357-359
eplerenone for, 369-370
eprosartan for, 372-373, 1002
felodipine for, 402-403, 1014
fosinopril for, 435-437, 1002
guanfacine for, 466-467, 1095
hydralazine for, 475-476, 1003, 1026
hydrochlorothiazide for, 476-478, 1018
isradipine for, 527-528, 1014
labetalol for, 534-536, 1003, 1012
losartan for, 570-571, 1002
methyldopa/methyldopate for, 605-607
metoprolol for, 617-619, 993, 1012
minoxidil for, 634-635, 1003, 1026
moexipril for, 642-643
nadolol for, 654-655, 993, 1012
nifedipine for, 675-676, 993, 1014
nitroprusside for, 682-683, 1003, 1043
olmesartan for, 693-694
phentolamine for, 749-750, 991
pindolol for, 755-756, 1012
prazosin for, 771-772, 1003
propranolol for, 791-793, 993, 1000, 1012
quinapril for, 803-805, 1002
ramipril for, 810-812, 1002
terazosin for, 890-891, 1003
timolol for, 912-913, 1012, 1045, 1046-1047
trandolapril for, 928-930, 1002
valsartan for, 956-957, 1002
verapamil for, 963-965, 993, 1000, 1014
Hypertension, pulmonary arterial
bosentan for, 150-151, 1026
Hyperthyroidism
propylthiouracil for, 793-795
Hypothyroidism
levothyroxine for, 551-553, 1025
thyroid USP for, 904-905, 1025

I

Influenza
ribavarin for, 818-819
zanamivir for, 980-981
Insomnia
triazolam for, 939-941, 1011
zolpidem for, 988-989, 1123
Iron deficiency anemia
ferrous sulfate for, 408-410
iron dextran for, 522-523

K

Kaposi's sarcoma
interferon alfa-2B for, 1005

L

Legionnaire's disease
erythromycin for, 379-380
Leprosy
clofazimine for, 1090
Leukemia, acute myeloid
dactinomycin for, 280-281, 1005, 1042
idarubicin for, 493-495, 1043
Leukemia, B-cell chronic lymphocytic
alemtuzumab for, 56-57, 1005
chlorambucil for, 214-216, 1005
cyclophosphamide for, 270-272, 1005, 1042
mechlorethamine for, 581-582, 1005
Leukemia, chronic myelocytic
busulfan for, 162-164, 1005, 1042
cytarabine for, 275-277, 1005, 1042
hydroxyurea for, 485-487
imatinib for, 496-497, 1005
mechlorethamine for, 581-582, 1005
Leukemia, hairy cell
pentostatin for, 736-738, 1005, 1043
Leukemia, meningeal
cytarabine for, 275-277, 1005, 1042
methotrexate for, 603-605, 1005, 1043, 1121
thiotepa for, 1005, 1100
Lipidemia
atorvastatin for, 117-118
cholestyramine for, 229-230
colestipol for, 265-266
fenofibrate for, 403-404
gemfibrozil for, 453-454
pravastatin for, 770-771

M

M. avium
rifabutin for, 820-821, 1008
Melanoma
dacarbazine for, 277-279, 1005, 1042
Menopause
estradiol for, 385-387
estrogens, conjugated for, 387-389
Migraine
almotriptan for, 61-62
eletriptan for, 355-356
frovatriptan for, 438-439
propranolol for, 791-793, 993, 1000, 1012
sumatriptan for, 875-876
Multiple sclerosis
cyclophosphamide for, 270-272, 1005, 1042
imipramine for, 499-501, 997
interferon beta-1b for, 516-517
tizanidine for, 917-918
Myasthenia gravis
cyclophosphamide for, 270-272, 1005, 1042
prednisone for, 774-775, 1017
pyridostigmine for, 798-800, 1015
Myocardial infarction
aspirin for, 111-113, 1024
heparin for, 470-472, 995, 1043
morphine for, 646-648, 1023, 1043, 1117, 1123
streptokinase for, 863-864, 1024, 1043

N

Narcolepsy
modafinil for, 1096

O

Obsessive-compulsive disorder
clomipramine for, 250-251, 997
sertraline for, 846-847, 997
Organ transplantation
azathioprine for, 123-124, 1019
basiliximab for, 129-130, 1019, 1042
cyclosporine for, 272-274, 1019
muromonab-CD3 for, 650-651, 1019
sirolimus for, 849-851, 1019
tacrolimus for, 878-879, 1019
Osteoarthritis
diclofenac for, 1022, 1046, 1047
ibuprofen for, 491-492, 1022
ketoprofen for, 531-533, 1022
naproxen for, 662-664, 1022

P

Paget's disease
calcitonin for, 166-168
tiludronate for, 910-911
Parkinsonism
amantadine for, 67-68, 1087
benztropine for, 133-135, 994, 1006, 1016
biperiden for, 141-142, 994, 1006, 1016
bromocriptine for, 152-153, 1006
carbidopa-levodopa for, 179-181, 1006
levodopa for, 549-550, 1006
pramipexole for, 769-770, 1006
ropinirole for, 832-833
selegiline for, 843-844, 1006
trihexyphenidyl for, 943-944, 1006, 1016
Peptic ulcer disease
aluminum hydroxide for, 66-67, 993
cimetidine for, 234-236, 1019
misoprostol for, 637
Pneumonia, fungal
amphotericin B for, 89-91
ketoconazole for, 530-531, 1001
Pneumonia, mycoplasma
erythromycin for, 379-380
tetracycline for, 896-898, 1004
Pneumonia, *Pneumocystis jiroveci*
pentamidine for, 732-733
Polyneuritis
riboflavin for, 819, 1026
Premature ventricular contractions
tocainide for, 920-921, 1000
Prostatic carcinoma
flutamide for, 427, 1005
Psoriasis
alefacept for, 1086
efalizumab for, 1093
methotrexate for, 603-605, 1005, 1043, 1121
Pulmonary embolism
enoxaparin for, 361-363, 995, 1043
heparin for, 470-472, 995, 1043
streptokinase for, 863-864, 1024, 1043
warfarin for, 976-977, 995, 1043

R

Renal graft rejection
cyclosporine for, 272-274, 1019
Rheumatoid arthritis
anakinra for, 97-98
aspirin for, 111-113, 1024
celecoxib for, 190-192, 1022, 1042
hydroxychloroquine for, 484-485, 1095
ibuprofen for, 491-492, 1022
methotrexate for, 603-605, 1005, 1043, 1121
Rhinitis, seasonal allergic
desloratadine for, 295, 1001
flunisolide for, 1048-1049

S

Schizophrenia
aripiprazole for, 105-107
chlorpromazine for, 224-227, 1007
clozapine for, 258-260
quetiapine for, 802-803, 1007
Septicemia
aztreonam for, 1089
cephalosporins—1st generation for, 192-196
cephalosporins—2nd generation for, 196-202
cephalosporins—3rd generation for, 202-210
drotrecogin alfa for, 348-349, 1024
ertapenem for, 377-379, 1004
imipenem/cilastatin for, 497-499, 1004
metronidazole for, 619-620
piperacillin for, 758-759, 1004
ticarcillin for, 906-908
tobramycin for, 918-920, 1003
Status epilepticus
diazepam for, 305-307, 996, 1011, 1117, 1123
Streptococcal sore throat
penicillin for, 729-732
Supraventricular tachycardia
amiodarone for, 79-81, 1000, 1042, 1121

T

Thrombosis, deep vein
ardeparin for, 995, 1042
dalteparin for, 281-282, 995, 1042
danaparoid for, 282-284, 995, 1042
desirudin for, 294, 995
enoxaparin for, 361-363, 995, 1043
fondaparinux for, 430-431, 995
streptokinase for, 863-864, 1024, 1043
warfarin for, 976-977, 995, 1043
Tuberculosis, pulmonary
ethambutol for, 390-391, 1008
isoniazid for, 524-525, 1008
rifampin for, 821-822, 1008
streptomycin for, 864-866, 1008

V

Ventricular fibrillation
amiodarone for, 79-81, 1000, 1042, 1121
bretylium for, 151-152, 1000, 1042
Ventricular tachycardia
amiodarone for, 79-81, 1000, 1042, 1121
bretylium for, 151-152, 1000, 1042
flecainide for, 415-416, 1000
tocainide for, 920-921, 1000

Z

Zollinger-Ellision syndrome
cimetidine for, 234-236, 1019
famotidine for, 399-401, 1019
ranitidine for, 812-813, 1019

Index

A

abacavir, 33-34, 1009
abarelix, 34-35
abatacept, 35, 1027-1028
Abbokinase, 950-951
Abbokinase Open-Cath, 950-951
Abbreviations, 1118-1120
abciximab, 1042, 1086
Abelcet, 89-91
Abenol, 38-39
Abilify, 105-107
Abraxane, 713-715
Abreva, 1054
Absorbine Antifungal Foot Powder, 1050, 1051-1052
Absorbine Athlete's Foot Cream, 1050, 1051-1052
acarbose, 35-36
Accolate, 977-978
AccuNeb, 52-54
Accupril, 803-805
Accurbron, 898-899
Accuretic 10/12.5, 1056
Accuretic 20/12.5, 1056
Accuretic 20/25, 1056
acebutolol, 36-38, 1000, 1012
Acel-Imune, 1105
Aceon, 740-741
Acephen, 38-39
Aceta, 38-39
Acetadote, 42-43
acetaminophen, 38-39
Aceta w/Codeine, 1056
acetazolamide, 39-42, 996, 1018
acetylcholine, 1045, 1047
acetylcysteine, 42-43, 1009
acetylsalicylic acid, 111-113
Achromycin V, 896-898
acidophilus, 1111
Acid X, 1056
Aciphex, 808-809
acrivastine/pseudoephedrine, 1102
Actagen C Cough Syrup, 1056
ACTH, 1090
Acti-B_{12}, 971-972
Actidose-Aqua, 43-44
Actifed, 1056
Actifed Allergy, Daytime, 1056
Actifed Allergy, Nighttime, 1056
Actifed Cold and Allergy, 1056
Actifed Cold and Sinus, 1056
Actifed Plus, 1056
Actifed Plus ES Caplets, 1056
Actifed Sinus Daytime, 1056
Actifed Sinus Nighttime, 1056
Actifed Syrup, 1056
Actifed with Codeine, 1056
Actifed with Codeine Cough Syrup, 1056
Actimmune, 517-518
Actimol, 38-39
Actiocort, 1050
Actiprofen, 491-492
Actiq, 405-407
Actisite (dental product), 896-898
Activase, 64-66
Activase rt-PA, 64-66
activated charcoal, 43-44
Activella Tablets, 1056
Actonel, 826-827
Actos, 756-758
Actron, 531-533
Acular, 533-534, 1046, 1047
Acuprin, 111-113
acyclovir, 44-46, 1009
acyclovir (topical), 1052-1053
Adalat, 675-676
Adalat CC, 675-676
adalimumab, 47
Adavite, 649-650
Adderall 5 mg, 1056
Adderall 10 mg, 1056
Adderall 20 mg, 1056
Adderall 30 mg, 1056-1057
Adderall XR 10 mg, 1057
Adderall XR 20 mg, 1057
Adderall XR 30 mg, 1057
adefovir dipivoxil, 47-48, 1004
Adenocard, 48-49
Adenoscan, 48-49
adenosine, 48-49, 1000, 1042
Adovate, 1049, 1050
Adrenalin, 366-367
Adrenalin (nasal), 1047, 1048-1049
ADRENERGIC AGONISTS, 1042, 1121
ADRENERGIC ANTAGONISTS, 1042, 1121
Adriamycin PFS, 343-345
Adriamycin RDF, 343-345
Adrucil, 419-421
Adsorbocarpine, 1045, 1047
Advair Diskus 100, 1057
Advair Diskus 250, 1057
Advair Diskus 500, 1057
Advicor 500, 1057
Advicor 750, 1057
Advicor 1000, 1057
Advil, 491-492
Advil Cold & Sinus Caplets, 1057
Advil Migraine, 491-492
Aeroseb-Dex, 1049, 1050
Aeroseb-HC, 1050
Afrin, 796-797
Afrin No-Drip 12-Hour, 1048-1049
Afrin No-Drip 12-Hour Extra Moisturizing, 1048-1049
Afrin Severe Congestion With Menthol, 1048-1049
Afrin Sinus With Vapornase, 1048-1049
Afrin 12 Hour Original, 1048-1049
Afrin 12-Hour Original Pump Mist, 1048-1049
Aftate for Athlete's Foot, 1050, 1051-1052
Aftate for Jock Itch, 1050, 1051-1052
agalsidase beta, 1086
Agenerase, 95-96
Aggrastat, 916-917
Aggrenox, 1057
Agrylin, 96-97
AHF, 101-102
A-hydroCort, 480-482
Airet, 52-54
Akarpine, 1045, 1047
AK Beta, 1045, 1046-1047
AK-Chlor, 1044, 1047

AK-Cide Ophthalmic Suspension/Ointment, 1057
AK-Con, 1046, 1047
AK-Dex, 1045, 1047
AK-Dilate, 1046, 1047
Akineton, 141-142
AK-Nefrin, 1046, 1047
Akne-Mycin, 1052
AK-Pentolate, 1045, 1047
AK-Pred, 1045, 1047
AKPro, 1046, 1047
AK-Sulf, 1044, 1047
AKTob, 1045-1047
Ala-Cort, 1050
alatrofloxacin, 49-51
alatrofloxacin/ trovafloxacin, 1004
Alavert, 567-568
Alazine, 475-476
Albalon, 1046, 1047
albumin, normal serum 5%/25%, 51-52
Albuminar 5%, 51-52
Albuminar 25%, 51-52
Albutein 5%, 51-52
Albutein 25%, 51-52
albuterol, 52-54, 1013
Alcaine, 1044, 1047
alclometasone, 1049, 1050
Alconefrin 12, 1048-1049
Aldactazide 25/25, 1057
Aldactazide 50/50, 1057
Aldactone, 860-861
aldesleukin, 54-56, 1042
Aldoclor-150, 1057
Aldoclor-250, 1057
Aldomet, 605-607
Aldoril 15, 1057
Aldoril 25, 1057
Aldoril D30, 1057
Aldoril D50, 1057
alefacept, 1086
alemtuzumab, 56-57, 1005
alendronate, 57-58
Aleve, 662-664
Aleve Cold & Sinus, 1057
alfalfa, 1111
alfentanil, 1086
alfuzosin, 58-59
Alimta, 727-729
Alinia, 679-680
alitretinoin, 59-60
Alka-Mints, 169-170
Alka-Seltzer Cold, 1057
Alka-Seltzer Effervescent, Original, 1057
Alka-Seltzer Plus Cold & Cough Effervescent Tablets, 1057
Alka-Seltzer Plus Cold & Flu Liqui-Gels, 1057
Alka-Seltzer Plus Cold Liqui-Gels, 1057
Alka-Seltzer Plus Flu Liqui-Gels, 1057
Alka-Seltzer Plus Night-Time Cold Effervescent Tablets, 1057
Alka-Seltzer Plus Night-Time Cold Liqui-Gels, 1058
Alkeran, 587-588
Allay, 478-480
Allegra, 410-411
Allegra-D, 1058
Aller-Chlor, 223-224
Allercon Tablets, 1058
Allercort, 1050
Allerdryl, 322-324
Allerest Eye Drops, 1046, 1047
Allerest Headache Strength Advanced Formula, 1058
Allerest Maximum Strength Tablets, 1058
Allerest No-Drowsiness, 1058
Allerest Sinus Pain Formula, 1058
Allerfrim Syrup, 1058
Allerfrim Tablets, 1058
Allergy Drops, 1046, 1047
AllerMax, 322-324
Allermed, 322-324, 796-797
All-Nite Cold Formula Liquid, 1058
alloprim, 60-61
allopurinol, 60-61
Almoate Magonate, 567-578
almotriptan, 61-62
aloe, 1111
Aloe Extra Burn Relief, 1053
Alomide, 1046, 1047
Alophen, 748-749
Alor 5/500, 1058
Alora, 385-387
Aloxi, 716
ALPHA-ADRENERGIC BLOCKERS, 991
ALPHA-ADRENERIC BLOCKERS, OPHTHALMIC, 1044, 1047
Alphaderm, 1050
Alphagan P, 1046, 1047
Alphamin, 971-972
Alphanate, 101-102
Alpha Nine SD, 397-398
Alpha-Tamoxifen, 880-881
Alphatrex, 1049, 1050
alprazolam, 62-64, 1011
alprostadil, 1087
Alramucil, 797-798
Alrex, 1045, 1047
Altace, 810-812
Altarussin, 466
alteplase, 64-66, 1024, 1042
AlternaGEL, 66-67
Alti-Bromocriptine, 152-153
Altocor, 571-572
altretamine, 1005, 1087
Alu-Cap, 66-67
Alugel, 66-67
Aluminet, 66-67
Aluminett, 66-67
aluminum hydroxide, 66-67, 993
Alupent, 596-597
Alu-Tab, 66-67
amantadine, 67-68, 1006, 1009, 1087
amantadine HCl, 67-68
Amaphen, 1058
Amaride, 459-460
Ambenyl Cough Syrup, 1058
Ambien, 988-989
AmBisome, 89-91
amcinonide, 1049, 1050
Amcort, 936-938
Amen, 583-584
Amerge, 664-665
Americaine Anesthetic, 1053
A-Methapred, 610-612
amethopterin, 603-605
Amicar, 75-76
amifostine, 69-70
Amigesic, 838-839
amikacin, 70-72, 1003
amikacin sulfate, 70-72
Amikin, 70-72
amiloride, 72-73, 1018
Amiloride HCl, 72-73
Aminess, 73-75
amino acid, 73-75
aminocaproic acid, 75-76, 1087
Aminofen, 38-39
aminoglutethimide, 1087
aminolevulinic acid, 1088
Amino-Opti-E, 973-974
aminophylline (theophylline ethylenediamine), 76-79, 1013
Aminosyn, 73-75
amiodarone, 79-81, 1000, 1042, 1121
Amitiza, 1041
Amitone, 169-170
amitriptyline, 81-82, 997

amitriptyline HCl, 81-82
amlodipine, 83-84, 993, 1014
ammonium chloride, 1088
amoxapine, 84-85, 997
amoxicillin, 85-87
amoxicillin/clavulanate, 87-89, 1004
Amoxil, 85-87
AMPHETAMINES, 1123, 1117
Amphojel, 66-67
Amphotec, 89-91
amphotericin B, 1001
amphotericin B (topical), 1050, 1051-1052
amphotericin B cholesteryl, 89-91
amphotericin B deoxycholate, 89-91
amphotericin B lipid based, 89-91
amphotericin B liposome, 89-91
ampicillin, 91-93
ampicillin/sulbactam, 93-95, 1004
Ampicin, 91-93
amprenavir, 95-96
amyl nitrite, 993, 1026, 1088
ANABOLIC STEROIDS, 1123
Anacin, 1058
Anacin w/Codeine, 1058
Anacin Maximum Strength, 1058
Anacin PM (Aspirin Free), 1058
Anacobin, 971-972
Anaflex, 838-839
Anafranil, 250-251
anagrelide, 96-97
Ana-Guard, 366-367
anakinra, 97-98
Anandron, 676-677
Anaplex HD Syrup, 1058
Anaplex Liquid, 1058
Anaprox, 662-664
Anaprox DS, 662-664
Anaspaz, 488-489
anastrozole, 98-99, 1005
Anatuss LA, 1058
Anbesol Maximum Strength, 1053
Ancalixir, 746-748
Ancef, 192-196
Andro-Cyp, 895-896
Androderm, 895-896
AndroGel 1%, 895-896
Andro LA, 895-896
Andronate, 895-896
Andropository, 895-896
androstanolone, 1123
Andryl, 895-896
Anectine, 867-868
Anectine Flo-Pack, 867-868
Anestacon, 1053
ANESTHETICS, GENERAL/LOCAL, 991, 1042, 1121
ANESTHETICS, OPHTHALMIC, 1044, 1047
ANESTHETICS, TOPICAL, 1053
Anexate, 418-419
Anexsia, 478-480
Anexsia 5/500, 1058
Anexsia 7.5/650, 1058
angelica, 1111
Angiomax, 146-147
anise, 1111
anisoylated plasminogen, 99-101
anistreplase, 99-101, 1024, 1042
Anolor DH, 478-480
ANOREXIANTS, 1123
ANTACIDS, 992-993
Antagon, 448-449
ANTIANGINALS, 993
ANTICHOLINERGICS, 994
ANTICOAGULANTS, 994-995
ANTICONVULSANTS, 995-996
ANTIDEPRESSANTS, 996-997
ANTIDIABETICS, 997-998
ANTIDIARRHEALS, 998-999, 1117
Antidiarrheals with opium, 1117
ANTIDYSRHYTHMICS, 999-1000
ANTIFUNGALS, SYSTEMIC, 1000-1001
ANTIFUNGALS, TOPICAL, 1050-1052
ANTIFUNGALS, VAGINAL, 1054-1055
antihemophilic factor VIII (AHF), 101-102, 1042
Antihist-1, 246-247, 1103
ANTIHISTAMINES, 1001
ANTIHISTAMINES, LESS FREQUENTLY USED, 1102-1105
ANTIHISTAMINES, OPHTHALMIC, 1044, 1047
ANTIHYPERTENSIVES, 1002-1003
ANTIINFECTIVES, 1003-1004
ANTIINFECTIVES, OPHTHALMIC, 1044-1045, 1047
ANTIINFECTIVES, OTIC, 1055
ANTIINFECTIVES, TOPICAL, 1052
ANTIINFLAMMATORIES, NONSTEROIDAL, 1021-1022
ANTINEOPLASTICS, 1004-1005
ANTIPARKINSONIAN AGENTS, 1005-1006
ANTIPSYCHOTICS, 1006-1007
ANTITUBERCULARS, 1007-1008
Anti-tuss, 466
ANTITUSSIVES/ EXPECTORANTS, 1008-1009, 1117
Antivert, 582-583
ANTIVIRALS/ANTI-RETROVIRALS, 1009-1010
ANTIVIRALS/ANTI-RETROVIRALS, TOPICAL, 1052-1053
Antrizine, 582-583
Anturan, 872-873
Anturane, 872-873
Anusol HC, 1050
Anzemet, 334-335
Apacet, 38-39
APAP, 38-39
Apidra, 510-512
Apo-Acetaminophen, 38-39
Apo-Acetazolamide, 39-42
Apo-Allopurinol, 60-61
Apo-Alpraz, 62-64
Apo-Amitriptyline, 81-82
Apo-Amoxi, 85-87
Apo-ASA, 111-113
Apo-Asen, 111-113
Apo-Atenolol, 114-116
Apo-Benztropin, 133-135
Apo-Bromocriptine, 152-153
Apo-C, 108-109
Apo-Cal, 169-170
Apo-Carbamazepine, 177-179
Apo-Cephalex, 192-196

APO-Chlorazepate, 256-257
Apo-Chlordiazepoxide, 218-219
Apo-Chlorthalidone, 227-228
Apo-Cimetidine, 234-236
Apo-Cloxi, 257-258
Apo-Desipramine, 292-293
Apo-Diazepam, 305-307
Apo-Dilo, 308-309
Apo-Diltiaz, 318-319
Apo-Dimenhydrinate, 319-321
Apo-Dipyridamole, 325-326
Apo-Doxy, 345-346
Apo Erythro, 379-380
Apo-Erythro-ES, 379-380
Apo-Erythro-s, 379-380
Apo-Ferrous Sulfate, 408-410
Apo-Fluphenazine, 423-425
Apo-flurazepam, 425-427
Apo-Folic, 428-429
Apo-Furosemide, 440-443
Apo-Glyburide, 460-462
Apo-Haloperidol, 468-470
Apo-Hydrol, 476-478
Apo-hydroxyzine, 487-488
Apo-Ibuprofen, 491-492
Apo-Imipramine, 499-501
Apo-Indomethacin, 507-508
Apo-ISDN, 526-527
Apo-K, 767-769
Apo-Keto, 531-533
Apo-Keto-E, 531-533
Apokyn, 102-103
Apo-Lorazepam, 568-570
Apo-methyldopa, 605-607
Apo-Metoclop, 613-615
Apo-Metronidazole, 619-620
apomorphine, 102-103, 1006
Apo-Napro-Na, 662-664
Apo-Napro-Na DS, 662-664
Apo-Naproxen, 662-664
Apo-Nifed, 675-676
Apo-Nitrofurantoin, 680-681
Apo-Oxazepam, 704-706
Apo-Pen-VK, 729-732
Apo-Perphenazine, 741-744
Apo-Piroxicam, 762-763
Apo-Prednisone, 774-775
Apo-Primidone, 775-776
Apo-Propranolol, 791-793
Apo-Quinidine, 805-807
Apo-Ranitidine, 812-813
Apo-Selegiline, 843-844
Apo-Sulfamethoxazole, 869-870
Apo-Sulfatrim, 945-947
Apo-Sulfatrim DS, 945-947
Apo-Sulin, 874-875
Apo-Tetra, 896-898
Apo-Thioridazine, 902-904
Apo-Timol, 912-913
Apo-Timop, 1045, 1046-1047
Apo-Triazo, 939-941
Apo-Trifluoperazine, 941-943
Apo-Trihex, 943-944
Apo-Verap, 963-965
Apo-Zidovudine, 981-983
apraclonidine, 1046, 1047
aprepitant, 103-104
Apresazide 25/25, 1058
Apresazide 50/50, 1058
Apresoline, 475-476
Apri, 1058
APSAC, 99-101
Aptivus, 916, 1039-1040
Aquachloral, 213-214
AquaMEPHYTON, 754-755
Aquaphyllin, 898-899
Aquasol A, 969-970
Aquasol E, 973-974
Ara-C, 275-277
Aralen HCl, 219-220
Aralen Phosphate, 219-220
Aranesp, 286-287
Arava, 541-542
ardeparin, 995, 1042
Aredia, 716-718
Arestin, 632-634
argatroban, 995, 104-105, 1042
Argatroban, 104-105
Aricept, 335-336
Arimidex, 98-99
aripiprazole, 105-107, 1007
Aristocort, 936-938, 1050
Aristocort Forte, 936-938
Aristospan Intra-Articular, 936-938
Aristocort Intralesional, 936-938
Arixtra, 430-431
Arm-a-Med, 596-597
Armour Thyroid, 904-905
Aromasin, 395-396
Arranon, 665, 1032-1033
Arrestin, 944-945
arsenic trioxide, 107, 1005, 1042
Artane, 943-944
Artane Sequels, 943-944
Arthrinol, 111-113
Arthrisin, 111-113
Arthritis Foundation Pain Reliever Aspirin-Free, 38-39
Arthritis Pain Formula, 1058
Arthropan, 230-231
Arthrotec, 1058
Articulose-50, 772-774
Articulose L.A., 936-938
Artria S.R., 111-113
A.S.A., 111-113
Asacol, 595-596
ascorbic acid (vitamin C), 108-109, 1026
Ascorbicap, 108-109
Ascriptin, 1058-1059
Ascriptin A/D, 1059
Asendin, 84-85
Asmalix, 898-899
asparaginase, 109-111, 1005, 1042
A-Spas S/L, 488-489
Aspergum, 111-113
aspirin, 111-113, 1024
Aspirin, 111-113
Aspirin-Free Anacin, 38-39
Aspirin-Free Bayer Select Allergy Sinus, 1059
Aspirin Free Excedrin, 1059
Aspirin Free Excedrin Dual, 1059
Aspirin-Free Pain Relief, 38-39
Aspir-Low, 111-113
Aspirtab, 111-113
Astelin, 1047, 1048-1049
AsthmaHaler Mist, 366-367
AsthmaNefrin (racepinephrine), 366-367
astragalus, 1111
Astramorph, 646-648
Astramorph PF, 646-648
Astrin, 111-113
Atacand, 173-174
Atacand HCT 16, 1059
Atacand HCT 32, 1059
Atamet, 179-181
Atarax, 487-488
Atasol, 38-39
atazanvir, 113-114, 1009
atenolol, 114-116, 993, 1012
Atgam, 574-575
Ativan, 568-570
Atolone, 936-938
atomoxetine, 116-117
atorvastatin, 117-118
atovaquone, 118-119

atracurium, 1021, 1088
Atretol, 177-179
Atro-Pen, 119-121
atropine, 119-121, 994, 1000, 1013, 1016, 1042
atropine (ophthalmic), 1045, 1047
Atropine-1, 1045, 1047
Atropine Care, 1045, 1047
atropine sulfate, 119-121
Atropine Sulfate Ophthalmic, 1045, 1047
Atropisol, 1045, 1047
Atrovent, 518-519
A/T/S, 1052
attapulgite, 121-122
Attenuvax, 1108
A-200 Shampoo, 1056
Augmentin, 87-89
Augmentin 125 Chewable, 1059
Augmentin 125 mg/5 ml Suspension, 1059
Augmentin 200 Chewable, 1059
Augmentin 200 mg/5 ml Suspension, 1059
Augmentin 250, 1059
Augmentin 250 Chewable, 1059
Augmentin 250 mg/5 ml Suspension, 1059
Augmentin 400 Chewable, 1059
Augmentin 400 mg/5 ml Suspension, 1059
Augmentin 500, 1059
Augmentin 875, 1059
Augmentin ES-600, 87-89
Augmentin XR, 87-89
Auralgan Otic Solution, 1059
auranofin, 1088
Auro-Dri, 1055
aurothioglucose/gold sodium thiomalate, 1088-1089
Avalide, 1059
Avalide 300, 1059
Avandamet, 1059
Avandia, 834-835
Avapro, 519-520
Avastin, 138-139
Avelox, 648-649
Avelox IV, 648-649
Aventyl, 686-687
Avinza, 646-648
Avirax, 44-46
Avonex, 516-517
Axert, 61-62
Axid, 684-685
Axid AR, 684-685
Ayercillin, 729-732
azacitidine, 122-123, 1042
azatadine, 1102
azathioprine, 123-124, 1019
Azdone, 478-480
azelaic acid, 1052
azelastine, 125, 1044, 1047, 1048-1049
Azelex, 1052
Azidothymidine, 981-983
azithromycin, 125-127, 1003
Azmacort, 936-938
Azo-Gantanol, 1059
Azo-Gantrisin, 1059
Azopt, 1045, 1046, 1047
AZO-Standard, 744
Azo-Sulfamethoxazole, 1059
Azo-Sulfisoxazole, 1059
AZT, 981-983
aztreonam, 1089
Azulfidine, 870-872
Azulfidine EN-tabs, 870-872

B

Baby Anbesol, 1053
Bacitin, 1052
bacitracin, 1052, 1089
Bacitracin, 1052
baclofen, 127-128
Bactine, 1050
Bactocill, 700-702
Bactrim, 945-947, 1059
Bactrim DS, 1050-1060
Bactrim I.V., 945-947, 1060
Bactroban, 1052
Balminil DM, 303
balsalazide, 128-129
Bancap HC, 478-480, 1060
Banesin, 38-39
Banophen, 322-324
Baraclude, 364, 1028-1029
Barbita, 746-748
BARBITURATES, 996, 1010, 1117, 1123
Baridium, 744
Barriere-HC, 1050
Basalgel, 66-67
Basaljel, 66-67
basiliximab, 129-130, 1019, 1042
Bayer Aspirin, 111-113
Bayer Plus, Extra Strength, 1060
Bayer Select Chest Cold, 1060
Bayer Select Flu Relief, 1060
Bayer Select Head Cold, 1060
Bayer Select Ibuprofen Pain Relief, 491-492
Bayer Select Maximum Strength Headache, 1060
Bayer Select Maximum Strength Menstrual, 1060
Bayer Select Maximum Strength Night-Time Pain Relief, 1060
Bayer Select Maximum Strength Sinus Pain Relief, 1060
Bayer Select Night Time Cold, 1060
Bay Gam, 501-502
BayHep B, 473
BCG vaccine, 1105
BCNU, 184-186
Beben, 1049, 1050
Beclodisk, 130-131
Becloforte Inhaler, 130-131
beclomethasone, 130-131, 1017
beclomethasone (nasal), 1048-1049
Beclovent, 130-131
Beclovent Rotocaps, 130-131
Beconase AQ Nasal, 1048-1049
Beconase Inhalation, 1048-1049
Bedoz, 971-972
Beepen-VK, 729-732
Beesix, 800-801
Bellatal, 1060
Bellergal-S, 1060
Bel-Phen-Ergot-SR, 1060
Benadryl, 322-324
Benadryl 25, 322-324
Benadryl Allergy Decongestant Liquid, 1060
Benadryl Allergy/Sinus Headache Caplets, 1060
Benadryl Decongestant Allergy, 1060
Benadryl Kapseals, 322-324
Benahist 10, 322-324

Entries can be identified as follows: generic name, Trade Name, DRUG CATEGORY, *Combination Product.*

Benahist 50, 322-324
Ben-Allergin-50, 322-324
benazepril, 131-133, 1002
Benefix, 397-398
Benemid, 777-778
Benicar, 693-694
Benoject-10, 322-324
Benoject-50, 322-324
Benuryl, 777-778
Benylin Cough, 322-324
Benylin DM, 303
Benylin-E, 466
Benylin Expectorant Liquid, 1060
Benylin Multi-Symptom Liquid, 1060
BenzaClin, 1060
Benzacot, 944-945
Benzamycin, 1060
benzaphetamine, 1123
benzazocines, 1123
Benzedrex Inhaler, 1048-1049
benzocaine, 1053
BENZODIAZEPINES, 1010-1011, 1123
benzonatate, 133, 1009, 1089
benzoyl peroxide, 1089
benztropine, 133-135, 994, 1006, 1016
benztropine mesylate, 133-135
bepridil, 993
beractant, 1089
BETA-ADRENERGIC BLOCKERS, 993, 1011-1012, 1045, 1046-1047
Betaclinron E-R, 791-793
Betacort, 1049, 1050
Betagen, 1045, 1046-1047
Betalin S, 900
Betaloc, 617-619
Betaloc Durules, 617-619
betamethasone, 135-137, 1017
betamethasone (augmented), 1049, 1050
betamethasone (topical), 1049, 1050
Betapace, 857-858
Betapace AF, 857-858
Betaseron, 516-517
Betatrex, 1049, 1050
Beta-Val, 1049, 1050
Betaxin, 900
betaxolol, 1045, 1046-1047
Betaxon, 1045, 1046-1047
bethanechol, 137-138, 1015
bethanechol chloride, 137-138
Bethaprim, 945-947
Bethovate, 1049, 1050
Betimol, 1045, 1046-1047
Betnelan, 135-137
Betnesol, 135-137
Betoptic, 1045, 1046-1047
Betoptic S, 1045, 1046-1047
bevacizumab, 138-139, 1042
bexarotene, 139-140
Biamine, 900
Biavax II, 1109
Biaxin, 244-246
Biaxin XL, 244-246
bicalutamide, 140-141
Bicillin L-A, 729-732
BiCNU, 184-186
Bidhist, 153-155
BiDil Isosorbide, 1060
bilberry, 1111
bimatoprost, 1046, 1047
BioCal, 169-170
Biocef, 192-196
Bioclate, 101-102
Biozene, 1053
biperiden, 141-142, 994, 1006, 1016
bisacodyl, 142-143, 1020
Bisacolax, 142-143
Bisaco-Lax, 142-143
Bisc-Evac, 142-143
Bisco-Lax, 142-143
Bismatrol, 143-144
Bismatrol Extra Strength, 143-144
Bismed, 143-144
bismuth subsalicylate, 143-144, 993, 999
bisoprolol, 144-146
bitolterol, 1089
bivalirudin, 146-147, 1042
black cohosh, 1111
Black Draught, 845
Blenoxane, 147-149
bleomycin, 147-149, 1005, 1042
Bleph-10, 1044, 1047
Bleph-10 S.O.P., 1044, 1047
Blephamide Ophthalmic Suspension/Ointment, 1060
Blis-To-Sol, 1050, 1051-1052
Blocadren, 912-913
Boil-Ease, 1053
Bonamine, 582-583
Bonine, 582-583
boric acid, 1055
bortezomib, 149-150, 1005
bosentan, 150-151, 1026
B&O Supprettes No. 15A Supps, 1059
B&O Supprettes No. 16A Supps, 1059
BranchAmin, 73-75
Breeze Mist, 1050, 1051-1052
Breeze Mist Antifungal, 1050, 1051-1052
B_{12} Resin, 971-972
Brethine, 893-894
Bretylate, 151-152
bretylium, 151-152, 1000, 1042
bretylium tosylate, 151-152
Bretylol, 151-152
Brevibloc, 383-384
Bricanyl, 893-894
brimonidine, 1046, 1047
brinzolamide, 1045, 1046, 1047
Brogan, 944-945
Bromfed Capsules, 1060
Bromfed-PD Capsules, 1060
Bromfed Talets, 1060
Bromfenac, 153-155
Bromfenex, 1061
Bromfenex PD, 1061
bromocriptine, 152-153, 1006
Bromo-Seltzer, 1061
brompheniramine, 153-155, 1001
BRONCHODILATORS, 1012-1013
Broncho-Grippol-DM, 303
Bronitin Mist, 366-367
Bronkaid Mist, 366-367
Bronkodyl, 898-899
Brove X, 153-155
Brove X CT, 153-155
buckthorn, 1112
Bucladin-S Softabs, 1102
buclizine, 1102
budesonide, 155-156, 1001
budesonide (nasal), 1048-1049
Bufferin, 1061
Bufferin AF Nite-Time, 1061
bumetanide, 156-158, 1018
Bumex, 156-158
Buminate 5%, 51-52
Buminate 25%, 51-52
Buprenex, 158-159
buprenorphine, 158-159, 1023

bupropion, 160-161, 997
Burn-O-Jel, 1053
BuSpar, 161-162
buspirone, 161-162
busulfan, 162-164, 1005, 1042
Busulfex, 162-164
butenafine, 1050, 1051-1052
Butibel, 1061
butoconazole, 1054-1055
butorphanol, 164-166, 1023
Bydramine, 322-324
Byetta, 1029-1030

C

cabergoline, 166, 1006, 1089-1090
Caduet, 1061
Cafatine PB, 1061
Cafergot, 1061
Cafergot Suppositories, 1061
Caladryl, 1061
Calan, 963-965
Calan SR, 963-965
Calcarb, 169-170
Calcet, 1061
Calci-Chew, 169-170
Calciferol, 972-973
Calcijex, 168-169
Calcilac, 169-170
Calcilean, 470-472
Calcimir, 166-168
Calciparine, 470-472
Calcite, 169-170
calcitonin (human), 166-168
calcitonin (salmon), 166-168
calcitriol, 168-169
calcium carbonate, 169-170, 993
CALCIUM CHANNEL BLOCKERS, 993, 1013-1014
calcium chloride, 170-172
calcium gluceptate, 170-172
calcium gluconate, 170-172
calcium lactate, 170-172
calcium polycarbophil, 172-173, 1020
Caldecort Anti-Itch, 1050
Caldesene, 1050, 1051-1052
Calglycine, 169-170
Calm-X, 319-321
Calmylin Expectorant, 466
Cal-Plus, 169-170
Calsan, 169-170
Caltrate 600, 169-170
Caltrate 600+D, 1061
Caltrate Jr., 169-170
Cama Arthritis Pain Reliever, 1061
Campath, 56-57
Camptosar, 520-522
Canadian controlled substance chart, 1123-1124
Canadian immunization schedules, 1125
CANADIAN MEDICATIONS, HIGH-ALERT, 1121
Canafed, 796-797
Canasa, 595-596
candesartan, 173-174, 1002
Canesten, 1054-1055
Canestew, 1050, 1051-1052
capecitabine, 174-175, 1005
Capital w/Codeine, 1061
Capoten, 175-177
Capozide 25/15, 1061
Capozide 25/25, 1061
Capozide 50/15, 1061
Capozide 50/25, 1061
capsicum peppers, 1112
captopril, 175-177
Carafate, 868-869
carbachol, 1045, 1047
Carbacot, 601-602
carbamazepine, 177-179, 996
Carbastat, 1045, 1047
Carbatrol, 177-179
Carbex, 843-844
carbidopa-levodopa, 179-181, 1006
Carbolith, 562-564
CARBONIC ANHYDRASE INHIBITORS, 1045, 1047
carboplatin, 181-182, 1005, 1042
carboprost, 182-183
Carboptic, 1045, 1047
Cardec DM Syrup, 1061
Cardene, 671-673
Cardene IV, 671-673
Cardene SR, 671-673
CARDIAC GLYCOSIDES, 1014
CARDIOPLEGIC SOLUTIONS, 1042, 1121
Cardioquin, 805-807
Cardizem, 318-319
Cardizem CD, 318-319
Cardizem LA, 318-319
Cardizem SR, 318-319
Cardura, 339-340
carimune NF, 501-502
carisoprodol, 183-184
Carmol HC, 1050
carmustine, 184-186, 1005, 1042
carteolol, 186-187, 1012, 1045, 1046-1047
Carteolol HCl, 1045, 1046-1047
Carter's Little Pills, 142-143
Cartrol, 186-187
carvedilol, 187-189
cascara sagrada/cascara sagrada aromatic fluid extract/cascara sagrada fluid extract, 189-190, 1020
Casodex, 140-141
Cataflam, 308-309
Catapres, 253-255
Catapres-TTS, 253-255
Cathflo, 64-66
CCNU, 565-566
CdA, 1090
Cebid, 108-109
Ceclor, 196-202
Ceclor CD, 196-202
Cecon, 108-109
Cecore 500, 108-109
Cedax, 202-210
Cedocard-SR, 526-527
CeeNU, 565-566
cefaclor, 190, 196-202, 1003
cefadroxil, 190, 192-196, 1003
Cefadyl, 192-196
cefazolin, 190, 192-196, 1003
cefdinir, 190, 202-210, 1003
cefditoren, 1003
cefditoren pivoxil, 190, 202-210
cefepime, 190, 202-210, 1003
cefixime, 190
Cefizox, 202-210
cefmetazole, 190, 196-202, 1003
Cefobid, 202-210
cefonicid, 1003
cefoperazone, 190, 202-210, 1003
Cefotan, 196-202

Entries can be identified as follows: generic name, Trade Name, DRUG CATEGORY, *Combination Product.*

cefotaxime, 190, 202-210, 1004
cefotetan, 190, 196-202
cefoxitin, 190, 196-202
cefpodoxime, 190, 202-210
cefprozil, 190, 196-202, 1004
ceftazidime, 190, 202-210
ceftibuten, 190, 202-210, 1004
Ceftin, 196-202
ceftizoxime, 190, 202-210
ceftriaxone, 190, 202-210
cefuroxime, 190, 196-202, 1004
Cefuroxime, 196-202
Cefzil, 196-202
Celebrex, 190-192
celecoxib, 190-192, 1022, 1042
Celestoderm, 1049, 1050
Celestone, 135-137
Celexa, 242-244
CellCept, 651-653
Cel-U-Jec, 135-137
Cemill, 108-109
Cenafed, 796-797
Cenafed Plus Tablets, 1061
Cena-K, 767-769
Cenestin, 387-389
Cenocort A-40, 936-938
Cenocort Forte, 936-938
Cenolate, 108-109
cephalexin, 190, 192-196, 1004
CEPHALOSPORINS—1st GENERATION, 192-196
CEPHALOSPORINS—2ND GENERATION, 196-202
CEPHALOSPORINS—3RD GENERATION, 202-210
cephapirin, 192-196, 210, 1004
cephradine, 192-196, 210, 1004
Cephulac, 536-537
Ceptaz, 202-210
Cerebyx, 437-438
Cerubidine, 288-290
Cervidil Vaginal Insert, 321-322
C.E.S., 387-389
Cetacort, 1050
Cetamide, 1044, 1047
Cetane, 108-109
Cetapred Ophthalmic Ointment, 1061
cetirizine, 210-211, 1001
cetrorelix, 211
Cetrotide, 211
cetuximab, 212-213, 1005
Cevalin, 108-109
Cevi-Bid, 108-109
Ce-Vi-Sol, 108-109
chamomile, 1112
Charco-Aid 2000, 43-44
CharcoCaps, 43-44
Chemet, 866-867
CHEMOTHERAPEUTIC AGENTS, 1042, 1121
Cheracol D Cough Formula Syrup, 1061
Cheracol Syrup, 1061
Chibroxin, 1044, 1047
Children, immunization schedules for, 1125
Children's Advil, 491-492
Children's Cepacol Liquid, 1061
Children's Chloraseptic, 1053
Children's Congestion Relief, 796-797
Children's Daramamine, 319-321
Children's Feverall, 38-39
Children's Hold, 303
Children's Motrin, 491-492
Children's Nostril, 1048-1049
Children's Silfedrine, 796-797
Chlo-Amine, 223-224
chloral hydrate, 213-214, 1117
chlorambucil, 214-216, 1005
chloramphenicol, 216-217
Chloramphenicol, 1044, 1047
chloramphenicol (ophthalmic), 1044, 1047
chloramphenicol (otic), 1055
Chlorate, 223-224
chlordiazepoxide, 218-219, 1011, 1117
chlordiazepoxide HCl, 218-219
Chloromag, 576-578
Chloromycetin, 216-217
Chloromycetin Ophthalmic, 1044, 1047
Chloromycetin Otic, 1055
Chloroptic, 1044, 1047
Chloroptic S.O.P., 1044, 1047
chloroquine, 219-220
chloroquine phosphate, 219-220
chlorothiazide, 220-223, 1018
Chlorpazine, 781-783
Chlorphed, 153-155
chlorpheniramine, 223-224, 1001
chlorpheniramine maleate, 223-224
Chlorpromanyl, 224-227
chlorpromazine, 224-227, 1007
chlorpromazine HCl, 224-227
chlorpropamide, 998, 1090
chlorthalidone, 227-228, 1018
Chlor-Trimeton, 223-224
Chlor-Trimeton Allergy 4 Hour Decongestant, 1061
Chlor-Trimeton 12 Hour Relief Tablets, 1061
Chlor-Tripolon, 223-224
Cholac, 536-537
cholecalciferol, 229, 972-973
Choledyl SA, 707-708
cholera vaccine, 1105
cholestyramine, 229-230
choline/magnesium salicylates, 230-231
CHOLINERGIC BLOCKERS, 1015-1016, 1045, 1047
CHOLINERGICS, 1015, 1045, 1047
choline salicylate, 230-231, 1024
chondroitin, 1112
Chooz, 169-170
Chromagen, 1061
chromium, 926-927, 1112
Chronulac, 536-537
Cialis, 879-880
Cibacalcin, 166-168
ciclopirox, 1050, 1051-1052
cidofovir, 232-233, 1009
Cidomycin, 456-458
cilastatin, 233
cilostazol, 233-234
Ciloxan, 1044, 1047
cimetidine, 234-236, 1019
cinacalcet, 236-237
Cin-Quin, 805-807
Cipro, 237-239
ciprofloxacin, 237-239, 1004
ciprofloxacin (ophthalmic), 1044, 1047
Cipro HC Otic, 1062
Cipro IV, 237-239
Cipro XR, 237-239

cisatracurium, 240
cisplatin, 240-242, 1005, 1042
citalopram, 242-244, 997
Citrate of Magnesia, 576-578
Citroma, 576-578
Citromag, 576-578
Citrovorum Factor, 544-545
cladribine (CdA), 1005, 1090
Claforan, 202-210
Clarinex, 295
Clarinex Reditabs, 295
clarithromycin, 244-246, 1003
Claritin, 567-568
Claritin-D 12 Hour, 1062
Claritin-D 24-Hour, 1062
Claritin Non-Drowsy Allergy, 567-568
Claritin Reditabs, 567-568
clavulanate, 246
Clavulin, 87-89
Clear Eyes, 1046, 1047
Clear Eyes ACR, 1046, 1047
Clear Nicoderm CQ, 673-674
clemastine, 246-247, 1103
Cleocin HCl, 247-249
Cleocin Pediatric, 247-249
Cleocin Phosphate, 247-249
Cleocin T, 1052
Climara, 385-387
Clinagen LA, 385-387
Clindagel, 1052
ClindaMax, 1052
clindamycin (topical), 1052
clindamycin HCl, 247-249
clindamycin palmitate, 247-249
clindamycin phosphate, 247-249
Clindets, 1052
Clindex, 1062
Clinoril, 874-875
clioquinol, 1050, 1051-1052
clobetasol, 1049, 1050
clocortolone, 1049, 1050, 1090
Cloderm, 1049, 1050
clofazimine, 1090
Clomid, 249-250
clomiphene, 249-250
clomiphene citrate, 249-250
clomipramine, 250-251, 997
Clomycin Ointment, 1062
clonazepam, 251-252, 996, 1011
clonidine, 253-255, 1002
clonidine HCl, 253-255
clopidogrel, 255-256
clorazepate, 256-257
Clotrimaderm, 1050, 1051-1052
clotrimazole, 1050, 1051-1052, 1090
Clotrimazole, 1050, 1051-1052, 1054-1055
clotrimazole (vaginal), 1054-1055
cloxacillin, 257-258, 1004
Cloxapen, 257-258
clozapine, 258-260
Clozaril, 258-260
CMT, 230-231
coagulation factor VIIa, recombinant, 260-261, 1042
Co-Apap, 1062
Cobex, 971-972
Cobolin-M Crystamine, 971-972
cocaine, 1117, 1123
codeine, 261-262, 1009, 1023, 1123
Codeprex, 1062
Codiclear DH Syrup, 1062
Codimal, 1062
Codimal DH Syrup, 1062
Codimal DM Syrup, 1062
Codimal-LA, 1062
Codimal PH Syrup, 1062
coenzyme Q10, 1112
Cogentin, 133-135
Co-Gesic, 478-480, 1062
Cognex, 877-878
Colace, 332-333
Colazal, 128-129
ColBenemid, 1062
colchicine, 263-264, 1121
Coldrine, 1062
colesevelam, 264-265
Colestid, 265-266
colestipol, 265-266
Collyrium Fresh, 1046, 1047
Col-Probenecid, 1062
Coly-Mycin S Otic Suspension, 1062
COMBINATION PRODUCTS, 1056-1085
CombiPatch 0.05/0.14, 1062
CombiPatch 0.05/0.25, 1062
Combipres 0.1, 1062
Combipres 0.2, 1062
Combipres 0.3, 1062
Combisor, 1062
Combivent, 1062
Combivir, 1062
Comfort Eye Drops, 1046, 1047
Compa-Z, 781-783
Compazine, 781-783
Compoz, 322-324
Comtan, 363-364
Comtrex Allergy-Sinus, 1062
Comtrex Liquid, 1063
Comtrex Maximum Strength, 1063
Comtrex Maximum Strength Multi-Symptoms Cold, Flu Relief, 1063
Comtrex Maximum Strength Non-Drowsy Caplets, 1063
Concentrated Multiple Trace Elements, 926-927
Concerta, 608-610
Congess SR, 1063
Congest, 387-389
Congestac, 1063
Congestion Relief, 796-797
conivaptan, 1041
conjugated estrogens, 387-389
Constilac, 536-537
Constulose, 536-537
Contac Allergy 12 Hour, 1103, 246-247
Contac Cough & Chest Cold Liquid, 1063
Contac Cough & Sore Throat Liquid, 1063
Contac Day Allergy/Sinus, 1063
Contac Day Cold and Flu, 1063
Contac Night Allergy Sinus, 1063
Contac Night Cold and Flu Caplets, 1063
Contac Non-Drowsy Maximum Strength 12 Hour, 1063
Contac Severe Cold & Flu Nighttime Liquid, 1063
ConTE-PAK-4, 926-927
contraceptives, 266-267
Contranzine, 781-783

Entries can be identified as follows: generic name, Trade Name, DRUG CATEGORY, *Combination Product.*

Controlled substance chart, 1117
Controlled substance chart, Canadian, 1123-1124
Copaxone, 458-459
copper, 926-927
Cordarone, 79-81
Cordran, 1049, 1050
Cordran SP, 1049, 1050
Coreg, 187-189
Corgard, 654-655
Coricidin, 1063
Coricidin D Cold, Flu & Sinus, 1063
Coricidin D Tablets, 1063
Coricidin HBP Congestion & Cough Softgels Capsules, 1063
Coricidin HBP Cough and Cold, 1063
Coricidin HBP Maximum Strength Flu, 1063
Corlopam, 404-405
Cormax, 1049, 1050
Coronex, 526-527
Correctol, 748-749
Correctol Extra Gentle, 332-333
Cortacet, 1050
Cortaid, 1050
Cortate, 1050
Cort-Dome, 1050
Cortef, 480-482, 1050
Cortenema, 480-482
Corticaine, 1050
CORTICOSTEROIDS, 1016-1017
CORTICOSTEROIDS, OPHTHALMIC, 1045, 1047
corticotropin (ACTH), 1090
Corticreme, 1050
Cortifair, 1050
Cortifoam, 480-482
cortisone, 268-269, 1017
Cortisporin Ophthalmic Ointment, 1063
Cortisporin Ophthalmic/Otic Suspension, 1063
Cortisporin Topical Cream, 1063
Cortisporin Topical Ointment, 1064
Cortizone, 1050
Cortoderm, 1050
Cortone, 268-269
cortone acetate, 268-269
Cortril, 1050
Corvert, 492-493
Coryphen, 111-113
Corzide 40/5, 1064
Corzide 80/5, 1064
Cosmegen, 280-281
Cosopt, 1064
cosyntropin, 1091
Cotazym, 718-719
Cotazym-65B, 718-719
Cotazym Capsules, 718-719
Cotazym E.C.S. 8, 718-719
Cotazym E.C.S. 20, 718-719
Cotazym-S, 718-719
Cotrim, 945-947
cotrimoxazole, 269, 945-947
Cough-X, 1064
Coumadin, 976-977
Covera-HS, 963-965
Cozaar, 570-571
Creon, 718-719, 1064
Creo-Terpin, 303
Crestor, 836-837
Crinone, 783-784
Crixivan, 506-507
crotamiton, 1091
Cruex, 1050, 1051-1052
C-Span, 108-109
Cubicin, 285-286
Curretab, 583-584
Cutivate, 1049, 1050
Cyanabin, 971-972
cyanocobalamin, 971-972
Cyanoject, 971-972
cyclizine, 1103
cyclobenzaprine, 269-270
cyclobenzaprine HCl, 269-270
Cyclocort, 1049, 1050
Cycloflex, 269-270
Cyclogyl, 1045, 1047
Cyclomen, 282-284
Cyclomydril Ophthalmic Solution, 1064
cyclopentolate, 1045, 1047
Cyclopentolate HCl, 1045, 1047
cyclophosphamide, 270-272, 1005, 1042
cyclosporine, 272-274, 1019
Cycrin, 583-584
Cymbalta, 349-350
Cyomin, 971-972
cyproheptadine, 274-275, 1001
cyproheptadine HCl, 274-275
Cystospaz, 488-489
Cystospaz-M, 488-489
cytarabine, 275-277, 1005, 1042
Cytomel, 557-559
Cytosar, 275-277
Cytosar-U, 275-277
cytosine arabinoside, 275-277
Cytotec, 637
Cytovene, 446-448
Cytoxan, 270-272

D

dacarbazine, 277-279, 1005, 1042
daclizumab, 279-280, 1042
Dacodyl, 142-143
dactinomycin, 280-281, 1005, 1042
Dalacin C, 247-249
Dalacin C Palmitate, 247-249
Dalacin C Phosphate, 247-249
Dalalone, 297-299
Dalalone DP, 297-299
Dalalone LA, 297-299
Dallergy Caplets, 1064
Dallergy-D Syrup, 1064
Dallergy Syrup, 1064
Dallergy Tablets, 1064
Dalmane, 425-427
dalteparin, 281-282, 995, 1042
Daltose, 973-974
Damason-P, 478-480, 1064
Damazide, 39-42
danaparoid, 282-284, 995, 1042
danazol, 282-284
Danocrine, 282-284
Dantrium, 284-285
dantrolene, 284-285
Dapa, 38-39
Dapacin, 38-39
dapiprazole, 1044, 1047
dapsone (DDS), 1091
daptomycin, 285-286, 1004
Daraprim, 801-802
darbepoetin alfa, 286-287
Darvocet-N 100, 1064
Darvon, 790-791
Darvon Compound-65, 1064
Darvon-N, 790-791
Darvon-N w/A.S.A., 1064
Darvon-N Compound, 1064
Datril, 38-39
daunorubicin, 288-290, 1005, 1042
daunorubicin citrate liposome, 288-290
DaunoXome, 288-290
Dayalets, 649-650
Daypro, 703-704

DC Softgels, 332-333
DDAVP, 295-297
ddC, 978-979
ddI, 311-312
DDS, 1091
Decadron, 297-299
Decadron-LA, 297-299
Decadron Phosphate, 297-299, 1045, 1047
Deca-Durabolin, 661-662
Decaject, 297-299
Decaject-LA, 297-299
Decaspray, 1049, 1050
Decofed Syrup, 796-797
Deconamine, 1064
Deconamine CX, 1064
Deconamine SR, 1064
Deconamine Syrup, 1064
DECONGESTANTS/ VASOCONSTRICTORS, NASAL, 1047-1049
DECONGESTANTS/ VASOCONSTRICTORS, OPHTHALMIC, 1046, 1047
Decylenes, 1050, 1051-1052
DeFed-60, 796-797
Defen-LA, 1064
deferoxamine, 1091
Deficol, 142-143
Defy, 1045-1047
Degest 2, 1046, 1047
Dehist, 153-155
Delatest, 895-896
Delatestryl, 895-896
delavirdine, 290-291, 1009
Delcort, 1050
Delestrogen, 385-387
Delsym, 303
Delta-Cortef, 772-774
Delta-D, 972-973
Deltasone, 774-775
Delta-Tritex, 1050
Del-Vi-A, 969-970
demecarium, 1045, 1047
demeclocycline, 1091
Demerol, 590-592
DemiCort, 1050
Demi-Regroton, 1064
Demulin 1/20, 1064
Demulin 1/35, 1064
Denavir, 1052-1053
denileukin diftitox, 291-292
Dentipatch, 1053
Depacon, 954-955
Depakene, 954-955
Depakote, 954-955
Depakote ER, 954-955
depAndro, 895-896
depGynogen, 385-387
dep Medalone, 610-612
Depo Cyt, 275-277
Depo-Estradiol, 385-387
Depogen, 385-387
Depoject, 610-612
Depo-Medrol, 610-612
Deponit, 681-682
Depopred, 610-612
Depo-Predate, 610-612
Depo-Provera, 583-584
Depotest, 895-896
Depo-Testadiol, 1064
Depo-Testosterone, 895-896
Dermacort, 1050
Derma Flex, 1053
Dermatop, 1050
Dermoplast, 1053
Dermovate, 1049, 1050
Dermtex HC, 1050
Deronil, 297-299
Desenex, 1050, 1051-1052
Desenex Maximum Strength, 1050, 1051-1052
desipramine, 292-293, 997, 1091
desipramine HCl, 292-293
desirudin, 294, 995
desloratadine, 295, 1001
desmopressin, 295-297
Desogen, 1064
desonide, 1049, 1050
Desonide, 1049, 1050
Des Owen, 1049, 1050
desoximetasone, 1049, 1050
desoxyephedrine, 1047, 1048-1049
desoxyribonuclease, 297
Desyrel, 932-934
Desyrel Dividose, 932-934
Detensol, 791-793
Detrol, 922-923
Detrol LA, 922-923
Dexacen-4, 297-299
Dexacen LA-8, 297-299
Dexacidin Ophthalmic Ointment/Suspension, 1064
dexamethasone, 297-299, 1017, 1045, 1047
dexamethasone (topical), 1049, 1050
dexamethasone acetate, 297-299
Dexamethasone Ophthalmic Suspension, 1045, 1047
dexamethasone sodium phosphate, 297-299
Dexasone, 297-299
Dexasone-LA, 297-299
Dexasporin Ophthalmic Ointment, 1064-1065
Dexchlor, 1103
dexchlorpheniramine, 1103
dexclorpheniramine maleate, 1103
Dexedrine, 301-302
Dexedrine Spansule, 301-302
DexFerrum, 522-523
dexmedetomidine, 299
dexmethylphenidate, 300-301
Dexon, 297-299
Dexone, 297-299
Dexone LA, 297-299
dextroamphetamine, 301-302
dextromethorphan, 303, 1009
dextrose, hypertonic, 1042, 1121
dextrose (D-glucose), 304-305
Dextrostat, 301-302
Dey-Lute, 596-597
d4T, 861-863
DHC Plus, 1065
DHE 45, 375-376
DHT Intensol, 316-317
DiaBeta, 460-462
Diabetic Tussin EX, 466
Dialose DOK, 332-333
Dialose Plus, 1065
Dialume, 66-67
DIALYSIS SOLUTIONS, 1042, 1121
Diamox, 39-42
Diamox Sequels, 39-42
Diar Aid, 121-122
Diasorb, 121-122
Diazemuls, 305-307
diazepam, 305-307, 996, 1011, 1117, 1123
diazoxide, 307-308, 1003
diazoxide parenteral, 307-308
dibucaine, 1053
Dibucaine, 1053
Dicarbosil, 169-170
diclofenac, 1022, 1046, 1047
diclofenac potassium, 308-309
diclofenac sodium, 308-309
dicloxacillin, 309-311, 1004

Entries can be identified as follows: generic name, Trade Name, DRUG CATEGORY, *Combination Product.*

dicloxacillin sodium, 309-311
dicyclomine, 1092
didanosine, 311-312, 1009
dideoxycitidine, 978-979
dideoxyinosine, 311-312
Didronel, 391-392
Didronel IV, 391-392
difenoxin/atropine, 312, 324-325
diflorasone, 1049, 1050
Diflucan, 416-417
diflunisal, 1092
Di-Gel Advanced Formula, 1065
Di-Gel Liquid, 1065
Digibind, 315-316
DigiFab, 315-316
digoxin, 313-315, 1000, 1014, 1042
digoxin immune Fab (ovine), 315-316
Dibistine DH Liquid, 1065
dihydroergotamine, 316, 375-376
Dihydroergotamine Sandoz, 375-376
dihydrotachysterol, 316-317
1,25-dihydroxycholecalciferol, 168-169
Dilacor-XR, 318-319
Dilantin, 752-754
Dilantin-125, 752-754
Dilantin Infatab, 752-754
Dilantin Kapseals, 752-754
Dilatrate-SR, 526-527
Dilaudid, 482-484
Dilaudid Cough Syrup, 1065
Dilaudid-HP, 482-484
Dilor, 352-353
Dilor-G, 1065
Diltia XR, 318-319
diltiazem, 318-319, 993, 1014, 1042
dimenhydrinate, 319-321
Dimentabs, 319-321
dimercaprol, 1092
Dimetane, 153-155
Dimetane Decongestant, 1065
Dimetane-DX Cough Syrup, 1065
Dimetane Extentabs, 153-155
Dimetapp Allergy Liqui-Gels, 153-155
Dimetapp DM Elixir, 1065
Dimetapp Long Acting Cough Plus Cold Syrup, 1065
Dimetapp Sinus, 1065
Dinate, 319-321
dinoprostone, 321-322
Diocaine, 1044, 1047
Dioeze, 332-333
Dioval, 385-387
Diovan, 956-957
Diovan 80 HCT, 1065
Diovan 160 HCT, 1065
Dipetum, 694-695
Diphenadryl, 322-324
Diphen Cough, 322-324
Diphenhist, 322-324
diphenhydramine, 322-324, 1001, 1009
diphenhydramine HCl, 322-324
diphenoxylate with atropine, 324-325
Diphenylan, 752-754
Diphenylhydantoin, 752-754
diphtheria, pertussis, and tetanus (DPT) vaccine, 1125
diphtheria and tetanus toxoids, adsorbed, 1105
diphtheria and tetanus toxoids and acellular pertussis vaccine, 1105
diphtheria and tetanus toxoids and whole-cell pertussis vaccine (DPT, DTP), 1105
dipivefrin, 1046, 1047
Diprivan, 788-790
Diprolene, 1049, 1050
Diprolene AF, 1049, 1050
Diprosone, 1049, 1050
dipyridamole, 325-326, 993, 1026
dirithromycin, 327-328
Disalcid, 838-839
Disonate, 332-333
Disoprofol, 788-790
disopyramide, 328-329, 1000
Di-Sosul, 332-333
disulfiram, 1092
Ditropan, 708-709
Ditropan XL, 708-709
DIURETICS, 1017-1018
Diurigen w/Reserpine, 1065
Diuril, 220-223
Diutensin-R, 1065
divalproex sodium, 329, 954-955
Dixarit, 253-255
Doan's PM Extra Strength, 1065
dobutamine, 329-330
Dobutamine, 329-330
Dobutrex, 329-330
docetaxel, 330-332
docosanol, 1054
Dr. Caldwell Dosalax, 845
docusate, 1020
docusate calcium, 332-333
docusate sodium, 332-333
dofetilide, 333-334
Dolacet, 478-480, 1065
Dolagesic, 478-480
dolasetron, 334-335
Dolene, 790-791
Dolophine, 598-600
donepezil, 335-336
dong quai, 1112
Donnamar, 488-489
Donnatal, 1065
Donnatal Elixir, 1065
Donnatal Extentabs, 1065
Donnazyme, 1065
Dopamet, 605-607
dopamine, 336-337, 1042
dopamine HCl, 336-337
Dopar, 549-550
Dopram, 337-339
Dorcol Children's Cold Formula Liquid, 1065
Dorcol Children's Decongestant, 796-797
Dormin, 322-324
Doryx, 345-346
dorzolamide, 1045, 1046, 1047
DOS Diocto, 332-333
Dostinex, 166
doxacurium, 1092
doxapram, 337-339
doxazosin, 339-340, 1003
doxepin, 340-342, 997
doxepin HCl, 340-342
doxercalciferol, 342
Doxidan, 1065
Doxil, 343-345
Doxine, 800-801
doxorubicin, 343-345, 1005, 1043
doxorubicin liposome, 343-345
Doxy, 345-346
Doxycin, 345-346
doxycycline, 345-346, 1004
DPH, 752-754
DPT, 1105, 1125
Dramamine, 319-321
Dramamine Less Drowsy Formula, 582-583
Dramanate, 319-321
Drenison 1/4, 1049, 1050
Drenison Tape, 1049, 1050
Dri/Ear, 1055
Drisdol, 972-973
Dristan, 1048-1049
Dristan Cold, 1065

Dristan Cold Maximum Strength Caplets, 1065-1066
Dristan Cold Multi-Symptom Formula, 1066
Dristan Sinus, 1066
Drixoral Allergy Sinus, 1066
Drixoral Cold & Allergy, 1066
Drixoral Cold & Flu, 1066
Drixoral Nasal Decongestant, 1066
Drixoral Non-Drowsy Formula, 796-797
droperidol, 347-348, 992, 1043
drotrecogin alfa, 348-349, 1024
Droxia, 485-487
DRUGS, HIGH ALERT, 1042-1043
DRUGS, RARELY USED, 1086-1101
DRUGS, RECENT APPROVALS OF, 1041
D-S-S, 332-333
DT, 1066
DTaP, 1105
DTIC, 277-279
DTIC-Dome, 277-279
DTP, 1066, 1105
DTwP, 1105
Duagen, 351
Dulcagen, 142-143
Dulcolax, 142-143
duloxetine, 349-350
Duocet, 478-480
DuoNeb, 1066
Duphalac, 536-537
Duracillin A.S., 729-732
Duraclon, 253-255
Dura-Estrin, 385-387
Duragan, 385-387
Duragesic, 407-408
Duralith, 562-564
Duralone, 610-612
Duramist Plus, 1048-1049
Duramorph, 646-648
Dura-test, 895-896
Duration, 1048-1049
Dura-Vent/DA, 1066
Duricef, 192-196
dutasteride, 351
Duvoid, 137-138
Dyazide, 1066
Dycill, 309-311
Dyflex-200, 352-353
Dylline, 352-353
Dylline-GG Tablets, 1066
Dymenate, 319-321
Dynabac, 327-328
Dynacin, 632-634
DynaCirc, 527-528
DynaCirc CR, 527-528
Dynafed, 796-797
Dynafed Asthma Relief, 1066
Dynafed Plus Maximum Strength, 1066
Dynapen, 309-311
dyphylline, 352-353, 1013
Dyphylline-GG Elixir, 1066
Dyrenium, 938-939

E

Ear Dry, 1055
Easprin, 111-113
E-base, 379-380
echinacea, 1112
EC-Naprosyn, 662-664
E-Complex-600, 973-974
econazole, 1050, 1051-1052
Econopred, 1045, 1047
Econopred Plus, 1045, 1047
ecothiophate, 1045, 1047
Ecotrin, 111-113
Ectosonel, 1049, 1050
E-Cypionate, 385-387
edetate calcium disodium, 1092-1093
edetate disodium, 1093
ED-INSOL, 408-410
edrophonium, 353-354, 1015
ED-SPAZ, 488-489
Edur-Acin, 670-671
EES, 379-381
efalizumab, 1093
efavirenz, 354-355
E-Ferol, 973-974
Effer-K, 767-769
Effexor, 962-963
Effexor XR, 962-963
Efidac/24, 796-797
Efudex, 419-421
8-Hour Bayer Timed Release, 111-113
E-200 I.U. Softgels, 973-974
ELA-Max, 1053
Elase, 411-412
Elase Ointment, 1066
Eldepryl, 843-844
Elestat, 1044, 1047
eletriptan, 355-356
Elidel, 1054
Elitek, 814
Elixomin, 898-899
Elixophyllin, 898-899
Elixophyllin GG Liquid, 1066
Ellence, 367-369
Elocon, 1050
E-Lor, 1066
Eloxitan, 702-703
Elspar, 109-111
Eltor, 796-797
Eltroxin, 551-553
Emadine, 1044, 1047
Embeline E 0.05%, 1049, 1050
emedastine, 1044, 1047
Emend, 103-104
Emex, 613-615
Eminase, 99-101
EMLA Cream, 1066
Emo-Cort, 1050
Empirin, 111-113
Empirin w/Codeine #3, 1066
Empirin w/Codeine #4, 1066
Empracet-60, 1066
emtricitabine, 356-357, 1009
Emtriva, 356-357
E-Mycin, 379-380
enalapril, 1002
enalapril/enalaprilat, 357-359
Enbrel, 389-390
Endep, 81-82
Endocervical Gel, 321-322
Endocet, 709-710, 1066
Endocodone, 709-710
Endodan, 709-710, 1066
Enduronyl, 1066
Enduronyl Forte, 1067
Ener-B, 971-972
enfuvirtide, 359-360, 1010
Engerix-G, 1106
Enjuvia, 387-389
Enlon, 353-354
enoxacin, 360-361, 1004
enoxaparin, 361-363, 995, 1043
entacapone, 363-364
entecavir, 364, 1028-1029
Entex PSE, 1067
Entocort EC, 155-156
Entrophen, 111-113
Enulose, 536-537
ephedrine, 364-365, 1013, 1043
ephedrine (nasal), 1047, 1048-1049
ephedrine sulfate, 364-365
EPIDURAL/INTRATHECAL MEDICATIONS, 1042, 1121

Entries can be identified as follows: generic name, Trade Name, DRUG CATEGORY, *Combination Product.*

Epifoam, 1050
Epifoam Aerosol Foam, 1067
Epifrin, 1046, 1047
E-Pilo-1 Ophthalmic Solution, 1066
E-Pilo-2 Ophthalmic Solution, 1066
E-Pilo-4 Ophthalmic Solution, 1066
E-Pilo-6 Ophthalmic Solution, 1066
Epimorph, 646-648
Epinal, 366-367
epinastine, 1044, 1047
epinephrine, 366-367, 1013, 1043
epinephrine (nasal), 1047, 1048-1049
epinephrine/epinephryl borate, 1046, 1047
Epinephrine Pediatric, 366-367
EpiPen, 366-367
EpiPen Jr., 366-367
epirubicin, 367-369, 1005, 1043
Epitol, 177-179
Epitrate, 366-367
Epival, 954-955
Epivir, 537-539
Epivir-HBV, 537-539
eplerenone, 369-370
EPO, 370-372
epoetin, 370-372
Epogen, 370-372
Eppy, 1046, 1047
Eppy/N, 366-367
Eprex, 370-372
eprosartan, 372-373, 1002
epsilon-aminocaproic acid, 75-76
Epsom Salt, 576-578
eptifibatide, 373-374, 1043
Epzicom, 1067
Equagesic, 1067
Equalactin, 172-173
Equetro, 177-179
Equilet, 169-170
Eramycin, 379-380
Erbitux, 212-213
ergocalciferol, 374, 972-973
Ergomar, 375-376
Ergometrine, 374-375
ergonovine, 374-375
Ergostat, 375-376
ergotamine, 375-376
ergotrate, 374-375
Eridium, 744
erlotinib, 376-377
Ertaczo, 1050, 1051-1052
ertapenem, 377-379, 1004
Erybid, 379-380
Eryc, 379-380
Eryderm, 1052
Erygel, 1052
Ery Ped, 379-380
Ery-Tab, 379-380
Erythrocin, 379-380
Erythromid, 379-380
erythromycin (ophthalmic), 1044, 1047
Erythromycin (ophthalmic), 1044, 1047
erythromycin (topical), 1052
Erythromycin (topical), 1052
erythromycin base, 379-380
Erythromycin Base Filmtab, 379-380
Erythromycin Delayed-Release, 379-380
erythromycin estolate, 379-380
erythromycin ethylsuccinate, 379-380
erythromycin gluceptate, 379-380
erythromycin lactobionate, 379-380
erythromycin stearate, 379-380
Eryzole, 1067
escitalopram, 381-382, 997
Esclim, 385-387
Esgic-Plus, 1067
Esidrix, 476-478
Esimil, 1067
Eskalith, 562-564
Eskalith CR, 562-564
esmolol, 383-384, 1000, 1012
esomeprazole, 384-385
Espotabs, 748-749
Estrace, 385-387
Estraderm, 385-387
estradiol, 385-387
estradiol cypionate, 385-387
estradiol topical emulsion, 385-387
estradiol transdermal system, 385-387
estradiol vaginal ring, 385-387
estradiol vaginal tablet, 385-387
estradiol valerate, 385-387
Estragyn LAS, 385-387
Estra-L, 385-387
estramustine, 1093
Estrasorb, 385-387
Estratest, 1067
Estratest HS, 1067
Estring, 385-387
Estro-Cyp, 385-387
Estrofem, 385-387
estrogens, conjugated, 387-389
estrogens, conjugated synthetic B, 387-389
Estroject-LA, 385-387
Estro-L.A., 385-387
Estro-span, 385-387
etanercept, 389-390
ethambutol, 390-391, 1008
Ethmozine, 644-646
ethosuximide, 1093
Ethyol, 69-70
Etibi, 390-391
etidronate, 391-392
etodolac, 392-394, 1022
etomidate, 992, 1093
etoposide (VP-16), 394-395, 1005, 1043
Etrafon, 1067
Etrafon 2-10, 1067
Etrafon A, 1067
Etrafon Forte, 1067
Euglucon, 460-462
Eulexin, 427
Evac-U-Gen, 748-749
Evac-U-Lax, 748-749
Evalose, 536-537
Everone, 895-896
Evista, 809-810
E-Vitamin Succinate, 973-974
Excedrin IB, 491-492
Excedrin Migraine, 1067
Excedrin P.M., 1067
Excedrin P.M. Liquigels, 1067
Excedrin Sinus Extra Strength, 1067
Exdol, 38-39
Exelon, 831
exemestane, 395-396
exenatide, 1029-1030
Ex-Lax, 332-333, 748-749
Ex-Lax Gentle, 845
Exsel, 1050, 1051-1052
Extra Strength Gas-X, 848
Extra Strength Maalox Anti-Gas, 848
Extra Strength Maalox GRF Gas Relief Formula, 848
Exubera, 509, 1030-1031
eyebright, 1112
20/20 Eye Drops, 1046, 1047

Eyesine, 1046, 1047
ezetimibe, 396

F

Factive, 454-455
factor IX complex (human)/factor IV, 397-398, 1043
famciclovir, 398-399, 1010
famotidine, 399-401, 1019
Famvir, 398-399
Fansidar, 801-802, 1067
Fareston, 925-926
Faslodex, 439-440
fat emulsions, 401-402
FDA DRUG APPROVALS, RECENT, 1041
FDA pregnancy categories, 1116
Fe^{50}, 408-410
Fedahist, 1067
Fedahist Expectorant Syrup, 1067
Fedahist Gyrocaps, 1067
Fedahist Timecaps, 1067
Feen-a-Mint, 142-143
Feen-A-Mint Pills, 748-749, 1067
felbamate, 996, 1093
Feldene, 762-763
felodipine, 402-403, 1014
Fem-1, 1067
Femara, 543-544
Fembrt 1/5, 1067
FemEtts, 38-39
Femiron, 408-410
Femizole-M, 1054-1055
Femogex, 385-387
FemPatch, 385-387
Femstat-3, 1054-1055
Fenicol, 1044, 1047
fenofibrate, 403-404
fenoldopam, 404-405, 1003
fenoprofen, 1094
fentanyl, 405-407, 992, 1023, 1043
Fentanyl Oralet, 405-407
fentanyls, 1123
fentanyl transdermal, 407-408, 992, 1023
Feosol, 408-410
Feostat, 408-410
Feostat Drops, 408-410
Feratab, 408-410
Fer-gen-sol, 408-410
Fergon, 408-410
Fer-Iron Drops, 408-410
Fero-Grade, 408-410
ferric gluconate complex, 408-410
Ferrlecit, 408-410
Ferro-Sequels, 1067
ferrous fumarate, 408-410
ferrous gluconate, 408-410
ferrous sulfate, 408-410
ferrous sulfate, dried, 408-410
Fertinic, 408-410
feverfew, 1112
fexofenadine, 410-411, 1001
Fiberall, 172-173, 797-798
Fiberall Natural Flavor and Orange Flavor, 797-798
FiberCon, 172-173
Fiber-Lax, 172-173
fibrinolysin/desoxyribonuclease, 411-412
filgrastim, 412-413
Finacea, 1052
finasteride, 413-414
Fioricet, 1067
Fioricet w/Codeine, 1067
Fiorinal, 1067
Fiorinal w/Codeine, 1067-1068
Flagyl, 619-620
Flagyl ER, 619-620
Flagyl IV, 619-620
Flagyl IV RTU, 619-620
Flamazine, 1052
Flarex, 1045, 1047
Flatulex, 848
flavocoxid, 414-415
Flavorcee, 108-109
flavoxate, 1094
flax, 1112
Flebogamma 5%, 501-502
flecainide, 415-416, 1000
Fleet Enema, 853
Fleet Laxative, 142-143
Fletcher's Castoria, 845
Flexeril, 269-270
Flomax, 881-882
Flonase, 1048-1049
Florinef, 417-418
Florone, 1049, 1050
Floxin, 690-691
floxuridine, 1094
fluconazole, 416-417, 1001
fludarabine, 1005, 1094
fludrocortisone, 417-418, 1017
Flumadine, 825-826
flumazenil, 418-419
flunisolide, 1048-1049
flunitrazepam, 1123
Fluocin, 1049, 1050
fluocinolone, 1049, 1050
Fluogen, 1107
fluorometholone, 1045, 1047
Fluor-Op, 1045, 1047
fluorouracil, 419-421, 1005, 1043
fluoxetine, 421-423, 997
fluphenazine, 1007
fluphenazine decanoate, 423-425
fluphenazine hydrochloride, 423-425
flurandrenolide, 1049, 1050
flurazepam, 425-427, 1011
flurbiprofen, 1046, 1047
FluShield, 1107
flutamide, 427, 1005
Flutex, 1050
fluticasone, 1048-1049, 1050
fluvastatin, 428-429
Fluviral, 1107
Fluvirin, 1107
Fluzone, 1107
FML, 1045, 1047
FML Forte, 1045, 1047
FML S.O.P., 1045, 1047
FML-S Ophthalmic Suspension, 1068
Focalin, 300-301
Focalin XR, 300-301
Foille, 1053
FoilleCort, 1050
Foille Plus, 1053
Folate, 428-429
folic acid (vitamin B_9), 429-430
Folinic Acid, 544-545
Folvite, 428-429
fomivirsen, 1044, 1047
fondaparinux, 430-431, 995
Foradil Aerolizer, 431-432
formoterol, 431-432, 1013
Fortamet, 597-598
Fortaz, 202-210
Forteo, 894
Fortovase, 839-840
Fosamax, 57-58
fosamprenavir, 434-435, 1010
foscarnet, 432-434, 1010
Foscavir, 432-434
fosinopril, 435-437, 1002
fosphenytoin, 437-438, 996
Fowler's Diarrhea Tablets, 121-122
Fragmin, 281-282
FreAmine, 73-75

Entries can be identified as follows: generic name, Trade Name, DRUG CATEGORY, *Combination Product.*

FreAmine III, 73-75
Frova, 438-439
frovatriptan, 438-439
5-FU, 419-421
fulvestrant, 439-440, 1005
Fungizone, 89-91, 1050, 1051-1052
Fungoid Tincture, 1050, 1051-1052
Furacin, 1052
Furadantin, 680-681
furosemide, 440-443, 1018
Furoside, 440-443
Fuzeon, 359-360

G

gabapentin, 443-444, 996
Gabitril, 906
galantamine, 444-445
gallamine, 1094
gallium, 445-446
galsulfase, 446, 1030
Gamimune N, 501-502
Gamma-Gard S/D, 501-502
gamma globulin, 501-502
Gammar-PIV, 501-502
Gamulin Rh, 817-818
Gamunex, 501-502
ganciclovir, 446-448, 1010
ganciclovir (ophthalmic), 1044, 1047
Ganidin NR, 466
ganirelix, 448-449
Ganite, 445-446
Gantanol, 869-870
Gantrisin, 873-874, 1045-1047
Gantrisin Pediatric, 873-874
Garamycin, 456-458
Garamycin Ophthalmic, 1044, 1047
garlic, 1113
Gas-Ban, 1068
Gas-Ban DS Liquid, 1068
Gas Relief, 848
Gastrosed, 488-489
Gas-X, 848
gatifloxacin, 449-451, 1044, 1047
Gaviscon, 1068
Gaviscon Liquid, 1068
GBH, 555-556
G-CSF, 412-413
gefitinib, 451, 1005
Gelprin, 1068
Gelusil, 1068
gemcitabine, 451-453, 1005
gemfibrozil, 453-454
gemifloxacin, 454-455, 1004
gemtuzumab, 455-456, 1043
Gemzar, 451-453
Genac Tablets, 1068
Genahist, 322-324
Gen-Allerate, 223-224
Genapap, 38-39
Genaphed, 796-797
Genasal, 1048-1049
Genaspor, 1050, 1051-1052
Genasyme, 848
Genatuss DM Syrup, 1068
Gencalc, 169-170
Genebs, 38-39
Geneye, 1046, 1047
Geneye Extra, 1046, 1047
Gen-Glyben, 460-462
Gengraf, 272-274
Genifiber, 797-798
Gen-K, 767-769
Genoptic Ophthalmic, 1044, 1047
Genoptic S.O.P., 1044, 1047
Genotropin, 855-856
Genpril, 491-492
Gen-Salbutamol, 52-54
Gen-Selegiline, 843-844
Gentacidin, 1044, 1047
Gentak, 1044, 1047
gentamicin, 456-458, 1003
gentamicin (ophthalmic), 1044, 1047
gentamicin (topical), 1052
Gentamicin (topical), 1052
Gentamicin Ophthalmic, 1044, 1047
Gentamicin Sulfate, 456-458
Gentlax, 845
Gen-Triazolam, 939-941
Geodon, 984-986
Geridium, 744
ginger, 1113
ginkgo, 1113
ginseng, 1113
glatiramer, 458-459
Glaucon/Epinal, 1046, 1047
Gleevec, 496-497
Gliadel, 184-186
glimepiride, 459-460
glipizide, 459-460, 998
GLUCOCORTICOIDS, TOPICAL, 1049-1050
Glucophage, 597-598
Glucophage XR, 597-598
D-glucose, 304-305
Glucose, 304-305
Glucotrol, 459-460
Glucotrol XL, 459-460
Glucovance 1.25, 1068
Glucovance 5, 1068
glutethimide, 1117
Glutose, 304-305
glyburide, 460-462, 998
glycerin, 1020, 1094
GLYCOPROTEIN IIB/IIIA INHIBITORS, 1042, 1121
glycopyrrolate, 462-463, 994, 1016
Gly-Cort, 1050
Glynase PresTab, 460-462
Glysėt, 630-631
G-mycin, 456-458
goldenseal, 1113
Gordo-Vite E, 973-974
goserelin, 464, 1005
granisetron, 465-466
Granulex Aerosol, 1068
granulocyte colony stimulator, 412-413
Gravol, 319-321
Gravol L/A, 319-321
green tea, 1113
griseofulvin, 1001
griseofulvin microsize/ultramicrosize, 1094-1095
guaifenesin, 466, 1009
Guaifenesin NR, 466
Guaifenex LA, 466
Guaifenex PSE 60, 1068
Guaifenex PSE 120, 1068
Guaituss AC, 1068
guanfacine, 466-467, 1002, 1095
Guiatuss, 466
G-Well, 555-556
Gynazol-1, 1054-1055
Gynecort, 1050
Gyne-Lotrimin 3, 1054-1055
Gyne-Lotrimin 7, 1054-1055
Gynergen, 375-376
Gyne-Trosyd, 1054-1055
Gynogen LA, 385-387

H

Habitrol, 673-674
haemophilus b conjugate vaccine, diphtheria CRM_{197} protein conjugate (HbOC), 1106
haemophilus b conjugate vaccine, meningococcal protein conjugate (PRP-OMP), 1106
Haemophilus influenzae type b (Hib) vaccine, 1125

halcinonide, 1049, 1050, 1095
Halcion, 939-941
Haldol, 468-470
Haldol Concentrate, 468-470
Haldol Decanoate, 468-470
Haldol LA, 468-470
Halenol, 38-39
Haley's M-O Liquid, 1068
Halfprin, 111-113
halobetasol, 1049, 1050
Halofed, 796-797
Halog, 1049, 1050
Halog-E, 1049, 1050
haloperidol, 468-470, 1007
haloperidol decanoate, 468-470
Haloperidol Intensol, 468-470
haloperidol lactate, 468-470
haloprogin, 1050, 1051-1052
Halotex, 1050, 1051-1052
Halotussin-DM Sugar Free Liquid, 1068
Haltran, 491-492
harmaline, 1123
Havrix, 1106
HbOC, 1106
HCTZ, 476-478
Head and Shoulders Intensive Treatment, 1050, 1051-1052
Hectorol, 342
Helidac, 1068
Helixate FS, 101-102
Hemabate, 182-183
Hemate P, 1068
Hemocyte, 408-410
Hemofil M, 101-102
Hepalean, 470-472
heparin, 470-472, 995, 1043
heparin, low molecular weight, 1121
heparin, unfractionated, 1121
heparin Leo, 470-472
heparin sodium, 470-472
HepatAmine, 73-75
hepatitis A vaccine, inactivated, 1106
hepatitis B immune globulin, 473
hepatitis B vaccine, 1125
hepatitis B vaccine, recombinant, 1106
Hep-Lock, 470-472
Hep-Lock U/P, 470-472
Hepsera, 47-48
Heptalac, 536-537
HERBAL PRODUCTS, 1111-1115
Herceptin, 931-932
heroin, 1117, 1123
Herplex, 1044, 1047
Hespan, 473-475
hetastarch, 473-475
Hexadrol, 297-299
Hexadrol Phosphate, 297-299
Hexit, 555-556
Hib, 1125
HibTITER, 1106
Hi-Cor, 1050
HISTAMINE H_2 ANTAGONISTS, 1018-1019
Histanil, 785-786
HIVID, 978-979
HMS, 1045, 1047
Hold DM, 303
homatropine, 1045, 1047
Homatropine HBr, 1045, 1047
hops, 1113
Humalin 30/70, 510-512
Humalog, 510-512
Humalog Mix 50/50, 1068
Humalog Mix 75/25, 1068
Humate-P, 101-102
Humatrope, 855-856
Humegon, 589-590
Humibid DM Sprinkle Caps, 1068
Humibid DM Tablets, 1068
Humira, 47
Humorsol, 1045, 1047
Humulin 50/50, 510-512
Humulin 70/30, 510-512
Humulin L, 510-512
Humulin N, 510-512
Humulin R, 510-512
Humulin U Ultralente, 510-512
Hurricaine, 1053
hyaluronidase, 1095
Hyate:C, 101-102
Hybolin Decanoate, 661-662
Hycamtin, 924-925
HycoClera Tuss, 1068
Hycodan, 478-480, 1068
Hycodan Syrup, 1068
Hycomed, 478-480
Hycomine Compound, 1068-1069
Hyco-Pap, 478-480
Hycort, 1050
Hycotuss Expectorant Syrup, 1069
Hydeltrasol, 772-774
Hydeltra-T.B.A., 772-774
Hydergine, 1069
Hyderm, 1050
Hydracet, 478-480
hydralazine, 475-476, 1003, 1026
hydralazine HCl, 475-476
Hydramine, 322-324
Hydramyn, 322-324
Hydrate, 319-321
Hydrated Magnesium Silicate, 121-122
Hydrea, 485-487
Hydril, 322-324
Hydrobexan, 971-972
Hydrocet, 1069
Hydro-Chlor, 476-478
hydrochlorothiazide, 476-478, 1018
Hydrocil Instant, 797-798
Hydro Cobex, 971-972
hydrocodone, 478-480, 1009
hydrocodone/acetaminophen, 478-480
hydrocodone/aspirin, 478-480
hydrocodone/ibuprofen, 478-480
hydrocortisone, 480-482, 1017
hydrocortisone (topical), 1050
hydrocortisone acetate, 480-482
hydrocortisone cypionate, 480-482
hydrocortisone sodium phosphate, 480-482
hydrocortisone sodium succinate, 480-482
Hydrocortone, 480-482
Hydrocortone Acetate, 480-482
Hydrocortone Phosphate, 480-482
Hydro-Crysti-1000, 971-972
Hydro-Crysti-12, 971-972
Hydrodiuril, 476-478
Hydrogesic, 478-480, 1069
hydromorphone, 482-484, 1023, 1043
Hydromorphone HCl, 482-484
Hydropres-50, 1069
Hydroserpine, 1069
Hydrostat IR, 482-484

Hydro-Tex, 1050
Hydroxo-12, 971-972
hydroxocobalamin (vitamin $B_{12}a$), 971-972
hydroxyamphetamine HBr, 1046, 1047
hydroxychloroquine, 484-485, 1095
Hydroxycobalamin, 971-972
hydroxyurea, 485-487
hydroxyzine, 487-488
Hygroton, 227-228
hyoscyamine, 488-489, 994
Hyperstat IV, 307-308
HYPOGLYCEMICS, ORAL, 1042, 1121
HypoRho-D, 817-818
HypoRho-D Mini-Dose, 817-818
Hyrexin-50, 322-324
Hytakerol, 316-317
Hytinic, 408-410
Hytone, 1050
Hytrin, 890-891
Hytuss, 466
Hytuss 2X, 466
Hyzaar, 1069

I

ibritumomab tiuxetan, 490, 1005
ibuprofen, 491-492, 1022
ibutilide, 492-493, 1000, 1043
Icar, 408-410
Idamycin, 493-495
Idamycin PFS, 493-495
idarubicin, 493-495, 1043
idoxuridine-IDU, 1044, 1047
Ifex, 495-496
ifosfamide, 495-496, 1043
IG, 501-502
IGIM, 501-502
IGIV, 501-502
IL-2, 54-56
Iletin II Regular, 510-512
Iletin II U-500, 510-512
Iletin NPH, 510-512
Illetin II NPH, 510-512
Ilosone, 379-380
Ilotycin, 1044, 1047
Ilozyme, 718-719
imatinib, 496-497, 1005
Imdur, 526-527
Imferon, 522-523
imipenem/cilastatin, 497-499, 1004
imipramine, 499-501, 997
Imipramine HCl, 499-501
Imitrex, 875-876
immune globulin (IGIV), 501-502
Immunization schedules, Canadian, 1125
IMMUNOSUPPRESSANTS, 1019
Imodium, 566-567
Imodium A-D, 566-567
Imodium A-D Caplet, 566-567
Imodium Advanced, 1069
IMOVax Rabies, 1109
IM-OVax Rabies I.D., 1109
Impril, 499-501
Imuran, 123-124
inactivated polio vaccine/oral polio vaccine, 1125
inamrinone, 503-504, 1043
Inapsine, 347-348
Increlex, 596, 1031-1032
Indameth, 507-508
indapamide, 504-506, 1018
Inderal, 791-793
Inderal LA, 791-793
Inderide 40/25, 1069
Inderide 80/25, 1069
Inderide LA 80/50, 1069
Inderide LA 120/50, 1069
Inderide LA 160/50, 1069
indinavir, 506-507, 1010
Indochron E-R, 507-508
Indocid, 507-508
Indocin, 507-508
Indocin IV, 507-508
Indocin PDA, 507-508
Indocin SR, 507-508
indomethacin, 507-508, 1022
Infants, immunization schedules for, 1125
InFed, 522-523
Infergen, 515-516
Inflamase Forte, 1045, 1047
Inflamase Mild, 1045, 1047
infliximab, 508-509
influenza virus vaccine, trivalent, 1107
influenza virus vaccine, trivalent A and B (whole virus/split virus), 1107
Infumorph, 646-648
INH, 524-525
Innohep, 914-915
Innovar, 1069
Inocor, 503-504
INOTROPIC MEDICATIONS, 1042, 1121
Insomnal, 322-324
Inspra, 369-370
Insta-Glucose, 304-305
insulin, 1043, 1121
insulin, inhaled, 509, 1030-1031
insulin, isophane suspension (NPH), 510-512
insulin, isophane suspension and regular insulin, 510-512
insulin, lispro, 998
insulin, regular, 510-512, 998
insulin, regular concentrated, 510-512, 998
insulin, zinc suspension (Lente), 510-512, 998
insulin, zinc suspension extended (Ultralente), 510-512, 998
insulin aspart, 510-512, 998
insulin detemir, 510-512
insulin glargine, 510-512, 998
insulin glulisine, 510-512, 998
insulin lispro, 510-512
insulins, 510-512
Integrilin, 373-374
Interferon β-1b, 516-517
interferon alfa-2a/interferon alfa-2b, 513-514, 1005
interferon alfacon-1, 515-516
interferon alfa-n 1 lymphoblastoid, 514-515
interferon gamma-1b, 517-518
interleukin-2, 54-56
Intralipid 10%, 401-402
Intralipid 20%, 401-402
INTRATHECAL/EPIDURAL MEDICATIONS, 1042, 1121
Intropin, 336-337
Invanz, 377-379
Invirase, 839-840
iodide, 926-927
Iofed, 1069
Iofed PD, 1069
IPOL, 1108
ipratropium, 518-519, 1013
Iprivask, 294
irbesartan, 519-520, 1002
Ircon, 408-410
Iressa, 451
irinotecan, 520-522, 1005, 1043

iron, carbonyl, 408-410, 522
iron dextran, 522-523
iron polysaccharide, 408-410, 523
iron sucrose, 523-524
ISDN, 526-527
ISMO, 526-527
Iso-Bid, 526-527
Isonate, 526-527
isoniazid, 524-525, 1008
Isopap, 1069
isophane insulin suspension (NPH) and insulin mixtures, 510-513
isoproterenol, 1013, 1095
Isoptin, 963-965
Isoptin SR, 963-965
Isopto Atropine, 1045, 1047
Isopto Carbachol, 1045, 1047
Isopto Carpine, 1045, 1047
Isopto Cetamide, 1044, 1047
Isopto Fenical, 1044, 1047
Isopto Frin, 1046, 1047
Isopto Homatropine, 1045, 1047
Isopto Hyoscine, 1046, 1047
Isorbid, 526-527
Isordil, 526-527
isosorbide, 993
isosorbide dinitrate, 526-527
Isosorbide dinitrate, 526-527
isosorbide mononitrate, 526-527
Isotamine, 524-525
Isotrate, 526-527
Isotrate ER, 526-527
isotretinoin, 1096
isradipine, 527-528, 1014
Itch-X, 1053
itraconazole, 528-529, 1001
Iveegam, 501-502

J

Japanese encephalitis virus vaccine, inactivated, 1107
Jenamicin, 456-458
JE-VAX, 1107

K

K+10, 767-769
Kabikinase, 863-864
Kabolin, 661-662
Kadian, 646-648
Kaletra Capsules, 1069
Kaletra Solution, 1069
Kalium Durules, 767-769
kanamycin, 1003, 1096
Kaochlor, 767-769
Kaochlor Eff, 767-769
Kaochlor S-F, 767-769
kaolin/pectin, 999
Kaon, 767-769
Kaon-Cl, 767-769
Kaopectate, 121-122
Kaopectate Advanced Formula, 121-122
Kaopectate II Caplets, 566-567
Kaopectate Maximum Strength, 121-122
Karacil, 797-798
kava, 1113
Kay-Ciel, 767-769
Kayexelate, 854-855
Kaylixir, 767-769
K+care, 767-769
K+Care ET, 767-769
KCl, 767-769
K-Dur, 767-769
Keflex, 192-196
Keftab, 192-196
K-Electrolyte, 767-769
Kenac, 1050
Kenacort, 936-938
Kenaject-40, 936-938
Kenalog, 936-938, 1050
Kenalog-10, 936-938
Kenalog-40, 936-938
Kenonel, 1050
Keppra, 548
ketamine, 1043
Ketek, 883-884
ketoconazole, 530-531, 1001
ketoconazole (topical), 1051-1052
ketoprofen, 531-533, 1022
Ketoprofen, 531-533
ketorolac, 533-534, 1022
ketorolac (ophthalmic), 1046, 1047
ketotifen, 1044, 1047
K-Exit, 854-855
Key-Pred 25, 772-774
Key-Pred 50, 772-774
Key-Pred-SP, 772-774
K-G Elixir, 767-769
khat, 1113
K-Ide, 767-769
Kidrolase, 109-111
Kineret, 97-98
Kionex, 854-855
K-Lease, 767-769
K-Long, 767-769
Klonopin, 251-252
K-Lor, 767-769
Klor-Con, 767-769
Klor-Con EF, 767-769
Klorvess, 767-769
Klorvess Effervescent Granules, 767-769
Klotrix, 767-769
K-Lyte, 767-769
K-Lyte/Cl, 767-769
K-Lyte/Cl powder, 767-769
K-Lyte DS, 767-769
K-med, 767-769
K-Norm, 767-769
Koate-DVI, 101-102
Koffex, 303
Kogenate, 101-102
Kogenate FS, 101-102
Kolyum, 767-769
Konsyl, 797-798
Konsyl Orange, 797-798
Konyne 80, 397-398
Kristalose, 536-537
K-Sol, 767-769
K-Tab, 767-769
Ku-Zyme HP, 718-719
K-Vescent, 767-769
Kwell, 555-556
Kytril, 465-466

L

LA-12, 971-972
labetalol, 534-536, 1003, 1012
Lacti-Care-HC, 1050
Lactinex, 1069
Lactulax, 536-537
lactulose, 536-537, 1020
Lactulose PSE, 536-537
Lamictal, 539-540
Lamictal Chewable Dispersible, 539-540
Lamisil, 891-892, 1050, 1051-1052
lamivudine (3TC), 537-539
lamotrigine, 539-540, 996
Lanacaine, 1053
Lanacort, 1050
Laniazid, 524-525
Lanophyllin, 898-899
Lanoxicaps, 313-315
Lanoxin, 313-315
lansoprazole, 540-541
Lantus, 510-512
Largactil, 224-227
Larodopa, 549-550
laronidase, 1096
Lasix, 440-443

Entries can be identified as follows: generic name, Trade Name, DRUG CATEGORY, *Combination Product.*

Lasix Special, 440-443
latanoprost, 1046, 1047
LAXATIVES, 1020
Laxit, 142-143
Lax-Pills, 748-749
L-Dopa, 549-550
leflunomide, 541-542
Lemoderm, 1050
lemon balm, 1113
lenalidomide, 1041
Lenoltec w/Codeine No. 1, 1069
Lente Iletin II, 510-512
Lente L, 510-512
lepirudin, 542-543, 995, 1043
Lescol, 428-429
letrozole, 543-544
leucovorin, 544-545
leucovorin calcium, 544-545
Leukeran, 214-216
Leukine, 840-842
leuprolide, 545-547, 1005, 1043
Leupron Depo PED, 545-547
levalbuterol, 547-548, 1013
Levaquin, 550-551
Levate, 81-82
Levemir, 510-512
levetiracetam, 548
Levitra, 958-959
Levlite, 1069
levobetaxolol, 1045, 1046-1047
levobunolol, 1045, 1046-1047
levobupivacaine, 1096
levocabastine, 1046, 1047
levodopa, 549-550, 1006
levofloxacin, 550-551, 1004, 1044, 1047
Levo-T, 551-553
Levothroid, 551-553
levothyroxine (T_4), 551-553, 1025
levothyroxine sodium, 551-553
Levoxyl, 551-553
Levsin, 488-489
Levsinex, 488-489
Levsin PB Drops, 1069
Levsin w/Phenobarbital, 1069
Lexapro, 381-382
Lexiva, 434-435
Lexxel 1, 1069
Lexxel 2, 1069
Librax, 1069
Librium, 218-219
Licon, 1049, 1050
licorice, 1113
Lida-Mantel-HC-Cream, 1069-1070
Lidemol, 1049, 1050
Lidex, 1049, 1050
lidocaine, 1000, 1121
lidocaine (topical), 1053
lidocaine, parenteral, 553-555, 992, 1000, 1043
Lidocaine HCl Topical, 1053
Lidocaine Viscous, 1053
Lidopen Auto-Injector, 553-555
Limbitrol DS 10-25, 1070
Limbrel, 414-415
lindane, 555-556
linezolid, 556-557
Lioresal, 127-128
liothyronine (T_3), 557-559, 1025
liothyronine sodium, 557-559
liotrix, 559-560, 1025
Lipitor, 117-118
LIPOSOMAL DRUGS, 1042, 1121
Liposyn II 10%, 401-402
Liposyn II 20%, 401-402
Liposyn III 10%, 401-402
Liposyn III 20%, 401-402
Lipram-CR20, 718-719
Lipram-PN10, 718-719
Lipram-PN16, 718-719
Lipram-UL12, 718-719
Liqu-Char, 43-44
Liquibid, 466
Liquid-Cal, 169-170
Liquid-Cal-600, 169-170
Liquid Pred, 774-775
Liquiprin, 38-39
lisinopril, 560-562, 1002
lithium, 562-564
lithium carbonate, 562-564
Lithizine, 562-564
Lithonate, 562-564
Lithotabs, 562-564
Livostin, 1046, 1047
LKV Drops, 649-650
Lobac, 1070
LoCHOLEST, 229-230
LoCHOLEST Light, 229-230
Locoid, 1050
Lodine, 392-394
Lodine XL, 392-394
lodoxamide, 1046, 1047
Lodrane 24, 153-155
Lodrane XR, 153-155
Loestrin Fe 1/20, 1070
Loestrin Fe 1.5/30, 1070
Logen, 324-325
Lo Hist 12 Hour, 153-155
Lomanate, 324-325
lomefloxacin, 564-565, 1004
Lomotil, 324-325, 1070
Lomotil Liquid, 1070
lomustine, 565-566, 1005
Loniten, 634-635
Lonox, 324-325
Lo Ovral, 1070
loperamide, 566-567, 999
Loperamide, 566-567
loperamide solution, 566-567
Lopid, 453-454
lopidine, 1046, 1047
Lopresor, 617-619
Lopressor, 617-619
Lopressor HCT 50/25, 1070
Lopressor HCT 100/25, 1070
Lopressor HCT 100/50, 1070
Lopressor SR, 617-619
Loprox, 1050, 1051-1052
Lopurin, 60-61
Lorabid, 196-202
loracarbef, 196-202, 567
loratadine, 567-568, 1001
lorazepam, 568-570, 1011, 1123
Lorcet, 478-480
Lorcet 10/650, 1070
Lorcet HD, 1070
Lorcet Plus, 1070
Lortab, 478-480
Lortab 2.5/500, 1070
Lortab 5/500, 1070
Lortab 7.5/500, 1070
Lortab 10/500, 1070
Lortab ASA, 478-480, 1070
Lortab Elixir, 1070
Losapan, 575-576
losartan, 570-571, 1002
Losec, 696-697
Losec 1-2-3A, 1070
Losec 1-2-3M, 1070
Lotemax, 1045, 1047
Lotensin, 131-133
Lotensin HCT 5/6.25, 1070
Lotensin HCT 10/12.5, 1070
Lotensin HCT 20/12.5, 1070
Lotensin HCT 20/25, 1070
loteprednol, 1045, 1047
Lotrel 2.5/10, 1070
Lotrel 5/10, 1070
Lotrel 5/20, 1070
Lotrimin AF, 1050, 1051-1052
Lotrimin Ultra, 1050, 1051-1052

Lotrisone Topical, 1070
lovastatin, 571-572
Lovenox, 361-363
Lowsium, 575-576
Loxapac, 573-574
loxapine, 573-574, 1007
loxapine succinate, 573-574
Loxitane, 573-574
Loxitane-C, 573-574
Loxitane IM, 573-574
Lozide, 504-506
Lozol, 504-506
LSD, 1117, 1123
lubiprostone, 1041
Lufyllin, 352-353
Lufyllin-EPG Elixir, 1070-1071
Lufyllin-GG, 1071
Lumigan, 1046, 1047
Luminal, 746-748
Lunelle Monthly Contraceptive Injection, 1071
Lupron, 545-547
Lupron Depot, 545-547
Lupron Depot-3 month, 545-547
Luxiq, 1049, 1050
Lyderm, 1049, 1050
Lyme disease vaccine (recombinant OspA), 1107
LYMErix, 1107
lymphocyte immune globulin (antithymocyte), 574-575
Lyphocin, 957-958
Lyrica, 775, 1034-1036
Lysatec, 64-66
lysine, 1113

M

Maalox, 1071
Maalox Antacid Caplets, 169-170
Maalox Antidiarrheal Caplets, 566-567
Maalox Anti-Gas, 848
Maalox Daily Fiber Therapy, 797-798
Maalox GRF Gas Relief Formula, 848
Maalox Plus, 1071
Maalox Plus Extra Strength Suspension, 1071
Maalox Suspension, 1071
Macrobid, 680-681, 1071
Macrodantin, 680-681
Macugen, 723-724
mafenide, 1052
magaldrate, 575-576, 993
magic mushrooms, 1123
Magnaprin, 1071
Magnaprin Arthritis Strength, 1071
magnesium chloride, 576-578
magnesium citrate, 576-578
magnesium gluconate, 576-578
magnesium hydroxide, 576-578
magnesium oxide, 576-578, 993
magnesium salicylate, 1024
magnesium salts, 576-578, 1020
magnesium sulfate, 576-578, 996, 1043, 1121
Mag-Ox 400, 576-578
Magtrate, 576-578
maitake, 1114
Malarone, 1071
Malarone Pediatric, 1071
Mallamint, 169-170
Mallazine Eye Drops, 1046, 1047
Malog, 895-896
Malog-x, 895-896
manganese, 926-927
mannitol, 578-580, 1018
Maox, 576-578
Mapap, 38-39
Mapap Cold Formula, 1071
Maprax, 1071
Maranox, 38-39
Marcillin, 91-93
Marezine, 1103
marijuana, 1117
Marthritic, 838-839
Matulane, 779-781
Mavik, 928-930
Maxair, 761-762
Maxalt, 831-832
Maxalt-MLT, 831-832
Maxaquin, 564-565
Maxeran, 613-615
Maxidex, 1045, 1047
Maxiflor, 1049, 1050
Maximum Strength Allergy Drops, 1046, 1047
Maximum Strength Desenex Atifungal, 1050, 1051-1052
Maximum Strength Gas Relief, 848
Maximum Strength Mylanta Gas Relief, 848
Maximum Strength Phazyme, 848
Maxipime, 202-210
Maxitrol Ophthalmic Suspension/Ointment, 1071
Maxivate, 1049, 1050
Maxzide, 1071
Maxzide-25 MG, 1071
mazindol, 1117
measles, mumps, and rubella (MMR) vaccine, 1125
measles, mumps, and rubella vaccine, live, 1107
measles and rubella virus vaccine, live attenuated, 1107
measles virus vaccine, live attenuated, 1108
mebendazole, 580-581
mechlorethamine, 581-582, 1005
meclizine, 582-583
meclizine HCl, 582-583
Meda, 38-39
Medamint, 1053
MEDICATIONS, CANADIAN, HIGH-ALERT, 1121
Medi-Flu Liquid, 1071
Medigesic, 1071
Medihaler, 366-367
Medilax, 748-749
Medipren, 491-492
Medralone, 610-612
Medrol, 610-612
medroxyprogesterone, 583-584
medrysone, 1045, 1047
Med Tamoxifen, 880-881
Mefoxin, 196-202
Mega-C/A Plus, 108-109
Megace, 584-585
Megacillin, 729-732
megestrol, 584-585, 1005
melatonin, 1114
Mellaril, 902-904
Mellaril-5, 902-904
Mellaril Concentrate, 902-904
meloxicam, 585-587
melphalan, 587-588, 1005, 1043
memantine, 588-589
Menadol, 491-492
Menaval, 385-387
Meni-D, 582-583
meningococcal polysaccharide vaccine, 1108
Menomune-A/C/Y/W-135, 1108

Entries can be identified as follows: generic name, Trade Name, DRUG CATEGORY, *Combination Product.*

menotropins, 589-590
Mentex, 1050, 1051-1052
Mepergan Fortis, 1071
Mepergan Injection, 1071
meperidine, 590-592, 1023, 1043, 1117
meperidine HCl, 590-592
Mephyton, 754-755
meprobamate, 1117
Mepron, 118-119
mercaptopurine, 592-593, 1005
meropenem, 593-595, 1004
Merrem IV, 593-595
Meruvax II, 1109
mesalamine, 595-596
Mesasal, 595-596
mescaline, 1117, 1123
mescasermin, 596, 1031-1032
Mestinon, 798-800
Mestinon SR, 798-800
Mestinon Timespan, 798-800
Metadate CD, 608-610
Metadate ER, 608-610
Metaderm, 1049, 1050
Metaglip, 1071
Metamucil, 797-798
Metamucil Lemon Lime, 797-798
Metamucil Orange Flavor, 797-798
Metamucil Sugar Free, 797-798
Metamucil Sugar Free Orange Flavor, 797-798
metaproterenol, 596-597, 1013
metformin, 597-598, 998
methadone, 598-600, 1023, 1043, 1123
Methadose, 598-600
methamphetamine, 1123
Methergine, 607-608
Methidate, 608-610
methimazole, 600-601
methocarbamol, 601-602
methotrexate (amethopterin, mtx), 603-605, 1005, 1043, 1121
Methotrexate, 603-605
methyldopa, 1002
methyldopa/methyldopate, 605-607
methylergonovine, 607-608
Methylin, 608-610
Methylin ER, 608-610
methylphenidate, 608-610
methylprednisolone, 610-612, 1017
methylprednisolone (topical), 1050
methysergide, 612-613
Meticorten, 774-775
Metimyd Ophthalmic Suspension/Ointment, 1071
metipranolol, 1045, 1046-1047
metoclopramide, 613-615
metolazone, 615-617, 1018
metoprolol, 617-619, 993, 1012
MetroCream, 1052
MetroGel, 1052
MetroLotion, 1052
metronidazole, 619-620
Metronidazole, 619-620
metronidazole (topical), 1052
Mevacor, 571-572
mexiletine, 620-622, 1000
Mexitil, 620-622
Mezlin, 622-624
mezlocillin, 622-624, 1004
Miacalcin, 166-168
Miacalcin Nasal Spray, 166-168
mibefradil, 624-625, 1013
Micardis, 884-885
Micardis HCT 40, 1071
Micardis HCT 80, 1071
Micatin, 625-626, 1050, 1051-1052
Micatin Liquid, 625-626
miconazole, 625-626
miconazole (topical), 1050, 1051-1052
miconazole (vaginal), 1054-1055
miconazole nitrate, 625-626
MICRh$_o$GAM, 817-818
Microgestin Fe 1/20, 1071
Microgestin Fe 1.5/30, 1072
Micro-K, 767-769
Micro-LS, 767-769
Micronase, 460-462
MicroNefrin, 366-367
Microzide, 476-478
Midamor, 72-73
midazolam, 626-628, 992, 1011
midodrine, 628-629, 1026
Midol, Teen, 1072
Midol Maximum Strength Cramp Formula, 491-492
Midol Maximum Strength Multi-Symptom Menstrual Gelcaps, 1072
Midol PM, 1072
Midol PMS Maximum Strength Caplets, 1072
Midrin, 1072
Mifeprex, 629-630
mifepristone, 629-630
miglitol, 630-631, 998
miglustat, 1096
Migranal, 375-376
Milophene, 249-250
milrinone, 631-632, 1043
Mini-Gamulin R, 817-818
Minims Homatropine, 1045, 1047
Minipres, 771-772
Mini Thin Pseudo, 796-797
Minitran, 681-682
Minizide 1, 1072
Minizide 2, 1072
Minizide 5, 1072
Minocin, 632-634
minocycline, 632-634, 1004
minoxidil, 634-635, 1003, 1026
Miochol-E, 1045, 1047
Miostat, 1045, 1047
Mirapex, 769-770
mirtazapine, 635-636, 997
misoprostol, 637
Mithracin, 764-766
Mithramycin, 764-766
mitomycin, 637-639, 1005, 1043
mitotane, 1005, 1096
mitoxantrone, 639-641, 1005, 1043
Mitrolan, 172-173
Mivacron, 641-642
mivacurium, 641-642, 1021, 1043
M-M-R-II, 1071, 1107
MMR vaccine, 1125
Mobic, 585-587
modafinil, 1096
Modane, 142-143, 332-333, 748-749
Modane Bulk, 797-798
Modecate, 423-425
Modecate Concentrate, 423-425
Moditen HCl, 423-425
Moditen HCl-H.P., 423-425
Moduretic, 1072
moexipril, 642-643
molindone, 1007
Mol-Iron, 408-410
MOM, 576-578
mometasone, 1048-1049, 1050
Monafed, 466

Monistat, 625-626, 1054-1055
Monistat 1, 1054-1055
Monistat 3, 625-626, 1054-1055
Monistat 7, 625-626, 1054-1055
Monistat-Derm, 625-626, 1050, 1051-1052
Monistat Dual-Pak, 625-626, 1054-1055
Monistat I.V., 625-626
Monitan, 36-38
Monoclate-P, 101-102
Monodox, 345-346
Mono-Gesic, 838-839
Monoket, 526-527
Mononine, 397-398
Monopril, 435-437
Monopril-HCT 10, 1072
Monopril-HCT 20, 1072
montelukast, 643-644
moricizine, 644-646, 1000
morphine, 646-648, 1023, 1043, 1117, 1123
Morphine H.P., 646-648
morphine sulfate, 646-648
Morphitec, 646-648
M.O.S., 646-648
M.O.S.-S.R., 646-648
Motofen, 324-325
Motrin, 491-492
Motrin Children's Cold Suspension, 1072
Motrin IB, 491-492
Motrin IB Sinus, 1072
Motrin Junior Strength, 491-492
Motrin Migraine Pain, 491-492
moxifloxacin, 648-649, 1044, 1047
M-oxy, 709-710
6-MP, 592-593
M-R-Vax II, 1107
MS Contin, 646-648
MSIR, 646-648
M.T.E.-4, 926-927
M.T.E.-4 Concentrated, 926-927
M.T.E.-5, 926-927
M.T.E.-5 Concentrated, 926-927
M.T.E.-6, 926-927
M.T.E.-6 Concentrated, 926-927
M.T.E.-7, 926-927
mtx, 603-605
Mucinex, 1072
Mucine X, 466
Mucinex D, 1072
Mucinex DM, 1072
Mucomyst, 42-43
Mucosil, 42-43
MulTE-PAK-4, 926-927
MulTE-PAK-5, 926-927
Multi-75, 649-650
Multi-Day, 649-650
Multipax, 487-488
Multiple Trace Element, 926-927
Multiple Trace Element Neonatal, 926-927
Multiple Trace Element Pediatric, 926-927
multivitamins, 649-650, 1026
Mumpsvax, 1108
mumps virus vaccine, live, 1108
mupirocin, 1052
Murine Plus, 1046, 1047
Murocoll-2 Ophthalmic Drops, 1072
muromonab-CD3, 650-651, 1019
Mustargen, 581-582
Mutamycin, 637-639
Myambutol, 390-391
Mycelex-3, 1054-1055
Mycelex 7, 1054-1055
Myclo, 1050, 1051-1052, 1054-1055
Mycobutin, 820-821
Mycolog II Topical, 1072
mycophenolate, 651-653
My Cort, 1050
Mycostatin, 687-688, 1050, 1051-1052
2.5% Mydfrin, 1046, 1047
Mydriacyl, 1046, 1047
MYDRIATICS, 1045-1046, 1047
Myfortic, 651-653
Mykrox, 615-617
Mylanta, 1072
Mylanta AR, 399-401
Mylanta Double Strength Liquid, 1072
Mylanta Gas, 848
Mylanta Gelcaps, 1072
Mylanta Lozenges, 169-170
Mylanta Natural Fiber Supplement, 797-798
Myleran, 162-164
Mylicon, 848
Mylotarg, 455-456
Mymethasone, 297-299
Myproic acid, 954-955
Myrosemide, 440-443
Mysoline, 775-776
M-Zole 7 Dual Pack, 1054-1055

N

Nabi-HB, 473
nabumetone, 653-654, 1022
nadolol, 654-655, 993, 1012
Nadopen-V, 729-732
Nadostine, 687-688
nafarelin, 656
Nafazair, 1046, 1047
nafcillin, 656-658, 1004
nafcillin sodium, 656-658
Nafrine, 1048-1049
naftifine, 1050, 1051-1052
Naftin, 1050, 1051-1052
Naglazyme, 446, 1030
nalbuphine, 658-660, 1023, 1043
nalbuphine HCl, 658-660
Naldecon Senior DX Liquid, 1072
Naldecon Senior EX, 466
Nallpen, 656-658
naloxone, 660-661
naloxone HCl, 660-661
Namenda, 588-589
nandrolone, 661-662
naphazoline, 1046, 1047
naphazoline (nasal), 1047, 1048-1049
naphazoline HCl, 1046, 1047
Naphcon, 1046, 1047
Naphcon-A Ophthalmic Solution, 1072
Naphcon Forte, 1046, 1047
Naprelan, 662-664
Napron X, 662-664
Naprosyn, 662-664
Naprosyn-E, 662-664
Naprosyn-SR, 662-664
naproxen, 662-664, 1022
naproxen sodium, 662-664
naratriptan, 664-665
Narcan, 660-661
NARCOTICS/OPIATES, 1042, 1121
Nardil, 745-746
Naropin, 833-834
Nasacort AQ, 1048-1049
Nasahist-B, 153-155
NASAL AGENTS, 1047-1049
Nasal Decongestant Maximum Strength, 1048-1049
Nasalide, 1048-1049
Nasal Relief, 1048-1049
NASAL STEROIDS, 1048-1049
Nasarel, 1048-1049

Entries can be identified as follows: generic name, Trade Name, DRUG CATEGORY, *Combination Product.*

octreotide, 689-690
Ocu-Carpine, 1045, 1047
OcuClear, 1046, 1047
Ocufen, 1046, 1047
Ocuflox, 690-691, 1044, 1047
Ocupress, 1045, 1046-1047
Ocusert Pilo-20, 1045, 1047
Ocusert Pilo-40, 1045, 1047
Ocusulf-10, 1044, 1047
ofloxacin, 690-691, 1004, 1044, 1047
olanzapine, 692-693, 1007
olmesartan, 1002
olmesartan medoxomil, 693-694
olopatadine, 1044, 1047
olsalazine, 694-695
omalizumab, 695-696
omeprazole, 696-697
Omnicef, 202-210
Omnipen, 91-93
OMS Concentrate, 646-648
Oncaspar, 724-726
Oncovin, 967-968
ondansetron, 697-698
One-A-Day, 649-650
Onset, 478-480
Ontak, 291-292
Onxol, 713-715
Ony-Clear Tetterine, 1050, 1051-1052
Opcon, 1046, 1047
Opcon-A Ophthalmic Solution, 1073
Ophthaine, 1044, 1047
OPHTHALMIC PRODUCTS, 1044-1047
Ophthestic, 1044, 1047
OPIATES, 1022-1023, 1123
opium, 1117
Opticyl, 1046, 1047
Optigene 3, 1046, 1047
Optilets, 649-650
Optimine, 1102
OptiPranolol, 1045, 1046-1047
Optivar, 125, 1044, 1047
Orabase, 1053
Oracin, 1053
Ora-Jel, 1053
Oramorph SR, 646-648
Oraphen-PD, 38-39
Orapred, 772-774
Orasone, 774-775
Orazinc, 984
Orbenin, 257-258
Orencia, 35, 1027-1028
Oretic, 476-478
Orfadin, 1041
Organidin NR, 466
Orgaran, 282-284
Orimune, 1108
orlistat, 698-699
Ornade Spansules, 1073
Ornex, 1073
Ornex-DM, 303
Ornex No Drowsiness Caplets, 1073
Orphengesic, 1073
Orphengesic Forte, 1073
Ortho-cept, 1073
Orthocone OKT3, 650-651
Ortho/CS, 108-109
Ortho-cyclen, 1073
Ortho-Novum 7/7/7, 1073-1074
Ortho-Prefest, 1074
Orudis, 531-533
Orudis-E, 531-533
Orudis-KT, 531-533
Orudis-SR, 531-533
Oruvail, 531-533
Os-Cal 500, 169-170
oseltamivir, 699-700
Osmitrol, 578-580
Osteocalcin, 166-168
OTIC ANTIINFECTIVES, 1055
Otrivin, 1048-1049
Otrivin Pediatric Nasal, 1048-1049
Ovcon-50, 1074
Ovol, 848
oxacillin, 700-702, 1004
oxacillin sodium, 700-702
oxaliplatin, 702-703, 1005
oxaprozin, 703-704
oxazepam, 704-706, 1011
oxcarbazepine, 706-707
oxiconazole, 1050, 1051-1052
Oxistat, 1050, 1051-1052
oxtriphylline, 707-708, 1013
oxybutynin, 708-709
Oxycocet, 709-710, 1074
Oxycodan, 709-710
oxycodone, 709-710, 1023, 1043
oxycodone/acetaminophen, 709-710
oxycodone/aspirin, 709-710
Oxycontin, 709-710
OxyFast, 709-710
Oxyl R, 709-710
oxymetazoline, 1046, 1047
oxymetazoline (nasal), 1048-1049
oxymetazoline HCl, 1048-1049
oxymorphone, 710-712, 1023, 1043
oxytocin, 712-713, 1043
Oxytrol, 708-709
Oysco 500, 169-170
Oyst-Cal 500, 169-170
Oystercal 500, 169-170

P

P-A-C Analgesic, 1074
Pacerone, 79-81
paclitaxel, 713-715
Pain-X Topical, 1074
Palafer, 408-410
palivizumab, 715
palonosetron, 716
L-Pam, 587-588
Pamelor, 686-687
pamidronate, 716-718
Pamprin Maximum Pain Relief, 1074
Pamprin Multi-Symptom, 1074
Panacet 5/500, 1074
Panadol, 38-39
Panasal 5/500, 1074
Panasol, 478-480
Panasol-S, 774-775
panax ginseng, 1114
Pancet, 478-480
Pancrease Capsules, 718-719, 1074
Pancrease MT 4, 718-719
Pancrease MT 10, 718-719
Pancrease MT 16, 718-719
pancrelipase, 718-719
pancuronium, 719-720, 1021, 1043
pancuronium bromide, 719-720
Panectyl, 1104
Panglobulin NF, 501-502
Panlor, 478-480
Panmycin, 896-898
Panretin, 59-60
pantoprazole, 720-721
papaverine, 1026, 1097
papaya, 1114
paraldehyde, 1097
Paraplatin, 181-182
Paraplatin-AQ, 181-182
Parcopa, 1074
Paredrine, 1046, 1047
paregoric, 1117
Parepectolin, 121-122
paricalcitol, 721
Parlodel, 152-153
Parnate, 930-931
paromomycin, 1097
paroxetine, 722-723, 997
Parvolex, 42-43

Pastilles, 687-688
Patanol, 1044, 1047
Pathocil, 309-311
Paveral, 261-263
Pavulon, 719-720
Paxil, 722-723
Paxil CR, 722-723
PBZ, 1104
PBZ-SR, 1104
PCE, 379-380
PCP, 1123
PediaCare Allergy Formula, 223-224
PediaCare Children's Fever, 491-492
Pedia Care Cold-Allergy Chewable, 1074
Pedia Care Cough-Cold Liquid, 1074
Pedia Care Infant's Decongestant, 796-797
Pedia Care NightRest Cough-Cold Liquid, 1074
Pediacof Syrup, 1074
Pediapred, 772-774
Pediazole Suspension, 1074
Pedi-Pro, 1050, 1051-1052
Ped TE-PAK-4, 926-927
Pedtrice-4, 926-927
PedvaxHIB, 1106
pegaptanib, 723-724
pegaspargase, 724-726, 1043
Pegasys, 727
pegfilgrastim, 726-727
peginterferon alfa-2a, 727, 1004
PEG-L-asparaginase, 724-726
pegvisomant, 1097
Pelamine, 1104
pemetrexed, 727-729, 1005, 1043
Penbriten, 91-93
penciclovir, 1052-1053
pencillin G potassium, 1004
Penetrex, 360-361
penicillamine, 1096-1098
penicillin G, 729-732, 1004
penicillin G benzathine, 729-732, 1004
Penicillin G Potassium, 729-732
penicillin G procaine, 729-732, 1004
PENICILLINS, 1004
penicillin V, 1004
penicillin V potassium, 729-732
Penlac Nail Lacquer, 1050, 1051-1052
Pentacarinat, 732-733
Pentacort, 1050
Pentam 300, 732-733
pentamidine, 732-733
Pentamycin, 1044, 1047
Pentasa, 595-596
Pentazine, 785-786
pentazocine, 733-735, 1023, 1043, 1123
pentobarbital, 735-736, 1010, 1043
pentobarbital sodium, 735-736
pentostatin, 736-738, 1005, 1043
pentothal, 1123
pentoxifylline, 738-739
Pen-Vee K, 729-732
Pepcid, 399-401
Pepcid AC, 399-401
Pepcid Complete, 1074
Pepcid IV, 399-401
Pepcid RPD, 399-401
Pepto-Bismol, 143-144
Pepto-Bismol Maximum Strength, 143-144
Pepto Diarrhea Control, 566-567
Peptol, 234-236
Percocet, 709-710
Percocet 2.5/325, 1074
Percocet 5/325, 1074
Percocet 7.5/500, 1074
Percocet 10/650, 1074
Percodan, 709-710, 1074
Percodan-Demi, 709-710, 1074
Percogesic, 1074
Perdiem, 797-798
Perdiem Granules, 1074
Perdiem Plain, 797-798
perflutren lipid microsphere, 1098
pergolide, 739-740
Pergonal, 589-590
Periactin, 274-275
Peri-Colace, 1075
Peri-Colace Syrup, 1075
Peridol, 468-470
perindopril, 740-741
Periostat, 345-346
Permapen, 729-732
Permax, 739-740
permethrin, 1098
Permitil, 423-425
perphenazine, 741-744, 1007
Persantine, 325-326
Persantine IV, 325-326
Pertofrane, 292-293
Pertussin, 303
Pertussin ES, 303
Pethidine, 590-592
peyote, 1117, 1123
Pfizerpen, 729-732
Pharmacort, 1050
Phazyme, 848
Phazyme-95, 848
Phazyme-125, 848
Phenadoz, 785-786
Phenaphen w/Codeine No. 3, 1075
Phenaphen w/Codeine No. 4, 1075
Phenazine, 741-744
Phenazo, 744
Phenazodine, 744
phenazopyridine, 744
phencyclidine (PCP), 1123
phendimetrazine, 1098, 1117, 1123
Phendry, 322-324
phenelzine, 745-746, 997
Phenerbel-S, 1075
Phenergan, 785-786
Phenergan w/Codeine Syrup, 1075
Phenergan VC Syrup, 1075
Phenergan VC w/Codeine Syrup, 1075
Phenetron, 223-224
phenmetrazine, 1123
phenobarbital, 746-748, 996, 1010, 1043, 1117
phenobarbital sodium, 746-748
Phenolax, 748-749
phenolphthalein, 748-749, 1020
Phenoptic Relief, 1046, 1047
phenoxybenzamine, 1098
phentolamine, 749-750, 991
phenylalanine mustard, 587-588
phenylephrine, 751-752
phenylephrine (nasal), 1048-1049
phenylephrine (ophthalmic), 1046, 1047
phenylephrine HCl, 1046, 1047
Phenytex, 752-754
phenytoin, 752-754, 996, 1000
Pherazine DM Syrup, 1075
Phicon F, 1050, 1051-1052

Entries can be identified as follows: generic name, Trade Name, DRUG CATEGORY, *Combination Product.*

Phillips' Laxative Gelcaps, 1075
Phillips Magnesia Tablets, 576-578
Phillips Milk of Magnesia, 576-578
Phospholine Iodide, 1045, 1047
Phospho-soda, 853
Photofrin, 766-767
Phyllocontin, 76-79
physostigmine, 1015, 1098
phytonadione (vitamin K_1), 754-755, 1026
Pilagan, 1045, 1047
Pilocar, 1045, 1047
pilocarpine, 1045, 1047
Pilopine AT BEDTIME, 1045, 1047
Piloptic-½, 1045, 1047
Piloptic-1, 1045, 1047
Piloptic-2, 1045, 1047
Piloptic-3, 1045, 1047
Piloptic-4, 1045, 1047
Piloptic-6, 1045, 1047
Pilopto-Carpine, 1045, 1047
Pilostat, 1045, 1047
pimecrolimus, 1054
pindolol, 755-756, 1012
Pink Bismuth, 143-144
pioglitazone, 756-758, 998
pipecuronium, 1021, 1043, 1099
piperacillin, 758-759, 1004
piperacillin/tazobactam, 759-761
Pipracil, 758-759
pirbuterol, 761-762, 1013
piroxicam, 762-763, 1022
Pitocin, 712-713
Pitressin Synthetic, 959-960
plague vaccine, 1108
Plaquenil, 484-485
Plasbumin 5%, 51-52
Plasbumin 25%, 51-52
Plasmanate, 763-764
Plasma Plex, 763-764
plasma protein fraction, 763-764
Plasmatein, 763-764
Platinol, 240-242
Platinol-AQ, 240-242
Plavix, 255-256
Plenaxis, 34-35
Plendil, 402-403
Pletal, 233-234
plicamycin, 764-766, 1005, 1043
PMB-400, 1075
PMS-ASA, 111-113
PMS-Bismuth Subsalicylate, 143-144
PMS-Chloral Hydrate, 213-214
PMS-Cyproheptadine, 274-275
PMS-Diazepam, 305-307
PMS-Dimenhydrinate, 319-321
PMS Egozine, 984
PMS-Ferrous Sulfate, 408-410
PMS Hydromorphone, 482-484
PMS-Isoniazid, 524-525
PMS-Levothyroxine Sodium, 551-553
PMS Lindane, 555-556
PMS-Methylphenidate, 608-610
PMS-Nystatin, 687-688
PMS Perphenazine, 741-744
PMS-Piroxicam, 762-763
PMS-Primidone, 775-776
PMS-Propranol, 791-793
PMS Pyrazinamide, 798
PMS Sodium Polystyrene Sulfonate, 854-855
PMS-Sulfusalazine, 870-872
PMS-Thioridazine, 902-904
PMS-Trihexyphenidyl, 943-944
pneumococcal 7-valent conjugate vaccine, 1108
pneumococcal vaccine, polyvalent, 1108
Pneumomist, 466
Pneumopent, 732-733
Pneumovax 23, 1108
Pnu-Imune 23, 1108
Poladex, 1103
Polaramine, 1103
Polaramine Expectorant Liquid, 1075
polio vaccine, 1125
poliovirus vaccine (IPV), 1108
poliovirus vaccine, live, oral, trivalent (TOPV), 1108
Polycillin, 91-93
Polycillin-PRB Oral Suspension, 1075
Polycitra Syrup, 1075
Polygam, 501-502
Polygam SD, 501-502
Polygesic, 478-480
Poly-Histine Elixir, 1075
polymyxin B, 1044, 1047
Polymyxin B Sulfate Sterile, 1044, 1047
Polysporin Ophthalmic Ointment, 1075
Polysporin Topical Ointment, 1075
Polytrim Ophthalmic Solution, 1075
Poly-Vi-Sol, 649-650
Pontocaine, 1044, 1047, 1053
poractant alfa, 1043, 1099
porfirmer, 766-767, 1005
Portalac, 536-537
Posicor, 624-625
Potasalan, 767-769
potassium acetate/potassium bicarbonate, 767-769
potassium bicarbonate/potassium chloride, 767-769
potassium bicarbonate/potassium citrate, 767-769
potassium chloride, 767-769, 1121
potassium chloride/potassium bicarbonate/potassium citrate, 767-769
potassium gluconate, 767-769
potassium gluconate/potassium chloride, 767-769
potassium gluconate/potassium citrate, 767-769
potassium phosphates, 1121
Potassium-Rougier, 767-769
pralidoxime, 1099
Pralzine, 475-476
PrameGel, 1053
pramipexole, 769-770, 1006
pramlintide, 770, 1033-1034
pramoxine, 1053
Prandese, 35-36
Prandin, 816-817
Pravachol, 770-771
pravastatin, 770-771
Pravigard PAC, 1075
Prax, 1053
prazosin, 771-772, 1003
Precedex, 299
Precose, 35-36
Predaject-50, 772-774
Predalone 50, 772-774
Predalone-T.B.A., 772-774
Predcor-25, 772-774

Predcor-50, 772-774
PredForte, 1045, 1047
prednicarbate, 1050
Prednicen-M, 774-775
prednisolone, 772-774, 1017, 1045, 1047
Prednisolone Acetate, 772-774
Prednisol TBA, 772-774
prednisone, 774-775, 1017
Prefrin, 1046, 1047
pregabalin, 775, 1034-1036
Prelone, 772-774
Premarin, 387-389
Premarin Intravenous, 387-389
Premphase, 1075
Prempro, 1075
Premsyn PMS, 1075
Prepidil, 321-322
Pretz-D, 364-365, 1047, 1048-1049
Prevacid, 540-541
Prevalite, 229-230
Prevnar, 1108
Prevpac, 1075
Priftin, 822-823
Prilosec, 696-697
Primacor, 631-632
Primatene, 1075
Primatene Mist, 366-367
Primaxin 250 mg IV for Injection, 1075
Primaxin 500 mg IV for Injection, 1076
Primaxin IM, 497-499
Primaxin IV, 497-499
primidone, 775-776, 996
Principen, 91-93
Prinivil, 560-562
Prinzide 10-12.5, 1076
Prinzide 20-12.5, 1076
Prinzide 20-25, 1076
Privine, 1047, 1048-1049
ProAmatine, 628-629
Probampacin Oral Suspension, 1076
Pro-Banthine, 787-788
Proben-C, 1076
probenecid, 777-778
procainamide, 778-779, 1000
ProcalAmine, 73-75
Pro-Cal-Sof, 332-333
Procanbid, 778-779
procarbazine, 779-781, 1005
Procardia, 675-676
Procardia XL, 675-676
prochlorperazine, 781-783, 1007
Procrit, 370-372
Proctofoam-HC Aerosol Foam, 1076
Procytox, 270-272
Prodium, 744
Profenal, 1046, 1047
Profilnine/Alpha Nine, 397-398
progesterone, 783-784
Prograf, 878-879
Proleukin, 54-56
Prolixin, 423-425
Prolixin Decanoate, 423-425
promethazine, 785-786, 1001
promethazine HCl, 785-786
Prometh w/Codeine Syrup, 1076
Prometh VCW/Codeine Syrup, 1076
Prometrium, 783-784
Promine, 778-779
Pronestyl, 778-779
Pronestyl-SR, 778-779
Propacet 100, 1076
propafenone, 786-787, 1000
Propanthel, 787-788
propantheline, 787-788, 994
proparacaine, 1044, 1047
Propecia, 413-414
Propine, 1046, 1047
Proplex SX-T, 397-398
Proplex T, 397-398
propofol, 788-790, 992, 1043
propoxyphene, 790-791, 1023, 1043
propranolol, 791-793, 993, 1000, 1012
propranolol HCl, 791-793
propylhexadrine, 1048-1049
propylthiouracil, 793-795
Propyl-Thyracil, 793-795
Proscar, 413-414
Prostigmin, 667-668
Prostin/15M, 182-183
Prostin E Vaginal Suppository, 321-322
protamine, 795
Protectol, 1050, 1051-1052
Protenate, 763-764
Protilase, 718-719
Protonix, 720-721
Protonix IV, 720-721
Protopic, 878-879
Protostat, 619-620
Provazin, 781-783
Proventil, 52-54
Provera, 583-584
Prozac, 421-423
Prozac Weekly, 421-423
PRP-OMP, 1106
Prulet, 748-749
Pseudo, 796-797
Pseudo-Chlor, 1076
pseudoephedrine, 796-797
pseudoephedrine HCl, 796-797
Pseudogest, 796-797
Pseudo-Gest Plus, 1076
psilocin, 1123
psilocybin, 1123
Psorcon, 1049, 1050
Psorion, 1049, 1050
psyllium, 797-798, 1020
P.T.E.-4, 926-927
P.T.E.-5, 926-927
PTU, 793-795
Pulmicort, 155-156
Purinethol, 592-593
Purinol, 60-61
PVFK, 729-732
P-V-Tussin, 1076
P-V-Tussin Syrup, 1076
pyrazinamide, 798, 1008
Pyri, 800-801
Pyridiate, 744
Pyridium, 744
pyridostigmine, 798-800, 1015
pyridoxine (vitamin B_6), 800-801, 1026
pyridoxine HCl, 800-801
pyrimethamine, 801-802

Q

Quadrinal, 1076
Quelicin, 867-868
Quelidrine Cough Syrup, 1076
Questran, 229-230
Questran Light, 229-230
quetiapine, 802-803, 1007
Quibron, 1076
Quibron-300, 1076
Quibron-T Dividose, 898-899
Quibron-T/SR, 898-899
Quinaglute Dura-Tabs, 805-807
Quinalan, 805-807
quinapril, 803-805, 1002
Quinaretic, 1076
Quinate, 805-807
Quinidex Extentabs, 805-807
quinidine, 805-807, 1000

Entries can be identified as follows: generic name, Trade Name, DRUG CATEGORY, *Combination Product.*

quinidine gluconate, 805-807
quinidine polygalacturonate, 805-807
quinidine sulfate, 805-807
quinine, 807-808
Quinora, 805-807
Quinsana Plus, 1050, 1051-1052
Quintabs, 649-650
Quixin, 1044, 1047
QVAR, 130-131

R

rabeprazole, 808-809
rabies vaccine, adsorbed, 1109
rabies vaccine, HDCV, 1109
RADIOCONTRAST AGENTS, 1042, 1121
Radiostol, 972-973
Radiostol Forte, 972-973
raloxifene, 809-810
ramelteon, 812, 1036-1037
ramipril, 810-812, 1002
Ranexa, 1041
Raniclor, 196-202
ranitidine, 812-813, 1019
ranitidine bismuth citrate, 812-813
ranolazine, 1041
Rapamune, 849-851
rasburicase, 814
raspberry, 1114
Rauzide, 1076
Razadyne, 444-445
Razepam, 885-886
R&C Shampoo, 1076
Rebetron, 1076
Reclomide, 613-615
Recombinate, 101-102
Recombivax HB, 1106
red clover, 1114
Rederm, 1050
Redutemp, 38-39
ReFacto, 101-102
Refludan, 542-543
Regitine, 749-750
Reglan, 613-615
Regonol, 798-800
Regroton, 1076
Regulace, 1076
Regulax, 332-333
Regulax SS, 332-333
Reguloid Natural, 797-798
Reguloid Orange, 797-798
Reguloid Sugar Free Orange, 797-798
Reguloid Sugar Free Regular, 797-798
Relafen, 653-654
Relenza, 980-981
Reliable Gentle Laxative, 142-143
Relpax, 355-356
Remeron, 635-636
Remeron Soltab, 635-636
Remicade, 508-509
remifentanil, 814-816, 1023
Remodulin, 934-935
RenAmin, 73-75
Renedil, 402-403
Renese-R, 1076
repaglinide, 816-817, 998
Repan, 1076
Rep-Pred, 610-612
Repronex, 589-590
Requip, 832-833
Rescriptor, 290-291
Rescula, 1046, 1047
Resectisol, 578-580
reserpine, 1003, 1099
Respa-GF, 466
Respahist, 1076
Respaire-60, 1076
Respbid, 898-899
Restore, 797-798
Restore Sugar Free, 797-798
Restoril, 885-886
Resyl, 466
Retin-A, 935-936
retinoic acid, 817, 935-936
Retrovir, 981-983
Reversol, 353-354
Rev-Eyes, 1044, 1047
Revimine, 336-337
Revitonus, 900
Revlimid, 1041
Reyataz, 113-114
Rheaban, 121-122
Rheumatrex Dose Pack, 603-605
Rhinocort, 1048-1049
Rhinocort Aqua, 155-156, 1048-1049
Rh_o (D) globulin microdose IM, 817-818
Rh_o (D) immune globulin, standard dose IM, 817-818
Rh_o (D) immune globulin IV, 817-818
Rhodis, 531-533
RhoGAM, 817-818
rhu GM-CSF, 840-842
Rhulicort S-T Cort, 1050
Rhythmodan, 328-329
ribavarin, 818-819
riboflavin (vitamin B_2), 819, 1026
RID Mousse, 1076
RID Shampoo, 1077
rifabutin, 820-821, 1008
Rifadin, 821-822
Rifamate, 1077
rifampin, 821-822, 1008
rifapentine, 822-823
Rifater, 1077
rifaximin, 823-824
Rilutek, 824-825
riluzole, 824-825
Rimactane, 821-822
Rimactane/INH Dual Pack, 1077
rimantadine, 825-826, 1010
rimexolone, 1045, 1047
Riomet, 597-598
Riopan, 575-576
Riopan Extra Strength, 575-576
Riopan Plus Suspension, 1077
Riphenidate, 608-610
risedronate, 826-827
Risperdal, 827-828
Risperdal M-TAB, 827-828
risperidone, 827-828, 1007
Ritalin, 608-610
Ritalin LA, 608-610
Ritalin SR, 608-610
ritonavir, 828-829, 1010
Rituxan, 830
rituximab, 830, 1005
rivastigmine, 831
Rivotril, 251-252
rizatriptan, 831-832
RMS, 646-648
Robaxin, 601-602
Robaxisal, 1077
Robidex, 303
Robidone, 478-480
Robigesic, 38-39
Robinul, 462-463
Robinul-Forte, 462-463
Robitet, 896-898
Robitussin, 466
Robitussin Allergy & Cough Liquid, 1077
Robitussin Cold, Multi-Symptom Cold & Flu Tablets, 1077
Robitussin Cough Calmers, 303
Robitussin Cough & Cold Infant Drops, 1077
Robitussin Cough & Congestion Formula, 1077
Robitussin-DM Infant Drops, 1077
Robitussin-DM Liquid, 1077

Robitussin Flu Liquid, 1077
Robitussin Honey Cough & Cold Liquid, 1077
Robitussin Honey Flu Multi-Symptom Liquid, 1077
Robitussin Honey Flu Night-Time Syrup, 1077
Robitussin Honey Flu Non-Drowsy Syrup, 1077
Robitussin Maximum Strength Cough and Cold Syrup, 1077
Robitussin Night Relief Liquid, 1077
Robitussin Pediatric, 303
Robitussin Pediatric Cough & Cold Liquid, 1077
Robitussin Pediatric Night Relief Cough & Cold Liquid, 1077
Robitussin PM Cough & Cold Liquid, 1077
Robitussin Sugar Free Cough Liquid, 1077
Rocaltrol, 168-169
Rocephin, 202-210
Rodex, 800-801
Rofact, 821-822
Roferon-A/Intron-A, 513-514
Rogaine, 634-635
Rogitine, 749-750
Rolaids Calcium Rich, 169-170, 1077
Rolzine, 475-476
Romazicon, 418-419
Rondec, 1077
Rondec DM Drops, 1078
Rondec DM Syrup, 1078
Rondec Oral Drops, 1078
ropinirole, 832-833
ropivacaine, 833-834, 992
rosiglitazone, 834-835, 998
rosuvastatin, 836-837
RotaTeq, 837, 1037
rotavirus vaccine, 837, 1037
Roubac, 945-947
Rounax, 38-39
Rowasa, 595-596
Roxanol, 646-648
Roxanol Rescudose, 646-648
Roxanol-T, 646-648
Roxicet, 709-710, 1078
Roxicet 5/500, 1078
Roxicet Oral Solution, 1078
Roxicodone, 709-710
Roxicodone Supeudol, 709-710
Roxilox, 709-710
Roxiprin, 709-710, 1078
Roychlor, 767-769
Rozerem, 812, 1036-1037
rt-PA, 64-66
rubella and mumps virus vaccine, live, 1109
rubella virus vaccine, live attenuated (RA 27/3), 1109
Rubex, 343-345
Rulets, 649-650
Rum-K, 767-769
Ru-Tuss DE, 1078
Ru-Tuss Expectorant Liquid, 1078
Ru-Tuss with Hydrocodone Liquid, 1078
Ryna-C Liquid, 1078
Ryna Liquid, 1078
Rynatan, 1078
Rynatan Pediatric Suspension, 1078
Rynatuss, 1078
Rythmol, 786-787

S

S-2, 366-367
St. John's wort, 1114
St. Joseph Antidiarrheal, 121-122
St. Joseph Children's Supasa, 111-113
St. Joseph Cough Suppressant, 303
Saizen, 855-856
Salazopyrin, 870-872
Salbutamol, 52-54
Saleta Tablets, 1078
Salflex, 838-839
Salgesic, 838-839
SALICYLATES, 1023-1024
salmeterol, 837-838
Salmonine, 166-168
Salofulk, 595-596
salsalate, 838-839, 1024
Salsalate, 838-839
Salsitab, 838-839
Sal-Tropine, 119-121
Salutensin, 1078
Salutensin Demi, 1078
SAM-e, 1114
Sanctura, 948
Sandimmune, 272-274
Sandoglobulin, 501-502
Sandostatin, 689-690
Sandostatin LAR Depot, 689-690
SangCya, 272-274
Sansert, 612-613
saquinavir, 839-840, 1010
Sarafem, 421-423
sargramostim, 840-842
Sarna HC, 1050
S.A.S., 870-872
saw palmetto, 1114
Scabene, 555-556
scopolamine, 842-843, 994, 1016
scopolamine (ophthalmic), 1046, 1047
Scot-Tussin DM, 303
Scot-Tussin DM Liquid, 1078
Scot-Tussin Expectorant, 466
Scot-Tussin Original 5-Action Liquid, 1078
Scot-Tussin Senior Clear Liquid, 1078
SD-Deprenyl, 843-844
secobarbital, 1010, 1043, 1099, 1117, 1123
Sectral, 36-38
Sedapap-10, 1078
SEDATION AGENTS, 1042, 1121
Sedatives, 1123
Sedatuss, 303
selegiline, 843-844, 1006
selenium, 926-927, 1050, 1051-1052
Selenium Sulfide, 1050, 1051-1052
Selestoject, 135-137
Selsun, 1050, 1051-1052
Selsun Blue, 1050, 1051-1052
Semprex-D, 1078, 1102
Senexon, 845
senna, 1020, 1114
senna, sennosides, 845
Senna-Gen, 845
Senokot, 845
Senokot-S, 1078
Senokotxtra, 845
Senolax, 845
Sensamide IV, 613-615
Sensipar, 236-237
Septra, 945-947, 1078-1079
Septra DS, 945-947, 1079
Septra I.V. for Injection, 1079
Septra Suspension, 1079
Ser-A-Gen, 1079

Entries can be identified as follows: generic name, Trade Name, DRUG CATEGORY, *Combination Product.*

Ser-Ap-Es, 1079
Serevent, 837-838
Serophene, 249-250
Seroquel, 802-803
Serostim, 855-856
sertaconazole, 1050, 1051-1052
Sertan, 775-776
sertraline, 846-847, 997
Serutan, 797-798
Sesame Street Vitamins, 649-650
Seudotabs, 796-797
sevelamer, 1099-1100
siberian ginseng, 1114
sibutramine, 1100
Silace, 332-333
Siladril, 322-324
Silafed Syrup, 1079
Silaminic Cold Syrup, 1079
Silapap, 38-39
sildenafil, 847-848
Siltussin DAS, 466
Siltussin SA, 466
Silvadene, 1052
silver nitrate 1%, 1044, 1047
silver nitrate sulfacetamide sodium, 1044, 1047
silver sulfadiazine, 1052
simethicone, 848
Simulect, 129-130
simvastatin, 848-849
Sinarest Extra Strength, 1079
Sinarest No Drowsiness, 1079
Sinarest Sinus, 1079
Sine-Aid IB, 1079
Sine-Aid Maximum Strength, 1079
Sinemet, 179-181
Sinemet 10/100, 1079
Sinemet 25/20, 1079
Sinemet 25/100, 1079
Sinemet CR, 179-181
Sinemet CR 25-100, 1079
Sinemet CR 50-200, 1079
Sine-Off Maximum Strength No Drowsiness Formula Caplets, 1079
Sine-Off Sinus Medicine, 1079
Sinequan, 340-342
Sinequan Concentrate, 340-342
Sine-Relief, 1079
Sinex, 1048-1049
Singulair, 643-644
Sinustop Pro, 796-797
Sinutab, 1079
Sinutab Maximum Strength Sinus Allergy, 1079
Sinutab Maximum Strength Without Drowsiness, 1079
Sinutab Non-Drying, 1079
sirolimus, 849-851, 1019
Skelid, 910-911
Sleep-Eze 3, 322-324
Slo-bid Gyrocaps, 898-899
Slo-Mag, 576-578
Slo-Niacin, 670-671
Slo-Phyllin, 898-899
Slo-Phyllin GG Syrup, 1079
Sloprin, 111-113
Slow Fe, 408-410
Slow-K, 767-769
Slow-Salt-K, 1079
SMZ/TMP, 945-947
Soda Mint, 851-853
sodium bicarbonate, 851-853, 993
sodium biphosphate/ sodium phosphate, 853, 1020
sodium chloride, hypertonic, 1121
Sodium nitroprusside, 682-683
sodium polystyrene sulfonate, 854-855
Sodium Sulamyd, 1044, 1047
Sodium Sulfacetamide, 1044, 1047
Solage, 1079
Solarcaine, 1053
Solazine, 941-943
Solfoton, 746-748
solifenacin, 855, 994
Solu-Cortef, 480-482
Solu-Medrol, 610-612
Solurex, 297-299
Solurex-LA, 297-299
Soma, 183-184
Soma-Compound, 1080
Soma Compound w/Codeine, 1079
somatropin, 855-856
Sominex 2, 322-324
Somnol, 425-427
Sonata, 979-980
sorafenib, 857, 1037-1038
Sorbitrate, 526-527
Sotacar, 857-858
sotalol, 857-858, 1000
Soyacal 20%, 401-402
Span-FF, 408-410
sparfloxacin, 858-860, 1004
Spectazole, 1050, 1051-1052
Spec-T Lozenge, 1080
Spectracef, 202-210
Spiriva, 915-916
spironolactone, 860-861, 1018
Sporanox, 528-529
SPS, 854-855
SSD, 1052
SSD AF, 1052
Stadol, 164-166
Stadol NS, 164-166
Stagesic, 478-480
Stalevo 50, 1080
Stalevo 100, 1080
Stalevo 150, 1080
Statex, 646-648
Staticin, 1052
stavudine, 861-863, 1010
Stemetic, 944-945
Stemetil, 781-783
Sterapred, 774-775
STEROIDS, ANABOLIC, 1123
STEROIDS, NASAL, 1048-1049
Stievaa, 935-936
Stimate, 295-297
Storz sulf, 1044, 1047
Strattera, 116-117
Streptase, 863-864
streptokinase, 863-864, 1024, 1043
streptomycin, 864-866, 1003, 1008
Sublimaze, 405-407
succimer, 866-867
succinylcholine, 867-868, 1021, 1043
succinylcholine chloride, 867-868
Sucostrin, 867-868
sucralfate, 868-869
Sucrets Cough Control, 303
Sudafed, 796-797
Sudafed Cold & Allergy, 1080
Sudafed Cold & Cough Liquicaps, 1080
Sudafed Cold & Sinus, 1080
Sudafed Plus, 1080
Sudafed Severe Cold, 1080
Sudafed Sinus Maximum Strength, 1080
Sudafed 12 hour, 796-797
Sudal 60/500, 1080
Sudal 120/600, 1080
Sudex, 796-797
Sular, 678-679
Sulcrate, 868-869
Sulf-10, 1044, 1047
Sulfalax Calcium, 332-333
sulfamethoxazole, 869-870
Sulfamylon, 1052
sulfasalazine, 870-872, 1004

Sulfatrim, 945-947
Sulfimycin Suspension, 1080
sulfinpyrazone, 872-873
sulfisoxazole, 873-874, 1004
sulfisoxazole diolamine, 1045-1047
Sulftrin Triple Sulfa Vaginal Cream, 1080
Sulftrin Triple Sulfa Vaginal Tablets, 1080
sulindac, 874-875, 1022
Sulster, 1044, 1047
sumatriptan, 875-876
Sumycin, 896-898
sunitinib, 1041
Sunkist, 108-109
Suppress, 303
Suprazine, 941-943
Supres, 475-476
suprofen, 1046, 1047
Surfak, 332-333
Sus-Phrine, 366-367
Sustaire, 898-899
Sustiva, 354-355
Sutent, 1041
Suxamethonium, 867-868
Syllact, 797-798
Symadine, 67-68
Symbyax, 1080
Symlin, 770, 1033-1034
Symmetrel, 67-68
SYMPATHOMIMETICS, OPHTHALMIC, 1046, 1047
Synacort, 1050
Synagis, 715
Synalgos-DC, 1080
Synarel, 656
Syn-Clonazepam, 251-252
Synercid, 1080
Synflex, 662-664
Synflex DS, 662-664
Syn-Nadolol, 654-655
Synophylate-GG Syrup, 1080
Syn-Pindol, 755-756
Syntest D.S., 1080
Syntest H.S., 1080
Synthroid, 551-553

T

T_3, 557-559, 1025
T_3/T_4, 559-560
T_4, 551-553, 1025
Tab-A-Vite, 649-650
Tac-3, 936-938
Tac-40, 936-938
tacrine, 877-878
tacrolimus, 878-879, 1019
tacrolimus topical, 878-879
tadalafil, 879-880
Tagamet, 234-236
Tagamet HB, 234-236
Talacen, 1080
Talwin, 733-735
Talwin Compound, 1080
Talwin NX, 733-735, 1080
Tambocor, 415-416
Tamiflu, 699-700
Tamofen, 880-881
Tamone, 880-881
Tamoplex, 880-881
tamoxifen, 880-881, 1005
tamsulosin, 881-882
Tapanol, 38-39
Tapazole, 600-601
Tarabine PFS, 275-277
Tarceva, 376-377
Targretin, 139-140
Tarka 182, 1080
Tarka 241, 1080
Tarka 242, 1080-1081
Tarka 244, 1081
Tasmar, 921-922
Tavist, 246-247, 1103
Tavist Allergy/Sinus Headache, 1081
Tavist ND, 567-568
Tavist Sinus, 1081
Taxol, 713-715
Taxotere, 330-332
Tazicef, 202-210
Tazidime, 202-210
tazobactam, 882
3TC, 537-539
T-Cypionate, 895-896
Tebamide, 944-945
Tebrazid, 798
Tecnal, 1081
Teczem, 1081
Tedrigen, 1081
tegaserod, 882-883
Tegretol, 177-179
Tegretol CR, 177-179
Tegretol-XR, 177-179
Tegrin-LT Shampoo, 1081
Teldrin, 223-224
Teline, 896-898
telithromycin, 883-884, 1004
telmisartan, 884-885, 1002
Temaril, 1104
temazepam, 885-886, 1011
Temazepam, 885-886
Temodar, 886-888
Temovate, 1049, 1050
temozolomide, 886-888
Tempra, 38-39
tenecteplase, 888-889, 1025, 1043
Tenex, 466-467
teniposide, 1100
Ten-K, 767-769
tenofovir, 889-890, 1010
Tenoretic 50, 1081
Tenoretic 100, 1081
Tenormin, 114-116
Tensilon, 353-354
Tequin, 449-451
Terazol 7, 1054-1055
terazosin, 890-891, 1003
terbinafine, 891-892, 1050, 1051-1052
terbutaline, 893-894, 1013
terconazole, 1054-1055
Terfluzine, 941-943
teriparatide, 894
Terra-Cortril Ophthalmic Suspension, 1081
Terramycin w/Polymycin B Sulfate Ophthalmic Ointment, 1081
Tessalon, 133
Testa-C, 895-896
Testim, 895-896
Testoderm, 895-896
Testoderm TTS, 895-896
Testoderm with Adhesive, 895-896
Testoject-LA, 895-896
testolactone, 1005
Testone LA, 895-896
Testopel, 895-896
testosterone, 895-896
testosterone, long acting, 895-896
testosterone cypionate, 895-896
testosterone enenthate, 895-896
testosterone gel, 895-896
testosterone pellets, 895-896
testosterone transdermal, 895-896
Testred, 895-896
Testrin-PA, 895-896
tetanus toxoid, adsorbed/ tetanus toxoid, 1109
tetracaine, 992
Tetracaine, 1044, 1047
tetracaine (ophthalmic), 1044, 1047
tetracaine (topical), 1053
Tetracap, 896-898
tetracycline, 896-898, 1004
tetracycline HCl, 896-898

Tetracyn, 896-898
tetrahydrozoline, 1046, 1047
tetrahydrozoline (nasal), 1048-1049
tetrahydrozoline HCl, 1046, 1047
Tetralan, 896-898
Tetram, 896-898
Tetrasine, 1046, 1047
Tetrasine Extra, 1046, 1047
Tetrazol 3, 1054-1055
Teveten, 372-373
Texa-Cort, 1050
6-TG, 1005, 1100
T-Gen, 944-945
T-Gesic, 478-480, 1081
Thalitone, 227-228
Theo-24, 898-899
Theobid Duracaps, 898-899
Theochron, 898-899
Theoclear-80, 898-899
Theoclear LA, 898-899
Theodrine, 1081
Theo-Dur, 898-899
Theolair-SR, 898-899
theophylline, 898-899, 1013
theophylline ethylenediamine, 76-79
Theo-Sav, 898-899
Theospan-SR, 898-899
Theostat 80, 898-899
Theovent, 898-899
Theo-X, 898-899
Therabid, 649-650
Thera-Flu, Cold & Cough Powder, 1081
Thera-Flu, Flu, Cold, Cough & Sore Throat Maximum Strength Powder, 1081
Thera-Flu, Flu & Chest Congestion Non-Drowsy Powder, 1081
Thera-Flu Maximum Strength Flu, Cold & Cough Powder, 1081
Thera-Flu Non-Drowsy Flu, Cold & Cough Maximum Strength Powder, 1081
Thera-Flu Severe Cold & Congestion Night-Time Maximum Strength Powder, 1081
Thera-Flu Severe Cold & Congestion Non-Drowsy Maximum Strength Powder, 1081
Thera-Flu Severe Cold & Cough Powder, 1081
Thera-Flu Severe Cold Non-Drowsy Packet, 1081
Thera-Flu Severe Cold Non-Drowsy Tablets, 1081-1082
Thera-Flu Severe Cold Tablets, 1082
Theragram, 649-650
Therapy Bayer, 111-113
Therelax, 142-143
Thermazene, 1052
Thiamilate, 900
thiamine (vitamin B_1), 900, 1026
thiamine HCl, 900
thiethylperazine, 901-902
thiobarbiturates, 1123
thioguanine (6-TG), 1005, 1100
thiopental, 996, 1010, 1043, 1100
thioridazine, 902-904, 1007
thioridazine HCl, 902-904
thiotepa, 1005, 1100
thiothixene, 1007, 1101
Thorazine, 224-227
Thor-Prom, 224-227
THROMBOLYTICS/FIBRINOLYTICS, 1024-1025, 1042, 1121
Thyrar, 904-905
THYROID HORMONES, 1025
Thyroid Strong, 904-905
thyroid USP (desiccated), 904-905, 1025
Thyrolar, 559-560
tiagabine, 996
Tiazac, 318-319
Ticar, 906-908
ticarcillin, 906-908, 1004
ticarcillin/clavulanate, 908-909, 1004
TICE BCG, 1105
Ticlid, 909-910
ticlopidine, 909-910
Ticon, 944-945
Tigan, 944-945
tigecycline, 910, 1038-1039
Tijet-20, 944-945
Tikosyn, 333-334
Tilade, 665
tiludronate, 910-911
Timentin, 908-909
Timentin for Injection, 1082
Timolide 10/25, 1082
timolol, 912-913, 1012, 1045, 1046-1047
timolol maleate, 912-913
Timoptic, 912-913, 1045, 1046-1047
Timoptic-XE[3], 1045, 1046-1047
Tinactin, 1050, 1051-1052
Tindamax, 913-914
Ting, 1050, 1051-1052
tinidazole, 913-914
tinzaparin, 914-915, 995, 1043
tioconazole, 1054-1055
tiotropium, 915-916, 1013
Tipramine, 499-501
tipranavir, 916, 1039-1040
tirofiban, 916-917, 1043
tissue plasminogen activator, 64-66
Titralac, 169-170
Titralac Plus, 1082
tizanidine, 917-918
TNKase, 888-889
TOBI, 918-920
Tobra Dex Ophthalmic Suspension/Ointment, 1082
tobramycin, 918-920, 1003
tobramycin (ophthalmic), 1045-1047
tobramycin sulfate, 918-920
Tobrex, 1045-1047
tocainide, 920-921, 1000
Tocopherol, 973-974
Tofranil, 499-501
Tofranil PM, 499-501
tolcapone, 921-922, 1006
tolnaftate, 1050, 1051-1052
tolterodine, 922-923
Tonocard, 920-921
Topamax, 923-924
TOPICAL AGENTS, MISCELLANEOUS, 1054
TOPICAL ANESTHETICS, 1053
TOPICAL ANTIFUNGALS, 1050-1052
TOPICAL ANTI-INFECTIVES, 1052
TOPICAL ANTIVIRALS, 1052-1053
TOPICAL GLUCOCORTICOIDS, 1049-1050
Topicort, 1049, 1050
Topicort LP, 1049, 1050
topiramate, 923-924, 996
topotecan, 924-925, 1005, 1043
Toprol XL, 617-619
Topsyn, 1049, 1050

Toradol, 533-534
Torecan, 901-902
toremifene, 925-926
torsemide, 1018
Totacillin, 91-93
TOTAL PARENTERAL NUTRITION SOLUTIONS, 1042, 1121
t-PA, 64-66
T-Phy, 898-899
trace elements (chromium, copper, iodide, manganese, selenium, zinc), 926-927
Tracleer, 150-151
tramadol, 927-928
Trandate, 534-536
trandolapril, 928-930, 1002
Transderm-Nitro, 681-682
Transderm-Scop, 842-843
Transderm-V, 842-843
Tranxene-SD, 256-257
Tranxene-SD Half strength, 256-257
Tranxene T-tab, 256-257
tranylcypromine, 930-931, 997
trastuzumab, 931-932, 1043
Travamine, 319-321
Travasol, 73-75
Travatan, 1046, 1047
travoprost, 1046, 1047
trazodone, 932-934, 997
trazodone HCl, 932-934
Trazon, 932-934
Trelstar Depot, 947-948
Trental, 738-739
treprostinil, 934-935
tretinoin (vitamin A acid, retinoic acid), 935-936
Tretinoin LF IV, 935-936
Trexall, 603-605
Triacin-C Cough Syrup, 1082
Triad, 1082
Triadapin, 340-342
Triaderm, 1050
Trialodine, 932-934
Triam-A, 936-938
triamcinolone, 936-938, 1017, 1048-1049
triamcinolone acetonide, 936-938
triamcinolone (topical), 1050
Triam Forte, 936-938
Triaminic AM Cough & Decongestant Formula Liquid, 1082
Triaminic AM Decongestant Formula, 796-797
Triaminic Nite Light Liquid, 1082
Triaminic Sore Throat Formula Liquid, 1082
Triamolone 40, 936-938
Triamonide 40, 936-938
triamterene, 938-939, 1018
Trianide, 1050
Triavil 2-10, 1082
Triavil 2-25, 1082
Triavil 4-10, 1082
Triavil 4-25, 1082
Triavil 4-50, 1082
triazolam, 939-941, 1011
Triban, 944-945
Tricor, 403-404
Tricosal, 230-231
Triderm, 1050
Tridesilon, 1049, 1050
Tridil, 681-682
trifluoperazine, 941-943, 1007
trifluoperazine HCl, 941-943
trifluridine, 1045-1047
Triflurin, 941-943
Trihexane, 943-944
Trihexy-2, 943-944
Trihexy-5, 943-944
trihexyphenidyl, 943-944, 994, 1006, 1016
trihexyphenidyl HCl, 943-944
Tri-Hydroserpine, 1082
I-Triiodothyronine, 557-559
Trikacide, 619-620
Tri-Kort, 936-938
Trileptal, 706-707
Tri-Levlen, 1082
Trilisate, 230-231
Trilog, 936-938
Trilone, 936-938
Trimazide, 944-945
trimeprazine, 1104
trimethobenzamide, 944-945
trimethobenzamide HCl, 944-945
trimethoprim/ sulfamethoxazole (cotrimoxazole), 945-947
trimipramine, 997
Tr-Immunol, 1105
Trimox, 85-87
Trinalin Repetabs, 1082
Triostat, 557-559
Tripedia, 1105
tripelennamine, 1104
tripelennamine HCl, 1104
Triphasil, 1082
Triple Antibiotic Ophthalmic Ointment, 1082
Triposed Tablets, 1082
Triprolidine/ Pseudoephedrine Syrup (generic), 1082
Triprolidine/Pseudoephedrine Tablets (generic), 1082
Triptone Caplets, 319-321
triptorelin, 947-948
Trisenox, 107
Trisoject, 936-938
Tritec, 812-813
Trizivir, 1083
Tronothane, 1053
Trophamine, 73-75
Tropicacyl, 1046, 1047
tropicamide, 1046, 1047
Tropicamide, 1046, 1047
trospium, 948
trovafloxacin, 49-51
Trovan (oral), 49-51
Trovan IV, 49-51
Truphylline, 76-79
Trusopt, 1045, 1046, 1047
Truvada, 1083
Trymex, 1050
T-Statd, 1052
Tubarine, 949-950
tubocurarine, 949-950, 1021, 1043
Tubocuraine, 949-950
Tuinal 100 mg, 1083
Tuinal 200 mg, 1083
Tums, 169-170
Tums E-X Extra Strength, 169-170
turmeric, 1114
Tusibron-DM Syrup, 1083
Tussigon, 478-480
Tussionex Pennkinetic Suspension, 1083
Tussi-Organidin NR Liquid, 1083
Tusstat, 322-324
12-Hour Nasal, 1048-1049
Twilite, 322-324
Twin-K, 767-769
Twinrix, 1083
Two-Dyne, 1083
Tygacil, 910, 1038-1039
Tylenol, 38-39
Tylenol Allergy Sinus, Maximum Strength Gelcaps, 1083

Entries can be identified as follows: generic name, Trade Name, DRUG CATEGORY, *Combination Product.*

Tylenol Children's Cold, 1083
Tylenol Children's Cold Liquid, 1083
Tylenol Children's Cold Multi-Symptom Plus Cough Liquid, 1083
Tylenol Children's Cold Plus Cough Chewable, 1083
Tylenol Children's Cold Plus Cough Suspension, 1083
Tylenol Children's Flu Suspension, 1083
Tylenol w/Codeine Elixir, 1084
Tylenol w/Codeine No. 1, 1084
Tylenol w/Codeine No. 2, 1084
Tylenol w/Codeine No. 3, 1084
Tylenol w/Codeine No. 4, 1084
Tylenol Cold Complete Formula Tablets, 1083
Tylenol Cold & Flu Severe DayTime Liquid, 1083
Tylenol Cold Severe Congestion Tablets, 1083
Tylenol Cold & Sore Throat DayTime Liquid, 1083
Tylenol Flu Maximum Strength Non-Drowsy Gelcaps, 1083
Tylenol Flu NightTime Maximum Strength Liquid, 1083-1084
Tylenol Headache Plus, Extra Strength, 1084
Tylenol PM, Extra Strength, 1084
Tylenol Severe Allergy, 1084
Tylenol Sinus Maximum Strength, 1084
Tylox, 709-710, 1084
Typhim Vi, 1110
typhoid vaccine, oral, 1110
typhoid vaccine, parenteral, 1110
typhoid Vi polysaccharide vaccine, 1110
Tyrodone Liquid, 1084
Tyzine, 1048-1049
Tyzine Pediatric, 1048-1049

U

Ugesic, 478-480
Ultiva, 814-816
Ultracet, 1084
Ultralente U, 510-513
Ultram, 927-928
Ultrase MT 12, 718-719
Ultrase MT 20, 718-719
Ultravate, 1049, 1050
Ultrazine, 781-783
Unasyn, 93-95
Unasyn for Injection 3 g, 1084
undecylenic acid, 1050, 1051-1052
Uni-Bent Cough, 322-324
Unicaps, 649-650
Unicort, 1050
Uni-Dur, 898-899
Unipen, 656-658
Uniphyl, 898-899
Uniretic, 1084
Unituss HC Syrup, 1084
Univasc, 642-643
unoprostone, 1046, 1047
Urebeth, 137-138
Urecholine, 137-138
Uridon, 227-228
Urised, 1084
Uritol, 440-443
Urobak, 869-870
Urobiotic 250, 1084
Urodine, 744
Urogesic, 744
urokinase, 950-951, 1025, 1043
Uro-Mag, 576-578
Uroxatral, 58-59
Urozide, 476-478

V

VACCINES AND TOXOIDS, 1105-1110
Vagifem, 385-387
VAGINAL ANTIFUNGALS, 1054-1055
Vagistat-1, 1054-1055
valacyclovir, 951-952
Valcyte, 952-953
Valergen, 385-387
valerian, 1114
valganciclovir, 952-953, 1010
Valisone, 1049, 1050
Valium, 305-307
valproate, 954-955
valproate/valproic acid/ divalproex sodium, 996
valproic acid, 954-955
valrubicin, 955-956
valsartan, 956-957, 1002
Valstar, 955-956
Valtrex, 951-952
Vanacet, 478-480
Vanadom, 183-184
Vancenase AQ Nasal, 1048-1049
Vancenase Pocket Inhaler, 1048-1049
Vanceril, 130-131
Vanceril Double Strength, 130-131
Vancocin, 957-958
Vancoled, 957-958
vancomycin, 957-958
vancomycin HCl, 957-958
Vandone, 478-480
Vanquish, 1084
Vantin, 202-210
Vaponefrin (racepinephrine), 366-367
Vaprisol, 1041
Vaqta, 1106
vardenafil, 958-959
varicella virus vaccine, 1110
Varivax, 1110
Vaseretic 5-12.5, 1084
Vaseretic 10-25, 1084
Vasocidin Ophthalmic Ointment, 1084
Vasocidin Ophthalmic Solution, 1084
Vasoclear, 1046, 1047
Vasocon-A Ophthalmic Solution, 1084
Vasocon Regular, 1046, 1047
Vasoderm, 1049, 1050
VASODILATORS, 1025-1026
vasopressin, 959-960
Vasotec, 357-359
Vasotec IV, 357-359
VaZol, 153-155
Vectrin, 632-634
vecuronium, 960-962, 1021, 1043
Veetids, 729-732
Velban, 965-967
Velbe, 965-967
Velcade, 149-150
Velosef, 192-196
Velosulin BR, 510-513
venlafaxine, 962-963, 997
Venofer, 523-524
Venoglobulin-I, 501-502
Venoglobulin-S, 501-502
Ventodisk, 52-54
VePesid, 394-395
verapamil, 963-965, 993, 1000, 1014
verapamil HCl, 963-965
verapamil HCl SR, 963-965
Verazinc, 984
Verelan PM, 963-965
Vergan, 582-583
Vermox, 580-581
Versed, 626-628
Vesanoid, 935-936
VESIcare, 855
Vexol, 1045, 1047

Vfend, 974-975
Viadur, 545-547
Viagra, 847-848
Vibramycin, 345-346
Vibra-Tabs, 345-346
Vicks 44D Cough & Head Congestion Liquid, 1084
Vicks 44E Liquid, 1084
Vicks 44M Cold, Flu, & Cough LiquiCaps, 1084
Vicks 44 Non-Drowsy Cold & Cough LiquiCaps, 1085
Vicks Children's NyQuil Nighttime Cough/Cold Liquid, 1085
Vicks Cough Silencers, 1085
Vicks DayQuil Liquid, 1085
Vicks DayQuil Multi-Symptom Cold/Flu Relief Liquid, 1085
Vicks DayQuil Sinus Pressure & Pain Relief, 1085
Vicks Formula 44, 303
Vicks Inhaler, 1047, 1048-1049
Vicks Nyquil Liquicaps, 1085
Vicks Nyquil Multi-Symptom Cold Flu Relief Liquid, 1085
Vicks Pediatric Formula 44e Cough & Chest Congestion Relief Liquid, 1085
Vicks Pediatric Formula 44 m Multi-Symptom Cough & Cold Liquid, 1085
Vicks Sinex 12 Hour Long-Acting, 1048-1049
Vicks Sinex 12-Hour Ultra Fine Mist for Sinus Relief, 1048-1049
Vicodin, 478-480, 1085
Vicodin ES, 1085
Vicodin HP, 1085
VicodinTuss, 1085
Vicoprofen, 478-480, 1085
vidarabine, 1045-1047
Vidaza, 122-123
Videx, 311-312
Videx EC, 311-312
Vigamox, 1044, 1047
vinblastine, 965-967, 1005, 1043
vinblastine sulfate, 965-967
Vincasar PFS, 967-968
vincristine, 967-968, 1005, 1043
vincristine sulfate, 967-968
vinorelbine, 968-969, 1005, 1043
Vioforim, 1050, 1051-1052
Viokase, 718-719
Vira-A, 1045-1047
Viracept, 665-666
Viractin, 1053
Viramune, 669-670
Virazole, 818-819
Viread, 889-890
Viridium, 744
Virilon IM, 895-896
Viroptic, 1045-1047
Visine L.R., 1046, 1047
Visine Moisturizing, 1046, 1047
Visken, 755-756
Vistaril, 487-488
Vistide, 232-233
Vitabee 6, 800-801
Vita-Bob, 649-650
Vita-Kid, 649-650
vitamin A, 969-970, 1026
Vitamin A, 969-970
vitamin A acid, 935-936, 970
vitamin B, 670-671
vitamin B_1, 900, 970, 1026
vitamin B_2, 1026
vitamin B_6, 1026
Vitamin B_6, 800-801
vitamin B_9, 428-429
Vitamin B_9, 429-430
vitamin B_{12}, 971-972
vitamin B_{12}a, 971-972
vitamin C, 108-109, 1026
vitamin D, 972-973, 1026
vitamin D_2, 972-973
vitamin D_3, 972-973
Vitamin D_3 (1,25-dihydroxycholecalciferol), 168-169
vitamin E, 973-974, 1026
vitamin K_1, 754-755
VITAMINS, 1026
Vita-Plus E Softgells, 973-974
Vitec, 973-974
Vitrasert, 446-448, 1044, 1047
Vitravene, 1044, 1047
Vivelle, 385-387
Vivol, 305-307
Vivotif Berna Vaccine, 1110
V-Lax, 797-798
Voltaran, 308-309, 1046, 1047
Voltaren Rapide, 308-309
Voltaren XR, 308-309
voriconazole, 974-975, 1001
VP-16, 394-395
Vytorin, 1085

W

warfarin, 976-977, 995, 1043
warfarin sodium, 976-977
Warfilone, 976-977
Wehdryl, 322-324
Welchol, 264-265
Wellbutrin, 160-161
Wellbutrin SR, 160-161
Wellcovorin, 544-545
Wellferon, 514-515
Westcort, 1050
Westhroid, 904-905
Wigraine Suppositories, 1085
Winpred, 774-775
WinRho SD, 817-818
WinRho SDF, 817-818
wintergreen, 1115
Wycillin, 729-732
Wymox, 85-87

X

Xalatan, 1046, 1047
Xanax, 62-64
Xanax XR, 62-64
Xeloda, 174-175
Xenical, 698-699
Xifaxan, 823-824
Xigris, 348-349
Xolair, 695-696
Xopenex, 547-548
Xylocaine, 553-555, 1053
Xylocaine 10% Oral, 1053
Xylocaine Viscous, 1053
Xylocard, 553-555
xylometazoline, 1048-1049

Y

Yasmin 28, 1085
yellow fever vaccine, 1110
YF-Vax, 1110
yohimbe, 1115

Z

Zaditor, 1044, 1047
zafirlukast, 977-978

Entries can be identified as follows: generic name, Trade Name, DRUG CATEGORY, *Combination Product.*

Zagam, 858-860
zalcitabine, 978-979, 1010
zaleplon, 979-980
Zanaflex, 917-918
zanamivir, 980-981
Zantac, 812-813
Zantac-C, 812-813
Zantac EFFER-dose, 812-813
Zantac GELdose, 812-813
Zaroxolyn, 615-617
ZeaSob-AF, 1050, 1051-1052
Zebeta, 144-146
Zefazone, 196-202
Zelnorm, 882-883
Zemplar, 721
Zenapax, 279-280
Zerit, 861-863
Zestoretic 10/12.5, 1085
Zestoretic 20/2, 1085
Zestoretic 20/12.5, 1085
Zestril, 560-562
Zetia, 396
Zevalin, 490
Ziac 2.5, 1085
Ziac 5, 1085
Ziac 10, 1085
Ziagen, 33-34
zidovudine, 981-983, 1010
Ziks Cream, 1085
Zilactin-L, 1053
zileuton, 983-984
Zinacef, 196-202
zinc, 926-927
Zinc 15, 984
Zinc-220, 984
Zinca-Pak, 984
Zincate, 984
zinc sulfate, 984
ziprasidone, 984-986, 1007
Zithromax, 125-127
Zocor, 848-849
Zofran, 697-698
Zoladex, 464
zoledronic acid, 986-987
zolmitriptan, 987-988
Zoloft, 846-847
zolpidem, 988-989, 1123
Zometa, 986-987
Zomig, 987-988
Zomig-ZMT, 987-988
Zonegran, 989-990
zonisamide, 989-990, 996
Zonolon Topical Cream, 340-342
ZORprin, 111-113
Zosyn, 759-761
Zovirax, 44-46, 1052-1053
Zyban, 160-161
Zydone, 478-480, 1085
Zyflo, 983-984
Zyloprim, 60-61
Zymar, 1044, 1047
Zymase, 718-719
Zyprexa, 692-693
Zyprexa Zydis, 692-693
Zyrtec, 210-211
Zyvox, 556-557

2008 Update to Mosby's Drug Guide for Nurses
Seventh Edition

Following are the monographs for 23 drugs that have received FDA approval since the publication of *Mosby's Drug Guide for Nurses,* 7th edition. These monographs follow the same format as those in the book. They are arranged in alphabetical order by generic name, and trade names are given for all medications in common use. Each monograph contains the same subsections as those listed and described on pages x through xii of the preface to this book.

Drug Monographs in this Update

GENERIC	TRADE
anidulafungin	Eraxis
arformoterol	Brovana
conivaptan	Vaprisol
darunavir	Prezista
dasatinib	Sprycel
decitabine	Dacogen
deferasirox	Exjade
desonide	Desonate, Verdeso
idursulfase	Elaprase
kunecatechins	Veregen
lubiprostone	Amitiza
micafungin	Mycamine
nabilone	Cesamet
natalizumab	Tysabri
panitumumab	Vectibix
posaconazole	Noxafil
ranibizumab	Lucentis
ranolazine	Ranexa
rasagiline	Azilect
sitagliptin	Januvia
sunitinib	Sutent
telbivudine	Tyzeka
varenicline	Chantix

anidulafungin (Rx)

(a-nid-yoo-luh-fun'jin)

Eraxis

Func. class.: Antifungal, systemic

Chem. class.: Echinocandin

Pregnancy category C

Action: Inhibits fungal enzyme synthesis; causes direct damage to fungal cell wall

Therapeutic Outcome: Decreased symptoms of candida infection, negative culture

Uses: *Candida albicans, C. glabrata, C. parapsilosis, C. tropicalis*

Dosage and routes

Candidemia and other candida infections

Adult: **IV** Loading dose 200 mg on day 1, then 100 mg/day until 14 days or more since last positive culture

Esophageal candidiasis

Adult: **IV** Loading dose 100 mg on day 1, then 50 mg/day for at least 14 days and for at least 7 days after symptoms are resolved

Available forms: Powder for injection, lyophilized 50 mg

Adverse effects

Candiemia/other candida infections

CNS: **Convulsions,** dizziness, *headache*

CV: Deep vein thrombosis, **atrial fibrillation, right bundle branch block,** hypotension, **sinus arrhythmia, thrombophlebitis superficial, ventricular extrasystoles (rare)**

GI: *Nausea; anorexia; vomiting; diarrhea; increased AST, ALT*

META: Hypokalemia

Esophageal candidiasis

CNS: *Headache*

GI: *Nausea, anorexia, vomiting, diarrhea,* **hepatic necrosis**

HEMA: **Neutropenia, thrombocytopenia, leukopenia, coagulopathy**

INTEG: *Rash*

META: Hypocalcemia, hyperglycemia, hyperkalemia, hypernatremia, hypomagnesium (rare)

MS: *Back pain, rigors*

Contraindications: Hypersensitivity to this product, or other echinocandins

Precautions: Pregnancy **C,** severe hepatic, lactation, children

Pharmacokinetics

Absorption	Unknown
Distribution	Steady state after loading dose, protein binding 84%
Metabolism	Unknown
Excretion	Unknown
Half-life	Distribution 0.5-1 hr, terminal 40-50 hr

Pharmacodynamics

Onset	Unknown
Peak	Unknown
Duration	Unknown

Interactions

Individual drugs

CycloSPORINE: increased plasma concentrations

Drug/lab test

Increased: amylase, bilirubin, CPK, creatinine, ECG, QT prolongation, lipase

Decreased: platelets, magnesium, potassium, transferase, urea

NURSING CONSIDERATIONS

Assessment

- Assess for infection, clearing of cultures during treatment; obtain culture baseline and throughout; drug may be started as soon as culture is taken
- Monitor CBC (RBC, Hct, Hgb), differential, platelet count periodically; notify prescriber of results
- Monitor renal studies: BUN, serum uric acid, urine CCr, electrolytes before and during therapy
- Monitor hepatic studies before and during treatment: bilirubin, AST, ALT, alk phosphatase, as needed
- Assess for bleeding: hematuria, heme-positive stools, bruising or petechiae, mucosa or orifices; blood dyscrasias can occur
- Assess for GI symptoms: frequency of stools, cramping, if severe diarrhea occurs, electrolytes may need to be given

Nursing diagnoses

- Infection, risk for (uses)
- Injury, risk for (adverse reactions)
- Knowledge, deficient (teaching)

Implementation

IV route

- Reconstitute with provided dilutent 50 mg vial/5 ml (3.33 mg/ml), dilute with D_5 of 0.9% NaCl, only to a concentration of 0.5 mg/ml, run at no more than 1.1 mg/ml
- Do not use if cloudy or precipitated; do not admix

- Store at room temperature, away from light, do not freeze; diluted sol must be used within 24 hrs

Patient/family education

- Advise patient to notify prescriber if pregnancy is suspected or planned; use nonhormonal form of contraception while taking this product
- Instruct patient to avoid breastfeeding while taking this product
- Advise patient to inform prescriber of kidney or liver disease
- Advise patient to report bleeding
- Teach patient to report signs of infection: increased temp, sore throat, flu-like symptoms
- Teach patient to notify prescriber of nausea, vomiting, diarrhea, jaundice, anorexia, clay-colored stools, dark urine; heptatotoxicity may occur

Evaluation

Positive therapeutic outcome

- Decreased symptoms of candida infection, negative culture

arformoterol (Rx)

(ar-for-moe'ter-ole)

Brovana

Func. class.: Long–acting adrenergic β_2-agonist, sympathomimetic, bronchodilator

Pregnancy category C

Action: Causes bronchodilation by action on β_2 (pulmonary) receptors by increasing levels of cAMP, which relaxes smooth muscle; produces bronchodilation, CNS, cardiac stimulation, as well as increased diuresis and gastric acid secretion; longer acting than isoproterenol

Therapeutic Outcome: Absence of dyspnea, wheezing after 1 hr, improved airway exchange, improved ABGs

Uses: COPD, including chronic bronchitis, emphysema

Dosage and routes

COPD

Adult: NEB 15 mcg, bid, am, pm

Available forms: Inh sol 15 mcg/2 ml

Adverse effects

CNS: *Tremors, anxiety,* insomnia, headache, dizziness, stimulation, *restlessness,* hallucinations, flushing, irritability

CV: Palpitations, **tachycardia,** hypertension, angina, hypotension, **dysrhythmias**

EENT: Dry nose, irritation of nose and throat

GI: Heartburn, nausea, vomiting

MISC: Flushing, sweating, anorexia, bad taste/smell changes, hypokalemia, **anaphylaxis**

MS: Muscle cramps

RESP: Cough, wheezing, dyspnea, **bronchospasm,** dry throat

Contraindications: Hypersensitivity to sympathomimetics, this product, or racemic formoterol; tachydysrhyhmias, severe cardiac disease, heart block, children, actively deteriorating COPD

Precautions: Pregnancy **C,** lactation, cardiac disorders, hyperthyroidism, diabetes mellitus, hypertension, prostatic hypertrophy, narrow-angle glaucoma, seizures, hypoglycemia

Pharmacokinetics	
Absorption	Unknown
Distribution	Crosses placenta, protein binding 52-65%
Metabolism	Direct conjugation by CYP2D6, CYP2C19, extensively
Excretion	Urine 63%, feces 11%
Half-life	Terminal (COPD) 26 hr

Pharmacodynamics	
Onset	5 min
Peak	1-1 ½ hr
Duration	4-6 hr

Interactions

Individual drugs

Oxytoxics: increased severe hypotension

Theophylline: increased toxicity

Drug classifications

Adrenergics, MAOIs, tricyclics: increased action of arformoterol; do not use together

Nebulized bronchodilators: increased action of nebulized bronchodilators

Other β-blockers: decreased arformoterol action

Potassium-losing diuretics: increased ECG changes/hypokalemia

Drug/herb

Caffeine (cola nut, green/black tea, guarana, yerba maté, coffee, chocolate): increased stimulation

NURSING CONSIDERATIONS

Assessment

- Assess respiratory function: vital capacity, forced expiratory volume, ABGs; lung sounds, heart rate and rhythm, B/P, sputum (baseline and peak)

• Determine that patient has not received theophylline therapy or other bronchodilators before giving dose
• Assess patient's ability to self-medicate
• Asses for allergic reactions; anaphylaxis may occur
• Assess paradoxical bronchospasm; hold medication, notify prescriber if bronchospasm occurs

Nursing diagnoses
• Airway clearance, ineffective (uses)
• Knowledge, deficient (teaching)

Implementation
• Must be used by nebulization
• Store in refrigerator

Patient/family education
• Teach patient to use exactly as prescribed; that death has resulted from asthma with products similar to this one
• Advise patient not to use OTC medications; excess stimulation may occur

Evaluation
Positive therapeutic outcome
• Absence of dyspnea, wheezing after 1 hr, improved airway exchange, improved ABGs

conivaptan (Rx)
(kon-ih-vap′-tan)
Vaprisol
Func. class.: Vasopressin receptor antagonist

Pregnancy category C

Action: Dual arginine vasopressin (AVP) antagonist with affinity for V_{1A}, V_2 receptors. Level of circulating AVP in circulating blood is critical for regulation of water, electrolyte balance and is usually elevated in euvolemic/ hypervolemic hyponatremia.

Therapeutic Outcome: Correct serum sodium levels

Uses: Euvolemia hyponatremia in those hospitalized, not indicated for CHF

Dosage and routes
Adult: **IV** inf loading dose 20 mg given over 30 min, then cont **IV** over 24 hr; after 1 day, give for an additional 1-3 days as a cont inf of 20 mg/day total, can be titrated up to 40 mg/day if serum sodium is not rising at the desired rate; max time 4 days

Available forms: 5 mg/ml (20 mg) in single use ampule

Adverse effects
CNS: Headache, confusion, insomnia
CV: **Atrial fibrillation,** hypo/hypertension, orthostatic hypotension, phlebitis
GI: Nausea, vomiting, constipation, dry mouth
GU: Hematuria, polyuria, UTI, pollaklura
HEMA: Anemia
INTEG: Erythemia, inj site reaction
META: Dehydration, hyperglycemia, hypoglycemia, hypokalemia, hypomagnesia, hyponatremia
MISC: Oral candidiasis, pain, peripheral edema, pneumonia

Contraindications: Hypersensitivity, hypovolemia

Precautions: Pregnancy **C**, lactation, orthostatic disease, renal disease

Pharmacokinetics	
Absorption	Unknown
Distribution	Protein binding 99%
Metabolism	By CYP3A4
Excretion	Unknown
Half-life	Terminal 5 hr

Pharmacodynamics	
Onset	Unknown
Peak	Unknown
Duration	Unknown

Interactions
Individual drugs
Digoxin: decreased plasma concentration of conivaptan

Drug classifications
CYP3A4 inhibitors: increased plasma concentrations of conivaptan

NURSING CONSIDERATIONS
Assessment
• Monitor renal/hepatic function
• Assess frequent sodium volume status; overly-rapid correction of sodium concentration (>12 mEq/L per 24 hrs) may result in osmotic demyelination syndrome
• Assess neuro status: confusion, headache
• Assess CV status: atrial fibrillation, hyper/ hypotension, orthostatic hypotension; monitor B/P, pulse
• Monitor other electrolytes (magnesium and potassium)

Nursing diagnoses
• Injury, risk for (uses)
• Knowledge, deficient (teaching)

Implementation
IV route
- Withdraw 4 ml (20 mg) of conivaptan, add to 100 ml D_5W, gently invert several times to mix, give over 30 mins

Continuous IV infusion route
- Withdraw 4 ml (20 mg) of conivaptan, add to 250 ml D_5W, gently invert several times to mix, give over 24 hr; or 40 mg in 250 ml D_5W, gently invert several times to mix, give over 24 hrs

Patient/family education
- Advise patient to avoid pregnancy, breast-feeding while taking this product
- Advise patient to report neuro changes: headache, insomnia, confusion
- Teach patient administration procedure and expected result
- Advise patient to report inj site pain, redness, swelling

Evaluation
Positive therapeutic outcome
- Correction of serum sodium levels

darunavir (Rx)
(dar-ue'na-vir)
Prezista
Func. class.: Antiretroviral
Chem. class.: Protease inhibitor
Pregnancy category B

Action: Inhibits human immunodeficiency virus (HIV-1) protease; this prevents maturation of virus

Therapeutic Outcome: Decrease viral load, increase in CD4 counts

Uses: HIV-1 in combination with ritonavir and other antiretrovirals

Dosage and routes
Reduce dose in mild/moderate hepatic impairment and ketaconazole coadministration
Adult: PO 600 mg bid; if given with ritonavir 100 mg bid with food

Available forms: Tabs 300 mg

Adverse effects
CNS: *Headache, insomnia,* dizziness, somnolence
GI: *Diarrhea, abdominal pain, nausea, vomiting,* anorexia, dry mouth
GU: Nephrolithiasis
INTEG: Rash
MS: Pain
OTHER: Asthenia, **insulin-resistant hyperglycemia,** hyperlipidemia, **ketoacidosis,** lipodystrophy

Contraindications: Hypersensitivity

Precautions: Pregnancy **B,** hepatic/renal disease, lacation, children, history of renal stones, diabetes, hypercholesterolemia

Pharmacokinetics	
Absorption	Unknown
Distribution	Protein binding 95%
Metabolism	By CYP3A
Excretion	Feces 79.5%, urine 13.9%
Half-life	Terminal 15 hr

Pharmacodynamics	
Onset	Unknown
Peak	2.5-4 hr
Duration	Unknown

Interactions
Individual drugs
Atorvastatin, lovastatin, simvastatin: increased myopathy
Delavirdine, itracinazole, ketoconazole: increased darunavir levels
Clarithromycin, zidovudine: increased levels of both drugs
Efavirenz, fluconazole, nevirapine: decreased darunavir levels
Isoniazid: increased levels of isoniazid
❗Midazolam, pimozide, rifampin, triazolam: life-threatening dysrhythmias
Drug classifications
Anticonvulsants: decreased both drugs
❗Ergots: life-threatening dysrhythmias; do not use concurrently
Oral contraceptives: increased levels of oral contraceptives
Rifamycins: decreased darunavir levels
Drug/herb
St. John's wort: decreased darunavir levels; avoid concurrent use
Drug/food
Darunavir: increased absorption

NURSING CONSIDERATIONS
Assessment
- Assess for complaints of lower back, flank pain; indicates kidney stones
- Assess for signs of infection, anemia, the presence of other sexually transmitted diseases
- Monitor hepatic studies: ALT, AST, bilirubin, amylase; all may be elevated

- Monitor viral load, CD4 during treatment; viral load should be decreasing, CD4 increasing
- Assess bowel pattern before, during treatment; if severe abdominal pain with bleeding occurs, drug should be discontinued; monitor hydration
- Assess skin eruptions: rash, urticaria, itching
- Assess allergies before treatment, reaction of each medication; place allergies on chart

Nursing diagnoses
- Infection, risk for (uses)
- Knowledge, deficient (teaching)
- Noncompliance (teaching)

Implementation
- Give with food and ritonavir
- Give water to 1.5 L/day minimum to prevent nephrolithiasis

Patient/family education
- Instruct patient to take as prescribed; if dose is missed, take as soon as remembered up to 1 hr before next dose; do not double dose
- Advise patient that drug must be taken in equal intervals around the clock to maintain blood levels for duration of therapy
- ❗ Advise patient that hyperglycemia may occur; watch for increased thirst, weight loss, hunger, dry, itchy skin; notify prescriber
- Teach patient to increase fluids to prevent kidney stones; if stone formation occurs, treatment may need to be interrupted
- Teach patient that drug does not cure AIDS, only controls symptoms; do not donate blood

Evaluation
Positive therapeutic outcome
- Decreased viral load, increased CD4 counts

dasatinib (Rx)
(da-si'ti-nib)

Sprycel

Func. class.: Miscellaneous antineoplastic

Chem. class.: Protein-tyrosine kinase inhibitor

Pregnancy category D

Action: Inhibits BCR-ABL, SRC, LCK, YES, FYN, C-KIT, $EPHA_2$, and PDGFR-β tyrosine kinase created in chronic myeloid leukemia (CML)

Therapeutic Outcome: Decrease in number of leukemic cells or size of tumor

Uses: Treatment of chronic myeloid leukemia (CML), accelerated blast crisis, or chronic phase, and acute lymphoblastic leukemia (ALL)

Dosage and routes
Adult: PO 70 mg bid

Available forms: Tabs 20, 50, 70 mg

Adverse effects
CNS: **CNS hemorrhage,** headache, dizziness, insomnia, neuropathy, asthenia

CV: Dsyrhythmias, chest pain, CHF, pericardial effusion

GI: *Nausea,* **vomiting,** *anorexia, abdominal pain,* constipation, diarrhea, GI bleeding, muscositis, stomatitis

HEMA: **Neutropenia, thrombocytopenia, bleeding**

INTEG: *Rash, pruritus*

META: Fluid retention, edema

MISC: Increased/decreased weight

MS: Pain, arthralgia, myalgia

RESP: Cough, dyspnea, pulmonary edema/ hypertension, pneumonia, URI

Contraindications: Pregnancy **D,** hypersensitivity

Precautions: Lactation, children, elderly

Pharmacokinetics	
Absorption	Unknown
Distribution	Protein binding 96%
Metabolism	By CYP3A4
Excretion	Feces 85%, urine 4%
Half-life	Terminal 1.3-5 hr

Pharmacodynamics	
Onset	0.5-6 hr
Peak	Unknown
Duration	Unknown

Interactions
Individual drugs

Clarithromycin, erythromycin, itraconazole, ketoconazole, nefazodine, telithromycin: increased dasatinib concentrations

Drug classifications

CYP3A4 inducers (dexamethasone, phenytoin, carbamazepine, rifampin, phenobarbital), H_2 blockers (famotidine), proton pump inhibitors (omeprazole): decreased dasatinib concentrations

CYP3A4 substrates (alfentanil, cycloSPORINE, ergots, fentanyl, pimozide, quinidine, sirolimus, tacrolimus): altered action

Protease inhibitors: increased dasatinib concentrations

Simvastatin: increased concentrations of this product

Drug/herb

St. John's wort: decreased dasatinib concentration

NURSING CONSIDERATIONS

Assessment

- Monitor ANC and platelets; in chronic phase if ANC $<1 \times 10^9$/L and/or platelets $<50 \times 10^9$/L, stop until ANC $>1.5 \times 10^9$/L and platelets $>75 \times 10^9$/L; in accelerated phase/ blast crisis if ANC $<0.5 \times 10^9$/L and/or platelets $<10 \times 10^9$/L, determine whether cytopenia is related to biopsy/aspirate, if not, reduce dose by 200 mg, if cytopenia continues, reduce dose by another 100 mg; if cytopenia continues for 4 wk, stop drug until ANC $\geq 1 \times 10^9$/L
- Assess for renal toxicity: if bilirubin $>3 \times$ IULN, withhold until bilirubin levels return to $<1.5 \times$ IULN
- Assess for hepatotoxicity: monitor LFTs, before treatment and qmo; if liver transaminases $>5 \times$ IULN, withhold until transaminase levels return to $<2.5 \times$ IULN
- Monitor CBC, differential, platelet count weekly; withhold drug if WBC is $<3500/mm^3$, or platelet count $<100{,}000/mm^3$; notify prescriber of these results; drug should be discontinued
- Monitor for signs of fluid retention, edema: weigh, monitor lung sounds, assess for edema, some fluid retention is dose dependent

Nursing diagnoses

- Infection, risk for (adverse reactions)
- Nutrition: less than body requirements, imbalanced (adverse reactions)
- Knowledge, deficient (teaching)

Implementation

- Do not break, crush, or chew tab
- Give after meal and with large glass of water
- Give nutritious diet with iron, vitamin supplement
- Store at 25° C (77° F)

Patient/family education

- Instruct patient to report adverse reactions immediately: SOB, swelling of extremities, bleeding
- Teach patient reason for treatment, expected result

Evaluation

Positive therapeutic outcome

- Decrease in number of leukemic cells

decitabine (Rx)

(de-sit′-a-been)

Dacogen

Func. class.: DNA demethylation agent

Chem. class.: Cytosine analog

Pregnancy category D

Action: Incorporated into DNA and inhibits DNA methylation, halting growth of rapid proliferation of blasts

Therapeutic Outcome: Decreasing blast count

Uses: Treatment of naïve and experienced myelodysplasic syndrome

Dosage and routes

Adult: Cont **IV** First treatment cycle: 15 mg/m^2 over 3 hrs, q8 hrs × 3 days; subsequent treatment cycles: repeat above cycle q6 wks for at least 4 cycles; a partial or complete response may take more than 4 cycles

Available forms: Powder for injection, lyophilized 50 mg, in single dose vial

Adverse effects

CNS: *Headache, anxiety, dizziness, hypoesthesia, insomnia,* confusion

CV: *Edema, murmur, hypotension*

GI: *Nausea, anorexia, vomiting, diarrhea, constipation, stomatitis,* abdominal pain, dyspepsia

HEMA: **Neutropenia, thrombocytopenia, leukopenia, anemia**

INTEG: *Alopecia, ecchymosis, erythema, pallor, petechiae, pruritus, rash, swelling face, urticaria,* hematoma, cellulitis

META: *Decreased potassium, sodium, magnesium, albumin; increased bilirubin, increased/decreased glucose*

MS: *Myalgia, arthralgia, back pain, chest wall pain, pain in limbs*

RESP: *Cough, crackles, hypoxia, pharyngitis, pneumonia, pulmonary edema*

Contraindications: Pregnancy **D**, hypersensitivity to this product, severe neurotoxicity, severe blood dyscrasias, lactation, children

Precautions: Severe hepatic/renal disease, men (men should not father a child while receiving treatments or for 2 months after treatment ends)

Pharmacokinetics

Absorption	Unknown
Distribution	Protein binding <1%
Metabolism	Liver, granulocytes, intestinal epithelium, whole blood
Excretion	Unknown
Half-life	Terminal 0.2-0.8 hr

Pharmacodynamics

Onset	Unknown
Peak	Unknown
Duration	Unknown

Interactions

Drug classifications

Do not use with live virus vaccines

NURSING CONSIDERATIONS

Assessment

- Monitor CBC (RBC, Hct, Hgb), differential, platelet count weekly; withhold drug if WBC <4000/mm^3, platelets <75,000/mm^3, or RBC, Hct, Hgb is low; notify prescriber of results
- Monitor renal studies: BUN, serum uric acid, urine CCr, electrolytes before and during therapy
- Monitor temp q 4 hrs; fever may indicate beginning infection; no rectal temps
- Monitor hepatic studies before and during treatment: bilirubin, AST, ALT, alk phosphatase, as needed or monthly
- Assess for bleeding: hematuria, heme-positive stools, bruising or petechiae, mucosa or orifices daily; blood dyscrasias can occur
- Assess for dyspnea, crackles, unproductive cough, chest pain, tachypnea, fatigue, increased pulse, pallor, lethargy, personality changes
- Assess buccal cavity daily for dryness, ulceration, white patches, oral pain, bleeding, dysphagia
- Assess GI symptoms: frequency of stools, cramping; if severe diarrhea occurs, electrolytes may need to be given

Nursing diagnoses

- Injury, risk for (uses)
- Knowledge, deficient (teaching)

Implementation

- Use procedures for handling and disposal of drugs
- Rinse mouth tid-qid with water or club soda; brush teeth tid with soft toothbrush or cotton tipped applicator for stomatitis; use unwaxed dental floss
- Store at room temperature, away from light

Patient/family education

- Advise patient to report bleeding; not to use commercial mouthwashes, razors
- Teach patient to report signs of infection: increased temp, sore throat, flu-like symptoms
- Teach patient to report signs of anemia: fatigue, headache, faintness, shortness of breath, irritability
- Advise patient to avoid citric acid, rough textured foods, if stomatitis is present
- Teach patient to notify prescriber if pregnancy is suspected or planned; use contraception while taking this product
- Teach patient to avoid breastfeeding while taking this product
- Instruct patient not to operate machinery or perform other hazardous activities while taking this product
- Teach patient that men should not father a child while taking this product, pregnancy category (D)
- Teach patient to inform prescriber of kidney or liver disease
- Teach patient not to receive vaccinations while taking this product

Evaluation

Positive therapeutic outcome

- Decreased blast count

RARELY USED

deferasirox (Rx)

Exjade

Func. class.: Heavy metal chelating agent

Dosage and routes

Adult: PO 20-30 mg/kg/day; oral dispersion tablet is dissolved in water <1 gm in 3.5 oz; >1 gm in 7 oz or more; give on empty stomach at least 30 min before meals

Uses: Chronic iron overload

Contraindications: Hypersensitivity, lactation, children, severe hepatic/renal disease

---

RARELY USED

desonide (Rx)

Desonate, Verdeso

Func. class.: Topical antiinflammatory

Dosage and routes

Adult: TOP apply to affected area; do not use more than 4 consecutive weeks

Uses: Atopic dermatitis

Contraindications: Open wounds, burns

RARELY USED

idursulfase (Rx)

Elaprase

Func. class.: Enzyme replacement

Dosage and routes

Adult: **IV** inf 0.5 mg/kg/wk; dilute calculated volume of concentrated drug in 100 ml of 0.9% NaCl; use a 0.2 micron filter

Child > 5 yrs: **IV** inf 0.5 mg/kg/wk given over 1-3 hr

Uses: Mucopolysaccharidosis II (Hunter's Syndrome) (MPS-11)

Containdications: Hypersensitivity, IM/intrathecal administration

RARELY USED

kunecatechins (Rx)

Veregen

Func. class.: Topical keratolytic

Dosage and routes

Adult: TOP Apply ointment using a 0.5 cm strand applied to warts tid; continue treatment until complete clearance has occurred, max 16 wks

Uses: External genital/perianal warts

Contraindications: Hypersensitivity

lubiprostone (Rx)

(loo-bee-pros'-tone)

Amitiza

Func. class.: Miscellaneous gastrointestinal agent

Pregnancy category C

Action: Locally acting chloride channel activator, enhances a chloride rich intestinal fluid secretion without altering other electrolytes; increases motility in the intestine, increasing softening and passage of stool

Therapeutic Outcome: Decreased constipation

Uses: Chronic idiopathic constipation

Dosage and routes

Adult: PO 24 mcg bid with food

Available forms: Caps 24 mcg

Adverse effects

CNS: *Headache,* dizziness, depression, fatigue, insomnia

CV: Hypertension, chest pain

GI: *Nausea, abdominal pain, eructation,* abdominal distention, constipation, diarrhea, dry mouth, dyspepsia, flatulence, gastroenteritis viral, gastroesophageal reflux disease, vomiting, fecal incontinence, fecal urgency

GU: UTI

MISC: Chest pain, peripheral edema, influenza, pyrexia, viral infection

MS: Back pain, arthralgia, muscle cramps, pain in extremities

RESP: Bronchitis, cough, dyspnea, nasopharyngitis, sinusitis, URI

Contraindications: Hypersensitivity, GI obstruction

Precautions: Pregnancy **C**, lactation, children, diarrhea, inflammatory bowel disease

Pharmacokinetics	
Absorption	Unknown
Distribution	Protein binding 94%
Metabolism	Rapid in stomach, jejunum
Excretion	Unknown
Half-life	0.9-1.4 hr

Pharmacodynamics	
Onset	Unknown
Peak	1.14 hr
Duration	Unknown

Interactions

Drug classifications

Antidiarrheals, anticholinergics: decreased effects of lubiprostone

NURSING CONSIDERATIONS

Assessment

- Assess GI symptoms: nausea, abdominal pain
- Assess periodically, need for continued treatment

Nursing diagnoses

- Constipation (uses)
- Knowledge, deficient (teaching)

Implementation

- Give with foods, bid
- Store at room temperature

Patient/family education

- Teach patient to notify prescriber of GI symptoms, diarrhea, hypersensitivity reactions

Evaluation

Positive therapeutic outcome

- Decreased constipation

micafungin (Rx)

(my-ca-fun'gin)

Mycamine

Func. class.: Antifungal, systemic

Chem. class.: Echinocandin

Pregnancy category C

Action: Inhibits an essential component in fungal cell walls; causes direct damage to fungal cell wall

Therapeutic Outcome: Prevention of candida infection in HSTC; or decreased symptoms of candida infection, negative culture

Uses: Treatment of esophageal candidiasis; prophylaxis of candida infections in patients undergoing hepatopoietic stem cell transplantation (HSCT); susceptible candida species: *C. albicans, C. glabrata, C. krusei, C. parapsilosis, C. tropicalis*

Dosage and routes

Esophageal candidiasis

Adult: **IV** 150 mg/day, given over 1 hr

Prophylaxis of candida infections

Adult: **IV** 50 mg/day, given over 1 hr

Available forms: Powder for injection 50 mg, in single dose vials

Adverse effects

CNS: **Convulsions,** dizziness, *headache, somnolence*

CV: Flushing, hypertension, phlebitis

GI: Abdominal pain, *nausea, anorexia, vomiting, diarrhea, increased AST, ALT, alk phos, blood dehydrogenase, hyperbilirubinemia*

HEMA: **Neutropenia, thrombocytopenia, leukopenia, coagulopathy, anemia, hemolytic anemia**

INTEG: *Rash, pruritis, inj site pain*

META: Hypokalemia, hypocalcemia, hypomagnesemia

MS: *Rigors*

Contraindications: Hypersensitivity to this product or other echinocandins

Precautions: Pregnancy **C,** severe hepatic, lactation, children, elderly

Pharmacokinetics

Absorption	Unknown
Distribution	Protein binding 99%
Metabolism	Liver
Excretion	Feces, urine
Half-life	Terminal 14-20 hr

Pharmacodynamics

Onset	Unknown
Peak	Unknown
Duration	Unknown

Interactions

Individual drugs

Sirolimus, nifedipine: increased plasma concentrations; may need dosage reduction

NURSING CONSIDERATIONS

Assessment

- Assess for signs and symptoms of infection, clearing of cultures during treatment; obtain culture baseline and throughout drug may be started as soon as culture is taken (esophageal candidiasis); monitor cultures during HSCT, for prevention of candidia infections
- Monitor CBC (RBC, Hct, Hgb), differential, platelet count periodically; notify prescriber of results
- Monitor renal studies: BUN, urine CCr, electrolytes before and during therapy
- Monitor hepatic studies before and during treatment: bilirubin, AST, ALT, alk phosphatase, as needed
- Assess for bleeding: hematuria, heme-positive stools, bruising or petechiae, mucosa or orifices; blood dyscrasias can occur
- Assess for hypersensitivity: rash, pruritis, facial swelling; also for phelibits
- Assess for hemolytic anemia
- Assess GI symptoms: frequency of stools, cramping; if severe diarrhea occurs, electrolytes may need to be given

Nursing diagnoses

- Infection, risk for (uses)
- Injury, risk for (adverse reactions)
- Knowledge, deficient (teaching)

Implementation

- Do not use if cloudy or precipitated; do not admix product
- Flush line before and after administration with 0.9% NaCl

IV route

- For candida prevention, reconstitute with provided dilutent 0.9% NaCl without bacteriostatic product; 50 mg vial/5 ml (10 mg/ml), swirl to dissolve, do not shake; further dilute with 100 ml 0.9% NaCl, only; run over 1 hr
- For candida infection, reconstitute with provided diluent 50 mg/5 ml (10 mg/ml); further dilute 3 reconstituted vials in 100 ml of 0.9% NaCl, run over 1 hr
- Store at room temperature, away from light, do not freeze; discard unused solution

Patient/family education

- Advise patient to notify prescriber if pregnancy is suspected or planned; use nonhormonal form of contraception while taking this product
- Teach patient to avoid breastfeeding while taking this product
- Teach patient to inform prescriber of kidney or liver disease
- Teach patient to report bleeding, facial swelling, wheezing, difficulty breathing, itching, rash, hives, increasing warmth, flushing
- Instruct patient to report signs of infection: increased temp, sore throat, flu-like symptoms
- Advise patient to notify prescriber of nausea, vomiting, diarrhea, jaundice, anorexia, clay-colored stools, dark urine; heptatotoxicity may occur

Evaluation

Positive therapeutic outcome

- Prevention of candida infection in HSTC; or decreased symptoms of candida infection, negative culture

nabilone (Rx)

(nab'-ih-lohn)

Cesamet

Func. class.: Antiemetic

Chem. class.: Miscellaneous-cannabinoid

Pregnancy category C

Action: Orally, active cannabinoid, chemically related to marijuana; may decrease nausea by action on cannabinoid receptors in the CNS

Therapeutic Outcome: Decreased nausea and vomiting associated with chemotherapy

Uses: Prevention of nausea, vomiting associated with cancer chemotherapy, in those that have not responded to other treatment; not to be used on an as needed basis

Dosage and routes

Adult: PO 1-2 mg bid; give initial dose 1-3 hrs prior to chemotherapy; start with lower dose and increase as needed; may give dose of 1-2 mg the night before chemotherapy; may give 2-3 times daily during chemotherapy cycle

Available forms: Caps 1 mg

Adverse effects

CNS: *Headache, ataxia, drowsiness, dysphoria, euphoria, sleep disturbance, vertigo, asthenia, concentration difficulties, depression,* syncope, hallucinations

CV: Chest discomfort, **tachycardia,** orthostatic hypotension

GI: *Dry mouth,* nausea, *anorexia,* increased appetite

INTEG: Allergic reactions, rash, photosensitivity, pruritus

MS: Back, joint, muscle, neck pain

Contraindications: Hypersensitivity to this product or cannabinoids

Precautions: Pregnancy **C,** lactation, depression, mental disorders, severe heptic/renal disease, hypertension, tachycardia, CV disorders

Pharmacokinetics

Absorption	Rapid 10-20%
Distribution	Unknown
Metabolism	Liver
Excretion	Biliary system in feces
Half-life	Terminal 2 hr

Pharmacodynamics

Onset	Unknown
Peak	Unknown
Duration	Unpredictable, psychiatric symptoms may occur for up to 72 hr after treatment concludes

Interactions

Individual drugs

Disulfiram, possibly fluoxetine: hypomanic reaction

Naltrexone: increased action or nabilone

Theophylline: decreased metabolism of nabilone

Drug classifications

Anticholinergics (antihistamines, atropine, scopolamine): increased tachycardia, drowsiness

CNS depressants (alcohol, barbiturates, benzodiazepines, buspirone, lithium, muscle relaxants, opioids): increased drowsiness, CNS depression

Opioids: increased action of both drugs

Sympathomimetics (amphetamines, cocaine): increased hypertension, tachycardia, and possibly cardiotoxicity

Tricyclic antidepressants: increased tachycardia, hypertension, drowsiness

NURSING CONSIDERATIONS

Assessment

- Assess for absence of nausea and vomiting during chemotherapy
- Assess for CNS symptoms: headache, depression, ataxia, drowsiness, dysphoria,

euphoria, sleep disturbances, concentration difficulties

- Assess for CV symptoms, cardiac status: tachycardia, orthostatic hypotension, hypertension

Nursing diagnoses

- Nutrition: less than body requirements, imbalanced (uses)
- Injury, risk for (uses, adverse reactions)
- Knowledge, deficient (teaching)

Implementation

- Give PO, not to be used on an as needed basis
- Store capsules at room temperature, away from light and moisture

Patient/family education

- Teach patient that mood, behavioral changes may occur while taking this product
- Advise patient to notify prescriber if pregnancy is suspected
- Advise patient to avoid breastfeeding while taking this product
- Instruct patient not to use alcohol or other CNS depressants unless approved by prescriber
- Instruct patient not to operate machinery or perform other hazardous activities while taking this product

Evaluation

Positive therapeutic outcome

- Decreased nausea and vomiting associated with chemotherapy

natalizumab (Rx)

(na-ta-liz'-u-mab)

Tysabri

Func. class.: Multiple sclerosis agent, monoclonal antibody

Pregnancy category C

Action: Action not clearly understood; biologic response modifying properties mediated through specific receptors on cells, may be secondary of blockade of the interaction by inflammatory cells on vascular endothelial cells

Therapeutic Outcome: Decreased symptoms of multiple sclerosis

Uses: Ambulatory patients with relapsing-remitting multiple sclerosis that have not responded to other treatment

Investigational uses: Crohn's disease

Dosage and routes

***Adult:* IV** inf 300 mg q 4 wks, give over 1 hr, observe during and for 1 hr after infusion

Available forms: Single use vial, 300 mg/100 ml 0.9% NaCl

Adverse effects

CNS: *Headache, fatigue,* rigors, syncope, tremors, *depression,* **PML (progressive multifocal leukoencephalopathy), suicidal ideation**

CV: Chest discomfort, hyper/hypotension

GI: *Abdominal discomfort,* abnormal LFT, gastroentritis

GU: Amenorrhea, *UTI, irregular menses,* vaginitis, urinary frequency

INTEG: *Rash,* dermatitis, pruritus

MS: *Arthralgia*

RESP: *Lower RTI*

SYST: **Anaphylaxis, angioedema**

Contraindications: Hypersensitivity, immunocompromised individuals (HIV, AIDS, leukemia, lymphoma, transplants), PML, murine (mouse) protein allergy

Precautions: Pregnancy **C**, lactation, chronic progressive MS, depression, mental disorders, diabetes, TB, elderly, active infections

Pharmacokinetics	
Absorption	Unknown
Distribution	Unknown
Metabolism	Unknown
Excretion	Unknown
Half-life	Approximately 11 days

Pharmacodynamics	
Onset	Unknown
Peak	Unknown
Duration	Unknown

Interactions

Drug classifications

Do not use with vaccines

Immunosupressants, antineoplastics, immunomodulators: increased infection

NURSING CONSIDERATIONS

Assessment

- Monitor blood, renal, hepatic studies: CBC, differential, platelet counts, BUN, creatinine, ALT, urinalysis, for hypersensitivity reactions
- Assess CNS symptoms: headache, fatigue, depression, rigors, tremors
- Assess GI status: abdominal discomfort
- Assess mental status: depression, depersonalization, suicidal thoughts, insomnia

- Assess for multiple sclerosis symptoms; this product should only be used in patients that have not responded to other treatments
- Assess for anaphylaxis: shortness of breath, hives; swelling, tightness in throat, chest pain; usually within 2 hrs of infusion
- Monitor PML using gadolinium-enhanced MRI scan of the brain, possibly cerebrospinal fluid for JC viral DNA

Nursing diagnoses

- Mobility, physical, impaired (uses)
- Injury, risk for (uses, adverse reactions)
- Knowledge, deficient (teaching)

Implementation

- Give acetaminophen for fever, headache
- Give only after being enrolled in the TOUCH™ Prescribing Program

IV infusion

- Use only clear, colorless solution, without particulates
- Withdraw 15 ml from the vial using aseptic technique: inject conc. into 100 ml 0.9% NaCl; do not use other diluents; mix completely; do not shake; infuse immediately or refrigerate for up to 8 hrs; warm to room temp before using; flush with 0.9% NaCl before and after infusion; do not admix or use in same line with other agents
- Withhold product at first sign of PML
- Store solution in refrigerator; do not freeze or shake; protect from light; use within 8 hrs of preparation

Patient/family education

- Provide patient or family member with written, detailed information about the drug
- Teach female patients they may experience irregular menses, amenorrhea
- Advise patient to use sunscreen to prevent photosensitivity
- Instruct patient to notify prescriber if pregnancy is suspected
- Instruct patient to avoid breastfeeding while taking this product
- Instruct patient to notify prescriber of possible infection: sore throat, cough, increased temperature

Evaluation

Positive therapeutic outcome

- Decreased symptoms of multiple sclerosis

panitumumab (Rx)

(pan-i-tue'moo-mab)

Vectibix

Func. class.: Antineoplastic—miscellaneous

Chem. class.: Multikinase inhibitor, signal transduction inhibitor

Pregnancy category C

Action: Decreases growth and survival of cancer cells by competitive inhibition of EGF receptor

Therapeutic Outcome: Decrease in colon carcinoma progression

Uses: EGFR expressing metastatic colorectal cancer

Dosage and routes

Adult: **IV** inf 6 mg/kg over 60 min every 2 wks

Available forms: Sol for inj 20 mg/ml

Adverse effects

CNS: Fatigue, ocular toxicity

CV: Peripheral edema

GI: *Nausea, diarrhea, vomiting,* anorexia, mouth ulceration, abdominal pain, constipation

HEMA: Thrombophlebitis

INTEG: *Rash,* pruritus, **exfoliative dermatitis,** skin fissure

META: Hypocalcemia, hypomagnesemia, antibody formation

RESP: **Bronchospasm, cough,** dyspnea, **hypoxia, pulmonary fibrosis,** pneumonitis, wheezing

Contraindications: Hypersensitivity

Precautions: Pregnancy **C,** lactation, children, hepatic disease, acute bronchospasm, diarrhea, exfoliative dermatitis, hamster protein allergy, hypomagnesemia, hypotension, pulmonary fibrosis, sepsis

Pharmacokinetics	
Absorption	38%-49%, high-fat meal decreases absorption
Distribution	Protein binding 99.5%
Metabolism	Liver, oxidative metabolism by CYP3A4, glucuronidation by UGT1A9
Excretion	Feces 77%
Half-life	Elimination 7.5 day

Pharmacodynamics	
Onset	Unknown
Peak	3 hr
Duration	Unknown

NURSING CONSIDERATIONS
Assessment
- Monitor serum electrolytes periodically
- Assess for signs of infection: increased temperature
- Assess for signs of infusion reactions: bronchospasm, fever, chills, hypotension
- Assess for signs of ocular toxicity

Nursing diagnoses
- Infection, risk for (uses)
- Nutrition: less than body requirements, imbalanced (adverse reactions)
- Knowledge, deficient (teaching)

Implementation
- Give in hospital or clinic setting with full resuscitation equipment
- Give only as IV infusion using controlled IV infusion pump; do not give IV push or bolus; use low-protein binding 0.2 or 0.22 micron in-line filter; flush line with 0.9% NaCl before and after administration
- Give over 60 min through a peripheral line or in dwelling catheter; infuse doses of >1000 mg over 90 min
- Dilute in 100 ml of 0.9% NaCl; dilute doses >1000 mg in 150 ml of 0.9% NaCl; mix by inverting; do not exceed 10 mg/ml; use within 6 hrs if stored at room temp; can be stored between 2°-8° C for up to 24 hr
- Store unopened vials in refrigerator; do not shake; protect from direct sunlight; do not freeze

Patient/family education
- (Alert) Instruct patient to report adverse reactions immediately: difficulty breathing, mouth sores, skin rash, ocular toxicity
- Teach patient reason for treatment, expected results, adverse reactions

Evaluation
Positive therapeutic outcome
- Decrease in colon carcinoma progression

posaconazole (Rx)
(poe'sa-kon'a-zole)

Noxafil

Func. class.: Antifungal, systemic

Chem. class.: Triazole derivative

Pregnancy category C

Action: Inhibits a portion of cell wall synthesis; alters cell membranes and inhibits several fungal enzymes

Therapeutic Outcome: Decreased fever, malaise, rash, negative C&S for infecting organism

Uses: Prevention of aspergillus, candida infection, oropharyngeal candidiasis in the immunocompromised

Dosage and routes
Adult: PO 800 mg/day in 2-4 divided doses

Child: PO 100 mg tid

Available forms: Oral susp 200 mg/5 ml

Adverse effects
CNS: *Headache, dizziness,* insomnia, fever, rigors, weakness, anxiety

CV: Hypertension, hypotension, tachycardia, anemia

GI: *Nausea, vomiting, anorexia, diarrhea,* cramps, abdominal pain, flatulence, **GI bleeding, hepatotoxicity**

GU: Gynecomastia, impotence, decreased libido

INTEG: *Pruritus,* fever, *rash,* **toxic epidermal necrolysis**

MISC: *Edema, fatigue,* malaise, hypokalemia, tinnitus, **rhabdomyolysis**

Contraindications: Hypersensitivity to this product or other systemic antifungal or azoles, fungal meningitis, onchomycosis or dermatomycosis in cardiac dysfunction

Precautions: Pregnancy **C,** hepatic disease, cardiac disease, children, lactation

Pharmacokinetics	
Absorption	Well, enhanced by food
Distribution	Protein binding 98-99%
Metabolism	Liver
Excretion	Feces, 77% unchanged
Half-life	19-35 hr

Pharmacodynamics	
Onset	Unknown
Peak	4-11 hr
Duration	Unknown

Interactions
Individual drugs
(Alert) BusPIRone, busulfan, clarithromycin, cycloSPORINE, diazepam, digoxin, felodipine, indinavir, isradipine, niCARdipine, niFEDipine, nimodipine, phenytoin, quinidine, ritonavir, saquinavir, tacrolimus, warfarin: increased levels, toxicity

Didanosine: decreased posaconazole action

(Alert) Dofetilide, pimozide, quinidine: life-threatening reactions

Midazolam (oral), triazolam: increased sedation

Quinidine: increased tinnitus, hearing loss

Drug classifications
Antacids, H_2-receptor antagonists, rifamycins: decreased posaconazole action
Calcium channel blockers: Increased edema
Ergots: life-threatening reactions
Other hepatotoxic drugs: increased hepatotoxicity
Oral contraceptives: decreased effect, use other contraceptives
Oral hypoglycemics: increased severe hypoglycemia

Drug/herb
Gossypol: nephrotoxicity

Drug/food
Food increases absorption

NURSING CONSIDERATIONS
Assessment
- Assess for type of infection; may begin treatment prior to obtaining results
- Assess for infection: temp, WBC, sputum, baseline and periodically
- Monitor I&O ratio, potassium levels
- Monitor hepatic studies (ALT, AST, bilirubin) if on long-term therapy
- Assess for allergic reaction: rash, photosensitivity, uricaria, dermatitis
- Assess for hepatotoxicity: nausea, vomiting, jaundice, clay-colored stools, fatigue

Nursing diagnoses
- Infection, risk for (uses)
- Knowledge, deficient (teaching)

Implementation
- Give after shaking well; use calibrated measuring device; take only with a full meal or liquid nutritional supplements such as Ensure; rinse measuring device after each use
- Store in a tight container in refrigerator; do not freeze

Patient/family education
- Teach patient that long-term therapy may be needed to clear infection (1 wk-6 mo depending on infection)
- Advise patient to avoid hazardous activities if dizziness occurs
- Advise patient to take 2 hr before administration of other drugs that increase gastric pH (antacids, H_2-blockers, omeprazole, sucralfate, anticholinergics); to notify health care provider of all medications taken
- Teach the patient the importance of compliance with drug regimen; to use alternative method of contraceptive
- Teach patient to notify prescriber of GI symptoms, signs of hepatic dysfunction (fatigue, nausea, anorexia, vomiting, dark urine, pale stools)

Evaluation
Positive therapeutic outcome
- Decreased fever, malaise, rash, negative C&S for infecting organism

ranibizumab (Rx)
(ran-ih-biz'oo-mab)
Lucentis
Func. class.: Ophthalmic
Chem. class.: Selective vascular endothelial growth factor antagonist
Pregnancy category C

Action: Binds to receptor-binding site of active forms of vascular endothelial growth factor A (VEGF-A) that causes angiogenesis and cell proliferation

Therapeutic Outcome: Prevention of increasing neovascular macular degeneration

Uses: Macular degeneration (neovascular) (wet)

Dosage and routes
Adult: Intravitreal 0.5 mg (0.05 ml) qmo

Available forms: Sol for inj 0.5 mg/0.05 ml

Adverse effects
CNS: Dizziness, headache
EENT: Blepharitis, cataract, conjunctival hemorrhage/hyperemia, detachment of the retinal pigment epithelium, dry/irritation/pain in the eye, visual impairment, vitreous floaters, ocular infection
GI: Constipation, nausea
MISC: Hypertension, UTI, thromboembolism
RESP: Bronchitis, cough, sinusitis, URI

Contraindications: Hypersensitivity, ocular infections

Precautions: Pregnancy **C,** lactation, children, retinal detachment, increased intraocular pressure

Pharmacokinetics	
Absorption	Minimal
Distribution	None
Metabolism	None
Excretion	None
Half-life	Elimination 9 days

Pharmacodynamics	
Onset	Unknown
Peak	Unknown
Duration	Unknown

Interactions

Individual drugs

Verteporfin photodynamictherapy (PDT): increased severe inflammation

NURSING CONSIDERATIONS

Assessment

- Assess for eye changes: redness, sensitivity to light, vision change, intraocular pressure change; report to ophthalmologist immediately

Nursing diagnoses

- Knowledge, deficient (teaching)

Implementation

- Given by ophthalmologist via intravitreal injection
- Store in refrigerator; do not freeze
- Protect from light

Patient/family education

- Teach patient that if eye becomes red, sensitive to light, painful or if there is a change in vision, seek immediate care from ophthalmologist
- Teach patient reason for treatment, expected results

Evaluation

Positive therapeutic outcome

- Prevention of increasing neovascular macular degeneration

ranolazine (Rx)

(ruh-no'luh-zeen)

Ranexa

Func. class: Antianginal

Pregnancy category C

Action: Antiaginal, anti-ischmic; unknown, may work by inhibiting portal fatty-acid oxidation

Therapeutic Outcome: Decreased anginal pain and number of episodes

Uses: Chronic stable angina pectoris; use in those that have not responded to other treatment options; should be used in combination with other antianginals such as amlodipine, beta blockers, or nitrates

Dosage and routes

Adult: PO 500 mg bid and increased to 1000 mg bid based on response; max 1000 mg bid

Available forms: Ext rel tabs 500 mg

Adverse effects

CNS: Headache, dizziness
CV: Palpitations, **QT prolongation**
GI: Nausea, vomiting, constipation, dry mouth
MISC: Peripheral edema
RESP: Dyspnea

Contraindications: Preexisting QT prolongation, hepatic disease (Child-Pugh class A, B, C), hypersensitivity, hypokalemia, renal failure, torsade de pointes, ventricular dysrhythmia, ventricular tachycardia

Precautions: Pregnancy **C,** hypotension, lactation, children, geriatric, renal disease

Pharmacokinetics	
Absorption	Varied
Distribution	Protein binding 62%
Metabolism	By CYP3A, CYP2D6 (lesser)
Excretion	Urine 75%, feces 25%
Half-life	7 hr

Pharmacodynamics	
Onset	Unknown
Peak	2-5 hr
Duration	Unknown

Interactions

Individual drugs

Arsenic trioxide, chloroquine, droperidol, grepafloxacin, halofantrine, haloperidol, levomethadyl, methadone, pentamidine, chlorpromazine, mesoridazine, thioridazine, pimozide, probucol, sparfloxacin: increased QT prolongation and torsade de pointes
Digoxin, simvastatin: increased action of digoxin, simvastatin
Diltiazem, ketoconazole, dofetilide, paroxetine, quinidine, sotalol, thioridazine, verapamil, ziprasidone: increased ranolazine action

Drug classifications

Anti-retroviral protease inhibitors: increased ranolazine absorption, toxicity
Class IA/III antidysrhythmics: increased QT prolongation and torsade de pointes
CYP3A4 inhibitors (ketoconazole, fluconazole, itraconazole, IV miconazole, voriconazole, diltiazem, verapamil): increased ranzolazine action and QT prolongation; do not use concurrently
Macrolide antibiotics, protease inhibitors: increased ranolazine action
Macrolides (clarithromycin, erythromycin, troleandomycin): increased QTc interval

Drug/food

Do not use with grapefruit or grapefruit juice

NURSING CONSIDERATIONS

Assessment

- Assess cardiac status: B/P, pulse, respiration, ECG; watch for prolongation of QT

Nursing diagnoses

- Pain, acute (uses)
- Tissue perfusion, ineffective (uses)
- Knowledge, deficient (teaching)

Implementation
- Do not break, crush, or chew tabs; to take drugs as prescribed; do not double or skip dose
- Give bid, without regard to meals

Patient/family education
- Teach patient to avoid hazardous activities until stabilized on drug, dizziness is no longer a problem
- Advise patient to avoid OTC drugs, grapefruit juice, drugs prolonging QTc (quinidine, dofetilide, sotalol, erythromycin, thioridazine, ziprasidone or protease inhibitors, diltiazem, ketoconazole, macrolide antibiotics, verapamil) unless directed by prescriber
- Advise patient to comply in all areas of medical regimen
- Teach patient to notify prescriber of palpitations, fainting
- Teach patient to notify all health care providers of this drug use

Evaluation
Positive therapeutic outcome
- Decreased anginal pain and number of episodes

rasagiline (Rx)
(ra-sa'-ji-leen)
Azilect
Func. class.: Antiparkinson agent
Chem. class.: MAOI

Pregnancy category C

Action: Inhibits MAOI type B; may increase dopamine levels

Therapeutic Outcome: Improved symptoms in those with Parkinson's disease

Uses: Idiopathic Parkinson's disease monotherapy or with levodopa

Dosage and routes
Monotherapy
Adult: PO 1 mg daily

Adjunctive therapy
Adult: PO 0.5 mg daily, may be increased to 1 mg daily; change of levodopa dose in adjunct therapy; reduce levodopa dose may be needed

Hepatic dose
Adult: PO 0.5 mg in mild hepatic disease

Concomitant ciprofloxacin, other CYP1A2 inhibitors
Adult: PO 0.5 mg; plasma concentrations of rasagiline may double

Available forms: Tabs 0.5, 1 mg

Adverse effects
CNS: Drowsiness, hallucinations, depression, headache, malaise, paresthesia, vertigo, syncope
CV: Angina, **hypertensive crisis** (ingestion of tyramine products), orthostatic hypotension
GI: *Nausea,* diarrhea, dry mouth, dyspepsia
GU: Impotence, decreased libido
MISC: Conjunctivitis, fever, flu syndrome, neck pain, allergic reaction, alopecia
MS: Arthralgia, arthritis, dyskinesia, fall
RESP: Rhinitis

Contraindications: Hypersensitivity to this drug or MAOIs; lactation, pheochromocytoma

Precautions: Pregnancy **C**, psychiatric disorders, children, severe hepatic disorders

Pharmacokinetics	
Absorption	Well
Distribution	Protein binding >88-94%
Metabolism	Liver, CYP1A2
Excretion	Kidneys
Half-life	Unknown

Pharmacodynamics	
Onset	Unknown
Peak	Unknown
Duration	Unknown

Interactions
Individual drugs
Ciprofloxacin: increased levels of rasagiline up to 2-fold
◆ Meperidine: do not give; serious reaction including coma and death may occur

Drug classifications
◆ Analgesics, sympathomimetics: do not give; serious reaction including coma and death may occur
◆ Antidepressants (tricyclics, SSRIs, SNRIs, mirtazapine, cyclobenzaprine): increased severe CNS toxicity
CYP1A2 inhibitors (atazanavir, mexiletine, taurine): increased levels of rasagiline up to 2-fold
◆ MAOIs: increased hypertensive crisis

Drug/herb
◆ St. John's Wort: do not give

NURSING CONSIDERATIONS
Assessment
- Assess for Parkinson's symptoms: tremor, ataxia, muscle weakness and rigidity; baseline and periodically
- Assess mental status: hallucinations, confusion, notify prescriber

- Assess for hypertensive crisis: severe headache, blurred vision, seizures, chest pain, difficulty thinking, nausea/vomiting, signs of stroke; any unexplained severe headache should be considered to be hypertensive crisis
- Assess for increased dyskinesia and postural hypotension if used in combination with levodopa
- Assess for melanomas frequently, perform periodic skin exams by a dermatologist
- Monitor cardiac status: B/P, ECG; periodically during beginning treatment

Nursing diagnoses

- Mobility, physical, impaired (uses)
- Injury, risk for (uses, adverse reactions)
- Knowledge, deficient (teaching)

Implementation

- Give with meals to prevent nausea; continuing therapy usually reduces or eliminates nausea
- Give reduced dose of carbidopa/levodopa, cautiously

Patient/family education

- Advise patient to change positions slowly to prevent orthostatic hypotension
- Instruct patient to avoid hazardous activities until stabilized; dizziness can occur
- Advise patient to rinse mouth frequently, use sugarless gum to alleviate dry mouth
- Teach patient to take as prescribed, not to miss dose or double doses; take missed dose as soon as remembered, if several hours before next dose
- Teach patient to prevent hypertensive crisis by avoiding tyramine foods
- Teach patient to report sings of hypertensive crisis

Evaluation

Positive therapeutic outcome

- Improved symptoms in those with Parkinson's disease (decreasing tremors, ataxia, muscle weakness/rigidity)

sitagliptin (Rx)

(sit-a-glip'tin)

Januvia

Func. class.: Antidiabetic, oral

Chem. class.: Dipeptidyl-peptidase-4 inhibitor (DPP-4 inhibitor)

Pregnancy category C

Action: Slows the inactivation of incretin hormones; improves glucose homeostasis, improves glucose dependent insulin synthesis, lowers glucagon secretions and slows gastric emptying time

Therapeutic Outcome: Decrease in polyuria, polydipsia, polyphagia; clear sensorium; absence of dizziness; stable gait, blood glucose at normal level

Uses: Type 2 diabetes mellitus as monotherapy or in combination with other antidiabetic agents

Dosage and routes

Adult: PO 100 mg daily; may use with other antidiabetic agents (metformin, pioglitazone, rosiglitazone)

Available forms: Tabs 25, 50, 100 mg

Adverse effects

CNS: *Headache*

ENDO: Hypoglycemia

GI: *Nausea, vomiting,* abdominal pain

Contraindications: Hypersensitivity, diabetic ketoacidosis (DKA)

Precautions: Pregnancy **C,** hypersensitivity, elderly, GI obstruction, thyroid disease, surgery, hepatic/renal disease, trauma

Pharmacokinetics	
Absorption	Rapidly
Distribution	Unknown
Metabolism	Unknown
Excretion	Kidneys, 79% unchanged
Half-life	Terminal 12.4 hr

Pharmacodynamics	
Onset	Unknown
Peak	1-4 hr
Duration	Unknown

Interactions

Individual drugs

Cimetidine, fluoxetine: increased hypoglycemia
Cimetidine, disopyramide: increased sitagliptan level
Digoxin: increased levels of digoxin
Aripiprazole, clozapine, olanzapine, quetiapine, risperidone, ziprasidone, phenytoin, fosphenytoin: decreased antidiabetic effect

Drug classifications

Androgens, insulins, beta blockers, corticosteroids, salicylates, MAOIs, fibric acid derivatives: increased hypoglycemia
Thiazide diuretics, ACE inhibitors, protease inhibitors, sympathomimetics, phenothiazines, estrogens, progestins, oral contraceptives: decreased antidiabetic effect

Drug/herb

Alfalfa, aloe, basil, bay, bilberry, bitter melon, black catechu, buchu, burdock, coriander, dandelion, eyebright (po), fenugreek, garlic,

ginseng, glucomannan, glucosamine, goat's rue, gymnema, horehound, horse chestnut, jambul, myrrh, myrtle: increased antidiabetic effect
Bee pollen, blue cohosh, broom, chromium, elecampane, eucalyptus, gotu kola: decreased antidiabetic effect
Chromium, coenzyme Q-10, fenugreek: increased hypoglycemia
Glucosamine: increased hyperglycemia

NURSING CONSIDERATIONS

Assessment

- Assess for hypoglycemic reactions (sweating, weakness, dizziness, anxiety, tremors, hunger), hyperglycemic reactions soon after meals
- Monitor CBC (baseline, q3mo) during treatment; check LFTs periodically, AST, LDH, renal studies: BUN, creatinine during treatment; glycosylated hemoglobin A1c
- Monitor blood glucose (BG) as needed

Nursing diagnoses

- Nutrition: more than body requirements, imbalanced (uses)
- Knowledge, deficient (teaching)
- Noncompliance (teaching)

Implementation

- May be taken with or without food
- Give 100 mg daily
- Conversion from other antidiabetic agents; change may be made with gradual dosage change
- Store in tight container in cool environment

Patient/family education

- Teach patient to use regular self-monitoring of blood glucose using blood glucose meter
- Teach patient the symptoms of hypo/hyperglycemia; what to do about each
- Teach patient that drug must be continued on daily basis; explain consequence of discontinuing drug abruptly
- Advise patient to avoid OTC medications, alcohol, digoxin, exenatide, insulins, nateglinide, repaglinide and other drugs that lower blood sugar, unless approved by prescriber
- Teach patient that diabetes is a lifelong illness; that this drug is not a cure, only controls symptoms
- Teach patient that all food included in diet plan must be eaten to prevent hyper/hypoglycemia
- Teach patient to carry emergency ID

Evaluation

Positive therapeutic outcome

- Decrease in polyuria, polydipsia, polyphagia; clear sensorium; absence of dizziness; stable gait, blood glucose at normal level

sunitinib (Rx)

(soo-nit'-in-ib)
Sutent
Func. class.: Miscellaneous antineoplastic
Chem. class.: Protein-tyrosine kinase inhibitor

Pregnancy category D

Action: Inhibits multiple receptor tyrosine kinases (RTKs), some are responsible for tumor growth

Therapeutic Outcome: Decrease in size of tumor

Uses: Gastrointesitnal stromal tumors (GIST) after disease progression or intolerance to imatinib; advanced renal carcinoma

Dosage and routes

Adult: PO 50 mg daily × 4 wk, then 2 wks off; may increase or decrease dose by 12.5 mg; if administered with CYP3A4 inducers, give 87.5 mg daily; if given with CYP3A4 inhibitors give 37.5 mg daily

Available forms: Caps 12.5, 25, 50 mg

Adverse effects

CNS: **CNS hemorrhage**, headache, dizziness, insomnia, **seizures**, fatigue
CV: Hypertension, **left ventricular dysfunction**
GI: *Nausea,* **hepatotoxicity, vomiting, dyspepsia,** *anorexia, abdominal pain,* altered taste, constipation, stomatitis, mucositis, **pancreatitis**
HEMA: **Neutropenia, thrombocytopenia**
INTEG: *Rash,* skin discoloration, depigmentation of hair or skin, alopecia
MS: Pain, arthralgia, myalgia
RESP: Cough, dyspnea
SYST: **Bleeding,** electrolyte abnormalities

Contraindications: Pregnancy **D,** lactation, hypersensitivity

Precautions: Children, elderly, active infections

Pharmacokinetics

Absorption	Unknown
Distribution	Protein binding 95%
Metabolism	By CYP3A4
Excretion	Feces, small amount in urine
Half-life	Terminal 40-60 hr (sunitnib); active metabolite 80-110 hr

Pharmacodynamics	
Onset	Unknown
Peak	6-12 hr
Duration	Unknown

Interactions
Individual drugs
Acetaminophen: increased hepatotoxicity
Clarithromycin, erythromycin, itraconazole, ketoconazole: increased sunitinib concentrations
Dexamethasone, carbamazepine, phenobarbital, phenytoin, rifampin: decreased sunitinib concentrations
Simvastatin: increased plasma concentrations
Warfarin: increased plasma concentration; avoid use with warfarin, use low-molecular-weight anticoagulants instead
Drug classifications
Calcium channel blockers: increased plasma concentrations
Drug/herb
St. John's wort: decreased sunitinib concentration
Drug/food
Grapefruit juice: increased plasma concentrations

NURSING CONSIDERATIONS
Assessment
- Monitor ANC and platelets; if ANC <1 × 10^9/L and/or platelets <50 × 10^9/L, stop until ANC >1.5 × 10^9/L and platelets >75 × 10^9/L ; if ANC <0.5 × 10^9/L and/or platelets <10 × 10^9/L, reduce dose by 200 mg, if cytopenia continues, reduce dose by another 100 mg; if cytopenia continues for 4 wk, stop drug until ANC ≥1 × 10^9/L
- Assess CV status: hypertension, QT prolongation can occur; monitor LVEF (left ventricular ejection fraction) baseline periodically
- Assess for renal toxicity: if bilirubin >3 × IULN, withhold sunitinib until bilirubin levels return to <1.5 × IULN
- Monitor for hepatotoxicity: LFTs, before treatment and qmo; if liver transaminases >5 × IULN, withhold sunitinib until transaminase levels return to <2.5 × IULN
- Monitor CBC, differential, platelet count weekly; withhold drug if WBC is <3500/mm^3, or platelet count <100,000/mm^3; notify prescriber of these results; drug should be discontinued
- Assess for CHF: adrenal insufficiency in those experiencing trauma
- Assess for bleeding: epitaxis rectal, gingival, upper GI, genital and wound bleeding; tumor related hemorrhage may occur rapidly

Nursing diagnoses
- Injury, risk for (uses, adverse reactions)
- Knowledge, deficient (teaching)

Implementation
- Give with meal and large glass of water, to decrease GI symptoms
- Give nutritious diet with iron, vitamin supplement, low fiber, few dairy products
- Store at 25°C (77°F)

Patient/family education
- Advise patient to report adverse reactions immediately: SOB, bleeding
- Teach patient reason for treatment, expected result
- Teach patient that many adverse reactions may occur: high B/P, bleeding, mouth swelling, taste change, skin discoloration, depigmentation of hair/skin
- Teach patient to avoid persons with known upper respiratory infections; immunosuppression is common

Evaluation
Positive therapeutic outcome
- Decrease in size of tumor

telbivudine (Rx)
(tel-bi'vyoo-deen)
Tyzeka
Func. class.: Antiretroviral
Chem. class.: Nucleoside reverse transcriptase inhibitor (NRTI)
Pregnancy category B

Action: Inhibits replication of HBV DNA polymerase which inhibits HBV replication

Therapeutic Outcome: Decreased hepatitis B serology

Uses: Hepatitis B

Dosage and routes
Adult and adolescent >16 yr: PO 600 mg daily; max 600 mg daily

Available forms: Tabs 600 mg

Adverse effects
CNS: *Fever, headache, malaise,* weakness, *dizziness, insomnia*
EENT: Taste change, hearing loss, photophobia
GI: *Nausea, vomiting, diarrhea, anorexia,* abdominal pain, hepatomegaly
INTEG: *Rash*

MISC: Lactic acidosis
MS: Myalgia, arthralgia, muscle cramps
RESP: Cough

Contraindications: Hypersensitivity, lactation

Precautions: Pregnancy **B,** lactation, children, severe renal disease, impaired hepatic function, anemia, organ transplant, dialysis, HIV, lactic acidosis, obesity, alcoholism

Pharmacokinetics

Absorption	Unknown
Distribution	Steady state 5-7 days, protein binding 3.3%
Metabolism	Unknown
Excretion	Kidneys, unchanged
Half-life	Terminal 40-49 hr

Pharmacodynamics

Onset	Unknown
Peak	Unknown
Duration	Unknown

Interactions
Individual drugs
CycloSPORINE, erythromycin, hydrochloroquine, niacin, penicillamine, zidovudine: increased myopathy risk
Drug classifications
Any agent altering renal function: altered telbivudine levels
Azole antifungals, corticosteroids, fibric acid derivatives, HMG-CoA reductase inhibitors: increased myopathy risk

NURSING CONSIDERATIONS
Assessment
- Monitor liver function tests, hepatitis B serology, creatine kinase, periodically

Nursing diagnoses
- Infection, risk for (uses)
- Knowledge, deficient (teaching)

Implementation
- Give with or without food with a full glass of water
- Store at room temperature

Patient/family education
- Advise patient that GI complaints and insomnia may resolve after 3-4 wk of treatment
- Teach patient that drug does not cure hepatitis B and does not stop the spread to others
- Teach patient that follow-up visits must be continued
- Teach patient that serious drug interactions may occur if OTC products are ingested; check with prescriber before taking
- Advise patient that drug may cause dizziness; avoid hazardous activities until response is known
- Teach patient to report symptoms of cough, difficulty sleeping or excessive headache

Evaluation
Positive therapeutic outcome
- Decreased hepatitis B serology

varenicline (Rx)
(var-e-ni'kleen)
Chantix
Func. class.: Smoking cessation agent
Pregnancy category C

Action: Partial agonist for nicotine receptors; partially activates receptors to help curb cravings; occupies receptors to prevent nicotine binding

Therapeutic Outcome: Smoking cessation

Uses: Smoking deterrent

Dosage and routes
Adult: PO Therapy should begin one week prior to smoking stop date (i.e. take drug plus tobacco for 7 days); titrate for 1 wk, days 1 through 3, 0.5 mg daily; days 4 through 7, 0.5 mg bid; day 8 through end of treatment 1 mg bid; treatment is 12 wks and may repeat for another 12 wks

Available forms: Tabs 0.5, 1 mg

Adverse effects
CNS: Headache, agitation, dizziness, insomnia, abnormal dreams, fatigue, malaise
CV: **Dysrhythmias,** hypertension, palpitations, **tachycardia,** angina, hypotension, **MI**
EENT: *Blurred vision,* tinnitus
GI: *Nausea, vomiting,* anorexia, *dry mouth,* increased/decreased appetite, *constipation,* flatulence, GERD
GU: Erectile dysfunction, urinary frequency, menstrual irregularities
INTEG: Rash, pruritus
MISC: Weight loss or gain
RESP: Dyspnea, rhinorrhea

Contraindications: Hypersensitivity, eating disorders

Precautions: Pregnancy **C,** renal disease, recent MI, lactation, children <18 yr, geriatric

Pharmacokinetics	
Absorption	Unknown
Distribution	Steady state 4 days
Metabolism	Minimal
Excretion	Urine 92%, unchanged
Half-life	Elimination 24 hr

Pharmacodynamics	
Onset	Unknown
Peak	Unknown
Duration	Unknown

NURSING CONSIDERATIONS

Assessment

- Assess for renal function in elderly
- Assess for smoking cessation after 12 wk; if progress has not been made, drug may be used for an additional 12 wks
- Assess mental status: mood, sensorium, affect

Nursing diagnoses

- Coping, ineffective (uses)
- Knowledge, deficient (teaching)

Implementation

- Do not break, crush, or chew tabs
- Give increased fluids, bulk in diet if constipation occurs
- Give after eating with a full glass of water
- Give sugarless gum, hard candy, or frequent sips of water for dry mouth

Patient/family education

- Teach patient that treatment for smoking cessation lasts 12 wk and another 12 wk may be required
- Teach patient to use caution in driving, other activities requiring alertness; blurred vision may occur
- Advise patient to set a date to quit smoking and initiate treatment 1 wk prior to that date
- Teach patient how to titrate product
- Advise patient not to use with nicotine patches unless directed by prescriber; may increase B/P
- Advise patient to notify prescriber if pregnancy is suspected or planned
- Teach patient common side effects to be expected

Evaluation

Positive therapeutic outcome

- Smoking cessation